Exam Preparatory Manual for Undergraduates

MEDICINE

G Entrance 2020

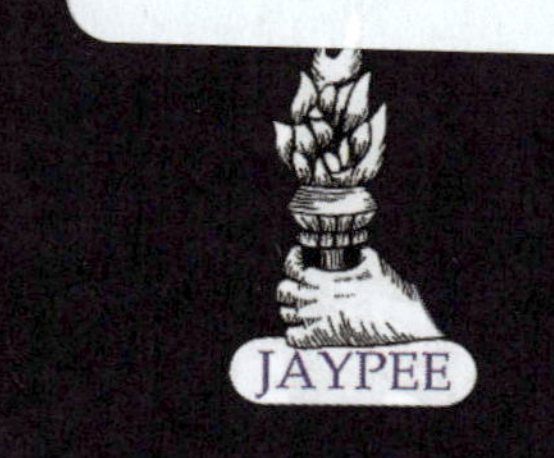

duates

PAN with HBSag Association
Ch. 9, Pg. 713

One required manifestation

- Recurrent oral ulceration: Aphthous or herpetiform, at least three times in 12 months, usually deep and multiple, and last for 10–30 days. This is the cardinal clinical feature.

plus

At least two of the following:

- Recurrent genital ulceration occurs in 60–80% of cases.
- Characteristic eye lesions: Anterior or posterior uveitis or retinal vasculitis or cells in vitreous on slit-lamp examination.
- Characteristic skin lesions: Erythema nodosum, pseudofolliculitis, papulopustular lesions and acneiform nodules.
- Positive pathergy test

Behcets disease case
Ch. 9, Pg. 715, Box 9.12

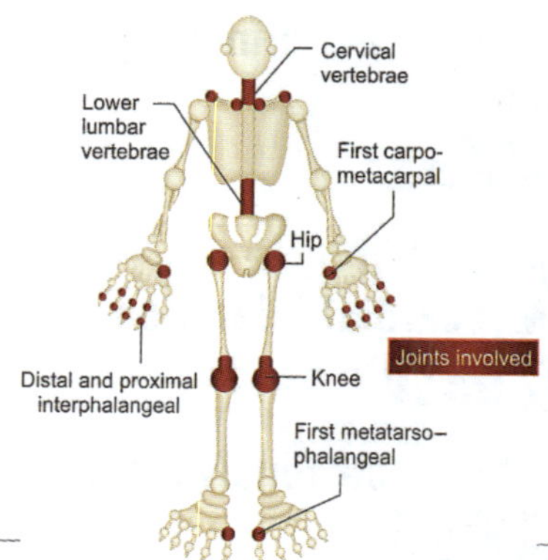

Osteoarthritis joint involvement case
Ch. 9, Pg. 718, Fig 9.11

Investigations in Systemic sclerosis- HRCT
Ch. 9, Pg. 720

Pegloticase in Gout

Minimal change disease- Patho
Ch. 13, Pg. 900

Renal transplant, 1-4 months infection - CMV
Ch. 13, Pg. 931

Symptom of Hyponatremia and Lithium toxicity
Ch. 14, Pg. 943

ABG interpretation– metabolic acidosis
Ch. 14, Pg. 963

Brocas Aphasia- location of brain
Ch. 15, Pg. 973

Wernickies Aphasia - case
Ch. 15, Pg. 986

RTA patient with papilledema- Raised ICT
Ch. 15, Pg. 1052

Headache with neck rigidity with CT image- SAH
Ch. 15, Pg. 995

Multiple sclerosis – pathology of slow conduction
Ch. 15, Pg. 998

Meningococcus – image
Ch. 15, Pg. 1012

Case of Sub acute combined degeneration

Salivary gland
Haptocorrin secreted by salivary glands
Gastric parietal cells intrinsic factor (IF)
Intrinsic factor (IF)
Pancreas
Intrinsic factor- B_{12} complex
Portal vein

Exam Preparatory Manual for Undergraduates

MEDICINE

Third Edition

Archith Boloor MBBS MD (Internal Medicine)
Additional Professor
Department of Medicine
Kasturba Medical College, Mangaluru
Manipal Academy of Higher Education
Karnataka, India
archithb@gmail.com

Ramadas Nayak MBBS MD (Pathology)
Professor
Department of Pathology
Yenepoya Medical College
Yenepoya (Deemed to be University)
Mangaluru, Karnataka, India

Forewords
Chakrapani M
M Venkatraya Prabhu

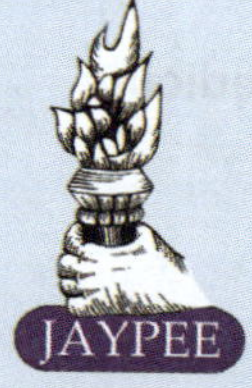

JAYPEE BROTHERS MEDICAL PUBLISHERS
The Health Sciences Publisher
New Delhi | London

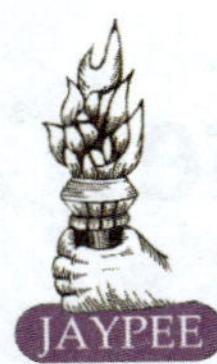

Jaypee Brothers Medical Publishers (P) Ltd

Headquarters
Jaypee Brothers Medical Publishers (P) Ltd
EMCA House, 23/23-B
Ansari Road, Daryaganj
New Delhi 110 002, India
Landline: +91-11-23272143, +91-11-23272703
+91-11-23282021, +91-11-23245672
Email: jaypee@jaypeebrothers.com

Corporate Office
Jaypee Brothers Medical Publishers (P) Ltd
4838/24, Ansari Road, Daryaganj
New Delhi 110 002, India
Phone: +91-11-43574357
Fax: +91-11-43574314
Email: jaypee@jaypeebrothers.com

Overseas Office
J.P. Medical Ltd
83 Victoria Street, London
SW1H 0HW (UK)
Phone: +44 20 3170 8910
Fax: +44 (0)20 3008 6180
Email: info@jpmedpub.com

Website: www.jaypeebrothers.com
Website: www.jaypeedigital.com

Inquiries for bulk sales may be solicited at: jaypee@jaypeebrothers.com

Exam Preparatory Manual for Undergraduates—Medicine

First Edition: 2017
Second Edition: 2018
Third Edition: 2021
Revised Reprint: 2021
Reprint: 2022
Reprint: January ***2023***

ISBN: 978-93-90595-22-8

Printed at: Samrat Offset Pvt. Ltd.

Dedicated to

All the health care workers,
the front-line essential workers and their families
who held their ground during these trying times

Contributing Authors

Madhav H Hande
Senior Resident
Department of Nephrology
Manipal Hospital, HAL Airport Road
Bengaluru, Karnataka, India

Mohamed Faizan Thouseef
Resident
Department of Internal Medicine
JN Medical College
KLE Academy of Higher Education and Research
Belgaum, Karnataka, India

Aashna Pankaj Gandhi
Resident
Department of Internal Medicine
Jawaharlal Nehru Medical College
KLE Academy of Higher Education and Research
Belgaum, Karnataka, India

Sheetal Raj M
Associate Professor
Department of Internal Medicine and Program
Director–Geriatric Medicine Fellowship
Kasturba Medical College, Mangaluru
Manipal Academy of Higher Education
Karnataka, India

Navyashree HC
Senior Resident
Department of Internal Medicine
Kasturba Medical College, Mangaluru
Manipal Academy of Higher Education
Karnataka, India

Athulya G Asokan
Associate Professor
Department of Internal Medicine
Pushpagiri Medical College and Research Centre
Tiruvalla, Kerala, India

Anudeep Padakanti
Senior Resident
Department of Oncology
MNJ Institute of Oncology and Regional Cancer Centre
Hyderabad, Telangana, India

Nikhil Kenny Thomas
Senior Resident
Department of Gastroenterology
PSG Institute of Medical Sciences and Research
Coimbatore, Tamil Nadu, India

Abu Thajudeen
Department of Internal Medicine
Kasturba Medical College, Mangaluru
Manipal Academy of Higher Education
Karnataka, India

Vivek K Koushik
Senior Resident
Department of Nephrology
Apollo Hospitals
Chennai, Tamil Nadu, India

Shriram Bhat Mudraje
Senior Resident
Department of Internal Medicine
Kasturba Medical College, Manipal
Manipal Academy of Higher Education
Karnataka, India

Thejus Bhaskar
Senior Resident
Department of Neurology
Bangalore Medical College
and Research Institute
Bengaluru, Karnataka, India

Mohammed Shaheen
Department of Internal Medicine
Kasturba Medical College, Mangaluru
Manipal Academy of Higher Education
Karnataka, India

Ashwini M
Senior Resident
Department of Internal Medicine
Kasturba Medical College, Mangaluru
Manipal Academy of Higher Education
Karnataka, India

Pranjal Sharma
Resident
Department of Internal Medicine
Kasturba Medical College, Mangaluru
Manipal Academy of Higher Education
Karnataka, India

Tejaswini Lakshmikeshava
Resident
Department of Internal Medicine
Kasturba Medical College, Mangaluru
Manipal Academy of Higher Education
Karnataka, India

Subraya Krishna Holla
Assistant Professor
Department of Internal Medicine
KS Hedge Medical Academy
NITTE University
(Deemed to be University)
Mangaluru, Karnataka, India

Sriraksha R Nayak
Consultant Psychiatrist
District Mental Health Programme
Uttara Kannada, Karnataka, India

Akshata Nayak U
Consultant Hematologist
AJ Institute of Medical Sciences and Research Centre
Mangaluru, Karnataka, India

GG Akshay Prabhu
Resident
Department of Internal Medicine
Kasturba Medical College, Mangaluru
Manipal Academy of Higher Education
Karnataka, India

Deepti Agarwal
Department of Internal Medicine
Kasturba Medical College, Mangaluru
Manipal Academy of Higher Education
Karnataka, India

Ishika Mahajan
Department of Internal Medicine
Kasturba Medical College, Mangaluru
Manipal Academy of Higher Education
Karnataka, India

Pradeep Krishna Chowdary
Senior Resident
Department of Cardiology
Government Medical College
Kozhikode, Kerala, India

Navjot Singh Dhillon
Department of Medicine
Kasturba Medical College, Mangaluru
Manipal Academy of Higher Education
Karnataka, India

Foreword to the Second Edition

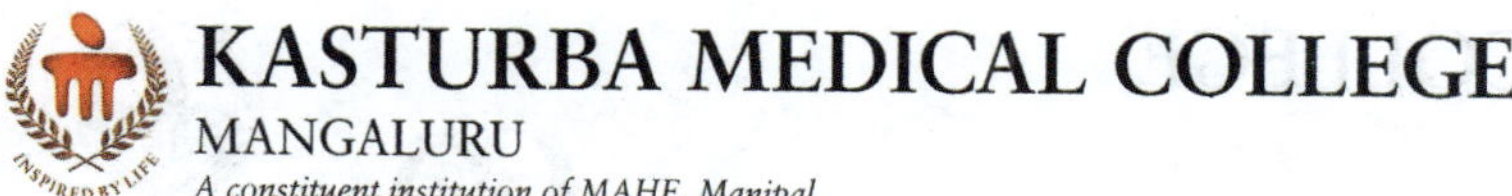

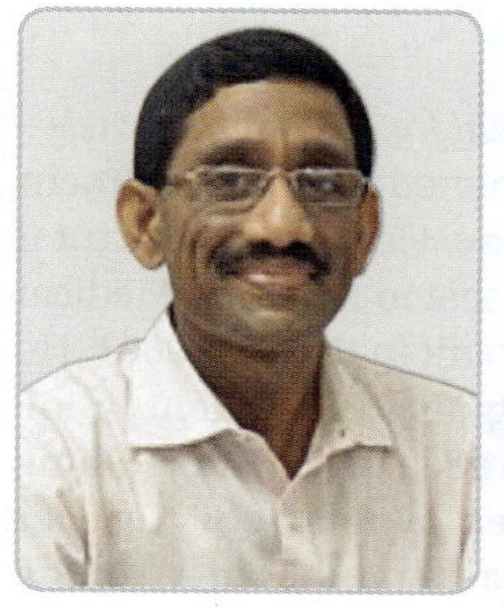

Internal medicine is expanding and evolving rapidly and there is a need for comprehensive yet simple textbook. Indian medical students have to be very competitive and up-to-date to excel in their fields. While a number of textbooks from foreign authors are available for the Indian students, they might not serve the purpose of preparing the students for the Indian examinations. A few Indian authors have accepted this challenge and have published textbooks oriented towards Indian medical examinations. Dr Archith Boloor realized this need many years ago and took up the challenge of publishing a textbook in internal medicine which was received well by the student community. Huge success of the first edition has prompted him to come out with the second edition of the book.

Dr Archith Boloor is an exceptionally gifted clinician and teacher. He has taken keen interest in medical education from his early days in the medical college and with more than a decade of experience in this field, he has been able to understand the needs of the students with regard to the medical examinations. He has received the Best Teacher Award at Kasturba Medical College, Mangaluru for many years.

The second edition of this compilation has seen qualitative improvements over the previous edition. While the contents of the book are comprehensive, presentation is simple. Clinical images, tables, boxes, algorithms and diagrams are simple and enhance the learning. This book will definitely be an essential learning tool for students of internal medicine.

Chakrapani M MD
Professor
Department of Medicine
Formerly, Head and Associate Dean
Kasturba Medical College, Mangaluru
Manipal Academy of Higher Education
Karnataka, India
chakrapani.m@manipal.edu

Foreword to the First Edition

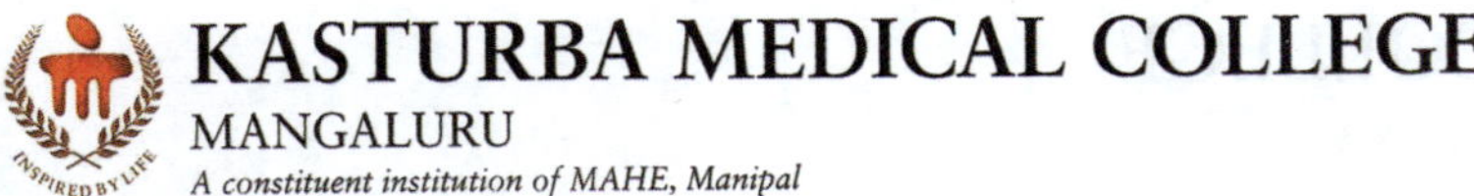

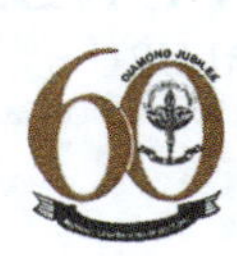

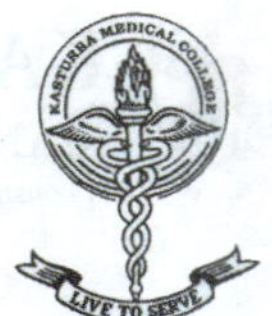

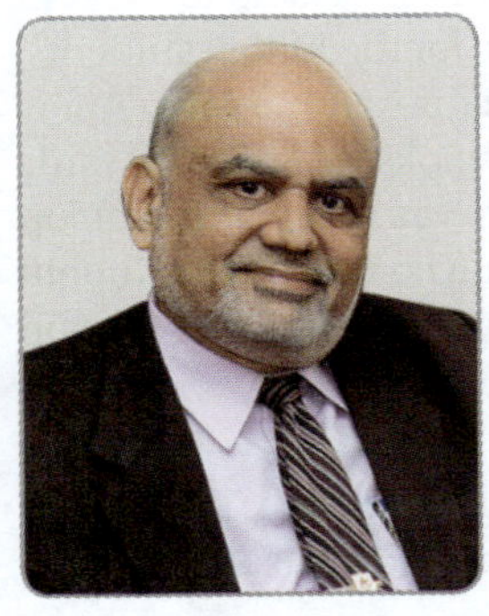

I am very proud to write a foreword to this book *Exam Preparatory Manual for Undergraduates—Medicine* written by Dr Archith Boloor, one of the outstanding students, trained in the Department of Medicine of our college of which I am faculty as Professor of Medicine. Coming from a rural background from outskirts of Mangaluru, Dr Boloor after getting a merit seat in Kasturba Medical College, Mangaluru for MBBS in 1998, completed his final MBBS with credit in the year 2003. He joined as a postgraduate student in the year 2005 and was the best outgoing PG student in the May 2008 examinations, a performance for which he was conferred gold medal. Soon after joining our department as a faculty, he had been committed teacher as proven by the Good Teacher Awards in the years 2013 and 2015 and Dr Patrick Pinto Memorial Best Teacher Award in 2014. The importance of these awards lies in that the selection is done by students which shows the efficacy of teaching. Not contented with this alone and trying to do better for the cause of students, I am pleased to know from him that he is writing a textbook *Exam Preparatory Manual for Undergraduates—Medicine* which is meant for training the students for internal medicine especially to face the final MBBS examination. Having taken part in several scientific meetings, continuing medical educations (CMEs) and conferences in internal medicine, here as a speaker and panelist give him credentials to write the book. I hope that this book will be different from other books. It will be student-centric rather than author-centric.

M Venkatraya Prabhu MD
Dean and Professor
Department of Medicine
Kasturba Medical College, Mangaluru
Manipal Academy of Higher Education
Karnataka, India
Email: *dean.kmcmlr@manipal.edu*
Website: *www.manipal.edu*

Preface to the Third Edition

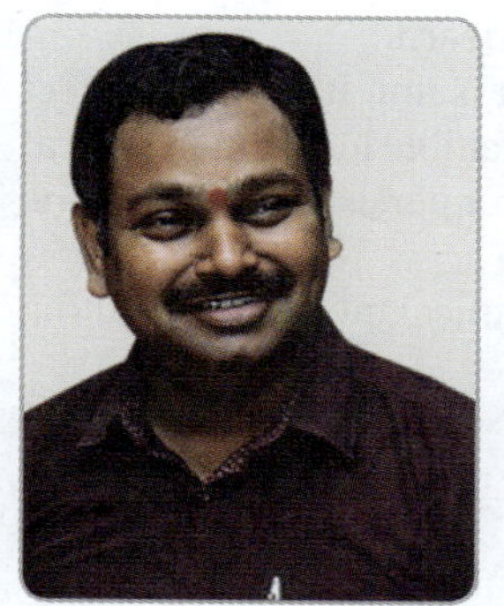

Third time's the charm they say. I don't know who said it, but I have always believed that three is a special number. In India, we train for three years in Internal Medicine; three is the time given to us by the system to become the doctors that can handle any crisis, convolution or conundrum. In statistics, we follow a Rule of Three; a simple trick to say that the confidence interval is 95% when all else fails. It takes three sets of three months: three trimesters to create a new life. This new life grows up, goes to school and finally comes to us in vivas; Bright eyed students who can confidently say three symptoms and three signs before they start with the umms and the aahs and the etceteras. The number three has a lot of significance in my life; both personal and professional. Three is a number as magical as can be; so it's only fitting that I feel just as magical and special now while I present to you – The third edition of my first book.

Learning medicine is not something that can be relegated to three short (or long) years. You are always going to be a lifelong student, you are always going to be an inexperienced teacher who doesn't know enough, and you are always going to be stuck after the third symptom. There's nothing wrong with it, it's just how we have conditioned ourselves. When I wrote this book for the first time, I tried to craft a medical text that can help you remember the threes; and know even more. The overwhelming response that the first edition of the book received was a lesson for me that my approach was headed in the right direction. Through a lot of welcome feedback, criticism and corrections; we worked to create this book, its third edition over the course of a raging pandemic.

The new edition of this book is different in the way that it is completely revamped, updated and reworked to suit the needs of the new CBME curriculum. The content is presented in the same reliable and easy-to-grasp fashion as the previous editions. All the tables and the guidelines are updated according to the latest revisions. I have a lot to be grateful to the universe for challenging me to produce new content in a new design for a new audience; especially when I'm used to my ways and my knick-knacks. The heart of my book is in the content that I have assimilated over the course of so many years. That heart remains beating; thankfully not in threes. But strong, regular, and powered by the thousands of students who continue to fulfil my experience as an author and as a teacher.

Medical literature has forever been governed by evidence and not by experience. So as always, this book is up for scrutiny, changes and suggestions. Hopefully, the book has been reviewed by enough of my colleagues and my students that we'll not have more than three changes for the next edition. But, life has a way of making things exciting for me; so I'm sure that I will have to work thrice as hard again for the next edition. Work that feels like a pleasant joy when I sit in a viva in the afternoon session at 3 PM, and the last three students list out three symptoms, three signs and three knick-knacks from my book.

Third time's the charm they say. I don't know who said it, but three is definitely a special number.

Archith Boloor

Preface to the First Edition

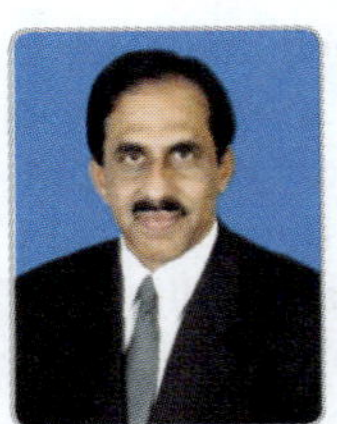

The glory of medicine is that it keeps moving forward, that there is always more to learn.

We look for medicine to be an orderly field of knowledge and procedure but it is not. It is an imperfect science, an enterprise of constantly changing knowledge, uncertain information, fallible individuals, and at the same time lives on the line. The gap between what we know and what we aim for persists. And this book is an attempt in bridging the gap.

This book is a first of its kind with an amalgamation of clinical pathology and clinical medicine, resulting in an integrated comprehensive manual.
Every attempt has been made by us to present information in a simplified text augmented with the use of colored illustrations, flowcharts, algorithms which help the reader to understand the concepts, recollect and make use of and thus acquire knowledge in the examinations as well as in clinical practice.

It is designed for use as a companion book for exam preparation for undergraduates. The main characteristics of this book are:

- Reader-friendly pattern
- Color coded as in etiology, management, etc.
- Includes management algorithms
- Key points are highlighted
- Question-answer format
- Covers all the questions appeared in university examinations till April 2016
- Extensively covers all theory and most clinical scenarios
- Management practices have been updated till September 2016
- Recent advances, newer drugs and upcoming sections of Geriatrics, Immunology, Clinical Pharmacology have been included
- Exclusive coverage of high yielding points which are important for answering MCQs.

This book consists of 23 chapters and is organized into systemwise chapters which are further divided into subsections. Each chapter starts with basic introduction and proceeds to individual disease discussions. The etiology of the diseases have been separately included. Also, important management sections are in separate colored tables, so that selective reading can be done. Important clinical examination-oriented questions have also been included under each section. Diagnostic procedures have been discussed separately. Radiological investigations and their abnormalities have been emphasized especially X-ray findings of specific diseases. Basic reading of ECGs have been covered with the common abnormalities encountered. Clear ECG images have been included for better understanding. Also, many tables comparing clinical situations/abnormalities will aid in better understanding and also help in answering a lot of questions in the clinics as well as viva voce. All common clinical cases (long, semi-long, and short) that you would encounter in your practical examination have been covered extensively to give the readers an edge over.

After many years of teaching undergraduates, we found that undergraduate students find it difficult to understand, remember and answer the questions during examinations in a satisfying way. There are many textbooks, but students face difficulty to refresh their knowledge during examinations. This encouraged us to write a book to fill the niche, to provide basic information to them in a nutshell. Most students are fundamentally 'visually-oriented.' As the saying goes 'a picture is worth a thousand words,' it encouraged us to provide many illustrations.

We recommend this book to all students for understanding the basic knowledge and refresh their knowledge during examinations. One of the aims of the students after getting undergraduate degree is to fetch a good ranking in the postgraduate entrance examination. Most graduates cannot answer multiple choice questions in entrance examination by just reading the usual textbooks in medicine. Our book lays specific importance on this aspect and answers to most commonly asked MCQs. This book provides sufficient information which would help postgraduates and practicing clinicians in the knowledge and management of cases.

Archith Boloor
Ramadas Nayak

Acknowledgments to the Third Edition

Third edition of my first book—It was an uphill task but with the pitching-ins of my colleagues all across India, the process was made smoother than I imagined. We were up against the pandemic—a crisis no one could have anticipated or prepared for; working as frontline health care workers, my peers and I still found the time to compile this edition, the experience of which has been infinitely memorable.

Firstly, I would like to thank my family, my mom and my sisters: The unwavering pillars of strength that have supported me throughout every challenge in my life. My friends, my colleagues and my well-wishers who have supported my work; this time was no exception. Lastly, my students: I thank all of them, each and every last one, because without their unrelenting urge to learn, I would not have the drive to teach.

I thank Dr Ramadas Nayak for inducting me into this field of medical writing, and also for the constant support.

The modifications that this book had to undergo to become a cohesive third edition undoubtedly needed lots of research and data. I am thankful to all of my friends whose contributions and knowledge flowed seamlessly and in very short notice. I would also like to place my sincerest gratitude to Dr Madhav H Hande, Dr Sheetal Raj, Dr Navyashree HC, Dr Mohammed Shaheen, Dr Shriram Bhat Mudraje, Dr Ashwini MV, Dr Pranjal Sharma, Dr Tejaswini Lakshmikeshava, Dr Mohamed Faizan Thouseef, Dr Aashna Pankaj Gandhi, Dr Athulya G Asokan, Dr Pradeep Krishna Chowdary, Dr Deepti Agarwal, Dr Sriraksha Nayak, Dr Thejus M, Akshata Nayak U, Dr Subraya Krishna Holla and Dr GG Akshay Prabhu for their contributions. Special thanks to Dr Ishika Mahajan and Dr Navjot Singh Dhillon for their timely help with the content especially the new tables, figures and flowcharts which have been added in this edition.

Thank you, Dr Nikhil Kenny Thomas, Dr Anudeep Padakanti, Dr Abu Thajudeen and Dr Vivek K Koushik for their encouragement, their contributions, and the sheer motivation they give me every day.

I convey my sincere thanks to Shri Jitendar P Vij (Group Chairman) for have been the guiding force behind all my works. Mr Ankit Vij (Managing Director), Mr MS Mani (Group President), Dr Madhu Choudhary (Publishing Head–Education), Ms Pooja Bhandari (Production Head), Ms Sunita Katla (Executive Assistant to Group Chairman and Publishing Manager), Mr Rajesh Sharma (Production Coordinator), Ms Seema Dogra (Cover Visualizer), Suhel Ahmed (Graphic Designer), Mr Deep Kumar (Typesetter) and Ms Neelam (Proofreader) of M/s Jaypee Brothers Medical Publishers (P) Ltd, New Delhi, India, for their help in the formatting and their well-received technical assistance and unwavering support during the process of developing this project.

I thank Dr M Venkatraya Prabhu and Dr Chakrapani M, my teachers, and guides for having written the forewords for the book.

I am grateful to my department, my college Kasturba Medical College, Mangaluru, Karnataka, India and my university, Manipal Academy of Higher Education (MAHE), Manipal for supporting my endeavors. I was made here, and every achievement of mine is made here as well.

A very special gratitude goes out to all my teachers, who are solely responsible for what I am today and for having ignited the passion of teaching and writing in me.

Lastly, I thank to Mother Goddess for guiding me through my life, and helping me understand the purpose of my existence. I pray for what was, what is and what will be.

Archith Boloor

Acknowledgments to the First Edition

'Writing this book has been an exercise in sustained knowledge gain, and for those who have played the larger role in our endeavor with constant encouragement and support; Well, you know who you are; Just a thanks would not suffice'.

After almost 6 years of working on it, we could not possibly come up with a full list of all the people who had helped, but we will try our best.

Dr Archith Boloor, thanks his family members namely his mother, Mrs Kumuda; sisters, Ms Arati, Ms Archana and Ms Aparna, his father and others. Dr Ramadas Nayak thanks Mrs Rekha Nayak and Dr Rakshatha Nayak who have patiently accepted his long preoccupation with this work.

We wish to express our gratitude to Dr Ramdas M Pai, Chancellor, Manipal University, Karnataka, India, for giving us an opportunity to be a part of this prestigious institution for nearly 20 years, to pursue our dreams and to grow to be the physician and teacher that we are today.

We are indebted to Dr HS Ballal (Pro-Chancellor), Dr H Vinod Bhat (Vice-Chancellor) and Dr V Surendra Shetty (Pro Vice-Chancellor) of Manipal University, Karnataka, India, for their support.

We are grateful to our beloved Dean, Dr M Venkatraya Prabhu, Kasturba Medical College, Mangaluru, Karnataka, India, for his constant support and encouragement and also for writing the foreword for the first edition.

We would like to express our gratitude to all colleagues in the Department of Medicine, Kasturba Medical College, Mangaluru, for their constant help at every juncture of our career. We would specially like to thank and acknowledge Dr Chakrapani M and Dr Damodar Shenoy, for mentoring Dr Archith to what he is today.

Dr Archith Boloor remains deeply indebted for his humble achievements, his passion for teaching and for instilling in him the tenacity to learn and achieve his goals to Dr Nagalakshmamma, Professor of Botany; Dr Ranjan Shetty and Dr Jayaraj Sindhur, his seniors, who are to him embodiments of the word 'Teacher'. He humbly lays down his gratitude to them for inspiring him.

We would like to express our gratitude to our students (both undergraduate and postgraduate), friends and colleagues who helped us at different stages of preparing the manuscript; to all those who provided the support, talked things over, read, offered comments and assisted in the editing, proofreading and designing of this book. Our heartfelt thanks to Dr Hasmukh Jain, Dr Raghavendra BS, Dr Sheetal Raj, Dr Athulya Roopak, Dr Kaushiki Kirty, Dr Vishnu B Chandran, Dr Joseph Samuel, Dr Jimmy Joseph, Dr Kolla Gautham, Dr Anudeep Reddy, and Dr M Harsha Sagar, for their timely and continued support.

A word of thanks would hardly suffice for our pillars of strength and our support system Dr Suresh Shetty B, Dr Jagadish Rao PP, Dr Abul Fazil, Dr Abhishek Gupta, Dr Veena Jasmine Pinto, Dr Akshata Nayak, Dr Nishita Shetty, Dr Sandip Ganguly, Dr Ruchi Romya Das, Dr Mamta Gupta, Dr Sahil Popli, Dr Pradeep Krishna Chowdary, Dr Yogesh Rasal, Dr Sravan Thumati, Dr Amrutraj, Dr Satish AV, Dr Sachin Vemula, Dr Neil Dominic Fernandes, Dr Mishaal Talish, and Dr Apurva Mittal.

Also, we convey our sincere thanks to Shri Jitendar P Vij (Group Chairman), Mr Ankit Vij (Managing Director), Ms Ritu Sharma (Director–Content Strategy), and Ms Chetna Malhotra Vohra (Associate Director–Content Strategy) of M/s Jaypee Brothers Medical Publishers (P) Ltd, New Delhi, India, for publishing the book in the same format as wanted, well in time.

We thank Ms Sunita Katla (Executive Assistant to Group Chairman and Publishing Manager), Ms Samina Khan (Executive Assistant to Director–Content Strategy), Mr Rajesh Sharma (Production Coordinator), Ms Seema Dogra (Cover Designer), Mr Laxmidhar Padhiary (Proofreader), Mr Rajesh Ghurkundi (Graphic Designer), and Mr Raj Kumar (DTP Operator) of M/s Jaypee Brothers Medical Publishers (P) Ltd, New Delhi, India.

We thank especially Mr Venugopal V (Associate Director—South) of Jaypee Brothers Medical Publishers (P) Ltd, Bengaluru Branch, Karnataka, for taking this book to every corner of Karnataka.

This book has been written for our students who have inspired us to take up this project; it is their questions that made us read and learn and compile this book. This is a book for you and I do not think we can finish without thanking you.

Lastly, we thank God Almighty, for making us what we are, guiding us through our life, and helping us in bringing this book to you all.

There are many more people we could thank, but constraints of space compel us to stop here.

Archith Boloor
Ramadas Nayak

Contents

Competency Table

Number	COMPETENCY The student should be able to	Core Y/N	Suggested learning methods	Suggested assessment methods	Chapter No.	Page No.
GENERAL MEDICINE						
IM1.1	Describe and discuss the epidemiology, pathogenesis clinical evolution and course of common causes of heart disease including: rheumatic/valvular, ischemic, hypertrophic inflammatory	Y	Lecture, small group discussion	Written/viva voce	7	406–564
IM1.2	Describe and discuss the genetic basis of some forms of heart failure	N	Lecture, small group discussion	Written	7	406–564
IM1.3	Describe and discuss the etiology microbiology pathogenies and clinical evolution of rheumatic fever, criteria, degree of rheumatic activity and rheumatic valvular heart disease and its complications including infective endocarditis	Y	Lecture, small group discussion	Written/viva voce	7	406–564
IM1.4	Stage heart failure	Y	Lecture, small group discussion	Written/viva voce	7	406–564
IM1.5	Describe, discuss and differentiate the processes involved in R versus L heart failure, systolic versus diastolic failure	Y	Lecture, small group discussion	Written/viva voce	7	406–564
IM1.6	Describe and discuss the compensatory mechanisms involved in heart failure including cardiac remodelling and neurohormonal adaptations	Y	Lecture, small group discussion	Written/viva voce	7	406–564
IM1.7	Enumerate, describe and discuss the factors that exacerbate heart, dietary factors drugs, etc.	Y	Lecture,small group	Written/viva voce	7	406–564
IM1.8	Describe and discuss the pathogenesis and development of common arrythmias involved in heart failure particularly atrial fibrillation	Y	Lecture, small group discussion	Written/viva voce	7	406–564
IM1.9	Describe and discuss the clinical presentation and features, diagnosis, recognition and management of acute rheumatic fever	Y	Lecture, small group discussion	Written/viva voce	7	406–564
IM1.10	Elicit document and present an appropriate history that will establish the diagnosis, cause and severity of heart failure including: presenting complaints, precipitating and exacerbating factors, risk factors exercise tolerance, changes in sleep patterns, features suggestive of infective endocarditis	Y	Bedside clinic	Skill assessment	6, 7	267–270 406–564
IM1.11	Perform and demonstrate a systematic examination based on the history that will help establish the diagnosis and estimate its severity including: measurement of pulse, blood pressure and respiratory rate, jugular venous forms and pulses, peripheral pulses, conjunctiva and fundus, lung, cardiac examination including palpation and auscultation with identification of heart sounds and murmurs, abdominal distension and splenic palpation	Y	Bedside clinic, DOAP session	Skill assessment	6, 7	267–270 406–564
IM1.12	Demonstrate peripheral pulse, volume, character, quality and variation in various causes of heart failure	Y	Bedside clinic, DOAP session	Skill assessment	7	406–564

Number	COMPETENCY The student should be able to	Core Y/N	Suggested learning methods	Suggested assessment methods	Chapter No.	Page No.
IM1.13	Measure the blood pressure accurately, recognize and discuss alterations in blood pressure in valvular heart disease and other causes of heart failure and cardiac tamponade	Y	Bedside clinic, DOAP session	Skill assessment	7	406–564
IM1.14	Demonstrate and measure jugular venous distension	Y	Bedside clinic, DOAP session	Skill assessment	7	406–564
IM1.15	Identify and describe the timing, pitch quality conduction and significance of precordial murmurs and their variations	Y	Bedside clinic, DOAP session	Skill assessment	7	406–564
IM1.16	Generate a differential diagnosis based on the clinical presentation and prioritise it based on the most likely diagnosis	Y	Bedside clinic, small group discussion	Skill assessment	7	406–564
IM1.17	Order and interpret diagnostic testing based on the clinical diagnosis including 12-lead ECG, chest radiograph, blood cultures	Y	Bedside clinic, DOAP session	Skill assessment	7	406–564
IM1.18	Perform and interpret a 12-lead ECG	Y	Bedside clinic, DOAP session	Skill assessment	7	406–564
IM1.19	Enumerate the indications for and describe the findings of heart failure with the following conditions including: 2D echocardiography, brain natriuretic peptide, exercise testing, nuclear medicine testing and coronary angiogram	N	Lecture, small group discussion, bedside clinic	Skill assessment	7	406–564
IM1.20	Determine the severity of valvular heart disease based on the clinical and laboratory and imaging features and determine the level of intervention required including surgery	Y	Small group discussion, lecture, bedside clinic	Written/skill assessment	7	406–564
IM1.21	Describe and discuss and identify the clinical features of acute and subacute endocarditis, echocardiographic findings, blood culture and sensitivity and therapy	Y	Bedside clinic, small group discussion, lecture	Skill assessment	7	406–564
IM1.22	Assist and demonstrate the proper technique in collecting specimen for blood culture	Y	DOAP session	Skill assessment	7	406–564
IM1.23	Describe, prescribe and communicate non-pharmacologic management of heart failure including sodium restriction, physical activity and limitations	Y	Lecture, small group discussion	Skill assessment	7	406–564
IM1.24	Describe and discuss the pharmacology of drugs including indications, contraindications in the management of heart failure including diuretics, ACE inhibitors, beta blockers, aldosterone antagonists and cardiac glycosides	Y	Lecture, small group discussion	Viva voce/written	7	406–564
IM1.25	Enumerate the indications for valvuloplasty, valvotomy, coronary revascularization and cardiac transplantation	Y	Lecture, small group discussion, bedside clinic	Viva voce/written	7	406–564
IM1.26	Develop document and present a management plan for patients with heart failure based on type of failure, underlying etiology	Y	Bedside clinic, skill assessment, small group discussion	Bedside clinic/skill assessment/written	7	406–564
IM1.27	Describe and discuss the role of penicillin prophylaxis in the prevention of rheumatic heart disease	Y	Bedside clinic, small group discussion	Written	7	406–564
IM1.28	Enumerate the causes of adult presentations of congenital heart disease and describe the distinguishing features between cyanotic and acyanotic heart disease	Y	Bedside clinic, small group discussion	Bedside clinic/skill assessment/written	7	406–564
IM1.29	Elicit document and present an appropriate history, demonstrate correctly general examination, relevant clinical findings and formulate document and present a management plan for an adult patient presenting with a common form of congenital heart disease	Y	Bedside clinic, small group discussion	Skill assessment/written	7	406–564

Number	COMPETENCY The student should be able to	Core Y/N	Suggested learning methods	Suggested assessment methods	Chapter No.	Page No.
IM2.1	Discuss and describe the epidemiology, antecedents and risk factors for atherosclerosis and ischemic heart disease	Y	Lecture, small group discussion	Written/viva voce	7	406–564
IM2.2	Discuss the etiology of risk factors both modifiable and non-modifiable of atherosclerosis and IHD	Y	Lecture, small group discussion	Written/viva voce	7	406–564
IM2.3	Discuss and describe the lipid cycle and the role of dyslipidemia in the pathogenesis of atherosclerosis	Y	Lecture, small group discussion	Written/viva voce	7	406–564
IM2.4	Discuss and describe the pathogenesis natural history, evolution and complications of atherosclerosis and IHD	Y	Lecture, Small group discussion	Written/viva voce	7	406–564
IM2.5	Define the various acute coronary syndromes and describe their evolution, natural history and outcomes	Y	Lecture, small group discussion	Written/viva voce	7	406–564
IM2.6	Elicit document and present an appropriate history that includes onset evolution, presentation risk factors, family history, comorbid conditions, complications, medication, history of atherosclerosis, IHD and coronary syndromes	Y	Bedside clinic, DOAP session	Skill assessment	7	406–564
IM2.7	Perform, demonstrate and document a physical examination including a vascular and cardiac examination that is appropriate for the clinical presentation	Y	Bedside clinic, DOAP session	Skill assessment	7	406–564
IM2.8	Generate document and present a differential diagnosis based on the clinical presentation and prioritise based on "cannot miss", most likely diagnosis and severity	Y	Bedside clinic, DOAP session	Skill assessment	7	406–564
IM2.9	Distinguish and differentiate between stable and unstable angina and AMI based on the clinical presentation	Y	Bedside clinic, DOAP session	Skill assessment	7	406–564
IM2.10	Order, perform and interpret an ECG	Y	Bedside clinic, DOAP session	Skill assessment	7	406–564
IM2.11	Order and interpret a chest X-ray and markers of acute myocardial infarction	Y	Bedside clinic, DOAP session	Skill assessment	7	406–564
IM2.12	Choose and interpret a lipid profile and identify the desirable lipid profile in the clinical context	Y	Bedside clinic, DOAP session	Skill assessment	7	406–564
IM2.13	Discuss and enumerate the indications for and findings on echocardiogram, stress testing and coronary angiogram	Y	Lecture, small group discussion	Written/viva voce	7	406–564
IM2.14	Discuss and describe the indications for admission to a coronary care unit and supportive therapy for a patient with acute coronary syndrome	Y	Lecture, small group discussion	Written/viva voce	7	406–564
IM2.15	Discuss and describe the medications used in patients with an acute coronary syndrome based on the clinical presentation	Y	Lecture, small group discussion	Written/viva voce	7	406–564
IM2.16	Discuss and describe the indications for acute thrombolysis, PTCA and CABG	Y	Lecture, small group discussion	Written/viva voce	7	406–564
IM2.17	Discuss and describe the indications and methods of cardiac rehabilitation	Y	Lecture, small group discussion	Written/viva voce	7	406–564
IM2.18	Discuss and describe the indications, formulations, doses, side effects and monitoring for drugs used in the management of dyslipidemia	Y	Lecture, small group discussion	Written/viva voce	7	406–564
IM2.19	Discuss and describe the pathogenesis, recognition and management of complications of acute coronary syndromes including arrhythmias, shock, LV dysfunction, papillary muscle rupture and pericarditis	Y	Lecture, small group discussion	Written/viva voce	7	406–564
IM2.20	Discuss and describe the assessment and relief of pain in acute coronary syndromes	Y	Lecture, small group discussion	Written/viva voce	7	406–564

Number	COMPETENCY The student should be able to	Core Y/N	Suggested learning methods	Suggested assessment methods	Chapter No.	Page No.
IM2.21	Observe and participate in a controlled environment an ACLS program	N	DOAP session	NA	7	406–564
IM2.22	Perform and demonstrate in a mannequin BLS	Y	DOAP session	Skill assessment	7	406–564
IM2.23	Describe and discuss the indications for nitrates, antiplatelet agents, gpIIb IIIa inhibitors, beta blockers, ACE inhibitors, etc., in the management of coronary syndromes	Y	Lecture, small group discussion	Written/viva voce	7	406–564
IM2.24	Counsel and communicate to patients with empathy lifestyle changes in atherosclerosis/ post-coronary syndromes	Y	DOAP session	Skill assessment	7	406–564
IM3.1	Define, discuss, describe and distinguish community acquired pneumonia, nosocomial pneumonia and aspiration pneumonia	Y	Lecture, small group discussion	Short note/viva voce	6	350–402
IM3.2	Discuss and describe the etiologies of various kinds of pneumonia and their microbiology depending on the setting and immune status of the host	Y	Lecture, small group discussion	Short note/viva voce	6	350–402
IM3.3	Discuss and describe the pathogenesis, presentation, natural history and complications of pneumonia	Y	Lecture, small group discussion	Short note/viva voce	6	350–402
IM3.4	Elicit document and present an appropriate history including the evolution, risk factors including immune status and occupational risk	Y	Bedside clinic, DOAP session	Skill assessment	6	350–402
IM3.5	Perform, document and demonstrate a physical examination including general examination and appropriate examination of the lungs that establishes the diagnosis, complications and severity of disease	Y	Bedside clinic, DOAP session	Skill assessment	6	350–402
IM3.6	Generate document and present a differential diagnosis based on the clinical features, and prioritise the diagnosis based on the presentation	Y	Bedside clinic, DOAP session	Skill assessment	6	350–402
IM3.7	Order and interpret diagnostic tests based on the clinical presentation including: CBC, chest X-ray PA view, Mantoux, sputum Gram stain, sputum culture and sensitivity, pleural fluid examination and culture, HIV testing and ABG	Y	Bedside clinic, DOAP session	Skill assessment	6	350–402
IM3.8	Demonstrate in a mannequin and interpret results of an arterial blood gas examination	Y	Bedside clinic, DOAP session	Skill assessment	6	350–402
IM3.9	Demonstrate in a mannequin and interpret results of a pleural fluid aspiration	Y	DOAP session	Skill assessment	6	350–402
IM3.10	Demonstrate the correct technique in a mannequin and interpret results of a blood culture	Y	DOAP session	Skill assessment	6	350–402
IM3.11	Describe and enumerate the indications for further testing including HRCT, viral cultures, PCR and specialized testing	Y	Bedside clinic, DOAP session	Skill assessment	6	350–402
IM3.12	Select, describe and prescribe based on the most likely etiology, an appropriate empirical antimicrobial based on the pharmacology and antimicrobial spectrum	Y	Bed side clinic, DOAP session	Skill assessment/written/ viva voce	6	350–402
IM3.13	Select, describe and prescribe based on culture and sensitivity appropriate empaling antimicrobial based on the pharmacology and antimicrobial spectrum	Y	Bedside clinic, DOAP session	Skill assessment/vritten/ viva voce	6	350–402
IM3.14	Perform and interpret a sputum Gram stain and AFB	Y	DOAP session	Skill assessment	6	350–402
IM3.15	Describe and enumerate the indications for hospitalization in patients with pneumonia	Y	Lecture, small group discussion	Short note/viva voce	6	350–402
IM3.16	Describe and enumerate the indications for isolation and barrier nursing in patients with pneumonia	Y	Lecture, small group discussion	Short note/viva voce	6	350–402

Number	COMPETENCY The student should be able to	Core Y/N	Suggested learning methods	Suggested assessment methods	Chapter No.	Page No.
IM3.17	Describe and discuss the supportive therapy in patients with pneumonia including oxygen use and indications for ventilation	Y	Lecture, small group discussion	Short note/viva voce	6	350–402
IM3.18	Communicate and counsel patient on family on the diagnosis and therapy of pneumonia	Y	DOAP session	Skill assessment	6	350–402
IM3.19	Discuss, describe, enumerate the indications and communicate to patients on pneumococcal and influenza vaccines	Y	Lecture, small group discussion	Short note/viva voce	6	350–402
IM4.8	Discuss and describe the pathophysiology, etiology and clinical manifestations of fever of unknown origin (FUO) including in a normal host, neutropenic host, nosocomial host and a host with HIV disease	Y	Lecture, small group discussion	Written	4	138–142
IM4.9	Elicit document and present a medical history that helps delineate the etiology of fever that includes the evolution and pattern of fever, associated symptoms, immune status, comorbidities, risk factors, exposure through occupation, travel and environment and medication use	Y	Bedside clinic, DOAP session	Skill assessment	1	30
IM5.1	Describe and discuss the physiologic and biochemical basis of hyperbilirubinemia	Y	Lecture, small group discussion	Written/viva voce	11	792–862
IM5.2	Describe and discuss the etiology and pathophysiology of liver injury	Y	Lecture, small group discussion	Written/viva voce	11	792–862
IM5.3	Describe and discuss the pathologic changes in various forms of liver disease	Y	Lecture, Small group discussion	Written/ Viva voce	11	792–862
IM5.4	Describe and discuss the epidemiology, microbiology, immunology and clinical evolution of infective (viral) hepatitis	Y	Lecture, small group discussion	Written/viva voce	11	792–862
IM5.5	Describe and discuss the pathophysiology and clinical evolution of alcoholic liver disease	Y	Lecture, small group discussion	Written/viva voce	11	792–862
IM5.6	Describe and discuss the pathophysiology, clinical evolution and complications of cirrhosis and portal hypertension including ascites, spontaneous bacterial peritonitis, hepatorenal syndrome and hepatic encephalopathy	Y	Lecture, small group discussion	Written/viva voce	11	792–862
IM5.7	Enumerate and describe the causes and pathophysiology of drug-induced liver injury	Y	Lecture, small group discussion	Written/ Viva voce	11	792–862
IM5.8	Describe and discuss the pathophysiology, clinical evolution and complications cholelithiasis and cholecystitis	Y	Lecture, small group discussion	Written/viva voce	11	792–862
IM5.9	Elicit document and present a medical history that helps delineate the etiology of the current presentation and includes clinical presentation, risk factors, drug use, sexual history, vaccination history and family history	Y	Bedside clinic, DOAP session	Skill assessment	11	792–862
IM5.10	Perform a systematic examination that establishes the diagnosis and severity that includes nutritional status, mental status, jaundice, abdominal distension ascites, features of portosystemic hypertension and hepatic encephalopathy	Y	Bedside clinic, DOAP session	Skill assessment	11	792–862
IM5.11	Generate a differential diagnosis and prioritise based on clinical features that suggest a specific etiology for the presenting symptom	Y	Bedside clinic, DOAP session	Skill assessment/ Viva voce	11	792–862
IM5.12	Choose and interpret appropriate diagnostic tests including: CBC, bilirubin, function tests, hepatitis serology and ascitic fluid examination in patient with liver diseases	Y	Bedside clinic, DOAP session	Skill assessment	11	792–862
IM5.13	Enumerate the indications for ultrasound and other imaging studies including MRCP and ERCP and describe the findings in liver disease	Y	Bedside clinic, small group discussion	Viva voce/written	11	792–862

Number	COMPETENCY The student should be able to	Core Y/N	Suggested learning methods	Suggested assessment methods	Chapter No.	Page No.
IM5.14	Outline a diagnostic approach to liver disease based on hyperbilirubinemia, liver function changes and hepatitis serology	Y	Bedside clinic, small group discussion	Viva voce/written	11	792–862
IM5.15	Assist in the performance and interpret the findings of an ascitic fluid analysis	Y	DOAP session	Documentation in logbook	11	792–862
IM5.16	Describe and discuss the management of hepatitis, cirrhosis, portal hypertension, ascites spontaneous, bacterial peritonitis and hepatic encephalopathy	Y	Written, small group discussion	Skill assessment/written/ viva voce	11	792–862
IM5.17	Enumerate the indications, precautions and counsel patients on vaccination for hepatitis	Y	Written, small group discussion	Written/viva voce	11	792–862
IM5.18	Enumerate the indications for hepatic transplantation	Y	Written, small group discussion	Written/viva voce	11	792–862
IM6.1	Describe and discuss the symptoms and signs of acute HIV seroconversion	Y	Lecture, small group discussion	Short note/viva voce	5	224–265
IM6.2	Define and classify HIV AIDS based on the CDC criteria	Y	Lecture, small group discussion	Short notes/viva voce	5	224–265
IM6.3	Describe and discuss the relationship between CDC count and the risk of opportunistic infections	Y	Lecture, small group discussion	Short notes/viva voce	5	224–265
IM6.4	Describe and discuss the pathogenesis, evolution and clinical features of common HIV related opportunistic infections	Y	Lecture, small group discussion	Short notes/viva voce	5	224–265
IM6.5	Describe and discuss the pathogenesis, evolution and clinical features of common HIV related malignancies	Y	Lecture, small group discussion	Short notes/viva voce	5	224–265
IM6.6	Describe and discuss the pathogenesis, evolution and clinical features of common HIV related skin and oral lesions	Y	Lecture, small group discussion	Short notes/viva voce	5	224–265
IM6.7	Elicit document and present a medical history that helps delineate the etiology of the current presentation and includes risk factors for HIV, mode of infection, other sexually transmitted diseases, risks for opportunistic infections and nutritional status	Y	Bedside clinic, DOAP session	Skill assessment	5	224–265
IM6.8	Generate a differential diagnosis and prioritise based on clinical features that suggest a specific etiology for the presenting symptom	Y	Bedside clinic, DOAP session, small group discussion	Skill assessment	5	224–265
IM6.9	Choose and interpret appropriate diagnostic tests to diagnose and classify the severity of HIV-AIDS including specific tests of HIV, CDC	Y	Bedside clinic, DOAP session, small group discussion	Written/ Skill assessment	5	224–265
IM6.10	Choose and interpret appropriate diagnostic tests to diagnose opportunistic infections including CBC, sputum examination and cultures, blood cultures, stool analysis, CSF analysis and chest radiographs	Y	Bedside clinic, DOAP session, small group discussion	Written/skill assessment	5	224–265
IM6.11	Enumerate the indications and describe the findings for CT of the chest and brain and MRI	N	Small group discussion, lecture, bedside clinic	Written/viva voce	5	224–265
IM6.12	Enumerate the indications for and interpret the results of: pulse oximetry, ABG, chest radiograph	Y	Bedside clinic, DOAP session, small group discussion	Written/skill assessment	5	224–265
IM6.13	Describe and enumerate the indications and side effects of drugs for bacterial, viral and other types of diarrhea	Y	Lecture, small group discussion	Written/viva voce	5	224–265
IM6.14	Perform and interpret AFB sputum	Y	DOAP session	Skill assessment	5	224–265
IM6.15	Demonstrate in a model the correct technique to perform a lumbar puncture	Y	Simulation	Skill assessment	5	224–265
IM6.16	Discuss and describe the principles of HAART, the classes of antiretrovirals used, adverse reactions and interactions	Y	Lecture, small group discussion	Written/viva voce	5	224–265
IM6.17	Discuss and describe the principles and regimens used in postexposure prophylaxis	Y	Lecture, small group discussion	Written/viva voce	5	224–265

Number	COMPETENCY The student should be able to	Core Y/N	Suggested learning methods	Suggested assessment methods	Chapter No.	Page No.
IM7.1	Describe the pathophysiology of autoimmune disease	Y	Lecture, small group discussion	Written/viva voce	9	683–733
IM7.2	Describe the genetic basis of autoimmune disease	N	Lecture, small group discussion	Written/viva voce	9	683–733
IM7.3	Classify cause of joint pain based on the pathophysiology	Y	Lecture, small group discussion	Written/viva voce	9	683–733
IM7.4	Develop a systematic clinical approach to joint pain based on the pathophysiology	Y	Lecture, small group discussion	Written/viva voce	9	683–733
IM7.5	Describe and discriminate acute, subacute and chronic causes of joint pain	Y	Lecture, small group discussion	Written/viva voce	9	683–733
IM7.6	Discriminate, describe and discuss arthralgia from arthritis and mechanical from inflammatory causes of joint pain	Y	Lecture, small group discussion	Written/viva voce	9	683–733
IM7.7	Discriminate, describe and discuss distinguishing articular from periarticular complaints	Y	Lecture, small group discussion	Written/viva voce	9	683–733
IM7.8	Determine the potential causes of join pain based on the presenting features of joint involvement	Y	Lecture, small group discussion	Written/viva voce	9	683–733
IM7.9	Describe the common signs and symptoms of articular and periarticular diseases	Y	Lecture, small group discussion	Written/viva voce	9	683–733
IM7.10	Describe the systemic manifestations of rheumatologic disease	Y	Lecture, small group discussion	Written/viva voce	9	683–733
IM7.11	Elicit document and present a medical history that will differentiate the etiologies of disease	Y	Bedside clinic, DOAP session	Skill assessment	9	683–733
IM7.12	Perform a systematic examination of all joints, muscle and skin that will establish the diagnosis and severity of disease	Y	Bedside clinic, DOAP session	Skill assessment	9	683–733
IM7.13	Generate a differential diagnosis and prioritise based on clinical features that suggest a specific etiology	Y	Bedside clinic, small group discussion	Skill assessment/written	9	683–733
IM7.14	Describe the appropriate diagnostic work up based on the presumed etiology	Y	Bedside clinic, small group discussion	Skill assessment/written	9	683–733
IM7.15	Enumerate the indications for and interpret the results of: CBC, anti-CCP, RA, ANA, DNA and other tests of autoimmunity	Y	Bedside clinic, small group discussion	Skill assessment/written	9	683–733
IM7.16	Enumerate the indications for arthrocentesis	Y	Small group discussion, lecture	Written/viva voce	9	683–733
IM7.17	Enumerate the indications and interpret plain radiographs of joints	Y	Bedside clinic, small group discussion	Skill assessment/written	9	683–733
IM7.18	Communicate diagnosis, treatment plan and subsequent follow up plan to patients	Y	DOAP session	Skill assessment/written	9	683–733
IM7.19	Develop an appropriate treatment plan for patients with rheumatologic diseases	Y	Bedside clinic, small group discussion	Skill assessment/written	9	683–733
IM7.20	Select, prescribe and communicate appropriate medications for relief of joint pain	Y	DOAP session	Skill assessment/written	9	683–733
IM7.21	Select, prescribe and communicate preventive therapy for crystalline arthropathies	Y	DOAP session	Skill assessment/written	9	683–733
IM7.22	Select, prescribe and communicate treatment option for systemic rheumatologic conditions	Y	DOAP session	Skill assessment/written	9	683–733
IM7.23	Describe the basis for biologic and disease modifying therapy in rheumatologic diseases	Y	Bedside clinic, small group discussion	Skill assessment/written	9	683–733
IM7.24	Communicate and incorporate patient preferences in the choice of therapy	Y	DOAP session	Skill assessment	9	683–733
IM7.25	Develop and communicate appropriate follow up and monitoring plans for patients with rheumatologic conditions	Y	DOAP session	Skill assessment	9	683–733
IM7.26	Demonstrate an understanding of the impact of rheumatologic conditions on quality of life, well being, work and family	Y	DOAP session	Skill assessment	9	683–733

Number	COMPETENCY The student should be able to	Core Y/N	Suggested learning methods	Suggested assessment methods	Chapter No.	Page No.
IM7.27	Determine the need for specialist consultation	Y	Small group discussion, lecture	Viva voce	9	683–733
IM8.1	Describe and discuss the epidemiology, etiology and the prevalence of primary and secondary hypertension	Y	Lecture, small group discussion	Written/viva voce	7	451–458
IM8.2	Describe and discuss the pathophysiology of hypertension	Y	Lecture, small group discussion	Written/viva voce	7	451–458
IM8.3	Describe and discuss the genetic basis of hypertension	N	Lecture, small group discussion	Written/viva voce	7	451–458
IM8.4	Define and classify hypertension	Y	Lecture, small group discussion	Written/viva voce	7	451–458
IM8.5	Describe and discuss the differences between primary and secondary hypertension	Y	Lecture, small group discussion	Written/viva voce	7	451–458
IM8.6	Define, describe and discuss and recognize hypertensive urgency and emergency	Y	Lecture, small group discussion	Written/viva voce	7	451–458
IM8.7	Describe and discuss the clinical manifestations of the various etiologies of secondary causes of hypertension	Y	Lecture, small group discussion	Written/viva voce	7	451–458
IM8.8	Describe, discuss and identify target organ damage due to hypertension	Y	Lecture, small group discussion	Written/viva voce	7	451–458
IM8.9	Elicit document and present a medical history that includes: duration and levels, symptoms, comorbidities, lifestyle, risk factors, family history, psychosocial and environmental factors, dietary assessment, previous and concomitant therapy	Y	Bedside clinic, DOAP session	Skill assessment	7	451–458
IM9.1	Define, describe and classify anemia based on red blood cell size and reticulocyte count	Y	Lecture, small group discussion	Written/viva voce	8	565–603
IM9.2	Describe and discuss the morphological characteristics, etiology and prevalence of each of the causes of anemia	Y	Lecture, small group discussion	Written/viva voce	8	565–603
IM9.3	Elicit document and present a medical history that includes symptoms, risk factors including GI bleeding, prior history, medications, menstrual history, and family history	Y	Bed side clinic, DOAP session	Skill assessment	8	565–603
IM9.4	Perform a systematic examination that includes: general examination for pallor, oral examination, DOAP session of hyperdynamic circulation, lymph node and splenic examination	Y	Bedside clinic, DOAP session	Skill assessment	8	565–603
IM9.5	Generate a differential diagnosis and prioritize based on clinical features that suggest a specific etiology	Y	Bedside clinic, DOAP session	Skill assessment/written	8	565–603
IM9.6	Describe the appropriate diagnostic work up based on the presumed etiology	Y	Bedside clinic, DOAP session	Skill assessment/written	8	565–603
IM9.7	Describe and discuss the meaning and utility of various components of the hemogram	Y	Lecture, small group discussion	Written/viva voce/skill assessment	8	565–603
IM9.8	Describe and discuss the various tests for iron deficiency	Y	Lecture, small group discussion	Written/viva voce/skill assessment	8	565–603
IM9.9	Order and interpret tests for anemia including hemogram, red cell indices, reticulocyte count, iron studies, B12 and folate	Y	Bedside clinic, DOAP session	Skill assessment/written	8	565–603
IM9.10	Describe, perform and interpret a peripheral smear and stool occult blood	P	Bedside clinic, DOAP session	Skill assessment/written	8	565–603
IM9.11	Describe the indications and interpret the results of a bone marrow aspirations and biopsy	Y	Lecture, small group discussion	Written/viva voce/skill assessment	8	565–603
IM9.12	Describe, develop a diagnostic plan to determine the etiology of anemia	Y	Lecture, small group discussion	Written/viva voce/skill assessment	8	565–603
IM9.13	Prescribe replacement therapy with iron, B12, folate	Y	Bedside clinic, DOAP session	Skill assessment/written	8	565–603

Number	COMPETENCY The student should be able to	Core Y/N	Suggested learning methods	Suggested assessment methods	Chapter No.	Page No.
IM9.14	Describe the national programs for anemia prevention	Y	Lecture, small group discussion	Written/viva voce	8	565–603
IM9.15	Communicate the diagnosis and the treatment appropriately to patients	Y	DOAP session	Skill assessment	8	565–603
IM9.16	Incorporate patient preferences in the management of anemia	Y	DOAP session	Skill assessment	8	565–603
IM9.17	Describe the indications for blood transfusion and the appropriate use of blood components	Y	Lecture, small group discussion	Written/viva voce/skill assessment	8	565–603
IM9.18	Describe the precautions required necessary when performing a blood transfusion	Y	Lecture, small group discussion	Written/ Viva voce/ Skill assessment	8	565–603
IM10.1	Define, describe and differentiate between acute and chronic renal failure	Y	Lecture, small group discussion	Written/viva voce	13	878–932
IM10.2	Classify, describe and differentiate the pathophysiologic causes of acute renal failure	Y	Lecture, small group discussion	Written/viva voce	13	878–932
IM10.3	Describe the pathophysiology and causes of pre renal ARF, renal and post renal ARF	Y	Lecture, small group discussion	Written/viva voce	13	878–932
IM10.4	Describe the evolution, natural history and treatment of ARF	Y	Lecture, small group discussion	Written/viva voce	13	878–932
IM10.5	Describe and discuss the etiology of CRF	Y	Lecture, small group discussion	Written/viva voce	13	878–932
IM10.6	Stage chronic kidney disease	Y	Lecture, small group discussion	Written/viva voce	13	878–932
IM10.7	Describe and discuss the pathophysiology and clinical findings of uremia	Y	Lecture, small group discussion	Written/viva voce	13	878–932
IM10.8	Classify, describe and discuss the significance of proteinuria in CKD	Y	Lecture, small group discussion	Written/viva voce	13	878–932
IM10.9	Describe and discuss the pathophysiology of anemia and hyperparathyroidism in CKD	Y	Lecture, small group discussion	Written/viva voce	13	878–932
IM10.10	Describe and discuss the association between CKD glycemia and hypertension	Y	Lecture, small group discussion	Written/viva voce	13	878–932
IM10.11	Describe and discuss the relationship between CAD risk factors and CKD and in dialysis	Y	Lecture, small group discussion	Written/viva voce	13	878–932
IM10.12	Elicit document and present a medical history that will differentiate the etiologies of disease, distinguish acute and chronic disease, identify predisposing conditions, nephrotoxic drugs and systemic causes	Y	Bedside clinic, DOAP session	Skill assessment	13	878–932
IM10.13	Perform a systematic examination that establishes the diagnosis and severity including determination of volume status, presence of edema and heart failure, features of uremia and associated systemic disease	Y	Bedside clinic, DOAP session	Skill assessment	13	878–932
IM10.14	Generate a differential diagnosis and prioritize based on clinical features that suggest a specific etiology	Y	DOAP session, small group discussion	Skill assessment/written/ viva voce	13	878–932
IM10.15	Describe the appropriate diagnostic work up based on the presumed etiology	Y	DOAP session, small group discussion	Skill assessment/written/ viva voce	13	878–932
IM10.16	Enumerate the indications for and interpret the results of: renal function tests, calcium, phosphorus, PTH, urine electrolytes, osmolality, anion gap	Y	DOAP session, small group discussion	Skill assessment/written/ viva voce	13	878–932
IM10.17	Describe and calculate indices of renal function based on available laboratories including fractional excretion of sodium (FENa) and creatinine clearance (CrCl)	Y	DOAP session, small group discussion	Skill assessment/written/ viva voce	13	878–932
IM10.18	Identify the ECG findings in hyperkalemia	Y	DOAP session, small group discussion	Skill assessment/written/ viva voce	13	878–932
IM10.19	Enumerate the indications and describe the findings in renal ultrasound	N	Lecture, small group discussion	Written/viva voce	13	878–932
IM10.20	Describe and discuss the indications to perform arterial blood gas analysis: interpret the data	Y	DOAP session	Documentation in logbook	13	878–932

Number	COMPETENCY The student should be able to	Core Y/N	Suggested learning methods	Suggested assessment methods	Chapter No.	Page No.
IM10.21	Describe and discuss the indications for and insert a peripheral intravenous catheter	Y	DOAP session, bedside clinic	Documentation in logbook	13	878–932
IM10.22	Describe and discuss the indications, demonstrate in a model and assist in the insertion of a central venous or a dialysis catheter	N	DOAP session	Skill assessment with model	13	878–932
IM10.23	Communicate diagnosis treatment plan and subsequent follow up plan to patients	Y	DOAP session	Skill assessment	13	878–932
IM10.24	Counsel patients on a renal diet	Y	DOAP session	Skill assessment	13	878–932
IM10.25	Identify and describe the priorities in the management of ARF including diet, volume management, alteration in doses of drugs, monitoring and indications for dialysis	Y	Lecture, small group discussion	Written/viva voce	13	878–932
IM10.26	Describe and discuss supportive therapy in CKD including diet, antihypertensives, glycemic therapy, dyslipidemia, anemia, hyperkalemia, hyperphosphatemia and secondary hyperparathyroidism	Y	Lecture, small group discussion	Written/viva voce	13	878–932
IM10.27	Describe and discuss the indications for renal dialysis	Y	Lecture, small group discussion	Written/viva voce	13	878–932
IM10.28	Describe and discuss the indications for renal replacement therapy	Y	Lecture, small group discussion	Written/viva voce	13	878–932
IM10.29	Describe discuss and communicate the ethical and legal issues involved in renal replacement therapy	Y	Lecture, small group discussion	Written/viva voce	13	878–932
IM10.30	Recognise the impact of CKD on patient's quality of life well being work and family	Y	Lecture, small group discussion, bedside clinic	Observation by faculty	13	878–932
IM10.31	Incorporate patient preferences in to the care of CKD	Y	Lecture, small group discussion, bedside clinic	Observation by faculty	13	878–932
IM11.1	Define and classify diabetes	Y	Lecture, small group discussion	Written/viva voce	3	94–132
IM11.2	Describe and discuss the epidemiology and pathogenesis and risk factors and clinical evolution of type 1 diabetes	Y	Lecture, small group discussion	Written/viva voce	3	94–132
IM11.3	Describe and discuss the epidemiology and pathogenesis and risk factors economic impact and clinical evolution of type 2 diabetes	Y	Lecture, small group discussion	Written/viva voce	3	94–132
IM11.4	Describe and discuss the genetic background and the influence of the environment on diabetes	N	Lecture, small group discussion	Written/viva voce	3	94–132
IM11.5	Describe and discuss the pathogenesis and temporal evolution of microvascular and macrovascular complications of diabetes	Y	Lecture, small group discussion	Written/viva voce	3	94–132
IM11.6	Describe and discuss the pathogenesis and precipitating factors, recognition and management of diabetic emergencies	Y	Lecture, small group discussion	Written/viva voce	3	94–132
IM11.7	Elicit document and present a medical history that will differentiate the etiologies of diabetes including risk factors, precipitating factors, lifestyle, nutritional history, family history, medication history, comorbidities and target organ disease	Y	Bedside clinic, DOAP session	Skill assessment	3	94–132
IM11.8	Perform a systematic examination that establishes the diagnosis and severity that includes skin, peripheral pulses, blood pressure measurement, fundus examination, detailed examination of the foot (pulses, nervous and deformities and injuries)	Y	Bedside clinic, DOAP session	Skill assessment	3	94–132

Number	COMPETENCY The student should be able to	Core Y/N	Suggested learning methods	Suggested assessment methods	Chapter No.	Page No.
IM11.9	Describe and recognize the clinical features of patients who present with a diabetic emergency	Y	Small group discussion, lecture	Written/viva voce	3	94–132
IM11.10	Generate a differential diagnosis and prioritise based on clinical features that suggest a specific etiology	Y	Small group discussion, lecture	Written/viva voce	3	94–132
IM11.11	Order and interpret laboratory tests to diagnose diabetes and its complications including: glucoses, glucose tolerance test, glycosylated hemoglobin, urinary microalbumin, ECG, electrolytes, ABG, ketones, renal function tests and lipid profile	Y	Bedside clinic, DOAP session	Skill assessment	3	94–132
IM11.12	Perform and interpret a capillary blood glucose test	Y	Bedside clinic, DOAP session	Skill assessment	3	94–132
IM11.13	Perform and interpret a urinary ketone estimation with a dipstick	Y	Bedside clinic, DOAP session	Skill assessment	3	94–132
IM11.14	Recognize the presentation of hypoglycemia and outline the principles on its therapy	Y	Small group discussion, lecture	Written/viva voce	3	94–132
IM11.15	Recognize the presentation of diabetic emergencies and outline the principles of therapy	Y	Small Group discussion, lecture	Written/viva voce	3	94–132
IM11.16	Discuss and describe the pharmacologic therapies for diabetes their indications, contraindications, adverse reactions and interactions	Y	Small group discussion, lecture	Written/viva voce	3	94–132
IM11.17	Outline a therapeutic approach to therapy of T2 diabetes based on presentation, severity and complications in a cost effective manner	Y	Small group discussion, lecture	Written/viva voce	3	94–132
IM11.18	Describe and discuss the pharmacology, indications, adverse reactions and interactions of drugs used in the prevention and treatment of target organ damage and complications of type II diabetes including neuropathy, nephropathy, retinopathy, hypertension, dyslipidemia and cardiovascular disease	Y	Lecture, small group discussion	Written/viva voce	3	94–132
IM11.19	Demonstrate and counsel patients on the correct technique to administer insulin	Y	DOAP session	Skill assessment	3	94–132
IM11.20	Demonstrate to and counsel patients on the correct technique of self-monitoring of blood glucoses	Y	DOAP session	Skill assessment	3	94–132
IM11.21	Recognize the importance of patient preference while selecting therapy for diabetes	Y	DOAP session	Faculty observation	3	94–132
IM11.22	Enumerate the causes of hypoglycemia and describe the counter hormone response and the initial approach and treatment	Y	Lecture, small group discussion	Written/viva voce	3	94–132
IM11.23	Describe the precipitating causes, pathophysiology, recognition, clinical features, diagnosis, stabilization and management of diabetic ketoacidosis	Y	Lecture, small group discussion	Written/viva voce	3	94–132
IM11.24	Describe the precipitating causes, pathophysiology, recognition, clinical features, diagnosis, stabilization and management of hyperosmolar non-ketotic state	N	Lecture, small group discussion	Written/viva voce	3	94–132
IM12.1	Describe the epidemiology and pathogenesis of hypothyroidism and hyperthyroidism including the influence of iodine deficiency and autoimmunity in the pathogenesis of thyroid disease	Y	Lecture, small group discussion	Written/viva voce	2	50–70
IM12.2	Describe and discuss the genetic basis of some forms of thyroid dysfunction	N	Lecture, small group discussion	Written/viva voce	2	50–70
IM12.3	Describe and discuss the physiology of the hypothalamopituitary—thyroid axis, principles of thyroid function testing and alterations in physiologic function	Y	Lecture, small group discussion	Short notes	2	50–70

Number	COMPETENCY The student should be able to	Core Y/N	Suggested learning methods	Suggested assessment methods	Chapter No.	Page No.
IM12.4	Describe and discuss the principles of radioiodine uptake in the diagnosis of thyroid disorders	Y	Lecture, small group discussion	Short notes/viva voce	2	50–70
IM12.5	Elicit document and present an appropriate history that will establish the diagnosis cause of thyroid dysfunction and its severity	Y	Bedside clinic	Skill assessment/short case	2	50–70
IM12.6	Perform and demonstrate a systematic examination based on the history that will help establish the diagnosis and severity including systemic signs of thyrotoxicosis and hypothyroidism, palpation of the pulse for rate and rhythm abnormalities, neck palpation of the thyroid and lymph nodes and cardiovascular findings	Y	Bed side clinic, DOAP session	Skill assessment	2	50–70
IM12.7	Demonstrate the correct technique to palpate the thyroid	Y	Bedside clinic, DOAP session	Skill assessment	2	50–70
IM12.8	Generate a differential diagnosis based on the clinical presentation and prioritise it based on the most likely diagnosis	Y	Bedside clinic, small group discussion	Short case	2	50–70
IM12.9	Order and interpret diagnostic testing based on the clinical diagnosis including CBC, thyroid function tests and ECG and radioiodine uptake and scan	Y	Bedside clinic, DOAP session	Skill assessment	2	50–70
IM12.10	Identify atrial fibrillation, pericardial effusion and bradycardia on ECG	Y	Bedside clinic, laboratory	Skill assessment	2	50–70
IM12.11	Interpret thyroid function tests in hypo- and hyperthyroidism	Y	Bedside clinic, laboratory	Skill assessment	2	50–70
IM12.14	Write and communicate to the patient appropriately a prescription for thyroxine based on age, sex, and clinical and biochemical status	Y	Skill assessment	Skill assessment	2	50–70
IM12.15	Describe and discuss the indications of thionamide therapy, radioiodine therapy and surgery in the management of thyrotoxicosis	Y	Bedside clinic, small group discussion	Short note/viva voce	2	50–70
IM13.1	Describe the clinical epidemiology and inherited and modifiable risk factors for common malignancies in India	Y	Lecture, small group discussion	Short note/viva voce	8, 12	605–638 873–875
IM13.2	Describe the genetic basis of selected cancers	N	Lecture, small group discussion	Short note/viva voce	8, 12	605–638 873–875
IM13.3	Describe the relationship between infection and cancers	Y	Lecture, small group discussion	Short note/viva voce	8, 12	605–638 873–875
IM13.4	Describe the natural history, presentation, course, complications and cause of death for common cancers	Y	Lecture, small group discussion	Short note/viva voce	8, 12	605–638 873–875
IM13.5	Describe the common issues encountered in patients at the end of life and principles of management	N	Lecture, small group discussion	Short note/viva voce	8, 12	605–638 873–875
IM13.6	Describe and distinguish the difference between curative and palliative care in patients with cancer	N	Lecture, small group discussion	Short note/viva voce	8, 12	605–638 873–875
IM13.7	Elicit document and present a history that will help establish the etiology of cancer and includes the appropriate risk factors, duration and evolution	Y	Bedside clinic	Skill assessment/short case	8, 12	605–638 873–875
IM13.8	Perform and demonstrate a physical examination that includes an appropriate general and local examination that excludes the diagnosis, extent spread and complications of cancer	Y	Bedside clinic	Skill assessment/short case	8, 12	605–638 873–875

Number	COMPETENCY The student should be able to	Core Y/N	Suggested learning methods	Suggested assessment methods	Chapter No.	Page No.
IM13.9	Demonstrate in a mannequin the correct technique for performing breast examination, rectal examination and cervical examination and Pap smear	Y	Bedside clinic	Skill assessment/short case	8, 12	605–638 873–875
IM13.10	Generate a differential diagnosis based on the presenting symptoms and clinical features and prioritise based on the most likely diagnosis	Y	Bedside clinic	Skill assessment/ short case	8, 12	605–638 873–875
IM13.11	Order and interpret diagnostic testing based on the clinical diagnosis including CBC and stool occult blood and prostate specific antigen	Y	Bedside clinic	Skill assessment/short case	8, 12	605–638 873–875
IM13.12	Describe the indications and interpret the results of chest X-ray, mammogram, skin and tissue biopsies and tumor markers used in common cancers	Y	Bedside clinic, small group discussion	Short note/viva voce	8, 12	605–638 873–875
IM13.13	Describe and assess pain and suffering objectively in a patient with cancer	Y	Bedside clinic, small group discussion	Short note/viva voce	8, 12	605–638 873–875
IM13.14	Describe the indications for surgery, radiation and chemotherapy for common malignancies	Y	Bedside clinic, small group discussion	Short note/viva voce	8, 12	605–638 873–875
IM13.15	Describe the need, tests involved, their utility in the prevention of common malignancies	Y	Bedside clinic, small group discussion	Short note/viva voce	8, 12	605–638 873–875
IM13.16	Demonstrate an understanding and needs and preferences of patients when choosing curative and palliative therapy	Y	Bedside clinic, small group discussion	Short note/viva voce	8, 12	605–638 873–875
IM13.17	Describe and enumerate the indications, use, side effects of narcotics in pain alleviation in patients with cancer	Y	Bedside clinic, small group discussion	Short note/viva voce	8, 12	605–638 873–875
IM13.18	Describe and discuss the ethical and the medicolegal issues involved in end of life care	Y	Bedside clinic, small group discussion	Short note/viva voce	8, 12	605–638 873–875
IM13.19	Describe the therapies used in alleviating suffering in patients at the end of life	Y	Bedside clinic, small group discussion	Short note/viva voce	8, 12	605–638 873–875
IM14.1	Define and measure obesity as it relates to the Indian population	Y	Lecture, small group discussion	Short note/viva voce	1	22–30
IM14.2	Describe and discuss the etiology of obesity including modifiable and non-modifiable risk factors and secondary causes	Y	Lecture, small group discussion	Short note/viva voce	1	22–30
IM14.3	Describe and discuss the monogenic forms of obesity	N	Lecture, small group discussion	Short note/viva voce	1	22–30
IM14.4	Describe and discuss the impact of environmental factors including eating habits, food, work, environment and physical activity on the incidence of obesity	Y	Lecture, small group discussion	Short note/viva voce	1	22–30
IM14.5	Describe and discuss the natural history of obesity and its complications	Y	Lecture, small group discussion	Short note/ Viva voce	1	22–30
IM14.6	Elicit and document and present an appropriate history that includes the natural history, dietary history, modifiable risk factors, family history, clues for secondary causes and motivation to lose weight	Y	Bedside clinic, skills laboratory	Skill assessment	1	22–30
IM14.7	Perform, document and demonstrate a physical examination based on the history that includes general examination, measurement of abdominal obesity, signs of secondary causes and comorbidities	Y	Bedside clinic, skills laboratory	Skill assessment	1	22–30
IM14.8	Generate a differential diagnosis based on the presenting symptoms and clinical features and prioritise based on the most likely diagnosis	Y	Bedside clinic, skills laboratory	Skill assessment/short note/viva voce	1	22–30
IM14.9	Order and interpret diagnostic tests based on the clinical diagnosis including blood glucose, lipids, thyroid function tests, etc.	Y	Bedside clinic, skills laboratory, small group discussion	Skill assessment/short note/viva voce	1	22–30

Number	COMPETENCY The student should be able to	Core Y/N	Suggested learning methods	Suggested assessment methods	Chapter No.	Page No.
IM14.10	Describe the indications and interpret the results of tests for secondary causes of obesity	Y	Bedside clinic, skills laboratory, small group discussion	Skill assessment/short note/viva voce	1	22–30
IM14.11	Communicate and counsel patient on behavioral, dietary and lifestyle modifications	Y	Bedside clinic, skills laboratory	Skill assessment	1	22–30
IM14.12	Demonstrate an understanding of patient's inability to adhere to lifestyle instructions and counsel them in a non- judgemental way	Y	Bedside clinic, skills laboratory	Skill assessment	1	22–30
IM14.13	Describe and enumerate the indications, pharmacology and side effects of pharmacotherapy for obesity	Y	Lecture, small group discussion	Short note/viva voce	1	22–30
IM14.14	Describe and enumerate the indications and side effects of bariatric surgery	Y	Lecture, small group discussion	Short note/viva voce	1	22–30
IM14.15	Describe and enumerate and educate patients, healthcare workers and the public on measures to prevent obesity and promote a healthy lifestyle	Y	Lecture, small group discussion	Short note/viva voce	1	22–30
IM15.1	Enumerate, describe and discuss the etiology of upper and lower GI bleeding	Y	Lecture, small group discussion	Short note/viva voce	10	735–789
IM15.2	Enumerate, describe and discuss the evaluation and steps involved in stabilizing a patient who presents with acute volume loss and GI bleed	Y	DOAP session, small group discussion, lecture	Written/viva voce/skill assessment	10	735–789
IM15.3	Describe and discuss the physiologic effects of acute blood and volume loss	Y	Lecture, small group discussion	Short note/viva voce	10	735–789
IM15.4	Elicit and document and present an appropriate history that identifies the route of bleeding, quantity, grade, volume loss, duration, etiology, comorbid illnesses and risk factors	Y	Bedside clinic	Skill assessment	10	735–789
IM15.5	Perform, demonstrate and document a physical examination based on the history that includes general examination, volume assessment and appropriate abdominal examination	Y	Bedside clinic, skills laboratory	Skill assessment	10	735–789
IM15.6	Distinguish between upper and lower gastrointestinal bleeding based on the clinical features	Y	Lecture, small group discussion	Short note/viva voce		
IM15.7	Demonstrate the correct technique to perform an anal and rectal examination in a mannequin or equivalent	Y	DOAP session	Skill assessment	10	735–789
IM15.8	Generate a differential diagnosis based on the presenting symptoms and clinical features and prioritise based on the most likely diagnosis	Y	Bedside clinic, skills laboratory	Skill assessment/short note/viva voce	10	735–789
IM15.9	Choose and interpret diagnostic tests based on the clinical diagnosis including complete blood count, PT and PTT, stool examination, occult blood, liver function tests, *H. pylori* test	Y	Bedside clinic, DOAP session, small group discussion	Skill assessment/ Short note/ Viva voce	10	735–789
IM15.10	Enumerate the indications for endoscopy, colonoscopy and other imaging procedures in the investigation of upper GI bleeding	Y	Lecture, small group discussion	Written/viva voce	10	735–789
IM15.11	Develop, document and present a treatment plan that includes fluid resuscitation, blood and blood component transfusion, and specific therapy for arresting blood loss	Y	Lecture, Small group discussion	Short note/viva voce	10	735–789
IM15.14	Describe and enumerate the indications, pharmacology and side effects of pharmacotherapy of pressors used in the treatment of upper GI bleed	Y	Lecture, Small group discussion	Short note/viva voce	10	735–789
IM15.15	Describe and enumerate the indications, pharmacology and side effects of pharmacotherapy of acid peptic disease including *Helicobacter pylori*	Y	Lecture, small group discussion	Short note/viva voce	10	735–789

Number	COMPETENCY	Core Y/N	Suggested learning methods	Suggested assessment methods	Chapter No.	Page No.
	The student should be able to					
IM15.16	Enumerate the indications for endoscopic interventions and surgery	Y	Lecture, small group discussion	Short note/viva voce	10	735–789
IM15.17	Determine appropriate level of specialist consultation	Y	Small group discussion	Short note/viva voce	10	735–789
IM15.18	Counsel the family and patient in an empathetic non-judgmental manner on the diagnosis and therapeutic options	Y	DOAP session	Skill assessment	10	735–789
IM16.1	Describe and discuss the etiology of acute and chronic diarrhea including infectious and non-infectious causes	Y	Lecture, small group discussion	Short note/viva voce	10	735–789
IM16.2	Describe and discuss the acute systemic consequences of diarrhea including its impact on fluid balance	Y	Lecture, small group discussion	Short note/viva voce	10	735–789
IM16.3	Describe and discuss the chronic effects of diarrhea including malabsorption	Y	Lecture, small group discussion	Short note/viva voce	10	735–789
IM16.4	Elicit and document and present an appropriate history that includes the natural history, dietary history, travel , sexual history and other concomitant illnesses	Y	Bedside clinic, skills laboratory	Skill assessment	10	735–789
IM16.5	Perform, document and demonstrate a physical examination based on the history that includes general examination, including an appropriate abdominal examination	Y	Bedside clinic, skills laboratory	Skill assessment	10	735–789
IM16.6	Distinguish between diarrhea and dysentery based on clinical features	Y	Lecture, small group discussion	Short note/viva voce	10	735–789
IM16.7	Generate a differential diagnosis based on the presenting symptoms and clinical features and prioritise based on the most likely diagnosis	Y	Bedside clinic, skills laboratory	Skill assessment/short note/viva voce	10	735–789
IM16.8	Choose and interpret diagnostic tests based on the clinical diagnosis including complete blood count, and stool examination	Y	Bedside clinic, skills laboratory, small group discussion	Skill assessment/short note/viva voce	10	735–789
IM16.9	Identify common parasitic causes of diarrhea under the microscope in a stool specimen	Y	DOAP session	Skill assessment	10	735–789
IM16.10	Identify *Vibrio cholerae* in a hanging drop specimen	Y	DOAP session	Skill Assessment	10	735–789
IM16.11	Enumerate the indications for stool cultures and blood cultures in patients with acute diarrhea	Y	Lecture, small group discussion	Written/viva voce	10	735–789
IM16.12	Enumerate and discuss the indications for further investigations including antibodies, colonoscopy, diagnostic imaging and biopsy in the diagnosis of chronic diarrhea	Y	Lecture, small group discussion	Written/viva voce	10	735–789
IM16.13	Describe and enumerate the indications, pharmacology and side effects of pharmacotherapy for parasitic causes of diarrhea	Y	Lecture, small group discussion	Short note/viva voce	10	735–789
IM16.14	Describe and enumerate the indications, pharmacology and side effects of pharmacotherapy for bacterial and viral diarrhea	Y	Lecture, small group discussion	Short note/viva voce	10	735–789
IM16.15	Distinguish based on the clinical presentation Crohn's disease from ulcerative colitis	Y	Lecture, small group discussion	Short note/viva voce	10	735–789
IM16.16	Describe and enumerate the indications, pharmacology and side effects of pharmacotherapy including immunotherapy	Y	Lecture, Small group discussion	Short note/viva voce	10	735–789
IM16.17	Describe and enumerate the indications for surgery in inflammatory bowel disease	Y	Lecture, Small group discussion	Short note/viva voce	10	735–789

Number	Competency The student should be able to	Core Y/N	Suggested learning methods	Suggested assessment methods	Chapter No.	Page No.
Topic: Headache Number of competencies: (14) Number of procedures that require certification: (NIL)						
IM17.1	Define and classify headache and describe the presenting features, precipitating factors, aggravating and relieving factors of various kinds of headache	Y	Lecture, small group discussion	Short note/viva voce	15	968–1068
IM17.2	Elicit and document and present an appropriate history including aura, precipitating aggravating and relieving factors, associated symptoms that help identify the cause of headaches	Y	Bedside clinic, small group discussion	Bedside clinic/skill assessment	15	968–1068
IM17.3	Classify migraine and describe the distinguishing features between classical and non-classical forms of migraine	Y	Bedside clinic, small group discussion	Bedside clinic/skill assessment	15	968–1068
IM17.4	Perform and demonstrate a general neurologic examination and a focused examination for signs of intracranial tension including neck signs of meningitis	Y	Bedside clinic, small group discussion	Bedside clinic/skill assessment	15	968–1068
IM17.5	Generate document and present a differential diagnosis based on the clinical features, and prioritize the diagnosis based on the presentation	Y	Bedside clinic, small group discussion	Bedside clinic/skill assessment	15	968–1068
IM17.6	Choose and interpret diagnostic testing based on the clinical diagnosis including imaging	Y	Lecture, small group discussion, bedside clinic	Skill assessment	15	968–1068
IM17.7	Enumerate the indications and describe the findings in the CSF in patients with meningitis	Y	Small group discussion, bedside clinic	Skill assessment	15	968–1068
IM17.8	Demonstrate in a mannequin or equivalent the correct technique for performing a lumbar puncture	Y	DOAP session	Skill assessment	15	968–1068
IM17.9	Interpret the CSF findings when presented with various parameters of CSF fluid analysis	Y	Small group discussion, bedside clinic	Skill assessment	15	968–1068
IM17.10	Enumerate the indications for emergency care admission and immediate supportive care in patients with headache	Y	Lecture, small group discussion	Written/viva voce	15	968–1068
IM17.11	Describe the indications, pharmacology, dose, side effects of abortive therapy in migraine	Y	Lecture, small group discussion	Written/viva voce	15	968–1068
IM17.12	Describe the indications, pharmacology, dose, side effects of prophylactic therapy in migraine	Y	Lecture, small group discussion	Written/viva voce	15	968–1068
IM17.13	Describe the pharmacology, dose, adverse reactions and regimens of drugs used in the treatment of bacterial, tubercular and viral meningitis	Y	Lecture, small group discussion	Written/viva voce	15	968–1068
IM17.14	Counsel patients with migraine and tension headache on lifestyle changes and need for prophylactic therapy	N	DOAP session	Skill assessment	15	968–1068
IM18.1	Describe the functional and the vascular anatomy of the brain	Y	Lecture, small group discussion	Written/viva voce	15	968–1068
IM18.2	Classify cerebrovascular accidents and describe the etiology, predisposing genetic and risk factors pathogenesis of hemorrhagic and non hemorrhagic stroke	Y	Lecture, small group discussion	Written/viva voce	15	968–1068
IM18.3	Elicit and document and present an appropriate history including onset, progression, precipitating and aggravating relieving factors, associated symptoms that help identify the cause of the cerebrovascular accident	Y	Bedside clinic	Skill assessment	15	968–1068
IM18.4	Identify the nature of the cerebrovascular accident based on the temporal evolution and resolution of the illness	Y	Bedside clinic, small group discussion	Skill assessment	15	968–1068

Number	Competency The student should be able to	Core Y/N	Suggested learning methods	Suggested assessment methods	Chapter No.	Page No.
IM18.5	Perform, demonstrate and document physical examination that includes general and a detailed neurologic examination as appropriate, based on the history	Y	Bedside clinic, DOAP session	Skill assessment	15	968–1068
IM18.6	Distinguish the lesion based on upper versus lower motor neuron, side, site and most probable nature of the lesion	Y	Bedside clinic, DOAP session	Skill assessment	15	968–1068
IM18.7	Describe the clinical features and distinguish, based on clinical examination, the various disorders of speech	N	Bedside clinic, DOAP session	Skill assessment	15	968–1068
IM18.8	Describe and distinguish, based on the clinical presentation, the types of bladder dysfunction seen in CNS disease	Y	Small group discussion, bedside clinic	Written/viva voce	15	968–1068
IM18.9	Choose and interpret the appropriate diagnostic and imaging test that will delineate the anatomy and underlying cause of the lesion	Y	Bedside clinic, DOAP session, small group discussion	Written/viva voce/skill assessment	15	968–1068
IM18.10	Choose and interpret the appropriate diagnostic testing in young patients with a cerebrovascular accident (CVA)	Y	Lecture, small group discussion	Written/viva voce	15	968–1068
IM18.11	Describe the initial supportive management of a patient presenting with a cerebrovascular accident (CVA)	Y	Lecture, small group discussion	Written/viva voce	15	968–1068
IM18.12	Enumerate the indications for and describe acute therapy of non-hemorrhagic stroke including the use of thrombolytic agents	Y	Lecture, small group discussion	Written/viva voce	15	968–1068
IM18.13	Enumerate the indications for and describe the role of antiplatelet agents in non-hemorrhagic stroke	Y	Lecture, small group discussion	Written/viva voce	15	968–1068
IM18.14	Describe the initial management of a hemorrhagic stroke	Y	Lecture, small group discussion	Written/viva voce	15	968–1068
IM18.15	Enumerate the indications for surgery in a hemorrhagic stroke	Y	Lecture, small group discussion	Written/viva voce	15	968–1068
IM18.16	Enumerate the indications describe and observe the multidisciplinary rehabilitation of patients with a CVA	Y	Lecture, small group discussion	Written/viva voce	15	968–1068
IM18.17	Counsel patient and family about the diagnosis and therapy in an empathetic manner	Y	DOAP session	Skill assessment	15	968–1068
IM19.1	Describe the functional anatomy of the locomotor system of the brain	Y	Lecture, small group discussion	Written/viva voce	15	968–1068
IM19.2	Classify movement disorders of the brain based on distribution, rhythm, repetition, exacerbating and relieving factors	Y	Lecture, small group discussion	Written/viva voce	15	968–1068
IM19.3	Elicit and document and present an appropriate history including onset, progression precipitating and aggravating relieving factors, associated symptoms that help identify the cause of the movement disorders	Y	Bedside clinic	Skill assessment	15	968–1068
IM19.4	Perform, demonstrate and document a physical examination that includes a general examination and a detailed neurologic examination using standard movement rating scales	Y	Bedside clinic	Skill assessment	15	968–1068
IM19.5	Generate document and present a differential diagnosis and prioritize based on the history and physical examination	Y	Bedside clinic	Skill assessment	15	968–1068
IM19.6	Make a clinical diagnosis regarding on the anatomical location, nature and cause of the lesion based on the clinical presentation and findings	Y	Bedside clinic	Skill assessment	15	968–1068

Number	Competency The student should be able to	Core Y/N	Suggested learning methods	Suggested assessment methods	Chapter No.	Page No.
IM19.7	Choose and interpret diagnostic and imaging tests in the diagnosis of movement disorders	Y	Bedside clinic, Small group session	Skill assessment/written/ viva voce	15	968–1068
IM19.8	Discuss and describe the pharmacology, dose, side effects and interactions used in the drug therapy of Parkinson's syndrome	Y	Lecture, small group discussion	Written/viva voce	15	968–1068
IM19.9	Enumerate the indications for use of surgery and botulinum toxin in the treatment of movement disorders	Y	Lecture, small group discussion	Written/viva voce	15	968–1068
IM22.1	Enumerate the causes of hypercalcemia and distinguish the features of PTH vs non PTH mediated hypercalcemia	N	Lecture, small group discussion	Written/viva voce	2	70–78
IM22.2	Describe the etiology, clinical manifestations, diagnosis and clinical approach to primary hyperparathyroidism	N	Lecture, small group discussion	Written/viva voce	2	70–78
IM22.3	Describe the approach to the management of hypercalcemia	N	Lecture, small group discussion	Written/viva voce	2	70–78
IM22.4	Enumerate the components and describe the genetic basis of the multiple endocrine neoplasia syndrome	N	Lecture, small group discussion	Written/viva voce	2	70–78
IM22.5	Enumerate the causes and describe the clinical features and the correct approach to the diagnosis and management of the patient with hyponatremia	Y	Lecture, small group discussion	Written/viva voce	14	934–966
IM22.6	Enumerate the causes and describe the clinical and laboratory features and the correct approach to the diagnosis and management of the patient with hyponatremia	Y	Lecture, small group discussion	Written/viva voce	14	934–966
IM22.7	Enumerate the causes and describe the clinical and laboratory features and the correct approach to the diagnosis and management of the patient with hypokalemia	Y	Lecture, small group discussion	Written/viva voce	14	934–966
IM22.8	Enumerate the causes and describe the clinical and laboratory features and the correct approach to the diagnosis and management of the patient with hyperkalemia	Y	Lecture, small group discussion	Written/viva voce	14	934–966
IM22.9	Enumerate the causes and describe the clinical and laboratory features of metabolic acidosis	N	Lecture, small group discussion	Written/viva voce	14	934–966
IM22.10	Enumerate the causes of describe the clinical and laboratory features of metabolic alkalosis	N	Lecture, small group discussion	Written/viva voce	14	934–966
IM22.11	Enumerate the causes and describe the clinical and laboratory features of respiratory acidosis	N	Lecture, small group discussion	Written/viva voce	14	934–966
IM22.12	Enumerate the causes and describe the clinical and laboratory features of respiratory alkalosis	N	Lecture, small group discussion	Written/viva voce	14	934–966
IM22.13	Identify the underlying acid-based disorder based on an ABG report and clinical situation	N	Lecture, small group discussion	Written/viva voce	14	934–966
IM23.1	Discuss and describe the methods of nutritional assessment in an adult and calculation of caloric requirements during illnesses	Y	Lecture, small group discussion	Written/viva voce	1	3–36
IM23.2	Discuss and describe the causes and consequences of protein caloric malnutrition in the hospital	Y	Lecture, small group discussion	Written/viva voce	1	22
IM23.3	Discuss and describe the etiology, causes, clinical manifestations, complications, diagnosis and management of common vitamin deficiencies	Y	Lecture, small group discussion	Written/viva voce	1	3–7

Number	Competency The student should be able to	Core Y/N	Suggested learning methods	Suggested assessment methods	Chapter No.	Page No.
IM23.4	Enumerate the indications for enteral and parenteral nutrition in critically ill patients	Y	Lecture, small group discussion	Written/viva voce	1	19–21
IM24.1	Describe and discuss the epidemiology, pathogenesis, clinical evolution, presentation and course of common diseases in the elderly	Y	Lecture, small group discussion	Written/viva voce	21	1199–1214
IM24.2	Perform multidimensional geriatric assessment that includes medical, psychosocial and functional components	Y	Bedside clinic, DOAP session	Skill assessment	21	1199–1214
IM24.11	Describe and discuss the etiopathogenesis,clinical presentation, identification, functional changes, acute care, stabilization, management and rehabilitation of the elderly undergoing surgery	Y	Lecture, small group discussion	Written/viva voce	21	1199–1214
IM24.18	Describe the impact of the demographic changes in ageing on the population	Y	Lecture, small group discussion	Written/viva voce	21	1199–1214
IM24.19	Enumerate and describe the social problems in the elderly including isolation, abuse, change in family structure and their impact on health	Y	Lecture, small group discussion	Written/viva voce	21	1199–1214
IM24.20	Enumerate and describe social interventions in the care of elderly including domiciliary discussion services, rehabilitation facilities, old age homes and state interventions	Y	Lecture, small group discussion	Written/viva voce	21	1199–1214
IM24.21	Enumerate and describe ethical issues in the care of the elderly	Y	Lecture, small group discussion	Written/viva voce	21	1199–1214
IM24.22	Describe and discuss the etiopathogenesis, clinical presentation, complications, assessment and management of nutritional disorders in the elderly	Y	Lecture, small group discussion	Written/viva voce	1	1 TO 36
IM25.1	Describe and discuss the response and the influence of host immune status, risk factors and comorbidities on zoonotic diseases (e.g. leptospirosis, rabies) and non-febrile infectious disease (e.g. tetanus)	Y	Lecture, small group discussion	Written	4	134–222
IM25.2	Discuss and describe the common causes, pathophysiology and manifestations of these diseases	Y	Lecture, small group discussion	Written	4	134–222
IM25.3	Describe and discuss the pathophysiology and manifestations of these diseases	Y	Lecture, small group discussion	Written	4	134–222
IM25.4	Elicit document and present a medical history that helps delineate the etiology of these diseases that includes the evolution and pattern of symptoms, risk factors, exposure through occupation and travel	Y	Bedside clinic, DOAP session	Skill assessment	6	267–271
IM25.5	Perform a systematic examination that establishes the diagnosis and severity of presentation that includes: general skin, mucosal and lymph node examination, chest and abdominal examination (including examination of the liver and spleen)	Y	Bedside clinic, DOAP session	Skill assessment	6	267–271
IM25.7	Order and interpret diagnostic tests based on the differential diagnosis including: CBC with differential, blood biochemistry, peripheral smear, urinary analysis with sediment, chest X-ray, blood and urine cultures, sputum Gram stain and cultures, sputum AFB and cultures, CSF analysis, pleural and body fluid analysis, stool routine and culture and QBC	Y	Bedside clinic, skill assessment	Skill assessment	4, 6	134–222, 267–271
IM25.8	Enumerate the indications for use of newer techniques in the diagnosis of these infections	N	Lecture, small group discussion	Written/ Viva voce	4	134–222

Number	Competency The student should be able to	Core Y/N	Suggested learning methods	Suggested assessment methods	Chapter No.	Page No.
IM25.9	Assist in the collection of blood and other specimen cultures	Y	DOAP session	Log book documentation	4	134–222
IM25.10	Develop and present an appropriate diagnostic plan based on the clinical presentation, most likely diagnosis in a prioritised and cost-effective manner	Y	Bedside clinic, skill assessment	Skill assessment	4	134–222
IM25.11	Develop an appropriate empiric treatment plan based on the patient's clinical and immune status pending definitive diagnosis	Y	DOAP session	Skill assessment	4	134–222
IM25.12	Communicate to the patient and family the diagnosis and treatment of identified infection	Y	DOAP session	Skill assessment	4	134–222
IM25.13	Counsel the patient and family on prevention of various infections due to environmental issues	Y	DOAP session	Skill assessment	1	30

CHAPTER 1

Nutrition and Environmental Medicine

NUTRITIONAL ASSESSMENT

Q. Discuss the methods of nutritional assessment in an adult.

Nutritional screening should include dynamic parameters rather than static ones, e.g., recent weight loss, current body mass index (BMI), recent food intake, and disease severity **(Table 1.1)**.

Nutritional Anthropometry

- Body weight and BMI
- Skinfold measurements: Subcutaneous fat tissues (SFTs) normally account for half of the entire body fat mass, and the measurement of SFT gives information on the energy stores of the body, mainly fat stores (i.e., triglycerides). Biceps, triceps, subscapular, and suprailiac skin-fold thickness are measured.
- Mid-upper arm muscle circumference (MAMC) reflects the muscle mass, while the mid-arm muscle area (MAMA) gives information about the muscle protein stores, as half of the body's proteins are stored in the skeletal muscles. The MAMA is calculated from the MAMC and the triceps SFT [MAMA = MAMC – (0.314 × SFT)].
- Assessment of body composition: Body composition describes the body compartments, such as fat mass, fat-free mass, muscle mass, and bone mineral mass. The methods used are bioelectrical independence analysis, creatinine height index, dual energy X-ray absorptiometry, magnetic resonance imaging (MRI), computed tomography (CT), dilution method, and neutron activation.
- Laboratory investigations: Complete blood count, lipid profile, electrolytes, albumin, transferrin, prealbumin/transthyretin (TTR), retinol-binding protein (RBP), insulin-like growth factor-1 (IGF-1).

TABLE 1.1: Nutritional screening.

Indications for nutritional screening			
➢ If BMI of the patient <20.5 kg/m² ➢ Significant loss of weight in the past 3 months ➢ Decreased food intake in the past week ➢ Critically ill patients			
Screening			
Nutritional status	*Score*	**Stress metabolism (severity of the disease)**	*Score*
None	0	*None*	0
Mild Weight loss >5% in 3 months Or 50–75% of the normal food intake in the last week	1	*Mild stress metabolism* Patient is mobile Increased protein requirement can be covered with oral nutrition *Hip fracture, chronic disease especially with complications, e.g., liver cirrhosis, chronic obstructive pulmonary disease (COPD), diabetes, cancer, chronic hemodialysis*	1
Moderate Weight loss >5% in 2 months Or BMI 18.5–20.5 kg/m² and reduced general condition Or 25–50% of the normal food intake in the last week	2	*Moderate stress metabolism* Patient is bedridden due to illness Highly increased protein requirement may be covered with oral nutritional supplement (ONS) *Stroke, hematologic cancer, severe pneumonia, extended abdominal surgery*	2
Severe Weight loss >5% in 1 month Or BMI <18.5 kg/m² and reduced general condition Or 0–25% of the normal food intake in the last week	3	*Severe stress metabolism* Patient is critically ill (intensive care unit) Very strongly increased protein requirement can only be achieved with (parenteral) enteral nutrition *APACHE-II >10, bone marrow transplantation, head traumas*	3
Total (A)		Total (B)	
		Age	
<70 years: 0 patient			
≥70 years: 1 patient			
TOTAL = (A) + (B) + Age			
≥3 points: Patient is at nutritional risk. Nutritional care plan should be set up *<3 points: Repeat screening weekly*			

Signs and Symptoms of Micronutrient Deficiencies

Signs and symptoms of micronutrient deficiencies have been shown in **Table 1.2**.

TABLE 1.2: Signs and symptoms of micronutrient deficiencies.

Vitamin deficiency	*Manifestation*
	Fat-soluble vitamins
Vitamin A (Retinol)	Night blindness, keratomalacia, Bitot's spots
Vitamin D (Ergocalciferol/ cholecalciferol)	Rickets/osteomalacia Bone pain, costochondral beading Proximal myopathy
Vitamin E (Tocopherol)	Hemolysis, posterior column signs, ataxia, muscle wasting, retinitis pigmentosa-like changes, night blindness
Vitamin K (Phylloquinone and other menaquinones)	Bruising, purpura, nose and GI bleeds
	Water-soluble vitamin (B-complex and vitamin C)
B_1 (Thiamine)	➢ Wernicke/Korsakoff ➢ Beriberi ➢ Nystagmus ➢ Sixth cranial nerve palsy ➢ Ataxia ➢ Acidosis ➢ Dementia ➢ Paresthesia ➢ Neuropathy ➢ Cardiac failure ➢ Anemia
B_2 (Riboflavin)	Ariboflavinosis Angular stomatitis, glossitis, magenta tongue
B_3 (Niacin)	Pellagra dermatitis of sun-exposed areas, dementia, poor appetite, difficulty sleeping, confusion, mouth sore
B_4 (Adenine)*	Immune dysfunction Aging
B_5 (Pantothenic acid)	Nausea, abdominal pain, paresthesia, burning feet
B_6 (Pyridoxine)	Poor appetite, lassitude, oxaluria
B_7 (Biotin)	Dermatitis, depression, lassitude, muscle pains, electrocardiogram abnormalities, blepharitis
B_8 (Inositol)*	Depression and other psychiatric manifestations
B_9 (Folic acid)	Macrocytic anemia, thrombocytopenia and megaloblastic bone marrow
B_{10} (PABA)*	Free radical damage Sun burns and skin rashes
B_{11} (Salicylic acid)*	Works in tandem with vitamin B_{12}
B_{12} (Cobalamin)	Subacute combined degeneration, macrocytic anemia, icterus, knuckle pigmentation
Vitamin C (Ascorbic acid)	Scurvy Poor wound healing, fatigue, limb pain, scorbutic rosary, difficulty sleeping, gingivitis, perifollicular purpura, hyperkeratosis
*** Note:** Vitamin B_4, B_8, B_{10}, and B_{11} are no longer labeled as vitamins, as they do not fit the official definition of vitamin.	
	Minerals
Iron	➢ Koilonychia ➢ Smooth tongue ➢ Anemia ➢ Esophageal web
Copper	➢ Microcytic hypochromic anemia, neutropenia, scurvy-like bone lesions, osteoporosis
Zinc	➢ Acrodermatitis enteropathica ➢ Peristomal/perinasal/perineal ➢ Erythema, thin hair, diarrhea, apathy, anorexia, growth failure, hypoglycemia ➢ Distorted or diminished taste (hypogeusia)
Chromium	Peripheral neuropathy, hyperglycemia
Selenium	Cardiomyopathy
Iodine	Goiter
	Others
Protein deficiency	Pitting edema Hair: Thinning, easily pluckable with dyspigmentation or flag sign, and change in texture to silken, sparse hair Dermatosis with desquamation of the so-called flaky-paint type, with or without hyperpigmentation

VITAMIN A

Q. Write a short essay/note on clinical features, diagnosis, and treatment of vitamin A deficiency.

- Vitamin A is the name given to a group of fat-soluble vitamins and includes **provitamin A carotenoids** and **preformed vitamin A.**
  - Provitamin A carotenoids—found in plants. For example, beta-carotene, alpha-carotene, and beta-cryptoxanthin. Sources—dark green and deeply colored fruits and vegetables.
  - Preformed vitamin A (retinol, retinal, retinoic acid, and retinyl esters) is the most active form of vitamin A; it is mostly found in animal sources of food and is also the form supplied by most supplements. Sources—liver, fish, milk, eggs, butter, cheese.
- **Vitamin A metabolism (Flowchart 1.1):**
  - Provitamin A (from plant sources) is cleaved to retinal before absorption. This step is subject to feedback regulation. Therefore, excessive intake of vitamin A from plant sources rarely causes toxicity.
  - Preformed vitamin A (from animal sources/supplements): This step is highly efficient and is not subject to feedback regulation. Therefore, excessive intake of vitamin A from animal sources can cause toxicity.
  - 50–85% of total body retinol is stored in the liver.
- **Functions of vitamin A:** Vitamin A has several metabolic roles. The main functions of vitamin A in humans are as follows:
  - **Maintenance of normal vision:** Vitamin A is essential for **dark adaptation** and its deficiency causes nyctalopia. Mainly controlled by retinaldehyde.
  - **Host resistance to infections:** Vitamin A deficiency causes keratinization of mucous membranes and thereby increases the risk of infections. RBP is a **negative "acute phase protein"**.
  - **Immune function:** Vitamin A has the ability to stimulate the immune system. Retinoids are required for normal growth, fetal development, fertility, hematopoiesis, and immune function.
  - **Control of cell growth and differentiation:** Vitamin A is needed for the maintenance of the surface linings of the eyes, growth and repair of epithelial cells, and integrity of the epithelial cells of the respiratory, urinary, and intestinal tracts. In vitamin A deficiency, mucus-secreting cells are replaced by keratin-producing cells and this process is known as squamous metaplasia.
  - **Regulation of lipid metabolism:** Fatty acid metabolism, including fatty acid oxidation in fat tissue and muscle, adipogenesis, and lipoprotein metabolism require vitamin A.
  - **Antioxidant:** Retinoids, beta-carotene, and some related carotenoids act as photoprotective and act as antioxidants.
  - **Other functions:** Vitamin A is involved in growth of bone, reproduction, embryonic development, and the regulation of adult genes.
  - **Tretinoin**, i.e., all-trans retinoic acid (ATRA) is also used to treat acute promyelocytic leukemia (APL), **isotretinoin** is used to treat psoriasis and 13-cis-retinoic acid is used in the treatment of acne.

FLOWCHART 1.1: Vitamin A metabolism.

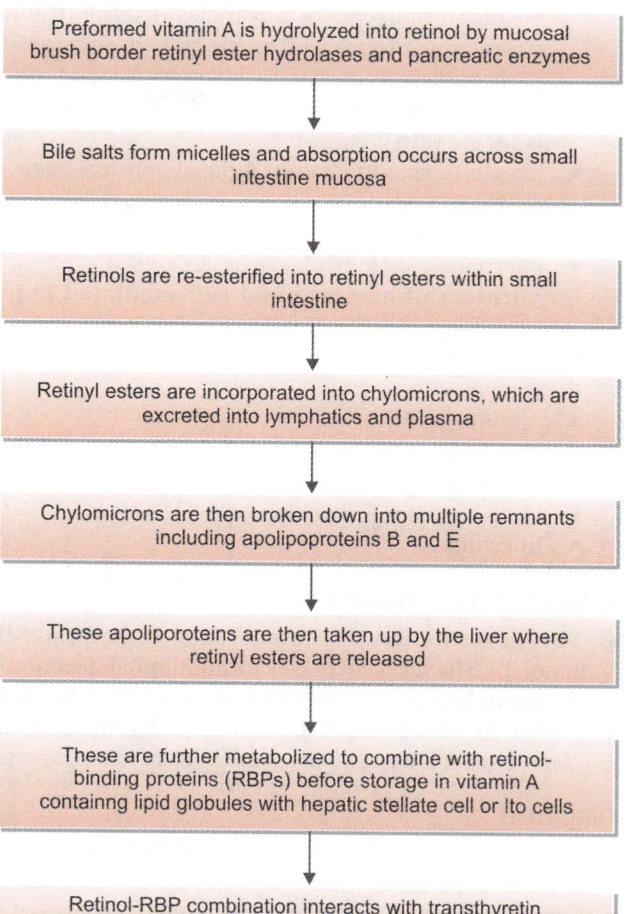

Vitamin A Deficiency (Table 1.3)

Clinical Features/Manifestations

- **Vision**
  - Xerophthalmia describes a spectrum of eye disease caused by vitamin A deficiency, which includes Bitot's spots, corneal xerosis and keratomalacia.
    - Bitot's spots **(Fig. 1.1)**: In young children with vitamin A deficiency, areas of abnormal squamous cell proliferation and keratinization of the conjunctiva known as Bitot's spots can be seen.

TABLE 1.3: Causes of vitamin A deficiency.

Primary causes	*Secondary causes*
➤ Prolonged dietary deprivation	➤ Sprue
➤ Vegetarians	➤ Cystic fibrosis
➤ Refugees	➤ Pancreatic insufficiency
➤ Chronic alcoholics	➤ Duodenal bypass
➤ Toddlers	➤ Chronic diarrhea
➤ Preschool children	➤ Bile duct obstruction
	➤ Giardiasis and cirrhosis

- ♦ Corneal xerosis refers to dryness of cornea.
- ♦ Keratomalacia: In advanced disease, the cornea becomes hazy and erosions can develop, finally leading to its destruction (keratomalacia).
- ▪ Night blindness (nyctalopia) and retinopathy.
- **Nonspecific skin changes**
  - Xerosis of skin in vitamin A deficiency has been shown in **Figure 1.2**.
  - Hyperkeratosis
  - Phrynoderma (follicular hyperkeratosis)
- **Impairment of humoral and cell-mediated immunity** causing increased susceptibility to infections.
- **Other features:**
  - Fatigue
  - Anemia
  - Diarrhea
  - Decreased growth rate
  - Decreased bone development
  - Infertility.

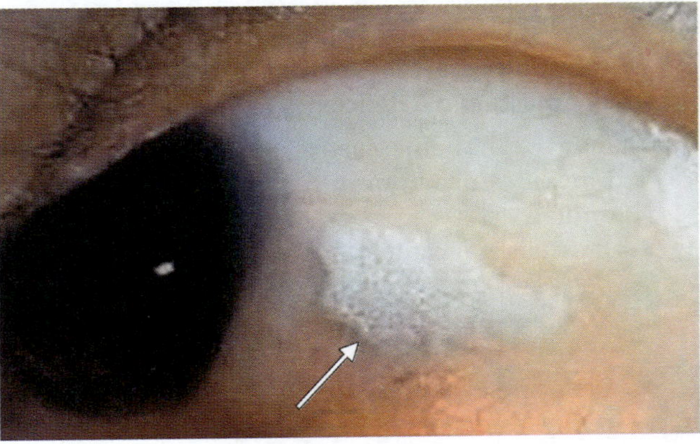

FIG. 1.1: Bitot's spot.

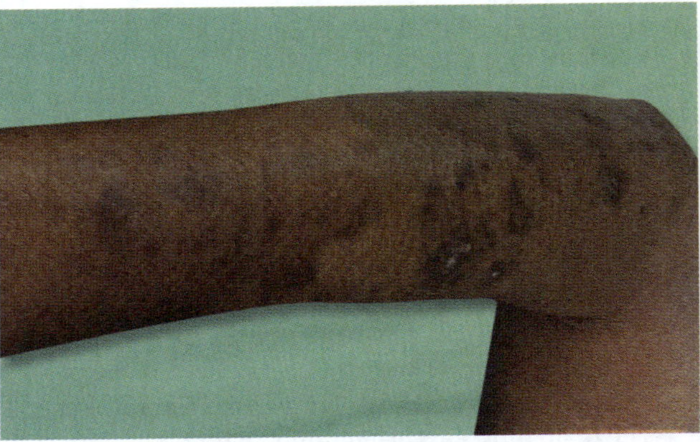

FIG. 1.2: Xerosis of skin in vitamin A deficiency.

Laboratory Investigations

- **Serum retinol level:** Normal range is 28–86 μg/dL (1–3 μmol/L). The level decreases in vitamin A deficiency.
- **Albumin levels** are indirect measures of vitamin A levels.
- **Complete blood count** (CBC) with differential count to be done, if there is a possibility of anemia, infection, or sepsis.

Diagnosis

- It is mainly on the basis of the **clinical features**. Response to replacement therapy is the best way for the diagnosis.
- Serum retinol levels <20 mg/dL suggest deficiency, or the ratio of retinol: RBP <0.8 suggests deficiency.

Prophylactic vitamin A at a dose of 2,00,000 IU every 6 months is to be given to all high-risk individuals. Patients with malabsorption syndrome need vitamin A supplements.

Treatment

- Xerophthalmia (irrespective of stage) should be treated with 2,00,000 IU of vitamin A in oily solution, usually contained in a soft-gel capsule. Three doses: day 0, day 1, and day 14.
- If child is suffering from measles give two capsules of 2,00,000 IU for 2 consecutive days.

Prevention

- *Children between 1 and 5 years of age:* 60,000 retinol activity equivalent (RAE) (2,00,000 IU) per oral every 6 months
- *Infants <6 months:* It can be given a one-time dose of 15,000 RAE (50,000 IU).
- *6–12 months of age:* It can be given a one-time dose of 30,000 RAE (1,00,000 IU).
- 1 retinol activity equivalent = 1 μg of retinol = 12 μg of beta-carotene = 24 μg of other provitamin A = 3.33 IU of retinol.

Vitamin A Toxicity

Q. Write short essay/note on hypervitaminosis A and its signs.

- **Types of toxicity:** Vitamin A toxicity can be **acute** (usually due to accidental ingestion by children) or **chronic**. Both types of toxicity cause **headache and increased intracranial pressure (pseudotumor cerebri).**
  - **Acute** toxicity also produces nausea and vomiting, vertigo, diplopia, bulging fontanels, seizures, exfoliative dermatitis. Single dose of 300 mg in adults and 100 mg in children can be harmful.
  - **Chronic** toxicity occurs with amounts higher than 10 times the RDA—causes changes in skin, hair (loss), and nails; liver and bone damage; double vision, ataxia, hyperlipidemia and vomiting.
- **Retinol is teratogenic** and incidence of birth defects in infants is high with vitamin A intakes of >3 mg a day during pregnancy (**spontaneous abortions** and **fetal malformations**, including microcephaly and cardiac anomalies).
- **Diagnosis is usually clinical**.
- Unless birth defects are present, adjusting the dose almost always leads to complete recovery. Recommended dietary allowances (RDAs)/adequate intake of fat-soluble vitamins for individuals **(Table 1.4A)**.
  - **Carotenemia** is common among infants and toddlers who eat large amounts of carrots and green leafy vegetables. It can be confused with jaundice, but discoloration of skin spontaneously resolves once the intake of carotenoid rich food is reduced.

TABLE 1.4A: Recommended dietary allowances (RDAs)/adequate intake of fat-soluble vitamins for different age group.

Age group	*Vitamin A (RAE*)*	*Vitamin D (μg/d)*	*Vitamin E (μg/d)*	*Vitamin K (μg/d)*
Infants	400–500	5	4–5	2–2.5
Children (1–13 yr)	300–600		6–11	30–60
>14 yr				
➤ Males	900	5–15	15	75–120
➤ Females	600–700		11–15	
Pregnancy	750–770	5	15	75–90
Lactation	1200–1300		19	

*1 RAE (retinol activity equivalents) = 1 μg retinol, 12 μg β-carotene; 1 μg calciferol = 40 IU vitamin D.

Dietary reference intake for water-soluble vitamins has been shown in **Table 1.4B**.

TABLE 1.4B: Dietary reference intake (DRI) for water-soluble vitamins.

	Thiamine (mg/day)		*Riboflavin (mg/day)*		*Niacin (mg/day)*		*Pantothenic acid (mg/day)*		*Vitamin B_6 (mg/day)*		*Biotin (μg/day)*		*Vitamin C (mg/day)*	
Life stage group	*RDA/AI*	*UL*	*RDA/AI*	*UL*	*RDA/AI*	*UL*	*RDA/AI*	*UL*	*RDA/AI*	*UL*	*RDA/AI*	*UL*	*RDA/AI*	*UL*
Infants														
0–6 months	0.2	ND	0.3	ND	2	ND	1.7	ND	0.1	ND	5	ND	40	ND
7–12 months	0.3	ND	0.4	ND	4	ND	1.8	ND	0.3	ND	6	ND	50	ND
Children														
1–3 years	0.5	ND	0.5	ND	6	10	2	ND	0.5	30	8	ND	15	400
4–8 years	0.6	ND	0.6	ND	8	15	3	ND	0.6	40	12	ND	25	650
Males														
9–13 years	0.9	ND	0.9	ND	12	20	4	ND	1	60	20	ND	45	1,200
14–18 years	1.2	ND	1.3	ND	16	30	5	ND	1.3	80	25	ND	75	1,800
19–30 years	1.2	ND	1.3	ND	16	35	5	ND	1.3	100	30	ND	90	2,000
31–50 years	1.2	ND	1.3	ND	16	35	5	ND	1.3	100	30	ND	90	2,000
51–70 years	1.2	ND	RDA	ND	16	35	5	ND	1.7	100	30	ND	90	2,000
>70 years	1.2	ND	1.3	ND	16	35	5	ND	1.7	100	30	ND	90	2,000
Females														
9–13 years	0.9	ND	0.9	ND	12	20	4	ND	1	60	20	ND	45	1,200
14–18 years	1	ND	1	ND	14	30	5	ND	1.2	80	25	ND	65	1,800
19–30 years	1.1	ND	1.1	ND	14	35	5	ND	1.3	100	30	ND	75	2,000
31–30 years	1.1	ND	1.1	ND	14	35	5	ND	1.3	100	30	ND	75	2,000
51–70 years	1.1	ND	1.1	ND	14	35	5	ND	1.5	100	30	ND	75	2,000
>70 years	1.1	ND	1.1	ND	14	35	5	ND	1.5	100	30	ND	75	2,000
Pregnancy														
14–18 years	1.4	ND	1.4	ND	18	30	6	ND	1.9	80	30	ND	80	1,800
19–30 years	1.4	ND	1.4	ND	18	35	6	ND	1.9	100	30	ND	85	2,000
31–50 years	1.4	ND	1.4	ND	18	35	6	ND	1.9	100	30	ND	85	2,000
Lactation														
14–18 years	1.4	ND	1.6	ND	17	30	7	ND	2	80	35	ND	115	1,800
19–30 years	1.4	ND	1.6	ND	17	35	7	ND	2	100	35	ND	120	2,000
31–50 years	1.4	ND	1.6	ND	17	35	7	ND	2	100	35	ND	120	2,000

Dietary reference intakes (DRIs) include the following measures describing optimal nutrient intake:
- **Recommended dietary allowance (RDA):** The level of dietary intake that is sufficient to meet the daily nutrient requirements of 97% of the individuals in a specific life stage group.
- **Adequate intake (AI):** An approximation of the average nutrient intake that sustains a defined nutritional state, based on observed or experimentally determined values in a defined population.
- **Upper tolerable level (UL):** The maximum level of daily nutrient intake that is likely to pose no risk of adverse health effects in almost all individuals in the specified life stage or gender group.

RDAs and AIs may both be used as goals for individual intake. The AI is used when there are insufficient data to determine the RDA for a given nutrient.

VITAMIN B COMPLEX

Thiamine (B_1)

- **Functions:** Thiamine is an important **water-soluble** vitamin.
  - Involved in **carbohydrate, fat, amino acid, glucose, and alcohol metabolism.**
  - Vitamin B_1 is **essential** for the **coenzyme**, thiamine pyrophosphate (TPP). It is required for the following reactions:

- Decarboxylation of pyruvate (glycolytic pathway) to acetyl CoA (Krebs cycle)
    - Transketolase in the hexose monophosphate (HMP/pentose) shunt pathway
    - Decarboxylation of alpha-ketoglutarate to succinate (Krebs cycle).
- Has an additional role in neuronal conduction.
- **Sources:** These vitamins can be produced by plants and some microorganisms. However, animals cannot synthesize them. In humans, the source is diet, though small amounts may be synthesized by intestinal bacteria.
- **Dietary sources:** Good dietary sources of thiamine are **whole wheat flour, unpolished rice, cereals, grains, beans, nuts and yeast**. There is little or no thiamine in milled rice and grains. Thus, thiamine deficiency is more common in individuals who consume mainly a rice-based diet.
- It is also present in **liver, meat, and eggs**.
- **Requirement:** Up to 30 mg of thiamine can be stored in body tissues. Required daily allowance (RDA) is **0.5–0.9 mg daily for children, 1.2 mg daily for adult men, and 1.1 mg daily for nonpregnant adult women**.
- Requirement increases with increased carbohydrate intake, pregnancy and lactation, smoking, alcoholism, prolonged antibiotic intake, serious or prolonged illness.
- It causes of thiamine deficiency are listed in **Box 1.1** and clinical syndromes of thiamine deficiency are mentioned in **Box 1.2**.

Box 1.1: Causes of thiamine deficiency.

Lack of thiamine intake
- Starvation state
- Food items like milled rice, raw freshwater fish, raw shellfish, and ferns that have a high level of *thiaminase*
- Food high in *anti-thiamine factor,* such as tea, coffee, and betel nuts
- Alcoholic state

Increased consumption states
- Diets high in carbohydrate or saturated fat intake
- Pregnancy and lactation
- Hyperthyroidism
- Fever—severe infection
- Increased physical exercise

Decreased absorption
- Chronic intestinal disease
- Alcoholism
- Malnutrition
- Gastric bypass surgery
- Malabsorption syndrome—celiac and tropical sprue

Increased depletion
- Diarrhea
- Peritoneal dialysis, hemodialysis, diuretic therapies
- Hyperemesis gravidarum

Box 1.2: Clinical syndromes of thiamine deficiency.

1. Wet beriberi—high cardiac output failure
2. Dry beriberi—peripheral neuropathy
3. Wernicke's encephalopathy
4. Korsakoff's psychosis
5. Leigh syndrome (progressive subacute necrotizing encephalomyopathy)

Consequences of Thiamine Deficiency

- Consequence of thiamine deficiency is **impaired glucose oxidation.**
- Cells **cannot metabolize glucose** aerobically to generate energy as ATP.
- **Neuronal cells** are **most susceptible**, because they depend almost exclusively on glucose for energy requirements.
- Causes an **accumulation of pyruvic and lactic acids**. This in turn produces **vasodilatation** and **increased cardiac output.**

Beriberi (Box 1.2)

Q. Write short essay/note on clinical features of beriberi/vitamin B_1 (thiamine) deficiency.

1. **Wet (cardiovascular) beriberi:** Wet beriberi is the term used for the **cardiovascular involvement** of thiamine deficiency.
    - First effects are **vasodilatation, tachycardia**, a wide pulse pressure, sweating, warm skin, and lactic acidosis.
    - Later, **congestive heart failure** develops, causing orthopnea, and pulmonary and peripheral edema. Marked cardiomegaly is present.
    - **Infantile beriberi** occurs in infants (usually by age 3–4 weeks) who are breastfed by **thiamine-deficient mothers.** Heart failure can develop suddenly and presents with edema, aphonia, tachycardia, tachypnea, and absent deep tendon reflexes. If prompt treatment is not given, death occurs quickly.
        - **Shoshin beriberi:** A more rapid form of wet beriberi is termed **acute fulminant cardiovascular beriberi.**
2. **Dry beriberi:** Dry beriberi usually manifests insidiously with **symmetrical peripheral neuropathy.**
    - **Early symptoms***:* There is bilateral and roughly symmetrical heaviness and stiffness of the legs.
    - **Later symptoms***:* These include weakness, numbness, and pins and needles (occurring in a stocking-glove distribution).
    - **Distribution of neuropathy:** They affect predominantly the lower limbs. They begin with paresthesias in the toes, burning in the feet (severe at night), muscle cramps in the calves, pains in the legs, and plantar dysesthesias.
    - **Physical signs***:* Calf muscle tenderness, difficulty rising from a squatting position, and decreased vibratory sensation in the toes. The ankle jerk reflexes are lost.
    - Deficiency may also cause **degeneration of thalamus, mammillary bodies, and cerebellum**.

    Biochemical tests
    - Measurement of thiamine, pyruvate, and lactate levels in blood or urine.
    - Erythrocyte thiamine transketolase activity.

Q. Write short essay/note on management/treatment of beriberi/vitamin B_1 (thiamine) deficiency.

Management
- Complete bed rest.
- 200 mg thiamine 3 times a day given till acute symptoms disappear, after that 10 mg/day till recovery.
- Parenteral thiamine produces marked diuresis (in wet beriberi), resulting in dramatic improvement in the symptoms.

Q. Write short essay/note on Wernicke's encephalopathy.

3. **Wernicke's encephalopathy:** It is an acute neuropsychiatric condition. Initially, it is reversible biochemical brain lesion caused by depletion of vitamin B_1 (thiamine). Its causes are listed in **Box 1.1.**
   Clinical features:
   - Wernicke's encephalopathy (WE) is a **triad of global confusion, ophthalmoplegia, and ataxia**, along with confusion. Impairment in the synthesis of one of the important enzymes of the **pentose phosphate pathway (erythrocyte transketolase)** may explain such a predisposition.
   - **Encephalopathy:** It is characterized by confusion, severe disorientation, indifference, and inattentiveness. There is also impaired memory and learning. If untreated patients will progress through stupor and coma to death.
   - **Oculomotor dysfunction:** Nystagmus, lateral rectus palsy, and lesions of the oculomotor, abducens, and vestibular nuclei resulting in conjugate gaze palsy.
   - **Gait ataxia:** Ataxia mainly involves stance and gait. It is probably due to a combination of polyneuropathy, cerebellar involvement, and vestibular dysfunction.

   Diagnosis: For confirmation of the diagnosis, measure the circulating thiamine concentration or transketolase activity in red cells using fresh heparinized blood. MRI may show **periventricular lesions** surrounding third ventricle, aqueduct and fourth ventricle with **petechial hemorrhages** in acute cases and atrophy of mammillary bodies in chronic cases.

Management
- Wernicke's disease is a medical emergency and requires immediate administration of thiamine.
- **Dosage:** 500 mg of thiamine intravenously, infused over 30 minutes, 3 times daily for 2 consecutive days and 250 mg intravenously or intramuscularly once daily for an additional 5 days, in combination with other B vitamins.
- Magnesium is often needed because it is a cofactor required for normal functioning of thiamine-dependent enzymes.
- Wernicke's encephalopathy may be precipitated by administration of intravenous glucose solutions to individuals with thiamine deficiency. In susceptible individuals, glucose administration should be preceded or accompanied by thiamine 100 mg IV.

4. ***Korsakoff's psychosis/syndrome***

Q. Write a short note on Korsakoff's psychosis/syndrome.

- Korsakoff's psychosis is caused by **deficiency of thiamine** with **involvement of central nervous system.**
- **Memory disturbances:** It is predominantly associated with **defect in retentive memory** (severe defect in storing new information and learning). Thus, there are **disturbances of short-term memory.** There are also marked deficits in anterograde and retrograde memory.
- Other features include apathy, an intact sensorium and relative preservation of long-term memory and other cognitive skills.
- **Confabulation:** It is a memory disturbance, characterized by the production of fabricated, distorted or misinterpreted memories about oneself or the world, without the conscious intention to deceive. Attention and social behavior are relatively maintained. Affected individuals can perform conversation that may seem normal to an unsuspecting spectator.
- The syndrome is common in **chronic alcoholics**. It may also be seen with thiamine deficiency due to **gastric disorders** (e.g., carcinoma, chronic gastritis, or persistent vomiting).

Treatment: Parenteral thiamine (100 mg IM daily for 7 days).

Thiamine metabolism dysfunction syndromes
- **Thiamine-responsive megaloblastic anemia**
  - Mutations in the *SLC19A2* gene (encodes thiamine transporter)
  - Syndrome of megaloblastic anemia, diabetes mellitus, and sensorineural deafness
  - Affects infants and adolescents.
- **Thiamine metabolism dysfunction syndrome type 2**
  - Mutations in the *SLC19A3* gene (encodes thiamine transporter)
  - Causes episodic encephalopathy
  - May be precipitated by a febrile episode.

Vitamin B_2 (Riboflavin)

- **Source:** Milk and eggs, meats, fish, green vegetables, yeast, and enriched foods (fortified cereals and breads).
- **Actions:**
  - Essential component of coenzymes involved in multiple cellular metabolic pathways like tricarboxylic acid (TCA) cycle and beta-oxidation of fatty acids.
  - Flavoproteins are involved in multiple redox reactions and function as electron transporters.

Deficiency

- **Diagnosis:**
  - **Erythrocyte glutathione reductase assay**—coefficient >1.4 indicates riboflavin deficiency.
  - Plasma, RBC or urine **riboflavin concentrations**.
- **Causes:**
  - Anorexia nervosa
  - Malabsorptive syndromes
  - Glutaric acidemia type 1
  - Multiple acyl-coenzyme A (CoA) dehydrogenase deficiency (MADD)
  - Brown-Vialetto-Van Laere syndrome (defect in riboflavin transporter)
  - Long-term use of barbiturates—can cause oxidation of riboflavin.
  - Lactose intolerance—because dairy products are a good source of riboflavin.
- **Features** of riboflavin deficiency include:
  - Cheilitis
  - Stomatitis
  - Glossitis
  - Normochromic anemia
  - Seborrheic dermatitis
- Pure deficiency of riboflavin is rare.
- **Therapeutic uses:**
  - Multiple CoA dehydrogenase deficiency
  - Lactic acidosis due to zidovudine/stavudine—responds to riboflavin
- **RDA:**
  - 0.5–0.9 mg daily in children
  - 1.3 mg daily for adult men
  - 1.1 mg daily for nonpregnant adult women

Vitamin B_3 (Niacin)

- **Sources:**
  - Yeast, meats (especially liver), grains, legumes, corn used in tortilla, and seeds.
  - Tryptophan can be converted to a niacin derivative in the liver. However, it requires approximately 60 mg of tryptophan to produce 1 mg of niacin, and this process requires vitamin B_6 (pyridoxine).
- **Actions:** NAD/NADP are co-factors for many enzymatic redox reactions.
- **RDA:** Dosed as a "niacin equivalent" (NE), in which 1 NE is equal to 1 mg of niacin, or 60 mg of dietary tryptophan. RDA is 6–12 mg daily in children, 16 mg for adult males, and 14 mg daily for nonpregnant adult females.

Pellagra

Q. Write short essay/note on clinical features and management of niacin deficiency (pellagra).

- **Vitamin B_3 niacin (nicotinamide) deficiency** causes a metabolic encephalopathy called **pellagra**. Causes of pellagra are listed in **Box 1.3**.
- It is found mostly in populations in which corn is the major source of energy in parts of China, Africa, and India. Pellagra means raw skin.

Box 1.3: Causes of pellagra.

- **Inadequate intake:** Maize or jowar (sorghum) diet, malnutrition, chronic alcoholism (who eat little), anorexia nervosa
- Generalized **malabsorption** (rare).
- **Drug-induced:**
  - Prolonged isoniazid therapy
  - Pyrazinamide
  - 6-mercaptopurine
  - 5-fluouracil
  - Azathioprine
  - Ethionamide
  - Carbamazepine
  - Phenytoin
  - Phenobarbitone.
- **Other disorders:**
  - **Hartnup's disease:** It is a rare genetic disorder, in which there is reduced absorption of basic amino acids including tryptophan by the gut.
  - **Carcinoid syndrome** and pheochromocytoma: In these conditions, tryptophan metabolism is diverted away from the formation of nicotinamide to form amine-producing pellagra-like symptoms.

Clinical Features

Pellagra has been easily remembered a disease of four **D**s namely: (1) **dermatitis;** (2) **diarrhea;** (3) **dementia (depression);** and (4) **death.** However, these features are not always observed and the mental changes are not a true dementia.

- **Skin manifestations:**
  - **Casal's necklace or collar rash:** Characteristic skin rash develops that is hyperpigmented and scaling that develops in skin areas exposed to sunlight. This rash forms a ring around the neck and is termed Casal's necklace **(Fig. 1.3)**.
  - **Dermatitis:** Lesions of the skin may progress to vesiculation, cracking (ulceration), exudation, and secondary infection. Symmetrical chronic thickening, dryness and pigmentation may be seen on the dorsal surfaces of the hands.

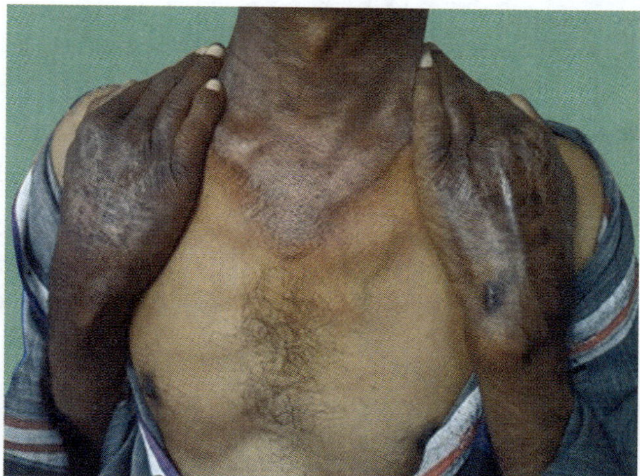

FIG. 1.3: Casal's necklace and dermatitis.

- **Gastrointestinal (GI) tract:**
  - **Diarrhea:** It may be in part due to proctitis and in part due to malabsorption. It is often a feature accompanied by anorexia, nausea, glossitis, and dysphagia indicating noninfective inflammation of the entire GI tract.
  - Other features include raw, painful, bright red tongue (glossitis), angular stomatitis, vaginitis, esophagitis, vertigo, and burning dysesthesias.
- **Dementia:**
  - This occurs in chronic severe deficiency and may also develop hallucinations and acute psychosis.
  - Milder deficiency may present with depression, apathy and sometimes thought disorders.
  - Other neurologic symptoms include insomnia, anxiety, disorientation, tremor, delusions, dementia, and encephalopathy.

Diagnosis

- Diagnosis in **endemic region** depends on the clinical features. Other vitamin deficiencies can also produce similar changes (e.g., angular stomatitis).
- **Dramatic improvement:** The response is usually rapid in the skin (within 24 hours), diarrhea and a striking improvement occurs in the patient's mental state **with nicotinamide** treatment.
- Niacin status can be assessed by measuring urinary N-methylnicotinamide, 2-pyridonenicotinamide or by measuring the erythrocyte NAD:NADP (ratio).

Management/Treatment

- **Nicotinamide:** 100–200 mg 3 times daily orally (approximately 300 mg daily) with a maintenance dose of 50 mg daily.
- **High-protein diet** with **adequate nutrients** and treatment of malnutrition.
- **Supplementation of other vitamin B** complex with **iron and folic acid** is also given, as other deficiencies are often likely to be present.
- In moderate-to-high doses (1–3 g a day), niacin is a well-established antihyperlipidemic agent.

Vitamin B_{12} and Folic Acid

Discussed in Chapter 8.

Vitamin B_5 (Pantothenic Acid)

- **Sources:**
  - Egg yolk, liver, kidney, broccoli, and milk
  - Pantothenic acid is also produced by **bacteria in the colon**
  - Main dietary source of pantothenic acid is in the form of **coenzyme A**.
- **Actions:** CoA is involved in **metabolism** of vitamins A, D, cholesterol, steroids, heme A, fatty acids, carbohydrates, amino acids, and proteins.
- **RDA:**
  - The recommended intake for pantothenic acid is expressed as **adequate intake (AI)** rather than recommended dietary allowance (RDA).
  - The AI is 2–4 mg daily for children and 5 mg daily for adult men and women.
- **Deficiency:** Pantothenic acid deficiency is very rare in humans.
- **Clinical manifestations:**
  - Paresthesias and dysesthesias, referred to as "**burning feet syndrome**"
  - Gastrointestinal disturbance, depression, muscle cramps, hypoglycemia, ataxia, etc.

- **Diagnosis:**
  - Blood, plasma, serum or urine pantothenic acid levels
  - **Urine levels** are most reliable indicator of dietary intake.

Management/Treatment

Oral pantothenic acid (vitamin B_5) - 5 mg/day.

Vitamin B_6 (Pyridoxine)

Vitamin B_6 consists of **pyridoxine, pyridoxamine, pyridoxal**, and the **phosphorylated derivatives** of each of these compounds.

- **Sources:**
  - Pyridoxine and pyridoxamine are predominantly found in plant foods.
  - Pyridoxal is most commonly derived from animal foods.
  - Meats, whole grains, vegetables, and nuts are the best sources.
- **Actions:**
  - Gluconeogenesis
  - Decarboxylation of amino acids
  - Conversion of tryptophan to niacin
  - Heme synthesis
  - Sphingolipid biosynthesis
  - Neurotransmitter synthesis
  - Steroid hormone modulation
  - Trans-sulfuration pathway by which homocysteine is converted into cystathionine and its subsequent conversion to cysteine.
- **RDA:**
  - 0.5–1 mg in children
  - 1.3 mg daily for young men and women
  - 1.7 mg daily for men older than 50 years
  - 1.5 mg daily for women older than 50 years

Deficiency

- Overt deficiency is rare.
- **Causes:**
  - **Drugs**—isoniazid, penicillamine, hydralazine, and levodopa/carbidopa
  - Associated with—asthma, diabetes, alcoholism, heart disease, pregnancy, breast cancer, Hodgkin's lymphoma, and sickle-cell anemia
- **Clinical manifestations:**
  - Nonspecific stomatitis, glossitis, cheilosis, irritability, confusion, and depression, and possibly peripheral neuropathy.
  - Severe deficiency is associated with **seborrheic dermatitis, microcytic anemia,** and **seizures**
  - A number of genetic syndromes affecting PLP-dependent enzymes such as homocystinuria, cystathioninuria, and xanthurenic aciduria mimic vitamin B_6 deficiency.
  - An inborn error of pyridoxine metabolism is responsible for **pyridoxine-dependent epilepsy.**
  - Cystathionine synthase is a PLP-dependent enzyme, which produces cystathionine from serine and homocysteine. As a result, vitamin B_6 insufficiency can lead to elevations in plasma homocysteine concentrations, a risk factor for the development of atherosclerosis and venous thromboembolism.
- **Diagnosis:**
  - **PLP concentrations** >30 nmol/L (>7.4 ng/mL) are normal.
  - **Erythrocyte transaminase activity**, with and without PLP added.
  - Urinary 4-pyridoxic acid excretion >3.0 mmol/day
  - Urinary excretion of xanthurenic acid is normally <65 mmol/day following a 2 g tryptophan load. **Increased xanthurenic acid excretion** suggests vitamin B_6 deficiency due to abnormal tryptophan metabolism.
- **Toxicity:** Peripheral neuropathy, dermatoses, photosensitivity, dizziness, and nausea have been reported with pyridoxine of over 250 mg/day.

Treatment:

- 50 mg/day in regular deficiency
- In case of deficiency secondary to certain drugs—higher doses of 100–200 mg/day are given.

Biotin

- **Sources:** Liver, egg yolk, soybean products, and yeast
- **Actions: Essential cofactor** for several carboxylase enzyme complexes involved in carbohydrate, amino acid, and lipid **metabolism.**
- **RDA:** The AI is 8–12 μg daily for children and 30 μg daily for adults.

Deficiency

- Deficiency is rare.
- **Causes:**
  - Long-term **parenteral nutrition**
  - Consumption of **large amounts of raw egg whites** (which contain avidin, a substance that binds to biotin and prevents its absorption), can also lead to biotin deficiency.
  - Secondary biotin deficiency can occur due to **lack of a specific enzyme** (**biotinidase**), which is required for release of protein-bound biotin to make it bioavailable.
- **Clinical manifestations:**
  - **Dermatitis** around the eyes, nose and mouth, conjunctivitis, alopecia
  - **Neurologic symptoms**, including changes in mental status, lethargy, hallucinations, and paresthesias
  - Myalgia, anorexia, and nausea
  - Multiple carboxylase deficiency—inherited defects of biotin metabolism
  - The **infantile form** is caused by a **deficiency of holocarboxylase synthetase** and presents in the first week of life with lethargy, poor muscle tone, and vomiting.
  - A **later-onset form** is caused by **biotinidase deficiency** and is associated with a slow but progressive loss of biotin in the urine, leading to organic aciduria; it is characterized by ataxia, ketoacidosis, dermatitis, seizures, myoclonus, and nystagmus.
- **Diagnosis:**
  - **Decreased urine biotin** concentrations
  - Increased urinary excretion of 3-hydroxyisovaleric acid after leucine challenge
  - Decreased activity of biotin-dependent enzymes in lymphocytes.

Treatment: Biotin in the dose of 10 mg/day.

VITAMIN C

Q. Write short essay/note on vitamin C and clinical features of scurvy.

- Vitamin C (ascorbic acid) is a **water-soluble** vitamin.
- **Sources:**
  - Citrus fruits, tomatoes, potatoes, brussel sprouts, cauliflower, broccoli, strawberries, cabbage, and spinach
  - Breast milk provides an adequate source of ascorbic acid for newborns and infants.
- **Metabolism:**
  - Ascorbic acid is absorbed in the **distal small intestine**.
  - Usual dietary doses of up to 100 mg/day are almost completely absorbed. As dietary concentrations increase, a smaller fraction is absorbed.
  - Pharmacologic dosing (>1,000 mg/day) can result in absorption rates of <50%
  - **Blood concentrations** of ascorbic acid are **regulated by renal excretion**. Excess amounts are filtered by renal glomeruli and reabsorbed via the tubules to a predetermined threshold.
  - **Dehydroascorbic acid** is the preferred form for **erythrocytes and leukocytes.**
  - The greatest concentrations of ascorbic acid are found in the **pituitary, adrenal, brain, leukocytes, and the eye.**
- **Functions:** These include:
  - **Formation of collagen** from procollagen. It is essential for **wound healing** and facilitates recovery from burns. It is needed for hydroxylation of proline to hydroxyproline (in protocollagen) and lysine to hydroxylysine (in mature collagen).
  - **Antioxidant properties:** Ascorbic acid is the **most active powerful reducing agent** controlling the redox potential within cells.
  - It is involved in intracellular electron transfer and supports **immune function**.
  - Promotes **absorption of nonheme iron**.
  - It is needed for the **formation of carnitine, hormones, neurotransmitters, and amino acids**.
  - Formation of **intercellular cement substances** in connective tissues, bones, and dentin, when defective, resulting in weakened capillaries with subsequent hemorrhage and defects in bone and related structures.
- **RDA:**
  - 15–45 mg daily in children
  - 75 mg/day for adult women
  - 90 mg/day for men
  - Pregnant or lactating women and the elderly have requirements up to 120 mg/day.

Deficiency of Vitamin C—Scurvy

- **Scurvy** is caused by deficiency of vitamin C.
- **Causes of vitamin C deficiency:**
  - Infants fed only on boiled cow's milk during the first year of life are at risk.
  - Individuals who do not eat vegetables such as elderly, people who live alone (singly) and chronic alcoholics.
  - Pregnant and lactating women and those with thyrotoxicosis require more vitamin C because of increased utilization.
  - **Individuals at risk of deficiency**:
    - Anorexia nervosa or anorexia from other diseases such as AIDS or cancer
    - Type 1 diabetes requires increased vitamin C
    - Patients undergoing peritoneal dialysis and hemodialysis
    - Diseases of small intestine such as Crohn's, Whipple's, and celiac disease.
  - **Types of scurvy:** Adult scurvy and infantile scurvy.
  - **Adult scurvy:** Early symptoms may be nonspecific, with malaise, weakness, lethargy and muscle pain (myalgias may be due to reduced production of carnitine).
    - **Bone disease:** More common in growing children and manifests after 1–3 months. It is characterized by **deranged formation of osteoid matrix and *bone pain*. Fractures, dislocations**, and tenderness of bones are common in children.
    - **Hemorrhages:** Hemorrhaging is a **hallmark** feature of scurvy and can occur in any organ. Hair follicles are one of the common sites of cutaneous bleeding. Marked tendency to bleed into the skin (easy **bruising, petechiae, ecchymosis, perifollicular hemorrhages**), bleeding into muscles, joints and underneath peritoneum. Bruising and hemorrhage may be spontaneous. Most commonly on the **legs and buttocks** where hydrostatic pressure is the greatest.
    - **Delayed/poor wound healing** and breakdown of old scars.
    - **Anemia:** It may cause high-output heart failure.
    - **Gums:** Inflamed spongy gums (**gum swelling**) friability, bleeding and infection with loosening of teeth; mucosal petechiae are common.
    - **Skin changes:** Roughness, keratosis of hair follicles with 'corkscrew' hair, perifollicular hemorrhages.
    - **Nails:** Splinter hemorrhages.
    - **Other features:** Emotional changes, shortness of breath.
- **Infantile scurvy (Barlow's disease):**
  - **Subperiosteal hemorrhage** into shafts of long bones.
  - **Scorbutic rosary** denotes enlargement of costochondral junctions, which are tender.
  - May be associated with **pectus excavatum**.
  - Retrobulbar, subarachnoid, and intracerebral **hemorrhages.**
  - Painful limbs giving rise to **'pseudoparalysis'**.
- **Laboratory investigations and diagnosis:**
  - Diagnosis is usually made **clinically** in a patient who has skin or gingival signs and is at risk of vitamin C deficiency.
  - **Plasma and leukocyte vitamin C** levels can be measured.
    - Leukocyte vitamin C levels are more reliable as recent treatment will improve plasma levels but tissues will still be deficient in vitamin C.
    - **Plasma vitamin C level** of <11 μmol/L (0.2 mg/100 mL).
    - **Anemia:** It can be normochromic, normocytic (due to bleeding), megaloblastic (due to reduced erythropoiesis) or microcytic hypochromic anemia (due to impaired iron absorption and impaired heme synthesis).
    - **Hess' capillary fragility** test can be checked by inflating a blood pressure cuff and looking for petechiae on the forearm.
    - **Bleeding time, clotting time, and prothrombin time:** To rule out other bleeding disorders.
  - **Imaging studies:** The findings include:
    - Loss of trabeculae results in a ground-glass appearance
    - Thinning of cortex
    - A line of calcified, irregular cartilage **(white line of Frankel)** may be visible at the metaphysis.
    - The epiphysis may be compressed and circular calcification surrounding epiphyseal center of ossification **(Wimberger's ring sign) (Fig. 1.4)**.

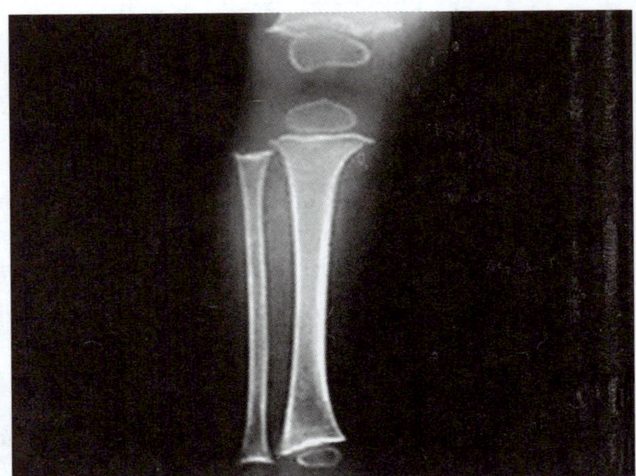

FIG. 1.4: X-ray of scurvy showing Frankel line and Wimberger's ring sign.

- **Toxicity:**
  - **Acute:** High doses >2 g of vitamin C—abdominal pain, diarrhea, nausea.
  - **Chronic:**
    - Increased prevalence of kidney stones.
    - Iron overload—can cause fatal arrhythmias.
    - Hemolysis in G6PD deficiency.
    - False-negative guaiac reactions and interference with tests for urinary glucose.
    - Interference with activity of certain drugs—like bortezomib in myeloma.

Management/Treatment

- **Ascorbic acid at 100 mg 3–5 times a day** until total of 4 g is reached, and then reduce the dose to 100 mg daily.
- **Encourage consumption of foods with high vitamin C.**
  - Citrus **fruits,** especially grapefruits and lemons.
  - **Vegetables**, including broccoli, green peppers, tomatoes, potatoes, and cabbage.
  - The recommended dose for adults is 120 mg daily, although a dose of 60 mg daily is all that is required to prevent scurvy.
  - Diets high in vitamin C may lower the incidence of certain cancers, particularly esophageal and gastric cancers.
  - Vitamin C supplementation can be useful in upper respiratory tract infections, Chediak-Higashi syndrome, and osteogenesis imperfecta.
  - There is inconclusive evidence of the protective role of vitamin C in the management of COVID-19 pneumonia.

VITAMIN D

Q. Write a short note on vitamin D.

- Vitamin D is a **fat-soluble secosteroid** responsible for enhancing **intestinal absorption of calcium, iron, magnesium, phosphate, and zinc.**
- **Physiology (Fig. 1.5)**
  - **Vitamin D_3 (Cholecalciferol)**
    - Produced in skin with direct sunlight. Cod liver oil is a rich source.
    - Preferred form of supplementation
  - **Vitamin D_2 (Ergocalciferol)**
    - Less effective as precursor to $1,25(OH)_2$-vitamin D
    - Hepatic conversion of vitamin D_3 to 25-OH-vitamin D (calcitriol)
    - Conversion of 25-OH-vitamin D to $1,25(OH)_2$-vitamin D (calcitriol)

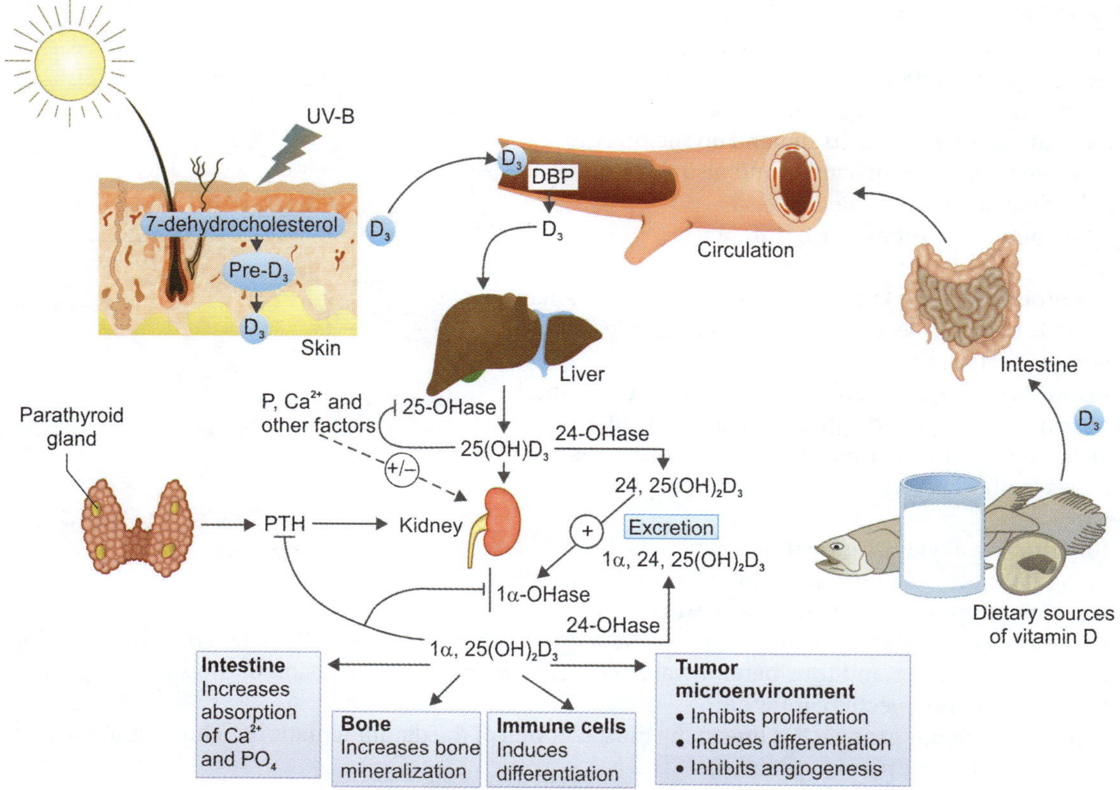

FIG. 1.5: Physiology of vitamin D.

- **Functions:** Vitamin D exists in two activated sterol forms. Its functions include:
  - **Regulation of plasma levels of calcium and phosphorus:** The main functions of 1,25-dihydroxyvitamin D on calcium and phosphorus homeostasis are:
    - **Stimulates intestinal absorption of calcium:** 1,25-dihydroxyvitamin D stimulates intestinal absorption of calcium in the duodenum through the interaction of 1,25-dihydroxyvitamin D with nuclear vitamin D receptor.
    - **Stimulates calcium reabsorption in the kidney:** 1,25-dihydroxyvitamin D increases calcium influx in distal tubules of the kidney.
    - **Interaction with PTH in the regulation of blood calcium.**
    - **Mineralization of bone:** Vitamin D plays a role in the **mineralization of osteoid matrix** and **epiphyseal cartilage** in both flat and long bones. Vitamin D stimulates osteoblasts to produce the calcium-binding protein osteocalcin, which is involved in the **deposition of calcium** during development of bone.
  - **Antiproliferative effects:** The vitamin D receptor (VDR) is expressed in the parathyroid gland, and $1,25(OH)_2$ D has an antiproliferative effect on parathyroid cells and it suppresses the transcription of the parathyroid hormone gene.
  - **Immunomodulatory:** Vitamin D is involved in the **innate and adaptive immune system.**

Vitamin D Deficiency

Q. Write briefly on clinical features, investigations, treatment, and prevention of rickets.

Causes of vitamin D deficiency are listed in **Box 1.4.** Diseases caused due to vitamin D deficiency are:

- **In children:** Deficiency of vitamin D in a growing child before the epiphyses has fused results in failure of growing bone to mineralize.
  - **Rickets:** Bone *softening* disease, deformity of *long bones* occurs.
- **In adults:**
  - **Osteomalacia:** Bone-thinning disorder, proximal muscle weakness, and bone fragility.
  - **Osteoporosis:** Decrease of bone mineralization and increased bone fragility.

Box 1.4: Causes of vitamin D deficiency.

- Impaired cutaneous production due to limited exposure to sunlight
- *Dietary absence*: Diets deficient in calcium and vitamin D
- Malabsorption
- Impaired hydroxylation by the liver to produce 25-hydroxyvitamin D
- Impaired hydroxylation by the kidneys to produce 1,25-dihydroxyvitamin D (vitamin D-dependent rickets type 1, chronic renal insufficiency)
- End-organ insensitivity to vitamin D metabolites [hereditary vitamin D-resistant rickets (HVDRR), vitamin D-dependent rickets type 2]

Rickets in Children (Fig. 1.6)

- In children, before the closure of epiphyses, vitamin D deficiency causes retardation of growth associated with an expansion of the growth plate known as **rickets.**
- **Gross skeletal changes in rickets** depend on the severity and duration of the vitamin D deficiency and also the stresses to which individual bones are subjected.
- **During the nonambulatory stage of infancy**
  - **Head:**
    - **Craniotabes:** The skull appears square and box-like, there is delayed closure of anterior fontanelle, frontal and parietal bossing.
    - **Frontal bossing:** Excess of osteoid produces frontal bossing and a squared appearance to the head.
    - Delayed eruption of primary teeth, enamel defects, and caries teeth.
  - **Chest:**
    - **Rachitic rosary:** Overgrowth of cartilage or osteoid tissue at the costochondral junction causes deformation of the chest producing the **'rachitic rosary'.**
    - **Pigeon breast/chest deformity:** The weakened metaphyseal areas of the ribs are subject to the pull of the respiratory muscles and thus bend inward. This creates anterior protrusion of the sternum producing **pigeon breast deformity** (pectus carinatum).
    - **Harrison's sulcus/groove:** It is due to the muscular pull of the diaphragmatic attachments to the lower ribs.
    - Respiratory infections and atelectasis.
- **During the ambulatory stage**
  - This occurs when an ambulating child develops rickets. It is characterized by deformities affecting the spine, pelvis, and tibia. Scoliosis, kyphosis, and lumbar lordosis are characteristic.

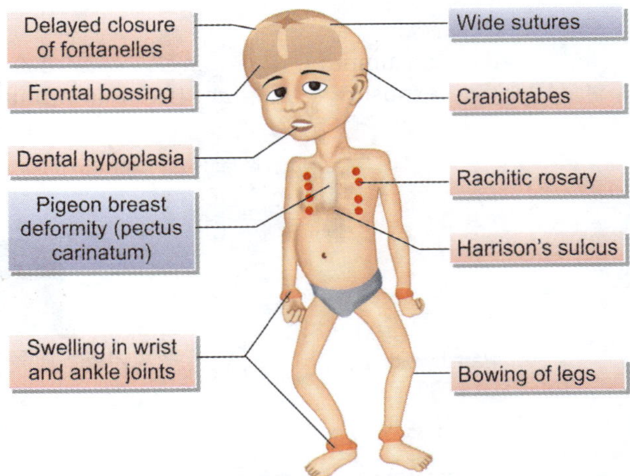

FIG. 1.6: Features of rickets.

- **Bowing of the legs:** Due to affection of tibia, knock knees, anterior curving of legs.
- **Extra skeletal manifestations**
  - **Seizures and tetany:** Secondary to hypocalcemia in vitamin D deficiency rickets.
  - **Hypotonia and delayed motor development:** In rickets developing during infancy.
  - Protuberant abdomen, bone pain, waddling gait, and fatigue.
- **Asymptomatic:** Detected on radiological evaluation.
- **Investigations**
  - **Wrist radiograph:** Findings include:
    - Lower ends of the shaft of radius and ulna become splayed.
    - Epiphyseal surfaces—fuzzy and ill-defined.
    - Unossified zone between shaft and radial epiphysis gets widened ('saucer' deformity).

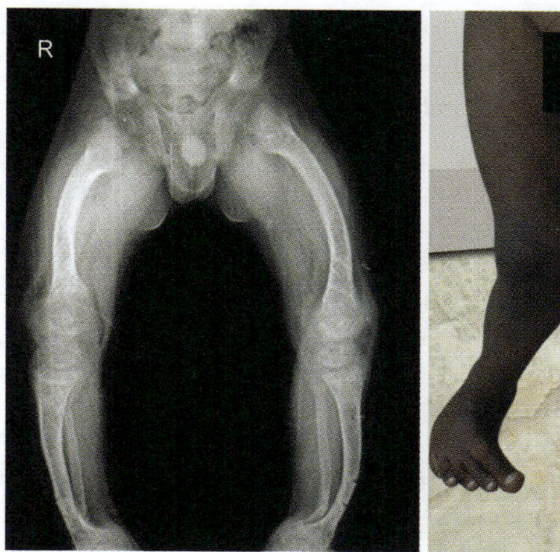

FIG. 1.7: X-ray of rickets showing splaying of epiphyses and bow legs.

- **Figure 1.7** shows a child with bow legs and X-ray **showing splaying, fraying and cupping of metaphysis.**
  - **Blood:**
    - **Serum calcium:** Low.
    - **Serum phosphate:** Low (due to associated secondary hyperparathyroidism).
    - **Serum alkaline phosphatase:** Increased due to increased osteoblast activity.
    - **Plasma 25-hydroxyvitamin D_3 level: Low** in most of the cases.

Comparison of conditions involving bone metabolism is presented in **Table 1.5**.

TABLE 1.5: Comparison of conditions involving bone metabolism.

Condition	*Calcium*	*Phosphorus*	*Vitamin D*	*ALP*	*Parathormone*	*Bone*
Rickets/Osteomalacia	Decreased	Decreased	Low	Elevated	Elevated	Softening, Looser's zones
Osteopenia	Normal	Normal	Normal	Normal/decreased	Normal	Decrease bone mass
Osteoporosis	Normal	Normal	Normal/ decreased	Normal/mild elevation	Normal	Degeneration of bone matrix
Hyperparathyroidism	Increased	Decreased	Normal	Elevated	Elevated	Brown tumor. lytic lesions
Paget's disease	Normal	Normal	Normal	Variable	Variable	Osteolytic/sclerotic lesion

- **Prevention:**
  - Adequate consumption of vitamin D (1,000–5,000 IU/day)
  - Adequate exposure to sunlight (from 30 minutes to 2 hours/week for infants).

Treatment of rickets
- Treat the underlying cause.
- Supplementation diet with calcium and vitamin D.
- **For nutritional deficiency** of vitamin D: Ergocalciferol, 1,50,000–6,00,000 IU orally or intramuscularly as a single dose. Or give Ergocalciferol in a dose of 2,000 IU every day.

Osteomalacia

Q. Discuss the causes, clinical features, investigations, and treatment in case of osteomalacia.

- Vitamin D deficiency in **adults** is accompanied by hypocalcemia and hypophosphatemia which result in **impaired mineralization of bone matrix** proteins, a condition known as osteomalacia.
- Thus, it is a disorder of mineralization of the organic matrix of the skeleton in adults when the **epiphyseal growth plates have closed**. In contrast, in rickets, the growing skeleton is involved.

Causes of osteomalacia are listed in **Box 1.5.**

Box 1.5: Causes of osteomalacia.

- **Nutritional abnormalities:** Dietary deficiency of vitamin D, parenteral nutrition
- **Malabsorption:** Tropical sprue, celiac disease, hepatobiliary diseases, pancreatic insufficiency
- **Disorders of vitamin D metabolism:** Vitamin D dependency type I and type II, anticonvulsants, chronic renal failure
- **Acidosis:** Distal renal tubular acidosis (type I)
- **Phosphate depletion:** Use of nonabsorbable antacids, tumor associated osteomalacia
- **Others:** Multiple myeloma, nephrotic syndrome, lead poisoning, inadequate sun exposure

Clinical Features

- **Bone pains, muscle weakness, fractures** of bones with minor trauma.
- Pain in the hip may cause **antalgic gait**.
- **Weakness of proximal muscle** results in waddling gait and may resemble primary muscle disease.
- **Collapse of vertebrae** causes local pain and deformity.
- Softening of skeleton may produce deformities such as **kyphosis, coxa vara, pigeon chest** and **triradiate pelvis** with a narrow pubic arch.

Laboratory Investigations

Blood (same as for rickets).
Urinary excretion of calcium: Reduced.

Radiological Findings

- **Bone density:** Reduced (osteopenia), diffuse demineralization.
- **Epiphyseal growth plate:** Increased in thickness, cupped and hazy at the metaphyseal border.
- **Cortical thinning:** Due to secondary hyperparathyroidism.
- **Other features:** Presence of nontraumatic fractures, radiolucent bands called pseudo-fractures **(Looser's zones) (Fig. 1.8).**
- **Bone scan** may be normal or show discrete foci of increased radionuclide uptake.
- **Bone mineral density** as assessed by dual-energy X-ray absorptiometry (DEXA) is reduced at spine, hip and forearm, with the maximum deficits at the cortical-rich bone in the forearms.

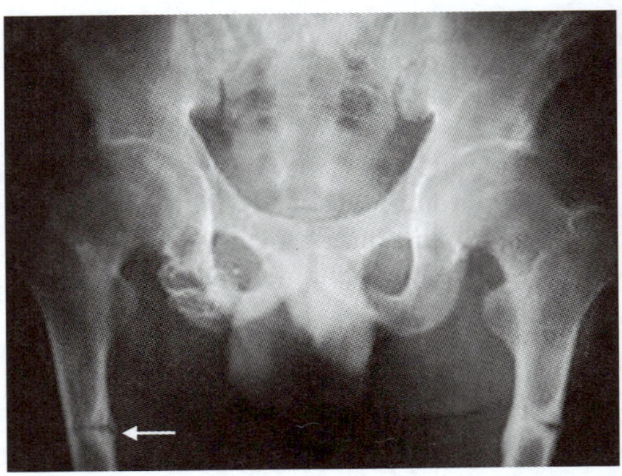

FIG. 1.8: X-ray shows Looser zones (arrow) and osteopenia.

Treatment of osteomalacia
- **Treat the underlying cause** wherever possible.
- **Dietary deficiency:** It is corrected by 1,000–4,000 IU of vitamin D_2 (ergocalciferol) or vitamin D_3 (cholecalciferol) for 3 months. This is followed by lower doses as maintenance. Vitamin D should be taken with fatty diet for maximum absorption.
- **Osteomalacia due to malabsorption:** Give 50,000–1,00,000 IU of vitamin D + calcium supplementation. Small doses of calcitriol (0.5–1.0 µg daily) also effective.
- **Chronic renal failure:** Calcitriol with weekly monitoring of calcium level.

Role of Vitamin D in Health and Disease

It has been shown in **Table 1.6.**

TABLE 1.6: Role of vitamin D in health and disease.

Parathyroid hormone	➤ Hypovitaminosis D causes secondary hyperparathyroidism which increases the risk of MI, HTN, and stroke
Malignancy	➤ Transcription of oncogenes involved in cell differentiation and proliferation is controlled: (c-myc, c-fos, c-sis) ➤ There is an inverse relationship between sun exposure and cancer mortality ➤ 10 ng/mL rise in vitamin D level of associated with—17% reduction in cancer incidence, 29% reduction in all cancer mortality, and 45% reduction in GI cancer mortality
Nervous system function	➤ Vitamin D modulates neurotransmitter and neurological function ➤ Has anticonvulsant and antidepressant effect ➤ 50% of multiple sclerosis patients are vitamin D deficient ➤ Seizures are common with vitamin D deficiency
Anti-inflammatory function	➤ Suppresses and may prevent autoimmune diseases ➤ Seems to reduce severity and frequency of childhood pneumonias
Calcium homeostasis	➤ Calcium absorption increases as 25(OH) vitamin D blood levels increase
Cardiovascular function	➤ Risk of myocardial infarction doubles in patients with vitamin D deficiency ➤ Heart failure patients have much lower vitamin D levels ➤ HTN patients given UV light treatments 3 times/week for 6 weeks have shown mild decrease in BP
Diabetes type 1	➤ Infants and children who were supplemented with had decreased incidence of DM type 1 by 80%
Diabetes type 2	➤ Low vitamin D levels associated with insulin resistance and β-cell dysfunction ➤ Postprandial glucose and insulin sensitivity are better in healthy adults with highest vitamin D levels ➤ Highest vitamin D levels associated with 60% improvement in insulin sensitivity
Respiratory system	➤ Vitamin D supplementation provides significant protective effect against influenza ➤ It is also associated with decrease in FEV1 ➤ Increased incidence of rhino-bronchial atopy
Osteoarthritis (OA)	➤ Vitamin D deficiency hastens the progression of OA hip and knee
Mood disorders	➤ Vitamin D supplementations improves general mood and hastens recovery in seasonal affective mood disorders
Polycystic ovary syndrome	➤ Deficiency exists in 60% of cases with normalization of menses and/or fertility within 3 months of supplementation
Pain	➤ Persistent, nonspecific musculoskeletal pain in 93% of patients had vitamin D deficiency ➤ Low back pain patients (53%) have vitamin D deficiency
Autoimmune disease	➤ Vitamin D insufficiency in half of the patients with fibromyalgia + SLE, Graves' disease, ankylosing spondylitis and rheumatoid arthritis
Falls in the elderly	➤ Vitamin D deficiency reported to affect predominantly the weight-bearing antigravity muscles of the lower limb, which are necessary for postural balance and walking ➤ Improvement in lower extremity muscle strength and balance with vitamin D supplementation thought to explain the reduced number of fall-related fractures

Hypervitaminosis D

Q. Write a short answer on hypervitaminosis D.

- Hypervitaminosis D causes hypercalcemia, which manifests as:
  - Nausea and vomiting
  - Excessive thirst and polyuria
  - Severe itching
  - Joint and muscle pains
  - Disorientation and coma
  - Metastatic calcifications

Treatment of hypervitaminosis: Hydration and treatment of hypercalcemia.

VITAMIN E (ALPHA TOCOPHEROL)

- **Sources:** Almonds, vegetable oils, and cereals
- **Actions:**
  - Acts as free radical scavenger and **antioxidant**
  - **Protects** LDL and PUFA in **membranes from oxidation**
  - **Inhibits prostaglandin synthesis**, activities of phospholipase A2, and protein kinase C.

Deficiency

- **Causes:**
  - Pancreatic exocrine insufficiency
  - Cholestatic liver disease
  - Extensive resection or disease affecting small intestine
  - Ataxia with vitamin E deficiency, due to a mutation in the gene encoding hepatic alpha-tocopherol transfer protein (*TTPA*)
  - Abetalipoproteinemia, due to mutations in the microsomal triglyceride transfer protein.
- **Diagnosis:**
  - **Alpha-tocopherol levels** of <0.5 mg/dL (5 µg/mL or 11.5 µmol/L)—deficiency.
  - For patients with marked hyperlipidemia, effective serum vitamin E level = alpha-tocopherol (mg)/total lipids (g); where total lipids = cholesterol + triglycerides.
  - A normal result is >0.8 mg.
- **Clinical manifestations:**
  - **Spinocerebellar syndrome**—ataxia, hyporeflexia, and loss of proprioceptive and vibratory sensation.
  - Ophthalmoplegia, skeletal myopathy, pigmented retinopathy.
  - Brown bowel syndrome (**intestinal lipofuscinosis**) is a brown pigmentation of the bowel that occasionally presents with bowel dilatation and pseudo-obstruction (due to lipofuscin accumulation within the smooth muscle mitochondria).
  - Life span of red blood cells is shortened.
  - In premature infants, vitamin E deficiency may cause a **hemolytic anemia**.

Treatment:
- For infants and children: 17–35 mg/kg/day of RRR-alpha-tocopherol.
- For adults: 800–1200 mg/day.

VITAMIN K

- **Sources:**
  - Dietary vitamin K_1 (**phylloquinone**) is found in green vegetables like spinach and broccoli, and in some oils.
  - Vitamin K_2 (**menaquinone**) is found in bacterial flora, meat (especially liver), cheeses, fermented soybeans, and eggs.
- **Actions:**
  - **Coagulation**: Vitamin K is essential for activity of several carboxylase enzymes within hepatic cells, and therefore is necessary for the activation of coagulation factors **VII, IX, X, and prothrombin.**
  - Activation of proteins C and S
  - Reversal of coumarin-like anticoagulants
  - Bone formation
  - Coronary vascular calcification

Deficiency

- **Causes:**
  - Cystic fibrosis
  - Primary biliary cholangitis
  - Primary sclerosing cholangitis
  - Biliary atresia
  - Familial intrahepatic cholestasis and other inherited disorders associated with cholestasis
  - Malabsorption syndromes
  - Liver failure
  - Medications: 2nd, 3rd generation cephalosporins, orlistat
  - Very high doses of vitamin E can cause vitamin K deficiency
- **Clinical manifestations:**
  - Easy bruising
  - Mucosal bleeding
  - Splinter hemorrhages
  - Melena
  - Hematuria
  - Other manifestations of impaired coagulation.
- **Diagnosis:**
  - Symptomatic patients with mild deficiency—only PT is elevated; in severe deficiency—both PT and aPTT are elevated.
  - Levels of PIVKA-II (**protein induced in vitamin K absence or antagonist-II**, also known as des-gamma-carboxy prothrombin) are **more sensitive** than PT in detecting vitamin K deficiency. PIVKA-II is also elevated in the presence of vitamin K antagonist (VKA) drugs or certain tumors such as hepatocellular carcinoma.
  - Measuring **vitamin K-dependent factors** (i.e., prothrombin, factors VII, IX, X, or protein C). In patients who are vitamin K deficient, levels of these factors often are **<50%** of normal.
  - Phylloquinone levels can also be measured directly but are impractical for clinical use.

Treatment:
- Vitamin K can be administered in doses of **1–25 mg** (usually 10 mg) via oral, intramuscular, subcutaneous, or intravenous routes.
- When vitamin K deficiency occurs in patients who are also receiving coumarin-like anticoagulants, doses of vitamin K should be minimized in order to prevent refractoriness to further anticoagulation.

Box 1.6: Classification of trace elements.

Essential trace elements	Trace elements that are probably essential	Potentially toxic elements with possible essential functions in low doses
• Iodine • Zinc • Selenium • Copper • Molybdenum • Chromium • Cobalt • Iron	• Manganese • Nickel • Silicon • Boron • Vanadium	• Fluoride • Lead • Cadmium • Mercury • Arsenic • Lithium • Tin • Aluminum

TRACE ELEMENTS

- The term 'trace' is used for concentrations of elements **not exceeding 250 µg/g of extracellular matrix.**
- Trace elements are **naturally occurring, homogeneous, inorganic substances** required in humans in amounts <100 mg/day.
- Classification of trace elements is presented in **Box 1.6**.
- There are about 15 trace elements of which only **10 are essential** nutrients in humans.
- These include: Iron, zinc, copper, chromium, selenium, iodine, fluorine, manganese, molybdenum, and cobalt.

Iron

Q. Write a short note on daily requirement of iron and important dietary sources of iron.

- **Most essential** trace element.
- **Deficiency state:**
  - **Asymptomatic**
  - **Anemia** (*refer* Chapter 8), weakness, headache, irritability, and varying degrees of fatigue and exercise intolerance.

The causes of iron overload have been shown in **Table 1.7**.

TABLE 1.7: Causes of iron overload.

Cause
Increased intake
➤ Transfusional overload (e.g., in inherited bone marrow failure syndromes, hemolytic anemias, myelodysplastic syndrome, aplastic anemia)
➤ Iron-loaded diet (e.g., "African iron overload")
➤ Repeated heroin infusions (e.g., to treat acute intermittent porphyria)
Increased absorption (with normal intake)
➤ Hereditary hemochromatosis due to HFE mutation (e.g., C282Y/C282Y; C282Y/H63D)
➤ Hereditary hemochromatosis due to rare mutations (e.g., ferroportin, hemojuvelin, hepcidin, ceruloplasmin)
➤ Thalassemia major or intermedia
➤ Sideroblastic anemia (inherited or acquired)
➤ Inherited anemias (e.g., CDA, DBA)
➤ Gestational alloimmune liver disease (GALD)
➤ Chronic liver disease, especially alcoholic liver disease, chronic hepatitis, and nonalcoholic fatty liver disease (NAFLD)

(HFE: hereditary hemochromatosis gene; CDA: congenital dyserythropoietic anemia; DBA: Diamond-Blackfan anemia).

Acute Iron Poisoning

- Develops when iron level **exceeds 60 mg/kg elemental iron.**
- **Clinical features:**
  - Vomiting, abdominal pain, bloody diarrhea, shock, dehydration, cyanosis, acidosis, and coma
  - Can cause **hepatotoxicity** and bowel obstruction
  - **Cardiomyopathy**, heart failure, and/or arrhythmias
  - **Diabetes mellitus**
  - Hypogonadism, decreased libido, and impotence
  - Skin involvement with hyperpigmentation (the bronze color in "**bronze diabetes**")
  - **Arthropathy,** especially involving the second and third metacarpophalangeal joints, and often with chondrocalcinosis.

Treatment

- **Gastric lavage** with sodium bicarbonate solution.
- **Desferrioxamine** 15 mg/kg/h IV, increased to maximum dose of 35 mg/kg/h.
- Correction of acidosis and shock.
- Extracorporeal removal with **exchange transfusion or continuous venovenous hemofiltration.**
- **Phlebotomy** can be done if no significant anemia present.

FLUOROSIS

Q. Write short note on fluorosis and its radiological signs.

- Fluorine's **ionic form** is known as fluoride.
- It is a component of **bone mineral** and alters its physical characteristics.
- Fluoride helps to **prevent dental caries**, because it increases the resistance of the enamel to acid attack.
- Requirement in adults is between 1.5 and 4 mg/day and 96% of fluorides in the body found in **bone and teeth.**
- **Deficiency:** Intake of <0.1 mg/day in infants and <0.5 mg/day in children predisposes to an increased incidence of dental caries.
- **Toxicity:** Results in **fluorosis.** This develops when fluoride content in the water is high (>3–5 ppm).
  - **Acute** ingestion of >30 mg/kg body weight usually manifests with GI symptoms such as diarrhea, vomiting leading to renal failure and may cause death.
  - **Dental fluorosis:** It is characterized by mottling of teeth where the enamel loses its luster, teeth appear chalky white with transverse yellow bands. It becomes rough, pigmented, pitted and brittle (fluoride teeth).
  - **Skeletal fluorosis:** Its features are:
    - **Sclerosis of bones** (especially of spine, pelvis, and limbs).
    - **Calcification** of ligaments, interosseous membrane **(Fig. 1.9)**, and tendinous insertions.
    - **Osteoporosis with** brittle bones.
    - **Severe pain and stiffness** in joints, stiffness in neck and backbone, bow legs. Other features are weakness, anemia, and weight loss.

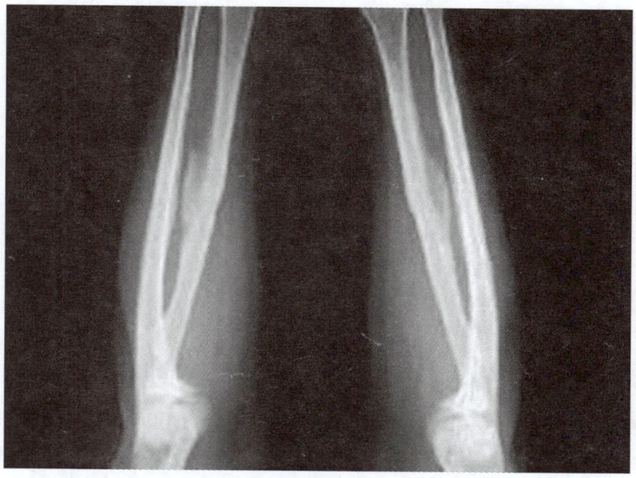

FIG. 1.9: X-ray of fluorosis showing calcification of interosseous membrane.

Angular Stomatitis

Q. Write a short note on angular stomatitis.

- **Angular stomatitis** refers to **cracking of the epithelium at the edge of the lips.**
- It presents with **erythema, maceration, scaling, and fissuring** at the corners of the mouth.
- Most commonly **bilateral** and **very painful.**
- **Causes of angular stomatitis** have been shown in **Box 1.7.**

Box 1.7: Causes of angular stomatitis.

- Iron deficiency anemia
- Secondary infection of *Candida albicans, Staphylococcus*
- **Vitamin deficiency:**
  - Riboflavin (B_2) deficiency
  - Pyridoxine (B_6) deficiency
  - Niacin deficiency (pellagra)
- Herpes labialis at the angle of mouth
- Angular stomatitis is associated with cheilosis in niacin deficiency and pellagra

ENTERAL AND PARENTERAL NUTRITION SUPPORT

Some form of **nutritional support** is needed for **patients who cannot eat, should not eat, will not eat or cannot eat enough.**

Indications for Nutritional Support

- **Severely malnourished patients** on admission to hospital.
- **Moderately malnourished** patients who are **not expected to eat for >3–5 days** (because of their physical illness).
- **Normally nourished** patients **not expected to eat for >5 days** or to eat less than half their intake for >8–10 days.

Types of Nutritional Support

- **Enteral nutrition** should be used, if the GI tract is functioning normally.
- **Parenteral nutrition**.

Q. Discuss the advantages and problems associated with enteral nutrition.

Enteral Nutrition

- **Prerequisite:** Must have **functioning GI tract**. Patients who are not able to swallow may need artificial nutritional support (e.g., after acute stroke or throat surgery, or long-term neurological disorders such as motor neuron disease and multiple sclerosis).
- Whenever possible, the enteral route is **preferred** and to be used.
- *Advantages and disadvantages of enteral nutrition have been shown in* ***Table 1.8.***
- *Methods of enteral nutrition have been shown in* ***Table 1.9.***
- **Complications of enteral feeding:**
  - **Access problems** (e.g., tube obstruction)
  - **Administration problems** (e.g., aspiration pneumonia)
  - **Gastrointestinal complications** (e.g., diarrhea)
  - **Metabolic complications** (e.g., overhydration).

TABLE 1.8: Advantages and disadvantages of enteral nutrition (EN).

Advantages	*Disadvantages*
➢ Intake easily/accurately monitored ➢ Provides nutrition when oral intake is not possible or adequate ➢ Less cost than parenteral nutrition ➢ Readily available ➢ Reduces risks associated with disease state ➢ Preserves gut integrity and immunologic function ➢ Decreases likelihood of bacterial translocation ➢ Increased compliance with intake ➢ Decreases the risk of multiorgan failure in ICU patients	➢ *Mechanical complications:* - Tube migration - Increased risk of bacterial contamination - Tube obstruction - Pneumothorax ➢ Costs more than oral diets ➢ Less palatable ➢ *Labor:* (1) Intensive assessment; (2) administration; (3) tube patency; and (4) site care; monitoring

TABLE 1.9: Methods of enteral nutrition.

Tube feeding <4 weeks	*Tube feeding >4 weeks*
➢ Nasogastric ➢ Nasoduodenal ➢ Nasojejunal ➢ Oro-gastric	➢ Enterostomy ➢ Gastrostomy ➢ Jejunostomy

- **Rate and method of delivery***
  - **Bolus:** 300–400 mL rapid delivery via syringe several times daily
  - **Intermittent:** 300–400 mL, over 20–30 minutes, several times/day via gravity drip or syringe
  - **Cyclic:** Via pump usually at night
  - **Continuous:** Via gravity drip or infusion pump

  *Determined by medical status, feeding route and volume, and nutritional goals.
- **Types of enteral formulations:**
  - **Standard polymeric formulas:**
    - Isotonic to serum
    - Caloric density of approximately 1 kcal/mL
    - Lactose-free
    - Protein content of about 40 g/1,000 mL (40 g/1,000 kcal)
    - Nonprotein calorie to nitrogen ratio of approximately 130
    - Mixture of simple and complex carbohydrates
    - Long-chain fatty acids (although some are now including medium-chain and omega-3 fatty acids)
    - Essential vitamins, minerals, and micronutrients
  - **Polymeric formulas** with fiber
  - **Immune-enhancing** formulas
  - **Protein-enriched** formulas
  - **Concentrated formulas:** Useful for patients requiring volume restriction
  - **Predigested** (elemental and semi elemental—previously called): Useful in thoracic duct leak, chylothorax, chylous ascites, malabsorption syndromes, nontolerance to standard enteral feeds (e.g., persistent diarrhea)
  - **Critical illness:** Special formulations for certain critical illnesses, have not proved beneficial over the others.
- **Contraindications to enteral feeding:** The intestinal tract cannot be used effectively in some patients because of the following:
  - Persistent nausea or vomiting
  - Postprandial abdominal pain or diarrhea
  - Mechanical obstruction or severe hypomotility
  - Malabsorption
  - Presence of high-output fistula

Parenteral Nutrition

Parenteral nutrition should be considered if **energy intake cannot**, or it is anticipated that it cannot be met by **enteral nutrition** (<50% of daily requirements) for >**7–10 days**.

Q. Discuss the indications, types and complications associated with total parenteral nutrition.

Central access: Total parenteral nutrition (TPN) both long, and short-term placement.

- The **infusion of hyperosmolar** (usually >1,500 mOsm/L) nutrient solutions requires a **large-bore, high-flow vessel** to minimize vessel irritation and damage.
- Percutaneous subclavian vein catheterization and peripherally inserted central venous catheterization (PICC) are the most commonly used techniques for **central parenteral nutrition (CPN)** access.
- The internal jugular, saphenous, and femoral veins are also used, although they are less desirable because of decreased patient comfort and difficulty in maintaining sterility.
- **Tunneled catheters** are preferred in patients who are likely to receive >8 weeks of TPN to reduce the risk of mechanical failure.
- **CPN macronutrient solutions:**
  - Crystalline amino acid solutions
  - Branched-chain amino acids for patients of hepatic encephalopathy, renal insufficiency
  - Glucose (dextrose) solutions
  - Lipid emulsions

Peripheral parenteral nutrition (PPN): Peripheral parenteral nutrition is often considered to have limited usefulness because of the high risk of thrombophlebitis.

*Advantages and disadvantages of parenteral nutrition have been shown in **Table 1.10**.*

*Indications for total parenteral nutrition have been shown in **Box 1.8**.*

*Complications of parenteral nutrition have been shown in **Table 1.11**.*

TABLE 1.10: Advantages and disadvantages of parenteral nutrition.

Advantages	*Disadvantages*
➢ Provides nutrients when <2–3 feet of small intestine remains ➢ Allows nutrition support when GI intolerance prevents oral or enteral support	➢ Economic impact ➢ Time-consuming ➢ Inconvenient ➢ Activities and work must be planned around feedings

Box 1.8: Indications of parenteral nutrition.

- Nonfunctioning GIT
- Nil per oral (NPO) >5 days
- GI fistula
- Acute pancreatitis
- Short bowel syndrome
- Malnutrition with >10–15% weight loss
- Nutritional needs not met; patient refuses food

Refeeding Syndrome

- **Definition:** Refeeding syndrome is a syndrome consisting of metabolic disturbances that occur as a result of reinstitution of nutrition to patients who are starved or severely malnourished.
- **Time of occurrence:** Usually occurs **within 4 days** of restarting nutritional support.

TABLE 1.11: Complications of parenteral nutrition.

	First 48 hours	*First 2 weeks*	*3 months onward*
Mechanical	➢ Malposition ➢ Hemothorax/pneumothorax ➢ Air embolism ➢ Blood loss ➢ Puncture of subclavian/carotid artery	➢ Catheter displacement ➢ Thrombosis ➢ Air embolism ➢ Occlusion	➢ Tear of catheter ➢ Catheter thrombosis ➢ Air embolism ➢ Blood loss
Metabolic/GI	➢ Fluid overload ➢ Hypoglycemia, hypophosphatemia, Hypokalemia, hypomagnesemia ➢ Refeeding syndrome	➢ Hypoglycemic coma ➢ Acid-base and electrolyte imbalance	➢ Deficiency of essential fatty acids, vitamins or trace element ➢ Metabolic bone disease ➢ Liver disease
Infectious		➢ Catheter-induced sepsis ➢ Exit site infection	➢ Tunnel infection ➢ Catheter-induced sepsis ➢ Exit site infection

- **Mechanism**
  - When nutritional support is given to a starved or severely malnourished patient, there is a **rapid change from a catabolic to an anabolic state.**
  - Administration of carbohydrates stimulates **release of insulin**. This causes cellular uptake of phosphate, potassium, and magnesium and may lead to significant falls in their levels in the serum. This results in electrolyte imbalance and can produce serious consequences (e.g., cardiac arrhythmias).
- **Clinical features**
  - Initial features may be **nonspecific**.
  - **Later:** Rhabdomyolysis, leukocyte dysfunction, respiratory and cardiac failure, hypotension, arrhythmias, seizures, coma, and sudden death.

Treatment of refeeding syndrome

- Start nutrition at **5–10 kcal/kg/day,** and **increase levels gradually**.
- Provide **thiamine, multivitamins and trace elements**.
- In thiamine-deficient patients, Wernicke's encephalopathy can be precipitated by refeeding with carbohydrates. This is prevented by providing thiamine before starting nutritional support.
- Restore the **circulatory volume**. Monitor fluid balance and clinical status.
- Replace **PO_4, K, and Mg.**

PROTEIN–ENERGY MALNUTRITION

Protein–energy malnutrition (PEM) **or protein–calorie malnutrition** includes marasmus, kwashiorkor and intermediate states of marasmus-kwashiorkor.

Marasmus

Q. Write a short note on marasmus.

- *Marasmus* is the childhood form of **starvation**.
- It develops **due to inadequate intake of protein and calories.**
- It is characterized by **emaciation** with apparent muscle wasting and loss of body fat.
- There is **no edema.**
- The hair is thin and dry.
- The marasmic child does not appear as apathetic or anorexic as with kwashiorkor.
- **Diarrhea** is frequent and there may be signs of infection.

Kwashiorkor

- Kwashiorkor develops due to an **inadequate protein intake with reasonable caloric** (energy) intake.
- *Kwashiorkor* occurs in a **young child displaced from breastfeeding by a new baby**.
- It may be **precipitated by infections** (e.g., measles, malaria, and diarrheal illnesses).
- Child appears **apathetic and lethargic with severe anorexia.**
- **Edema:** In kwashiorkor, marked protein deprivation causes **hypoalbuminemia** leading to **generalized or dependent edema.**
- **Skin lesions:** Children with kwashiorkor have characteristic *skin lesions*. This consists of alternating zones of hyperpigmentation, and hypopigmentation, producing **'flaky paint' appearance**.
- **Hair changes:** The hair is **dry and sparse**. There may be loss of color or alternating bands of pale and darker hair (**flag sign**).
- **Other features:** The other features that differentiate kwashiorkor from marasmus are:
  - Abdomen is distended due to **hepatomegaly** (presence of enlarged, fatty liver) and/or **ascites.**
  - Development of apathy, listlessness, and **loss of appetite**.
  - Likely presence of **vitamin deficiencies.**
  - Defects in immunity and secondary **infections.**

Treatment of PEM
- Provision of **protein and energy supplements.**
- Control of infection.

OBESITY

Q. Describe the risk factors, clinical features, complications, and management of obesity.

Q. Describe and discuss the etiology of obesity including modifiable and nonmodifiable risk factors and secondary causes.

- **Definition:** Obesity is defined as an accumulation of **excess body fat (adipose tissue)** that is of **sufficient magnitude to impair health.** Latin word 'obesus' meaning stout, fat, plump.
- **Measurement of obesity**
  - Body mass index—weight/height^2 in kg/m^2
  - Anthropometry—skinfold thickness
  - Densitometry—underwater weighing
  - CT/MRI imaging
  - Electrical impedance
- **Classification of overweight and obesity by BMI (Table 1.12)**

TABLE 1.12: Nutritional status based on the WHO and "Asian criteria" values.

Nutritional status	*WHO criteria BMI cut off*	*"Asian criteria" BMI cut off*
Underweight	<18.5	<18.5
Normal	18.5–24.9	18.5–22.9
Overweight	25–29.9	23–24.9
Pre-obese	–	25–29.9
Obese	>30	>30
Obese type-1 (obese)	30–40	30–40
Obese type-2 (morbid obese)	40.1–50	40.1–50
Obese type 3 (super obese)	>50	>50

- **Types of obesity according to body fat distribution:** The distribution of the stored fat is important in obesity and accordingly obesity is divided into:
  - **Central (abdominal, visceral, android or apple-shaped) obesity**:
    - This type of obesity shows **increased accumulation of fat in the trunk** and in the **abdominal cavity** (in the mesentery and around viscera).
    - It is associated with a **greater risk** for several diseases (e.g., type 2 diabetes, the metabolic syndrome, and cardiovascular disease) than generalized obesity.
    - **Increased Waist: Hip ratio—** >0.9 in females, >1 in males is abnormal.

- Hypothesis—intra-abdominal adipocytes are more lipolytically active than others—release free fatty acids into portal circulation—cause adverse metabolic reactions, especially on the liver.

- **Generalized ('gynoid' or 'pear-shaped') obesity:** This type is characterized by excess accumulation of **fat diffusely in the subcutaneous tissue**.

Etiology (Table 1.13)

- Accumulation of fat in obesity can be considered by the result of **caloric imbalance** between the energy consumption (**intake** of calories) in the diet and **energy expenditure** through exercise and bodily functions.
- However, the pathogenesis of obesity is complex and incompletely known.

TABLE 1.13: Etiology and risk factors of obesity.

Genetic aspects	*Environmental factors*
➢ Obesity is a **polygenic disorder**, with small contributions from a number of different genes. ➢ Single-gene (**monogenic forms**) disorders are rare and produce severe childhood obesity—mutations in the leptin gene and leptin receptor gene, mutations of *POMC* (pro-opiomelanocortin), *Mc4R* (melanocortin-4 receptor) *genes*	➢ **Food:** Many environmental factors can influence food intake ➢ Increased consumption of energy-dense foods, larger food portion size, and increased variety of food, increased availability, reduced cost and increased caloric beverages (soft drinks, juices) promote obesity
➢ A few **genetic conditions in which obesity** is a feature including the Prader–Willi and Laurence–Moon–Biedl syndromes	➢ **Physical activity:** (1) exercise (fitness and sports-related activities); (2) work-related physical activity; and (3) non-exercise, nonemployment (spontaneous) activity. ➢ Increased sedentary behavior, reduced activities of daily living and decreased physical activity promote obesity
Reversible causes of obesity and weight gain Minority of patients presenting with obesity have specific cause which can be identified and treated **(Table 1.14)**. Compared to idiopathic obesity, these patients have short history of marked weight gain	

TABLE 1.14: Potentially reversible causes of obesity and weight gain.

Endocrine factors	
➢ Hypothyroidism ➢ Cushing's syndrome ➢ Insulinoma	➢ Stein–Leventhal syndrome ➢ Hypothalamic damage (e.g., due to trauma, tumor)
Drug induced	
➢ **Psychiatric and neurologic medications:** Atypical antipsychotics (e.g., olanzapine) pizotifen, sodium valproate, flunarizine ➢ **Steroid hormones:** Progestational steroids, corticosteroids, hormonal contraceptives	➢ **Antidiabetic agents:** insulin (most forms), sulfonylureas, thiazolidinediones ➢ **Antihypertensive agents:** α- and β-adrenergic receptor blockers

Q. Describe and discuss the monogenic and polygenic forms of obesity.

Monogenic and Polygenic Obesity (Table 1.15)

TABLE 1.15: Features of monogenic and polygenic obesity.

Feature	*Monogenic obesity*	*Polygenic obesity*
Genes	➢ LEP (Leptin) ➢ LEPR (Leptin Receptor) ➢ POMC (Pro-opiomelanocortin), ➢ PCSK1 (Prohormone convertase 1/3) ➢ MC4R (Melanocortin 4 receptor) ➢ SIM1 (Single-Minded Homolog 1)	➢ PPARG (Peroxixome proliferator-activator receptor γ) ➢ Adiponectin (ADIPOQ) ➢ FTO (Fat-mass and Obesity associated gene) ➢ LEP (Leptin)
Mutation	Autosomal loss-of-function mutation, usually dominant or co-dominant More severe in homozygous individuals	
Features	➢ High BMI ➢ Compulsive hyperphagia ➢ Endocrinal abnormalities ➢ Developmental delay	Influenced by environmental external factors like exposure to physical, chemical or biological agents, diet

Adipocyte and Adipose Tissue (Figs. 1.10 and 1.11)

- Adipose tissue consists of adipocytes and stromal/vascular component (preadipocytes, macrophages, fibroblasts, collagen tissue).
- Adipose mass increases by:
  - Enlargement of adipose cells through lipid deposition
  - Increase in number of adipocytes
  - Increase in number of infiltrating macrophages.

Pathogenesis (Fig. 1.12)

Peripheral Afferent System

- Peripheral afferent system can be further subdivided into **peripheral appetite suppressing signals** and **peripheral appetite stimulant signals.**
- *Peripheral appetite suppressing signals*
  - **Leptin (Greek term leptos, meaning 'thin'):** Leptin is a **hormone secreted by fat cells** and it stimulates POMC (pro-opiomelanocortin)/CART (cocaine and amphetamine-regulated transcript) pathway **(Fig. 1.13)** and inhibits NPY/AgRP pathway causing **appetite** to be **suppressed** (anorexigenic). Increased leptin **stimulates physical activity**, heat **production** (thermogenesis), and **energy expenditure**.
  - **Adiponectin:** It is a hormone **(fat-burning molecule)** and the 'guardian angel against obesity,' and is produced mainly by fat cells (adipocytes). Its levels are lower in obese.

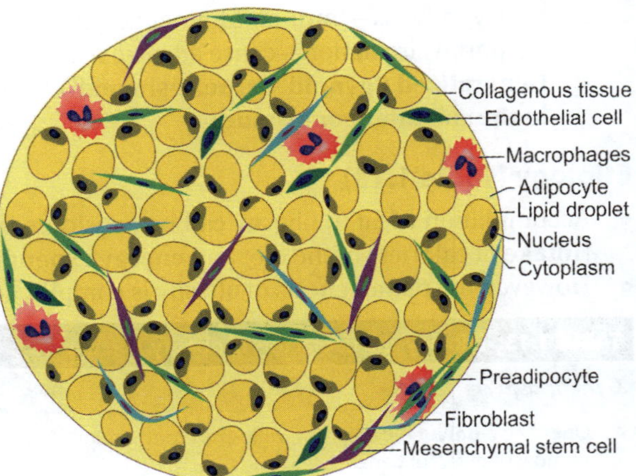

FIG. 1.10: Adipose tissue.

	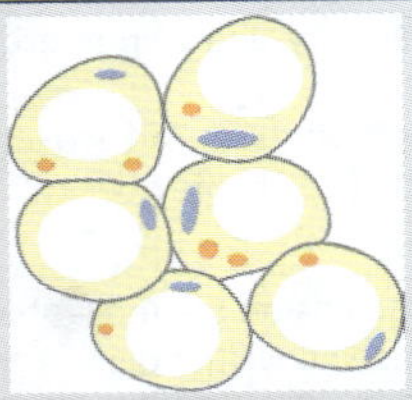 *White adipose tissue*	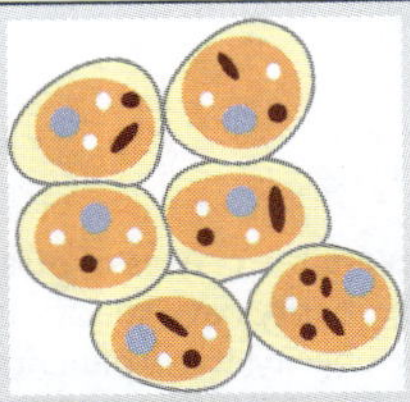 *Brown adipose tissue*	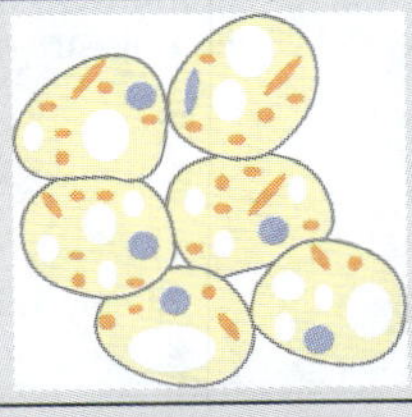 *Beige adipose tissue*
Localization	➢ Subcutaneous ➢ Intra-abdominal ➢ Epicardial ➢ Gonadal	➢ Interscapular ➢ Paravertebral ➢ Perirenal ➢ Cervical ➢ Supraclavicular	Emerges in white adipose tissue depots with appropriate stimuli
Morphology	Spherical	Elliptical and smaller than white	Spherical
Cell composition	➢ Single lipid droplet ➢ Few mitochondria ➢ Flattened peripheral nucleus ➢ Little endoplasmic reticulum	➢ Multiple small lipid droplets ➢ Large number of mitochondria ➢ Oval central nucleus	➢ Unilocular morphology but small lipid droplets after stimulation ➢ Mitochondria appear after stimulation
Function	Storing energy	➢ Expending energy and heat production (nonshivering thermogenesis)	Thermogenic potential
Uncoupling protein	Undetectable	Positive	Positive after stimulation

FIG. 1.11: Features of adipose tissue.

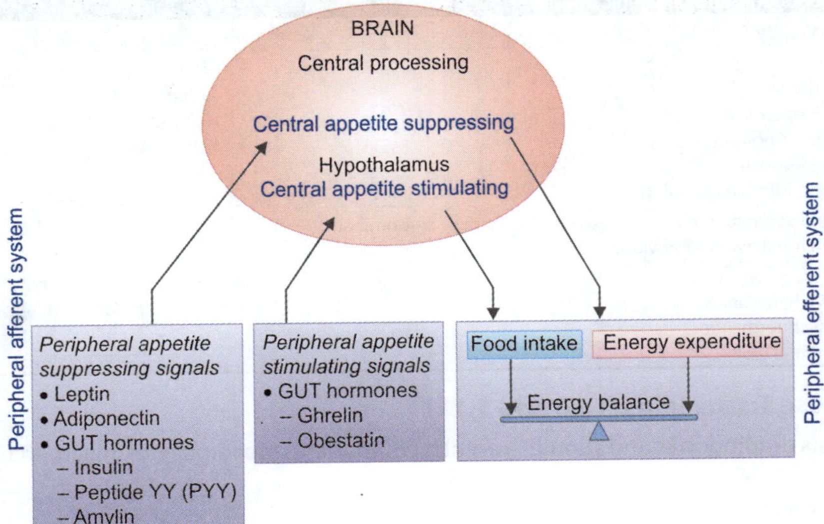

FIG. 1.12: Regulation of energy balance. Peripheral afferent system (appetite suppressing and stimulating signals) influences the activity of the hypothalamus, which is the central regulator of appetite and satiety. Signals from hypothalamus in turn act on peripheral efferent system (food intake and energy expenditure).

- **Resistin**: Primarily produced by macrophages and not fat cells. It **causes insulin resistance.**
- **Gut hormones:** These include peptide YY (PYY), pancreatic polypeptide, insulin, and amylin.
  - **Insulin:** It is **secreted by cells of the pancreas** and acts centrally to **activate the appetite suppressing pathway**.
  - **Peptide YY:** It is **secreted by the endocrine cells** (L cells) in the ileum and colon. It **reduces appetite**. Other peripheral **appetite suppressing** signals include glucagon like peptide 1 (**GLP1**) and oxyntomodulin.
  - **Amylin:** It is a peptide secreted with insulin from pancreatic β-cells.

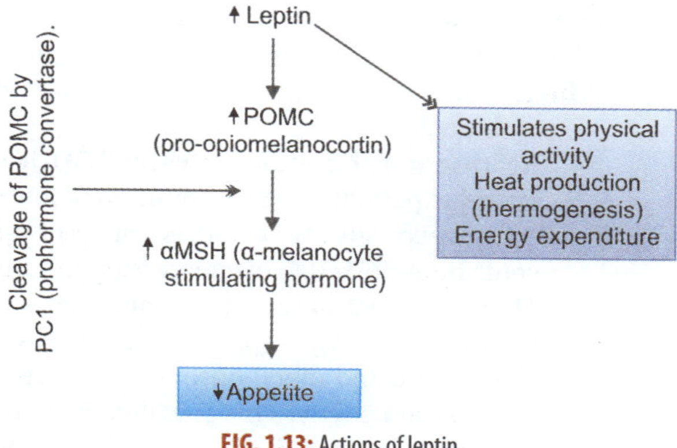

FIG. 1.13: Actions of leptin.

- *Peripheral appetite-stimulating signals*
  - **Gut hormones:**
    - **Ghrelin:** It is produced by the **oxyntic cells of the fundus of the stomach** and in the **arcuate nucleus of the hypothalamus**. Ghrelin **increases food intake** (orexigenic effect) and **stimulates appetite** by activating the central appetite stimulating NPY/AgRP pathway.
    - **Obestatin:** It is a peptide produced by the **same gene that encodes ghrelin**. It counteracts the **increase in food intake induced by ghrelin**.
  - **Retinol-binding protein 4 (RBP4):** Secreted by fat cells. Its actions counteract with those of insulin. Raised levels of RBP4 found in type 2 diabetes mellitus.

TABLE 1.16: Examples of central nervous system regulators of energy balance.

Central anabolic (increased intake) regulators	*Central catabolic (decreased intake) regulators*
Neuropeptide Y	α-Melanocyte-stimulating hormone
Agouti-related protein	Corticotropin-releasing hormone
Melanin-concentrating hormone	Thyrotropin-releasing hormone
Hypocretins and orexins	Cocaine- and amphetamine-regulated transcript (CART)

Central Processing (Table 1.16)

The arcuate nucleus of the hypothalamus processes and integrates neurohumoral peripheral afferent signals and generates efferent signals. It consists of:

- *Central appetite-suppressing (anorexigenic pathway or leptin melanocortin pathway):* In this pathway, **POMC/CART neurons enhance energy expenditure** and weight loss through the production of the anorexigenic (suppresses appetite) neuro-peptides mainly α-MSH (α-melanocyte-stimulating hormone) by cleavage of POMC by PC1 (prohormone convertase).
- *Central appetite-stimulating (orexigenic) pathway:* It consists of:
  - NPY (neuropeptide Y)/AgRP (agouti-related peptide) containing neurons promote food intake (orexigenic effect) and weight gain, through the activation of Y1/5 receptors in secondary neurons.
  - Secondary neurons in turn release factors such as melanin-concentrating hormone (MCH) and orexin, which stimulate appetite. This pathway also decreases energy expenditure.

Peripheral Efferent System

- It is organized into two pathways namely anabolic and catabolic that control food intake and energy expenditure, respectively.
- **Energy intake (food intake)**
  - **Food:** The increase in obesity can be related to the type of food consumed (i.e., food-containing sugar and fat) and also psychological factors.
  - **Control of appetite:** Signals may affect different aspects of eating behavior. For example:
    - **Ghrelin** (peptide produced by the stomach) **increases hunger but does not affect satiation or satiety.**
    - **Cholecystokinin causes satiation**, but has **no effect on satiety**.
    - **Leptin acts on multiple pathways**, its deficiency causes increased hunger and reduced satiation and satiety.
  - Following a meal, substances such as cholecystokinin (CCK), bombesin, and glucagon-like peptide-1 (GLP-1) are released from the small intestine, and glucagon and insulin from the pancreas. These hormones are involved in the control of satiety. The control of appetite is extremely complex. Many transmitters in the central nervous system affect appetite:
    - **Appetite inhibitors:** Dopamine, serotonin, γ-aminobutyric acid
    - **Appetite stimulators:** Opioids

- **Energy expenditure**
  - It can be divided into resting (or basal) metabolic rate, the thermic effect of food, and physical activity energy expenditure.
    - **Resting basal metabolic rate (BMR):** BMR is the energy expenditure and accounts for about 70% of daily energy expenditure, whereas active physical activity contributes to 5–10% of energy expenditure.
    - **Thermic effect of food (thermogenesis):** About 10% of ingested energy is spent in the process of digestion, absorption, and metabolism of nutrients irrespective of physical activity. This is called as dietary-induced thermogenesis which is lower in obese individuals.
    - **Physical activity:** Obese individuals tend to spend more energy during physical activity as they have a larger mass to move.

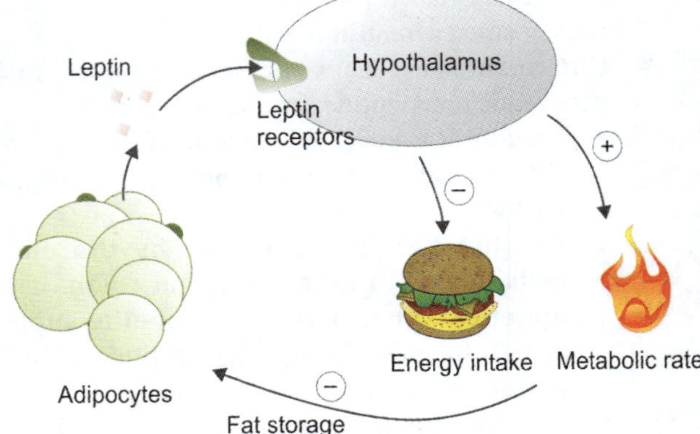

FIG. 1.14: Lipostat/adipostat—body weight "set point" in hypothalamus.

Theory of Body Weight 'Set Point' in Hypothalamus (Fig. 1.14)

Pathologic Consequences of Obesity (Complications of Obesity)

Q Describe the pathogenesis of obesity and its consequences.

Morbidity and mortality: Obesity is associated with an **increase** in mortality and morbidity. Obese individuals are at risk of early death, mainly from diabetes, coronary heart disease, and cerebrovascular disease.

Box 1.9: Consequences of insulin resistance.

- **Muscle:** Hyperglycemia and diabetes mellitus
- **Kidneys:** Salt retention and hypertension
- **Ovaries:** Increase testosterone and polycystic ovary syndrome (PCOS)
- **Heart:** Increase plasminogen activator inhibitor-1 (PAI-1) and acute coronary syndrome
- **Cancers:** Colon, prostate, breast
- **Sympathetic system:** Increased cytokines and blood pressure

Metabolic Complications of Obesity

- Central obesity or upper body fat distribution is associated with increased concentration of FFA (free-fatty acid), which can produce several metabolic complications of obesity.
- **Insulin resistance and type 2 diabetes mellitus**
  - Insulin resistance is the decrease/failure of response of target (peripheral) tissues to insulin action.
  - Insulin resistance can develop in obesity and may produce type 2 diabetes mellitus.
  - **Central/upper body/visceral obesity** is found in >80% of patients with **type 2 diabetes.**
  - **Causes of insulin resistance in obesity:**
    - **Obese individuals** have **excess** circulating **FFAs** and there is an **inverse correlation between fasting plasma FFAs and insulin sensitivity**. Central obesity is associated with **insulin resistance. Excess intracellular FFAs increase gluconeogenesis.**
    - **Adipokines: Adipose tissue** acts as a functional endocrine organ and **secretes variety of proteins** into the systemic circulation, which are **termed adipokines** (or adipose cytokines). **In obesity, adiponectin (one of the adipokines) levels are reduced,** which contributes to insulin resistance.
  - **Consequences of insulin resistance (Box 1.9).**

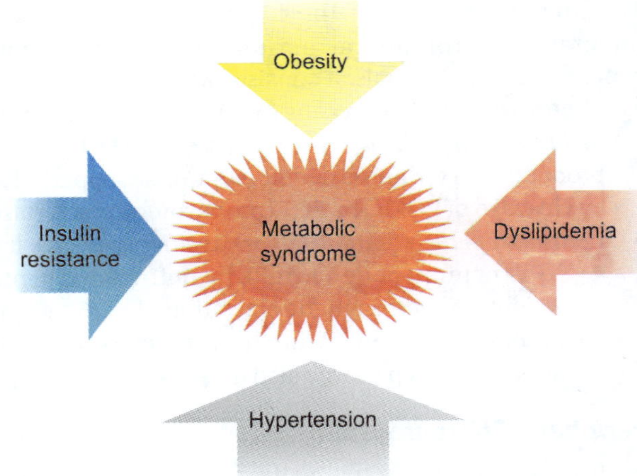

FIG. 1.15: Obesity and metabolic syndrome.

- **Dyslipidemia**
  - Upper body obesity and type 2 diabetes mellitus are associated with an atherogenic lipid profile. Dyslipidemia includes **increased triglycerides, increased low-density lipoprotein (LDL) cholesterol with very low-density lipoprotein (VLDL) cholesterol**, decreased **high-density lipoprotein (HDL)** cholesterol, and decreased levels of the vascular protective adipokine adiponectin.
  - Dyslipidemia increases the risk of cardiovascular diseases (**atherosclerosis, cardiomyopathy**) in the metabolic syndrome **(Fig. 1.15)**.
- **Endocrine manifestations of obesity**
  - Reproductive disorders associated with obesity are listed in **Table 1.17**.
- **Mechanical complications of obesity**

Osteoarthritis: Extremity degenerative joint disease (osteoarthritis) and also gout.

- **Venous stasis/varicose veins.**
- **Acanthosis nigricans:** Reflects the severity of underlying insulin resistance.
- **Increased friability of skin:** It may be seen especially in skinfolds, thereby increasing the risk of fungal and yeast infections.
- **Urinary incontinence.**
- **Pulmonary disease**
  - These include reduced chest wall compliance, increased work of breathing, increased minute ventilation (due to increased metabolic rate), and decreased functional residual capacity and expiratory reserve volume.
  - **Obstructive sleep apnea:** Sleep apnea is common in patients with severe obesity. Sleep apnea can be obstructive (most common), central, or mixed and is often associated with an increased risk of hypertension, right heart failure and sudden death. Obesity hypoventilation syndrome is also known as **Pickwickian syndrome**.
  - **Obesity and asthma:** Reduced TLC (total lung capacity), reduced RV (residual volume) and FRC (functional residual capacity).
- **Obesity and cancer (Table 1.18)**
  - Obesity is the biggest preventable cause of cancer after smoking.
  - Accounts for 14% of cancer deaths in men and 20% in women.
- **Gastrointestinal disorders:** Following are more prevalent in obese patients:
  - **Gastroesophageal reflux disease**
  - **Gallstones:** Obesity is associated with increased secretion of cholesterol in the bile, supersaturation of bile, and a higher incidence of gallstones, especially cholesterol gallstones.
  - **Fatty liver (steatosis) and nonalcoholic steatohepatitis: Nonalcoholic fatty liver disease (NAFLD)** can progress to hepatic cirrhosis and rarely to hepatocellular carcinoma.
- **Obesity and retinal disease**
  - Overweight diabetics are twice more likely to develop retinopathy than nonobese.
  - Waist to hip ratio was only second to glycemic control in its importance in preventing retinopathy in studies.
  - Conditions and complications associated with obesity are summarized in **Table 1.19**.

Clinical Assessment, Investigations, and Diagnosis

Aims of assessing of obesity are to:

1. **Evaluate and quantify severity of obesity:** Severity of obesity can be quantified using the BMI (*refer* **Table 1.12**).
2. **Exclude an underlying cause**
3. **Identify complications**
4. **Prepare a management plan**

Appearance of a patient with morbid obesity is shown in **Figure 1.16**.

TABLE 1.17: Endocrine manifestations of obesity.

Men	*Women*
➤ Plasma testosterone and SHBG are reduced ➤ Increase estrogen ➤ Gynecomastia seen ➤ Secondary sexual characters preserved	➤ Increased androgen ➤ Decrease SHBG ➤ PCOS ➤ Not only fertility but their chances of IVF success reduce

(SHBG: sex hormone-binding globulin; PCOS: polycystic ovary syndrome)

TABLE 1.18: Obesity and related cancers.

Males	*Females*
Esophagus	Gallbladder
Colon	Bile ducts
Rectum	Breasts
Pancreas	Endometrium
Liver	Cervix
Prostate	Ovaries

TABLE 1.19: Conditions and complications associated with obesity.

Risk factors/system involved	*Outcomes*
Metabolic syndrome	
Type 2 diabetes	Coronary heart disease, ischemic heart disease
Hypertension	Stroke
Hyperlipidemia	Diabetes complications
Cardiovascular	Heart failure
Gastrointestinal	Gastroesophageal reflux disease, hiatus hernia
Hepatobiliary	Liver fat accumulation, nonalcoholic steatohepatitis, cirrhosis, gallstones
Pulmonary disease	Exertional dyspnea, breathlessness
Restricted ventilation Obesity hypoventilation syndrome (Pickwickian syndrome)	Obstructive sleep apnea
Mechanical effects of weight **Endocrine manifestations** (Increased peripheral steroid interconversion in adipose tissue)	Urinary incontinence, osteoarthritis of knees and hips, varicose veins, back strain Menstrual abnormalities Hormone-dependent cancers (breast, uterus) Polycystic ovarian syndrome (infertility, hirsutism)
Increased morbidity and mortality	
Psychological problems	Lack self-confidence, depression, more physical and sexual abuse, lack of attention, low education, and low self-esteem
Others	Accident-proneness, socioeconomic disadvantage (lower income, less likely to be promoted), postoperative problems, increased cancer risk (e.g., colorectal cancer), skin infections (groin and submammary candidiasis; hidradenitis)

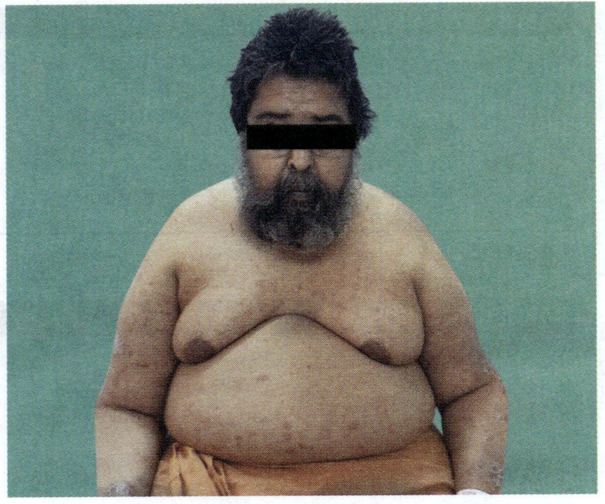

FIG. 1.16: Appearance of a patient with morbid obesity.

TABLE 1.20: Types of diet in the treatment of obesity.

Fixed energy diet	*Low-calorie diet*	*Very low-calorie diet (VLCD)*
➢ 1,200–1,800 kcal ➢ Intake is limited by controlling portion sizes, menu choice and composition ➢ Minimal self-monitoring ➢ Lack of compliance to this rigid pattern	➢ 800–1,000 kcal ➢ Applicable to most of the patients ➢ Fewer restrictions than VLCD ➢ Supplementation of vitamins and minerals ➢ Reduction of 6–7 kg observed over a year	➢ 400–600 kcal ➢ Even below one's basal metabolic rate ➢ Used for period of 1–2 months under medical supervision ➢ 45–70% protein, 30–50% carbohydrates, and 2 g fat ➢ Supplementation of vitamins, minerals, and trace elements ➢ Greater weight loss compared to restrictive diets

Q. Describe and enumerate the indications, pharmacology, and side effects of pharmacotherapy for obesity.

Management

- **Goal:**
  - Initially to reduce weight by about 10% from baseline
  - Reduce weight of about 0.5–1 kg/week for 6 months.
- **Life style modification diet (Table 1.20)**
  - Low calorie diet, low in saturated fats, low density foods, normal protein intake and increased fibers in diet.
  - 1,000 kcal deficit produces 1 kg weight loss per week. No matter what the calorie intake is the constituents remain in same proportion (i.e., carbohydrates 55%, fat 30%, and protein 15%).
  - **Total fasting: Not recommended**. There is diuresis, natriuresis, and all deficiencies.
  - *Refeeding syndrome:* Severe and potentially fatal electrolyte, fluid and metabolic abnormalities when feeding is resumed.
  - **Physical activity:** Regular physical activity enables to maintain loss of weight. Has to be done under supervision. Moderate exercise to be done for 30–45 minutes and 3–5 days/week.
  - **Behavioral modification:** (1) Useful as adjunct to diet and physical exercise; (2) Patient often needs motivation to lose weight.
- **Drug therapy (pharmacotherapy):** Lifestyle modification should be considered before starting drug therapy.
  - *Centrally acting drugs*
    - **Sibutramine**
      - **Mechanism of action:** Centrally acting, mono-amine reuptake inhibitor (primarily serotonin and norepinephrine). By sympathetic stimulation, it prevents decrease in BMR. It reduces appetite.
      - **Dose:** 10–15 mg once daily.
      - **Side effects:** Hypertension, tachycardia, sweating, dizziness, and headache.
      - **Contraindications:** Coronary artery disease, cardiac arrhythmias, uncontrolled hypertension.
    - **Rimonabant**
      - **Mechanism of action:** Endocannabinoid 1 (CB1) receptor blocker. It has both central and peripheral actions and reduces weight and weight-related metabolic factors.
      - **FDA approval:** BANNED
      - **Side effects:** Depression, anxiety, suicidal tendencies.
  - *Peripherally acting drugs*
    - **Orlistat**
      - **Mechanism of action:** Nonsystemic reversible inhibitor of gastric and pancreatic lipases by forming a covalent bond with serine residue. It acts on stomach and intestine.
      - **Dose:** 120 mg BD or TID with meals.
      - **FDA approval:** For adults and adolescents as well as children.
      - **Side effects:** Flatulence, defecation increases, oily evacuation, rectal leakage, steatorrhea.
    - **Olestra:** Olestra is synthesized using a sucrose molecule, which can support from 6 to 8 fatty acid chains arranged radially like an octopus. Too large to move through the intestinal wall and be absorbed. Same taste and mouth feel as fat. Approval as a food additive up to 35% replacement of fats in home cooking and 75% in commercial uses.

- **Others:**
  - **Phentermine:** Amphetamine like drug, acts centrally to reduce appetite. It has low addictive potential, modest efficacy and CVS side effects.
  - **Metformin:** Decreases appetite and thereby reduces weight. Since most DM 2 patients are obese, this is a good choice in DM 2.
  - **Tesofensine (TE)** is a norepinephrine, dopamine, and serotonin reuptake inhibitor. Primarily used as an appetite suppressant.
  - **Betahistine:** Stimulates the histamine-1 receptor and reduces the craving not only for food in general but for fatty foods in particular. Not approved by FDA.
  - **Amylin (pramlintide):** Part of the endocrine pancreas and contributes to glycemic control. Functions as a synergistic partner to insulin.
  - **Liraglutide,** a GLP-1 agonist (1.8 or 3 mg daily), is an option for overweight or obese patients.
  - **Lorcaserin,** serotonin agonist approved by FDA
  - **Combination therapy:**
    - Phentermine-topiramate
    - Bupropion-naltrexone

- *Bariatric surgical techniques:* Divided into three groups:
  1. **Malabsorptive procedures:** Induce decreased absorption of nutrients by shortening the functional length of the small intestine (e.g., biliopancreatic diversion and Roux-en-Y gastric bypass). These procedures cause deficiency of nutrients, malnutrition and in some cases, anastomotic leaks and the dumping syndrome (e.g., with the duodenal switch).
  2. **Restrictive procedures:** Reduce the storage capacity of the stomach and as a result early satiety arises, leading to a decreased caloric intake (e.g., adjustable gastric banding, vertical banded gastroplasty and sleeve gastroplasty).
  3. **Restrictive plus malabsorptive procedures** (e.g., duodenal switch, Roux-en-Y gastric bypass, intragastric balloon).
- **Liposuction:** It is the removal of large amounts of fat by suction (liposuction). It does not deal with the underlying cause and weight regain frequently occurs. There is no reduction in cardiovascular risk factors with the procedure.
- *Others:*
  - Electrical stimulation (vagal blockade) systems
  - Hydrogels**: Hydrogels are orally administered products, taken twice daily before meals, which expand in the stomach and intestines to create a sensation of satiety. They are not systemically absorbed, and are eliminated through the** feces.
  - Dietary supplements: Although over-the-counter dietary supplements are widely used by individuals attempting to lose weight—like ephedra, green tea, chromium, chitosan, and guar gum. These are not recommended and are inadequate and unsafe methods to lose weight.

Various surgical options for the treatment of obesity are shown in **Figures 1.17A to C**.

Q. Describe and enumerate the indications and side effects of bariatric surgery.

Bariatric Surgery

- **Indications:**
  - **BMI ≥40 kg/m²** without comorbid illness
  - BMI 35.0–39.9 kg/m² with at least one serious comorbidity like:
    - Type 2 diabetes
    - Obstructive sleep apnea (OSA)
    - Hypertension
    - Hyperlipidemia
    - Obesity hypoventilation syndrome (OHS)
    - Pickwickian syndrome (combination of OSA and OHS)
    - Nonalcoholic fatty liver disease
    - Nonalcoholic steatohepatitis (NASH)
    - Pseudotumor cerebri
    - Gastroesophageal reflux disease
    - Asthma
    - Venous stasis disease
    - Severe urinary incontinence
    - Debilitating arthritis
    - Impaired quality of life
    - Disqualification from other surgeries as a result of obesity (i.e., surgeries for osteoarthritic disease, ventral hernias, or stress incontinence)
  - **BMI between 30.0–34.9 kg/m²** and one of the following comorbid conditions like:
    - Uncontrollable type 2 diabetes
    - Metabolic syndrome

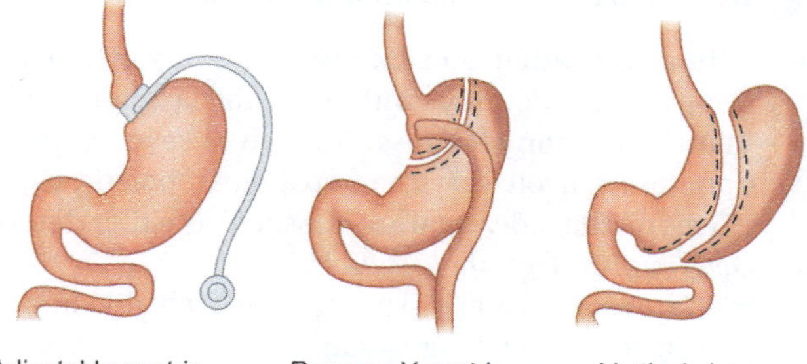

FIGS. 1.17A TO C: Various surgical options for the treatment of obesity.

- **Contraindications:**
  - Untreated major depression or psychosis
  - Uncontrolled and untreated eating disorders (e.g., bulimia)

- Drug and alcohol abuse
- Severe cardiac disease, in which anesthesia may be dangerous and contraindicated
- Severe coagulopathy
- Compliance issues with long-term nutritional replacement (e.g., vitamins)

- **Adverse effects:**
  - **During the procedure:**
    - Hemorrhage
    - Infections
    - Gastrointestinal leaks
    - Anesthesia-related complications
  - **Postoperative:**
    - Bowel obstruction
    - Dumping syndrome
    - Gallstones
    - Hernias
    - Malnutrition, hypoglycemia
    - Gastroesophageal reflux disease
    - Repeat surgery may be required.

ENVIRONMENTAL DISEASES

Radiation Exposure

Types of Radiation

- **Ionizing radiation:** Used in X-rays, computed tomography (CT), radionuclide scans and radiotherapy. Radiations interact with atoms, and release energy and results in ionization which can cause molecular damage.
  - **Penetrating radiation:** It includes uncharged neutrons or high-energy electromagnetic radiations such as X-rays and gamma (γ) rays. It affects the skin and deeper tissues.
  - **Nonpenetrating radiation:** It includes charged subatomic alpha (α) and beta (β) particles.
- **Nonionizing radiations:** Ultraviolet (UV) rays of sunlight visible light, laser, infrared and microwave. It affects only skin. Nonionizing UV is used for therapy in skin diseases and laser therapy for diabetic retinopathy.
- **Sources:** Background radiation, medical exposure, industrial exposure, and accidental or deliberate nuclear events.

Effects of Radiation Exposure

Q. Write short essay/note on effects of radiation exposure.

Radiation Sickness

Q. Write short note on radiation sickness.

- **Mild acute radiation sickness:** It is characterized by nausea, vomiting, and malaise following doses of about 1 Gy. Lymphopenia develops within several days, followed 2–3 weeks later by a reduction in all WBCs and platelets.
- **Acute radiation sickness:** It involves several systems and the extent of damage depends on the dose of radiation. Commonly involved systems are hematopoietic, GI, central nervous system, and skin.
- Effects on the individual are classified as either **deterministic or stochastic**.
- *Deterministic (threshold) effects*
  - **Nature of tissue:** Tissues with actively dividing cells (labile cells), such as bone marrow and GI mucosa, are more sensitive to ionizing radiation.
  - **Hemopoietic system:** Lymphocyte depletion is the most sensitive indicator of bone marrow injury. After exposure to a fatal dose, aplasia of the bone marrow is a most common cause of death.
  - **Gastrointestinal mucosal toxicity:** May cause death due to severe diarrhea, vomiting, dehydration, and sepsis.
  - **Gonads:** Highly radiosensitive and may cause temporary or permanent sterility.
  - **Eye:** Cataracts.
  - **Skin:** Radiation dermatitis (radiation burns) characterized by skin erythema, purpura, blistering, and secondary infection may occur. Complete loss of body hair develops after an exposure >5 Gy.
  - **Lung:** Acute inflammatory reactions and pulmonary fibrosis.
  - **Central nervous system syndrome:** Exposure of >30 Gy causes nausea, vomiting, disorientation, and coma. Death due to cerebral edema can follow within 36 hours. It may also cause **permanent neurological deficit.**
  - **Bone necrosis and lymphatic fibrosis** occur following regional irradiation, particularly for breast cancer.
  - **Thyroid gland** due to its capacity to concentrate iodine is responsible for its susceptibility to damage even after exposure to relatively low doses of radioactivity.

- *Stochastic effects:* Stochastic (chance) effect is directly proportional to the dose of radiation.
  - **Carcinogenesis:** It represents a stochastic effect. With acute exposures, leukemias (e.g., acute myeloid leukemia) may develop after a latent period of 2–5 years and solid tumors (e.g., skin, thyroid and salivary glands) after a latent period of about 10–20 years. Thereafter, the incidence of cancer increases with time. Cancer risk depends on the amount of radiation received, the time to accumulate the total dose and the interval following exposure.
  - **Teratogenic effects.**

Management of radiation exposure

- **Large-dose exposures:** Maintain adequate hydration, control of sepsis, and the management of marrow aplasia. Associated injuries such as thermal burns require treatment.
- **Internal exposure to radioisotopes:** White cell colony stimulation and hematopoietic stem cell transplantation may be required for marrow aplasia.
  - 137-cesium—chelation with Prussian blue
  - Radioactive iodine—supersaturated potassium iodide to block thyroid deposition
  - Plutonium, yttrium—chelation with diethylenetriaminepenta-acetic acid (DTPA)
  - Strontium—oral calcium or aluminum phosphate solutions can block absorption of strontium
- A cumulative risk of cancer following repeated imaging procedures has been well known and reduction of X-ray exposures should be made, whenever possible.

High Altitude

Illnesses at High Altitude

Q. Write short essay/note on mountain sickness.

- For normal individuals, ascent to altitudes up to 2,500 m or travel in a pressurized aircraft cabin is harmless.
- **Above 2,500 m** high-altitude illnesses may develop in **healthy individuals**, and **above 3,500 m** symptoms commonly develop.
- **Sudden ascent to altitudes above 6,000 m** (e.g., by aviators, balloonists and astronauts) may cause **decompression sickness.**
- The clinical features of decompression sickness are similar to in divers and even cause loss of consciousness.
- However, most high-altitude illness develops in travelers and mountaineers.

High-altitude physiology

- **Hypobaric hypoxia**—pressure gradient as well as oxygenation decreases with increase in altitude.
- **Acclimatization—**complex physiological processes occurring in the body in response to acute hypobaric hypoxia; adaptation—different from acclimatization as it occurs in individuals living chronically in high-altitude areas.
- **Ventilation**—hypoxia stimulates peripheral chemoreceptors causing increase in minute ventilation called hypoxia ventilation response (HVR).
- **Arterial blood gases**—hyperventilation leads to decreased pCO_2 and increased pH—respiratory alkalosis. This is sensed by the central chemoreceptors and ventilation is inhibited.
- **Renal compensation**—within 24–48 hours, kidney starts excreting bicarbonate; therefore, decreasing pH so as to allow ventilation that leads to alkalosis.
- **Circulatory changes**—increased cardiac, pulmonary, and cerebral blood flow.
- **Hematological changes**—rise in Hb to increase oxygen carrying capacity of blood.

Acute Mountain Sickness

- Acute mountain sickness (AMS) is a syndrome characterized by **headache, fatigue, anorexia, nausea, and vomiting, difficulty sleeping or dizziness**.
- Ataxia and peripheral edema may be present.
- **Etiology:** Not fully understood. Probably hypoxemia increases cerebral blood flow and intracranial pressure.
- **Symptoms:** Develop within 6–12 hours of an ascent and vary in severity from trivial to completely incapacitating.

Treatment of acute mountain sickness

- **Mild cases** require **rest and simple analgesics**.
- Symptoms usually resolve after 1–3 days at a stable altitude, but may recur with further ascent. Occasionally, it may then progress to cerebral edema.
- Supplemental oxygen may help.
- **If the symptoms persist**, it indicates the need to descend but may respond to **acetazolamide** (carbonic anhydrase inhibitor) that produces a metabolic acidosis and stimulates ventilation. Acetazolamide is used as a prophylaxis, if a rapid ascent is planned.
- Hyperbaric therapy

Chronic Mountain Sickness (Monge's disease)

- It occurs on long exposure to high altitude.
- **Symptoms: Headache,** poor concentration, and signs of **polycythemia.**
- **Physical examination:** Cyanosis and clubbing of fingers.

Treatment of high-altitude cerebral edema

- Improve oxygenation
- Descent is needed, and if descent is not possible, oxygen therapy in a portable pressurized bag is useful
- Dexamethasone: 8 mg immediately and 4 mg four times daily
- Supplemental oxygen
- Hyperbaric therapy

High-altitude Cerebral Edema

- High-altitude cerebral edema (HACE) is a **rare, life-threatening** condition and usually preceded by AMS.
- **Symptoms: Ataxia and altered consciousness**. In addition to features of AMS, the patient also develops confusion, disorientation, visual disturbance, lethargy and can lead to loss of consciousness.
- **Signs: Papilledema and retinal hemorrhages** are common. Focal neurological signs may be detected.

High-altitude Pulmonary Edema

Q. Write short essay/note on high-altitude pulmonary edema.

- High-altitude pulmonary edema (HAPE) is a life-threatening condition.
- **Time of occurrence:** It usually occurs in the first 4 days after ascent above 2,500 m. Unlike HACE, HAPE may develop *de novo* without the preceding signs of AMS.
- **Types:** classic HAPE—acute ascent in those residing at low altitude, re-entrant HAPE—acute ascent in those residing at high altitude after residing at low altitude.
- **Symptoms:**
  - Initially, **dry cough, exertional dyspnea** and **extreme fatigue**. Later, the cough becomes wet and may be with **blood-stained sputum**.
  - **Tachycardia** and **tachypnea** develop at rest. **Crepitations** may be heard in both lung fields. It may lead to severe hypoxemia, pulmonary hypertension.
- **Investigations:**
  - **Radiologically,** show **diffuse alveolar edema**.
  - Decreased arterial oxygen saturation.

Treatment of high-altitude pulmonary edema

- **Reversal of hypoxia** with **immediate descent** and **oxygen administration.**
- **Nifedipine** (20 mg four times daily) is given to reduce pulmonary arterial pressure. If there is delay in descent, oxygen therapy in a portable pressurized bag should be given.
- **Other treatment options:** Hyperbaric therapy, positive airway pressure, tadanafil/sildenafil, dexamethasone, salmeterol.

High-altitude retinal hemorrhage

- It may be found in about **30% of trekkers** at 5,000 m and is **usually asymptomatic** and **resolve spontaneously**.
- **Visual defects** can develop when the hemorrhage involves the macula.
- There is **no specific treatment**.

Venous thrombosis

- Can develop at **altitudes over 6,000 m**.
- **Risk factors** are dehydration, inactivity, cold and use of oral contraceptive pill at high altitude.

Refractory cough

- **Cough** is common at high altitude and usually benign.
- Causes include **breathing of dry, cold air** and **increased mouth breathing**.
- It may be similar to cough that occurs in early HAPE.

HEAT-RELATED ILLNESS

Q. Write short essay/note on causes and clinical features of hyperthermia.

Hyperthermia

- **Definition:** Hyperthermia is defined as an **elevation of the core body temperature** above the normal diurnal range of 36–37.5°C due **to failure of thermoregulation**.
- A **temperature above 40°C** (or 104°F) is generally considered as **severe hyperthermia**.

Heat-related illnesses are listed in **Box 1.10**.

Box 1.10: Heat-related illnesses.

- Heat cramps
- Heat edema
- Heat exhaustion
- Exertional heat injury
- Heatstroke

- **Pathophysiology (Flowchart 1.2):**
  - Temperature elevation is accompanied by an increase in oxygen consumption and metabolic rate, resulting in hyperpnea and tachycardia.
  - Above 42°C (108°F), oxidative phosphorylation becomes uncoupled, and a variety of enzymes cease to function.
  - A cytokine-mediated systemic inflammatory response develops, and production of heat shock proteins is increased.
  - Blood is shunted from the splanchnic circulation to the skin and muscles, resulting in GI ischemia and increased permeability of the intestinal mucosa.
  - Hepatocytes, vascular endothelium, and neural tissue are most sensitive to increased core temperatures, but all organs may ultimately be involved.
  - In severe cases, patients develop multiorgan system failure and disseminated intravascular coagulation (DIC).

FLOWCHART 1.2: Pathophysiology.

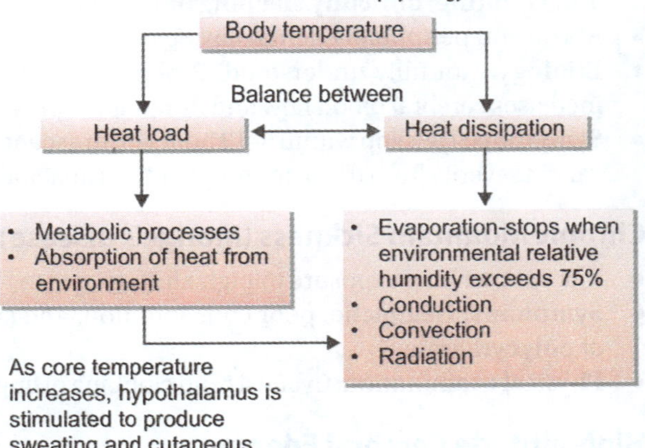

Heatstroke

Q. Write short essay/note on heatstroke.

Types of Heatstroke

- **Classic/Nonexertional**
  - "Summer Heat Waves"
  - No sweat in 84–100% of patients
  - More insidious onset
  - Usually affects elderly and debilitated patients with chronic underlying disease
  - Rhabdomyolysis and acute renal failure (ARF) rare.
- **Exertional**
  - Young, healthy, laborers, athletes, military recruits who over **exert themselves in high ambient** (temperatures or in a hot environment) to which they are **not acclimatized.**
  - Rhabdomyolysis and ARF common.
  - Usually have predisposing factor.

Predisposing Factors

- **Increased heat production:** Hyperthyroidism, exercise, sepsis.
- **Impaired heat loss** (impaired sweating)
  - **Drugs:** Anticholinergics, anti-Parkinsonian drugs, antihistamines, butyrophenones, phenothiazines, tricyclics.
  - **Abnormal sweat glands:** Examples: (1) sweat gland injury following acute heatstroke, barbiturate poisoning; (2) cystic fibrosis; and (3) healed thermal burn.
  - **Salt and water depletion:** diuretic induced.
  - Hypokalemia
- **Impaired voluntary mechanisms**: Coma, physical disability, mental illness
- **Impaired delivery of blood to peripheral circulation:** Cardiovascular disease, hypokalemia (decreased muscle blood flow), dehydration.
- **Others:** Elderly, high ambient temperature and humidity, poor ventilation, lack of acclimatization, obesity, fatigue, diabetes mellitus, malnutrition, and alcoholism.

Clinical Features

- It may develop without any warning prodrome prior to development of nonexertional heatstroke (classic heatstroke).
- As thermoregulatory mechanisms fail **body temperature rises rapidly** and patient can **deteriorate rapidly** from apparent baseline health to coma or mentally dull state.
- **Three cardinal signs are:**
  - **CNS dysfunction**
  - **Hyperpyrexia** (core temperature >40°C)
  - **Hot dry skin**. Pink or ashen depending on circulatory state. However, it may be clammy and sweat.

  Clinical features of heat exhaustion and heatstroke are depicted in **Figure 1.18.**

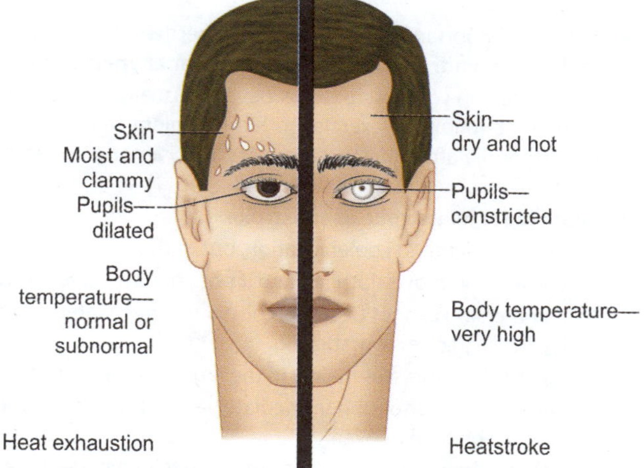

FIG. 1.18: Clinical features of heat exhaustion and heatstroke.

- **Central nervous system**
  - **Direct thermal toxicity** causes cell death, cerebral edema, and local hemorrhage. Irritability or irrational behavior may precede the development of either form of heatstroke.
  - **Confusion, aggressive behavior, delirium, convulsions,** and pupillary abnormalities may progress rapidly to coma.
  - ± decorticate posturing, fecal incontinence, flaccidity or hemiplegia (however, focal signs are unusual).
  - **Cerebellar signs**, including **ataxia and dysarthria**
  - **Hypothalamic damage** may exacerbate heatstroke by further impairing sweating and heat loss.
  - Lumbar puncture may show increased protein, xanthochromia, and slight increase in lymphocytes.
- **Cardiovascular system**
  - **Tachycardia, dysrhythmias**
  - Hypotension or normotensive with wide pulse pressure.
  - Hyperdynamic-hemodynamic profile.

- **Myocardial pump failure:** Myocardial damage and frank infarction frequent even in patients with normal coronaries due to the effect of heat on myocytes and coronary hypoperfusion secondary to hypovolemia.

- **Respiratory system**
  - **Extreme tachypnea** with respiratory rate up to 60/minute.
  - Crackles and cyanosis—signs of **pulmonary edema**
  - Direct thermal injury to pulmonary vascular endothelium may lead to cor pulmonale or **acute respiratory distress syndrome (ARDS).**
- **Metabolic**
  - Dehydration leading to raised urea and creatinine, and hemoconcentration.
  - Sweating results in **low levels of Na, Mg, K**, during early phase of the illness. Hypokalemia decreases sweat secretion and therefore exacerbates the condition.
  - **Rhabdomyolysis** resulting in hyperkalemia, hypocalcemia, and renal failure.
  - **Metabolic acidosis and respiratory alkalosis common.**
- **Splanchnic**
  - Ischemic intestinal ulceration common. May lead to hemorrhage.
  - Hepatic damage common. In 5–10%, hepatic necrosis may be severe enough to cause death.
- **Renal**
  - As a direct result of heat potentiated by dehydration and **rhabdomyolysis**.
  - **Acute renal failure** 5–6 times more common in patients with exertional heatstroke in whom it occurs in 30–35%.
- **Hematological**
  - **Anemia and bleeding:** Result from direct inactivation of platelets and clotting factors by heat, liver failure, and platelet aggregation due to heat.
  - **Disseminated intravascular coagulation:** Due to activation of clotting cascade by damaged vascular endothelium. Latter may be damaged as a direct result of heat.

Box 1.11: Investigations in heatstroke.

- Temperature recording
- Electrolytes, urea, creatinine, calcium
- Liver function tests
- Creatine phosphokinase (CPK)
- Arterial blood gas (ABG)
- ECG monitoring
- Urine output
- Full blood count (FBC), clotting, fibrinogen, FDP, D-dimer: Anemia frequent, platelets low/normal, lymphocytosis
- Test urine for myoglobin

Investigations

See **Box 1.11**.

Management

- The most important causes of severe hyperthermia [>40°C (104°F)] due to a **failure of thermoregulation** are **heatstroke, neuroleptic malignant syndrome (NMS), and malignant hyperthermia** [Other differentials refer **(Box 1.12)**].
- The context in which symptoms develop usually suggests the etiology (e.g., exertional heatstroke following exercise in high ambient temperature and humidity; malignant hyperthermia after anesthetic agents; NMS among patients treated with antipsychotic medications).
- **First aid for heatstroke or sunstroke**
  - Remove victim to cooler location, out of the sun.
  - Loosen or remove clothing, and if possible, immerse the victim in very cool water.
  - If immersion cannot be done, cool victim with water, or wrap in wet sheets and fan to facilitate quick evaporation.
  - Use cold compresses mainly in the region of the head and neck, armpits and groin.
  - Seek medical attention immediately—continue first aid to lower temperature. Until medical help takes over.
  - Not to administer any medication to lower fever because it is not useful and may be in fact cause more harm.
  - Do not use an alcohol rub.
  - Do not give anything by mouth including water until the condition has been stabilized.
- **In hospital care:** Usually treat the heatstroke in a critical care unit. Various cooling methods are listed in **Box 1.13**.
- **Supportive**
  - **IV volume replacement.**
  - If inotrope required dobutamine probably drug of choice.
  - **Urgent treatment of hyperkalemia.**

Box 1.12: Differential diagnosis of heatstroke.

- Acute CNS infection
- Cocaine, amphetamine, antihistamine overdosage
- Cerebral malaria
- Severe sepsis
- Thyroid storm
- Drug toxicity

Box 1.13: Various cooling methods that can be carried out in heatstroke.

- Evaporative
- Immersion
- Strategic ice packs
- Ice cold IV fluids
- Ice packing
- Cooling blankets
- Gastric lavage
- Peritoneal lavage
- Cardiac bypass
- Endovascular cooling
- Catheters

- **Do not treat hypocalcemia per se;** only give calcium, if ECG changes of severe hyperkalemia occur as calcium may exacerbate rhabdomyolysis.
- Small dose of mannitol may benefit patients with rhabdomyolysis, intravenous lorazepam for shivering.

- **Avoid following medications**
  - **Acetylsalicylic acid (ASA):** Uncouples oxidative phosphorylation and increases temperature.
  - **Paracetamol:** Increases hepatic dysfunction and may create toxicity.
  - **Dantrolene** is not effective, but good for malignant hyperthermia.

Hypothermia

- **Definition:** Hypothermia is defined as a core temperature below 35°C (95°F).
  - **Mild hypothermia:** Core temperature 32–35°C (90–95°F).
  - **Moderate hypothermia:** Core temperature 28–32°C (82–90°F).
  - **Severe hypothermia:** Core temperature below 28°C (82°F).
- Primary hypothermia happens because of overwhelming cold exposure. Heat production in itself is normal.
- **Secondary hypothermia:** Hypothyroidism, Addison's disease, malnutrition, burns, hypothalamic abnormalities, sepsis, thiamine deficiency, alcohol intoxication, hypoglycemia, etc.

Clinical Symptoms

See **Table 1.21**.

TABLE 1.21: Clinical symptoms of hypothermia (HT).

Stage	*Features*
Mild (HT I)	Normal mental status with shivering. Estimated core temperature 32–35°C (90–95°F) ➢ Increased metabolic rate ➢ Maximum shivering thermogenesis, "cold diuresis" ➢ Amnesia/dysarthria/ataxia ➢ Loss of coordination ➢ Tachycardic, tachypneic
Moderate (HT II)	Altered mental status without shivering. Estimated core temperature 28–32°C (82–90°F) ➢ Stupor ➢ No shivering ➢ Bradycardic/atrial fibrillation ➢ Decreased BP and RR ➢ Pupils dilated (<30°C)
Severe (HT III)	Unconscious Estimated core temperature 24–28°C (75–82°F)
Severe (HT IV)	Apparent death. Core temperature 13.7–24°C (56.7–75°F) (resuscitation may be possible) ➢ Coma ➢ No corneal or oculocephalic reflexes ➢ Decreased BP ➢ Ventricular fibrillation (maximum risk: 22°C) ➢ Apnea ➢ Asystole ➢ Areflexia/fixed pupils ➢ Flat EEG (19°C)
Death (HT V)	Due to irreversible hypothermia. Core temperature <9–13.7°C (48.2–56.7°F) (resuscitation not possible).

Investigations

- These include: Blood glucose, renal function tests, electrolytes including calcium, CPK, TSH, ABG, complete hemogram, X-ray chest, and ECG.
- **Electrocardiographic changes**
  - Hypothermia causes characteristic ECG changes because of slowed impulse conduction through potassium channels. This results in prolongation of all the ECG intervals, including RR, PR, QRS, and QT.
  - Elevation of the J point (only if the ST segment is unaltered), producing a characteristic **J or Osborn wave (Fig. 1.19)**. The height of the Osborn wave is roughly proportional to the degree of hypothermia.

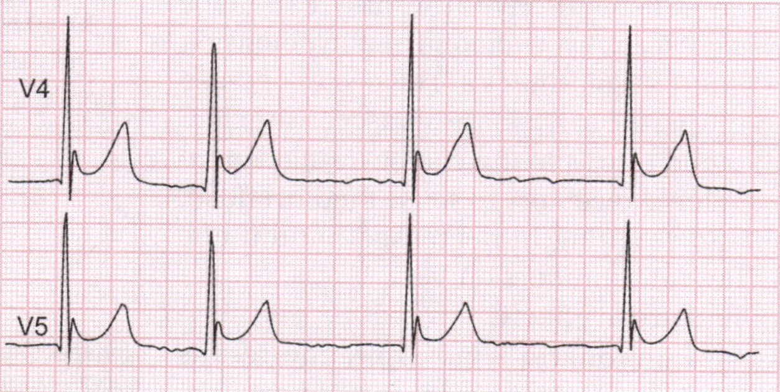

FIG. 1.19: ECG of Osborn wave.

Management

- **Evaluation and support of the airway, breathing, and circulation.**
- **Prevention of further heat loss.**
- **Initiation of rewarming** appropriate to the degree of hypothermia. Various rewarming methods are:
  - **Passive rewarming:**
    - **Endogenous heat production:** Shivering, metabolic rate, TSH, sympathetic activity.
    - Involves decreasing heat loss—remove from cold environment, remove wet clothes, provide blanket.
  - **Active external rewarming and active internal (core) rewarming (Table 1.22)**
- **Treatment of complications:** Careful attention to potential complications, including hypotension during active rewarming, arrhythmia, hyperkalemia, hypoglycemia, rhabdomyolysis, bladder atony, and bleeding diathesis.

TABLE 1.22: Methods of active external rewarming and active internal (core) rewarming.

Active external rewarming	*Active internal (core) rewarming*
➢ Heat to body surfaces ➢ Heating blankets (fluid-filled) ➢ Air blankets ➢ Radiant warmers ➢ Immersion in hot bath ➢ Water bottles/heating pads ➢ Less effective than internal rewarming, if vasoconstricted. Concern about after drop. ➢ *Rewarming rates:* 1–2.5°C/h	➢ Warm IV fluids ➢ Warm, humid oxygen ➢ Peritoneal lavage ➢ Gastric/esophageal lavage ➢ Bladder/rectal lavage ➢ Pleural/mediastinal lavage ➢ Microwaves (diathermy) ➢ Extracorporeal circulatory rewarming

DROWNING (SUBMERSION INJURIES)

Q. Write a short essay on near drowning in fresh water.

- **Drowning:** Asphyxiation caused by submersion in a liquid that causes interruption of the body's oxygen absorption.
- **Near drowning:** Term formerly used to describe victim's survival at least 24 hours after submersion.
- Salt versus fresh water is no longer emphasized as degree of pulmonary insult is determined by quantity aspirated.
- **Wet drowning:** Aspiration of water into airways and lungs (85%). 1-3 cc of aspirated water will lead to destruction of surfactant, alveolar instability, noncardiogenic pulmonary edema, and impaired gas exchange.
- **Dry drowning:** Severe parasympathetically mediated laryngospasm (15%).
- Aspiration of >11 mL/kg of body weight must occur before blood volume changes occur, and >22 mL/kg before electrolyte changes take place.
- It is unusual for nonfatal drowning victims to aspirate >3–4 mL/kg.
- Both types result in common pathway of hypoxia which leads to acidosis, cardiac arrest, and brain death.

Pathophysiology of Drowning

Risk Factors for Drowning (Box 1.14)

Three peaks in incidence:
1. Toddlers
2. Adolescents
3. Elderly

Various stages of drowning are shown in **Flowchart 1.3**.

Box 1.14: Risk factors for drowning.

- Drug and alcohol intoxication
- Cardiac arrest
- Hypoglycemia
- Seizure
- Suicidal or homicidal behavior
- Child abuse
- Inadequate adult supervision
- Inability to swim or overestimation of swimming capabilities
- Risk-taking behavior
- Hypothermia, which can lead to rapid exhaustion or cardiac arrhythmias
- Undetected primary cardiac arrhythmia: Cold water immersion and exercise can cause fatal arrhythmias in patients with the congenital long QT syndrome type 1. Similarly, mutations in the cardiac ryanodine receptor (RyR)-2 gene, which is associated with familial polymorphic VT in the absence of structural heart disease or QT prolongation, have been identified in some individuals with unexplained drowning
- Hyperventilation prior to a shallow dive: Swimmers commonly hyperventilate in order to prolong the duration of underwater swimming, and by so doing they reduce the arterial partial pressure of carbon dioxide ($PaCO_2$) while the content of oxygen (CaO_2) does not increase appreciably. As the individual swims, oxygen is consumed and the partial pressure of oxygen (PaO_2) falls to 30–40 mm Hg before the $PaCO_2$ rises sufficiently to trigger the urge to breathe. This can lead to cerebral hypoxia, seizures, and loss of consciousness, which can result in drowning.

Signs and Symptoms

- About 70% of patients develops signs within 7 hours.
- Alertness, agitation, coma.
- Cyanosis, coughing, and pink frothy sputum (pulmonary edema).
- Tachypnea, tachycardia.
- Low-grade fever.
- Rales, rhonchi, and less often wheezes.
- Signs of associated trauma to the head and neck should be sought.
- Persons with hypothermia can have significant hypovolemia and hypotension due to a "cold diuresis". This occurs because during the early phase of vasoconstriction, blood moves to the core, causing central volume receptors to sense fluid overload, and resulting in decreased antidiuretic hormone production.
- **End organ effects:**
  - **Pulmonary:** Fluid aspiration results in varying degrees of hypoxemia, noncardiogenic pulmonary edema—ARDS.
  - **Neurologic:** Hypoxemia and ischemia cause neuronal damage, which can produce cerebral edema and elevations in intracranial pressure which can progress into hypoxic ischemic encephalopathy.
  - **Cardiovascular:** Arrhythmias secondary to hypothermia and hypoxemia like sinus tachycardia, sinus bradycardia, and atrial fibrillation.
  - **Acid-base and electrolytes:** A metabolic and/or respiratory acidosis is often observed. Rarely drowning in concentrated seawater can produce life-threatening hypernatremia, hypermagnesemia, and hypercalcemia due to absorption of swallowed seawater.

FLOWCHART 1.3: Various stages of drowning.

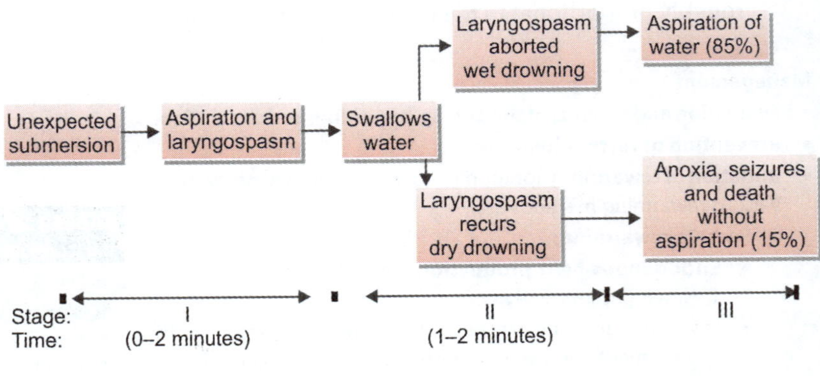

- **Renal:** Renal failure due to acute tubular necrosis resulting from hypoxemia, shock, hemoglobinuria, or myoglobinuria is rare.

Poor prognostic signs of drowning are listed in **Box 1.15**.

Box 1.15: Poor prognostic signs of drowning.

- Duration of submersion >5 minutes (most critical factor)
- Time to effective basic life support >10 minutes
- Resuscitation duration >25 minutes
- Glasgow coma scale <5 (i.e., comatose)
- Persistent apnea and requirement of cardiopulmonary resuscitation in the emergency department
- Arterial blood pH <7.1 upon presentation

Management

- It includes prehospital care, emergency department (ED) care, and inpatient care.
- **Ventilation is the most important** initial treatment of submersion injury.
- The Heimlich maneuver or other postural drainage techniques to remove water from the lungs are of no proven value, and rescue breathing should not be delayed in order to perform these maneuver.
- Standard CPR protocol needs to be followed.
- Identify spine injuries and other major organ injuries and manage accordingly.
- *Supportive care:* Renal failure, shock, infections, etc.

CHAPTER

2

Endocrinology

DISORDERS OF PITUITARY AND HYPOTHALAMUS

Pituitary Hormones and Their Principal Actions (Table 2.1)

Q. Write short essay/note on:
- **Pituitary hormones and their principal actions.**
- **List the hormones of anterior pituitary.**

TABLE 2.1: Pituitary hormones and principal actions.

<table>
<tr><th>Hormone</th><th colspan="2">Actions</th></tr>
<tr><td colspan="3">Anterior Pituitary Hormones</td></tr>
<tr><td>Thyroid-stimulating hormone (TSH)</td><td colspan="2">Synthesis and secretion of thyroxine (T_4) and tri-iodothyronine (T_3)</td></tr>
<tr><td>Growth hormone (GH)</td><td colspan="2">Growth induction</td></tr>
<tr><td rowspan="2">Follicle-stimulating hormone (FSH)
Luteinizing hormone (LH)</td><td colspan="2">Sex-steroid production, follicle growth, germ-cell maturation</td></tr>
<tr><td>Males:
➢ FSH and LH: Spermatogenesis
➢ FSH: Stimulates Sertoli cells to secrete androgen binding protein (ABP), transferrin, plasminogen activator, and inhibin
➢ LH: Stimulates Leydig cells to produce testosterone</td><td>Females:
➢ FSH and LH are necessary for the development of corpus luteum during the luteal phase of menstrual cycle
➢ FSH promotes growth and development of ovarian follicles during the follicular phase of menstrual cycle
➢ LH (LH surge) induces ovulation</td></tr>
<tr><td>Prolactin (PRL)</td><td colspan="2">Controls milk production by breasts</td></tr>
<tr><td>Adrenocorticotrophic hormone (ACTH)</td><td colspan="2">Controls cortisol release from adrenal cortex and skin pigmentation</td></tr>
<tr><td colspan="3">Posterior Pituitary Hormones</td></tr>
<tr><td>Arginine vasopressin (AVP)</td><td colspan="2">Promotes reabsorption of water by renal tubules</td></tr>
<tr><td>Oxytocin</td><td colspan="2">Promotes uterine contraction and expression of milk from the breasts</td></tr>
</table>

Hypopituitarism

Q. Write short essay/note on hyposecretion of anterior pituitary hormones/hypopituitarism/panhypopituitarism.

Definition

- Hypopituitarism is defined as **combined deficiency (partial or complete) of any of the anterior pituitary hormones**.
- Panhypopituitarism is defined as **deficiency of all anterior pituitary hormones**. It may be due to selective or multiple deficiencies of pituitary hormones or diseases of the hypothalamus.

Etiology

See **Box 2.1**.

Box 2.1: Various causes of hypopituitarism.

"Nine I's": **Invasive, Infarction, Infiltrative, Injury, Immunologic, Iatrogenic, Infectious, Idiopathic, and Isolated.**

- **Isolated** hormone **deficiencies**
- **Invasive tumors:** Pituitary adenomas, cysts, metastasis, and hypothalamic tumors
- **Injury:** Surgery, irradiation, and stalk section
- **Infarction:** Sheehan's syndrome (postpartum pituitary necrosis), diabetic antepartum necrosis, and carotid aneurysm
  - **Cerebrovascular accident (CVA):** Ischemic stroke, subarachnoid hemorrhage, and pituitary apoplexy
- **Inflammatory diseases:** Granulomatous disease and autoimmune (lymphocytic) hypophysitis
- **Infiltrative diseases:** Hemochromatosis, amyloidosis, sarcoidosis, Langerhans' cell histiocytosis
- **Injury:** Head trauma
- **Immunologic:** Lymphocytic hypophysitis
- **Infections:** Meningitis, tuberculosis, syphilis, fungal infection such as *Candida* and Hantavirus. More likely immunocompromised patients such as HIV and high-dose steroids
- **Idiopathic**
- **Developmental defects** (Kallmann syndrome) and **genetic diseases** such with mutations detected in:
  - ROBOS guidance receptors (ROBOS) determine axonal guidance in the central nervous system.
  - BMP4 induces Rathke's pouch formation, which is necessary for anterior pituitary development.
  - *HESX1, LHX3,* and *LHX4* transcription factors that are important for pituitary organogenesis and early differentiation of pituicytes.
  - PROP-1, which is necessary for the differentiation of a cell type that is a precursor to somatotroph, lactotroph, thyrotroph, and gonadotroph cells.
  - PIT-1 (called POU1F1 in the human), which acts temporally just after PROP-1 and is necessary for the differentiation of a cell type that is a precursor of somatotroph, lactotroph, and, to a lesser degree, thyrotroph cells.
  - TPIT, which is required for specific differentiation of the corticotroph cells.

Clinical Features (Table 2.2)

- The presentation is highly variable and depends on the underlying cause/lesion.
- Symptoms and signs depend on the degree of hypothalamic and/or pituitary deficiencies. Mild deficiencies may be asymptomatic.
- **Hypopituitarism secondary to pituitary tumors:** Symptoms are due to mass effects (e.g., headache, visual impairment, electrolyte alterations, and disorders of the autonomic nervous system produced by hypothalamic involvement). As the lesions progress, there is a sequential loss of hormone secretion.
- Prolactin (PRL) deficiency is rare, except for complete destruction of pituitary or genetic syndromes.
- The order of diminished trophic hormone reserve function by pituitary compression usually follows the order
  GH > FSH > LH > TSH > ACTH.
- Longstanding panhypopituitarism produces a classic picture of **pallor with hairlessness ("alabaster skin").**

TABLE 2.2: Clinical features due to deficiencies of various pituitary hormones.

Deficiency	*Features*
GH *(earliest to be lost)*	➢ Decreased growth in children but may be clinically occult in adult patients ➢ Associated with a decreased sense of well-being, lethargy, muscle weakness, and increased fat mass with a decrease in lean body mass
LH and FSH	➢ Hypogonadism may precede the clinical appearance of a hypothalamic-pituitary lesion ➢ Leads to loss of libido and impotence in males, and oligomenorrhea or amenorrhea in females ➢ In both sexes, infertility and osteoporosis occur, axillary and pubic hair becomes sparse, and the skin becomes fine and wrinkled ➢ In males, there may be gynecomastia and decreased frequency of shaving
ACTH	➢ Weakness, nausea, vomiting, anorexia, decreased libido, weight loss, fever, tachycardia, and postural hypotension may occur. Severe forms of deficiency cause death due to vascular collapse. Plasma electrolytes are normal (relative preservation of mineralocorticoid production) ➢ Depigmentation and diminished tanning may develop due to ACTH insufficiency
TSH	Secondary hypothyroidism is usually less severe than primary hypothyroidism, and goiter is absent. Cold intolerance, dry skin, mental dullness, bradycardia, delayed relaxation phase of the deep tendon reflexes, constipation, weight gain, hoarseness, and anemia are seen
PRL	Failure of lactation (postpartum)

(ACTH: adrenocorticotropic hormone; FSH: follicle-stimulating hormone; GH: growth hormone; LH: luteinizing hormone; PRL: prolactin; TSH: thyroid-stimulating hormone)

Laboratory Investigations

- **Demonstration of low levels of trophic pituitary hormones:** Biochemical diagnosis of pituitary insufficiency is made by demonstration of low levels of trophic pituitary hormones along with low levels of target hormones.
  - **Low free thyroxine (T_4)** with **low or inappropriately normal TSH** level suggests **secondary hypothyroidism**.
  - **Low early morning (8-9 AM) cortisol,** about ≤3 μg/dL, with **low or inappropriately normal ACTH.**
  - **Low testosterone level without elevation of gonadotrophins** (LH and FSH) suggests **hypogonadotropic hypogonadism.**
  - **Low IGF-1 (insulin-like growth factor-1)** level indicates **GH deficiency.**

- **Provocation tests:** These may be necessary to **assess pituitary reserve**.
  - **GH reserve:** GH response to insulin-induced hypoglycemia, L-dopa, arginine, growth hormone-releasing hormone (GHRH), or growth hormone-releasing peptides (GHRPs). Insulin-induced hypoglycemia (also known as **insulin tolerance test**) is the **gold standard test**.
  - **Thyrotropin-releasing hormone (TRH) reserve: TRH** stimulates **prolactin secretion**. In the presence of optimal levels of TRH, exogenous administration of TRH will not raise levels of prolactin. In the absence of a TRH reserve, exogenous administration of TRH will elevate serum prolactin levels.
  - **ACTH reserve:** It is assessed by measuring ACTH and cortisol levels during insulin-induced hypoglycemia. Corticotropin-releasing hormone (CRH) administration induces ACTH release, and administration of synthetic ACTH (cosyntropin) causes adrenal cortisol release. It is an **indirect indicator** of **pituitary ACTH reserve**.
  - **Metyrapone test:** Metyrapone **blocks 11-beta-hydroxylase**, the enzyme that catalyzes the conversion of 11-deoxycortisol to cortisol, resulting in a reduction in cortisol secretion. If the hypothalamo-pituitary-adrenal axis is normal, the ensuing fall in serum cortisol should cause an increase in ACTH secretion and therefore an increase in adrenal steroidogenesis and 11-deoxycortisol.
    - In normal subjects, administration of 750 mg of metyrapone orally every 4 hours for 24 hours results in a decline in 8 AM serum cortisol to <7 μg/dL and an elevation in 8 AM serum 11-deoxycortisol to ≥10 μg/dL at the end of the 24 hours. In patients who have decreased ACTH reserve due to hypothalamic or pituitary disease, the serum 11-deoxycortisol concentration will be <10 μg/dL and the serum cortisol < 7 μg/dL at the end of 24 hours.
  - **TSH reserve:** TSH response to TRH.
- **Surgical biopsy of tumor:** Usually done as part of a therapeutic operation of tumors. Histological examination of pituitary tumors will help in **identifying the type of tumor**. Immunohistochemistry useful in confirming their secretory capacity.
  - **Chromophobe** (usually nonfunctioning)
  - **Acidophil** (typically prolactin- or growth-hormone secreting)
  - **Basophil** (typically ACTH-secreting).

Management: It is by replacement of deficient hormones (**Box 2.2**).

Box 2.2: Replacement therapy for adult hypopituitarism.

Adrenocorticotropic hormone

Hydrocortisone 15–25 mg daily in divided doses. Mineralocorticoid replacement not needed.

Follicle-stimulating hormone/Luteinizing hormone

Female Patients (any one)

- Conjugated estrogen 0.65 mg/day
- Micronized estradiol 1 mg/day
- Ethinyl estradiol 0.02–0.05 mg/day
- Estradiol skin patch 4–8 mg twice weekly
- Estradiol plus testosterone

Male Patients (any one)

- Testosterone enanthate 200 mg IM every 2–3 weeks
- Testosterone skin patch 2.5–5.0 mg/day; can increase dose up to 7.5 mg/day
- Testosterone gel 3–6 g daily

Growth hormone

- *Adults*: Recombinant human GH (rhGH) starting dose 2–5 μg/kg subcutaneously daily. This weight-based recommendation is for the starting dose only. The goal should be to start with low doses and increase gradually until the serum IGF-1 concentration is normal.
- *Children*: Recombinant human GH (rhGH) is 0.16–0.24 mg/kg/week, divided into once daily injections. Further adjustments of GH dose based on growth response, serum insulin-like growth factor-1 (IGF-1) levels, and body weight

Thyroid-stimulating hormone

L (levo)-thyroxine dose of 1.6 μg/kg daily and adjusting dose according to serum free T_4 levels in upper half of reference range.

Vasopressin

- Intranasal desmopressin-rhinal tube 5–20 μg twice daily
- Oral DDAVP (desmopressin) 300–600 μg daily, usually in divided doses

Prolactin

Recombinant human prolactin (r-hPRL), although not commercially available, has been used experimentally.

Sheehan's Syndrome

Q. Write a short note on Sheehan's syndrome.

Sheehan's syndrome is a potentially life-threatening complication due to **infarction of pituitary gland following postpartum hemorrhage**.

Mechanism

During pregnancy, the pituitary gland is enlarged and is more vulnerable to ischemia. Postpartum hemorrhage and consequent systemic hypotension can cause pituitary infarction.

Clinical Features

- Earliest symptom is **failure to lactate**.
- **Failure to regain menstruation after delivery**
- **Other symptoms of hypopituitarism:** They appear over months or years. Few patients may present acutely (hypotension, hyponatremia, and hypothyroidism).
- Coma and death can occur in severe cases.

Diagnosis

- Refer laboratory findings of hypopituitarism.
- **MRI:** In early stages, it may show hypertrophied pituitary. Later stages, atrophic pituitary and empty sella.

Treatment of Sheehan's syndrome

Control of hemorrhage and volume replacement. Administration of deficient hormones.

Empty Sella Syndrome

Q. Write a short note on empty sella syndrome.

- Often an **incidental MRI** finding **(Fig. 2.1)**.
- In this condition, **herniation of arachnoid diverticulum** through an incomplete diaphragm sellae results in symmetrically ballooned sella, which gets filled up with cerebrospinal fluid (CSF).
- Usually have **normal pituitary function**, implying that the surrounding rim of pituitary tissue is fully functional.
- An empty sella can be a primary congenital weakness of the diaphragm or secondary subsequent to infarction of a pituitary adenoma or to surgical or radiation-induced damage to the sellar diaphragm.
- **Hypopituitarism** may develop insidiously.
- Common in obese, multiparous women with chronic headache.
- Rarely, functional pituitary adenomas may arise within the rim of pituitary tissue, and these are not always visible on MRI.

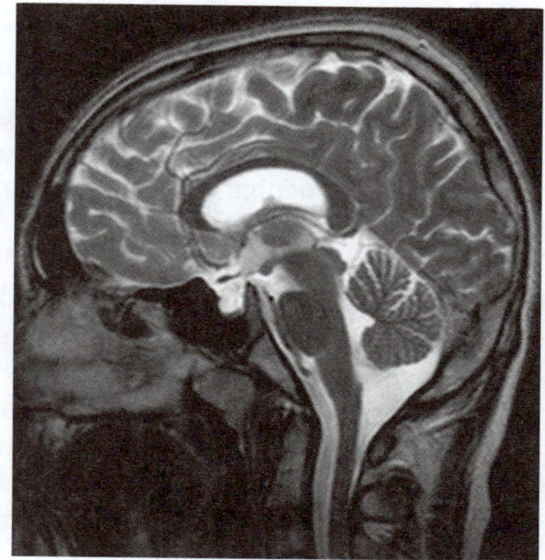

FIG. 2.1: MRI image of empty sella.

Kallmann Syndrome

Q. Write a short note on Kallmann syndrome.

- It is due to **defective hypothalamic gonadotropin-releasing hormone synthesis**.
- Olfactory bulb agenesis or hypoplasia is associated with **anosmia or hyposmia**.
- Conditions associated with this are color blindness, optic atrophy, cleft palate, renal abnormalities, cryptorchidism, and neurologic abnormalities like synkinesis or mirror movements.
- The deficiency **prevents progression through puberty** due to **low LH and FSH levels and sex steroids.**
- **Males**: Delayed puberty and hypogonadism, including micropenis. Replacement by human chorionic gonadotropin (hCG) or testosterone for a long-term is needed.
- **Female:** It manifests as **primary amenorrhea** and failure of secondary sexual development. Long-term treatment with estrogen and progestin is warranted.

TABLE 2.3: Indications and side effects of growth hormone therapy.

Indications	*Side effects*
GH (growth hormone) deficiency	Edema
Intrauterine growth retardation (IUGR)	Arthralgia
Non-GH deficient short stature FSS (familial short stature), CGD (constitutional growth delay)	Myalgia, muscle stiffness
Chronic renal failure	Paresthesia
Burns	Carpal tunnel syndrome
Steroid therapy	Hypertension
Osteoporosis	Melanocytic nevi
HIV-associated cachexia	Hypothyroidism
Sports abuse	

Growth Hormone Therapy (Table 2.3)

Q. Lists the indications and side effects of growth hormone therapy.

- **Route of administration of GH:** Subcutaneously after 8.00 PM, 3-7 times a week (0.15-0.3 mg/kg/week).
- Effect is dose-dependent and the response is better if started earlier. Average increment in height = 10 cm/year.
- Better response in classic growth hormone deficiency (GHD).

Pituitary Apoplexy

Q. Write a short note on pituitary apoplexy.

Pituitary apoplexy is a rare life-threatening endocrine **emergency** characterized by a sudden onset of headache, visual symptoms, altered mental status, and hormonal dysfunction due to **acute hemorrhage** or **infarction** of a pituitary gland.

Clinical Features

- Sudden severe headache, double vision, and sudden severe visual loss.
- Cardiovascular collapse, change in consciousness, neck stiffness, and sometimes hypoglycemia. Sometimes acute life-threatening hypopituitarism.
- GnRH deficiency is most common. Acute adrenal insufficiency is common due to loss of ACTH. TSH deficiency occurs in half of the patients.
- The condition can evolve over 1-2 days.
- **CT/MRI findings:** Pituitary imaging without contrast (CT or MRI) usually reveals signs of intrapituitary or intra-adenoma hemorrhage, "**pituitary ring sign**" on T1-weighted MRI, stalk deviation and compression of normal pituitary tissue and, in severe cases, signs of parasellar subarachnoid hemorrhage (**Fig. 2.2**).

Management of Pituitary Apoplexy

- **Initial management: Conservative** with careful monitoring of fluid and electrolyte balance along with immediate replacement of deficient hormones, in particular corticosteroids. Close monitoring of vision. High-dose corticosteroids and supportive treatment needed.
- **Surgical decompression:** If there is a rapid deterioration in visual acuity and fields, surgical decompression of the optic chiasm may be required.

Pituitary Tumors

Q. Write short essay/note on clinical manifestation, investigations, and management of pituitary tumors.

Pituitary tumors are the most common cause of pituitary disease, and most of them are benign pituitary adenomas.

Classification

- Pituitary tumors are classified depending on the tumor size into **microadenomas** (<1 cm in diameter) and **macroadenomas** (exceed 1 cm in diameter).
- Pituitary adenomas may be **functional** (i.e., associated with hormone excess and clinical manifestations thereof) or **nonfunctional** (i.e., without clinical symptoms of hormone excess). Nonfunctional tumors detected incidentally during MRI/CT examination or at autopsy are called as pituitary **incidentalomas**.

Various tumors of pituitary are listed in **Table 2.4**.

Other tumors of pituitary are listed in **Box 2.3**.

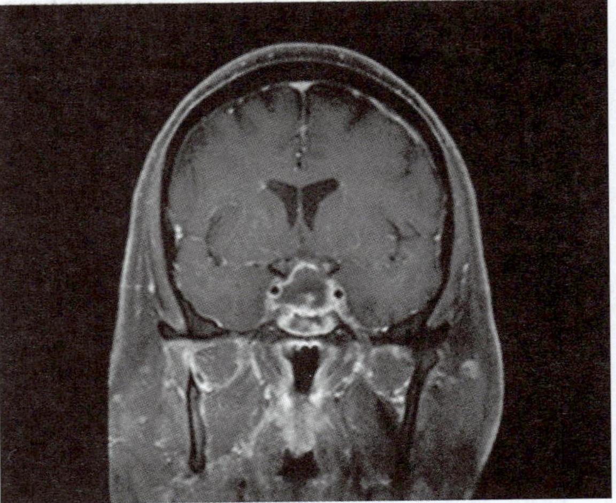

FIG. 2.2: CT/MRI findings: Pituitary imaging.

TABLE 2.4: Pituitary tumors, hormone produced and their associated disorder.

Pituitary adenomas	*Hormone produced*	*Associated disorder*
Lactotroph adenoma (Prolactinoma)	Prolactin	Hypogonadism, galactorrhea, and amenorrhea (in females)
Somatotroph adenoma	Growth hormone	Acromegaly (adults) and gigantism (children)
Corticotroph adenoma	Adrenocorticotropic hormone (ACTH) and other POMC-derived peptides	Cushing's disease
Gonadotroph adenoma	Follicle-stimulating hormone (FSH) and luteinizing hormone (LH)	Mass effects, hypopituitarism
Thyrotroph adenoma	Thyroid-stimulating hormone (TSH)	Hyperthyroidism
Mammosomatotroph adenoma	Prolactin, GH	Combined features of GH and prolactin excess
Nonfunctioning/null cell adenoma	None	Mass effects, hypopituitarism

Box 2.3: Other tumors of pituitary.

- Craniopharyngioma
- Metastatic tumors
- As a component of multiple endocrine neoplasia type I (MEN-I), which includes parathyroid, pancreatic, and pituitary (usually prolactinoma) tumors

Clinical Features

The signs and symptoms may be due to mass effects and endocrine abnormalities.

- **Mass effects:** Mass effects of the enlarging tumor can produce specific signs and symptoms of hypofunction by pressure effect on surrounding normal pituitary tissue (see hypopituitarism). The mass effect on the neighboring structures causes:
  - **Due to stretching of the diaphragm sellae or by invasion of bone:** It causes **headache** and is common (especially in patients with macroadenomas) but non-specific.
  - **Due to pressure effects on optic chiasma, nerve or tract: Visual field abnormalities** which include loss of acuity and optic atrophy (superior temporal quadrantanopia or temporal hemianopia).
  - **Due to lateral extension into cavernous sinus** with subsequent compression of cranial nerve which produces **palsies** of cranial **nerves III, IV, and VI.** This results in diplopia and strabismus and facial numbness.
  - **Due to mass effects on hypothalamus:** Obesity, disturbances of sleep, thirst, appetite, temperature regulation, and diabetes insipidus (DI).
  - **Others:** Anosmia (frontal lobe involvement), vomiting, papilledema (raised intracranial tension).
  - **Occasionally**, pituitary tumors infarct or bleeding into produces "**pituitary apoplexy**".
- **Clinical features due to secretion of hormones** (**Table 2.4**).

Investigations

- **Plain radiograph of the pituitary fossa (skull):** It may show one or more of the following:
  - Enlargement of sella turcica
  - Calcification of suprasellar region
  - Erosion of clinoid process
  - Double floor of the sella.
- **CT scan with contrast enhancement:** More sensitive to detect bony erosions and presence of calcification.
- **Magnetic resonance imaging (MRI) of the pituitary:** MRI with gadolinium **(imaging method of choice)** is superior to CT scanning and shows pituitary mass. In situations in which the use of gadolinium is contraindicated, such as renal impairment or pregnancy, MRI without gadolinium may still be helpful. Small lesions within the pituitary fossa

(small pituitary microadenomas) are very common. Such small lesions are sometimes detected during MRI scanning of the head for other reasons and are called **"pituitary incidentalomas"**.

- **Visual field plotting** by automated computer perimetry or Goldmann perimetry.
- **Functional assessment of the pituitary gland:** By hormonal assays and include prolactin (lactotroph adenomas), IGF-1 (somatotroph adenomas), 24-hour urinary-free cortisol (corticotroph adenomas), plasma corticotropin (ACTH), FSH, LH, free T_4, and thyroid function tests.

Treatment of pituitary tumors

Surgery

- Surgery (except for prolactinomas) is the **primary mode of treatment** for pituitary tumors that warrant intervention.
- Surgery via the **trans-sphenoidal** adenomectomy or hypophysectomy is the treatment of choice.
- Very large tumors are removed via the open **transcranial** (usually transfrontal) route. It is usually performed by an endoscopic or endonasal approach.

Medical therapy

Somatostatin analogs and/or dopamine agonists: Octreotide is administered postresection. Drug therapy with dopamine agonists such as bromocriptine and cabergoline are effectively used in the management of prolactinomas. They induce a rapid fall in PRL levels and can decrease the size of tumor and possibly avoid surgery.

Radiation therapy

It is usually **used as adjunctive therapy after surgery** or when surgery is impracticable or incomplete or in **combination with medical therapy**. Includes **external radiotherapy, or implantation of Yttrium** in the pituitary fossa, or gamma knife or a modified linear accelerator.

- It suppresses the tumor growth and reduces its secretory capacity.
- **Gamma knife** (stereotactic radiosurgery) involves precise delivery of large single high-energy dose directly to the tumor under stereotactic surgery and is particularly useful for residual tumor in the cavernous sinus.

Acromegaly

Q. Write short essay/note on acromegaly and its major clinical signs.

- **Growth hormone (GH)** is required for proper growth and development. It directly affects metabolism of fat and indirectly effects bone growth.
- Acromegaly results from **persistent hypersecretion** of growth hormone (GH). Excess GH stimulates hepatic secretion of **insulin-like growth factor-1 (IGF-1)**, which causes most of the clinical manifestations of acromegaly.
- Excess secretion of GH prior to closure of epiphyseal growth plates in long bone before onset of puberty causes **pituitary gigantism**. Excess secretion **after puberty** causes **acromegaly**.
- Males and females are equally affected.

Etiology of Acromegaly

Excess of growth hormone (GH excess) after puberty may be due to**:**

- **Pituitary tumor (somatotrope pituitary adenoma)** is the **most common cause**. Acromegaly is caused by growth hormone (GH) secretion usually from a macroadenoma of pituitary gland. Few adenomas secrete both GH as well as prolactin.
- **Other tumors:** In a few patients, acromegaly is caused by tumors of the **pancreas, lungs, and adrenal glands** (either because they produce GH themselves or, more frequently they produce GHRH, the hormone that stimulates the pituitary to make GH).

Clinical Features (Figs. 2.2A to C and Table 2.5)

Clinical features are due to increased GH (growth hormone) and IGF-1 (insulin-like growth factor-1).

Investigations

- **Biochemical investigations**
  - **Insulin-like growth factor-1 (IGF-1) levels:** It is the **single best test** useful in diagnosis. IGF-1 is almost always elevated in acromegaly **(Flowchart 2.1)**.
  - **GH levels:** Confirmed by assessment of GH secretion. Basal fasting GH levels are >10 ng/mL (465 pmol/L) (normal, 1–5 ng/mL, 46–232 pmol/L) in >90% of patients and range from 5 ng/mL (232 pmol/L) to >500 ng/mL (23,000 pmol/L), with a mean of approximately 50 ng/mL (2,300 pmol/L).
  - **Oral glucose tolerance test:** The **most specific dynamic test** for establishing the diagnosis of acromegaly. GH levels are measured before and 2 hours after an OGTT. In normal subjects, serum GH concentrations fall to 1 ng/mL or less within 2 hours of ingestion of 75 g glucose. **The criterion for the diagnosis of acromegaly is a GH concentration of >1 ng/mL.** Some patients may show a paradoxical rise and about 25% of patients with acromegaly have a positive diabetic glucose tolerance test.
  - **Serum insulin-like growth factor binding protein-3 (IGFBP-3)** concentrations are elevated in patients with acromegaly.

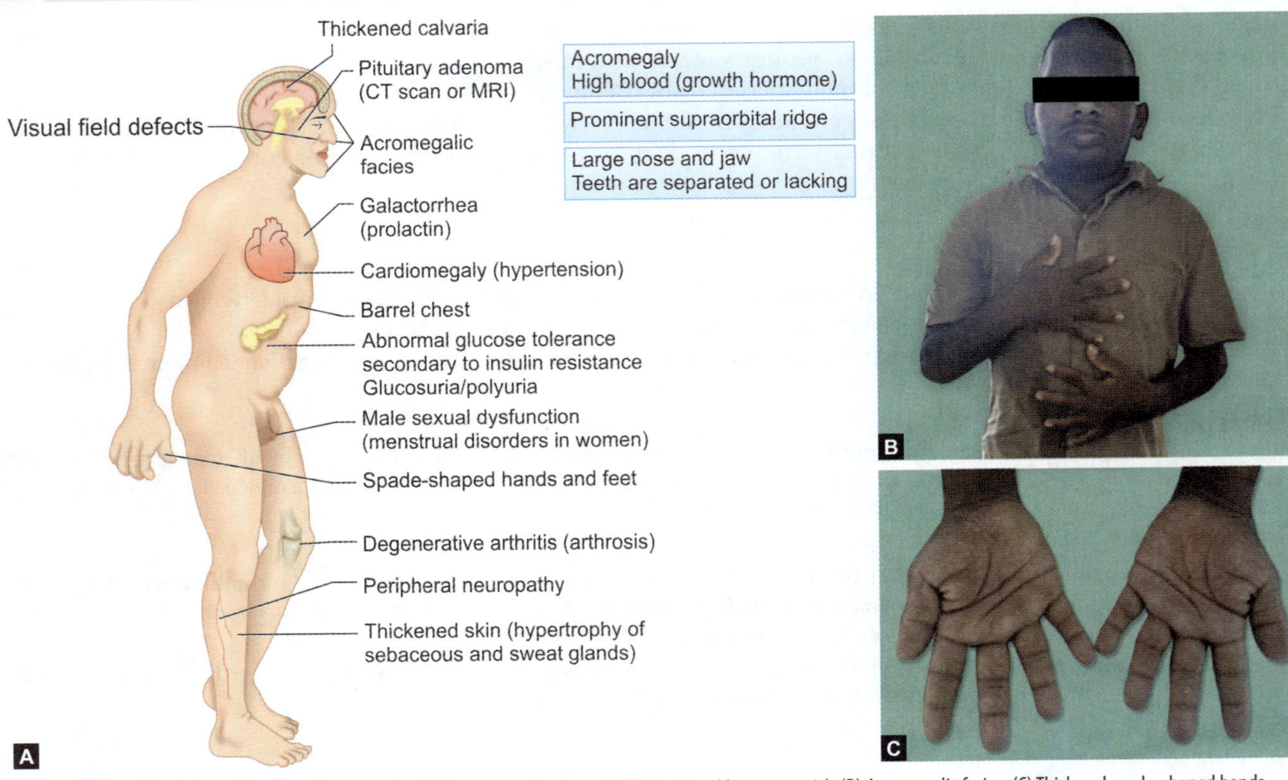

FIGS. 2.2A TO C: Clinical features of acromegaly. (A) Summary of various clinical features (diagrammatic); (B) Acromegalic facies; (C) Thick and spade-shaped hands.

TABLE 2.5: Various systems involved in acromegaly and presenting features.

System/tissue involved	*Features*
Local tumor effects	Pituitary enlargement, visual-field defects, cranial nerve palsy, headache
Somatic systems	Acral enlargement including thickness of soft tissue of hands and feet
Musculoskeletal system and neurological	Gigantism, prognathism, jaw malocclusion, widely spaced teeth, arthralgias and arthritis, carpal tunnel syndrome, acroparesthesia, proximal myopathy, hypertrophy of frontal bones, osteoporosis
Skin and integumental	Skin tags, acanthosis nigricans, increased sweat and sebum resulting in moist and oily skin, enlargement of lips, nose, and tongue, and increased heel pad thickness
Gastrointestinal system	Macroglossia, colonic polyps, visceromegaly, and pancreatic cancer
Cardiovascular system	Left ventricular hypertrophy, asymmetric septal hypertrophy, cardiomyopathy, hypertension, congestive heart failure, and coronary artery disease
Pulmonary system	Sleep disturbances, sleep apnea (central and obstructive), and narcolepsy
Visceromegaly	Tongue, thyroid gland, salivary glands, liver, spleen, kidney, and prostate
Reproduction	Menstrual abnormalities, galactorrhea, decreased libido, impotence, low levels of sex hormone-binding globulin, and gynecomastia
Multiple endocrine neoplasia type 1	Hyperparathyroidism, pancreatic islet cell tumors
Carbohydrate metabolism	Impaired glucose tolerance, insulin resistance and hyperinsulinemia, and diabetes mellitus
Lipid	Hypertriglyceridemia
Mineral	Hypercalciuria, increased levels of 25-hydroxyvitamin D_3, urinary hydroxyproline levels increased
Electrolyte	Low renin levels, increased aldosterone levels
Thyroid	Low thyroxine binding globulin levels, goiter

- **Thyrotropin-releasing hormone (TRH),** in a dose of 500 µg intravenously, raises serum GH concentrations by 50% or more in approximately one-half of patients with acromegaly, with peak values occurring at 20-30 minutes of administration.
- **L-DOPA** (500 mg orally) reduces serum GH concentrations by 50% or more in approximately one-half of patients with acromegaly, while it raises the GH concentration in normal subjects.
- **Postprandial plasma glucose** may be **elevated** and serum insulin is increased in 70% of patients.

- **Prolactin:** Shows mild-to-moderate elevation in about 30% of patients due to **cosecretion of prolactin** from the tumor.
- **Others:** Elevated serum phosphorus.

- **Radiological investigations**
  - **MRI of pituitary**: If the biochemical tests are abnormal and GH hypersecretion is confirmed, MRI will almost always reveal and localize the pituitary adenoma usually a somatotroph adenoma (most common cause of acromegaly). If the MRI is normal, abdominal, chest imaging or DOTATATE positron emission tomography (PET) scan should be performed to look for an ectopic source of hormone secretion.
  - **X-ray (Figs. 2.3A to C):**
    - **Plain films of skull:** Shows **sellar enlargement** in 90% of cases. Other findings may be **thickening of the calvarium, enlargement of the frontal and maxillary sinuses**, and **enlargement of the jaw**.
    - **Radiographs of the hand:** Shows increased **soft tissue bulk, "arrowhead" tufting** of the distal phalanges, **increased width of intra-articular cartilages**, and **cystic changes** of the carpal bones.
    - **Radiographs of the feet:** Shows similar changes to that of hand, and there is **increased thickness of the heel pad** (normal heel pad thickness < 22 mm).
    - **X-ray of spine: Scoliosis, calcification of spinal ligaments.**
- **Pituitary function:** Partial or complete anterior hypopituitarism is common.
- **Visual field examination:** Defects are common (e.g., bitemporal hemianopia)

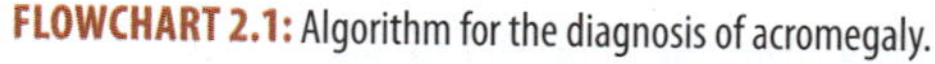
FLOWCHART 2.1: Algorithm for the diagnosis of acromegaly.

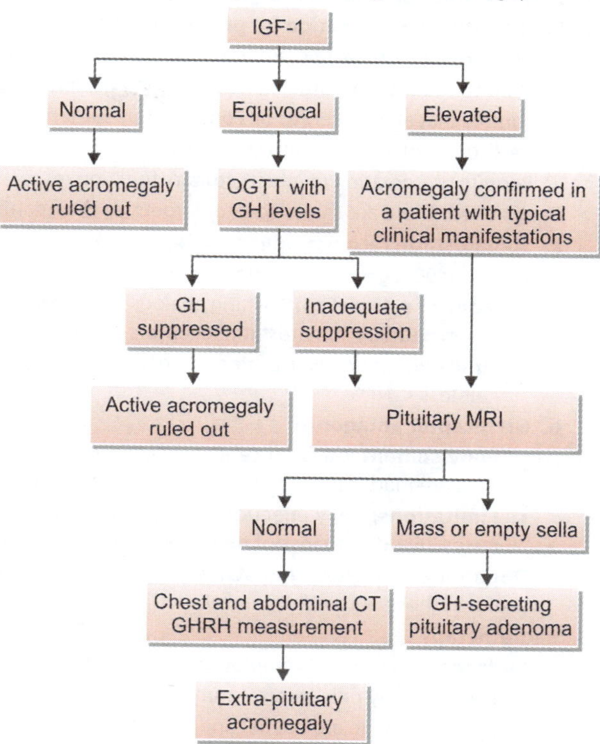

(IGF-1: insulin growth factor-1; GH: growth hormone; OGTT: oral glucose tolerance test; GHRH: growth hormone -releasing hormone)

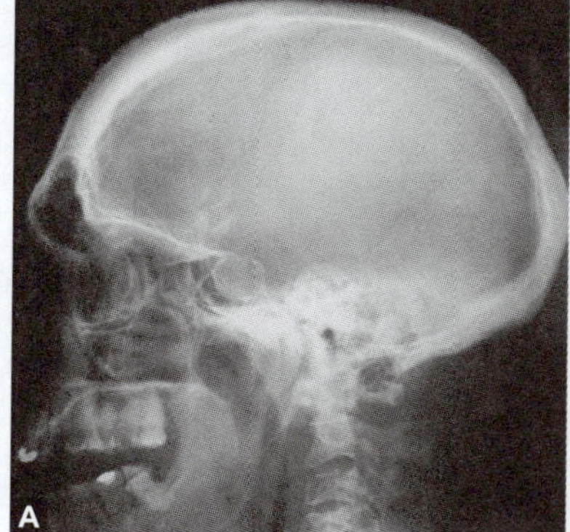

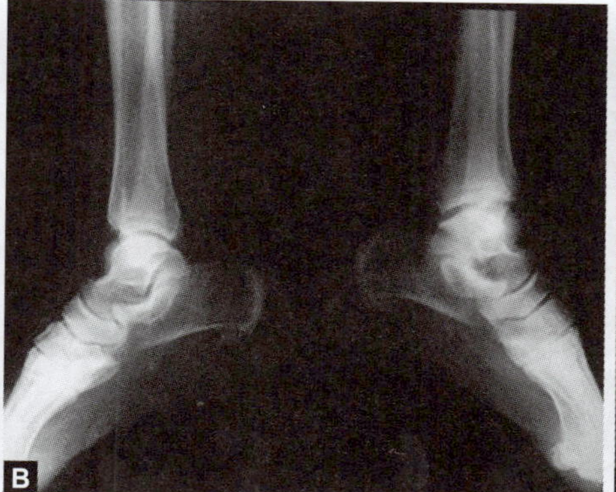

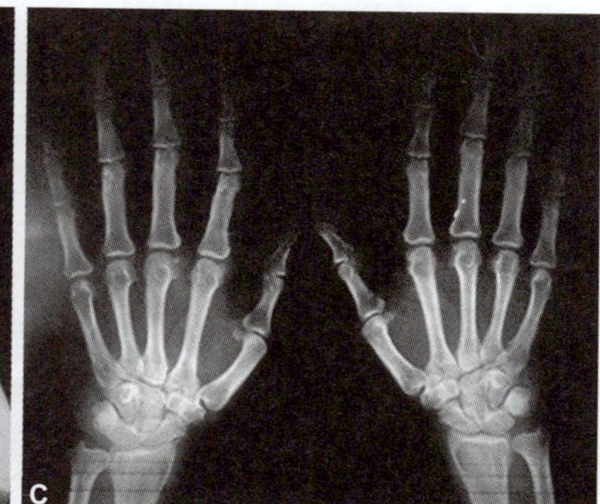

FIGS. 2.3A TO C: X-ray findings in acromegaly. (A) Lateral X-ray skull showing sellar enlargement, thickening of the calvarium, enlargement of the frontal and maxillary sinuses, and enlargement of the jaw; (B) X-ray ankle shows increased thickness of the heel pad in acromegaly; (C) X-ray of hand showing increased soft tissue bulk, "arrowhead" tufting of the distal phalanges.

Treatment of Acromegaly

- Untreated acromegaly is associated with markedly reduced survival.
- Most deaths are due to **heart failure, coronary artery disease, and hypertension** related causes. Patients with acromegaly have an increased risk for cancer (i.e., carcinoma colon).
- Treatment is indicated in all except the elderly or those with minimal abnormalities.
- **Aim of therapy:**
  - To lower the serum IGF-1 concentration to within the normal range for the patient's age and gender.
  - Control adenoma size and reduce mass effects.
  - Alleviate symptoms such as headaches, vision loss without causing hypopituitarism.
  - Reverse metabolic abnormalities such as diabetes mellitus.
  - To lower the serum growth hormone (GH) concentration to <1 μg/L

1. **Surgery: Trans-sphenoidal surgical removal** of pituitary adenoma is the first-line therapy.
2. **Medical therapy: Indication for primary medical management (Flowchart 2.2):** Patients
   - With no risk of visual impairment from the tumor
   - Unfit candidates for surgery and those who decline surgery
   - Tumors that are unlikely to be controlled by surgery
   - Persistence of acromegaly after surgery
   - Require preservation of intact pituitary function (especially fertility).

   Drugs used: There are three receptor targets for the treatment of acromegaly.

   a. **Somatostatin receptor ligands (SRL)**
      - About 90% growth-hormone secreting adenomas express somatostatin receptor subtypes (SSTR), SSTR2, and SSTR5.
      - **Mode of action:** Somatostatin analogs (**Octreotide, Pasireotide or Lanreotide**) are more effective than dopamine agonists and act on pituitary somatostatin receptors to produce inhibition of GH and IGF-1.
      - **Limitations:** Costly, transient diarrhea, nausea, and abdominal discomfort due inhibition of motor activity, gallstones, and hair loss < 10%.

   b. **GH receptor antagonist**
      - **Pegvisomant** is a GH receptor antagonist, blocks peripheral IGF-1 action in almost all patients, and is indicated in patients who are inadequately controlled with other modalities or in patients experiencing clinically significant drug side effects.
      - **Limitations:** Daily injection, costly, acts on peripheral tissues, and neither affects pituitary tumor nor secretion of GH, GH raises 76% due to loss of negative feedback by lower IGF-1 levels, and LFTs to be monitored due to elevated levels of AST.

   c. **Dopamine receptor agonists:** Act on D_2 receptors. **Bromocriptine or cabergoline** are dopamine receptor agonists and are useful in those with mildly elevated IGF-1.
3. **Radiotherapy**
   - **Indications:** It is usually employed as second-line treatment
     - If acromegaly persists after surgery
     - In patients who are not fit candidates for surgical therapy
     - In whom medical therapy fails.
   - External radiotherapy or implantation of Yttrium into the gland.
   - Stereotactic radiosurgery (gamma knife and cyber knife).
4. **Others:** Treatment of associated conditions such as diabetes, hypertension, and hyperlipidemia.

FLOWCHART 2.2: Management of the patient with acromegaly.

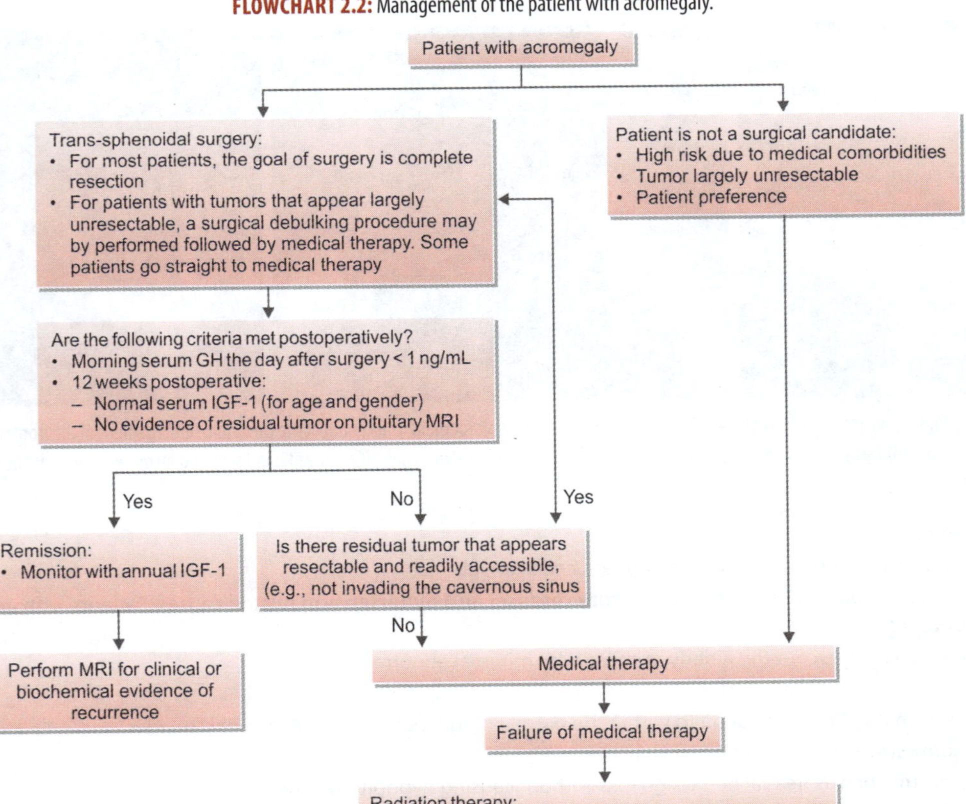

(IGF-1: insulin growth factor-1; GH: growth hormone)

Prolactinoma

Q. Write short essay/note on:
- **Prolactinoma and hyperprolactinemia.**
- **Causes, clinical features, investigations, and treatment of hyperprolactinemia.**

- **Prolactinoma** is a pituitary tumor that produces prolactin.
- Most common functional pituitary tumor. Most of these tumors are microadenomas.
- Elevated level of plasma prolactin is known as **hyperprolactinemia.**

Causes of Hyperprolactinemia (Box 2.4)

Box 2.4: Causes of hyperprolactinemia.

Physiological
- Pregnancy
- Stress
- Nursing
- Nipple stimulation

Pathological

A. **Drug-induced:** Estrogens, opiates, dopamine-receptor antagonists (phenothiazines, butyrophenones, metoclopramide), and dopamine-depleting agents (reserpine and methyldopa)

B. **Disease states**
- Pituitary adenomas (lactotroph, somatotroph-lactotroph, and stalk compression by chromophobe tumors)
- Hypothalamic and stalk disease (craniopharyngiomas, irradiation, granulomas, and stalk section/compression)
- Primary hypothyroidism
- Miscellaneous (cirrhosis, chronic renal failure, and seizures)

Clinical features

Hyperprolactinemia stimulates **milk production in the breast** and **inhibits GnRH and gonadotropin secretion**. It usually presents with:
- **Hypogonadism, decreased libido, infertility**, and **galactorrhea** (spontaneous or expressible) in both sexes.
- **In females: Amenorrhea, oligomenorrhea,** and **osteoporosis.**
- **In males: Hypogonadotropic hypogonadism** leading to loss of libido, impotence, infertility, gynecomastia, and rarely galactorrhea.
- A sufficiently large macroadenoma usually produces visual field defects and headache.

Investigations

The investigation of prolactinomas is the same as for other pituitary tumors discussed above.
- **Normal range for serum prolactin is approximately 5-20 μg/L.**
- The diagnosis of hyperprolactinemia is made by a serum prolactin concentration that is well above the normal range > **20 μg/L in men and postmenopausal women** and **>30 μg/L in premenopausal women.**
- Serum PRL over 150 μg/L in a nonpregnant woman is generally due to pituitary adenoma; a level of over 300 μg/L is almost diagnostic of tumor (even in a nursing mother).
  - **Hook effect**: Caution should be exercised in interpreting serum prolactin concentrations between 20 and 200 μg/L in the presence of a macroadenoma because of possible artifactually low values due to the «hook effect». This effect occurs when a very high serum prolactin, e.g., 5,000 μg/L, saturates both the capture and signal antibodies used in immunoradiometric and chemiluminescent assays, preventing the binding of the two in a «sandwich». The result is an apparent prolactin concentration that is only modestly elevated, suggesting that the macroadenoma is clinically nonfunctioning. The artifact can be avoided by repeating the assay using a 1:100 dilution of serum.
  - **Macroprolactin**: Macroprolactin is native prolactin that is bound to IgG. This causes hyperprolactinemia through decreased prolactin clearance.
- **Visual fields** should be checked.
- **Primary hypothyroidism** must be excluded.
- **Anterior pituitary function** should be assessed if there is evidence of hypopituitarism or radiological evidence of a pituitary tumor.
- **MRI or contrast-enhanced CT scan of the pituitary:** It is needed if there are any clinical features suggestive of a pituitary tumor. It is desirable when prolactin is significantly elevated (above 1,000 mU/L). It can easily delineate macroprolactinoma (tumors above 10 mm diameter), but microprolactinoma (smaller ones) may be more difficult to delineate.

Treatment of prolactinoma

Hyperprolactinemia is usually treated to **prevent the long-term effects of estrogen or testosterone deficiency.**
- **Medical treatment by dopamine agonists:**
  - **Cabergoline** is the first choice with a dose of 0.25–0.5 mg twice a week.
  - **Bromocriptine** (1.25–2.5 mg twice daily) reduces the secretion of prolactin as well as size of pituitary tumor.
  - **Quinagolide:** Initial: 0.025 mg once daily for 3 days followed by 0.05 mg once daily for 3 days. Maintenance (beginning on day 7): 0.075 mg once daily
- **Treatment of men:** Testosterone.
- **Treatment of women:** Estradiol.
- **Trans-sphenoidal removal:** It is indicated if dopamine agonists fails or in the presence of a large, invasive tumor.
- **External radiotherapy:** Rarely necessary.
- **Asymptomatic patients** who do not require restoration of pregnancy give estrogens to prevent bone loss and should be regularly monitored.

Diabetes Insipidus (DI)

Q. Write a short note on diabetes insipidus (DI) and its diagnosis.

- Diabetes insipidus (DI) is a disorder in which **polyuria** due to **decreased collecting tubule water reabsorption** is induced by either **decreased secretion of antidiuretic hormone** (ADH; central DI) or **resistance to its renal effects** (nephrogenic DI).
- It is characterized by the persistent passage of **excessive amounts of dilute urine** and thirst.

Types of Diabetes Insipidus (DI)

- **Primary deficiency** (neurogenic, pituitary, hypothalamic, cranial or central DI): It is due to agenesis or destruction of neurohypophysis.
- **Secondary deficiency:** It is due to inhibition of ADH secretion (primary polydipsia).
- **Deficient action of ADH** (nephrogenic DI)
- Transient **diabetes insipidus of pregnancy** produced by accelerated metabolism of vasopressin by **vasopressinases** released from the placenta (gestational DI).

Causes of Diabetes Insipidus (Table 2.6)

Clinical features

- **Polyuria and polydipsia:** The urine output may range from 2 L/day with mild partial DI to over 10-15 L/day in patients with severe disease, nocturia, and compensatory excessive thirst (polydipsia) are the most marked symptoms.
- **Other features:** Change in mentation, insomnia, and weight loss.
- Skin, mucous membranes cool.
- If left untreated changes in LOC (loss of consciousness), tachycardia, tachypnea, and hypotension (shock-like symptoms), but unlike hypovolemic shock, urine output is increased.
- Patients with nephrogenic DI may also have manifestations related to underlying cause such as lithium toxicity, hypercalcemia, and hypokalemia.
- It can lead to **hypernatremia**, restlessness, agitation, diminished deep tendon reflexes, and seizures.

TABLE 2.6: Causes of diabetes insipidus (DI).

Central DI	*Nephrogenic DI*
1. **Idiopathic** (30–50%) 2. **Neoplastic or infiltrative lesions of hypothalamus** (pituitary tumors with suprasellar extension, metastases, leukemia, histiocytosis, craniopharyngioma, lymphoma, sarcoidosis, germinomas, and pinealomas) 3. **Pituitary or hypothalamic surgery** 4. **Severe head injury,** usually associated with skull fracture 5. **Hypoxic encephalopathy** 6. **Ruptured cerebral aneurysms** 7. **Infections** (e.g., encephalitis, TB, etc.) 8. **Autoimmune:** Associated with thyroiditis 9. **Postsupraventricular tachycardia** 10. **Anorexia nervosa** 11. **Familial:** - Autosomal dominant familial neurohypophyseal DI (FNDI) due to mutations in the gene encoding ADH - X-linked inheritance **Wolfram syndrome** (also known as **DIDMOAD** syndrome) characterized by DI, DM, optic atrophy and deafness, - Septo-optic dysplasia ***Proprotein convertase subtilisin/kexin-type 1 (PCSK1) gene deficiency***	1. **Primary/congenital or familial:** - X-linked recessive vasopressin receptor V2 mutation - Autosomal dominant or autosomal recessive aquaporin-2 gene mutation - Autosomal recessive Bardet–Biedl syndrome - Bartter syndrome - Nephronophthisis - Cystinosis - Familial hypomagnesemia with hypercalciuria and nephrocalcinosis (FHHNC) - Autosomal recessive ARC syndrome (arthrogryposis-renal dysfunction-cholestasis) 2. **Acquired:** Chronic pyelonephritis, hypokalemia, hypercalcemia, sickle cell disease, protein deprivation drug-induced (lithium, cidofovir, foscarnet, ifosfamide, ofloxacin, orlistat, demeclocycline, didanosine, amphotericin B, aminoglycosides, cisplatin, rifampicin, colchicine), amyloidosis, other renal diseases (chronic renal failure, obstructive uropathy, polycystic disease), Sjögren's syndrome, postsurgery for craniopharyngioma, and pregnancy

Complications

- Hypernatremia, dehydration, and their neurological sequelae
- Growth retardation
- Hydronephrosis (due to excessive urine output)

Investigation and diagnosis

- **Careful history, examination**
- Document presence of **polyuria** (usually 2-15 L/24 hours).
- **Measurement of osmolality of plasma and urine:** It establishes the diagnosis.
  - Normally, plasma osmolality is <295 mOsml/kg and urine osmolality (random specimen) is 50-1,200 mOsml/kg.
  - In patients with DI and excess urine free water, there is **high or high normal plasma osmolality** (>295 mOsml/kg) and **low urine osmolality** (50–150 mOsml/kg).
  - In primary polydipsia, plasma osmolality tends to be low and may be lower than urinary osmolality.

- **Urine:**
  - **High 24 hours urine volumes.** If the volume is <2 L, there is no need for further investigation.
  - **Clear and of low specific gravity** of urine.
  - **Low urine osmolality** and usually less than that of plasma osmolality.
- **Serum sodium is high or high normal** (hypernatremia) and indicates loss of water.
- **MRI of pituitary and hypothalamus** to identify hyperintensities in the posterior pituitary or thickening of the pituitary stalk can help determine the cause of CDI.

Q. Write a short note on water deprivation test.

- **Water deprivation test (Miller-Moses Test) (Fig. 2.4):**
  - **Indication**
    - Diagnosis or exclusion of diabetes insipidus
    - To differentiate CDI and NDI
    - To differentiate diabetes insipidus from primary polydipsia
  - **Procedure**
    - Should be done in the morning under observation with 8 hours fasting. No fluids (water deprivation) from 07:30 hours.
    - Measure plasma and urine osmolality, urine volume and weight hourly for up to 8 hours.
    - Abandon fluid deprivation if weight loss is >5%.
    - If plasma osmolality > 300 mOsm/kg and/or urine osmolality < 600 mOsm/kg, ADH (vasopressin) is given in the dose of 2 μg IM at end of test. Allow free intake of fluids but measure urine osmolality for 2–4 hours.
  - **Normal response:**
    - Withholding fluid in normal individuals, the **plasma osmolality remains within normal range** (275–295 mOsm/kg) while **urine osmolality rises** above 600 mOsm/kg (800–1,200 mOsm/kg).
    - **Urine osmolality is greater than plasma osmolality after restriction of water.**
    - Urine osmolality increases minimally (<10%) after exogenous ADH.
  - **Primary polydipsia**
    - Patients with primary polydipsia start with low normal plasma osmolality (280 mOsm/kg).
    - **Urine/plasma osmolality ratio rises to >2 after dehydration (water deprivation).**
  - **Central diabetes insipidus**
    - After water restriction in patients with DI, the **plasma osmolality rises above normal** (>300 mOsm/kg) **without rise in urine osmolality** (<600 mOsm/kg) or specific gravity of urine. (Normally urine osmolality rises to 1,000–1,200 mOsml/kg after water restriction). Urine osmolality remains less than plasma osmolality and urine/plasma osmolality ratio remains <1.5.
    - After ADH is given, urine osmolality increases 100% in complete CDI and over 50% in partial CDI.
  - **Nephrogenic diabetes insipidus**
    - Urine osmolality remains less than plasma osmolality.
    - After ADH, urine osmolality increases by <50%.

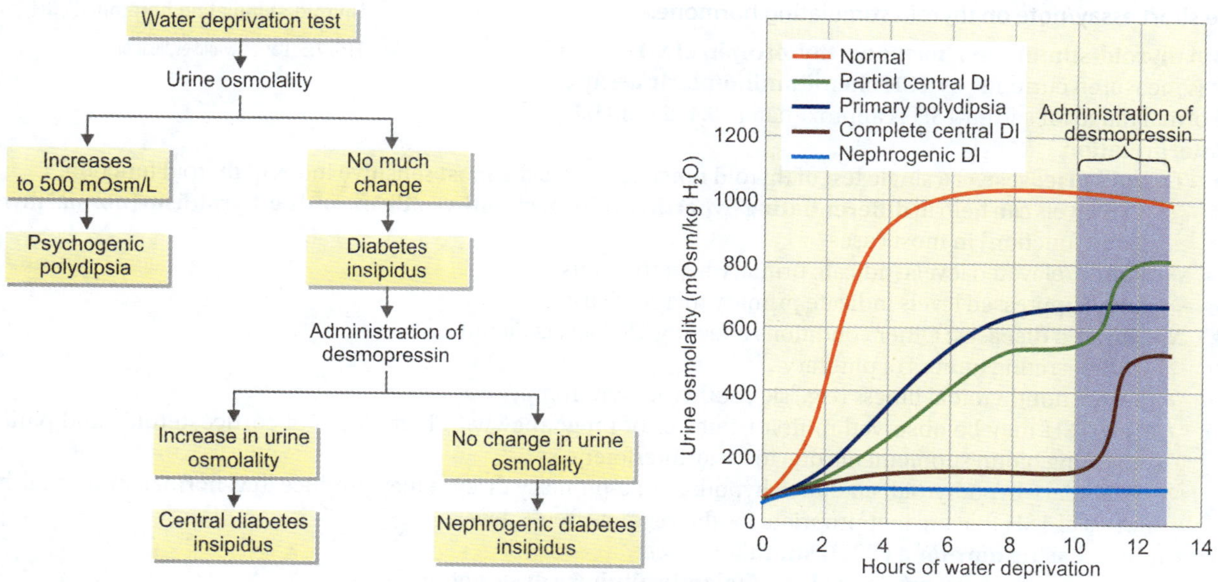

FIG. 2.4: Water deprivation test and its interpretation.

- Alternative to water deprivation test is by **infusing hypertonic (5%) saline and measures ADH secretion** in response to increasing plasma osmolality.

Treatment

- **Goals of treatment**
  - **Balance fluid intake with output:** In acute cases, rapidly replace fluid and in chronic cases with slow replacement to prevent cerebral edema.
  - Daily weights, accurate intake/output monitoring, urine specific gravity, and osmolality.
- **Drugs**
  - **Desmopressin (DDAVP):** Drug of choice, initial dose of 5 µg (rhinal tube) or 10 µg (metered spray) by intranasal route is given at bedtime. This dose is titrated up, in 5 µg increments as needed, depending on the response of the nocturia and then additional daytime doses are added. The typical daily maintenance dose is 5–20 µg once or twice daily.
  - **Chlorpropamide:** Increases the renal responsiveness to vasopressin. Hypoglycemia may develop.
  - **Carbamazepine:** It is an alternate drug which enhances ADH release and raises the sensitivity of the collecting duct to it.
  - **Clofibrate:** It is a lipid lowering agent which stimulates residual ADH production in the hypothalamus, therefore, increasing ADH release from the posterior pituitary.
  - **Nonsteroidal anti-inflammatory drugs (NSAIDs):** Work by inhibiting renal prostaglandin synthesis which are ADH antagonists and also, they decrease the glomerular filtration rate by prostaglandin-mediated effect of afferent arteriole dilation.
- **Treatment of nephrogenic DI**
  - Provision of adequate fluids especially in cases of impaired thirst, calorie and decreased dietary solute such as low sodium diet.
  - Correct the underlying cause.
  - **Thiazide diuretics:** These (e.g., hydrochlorothiazide 25 mg once or twice daily with a low sodium diet) are the first-line therapy in nephrogenic DI.
  - **Amiloride** (potassium-sparing diuretic)**: Additive effect** with thiazide diuretic and may be particularly beneficial in patients with **reversible lithium nephrotoxicity** by possibly allowing lithium to be continued.
  - **Exogenous ADH (DDAVP)**
  - **NSAIDs:** Indomethacin

THYROID DISORDERS

Thyroid Function Tests (TFTs)

Q. Write short essay/note on various thyroid function tests.

- **Indications for thyroid function tests**
  - Screening for thyroid dysfunction
  - Surveillance: Women with postpartum thyroiditis, postneck irradiation
  - Monitoring: Treatment of hyperthyroidism and hypothyroidism

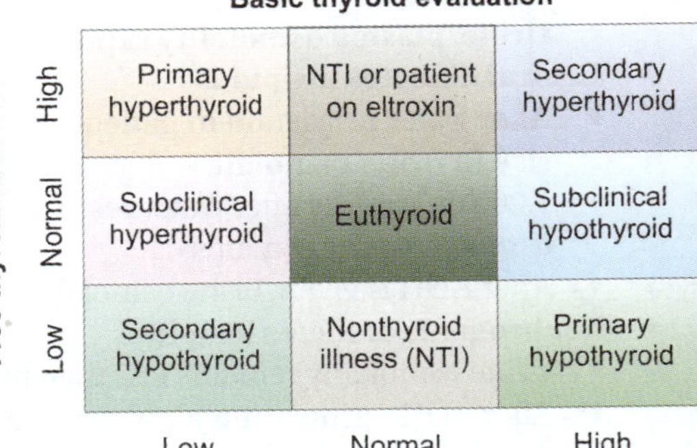

FIG. 2.5: Basic thyroid evaluation.

Various Thyroid Function Tests (Fig. 2.5)

Q. Write short essay/note on thyroid stimulating hormone.

- **Serum thyroid-stimulating hormone/thyrotropin (TSH)**
  - It is measured currently by **TSH chemiluminometric assays**.
  - Normal range for serum TSH is approximately **0.4–5.0 mU/L**.
  - **Interpretation**
    - **Thyroid diseases:** As a single test of thyroid function TSH is the most sensitive index of thyroid function.
      - TSH levels can help in **differentiating hyperthyroidism, hypothyroidism, and euthyroidism** (normal thyroid gland function) in most cases.
      - Raised/elevated levels indicate primary hypothyroidism.
      - Low/suppressed levels indicate primary thyrotoxicosis.
    - **Nonthyroid diseases:** Other conditions affecting TSH levels include:
      - TSH-secreting tumors of pituitary
      - Severe nonthyroidal illness (e.g., sick euthyroid syndrome)
      - Low TSH may be observed in first trimester of pregnancy with high doses of corticosteroids and patients ingesting biotin supplements due to assay interference.
      - Secondary hypothyroidism due to hypothalamic-pituitary disease may produce low, normal, or normal-high levels of TSH that are inappropriate for the very low free T_4 level.
- **Thyrotropin releasing hormone (TRH) stimulation test**
  - It may be used in the investigation of **hypothalamic pituitary dysfunction**.
  - Serum TSH is measured before and after the intravenous administration of TRH.

- **Use:** To differentiate secondary or tertiary hypothyroidism.
  - Secondary hypothyroidism (pituitary disease): TRH administration does not produce increase in TSH.
  - Tertiary hypothyroidism (hypothalamic disease): TRH administration produces delayed increase in TSH.
  - In primary hypothyroidism, TRH administration produces a prompt increase in TSH.

- **Serum free T_3 (tri-iodothyronine fT_3) and free T_4 (free thyroxine/fT_4)**
  - Advantage of this test compared to the measurement of total T_3 and T_4 is that these are **not influenced by changes in the thyroid hormone-binding globulins (TBG), prealbumin and albumin**. Its level reflects secretory activity.
  - **Primary thyrotoxicosis:** fT_3 and fT_4 levels are elevated.
  - **T_3-thyrotoxicosis:** fT_4 levels are normal and fT_3 levels are elevated.
  - **On T_4 therapy:** fT_4 levels are elevated and fT_3 levels are normal.
- **Total serum thyroxine (tT_4)**
  - Measured by automated competitive binding chemiluminometric assays.
  - Its levels are altered by factors that affect the concentration of TBG.
  - **Normal ranges: 4.6–11.2 µg/dL.**
  - **Increased:** In hyperthyroidism, during pregnancy, estrogen therapy, tamoxifen use and as a congenital anomaly.
  - **Decreased:** In hypothyroidism, nephritic syndrome, androgen therapy, liver failure, or drugs (e.g., salicylates, sulfonylureas, and phenytoin).
- **Total serum tri-iodothyronine (tT_3)**
  - Measured by automated competitive binding chemiluminometric assays.
  - Its levels are subject to the same limitations as for tT_4 in relation to TBG.
  - **Normal range: 75–195 ng/dL.**
- **T_3 resin uptake, free T_4 index (FTI), effective T_4 ratio**
  Nowadays, above three tests (4, 5, and 6) are not used.
- **Reverse T_3 (rT_3)**
  - Reverse T_3 (rT_3) is mainly an **inactive metabolite of T_4** in peripheral tissues.
  - It has **extremely limited utility** for assessing **rare conditions** such as consumptive hypothyroidism, MCT8 or SBP2 mutations, or possibly distinguishing central hypothyroidism from nonthyroidal illness in critically ill hospitalized patients.
- **Thyroglobulin (Tg)**
  - It is synthesized by follicular cells, secreted into the lumen of the thyroid follicle, stored as a colloid and is involved in iodination/synthesis of thyroid hormones.
  - **Use:** To predict the **outcome of therapy** for hyperthyroidism.
    - **Increased:** Well-differentiated thyroid carcinoma, hyperthyroidism
    - **Decreased:** Total thyroidectomy or destruction of thyroid by radiation.
- **Uptake of radioactive iodine (RAIU) or technetium**
  - The iodine uptake activity of thyroid can be measured by administering orally a low/trace dose of radioactive iodine **^{131}I or ^{121}I** and the radioactivity over the thyroid is measured after 4 hours, using a counter over the neck.
  - Pregnancy and breastfeeding are **absolute contraindications** to radionuclide imaging. However, in the unusual instance where radioiodine uptake measurement is felt to be essential for a definitive diagnosis in a lactating woman, breast milk can be pumped and discarded for 5 days after ingestion of I^{123}, then breastfeeding may be resumed; breastfeeding should not be resumed if the I^{131} isotope is used for determining the uptake.
  - The **amount of radioactivity that is taken up** by the thyroid gland is known as radioactive iodine uptake (RAIU). Alternatively, thyroid uptake is measured by giving **technetium-99m (^{99m}Tc) intravenously**.
  - **Uses of radioactive iodine uptake (RAIU)**
    - Evaluation of hyperthyroidism
    - Differentiate Graves's disease from toxic goiter
    - Function of a thyroid nodule as hot or cold
  - **Interpretation: Normal uptake ranges from 10% to 35% in 24 hours.**
    - **Uptake increased: Overactive** thyroid gland synthesizing excess T_3 shows increased uptake of iodine. A very high RAIU is seen in hyperthyroidism (e.g., Graves' disease, toxic multinodular goiter, toxic adenoma and early thyroiditis). Iodine/enzyme deficiency may show increased uptake even in the absence of thyrotoxicosis.
    - **Uptake decreased:** Low RAIU is seen in hypothyroidism and late thyroiditis. Excess iodine may show diminished uptake even in the presence or thyrotoxicosis. Acute autoimmune thyroiditis may manifest as low iodine uptake thyrotoxicosis.
  - **Use:** To determine **the functional activity and morphology** of the thyroid gland.
    - **Very useful in determining the activity of a solitary thyroid nodule.** Functional nodule appears as a "hot" nodule, and a nonfunctional appears as a "cold" nodule.
    - **Useful in follow-up of patients with treated thyroid cancer.**
    - **Detection of ectopic thyroid tissue:** Confirmation of a mass on the tongue as lingual thyroid in the midline of the neck as thyroglossal duct, or in the mediastinum as substernal goiter.

- **Ultrasound of thyroid gland:** Look for **nodularity, vascularity, shape, microcalcifications, lymph nodes status,** and for **guided FNAC.**
- **Thyroid auto-antibody tests:** The different types of thyroid autoantibodies responsible for the autoimmune thyroid disorders are:
  - **Anti-microsomal antibody**
    - **Antithyroid peroxidase (TPO) antibody (TPOAb):** They are involved in the tissue destructive process associated with hypothyroidism in Hashimoto and atrophic thyroiditis.
  - **Antithyroglobulin (Tg) antibody:** May be present in Hashimoto's thyroiditis and Graves' disease.
  - **TSH receptor (TR) antibody (TRAb):** Classified as **stimulating, blocking, or neutral.**
    - Stimulating antibodies (thyroid-stimulating immunoglobulins, TSI) cause Graves' disease.
    - Thyroid receptor-blocking antibodies can cause hypothyroidism.
    - Neutral antibodies bind the receptor but do not stimulate or block function.
- **Tests to determine etiology of thyroid disease**
  - **Calcitonin:** It is secreted by parafollicular C-cells and is increased in medullary carcinoma of thyroid.
  - **Fine-needle aspiration cytology/excision biopsy:** It is helpful in diagnosis thyroid diseases.

Thyrotoxicosis

Q. Discuss the etiology, clinical features, investigations (laboratory diagnosis), complications and management of hyperthyroidism/thyrotoxicosis.

Q. Discuss the etiopathogenesis, clinical features, investigations, diagnosis, and management/treatment modalities of Graves' disease.

Definition

- **Thyrotoxicosis** is a state of **circulating thyroid hormone excess** (with hypermetabolic state) caused by exposure to **excessive levels of thyroid hormone** (free T_3 and T_4).
- This increase in circulating hormone may be either from destruction of thyroid gland or from ectopic source.
- **Hyperthyroidism** (thyroid overactivity): It is the **clinical consequence due to the excessive circulating thyroid hormone due to excessive thyroid function**/hyperfunction and is the **most common cause of thyrotoxicosis**. Its causes are listed in **Table 2.7A**.

TABLE 2.7A: Causes of hyperthyroidism.

Primary hyperthyroidism	*Thyrotoxicosis without hyperthyroidism*	*Secondary hyperthyroidism*
➢ Graves' disease ➢ Toxic multinodular goiter ➢ Toxic adenoma (Plummer's disease) ➢ Iodine excess (Jod-Basedow) ➢ Activating mutation of TSH receptor	➢ Subacute thyroiditis ➢ Hashitoxicosis ➢ Amiodarone induced ➢ Radiation induced ➢ Thyrotoxicosis factitia ➢ Struma ovarii ➢ Infarction of thyroid gland	➢ TSH secreting pituitary adenoma ➢ hCG-mediated hyperthyroidism (hyperemesis gravidarum, trophoblastic disease) ➢ Gestational thyrotoxicosis

Etiology (Table 2.7B) and Pathogenesis of Hyperthyroidism

Q. Write short essay/notes on causes of hyperthyroidism.

Few of the causes of hyperthyroidism/thyrotoxicosis are discussed below.

1. **Graves' disease**
   - Graves' disease is the **most common form** of thyrotoxicosis. It is characterized by one or more of the following features:
     - Thyrotoxicosis
     - Goiter
     - Orbitopathy (exophthalmos) **(Box 2.5)**
     - Dermopathy (pretibial myxedema).
   - **Age, gender, and genetic susceptibility:**
     - It may occur at any age with a peak incidence between **20 and 40 years** of age.
     - The diseases cluster in families and are **more common in women**.
     - The concordance rate in monozygotic twins is 20-40%.
     - Associated with certain alleles of CTLA-4
     - Associated with certain alleles of HLA on Chromosome 6 namely, HLA-DRB1*08 and DRB3*0202.
     - HLA-DRB1*07 is found to be protective.
   - **Autoantibodies:**
     - It is an autoimmune disorder with autoantibodies.
     - **TSI or TSH-receptor antibodies of the stimulating type (TRAb):** IgG type of antibodies directed against the TSH receptors on the follicular cell of thyroid. They stimulate thyroid hormone production and enlargement of thyroid.

- ♦ **T cells:** Activated T cells release cytokines and increase the secretion of thyroid-specific autoantibodies from B cells. The current concept is that thyroid-specific T cells in Graves' disease primarily act as helper (CD4+ Th1) cells.
- **Histology:** Characterized by **follicular hyperplasia, intracellular colloid droplets, cell scalloping,** a reduction in follicular colloid, and a patchy (multifocal) **lymphocytic infiltration.**
- **Ophthalmopathy and dermatopathy:** Observed in Graves' disease is due to **immunologically mediated** activation of fibroblasts in the **extraocular muscles and skin**. This along with accumulation of **glycosaminoglycans** and **trapping of water causes edema** initially. Later fibroblasts cause fibrosis.
- **Hyperthyroidism may be triggered by viral or bacterial infections**. *E. coli* and *Yersinia enterocolitica* possess cell membrane TSH receptors. The antibodies produced against these micro-organisms can cross-react with the TSH receptors (molecular mimicry).
- **Other mediating mechanisms**: Bystander activation and thyroid cell HLA-antigen expression.
- **Other precipitating causes**:
  - ♦ Thyroid injury by radiation and drugs
  - ♦ Stress
  - ♦ Smoking
  - ♦ Sex steroids
  - ♦ Pregnancy
  - ♦ Fetal microchimerism
  - ♦ Iodine and iodine-containing drugs such as amiodarone.
  - ♦ Alemtuzumab, a monoclonal antibody against CD52, has been associated with a 10-15% incidence of new-onset Graves' disease.

TABLE 2.7B: Causes of hyperthyroidism.

Hyperthyroidism with a normal or high radioiodine uptake
Autoimmune thyroid disease
Graves' disease
Hashitoxicosis
Autonomous thyroid tissue (uptake may be low if recent iodine load led to iodine-induced hyperthyroidism)
Toxic adenoma
Toxic multinodular goiter
TSH-mediated hyperthyroidism
TSH-producing pituitary adenoma
Non-neoplastic TSH-mediated hyperthyroidism
Human chorionic gonadotropin-mediated hyperthyroidism
Hyperemesis gravidarum
Trophoblastic disease
Hyperthyroidism with a near absent radioiodine uptake
Thyroiditis
Subacute granulomatous (de Quervain's) thyroiditis
Painless thyroiditis (silent thyroiditis, lymphocytic thyroiditis)
Postpartum thyroiditis
Amiodarone (also may cause iodine-induced hyperthyroidism)
Radiation thyroiditis
Palpation thyroiditis
Exogenous thyroid hormone intake
Excessive replacement therapy
Intentional suppressive therapy
Factitious hyperthyroidism
Ectopic hyperthyroidism
Struma ovani
Metastatic follicular thyroid cancer

Box 2.5: Thyroid orbitopathy (eye signs) **(Table 2.8 and Figs. 2.6A to D).**

- An **autoimmune disease** of the retro-ocular tissues occurring in patients with Graves' disease. Although it has often been referred to as Graves' ophthalmopathy, or thyroid eye disease (TED), it is **primarily a disease of the orbit** and is better termed **Graves' orbitopathy**.
- The ophthalmopathy causes **abnormal protrusion of the eyeball (exophthalmos)**.
- **Sympathetic overactivity** may produce the characteristic **wide, staring gaze, and** can also be the reason for **lid lag**.
- It is observed in about **50%** of the patients when first seen. It may precede Graves' disease by many years or may develop even after successful treatment of Graves' disease.
- The volume of both the extraocular muscles and retro-ocular connective tissue is increased due to **fibroblast proliferation, inflammation** and the accumulation of **hydrophilic glycosaminoglycans** (GAG), mostly hyaluronic acid.
- **Pathogenesis of orbitopathy:**
  - The main autoantigen is the **thyroid-stimulating hormone receptor (TSHR)**, which is expressed primarily in the thyroid but is also expressed in adipocytes, fibroblasts, and a variety of additional sites.
  - TSHR antibodies and T-cells activate **retro-ocular fibroblast** and **adipocyte TSHR and IGF-1 receptors,** initiating a **retro-orbital inflammatory environment**.
  - GAG secretion by fibroblasts is increased by thyroid-stimulating antibodies and activated T cells (via cytokine secretion), implying that both **B and T cell activation** are integral to this process.
  - The accumulation of hydrophilic GAG in turn leads to **fluid accumulation, muscle swelling**, and an **increase in pressure within the orbit.**
  - These changes, together with retro-ocular adipogenesis, displace the eyeball forward leading to extraocular muscle dysfunction and impaired venous drainage.
- **Symptoms:** There may not be any ocular symptoms, but the patient may be distressed by the appearance. However, the following symptoms can prevail:
  - A gritty or foreign object sensation in the eyes
  - Excessive tearing, often made worse by exposure to cold air, wind, or bright lights
  - Eye or retro-ocular discomfort or pain

- Blurring of vision
- Diplopia
- Color vision desaturation
- Loss of vision in severe cases

- **Signs**
  - Exophthalmos (proptosis) often asymmetric but can be symmetric
  - Lid lag
  - Lid retraction
  - Periorbital edema
  - Corneal ulcers
  - Chemosis
  - Ophthalmoplegia
  - Visual field defects
  - Papilledema.
- **Treatment**
  - **Reversal of hyperthyroidism:**
    - Rapid amelioration of symptoms, with a **beta-blocker** and decreasing thyroid hormone synthesis with a **thionamide** or **surgery**.
    - Reduction of thyroid hormone synthesis **decreases eyelid retraction and stare**. (If hypothyroidism develops during the course of therapy, more fluid retention can occur and may have an adverse effect on the orbitopathy).
    - For patients with active and moderate-to-severe or sight-threatening orbitopathy, thionamides or surgery are the preferred treatment modalities, as this is usually followed by a fall in serum thyrotropin receptor antibody (TRAb) concentrations, suggesting a waning of autoimmunity. **Radioiodine therapy** leads to the development or worsening of orbitopathy as it is associated with a sustained increase in TRAb, hence **contraindicated**.
    - Patients with active and mild orbitopathy may still be candidates for thionamides, radioiodine, or surgery. If radioiodine is chosen, glucocorticoids should be administered concurrently for those with risk factors for progression.
  - **Smoking cessation:** Increases the incidence of symptomatic Graves' orbitopathy, increases the risk of worsening orbitopathy after radioiodine therapy and also renders patients more refractory to anti-inflammatory therapy.
  - **Local measures: Eye shades, artificial tears, and lubricants** such as methylcellulose or petroleum jelly, raising head end of bed at night, **eye patching** and **prisms** for diplopia.
  - **Medical**:
    - **Selenium** 100 µg twice daily may improve symptoms in patients with mild Graves' orbitopathy. It has an antioxidant role and also decreases inflammatory activity.
    - **Glucocorticoids** are the **mainstay** of **immunomodulatory therapy** for moderate-to-severe Graves' orbitopathy. For patients with moderate symptoms, a trial of oral (**prednisone**, 30 mg/day for 4 weeks) or IV (**methylprednisolone**, 500 mg once weekly for weeks 1–6, then 250 mg once weekly for weeks 7–12 with cumulative dose 4.5–5 g over 12 weeks) can be tried. For more severe or progressive cases, initial IV therapy is appropriate.
    - **Teprotumumab,** an **IGF-1 receptor inhibitor**, was approved for the treatment of Graves' orbitopathy by the Food and Drug Administration (FDA) in February 2020. It is administered every 3 weeks as an IV infusion (10 mg/kg initial dose, then 20 mg/kg) for a total of eight infusions. Teprotumumab is **contraindicated** during pregnancy.
    - **Mycophenolate mofetil** is under investigation for the treatment of Graves' orbitopathy, either alone or in combination with glucocorticoids.
    - **Tocilizumab** targets IL-6 is being investigated for the treatment of patients with Graves' orbitopathy who are not improving with glucocorticoids.
    - **Rituximab** reported to be as effective as glucocorticoids without the glucocorticoid-related side effects induces a fall in thyrotropin receptor antibody (TRAb) levels and depletion of B cells in the retro-orbital tissues.
  - **Orbital decompression surgery: Indicated in** optic neuropathy caused by enlarged extraocular muscles not responsive to high-dose corticosteroids, severe orbital inflammation, excessive proptosis leading to exposure keratitis, corneal ulceration, or debilitating cosmetic defect, pain relief, and progressive orbitopathy not responding to other measures.
  - **Other surgeries:**
    - Fat decompression surgery, bilateral lateral tarsorrhaphy, surgical recession of Müller's muscle and the levator to correct upper lid retraction.
    - For patients requiring both strabismus surgery and orbital decompression, the **decompression** should be **performed first**, followed by strabismus surgery.

2. **Treatment-induced hyperthyroidism.**
   Drugs include iodine, amiodarone, iodine-containing contrast media, interferon-alpha, and rarely, lithium.
   - **Iodine-induced hyperthyroidism**
     - It develops following excess intake of iodine in diet or exposure to radiographic contrast media or iodine medication.
     - **Jod-Basedow phenomenon:** In states of iodine deficiency, thyroid nodules can develop, some of which can be autonomous functioning nodules. On supplementation of iodine, there is an increase in production of thyroxine, leading to **thyrotoxicosis**. Usually develops in patients with autonomously functioning thyroid gland (e.g., nodular

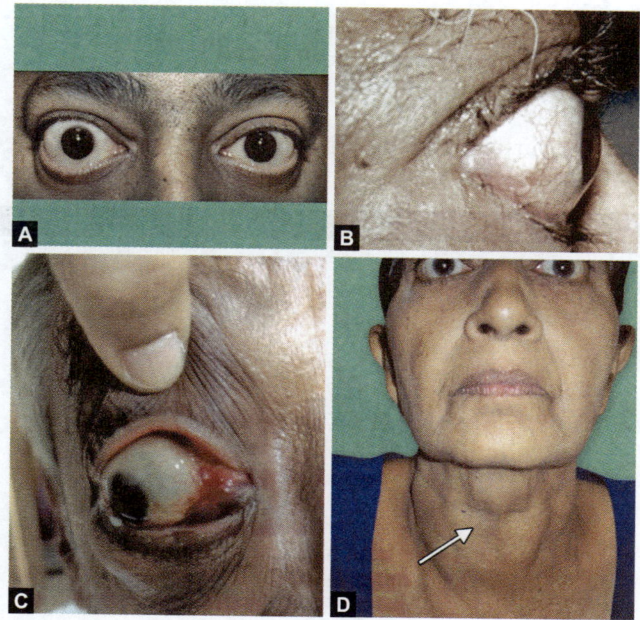

FIGS. 2.6A TO D: (A and B) Exophthalmos (front and side view); (C) Infiltration of extraocular muscles in hyperthyroidism; (D) Eye signs and enlarged nodular goiter (arrow).

TABLE 2.8: Eye signs of thyrotoxicosis.

Eye signs	*Description*
Dalrymple sign	Rim of sclera is seen all around the cornea on looking straightforward
Rosenbach's sign	Fine tremor of the upper eyelids on slight closure of the eye
Joffroy's sign	Lack of wrinkling of the forehead when a patient looks upward
Möbius sign	Lack of convergence on looking to near object
Von Graefe's sign (lid lag)	Lagging of the upper eyelid on looking downward without moving the head
Stellwag's sign	Staring look with infrequent blinking
Vigouroux sign	Eyelid fullness
Grove sign	Resistance to pulling down the retracted upper lid
Ballet sign	Restriction of one or more extraocular muscles
Kocher sign	Staring look (upper sclera visible)
Naffziger's sign	Standing behind, patient's neck is extended and examiner looks from behind along the superior orbital margin of the patient. Eyeball is seen beyond the superior orbital margin in exophthalmos

goiter/Graves' disease). It can also occur in endemic goiter and with iodine. Takes place due to a loss in the negative feedback mechanism of the circulating hormones on the thyroid gland.

- It is characterized by suppressed serum TSH level with normal levels of circulating thyroid hormone.
- **Wolff-Chaikoff effect**: Autoregulation by the follicular cells protects the gland from the wide variations in the amount of iodide intake. Sometimes, excess exposure and uptake of iodide by the gland can inhibit organification of iodide, thereby diminishing hormone biosynthesis, resulting in **hypothyroidism or myxedema.**

TABLE 2.9: Amiodarone-induced hyperthyroidism (AIT).

Type I AIT	*Type II AIT*
➢ It develops in patients with pre-existing multinodular goiter or latent Graves' disease. ➢ There is hyperthyroidism with increased synthesis of T_4 and T_3 and is triggered by the high iodine content of amiodarone. ➢ Jod-Basedow effect (refer above) occurs in patients with underlying thyroid disease.	➢ It is not associated with previous thyroid disease. ➢ It is due to a direct cytotoxicity of amiodarone on thyroid follicular cells leading to a destructive thyroiditis with release of T_3 and T_4. ➢ It produces a hyperthyroid phase which may last several weeks to months and may later progress to hypothyroid phase and eventual recovery in most but not all patients.

- **Amiodarone-induced hyperthyroidism (AIT):** Amiodarone is a class III antiarrhythmic drug. A 200-mg formulation of the drug contains 75 mg iodine. It can also induce hyperthyroidism which can be **(Table 2.9)**:

3. **Thyrotoxicosis factitia**
   - Exogenous hyperthyroidism is due to the **surreptitious ingestion of thyroid hormone**, it is termed as "thyrotoxicosis factitia".
   - Patients are **clinically thyrotoxic** without eye signs of Graves.
   - High doses of thyroxine lead to TSH suppression and causes shrinkage of the thyroid.
   - Find cause or contamination and treat symptomatically.
4. **Toxic multinodular goiter (Plummer's disease)**
   - Result of **diffuse hyperplasia of thyroid follicular cells** whose functional capacity is independent of regulation by TSH.
   - Goiter will be nodular.
   - Constitutes 14% of thyrotoxicosis cases.
   - Commonly occurs in elderly women (>50 years).
   - T_3 (greater), T_4 raised, and TSH undetectable.
5. **Toxic solitary adenoma/nodule**
   - Constitutes <5% of all thyrotoxicosis (hyperthyroidism) cases and the solitary nodule is follicular adenoma.
   - Usually occurs in female >40 years of age.
   - Suspected thyroid nodules merit close attention in the pediatric population because such nodules are much more likely to be malignant in children than they are in adults.

Clinical Features of Thyrotoxicosis (Table 2.10)

Q. Write short essay/notes on clinical features/signs/manifestations of thyrotoxicosis/hyperthyroidism.

Q. Write a short note on cardiac complications of hyperthyroidism.

- **Classic symptoms** include heat intolerance, tremor, palpitations, anxiety, weight loss, increased appetite increased frequency of bowel movements, and shortness of breath.

TABLE 2.10: Clinical features of thyrotoxicosis.

Organ/System involved	*Symptoms/Signs*	
Thyroid	Diffuse or nodular enlargement Warmth	Bruit (due to increased vascularity)
Gastrointestinal system	**Weight loss despite increased appetite** Vomiting Abdominal pain Increased gut motility Hyperdefecation and diarrhea	Malabsorption Steatorrhea Dysphagia due to goiter. Celiac disease is also more prevalent in patients with Graves' disease.
Cardiovascular system	Tachycardia Exertional dyspnea Palpitations Hyperdynamic precordium Pulmonary hypertension Angina	**Sinus tachycardia, atrial fibrillation** Wide pulse pressure Lowering of diastolic blood pressure Cardiac failure Cardiomyopathy Means-Lerman scratch (scratchy midsystolic murmur)
Neuropsychiatric system	Nervousness **Irritability** Psychosis Emotional lability Fine **tremors** Agitation Depression Inability to concentrate	Insomnia Hyperreflexia Cognitive impairments Poor orientation and immediate recall Amnesia Constructional difficulty Proximal myopathy Bulbar myopathy Ill-sustained clonus
Respiratory system	Increased ventilation: hypoxemia and hypercapnia Respiratory muscle weakness Decreased lung volume	Large goiter causing tracheal obstruction, exacerbation of asthma, and rise in pulmonary arterial systolic pressure.
Metabolic/Endocrine	Increased bone resorption—osteoporosis Periosteal new bone formation (**thyroid acropachy**)	Dyslipidemia Hyperglycemia
Hematologic	Normocytic normochromic anemia. Graves' hyperthyroidism may be associated with autoimmune hematologic disorders such as immune thrombocytopenia (ITP) and pernicious anemia	Maybe prothrombotic, excess thyroid hormone was associated with a rise in prothrombotic factors, including factors VIII, IX, fibrinogen, von Willebrand factor, and plasminogen activator inhibitor-1
Skin/integumentary system	Soft, warm, moist, and smooth skin due to decrease in keratin layer Increased sweating Pruritus, hives Onycholysis and softening of nails Palmar erythema Spider naevi Hyperpigmentation	Vitiligo Alopecia areata Clubbing Infiltrative dermopathy occurs only in patients with Graves' hyperthyroidism. The most common site is the skin overlying the shins, where it presents as raised, hyperpigmented, violaceous, orange-peel-textured papules **[Pretibial Myxedema (Box 2.6)].**
Urinary	Urinary frequency	Nocturia
Sex hormones	**Women:** Oligomenorrhea, amenorrhea, and anovulatory infertility	**Men:** Gynecomastia, reduced libido, erectile dysfunction, and abnormal/decreased spermatogenesis.
General	**Heat intolerance** Fatigue Gynecomastia	Apathy Thirst Thymic enlargement in Graves' disease.
Eyes (classically seen in Graves' disease)	Stare Lid lag **Exophthalmos** Proptosis	Extraocular diplopia Exposure keratitis Lagophthalmos

Note: Bold words indicate symptoms of greater discriminant value.

- **Elderly** patients present with anorexia, apathy, fatigue, weight loss, and dominant cardiovascular and myopathic features **(apathetic hyperthyroidism)**.
- **Younger** patients present predominantly with neurological manifestations.
- **Children** present with excessive height or excessive growth rate, or with behavioral problems (e.g., hyperactivity), and weight gain rather than loss.

Box 2.6: Pretibial myxedema (infiltrative dermopathy).

Q. Write short essay/notes on pretibial myxedema.

- Formerly used to occur in 5% of patients with only Graves' disease and 15% of patients with both Graves' disease and ophthalmopathy. However, the **incidence has declined** due to early diagnosis and treatment of Graves' disease.
- Characterized by **bilateral, asymmetric, nonpitting, scaly thickening, and induration of the skin.**
- Lesion may be **violaceous or slightly pigmented** (yellow-brown) and often have a peau d'orange appearance.
- The most frequent location is over the **lower limbs**, especially the pretibial areas or the dorsum of the foot. Rarely, the fingers and hands, elbows, arms, or face are affected (**Fig. 2.7**).
- Rarely, lesions progress to involve the legs, feet, or hands completely, resulting in a form reminiscent of elephantiasis.
- Occurs due to **deposition of glycosaminoglycans** especially hyaluronic acid, secreted by fibroblasts under the stimulation of local cytokines arising from a lymphocytic infiltration.
- **Treatment of pretibial myxedema**
  - Some patients do not seek treatment as they are asymptomatic.
  - **Indications:** Pruritus, local discomfort, the unsightly appearance of the lesions, or progression of lesions.
  - **Nonpharmacologic** includes minimizing risk factors, such as avoiding tobacco, reducing weight, normalizing thyroid function and in severe cases, physiotherapy. Normalization of thyroid function does not necessarily improve pretibial myxedema.
  - **Pharmacologic**
    - Topical 0.025% **fluocinolone acetonide** under plastic wrap.
    - **Intralesional corticosteroids** if there is no improvement with topical treatment after 4–12 weeks, using **triamcinolone acetate** dose calculated according to 8 mg per 2 cm—diameter circle area at each session, but the total dose was not >100 mg at each session in a patient.
    - **Pentoxifylline** may be helpful in resistant cases.

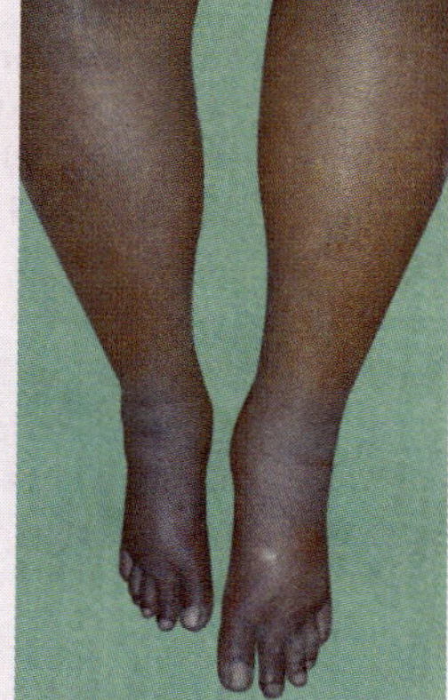

FIG. 2.7: Nonpitting pedal edema-myxedema.

Box 2.7 lists the other disorders associated with Graves' disease.

Box 2.7: Other disorders associated with Graves' disease.

- **Autoimmune disorders**
  - **Endocrine:** Addison's disease, type 1 diabetes mellitus (DM), Hashimoto's thyroiditis, primary gonadal failure, hypophysitis
  - **Nonendocrine:** Celiac disease, pernicious anemia, myasthenia gravis, immune thrombocytopenic purpura, rheumatoid arthritis, vitiligo, and alopecia areata
- **Others:** Hypokalemic periodic paralysis and mitral valve prolapse

Subclinical hyperthyroidism

- **Clinical manifestations (Box 2.8).**

Box 2.8: Clinical manifestations of subclinical hyperthyroidism.

Bone disease
- Decreased bone density, especially in postmenopausal women
- Increased fracture risk
- Biochemical markers of increased bone resorption
  - Increased urinary pyridinoline and deoxypyridinoline excretion
  - Increased urinary hydroxyproline excretion

Heart disease
- Increased incidence of atrial fibrillation
- Increased heart rate and incidence of atrial premature beats
- Increased cardiac contractility
- Increased left ventricular mass index and septal and posterior wall thickness

Laboratory abnormalities
- Decrease in serum total and low-density lipoprotein low-density lipoprotein (LDL) cholesterol concentrations
- Increased serum concentrations of hepatic enzymes and creatine kinase
- Increased serum concentration of sex hormone-binding globulin (SHBG)

Other
- Decreased time asleep at night
- Improved mood

- **Laboratory findings:** Serum levels of free T_4 and T_3 are within normal limits. Serum TSH levels is subnormal (<0.5 mU/L).

Investigations of Graves' Disease

- **TSH levels: Very low or undetectable**. This is performed as the primary test and normal level excludes thyrotoxicosis.
- **Serum T_3 and T_4 levels:** Raised in most cases. T_3 thyrotoxicosis is associated with raised T_3 levels and normal T_4 level.
- **Absence of TSH response** following intravenous **TRH**.
- **^{131}I uptake by the thyroid gland:** It may be increased but not necessary to perform in most of the patients.
- **TSH receptor antibody (TRAb):** Present in most cases.
- Few patients may show minor LFT abnormalities, mild hypercalcemia, and glycosuria.

Q. Write short essay/notes on drugs used in thyrotoxicosis.

Q. Write short essay/notes on adverse effects of antithyroid drugs.

Management of Hyperthyroidism of Graves' Disease

- The therapeutic approach to Graves' hyperthyroidism consists of both **rapid amelioration** of symptoms with a beta-blocker and measures aimed at **decreasing thyroid hormone synthesis**: the administration of a thionamide, radioiodine ablation, or surgery.
- **Symptom control:** Beta-blocker, **Propranolol** (drug of choice) in the dose of 20–40 mg 6 hourly or **Atenolol** 25–50 mg/day to reduce symptoms for immediate relief **due to sympathetic overactivity** such as anxiety, palpitation, increased bowel activity, lid retraction, finger tremors.
- **Decrease thyroid hormone synthesis:** There are 3 treatment options for Graves' disease. All three options are effective, but all three options have significant side effects. There is no consensus as to the "best" treatment: (i) Antithyroid drugs (thionamides), (ii) Radioiodine and (iii) Surgery.

1. **Antithyroid drugs (ATD)** may be used initially to control hyperthyroidism (in addition to beta-blockers) prior to definitive therapy with radioiodine or surgery; they may be prescribed for 1–2 years to attain a remission, or may be used long-term.
   - **Indications:** Primary therapy in **pregnancy**, in **children** and **adolescents** and **severe Graves' disease with eye changes**.
   - The drugs include: **Thionamides: Methimazole, Propylthiouracil, and Carbimazole**
   - **Mechanism of action:** Inhibit the function of **thyroid peroxidase (TPO) enzyme** and prevent binding of iodine to tyrosine (prevents iodination and organification).
     - **Methimazoleis the primary drug used to treat hyperthyroidism. Dose:**
       - Free T_4 1–1.5 times upper limit of normal: begin treatment with 5–10 mg once daily.
       - Free T_4 1.5–2 times upper limit of normal: begin treatment with 10–20 mg once daily.
       - Free T_4 2–3 times upper limit of normal: begin treatment on 20–40 mg daily in divided doses.
       - The dose is tapered to maintenance levels (5–10 mg/day) as the patient improves.
     - **Propylthiouracil:** Preferred during the first trimester of pregnancy. **Dose:** 300 mg daily in 3 equally divided doses; 400 mg daily in patients with severe hyperthyroidism and/or very large goiters; usual maintenance: 100–150 mg daily in 3 divided doses.
     - **Carbimazole:** It has additional immunosuppressive action.
       - **Dose:** Initially 20–60 mg daily given in 2–3 divided doses and maintenance 5–15 mg daily or alternatively 20–60 mg daily.
       - **Total duration of treatment:** 18–24 months.
       - **Adverse effects:** Rashes, urticaria, fever, arthralgia, blood dyscrasias **(agranulocytosis),** hepatotoxicity, aplasia cutis in neonates.
   - **Advantages:**
     - No surgical risk, scar, or chances of injury to parathyroid or recurrent laryngeal nerve.
     - Hypothyroidism, if induced, is reversible.
     - Can be used even in children and young adults.
   - **Disadvantages:**
     - Prolonged (often lifelong) treatment is needed and relapse rate is high.
     - Not practicable in uncooperative patient.
2. **Radioiodine ablation:** Preferred as **definitive therapy** of hyperthyroidism in nonpregnant patients except in patients with moderate or severe orbitopathy and chronic smokers. Administered as a capsule I^{131}, induces extensive tissue damage by emitting gamma-radiation from within the follicles, resulting in ablation of the thyroid within 6–18 weeks.
   - **Dose:** 185–555 MBq
   - **Indications:** (i) Patients **above 40 years of age,** (ii) young patients with a short life-span due to some other reason, and (iii) young individuals who are sterilized.
   - **Complication: Hypothyroidism**, infertility, and secondary cancers.
3. **Surgery: Subtotal thyroidectomy** is the **treatment of choice**. Surgical treatment is reserved for multinodular goiter (MNG) with following features:
   - Severe hyperthyroidism in children.
   - Pregnant women who cannot tolerate antithyroid drugs.
   - Large goiters with severe ophthalmopathy or with pressure symptoms.
   - Patients who require quick normalization of thyroid function
   - **Preparation for thyroidectomy:** It includes pretreatment with propranolol or atenolol, methimazole 5–40 mg depending on severity and potassium iodide (to decrease vascularity and make the gland firm) 8 mg iodide per drop, 5–7 drops three times daily for 2 weeks before surgery.
   - **Postoperative complications:** Hypothyroidism, hypoparathyroidism, hypocalcemia, and damage to recurrent laryngeal nerve.

- **Adjunctive therapies:**
  - **Oral radiocontrast agents: Sodium ipodate** and **iopanoic acid** are potent inhibitors of the peripheral conversion of T_4 to T_3. **Dose:** A dose of 500–1,000 mg/day in combination with methimazole can rapidly ameliorate severe hyperthyroidism and can also be used to prepare a hyperthyroid patient for early surgery.

- **Iodine elixirs:** Up to 10 drops of **saturated solution of potassium iodide** [SSKI, 50 mg iodide per drop (0.05 mL)] daily for 7–10 days is used perioperatively to reduce gland vascularity.
- **Glucocorticoids** inhibit peripheral T_4 to T_3 conversion and in patients with Graves' hyperthyroidism reduce thyroid secretion (**Table 2.11**).
- **Cholestyramine**, given in a dose of 4 g four times daily with methimazole, lowers serum T_4 and T_3 concentrations more rapidly than methimazole alone.
- **Potassium perchlorate:** It reduces uptake of iodine. It is more toxic and produces red cell aplasia. It is used only as temporary measure in iodine-induced thyrotoxicosis or when other therapy is not acceptable.
- **Lithium:** Blocks thyroid hormone release, but its use has been limited by its toxicity.
- **Rituximab:** May induce a sustained remission in patients with Graves' disease and induces low TSH-receptor antibodies (TRAb) levels, but its cost and side effects limit its utility

• **Skeletal Health:** Advised to **ingest 1,200–1,500 mg elemental calcium** daily through diet or supplements.

TABLE 2.11: Treatment of Graves' hyperthyroidism.

Therapy	*Advantages*	*Disadvantages*
Thionamides	Chance of permanent remission Some patients avoid permanent hypothyroidism Lower initial cost	Minor side effects - Rash, hives, arthralgias, transient granulocytopenia, gastrointestinal symptoms Major side effects - Agranulocytosis, vasculitis (lupus-like syndrome), hepatitis Risk of fetal goiter, hypothyroidism, and birth defects if pregnant Requires more frequent monitoring
Radioiodine	Permanent resolution of hyperthyroidism	Permanent hypothyroidism Patient must take radiation precautions for several days after treatment, avoiding contact with young children and pregnant women Development or worsening of Graves ophthalmopathy Rare radiation thyroiditis Patient concerns about long-term oncogenic effects of radiation
Surgery	Rapid, permanent cure of hyperthyroidism	Permanent hypothyroidism Risks for iatrogenic hypoparathyroidism and recurrent laryngeal nerve damage Risks associated with general anesthesia High cost

Approach for the hyperthyroidism is presented in **Flowchart 2.3**.

FLOWCHART 2.3: Approach to diagnosis in hyperthyroidism.

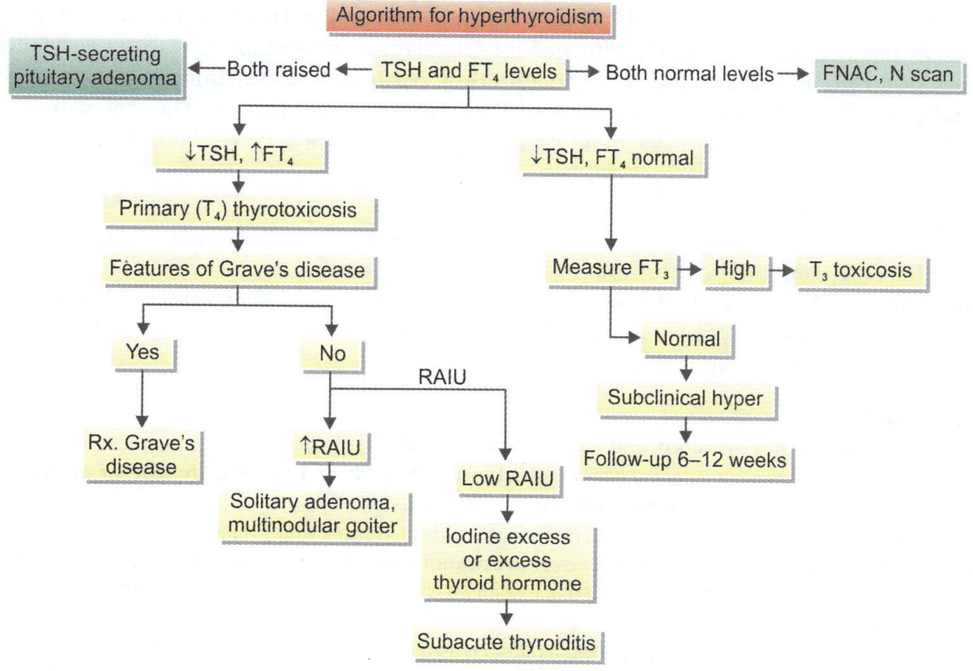

[FT_4: free T_4 (tetrahydrothyronine); FT_3: free T_3 (triiodothyronine); TSH: thyroid-stimulating hormone; RAIU: radioactive iodine uptake]

Hyperthyroid Crisis/Thyrotoxic Crisis/Thyroid Storm

Q. Write short essay/note on hyperthyroid crisis/thyrotoxic crisis/thyroid storm/thyroid crisis.

It is a rare **life-threatening** medical emergency that develops as **complication of thyrotoxicosis** which is associated with a mortality of 10-30%.

Causes of Hyperthyroid Crisis

- Thyroid storm can develop in patients with longstanding untreated hyperthyroidism (Graves' disease, toxic multinodular goiter, and solitary toxic adenoma), it is often precipitated by an acute event:
  - **Severe infections** in a patient with previously undetected or inadequately treated hyperthyroidism/thyrotoxicosis.
  - **Following surgery:** May develop **following subtotal thyroidectomy** in an ill-prepared patient or some other surgery in an undetected hyperthyroidism/thyrotoxicosis.
  - **Following radiotherapy:** May occur within a few days of ^{131}I therapy in an inadequately prepared patient. This is because of a transient rise in serum thyroid hormone levels caused due to acute damage by irradiation.
  - **Other precipitating factors:**
    - Cerebrovascular accidents
    - Diabetic ketoacidosis
    - Acute coronary syndrome
    - Use of iodine contrast agent
    - Acute iodine load
    - Parturition
    - Sudden withdrawal of antithyroid medications
    - Stress
    - Major trauma.
- It is unclear why certain factors result in the development of thyroid storm. Hypotheses include a **rapid rate of increase** in **serum thyroid hormone** levels, **increased responsiveness to catecholamines**, or **enhanced cellular responses to thyroid hormone**. One study found that while the total T_4 and T_3 levels were similar to those seen in uncomplicated patients, the free T_4 and free T_3 concentrations were higher in patients with thyroid storm.

Clinical Features

- The clinical manifestations are due to **marked hypermetabolism** and **excessive adrenergic response.**
- **Hyperpyrexia** from 104°F to 106°F is common and is associated with flushing and sweating.
- **Marked tachycardia** rates that can exceed 140 beats/min, often with **atrial fibrillation** and high pulse pressure, hypotension, occasionally congestive heart failure occurs. A fatal outcome is associated with heart failure and shock.
- **Central nervous system symptoms** include marked **agitation, restlessness, delirium**, psychosis, stupor, and coma.
- **Gastrointestinal symptoms** include nausea, vomiting, diarrhea, abdominal pain, and hepatic failure with jaundice.
- **Physical examination** may reveal goiter, ophthalmopathy (in the presence of Graves' disease), lid lag, hand tremor, and warm and moist skin.

Laboratory Findings

- **Low TSH** and **high free T_4 and/or T_3** concentrations
- Nonspecific laboratory findings may include—mild hyperglycemia secondary to a catecholamine-induced inhibition of insulin release and increased glycogenolysis, mild hypercalcemia due to hemoconcentration and enhanced bone resorption, abnormal liver function tests, leukocytosis, or leukopenia.

Treatment of Hyperthyroid Crisis

- Patients should be admitted in ICU, **rehydrated,** and given **antibiotics** if there is infection.
- **Control hyperthermia:** Aggressively by external cooling. **Acetaminophen should be used instead of aspirin** since the latter can increase serum free T_4 and T_3 concentrations by interfering with their protein binding
- **Propranolol:** Either orally (60–80 mg every 4–6 hours) or intravenously (1–5 mg 4 times daily). It also blocks peripheral conversion of T_4 to T_3. The Japanese guidelines recommend **esmolol** over **propranolol** because of increased mortality in patients with congestive heart failure treated with propranolol. In patients with reactive airways disease, cardio-selective beta-blockers such as **metoprolol** or **atenolol** could be considered.
- **Propylthiouracil** 200 mg orally every 4 hours (preferred as it decreases T_4 to T_3 conversion) or **methimazole** (20 mg orally every 4–6 hours) **or carbimazole** (inhibit the synthesis of new thyroid hormone) 15–30 mg stat followed by 15 mg TID. In an unconscious or uncooperative patient, carbimazole can be administered rectally with good effect.
- **Lugol's iodine:** 10 drops TID about 1 hour after the first dose of thionamide.
- **Sodium iopodate:** 500 mg/day orally will restore serum T_3 levels to normal within 48–72 hours. This is a radiographic contrast medium which inhibits the release of thyroid hormones and also reduces the conversion of T_4 to T_3. Hence, more effective than potassium iodide or Lugol's solution.

- **IV hydrocortisone:** 100 mg every 8 hours.
- **Bile acid sequestrant, cholestyramine:** 4 g orally QID to reduce enterohepatic recycling of thyroid hormones.
- **Benzodiazepines:** For agitation.
- **Digoxin:** To control cardiac failure and atrial fibrillation (AF).
- **Plasmapheresis** has been tried when traditional therapy has not been successful, it removes cytokines, antibodies, and thyroid hormones from plasma.
- **Lithium** has also been given to acutely block the release of thyroid hormone. However, its renal and neurologic toxicity limit its utility.

Hypothyroidism

Q. Describe the etiology, clinical features, diagnosis, and management of primary hypothyroidism/spontaneous atrophic hypothyroidism?

- Hypothyroidism is a **clinical syndrome resulting from a deficiency of thyroid hormones.** It results in a generalized slowing down of metabolic processes.
- **Infants and children:** Hypothyroidism results in marked **slowing of growth and development** with serious permanent consequences including **mental retardation**, when it occurs in infancy **(cretinism)**.
- **Adults:** Hypothyroidism causes a **generalized decrease in metabolism** with slowed heart rate, diminished oxygen consumption, and deposition of glycosaminoglycans in intracellular spaces, particularly in skin and muscle, producing in extreme cases the clinical picture of **myxedema**.

Classification and Etiology (Table 2.12)

TABLE 2.12: Etiology of hypothyroidism.

Primary	*Secondary*	*Tertiary*
➢ Dyshormonogenesis **(Pendred syndrome)** ➢ Hashimoto's thyroiditis (chronic autoimmune thyroiditis) ➢ Radioactive iodine therapy ➢ External neck irradiation ➢ Subtotal thyroidectomy for Graves' disease, nodular goiter, or thyroid cancer ➢ Excessive iodide intake (radiocontrast dyes) ➢ Subacute thyroiditis (usually transient) ➢ Postpartum thyroiditis ➢ Iodide deficiency ➢ Drugs: Lithium, interferon-alfa, amiodarone, PTU, methimazole, ethionamide, ipilimumab, pembrolizumab, and nivolumab ➢ Environmental exposures: polybrominated diphenyl ethers (fire retardant) ➢ Infiltrative diseases: fibrous thyroiditis (Reidel's thyroiditis), hemochromatosis, scleroderma, leukemia, and cystinosis	➢ Hypopituitarism due to pituitary adenoma ➢ Pituitary ablative therapy ➢ Pituitary destruction ➢ Sheehan syndrome ➢ Trauma ➢ Hypophysitis ➢ Nonpituitary tumors such as craniopharyngiomas ➢ Infiltrative diseases ➢ Inactivating mutations in the gene for either TSH or the TSH receptor	➢ Hypothalamic dysfunction (rare) ➢ Mutations in the gene for the TRH receptor ➢ Hypothalamic damage results from – Tumors – Trauma – Radiation therapy – Infiltrative diseases ➢ Rarely peripheral resistance to the action of thyroid hormone

Q. Write short essay/note on causes of hypothyroidism and treatment.

- **Primary hypothyroidism:** Due **intrinsic disorder of the thyroid gland**. Accounts for over 95% of cases of hypothyroidism. There are **two** degrees of primary hypothyroidism:
  1. **Subclinical hypothyroidism**, defined as a **high serum TSH** concentration in the presence of **normal serum free T_4 and T_3** concentrations.
  2. **Overt hypothyroidism**, defined as a **high serum TSH** concentration in the presence of a **low serum free T_4** concentration.
- **Central hypothyroidism:** It is rare and is caused due to **failure of TSH and TRH production** due to disease of anterior pituitary (**secondary hypothyroidism**) or hypothalamus (**tertiary hypothyroidism**).
- ***Hashimoto's thyroiditis (chronic autoimmune thyroiditis)***
  - **Most common cause** of primary hypothyroidism in iodine sufficient areas of the world.
  - Organ-specific **autoimmune disorder** of thyroid characterized gradual thyroid failure with or without goiter formation by lymphoid infiltration of thyroid leading to apoptosis, fibrosis, and atrophy.
  - The two major forms of Hashimoto's thyroiditis are **goitrous autoimmune thyroiditis** and **atrophic autoimmune thyroiditis** (often called **primary myxedema**), with the common pathologic feature being lymphocytic infiltration, and follicular destruction.
  - Patients have **TRAb** that block the effects of endogenous TSH, antibodies to TPO and thyroglobulin.
  - The cause of Hashimoto's thyroiditis is thought to be a combination of **genetic susceptibility** and **environmental factors**.
  - Several mechanisms have been proposed for the pathogenesis of Hashimoto's thyroiditis. These include **molecular mimicry** and **bystander activation** including the involvement of thyroid cell expression of HLAs and activation of thyroid cell apoptosis by a Fas ligand-Fas interaction.

- It may be observed in **some patients of Graves' disease** treated with antithyroid drugs 10–20 years earlier.
- Patients have **high-risk of** developing **other autoimmune disorders** such as type 1 diabetes mellitus, pernicious anemia and Addison's disease.

- ***Postpartum thyroiditis***
    - It is a **destructive thyroiditis** induced by an **autoimmune mechanism** within **1 year of parturition.**
    - It may produce **transient hyperthyroidism** alone, **transient hypothyroidism** alone or the **two sequentially** and then **recovery.**
    - Thyroid biopsies in women with postpartum thyroiditis show **lymphocytic infiltration**, with occasional **germinal centers**, and **disruption and collapse of thyroid follicles** (lymphocytic thyroiditis).
    - **Laboratory assessment** of thyroid function should be performed at **3 and 6 months postpartum** in women at high-risk for developing postpartum thyroiditis, including women with **type 1 diabetes mellitus**, a history of **postpartum thyroiditis after a previous pregnancy** and **history of high serum antithyroid peroxidase antibody concentrations** prior to pregnancy.

TABLE 2.13: Clinical features of hypothyroidism.

System involved	*Symptoms/Signs*	
General	Lethargy Somnolence **Weight gain** **Goiter (iodine deficiency, Hashimoto's thyroiditis)**	**Cold intolerance** Hoarse voice Pallor Cognitive dysfunction
Thyroid	Enlargement of the gland	
Gastrointestinal	Reduced appetite Constipation Decreased taste Gastric atrophy Celiac disease	Ileus Macroglossia Nonalcoholic fatty liver disease Ascites
Cardiorespiratory	Angina **Bradycardia** **Diastolic hypertension** Cardiac failure **Pericardial effusion** Pleural effusion Dyslipidemia	Hyperhomocysteinemia Fatigue Shortness of breath on exertion Rhinitis Hypoventilation Reduced pulmonary responses to hypoxia and hypercapnia
Neuromuscular	Aches and pains Muscle stiffness Delayed relaxation of tendon reflexes **(Woltman's sign)*** Carpal tunnel syndrome **Depression** Psychosis	Cerebellar **ataxia** Deafness Myotonia Proximal myopathy Pseudohypertrophy of muscles Hashimoto encephalopathy
Skin	**Myxedema** (nonpitting edema of the skin of hands, feet and eyelids) Dry flaky skin and hair Alopecia Brittle nails Vitiligo	Purplish lips Malar flush Carotenemia Erythema ab igne Xanthelasmas Madarosis (thinning of lateral one-third of eyebrows)
Reproductive	**Pubertal delay** **Menorrhagia** Infertility	Galactorrhea (hyperprolactinemia) Impotence
Hematological	Macrocytosis Normochromic, normocytic hypoproliferative Anemia	Hypothyroidism associated hypocoagulable state
Renal	Impaired GFR Renal dysfunction Raised creatinine	
Miscellaneous	➢ Obstructive sleep apnea: Mostly due to macroglossia ➢ Hyponatremia	

Note: Bold words indicate symptoms of greater discriminant value. * Woltman's sign (hung up ankle jerk) is due to decreased myosin ATPase activity and decreased rate of reaccumulation of calcium in the sarcoplasmic reticulum.

Clinical Features (Table 2.13)

Q. Write short essay/note on clinical features of hypothyroidism.

- Depends on the duration and severity of the hypothyroidism.
- **Consequence of prolonged hypothyroidism:**
    - **Infiltration of many body tissues** by the mucopolysaccharides, hyaluronic acid and chondroitin sulfate.
    - **Infiltration of the dermis** produces nonpitting edema (myxedema).
    - The term myxedema refers to the **accumulation of mucopolysaccharides in the subcutaneous tissues.** It is most marked in the skin of the hands, feet, and eyelids.
    - **Myxedema facies:** It is a **peculiar facial appearance** characterized by:
        - Striking **periorbital puffiness** (due to myxedema)
        - Scanty eyebrows
        - **Facial pallor** (due to vasoconstriction and anemia), or a **lemon-yellow tint to the skin** (due to **carotenemia** produced by reduced conversion of carotene to vitamin A)
        - Purplish lips and malar flush.
- **Most cases** of hypothyroidism are **not clinically obvious** and should be kept in mind when individuals complain of non-specific symptoms such as tiredness, weight gain, depression or carpal tunnel syndrome.
- Many cases are diagnosed on biochemical screening.

Investigations of Primary Hypothyroidism (Flowchart 2.4)

Majority of hypothyroidism results from an intrinsic disorder of the thyroid gland (primary hypothyroidism).

- **Serum TSH:** It is the investigation of choice. **High** TSH level **confirms primary hypothyroidism.**
- **Serum T_4 levels: Low** level confirms the hypothyroid state.

FLOWCHART 2.4: Algorithm for hypothyroidism.

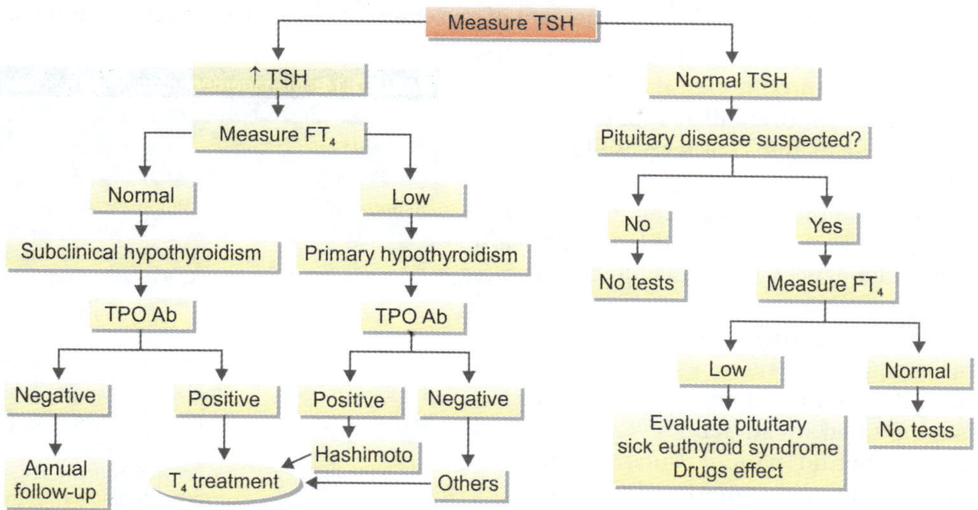

[T_4: free T_4 (tetrahydrothyronine); TPOAb: thyroid peroxidase antibodies; TSH: thyroid-stimulating hormone]

- **Thyroid and other organ-specific antibodies** may be found.
- **Other abnormalities:**
  - **Increased serum aspartate transferase** from muscle and/or liver
  - Increased serum lactate dehydrogenase (LDH) and **creatine kinase** (CK): With associated myopathy
  - **Hypercholesterolemia and hypertriglyceridemia**
  - **Hyponatremia:** Due to an increase in ADH and impaired free water clearance.
  - **Anemia:** Usually normochromic and normocytic
- **Electrocardiogram (ECG):** Demonstrates sinus bradycardia, low voltage QRS complexes, and ST segment and T wave abnormalities.
- **Chest radiograph:** May reveal enlarged cardiac shadow.

Q. Write short essay/note on treatment of hypothyroidism (drug, dose, and duration of therapy).

Treatment of Hypothyroidism

- Hypothyroidism is treated with $\mathbf{T_4}$.
- Replacement therapy with **levothyroxine sodium** is given for life as a once daily dosage **(1.6–2.3 µg/kg/day).**
- **Initial dose**: It depends upon the severity of the deficiency as well as on the age and fitness of the patient.
  - **For young healthy patients**—1.6 µg/kg/day.
  - **For older patients or those with coronary heart disease**—25–50 µg/day
- **Timing:** Should be taken on an empty stomach with water, ideally an hour before breakfast.
- The patient with symptomatic improvement should be re-evaluated with serum TSH measured in 4–6 weeks. If the TSH remains above the reference range, the dose of T_4 can be **increased by 12–25 µg/day in older patients** and in younger patients, it can be increased by a higher dose. The patient will require a repeat TSH measurement in 6 weeks.
- **For patients with heart disease:** 12.5–25 µg/day and increase by 12.5–25 µg/day, if needed, at 6–8 weeks intervals. Few patients with ischemic heart disease may develop angina or worsen with therapy. They require β-blockers, vasodilators or coronary artery bypass graft (CABG) or angioplasty.
- **Dosage adjustments**
  - **Age:** In elderly start with half dose.
  - **Severity and duration of hypothyroidism:** Increase the dose in severe cases
  - **Weight:** 0.5 µg/kg/day increase up to 3.0 µg/kg/day
  - **Malabsorption:** Requires increased dose
  - **Concomitant drug therapy:** Thyroxine only to be taken on empty stomach
  - **Pregnancy:** 25–50% increase in dose, safe in lactating mother
  - **Presence of cardiac disease:** Start low dose or alternate day treatment.
- **Monitoring**
  - **Goal:** It is to **normalize TSH level** regardless of cause of hypothyroidism and to **restore $\mathbf{T_4}$ within the normal range**.
  - **Adequacy of replacement: Assessed clinically** and by **thyroid function tests** after 6 weeks on a steady dose.
  - Complete suppression of TSH should be avoided because it may cause atrial fibrillation and osteoporosis.
  - Lifelong therapy is needed.

Myxedema Coma

Q. Write short essay on clinical features and management of myxedema coma and myxedema madness.

- Myxedema coma is a **very rare and life-threatening medical emergency** with a high mortality rate that develops as a **complication of severe hypothyroidism (Table 2.14)**.
- The **hallmarks** of myxedema coma are **decreased mentation** and **hypothermia.**
- Other features are bradycardia, hyponatremia, hypoglycemia, hypotension, puffiness of the hands and face, puffy nose, swollen lips, enlarged tongue, hypoventilation, and features of the precipitating cause/illness.
- **Epidemiology and precipitating factors:**
  - It can occur as the culmination of severe longstanding hypothyroidism with **older women** being most affected.
  - It can be precipitated by an acute event in a poorly controlled hypothyroid patient, such as infection, myocardial infarction, hypothermia, surgery, drugs (amiodarone, β-blockers, diuretics, anesthetic agents, barbiturates, lithium, narcotics, and phenothiazines), cardiac failure, hypoxia, hyponatremia, and hypercapnia.
- **Warning signs:** Presence of cool pale skin (due to **hypothermia**—body temperature may be as low as 25°C), absence of mild diastolic hypertension, and altered sensorium.
- **Laboratory findings**
  - Serum **free T_4 is low**, **serum TSH** is usually **high** but sometimes only slightly elevated.
  - Serum **cortisol**, maybe low in patients with central hypothyroidism with associated hypopituitarism and secondary adrenal insufficiency.
  - **Serum creatine phosphokinase** mostly markedly raised.
  - **Hyponatremia**

TABLE 2.14: Management of myxedema coma.

Treatment must be started before biochemical confirmation of the diagnosis.

Abnormality	*Treatment*
Hypothyroidism	Initial intravenous dose of 200–400 μg T_4, followed by daily IV dose of 50–100 μg until oral dose is possible. Total serum T_4 should increase by 2–4 μg/dL IV T_3, initially 5–20 μg, followed by 2.5–10 μg every 8 hours
Hypocortisolemia	IV hydrocortisone 100 mg every 8 hours
Hypoventilation	Intubation and mechanical ventilation
Hypothermia	Gentle warming of patient with blankets (passive rewarming) No active rewarming as it increases the risk for vasodilation and further hypotension.
Hyponatremia	Mild fluid restriction, 3% saline
Hypotension	Cautious volume expansion with crystalloid or whole blood and vasopressors.
Hypoglycemia	Glucose administration
Precipitating event	Identification and elimination by specific treatment (liberal use of empirical antibiotics)
Other measures	Monitor cardiac output and pressures Whenever needed, cautious use of intravenous fluids, high-flow oxygen or assisted ventilation

Myxedema Madness

- Patient presents with **hypothermia** and neuropsychiatric manifestations.
- **Neuropsychiatric manifestations:** Include:
  - Depression is common in hypothyroidism.
  - Rarely, elderly patient with severe hypothyroidism may become **frankly demented, psychotic, confused, disoriented,** sometimes with **striking delusions and hallucinations**.
- It may develop shortly after starting T_4 replacement.
- **Laboratory findings:**
  - Hypoglycemia and hyponatremia, increased CO_2, decreased WBC count and Hct, increased CPK.
  - Reduced ECG voltage, blood gases often reveal respiratory acidosis, hypoxia and hypercapnia.
  - **EEG**: Slow waves with decreased amplitude, triphasic waves may be present.
  - **CSF analysis**: Elevated protein levels (<100 mg/dL).

Sick Euthyroid Syndrome/Nonthyroid Illness State (NTIS)

Q. Write a short note on sick euthyroid syndrome.

- Nonthyroidal illness influences thyroid hormone production and action at multiple levels, including H-P-T axis, thyroid hormone transport, and metabolism.
- Changes in thyroid function in the setting of **systemic illness, surgery, or fasting not caused by primary thyroid or pituitary dysfunction** are referred to as the nonthyroidal illness syndrome (also called "sick euthyroid syndrome"). Also called "**low-T_3 syndrome**", due to the most common abnormality, a decreased level of serum total T_3.
- Measurement of serum T_4 concentration can be normal, low or elevated.
- Serum TSH, is usually normal but can be influenced by nonthyroidal illness.
- Conditions associated with euthyroid sick syndrome include **malnutrition, HIV, anorexia nervosa, trauma, myocardial infarction, chronic renal failure, diabetic ketoacidosis, cirrhosis, and sepsis**.
- Treatment with thyroxine is not recommended.

Subclinical Thyroid Diseases

Q. Write a short note/essay on subclinical thyroid diseases.

Q. Write a short note on subclinical hypothyroidism.

Subclinical Hypothyroidism

- **Subclinical hypothyroidism is defined as an increased serum TSH in the presence of a normal serum free T_4.**
- Prevalent in women and elderly persons.
- Common causes of subclinical hypothyroidism (**Box 2.8**)

Clinical consequences

- Progression to **overt hypothyroidism** (2–4% yearly)
- Risk of **CV disease** especially when TSH > 10 mU/L: Diastolic dysfunction, diastolic hypertension, increase in LDL-C, increased hsCRP, alteration in coagulation parameters, and endothelial dysfunction
- **Decreased fertility**
- **Nonalcoholic fatty liver disease (NAFLD)**
- Neuropsychiatric manifestations and increased risk for **Alzheimer disease.**

Indication for treatment with levothyroxine:

- Patients with serum TSH > 10.0 mU/L
- Patients <65–70 years, asymptomatic with TSH ≥ 7 mU/L
- Patients <65–70 years, symptomatic with TSH from *upper limit of normal* to 6.9 mU/L.
- Patients who are infertile, ovulatory dysfunction or planning for pregnancy.
- Symptoms or signs of hypothyroidism
- Goiter
- High serum anti-TPO antibodies.
- High vascular risk including ischemic heart disease, diabetes, dyslipidemia.

Box 2.8: Common causes of subclinical hypothyroidism.

- Iatrogenic
- Hashimoto's thyroiditis
- Postpartum thyroiditis, painless thyroiditis
- Thyroid infiltration (amyloidosis, sarcoidosis, hemochromatosis, etc.)
- Medications: Amiodarone, lithium, interferon, and sorafenib
- Partial thyroidectomy
- Head and neck radiation

Subclinical Hyperthyroidism (Box 2.9)

Q. Write a short note on subclinical hyperthyroidism.

- Defined as **normal** serum free T_4 and T_3 in the presence of **subnormal** TSH (<0.5 mU/L).
- Prevalence between 0.7 and 12.4%
- Natural course: 40-60% normalize. About 0.5-8% progresses to overt hyperthyroidism.
- **Effects of subclinical hyperthyroidism**
- **Cardiac effects** of subclinical hyperthyroidism (**Box 2.10**).
- **Noncardiac effects**:
  - Osteoporosis
  - Decreased Bone mineral density
  - Increased risk of fractures
  - Muscle weakness
  - Dementia, etc.

Box 2.9: Causes of subclinical hyperthyroidism.

- Iatrogenic (exogenous subclinical hyperthyroidism)
- Autonomously functioning thyroid adenomas and multinodular goiters (endogenous subclinical hyperthyroidism)
- Graves' disease (endogenous subclinical hyperthyroidism)
- Thyroiditis
- Euthyroid patients with Graves' orbitopathy
- Early Graves'
- Graves' disease in remission
- High hCG

Box 2.10: Cardiac effects of subclinical hyperthyroidism.

- Resting tachycardia
- Coronary heart disease
- Heart failure
- Atrial fibrillation
- Left ventricular hypertrophy
- Increase LV mass index
- Increase cardiac workload
- Diastolic dysfunction (impaired relaxation)
- Increased systolic function at rest
- Impaired systolic response to exercise

Thyroiditis

Q. Write a short note on causes of thyroiditis.

- It is a heterogeneous group of **inflammatory disorders involving the thyroid gland.**
- Etiologies range from autoimmune to infectious origins.
- The clinical course may be **acute, subacute, or chronic.**

Causes of Thyroiditis

See **Table 2.15.**

TABLE 2.15: Causes of thyroiditis.

Type	*Causes*
Acute	**Bacterial infections**: *Staphylococcus, Streptococcus, Enterobacter* **Fungal infections**: *Aspergillus, Candida, Histoplasma* **Radiation:** After ^{131}I treatment **Drugs:** Amiodarone (may also be subacute or chronic)
Subacute	Viral or granulomatous (de Quervain's) thyroiditis Silent thyroiditis (includes postpartum thyroiditis) Mycobacterial infection **Drug induced:** Interferon, amiodarone
Chronic	**Autoimmune:** Hashimoto's thyroiditis and Riedel's thyroiditis **Parasitic thyroiditis:** Echinococcosis, strongyloidiasis, cysticercosis **Traumatic:** Palpation thyroiditis

Subacute Thyroiditis (De Quervain's Thyroiditis)

Q. Write a short note on subacute thyroiditis (de Quervain's thyroiditis/granulomatous thyroiditis).

- A spontaneously remitting, painful, subacute inflammatory disease of the thyroid characterized by transient inflammation of the thyroid gland.
- Most prevalent in the temperate zone.
- Strongly associated with HLA-B35
- **Gender and age:** Affect women more often than men (3 to 5:1). It is most common in young adults and middle age.

Clinical Features

- **Prodromal viral symptoms:** These are often preceded by a viral infection (e.g., Coxsackie, mumps, adenovirus, measles) of upper respiratory tract. Prodromal symptoms include fever, malaise and pain in the neck with tachycardia, and local thyroid tenderness.
- **Anterior neck pain** in the region of thyroid is the **presenting symptom** is majority of cases and occurs abruptly and may be sometimes unilateral.
  - It **may radiate to the ear, mandible, or occiput**.
  - Pain may shift to the contralateral lobe (**creeping thyroiditis**).
  - Pain may be **aggravated** by **moving the head, swallowing, or coughing**.
- **Functional impairment: Initially** there is **hyperthyroidism followed by euthyroidism** and **later** followed by a period of **hypothyroidism.** Finally, **full recovery occurs in 4–6 months**. In about 5% of cases hypothyroidism may persist.
- **Signs: Enlarged diffusely or asymmetrically** and **tender thyroid gland**.

Laboratory Findings

- **Mildly elevated** serum free T_4 and T_3 and **low** serum TSH
- **Erythrocyte sedimentation rate (ESR):** Elevated (>50 mm/h may exceed 100 mm/h)
- **CRP** may be **elevated**
- **High** serum thyroglobulin
- **Mild** anemia
- **Leukocyte counts:** Normal or slightly elevated
- **Serum IL-6 and Tg concentrations:** Increased during the thyrotoxic phase.
- **Thyroid radionuclide uptake** is reduced or absent.
- **Thyroid antibodies** are **transiently detectable** at low titers in a minority of patients.

Treatment

- **Mild cases:** Salicylates (**aspirin** 2,600 mg daily) or NSAIDS (**naproxen** 500–1000mg daily in 2 divided doses or **ibuprofen** 1,200–3,200 mg daily in 3–4 divided doses) relieve pain and tenderness
- **Severe cases:** Corticosteroids (**prednisone** 40 mg/day) have a more dramatic and rapid effect.
- Symptoms of thyrotoxicosis should be managed with β-adrenergic blocking agents (**propranolol** 40–120 mg, **propranolol LA** 80 mg daily or 25–50 mg **atenolol** daily)
- If TSH > 10 mU/L or associated with symptoms, 50–100 mg of **levothyroxine** for 6–8 weeks.

Hashimoto's Thyroiditis

Q. Write short essay/note on Hashimoto's (autoimmune) thyroiditis.

- Organ-specific **autoimmune disorder** of thyroid characterized gradual thyroid failure with or without goiter formation by lymphoid infiltration of thyroid leading to apoptosis, fibrosis and atrophy with high titers of circulating:
  - **Antithyroid peroxidase (TPO) antibody (TPOAb)** in 95% patients.
  - **Antithyroglobulin (Tg) antibody** in 60–80% patients.
- **Most common cause** of primary hypothyroidism in iodine sufficient areas of the world.
- The two major forms of Hashimoto's thyroiditis are **goitrous autoimmune thyroiditis** and **atrophic autoimmune thyroiditis** (often called **primary myxedema**).
- **Age and gender:** Most often diagnosed between 50 and 60 years of age, more frequent in women than in men with a sex ratio of approximately 7:1.
- **Association with other autoimmune diseases:** Often associated with ulcerative colitis or type 1 diabetes mellitus, pernicious anemia and Addison's disease.

Pathology

- **Lymphocytic infiltration** (lymphoid follicles with germinal center)
- Fibrosis

- Follicular cell hyperplasia
- Presence of **oxyphil cells** (Ashkenazy cells/Hürthle cells).

Clinical Features

- **Most** patients are **asymptomatic.**
- Some may have a feeling of tightness or fullness in the neck.
- Neck pain and tenderness are rare.
- **Hypothyroidism, the most common cause** of **goitrous hypothyroidism**. About 25% present with hypothyroidism and remaining are at a higher risk of developing in future years.
- **Hashitoxicosis** is seen in the acute phase.
- Chronic autoimmune thyroiditis is a **component of type 2 autoimmune polyglandular syndrome**
- **Physical examination:** Diffuse enlargement of thyroid with firm or rubbery consistency.

Investigations

Q. **Investigations and treatment of Hashimoto's thyroiditis.**

- **Thyroid function tests:** Show features of **hypothyroidism**
- **Antithyroid peroxidase (TPO) antibody (TPOAb)** in 95% patients
- **Antithyroglobulin (Tg) antibody** in 60–80% patients
- **Antinuclear factor (ANF)** may be found in patients below the age of 20 years
- **Ultrasound of thyroid:** Reduced echogenicity
- **Fine-needle aspiration cytology (FNAC) of thyroid.**

Complication

An increased risk for **thyroid lymphoma** (rare).

Treatment

Levothyroxine (150–200 µg/day) is indicated for the treatment of hypothyroidism and it may produce shrinkage of goiter. The dose of thyroxine should be sufficient enough to suppress serum TSH to low but detectable levels.

Riedel's Thyroiditis (Sclerosing Thyroiditis/Ligneous Thyroiditis/Invasive Fibrous Thyroiditis)

- Rare, chronic inflammatory disorder of unknown etiology.
- Characterized by **dense fibrosis** of the **thyroid gland and adjacent perithyroidal tissues** (parathyroid glands, the recurrent laryngeal nerve and trachea), and extra cervical areas (fibrous mediastinitis, retroperitoneal fibrosis, retro-orbital fibrosis, sclerosing cholangitis, and pancreatitis).
- **Women** are four times more likely than men to be affected, and it most commonly occurs between the ages of **30 and 50 years**.

Clinical Features

- Usually present with a long history of a **painless, progressively increasing anterior neck mass.**
- Most patients are euthyroid.
- **Pressure symptoms:**
  - Dysphagia
  - Cough
  - Hoarseness
  - Stridor
  - Attacks of suffocation may be present.
  - Local obstructive pneumonia
  - Superior vena cava syndrome
- **Physical examination:** A **stony-hard or woody thyroid** mass which varies in size from small to very large. It may involve one or both lobes and is **fixed to surrounding structures.**

Investigations

- **Thyroid function test:** 25-67% have subclinical or overt hypothyroidism.
- **Thyroid antibodies:** May be found in about 45% of patients.
- **Serum calcium:** May be low due to parathyroid invasion.
- **Imaging:**
  - **USG** shows heterogeneous **hypoechoic lesions** that may infiltrate the perithyroid muscles
  - **Doppler** shows absence of vascular flow in the Riedel's regions.

    - **CT/MRI** shows extent of fibrosis.
    - Riedel's thyroiditis is hypermetabolic on **FDG-PET**.
- The differential diagnosis based on **FNAC** includes su**bacute thyroiditis, a fibrosing variant of Hashimoto's thyroiditis, radiation-induced thyroiditis, and malignancy, specifically a paucicellular variant of anaplastic cancer.**
- **Definitive diagnosis** can be established pathologically only by **open biopsy**, since FNAC may be difficult to interpret due to insufficient thyroid epithelial cells but may reveal mononuclear cells and fibrous tissue.

Treatment
- If untreated, this condition may stabilize or regress.
- **Glucocorticoids** has reduced enlargement and induced softening of mass in a few patients; however, therapy is long- term and it recurs when steroids are tapered.
- **Tamoxifen** 10–20 mg twice daily
- **Rituximab** intravenous 375 mg/m^2 monthly for 3 months
- **Mycophenolate mofetil** 1 g twice daily
- **Surgery:** Indicated to relieve tracheal and esophageal compression or to rule out malignancy. Surgery should be limited to relieve the obstruction and extensive resection is not indicated to avoid injury to adjacent adhering structures.
- **Radiation:** Low dose in cases refractory to other treatment.

Goiter

Goiter is the enlargement of thyroid gland.

Classification (Table 2.16)

TABLE 2.16: Classification of goiter.

Diffuse	*Nodular*
➢ **Simple (nontoxic):** Physiological (puberty, pregnancy), iodine deficiency (endemic goiter) ➢ **Toxic goiter:** Graves' disease ➢ **Autoimmune/inflammatory:** Hashimoto's thyroiditis, de Quervain's thyroiditis, Riedel's thyroiditis ➢ Dyshormonogenesis, goitrogens (e.g., sulfonylureas)	➢ Multinodular goiter, toxic multinodular goiter (Plummer's disease) ➢ Solitary nodular fibrotic (Riedel's thyroiditis) ➢ Cysts ➢ **Tumors:** – Benign: Adenomas – Malignant: Carcinoma and lymphomas ➢ **Miscellaneous:** Sarcoidosis and tuberculosis

Simple (Nontoxic) Goiter

- Diffuse nontoxic (simple) goiter is characterized by the **diffuse enlargement of the thyroid gland without any nodularity**.
- This includes: **Simple hyperplastic goiter (colloid goiter)**
- **Causes:**
    - Physiological in pregnancy, puberty
    - Iodine deficiency.
- **Appearance:** Large, smooth firm, and nontender goiter
- **Effect:** Euthyroid and pressure effect.

Risk Factors for Malignancy in Goiter

- Solitary thyroid nodules in patients >60 or <30 years of age
- Irradiation of the neck or face during infancy or teenage years
- Past history of surgery
- Presence of cervical lymphadenopathy
- Symptoms of pain or pressure (especially a change in voice)
- Male sex
- Large nodules (>3 or 4 cm)
- Growth of nodule

Diffuse Nontoxic (Simple) Goiter

Q. Write short essay/note on clinical features, investigations and treatment of goiter/multinodular goiter.

Diffuse nontoxic (simple) goiter is characterized by the diffuse enlargement of the thyroid gland without any nodularity (**Flowchart 2.5**).

FLOWCHART 2.5: Algorithm for approach to goiter and its treatment modality.

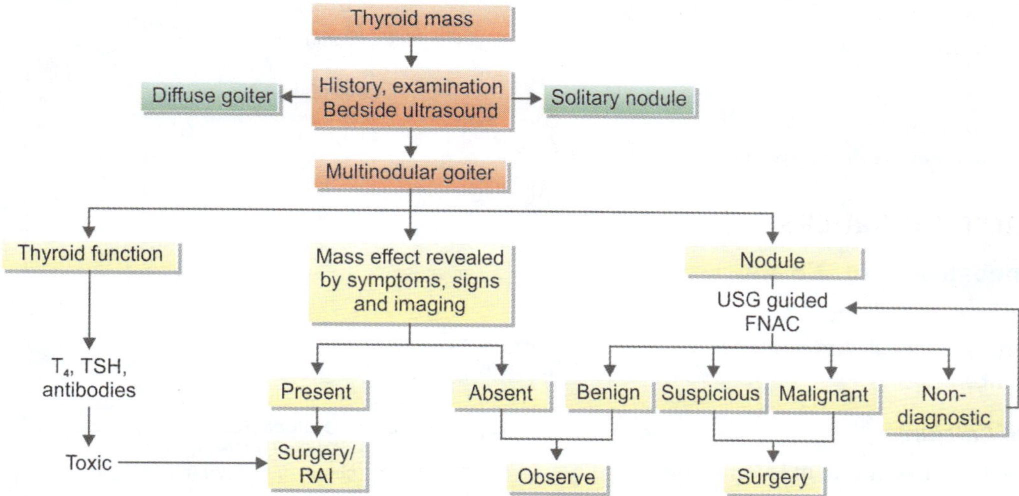

(FNAC: fine-needle aspiration cytology; RAI: radioactive iodine therapy; TSH: thyroid-stimulating hormone)

Etiology

- Types:
  - **Endemic**
  - **Sporadic**
- **Endemic goiter**
  - This term is used when goiters are present in >10% of the population in a given region. The causes are:
    - **Deficiency of iodine:** This may be due to low iodine in the soil, water and food.
      Consequences of iodine deficiency: Decreased synthesis of thyroid hormone and causes compensatory increase in TSH. This leads to **follicular cell hypertrophy** and **hyperplasia** and goitrous enlargement.
    - **Goitrogens:** These are substances ingestion of which **interferes with thyroid hormone synthesis**. Goitrogenic substances include vegetables which belong to Brassicaceae (Cruciferae) family such as cabbage, cauliflower, Brussels sprouts, and turnips and cassava root which contain a thiocyanate that inhibits iodide transport within the thyroid. Consumption of this may worsen the concurrent iodine deficiency.
- **Sporadic goiter**
  - Less frequent than endemic goiter
  - Age: Puberty or in young adult life
  - Sex: Female preponderance.
  - Causes: In most cases of sporadic goiter the cause is not known.

Clinical Features

- **Endemic goiter:**
  - Diffuse enlargement of the thyroid with euthyroid state in the initial stage. This is called as simple goiter.
  - But later they may develop hypothyroidism.
  - In children and adults, endemic goiter may be present with features of hypothyroidism and mental retardation.
- **Cretinism:**
  - Iodine deficiency may produce severe hormone-induced physiological damage to fetus and newborn and cause cretinism.
  - Stunting
  - Deaf-mutism
  - Malformed limbs
  - Spastic motor disorders
  - Goiter
  - Mental impairment.

Investigations (Flowchart 2.5)

- Serum inorganic iodide: Reduced
- Urinary iodide excretion: Low < 50 µg/day.
- Serum T_4: Normal

- Serum T_3: May be normal or raised due to increased conversion of T_4 to T_3
- TSH: May be normal or mildly raised.

Treatment
- Early stages: Supplementation with iodine.
- Later may need suppressive therapy with T_4.

PARATHYROID DISORDERS

Calcium Homeostasis (Fig. 2.8 and Table 2.17)

Q. Write a short note on calcium homeostasis and its importance.

Distribution of Calcium

- Calcium weight is 400 mg/kg in infants and 950 mg/kg in adults.
- **Blood Ca^{++} level:** 8.5–10.2 mg/dL. Usually 10 mg/100 mL (so 500 mg total in plasma = 0.5 g).
- About 99% of total body calcium in the **bone.**
- Remaining 1% in **intracellular fluid (ICF), extracellular fluid (ECF), and cell membranes**.
- It can be divided in three components:
  - i. 45% ionized
  - ii. 40% bound to albumin
  - iii. 15% complex with anions (citrate and phosphate).

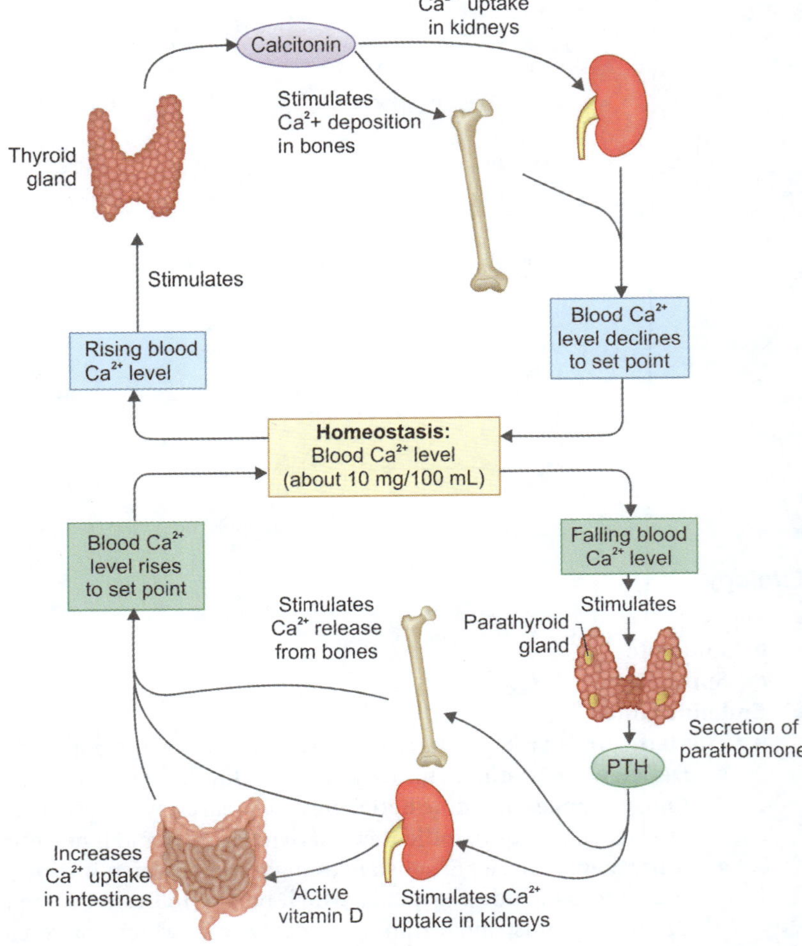

FIG. 2.8: Calcium metabolism.

Importance of Ionized Calcium

Ionized calcium (Ca^{++}) is physiologically important because:
- One of the major intracellular messengers
- Precise levels are necessary for muscle contraction (cardiac and skeletal)
- Responsible for exocytosis of secretory granules in neuronal synapses.
- Serves as second messenger in many cells.
- Necessary for blood clotting.

Regulation of Calcium Levels

- It occurs in three different organs namely:
  - i. **Small intestine:** Dietary Ca^{++} is absorbed in an active transcellular pathway in the duodenum and proximal jejunum. Paracellular calcium transport occurs throughout the length of the intestine.
  - ii. **Kidney:** Ionized Ca^{++} is filtered through the nephron, and can be excreted in the urine.
  - iii. **Bone:** Major storage site for Ca^{++}.
- **Calcium cycling in bone tissue:** Two processes that go on continuously and include bone formation and bone resorption.
  - Calcium phosphate crystals are called **"hydroxyapatite"**. The surfaces of crystals can exchange Ca^{++} and phosphate ions with extracellular fluid.

TABLE 2.17: Hormonal regulators of calcium homeostasis.

Calcitonin (CT)	*Parathormone (PTH)*	*Vitamin D (1, 25 vitamin D_3)*
➢ Secreted from the parafollicular/C-cells in the thyroid gland. ➢ Actions: – Lowers Ca^{++} in blood. – Promotes deposition of Ca^{++} into bone. – It inhibits bone resorption by osteoclasts. ➢ **Control of secretion:** Increased plasma Ca^{++} stimulates C-cells to synthesize and release calcitonin.	➢ Secreted from cells of the parathyroid glands (chief cells). ➢ **Actions:** – Increases Ca^{++} in the blood – Increases Ca^{++} resorption from the bone – Stimulates the osteoclasts – Increases the number of osteoclasts – Increases Ca^{++} resorption from the pre-urine filtrate in the nephron.	➢ **Actions:** Vitamin D increases: – Calcium absorption from intestine. – PO_4 absorption from intestine. – Renal reabsorption of Ca and PO_4. – Bone resorption from old bone and mineralize new bone (net resorption). ➢ **Overall effect:** Increases serum Ca and PO_4.

- **Osteoblasts:** Synthesize a collagen matrix that holds calcium phosphate in crystallized form. Once surrounded by bone, osteoblast becomes osteocyte.
- **Osteoclasts:** They break down bone (removes Ca^{++} from bone). Change local pH, causing Ca^{++} and phosphate to dissolve from crystals into extracellular fluids.

Hyperparathyroidism

Q. Write a short essay on clinical features, investigations, and management of primary hyperparathyroidism.

Q. Write a short essay on classification of hyperparathyroidism.

Classification and Causes of Hyperparathyroidism (Table 2.18)

TABLE 2.18: Classification and causes.

Type	*Calcium*	*PTH*	*Causes*
Primary Autonomous secretion of PTH by parathyroid	Raised	Raised	Single adenoma (90%), multiple adenomata, nodular hyperplasia and carcinoma of parathyroid
Secondary Parathyroid hyperplasia with increased PTH secretion in an attempt to compensate for prolonged hypocalcemia	Low	Raised	Chronic renal failure, malabsorption, osteomalacia, and rickets
Tertiary Adenoma formation and autonomous PTH secretion. Occurring in cases of secondary hyperparathyroidism	Raised	Raised	Chronic secondary hyperparathyroidism Postrenal transplantation

Clinical Features of Hyperparathyroidism

- The most common clinical presentation of primary hyperparathyroidism (>70%) is asymptomatic hypercalcemia detected by routine biochemical screening
- **Classical symptoms of primary hyperparathyroidism** are described by the adage "*moans, bones, stones, abdominal groans*". However, nowadays only few patients present in this way
  - **Moans:** Psychiatric manifestations—lethargy, fatigue, depression, memory loss, psychoses, neuroses, paranoia, confusion, stupor, and coma
  - **Bones:** Arthritis, osteomalacia, and osteitis
  - **Stones:** Renal stones, uremia, polydipsia, and polyuria
  - **Abdominal groans:** Constipation, nausea, vomiting, peptic ulcers, indigestion, and pancreatitis
- **Nonspecific symptoms**: About 50% of patients are asymptomatic while others have nonspecific symptoms. These include: anorexia, nausea, vomiting, constipation, weakness, fatigue, lassitude, tiredness, generalized aches, weight loss, pain, drowsiness, poor concentration, memory loss, and depression.
- **Manifestations of hyperparathyroidism:** Involve primarily the **kidneys** and the **skeletal system**.
  - **Renal manifestations:** Due either to deposition of calcium in the renal parenchyma or to recurrent nephrolithiasis.
    - **Recurrent renal calculi** (usually composed of either calcium oxalate or calcium phosphate)
    - **Nephrocalcinosis:** Deposition of calcium salts in the renal parenchyma.
    - Polyuria and polydipsia
    - Loss of renal function with uremia, hypokalemia, hyperuricemia, hyperchloremic acidosis, and dilute urine.
  - **Skeletal manifestations**
    - Bone pain, osteopenia, osteoporosis, fractures, and deformity due to osteitis fibrosa cystica (10–25% of patients)
    - Localized bone swelling/brown tumor (e.g., mandible).
  - **Other manifestations**
    - Hypertension is a common feature.
    - Calcification of cornea (observed by slit-lamp examination), arterial walls, and soft tissues of hand.
    - Peptic ulcers
    - Myopathy
  - A family history of hypercalcemia or primary hyperparathyroidism secondary to a parathyroid adenoma raises the possibility of multiple endocrine neoplasia (MEN) syndrome. Features of multiple endocrine neoplasia syndromes are presented in **Box 2.11**.

Investigations

- **Biochemical investigations:** Estimation of several fasting serum calcium and phosphate samples should be done.
- **Hallmark of primary hyperparathyroidism:**
  - **Hypercalcemia** and **hypophosphatemia** with **detectable or elevated intact PTH levels** during hypercalcemia. When this combination is present in an asymptomatic patient then further investigation is usually unnecessary. Established hypercalcemia in more than one serum measurement accompanied by elevated immunoreactive PTH (iPTH) is characteristic.

- Serum concentrations of 1,25 dihydroxy vitamin D may therefore be at upper limits of normal or elevated.
- **Correction of serum calcium concentrations:** It should be corrected to the prevailing serum albumin concentration. Calcium level is corrected for low albumin levels by adding 0.8 mg/dL to the total serum calcium level for every 1.0 g/dL by which the serum albumin concentration is lower than 4 g/dL.
- May be associated with **mild hyperchloremic acidosis**.
- **Calcium/creatinine (Ca/Cr) clearance ratio (Fig. 2.9):** [24-hour urine Ca x serum Cr] ÷ [serum Ca x 24-hour urine Cr]

- **Urine investigations**
  - **Hypercalciuria (24 hours urinary calcium)** (>200-300 mg/24 hours): Observed in ~30% of patients.
  - **Increased markers of bone resorption:** These include urinary pyridinoline, deoxypyridinoline, and N-telopeptide of collagen.
- **ECG findings**
  - Shortened QT interval
  - Rarely cardiac arrhythmias
  - Rarely ST-segment elevation
- **Radiological abnormalities**
  - Most sensitive and specific radiologic finding of **osteitis fibrosa cystica** is **subperiosteal resorption of cortical bone**, best seen in high-resolution films of the phalanges.
  - A similar process in the **skull** leads to a **salt-and-pepper appearance**.
  - Bone cysts or **brown tumors** may be evident as osteolytic lesions.
  - The other important skeletal consequence of hyperparathyroidism is **osteoporosis**. Unlike other osteoporotic disorders, hyperparathyroidism often results in the preferential loss of cortical bone.
  - Dental films may disclose loss of the lamina dura of the teeth, but this is a nonspecific finding also seen in periodontal disease.
  - **Nephrocalcinosis:** Appears as scattered opacities within the renal outline.
  - **Soft tissue calcification:** For example, calcification of arterial wall.
  - **Dual-energy X-ray absorptiometry (DEXA) and CT scan:** Reveal reduced bone density.
- **Investigations for localization of the tumor:** Parathyroid imaging is generally indicated only for patients who have undergone previous parathyroid surgery. Investigations to localize the tumor include:
  - **High-resolution ultrasonography**, **CT scanning** and **subtraction imaging** and **scintigraphy** with technetium 99m sestamibi.
  - **Selective neck vein catheterization** with PTH estimation.

Box 2.11: Features of multiple endocrine neoplasia (MEN) syndromes.

MEN 1 (Wermer's syndrome)
- Parathyroid hyperplasia (very common)
- Pancreatic tumors (benign or malignant)
  - Gastrinoma
  - Insulinoma
  - Glucagonoma
  - VIPoma
- Pituitary tumor
  - Growth hormone-secreting
  - Prolactin-secreting
  - Adrenocorticotropic hormone (ACTH)-secreting
- Other tumors: Lipomas, carcinoids, adrenal, and thyroid adenomas

MEN 2A (Sipple syndrome)
- Medullary carcinoma of the thyroid
- Pheochromocytoma (benign or malignant)
- Parathyroid hyperplasia

MEN 2B
- Medullary carcinoma of the thyroid
- Pheochromocytoma
- Mucosal neuromas and ganglioneuromas
- Marfanoid habitus
- Hyperparathyroidism (very rare)

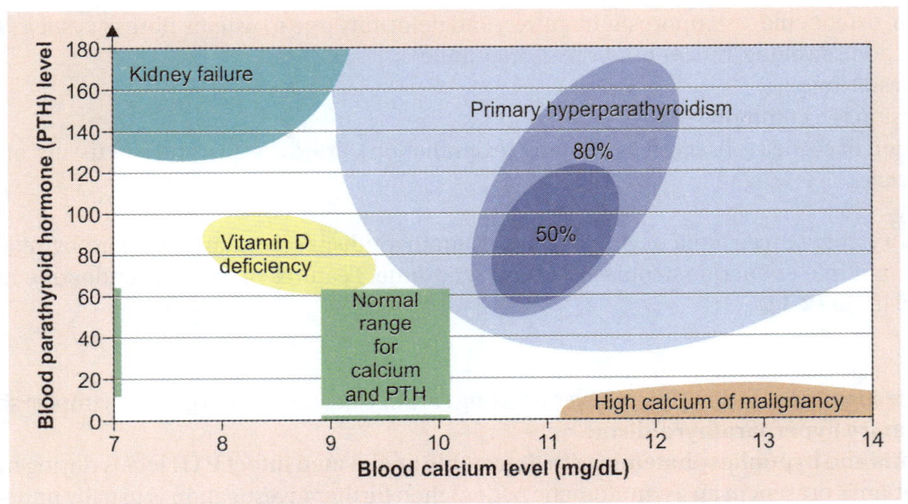

FIG. 2.9: Graphic representation of relationship between calcium and parathormone.

Diagnosis of primary hyperparathyroidism has been shown in **Flowchart 2.6.**

FLOWCHART 2.6: Diagnosis of primary hyperparathyroidism.

- Hypercalcemia
  - Measures intact PTH, with repeat calcium
    - Hypercalcemia and elevated PTH → Primary hyperparathyroidism
    - Hypercalcemia and PTH low (<20 pg/mL) → Rarely PHPT: Evaluate for non-PTH-mediated causes of hypercalcemia
    - Hypercalcemia and PTH mid-upper normal or minimally elevated → PHPT versus FHH
      - Measures 24-hour urinary calcium excretion
        - Normal (>100 but <200 to 300 mg/day, Ca/Cr 0.01 to 0.02) → Likely PHPT with vitamin D deficiency or extremely low calcium intake, FHH still possible
          - Measures serum 25-hydroxyvitamin D
            - Normal (>20 ng/mL) → Likely PHPT, FHH possible → Diagnosis may be established with one or more of the following (see below)
            - Low (≤20 ng/mL) → PHPT with vitamin D deficiency versus FHH → Replete vitamin D
        - Low (<100 mg/day, Ca/Cr <0.01) → Likely FHH, PHPT with vitamin D deficiency or extremely low calcium intake is possible
          - Measures serum 25-hydroxyvitamin D
            - Low (≤20 ng/mL) → FHH versus PTH with vitamin D deficiency → Replete vitamin D
            - Normal (>20 ng/mL) → FHH
        - Normal to elevated (>200 to 300 mg/day, Ca/Cr >0.02) → PHPT
- Replete vitamin D
  Reassess urinary calcium excretion
  when vitamin D normal
  - Normal (>100 but <200 to 300 mg/day, Ca/Cr 0.01 to 0.02) → PHPT versus FHH → Diagnosis may be established with one or more of the following:
    - Family screening for FHH
    - Monitor serum calcium and PTH
    - Sequence the CaSR (where available) for FHH mutation
  - Low (<100 mg/day, Ca/Cr <0.01) → FHH
  - Normal to elevated (>200 to 300 mg/day, Ca/Cr >0.02) → PHPT

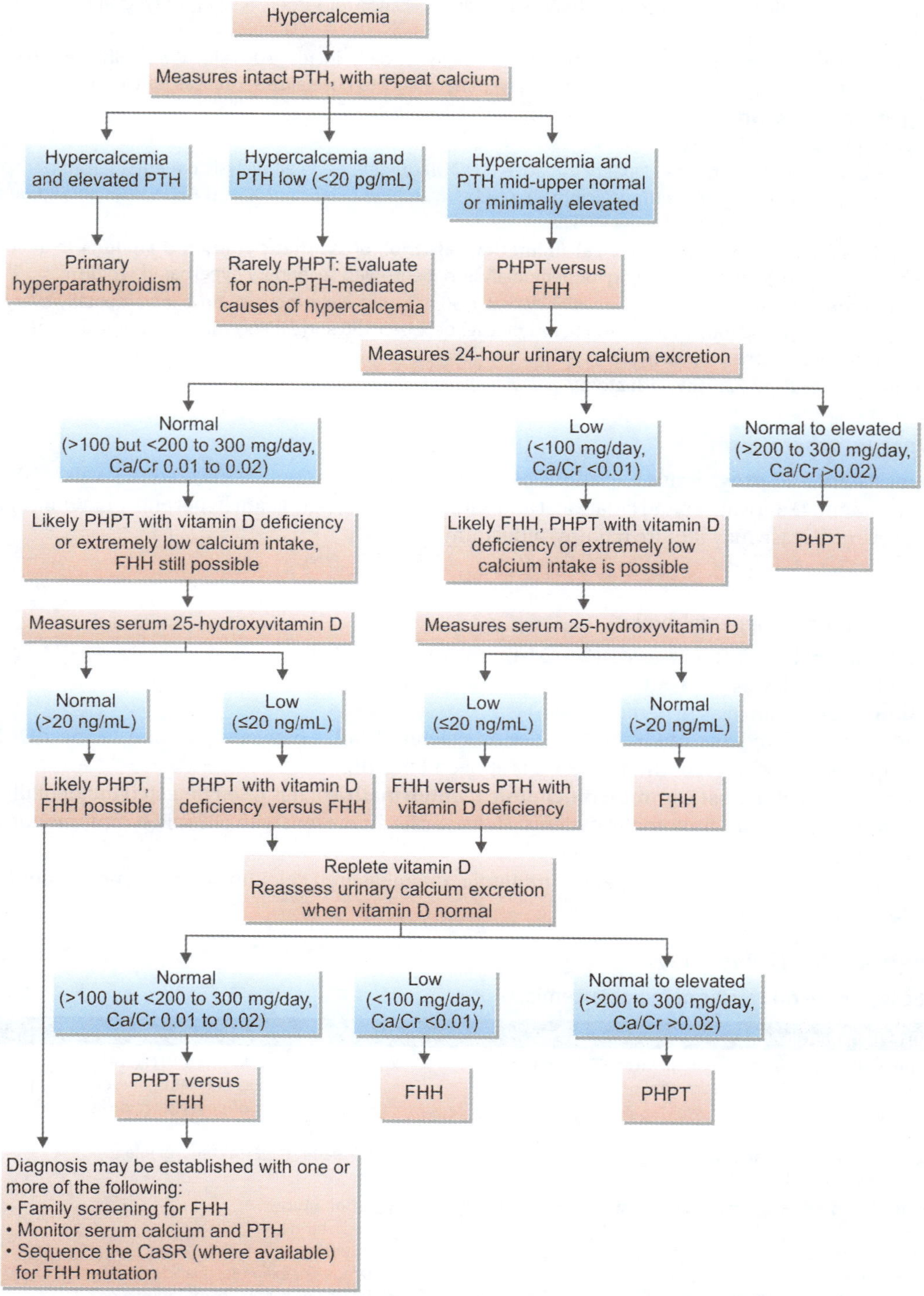

(FHH: familial hypocalciuric hypercalcemia; PTH: parathyroid hormone; PHPT: primary hyperparathyroidism)

Treatment

- **Primary hyperparathyroidism**
  - Patients with **symptomatic** primary hyperparathyroidism should undergo **parathyroid surgery** which is the only definitive therapy.
  - Guidelines for surgery in asymptomatic primary hyperparathyroidism: Any **ONE** of the following criteria:
    - Serum calcium: >1 mg/dL above the upper limit of normal.
    - BMD by DXA: T-score <–2.5 at lumbar spine, total hip, femoral neck, or distal one-third radius.
    - Vertebral fracture by radiograph, CT, MRI, or VFA.
    - Creatinine clearance <60 mL/min
    - 24-hour urine for calcium >400 mg/day and increased stone risk by biochemical stone risk analysis.

- Presence of nephrolithiasis or nephron-calcinosis by radiograph, ultrasound, or CT.
- Age < 50 years
  - For patients who are **unable to have surgery** and whose primary indication for surgery is symptomatic and/or severe hypercalcemia, **Cinacalcet** is preferred over bisphosphonates.
  - **Cinacalcet:** In primary hyperparathyroidism, initially: Oral, 30 mg twice daily; increase dose incrementally every 2–4 weeks (to 60 mg twice daily, 90 mg twice daily, and 90 mg 3 or 4 times daily) as necessary to normalize serum calcium levels.
- **Secondary hyperparathyroidism**
  - Treatment of chronic kidney disease (CKD)
  - According to Kidney Disease Outcomes Quality Initiative (KDOQI) guidelines, in all dialysis patients, serum phosphate should be maintained between 3.5–5.5 mg/dL, serum calcium should be maintained <9.5 mg/dL and PTH values should be maintained less than two to nine times the upper limit for the PTH assay.
  - Treatment options for increased PTH include **calcimimetics, calcitriol, or synthetic vitamin D analogs**. In a recent update, oral calcitriol is comparable to IV vitamin D analog for hemodialysis patients with secondary hyperparathyroidism.
  - **Cinacalcet**: In secondary hyperparathyroidism, initially orally: 30 mg once daily; increase dose incrementally every 2 to 4 weeks as necessary to maintain intact parathyroid hormone (iPTH) level between 150 and 300 pg/mL. May be used alone or in combination with vitamin D and/or phosphate binders.
- **Tertiary hyperparathyroidism: Parathyroidectomy**

Refractory Hyperparathyroidism

- Defined as **persistent** and **progressive** elevations of serum PTH, that cannot be lowered to levels < 600 pg/mL despite treatment with vitamin D derivatives and cinacalcet and without causing significant hyperphosphatemia or hypercalcemia.
- Patients with severe disease may require parathyroidectomy.

Hypercalcemia

Q. Write short essay/note on hypercalcemia.

- Normal serum calcium level is **8–10 mg/dL** (2.0–2.5 mmol/L)
- Normal ionized calcium levels are **4–5.6 mg/dL** (1–1.4 mmol/L).
- **Raised calcium level** is known as hypercalcemia.
- Hypercalcemia is considered as **mild** if the total serum calcium level is between 10.5 and 12 mg/dL (2.6–3 mmol/L), **moderate** 12–14 mg/dL and **severe** when the level is above 14 mg/dL.
- Hypercalcemia is one of the **most common biochemical abnormalities**. It is often detected incidentally during routine biochemical investigation in asymptomatic patients. However, it can present with chronic symptoms and occasionally as an acute emergency.
- In patients with hypoalbuminemia or hyperalbuminemia, the measured calcium concentration should be corrected in view of the albumin abnormality.

Causes of Hypercalcemia (Table 2.19)

Q. Write short essay/note on causes of hypercalcemia.

TABLE 2.19: Causes of hypercalcemia.

Parathyroid hormone related with normal or elevated PTH levels ➢ Primary hyperparathyroidism (the most common) or tertiary hyperparathyroidism ➢ MEN syndromes ➢ Lithium therapy—induced hyperparathyroidism ➢ Familial hypercalciuric hypercalcemia	**Vitamin D related with low PTH levels** ➢ Vitamin D intoxication: Iatrogenic or self-administered excess ➢ Granulomatous diseases (sarcoidosis, tuberculosis, and berylliosis) ➢ Lymphoma ➢ Idiopathic hypercalcemia of infancy
Malignancy related with Low PTH levels (second most common cause) ➢ Multiple myeloma ➢ PTH related protein secretion: Tumors of lung and kidney ➢ Secondary deposits in bone: Breast carcinoma ➢ Production of osteoclastic factors by tumors	**High bone turnover** ➢ Long-term immobilization ➢ Hyperthyroidism ➢ Drugs: For example, thiazide diuretics, etc. ➢ Paget's disease with immobilization
Associated with renal failure ➢ Secondary hyperparathyroidism ➢ Aluminum toxication	**Excessive calcium intake** ➢ Milk-alkali syndrome ➢ Parenteral nutrition

(PTH: parathyroid hormone)

Clinical Features

(Refer clinical features of hyperparathyroidism above).

Q. Write a short essay/note on the management of hypercalcemia.

Management: Treatment of acute hypercalcemia:

- **Adequate rehydration and volume expansion** are essential, usually at least 4–6 L of 0.9% saline on day 1, and 3–4 L for several days thereafter.
- Diuretics after correction of volume (not recommended in the present day due to potential complications and the availability of drugs that inhibit bone resorption, which is primarily responsible for the hypercalcemia). For example, **furosemide** 40–160 mg/day or **ethacrynic acid** 50–200 mg/day. Forced diuresis with 4–6 L of intravenous fluid/day and furosemide 2 hourly.
- Sodium, potassium, and magnesium should be supplemented. Saline decreases concomitant reabsorption of sodium and calcium in both the proximal and distal renal tubules, and enhances urinary excretion of calcium.
- **Intravenous bisphosphonate** is the treatment of choice for hypercalcemia of malignancy or of undiagnosed cause. Concurrent administration of **zoledronic acid** 4 mg IV over 15 minutes or **pamidronate** 60–90 mg over 2 hours.
- **Calcitonin** (4 IU/kg IV 6-hourly), tachyphylaxis develops after 24–48 hours.
- **Prednisolone** (20–40 mg daily) is effective in few instances (e.g., in myeloma, lymphoma, sarcoidosis, and vitamin D excess).
- Oral phosphate (sodium cellulose phosphate) 5 g three times daily.
- **Denosumab**: For hypercalcemia refractory to ZA or in patients in whom bisphosphonates are contraindicated due to severe renal impairment. Starting dose 120 mg every 4 weeks.
- **Cinacalcet**: Reduces the serum calcium in patients with severe hypercalcemia due to parathyroid carcinoma and in hemodialysis patients with an elevated calcium-phosphorous product and secondary hyperparathyroidism.
- **Dialysis**: Treatment of last resort, HD with little or no calcium in the dialysis fluid.

Hypoparathyroidism

Q. Write a short note on causes and general management of hypoparathyroidism.

- Deficient secretion of PTH which manifests itself biochemically by:
  - Hypocalcemia
  - Hyperphosphatemia
  - Diminished or absent circulating iPTH and
  - Clinically the symptoms of neuromuscular hyperactivity.

Causes of Hypoparathyroidism

- **Surgical hypoparathyroidism:** It is the most common. It may be due to the removal of the parathyroid glands or due to interruption of blood supply to the parathyroid glands. Postparathyroidectomy (**hungry bone syndrome**)
- **Idiopathic hypoparathyroidism**
  - Occurs at an **early age** (genetic origin) with autosomal recessive mode of transmission "multiple endocrine deficiency-autoimmune-candidiasis (**MEDAC**) syndrome".
  - "Juvenile familial endocrinopathy"—"Hypoparathyroidism—Addison's disease—mucocutaneous candidiasis (HAM) syndrome"
  - Circulating antibodies for the parathyroid glands and the adrenals are frequently present.
  - Other associated disease: Pernicious anemia, ovarian failure, autoimmune thyroiditis, and diabetes mellitus.
- **Infantile hypoparathyroidism**
- **Infiltrative diseases**: Granulomatous, iron overload, and metastases
- **Radiation-induced destruction**
- **Human immunodeficiency virus (HIV)**
- **Pseudohypoparathyroidism** (resistance to PTH)
- **Functional hypoparathyroidism:** In patients who has chronic hypomagnesemia of various causes. Magnesium is necessary for the PTH release from the glands and also for the peripheral action of the PTH.
- **DiGeorge syndrome** is a familial condition where the hypoparathyroidism is associated with intellectual impairment, cataracts and calcified basal ganglia, and occasionally with specific autoimmune disease.
- **Malabsorption syndrome:** Presumably secondary to decreased calcium level and may lead to steatorrhea with longstanding untreated disease.

Clinical Features

- **Acute**:
  - Neuromuscular irritability (**Tetany**)
  - Paresthesia (perioral and extremities)
  - Muscle twitching

- Carpopedal spasm
- Trousseau's sign **(Fig. 2.10B)**
- Chvostek's sign **(Fig. 2.10A)**
- Seizures
- Laryngospasm
- Bronchospasm
- Prolonged QT interval
- Hypotension, heart failure, and arrhythmia
- Papilledema
- **Chronic:**
  - Ectopic calcification (basal ganglia)
  - Extrapyramidal signs
  - Parkinsonism
  - Dementia
  - Subcapsular cataracts
  - Abnormal dentition
  - Dry skin

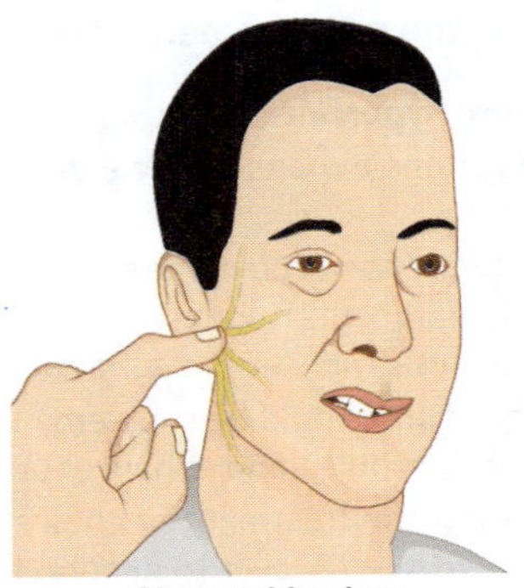

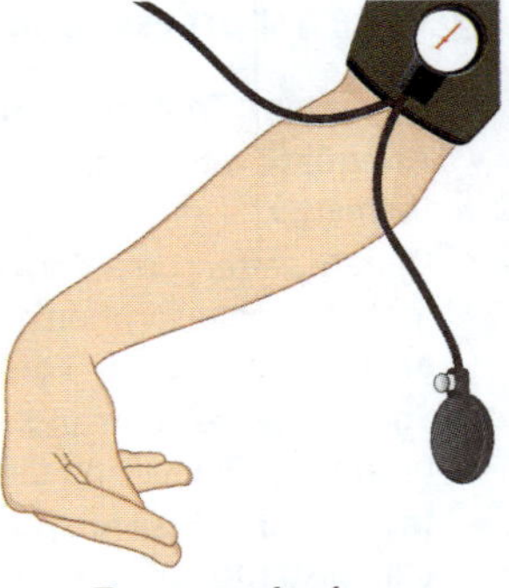

FIGS. 2.10A AND B: Chvostek's sign and Trousseau's sign.

Treatment
- To effectively treat hypocalcemia in patients with magnesium deficiency, hypomagnesemia should be corrected first.
- **Acute cases**:
  - **Symptomatic: IV calcium** (initially, 10 mL ampule of 10% **calcium gluconate** in 50 mL of 5% dextrose infused over 10–20 minutes, followed by an intravenous infusion of calcium gluconate) with oral **calcitriol** (0.5 μg two times daily).
  - **Asymptomatic:** IV calcium if serum corrected calcium is ≤7.5 mg/dL. Oral calcium (1–4 g of **calcium carbonate** daily in divided doses) should be initiated as soon as the patient is able to take supplements orally.
- **Chronic cases:**
  - **Calcium: Calcium carbonate** or **calcium citrate** 1,000–2,000 mg daily in divided doses.
  - **Vitamin D:**
    - **Calcitriol** (drug of choice)**:** Initial: 0.25–0.5 μg daily and maintenance: 0.5–2 μg daily.
    - **Alfacacidol:** Initial 0.25 μg daily and maintenance 0.5–1 μg daily
    - **Dihydrotachysterol:** 0.2–1.2 mg daily.
  - **Hydrochlorothiazide:** If needed for hypercalciuria, 12.5–50 mg daily
  - Second-line therapy by subcutaneous **recombinant human PTH**.

Tetany

It is characterized by **neuromuscular irritability** manifested clinically by **sensory, muscular dysfunction** and **autonomic manifestations**.

Causes of Tetany (Fig. 2.11 and Table 2.20)

Q. Write a short essay/note on causes of tetany/hypocalcemia.

- Tetany is caused due to **hypocalcemia** or **alkalosis** or **hypomagnesemia**.
- Respiratory alkalosis alone (e.g., hyperventilation) can cause tetany, even in the absence of underlying hypocalcemia.
- Tetany is unusual among patients with chronic renal failure and hypocalcemia (occasionally severe) because of the protective effect of concurrent metabolic acidosis.
- Occurs when there is acute fall in **serum ionized calcium to <4.3 mg/dL** and **total calcium concentration to 7-7.5 mg/dL**.

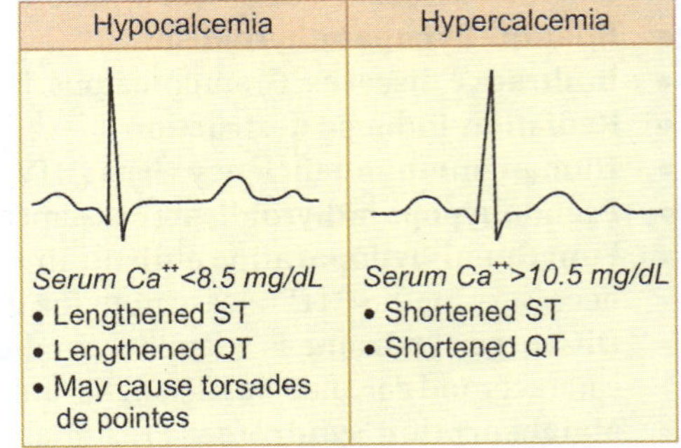

FIG. 2.11: ECG changes in hypo/hypercalcemia.

Clinical Features

Q. Write a short essay/note on clinical features of tetany.

- Symptoms begin with **perioral and acral paresthesia** leading to hyperventilation—respiratory alkalosis—exacerbation of paresthesia.
- **Motor symptoms:** Stiffness, clumsiness, myalgia, muscle spasms, cramps, carpal spasm, spasm of the respiratory muscles, and laryngismus stridulus.
- **Autonomic manifestations** are diaphoresis, bronchospasm, and biliary colic.

TABLE 2.20: Causes of tetany.

Due to hypocalcemia	
Increased phosphate levels ➢ Chronic renal failure (common) ➢ Phosphate therapy	**Vitamin D deficiency** ➢ Osteomalacia/rickets ➢ Vitamin D resistance
Hypoparathyroidism ➢ Surgical—after neck exploration (thyroidectomy, parathyroidectomy—common) ➢ Congenital deficiency (DiGeorge syndrome) ➢ Idiopathic hypoparathyroidism (rare) ➢ Severe hypomagnesemia	**Others** ➢ Acute pancreatitis (quite common) ➢ Citrated blood in massive transfusion (not uncommon) ➢ Low plasma albumin, e.g., malnutrition, chronic liver disease ➢ Malabsorption, e.g., celiac disease
Resistance to PTH Pseudohypoparathyroidism	**Drugs** ➢ Calcitonin ➢ Bisphosphonates
Due to alkalosis	
➢ Repeated vomiting of gastric juice ➢ Excessive intake of oral alkali	➢ Hyperventilation, e.g., hysteria ➢ Primary hyperaldosteronism
Due to hypomagnesemia	

Q. Write a short note on Chvostek's sign and Trousseau's sign (*Refer* FIGS. 2.10A AND B).

- **The classic physical findings in patients with neuromuscular irritability due to latent tetany are:**
  - **Chvostek's sign:** It is elicited by tapping the skin over the facial nerve in front of the external auditory meatus. It causes an **ipsilateral contraction of the facial muscles**, but up to 10% of normal population has a positive test.
  - **Trousseau's sign:** Inflate BP cuff on arm to 20 mm Hg > systolic BP for 3 minutes and watch for **carpopedal spasm** [flexion at the wrist, flexion at the metatarsophalangeal (MP) joints, extension of the interphalangeal (IP) joints adduction thumbs/fingers]. It may also be induced by voluntary hyperventilation for 1-2 minutes after release of the cuff.

Q. Write a short essay/note on management of tetany.

Treatment
- **Control of tetany**
  - **Calcium gluconate:** Slow intravenous (over 10 minutes) injection of 20 mL of 10% solution of calcium gluconate is rapidly effective in controlling the tetany.
  - **Magnesium:** If tetany is not relieved by above treatment, administration of magnesium may be necessary.
- **Correction of alkalosis**
  - If alkalosis is due to persistent vomiting, treat with **intravenous isotonic saline and potassium**.
  - In alkalosis is due to alkali excess, it should be withdrawn. If needed, ammonium chloride 2 g 4 hourly orally will control tetany.
- **Hysterical hyperventilation:** It may be controlled by **rebreathing expired air from a suitable bag** or inhalation of 5% carbon dioxide in oxygen.

Pseudohypoparathyroidism (PHP)

- PHP is an inherited disorder of **target-organ unresponsiveness to PTH.**
- It mimics hormone-deficient forms of hypoparathyroidism, with **hypocalcemia and hyperphosphatemia**, but the **PTH level is elevated.**

Clinical Features

- **PHP type IB** is a disorder of isolated resistance to PTH, which presents with the biochemical features of hypocalcemia, hyperphosphatemia, and secondary hyperparathyroidism.
- **PHP type IA** has, in addition to these biochemical features, a characteristic somatic phenotype known as **Albright's hereditary osteodystrophy (AHO) (Figs. 2.12A to C).** This consists of short stature, round face, short neck, brachydactyly, shortened metatarsals, subcutaneous ossifications, and mental retardation. Due to shortening of the metacarpal bones—most often the fourth and fifth metacarpals—affected digits have a dimple, instead of a knuckle, when a fist is made.
- Certain individuals in families with PHP inherit the somatic phenotype of AHO without any disorder of calcium metabolism; this state is called **pseudopseudohypoparathyroidism or PPHP.**

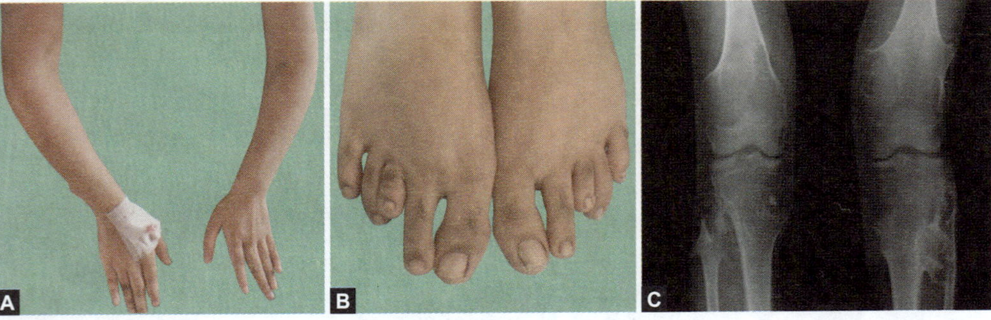

FIGS. 2.12A TO C: Albright's hereditary osteodystrophy (AHO): (A) Brachydactyly; (B) Shortened metatarsals; (C) X-ray of knee region.

ADRENAL GLAND DISORDERS

Hormones Secreted by the Adrenal Gland (Table 2.21)

Q. Write a short note on hormones secreted by the adrenal gland.

TABLE 2.21: Various hormones secreted by adrenal gland.

Site	*Category*	*Hormone produced*
Adrenal cortex		
➢ Zona glomerulosa	Mineralocorticoid	Aldosterone
➢ Zona fasciculata	Glucocorticoid	Cortisol
➢ Zona reticularis	Androgens	➢ Dehydroepiandrosterone sulfate ➢ Dehydroepiandrosterone ➢ Androstenedione
Adrenal medulla		
	Catecholamines	➢ Adrenaline ➢ Noradrenaline

Cushing's Syndrome

Q. Write a short essay on causes, clinical features, investigations, and management of Cushing's syndrome.

- **Cushing's syndrome** is the term used to describe the **clinical state of increased free circulating glucocorticoid.**
- It occurs most often following the therapeutic administration of synthetic steroids or ACTH.

Q. Write a short essay on Cushing's disease.

- **Cushing's disease** results from **corticosteroid excess** due to **pituitary dependent bilateral adrenal hyperplasia**.
- The pituitary tumors producing Cushing's disease are usually microadenomas (<10 mm in size) which usually do not cause symptoms by local mass effect.
- It usually develops sporadically but may be a component of multiple endocrine neoplasia type 1.
- All the spontaneous forms of the syndrome are rare.

TABLE 2.22: Causes of Cushing's syndrome.

ACTH-dependent causes	*ACTH-independent causes*
➢ ACTH-secreting pituitary tumor **(Cushing's disease)—**68% ➢ Nonpituitary ACTH-secreting neoplasm (ectopic ACTH syndrome)—12% ➢ CRH-secreting neoplasm (ectopic CRP syndrome)—<1%	➢ Adrenal adenoma—10% ➢ Adrenal carcinoma—8% ➢ Micronodular hyperplasia— <1% ➢ Macronodular hyperplasia— <1% ➢ McCune-Albright syndrome ➢ Iatrogenic (use of corticosteroids)

(ACTH: adrenocorticotropic hormone)

Causes of Cushing's Syndrome (Table 2.22)

Common causes of ectopic ACTH secretion (Box 2.12)

A **Cushingoid appearance** can be caused by excess alcohol consumption (pseudo-Cushing's syndrome)—the pathophysiology is poorly understood.

Box 2.12: Common causes of ectopic ACTH secretion.

Types of tumor	*Percentage*
Small cell carcinoma of the lung	50%
Endocrine tumors of foregut origin	35%
• Thymic carcinoid	
• Pancreatic islet cell tumor	
• Medullary carcinoma thyroid	
• Bronchial carcinoid	
Pheochromocytoma	5%
Ovarian tumors	2%

(ACTH: adrenocorticotropic hormone)

Clinical Features (Figs. 2.13 and 2.14, Box 2.13, and Table 2.23)

Q. Write a short essay on major signs of Cushing's syndrome.

- Systemic fungal infections and tinea versicolor may develop in untreated patients.
- Higher risk of coronary artery disease and venous thrombosis.
- The predominant clinical features of Cushing's syndrome are those of glucocorticoid excess.
- Skin pigmentation occurs only with ACTH-dependent causes.
- Impaired glucose tolerance or frank diabetes is common, especially in the ectopic ACTH syndrome.

Box 2.13: Mnemonic for Cushing's syndrome.

C-Central obesity, **C**ollagen fiber weakness, and **C**omedones (acne)
U-Urinary free cortisol increased along with glucose
S-Striae and **S**uppressed immunity
H-Hypercortisolism, **H**ypertension, **H**yperglycemia, and **H**ypercholesterolemia
I-Iatrogenic due to administration of corticosteroids
N-Noniatrogenic and **N**eoplasms
G-Glucose intolerance and **G**rowth retardation

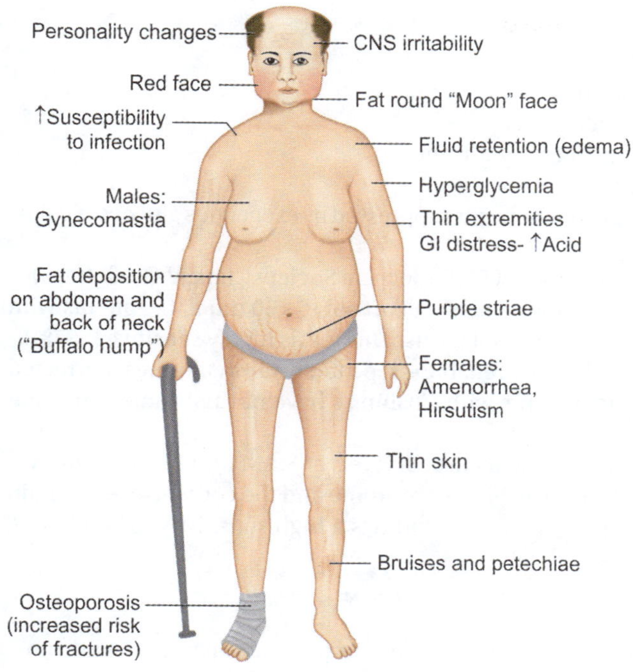

FIG. 2.13: Clinical features of Cushing's syndrome.

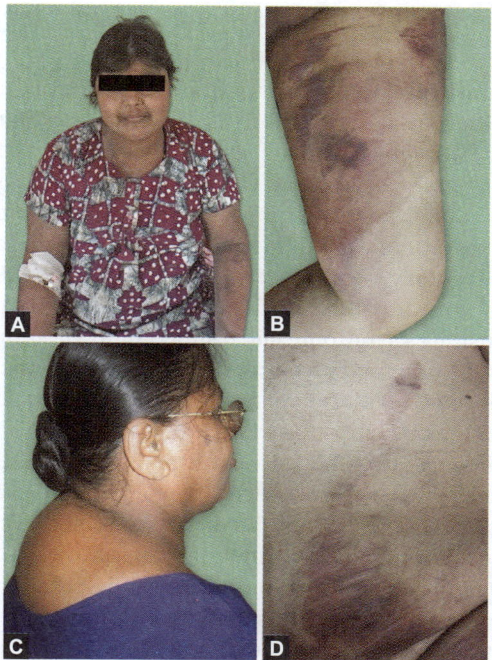

FIGS. 2.14A TO D: Features of Cushing's syndrome: (A) Cushing's habitus, obesity and moon facies; (B) Buffalo hump; (C and D) Pigmented striae.

TABLE 2.23: Clinical features of Cushing's syndrome (% prevalence).

Clinical features	*Cause*
General	
Weight gain/obesity (90%)	Accumulation of fat and retention of fluid
Central obesity ("lemon on match-stick")	Centripetal distribution of fat
Buffalo hump	Fat accumulation at the lower part of neck
Moon face	Rounded plethoric appearance
Hypertension (85%)	Increase in plasma volume and sodium retention
Skin	
Hirsutism (70–75%)	Increased secretion of adrenal androgen
Plethoric appearance	Thinning of the skin
Purplish striae over abdomen, buttocks and thighs	Thinning of the skin from collagen breakdown
Bruising	Thinning of blood vessels from collagen breakdown
Musculoskeletal	
Back pain (80%)	Osteopenia, osteoporosis and vertebral compression fractures
Muscle weakness (65%)	Proximal myopathy and **hypokalemia**. Loss of protein in muscle
Gonadal dysfunction	
Menstrual disorders (oligomenorrhea, amenorrhea) (70–85%)	Gonadal dysfunction
Decreased libido and impotence	
Neuropsychiatric	
Emotional lability, depression, euphoria, psychosis, irritability (85%)	
Metabolic	
Glucose intolerance (75%)	Metabolic abnormalities
Diabetes (20%)	
Hyperlipidemia (70%)	
Polyuria (30%)	
Kidney stones (15%)	

- Hypokalemia due to the mineralocorticoid activity of cortisol is common with ectopic ACTH secretion
- Proximal muscle weakness, sleep apnea, osteoporosis, and hypertension are common features of the disease.

Features of Cushing's syndrome due to ectopic ACTH secretion

- Impaired glucose tolerance due to gluconeogenesis
- Hypokalemic alkalosis due to the mineralocorticoid activity of cortisol
- Skin pigmentation

Investigations in Cushing's syndrome (Flowchart 2.7)

- There are two phases of the investigation:
  i. **Confirmation** of the presence or absence of Cushing's syndrome.
  ii. **Differential diagnosis** of its cause (e.g., pituitary, adrenal or ectopic).
    - Most obese, hirsute, hypertensive patients do not have Cushing's syndrome.
    - Some cases of mild Cushing's have relatively subtle clinical signs.
    - Confirmation rests on demonstrating inappropriate cortisol secretion, not suppressed by exogenous glucocorticoids.
    - Random cortisol measurements are of no value.
- **Confirmatory tests to establish the presence of Cushing's syndrome** (2008 Endocrine Society Clinical Guidelines)
  - **48-hour low-dose dexamethasone test:** Normal individuals suppress plasma cortisol to <50 nmol/L. Patients with Cushing's syndrome fail to show complete suppression of plasma cortisol levels. This test is highly sensitive (>97%).
  - **24-hour urinary free cortisol measurements:** This is simple, but less reliable—repeatedly normal values (corrected for body mass) render the diagnosis most unlikely, but some patients with Cushing's have normal values on some collections (approximately 10%).
  - **Plasma cortisol levels:** In normal individuals, measurement of plasma cortisol levels at 8 AM and 12 midnight will show the lowest levels at midnight. This circadian rhythm is lost in Cushing's syndrome and the cortisol levels remain the same throughout the day. A midnight level below 1.8 μg/dL is normal, and has a high sensitivity for excluding Cushing's syndrome. However, it has a low specificity.
  - **Overnight 1 mg dexamethasone suppression test**
  - **Low dose dexamethasone suppression test**
  - **Late-night salivary cortisol** (two measurements)**:** It may be used as a screening test for Cushing's syndrome. Concentration of cortisol in saliva is highly correlated with free plasma cortisol, irrespective of salivary flow rates and stable at room temperature for 1 week.
- **Tests that establish the cause of Cushing's syndrome:**
  - The first step in the evaluation is to distinguish whether hypercortisolism is **ACTH dependent or ACTH independent** (primary adrenal disease) by measuring ACTH, best performed by **two-site immunoradiometric assay (IRMA). Plasma ACTH level at 8 AM (Table 2.24)**.
  - **Imaging for ACTH Independent conditions (primary adrenal disease):** The next procedure after ruling out ACTH dependency is **CT** of the adrenal glands to look for adrenal mass.
    (Note: Bilateral hyperplasia or bilateral macronodular adrenal hyperplasia may be seen with ACTH-dependent disease)
  - In patients with **ACTH dependent Cushing's**, the final stage of the diagnostic evaluation is to determine the source of ACTH by

TABLE 2.24: Interpretation of plasma ACTH level at 8 AM.

Level of plasma ACTH	*Probable source of ACTH as*
Normal levels (20–80 ng/L)	Pituitary
Intermediate values (80–300 ng/L)	Pituitary dependent disease or ectopic ACTH syndrome
Very high levels (>300 ng/L)	Ectopic ACTH syndrome
Low ACTH (<10 ng/L)	Adrenal tumors, macronodular adrenal hyperplasia or exogenous steroid administration

(ACTH: adrenocorticotropic hormone)

FLOWCHART 2.7: Algorithm of Cushing's syndrome.

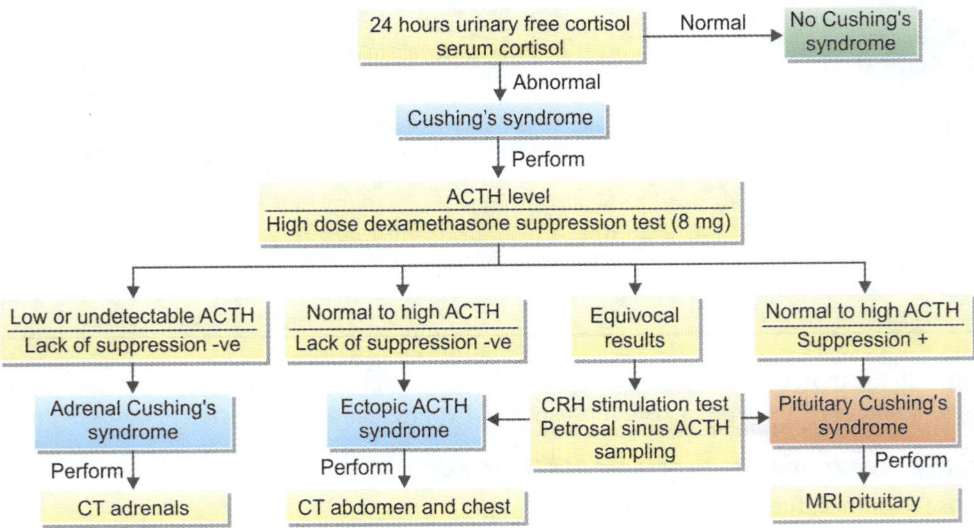

(ACTH: adrenocorticotropic hormone; CRH: corticotropin-releasing hormone)

- **High-dose dexamethasone suppression test (Table 2.25)**
  - 8 mg dexamethasone given orally at 11 PM, blood sample drawn at 8 AM the next day for serum cortisol
  - Usually <5 µg/dL in most patients with Cushing's disease.
- **CRH stimulation test:** Patients with Cushing's have ACTH and cortisol increases within 45 minutes after the IV administration of CRH.
  - Increased in pituitary dependent disease
  - Unchanged in ectopic ACTH syndrome and tumors of adrenal gland.

TABLE 2.25: Tests in Cushing's syndrome.

Test and protocol	*Measure*	*Normal test result or positive suppression*	*Use and explanation*
Dexamethasone (for Cushing's)			
Overnight			
Take 1 mg on going to bed at 23:00 h	Plasma cortisol at 09:00 h next morning	Plasma cortisol <100 nmol/L	Outpatient screening test. Some 'false positives'
'Low-dose'			
0.5 mg 6-hourly Eight doses from 09:00 h on day 0	Plasma cortisol at 09:00 h on days 0 and +2	Plasma cortisol < 50 nmol/L on second sample	For diagnosis of Cushing's syndrome
'High-dose' used in differential diagnosis			
2 mg 6-hourly Eight doses from 09:00 h on day 0	Plasma cortisol at 09:00 h on days 0 and +2	Plasma cortisol on day +2 less than 50% of that on day 0 suggests pituitary-dependent disease	Differential diagnosis of Cushing's syndrome Pituitary-dependent disease suppresses in about 90% of cases

- **Vasopressin stimulation test:** Stimulates ACTH in most patients with Cushing's disease.
- **Petrosal venous sinus catheterization:** ACTH is measured in petrosal and peripheral venous plasma before and within 10 minutes after administration of CRH.
- **Plasma potassium levels**
  - **Normal** in **pituitary dependant disease** and tumors of adrenal gland.
  - **Low** (3.5 mmol/L) in **ectopic ACTH syndrome**.

- **Other investigations**
  - **Biochemical investigations:** Blood glucose, cholesterol, and LDL may be raised.
  - **Radiological investigations**
    - **Plain radiograph** of the skull. Radiograph of chest to detect lung cancer.
    - **CT scan** of anterior mediastinum, upper abdomen and pancreas to rule out tumors.
    - **CT/MRI** head and MRI abdomen.

Management

- **Exogenous Cushing's syndrome:** Taper and withdraw the glucocorticoid.
- **Cushing's disease**
  - **Treatment of choice:** Trans-sphenoidal adenomectomy when there is clear circumscribed microadenoma. In the remaining patients subtotal resection of anterior pituitary.
  - **Radiotherapy and radiosurgery:** For recurrent or residual ACTH-secreting tumors. External pituitary irradiation alone is slow-acting and useful in only 50–60% of cases.
  - **Medical therapy to reduce ACTH:** Needed when surgery is delayed, contraindicated, or unsuccessful. "Block and replace strategy" with **Ketoconazole** 200 mg TID and increased to 400 mg TID. If ketoconazole is unsuccessful in controlling cortisol secretion, it should be maintained at a total dose of 1,200 mg/day and **metyrapone** or **mitotane** (adrenolytic) should be added.
  - Pituitary targeted therapies have been tried. Only the somatostatin analog, **pasireotide**, and the dopamine agonist, **cabergoline** (and the combination of the two), have shown potential benefit.
  - **Bilateral adrenalectomy:**
    - Bilateral total adrenalectomy with lifelong daily glucocorticoid and mineralocorticoid replacement therapy is the final definitive cure.
    - Done if the diagnosis is uncertain.
    - Followed by pituitary irradiation with Yttrium-90 implantation to prevent the development of Nelson's syndrome.
    - Prednisolone and fludrocortisones should be given postoperatively for a variable length of time.
- **Adrenal tumors**
  - **Surgical resection**
    - **Adrenal adenomas:** Surgical removal. Postoperatively, prednisolone is given as a replacement therapy till the contralateral adrenal, hypothalamus, and pituitary recovers.
    - **Adrenal carcinomas:** Surgical resection, irradiation of tumor bed, and administration of adrenolytic drug (mitotane).
  - **Medical adrenalectomy:** Medications that inhibit steroidogenesis include ketoconazole, metyrapone, mitotane, aminoglutethimide, and octreotide.

- **Ectopic ACTH syndrome**
  - Surgical excision of benign tumors (e.g., bronchial carcinoid).
  - Radiotherapy and chemotherapy: For malignant tumors.
- Recurrent tumors may be treated with ketoconazole, metyrapone, or aminoglutethimide.

Nelson's Syndrome

Q. Write a short note on Nelson's syndrome.

- Nelson's syndrome is **increased pigmentation** (high levels of ACTH) associated with an enlarging pituitary tumor **postbilateral adrenalectomy.**
- It occurs in about 20% of cases after bilateral adrenalectomy for Cushing's disease.
- The syndrome is **rare** now that adrenalectomy is an uncommon primary treatment, and its incidence may be reduced by **pituitary radiotherapy** soon after adrenalectomy.
- **Treatment:** Nelson's adenoma may be treated by **pituitary surgery and/or radiotherapy.**

Hyperaldosteronism/Conn's syndrome

Q. Write short essay on:
- **Etiology, clinical features, diagnosis, and management of primary hyperaldosteronism.**
- **Conn's syndrome.**

Excessive production of the aldosterone hormone is called hyperaldosteronism.

Classification

- **Primary hyperaldosteronism:** Develops due to an **abnormality in the zona glomerulosa** of the adrenal gland.
- **Secondary hyperaldosteronism:** Develops due to the **stimulation of aldosterone secretion** by angiotensin II following activation of renin-angiotensin system.

Primary hyperaldosteronism

Etiology

- Adrenal adenoma **(Conn's syndrome)**
- Bilateral hyperplasia of zona glomerulosa/bilateral adrenal hyperplasia
- Idiopathic
- ACTH dependent (glucocorticoid-responsive or dexamethasone-suppressible): This is characterized by secretion of aldosterone under ACTH control. Therefore, treatment consists of **administration of glucocorticoids** to suppress release of ACTH.

Consequences

Excess secretion of aldosterone results in **sodium retention, potassium loss, and metabolic alkalosis.**

Clinical features

- **Hypertension:** Most important clinical consequence of hyperaldosteronism.
- **Tetany** due to metabolic alkalosis
- **Muscle weakness** due to hypokalemia.
- **Polyuria and polydipsia** due to nephrogenic DI.

Investigations

- **Investigation for diagnosis**
  - **Hypokalemia:** However, normal serum potassium does not exclude the diagnosis.
  - **Urinary potassium loss:** Levels > 30 mEq/day during hypokalemia are inappropriate.
  - **Plasma aldosterone concentration (PAC):** Elevated (>10 ng/dL) and is not suppressed with 0.9% saline infusion (2 L over 4 hours, 8 AM to 12 PM, ideally when the patient is seated) or fludrocortisone administration.
  - **Suppressed plasma renin activity (PRA)** or immunoreactivity.
  - **PAC: PRA ratio** *[Plasma aldosterone: renin ratio (ARR)]*: Used as the screening test for primary hyperaldosteronism. A level above 20 is abnormal when plasma aldosterone is measured in ng/dL and PRA is measured in ng/mL/min.
  - **Confirmatory aldosterone suppression test**
    - **Oral salt loading test:** After controlling hypertension and hypokalemia, a high sodium diet (5,000 g sodium diet) should be given for 3 days. On the third day of this diet, a 24-hour urine specimen is collected for measurement of aldosterone, sodium, and creatinine. The 24-hour sodium excretion should be >4,600 mg to indicated proper sodium loading. Urine aldosterone excretion > 12 μg/day indicates hyperaldosteronism.
    - **Oral captopril test:** In primary hyperaldosteronism, this test does not produce any significant decrease in PAC.

- **Investigation for differential diagnosis**
  - **CT/MRI scanning:** To detect adenoma and hyperplasia. Scanning of the adrenal with selenium-75 cholesterol to detect an adenoma.
  - **Adrenal vein catheterization:** To detect hypersecretion of aldosterone.
    - Unilateral hypersecretion in adenoma.
    - Bilateral hypersecretion in hyperplasia.
  - **Dexamethasone suppression**
    - Lowers plasma aldosterone transiently in adenoma.
    - Prolonged suppression in glucocorticoid sensitive hyperaldosteronism.
  - **Measurement of 18-OH-cortisollevels.**
    - Very high levels observed in adenomas and glucocorticoid-responsive hyperplasia.
    - Slightly raised in idiopathic hyperplasia.

Management of primary hyperaldosteronism

- Potassium (K^+) supplementation
- Unilateral disease: Laparoscopic adrenalectomy, bilateral if multiple tumors are present. Surgery is the definitive treatment in unilateral disease.
- In patients with bilateral hyperaldosteronism, mineralocorticoid therapy is administered.
- **Aldosterone antagonists: Spironolactone and eplerenone** are useful in patients where surgery cannot be performed. High dose of spironolactone (up to 400 mg/day) may be required. A few patients may develop gynecomastia with spironolactone and the incidence is lower with eplerenone. Amiloride (10–40 mg/day) may also be tried.

Secondary Hyperaldosteronism

Q. Write a short note on secondary hyperaldosteronism.

- Secondary hyperaldosteronism is **secondary to an extra-adrenal** cause.
- The aldosterone release occurs in response to **activation of the renin-angiotensin system**. It is characterized by *increased levels of plasma renin* that stimulates the zona glomerulosa.

Causes of secondary hyperaldosteronism (Table 2.26)

TABLE 2.26: Causes of secondary hyperaldosteronism.

Physiological	*Pathological*
➢ **Salt depletion:** Inadequate intake or excessive loss through kidney or gastrointestinal tract ➢ Pregnancy (due to estrogen-induced increases in plasma renin substrate)	➢ **Inadequate renal perfusion**: Excessive diuretic therapy, nephrotic syndrome, liver failure, congestive cardiac failure, Bartter's syndrome accelerated or malignant phase of hypertension, severe renal artery stenosis ➢ Renin-secreting renal tumor (very rare)

Adrenocortical Insufficiency

Classification and Causes (Box 2.14 and Table 2.27)

Q. Write a short essay/note on classification and causes of adrenocortical insufficiency.

Q. Write a short essay/note on etiology and clinical features of Addison's disease.

Adrenocortical insufficiency, or hypofunction, may be due to **primary adrenal disease** (primary hypoadrenalism) or **decreased stimulation of the adrenals** due to a deficiency of ACTH (secondary hypoadrenalism).

Box 2.14: Three-step process in the investigation of adrenocortical insufficiency.

- Confirm adrenal insufficiency by demonstrating inappropriately low cortisol secretion.
- Determine whether the cortisol deficiency is primary or central AI.
- Determine the cause of the underlying disorder.

TABLE 2.27: Causes of adrenocortical insufficiency.

Primary (adrenal causes)		*Secondary (inadequate ACTH)*
➢ **Autoimmune adrenal insufficiency**: Isolated adrenal insufficiency, polyglandular autoimmune syndrome type 1 and 2 ➢ **Metastatic malignancy:** Lung, breast, stomach, colon carcinomas, or lymphoma ➢ **Adrenal hemorrhage** – Waterhouse–Friderichsen syndrome – Anticoagulation therapy ➢ **Infectious**: Tuberculosis, CMV, disseminated fungal infection (histoplasmosis, coccidioidomycosis), HIV, syphilis and African trypanosomiasis	➢ **Adrenal infarction:** APLA, SLE ➢ Adrenoleukodystrophy and adrenomyeloneuropathy ➢ **Infiltrative disorders**: Amyloidosis, hemochromatosis, and sarcoidosis ➢ Bilateral adrenalectomy ➢ Congenital adrenal hyperplasia ➢ Familial glucocorticoid deficiency and hypoplasia ➢ **Drugs:** Ketoconazole, fluconazole, metyrapone, aminoglutethimide, mitotane, etomidate, rifampin, and cyproterone acetate ➢ Kearns–Sayre syndrome	➢ Exogenous glucocorticoid therapy ➢ Hypopituitarism: Selective removal of pituitary ➢ Pituitary apoplexy ➢ Granulomatous disease of pituitary (tuberculosis, sarcoidosis, and eosinophilic granuloma) ➢ Secondary tumor deposits in pituitary (breast and bronchus) ➢ Postpartum pituitary infarction (Sheehan's syndrome) ➢ Pituitary irradiation

(ACTH: adrenocorticotropic hormone; APLA: antiphospholipid antibody; CMV: cytomegalovirus; HIV: human immunodeficiency virus; SLE: systemic lupus erythematosus)

Addison's Disease

Addison's disease or chronic adrenocortical insufficiency is an uncommon disorder resulting from **progressive destruction of the entire adrenal cortex.**

Clinical features of Addison's disease (Table 2.28 and Figs. 2.15A and B)

Q. Write a short essay/note on major clinical signs of Addison's disease.

- Clinical features are produced due to the **deficiency of glucocorticoid, mineralocorticoid, and androgen** as well as **excess of ACTH.**
- Fatigue and weight loss are the most prominent symptoms.

FIGS. 2.15A AND B: (A) Pigmentation of palms; (B) Oral pigmentation in Addison's disease.

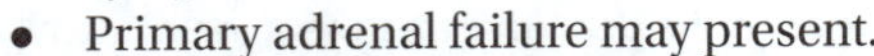

- Primary adrenal failure may present.
  - **Acute:** Hypotension and acute circulatory failure with shock out of proportion to severity of current illness, dehydration, an "acute abdomen", unexplained hypoglycemia, and unexplained fever (Addisonian crisis)

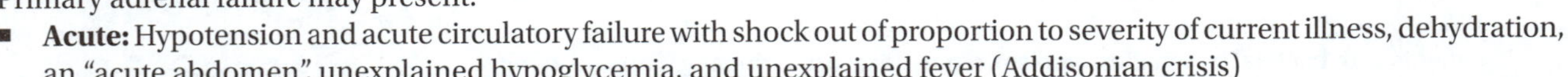

  - **Chronic**: Vague features of ill health, sometimes including gastrointestinal symptoms, features suggestive of postural hypotension and salt craving.
- Skin pigmentation is nearly always present in primary adrenal insufficiency (but not in secondary).
- **Cardinal features of Addison's disease:** Hypotension, pigmentation and previous history of acute adrenal crisis following stress, or slow recovery from illness.
- **Other autoimmune diseases associated with Addison's disease:** Hashimoto's thyroiditis, primary atrophic hypothyroidism, pernicious anemia, type 1 diabetes mellitus, primary ovarian failure, and hypoparathyroidism.

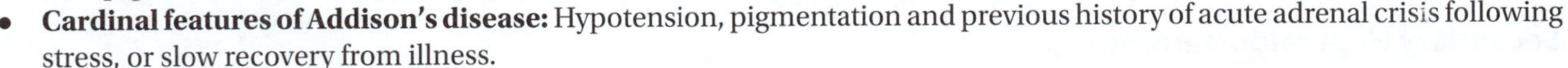

  - **Type I polyglandular autoimmune syndrome** is the combination of adrenal insufficiency, hypoparathyroidism, and chronic mucocutaneous candidiasis.
  - **Type II polyglandular autoimmune syndrome/Schmidt syndrome** is the association of Addison's disease and Hashimoto's thyroiditis.

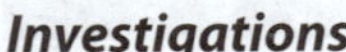

Investigations

Q. Write a short essay/note on biochemical abnormality in Addison's disease.

- **Early morning (6 AM) cortisol level**
  - Normally, levels are 10-20 μg/dL
  - Levels <3 μg/dL is suggestive of adrenal insufficiency.
  - Levels >11 μg/dL exclude AI
  - Random cortisol in ill patient 20 μg/dL reassuring.
- **Morning salivary cortisol concentration**
  - Levels below 1.8 ng/mL is highly suggestive of adrenal insufficiency.
  - Levels above 5.8 ng/mL rule out adrenal insufficiency.
- **Plasma ACTH level:** Elevated in adrenal insufficiency.
- **ACTH stimulation test:** There is failure of rise in plasma cortisol level following the administration of 0.25 mg (standard high dose test) of synthetic ACTH (cosyntropin)
  - Low dose test (1 μg)
    - Baseline and 30-minute cortisol levels

TABLE 2.28: Clinical features of adrenocortical insufficiency.

Glucocorticoid deficiency	*Mineralocorticoid deficiency*	*Adrenal androgen deficiency*	*ACTH excess*
Fasting hypoglycemia	Hypotension	Decreased axillary hair in females	Pigmentation of exposed areas, pressure areas (elbows, knees and knuckles, palmar creases, mucous membranes, conjunctive and recently acquired scars, perineum, axillae and areolae of breasts) [increased production of pro-opiomelanocortin (POMC), that is cleaved into ACTH and melanocyte-stimulating hormone (MSH)
Increased insulin sensitivity	Dizziness	Decreased pubic hair in females	
Muscle weakness	Salt craving	Loss of libido in females	
Morning headache	Weight loss and anorexia	Asymptomatic-during prepuberty	
Fatigue, malaise, weakness, weight loss, anorexia, nausea, vomiting, diarrhea or constipation, and postural hypotension	Electrolyte anomalies (hyponatremia, hyperkalemia, and metabolic acidosis)		

(ACTH: adrenocorticotropic hormone)

- More physiological ACTH level/stimulation
- Useful in central AI
- Useful for assessing recovery after chronic steroid treatment.
- High dose (250 μg) test
  - Baseline, 30- and 60-minute levels
  - Stronger stimulation than 1 μg test.
- **Metyrapone test:** Useful to detect partial ACTH deficiency and partial secondary adrenal insufficiency.
- **Insulin-induced hypoglycemia test:** Insulin at a dose of 0.15 U/kg is administered to achieve hypoglycemia of 35 mg/dL or less. Cortisol levels are measured at 0, 30, and 45 minutes.
- **Corticotropin-releasing hormone test:** To differentiate between secondary and tertiary adrenal insufficiency.
- **Other investigations:** PRA is high and plasma aldosterone levels are low or normal.
- **Radiograph:** In patients with tuberculous adrenalitis: Chest radiograph may show evidences of pulmonary tuberculosis and plain radiograph of abdomen, CT scan, and MRI scan may show calcification in the adrenal gland.
- **Adrenal autoantibodies:** ACA—adrenal cortex antibody and anti-21-OH-hydroxylase antibody
- Elevated blood urea, hyponatremia, and hyperkalemia.
- **Blood sugar:** Low levels.
- **Peripheral blood:** Mild anemia and mild eosinophilia.
- **Central AI**: Evaluate for secretion of other pituitary hormones.

Management of primary adrenal insufficiency

- **Acute treatment:**
  - Normal saline for volume resuscitation
  - Look for/treat hypoglycemia by 25% dextrose
  - **Steroids:**
    - Loading dose: 50–100 mg/m² **hydrocortisone** IV/IM
    - Continue hydrocortisone with 50–100 mg/m²/day, divided 6th or 8th hourly
- **Long-term treatment:**
  - Daily glucocorticoid replacement (hydrocortisone): 10–15 mg/m²/day in divided doses.
  - Daily mineralocorticoid replacement: Fludrocortisone 0.05–0.2 mg daily
  - Relative steroid potencies **(Table 2.29)**
- **Stress conditions**
  - Primary goal is to avoid serious consequences of an adrenal crisis
  - Always wear identification
  - Illness:
    - Minor stress (e.g., sore throat, rhinorrhea, temperature < 38°C) may not require increase in dose.
    - Moderate stress (e.g., severe URTI)—double the glucocorticoid (GC) replacement dose
    - Major stress (e.g., T > 38°C and/or vomiting), three to four times the GC replacement dose.
  - **Surgery:**
    - During general anesthesia, ± surgery, the GC requirement increases greatly.
    - Dose equivalent to 100–150 mg hydrocortisone for major surgical procedures in divided doses.
    - Stress dosing is generally continued until the patient can tolerate oral intake, is afebrile, and is hemodynamically stable.
- Tuberculous adrenalitis causing Addison's disease is treated with **anti-tuberculous chemotherapy.**

TABLE 2.29: Anti-inflammatory action of steroids compared to hydrocortisone.

Type of steroid	*Activity*
Short acting	
Hydrocortisone	1
Cortisone acetate	0.8
Intermediate acting	
Prednisone	4
Prednisolone	4
Methylprednisolone	5
Triamcinolone	5
Long acting	
Dexamethasone	30
Betamethasone	30

Acute Adrenal Crisis/Addisonian Crisis

Q. Write a short note on acute adrenal crisis.

- Acute adrenal crisis is a state of **acute adrenocortical insufficiency** and occurs in patients with **Addison's disease** who are exposed to the **stress** of infection, trauma, surgery, or dehydration due to salt deprivation, vomiting, or diarrhea.
- **Other causes:** Acute adrenal crisis can also develop after:
  - Bilateral adrenal infarction
  - Bilateral adrenal hemorrhage: Adrenal hemorrhage and often death may occur following meningococcemia (**Waterhouse-Friderichsen syndrome**).
- It is rare with secondary adrenal insufficiency.

Clinical Features

- **Major manifestations:**
  - Shock (out of proportion to severity of illness)
  - **Nonspecific symptoms:** Weakness, fatigue, lethargy, anorexia, nausea, vomiting, abdominal pain, confusion or coma.
  - Abdominal tenderness "acute abdomen" and unexplained fever.
- **Crisis in patients with long-standing adrenal insufficiency:** Shows features of chronic adrenal insufficiency and may show hyperpigmentation (due to chronic ACTH hypersecretion), weight loss, and serum electrolyte abnormalities.

Laboratory Findings

- Hyponatremia
- Hyperkalemia
- Hypercalcemia
- Azotemia
- Lymphocytosis
- Eosinophilia
- Hypoglycemia.

Management

- Establish IV access with a large bore needle.
- Withdraw blood for serum electrolytes, glucose and routine plasma cortisol and ACTH. **Do not wait for results.**
- IV infusion of 2–3 L normal saline bolus. Avoid iatrogenic fluid overload.
- IV **hydrocortisone** 100 mg, followed by 50 mg IV every 6 hours OR 200 mg/day IV infusion.
- After initial stabilization, continue IV NS at a slower rate for next 24–48 hours.
- Search and manage possible precipitating cause.
- In case patient is not a known case of AI, do short ACTH stimulation test.
- Determine the type of AI.
- Taper parenteral glucocorticoid over 1–3 days to oral maintenance dose.
- Start mineralocorticoid replacement with **fludrocortisone** 0.1 mg by mouth daily when saline infusion is stopped.

Equivalent doses of glucocorticoids (Table 2.30)

- Compared to hydrocortisone, prednisolone has only 25% of mineralocorticoid activity (**Table 2.31**).
- Both dexamethasone and betamethasone have negligible mineralocorticoid activity.

TABLE 2.30: Equivalent doses of glucocorticoids (anti-inflammatory potency).

Hydrocortisone (cortisol)	20 mg	Methylprednisolone	4 mg
Cortisone acetate	25 mg	Betamethasone	0.75 mg
Prednisolone	5 mg	Dexamethasone	0.75 mg

Steroid Therapy

Common Indication and Contraindications of Steroids (Table 2.31)

Q. Write a short note on the use and abuse of steroids/the present role of steroid therapy.

TABLE 2.31: Common indications and contraindications of steroids.

Common indications of steroids	
➤ Bronchial asthma ➤ Raised intracranial tension ➤ Cerebral edema ➤ Connective tissue diseases—rheumatoid arthritis and systemic lupus erythematosus ➤ Nephrotic syndrome ➤ Adrenal insufficiency ➤ Shock and septicemia ➤ Transplant rejection and graft versus host disease	➤ Leukemia, lymphoma, ➤ As an adjunct in chemotherapy ➤ Carditis (e.g. rheumatic carditis) ➤ Demyelinating diseases ➤ Tuberculosis of pericardium and tuberculous meningitis ➤ Bone marrow transplantation ➤ Psoriasis and inflammatory bowel disease ➤ Eye conditions: Scleritis and chorioretinitis

Common Contraindications for Steroids

- Active tuberculosis
- Peptic ulcer
- Diabetes
- Uncontrolled hypertension
- Active infection

Side Effects of Corticosteroids Therapy (Table 2.32)

Q. Write a short note on the complications of corticosteroid therapy.

TABLE 2.32: Adverse effects of glucocorticoids.

Immune system	***Bones***
➢ Increased susceptibility to infections, reactivation of latent tuberculosis ➢ Lymphopenia ➢ Suppression of inflammation impaired wound healing ➢ Suppression of delayed hypersensitivity reaction	➢ Osteoporosis ➢ Avascular necrosis ➢ Bone pains ➢ Fracture
Gastrointestinal tract	***Endocrine***
➢ Gastric erosions ➢ Peptic ulceration ➢ Masked perforation ➢ Hemorrhage from stomach and duodenum ➢ Pancreatitis	➢ Growth retardation ➢ Menstrual irregularities ➢ Hypothalamic-pituitary-adrenal axis suppression ➢ Impotence ➢ Acute adrenal insufficiency, Cushingoid features
Skin	***Metabolic***
➢ Acne rubeosis steriodica ➢ Hirsutism ➢ Striae ➢ Ecchymoses ➢ Thin and fragile skin ➢ Panniculitis (on withdrawal)	➢ Glucose intolerance or frank diabetes mellitus ➢ Weight gain ➢ Hyperlipidemia ➢ Hypokalemia ➢ Alkalosis ➢ Fluid and salt retention ➢ Negative nitrogen balance-muscle wasting
Psychiatric	***Cardiovascular***
➢ Depression ➢ Insomnia ➢ Euphoria ➢ Steroid psychosis	➢ Hypertension ➢ Fluid retention ➢ Accelerated atherosclerosis ➢ Ischemic heart disease (IHD)

Muscles	***Eye***	***Neurological***
➢ Myopathy	➢ Cataract ➢ Glaucoma	➢ Pseudotumor cerebri

Measures to Reduce the Side Effects of Corticosteroids Therapy

Q. Write a short note on measures to minimize the side effects of corticosteroid.

Side effects of steroids can be reduced by administering them with the following rules:
- Lowest required dose
- On alternate days rather than daily
- As a single dose than in divided doses
- In the morning
- For the shortest required duration
- For indications only
- Only under medical supervision
- Monitor intake of calories to prevent weight gain
- Reduce intake of sodium
- Use H_2 receptor blockers or proton-pump inhibitors
- Provide high calcium intake and pump inhibitors
- Use bisphosphonates

Waterhouse–Friderichsen Syndrome

Q. Write a short note on Waterhouse–Friderichsen syndrome.

- It is characterized by an **acute hemorrhagic** infarction **(destruction) of both the adrenal glands** and is usually associated with fulminant **meningococcal septicemia**.
- It produces cutaneous petechiae, vasomotor collapse, and shock.
- Can occur at any age but is more common in children.
- **Abrupt in onset** and profound prostration occurs within a few hours.
- It produces petechiae, purpuric lesion, and hemorrhage into the skin.

Management: Prompt recognition and appropriate therapy, intravenous fluids, high dose antibiotics (penicillin, cephalosporins, and sulfonamides), vasopressors, inotropes, plasma transfusion, steroids must be instituted immediately, or death follows within hours to a few days due to cardiac and/or respiratory failure.

Pheochromocytoma

Q. Write a short essay/note on clinical features, diagnosis, and treatment of pheochromocytoma.

- Pheochromocytoma is a very rare tumor of the sympathetic nervous system composed of chromaffin cells that secretes catecholamines.
- Important because they are a rare cause of surgically correctable hypertension.

- **Paraganglioma:** Pheochromocytomas that develop in **sympathetic ganglia** are known as paragangliomas.
- It arises from both sympathetic and parasympathetic paraganglia, located anywhere from the base of the skull to the pelvis.
- Paragangliomas typically occur in the head and neck but are also found in the thorax, pelvis, and bladder.
- Traditionally, the features of pheochromocytomas have been summarized by the "rule of 10s" **(Box 2.15)**.
- **Neurofibromatosis type 1 (Von Recklinghausen's disease)** is associated with an increased incidence of pheochromocytoma.

Box 2.15: Rule of 10s' for pheochromocytoma.

10%	Extra-adrenal (closer to 15%)
10%	Abdominal
10%	Occur in children
10%	Familial (now modified as closer to 25%)
10%	Sporadic are bilateral or multiple (more if familial)
10%	Not associated with hypertension
10%	Malignant
10%	Discovered incidentally
10%	Recur (more if adrenal)

Clinical Features (Table 2.33)

- The classic triad of symptoms in patients with a pheochromocytoma consists of episodic headache, sweating, and tachycardia
- **5 Ps:** *Pressure (90%), Pain (80%), Perspiration (70%), Palpitations (65%), and Pallor (42%)*
- **Paroxysmal hypertension:**
  - Characterized by episodes of **pallor or flushing, headache sweating, palpitations, and anxiety** (fear of death).
  - Paroxysms last 10–60 minutes duration, daily to monthly
  - **Paroxysms are spontaneous or precipitated by:**
    - Diagnostic procedures, intra-arterial contrast
    - Drugs (opioids, unopposed beta-blockade, anesthesia induction, histamine, ACTH, glucagon, and metoclopramide)
    - Strenuous exercise, movement that increases intra-abdominal pressure (lifting and straining)
    - Micturition (bladder paraganglioma)
- Sustained hypertension is more common than paroxysmal hypertension.
- **Complications of hypertension:** Stroke, myocardial infarction, cardiomyopathy, and left ventricular failure.
- **Gastrointestinal symptoms:** Abdominal pain, vomiting, constipation, and weight loss.
- **Hypercalcemia:** Observed in associated MEN2 hyperparathyroidism
- **Mild glucose intolerance**
- Lipolysis and weight-loss

TABLE 2.33: Familial pheochromocytoma.

MEN 2a	50% pheochromocytoma (usually bilateral), medullary carcinoma of thyroid, and hyperparathyroidism
MEN 2b	50% pheochromocytoma (usually bilateral), medullary carcinoma of thyroid, mucosal neuroma, and marfanoid habitus
Von Hippel–Landau	50% pheochromocytoma (usually bilateral), retinoblastoma, cerebellar hemangioma, nephroma, and renal/pancreas cysts
NF1 (Von Recklinghausen's)	2% pheochromocytoma (50% if NF-1 and HTN) Café-au-lait spots, neurofibroma, and optic glioma
Familial paraganglioma	
Familial pheochromocytoma and islet cell tumor	
Other: Tuberous sclerosis, Sturge–Weber, ataxia-telangiectasia, Carney's triad (pheochromocytoma, gastric leiomyoma, and pulmonary chondroma)	

(HTN: hypertension; NF-1: neurofibromatosis type 1)

Investigations (Table 2.34)

- **Plasma metanephrine** is the most sensitive test.
- **Other investigations**
  - **Chromogranin A:** It is a major secretory protein present in the soluble matrix of chromaffin granules and is elevated.
  - **Provocative** (glucagon provocative test) and adrenolytic (clonidine, phentolamine test) tests: Rarely necessary.
  - **CT/MRI scan:** To localize tumor.
  - **Scintigraphy:** Useful for localization of tumor and includes:
    - MIBG (^{123}I-labeled meta-iodobenzylguanidine) scintigraphy
    - Somatostatin receptor scintigraphy using 111indium-labeled diethylenetriaminepentaacetic acid octreotide scan.
    - (^{18}F) fluro-dihydroxyphenylalanine (DOPA) PET scan.
  - **Plasma noradrenaline:** Selective venous sampling and estimation of plasma noradrenaline level may be useful in localizing the tumor in difficult cases.

TABLE 2.34: Laboratory findings in pheochromocytoma.

Investigation	*Level*	*Sensitivity*	*Specificity*
24-hour urine vanillylmandelic acid (VMA)	Raised	63%	94%
24-hour urine metanephrines and normetanephrines	Raised	76%	94%
24-hour urine free catecholamines	Raised	83%	88%
24-hour urine free catecholamines + metanephrines	Raised	90%	98%
Plasma catecholamines	Raised	85%	80%
Plasma metanephrines	Raised	99%	89%

Management

- **Excision of the tumor** is the main treatment.
- Special care has to be taken preoperatively, intraoperatively, and postoperatively.
- **Preoperative preparation regimens**
  - Combined α + β-**blockade** to be given at least 2 weeks preoperatively to control the hypertension. Antihypertensive agents used are: **phenoxybenzamine** (preferred drug for preoperative preparation). Initial dose is 10–20 mg in divided doses every 2–3 days as needed, final dose will be 20–100 mg/day. Other drugs used are selective α1-blocker (prazosin, terazosin, or doxazosin).
  - Beta-blockers should never be started first. Drugs such as **propranolol** or **metoprolol** are used. Dose should be adjusted to control tachycardia. Typical maximum doses in this setting are 120 mg of propranolol or 200 mg of metoprolol.
  - **High sodium diet**—patients are encouraged to start a diet high in sodium content (>5,000 mg daily) on the second or third day because of the catecholamine-induced volume contraction and the orthostasis associated with alpha-adrenergic blockade.
  - **If uncontrolled add:**
    - Metyrosine
    - Calcium channel blockers: **Nicardipine** and **amlodipine** are most commonly used in this setting; starting dose of nicardipine is 30 mg twice daily of the sustained-release preparation and the starting dose of amlodipine is 2.5 or 5 mg administered once daily.
    - Avoid diuretics as ECF volume is already contracted.
- **Intraoperative** blood pressure needs to carefully monitored and controlled.
- **Postoperative** hypotension can be avoided by adequate fluid replacement and hypoglycemia (10–15% of patients) due to removal of catecholamine suppression of insulin secretion by glucose infusion. Postoperatively patients may become hypertension free.
- **If tumor cannot be excised:**
  - Long-term treatment with α- and β-adrenoreceptors blocking drugs (phenoxybenzamine and propranolol, or labetalol) is advocated.
  - β-blockers should never be given alone.
  - Patients can also be subjected to nuclear medicine treatment.

GONADAL DISORDERS (TABLES 2.35 AND 2.36)

Male Hypogonadism

- **Primary hypogonadism,** if the serum testosterone and/or the sperm count are below normal and the serum LH and/or FSH concentrations are above normal.
- **Secondary hypogonadism,** if the serum testosterone concentration and/or the sperm count are below normal and the serum LH and/or FSH concentrations are normal or low.

TABLE 2.35: Specific abnormalities of sexual development.

First trimester	Ambiguous genitalia in deficient testosterone production Female external genitalia in complete lack of testosterone production Incomplete testosterone deficiency or androgen action causes partial virilization
Third trimester	Micropenis Bilateral cryptorchidism
Prepubertal	Failure to undergo/complete puberty
Adult	Decreased energy/libido Infertility

TABLE 2.36: Androgen deficiency symptoms.

Musculoskeletal	Decreased vigor and physical energy Diminished muscle strength
Sexuality	Decreased interest in sex Reduction in frequency of sexual activity Poor erectile function/arousal Loss of nocturnal erections Reduced quality of orgasm Reduced volume of ejaculate
Mood disorder and cognitive function	Irritability and lethargy Decreased sense of well-being, lack of motivation Low mental energy, difficulty with short-term memory Depression Low self-esteem, insomnia, and nervousness
Vasomotor and nervous	Hot flushes and sweating

Q. Discuss the causes and approach to male hypogonadism.

Classification and Causes of Male Hypogonadism (Table 2.37)

TABLE 2.37: Classification and causes of male hypogonadism.

Hypothalamic-Pituitary Disorders	***Defects in Androgen Action***
Panhypopituitarism LH and FSH deficiency ➢ With normal sense of smell ➢ With hyposmia or anosmia (Kallmann's syndrome) ➢ With complex neurologic syndromes Prader–Willi syndrome < Laurence–Moon, Bardet–Biedl syndromes < Möbius' syndrome < Lowe's syndrome	Complete androgen insensitivity (testicular feminization) Incomplete androgen insensitivity

Contd...

Contd...

Gonadal Abnormalities	
Klinefelter's syndrome	Anorexia nervosa
Other chromosomal defects (XX male, XY/XXY, XX/XXY, XXXY, and XYY)	Diabetes mellitus
Bilateral anorchia (vanishing testes syndrome)	Hepatic cirrhosis
Cryptorchidism	HIV
Noonan's syndrome	Mumps
Myotonic dystrophy	Obesity
Adult seminiferous tubule failure < adult Leydig cell failure	Malignant tumors of testes
Secondary hypogonadism	Infiltrative diseases—hemochromatosis
Hyperprolactinemia	Chronic orchitis: TB, leprosy, and syphilis
Glucocorticoid treatments	Pituitary apoplexy
Chronic and systemic illness	Trauma and testicular torsion
	Idiopathic

Physical Signs

- Diminished muscle mass
- Loss of body hair
- Abdominal obesity
- Gynecomastia
- Testes frequently normal, occasionally small

Prepubertal onset: Eunuchoidism

- Lack of adult male hair distribution
  - Sparse axillary and pubic hair
  - Lack of temporal hair recession
- High-pitched voice
- Infantile genitalia: Small penis, testes, and scrotum
- Fat deposition in pectoral, hip, thigh, and lower abdomen
- Eunuchoidal proportion
  - Arm span > height > 5 cm
  - Upper/lower segment ratio < 1

Investigations

- Serum testosterone: 8.00 AM
- Serum FSH and LH
- **Semen analysis:** Normally, >40% of the sperm ejaculated are motile, >32% have rapid forward progression, and >4% have normal morphology.
- Others: Peripheral leukocyte karyotype, other pituitary hormones, serum prolactin, iron saturation, and MRI brain.

Treatment

Treatment of Primary Hypogonadism

- Testosterone replacement for men who are hypogonadal only with signs and symptoms with subnormal morning serum testosterone.
- Treatment of the underlying disease

Q. Write a short note on testosterone replacement.

Testosterone replacement

- **Transdermal testosterone** is started in gel form.
- Intramuscular preparations—**testosterone enanthate** (100–200 mg IM q 2 weeks)
  - Oral agent—**testosterone undecanoate** (initial 120–160 mg/day in 2 divided doses for 2–3 weeks; usual maintenance dose: 40–120 mg/day), however parenteral formulations are preferred as adverse effects of oral preparation are hypertension and cardiovascular events.
  - **Undesirable effects:** BPH, prostatic cancer, dyslipidemia, polycythemia, and transaminitis.
- **Treatment of secondary hypogonadism**
  - GnRH pulsatile infusion
  - hCG

Impotence

Q. What is impotence? Discuss briefly.

- **Definition: Male sexual dysfunction** is termed "impotence".
- **Manifestations:**

- Loss of desire
- Inability to obtain and maintain erection
- Premature ejaculation
- Absence of emission
- Inability to achieve orgasm.

Causes of Male Infertility (Box 2.16)

Erectile impotence may be due to various causes, but majority are of psychological origin. In each case of erectile impotence, it is necessary to rule out the organic causes (**Table 2.38**).

Box 2.16: Causes of male infertility.

- **Endocrine**
  - Hypothalamic-pituitary disorders
  - Testicular disorders
  - Defects of androgen action
  - Hyperthyroidism
  - Hypothyroidism
  - Adrenal insufficiency
  - Congenital adrenal hyperplasia
- Systemic illness
- Defects in spermatogenesis
- Immotile cilia syndrome
- Drug-induced
- **Ductal obstruction**
  - Congenital
  - Acquired seminal vesicle disease
  - Prostatic disease
  - Varicocele
- Retrograde ejaculation
- Antibodies to sperm or seminal plasma
- Anatomic defects of the penis
- Poor coital technique
- Sexual dysfunction
- Idiopathic

Gynecomastia

Q. Write a short note on gynecomastia.

- It is clinically defined as the presence of a rubbery or firm mass concentrically extending from the nipples in a male secondary to proliferation of both **stromal and epithelial component of the glands**.
- It must be differentiated from pseudogynecomastia **(lipomastia)** seen in obese individuals, which is characterized by **only fat deposition** without glandular proliferation.

Causes of Gynecomastia (Table 2.39)

Clinical features

- **Enlargement of breast:** The principal complaint is unilateral or bilateral concentric enlargement of breast glandular tissue.
- **Breast pain:** Present in one-fourth of patients and objective tenderness in about 40%.
- A complaint of nipple discharge can be elicited in 4% of cases.
- Patients with gynecomastia may have a slightly increased risk of development of breast carcinoma.

Treatment

- **Medical treatment:**
  - The **underlying disease** should **be corrected** if possible, and offending drugs should be discontinued.
  - **Antiestrogens or selective estrogen receptor modulators**, such as tamoxifen or raloxifene, have been found useful in relieving pain and reversing gynecomastia in some patients. Aromatase inhibitors have also been tried but are not as beneficial as tamoxifen.
- **Surgical treatment: Reduction mammoplasty** should be considered for cosmetic reasons.
- **Radiotherapy:**
  - Patients with **prostatic carcinoma** may receive low-dose radiation therapy (900c Gy or less) to the breasts before initiation of estrogen therapy. This may prevent or diminish the gynecomastia that usually results from such therapy.
  - Radiotherapy should not be given to other patients with gynecomastia.

TABLE 2.38: Organic causes of erectile dysfunction.

Neurologic	***Urogenital***	***Drugs***
Anterior temporal lobe lesions	Trauma	Antiandrogens
Spinal cord lesions	Castration	Estrogens
Autonomic neuropathy	Priapism	5-α-reductase inhibitors
Vascular	Peyronie's disease	GnRH agonists
Leriche's syndrome	***Systemic illness***	Antihypertensives
Pelvic vascular insufficiency	Cardiac insufficiency	Diuretics
Sickle cell disease	Cirrhosis	Psychotropic agents
Endocrine	Uremia	Tranquilizers
Diabetes mellitus	Respiratory insufficiency	Monoamine oxidase inhibitors
Hypogonadism	Lead poisoning	Tricyclic antidepressants
Hyperprolactinemia	***Postoperative***	Tobacco
Adrenal insufficiency	Aortoiliac or aortofemoral reconstruction	Alcohol
Feminizing tumors	Lumbar sympathectomy	Cocaine
Hypothyroidism	Perineal prostatectomy	
Hyperthyroidism	Retroperitoneal dissection	

TABLE 2.39: Causes of gynecomastia.

Physiologic		***Neoplasms***
➤ Neonatal ➤ Pubertal ➤ Involutional		➤ Testicular germ cell ➤ Leydig cell tumors ➤ hCG-secreting nontrophoblastic neoplasms
Drug-induced		***Systemic diseases***
➤ Androgens and anabolic steroids ➤ Chorionic gonadotropin ➤ Estrogens and estrogen agonists ➤ Growth hormone ➤ Cyproterone ➤ Flutamide ➤ Isoniazid ➤ Ketoconazole ➤ Metronidazole ➤ Cimetidine, ranitidine ➤ Omeprazole ➤ Chemotherapeutic agents (especially alkylating agents) ➤ Amiodarone ➤ Captopril	➤ Reserpine ➤ Spironolactone ➤ Verapamil ➤ Psychoactive agents ➤ Diazepam ➤ Haloperidol ➤ Phenothiazines, ➤ Tricyclic antidepressants ➤ Alcohol ➤ Amphetamines ➤ Heroin ➤ Marijuana ➤ Highly active antiretroviral therapy ➤ Phenytoin ➤ Penicillamine	➤ Hepatic cirrhosis ➤ Uremia ***Endocrine*** ➤ Primary hypogonadism with Leydig cell damage ➤ Hyperprolactinemia ➤ Hyperthyroidism ➤ Androgen receptor disorders ➤ Excessive aromatase activity ***Idiopathic***

(hCG: human chorionic gonadotropin)

Short Stature (Tables 2.40 and 2.41)

Q. Write a short note on short stature and its differential diagnosis.

- Short stature is defined as a height that is **below the 3rd percentile** OR **two or more standard deviations below** the mean for chronological age and gender for a given population.

TABLE 2.40: Differential diagnosis of short stature.

Causes	***Characteristic findings***
GH deficiency	Frontal bossing, high-pitched voice, and central obesity
Hypothyroidism	Immature facies, dry skin, and coarse hair
Cushing's syndrome	Central obesity, striae, and hypertension
Gonadal dysgenesis	Webbed neck, multiple pigmented naevi, delayed sexual development, and shield chest
Pseudohypoparathyroidism	Moon facies, mental retardation, obesity, and short metacarpals
Bone-cartilage dysplasia	Abnormal proportions and macrocephaly
Russell-Silver dwarfism	Small at birth, pointed facies, and asymmetry
Other causes	Turner's syndrome, IUGR, premature birth, cyanotic congenital heart diseases, chronic liver disease, chronic pulmonary or kidney disease, undernutrition, uncontrolled type 1 diabetes mellitus, rickets, and malabsorption

(GH: growth hormone; IUGR: intrauterine growth retardation)

TABLE 2.41: Causes of short stature.

Nonendocrine causes	***Endocrine disorders***
➤ Constitutional short stature ➤ Familial short stature ➤ Genetic short stature ➤ Intrauterine growth retardation and SGA syndromes of short stature ➤ Turner's syndrome and its variants ➤ Noonan's syndrome (**Fig. 2.16A**) ➤ Prader–Willi syndrome ➤ Laurence–Moon and Bardet–Biedl syndromes ➤ Chronic disease ➤ Cardiac disorders (left-to-right shunt and congestive heart failure) ➤ Pulmonary disorders (cystic fibrosis and asthma) ➤ Gastrointestinal disorders: Malabsorption (e.g., celiac disease) ➤ Hematologic disorders ➤ Sickle-cell anemia ➤ Thalassemia ➤ Renal disorders ➤ Renal tubular acidosis ➤ Chronic uremia ➤ Immunologic disorders ➤ Connective tissue disease ➤ Juvenile rheumatoid arthritis ➤ Chronic infection (TB) ➤ Malnutrition ➤ Voluntary dieting ➤ Anorexia nervosa ➤ Cancer chemotherapy	➤ GH deficiency and variants ➤ Congenital GH deficiency ➤ With midline defects ➤ With other pituitary hormone deficiencies ➤ Isolated GH deficiency ➤ Pituitary agenesis ➤ Acquired GH deficiency ➤ Hypothalamic-pituitary tumors ➤ Histiocytosis X ➤ Central nervous systemic infections ➤ Head injuries ➤ GH deficiency following cranial irradiation ➤ Central nervous system vascular accidents ➤ Hydrocephalus ➤ Empty Sella syndrome ➤ Abnormalities of GH action ➤ GH insensitivity (Laron's dwarfism) ➤ Pygmies ➤ Psychosocial dwarfism ➤ Hypothyroidism ➤ Glucocorticoid excess (Cushing's syndrome) ➤ Pseudohypoparathyroidism ➤ Disorders of vitamin D metabolism ➤ Diabetes mellitus, uncontrolled ➤ Diabetes insipidus, untreated

- A **growth velocity that is below the 5th percentile** for age and gender is called **growth deceleration** (e.g., <5 cm/year after the age of 5 years).
- **Dwarfism** is defined as **short stature for the age** of the patient.
- Most common causes of dwarfism are **familial short stature** and **constitutional delay of growth and puberty.**

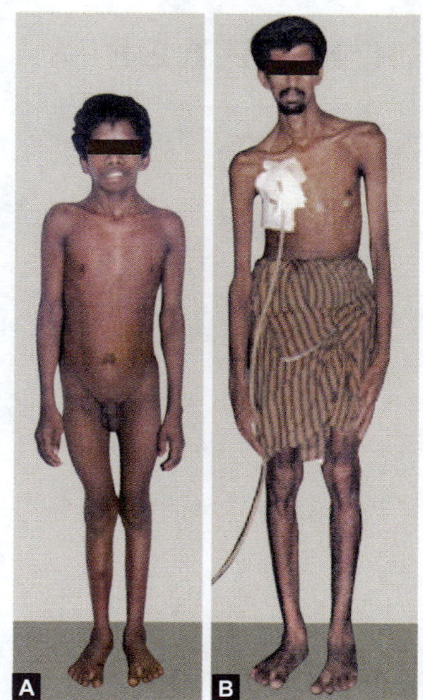

FIGS. 2.16A AND B: (A) Short stature in Noonan syndrome; (B) Tall stature in Marfan syndrome.

Proportionate Short Stature

- Limbs proportionate to trunk
- Seen in most cases of familial short stature

Disproportionate Short Stature

- Limbs disproportionately short compared to trunk
- Seen mostly in cases of skeletal dysplasia

Growth failure: Growth rate below the rate considered appropriate for sex and age.

Tall Stature (Table 2.42)

Tall stature is defined as **height above 97th percentile** for chronological age and sex or **more than 2 SD** above the mean for a defined population.

TABLE 2.42: Causes of tall stature.

Nonendocrine causes	*Endocrine disorders*
➢ Constitutional tall stature ➢ Genetic tall stature ➢ Cerebral gigantism ➢ Homocystinuria ➢ Marfan's syndrome (**Fig. 2.16B**) ➢ Beckwith–Wiedemann syndrome ➢ XYY and XYYY syndromes, Klinefelter's syndrome ➢ Syndromes of tall stature	➢ Pituitary gigantism ➢ Sexual precocity ➢ Thyrotoxicosis ➢ Infants of diabetic mothers

Q. How do we calculate height of child based on parental height?

Estimated adult height of a child calculated on the basis of parental height using the following formulas:

- ♂: [(Paternal height + Maternal height)/2] + 2.5″ (6.5 cm)
- ♀: [(Paternal height + Maternal height)/2] - 2.5″ (6.5 cm)

CHAPTER

3

Diabetes Mellitus

INTRODUCTION

Q. Define and classify diabetes mellitus (DM).

Definition

Diabetes mellitus (DM) is a metabolic cum vascular syndrome of multiple etiologies characterized by chronic hyperglycemia with disturbances of carbohydrate, fat, and protein metabolism resulting from defects in insulin secretion, insulin action, or both leading to changes in both small blood vessels (microangiopathy) and large blood vessels (macroangiopathy).

The International Diabetes Federation (IDF) estimated that in 2015, 415 million people worldwide were diagnosed with DM. This number is expected to go up to 642 million by 2040.

China and India have the largest number of diabetics (109.6 million and 69.2 million, respectively) with the prevalence in Southeast Asia second only to the Western Pacific. β-cell dysfunction may play a more prominent role in the pathogenesis of type 2 diabetes in population or subgroups where low body mass index (BMI) coexists with a high prevalence of the disease, as seen in Southeast Asia, the type 2B, or the Asian-Indian phenotype.

CLASSIFICATION AND ETIOLOGY

Diabetes mellitus is classified according to etiopathogenesis that leads to hyperglycemia into different groups (**Table 3.1 and Fig. 3.1**), but **majority of cases fall into one of two** broad classes namely: **Type 1** (not type I) and **Type 2** (not type II).

- **Type 1 DM**: In this, there is **absolute (complete or near-total) deficiency of insulin**. It is subdivided into two subtypes namely **type 1A**, which is due to **autoimmune** destruction of β-cells and **Type 1B**, where the cause of β-cell destruction is **unknown**.
- **Type 2 diabetes mellitus (T2DM)**: It constitutes a **heterogeneous group** characterized by variable degrees of **insulin resistance, impaired insulin secretion, and increased glucose production**. It also develops due to several genetic and metabolic syndromes.
  - **Risk categories**: Type 2 diabetes mellitus is usually preceded by a period of abnormal glucose homeostasis classified as **impaired fasting glucose (IFG) or impaired glucose tolerance (IGT)**.

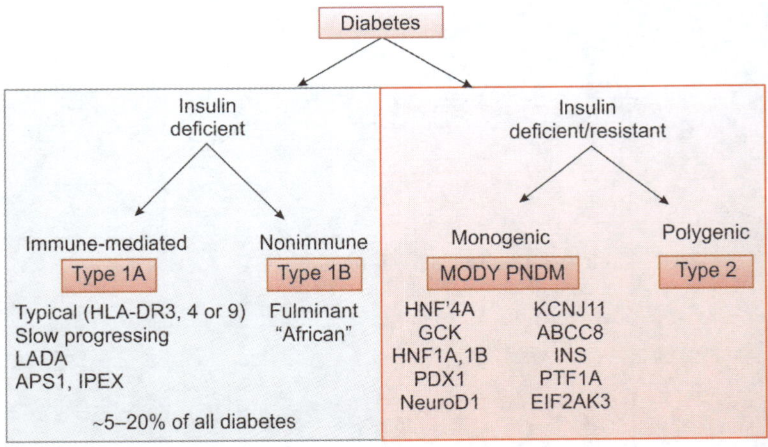

FIG. 3.1: Types of diabetes mellitus.

(ABCC8: ATP-binding cassette transporter subfamily C member 8; APS1: autoimmune polyendocrine syndrome type 1; EIF2AK3: eukaryotic translation initiation factor 2-alpha kinase 3; GCK: glucokinase; HNF4: hepatocyte nuclear factor 4; HLA: human leukocyte antigen; IPEX: immune dysregulation, polyendocrinopathy, enteropathy, X-linked; INS: insulin; KCNJ11: potassium inwardly rectifying channel subfamily J member 11; LADA: latent autoimmune diabetes in adults; MODY: maturity-onset diabetes of the young; NeuroD1: neurogenic differentiation 1; PDX1: pancreatic and duodenal homeobox 1; PNDM: permanent neonatal diabetes mellitus; PTF1A: pancreas transcription factor 1 subunit alpha)

TABLE 3.1: Classification of diabetes mellitus.

- **Type 1 diabetes** (destruction of β-cell usually leading to absolute deficiency of insulin):
  - Type 1A: Immune-mediated
  - Type 1B: Idiopathic
- **Type 2 diabetes** (may range from predominantly insulin resistance with relative insulin deficiency to a predominantly insulin secretory defect with insulin resistance)
- **Other specific types of diabetes:**
  - **Genetic defects of β-cell development or function characterized by mutations in:**
    - Hepatocyte nuclear factor 4α (HNF4α) and maturity-onset diabetes of the young 1 (MODY 1)
    - Glucokinase (MODY 2)
    - HNF1α (MODY 3)
    - Insulin promoter factor 1 (MODY 4)
    - Hepatocyte nuclear factor 1β (MODY 5)
    - Neurogenic differentiation factor 1 (MODY 6)
  - **Genetic defects in insulin action**: Type A insulin resistance, Leprechaunism, Rabson–Mendenhall syndrome, and lipodystrophy syndromes
  - **Exocrine pancreatic defects**: Pancreatitis, pancreatectomy, hemochromatosis, pancreatic neoplasm, cystic fibrosis, and fibrocalculous pancreatopathy
  - **Endocrinopathies**: Acromegaly, Cushing syndrome, hyperthyroidism, pheochromocytoma, and glucagonoma
  - **Infections**: Cytomegalovirus, Coxsackie B virus, and congenital rubella (Hepatitis C virus infection has been associated with an increased incidence of diabetes, but it is uncertain if there is a direct relationship)
  - **Drugs or chemical-induced:** Glucocorticoids, pentamidine, nicotinic acid, thyroid hormone, diazoxide, β-adrenergic agonists, thiazides, phenytoin, α-interferon, asparaginase, and tacrolimus
  - **Genetic** syndromes **sometimes associated with diabetes**: Down syndrome, Klinefelter syndrome, Turner syndrome, Wolfram syndrome, DIDMOAD (diabetes insipidus, diabetes mellitus, optic atrophy, and deafness), Friedreich's ataxia, Huntington's disease, Laurence–Moon–Biedl syndrome, myotonic dystrophy, porphyria, and Prader–Willi syndrome
  - Uncommon forms of immune-mediated diabetes: "Stiff-man" syndrome and anti-insulin receptor antibodies
- **Gestational diabetes mellitus (GDM)**
- **Latent autoimmune diabetes in adults (LADA)**

FEATURES OF CURRENT CLASSIFICATION OF DIABETES MELLITUS

- The terms insulin-dependent diabetes mellitus (IDDM) and noninsulin-dependent diabetes mellitus (NIDDM) are no longer used now because many patients with T2DM eventually need insulin for control of hyperglycemia.
- The age or treatment modality is not a criterion for classification. Type 1 DM most often occurs in younger patients before the age of 30 years and an autoimmune destruction of P-cell can start at any age. However, about 10% of patients above the age of 30 years have type 1 DM. T2DM usually develops with increasing age. However, it is now being diagnosed more frequently in children and young adults (particularly in obese adolescents).

METABOLIC EFFECTS OF LACK OF INSULIN (TABLE 3.2)

TABLE 3.2: Functions of insulin and metabolic effects of insulin deficiency.

Functions of insulin	*Consequences of insulin deficiency*
Functions that decreases blood glucose level	**Insulin deficiency increases the blood glucose level**
➢ Increases activity of glycolytic enzymes	➢ Decreased activity of glycolytic enzymes
➢ Increases glycogen synthesis	➢ Glycogen breakdown into glucose increases (gluconeogenesis)
➢ Increases uptake of glucose by skeletal and cardiac muscle	➢ Decreased glucose transport into skeletal and cardiac muscle
➢ Decreases activity of gluconeogenic enzymes	➢ Increased activity of gluconeogenic enzymes (gluconeogenesis)
Lipid metabolism: Increases lipid synthesis	Lipolysis (raised plasma free fatty acids) and ketogenesis
Protein metabolism: Enhances tissue uptake of amino acids and accelerates protein synthesis	Decrease in tissue uptake of amino acids and reduced protein synthesis
Other functions	
➢ Increases transmembrane K^+ transport	➢ Decrease in movement of K^+ into the cell
➢ Decreases cyclic adenosine monophosphate (AMP) level in adipose tissue and liver	➢ Increased cyclic AMP levels in adipose tissue and liver

ETIOPATHOGENESIS OF TYPE 1 DIABETES MELLITUS

Q. Describe and discuss the epidemiology, pathogenesis, risk factors, and clinical evolution of type 1 diabetes.

Q. Describe and discuss the genetic background and the influence of the environment on diabetes.

It accounts for ~ **5–10%** of all cases.

Age: Most common in **childhood (younger than 20 years** of age). Since, it can develop at any age; the term "juvenile diabetes" should be avoided.

Etiology

- **Autoimmune disease** is characterized by:
  - **Pancreatic β-cell destruction**
  - **Absolute deficiency of insulin**
- **Idiopathic:** It is a rare form in which there is no evidence for autoimmunity.

Pathogenesis of Type 1 Diabetes Mellitus (Fig. 3.2)

- It is an **autoimmune disease** that involves interplay of both genetic susceptibility and environmental factors.
  Genetic susceptibility: Incidence of type 1 diabetes is greater in twins of affected individuals than in the general population and greater in monozygotic than in dizygotic twins.
- **Human leukocyte antigen (HLA) genes**: About 95% of patients with type 1 diabetes have either **HLA-DR3 or HLA-DR4, or both**, compared with the general population.
  Environmental factors: **Viral infections may trigger islet cell destruction** and associations have been found between type 1 diabetes and infection with ***mumps, rubella, Coxsackie B, or cytomegalovirus***. Environmental event initiates the process in genetically susceptible individuals. Relative deficiency of vitamin D may also be responsible.
  Mechanisms of β-cell destruction (Fig. 3.2): The autoimmune damage starts many years before the disease becomes clinically evident. An inflammatory response in the pancreas called **"insulitis"** develops and there is infiltration of the islets with activated T lymphocytes.
- **Phases in the development of diabetes mellitus**:
  - **Phase with normal glucose tolerance**: In most of the patients, islet cell autoantibodies appear much earlier than overt diabetes. β-cell mass and insulin secretion progressively decrease; however, normal levels of blood glucose are maintained.
  - **Phase of impaired glucose intolerance**: Features of diabetes do not become evident even with destruction of 70–80% of β-cells. At this point, residual functional β-cells cannot maintain glucose tolerance and patient develops glucose intolerance.
  - **Phase of frank diabetes**: Stress, infection, or puberty may be associated with increased insulin requirements and may trigger the *transition* from glucose intolerance to frank diabetes.
  - ***Honeymoon phase****: After the initial clinical presentation of frank type 1 DM, a phase may occur during which time patient is euglycemic with modest doses of insulin or rarely without insulin for some time. This is referred to as honeymoon phase. This usually lasts for a few months after which the patient develops frank DM again.*
    - **Hyperglycemia and ketosis** occur after **>90% of the β-cells have been destroyed** by an autoimmune process.
    - **Immunologic markers**: These include autoantibodies against islet cell, insulin, glutamic acid decarboxylase (GAD65), zinc transporter 8 (ZnT8), and tyrosine phosphatase such as insulinoma-associated protein-2 (IA-2) and IA-2p. One or more of these autoantibodies are detected in 85–90% of individuals when fasting hyperglycemia is initially detected.

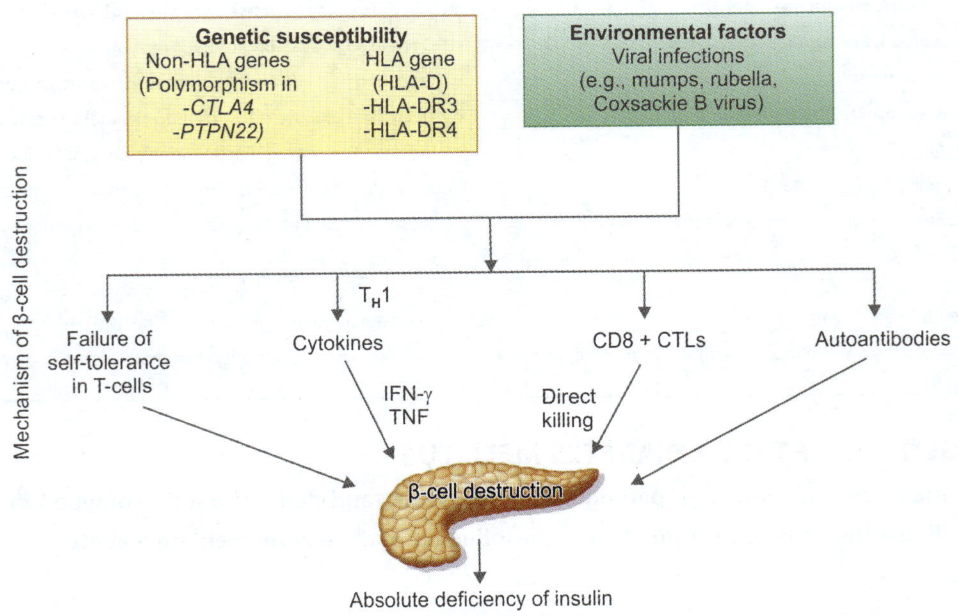

FIG. 3.2: Pathogenesis of type 1 diabetes mellitus.
(CTLs: cytotoxic T lymphocytes; HLA: human leukocyte antigen; IFN-γ: interferon-γ; TNF: tumor necrosis factor)

- Type 1 DM can be associated with various autoimmune disorders as outlined in **Table 3.3**.
- **Slow-burning variant of type 1 DM**: It is characterized by slower progression to insulin deficiency and develops in later life and is sometimes called **latent autoimmune diabetes in adults (LADA)**. LADA may be difficult to distinguish from T2DM.

TABLE 3.3: Various autoimmune disorders that can be associated with type 1 diabetes mellitus (DM).

Autoimmune diseases	*Autoantibody types*	*Autoantibody percentage*	*Disease prevalence (%)*
Addison's disease	21-hydroxylase	1.5	0.5
Celiac disease	Transglutaminase	12	6
Pernicious anemia	Parietal cell	21	2.6
Thyroiditis or Graves' disease	Peroxidase or thyroglobulin	25	4

PATHOGENESIS OF TYPE 2 DIABETES MELLITUS (FIG. 3.3)

Q. Describe and discuss the epidemiology, pathogenesis, risk factors, and clinical evolution of type 2 diabetes.

Type 2 diabetes is a **multifactorial disease**. The four major factors are: (1) **increasing age**, (2) **obesity**, (3) **ethnicity**, and (4) **family history**.

Type 2 diabetes is associated with central obesity, hypertension, hypertriglyceridemia, and decreased high-density lipoprotein (HDL) cholesterol (metabolic syndrome).

- **Environmental factors** play a role and include:
  - **Sedentary lifestyle**
  - **Dietary habits and associated obesity**: Overeating, obesity, and underactivity are associated with the development of T2DM.
- **Genetic factors**: It is much more significant in T2DM than in type 1 DM.
  - Type 2 diabetes has a **concordance rate of 35–60% in monozygotic twins compared with 17–30% in dizygotic twins.**
  - Lifetime risk for type 2 diabetes in an offspring is more than double, if **both parents** are **affected.**
  - Diabetogenic genes have been found.
- In contrast to type 1 DM, in T2DM, there is no HLA relationship and there is no evidence of an autoimmune basis. Pancreatic β-cell mass is intact in T2DM, in contrast to type 1 DM. The β-cell mass is increased.

Characteristics of Type 2 Diabetes Mellitus

These include: (1) insulin resistance, (2) abnormal/impaired insulin secretion/action, (3) increased hepatic production of glucose, and (4) abnormal fat metabolism.

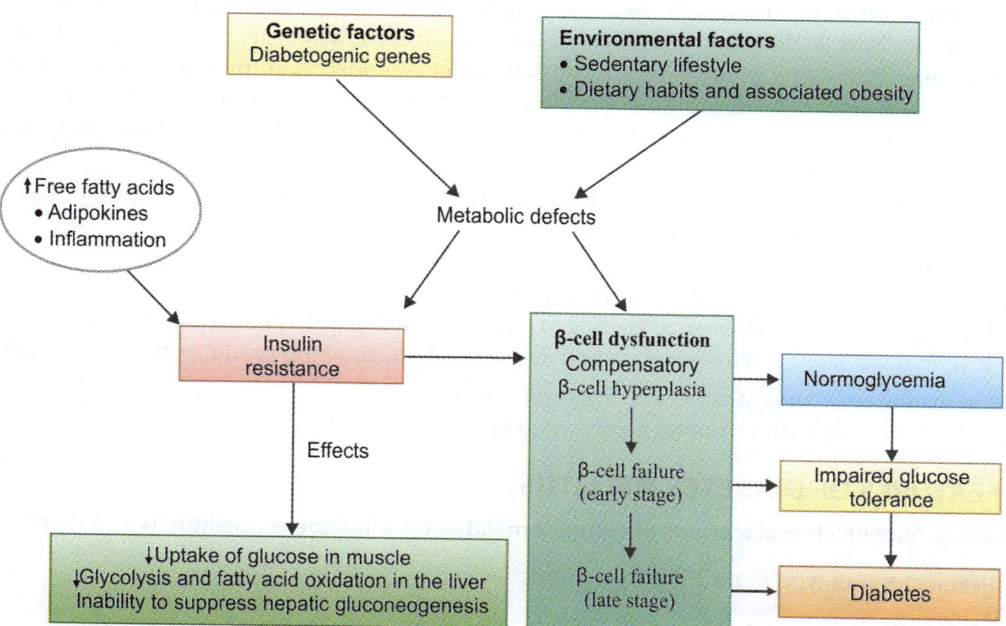

FIG. 3.3: Pathogenesis of type 2 diabetes. Insulin resistance associated with obesity is induced by free fatty acids, adipokines, and chronic inflammation in adipose tissue. Insulin resistance causes β-cells of pancreas to undergo compensatory hyperplasia and the resulting hypersecretion of insulin maintains normoglycemia. However, at some point, β-cell compensation is followed by β-cell failure and diabetes develops.

Genome-wide association studies (GWASs) have linked aberrations in >40 different genes with an increased risk of T2DM. These genes are involved in the regulation of various biological processes including cellular development, differentiation, and physiological functions.

Epigenetics and deoxyribonucleic acid (DNA) methylation play an important role in the pathogenesis of T2DM including insulin production, β-cell secretion, and resistance. This regulation can either occur by affecting the DNA methylation of the insulin gene itself or by affecting the DNA methylation status of other genes that regulate insulin production, secretion, and sensing.

INSULIN RESISTANCE

Q. Write short essay/note on insulin resistance.

- Insulin resistance is **the decrease/failure of target (peripheral) tissues to insulin action.**
- Main factors in the development of insulin resistance are combination of genetic susceptibility and **obesity**. The obesity accompanying T2DM is central obesity and central adipose tissue is more "lipolytic" than peripheral sites. Insulin resistance is induced by free fatty acids (FFAs), adipokines, and chronic inflammation in adipose tissue.
- **Consequences of insulin resistance**:
  - **Decreased uptake of glucose in muscle** results in postprandial hyperglycemia. The defects in the uptake are due to defect in the receptors present in target tissues and usually at the postreceptor level.
  - **Reduced glycolysis** and **fatty acid oxidation** in the liver.
  - **Inability to suppress hepatic gluconeogenesis.**
- **Abnormalities of insulin secretion and action**:
- **β-cell dysfunction**: Abnormalities (abnormal/impaired) of insulin secretion develops early in the course of type 2 diabetes and is due to β-cell dysfunction. β-cell dysfunction is multifactorial in origin. In type 2 diabetes, β-cell dysfunction manifests as **inadequate insulin secretion by the pancreatic β-cells (relative insulin deficiency)** in association with insulin resistance and hyperglycemia.
- **Compensatory β-cell hyperplasia**: Pancreatic β-cells **initially respond** to long-term demands of peripheral insulin resistance **by undergoing compensatory hyperplasia leading to increased insulin secretion (hypersecretion)**. Thus, the hyperinsulinemic state can compensate for peripheral resistance and maintain normal blood glucose for years.
  - **β-cell failure (early stage)**: However, at some point, β-cells exhaust their capacity to adapt. β-cell compensation cannot maintain normal blood sugar level. In this stage, the patient develops IGT.
  - **β-cell failure (late stage)**: The early stage of cell failure is followed by decreased insulin secretion, hyperglycemia, and frank diabetes develops.
- **Increased hepatic production of glucose**: Relative lack of insulin is associated with increased production of glucose from the liver (due to inadequate suppression of gluconeogenesis) and reduced glucose uptake by peripheral tissues. Increased hepatic glucose output produces fasting hyperglycemia.
- **Abnormal fat metabolism**: Insulin resistance in adipose tissue causes lipolysis and increased production of free fatty acid from adipocytes. This leads to increased synthesis of lipid [very-low-density lipoprotein (VLDL) and triglyceride] in hepatocytes. Deposition of fat in the liver is a common association with central obesity and is increased by insulin resistance and/or deficiency. The deposition of fat/lipid or steatosis in the liver may result in nonalcoholic fatty liver disease (NAFLD). This is also responsible for the dyslipidemia observed in T2DM (i.e., **raised triglycerides, decreased HDL, and raised small dense LDL**).

  Hyperglycemia (**glucotoxicity**) and elevated free fatty acid levels (**"lipotoxicity"**) and dietary fat may also cause further β-cell loss and deterioration of glucose homeostasis.
- Phases of insulin resistance:
  - Phase 1: Normal plasma glucose due to compensatory increase in insulin secretion.
  - Phase 2: Worsening of insulin resistance leading to postprandial hyperglycemia despite elevated insulin secretion.
  - Phase 3: Insulin resistance remains constant and decline in β-cell function produces fasting hyperglycemia.

Clinical findings in insulin resistance: Acanthosis nigricans and skin tags.
Pathophysiology of T2DM—the **ominous octet** is presented in **Figure 3.4**.

CLINICAL FEATURES OF DIABETES MELLITUS

Q. Write short essay/note on clinical features of diabetes mellitus/type 1 diabetes mellitus/type 2 diabetes mellitus.

Usually, the clinical features of type 1 and T2DM are distinctive.

Type 1 Diabetes Mellitus

- **Age**: Usually begins before the age of 30 years, but can occur at any age.
- Weight is normal to lean (wasted).

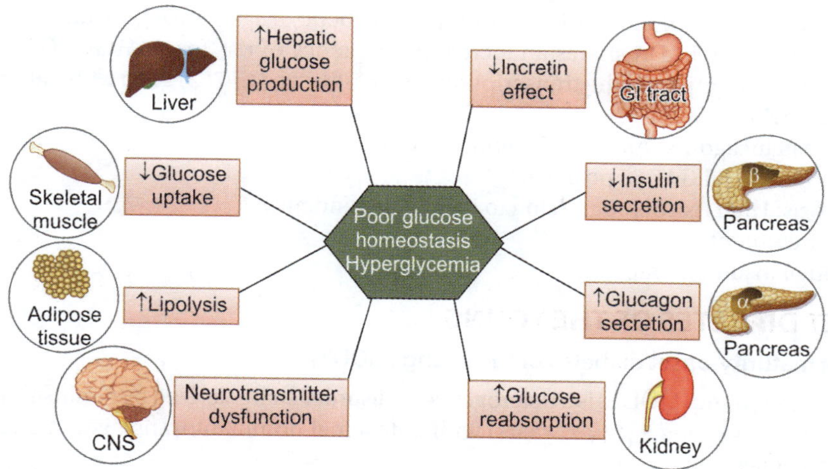

FIG. 3.4: Pathophysiology of type 2 diabetes mellitus—the ominous octet. Multiple drugs in combination may be needed to improve glucose homeostasis. The treatment should target the underlying pathophysiology.
(CNS: central nervous system)

- **Classical triad of diabetes**: The onset of symptoms may be abrupt with **polyuria, polydipsia, and polyphagia** to metabolic derangements. Weight loss may develop over days or weeks.
- Diabetic ketoacidosis (DKA) may be the initial presentation in approximately 25% of adults with newly diagnosed type 1 diabetes.
- **Insulin requirement**: In the initial 1 or 2 years, the exogenous insulin required may be minimal because of endogenous insulin secretion. But later, its requirement suddenly increases.
- Characteristically, the **plasma insulin is low** and **C-peptide levels are low** and unmeasurable. *Glucagon levels are raised and suppressible with insulin.*

Type 2 Diabetes Mellitus

- **Age**: Usually begins in older **above the age of 40 years** and frequently in **obese individuals**. Due to increase in obesity and sedentary lifestyle, it is now detected also in children and adolescents.
- **Presentation**: The symptoms develop gradually over a period of months to years. Examples are **polyuria, polydipsia, nocturia, blurred vision, unexplained weakness, or weight loss**.
- Polyuria occurs when the serum glucose concentration rises significantly above 180 mg/dL, exceeding the renal threshold for glucose reabsorption, which leads to increased urinary glucose excretion.
- Glycosuria causes osmotic diuresis (i.e., polyuria) and hypovolemia, which, in turn, can lead to polydipsia.
- In **asymptomatic individuals**, the **diagnosis is made after routine blood** (hyperglycemia) or **urine testing (glycosuria)**.
- Patients may complain of symptoms such as lack of energy, blurring of vision (due to glucose-induced changes in refraction), or pruritus vulvae or balanitis caused by *Candida* infection.
- Many patients may present with one of the chronic complications of diabetes and are found to be diabetic on investigations. These include: staphylococcal skin infections, retinopathy, polyneuropathy, erectile dysfunction, and arterial disease (myocardial infarction or peripheral gangrene).
- Adults with type 2 diabetes can present with a hyperosmolar hyperglycemic state (HHS) characterized by marked hyperglycemia, severe dehydration, and obtundation, but without ketoacidosis. DKA as the presenting symptom of type 2 diabetes is also uncommon in adults.
- **Insulin levels in the plasma are normal to high**. Glucagon levels are raised, but resistant to insulin.

LATENT AUTOIMMUNE DIABETES IN ADULTS

Q. Write short note on LADA.

- Latent autoimmune diabetes in adults is a form of **autoimmune type 1 diabetes**, which is diagnosed in individuals who are older than the usual age of onset of type 1 diabetes. Often, LADA is mistaken for **type 2 diabetes** based on their age at the time of diagnosis.
- Alternate terms for "LADA" include late-onset autoimmune diabetes of adulthood, "slow-onset type 1" diabetes, and "type 1.5 diabetes".

Features of Latent Autoimmune Diabetes in Adults

- Age: Usually ≤25 years of age.
- Clinical presentation: Similar to nonobese type 2 diabetes.

- Initial control achieved with diet alone or diet plus oral antidiabetic drugs (OADs). Insulin dependency occurs within months (rarely can take years). LADA shares an increased frequency of risk for an HLA-DQB1 genotype than patients with type 1 diabetes and for a variant in the transcription factor 7-like 2 (*TCF7L2*) gene with patients with type 2 diabetes.
- Other features of type 1 DM:
  - Low fasting and postglucagon-stimulated C-peptide levels
  - Islet cell antibody (ICA) and GAD65 positive.
- Importance of diagnosis: High risk of progression to insulin dependency.
  - Avoid metformin treatment
  - Early introduction of insulin therapy.

MATURITY-ONSET DIABETES OF THE YOUNG

Q. Write short essay on maturity-onset diabetes of the young (MODY).

Maturity-onset diabetes of the young (MODY) is a heterogeneous disorder characterized by noninsulin-dependent monogenic form of diabetes diagnosed at a young age (<25 years) with autosomal dominant transmission and lack of autoantibodies accounting for 2–5% of diabetes.

- **Mutations** in several **transcription factors** or in **glucokinase** result in insufficient insulin release from pancreatic β-cells causing MODY. Almost 11 subtypes of MODY are identified based on the mutated gene.
- MODY can **occur at any age**. About 70% forms of MODY are MODY 3 (hepatic transcription factor 1 gene) and 10% MODY 2 (glucokinase gene).

Features of Maturity-onset Diabetes of the Young

- Age: Young onset of diabetes <25 years of age
- Strong family history of early-onset diabetes (2–3 generations affected)
- Evidence of macrovascular complications in earlier generation
- Sulfonylurea sensitivity and noninsulin dependence (not requiring insulin even after 5 years of diagnosis)
- Absence of insulin resistance phenotype: Normal blood pressure, triglycerides, and HDL.

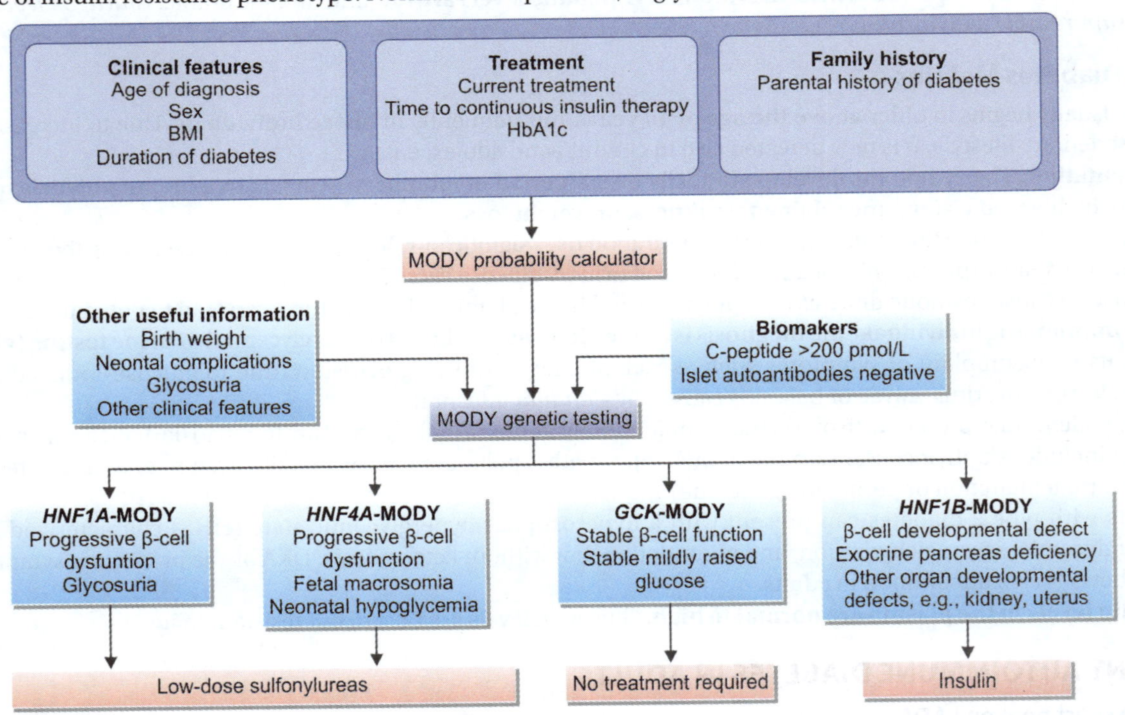

FIG. 3.5: Features of MODY

(BMI: body mass index; GCK: glucokinase; HbA1c: glycated hemoglobin; HNF1A: hepatocyte nuclear factor 1 alpha; MODY: maturity-onset diabetes of the young)

Subtypes of Maturity-onset Diabetes of the Young (Table 3.4)

Differences between type 1 DM, T2DM, and MODY are listed in **Table 3.5**.

Q. Write short note on fibrocalculous pancreatic diabetes (FCPD).

Fibrocalculous Pancreatic Diabetes

- Pancreatogenic diabetes is classified by the American Diabetes Association (ADA) and by the World Health Organization as **type 3c diabetes mellitus (T3cDM)**.

TABLE 3.4: Types of maturity-onset diabetes of the young (MODY).

MODY types	Defective chromosomes	Mutation in	Phenotypic features
1.	20q	Hepatocyte nuclear factor 4α (HNF4α)	Adolescent/early adult: Progressive in insulin secretory defect
2.	7p	Glucokinase (GCK) gene	Since birth: Stable mild fasting hyperglycemia
3.	12q	HNF1α	Adolescent/early adult: Progressive insulin secretory defect
4.	13q	Insulin promoter factor-1 (IPF-1)	Early adult: Very rare, mild diabetes
5.	17q	HNF1β	Adolescent: Progressive diabetes
6.	2q	NeuroD1	Early adult: Rare
7.	2p	KLF11	Early adult: Pancreatic atrophy
8.	9q	Carboxyl ester lipase (CEL)	Early adult: Rare
9.	7q	PAX4	Early adult: Rare
10.	11p	INS	Rare
11.	8p	BLK	Rare

(BLK: B lymphocyte kinase; NeuroD1: neurogenic differentiation 1; PAX4: paired box gene 4; KLF11: Krüppel-like factor 11)

TABLE 3.5: Differences between type 1 DM, type 2 DM, and MODY.

Features	Type 1 DM	Type 2 DM	MODY
Frequency	Common	Increasing	2–5% of type 2 DM
Genetics	Polygenic	Polygenic	Monogenic autosomal dominant
Family history	<15%	>50%	100%
Ethnicity	Different races	Different races	Asians, Polynesians, and indigenous Australians
Age of onset	Throughout childhood	Postpuberty	<25 years
Severity of onset	Acute and severe	Mild	Mild/asymptomatic
Ketosis/diabetic ketoacidosis	Common	Uncommon	Rare
Obesity association	–	>90%	±
Acanthosis nigricans and metabolic syndrome	Absent	Common	Absent
Autoimmunity	Positive	Negative	Positive
Pathophysiology	β-cell destruction	Insulin resistance and relative insulinopenia	β-cell dysfunction

(DM: diabetes mellitus; MODY: maturity-onset diabetes of the young)

- Prevalence of 5–10% among all patients with DM.
- Seen almost exclusively in developing countries, FCPD is characterized by a triad of abdominal pain, steatorrhea, and diabetes.
- Genes implicated are serine protease inhibitor Kazal type 1 (*SPINK1*), *cathepsin B*, and cystic fibrosis transmembrane conductance regulator (*CFTR*).
- 70% are males in their second and third decades.
- Classically, patients are malnourished with low BMI, but very high insulin requirements. While the presence of microvascular complications are similar as in other types of diabetes, the presence of macrovascular complications are rare, believed to be due to young age, lean body, and low lipid levels.
- Risk of pancreatic cancer is very high in this population.

DIAGNOSIS OF DIABETES MELLITUS

Q. Discuss the diagnostic criteria for diabetes mellitus.

- Classical symptoms: Diabetes may present with polyuria, polydipsia, and polyphagia. There may significant weight loss, despite polyphagia.
- Symptoms due to depressed immune status: Diabetes is associated with immune dysfunction. It may result in activation of pulmonary tuberculosis, nonhealing of wounds, candidial pruritus vulvae or balanitis, recurrent styes, and recurrent urinary tract infections.

- End-organ involvement: Some patients may present with symptoms of end-organ involvement such as retinopathy, nephropathy, or neuropathy.
- Risk factors of DM: Some patients may have identifiable risk factors such as obesity, pregnancy, and first-degree relatives of known diabetics.

Normal Glucose Levels

- Normally, the **blood glucose levels** are maintained in a very narrow range of **70–120 mg/dL**.
- Glycemia can be classified into three categories: (1) euglycemia (normal), (2) prediabetes (impaired), and (3) diabetes (**Table 3.6**).

Prediabetes: It is defined as condition in which there is **IGT**, but elevated **blood sugar does not reach the criterion accepted for an outright diagnosis of diabetes**. Prediabetes may be either IFG based upon a fasting plasma glucose (FPG) result or IGT based upon the fasting and 2-hour oral glucose tolerance test (OGTT) results. Recently, the term "prediabetes" has been changed to **"categories of increased risk for diabetes"**. The criteria for diagnosis are:

TABLE 3.6: WHO criteria: Levels of blood glucose in normal, prediabetes, and diabetes in glucose tolerance test.

	Euglycemic	*Prediabetes (impaired glucose tolerance)*	*Diabetes*
Fasting glucose level	<100 mg/dL	>100 mg/dL but <126 mg/dL	>126 mg/dL on more than one occasion
2-hour OGTT (75 g anhydrous glucose in water)	<140 mg/dL	>140 mg/dL but <200 mg/dL	>200 mg/dL

(OGTT: oral glucose tolerance test)

Q. Write short note/essay on impaired fasting glucose (IFG).

Impaired fasting glucose: **Fasting glucose** level is **>100 mg/dL but <126 mg/dL** (whole-blood glucose ≥88 mg/dL but <110 mg/dL). This diagnostic category does not need glucose tolerance test. It is not a distinct clinical entity, but individuals have the future risk of frank diabetes and cardiovascular disease.

Q. Write short note/essay on impaired glucose tolerance (IGT).

- **Impaired glucose tolerance**: **GTT** values **>140 mg/dL but <200 mg/dL** (whole-blood glucose between 125 and 175 mg/dL 2 hours after oral glucose load). IGT is not a disease, but a risk factor for future diabetes and cardiovascular disease. This is heterogeneous group of people who are obese, have fatty liver, and are on medication, which can alter glucose tolerance. IGT patients have the same risk of cardiovascular disease as those with frank diabetes, but microvascular complications are rare.
  - Additionally, glycated hemoglobin (HbA1c) in the range of **5.7–6.4%** is also included in "prediabetes".
    Risks in prediabetes: (1) **Progression to frank diabetes** over time and (2) **cardiovascular disease**.
  - Impaired fasting glucose and IGT are associated with the **metabolic syndrome**.
- **Medical nutrition therapy** aimed at reducing 5–10% loss of body weight and exercise has been found to prevent or delay the development of diabetes in individuals with IGT. However, no drug therapy is recommended at present. Acarbose and metformin have been tried in prediabetes.

Diagnostic Criteria for Diabetes Mellitus

Q. Write short essay/note on oral glucose tolerance test: WHO diagnostic criteria.

WHO Diagnostic Criteria for Diabetes Mellitus (Box 3.1)

Q. Write short note on World Health Organization (WHO) diagnostic criteria for diabetes mellitus.

Box 3.1: WHO criteria for the diagnosis of diabetes mellitus.

- Fasting plasma glucose >126 mg/dL (7.0 mmol/L)
- Random plasma glucose >200 mg/dL (11.1 mmol/L) with classical signs and symptoms
- One abnormal laboratory value is diagnostic in symptomatic individuals:
  - Two values are needed in asymptomatic individuals
  - The glucose tolerance test is only required for borderline cases and for diagnosis of gestational diabetes
- HbA1c > 6.5 (48 mmol/mol).

(HbA1c: glycated hemoglobin: WHO: World Health Organization)

Criteria for Diagnosis of Diabetes (American Diabetes Association) (Box 3.2)

Q. Write short note/essay on American Diabetes Association (ADA) criteria for the diagnosis of diabetes mellitus.

Q. Write short note/essay on differential diagnosis of glycosuria.

Differential diagnosis of glycosuria (Box 3.3):

- Normal renal threshold is blood glucose level of 180 mg/dL and at this level, there is no glycosuria. If the blood sugar level exceeds the renal threshold (usually >180–200 mg/dL), the excess glucose will not be reabsorbed into the blood and will be eliminated in the urine as in cases of DM. The presence of detectable amounts of **glucose in urine** is termed as **glycosuria**.
- When there is glycosuria, it should be determined whether it is secondary to hyperglycemia (DM) or renal glycosuria or alimentary (lag storage) glycosuria or any other causes (nondiabetic glycosuria).

Renal glycosuria

Q. Write short note/essay on renal glycosuria and Marble's criteria for diagnosis of renal glycosuria.

- **Definition**: Renal glycosuria is the excretion of glucose in the urine at normal blood glucose concentrations in the absence of any signs of generalized proximal renal tubular dysfunction. There is decreased renal threshold below the normal level of 180 mg/dL for glucose. Renal glycosuria is a benign condition transmitted as an autosomal dominant disorder.
- Diagnosis of renal glycosuria: It is based on the Marble's criteria (**Box 3.4**).

Alimentary (lag storage) glycosuria

Q. Write short note/essay on alimentary (lag storage) glycosuria.

- Alimentary glycosuria is characterized by a transient abnormal rise in blood glucose level following moderate amount of a meal (which normally does not cause appearance of glucose in the urine) and appearance of glucose in the urine. It develops because the blood sugar level exceeds the normal renal threshold (180 mg/dL).
- **Conditions associated** with alimentary glycosuria:
    - Glucose tolerance test reveals a peak at 1 hour above renal threshold (which causes glycosuria), but the fasting and postprandial (i.e., 2 hours after meal) glucose values are normal.
    - Following gastric surgery (e.g., gastrectomy or gastrojejunostomy) with rapid gastric emptying time.
    - Hyperthyroidism
    - Liver diseases
    - Some normal individuals.

Box 3.2: Criteria for diagnosis of diabetes (American Diabetes Association, 2016).

Typical symptoms of diabetes mellitus (DM) (polyuria, polydipsia, and weight loss) + random plasma glucose **≥200 mg/dL** (symptoms of diabetes + random whole-blood glucose >175 mg/dL)

Or

Fasting plasma glucose **≥126 mg/dL** (fasting whole-blood glucose ≥110 mg/dL)

Or

2-hour plasma glucose **≥200 mg/dL** during an oral glucose tolerance test (OGTT) (whole blood ≥175 mg/dL during an oral 75-g glucose tolerance test)

Or

Glycated hemoglobin (HbA1c) **≥6.5%**

Box 3.3: Differential diagnosis of glycosuria.

Glycosuria with hyperglycemia:

- Endocrine disorders: Diabetes mellitus, acromegaly, Cushing's syndrome, hyperthyroidism, hyperadrenocorticism, functioning α- or β-cell pancreatic tumors, and pheochromocytoma
- Nonendocrine diseases: Increased intracranial tension (brain tumor or hemorrhage), liver disorders, drugs (e.g., corticosteroids, adrenocorticotropic hormones, thiazides), and alimentary glycosuria

Glycosuria without hyperglycemia: Renal glycosuria and pregnancy

Box 3.4: Marble's criteria for the diagnosis of renal glycosuria.

- Constant glycosuria with little fluctuation related to diet
- Normal oral glucose tolerance test (OGTT)
- Identification of urinary reducing substance as glucose
- Normal storage and utilization of carbohydrates

Oral Glucose Tolerance Test

Q. Write short essay/note on oral glucose tolerance test (OGTT).

Indication: It is not recommended for routine diagnosis of either type 1 or T2DM. This is because FPG identifies the abnormal glucose metabolism.

- In patients where the FPG is in the range of IFG (100–125 mg/dL)
- Diagnosis of gestational DM
- Uncertainty about the diagnosis of diabetes.

Preparation of the patient: Patient should be taking an unrestricted carbohydrate diet for at least 3 days or more prior to the test because carbohydrate-restricted diet reduces glucose tolerance. Patient should be with normal physical activity.

- Oral glucose tolerance test is performed in the morning after patient has fasted overnight (at least 8 hours).
- The patient should rest for at least half an hour before starting the test and refrain from smoking, tea/coffee, or exercise during the test.

Test: A fasting venous sample of blood is drawn to estimate the glucose level.

- Patients are given 75 g of anhydrous glucose dissolved in 250–300 mL of water orally over 5 minutes. Dose in children is 1.75 g of glucose/kg body weight up to a maximum of 75 g. Time of starting glucose is taken as 0 hour.

- A single venous sample of blood is drawn 2 hours after the glucose administration and glucose level is estimated (previously, blood samples were collected at 0.5 hour, 1 hour, 1.5 hour, and 2 hours).
- The criteria for IGT are discussed earlier.

MANAGEMENT OF DIABETES MELLITUS

Q. Long essay on:
- **Treatment and monitoring the control of uncomplicated diabetes mellitus.**
- **Diagnosis and management of type 1 diabetes mellitus (DM)/type 2 DM.**
- **Diagnosis and treatment of obese patient with type 2 diabetes mellitus (DM).**

Diet and Lifestyle Management

Q. Write short essay/note on:
- **Dietary management of diabetes mellitus.**
- **Medical nutrition therapy in diabetes.**

Aims of dietary management are given in **Box 3.5**.

Box 3.5: Aims of dietary management in diabetes.

- Achieve good glycemic control
- Reduce hyperglycemia and avoid hypoglycemia
- Reduce the risk of diabetic complications
- Weight management:
  - Weight maintenance for type 1 diabetes mellitus (DM) and nonobese type 2 DM
  - Weight loss for overweight and obese type 2 DM
- Maintain adequate intake of nutrition
- Avoid atherogenic diets or restrict diet for those aggravate complications (e.g., avoid high-protein diet in nephropathy)

Medical Nutrition Therapy

Medical nutrition therapy (MNT) should optimally manage the "**ABCs**" of diabetes control: Hb**A**1c, **B**lood pressure, and LDL **C**holesterol.

Medical nutrition therapy for diabetes **has to be individualized** with consideration given to eating habits and lifestyle factors. There must be flexibility in use of ordinary foods for patients and families. The best diet advised is the Mediterranean diet.

Medical nutrition therapy can reduce the HbA1c levels by **0.6–1.4%** if strictly adhered to:

- A **regular pattern of meals** (and snacks) is important to maintain a constant daily intake of carbohydrate and protects against hypoglycemia. Mild deviations in one or two meals do not matter. It is overall long-term dietary pattern that is important.
- Diet in the management of diabetes **varies with the type of disease**.
- In **insulin-dependent** patients and those on intensive insulin regimens, since adjustment of insulin can cover wide variations, the composition of the **diet is not of critical importance**.
- In **noninsulin-dependent** patients, who are not on exogenous insulin, **rigorous adherence to diet** is needed, as the endogenous insulin reserve is limited. The increased demand produced by excess calories or increased intake of rapidly absorbed carbohydrate cannot be met.
- **Caloric content of the diet**: It is first decision to be taken based on the need to gain, lose, or maintain current weight. **Two basic types of diet** used in the treatment of diabetes are: (i) **low-calorie weight reducing diets** and (ii) **weight maintenance diets.** Dietary prescriptions, should be such that there is daily deficit of 500 kcal, provide a realistic diet and produce a weekly weight loss of around 0.5 kg. Calorie recommendations for adults carrying out "average" activity are 36 kcal/kg for men and 34 kcal/kg for women. Recommended diabetic diet should aim at achieving a BMI of 22 kg/m^2. If weight loss cannot be achieved, weight maintenance (rather than gain) is an important goal.
- **Low glycemic index of pulses and pulse-incorporated cereal foods**—including grams and pulses in rice or wheat-based starchy high glycemic index diets reduces the glycemic index and brings satiety along with adequate supply of calories. Meals with mixed sources of cereals, pulses, and legumes contribute to regulation of insulin and glycemic responses.
- **Protein requirement**: Minimal protein requirement for good nutrition is about **0.9 g/kg of body weight/day** (acceptable range is 1.0–1.5 g/kg/day) and should constitute **10–15% of the total calorie intake**. Very low protein diets may retard the progression of diabetic nephropathy. Protein content should be limited to 0.8 g/kg/day or about 10% of daily calories, once nephropathy develops.
- **Fat**: The calories required through carbohydrate and fat must be determined individually. **Restriction of fat** is necessary **if weight loss is desired** because of the high energy value of fat compared to protein and carbohydrate. An **average recommendation** of fat for nonobese diabetic patients and those without hyperlipidemias is **30% or less of total calories** with 10% each as saturated, monounsaturated, and polyunsaturated fats. Monounsaturated fats improve plasma lipid profile with reduction in total and LDL cholesterol without lowering HDL cholesterol in T2DM patients.
- **Carbohydrate**: After choosing the protein and fat content, the remaining calories are to be derived from carbohydrate. It should **constitute 50–55% of the daily caloric intake**, of which significant amount should be in the form of nonstarch polysaccharide, as dietary fiber. Foods with higher fiber content have a lower glycemic index. **Restrict mono- and**

disaccharides (fructose, sucrose, and glucose). The nonnutritive sweeteners such as saccharin, aspartame, sucromate, and acesulfame K are used to reduce energy intake without loss of palatability.
- **Fiber and diabetes mellitus**—increasing the intake of dietary fibers is known to have a favorable effect on the overall metabolic health. Fiber-rich foods contain complex carbohydrates that are resistant to digestion and thereby reduce glucose absorption and insulin secretion.
- **Alcohol consumption**: It accounts for extra calories and has tendency to inhibit gluconeogenesis. Thus, it may potentiate the hypoglycemic action of sulfonylureas and insulin. In addition, alcohol predisposes toward the development of lactic acidosis in patients taking metformin. Hence, it should be best avoided.

Recommended intake of various nutrients in diabetic patients is presented in **Table 3.7**.

Pattern of distribution of calories is presented in **Table 3.8**.

TABLE 3.7: Recommended intake of various nutrients in diabetic patients.

Nutrients	Recommended intake
Carbohydrate	~50–60% of total calories
Protein	15–20% of total calories
Total fat	25–35% of total calories
Saturated fat	<10% of total calories (<7% in dyslipidemia)
Polyunsaturated fat	~10% of total calories
Monounsaturated fat	Up to 20% of total calories
Cholesterol	<300 mg/day (<200 mg/day in dyslipidemia)
Total calories	➢ Adjust based on age, weight, and height ➢ Sedentary individuals: 30 kcal/kg/day ➢ Moderately active individual: 35 kcal/kg/day ➢ Heavily active individuals: 40 kcal/kg/day

TABLE 3.8: Pattern of distribution of calories.

Percentage of total calories (%)	Provision for
20	Breakfast
35	Lunch
15	Late evening feed
30	Dinner

Exercise

Advantages: Exercise **improves insulin sensitivity, reduces fasting and postprandial glucose**, and has **metabolic, cardiovascular, and psychological benefits** in diabetic patients.

Based on all available evidence, the ADA and the IDF recommend a total of at least 150 minutes of moderate-intensity physical activity per week that can be a combination of aerobic activities (such as walking or jogging) or resistance training

Aerobic exercise—adults with diabetes are encouraged to decrease sedentary time and to perform 30–60 minutes of moderate-intensity aerobic activity on most days of the week. Shorter-duration, intensive exercise may be appropriate for physically fit individuals

Resistance training—in the absence of contraindications (e.g., moderate-to-severe proliferative retinopathy, severe coronary artery disease), people with type 2 diabetes should also be encouraged to perform resistance training (exercise with free weights or weight machines) at least twice per week.

Goals of therapy are presented in **Table 3.9**.

TABLE 3.9: Treatment goals for adults with diabetes.

Index	Goal
Glycemic control [glycated hemoglobin (HbA1c)]	<7.0%
Preprandial capillary plasma glucose	3.9–7.2 mmol/L (70–130 mg/dL)
Peak postprandial capillary plasma glucose	<10.0 mmol/L (<180 mg/dL)
Blood pressure	<130/80 mm Hg
Lipids	
➢ Low-density lipoprotein	<2.6 mmol/L (100 mg/dL)
➢ High-density lipoprotein	>1 mmol/L (40 mg/dL) in men and >1.3 mmol/L (50 mg/dL) in women
➢ Triglycerides	<1.7 mmol/L (150 mg/dL)

Cardiovascular Risk Factor Management

In addition to glycemic control, vigorous cardiac risk reduction (smoking cessation; blood pressure control; reduction in serum lipids with a statin; diet, exercise, and weight loss or maintenance; and antiplatelet therapy aspirin for those with established atherosclerotic cardiovascular disease) should be a top priority for all patients with type 2 diabetes.

ORAL HYPOGLYCEMIC (GLUCOSE-LOWERING) DRUGS

Q. Discuss and describe the pharmacologic therapies for diabetes, their indications, contraindications, adverse reactions, and interactions of drugs used in diabetes.

Agents used for treatment of type 1 and type 2 diabetes are listed in **Table 3.10**.

Based on their mechanisms of action, oral hypoglycemic drugs are subdivided into agents that increase insulin secretagogues, reduce glucose production, increase insulin sensitivity, enhance glucagon-like peptide-1 (GLP-1) action, or promote urinary excretion of glucose. Various categories of oral hypoglycemic drugs are listed in **Table 3.10**.

TABLE 3.10: Agents used for treatment of type 1 and type 2 diabetes.

	Mechanism of action	*Examples*	*HbA1c reduction (%)*	*Specific advantages*	*Specific disadvantages*
Oral					
Biguanides	Hepatic glucose production	Metformin	1–2	Weight neutral/mild weight loss do not cause hypoglycemia, inexpensive	Diarrhea, nausea, lactic acidosis, and vitamin B_{12} deficiency (0.5%)
Insulin secretagogues: Sulfonylureas	Insulin secretion	Glibenclamide (glyburide), glipizide, gliclazide, and glimepiride	1–2	Inexpensive	Hypoglycemia, weight gain, and sulfonamide allergies
Insulin secretagogues: Nonsulfonylureas	Insulin secretion	Repaglinide, nateglinide, and mitiglinide	1–2	Short onset of action, lower postprandial glucose	Hypoglycemia
Insulin secretagogues: Dipeptidyl peptidase-4 inhibitors	Prolong endogenous GLP-1 action	Saxagliptin, sitagliptin, vildagliptin, linagliptin, teneligliptin, and evogliptin	0.5–0.8	Do not cause hypoglycemia	Nasopharyngitis, meniscus lesions, headache, contact dermatitis, osteoarthritis, and tremor
α-glucosidase inhibitors	↓GI glucose absorption	Acarbose, miglitol, and voglibose	0.5–0.8	Reduce postprandial glycemia	GI flatulence, liver function abnormalities, and contraindicated in kidney disease, inflammatory bowel disease
Thiazolidinediones *Contraindication: CHF and liver disease*	↓ Insulin resistance and ↑ glucose utilization	Rosiglitazone and pioglitazone	0.5–1.4	Lower insulin requirements	Peripheral edema, CHF, weight gain, fractures, macular edema; rosiglitazone may increase cardiovascular risk
Sodium-glucose cotransporter 2 (SGLT2) inhibitors	Help eliminate glucose in the urine	Canagliflozin, dapagliflozin, empagliflozin, and remogliflozin	0.4–1.1	No hypoglycemia and weight loss	Genital and urinary infections
Bile acid sequestrants					
Bile acid sequestrants *Contraindications: Elevated plasma triglycerides*	Bind bile acids, mechanism of glucose lowering is not known	Colesevelam	0.5		Constipation, dyspepsia, abdominal pain, nausea, triglycerides interfere with absorption of other drugs, and intestinal obstruction
Parenteral					
Insulin	↑Glucose utilization, ↓hepatic glucose production, and other anabolic actions	*Refer* **Table 3.14**	Not limited	Known safety profile	Injection, weight gain, and hypoglycemia
GLP-1 receptor agonists *Contraindications: Renal disease, agents that also slow GI motility*	↑Insulin, ↓glucagon, slow gastric emptying, and satiety	Exenatide and liraglutide	0.5–10	Weight loss, do not cause hypoglycemia	Injection, nausea, risk of hypoglycemia with insulin secretagogues, pancreatitis, and renal failure
Amylin agonists *Contraindication: Agents that also slow GI motility*	Slow gastric emptying, ↑glucagon	Pramlintide	0.25–0.5	Reduce postprandial glycemia and weight loss	Injection, nausea, and risk of hypoglycemia with insulin
Medical nutrition therapy and physical activity	↓Insulin resistance, ↑insulin secretion	Low-calorie, low-fat diet and exercise	0.6–1.4	Other health benefits	Compliance difficult, long-term success low

(CHF: congestive heart failure; GI: gastrointestinal; GLP-1: glucagon-like pepetide-1; HbA1c: glycated hemoglobin)

Biguanides-Metformin

Q. Write short essay/note on metformin.

- It activates cyclic adenosine monophosphate (AMP) kinase and inhibits mitochondrial glycerol-3-phosphate dehydrogenase.
- It reduces both fasting level of blood glucose and the degree of postprandial hyperglycemia in patients with type 2 diabetes, but has no effect on normal subjects. It is thought to act by inhibiting the hepatic gluconeogenesis.
- Metformin is known to downregulate the hepatic glucose production, acts on the gut to increase glucose utilization, enhances insulin, increases GLP-1, and alters the microbiome.
- Reduces HbA1c by 1.5–2%.

Profiles of antidiabetic medications

	MET	GLP-1RA	SGLT2I	DPP-4i	AGI	TZD (moderate dose)	SU / GLN	COLSVL	BCR-QR	Insulin	PRAML
Hypo	Neutral	Neutral	Neutral	Neutral	Neutral	Neutral	Moderate/ severe (SU) / Mild (GLN)	Neutral	Neutral	Moderate-to-severe	Neutral
Weight	Slight loss	Loss	Loss	Neutral	Neutral	Gain	Gain	Neutral	Neutral	Gain	Loss
Renal/GU	Contra-indicated if eGFR <30 mL/min/ 1.73 m²	Exenatide not indicated CrCl <30; Possible benefit of liraglutide	Not indicated for eGFR <45 mL/ min/1.73 m²; Genital myocotic infections; Possible CKD benefit	Dose adjustment necessary (Except linagliptin); Effective in reducing albuminuria	Neutral	Neutral	More hypo risk	Neutral	Neutral	More hypo risk	Neutral
GI Sx	Moderate	Moderate	Neutral	Neutral	Moderate	Neutral	Neutral	Mild	Moderate	Neutral	Moderate
Cardiac: CHF	Neutral	See #1	See #2	See #3	Neutral	Moderate	Neutral	Neutral	Neutral	CHF risk	Neutral
Cardiac: ASCVD	Neutral	See #1	See #2	See #3	Neutral	May reduce stroke risk	Possible ASCVD risk	Benefit	Safe	Neutral	Neutral
Bone	Neutral	Neutral	Neutral	Neutral	Neutral	Moderate fracture risk	Neutral	Neutral	Neutral	Neutral	Neutral
Ketoacidosis	Neutral	Neutral	DKA can occur in various stress settings	Neutral	Neutral	Neutral	Neutral	Neutral	Neutral	Neutral	Neutral

- Few adverse events or possible benefits
- Use with caution
- Likelihood of adverse effect

1. Liraglutide ---FDA approved for prevention of MACE events.
2. Empagliflozin---FDA approved to reduce CV mortality. Canagliflozin---FDA approved to reduce MACE events
3. Possible increased hospitalizations for heart failure with alogliptin and sexagliptin

FIG. 3.6: Profile of antidiabetic agents.

(ASCVD: atherosclerotic cardiovascular disease; CHF: congestive heart failure; CKD: chronic kidney disease; CrCl: creatinine clearance; DKA: diabetic ketoacidosis; DPP-4i: dipeptidyl peptidase-4 inhibitor; eGFR: estimated glomerular filtration rate; FDA: Food and Drug Administration; GLP-1RA: glucagon-like peptide-1 receptor agonist; MACE: major adverse cardiovascular event; MET: metformin; SGLT2i: sodium-glucose cotransporter 2 inhibitor; SU: sulfonylurea; TZD: thiazolidinedione)

- It is particularly useful in obese patients or those patients who are not responding optimally to maximal doses of sulfonylureas.
- Hypoglycemia does not occur with therapeutic doses of metformin, which permits its description as a "euglycemic" drug rather than an oral hypoglycemic agent (OHA).
- Metformin is not indicated for patients with type 1 diabetes.

Contraindications for metformin are given in **Box 3.6**.

Box 3.6: Contraindications for metformin.

- Malabsorption or GI disturbances/GI intolerance
- Low BMI <21 kg/m², marked weight loss
- Organ failure: Creatinine: >1.4 mg/dL, eGFR <30 mL/min/1.73 m²
  - Liver failure: Acute/chronic
  - Cardiac failure, hypotension/sepsis
- Active vitamin B_{12} deficiency
- Metabolic acidosis

(BMI: body mass index; eGFR: estimated glomerular filtration rate; GI: gastrointestinal)

Insulin Secretagogues (Table 3.11)—Agents that Affect the ATP-sensitive K⁺ Channel

Sulfonylureas

Q. Write short essay/note on sulfonylureas and name newer sulfonylureas.

They specifically bind to a receptor that closes an ATP-sensitive potassium channel of the pancreatic β-cell, thus depolarizing the cell membrane. This results in an influx of extracellular calcium through voltage-gated calcium channels, which causes insulin granules to move toward the cell surface, facilitating exocytosis. Thus, sulfonylureas have an insulinotropic effect on pancreatic β-cells.

The sulfonylureas are most appropriate for use in nonobese mild type 2 diabetes. In obese mild diabetics and others with peripheral insensitivity to levels of circulating insulin, primary emphasis should be on weight reduction. However, concerns of modest weight gain and moderate-to-severe hypoglycemia and cardiovascular risk limit their clinical benefits. As a consequence of closure of cardiac KATP channel, the use of sulfonylureas have also been related to adverse cardiovascular effects due to impaired hypoxic coronary vasodilation during increased oxygen demands such as acute myocardial ischemia.

They can reduce fasting sugars by 40–70 mg/dL and HbA1c by 1-2% by immediate action.

First generation: Tolbutamide and chlorpropamide.

Second generation: Glibenclamide (glyburide), glipizide, gliclazide, and glimepiride.

Third generation: Glimepiride.

- Glibenclamide should be taken about half an hour before meals, since rapid absorption is delayed when the drug is taken with food. Most sulfonylureas act via the 140 kDa part of the receptor while glimepiride acts via 65 kDa part of the receptor, hence has better cardiovascular safety.
- Sulfonylureas, particularly gliclazide-modified release (MR) and glimepiride, have a lower risk of hypoglycemia and are preferred in South Asian T2DM patient.

Contraindications to Sulfonylureas

Hypersensitivity, renal insufficiency is a relative contraindication (glipizide and gliclazide are preferred, glibenclamide is avoided), hepatic insufficiency, type 1 DM, and DKA.

TABLE 3.11: Properties of insulin secretagogues.

Class/Genetic name	*Daily dosage in milligrams (mg)*	*Duration of action in hours*
Sulfonylureas		
Glimepiride	1–8	24
Glipizide	5–40	12–18
Glipizide (extended release)	5–20	24
Glyburide/glibenclamide	1.25–20	12–24
Glyburide (micronized)	0.75–12	12–24
Nonsulfonylureas (Meglitinides)		
Repaglinide	0.5–16	2–6
Nateglinde	180–360	2–4
Glucagon-like peptide-1 (GLP-1) agonist		
Exenatide	0.01–0.02	4–6
Liraglutide	0.6–1.8	12–24
Dipeptidyl peptidase-4 inhibitors		
Saxagliptin	2.5–5	12–16
Sitagliptin	100	12–16
Vildagliptin	50–100	12–24

Nonsulfonylureas—Meglitinides

- **Repaglinide and nateglinide** are not sulfonylureas, but interact with the ATP-sensitive potassium channel. Owing to their short half-life, these are given with each meal or immediately before to reduce meal-related glucose excursions.
- **Advantages of meglitinides**: Flexibility in mealtime dosing—"Ramzan" drug, no significant increase in body weight, can be utilized in mild-to-moderate renal failure, and lesser hypoglycemia.

Agents that Enhance Glucagon-like Peptide-1 Receptor Signaling—Incretin-based Therapy

- The **incretin effect** is defined as the increased stimulation of insulin secretion caused by oral administration of glucose.
  - Two intestinal peptide hormones (incretin hormones) namely—**glucose-dependent insulinotropic polypeptide (GIP)** and **GLP-1** have a potentiating effect on secretion of insulin by pancreas. In response to food, GIP is secreted by the K-cells in the duodenum and GLP-1 by the L-cells of the ileum.
  - These hormones act on their receptors present on islet cells of pancreas and stimulate insulin secretion in response to food. This stimulation of insulin secretion by the gut is referred to as the intestinal secretion of insulin or incretin effect.
  - **The insulin secretion is markedly greater in response to an oral than to an intravenous glucose challenge**.
- **Glucagon-like peptide-1 analogs**:
  - The injectable GLP-1 analogs such as liraglutide, exenatide, lixisenatide, dulaglutide, and albiglutide imitate the effects of endogenous GLP-1, thereby stimulating pancreatic insulin secretion in a glucose-dependent fashion, suppressing pancreatic glucagon output, slowing gastric emptying, and decreasing appetite.
  - Their main advantage is weight loss, which can be significant in some of the patients.
  - Limiting side effects of these agents are nausea and vomiting, particularly early in the course of treatment.
  - Chances of pancreatitis and pancreatic and thyroid cancer are a matter of concern.

Dipeptidyl peptidase-4 inhibitors, Gliptins

Q. Write short note on dipeptidyl peptidase-4 (DPP-4) inhibitors/vildagliptin.

- An alternative approach to the use of GLP-1 analogs is to inhibit DPP-4 to conserve endogenous GLP-1. DPP-4 enhances the incretin effect.
- The enzyme DPP-4 rapidly inactivates GLP-1. Inhibition of this enzyme, thus, potentiates the effect of endogenous GLP-1 secretion.
- **Drugs available: Linagliptin (5 mg OD), saxagliptin (5 mg OD), alogliptin, sitagliptin (100 mg OD), vildagliptin (50 mg OD/BD), teneligliptin (20–40 mg), and evogliptin (5 mg OD)** are oral agents. They are most effective in the early stages of T2DM when insulin secretion is relatively preserved. They are recommended for second-line use in combination with metformin or a sulfonylurea.
- They have a moderate effect in lowering blood glucose and risk of hypoglycemia is low.
- **Side effects**: Adverse effects (AEs) such as constipation, nasopharyngitis, urinary tract infection, myalgia, arthralgia, headache, and dizziness are the commonly reported AEs with the use of these agents. Worsening of heart failure and rare risk for pancreatitis have been reported.
- **Teneligliptin** is a newer, more potent DPP-4 inhibitor which is safe in renal failure.

α-Glucosidase Inhibitors

Q. Write short essay/note on α-glucosidase inhibitors/acarbose.

Drugs in this group: Acarbose, miglitol, and voglibose.

Mechanism of action: α-glucosidase is an enzyme present on the brush border of the small intestine. It is needed for the breakdown of oligosaccharides (carbohydrates) into simple sugars (before carbohydrates can be absorbed) in the intestinal lumen.

- α-glucosidase inhibitors **reduce glucose absorption** by inhibiting the enzyme α-glucosidase. This result in poor absorption of carbohydrates, thereby reduces postprandial hyperglycemia.
- They neither affect glucose utilization nor insulin secretion.

Indications: They are useful in the management of patients who develop **significant postprandial hyperglycemia** but otherwise have relatively well-controlled blood glucose levels.

- **Dosage**: Dose of both acarbose and miglitol is 25 mg which is first started with a single dose taken just before evening meal. This can be gradually increased to 50 mg with each meal. Dose of voglibose is 0.2–0.3 mg just before each meal.
- **Major side effects**: These drugs are poorly tolerated and may produce diarrhea, flatulence, and abdominal distension. They are due to increased delivery of unabsorbed oligosaccharides to the large intestine where it undergoes fermentation.
- **Advantages**: They are not as potent as other oral hypoglycemic drugs in lowering the HbA1c, but they are unique because it reduces the postprandial glucose rise even in patients with type 1 DM. They do not produce hypoglycemia.

Thiazolidinediones

Q. Write short essay/note on thiazolidinediones.

Drugs in this group: Thiazolidinediones (more conveniently known as the "glitazones") include **pioglitazone**, rosiglitazone, and troglitazone. Troglitazone and rosiglitazone are withdrawn due to increased incidence of liver failure and increased cardiovascular risk, respectively, in patients using it.

Mechanism of action: Thiazolidinediones reduce insulin resistance by binding to **peroxisome proliferator-activated receptor γ (PPARγ)**.

- Highest levels of the PPARγ receptor are found in adipocytes. PPARγ is a nuclear receptor, which regulates transcription of large numbers of genes including those involved in lipid metabolism (promote adipocyte differentiation, reduce hepatic fat accumulation, and promote fatty acid storage) and insulin action.

Pioglitazone

Q. Write short note on side effects of pioglitazone.

- **Dosage of pioglitazone**: 15–45 mg/day
- **Combination therapy**: It can be combined with metformin and sulfonylureas
- **Side effects**: It include:
  - Weight gain of 2–3 kg (due to fluid retention as well as increase in adiposity), fluid retention, and heart failure
  - Mild anemia and osteoporosis (increased propensity to bone fractures) and bladder carcinoma
- Maximum effect may be seen only after 3–4 weeks
- Conversely, pioglitazone is known to exert pleotropic effects on cardiovascular event; pioglitazone improves endothelial dysfunction, lowers hypertension, improves dyslipidemia, and lowers circulating levels of inflammatory cytokines and prothrombotic factors
- **Precautions**: Liver function should be periodically monitored as liver dysfunction may develop. It is contraindicated in liver disease and congestive cardiac failure.

Sodium-glucose Cotransporter 2 Inhibitors

- For example, dapagliflozin (5–10 mg/day), remogliflozin (100 mg BD), empagliflozin (25 mg/day), ertugliflozin, and canagliflozin (100–300 mg/day).
- Sodium-glucose cotransporters (SGLTs) are found in the intestinal mucosa of the small intestine and the proximal tubules of the nephrons.
- They provide insulin-independent glucose lowering by blocking glucose reabsorption in the proximal renal tubule. The capacity of tubular cells to reabsorb glucose is reduced by SGLT2 inhibitors leading to increased urinary glucose excretion and consequently, correction of the hyperglycemia.
- The AEs of SGLT2 inhibitors may include fatigue, hypoglycemia, increased urine output, increased hematocrit, and **mycotic genital or urinary tract infections.**
- Other side effects include hypotension, acute kidney injury, bone fracture, and autoamputations.

- Bring about a reduction in HbA1c by 0.7–1%.
- Dose reduction is needed in renal insufficiency.

SGLT2 inhibitors are especially useful in patients with heart failure and comorbid type 2 diabetes (T2D) by **reducing the risk of heart failure events** and improve life expectancy among patients with HFrEF.

Other Drugs Used in Diabetes

- **Amylin agonist**: **Pramlintide** is a synthetic pancreatic hormone amylin. It is to be injected before each meal.
- **Bile acid-binding resins**: **Colesevelam** is a bile acid sequestrants and acts in the GI tract to reduce glucose absorption. Side effects can include constipation, nausea, and dyspepsia.
- **Dopamine agonist**: **Bromocriptine** is an ergot-derived dopamine agonist that has been used for the treatment of hyperprolactinemia and Parkinson's disease. A quick-release formulation of bromocriptine is used for the treatment of T2DM. Bromocriptine (up to 4.8 mg daily) as monotherapy or as adjunctive therapy to sulfonylureas was minimally effective in reducing HbA1c. Common side effects include nausea, vomiting, dizziness, and headache.

Hydroxychloroquine: 400 mg once daily, reduces HbA1c by 0.5–0.6%. Mechanism of action is impairing insulin degradation.

Lipase Inhibitors (Orlistat)

It produces weight loss which improves glucose tolerance and slows the rate of progression to type 2 diabetes.

Drugs in Pipeline

- Glucokinase activators: Piragliatin
- Dual PPAR (α and γ) agonists: Aleglitazar
- Chromium (Cr), sodium tungstate, vanadium, proxyfan, and β-sitosterol
- S-Allylcysteine (a natural constituent of fresh garlic)
- Otelixizumab and teplizumab—anti-CD3 monoclonal antibody, are known to stimulate C-peptide levels and reduce insulin requirement in type 1 diabetes
- Recombinant human GAD vaccine—for LADA
- Glimins—Imeglimin is the first in a new tetrahydrotriazine-containing class of oral antidiabetic agents, the glimins. It has been shown to act on the liver, muscle, and pancreatic β-cells to uniquely target the key defects of type 2 diabetes.
- **A bionic or "artificial" pancreas** is an external device or system of devices that mimics the glucose regulating function of a healthy pancreas. Such systems monitor glucose levels and automatically provide insulin and potentially other blood-glucose stabilizing hormones to the body.

INSULIN TREATMENT

Q. Write short essay/note on:
- **Role of insulin in the management of diabetes/insulin therapy.**
- **Classify insulins. Give a brief account of the commonly used insulins.**
- **Insulin indication and types/indications for short-, intermediate-, and long-acting insulins.**

Insulin is necessary for all patients with type 1 DM and many patients with T2DM. Goals of insulin therapy are mentioned in **Box 3.7**.

Box 3.7: Goals of insulin therapy.

- Elimination of primary symptoms of hyperglycemia and glycosuria
- Prevention of diabetic ketoacidosis (DKA) and hyperosmolar coma
- Restoration of lost lean body mass
- Improvement of physical performance and sense of well-being
- Reduction of frequent infections
- During pregnancy: Decrease fetal malformation, maternal and fetal morbidity
- Delay, arrest, or prevent macrovascular or microvascular complications

General Indications for Insulin Therapy (Table 3.12)

TABLE 3.12: Indications for insulin therapy.

➢ Type 1 DM ➢ Diabetic ketoacidosis (DKA) ➢ Hyperosmolar hyperglycemic state	Diabetes under following conditions: ➢ Pregnancy (preferably prior to pregnancy) ➢ Acute severe illness needing hospitalization ➢ Perioperative/intensive care unit setting ➢ Patients with acute coronary syndrome [myocardial infarction (MI)] ➢ Patients on high-dose corticosteroids ➢ Inability to tolerate or contraindication to oral antiglycemic agents ➢ Newly diagnosed type 2 diabetes with significantly elevated blood glucose levels (patients with severe symptoms or DKA) ➢ Patient no longer achieving therapeutic goals on combination of antiglycemic therapy

Insulin Preparations

Classification of Insulin Preparations (Table 3.13)

TABLE 3.13: Various ways of classification of insulin preparations.

Basis of classification	*Types*
Source	Bovine, porcine, and human insulins
Purity	Conventional, single peak, and monocomponent insulins
Time course of action	Rapid-, intermediate-, and long-acting insulins
Strength	40 and 100 units/mL
Newer insulin analogs	Glargine, detemir, etc.
Bolus insulin (mealtime or prandial)	Regular insulin, lispro, aspart, and glulisine
Basal insulin	Isophane insulin (NPH), glargine, and detemir

Properties of Various Insulin Preparations

The commonly used insulin preparations and their duration of action are presented in **Table 3.14**.

TABLE 3.14: Duration of action (in hours) of various insulin preparations.

Classes	*Types*	*Onset of effect (hours)*	*Peak effect (hours)*	*Effective duration of action (hours)*
Rapid acting	Insulin analogs: Lispro, aspart, and glulisine	<0.25	0.5–1.5	2–4
Short acting	Regular (crystalline, soluble, and plain)	0.5–1	2–3	3–6
	Semilente	0.5–1	2–6	10–12
Intermediate acting	Isophane insulin (NPH)	2–4	4–10	10–16
	Lente (excess zinc ions)[#]	1–3	6–12	18–24
Long acting	Protamine zinc insulin (PZI)	2–4	14–24	36
	Ultralente	2–4	18–24	36
	Insulin analogs: Glargine and detemir	1–4	None	18–24

[#]Lente (intermediate acting) insulin is mixtures of semilente and ultralente in the ratio of 30:70, respectively.

INSULIN ANALOGS/NEWER INSULINS (TABLE 3.15 AND FIG. 3.7)

Q. Write short note on human insulin analogs and advantages of newer insulins/insulin analogs.

Insulin analogs are prepared by modifying human insulin and have replaced soluble and isophane insulins, especially type 1 diabetes mellitus. Insulin analogs have more flexibility and convenience. In contrast to soluble insulin (which should be injected 30 minutes before eating), rapid-acting insulin analogs can be given immediately before, during, or even after meals. Long-acting insulin analogs (better than isophane insulin) maintain "basal" insulin levels for up to 24 hours and may be given once daily.

TABLE 3.15: Insulin analogs.

Short acting	*Long acting*
Lispro	Glargine
Aspart	Detemir
Glulisine	Degludec

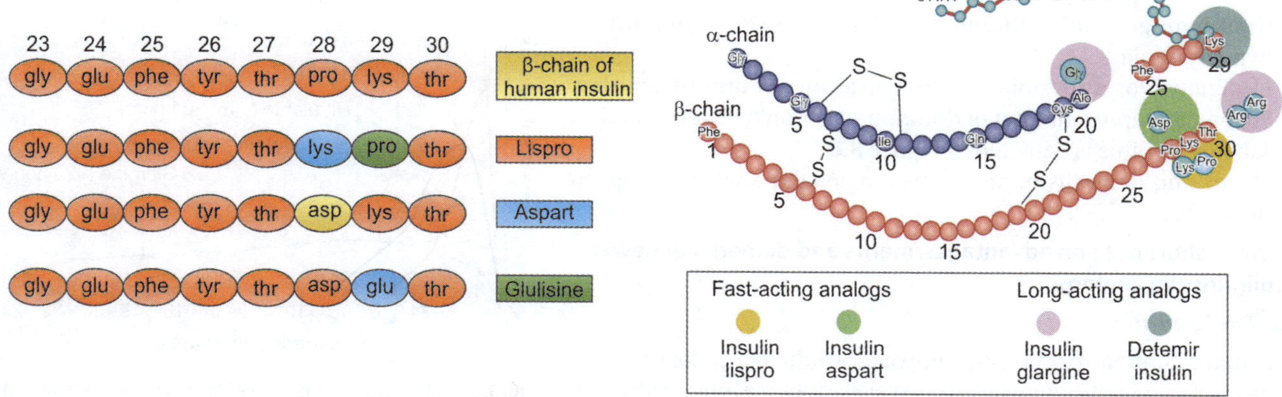

FIG. 3.7: Amino acid structure of insulin and insulin analogs.

Patients on regular insulin regimens may develop repeated episodes of hypoglycemia between meals (during some part of the day) and particularly at night. Insulin analogs are useful in such patients. The various preparations include:

Insulin Lispro

- It is first human insulin analog produced by recombinant DNA technology utilizing a nonpathogenic strain of *Escherichia coli (E. coli)*.
- Glucose-lowering activity: More rapid onset of action (<15 minutes), early peak (60–90 minutes), and a shorter duration of glucose-lowering activity (<5 hours).
- Disadvantages: Because of its short duration of action.
- Patient needs to take this insulin analog just before or after meals.
- **Patients need** additional use of longer-acting insulin to maintain glucose control.

Insulin Aspart and Insulin Glulisine

They are also short-acting insulin analogs similar to lispro.

Insulin Glargine:

- **It is a human "peakless" bioengineered insulin analog that has a long duration of action and has an acidic pH.**
- **Glucose-lowering activity**: After a lag time of 4–6 hours, the flat peakless effect lasts for 24 hours.
- **Mechanism of action**: After injection into the subcutaneous tissue, **acidic form of insulin becomes neutral and forms microprecipitate**. They **release small amounts** of insulin **very slowly**. It results in a relatively constant concentration for 24 hours without a pronounced peak.
- **Advantages**: It is given **once daily** as subcutaneous injection generally at bedtime. **Hypoglycemia** does not develop.
- **Disadvantages**: As insulin glargine is in acid form, it may cause **increased pain at the injection site**. Its acid nature also **limits its ability to mix with other insulins**.

Insulin Detemir

It is a long-acting, basal soluble human insulin analog and has a neutral pH.

Advantages:

- Because of its neutral pH, it causes **least pain** at the site of injection.
- It binds to albumin via its fatty acid chain which allows this analog to remain liquid and soluble following injection. It has **prolonged mode of action** due to its attachment to fatty acid.
- **Neither renal nor hepatic impairment exerts influence** over its pharmacological effects.
- **No gain of weight.**
  - It is effective when administered once or twice daily and **combined with** the basal **soluble analog** insulin and/ or with **oral hypoglycemic drugs** or **premeal short-acting insulin regimen**. Insulin detemir and the rapid-acting analog insulin aspart or lispro closely mimic near-normal insulin profiles and **improve glycemic control than more conventional insulin therapy**.

Insulin Degludec

- **It is a long-acting (>40 hours) human insulin analog.**
- **It forms** soluble multihexamers at the site of subcutaneous injection and releases monomers slowly to give an ultra-long peakless pharmacokinetic (PK) profile. It reduces variability of concentration in the plasma with once-daily regimen.

Advantages of Degludec:

- **Peakless insulin**
- Excellent improvement in HbA1c and superior FPG reduction
- Less hypoglycemia. Reduction of up to 36% in nocturnal hypoglycemia
- Flexibility: Dosing flexibility: **administration any time on any day.**

Schematic representation of duration of action of insulin profiles in diabetes mellitus is depicted in **Figure 3.8**.

Merits and demerits of newer insulin/insulin analogs are given in **Table 3.16**.

Q. Write short note on advantages/merits and demerits of newer insulin/insulin analogs.

Inhaled Insulin

- Inhaled human insulin powder was introduced in 2006 and its absorption was through the alveolar surface in the lungs. However, because of adverse effects and cost, it was withdrawn in 2007.

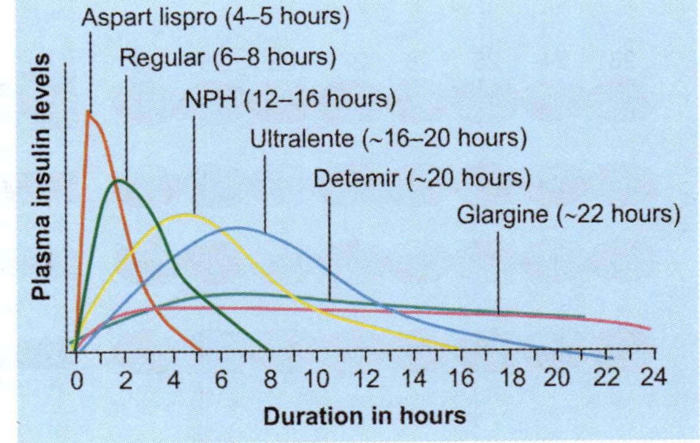

FIG. 3.8: Insulin therapy in diabetes mellitus. Schematic representation of duration of action of insulin profiles.

TABLE 3.16: Merits and demerits of newer insulin/insulin analogs.

Merits	*Demerits*
➢ Better mimicking of physiological insulin secretion ➢ Better control of glucose levels in the fasting, interdigestive, and postprandial period ➢ Lesser risk of hypoglycemia (especially nocturnal) ➢ No need to be injected half an hour before meals ➢ More predictable action profile independent of dose/site of injection/exercise ➢ Greater flexibility with short-acting analogs ➢ Compliance is improved with long-acting analogs as once a day insulin	➢ No significant different in adverse effects when compared to standard insulins ➢ Worsening retinopathy with lispro [homologous to insulin-like growth factor-1 (IGF-1)] ➢ Carcinogenicity: Concerns over glargine carcinogenicity ➢ High cost

TABLE 3.17: Insulin regimens.

Once-daily insulin regimen	Long-acting peakless insulin + oral hypoglycemic agents
Twice-daily insulin regimen	Intermediate insulin (NPH) given twice daily
Sliding scale—premixed/split—mix regimen	Combination of premixed insulin (30:70/50:50) given twice daily or combination of short- and long-acting analogs given three to four times a day
Basal-bolus regimen/multiple daily injection therapy	➢ Basal long-acting or intermediate-acting insulin (NPH, detemir/glargine) once daily usually at night and ➢ Bolus-separate injections of short- or rapid-acting insulin (regular, aspart/lispro/glulisine) at each meal
Continuous subcutaneous insulin infusion/insulin pump therapy	➢ Pump delivers a constant feed of insulin into the body via a cannula subcutaneously ➢ At meal times, an increased burst (bolus) of insulin can be delivered

- Inhalation was done with each meal along with single injection of long-acting insulin to provide basal levels of insulin.
- **Side effects**: Cough, dry mouth, sore throat and shortness of breath, and hypoglycemia.
- Example: Afrezza.

Insulin Regimens (Table 3.17)

Three insulin regimens include: (i) conventional insulin therapy, (ii) multiple subcutaneous injections (MSI), and (iii) continuous subcutaneous insulin infusion (CSII). The choice of regimen depends on the degree of glycemic control desired, the severity of insulin deficiency, the patient's lifestyle, and their ability to adjust the insulin dose. Most of type 1 diabetes requires two or more injections of insulin daily. In type 2 diabetes, insulin is usually started as once-daily long-acting insulin, either alone or in combination with OHAs.

Conventional insulin therapy: It is the simplest regimen and used commonly. In this regimen, **intermediate-acting insulin** (lente), with **or without the addition of small amounts of regular insulin**, is injected subcutaneously **once or twice** per day.

- **Insulin mixtures**: In this, intermediate-acting insulin along with small doses of regular insulin is administered to achieve better euglycemic status.
- **Split-lente regimen**: If the total daily requirement of insulin exceeds 50 or 60 units or when there is a need for better control, the intermediate-acting insulin (lente) is administered in two doses/day. Two-thirds of the total required dose is taken before breakfast (7–8 AM) and the remaining one-third before dinner (7–8 PM).

Multiple subcutaneous injections: Insulin is injected subcutaneously several times a day into the anterior abdominal wall, upper arms, outer thighs, and buttocks.

- In this regimen, **intermediate- or long-acting insulin** is administered in the evening as a **single dose**/day together **with regular insulin prior to each meal**.
- It achieves overall control and may reduce the rate of development of long-term complications.
- **Commonly used schedule**: Calculate the total daily dose of insulin required at 0.6–0.7 units/kg body weight.
  - **25% of the calculated dose** is administered as **intermediate-acting insulin at bedtime.**
  - **75% of the calculated dose** is administered as **regular insulin in three divided doses** (40% before breakfast, 30% before lunch, and 30% before dinner).

Continuous subcutaneous insulin infusion/alternative insulin therapies: "Open-loop" systems are small battery-powered portable insulin pumps which provide continuous subcutaneous, intraperitoneal, or intravenous infusion of insulin.

- In this regimen, a **small battery-driven insulin pump** is worn externally and connected to a butterfly needle, which is inserted into the anterior abdominal wall.
- It mimics the physiological basal plus prandial pattern of insulin secretion and can achieve excellent glycemic control. The rate of insulin infusion can be programmed to match the patient's diurnal variation in requirements. About **40% of the total daily required dose** is given **at basal rate; the remainder is given as preprandial boluses.**
- **Advantages**:
  - Ease of taking multiple boluses, if desired.
  - Availability to program the basal rate of insulin delivery, especially useful in dawn phenomenon.
  - Improved control over multiple dose insulin (MDI).
  - Reduced risk of severe hypoglycemia and hypoglycemic attacks can be easily treated.

- **Disadvantages**:
  - Needs a high degree of patient motivation
  - Expensive—high cost
  - Infection at infusion sites
  - High incidence of ketoacidosis
  - Hypoglycemia, especially nocturnal and may be fatal
  - Risk of mechanical malfunctioning.
- **Artificial pancreas project** aims to close the loop by using miniaturized glucose sensors to communicate wirelessly with the insulin pump. This would automatically adjust its insulin rate. However, this is not used in clinical practice at present.

Insulin Delivery Systems

Q. Write short note on newer insulin delivery device.

- **Insulin syringes**: These are available as disposable plastic syringe in various sizes (i.e., 40 U/mL or 100 U/mL). Insulin can be administered using a fine needle (can be reused several times). They can be used easily and has enhanced accuracy.
- **Insulin pen**: An insulin pen holds a prefilled cartridge contain desired type of insulin and has a fine disposable needle that can be changed for each injection. It is suitable for multiple dosing.
- **Implanted insulin pump therapy**: Controlled pumps can be implanted in the peritoneal cavity. Insulin released into the peritoneal cavity is mostly absorbed and delivered into the splanchnic system.
- **External insulin pump therapy**: Portable insulin infusion pump or CSII is alternative insulin delivery devices (refer above).

Complications of Insulin Therapy

Q. Write short essay/note on adverse/side effects (complications) of insulin therapy.

- **Hypoglycemia during insulin treatment**: It is the most common complication of insulin therapy and causes anxiety for both patients and relatives. It occurs due to imbalance between injected insulin and a patient's normal diet, activity, and basal insulin requirement. The risk of hypoglycemia is more before meals, during the night, and during exercise. Irregular eating habits, unusual exertion, and alcohol excess may precipitate hypoglycemic episodes.
- **At the injection site**:
  - A **shallow injection** causes intradermal (rather than subcutaneous) delivery of insulin resulting in **painful, red lesions** or even scarring. Abscess at injection site is extremely rare.
  - **Local allergic reactions:** It may occur at the injection site early in therapy. These include local itching, erythematous and indurated lesions, and discrete subcutaneous nodules. They usually resolve spontaneously.
  - **Fatty lumps, called as lipohypertrophy,** may develop due to overuse of a single injection site due to lipogenic effects of the injected insulin. It may occur with any type of insulin.
  - **Insulin resistance and anti-insulin antibodies**: Most common cause of mild insulin resistance is obesity. Insulin resistance may be associated with antibodies directed against the insulin receptor.
- **Weight gain**: Many patients may gain weight on insulin treatment, especially if the insulin dose is increased inappropriately. This may be prevented by diet restriction, exercise, and addition of metformin.
- Generalized allergic (urticaria and anaphylactic) reactions are very rare.

Pancreatic Transplantation

Q. Write short note on pancreatic transplantation.

Other option available in patients with type 1 diabetes mellitus includes whole-pancreas transplantation and islet cell transplantation. Both transplantation can restore normoglycemia without exogenous insulin therapy and survival rates of these patients are consistent with other organ transplantation procedures.

- Whole-pancreas transplantation: At present, it is usually performed only in patients with end-stage renal failure who require a combined pancreas/kidney transplantation and in whom diabetes control is particularly difficult (e.g., because of recurrent hypoglycemia).
- Transplantation of isolated pancreatic islets: It is performed by harvesting pancreatic islets from cadavers (two or three pancreata are usually necessary). These islets cells are injected into the portal vein and they seed themselves into the liver.
- Management of type 1 diabetes, nonobese type 2 diabetes, and obese type 2 diabetes are summarized in **Boxes 3.8 to 3.10**, respectively.

Box 3.8: Summarized management of type 1 diabetes.

- **Insulin therapy**: Oral hypoglycemic agents (OHAs) are ineffective and patient should be started on insulin therapy. It can be split-dose insulin therapy or intensive insulin therapy
- Usually need multiple injections for acceptable glycemic control

Box 3.9: Summarized management of nonobese type 2 diabetes.

- **Lifestyle modification**: If hyperglycemia is mild, following diabetic diet can occasionally restore normal metabolic control
- **Monotherapy**: When diet therapy is not sufficient, a trial of sulfonylurea is often effective in reducing sugar levels
- **Two-drug therapy**: Next step involved combination therapy with metformin, thiazolidinedione/dipeptidyl peptidase-4 inhibitors/glucagon-like peptide-1 receptor agonists/sodium-glucose cotransporter 2 inhibitors can be the next addition for sugar control
- **Insulin therapy**: When patient fails the combination of these three drugs, insulin therapy is indicated. Usually, patients have enough baseline insulin to allow use of single long-acting insulin to take care of sugar control

Box 3.10: Summarized management of obese type 2 diabetics.

- **Weight reduction**: First step is weight reduction to improve tissue sensitivity to insulin
- **Monotherapy**: Among oral hypoglycemic agents (OHAs), monotherapy with **α-glucosidase inhibitors or metformin** may be started, as they are not associated with weight gain or drug-induced hypoglycemia
- **Two-drug therapy**: If metformin therapy is inadequate, **sulfonylurea may be added**
- **Three-drug therapies**: If this combination of metformin and sulfonylurea is ineffective in controlling sugar levels, then **addition of thiazolidinediones**/dipeptidyl peptidase-4 inhibitors/glucagon-like peptide-1 receptor agonists/sodium-glucose cotransporter 2 inhibitors should be considered
- **Insulin therapy** should be instituted, if the combination of these three drugs fails to restore euglycemia. Generally, the sulfonylurea is discontinued when insulin therapy is instituted but the patient can stay on the metformin and thiazolidinediones. Usually, patients have enough baseline insulin to allow use of single long-acting insulin to take care of sugar control

Metabolic Surgery

It is a recommended treatment option for adults with type 2 diabetes and (1) a BMI of 40 kg/m^2 (or 37.5 kg/m^2 or over in people of Asian ancestry) or (2) a BMI of 35.0–39.9 kg/m^2 (32.5–37.4 kg/m^2 in people of Asian ancestry) who do not achieve durable weight loss and improvement in comorbidities with reasonable nonsurgical methods.

Algorithm of therapy for T2DM is depicted in Flowchart 3.1.

GLYCOSYLATED HEMOGLOBIN AND FRUCTOSAMINE

Q. Write short essay/note on glycosylated hemoglobin (HbA1c).

Glycosylated Hemoglobin

- **HbA1 is a minor component of adult hemoglobin A (HbA) and its important subgroup is HbAlc. HbAlc has an irreversibly attached glucose and is known as glycosylated hemoglobin.**
- **Normal level: Glycosylated hemoglobin is expressed as a percentage of the normal hemoglobin (standardized range 4–6.1%). In general, the goal of diabetic treatment is to obtain a value below 7%. It should be as close to normal (<6%) as possible without significant hypoglycemia**.
- **Significance**: The percentage of HbA1c can be measured and its value provides an excellent assessment of overall state of **glycemic control during the preceding 3 months**.
- **Factors that influence HbA1c level**:
  - **Blood glucose level**: The level of HbA1c is dependent on the prevailing glucose level in the blood (exposure of the red cell to glucose). If young red blood cells (RBCs) are exposed to extremely high blood glucose (>400 mg/dL) for several hours, HbA1c level increases. Thus, in patients with DM, it is useful in assessing the blood glucose control; higher the count, poorer is the control.
  - **Disease associated with altered RBC survival**: Glycation of hemoglobin occurs only when the RBC circulates in serum. Older RBCs have more HbA1c than reticulocytes. Total HbA1c reflects the mixture of both old and younger RBCs. In patients with hemolytic anemia such as thalassemia, the measured HbA1c level will be lower, independent of glycemia. Conversely, if the circulating RBCs are older (e.g., aplastic anemia), then measured HbA1c level will be higher, regardless of glycemic status.
- Although the HbA1c level provides a rapid assessment of glycemic control, blood glucose level should also be tested to know the control.

Glycosylated Plasma Proteins (Fructosamine)

- It may also be measured as an index of diabetic control. It measures glycation of all serum proteins and the major component being **glycosylated albumin**. Since albumin accounts for most of the protein in blood, the measurement of fructosamine, for practical purposes, measures glycated albumin. As albumin has a turnover of about 2 weeks, fructosamine reflects **glycemia over the preceding 2–3 weeks** (shorter period).
- It is **useful in diabetic patients with anemia or hemoglobinopathy and in pregnancy** (when hemoglobin turnover is changeable).

FLOWCHART 3.1: Stepwise approach for the management of type 2 diabetes.

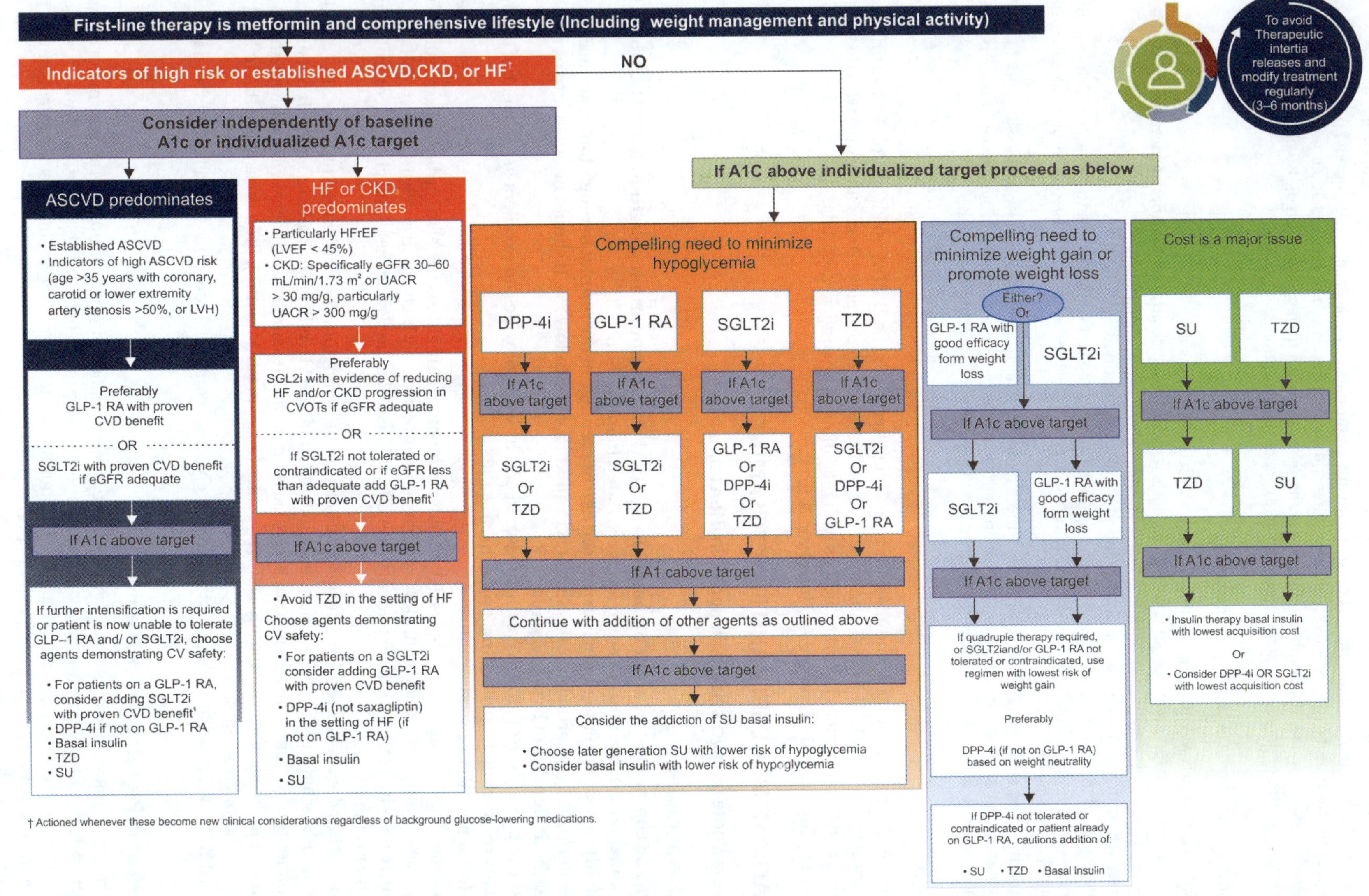

(ASCVD: atherosclerotic cardiovascular disease; CKD: chronic kidney disease; DPP-4i: dipeptidyl peptidase-4 inhibitor; eGFR: estimated glomerular filtration rate; GLP-1-RA: glucagon-like peptide-1 receptor agonist; SGLT2i: sodium-glucose cotransporter 2 inhibitor; SU: sulfonylurea; TZD: thiazolidinedione)

Source: American Diabetes Association (ADA). (2019). Standards of Medical Care in Diabetes—2020 Abridged for Primary Care Providers. [online] Available from https://clinical.diabetesjournals.org/content/diaclin/early/2019/12/18/cd20-as01.full.pdf. [Last accessed December, 2020].

COMPLICATIONS OF DIABETES

Classification of complications of diabetes is presented in **Table 3.18**.

Q. Write short essay/note on:
- **Classify and enumerate the complications of diabetes.**
- **Chronic complications of diabetes mellitus.**

Acute Complications of Diabetes (Table 3.18)

Q. Write short essay/note on acute complications of diabetes mellitus.

TABLE 3.18: Complications of diabetes.

Acute metabolic complications
➢ Diabetic ketoacidosis (DKA) ➢ Hyperosmolar hyperglycemic state (hyperosmolar nonketotic diabetic coma) ➢ Lactic acidosis ➢ Hypoglycemia
Chronic (long-term) complications
A. Vascular complications ➢ **Microvascular** – Ophthalmic ◆ Diabetic retinopathy (nonproliferative and proliferative) ◆ Cataract ◆ Glaucoma – Peripheral neuropathy: ◆ Sensory ◆ Motor ◆ Sensory motor ◆ Autonomic neuropathy – Renal: ◆ Nephropathy: Microalbuminuria, macroalbuminuria ◆ Chronic kidney disease – Foot disease ➢ **Macrovascular:** – Coronary artery disease – Peripheral vascular disease – Cerebrovascular disease
B. Nonvascular complications: ➢ Gastroparesis ➢ Infections ➢ Skin changes (dermatological complications) ➢ Hearing loss

DIABETIC KETOACIDOSIS

Q. Describe the precipitating causes, pathophysiology, recognition, clinical features, diagnosis, stabilization, and management of diabetic ketoacidosis.

Diabetic ketoacidosis, a medical emergency, is a state of metabolic decompensation, which occurs due to a severe deficiency of insulin. It is **more common and marked in type 1 diabetes** and is rare but may also occur in type 2 diabetes. It is usually seen in previously undiagnosed DM. Precipitating factors are listed in **Box 3.11**.

Box 3.11: Precipitating factors of diabetic ketoacidosis (DKA) in a known patient with diabetes mellitus (DM).

- Infections (pneumonia, urinary tract infections, sepsis, and gastroenteritis)
- Acute pancreatitis
- Alcohol intoxication
- Inadequate insulin
- Infarction (cerebral, coronary, mesenteric, and peripheral)
- Severe stress (e.g., physical, emotional)
- Hyperthyroidism, pheochromocytoma
- Drugs (e.g., thiazides, corticosteroids, cocaine)
- Pregnancy

Mechanism/pathogenesis (Fig. 3.9)

Cardinal biochemical features of DKA: (1) hyperglycemia, (2) hyperketonemia (and ketonuria), and (3) metabolic acidosis. DKA develops due to the combined effects by: (1) relative or absolute insulin deficiency and (2) counterregulatory glucagon

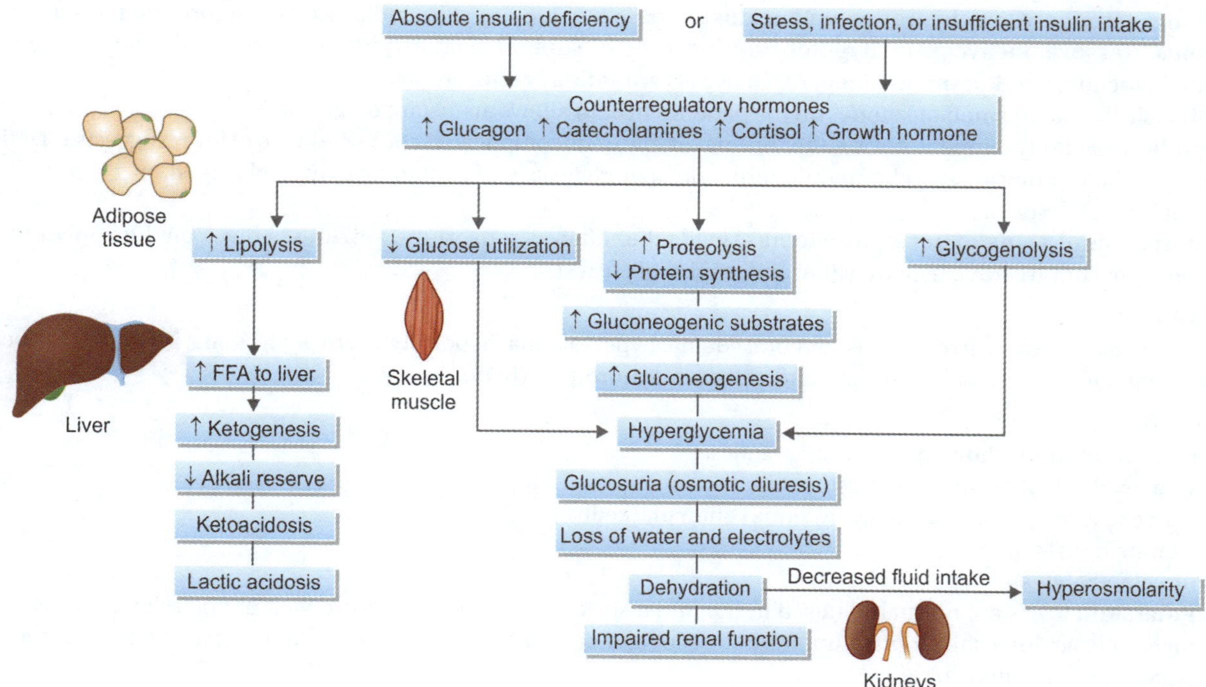

FIG. 3.9: Pathogenesis of diabetic ketoacidosis.
(FFA: free fatty acid)

excess. Other hormones such as catecholamines (e.g., epinephrine), cortisol, and growth hormone are also being produced in excess.

Consequences of insulin deficiency and glucagon excess:

- **Severe hyperglycemia**: The blood glucose levels of 500–700 mg/dL.
- **Diuresis and dehydration**: Hyperglycemia causes a hyperosmolar state, which induces an **osmotic diuresis** leading to volume depletion and **dehydration** (characteristic features of ketoacidosis). There is loss of electrolyte, particularly of sodium and potassium.

Q. Write short essay/note on ketone bodies.

- **Activation of the ketogenic machinery**:
  - **Lipolysis**: Insulin deficiency stimulates lipoprotein lipase, which breaks down fat stores (lipolysis) and increases the FFAs levels in the plasma.
  - **Generation of ketone bodies in liver**: In DKA, hyperglucagonemia (excess of glucagon) alters hepatic metabolism of FFA to favor ketone body formation. This is through activation of the enzyme **carnitine palmitoyltransferase 1**. The FFAs are esterified to fatty-acyl coenzyme A in the liver. In the mitochondria of liver cells, fatty-acyl coenzyme A molecules are oxidized to ketone bodies (**acetoacetic acid**, **β-hydroxybutyric acid**, and minor amount of acetone). These ketone bodies accumulate in the body fluids.
- **Ketonemia and ketonuria**: When the **rate of production of ketone bodies exceeds the rate of utilization** by peripheral tissues, it results in **ketonemia** and **ketonuria**.
- **Metabolic acidosis**: Acetoacetic acid and β-hydroxybutyric acid are strong acids and are responsible for the acidotic state. If the excretion of ketone bodies in the urinary is compromised by dehydration, it results in **systemic metabolic ketoacidosis (high anion gap)**.

Clinical features of diabetic ketoacidosis:

- DKA may present as the initial symptom complex that leads to a diagnosis of type 1 DM for the first time, but more commonly, it develops in patient with already diagnosed DM.
- Clinical features of DKA are those of uncontrolled diabetes with acidosis. Patients typically present with **polyuria, polydipsia**, and other symptoms of progressive hyperglycemia.
- **Other clinical features** include **nausea, vomiting, weakness, weight loss**, lethargy, anorexia, leg cramps, blurred vision, and shortness of breath. Vomiting is an ominous symptom because it precludes oral replacement of fluid losses; severe volume depletion may follow quickly.
- **Abdominal pain** is classically periumbilical and sometimes may be so severe that may be confused with a surgical acute abdomen (such as acute pancreatitis or ruptured viscus).

Physical findings in diabetic ketoacidosis:

- Findings secondary to **dehydration and acidosis**: These include **dry skin** and mucous membranes, **reduced jugular venous pressure, tachycardia, hypotension** (postural or supine), cold extremities/peripheral cyanosis, depressed mental function, and **Kussmaul (deep, rapid hyperventilation) respirations**.
- **Fruity** (sickly-sweet) **smell** of ketones on the patient's **breath** allows an instant diagnosis.
- **Hypothermia**: Body temperature is either normal or low in uncomplicated DKA. Presence of fever suggests infection.
- Mental apathy, confusion, psychomotor retardation, hyporeflexia, and hypotonia may be observed.
- Abdominal tenderness.
- **Symptoms and signs of cerebral edema**: Headache, altered sensorium, seizures, bowel/bladder incontinence, papilledema, bradycardia, hypertension, and respiratory arrest.

Complications

Acute gastric dilatation/erosive gastritis, cerebral edema, hyperkalemia/hypokalemia, hypoglycemia, infections, myocardial infarction, mucormycosis, and acute respiratory distress syndrome (ARDS).

Investigations:

- **Urine examination**: Shows glucose and ketones.
- **Plasma levels** of following is to be estimated:
  - **Glucose** levels are raised (hyperglycemia) often markedly
  - **Ketone bodies** are raised.
- **Serum electrolytes**:
  - **Potassium** levels are normal or raised in the initial stages despite a total body deficit of potassium. This is because metabolic acidosis shifts potassium from intracellular compartment to extracellular compartment. The levels drop once the treatment is started.
  - **Sodium** levels are usually low, particularly if the patient has repeated vomiting and continued to drink water (pseudohyponatremia).

- **Bicarbonate** levels are low. Value <12 mmol/L indicates severe acidosis.
- **Phosphorus** level may be high initially despite a total body deficit of phosphorus.

- **Blood**:
  - **Leukocytosis** invariably occurs in DKA; this represents a stress response and may not necessarily indicate infection.
  - **Arterial blood gas (ABG):** Reveals high anion gap metabolic acidosis.
  - Blood urea nitrogen (BUN) is usually raised due to prerenal failure produced from volume depletion.
  - **Infection screen:** Full blood count, blood and urine culture, C-reactive protein, and chest X-ray.
  - **Serum amylase** may be elevated.
- **Electrocardiogram (ECG): To rule out myocardial infarction.**

Diagnostic criteria for DKA (Table 3.19)

Diagnostic criteria for DKA include plasma glucose >250 mg/dL, arterial pH <7.3, serum bicarbonate <15 mEq/L, ketonemia and/or ketonuria, and anion gap of >12 mEq/L (usually present in DKA).

TABLE 3.19: Diagnostic criteria for diabetic ketoacidosis and the hyperosmolar hyperglycemic state.

Features	*Diabetic ketoacidosis (DKA)*			*Hyperosmolar hyperglycemic state (HHS)*
	Mild	*Moderate*	*Severe*	
Mental status	Alert	Drowsy	Stupor or coma	Stupor or coma
Urine or serum ketone bodies	Positive	Positive	Positive	Negative to trace
Plasma glucose level (mg/dL)		>250		>600
Effective serum osmolality (mOsm/kg)		Variable		>320
Arterial pH	7.25–7.30	7.00–7.24	<7.00	>7.30
Serum bicarbonate (mEq/L)	15–18	10–15	<10	>15
Anion gap (mEq/L)	>10	>12	>12	<12

Management:

Goals of therapy of diabetic ketoacidosis are given in **Box 3.12**.

Fluid resuscitation (Flowchart 3.2):

It is a critical part of treating patients with DKA as it is a state of severe dehydration.

- Intravenous solutions to replace extravascular and intravascular fluids and electrolyte losses. The usual fluid deficit is minimum 3–5 L and should be replaced intravenously. They dilute levels of both the glucose and the circulating counterregulatory hormones.
- Fluid itself leads to correction of acidosis to some extent.

Insulin recommendations (Flowchart 3.3)

Short-acting insulin is administered to reverse acidosis and treat hyperglycemia.

Potassium repletion (Flowchart 3.4)

Correction of acid-base balance (Flowchart 3.5):

Its role is controversial and usually not practiced.

Phosphorus repletion: A sharp drop of serum phosphorus can also occur during insulin treatment and no treatment is usually necessary.

Complications of DKA: Mortality is <10%. Death occurs due to infection, thrombosis, cerebral edema, and shock.

Criteria for resolution of DKA are mentioned in **Box 3.13**.

Box 3.12: Goals of therapy of diabetic ketoacidosis.

- Rehydration
- Reduction of hyperglycemia
- Correction of electrolyte imbalance
- Correction of acid-base imbalance
- Investigation and correction of precipitating factors
- Treatment of complications

FLOWCHART 3.2: Fluid resuscitation.

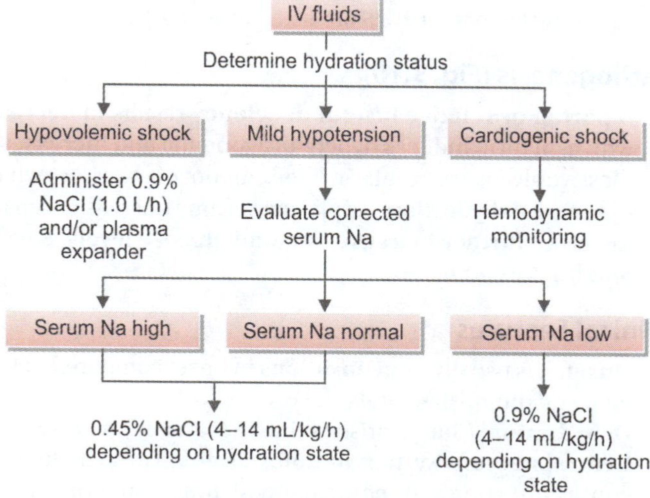

(IV: intravenous; NaCl: sodium chloride)

HYPEROSMOLAR HYPERGLYCEMIC STATE

Q. Describe the precipitating causes, pathophysiology, recognition, clinical features, diagnosis, stabilization, and management of hyperosmolar nonketotic state.

- It is **metabolic emergency**, which usually occurs as a complication of **uncontrolled T2DM**. Patients usually present in **middle or later life** (presently it is increasingly seen in younger adults), often with previously undiagnosed diabetes.
- This syndrome has a high mortality rate (>50%).

FLOWCHART 3.3: Insulin recommendations.

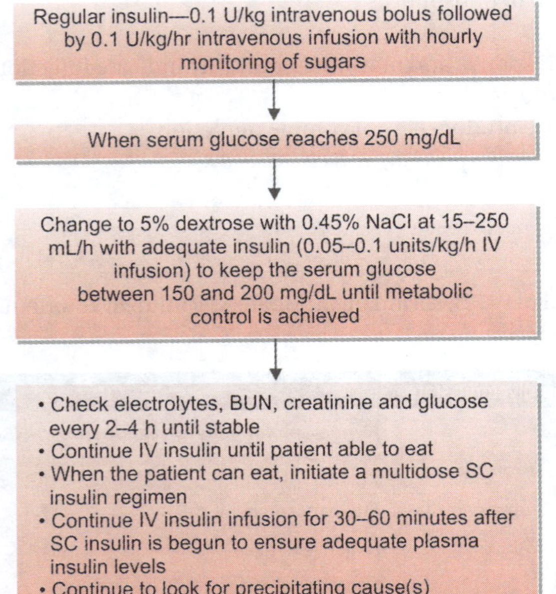

(BUN: blood urea nitrogen; IV: intravenous; NaCl: sodium chloride; SC: subcutaneous)

FLOWCHART 3.4: Potassium repletion.

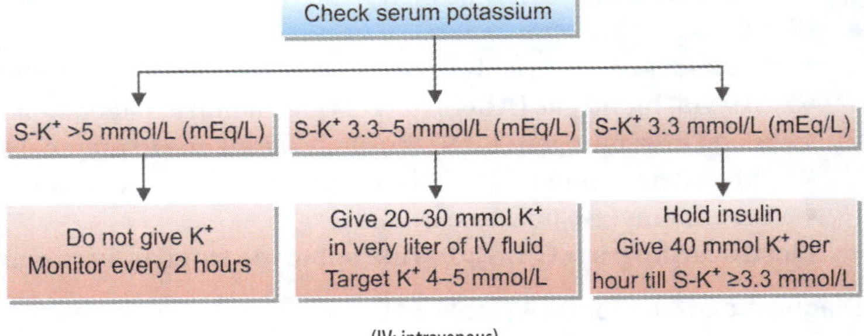

(IV: intravenous)

FLOWCHART 3.5: Correlation of acid-base balance.

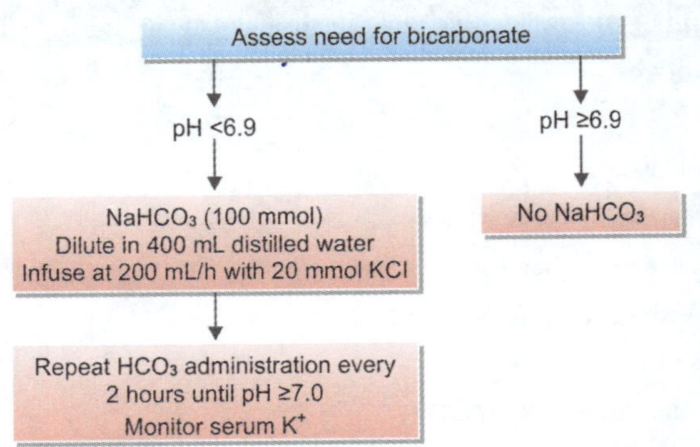

Box 3.13: Criteria for resolution of diabetic ketoacidosis (DKA).

- Glucose <200 mg/dL
- Serum bicarbonate ≥18 mEq/L
- Venous pH of >7.3
- Plasma osmolality effectively has fallen below 315 mOsmol/kg
- The patient is able to eat

Characteristics of Hyperosmolar Hyperglycemic State

It is a syndrome characterized by:
- **Severe hyperglycemia** [>30 mmol/L (600 mg/dL)]
- **Hyperosmolality** (serum osmolality >320 mOsm/kg)
- Extreme **dehydration in the absence of significant hyperketonemia** (<3 mmol/L) **or ketoacidosis** (pH >7.3, bicarbonate >15 mmol/L).

Precipitating factors for HHS are listed in **Box 3.14**.

Box 3.14: Precipitating factors for hyperosmolar hyperglycemic state (HHS).

- Infections
- Physical and emotional stress
- Inadequate fluid intake
- Cerebrovascular accidents
- Myocardial infarction
- Concurrent medication, e.g., thiazide diuretics, steroids, immunosuppressive agents, phenytoin, and osmotic agents like mannitol
- Peritoneal dialysis and hemodialysis
- Tube feeding of high-protein formulas/consumption of glucose-rich fluids/parenteral nutrition

Pathogenesis (Fig. 3.10)

- A **partial or relative insulin deficiency** results in **decreased utilization of glucose** by skeletal muscle, fat, and liver, which, in turn, induces hyperglucagonemia and **increases hepatic glucose output**.
- Massive glycosuria results in large amount of water loss which along with decreased intake due to associated illness results in **severe dehydration**. As plasma volume decreases, renal insufficiency develops and limits the renal glucose loss. This increases **further increase in blood glucose levels**. **Severe hyperosmolality** develops that causes **mental confusion and finally coma**.

Clinical Features

- **Onset**: It is usually more **insidious** in onset compared to DKA. It presents with a several-week history of polyuria, weight loss, and diminished oral intake.
- **Dehydration**: Characteristic **clinical features** on presentation are **due to volume depletion and extreme dehydration**.
- **Central nervous system manifestations**: These include alteration in the level of consciousness ranging from mental confusion, stupor, or coma, **convulsions** (sometimes Jacksonian in type), hemiballism/hemichorea, and transient hemiplegia. Impairment of consciousness is directly related to the degree of hyperosmolality.
- Milder gastrointestinal (GI) symptoms
- Infections, particularly pneumonia or pyelonephritis and gram-negative sepsis are very common.
- Hyperosmolar state may predispose to stroke or myocardial infarction.
- Bleeding and acute pancreatitis may accompany HHS.

Physical examination: Shows severe dehydration, hyperosmolality, hypotension, tachycardia, and altered mental status.

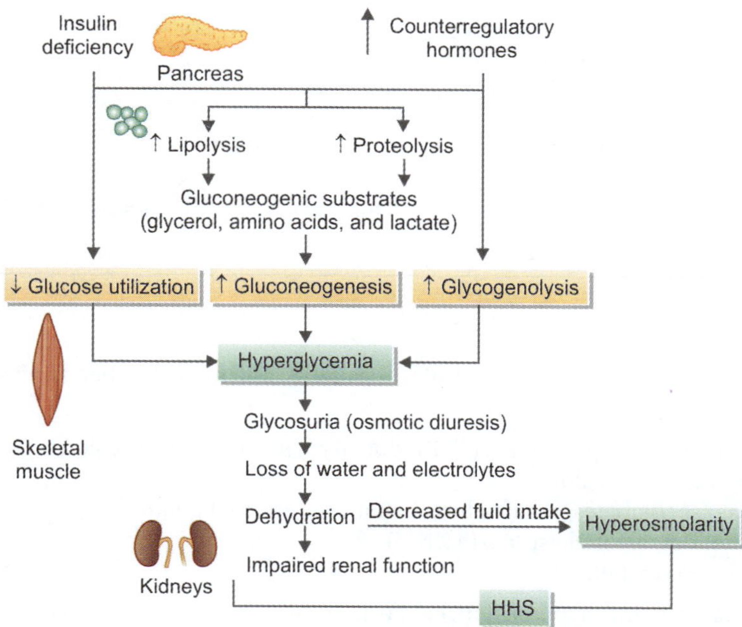

FIG. 3.10: Pathogenesis of hyperosmolar hyperglycemic state (HHS).

Laboratory Findings

- **Plasma glucose**: Markedly raised and usually **around 1,000 mg/dL** (range 600–2,400 mg/dL)
- **Serum osmolarity**: Usually extremely high
- **Prerenal azotemia** with raised blood urea nitrogen (BUN) and creatinine
- **Plasma bicarbonate**: A mild metabolic acidosis with **marginal decrease** in plasma bicarbonate (about 20 mmol/L) is seen. Marked decrease in plasma bicarbonate (<10 mmol/L) indicates lactic acidosis.
- **Diagnostic criteria for HHS (*refer* Table 3.19).**

Management

- **Fluid replacement**: The average fluid deficit is much higher than DKA and is about 10 L. It should be corrected intravenously. Initially, 2–3 L isotonic (0.9%) saline should be administered over 1–2 hours. Subsequently, half-strength (0.45%) saline should be given. Once the plasma glucose reaches 300 mg/dL, use 5% dextrose-saline solution. Central venous pressure (CVP) should be monitored in patients with cardiac disease.
- **Insulin**: Regular insulin should be administered as low-dose intravenous infusion as in DKA. The goal is to achieve the plasma glucose around 200 mg/dL.
- **Potassium supplementation** is needed early (as in DKA).
- **Lactic acidosis**: Treat with intravenous sodium bicarbonate.
- **Infections**: With suitable antibiotics.
- **Anticoagulants**: To prevent thrombosis.

Q. How will you differentiate between diabetic ketoacidosis (DKA) and hyperosmolar hyperglycemic state (HHS)?

Differentiate between DKA and HHS is described in Table 3.20.

TABLE 3.20: Differentiate between diabetic ketoacidosis and hyperosmolar hyperglycemic state.

Features	*Diabetic ketoacidosis (DKA)*	*Hyperosmolar hyperglycemic state (HHS)*
Clinical features		
Type of diabetes	Both type 1 or type 2 diabetes mellitus (DM)	Type 2 DM
Evolution/onset	Over hours	Over days
Fruity (acetone) odor of breath	Observed	Not present
Kussmaul's respiration	Seen	Not seen
Abdominal pain/tenderness	Present	Absent
Laboratory findings		
Plasma glucose level	>250 mg/dL	>600 mg/dL
Serum sodium	Normal or low (<140 mmol/L)	Usually high (>155 mmol/L)
Blood/urine ketones	Moderate ketonuria or ketonemia	Absent/Minimal ketonuria and ketonemia

Contd...

Contd...

Arterial pH	<7.3	>7.3
Serum bicarbonate	<15 mEq/L	>15 mEq/L
Serum osmolality	Variable	>320 mOsm/L
Anion gap	>12	Variable
Fluid deficit	6 liters	>10 liters
Mortality rate	1%	20–30%

LACTIC ACIDOSIS

This can be a complication of DM, usually seen in critically ill patients, and rarely has been linked to the use of metformin.

Classification of Lactic Acidosis

- **Type A:** Reduced tissue adenosine triphosphate (ATP) (due to reduced tissue perfusion)
- **Type B:** No evidence of reduced perfusion
  - **Type B1:** Systemic disease (diabetes, renal failure, hepatic failure, malignancy)
  - **Type B2:** Drugs (biguanides, alcohol, isoniazid (INH)
  - **Type B3:** Inborn errors of metabolism

Clinical features: Cyanosis, tachycardia, hypotension, cold extremities, altered sensorium, and hyperventilation.

Investigations: High anion gap metabolic acidosis and serum lactate >1 mEq/L.

Treatment: Hydration, intravenous (IV) bicarbonate is the drug of choice, and dialysis can also be done.

HYPOGLYCEMIA

Q. Enumerate the causes of hypoglycemia and describe the counter hormone response and the initial approach and treatment.

Whipple's triad: It is the most convincing documentation of hypoglycemia.

- **Symptoms** consistent with **hypoglycemia**
- **Low plasma concentration** of blood glucose ≥70 mg/dL (3.9 mmol/L) measured with a precise method (not a glucose monitor)
- **Relief of symptoms after the plasma glucose level is raised.**
  The ADA recommends a plasma glucose threshold of 54 mg/dL for the diagnosis of clinically significant hypoglycemia.

Causes/Etiology (Box 3.15)

Q. Write short essay/note on causes of hypoglycemia.

Significance: Hypoglycemia is a dangerous complication and more serious than hyperglycemia. Prolonged hypoglycemia may cause permanent damage to the brain.

Box 3.15: Causes of hypoglycemia in adults.

- Drugs: Insulin or insulin secretagogues, alcohol, and others
- Critical illness: Hepatic, renal or cardiac failure, sepsis, malaria, and inanition
- Hormone deficiency: Cortisol, glucagon, and epinephrine (in insulin-deficient diabetes)
- Nonislet cell tumor
- Endogenous hyperinsulinism: Insulinoma, functional β-cell disorders (nesidioblastosis), noninsulinoma pancreatogenous hypoglycemia, postgastric bypass hypoglycemia, insulin autoimmune hypoglycemia, antibody to insulin, antibody to insulin receptor, and insulin secretagogue
- Accidental, surreptitious, or malicious hypoglycemia

Pathogenesis

Whenever blood glucose level falls, three primary physiological defense mechanisms come into action:

- **Suppression of endogenous insulin release** from pancreatic β-cells
- **Increased release of glucagon** from pancreatic β-cells
- **Activation of the autonomic nervous system** with release of catecholamines.

In addition, stress hormones, such as cortisol, catecholamines (adrenaline and noradrenaline), and growth hormone (GH), are also increased in the blood.

Mechanism of Hypoglycemia in Diabetes

It may be due to:

- **Insulin excess** (exogenous in patient on insulin therapy)
- **Counterregulatory failure**:

- In type 1 DM, in the early stages itself, there is loss of capacity to increase glucagon release in response to hypoglycemia.
- Subsequently, many patients also lose the capacity to release catecholamines in response to hypoglycemia. This is due to diabetic autonomic neuropathy.

Clinical Features

- **Blood glucose level and symptom development**: Symptoms due to hypoglycemia usually occur with a plasma glucose at:
  - Level of 60 mg/dL in nondiabetic individuals
  - Higher levels (80 mg/dL) in poorly controlled diabetic patients
  - Lower levels in well-controlled diabetic patients.
- **Symptoms** fall into two main groups:
  - **Related to acute activation of the autonomic nervous system (neurogenic symptoms)**: These are produced by excessive secretion of adrenaline and symptoms include sweating, tremor, tachycardia, anxiety, and hunger. Adrenergic symptoms predominate when hypoglycemia is of rapid onset (e.g., insulin reactions).
  - Those **secondary to glucose deprivation of the brain (neuroglycopenia)**: It causes dizziness, headache, clouding of vision, blunted mental acuity and loss of fine motor skill, confusion, abnormal behavior, convulsions, and loss of consciousness. Central nervous system symptoms predominate when hypoglycemia is of gradual onset. Patients with long-standing diabetes may not develop warning adrenergic symptoms (**hypoglycemic unawareness**) due to severe neuropathy and are at a greater risk of central nervous dysfunction.
- **Daytime versus nocturnal hypoglycemia**:
  - **Daytime hypoglycemic episodes** present with sweating, nervousness, tremor, and hunger.
  - **Nocturnal hypoglycemic episodes** develop during sleep and present with night sweats, unpleasant dreams, and early morning headache. Frequently, nocturnal hypoglycemia is asymptomatic.

Management

- **Oral carbohydrate**: If hypoglycemia is detected early, it may be corrected by ingestion of carbohydrate (preferably in an easily absorbable form).
- **Intravenous dextrose**: It is given in serious hypoglycemia when there is impaired mental functions and prolonged hypoglycemia is anticipated (e.g., with depot insulin and oral sulfonylureas like chlorpropamide). 100 mL of 25% dextrose is administered. Oral carbohydrate should be given as soon as the patient is able to eat.
- **Glucagon**: Glucagon in the dose of 0.5–1 mg subcutaneously or intramuscularly may be given when there is severe hypoglycemia. It may be repeated if necessary after 10 minutes. Glucagon stimulates hepatic glycogenolysis, but it may not be effective in severe and prolonged hypoglycemia due to depot insulins. It should not be used for the treatment of hypoglycemia due to oral hypoglycemic drugs.
- **Octreotide**: It is useful for patients who develop recurrent hypoglycemia following dextrose infusion.
- **Other measures** are aimed at preventing recurrence of hypoglycemia. These include adjusting the dose of oral hypoglycemic drugs, changing the timing of insulin injections, adjustments in diet and physical activity/exercise, etc.

Somogyi Phenomenon

Q. Write short note on Somogyi phenomenon.

- The Somogyi phenomenon (posthypoglycemic hyperglycemia) is rebound hyperglycemia that follows an episode of hypoglycemia. It is due to counterregulatory hormone release.
- **Significance**: The correction of the morning hyperglycemia is by reducing and not increasing the evening dose of intermediate-acting insulin.

Clues to the Presence of Somogyi Phenomenon

- **Worsening of diabetic control** in the **presence of increasing insulin doses**. It manifests as morning fasting hyperglycemia in response to unrecognized nocturnal hypoglycemia.
- **Excessive hunger and weight gain** in presence of worsening hyperglycemia.
- **Nocturnal hypoglycemia**: Subtle manifestations such as mild nocturnal sweating, morning headache, and hypothermia.
- **Plasma glucose and urine glucose**: Shows wide fluctuations over short time intervals and not related to meals.
- **Confirmation of Somogyi phenomenon**: By documentation of hypoglycemia at 3 AM and hyperglycemia in the morning (fasting). Improvement in diabetic control after a decrease in the insulin dose.

Dawn Phenomenon

Q. Write short note on Dawn phenomenon.

- It is closely related to the Somogyi phenomenon in that there is fasting hyperglycemia without nocturnal hypoglycemia.
- **Mechanism**: Nocturnal surge of GH release or increased clearance of insulin in the mornings.
- **Confirmation**: Documenting of hyperglycemia at 3 AM and in the morning (fasting).
- **Significance**: Correction of the fasting hyperglycemia depends on increasing and not decreasing the insulin.

Differential diagnosis of morning hyperglycemia is mentioned in **Table 3.21**.

Q. List the differences in coma due to hypoglycemia and diabetic coma/ketoacidosis in type 1 diabetes mellitus (DM).

Differences between hypoglycemic and hyperglycemic/diabetic coma are presented in **Table 3.22**.

Causes of coma in diabetes are described in **Box 3.16**.

Q. Write short essay/note on the cause of coma in diabetes.

TABLE 3.21: Differences in diagnosis of morning hyperglycemia.

Features	*Dawn phenomenon*	*Somogyi effect*
Definition	Recurring early morning hyperglycemia	Early morning hyperglycemia due to treatment with excessive amount of exogenous insulin
Cause	Decrease of insulin secretion between 3 and 5 AM	Nocturnal hypoglycemia due to excessive dose of insulin
Diagnosis (3 AM and 5 AM glucose level)	High/normal plasma glucose level	Low plasma glucose level

Box 3.16: Causes of coma in a diabetic patient.

- Diabetic coma:
  - Ketosis producing diabetic ketoacidosis (DKA)
  - Nonketotic hyperglycemic-hyperosmolar coma (NKHHC)
  - Lactic acidosis (LA)
- Hypoglycemic coma (HC)
- Other comorbid conditions: Metabolic encephalopathies or infection related

TABLE 3.22: Differences between hypoglycemic and hyperglycemic/diabetic coma.

Features	*Hypoglycemic coma*	*Hyperglycemic coma*
Physical findings		
Volume of pulse	Full	Weak
Respiration	Shallow or normal	Rapid and deep (air hunger)
Blood pressure	Normal/may be raised	Decreased
Skin	Clammy, sweating	Dry
Tongue	Moist	Dry
Tissue turgor	Normal	Reduced
Eyeball tension	Normal	Reduced
Breath acetone	Not present	May be present
Reflexes	Brisk	Diminished
Laboratory findings		
Glucose in urine	Absent/Present (depends on time of last voiding)	Present
Plasma glucose level	Reduced	Raised >200 mg/dL
Plasma acetone	Negative	Usually present
Plasma bicarbonate	Normal	Low <20 mg/L
Plasma carbon dioxide (CO_2)	Normal	Diminished
Blood pH	Normal	<7.35

Chronic Complications of Diabetes

Q. Describe and discuss the pathogenesis and temporal evolution of microvascular and macrovascular complications of diabetes.

Pathogenesis of chronic complications of diabetes is multifactorial and includes: (1) hyperglycemia (glucotoxicity) is the main mediator, (2) insulin resistance, and (3) obesity.

Hyperglycemia

Effects of Hyperglycemia (Fig. 3.11)

These can be brought out by four **distinct metabolic pathways**.

1. **Formation of advanced glycation end products (AGEs)**: Increased intracellular glucose leads to **markedly increased** formation of AGEs. AGEs can **directly cross-link extracellular matrix proteins** and its consequences are:
   - **Basement membrane thickening**
   - **Trapping of LDL in the intima accelerating atherogenesis**
   - Glomerular dysfunction, endothelial dysfunction, and altered extracellular matrix composition.
2. **Activation of protein kinase C (PKC)**: In patients with hyperglycemia, intracellular hyperglycemia stimulates synthesis of diacylglycerol (DAG) from glycolytic intermediates. DAG activates intracellular PKC. PKC activation produces:
   - **Proangiogenic molecules** such as **vascular endothelial growth factor (VEGF)** causes **neovascularization** characteristic of **diabetic retinopathy**.
   - **Profibrogenic factors** [e.g., **transforming growth factor-β (TGF-β)**] results in **increased production of extracellular matrix and basement membrane material**.
   - Plasminogen activator inhibitor-1 (PAI-1) **reduces fibrinolysis and favors vascular occlusion** (by forming atherosclerotic plaques or thrombus).
3. **Disturbances in polyol pathways**: Some tissues (e.g., nerves, lenses, kidneys, and blood vessels) do not require insulin for glucose transport. Persistent hyperglycemia increases the intracellular glucose in these tissues and excess intracellular glucose is metabolized by the enzyme aldose reductase to sorbitol (polyol) to fructose.
   - This **reaction uses NADPH** (the reduced form of nicotinamide dinucleotide phosphate) as a cofactor.
   - NADPH is also necessary for the regeneration of reduced glutathione (GSH). GSH protects against injury by free radicals.
   - Reduced NADPH and decrease in GSH increase cells **susceptibility to oxidative stress**.

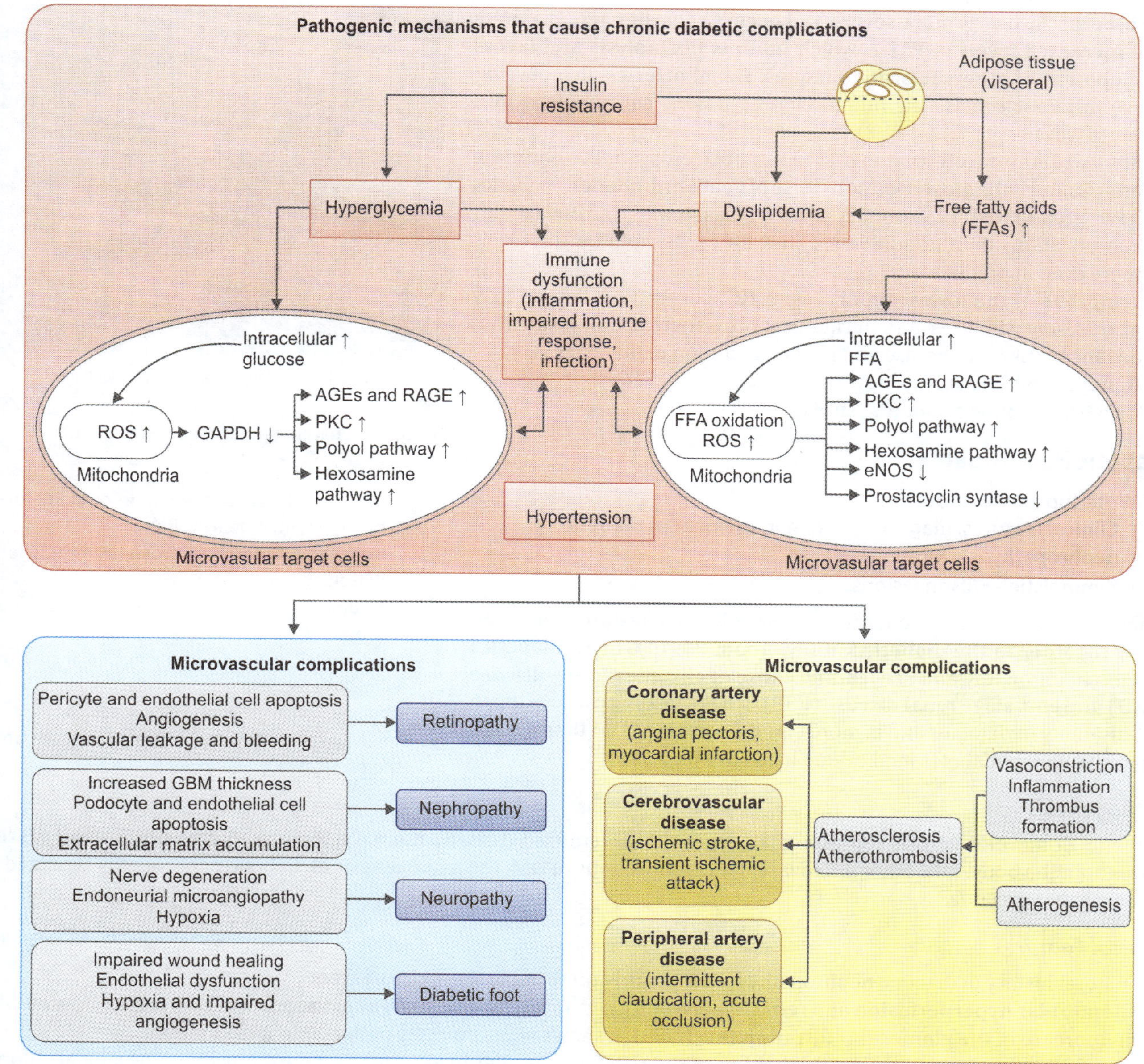

FIG. 3.11: Pathogenesis of chronic complications of DM due to hyperglycemia.
(AGEs: advanced glycation end products; DM: diabetes mellitus; eNOS: endothelial nitric oxide synthase; GAPDH: glyceraldehyde-3-phosphate dehydrogenase; GBM: glomerular basement membrane; PKC: protein kinase C; ROS: reactive oxygen species)

4. Hyperglycemia increases the flux through the **hexosamine pathway** and generates fructose-6-phosphate, which results in glycosylation of proteins such as endothelial nitric oxide synthase or by changes in gene expression of TGF-β or PAI-1.

Symptoms of Hyperglycemia (Box 3.17)

Box 3.17: Symptoms of hyperglycemia.

- Excessive thirst, dry mouth
- Polyuria, nocturia
- Tiredness, fatigue, lethargy, and weight loss
- Pruritus vulvae/balanitis due to genital candidiasis
- Blurring of vision
- Nausea, headache, mood changes, irritability, difficulty in concentrating, and apathy
- Hyperphagia (especially for sweet foods)

Cardiovascular Complications of Diabetes

Q. Write short essay/note on the cardiovascular complications of diabetes.

The lesions of large- and medium-sized muscular arteries are the **most common causes of mortality** in long-standing diabetes. These include:

Atherosclerosis: Diabetes is one of the major modifiable risk factor for atherosclerosis and other cardiovascular morbidities. The main cardiovascular complications of diabetes are accelerated atherosclerosis.

The **atherosclerosis is more severe and occurs at earlier age**. Diabetics have **increased levels** of **PAI-1**, which **inhibits fibrinolysis and favors development of atherosclerotic plaques. Renal arteries** also develop **severe atherosclerosis**. The atherosclerotic lesions can manifest in a variety of ways:

- **Myocardial infarction**: It is due to atherosclerosis of the coronary arteries and is the **most common cause of death in diabetics**. Diabetics have greater risk of coronary artery disease and cardiovascular complications than nondiabetics. Risk for cardiovascular disease is more even in prediabetics.
- **Gangrene of the lower/upper (Fig. 3.12) extremities**: Patient may also present with intermittent claudication. Gangrene may result from advanced vascular disease and is more common in diabetics.
- **Renal vascular insufficiency**.
- **Cerebrovascular accidents** (stroke).

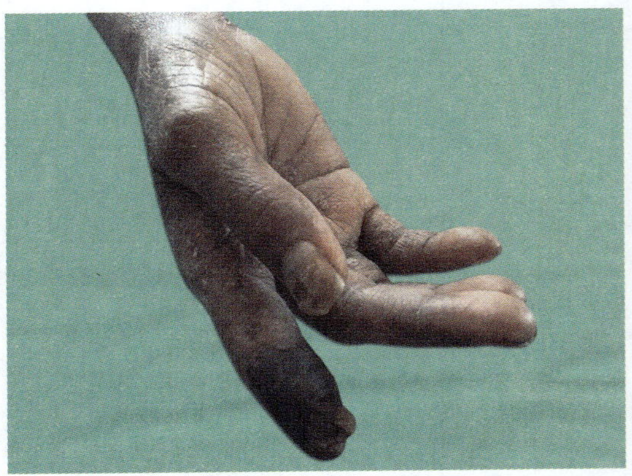

FIG. 3.12: Diabetic gangrene of right index finger.

Diabetic Nephropathy

Q. Write short essay/note on:
- **Clinical features, diagnosis, and management of diabetic nephropathy.**
- **Kimmelstiel–Wilson lesions.**

Diabetic nephropathy is the term used for **collective lesions that often occur together in the diabetic kidney**. About **30–40% of all diabetics** develop nephropathy and **are leading cause of chronic kidney disease (CKD) and end-stage renal disease (ESRD)**. It is a leading cause of death and disability in diabetes and is more common in type 1 DM than T2DM. Renal changes in diabetes mellitus are listed in **Box 3.18**.

Box 3.18: Renal changes in diabetes mellitus.

- Glomerular lesions:
  - Diffuse widespread thickening of glomerular basement membrane (GBM)
  - Nodular glomerulosclerosis (Kimmelstiel–Wilson nodules)
  - Insudative lesions: Fibrin caps and capsular drop
- Pyelonephritis: Acute and chronic including necrotizing papillitis
- Tubular lesions: Armanni–Ebstein lesions
- Renal vascular lesions (arteriosclerosis and atherosclerosis)

Pathogenesis

Diabetic glomerulosclerosis represents a part of the generalized diabetic microangiopathy that involves small vessels throughout the body. Like other microvascular complications of DM, the pathogenesis of diabetic nephropathy is related to chronic hyperglycemia.

Clinical Features

The natural history of diabetic nephropathy follows a fairly predictable sequence of events.

- **Glomerular hyperperfusion** and **renal hypertrophy** develop in the first years after the onset of DM. It is associated with an **increase of the glomerular filtration rate** (GFR). It shows nephromegaly (enlargement of kidneys).
- During the first 5 years of DM, **thickening of the GBM**, glomerular hypertrophy, and expansion of mesangial volume occur as the GFR returns to normal.
- **Microalbuminuria**: After 5–10 years, many patients start excreting **small amounts of albumin in the urine**. It is the **earliest manifestation** of diabetic nephropathy in which the urine has low amounts of albumin (>20 mg/day, but <300 mg/day). Microalbuminuria is defined as the **persistent elevation of the urinary albumin excretion of 20–300 mg/L** (or 20–200 μg/min) in an early morning urine sample. It is also a well-established marker for increased cardiovascular morbidity and mortality in either type 1 or type 2 diabetics. Normal individual excretes albumin <20 mg/day. It indicates early and possibly reversible glomerular damage. Type 2 diabetes is more likely to have microalbuminuria (or overt nephropathy) at diagnosis. This is because of the long duration of abnormal glucose metabolism in T2DM. Hence, patients with T2DM should be screened at the time of diagnosis for the presence of microalbuminuria.
- **Nephropathy with macroalbuminuria**: Without specific interventions, diabetics will develop **overt nephropathy with macroalbuminuria** (>300 mg of urinary albumin per day) usually associated with hypertension. From this stage, the renal disease is irreversible. There is a steady decline in GFR at a rate of about 1 mL/min/month. The stage of macroalbuminuria may progress to nephrotic syndrome.
- **End-stage renal disease**: The overt nephropathy may progress to ESRD. Patient develops azotemia, renal failure, and uremia.

Different stages of diabetic nephropathy are mentioned in **Table 3.23**.

TABLE 3.23: Classification of diabetic nephropathy.

Stages	***Urinary albumin (mg/g Cr) or urinary protein (g/g Cr)***	***GFR [estimated glomerular filtration rate (eGFR)] (mL/min/1.73 m²)***
Stage 1 (prenephropathy)	Normoalbuminuria (<30)	≥30
Stage 2 (incipient nephropathy)	Microalbuminuria (30–299)	≥30
Stage 3 (overt nephropathy)	Macroalbuminuria (≥300) or persistent proteinuria (>0.5)	≥30
Stage 4 (kidney failure)	Any albuminuria/proteinuria status	<30
Stage 5 (dialysis therapy)	Any status on continued dialysis therapy	

Causes of Microalbuminuria other than Diabetes

- **Essential hypertension**: In hypertensive patients, microalbuminuria **predicts cardiovascular morbidity and mortality**.

Screening for microalbuminuria: It can be done in a variety of ways. Microalbuminuria can be assessed by radioimmunoassay or by using special dipsticks.

- **Measurement of albumin-to-creatinine ratio**: This is most easily obtained with minimal collection errors. A ratio of >30 mg albumin/g creatinine is considered elevated on a spot urine test.
- **Albumin from a 24-hour urine sample**: Urinary albumin >30 mg/24 h is diagnostic.

Management

- **Prevention**: Control of glycemia can reverse microalbuminuria in some patients. Stop smoking and control dyslipidemia.
- **Management of diabetic nephropathy**:
  - Glycemic control: Insulin is the antidiabetic of choice and regular and rapid-acting insulin is preferred.
  - Biguanides are contraindicated if estimated glomerular filtration rate (eGFR) <30 mL/min/1.73 m². SGLT2 inhibitors can be used till eGFR >45 mL/min/1.73 m². Sulfonylureas, glitazones, and acarbose are avoided.
- Blood pressure (BP) control: Recommended BP <140/90 mm Hg. Angiotensin-converting enzyme (ACE) inhibitors and angiotensin receptor blockers (ARBs) are first line for BP control.
- Dietary modification: Protein restriction, as it reduces hyperfiltration and intraglomerular pressure. Up to 0.8 g/day is recommended by the ADA. Sodium restriction to <2,300 mg/day is also mandated.
- Miscellaneous: Treat UTI aggressively. Lipid lowering by HMG-CoA reductase inhibitors.

"Burnt-out" Diabetes: Patients with ESRD experience drastic reductions of insulin and OHA requirements due to decreased renal and hepatic insulin clearance, decline in renal gluconeogenesis, deficient catecholamine release, decreased food intake, protein energy wasting, and hypoglycemia due to dialysis.

Ophthalmologic Complications of Diabetes Mellitus

Q. Write short essay/note on ocular complications of diabetes mellitus.

Diabetes can produce different lesions in the eye. These include:

- **Diabetic retinopathy** (DR) (damage to the retina and iris) can lead to blindness.
- **Cataract** is denaturation of the protein and other components of the lens of the eye and leads to opacity of lens. Cataract develops early in diabetics than in the general population. Sustained very poor control of diabetes and ketosis can cause an acute cataract (snowflake cataract). Fluctuations in blood glucose level can cause refractive variability due to osmotic changes within the lens (the absorption of water into the lens can produce temporary hypermetropia). This clinically presents as fluctuating difficulty in reading and it resolves with control of the diabetes.
- **External ocular palsies**: The 6th and the 3rd cranial nerves (**Tolosa-Hunt syndrome**) are the most commonly affected. These nerve palsies usually recover spontaneously within 3–6 months.
- Glaucoma.

Diabetic Retinopathy (Figs. 3.13A and B)

Q. Write short essay/note on diabetic retinopathy.

Diabetic retinopathy is the most commonly diagnosed complication of DM. It is a microangiopathy due to prolonged hyperglycemia causing microaneurysms/hemorrhages/exudates and/or abnormal vessels on the retina. In developed countries, it is one of the most common causes of blindness between 30 and 65 years of age. Its prevalence increases with the duration of diabetes and develops in ~**60–80% of diabetics, about 15–20 years after diagnosis**.

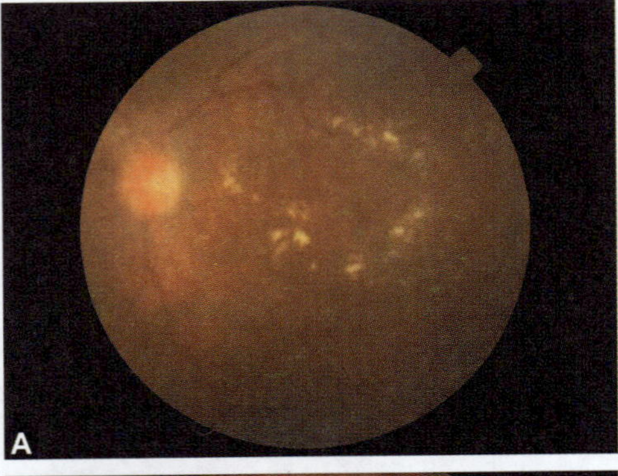

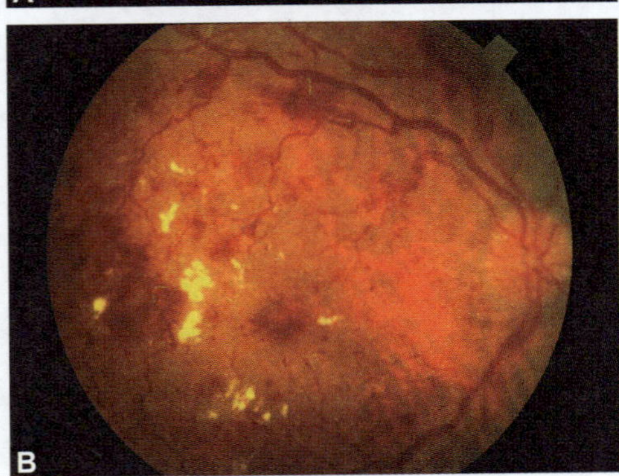

FIGS. 3.13A AND B: (A) Moderate nonproliferative diabetic retinopathy (NPDR) with hard exudates; (B) Proliferative diabetic retinopathy (PDR).

Box 3.19: Risk factors for diabetic retinopathy.

- Long duration of diabetes mellitus
- Poor glycemic control
- With nephropathy/renal disease
- Hypertension
- Hyperlipidemia
- Pregnancy
- Others: Obesity, smoking

TABLE 3.24: Features of diabetic retinopathy.

Nonproliferative diabetic retinopathy/ simple background (NPDR)	*Proliferative diabetic retinopathy (PDR)*
➢ Develops late in the first decade or early in the second decade ➢ Increased capillary permeability ➢ Marked retinal vascular microaneurysms, capillary closure, and dilatation ➢ Hemorrhages: Dot (capillary microaneurysms) and blot (leakage of blood into deeper retinal layers) ➢ Cotton-wool spots/cytoid bodies (caused by microinfarcts within the retina due to occluded vessels) ➢ Hard exudates (exudation of plasma rich in lipids and protein) ➢ Arteriovenous shunts and dilated veins	➢ New blood vessel formation/ neovascularization ➢ Preretinal or subhyaloid hemorrhage ➢ Vitreous hemorrhage ➢ More numerous microaneurysms and hemorrhages ➢ Changes in caliber of venous vessel ➢ Retinal fibrosis/scar (retinitis proliferans) ➢ Traction retinal detachment

Risk factors for diabetic retinopathy (Box 3.19)

Lesions of diabetic retinopathy: DR can be classified into two stages: (1) nonproliferative/simple background and (2) proliferative (**Table 3.24**).

Diabetic macular edema (DME): In addition to proliferative and nonproliferative DR, patients may also develop clinically significant macular edema (CSME). This can develop at any stage of DR and is characterized by increased vascular permeability and hard exudates in the central retina. CSME is the most common cause of loss of vision in DM.

Investigations

- **Fundus fluorescein angiography (FFA)**: In this, a fluorescent dye is injected into a vein of upper arm and photographed in transit through the retinal vessels. It helps to identify the extent of the potentially sight-threatening DR.
- **Optical coherence tomography (OCT)**: It is used to image the content of the layers of the retina at the macula and to measure retinal thickness. It helps in detecting macular edema and other macular abnormalities.

Treatment

- **Prevention**: By intensive glycemic, BP **control**, and lipid control in both type 1 or T2DM.
- **Screening**: Regular eye examinations in all patients with DM.
- Diabetic retinopathy is treated by **laser photocoagulation**.
- Proliferative retinopathy is usually treated with **panretinal laser photocoagulation**. **DME** by focal and grid therapy and pars plana vitrectomy is performed for the treatment of nonresolving vitreous hemorrhage and retinal detachment. Intravitreal hyaluronidase, chondroitinase, and plasmin have shown promise in clearing vitreous hemorrhage.
- **Vascular endothelial growth factor inhibitors** such as bevacizumab, ranibizumab, and aflibercept are useful as adjunct therapy to panretinal photocoagulation and/or vitrectomy for selected cases of proliferative diabetic retinopathy (PDR) and DME.

Diabetic Neuropathy

The presence of symptoms and/or signs of peripheral nerve dysfunction in people with diabetes after the exclusion of other causes.

Q. Write short essay/note on:
- **Different neurological complications/manifestations of diabetes mellitus.**
- **Classification, clinical manifestations, and management of diabetic neuropathy.**

Diabetes can involve the **peripheral nervous systems** in a number of ways.

Risk factors: Similar to other complications of DM, the development of neuropathy is related to the duration of diabetes and the degree of glycemic control. Other risk factors are greater BMI and smoking.

Classification of diabetic neuropathy: There are various classifications of diabetic neuropathy and one of them is presented in **Box 3.20**.

Box 3.20: Classification of diabetic neuropathy.

- **Diffuse neuropathy:**
  Distal symmetrical polyneuropathy (DSPN):
  - Small fiber
  - Large fiber
  - Mixed (most common)
- **Mononeuropathy (mononeuritis multiplex):**
  - Isolated cranial/peripheral nerve
  - Mononeuritis multiplex
- **Radiculopathy or polyradiculopathy:**
  - Radiculoplexus neuropathy
  - Thoracic radiculopathy
- **Nondiabetic neuropathies common in diabetes:**
  - Pressure palsies
  - Chronic inflammatory demyelinating polyneuropathy (CIDP)
  - Treatment-induced painful small fiber neuropathy

Polyneuropathy

Distal Symmetric Sensorimotor Polyneuropathy

- It is the most common form of diabetic neuropathy. It affects both **motor and sensory function** of the lower extremities. It can be divided into two types:
  1. **Asymptomatic**: It is a relatively asymptomatic form. It is diffuse, distal, usually involves the lower extremities, and later it may involve the upper extremities with a "**glove and stocking**" type of distribution.
  2. **Acute** painful **neuropathy**: It is a diffuse, painful neuropathy, and is less common. It presents with burning or crawling or dull aching sensation or excruciating, lancinating pain in the feet, shins, and anterior thighs. The pain is typically worse at night and pressure from bedclothes may be intolerable and partially relieved by movement. Hyperesthesia may be severe.
- In both forms, physical findings are: Loss of vibration sense, loss of tendon reflexes in the lower limbs (especially ankle jerk), and "glove and stocking" impairment of all sensation.
- With progression, patients may complain of a feeling of "walking on cotton wool" and loss of balance while washing the face ("wash-basin sign") or walking in the dark owing to impaired proprioception. It may be associated with involvement of other sensation such as joint position, touch, pain, and temperature, later leading to weakness and wasting of muscles.
- **Sequelae of neuropathy**: Involvement of motor nerves to the small muscles of the feet results in interosseous wasting. Unbalanced traction by the long flexor muscles results in a characteristic shape of the foot with a high arch and clawing of the toes. This can lead to abnormal distribution of pressure on walking, producing callus formation under the first metatarsal head or on the tips of the toes. Complications include unrecognized trauma, beginning as blistering due to an ill-fitting shoe, and neuropathic ulceration. Sometimes, **neuropathic arthropathy (Charcot's joints)** may develop in the ankle.

Asymmetrical Motor Diabetic Neuropathy (Diabetic Amyotrophy/Bruns–Garland Syndrome)

Q. Write short essay/note on diabetic amyotrophy.

- Usually develops in older individuals with diabetes.
- It presents with asymmetrical, severe, and progressive weakness and atrophy of the proximal (quadriceps) muscles of the lower limbs. It is associated with severe pain, mainly on the anterior aspect of the leg, and hyperesthesia and paresthesias.
- Sometimes, there may be marked wasting and weight loss ("neuropathic cachexia"). The patient may appear extremely ill and be unable to get out of bed. Tendon reflexes may be diminished or absent on the affected side(s).
- This neuropathy is probably due to the acute infarction of the lower motor neurons of the lumbosacral plexus. Other lesions of this plexus (e.g., neoplasms and lumbar disk disease) must be excluded, before a diagnosis is made.
- It is seen in patients with poor glycemic control and resolves with optimization of metabolic control.
- Management is mainly supportive.

Mononeuropathy and Mononeuritis Multiplex

Mononeuropathy characterized by dysfunction of isolated cranial or peripheral nerves is less common than polyneuropathy in DM.

- **Nerve involvement**: Diabetic mononeuropathy can involve a single **peripheral or cranial nerve** and affect either motor or sensory function. Usually, it affects 3rd, 6th, 4th (Tolosa–Hunt) or 7th (Bell's palsy) cranial nerves and the **femoral and sciatic nerves** (in order of frequency). Third nerve involvement is characterized by diplopia and normal pupillary constriction to light (pupil sparing). Rarely, other single nerves are involved and produce paresis and paresthesias in the thorax and trunk (truncal radiculopathies). Simultaneous involvement of more than one nerve (mononeuropathy multiplex) may also occur.
- **Presentation**: Unlike the gradual progression of distal symmetrical and autonomic neuropathies, the mononeuropathies present as **rapid, severe pain and motor weakness** in the distribution of a single nerve. However, eventually they recover.
- **Nerve compression palsies**: Mononeuropathies can present with or without nerve compression. Nerve compression is more common in diabetes. Compression may affect the median nerve (presents the clinical picture of **carpal tunnel syndrome**), lateral popliteal nerve (**foot drop**), or less commonly the ulnar nerve (**wrist drop**). Compression palsies may

be due to glycosylation and thickening of connective tissue and/or increased susceptibility of nerves affected by diabetic microangiopathy.

Autonomic Neuropathy (Table 3.25)

- Autonomic neuropathy may affect both the sympathetic and parasympathetic nervous systems.
- Diabetes mellitus-related autonomic neuropathy can involve one or more systems, including the cardiovascular, GI, genitourinary, sudomotor, and metabolic systems (**Table 3.25**).
- It may result in loss of awareness of hypoglycemia and can cause disabling postural hypotension.

TABLE 3.25: Clinical features of diabetic autonomic neuropathy.

System involved	*Clinical features*
Cardiovascular	Postural hypotension, resting tachycardia, fixed heart rate, impaired Valsalva maneuver, painless myocardial infarction, and sudden cardiac death
Gastrointestinal	Dysphagia (due to esophageal atony), abdominal fullness, nausea, vomiting, gastroparesis, nocturnal diarrhea, constipation, and fecal incontinence
Genitourinary	Difficulty in micturition, urinary incontinence, recurrent infection, impotence, erectile dysfunction, and retrograde ejaculation
Sudomotor	Gustatory sweating, nocturnal sweat without hypoglycemia, fissures in feet, and anhidrosis
Vasomotor	Feet feel cold (due to loss of skin vasomotor responses), dependent pedal edema (due to loss of vasomotor tone and increased vascular permeability)
Pupillary	Decreased pupil size, delayed or absent reflexes to light, resistance to mydriatics, and Argyll–Robertson pupil
Metabolic	Hypoglycemia unawareness

Management

Strict glycemic control, foot care

- **Mononeuropathies are usually self-limiting** and do not require any specific therapy. Explanation and reassurance about remission within months may be necessary.
- **Neuritic pain** of diabetic neuropathy may be treated with nonsteroidal anti-inflammatory drugs (opiates—tramadol, oxycodone), tricyclic antidepressants (amitriptyline, imipramine, duloxetine, venlafaxine mexiletine, valproate), and anticonvulsants (e.g., phenytoin, carbamazepine, gabapentin, or pregabalin). Duloxetine is an antidepressant, potent dual reuptake inhibitor of serotonin and noradrenaline is useful in refractory cases.
- Transepidermal nerve stimulation (**TENS**): Beneficial in some patients.
- Topical **capsaicin**-containing creams: May be occasionally beneficial.
- **Orthostatic/postural hypotension**: Responds to sleeping with the head of the bed raised, avoiding sudden upright position, full-length elastic support stockings, and increased salt intake. Rarely, fludrocortisone and α-adrenoceptor agonist (midodrine) are needed.
- **Gastroparesis**: Patient is advised to take frequent small meals and prokinetic agents. Dopamine antagonists (metoclopramide, domperidone), erythromycin, and gastric pacemaker; percutaneous enteral (jejunal) feeding may be necessary in some cases.
- **Diarrhea**: In diabetics, it often responds to diphenoxylate, loperamide, or broad-spectrum antibiotics (e.g., tetracyclines). Rarely, clonidine and octreotide may be needed.
- **Constipation**: It can be treated by stimulant laxatives (Senna).
- **Atonic bladder**: By intermittent self-catheterization.
- **Excessive sweating**: By anticholinergic drugs (propantheline, poldine, oxybutynin), clonidine, or topical antimuscarinic agent (glycopyrrolate cream).
- **Erectile dysfunction**: Treatment includes:
  - Psychological counseling; psychosexual therapy
  - Phosphodiesterase type 5 inhibitors: Oral therapy with sildenafil, vardenafil, and tadalafil
  - Dopamine agonist (apomorphine) through sublingual route
  - Prostaglandin E (alprostadil): Injected into corpus cavernosum or intraurethral administration of pellets
  - Vacuum tumescence devices
  - Implanted penile prosthesis.

Specific treatment to reverse neuropathy

- **α-lipoic acid**: It is a natural cofactor of dehydrogenase complex and is an antioxidant (redox-modulating agent). It may ameliorate both somatic and autonomic diabetic neuropathies.
- **Aldolase reductase inhibitors (e.g., epalrestat)**: They decrease the flux of glucose through polyol pathways, inhibit accumulation of sorbitol and fructose, and prevent reduction of redox potential. However, they are not effective.
- **Carnitine** may be useful in few cases.
- **Methylcobalamin** may provide some benefit.
- **Ruboxistaurin, a PKC-β inhibitor, is** an emerging treatment for diabetes microvascular complications.

Dermatological Complications of Diabetes Mellitus (Box 3.21)

Q. Write short note on dermatological complications of diabetes mellitus.

Musculoskeletal Complications of Diabetes Mellitus (Box 3.22)

Q. Write short note on musculoskeletal complications of diabetes mellitus.

Box 3.21: Dermatological complications of diabetes mellitus (DM).

- Skin infections: Due to immune dysfunction, e.g., carbuncles and furuncles and intertrigo (**Fig. 3.14**)
- Balanoposthitis (**Fig. 3.15**)
- Vaginal candidiasis/balanitis (**Fig. 3.16**): Due to immune dysfunction
- Diabetic ulcers: Due to peripheral neuropathy and ischemia
- Xanthomatoses: Due to hyperlipoproteinemia
- Necrobiosis lipoidica diabeticorum (NLD)
- Diabetic dermopathy (shin spots)
- Tight waxy skin and the dorsum of the hands with joint contractures in type 1 DM—digital sclerosis
- Acanthosis nigricans
- Acrochordons/skin tags: Marker of insulin resistance
- Granuloma annulare
- Diabetic blisters: Bullosis diabeticorum

Box 3.22: Musculoskeletal complications in diabetes.

- Diabetic muscle infarction: Painful muscle swelling, usually in thigh
- Neuropathic arthropathy (Charcot joint)
- Carpal tunnel syndrome
- Dupuytren's contracture
- Flexor tenosynovitis
- Adhesive capsulitis (frozen shoulder)
- Diabetic cheiroarthropathy—"prayer sign" and "tabletop test"
- Diabetic sclerodactyly

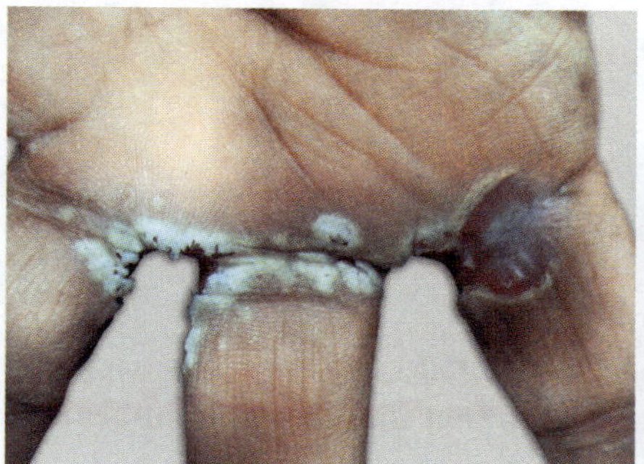

FIG. 3.14: Intertrigo (intertriginous dermatitis) characterized by inflammation of skinfolds.

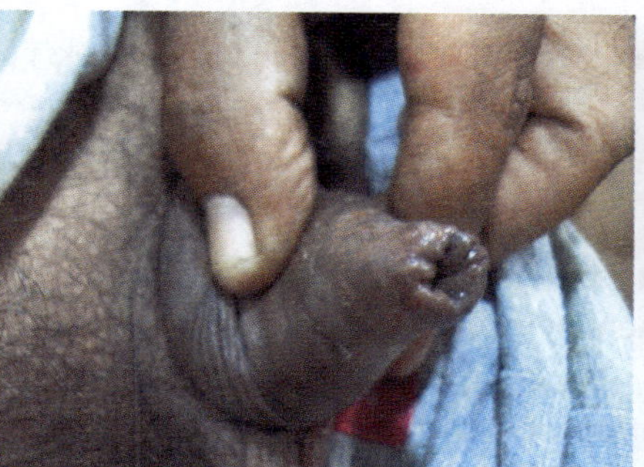

FIG. 3.15: Balanoposthitis.

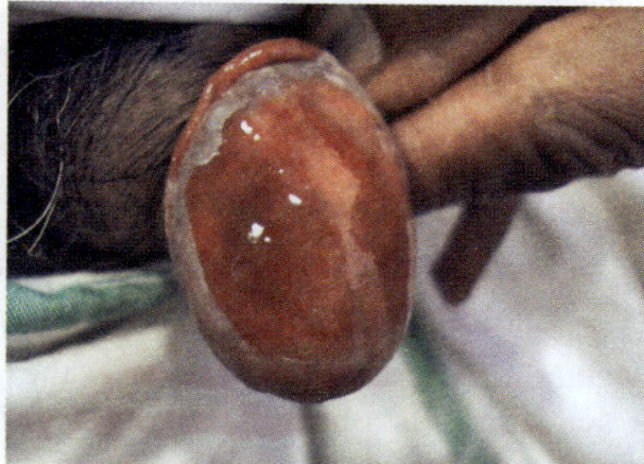

FIG. 3.16: Candida balanitis.

GESTATIONAL DIABETES MELLITUS

Q. Write short essay/note on gestational diabetes mellitus (GDM), its significance, and management.

Gestational diabetes mellitus (GDM) is defined as **glucose intolerance (diabetes) that develops or is first recognized during pregnancy**. Typically, it is asymptomatic and usually remits after delivery. However, there is an increased risk of type 2 diabetes in later life and maintaining a low body weight and keeping physically active can reduce this risk.

Risk factors for GDM, low-risk groups for GDM, and importance of diagnosis of GDM are mentioned in **Boxes 3.23 to 3.25**, respectively.

Box 3.23: Risk factors that predispose to gestational diabetes mellitus.

Women with:
- Previous history of gestational diabetes
- Obesity (overweight) and pregnancy at older age
- History of large for gestational age babies
- Ethnic groups at particular risk

Box 3.24: Low-risk groups for gestational diabetes mellitus.

Women with:
- Age below 25 years
- Normal weight before pregnancy
- Member of an ethnic group with a low prevalence of diabetes
- No diabetes in first-degree relatives
- No history of abnormal glucose tolerance or poor obstetrical outcome

Box 3.25: Importance of diagnosis of gestational diabetes mellitus (GDM).

Fetal risk with GDM:
- Fetal macrosomia
- Intrauterine fetal death
- Respiratory distress
- Hypoglycemic fetuses
- Polyhydramnios
- Hypocalcemia
- Increased incidence of shoulder dystocia
- Fetal hyperbilirubinemia
- Transient tachypnea of the newborn

Risk for offspring of women with GDM: Increased risk of obesity and diabetes

Risk for women with GDM: Increased risk of obesity and diabetes in future.
- Increased incidence of preeclampsia
- Cesarean section

Oral Glucose Tolerance Test

- Diagnosis is based on an OGTT performed at 24–28 weeks of gestation in women with moderate-to-high risk.
- **Method**: 100 g glucose is dissolved in 300–400 mL of water and consumed over 5 minutes. The quantity of glucose is more than usual glucose load of 75 g and is recommended because there is an increased turnover of glucose in pregnancy.

Criteria for Diagnosis of Gestational Diabetes Mellitus

See **Table 3.26.**

TABLE 3.26: Criteria for diagnosis of gestational diabetes mellitus.

Time (hour)	Upper limit of normal values (mg/dL)	
	Whole blood (O'Sullivan)	Plasma (Carpenter and Coustan)
0 (fasting)	85	95
1	160	180
2	140	155
3	125	140

(Two or more of these values must be abnormal).

Management

Aim

To normalize the maternal blood glucose and reduce excessive growth of fetus.

- **Insulin**: Initiate insulin therapy when target glucose levels exceed despite nutritional therapy. Insulin does not cross the placenta.
- **Dietary modification**: Reduce the consumption of quick-acting refined carbohydrate. Treatment for other patients with diet in the first instance, although most may require insulin at some stages during pregnanc y.
- Many oral hypoglycemic drugs cross the placenta and should be avoided because of the potential risk to the fetus. However, *metformin or glyburide/glibenclamide* is considered safe to use in pregnancy.

Follow-up

Though the sugar levels normalize after delivery, it is advised to repeat an OGTT 6 weeks postpartum.

METABOLIC SYNDROME

Q. Write short essay or note on:

- **Metabolic syndrome/insulin resistance syndrome and its components.**
- **Clinical diagnosis, risks, and treatment of insulin resistance syndrome (syndrome X).**

Metabolic syndrome (also known as the *insulin resistance syndrome, Reaven syndrome, dysmetabolic syndrome*, and *syndrome X* syndrome) is a proinflammatory, prothrombotic state that consists of a **cluster of clinical findings and laboratory abnormalities**.

- **Clinical findings**: Include obesity (central, abdominal, or visceral), increased sympathetic nervous system activity, and hypertension. Risk factors associated with metabolic syndrome are listed in **Table 3.27**. These clinical features include acanthosis nigricans, skin tags—acrochordons, ovarian hyperandrogenism [polycystic ovary syndrome (PCOS)], and lipodystrophy.
- **Laboratory abnormalities**: Cardiovascular risk factors and it includes hyperglycemia, dyslipidemia (high TGs, low HDL), glucose intolerance, insulin resistance (the common etiologic factor), and hyperinsulinemia (compensatory).
- **Pathogenesis**: The basic defect is insulin resistance.
  - Insulin resistance is **the decrease/failure of target (peripheral) tissues to insulin action**. Insulin is unable to produce its numerous actions in spite of unimpaired secretion from the P-cells.
  - **Main factors** in the development of insulin resistance are combination of genetic susceptibility and **obesity**. The obesity accompanying T2DM is central obesity and central adipose tissue is more "lipolytic" than peripheral sites. Insulin resistance is induced by FFAs, adipokines, and chronic inflammation in adipose tissue.
  - **Consequences of insulin resistance**:
    - **Decreased uptake of glucose in muscle** results in postprandial hyperglycemia. The defects in the uptake are due to defect in the receptors present in target tissues and usually at the postreceptor level.
    - **Reduced glycolysis** and **fatty acid oxidation** in the liver.
    - **Inability to suppress hepatic gluconeogenesis**.
- **Clinical diagnosis (Box 3.26)**: Individual on medical treatment for dyslipidemia or hypertension and those with isolated systolic or diastolic hypertension are included in the above criteria.

TABLE 3.27: Risks associated with metabolic syndrome.

➢ Cardiovascular diseases (atherosclerotic vascular disease, specifically coronary artery disease) ➢ Type 2 diabetes mellitus ➢ Nonalcoholic fatty liver disease	➢ Sleep disorders: Obstructive sleep apnea ➢ Polycystic ovary syndrome (PCOS) ➢ Hyperuricemia ➢ Chronic kidney disease ➢ Erectile dysfunctions

Box 3.26: Diagnostic criteria for metabolic syndrome.

Presence of at least three of the following:

- Abdominal obesity (waist circumference ≥88 cm in women and ≥102 cm in men
  - **Body mass index ≥30 kg/m^2 and/or waist-hip ratio ≥0.09 in men and ≥0.85 in women**
- Raised triglyceride (TG) levels (≥150 mg/dL) or on treatment for TG
- Reduced high-density lipoproteins (HDLs) cholesterol level (<40 mg/dL in males and <50 mg/dL in females) or on treatment for HDL
- Raised blood pressure (systolic ≥130 mm Hg or diastolic ≥85 mm Hg)
- Raised fasting glucose level (110–125 mg/dL); type 2 diabetes mellitus (DM) or impaired glucose tolerance and/or insulin resistance denoted by hyperinsulinemia relative to glucose levels

Management

Currently, there is no evidence that treatment of insulin resistance reduces mortality and morbidity in metabolic syndrome. However, treatment of insulin resistance consists of:

- Lifestyle changes and exercise
- Diet: Low in calories and high in fibers
- Reduction of weight
- Treatment and control of diabetes, hypertension, and lipid abnormalities.

CHAPTER

4

Infectious Diseases

COVID-19

Q. Discuss the epidemiology, clinical features, complications, and management of COVID-19.

At the end of 2019, a novel coronavirus was identified as the cause of a cluster of pneumonia cases in Wuhan, China. The WHO designated the disease COVID-19 and the virus is designated severe acute respiratory syndrome coronavirus 2 (SARS-CoV-2) **(Fig. 4.1)**.

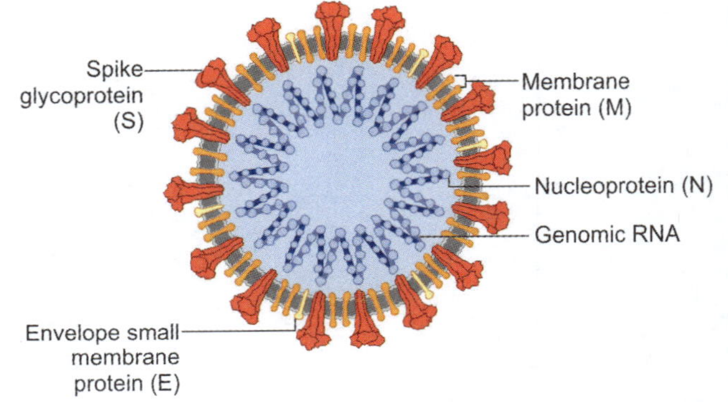

FIG. 4.1: Severe acute respiratory syndrome coronavirus-2 (CoV-2).

Transmission

1. Person-to-person:
   - Mainly via respiratory droplets
   - Direct contact with mucous membrane (eyes/nose/mouth)
2. Viral shedding and period of infectivity:
   - It can be transmitted prior to the onset of symptoms and throughout the course of illness, particularly early in the course.
   - Transmission can occur during incubation period (from asymptomatic individuals)
   - Duration of viral shedding is variable
3. Risk of transmission: Depends on:
   - Type and duration of exposure
   - Use of preventive measures
   - Amount of virus in respiratory secretions
   - Environmental contamination—it is a potential source, especially in hospitals. Period of infectivity is ~6 days
4. Risk of reinfection: Some antibodies are protective; not definitely established yet.

Pathogenesis

Binding of spike protein to ACE-2 receptors
↓
Uncoating
↓
Replication of viral genomic RNA by RNA-dependent RNA-polymerase
↓
Translation of viral proteins
↓
Viral assembly into vesicles in the Golgi apparatus
↓
Exocytosis

Clinical Features

- Incubation period: <14 days
- Majority are asymptomatic
- Spectrum of disease:
  - Mild—no/mild pneumonia
  - Severe—>50% lung involvement, dyspnea, and hypoxia seen
  - Critical—respiratory failure, shock, and multiple organ dysfunction syndrome (MODS)
  - Death
- Most common manifestation/pneumonia—fever, cough, dyspnea, and bilateral lung infiltrates on imaging.

- Fever
- Dry/wet cough
- Dyspnea (new or worsening)
- Anosmia or other smell abnormalities
- Ageusia or other taste abnormalities
- Sore throat
- Myalgia
- Conjunctivitis
- Fatigue
- Confusion
- Chest pain
- Nausea/vomiting
- Diarrhea
- Chills/rigor
- Headache
- Rhinorrhea
- Tachypnea
- Hypoxia

Complications

- Acute respiratory distress syndrome (ARDS)
- Cardiac arrhythmias
- Acute cardiac injury
- Shock
- Guillain-Barré syndrome
- Deep venous thrombosis (DVT) and pulmonary embolism
- Acute stroke
- Children—kawasaki disease and toxic shock syndrome. Multisystem inflammatory syndrome in children (MIS-C)
- Cytokine release syndrome
- Secondary infections—bacteremia, aspergillus, mucormycosis

Risk Factors for Severe Illness

Laboratories:
- Lymphopenia with N/L >3.5
- CRP >100
- Ferritin >300
- LDH >245
- D-dimer >1,000 ng/mL
- High AST/ALT
- High PT/INR
- High trop-T
- AKI
- Increased CPK

Comorbidities:
- Age >50 years
- DM
- HTN
- Lung disease (COPD, BA, post-TB, and sequelae)
- CKD
- CLD
- HIV
- Malignancy (hematologic and solid organ tumors)
- Immunosuppression
- Obesity

Clinically:
- Hypoxia—SpO_2 <94%
- HR >100 bpm
- RR >30 cpm
- SBP <90 mm Hg
- Altered mental status

Imaging

- Chest X-ray: Normal in early/mild disease. Consolidation and ground glass opacities (GGO) in **bilateral peripheral and lower lung zone distributions**.
- CT chest:
  - GGO: 83% cases
  - GGO with mixed consolidation
  - Pleural thickening
  - Interlobular septal thickening
  - Air bronchograms
- Less common findings:
  - Bronchiectasis
  - Pleural effusions
  - Pericardial effusion
  - Lymphadenopathy
  - Crazy pavement pattern (GGO with superimposed septal thickening)

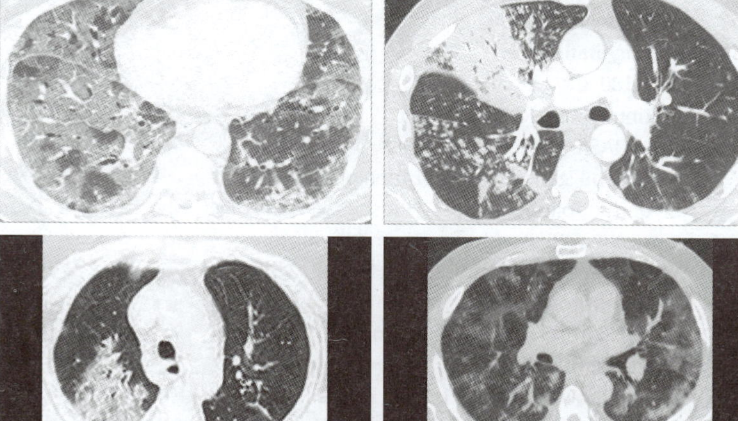

FIG. 4.2: Chest CT findings in COVID-19.

Chest CT Severity Score

20 lung regions evaluated on chest CT using a system attributing scores of 0, 1, and 2 if parenchymal opacification involved 0%, less than 50%, or equal or more than 50% of each region. The CT-SS is defined as the sum of the individual scored in the 20 lung segment regions, which may range from 0 to 40 points **(Fig. 4.2)**.

Diagnosis

1. Clinical suspicion:
   - New-onset fever/cough/dyspnea
   - History of contact with a COVID positive case/suspect within last 14 days
   - History of travel within last 14 days
   - History of work in healthcare settings
   - History of comorbidities/risk for severe illness
2. RT-PCR:
   - Preferred diagnostic test for COVID-19
   - Specimens—nasopharyngeal swab/nasal swab from both anterior nares/nasal or nasopharyngeal wash or aspirate/ oropharyngeal swab
   - RT-PCR positive for SARS-CoV-2 indicates COVID-19 disease present
   - Detectable SARS-CoV in upper respiratory tract specimens may persist for weeks after symptom onset
   - Prolonged viral detection does not indicate ongoing infectiousness
   - Single negative RT-PCR is sufficient to exclude COVID-19 in many individuals.
   - False-negative RT-PCR has been well-documented. If clinical suspicion remains, repeat test is performed 24–48 hours after initial testing.
   - Lower respiratory tract specimens (expectorated sputum, tracheal aspirate, and BAL fluid) for RT-PCR may be reserved for hospitalized patients. Induced sputum is not recommended for testing.
3. Serology—Detects SARS-CoV-2 antigens nucleocapsid or spike protein. Uncertain sensitivity and specificity.
4. Imaging—CXR/CT thorax, bilateral peripheral, and lower zone involvement
5. ECG
6. Blood tests:

Basic Investigations:
- CBC
- ESR and CRP
- LFT
- RFT
- RBS

Others:
- D-dimer
- Ferritin
- LDH
- PT/INR
- Trop-T
- Procalcitonin
- ABG

Treatment

- **Influenza-like illness (ILI)**—fever (>38°C) + cough with onset <10 days **not** requiring admission.
- **Severe acute respiratory infection (SARI)**—fever (>38°C) with cough with onset <10 days requiring admission.

1. General:
   - No dietary restriction
   - Good hydration
   - RBS <180
   - Continue ACE/ARBs, if present
   - Avoid NASIDs other than PCT
   - Avoid nebulization (aerosolization of the virus)
   - Oxygen supplementation—Hudson's/venturi/HFNC/NIV/mechanical ventilation
2. Category A (ICMR): Asymptomatic/mild symptoms:
   - Tablet oseltamivir 75 mg 1-0-1 × 5 days
   - Tablet azithromycin 500 mg 0-1-0 × 5 days
   - Tablet HCQ 400 mg stat → 100 mg 1-0-1 × 4 days
   - Tablet zinc 50 mg 0-1-0 × 7 days
   - Tablet vitamin C 500 mg 1-1-1 × 7 days
   - Injection enoxaparin 40 mg SC OD × 7 days (if D-dimer increased or CXR/CT suggestive of GGO)
3. Category B (ICMR): Symptomatic with mild-moderate pneumonia with no signs of severe disease, RR 15–30 cpm, SpO_2 90–94% at room air:
   - Category A treatment PLUS
   - IV antibiotics if indicated
   - Tablet N-acetylcysteine 600 mg 1-1-1 if cough +
   - Injection dexamethasone 6 mg 1-0-0 × 10 days or till discharge, whichever is shorter
   - Continuous SpO_2 monitoring
   - Oxygen via nasal prongs or Hudson's mask

4. Category C (ICMR): Symptomatic with severe pneumonia, RR > 30 CPM, SpO_2 <90% at room air or 90–94% with O_2, ARDS, and septic shock.
   - Category A and B treatment PLUS
   - If septic shock: Injection Sepsivac 0.3 mL I/D OD × days
   - NIV/MV
   - Inotropes, if required
   - Novel therapy as per clinical discretion: Discussed below

Drugs Approved for the Treatment of COVID-19

Remdesivir:
- Acts against RNA-dependent RNA polymerase of SARS-CoV-2
- Indicated in those on supplemental oxygen/mechanical ventilation/ECMO
- Contraindicated in deranged LFT, GFR <30 mL/min
- Should not be used concurrently with HCQ
- Pregnancy is not a contraindication

IL-6 pathway inhibitors—tocilizumab, sarilumab, and siltuximab:
- Observational data revealed decreased risks of intubation and/or death
- Associated with an increased risk of secondary infections

Hydroxychloroquine/chloroquine:
- Was recommended initially, but FDA revoked emergency use authorization in June 2020, due to increased arrhythmias
- Contraindications for HCQ:
  - QTc >500
  - Porphyria
  - Myasthenia gravis
  - Retinal pathology
  - Epilepsy
  - Hypokalemia <3

  Pregnancy is not a contraindication.

Convalescent plasma:
- High neutralizing antibody titers is hypothesized to have clinical benefit when given early in the course of disease, however recent studies have not shown significant benefit

Lopinavir/ritonavir:
- Though recommended initially, clinical trials have failed to demonstrate efficacy

Favipiravir:
- An RNA polymerase inhibitor
- Used in mild disease
- Dosage of favipiravir for adults is 1800 mg orally twice daily on 1st day followed by 800 mg orally twice daily, up to maximum of 14 days.

Ivermectin:
- In vitro activity against SARS-CoV-2, various clinical trials of ivermectin are underway

Bamlanivimab
- Recombinant neutralizing human IgG1-kappa monoclonal antibody directed against the spike (S) surface protein of SARS-CoV-2, derived from antigen specific B cells of a convalescent COVID-19 patient
- Binds to the receptor binding domain (RBD) of the S protein at a position overlapping the ACE-2 binding site
- Emergency use authorization (EUA) on 9th November 2020 for mild/moderate COVID-19 disease

Casirivimab and imdevimab:
- Casirivimab IgG1-kappa and imdevimab IgG1-lambda, recombinant human IgG1 monoclonal antibodies that bind simultaneously to the receptor binding domain of SARS CoV-2's spike protein, and thereby preventing the entry of virus into the host cells.
- EUA by FDA on November 21st 2020. Approved for treatment of mild-to-moderate COVID-19 in adults

Baricitinib:
- Janus kinase inhibitor used as a treatment for adults with moderate to severe rheumatoid arthritis

Foralumab:
- Anti CD3 monoclonal antibody which induces T regulatory cells, resulting in IL-10 mediated antiinflammatory effect

AZD7442:
- It is a combination of two long-acting antibodies (LAABs) derived from convalescent patients after SARS-CoV-2 infection? The LAABs were optimized with half-life extension and reduced Fc receptor binding

Other agents that have been proposed for COVID-19 therapy include the HCV antivirals sofosbuvir plus daclatasvir, the selective serotonin receptor blocker fluvoxamine, famotidine, colchicine, vitamin D, and zinc.

COVID-19 vaccines: The aim of the COVID-19 vaccine is to induce a protective immunity to, prevent symptomatic infection and further to prevent severe illness, hospitalization, and death.

Vaccine type	*Dosing*	*Efficacy against symptomatic COVID*
mRNA based vaccines		
Modern (mRna-1273)	0.5 mL per dose for 2 doses administered 28 days apart	94%
Pfizer-BioNTech (BNT162b2)	0.3 mL per dose for 2 doses administered 21 days apart	95%
Viral vector-based vaccines		
Chimpanzee adenovirus ChAdOx1 based Oxford/AstraZeneca (Vaxzevria, Covishield)	0.5 mL per dose for 2 doses 4-12 weeks apart. The WHO recommends a dosing interval of 8–12 weeks due to increased immunogenicity observed with longer dosing intervals.	70%
Human adenoviruses type 26 and type 5 based Sputnik V and Human adenovirus type 26 based Johnson & Johnson (Janssen)	0.5 mL per dose for 2 doses 3 weeks apart 0.5 mL as a single dose	92%
Inactivated/killed virus vaccines		
Bharat Biotech Covaxin	0.5 mL per dose for 2 doses 4–12 weeks apart	66%
Sinovac Biotech	0.5 mL per dose for 2 doses 2–4 weeks apart	50%
Subunit (spike-protein) vaccine		
Novavax	two doses administered 21 days apart	89%

PYREXIA (FEVER) OF UNKNOWN ORIGIN

Q. Define pyrexia of unknown origin (PUO). Discuss briefly your approach to a case of PUO or fever of unknown origin (FUO).

Q. Describe types, investigation, and differential diagnosis of a case of pyrexia of unknown origin.

Q. Mention the etiology of pyrexia of unknown origin and discuss the investigation in a case of pyrexia of unknown origin.

Definition

The definition of FUO (classical) was given by Petersdorf and Beeson in 1961. According to new classification, PUO is divided into four types:

1. **Classic pyrexia of unknown origin** (PUO) is classically defined as:
   - **Duration: Fever** of **at least 3 weeks duration.**
   - **Temperature: Daily temperature** persistently elevated **above 101°F** (38.3°C).
   - **Remains undiagnosed** despite after a thorough history-taking, physical examination, and the following obligatory (intelligent and intensive) investigations (or at least three outpatient visits or 3 days in hospital).
   - **No known immunocompromised state** (e.g., HIV or other immunosuppressing conditions).
2. **Nosocomial PUO:**
   - **Temperature:** Daily temperature persistently elevated **above 101°F** (38.3°C) developing on several occasions.
   - In a **hospitalized patient (>24 hours) who is receiving acute care but no fever or incubating on admission.**
   - It is mandatory that the cause of fever is not found at least on 3 days of intelligent investigations, including at least 2 days incubation of cultures.
3. **Neutropenic PUO:**
   - A temperature of >38.3°C (101°F) developing on several occasions
   - **Neutrophil count is below 500/mL** or is expected to fall to that level in 1 or 2 days
   - It is mandatory that the cause of fever is not found at least on 3 days of intelligent investigations, including at least 2 days incubation of cultures.
4. **HIV-associated PUO:**
   - A temperature of more than 38.3°C (101°F) developing on several occasions
   - Duration of fever is more than 4 weeks for outpatients or more than 3 days for hospitalized patients
   - **HIV infection confirmed**
   - It is mandatory that the cause of fever is not found at least on 3 days of intelligent investigations, including at least 2 days incubation of cultures.

Etiology

Classic PUO is usually not due to a rare disease, but due to atypical presentation of common diseases. Common causes of prolonged fever are:

Infections (40% Cases)

Most common infections causing PUO are **tuberculosis, malaria, typhoid, and HIV.** Other causes are:

1. **Bacterial:**
   - **Abscesses:** Most commonly in the subphrenic space, liver, right lower quadrant, retroperitoneal space or the pelvis in women.
   - **Tuberculosis (TB):** Disseminated tuberculosis occurring in **immunocompromised** patients, presents with more constitutional symptoms than localizing signs. **Chest X-ray** may be normal.
   - **Urinary tract infections (UTIs)** are rare causes. Perinephric abscesses occasionally fail to communicate with the urinary system resulting in a normal urinalysis.
   - **Infective endocarditis:** Culture-negative endocarditis occurs in 5–10% of endocarditis. The HACEK *(H. parainfluenzae, H. aphrophilus,* and *H. paraphrophilus), Actinobacillus actinomycetemcomitans, Cardiobacterium hominis, Eikenella corrodens,* and *Kingella spp.)* group are responsible for 5–10% cases of infective endocarditis and are the most common causes of gram-negative endocarditis in individuals without any abuse of intravenous drugs.
   - **Hepatobiliary infections: Cholangitis** may develop without local signs and with only mildly elevated or normal liver function tests especially in the elderly patients.
   - **Osteomyelitis**
   - **Brucellosis:** Should be considered in patients with persistent fever and a history of contact with cattle, swine, goats or sheep, or patients who consume raw milk products.
   - ***Borrelia recurrentis*** is responsible for tick borne relapsing fever.
   - Other spirochetal diseases that can cause PUO include *Spirillum minor* **(rat-bite fever),** *Borrelia burgdorferi* **(Lyme disease),** and *Treponema pallidum* **(syphilis).**
2. **Viral:**
   - **Herpes viruses,** such as ***Cytomegalovirus*** and ***Epstein–Barr virus*** (EBV) can cause prolonged febrile illnesses with constitutional symptoms without any significant organ manifestations, particularly in the elderly.
   - **HIV:** Prolonged fever may be the only manifestation in patients with advanced HIV infection.
3. **Fungi:** Immunosuppression, the use of broad-spectrum antibiotics, the presence of intravascular devices and total **parenteral nutrition** all predispose individual to disseminated fungal infections.
4. **Parasites:**
   - **Malaria**
   - **Toxoplasmosis:** It should be considered in febrile patients with lymph node enlargement.
   - **Trypanosoma,** leishmania, and **amoeba** species may rarely cause PUO.
5. **Rickettsial organisms:** *Coxiella burnetii* may cause chronic infections; chronic **Q fever** or Q fever endocarditis may be identified in patients with a PUO.
6. **Psittacosis:** Infection by the causative organism, *Chlamydophila* should be considered in a patient with PUO who has a history of contact with birds. **Lepidopterism** (fever with rash due to exposure to scales and toxic fluids of adult moths, butterflies or its caterpillars).

Neoplasms

Primary or metastatic neoplasms constitute 20% of cases of PUO (**Table 4.1**).

Collagen Vascular Disease/Autoimmune Disease

Constitute 20% of cases of PUO (**Table 4.1**).

Psychogenic Fevers

- **Habitual hyperthermia:** It is seen in young females, characterized by temperatures of 99–100.5°F that occurs regularly or intermittently for years. No organic cause can be found.
- **Afebrile PUO:** In this, patient always complaints of feverishness but the temperature recorded is always <38.3°C.
- **Exaggerated circadian rhythm:** Normal person usually have an evening rise of temperature which is not normally apparent. In this condition, it becomes evident.
- **Hysterical fever:** In this, the patient is thinks and believes that he is always having fever.

TABLE 4.1: Neoplasms and collagen vascular diseases causing PUO.

Neoplasms—primary or metastatic (20% cases)	*Collagen vascular disease/ autoimmune disease (20% cases)*
➢ **Hematological**	➢ Adult onset Still's disease, MAS/HLH
– Lymphoma	➢ Polymyalgia rheumatica
– Chronic leukemia	➢ Temporal arteritis
➢ **Nonhematological**	➢ Rheumatoid arthritis
– Renal cell cancer	➢ Rheumatic fever
– Hepatocellular carcinoma	➢ Inflammatory bowel disease
– Pancreatic cancer	➢ Reiter's syndrome
– Colon cancer	➢ Systemic lupus erythematosus
– Myelodysplastic syndrome	➢ Vasculitides
– Sarcomas	– Polyarteritis nodosa
– Atrial myxoma	– Giant cell arteritis
– Malignant histiocytosis	– Kawasaki disease

(PUO: pyrexia of unknown origin; MAS: macrophage activation syndrome; HLH: hemophagocytic lymphohistiocytosis)

- **Malignant hyperthermia:** It is a rare life-threatening condition triggered by exposure to certain drugs used for general anesthesia (especially all volatile anesthetics), nearly all gaseous anesthetics, and neuromuscular blocking agent like succinylcholine.
- **Neuroleptic malignant syndrome (NMS):** It is a rare, life-threatening, neurological disorder, most often caused by an adverse reaction to neuroleptic or antipsychotic drugs. It presents with muscle rigidity, fever, and autonomic instability.

Periodic Fevers

For example, familial Mediterranean fever.

Miscellaneous

Constitute 10% cases **(Table 4.2)**.

TABLE 4.2: Miscellaneous causes of PUO (10% cases).

➢ Drugs: Penicillin, phenytoin, captopril, allopurinol, erythromycin, cimetidine, etc. All drugs can cause fever except *Digitalis* ➢ Hyperthyroidism, pheochromocytoma, Addison's disease ➢ Alcoholic hepatitis ➢ Sarcoidosis ➢ Inflammatory bowel disease	➢ Deep venous thrombosis/ pulmonary thromboembolism ➢ Hemolytic anemia ➢ Thyroiditis ➢ Granulomatous hepatitis ➢ Cyclic neutropenia ➢ Kikuchi–Fujimoto disease ➢ CVA—intracranial bleeds

(PUO: pyrexia of unknown origin; CVA: cerebrovascular accidents)

Undiagnosed (10% Cases)

About 10–15% of patients remain undiagnosed despite extensive investigations and in 75% of these the fever resolves spontaneously. In the remainder, other signs and symptoms make the diagnosis clear.

Clinical Approach to PUO

History Taking

1. **Onset:**
   - **Acute:** Malaria and pyogenic infection
   - **Gradual:** TB and typhoid fever
2. **Character:** High-grade fever is seen in urinary tract infections (UTI), malaria, thrombosis, and drug fever.
3. **Pattern (Fig. 4.3):**
   - **Sustained/persistent:** Typhoid fever and drugs
   - **Intermittent fever:**
     - Daily spikes: Malaria, abscess, tuberculosis (TB), and schistosomiasis
     - Double quotidian, twice-daily spikes: Leishmaniasis, gonococcal endocarditis, and adult-onset Still's disease
     - Saddle back fever: Leptospirosis, dengue, and *Borrelia*
     - Relapsing/recurrent fever: Nonfalciparum malaria, brucellosis, and Hodgkin's lymphoma
4. **Antecedents:** Prior to onset of fever:
   - **Dental extraction:** Infective endocarditis
   - **Urinary catheterization:** UTI and bacteremia

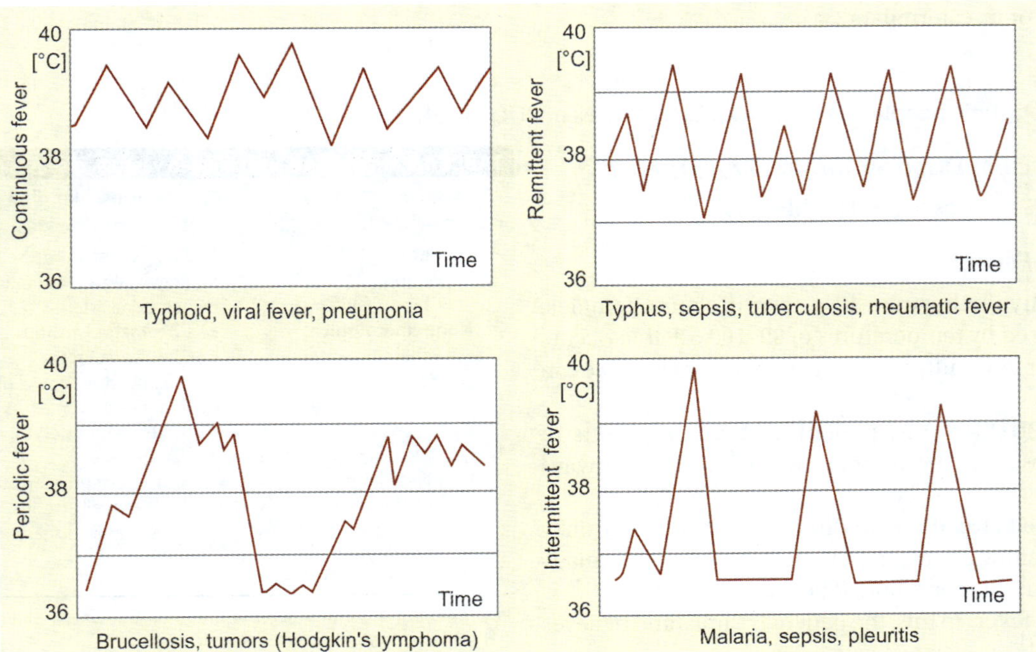

FIG. 4.3: Patterns/types of fever.

5. **Associated symptoms:**
   - **Chills and rigors:** Bacterial, rickettsial, and protozoal disease (malaria), influenza, lymphoma, leukemia, and drug-induced
   - **Night sweats:** TB and Hodgkin's lymphoma
   - **Loss of weight:** Malignancy and TB
   - **Cough and dyspnea:** Miliary TB, multiple pulmonary emboli, AIDS patient with *Pneumocystis pneumonia* (PCP), and *Cytomegalovirus* (CMV)
   - **Headache:** Giant cell arteritis, typhoid fever, sinusitis, meningitis, and drug fever
   - **Joint pain:** Rheumatoid arthritis, systemic lupus erythematosus (SLE), vasculitis, adult-onset Still's disease
   - **Abdominal pain:** Cholangitis, biliary obstruction, perinephric abscess, Crohn's disease, dissecting aneurysm, and gynecological infection
   - **Bone pain:** Osteomyelitis and lymphoma
   - **Sore throat:** Infectious mononucleosis, retropharyngeal abscess, and streptococcal infection
   - **Dysuria and rectal pain:** Prostatic abscess and UTI
   - **Altered bowel habit:** Inflammatory bowel disease (IBD), typhoid fever, schistosomiasis, and amebiasis
   - **Skin rash:** Gonococcal infection, polyarteritis nodosa (PAN), non-Hodgkin's lymphoma (NHL), dengue fever, and connective tissue disorders.
6. **Review past medical history:** Malignancy (e.g., leukemia, lymphoma, and hepatocellular carcinoma), HIV infection, diabetes mellitus, inflammatory bowel disease, collagen vascular disease [e.g., SLE and rheumatoid arthritis (RA)], giant cell arteritis, tuberculosis, and heart disease (e.g., valvular heart disease)
7. **Past surgical history:** Postsplenectomy/post-transplantation, prosthetic heart valve, catheter, AV fistula, and recent surgery/operation
8. **Drug history:**
   - **Immunosuppressive drug/corticosteroid**
   - **Anticoagulants**
   - **Before the fever: Drug fever** occur within 3 months after starting, taking drugs may cause hypersensitivity and low grade fever, usually associated with rash.
     - **Due to the allergic reaction,** direct effect of drug which impairs temperature regulation (e.g., phenothiazine), antiarrhythmic drug (e.g., procainamide and quinidine); antimicrobacterial agent (e.g., penicillin, cephalosporin, and hydralazine), and phenytoin.
   - **After the fever:** May modify clinical pictures and mask certain infection, e.g., subacute bacterial endocarditis (SBE) and antibiotic allergy.
9. **Family history:** Whether anyone in family has similar problem (e.g., tuberculosis and familial Mediterranean fever)
10. **Social history:**
    - **Travel:** Amebiasis, typhoid fever, malaria, and schistosomiasis
    - **Residential area:** Malaria, leptospirosis, and brucellosis
    - **Occupation:**
      - Farmers, veterinarian, and slaughter-house workers: Brucellosis
      - Workers in the plastic industries: Polymer-fume fever
      - Contact with domestic/wild animal/birds: Brucellosis, psittacosis (pigeons), leptospirosis, Q fever, and toxoplasmosis
    - **Diet history:**
      - Unpasteurized milk/cheese: Brucellosis
      - Poorly cooked pork: Trichinosis
    - **Intravenous drug user (IVDU):** HIV-AIDS-related condition and endocarditis
    - **Sexual orientation:** HIV, sexually transmitted disease (STD), and pelvic inflammatory disease (PID)
    - Close contact with TB patients

Physical Examination (Table 4.3)

TABLE 4.3: Various physical examination in pyrexia of unknown origin (PUO).

General	*Hands*	*Arms*
➢ Pattern of fever (continuous, intermittent, remitting, and relapsing) ➢ Patient is ill/not ill ➢ Weight loss (presence indicates chronic illness) ➢ Skin rash	➢ Stigmata of infective endocarditis ➢ Vasculitis changes ➢ Clubbing ➢ Presence of arthropathy ➢ Raynaud's phenomenon	➢ Drug injection sites (IVDU) ➢ Epitrochlear and axillary nodes (lymphoma, sarcoidosis, and focal infection) ➢ Skin rash and nodules ➢ Intravenous cannula—phlebitis

Contd...

Contd...

Head and neck		*Chest*
➢ Feel temporal arteries (tender and thickening) ➢ Eyes: Iritis/conjunctivitis (connective tissue disease—Reiter syndrome), jaundice (ascending cholangitis) ➢ Fundi: Choroidal tubercle (miliary TB), Roth's spot (infective endocarditis), and retinal hemorrhage (leukemia)	➢ Lymphadenopathy ➢ Butterfly rash: SLE ➢ Mucous membranes—petechiae ➢ Seborrheic dermatitis (HIV) ➢ Mouth ulcers (SLE) ➢ Buccal candidiasis ➢ Teeth and tonsils infection (abscess) ➢ Parotid enlargement ➢ Ears: Otitis media	➢ Bony tenderness: Sternum (acute leukemia) ➢ CVS: Changing murmurs (endocarditis) tumor plop (atrial myxoma), and rubs (pericarditis) ➢ Respiratory: Signs of pneumonia, TB, empyema, and lung carcinoma
Abdomen		***Others***
➢ Tenderness ➢ Hepatomegaly (abscess, hepatoma, and metastasis) ➢ Splenomegaly (hemopoietic malignancy, endocarditis, and malaria) ➢ Renal enlargement (renal cell carcinoma) ➢ Testicular enlargement (seminoma) ➢ Penis and scrotum: Discharge/rash ➢ Inguinal ligament: Lymphadenopathy	➢ **Per-rectal examination:** Mass/ tenderness in rectum/pelvis (abscess, carcinoma, and prostatitis) ➢ **Vaginal examination:** Collection of pelvic pus/pelvic inflammatory disease ➢ **Locomotor system:** Arthralgia/ arthritis, synovitis, ulcers, Raynaud's phenomenon	➢ **Nervous system** – Signs of meningism (chronic TB and meningitis) – Focal neurological signs (brain abscess, mononeuritis multiplex in polyarteritis nodosa)

Investigations (Tables 4.4 and 4.5)

TABLE 4.4: Laboratory investigations in pyrexia of unknown origin.

Stage 1: Screening tests	*Stage 2: Laboratory investigations*	*Stage 3: Laboratory investigations in PUO*
➢ Full blood count with peripheral smear ➢ ESR and CRP ➢ Renal function tests ➢ Liver function tests ➢ Blood culture ➢ Serum virology for HIV, dengue, *Leptospira*, and widal test ➢ Urinalysis and culture ➢ Blood culture ➢ Sputum culture and sensitivity ➢ Stool routine and occult blood ➢ Chest X-ray ➢ Mantoux test ➢ Ultrasound abdomen, pelvis, and neck (if adenopathy, thyroid) ➢ Malarial smear in endemic areas	➢ Repeat blood counts and chemistry ➢ Protein electrophoresis ➢ CT (chest, brain, abdomen, and pelvis) ➢ Autoantibody screen (ANA, RF, ANCA, and anti-ds DNA) ➢ ECG ➢ Thyroid function tests ➢ Bone marrow examination with culture ➢ Lumbar puncture ➢ Coagulation workup ➢ Serum ferritin (adult onset Still's disease) ➢ Consider PSA, CEA, and LDH ➢ Temporal artery biopsy ➢ Paul–Bunnell test and Brucella agglutination test ➢ Weil–Felix reaction	➢ Echocardiography ➢ PET scan (indium-labeled WBC scan) ➢ Intravenous urogram (IVU) ➢ Liver biopsy ➢ Exploratory laparotomy ➢ Bronchoscopy

TABLE 4.5: Various radiological investigations and its usefulness in PUO.

Radiological investigations	*Usefulness in the diagnosis of*
Chest X-ray	Tuberculosis, malignancy, and *pneumocystis* pneumonia
CT of abdomen or pelvis with contrast agent	Abscess and malignancy
MRI of brain	Malignancy and autoimmune disorders
PET scan	Malignancy and inflammation
Transthoracic or transesophageal echocardiography	Bacterial endocarditis
Gallium-67 scan	Infection, malignancy
Indium-labeled leukocytes	Occult septicemia
Technetium Tc 99m scan	Acute infection and inflammation of bone and soft tissue
Venous Doppler study	Venous thrombosis

Treatment
- Treat the underlying cause identified after investigations
- Use empirical broad-spectrum antibiotics
- Therapeutic trial of aspirin/steroids
- Naprosyn challenge for malignancy/lymphoma
- Empirical antitubercular treatment

BACTERIAL INFECTIONS

Streptococcal Infections

Streptococci are gram-positive cocci, 1 μm in diameter, nonmotile, and nonsporing. Many strains are capsulated.

Various products secreted by streptococci, which aid in their pathogenicity include *streptolysin O* and *S, deoxyribonucleases, hyaluronidase,* and *erythrogenic toxins.*

Streptococcal Pharyngitis

- Incubation period is 2–4 days.
- *Clinical features*: Presents with abrupt onset of sore throat, dysphagia, headache, malaise, anorexia, and fever. The posterior pharyngeal wall is red and edematous. The tonsils are enlarged, red, and covered with yellowish exudate, which can be easily removed with a swab. Anterior cervical lymph nodes are enlarged and tender.
- **Complications: Rheumatic fever** and **poststreptococcal glomerulonephritis** are two major immunologically triggered complications of streptococcal infection of the upper oropharyngeal regions.

Treatment

Pharyngitis responds readily to penicillin, erythromycin, cephalosporins (first generation given orally) or clindamycin 600–900 mg given 8th hourly.

Scarlet Fever

Characterized by the development of an **erythematous rash** on the second day of illness. The primary lesion is in the throat. The rash is seen over the neck and trunk, the palms and soles are generally spared. The rash blanches on pressure. The rash subsides with extensive desquamation after 4–5 days.

Treatment

Streptococcal lesions respond promptly to penicillin. A single intramuscular injection of benzathine penicillin G 600,000 units for children <25 kg and 1.2 million units for all others. Phenoxymethylpenicillin (penicillin V) 250 mg orally four times daily for 7–10 days is also equally effective. Erythromycin 250 mg 6 hourly for 7–10 days is given to patients allergic to penicillin. If suppuration develops, surgical drainage of the pus may be required.

Erysipelas

Acute spreading infection of the **skin and the subcutaneous tissue** by streptococci. Face is commonly affected. The disease sets in abruptly with malaise, chills, headache, and vomiting. The skin lesions are erythematous with clear advancing margins which may show vesicles. The part is tender and local lymph node enlargement may occur.

Streptococcal Impetigo

- It is inflammation of the skin characterized by isolated pustules which become crusted. Sites of predilection are around the mouth and nostrils.
- If left untreated they may ulcerate to produce shallow ulcers with crusts or scabs which may lead to pigmentation and scarring. This stage is called ecthyma.

Cellulitis

This is spreading inflammation of the subcutaneous tissue due to entry of the organism through the abrasions of the skin. There is pain, tenderness, erythema, fever, and often regional lymphadenopathy.

Lymphangitis

Acute lymphangitis may follow local trauma. This condition presents in the form of linear red streaks radiating from the site of entry to the draining lymph nodes.

Streptococcal Bacteremia

Irrespective of the focus of entry and primary lesion, streptococcal bacteremia gives rise to metastatic foci of infection, such as suppurative arthritis, osteomyelitis, peritonitis, endocarditis, meningitis, or visceral abscesses.

Necrotizing Fasciitis (Synonym: Streptococcal Gangrene) (Fig. 4.4A)

- This is a progressing destructive lesion of the subcutaneous tissue leading to necrosis of fascia and adipose tissue, but often sparing the skin. The organisms enter through trivial wounds, but within 24 hours the part is hot, swollen, tender, and edematous. The edema and violaceous hue spreads in all directions.

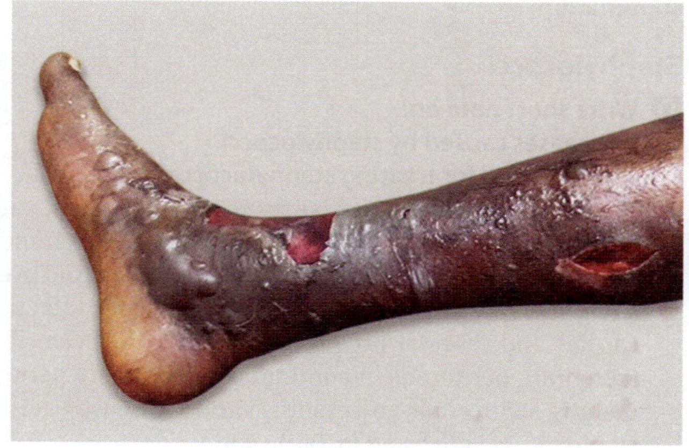

FIG. 4.4A: Necrotizing fasciitis—due to *Streptococcus*.

- It is more common in diabetes, immunocompromised individuals and those with local conditions impairing the vitality of the part, e.g., vascular occlusions, chronic edema, and infective lesions. Increase in the fascial compartmental pressure further jeopardizes the vascularity. Within 48 hours bullae develop, which progresses to gangrene within 4–5 days. The gangrenous area gets demarcated. General symptoms include severe prostration, toxemia, mental clouding, and delirium. If the diagnosis is missed, mortality is high.

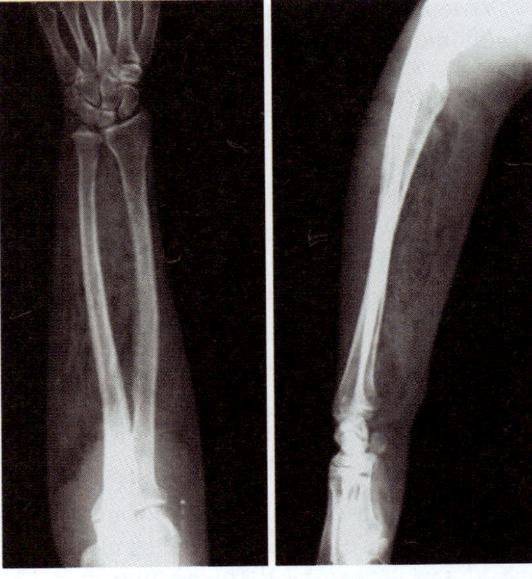

FIG. 4.4B: X-ray of hand showing gas in subcutaneous plane.

Streptococcal Myositis

- This is an uncommon lesion. Infection reaches the muscles by the bloodstream. Onset is with severe pain and swelling of muscles. Muscle compartment syndromes may develop. If unrecognized, mortality is over 80%.
- It should be differentiated from spontaneous gas gangrene **(Fig. 4.4B)**. Presence of superficial crepitus favors the diagnosis of gas gangrene (clostridial myonecrosis).

Treatment: Includes the administration of broad-spectrum antibiotics and early surgical debridement.

Pneumonia and Empyema

Streptococcal pneumonia usually follows a viral infection, and it manifests as bronchopneumonia. In many cases empyema develops as a complication.

Streptococcal Toxic Shock Syndrome

Infection by group A streptococcus may lead to vascular collapse and organ failure. M-protein which is a constituent of the cell wall is the virulence factor, which plays the major role in the pathogenesis of toxic shock syndrome. It forms large aggregates with fibrinogen, in blood and tissues. These activate polymorphonuclear leukocytes intravascularly and this leads to the production of toxic shock syndrome.

Other Pathogenic Strains of Streptococci

Group B streptococcus (Synonym: Streptococcus agalactiae)

This is a major pathogen found in the female genital tract, rectum, and also throat. **Chorioamnionitis, septic abortion,** and **puerperal sepsis** may occur during pregnancy. Urinary tract infection may occur in both sexes. Hematogenous spread may result in endocarditis, pneumonia, empyema, meningitis, and peritonitis. Immunocompromised hosts and elderly subjects are more susceptible.

Streptococcus viridans

Viridans streptococci account for more than 40% cases of **infective endocarditis.** *Streptococcus mutans* which colonizes dental plaques is an important cause of dental caries.

Enterococci

Causes urinary tract infections, biliary tract infections, septicemia, peritonitis, infective endocarditis, and abdominal suppuration.

Staphylococci

Q. Write short note on:
- **Diseases caused by staphylococci.**
- **Drugs used for treating staphylococcal septicemia.**

- ***Staphylococcus aureus:*** Causes pyogenic lesions, such as boils, carbuncles, wound infection, abscesses, impetigo, mastitis, osteomyelitis, pneumonia, septicemia, and pyemia.
- ***Coagulase negative staphylococci:*** It causes infection of cardiac and vascular prostheses, endocarditis, ventriculitis (cerebral), peritonitis in continuous ambulatory peritoneal dialysis, septicemia, and cystitis. Various diseases caused by staphylococci are listed in **Table 4.6**.

TABLE 4.6: Diseases caused by staphylococci.

Superficial Lesions ➢ Furuncle, carbuncle, impetigo, ecthyma, and sycosis barbae ➢ Follicular impetigo of Bockhart ➢ The scalded skin syndrome (Synonym: pemphigus neonatorum, Ritter's disease, and toxic epidermal necrolysis) **(Fig. 4.5)**	➢ Staphylococcal pneumonia ➢ Osteomyelitis/septic arthritis ➢ Staphylococcal bacteremia ➢ Staphylococcal food poisoning ➢ Endocarditis ➢ Toxic shock syndrome ➢ Tropical pyomyositis

- ***Staphylococcus epidermidis*** is a common infective agent in implanted prosthetic devices. Most of the infections are acquired from hospital.

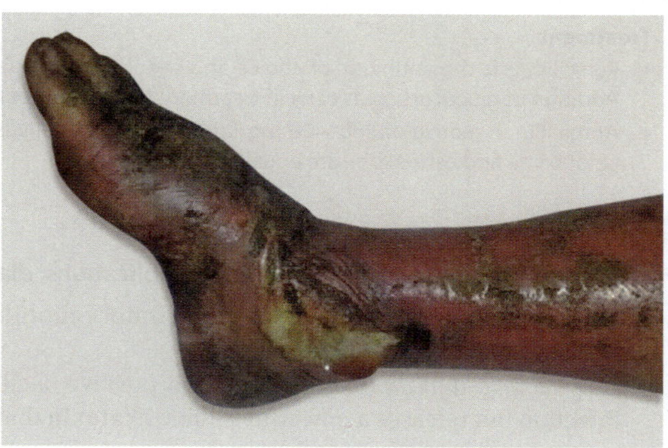

FIG. 4.5: Staphylococcal scalded skin syndrome.

Treatment of staphylococcal infections
- Antistaphylococcal antibiotics of the first choice:
  - Oxacillin (methicillin)
  - Cephalosporins of first generation (cefazolin and cephalothin)
- Antistaphylococcal antibiotics of the second choice: For MRSA/VRSA
  - Lincosamides (e.g., clindamycin), glycopeptides (vancomycin and teicoplanin), quinupristin/dalfopristin, chloramphenicol, minocycline, rifampin, trimethoprim sulfamethoxazole, fosfomycin, linezolid, daptomycin, tigecycline, and dalbavancin.
  - Oritavancin, telithromycin, ceftobiprole medocaril anti-MRSA and cephalosporin antibiotics.

Community-acquired Methicillin-resistant *Staphylococcus aureus* (CA-MRSA)

Q. Write short note on community-acquired methicillin-resistant *Staphylococcus aureus* (CA-MRSA).

- It is a type of staphylococcal bacteria that is resistant to certain antibiotics, such as methicillin, oxacillin, penicillin, and amoxicillin. It was first identified in 1968.
- The infection does not occur in individuals who are hospitalized or had any medical procedure. On the other hand, HA-MRSA occurs in the hospital setting.
- Outbreaks of CA-MRSA have occurred among categories such as: athletic teams (e.g., football, wrestling, rugby, and fencing), military barracks, correctional facilities, dormitories, daycares, and schools.
- **Factors that favor for MRSA transmission (5 Cs)**
  - **C**rowding
  - **C**ompromised skin (abrasions and cuts)
  - **C**ontaminated surfaces
  - Frequent and skin-to-skin **c**ontact
  - Lack of **c**leanliness
- **Feature:** It tends to cause more aggressive skin and soft-tissue infections, necrotizing pneumonia, septic shock and bacteremia.

Treatment of methicillin-resistant *Staphylococcus aureus* (MRSA) **(Table 4.7)**.

TABLE 4.7: Treatment of methicillin-resistant *Staphylococcus aureus.*

Drug	***Traditional dosage***
Doxycycline (mild cases oral)	100 mg IV or per oral 12 hourly
Trimethoprim sulfamethoxazole (mild cases oral)	160 mg per oral 12 hourly 2.5 mg/kg IV 12 hourly
Clindamycin	300–400 mg per oral 6 hourly 600–900 mg IV 8 hourly
Daptomycin	4 mg/kg IV per day 6 mg/kg IV per day
Linezolid	600 mg per oral or IV 12 hourly
Minocycline	100 mg IV or per oral 12 hourly
Quinupristin-dalfopristin	7.5 mg/kg IV 12 hourly
Telavancin	10 mg/kg IV per day
Tigecycline	100 mg IV (initial) then 50 mg IV 12 hourly
Vancomycin	1 g IV 12 hourly

Pneumococcal Infections

Diseases caused by pneumococci are listed in **Box 4.1.**

Box 4.1: Diseases caused by pneumococci.
- Pneumococcal pneumonia
- Extrapulmonary pneumococcal lesions
  - *Pneumococcal meningitis*
  - *Pneumococcal peritonitis*

Treatment of pneumococcal infections
- Pneumococci are generally susceptible to penicillin, but resistant strains are frequent. It is advisable to send the sputum for sensitivity tests before starting specific therapy. Benzyl penicillin is the drug of choice for uncomplicated pneumococcal infections.
- Multiple drug-resistant pneumococci respond to vancomycin 2 g/day given IV in divided doses or cefotaxime or ceftazidime. Levofloxacin is also effective.

Meningococcal Infections

Meningococcal Meningitis (Synonym: Cerebrospinal Fever)

- Meningococcemia may be fulminant or chronic.
- **Fulminant meningococcemia:** This is characterized by abrupt onset, severe constitutional disturbances, peripheral vascular collapse, shock, and sometimes myocarditis. In some cases the illness may progress rapidly so that toxemia and shock may occur within hours. These features are collectively called ***Waterhouse–Friderichsen syndrome.*** This syndrome is caused by hemorrhage into the adrenal glands resulting in acute adrenal failure. Toxic vasculitis aggravates the hypotension. Complications include endocarditis, allergic polyarthritis, pneumonia, and osteomyelitis.

Treatment

- Penicillin G is the antibiotic of choice and should be administered intravenously in a dose of 24 million units daily in divided doses. Addition of glucocorticoids early in treatment favors prompt recovery and prevents complications considerably.
- Ampicillin in a dose of 200–400 mg/kg body weight daily is also equally effective. The third-generation cephalosporins, especially cefotaxime and ceftriaxone are equally effective.

Diphtheria

Q. Discuss the clinical manifestations, complications, diagnosis, and management of diphtheria.

- Diphtheria is a nasopharyngeal (respiratory diphtheria) and/or skin infection (cutaneous diphtheria) caused by *Corynebacterium diphtheriae.*
- *Corynebacterium diphtheriae* is a gram-positive bacillus. *Corynebacterium diphtheriae* remains localized at the site of infection but releases a powerful soluble **exotoxin** that damages the heart muscle and the nervous system.

Mode of Transmission

- It is through airborne/droplet infection from active cases or carriers. Infection may also transmit through skin lesions.
- Incubation period: 2–7 days.

Pseudomembrane

The diagnostic pathologic feature is mucosal ulcers coated by pseudomembrane. The **pseudomembrane** has a well-defined edge which appears as wash-leather, elevated, firm, and grayish-green (black in advanced stages) adherent membrane. It is surrounded by a zone of inflammation.

Clinical Features

- Its manifestations may be local (due to the membrane) or systemic (due to exotoxin).
- Insidious in onset with a sore throat and fever being the usual manifestation. The fever is moderate but there is usually marked tachycardia.

Respiratory diphtheria

- **Pharyngeal diphtheria:** It is characterized by marked tonsillar and pharyngeal inflammation and the presence of a pseudomembrane. There may be regional often tender lymphadenopathy (cervical lymph nodes), and along with marked edema of submandibular areas produces the so-called **"bull-neck"** appearance (swelling of the neck). Pharyngeal diphtheria is associated with the greatest toxicity.
- **Laryngeal diphtheria:** It is usually represents extension of the membrane from the pharynx. Extension and sloughing of membranes may produce fatal airway obstruction. It usually presents with a husky voice, a brassy cough and later dyspnea and cyanosis due to respiratory obstruction.
- **Nasal diphtheria:** It is restricted to the nasal mucosa and is characterized by the presence of a unilateral, serosanguineous (frequently blood-stained) nasal discharge.

Cutaneous diphtheria

It is uncommon but occurs in individuals with poor personal hygiene and with burns. It produces round, deep, "punched-out" skin ulcers with undermined edges and is covered by a gray-yellow or gray-brown adherent membrane. The ulcers occur more commonly on the lower and upper extremities, head, and trunk. Constitutional symptoms are not common.

Complications

- **Airway (laryngeal) obstruction:** It may occur with advanced diphtheria. Airway obstruction may be either due to the sloughed pseudomembrane or extension of the pseudomembrane to the larynx or into the tracheobronchial tree (bronchopulmonary diphtheria). It is mainly observed in children because of their small airways.
- **Cardiac complications:** These include **myocarditis** with arrhythmias, cardiac failure, and ECG changes. They often develop weeks after initial episode of diphtheria. These are usually reversible.
- **Neurological complications** occur in 75% of cases.
  - **Palatal palsy** may develop after 10 days.
  - **Polyneuropathy** with weakness and paresthesia may develop 3–5 weeks after the onset of diphtheria.
  - **Paralysis of accommodation** may manifest as difficulty in reading small print.
  - Encephalitis can occur rarely.
- **Other complications** include pneumonia, renal failure, encephalitis, cerebral infarction, and pulmonary embolism.

Diagnosis

- **Clinical diagnosis**
- **Confirmation of diagnosis:**
  - Demonstration of *Corynebacterium diphtheriae* on methylene blue-stained preparations.
  - Bacterial culture of *Corynebacterium diphtheriae* on Loeffler's medium and toxin studies (Elek test).

Management

- Patients should be hospitalized with close monitoring of cardiac and respiratory function. Patient should be **isolated** and strict bed rest.
- **Diphtheria antitoxin** is the only specific treatment. It is produced from hyperimmune horse serum and it neutralizes circulating toxin.
  - It must be given as early in the course of diphtheria as possible without awaiting the result of a throat swab. Because any delay in administration can be dangerous because toxin once fixed to the tissues can no longer be neutralized by antitoxin.
  - **Dose:** It is administered intravenously over 60 minutes after an initial test dose to exclude any allergic reaction. 20,000 to 40,000 units for pharyngeal/laryngeal disease of <48 hours duration, 40,000 to 60,000 units for nasopharyngeal disease, and 80,000 to 120,000 units for >3 days of illness or diffuse neck swelling ("bull neck").
  - **Adverse reactions:** It can cause two types of reactions, an immediate anaphylactic reaction and delayed serum sickness. The immediate anaphylactic reaction is treated with adrenaline and an antihistamine.
- **Antibiotics** should be given concurrently to eliminate *C. diphtheriae* and thereby remove the source of toxin production. Benzylpenicillin (1,200 mg four times daily IV) or amoxicillin (500 mg three times daily) is given for 2 weeks. Patients allergic to penicillin are given erythromycin (500 mg four times daily for 14 days).
- **Tracheostomy** or intubation may be needed for respiratory distress.
- **Immunization:** Primary diphtheria does not produce immunity against infection. Hence, following recovery all sufferers should be immunized with diphtheria toxoid. Close contacts should be protected by erythromycin prophylaxis and also by immunization. Vaccines include DPT (diphtheria, pertussis, tetanus) and DT (diphtheria, tetanus).
- **Contact prophylaxis:** Single dose of penicillin G benzathine [600,000 units intramuscularly (IM)] or oral erythromycin (500 mg four times daily for 7–10 days).

Tetanus

Q. Write a short essay/note on tetanus.

Tetanus is due to infection by toxin secreting clostridium namely *Clostridium tetani.* The organism is found in soil derived from animal and human excreta.

Mode of infection: Infection enters the body through a contaminated wound (injury may be trivial). It can also develop as complication in intravenous drug misusers. Neonatal tetanus may develop following contamination of the umbilical stump, often after dressing the area (unhygienic practices) with dung (e.g., in many developing countries) or site of circumcision, causing tetanus neonatorum.

Pathogenesis: During circumstances unfavorable to the growth of *Clostridium tetani,* it forms spores and remain dormant for years in the soil. Spores germinate and organism multiplies only in the anaerobic conditions. Thus, it may multiply in areas of tissue necrosis or wherever the oxygen tension is reduced by the presence of other organisms (e.g., aerobic organism). *Clostridium tetani* is not invasive and remain localized. Its clinical manifestations are due to the potent neurotoxin (exotoxin) called tetanospasmin.

Incubation period: Varies from 2 days to several weeks after injury. Shorter the incubation period, the more severe the attack and the worse the prognosis.

Clinical Features

Q. Write a short essay/note on the clinical features of tetanus.

Generalized tetanus is the most common form of tetanus.

- **Lockjaw:** General malaise is rapidly followed by the most important symptom namely trismus. It is due to spasm of the masseter muscles, which causes difficulty in opening the mouth and in masticating.
- **Risus sardonicus:** When the tonic rigidity involve the muscles of the face, neck, and trunk, contraction of the frontalis and the muscles at the angles of the mouth produces characteristic grinning expression known as "risus sardonicus".
- **Opisthotonus:** Varying degree of rigidity develops in the muscles at the neck and trunk. The back is usually slightly arched ("opisthotonus") and the abdominal wall appears board-like.

- **Severe disease:**
  - If the disease is severe, **painful, violent, exhausting, and reflex spasms** (convulsions) develop, usually within 24–72 hours of the initial symptoms and lasts for a few seconds to 3–4 minutes. The interval between the first symptom and the first spasm is known as the "onset time".
  - The **spasms can be spontaneous or may be induced by stimuli** such as movement or noise or by light. Laryngeal spasm can impair respiration; esophageal and urethral spasm can produce dysphagia and urinary retention, respectively. Patients are mentally alert.
  - **Autonomic involvement** may produce cardiovascular complications (e.g., tachycardia, a labile blood pressure, sweating, and cardiac arrhythmias).
- **Death:** Spasms gradually increase in frequency and severity and death may occur from exhaustion, hypoxia, cardiac arrest, asphyxia, respiratory failure or aspiration pneumonia or exhaustion. Mild cases with rigidity usually recover.

Local tetanus is a milder form of the disease in which the pain, stiffness, increased tone or spasms of the muscles develop only near the infected wound. Prognosis is good and recovery usually occurs if treatment is commenced at this stage.

Cephalic tetanus: Uncommon but fatal. It usually develops due to entry of *C. tetani* through the middle ear. Cranial nerve abnormalities (e.g., seventh nerve) are usual.

Neonatal tetanus is usually develops due to infection of the umbilical stump. Characterized by failure to thrive, poor sucking, grimacing, and irritability followed by intense rigidity and spasms. Mortality is almost 100%. It can be prevented by immunizing all women of childbearing age and providing clean delivery facilities.

Investigations/Diagnosis

- Diagnosis is usually made on clinical grounds.
- *C. tetani:* Rarely possible to isolate from wounds (original locus of entry).

Differential diagnosis: Phenothiazine over dosage, strychnine poisoning, meningitis, and tetany.

Management/Treatment of Tetanus

Q. Write a short essay/note on the treatment of tetanus.

Suspected tetanus

- **Care of the wound:** Clean the wound and debrided if necessary, to remove the source of toxin.
- **Human tetanus immunoglobulin:** In the dose of 250 units should be given along with an intramuscular injection of tetanus toxoid. If the patient is already immunized a single booster dose of the tetanus toxoid is given; otherwise the full three dose course of adsorbed vaccine is given.

Established tetanus

Management of established disease should be started as soon as possible.

- **Prevent further toxin production:** Debridement of wound and antibiotics (see below).
- **General supportive medical and nursing care.** Patient is isolated in a quiet, well ventilated and darkened room. Maintain hydration and nutrition and treat secondary infections.
- **Control of spasm:** Nurse in a quiet room, avoid unnecessary stimuli. Benzodiazepines/IV diazepam is used to control spasms and sedate the patient. If spasms continue, paralyze patient and ventilate. Baclofen may be useful.
- **Intubation and mechanical ventilation:** If the airway is compromised.
- **Magnesium sulfate infusion:** Reduces the need for antispasmodics.
- **Antibiotics and antitoxin:** Given even in the absence of an obvious wound. Drug of choice is intravenous metronidazole. Other antibiotic include penicillin (Benzylpenicillin 600 mg IV four times daily) and cephalosporins.
- **Neutralization of absorbed toxin:** Human tetanus immunoglobulin (HTIG) 3,000–6,000 IU should is given by intramuscular injection to neutralize any circulating toxin. If HTIG is not available, immune equine tetanus immunoglobulin 10,000 IU should be given intramuscularly: but there is a high incidence of severe allergic reactions.
- If the patient recovers active immunization should be instituted, as immunity following tetanus is incomplete.

Anthrax

Q. Write short essay on anthrax.

- Anthrax is a zoonotic disease caused by *Bacillus anthracis.*
- *Bacillus anthracis* is a gram-positive bacillus with a central spore. It produces toxins and is responsible for the clinical features of disease **that** most closely correlated with its virulence.

Mode of Transmission

It is through direct contact (inoculation of the spores) with an infected animal particularly herbivores. Infection is most frequent as an occupational disease in farmers, butchers, and dealers in wool and animal hides. Spores of

Bacillus anthracis can also be ingested or inhaled. Deliberate release of anthrax spores is an important bioterrorist weapon.

Incubation period: 1–10 days.

Clinical Manifestations

It depends on the route of entry of the anthrax spores.

Cutaneous anthrax

Q. Write short essay on cutaneous anthrax and malignant pustule.

- It is the most common type of anthrax. It follows inoculation of spores into the subcutaneous of the exposed skin. Occupational exposure to anthrax spores during processing of hides and bone products results in cutaneous anthrax.
- Skin lesions **(Hide-porter's disease)** begin as a small, itching, erythematous, maculopapule on an edematous hemorrhagic base. The lesion is initially painless despite edema. It enlarges to form a vesicle filled with serosanguinous fluid and is surrounded by gross edema **("malignant pustule").** The vesicle ulcerates and dries to form a central depressed thick black **"eschar"** surrounded by blebs. Despite marked edema, pain is infrequent.
- It is self-limiting illness in the majority of patients, but occasionally perivascular edema and regional lymphadenopathy may be associated with marked toxemia.

Inhalational anthrax (Woolsorter's disease)

Q. Write short essay on inhalation anthrax and Woolsorter's disease.

- It is extremely rare and follows inhalation of spores into the lung producing **"Woolsorter's disease"**
- Bioterrorism-related anthrax also due to inhalation of spores.
- It begins with fever, nonproductive cough, dyspnea, headache, and retrosternal discomfort. Patient develops bronchopneumonia. Symptoms of septicemia may develop 3–14 days following exposure. Pleural effusions (hemorrhagic) are common and **meningitis** may occur.
- Chest X-ray shows bronchopneumonia, widening of the mediastinum, and pleural effusions.
- Without rapid and aggressive treatment at the onset of symptoms, the mortality ranges from 50 to 90%.

Gastrointestinal anthrax

- It is associated with ingestion of undercooked and contaminated meat products.
- The cecum is involved and it manifests as a severe gastroenteritis. The symptoms include nausea, vomiting, anorexia, and fever followed in 2–3 days by severe abdominal pain and bloody diarrhea.
- Toxemia, shock, and death may develop rapidly.

Diagnosis

- **Demonstrating the organism:** A stained smear of fluid taken from the edge of a skin lesion may demonstrate the organism. The organism may also be demonstrated in stools, laryngeal secretions, sputum, and CSF.
- **Culture** of blood and other body fluids: *Bacillus anthracis* can be cultured in mice, rabbits or guinea pigs.
- **Serological examination:** ELISAs for detecting antibodies to both the organism and a toxin.
- **Chest X-ray** may show mediastinal widening, bronchopneumonia, and pleural effusion.

Treatment

- **Systemic anthrax with meningitis:** Ciprofloxacin (400 mg TDS) plus meropenem plus linezolid/clindamycin.
- **Anthrax related to bioterrorism:** Ciprofloxacin is the drug of choice. Dose is 400 mg IV ciprofloxacin BID. Once the patient stabilizes, ciprofloxacin is given orally in a dose of 500 mg BID. Duration of treatment is 60 days.
- **Raxibacumab and obiltoxaximab:** 40–80 mg/kg human monoclonal antibody directed against the protective antigen has been shown in animal studies to improve survival in inhalation anthrax. Anthrax immunoglobulin is available to treat inhalational anthrax.

Prevention and Control

- **Prophylaxis:**
  - Ciprofloxacin (500 mg twice daily) is recommended for individuals with high risk of exposure to anthrax spores.
  - Doxycycline (100 mg BID) for 60 days.
- Vaccination of animals and persons at risk.
- When an infected animal dies, it should be burned and the area in which it was housed must be disinfected.

Plague

Q. Write short essay/note on plague.

- Plague is caused by a small gram-negative, nonmotile bacillus namely *Yersinia pestis.*
- 11 *Yersinia* species—three human pathogens namely *Y. pestis, Y. pseudotuberculosis, Y. enterocolitica.*

- One of three WHO quarantinable diseases.
- Plague is also called as **"black death"**. Historically, three plague pandemics have caused more than 200 million deaths, including the Black Death epidemic in 14th century Europe (Justinian 541 AD, Black Death 1,346, China 1,855).
- Used for biological warfare.

Source of Infection

The main reservoirs are woodland rodents (sylvatic rats) that spread infection to the domestic rat species *(Rattus rattus)* and finally infected rat fleas *(Xenopsylla cheopis)*. These fleas bite humans when there is a sudden reduction in the rat population.

Route of Infection

- **Rat flea bite:** Most common route in humans is after bite of a plague-infected rat flea.
- **Direct contact** with infected tissues or fluids from sick or dead plague-infected animals. Hunters and trappers can develop plague from handling rodents.
- **Droplet infection:** Plague pneumonia or by laboratory exposure.
- **Incubation period:** 3–6 days (shorter in pneumonic plague).

Clinical Features

Type of plague: Four clinical forms are recognized: bubonic, septicemic, pneumonic, and cutaneous.

Bubonic plague

- Most common form of the disease and occurs in about 90% of infected individuals.
- Onset is usually **acute/sudden,** with a high fever, rigor, chills, severe headache, dry skin, myalgia, nausea, vomiting and when severe, prostration. This is rapidly followed painful lymphadenopathy. Characteristically these lymph nodes are tender and suppurate in 1–2 weeks. Most common site for lymphadenopathy is the inguinal region or axilla. The swollen lymph nodes and surrounding tissue constitute the characteristic **"bubo"** called so because they are rarely fluctuant.
- Other manifestations include apathy, confusion, fright, anxiety, oliguria or anuria, tachycardia, toxemia, and hypotension. The spleen is usually palpable.
- Without treatment, complications, such as secondary septicemia, secondary pneumonia, and meningitis may occur. Mortality rate for untreated cases is 60%.

Septicemic plague

- It may be primary without signs of primary disease (primary septicemic plague) or secondary as a complication of untreated bubonic plague or pneumonic plague (secondary septicemic plague).
- Primary septicemic plague presents as an acute fulminant infection characterized by high fever, chills, and malaise, but without any lymph node enlargement. Elderly individuals are more prone. The patient is toxic and may develop gastrointestinal symptoms, such as nausea, vomiting, abdominal pain, and diarrhea. Patients may develop hypotension, septic shock, renal failure, ARDS, and disseminated intravascular coagulation (DIC).
- Gangrene of acral regions (tip of the nose or the fingers and toes) may develop due to thrombosis of small artery in advanced stages (hence named Black Death).
- Left untreated, it deteriorates rapidly and the mortality approaches 100%.

Pneumonic plague

- It may occur as a primary infection in the lung or as secondary infection (as a complication of the bubonic and septicemic plague—secondary pneumonia).
- Primary form: Develops within 1–6 days of exposure. It begins suddenly with features of a fulminant pneumonia. Patient develops malaise, high fever, vomiting, abdominal pain, diarrhea, and marked prostration. Soon followed by cough, dyspnea, copious blood-stained, frothy, highly infective sputum marked respiratory distress/failure, cyanosis, and septic shock. Without antibiotics, death occurs in almost all patients within 2 or 3 days.
- Chest X-ray: Shows bilateral infiltrates that may be nodular and progress to an ARDS-like picture.

Cutaneous plague

It presents either as a pustule, eschar or papule or an extensive purpura. It can develop necrosis and gangrene.

Investigations and Diagnoses

Diagnosis is based on clinical, epidemiological, and laboratory findings.

- **Demonstration of organism:** For rapid diagnosis, smears are prepared from blood, sputum, bubo aspirate (lymph node aspirate), and cerebrospinal fluid. They are stained with Gram, Giemsa or Wayson's stains (contains methylene blue), and examined under microscopy. *Y. pestis* is seen as bipolar staining coccobacilli, giving a "safety pin" appearance.
- **Culture of organism:** From blood, sputum, and bubo aspirates.

- **Serological diagnosis:** A presumptive diagnosis in an appropriate clinical setting is possible by a rapid antigen detection test (by immunofluorescence, using *Y. pestis* F1 antigen-specific antibodies).
- **Septicemic plague:** Often associated with laboratory findings of DIC.
- **Chest X-ray:** In pneumonic plague, it shows evidence of multilobar consolidation, cavities or bronchopneumonia.
- **Blood:** WBC count 20,000/mm² and/or thrombocytopenia in about 50% of patients.

Treatment/Management

If the diagnosis is suspected on clinical and epidemiological grounds, urgent treatment is required even before the results of culture studies are available.

1. **First choices**
   - **Streptomycin:** 30 mg/kg per day IM (up to a total dose of 2 g) in two divided doses for 10 days.
   - **Gentamicin** as effective OD dosing and less toxic.
2. **Second choices**
   - **Tetracyclines:** Doxycycline
   - **Fluoroquinolones:** Ciprofloxacin, levofloxacin, ofloxacin, and moxifloxacin
   - **Chloramphenicol:** 1st choice for meningitis ± aminoglycoside supportive treatment of ARDS, DIC, and shock

Prophylaxis

- **Control of rats and flea**
- Avoid handling and skinning of wild animal in endemic areas.
- **Prevention of human-to-human transmission:** Patients with plague pneumonia should be isolated until at least 4 days of antibiotic treatment have been administered. For the other types of the plague, patients should be isolated for the first 48 hours or until clinical improvement begins. Attendants must wear gowns, masks, and gloves and healthcare workers should use high-efficiency respirators.
- **Chemoprophylaxis:** Close contact with a patient with pneumonic plague should receive postexposure antibiotic prophylaxis (doxycycline 100 mg or ciprofloxacin 500 mg twice daily) for 7 days.
- **Vaccine:** A partially effective formalin-killed vaccine is available for those who travel to plague-endemic areas and individuals at occupational risk.

Botulism

Q. Write a short essay/note on botulism.

- Botulism is caused by neurotoxin (botulinum) produced by *Clostridium botulinum.*
- It produces a neurotoxin which is the most potent poison known and cause disease after ingestion of even picogram (as low as 0.05 g) amounts. There are seven types of toxins which are labeled as A to G.

Mode of Infection

- **Ingestion:** It can contaminate many foodstuffs, such as canned or bottled foodstuff, in which it can multiply. Most cases of botulism are due to consumption of contaminated food being served undercooked. Contaminated honey causes in infant botulism, in which the organism colonizes the gastrointestinal tract.
- **Inoculation:** Wound botulism can develop in injection drug-users.
- **Incubation period:** 2 hours to 8 days.

Classification

- **Food-borne botulism:** It occurs due to ingestion of toxin present in the contaminated food (fish and canned food) and it is the most common type of botulism.
- **Infantile botulism:** It develops due to ingestion of spores, which germinate in the gut and produce toxin.
- **Wound botulism:** It follows the contamination of wounds, street heroin injection contaminated with *C. botulinum.* Other types are inhalational and iatrogenic botulism.

Clinical Features

Food-borne botulism

- Initial symptoms are related to gastrointestinal symptoms, such as nausea and diarrhea. These are rapidly followed **neurotoxic effects** of toxin. The toxin causes **mainly bulbar and ocular palsies** (difficulty in swallowing, blurred or double vision, and ptosis), progressing to **symmetrical descending limb weakness,** diaphragmatic paralysis, respiratory paralysis, and death. **No sensory deficits** seen except blurring of vision.
- **Absence of fever** and patients are alert, remains responsive, though mild drowsiness may be present.
- Heart rate is normal or slow and blood pressure is normal.
- Parasympathetic dysfunction: Rare and may produce dry mouth, paralytic ileus, and dilated nonreactive pupils.

Infantile botulism

- Characterized by onset of constipation, followed by weakness in sucking, crying or swallowing. Later there is progressive bulbar and muscle weakness of the extremities.

Wound botulism

- It is similar to food-borne botulism except that GI upset does not occur.

Diagnosis

- Diagnosis of botulism is usually based on clinical features.
- **Detection of toxin:** In blood (foodborne) or stools (infant botulism) or in the contaminated food.
- Culture of organism from wound.

Differential Diagnosis

Guillain–Barré (GB) syndrome, myasthenia gravis, tick paralysis, diphtheria, and hypermagnesemia.

Treatment

- It is mainly general supportive care with mechanical ventilation, prevention of secondary infection, and administration of antitoxin (not available in India). Equine serum heptavalent botulism antitoxin and human-derived botulism immune globulin are available in United States.
- Antibiotics are of no much use. However, penicillin G and metronidazole are used. The overall mortality is high, but those who survive the acute paralysis fully recover.

Whooping Cough

Q. Describe the etiology, clinical features, complications, diagnosis, and management of whooping cough.

- Whooping cough (pertussis) is an acute infection of the respiratory tract caused by *Bordetella pertussis. Bordetella pertussis* is a gram-negative coccobacillus.
- The term pertussis means "violent cough" which is the most prominent feature of the illness.

Mode of spread: Pertussis is highly contagious and spreads by droplet infection.
Incubation period: 7–10 days.
Age group: Classic case is seen in childhood, with 90% occurring below 5 years of age.

Clinical Features

Catarrhal phase

This first stage is highly infectious characterized by upper respiratory catarrh with rhinitis, lacrimation (conjunctivitis), low-grade fever, and an unproductive cough. This stage lasts about 1–2 weeks.

Paroxysmal phase

It is called so because of the characteristic paroxysms of coughing.

- **Whoop:** During this stage, the cough becomes spasmodic, more frequent and severe with repetitive bouts of 5–10 coughs. The coughing paroxysms episode may be terminated by a **classic inspiratory audible whoop.** The whoop is due to rapid inspiration against a closed glottis at the end of a paroxysm. It is observed only in younger patients in whom the lumen of the respiratory tract is narrowed due to mucus secretion and mucosal edema. These paroxysms usually terminate in vomiting. Early paroxysmal stage is also infectious.
- **Other features** include conjunctival suffusion and petechiae and ulceration of the frenulum of the tongue. Lymphocytosis is observed.
- This stage lasts for about 2 weeks and may be associated with many complications **(Table 4.8)**.

Convalescence phase

It follows the paroxysmal phase during which slow resolution of whoop occurs. This phase can last 1–3 months, and cough may persist for several weeks to months.

TABLE 4.8: Complications of pertussis.

Respiratory	Other complications	
➢ Apnea (in children) ➢ Bronchopneumonia ➢ Atelectasis ➢ Bronchiectasis (sequelae) ➢ Rib fractures ➢ Pneumothorax	➢ Encephalitis ➢ Convulsions (due to cerebral anoxia) ➢ Conjunctival hemorrhage	➢ Subdural hematoma ➢ Direct inguinal hernia ➢ Rectal prolapse ➢ Weight loss

Complications

See **Table 4.8.**

Diagnosis

- **Clinical diagnosis** is not difficult if the classic symptoms, characteristic whoop and a history of contact with an infected individual are present.

- **Blood:** Peripheral blood may show lymphocytosis.
- **Culture of nasopharyngeal secretions** is the gold standard for diagnosis.
- *B. pertussis* DNA detection by PCR assay.
- Direct fluorescent antibody test.

Management

Antibiotics

- Erythromycin for 7–14 days is the recommended treatment.
- CDC recommends azithromycin for 5 days (500 mg day 1, followed by 250 mg day 2 through 5) or clarithromycin (500 mg twice daily for 7 days).
- Trimethoprim/sulfamethoxazole reduces pertussis transmission and is an alternative treatment for patients who are allergic to macrolides.
- Cough suppressants are not effective.
- Others: Steroids, antihistamines, β-agonists, and immunoglobulins are not beneficial.

Prevention

- **Isolation of patient:** Patients should be isolated to prevent contact with others, e.g., in hostels and boarding schools.
  - Catarrhal phase: If antibiotics have been given during catarrhal phase, patient is infectious until 5 days after starting antibiotics.
  - Paroxysmal phase: Patient is contagious till 3 weeks after the paroxysmal stage ends if not treated during catarrhal stage.
- **Chemoprophylaxis:** Risk of transmission of *B. pertussis* within households is high. Hence, close contacts of patients should receive macrolides, especially if they are not vaccinated.
- **Active immunization:** Pertussis is an easily preventable disease with active immunization by DPT vaccine. Immunity begins to decline 4–12 years after vaccination, and may make adolescent and adult susceptible to infection. Rarely, the vaccine can produce convulsions and neurological damage. Currently acellular effective vaccines with few adverse reactions are available. A triple vaccine containing tetanus toxoid, reduced diphtheria toxoid, and acellular pertussis (Tdap) is available for use in adolescents and adults.

Enteric Fever

Q. Describe the etiology, clinical features, investigations, diagnosis, complications, and treatment of typhoid fever.

Q. Write short note on enteric fever (typhoid and paratyphoid fever).

Enteric fever is the general term, which includes **both typhoid and paratyphoid** fever. It is an acute systemic illness characterized by fever, headache and abdominal discomfort.

Causative Agent

- Enteric fevers are caused by ***Salmonella typhi* and *Salmonella paratyphi*.** *Salmonella* are gram-negative, flagellate, motile, nonsporulating, and facultative anaerobic bacilli (rods). Boiling or chlorination of water and pasteurization of milk destroy the bacilli.
- Typhoid fever (enteric) is an **acute systemic disease** caused by infection with *Salmonella typhi* (also known as *Salmonella enterica serovar Typhi*). Paratyphoid fever is a clinically similar but milder disease caused by *Salmonella paratyphi* (Salmonella enterica serovar Paratyphi A, B or C).

Source of Infection

Humans are the only natural reservoir and include:

1. **Patient suffering from disease:** Infected urine, feces, or other secretions from patients.
2. **Chronic carriers of typhoid fever:** *S. typhi* or *S. paratyphi* **colonizes in the gallbladder, urinary bladder,** or biliary tree.

Mode of transmission: From **person-to-person contact.**

- **Ingestion** of **contaminated food** (especially dairy products) and shellfish or **water.** Chronic carriers, often food handlers transmit the disease.
- **Direct spread:** Rare by **finger-to-mouth contact** with feces (fecal-oral route), urine, or other secretions is rare.

Incubation period: Usually 10–14 days and for paratyphoid it is shorter.

Pathogenesis

- The typhoid bacilli *(Salmonella)* are **ingested through contaminated food or water are** able to **survive in gastric acid of the stomach and** reach mucosa of small intestine.
- In the small intestine, they penetrate the **ileal mucosa,** reach the submucosa and are **phagocytosed by the macrophages in the Peyer's patches.**

- They are **carried to** the **mesenteric lymph node** via lymphatics **and** enter the **bloodstream via** the **thoracic duct causing** bacteremia.
- They colonize reticuloendothelial tissues **(liver, gallbladder, spleen, and bone marrow),** and multiply further and re-enter bloodstream causing **massive bacteremia** (occurs towards the end of incubation period) and disease clinically manifests.
- In the intestine, the bacilli are localized to the **Peyer's patches and lymphoid follicles** of the terminal ileum. They cause inflammation, plateau-like elevations of Peyer's patches and necrosis, which results in characteristic **oval typhoid ulcers.**

Clinical Features

- Onset is gradual and nonspecific. Patients usually present with fever, anorexia, headache, abdominal pain, bloating, nausea, and vomiting.
- **Fever:** The temperature rises in a step-ladder fashion **(step-ladder fever)** to 40–41°C for 4 or 5 days in some cases. The hallmark of typhoid fever is continuous, persistent fever, often lasting 4–8 weeks in untreated patients.
- Early intestinal manifestations include constipation (especially in adults) or mild diarrhea (in children).

Physical findings

- In the early stages abdominal tenderness, hepatosplenomegaly, lymphadenopathy, and a scanty maculopapular rash ("rose spots") are found.
- **Rose spots** or "rose-red spots": These are small 2–4 mm, pale-red maculopapular lesions on the skin that fade/blanch on pressure appear on the chest and abdomen, which occur during first week and usually last only 2–3 days. They result from bacterial embolism and *Salmonella* can be cultured from the biopsy of these lesions.
- **Mild hepatosplenomegaly:** Spleen is soft and palpable (around the seventh to tenth day) may be accompanied by tender hepatomegaly.
- **Relative bradycardia:** The pulse is often slower than would be expected from the height of the fever.
- **Intestinal manifestations:** By the end of first week, constipation is succeeded by diarrhea and abdominal distension, with tenderness in the right iliac fossa. The stools are loose and greenish in color and characteristically described as "pea-soup" intestinal complications often develop in the third of fourth week of illness.
  - If untreated by the end of second week: Patient may be profoundly ill
  - By third week: Toxemia increases and patient may develop coma and die
  - The fouth week of the illness is characterized by gradual improvement.

Complications of Typhoid

See **Box 4.2.**

Q. Write short note on complications of typhoid fever.

Laboratory Diagnosis

See **Box 4.3.**

Q. Write short note on:
- **Laboratory diagnosis of typhoid fever.**
- **Widal test.**

Box 4.2: Complications of typhoid.

- **General complications:** Toxemia, dehydration, peripheral circulatory failure, and DIC.
- **Intestinal complications:** The most common intestinal complication is ileus. **Perforation** of typhoid ulcer and **hemorrhage from the ulcer** may occur at the end of the second week or during the third week of the illness.
- **Extraintestinal complications:**
  - **Neurological:** Delirium **(muttering delirium),** psychosis, **seizures,** coma vigil, catatonia, meningitis, encephalopathy, GB syndrome peripheral neuritis, and deafness.
  - **Miscellaneous: Myocarditis,** endocarditis, pericarditis, pneumonia, **cholecystitis,** pyelonephritis, glomerulonephritis, osteomyelitis, arthritis, periostitis, hepatitis, and thrombophlebitis. Patients with **sickle cell disease are susceptible to *Salmonella* osteomyelitis.**
- **Carrier state:** Persistence of bacilli in the **gallbladder or urinary tract** may result in passage of bacilli in the feces or urine and causes a "carrier state" which is the source of infection to others. After clinical recovery, about 5–10% will continue to excrete *S. typhi* for several months and they are termed convalescent carriers.

Box 4.3: Laboratory diagnosis of typhoid fever.

- **Total leukocyte count:** It shows **leukopenia with relative lymphocytosis. Eosinophils are usually absent.**
- **Isolation of Bacilli:**
  - **Blood culture:** This is the "Gold Standard" investigation for diagnosis of typhoid. The maximum positivity of blood culture is in **first week** of fever in 90% of patients and remains positive in second week till the fever subsides. Blood culture rapidly becomes negative on treatment with antibiotics. During early phase, bone marrow culture aspirate is more sensitive than blood culture, even after a brief prior antibiotic treatment.
  - **Stool cultures:** It is almost as valuable as blood culture and become positive in the **third week.**
  - **Urine culture:** It reveals the organism in approximately 25% of patients by **third week.**
- **Widal test/reaction:** Classic Widal test **measures** agglutinating **antibodies against** *O, H,* and **Vi antigens** of *S. typhi* and H antigens of *S. paratyphi* A and B, but **lacks sensitivity and specificity.** Widal test (immunological reactions) becomes positive from **end of the first week till fourth week.** There are many false-positive (anamnestic reaction) and occasional false-negative Widal reactions. Vi antigen is alone detected in the carrier state. The mean sensitivity, specificity, NPV, and PPV of Widal test remains below 80%. Therefore, Widal test should not be used as a diagnostic tool to rule out typhoid fever unless supported by invasive clinical pictures and other confirmatory tests.
- **Other serologic tests:** They are available for the rapid diagnosis of typhoid fever with a higher sensitivity.
- **Molecular methods:** PCR detects flagellin, somatic gene, and Vi gene.

Q. Write short note on:
- **Treatment and prevention of typhoid fever.**
- **Chronic carrier state in typhoid.**
- **New drugs with dosage and duration used to treat enteric fever.**

Treatment

- **General management:** These include bed rest, isolation, and maintenance of nutrition and fluid intake.
- **Antibiotic therapy:** Several antibiotics are effective in enteric fever and various drug regimens are presented in **Table 4.9**. It must be guided by culture and sensitivity report.
- **Multidrug resistant strains:** Certain strains of *S. typhi* (especially in India) are resistant to chloramphenicol, amoxicillin, and cotrimoxazole are called as multidrug resistant strains. These should be treated with ciprofloxacin.
- **NARST-nalidixic acid resistant *Salmonella typhi:*** Sometimes, strains that are sensitive to ciprofloxacin in vitro may not respond to ciprofloxacin. They are usually resistant to nalidixic acid when tested in vitro (NARST-nalidixic acid resistant *Salmonella typhi)*. These patients need treatment for longer duration with ciprofloxacin or with ceftriaxone.
- **Corticosteroids:** It is indicated in patients with severe toxemia, central nervous system manifestations, and DIC. Intravenous dexamethasone is given in the dose of 3 mg/kg as a loading dose, followed by 1 mg/kg every 6 hourly for 24 hours.
- **Treatment of complications:** Intestinal perforation and hemorrhage occur in the third or fourth week of illness are managed accordingly.

TABLE 4.9: Various antibiotic regimens in typhoid fever.

Drug	***Dosage and duration of treatment***
Ceftriaxone	75 mg/kg/day for 7–14 days
Chloramphenicol	3–4 g/day till the fever subsides, followed by 2 g/day, for a total duration of 14 days
Amoxicillin	4–6 g/day in four divided doses of 14 days
Cotrimoxazole	Trimethoprim 640 mg + sulfamethoxazole 3,200 mg in two divided doses daily for 14 days
Ciprofloxacin	500–750 mg twice daily for 14 days
Ofloxacin	400–800 mg/day for 14 days
Cefotaxime	50–75 mg/kg/day for 7–14 days
Cefixime	20 mg/kg/day for 10–14 days
Azithromycin	1 g once a day for 7 days
Aztreonam	50–100 mg/kg/day for 14 days

Carrier state in typhoid

- **Asymptomatic carrier state:** About 3–5% of patients develop long-term asymptomatic carrier state. Many carriers does not give history of typhoid fever and are probably had an undiagnosed mild infection.
- **Chronic carriers:** These carriers are usually older than 50 years and females with gallstones. *S. typhi* resides in the gallbladder, urinary bladder and even within the gallstones. They are intermittently excreted into the stool, thereby contaminating water or food. Vi antigen is positive in carriers.
- Chronic carriers should be given ciprofloxacin/ampicillin for 4 weeks. Cholecystectomy may be needed in some patients.

Prevention

Improved sanitation and living conditions: It is most important method to prevent typhoid fever. These measures include good hygiene, clean water, proper sewage disposal and proper water treatment. Travelers are advised to avoid drinking untreated water, ice in drinks, and eating ice creams.

Vaccination: Three available typhoid vaccines are:

- **Inactivated injectable:** Two in number
  - Heat-killed, phenol-extracted, whole-cell vaccine—because of several adverse reactions, this is not used at present.
  - Vi-polysaccharide-parenteral administration in individuals >2 years; single dose.
- **Oral live attenuated vaccines:** Ty21a, a live, attenuated vaccine containing the *S. typhi* strain Ty21a is oral administered in individuals >6 years; one capsule every other day for three doses.

Food Poisoning

Q. List the causes of food poisoning. Discuss briefly the manifestations, diagnosis, and management of food poisoning.

- Food poisoning is an **illness contracted by eating contaminated food.**
- In most cases, food that causes food poisoning is contaminated by bacteria, such as salmonella or *Escherichia coli (E. coli)*, or a virus, such as the norovirus. Some toxins can cause food poisoning within a short time. Vomiting is the main symptom of food poisoning.
- **Box 4.4** lists the food infection *versus* intoxication.
- Each year about 6.5–33 million foodborne illness occurs. Campylobacter cause 1–6 million cases/year. Salmonella causes 2–4 million illnesses/year. *E. coli* causes about 21,000 cases each year.

Box 4.4: Food infection versus intoxication.

- **Food infection**
  - Bacteria are consumed
  - Body reacts by raising temperature—fever
  - Longer incubation
- **Food intoxication**
  - Toxin contaminated food is eaten
  - Shorter incubation

Causes of Food Poisoning (Table 4.10)

TABLE 4.10: Causes of food poisoning.

Infective (bacteria or their toxins) ➢ Due to toxin: – Preformed toxins, e.g., *Staphylococcus aureus and Bacillus cereus* – Enterotoxins released in the intestine, e.g., *Vibrio cholerae, E. coli, Clostridium perfringens, and Clostridium difficile* ➢ Due to intestinal mucosal damage: – Invasion of mucosa, e.g., Rotavirus – Invasion and destruction of mucosa, e.g., *Shigella, Yersinia enterocolitica, Salmonella, Entamoeba histolytica, and Bacillus anthracis*
Noninfective ➢ Allergic type, e.g., shellfish ➢ Nonallergic type, e.g., scombrotoxin (fish) and fungi (Amanita Phalloides) ➢ Chemicals, e.g., detergents and pesticides

Various organism causing food poisoning and their symptoms are summarized in **Table 4.11**.

TABLE 4.11: Various organism causing food poisoning and their symptoms.

Organism	*Incubation*	*Symptoms*	*Foods*
Campylobacter jejuni	2–5 days	Diarrhea, vomiting, headache, fever, and muscle pain	Poultry, dairy products, and water
Salmonella enteriditis	12–36 hours	Abdominal cramps, headache, fever, nausea, and diarrhea	Poultry, meat, eggs and egg products, and sliced melons
Escherichia coli	3–4 days	Diarrhea, vomiting, and mild fever	Undercooked ground beef and unpasteurized cider
Listeria monocytogenes	3–70 days	Flu-like, meningitis, encephalitis, and spontaneous abortion	Unpasteurized milk, ice cream, ready-to-eat, and lunch meats
Clostridium perfringens	10–12 hours	Abdominal pain, nausea, diarrhea fever, headache, and vomiting usually absent	Stews, gravies, and beans
Clostridium botulinum (intoxication)	4 hours to 8 days	Vomiting; constipation; diplopia, dysphagia, dysarthria, paralysis, and death	Baked potatoes, fish, garlic/oil mixtures, and low-acid canned foods
Staphylococcus aureus (intoxication)	1–7 hours	Nausea, retching, abdominal cramps, and diarrhea	Ready-to-eat, reheated foods, dairy products, and protein foods
Bacillus cereus (intoxication)	30 minutes to 6 hours (emetic) or 6–15 hours (diarrheal)	Nausea, vomiting, and watery diarrhea	Rice products, starchy foods, casseroles, puddings, and soups
Hepatitis A	10–50 days	Sudden fever, vomiting, and jaundice	Water (ice), shellfish, ready-to-eat, fruit juices, and vegetables
Norwalk virus	10–50 hours	Nausea, diarrhea, headache, and mild fever	Water, shellfish, raw vegetables, and fruits
Rotavirus	1–3 days	Vomiting, diarrhea, and mild fever	Ready-to-eat, water, and ice
Giardia lamblia	3–25 days	Fatigue, nausea, weight loss, and abdominal cramps	Water, ice, and raw vegetables
Cryptosporidium parvum	1–12 days	Severe diarrhea, may have no symptoms	Water, raw foods, unpasteurized cider, and ready-to-eat

Clinical Feature and Diagnosis

The symptoms will be different depending on what type of contamination is responsible. Common symptoms of food poisoning are listed in **Box 4.5.**

Management
- The symptoms of food poisoning subside in 2–3 days.
- The goal of treatment is to replace fluids and electrolytes lost through vomiting and diarrhea. If dehydration is severe and cannot be managed at home, patient needs to be admitted, intravenous saline and supportive treatment (antiemetics, antipyretics, probiotics, and antimotility agents) advised.
- Antibiotics to be used sparingly only in infective cases.

Box 4.5: Common symptoms of food poisoning.
- Severe vomiting
- Diarrhea
- Headache
- Fever
- Abdominal pain
- Tiredness

Dysentery

Dysentery is defined as an acute inflammation of the large intestine (colitis) characterized by diarrhea with blood and mucus in the stools. Two causes are bacillary and amebic infections.

Bacillary Dysentery (Shigellosis)

Q. Write short essay on the etiology, clinical presentation, diagnosis, and management of acute bacillary dysentery.

Q. Write short essay on clinical features of Shigellosis.

- Bacillary dysentery is an acute **necrotizing infection** of the **distal small bowel and colon** caused mostly by one of ***Shigella*** species. *Shigella* species that cause colitis are classified into four major subgroups namely: *Dysenteriae* (most virulent), *flexneri, boydii,* and *sonnei.* Bacillary dysentery is one of the **most common causes of bloody diarrhea.** Other organisms causing bacillary dysentery include *E. coli* O157:H7, *Salmonella, Campylobacter,* etc.
- *Shigella* **produces toxin** (endotoxin as well as an exotoxin) that has cytotoxic, neurotoxic, and enterotoxic effects. When inflammation is severe, ileus, toxic megacolon, gross hemorrhage, and perforation may develop.
- **Source of infection: Humans** are the only natural reservoir.
- **Mode of transmission:** By **ingestion** through fecal-oral route or via fecally contaminated water and food. It can be acquired by oral contact with any contaminated surface (e.g., clothing, towels, and unwashed hands after defecation or skin surfaces) or flies.
- **Incubation period:** It ranges from **1 to 3 days.**

Clinical features

- **Severity of infection:** Disease severity varies from mild to severe. *S. sonnei* produces mild infection, *S. flexneri* infection is usually more severe, and *S. dysenteriae* may produce fulminating infection resulting in death within 48 hours.
- Symptoms start 24–48 hours after ingestion and usually presents as frequent small quantity of stools containing blood, mucus, and purulent exudate with little fecal material (dysentery). This is accompanied by fever, colicky abdominal pain, and tenesmus. Severe cases may show signs of systemic toxicity, dehydration and electrolyte disturbances.
- Physical examination may show tenderness over the colon in the left iliac fossa and hyperactive bowel sounds.

Complications

See **Table 4.12**.

TABLE 4.12: Complications of bacillary dysentery.

Intestinal	*Extraintestinal*
➢ Rectal prolapse ➢ Toxic megacolon ➢ Colonic perforation	➢ Bacteremia ➢ Meningismus and seizures ➢ Transient peripheral neuropathy ➢ Reiter syndrome ➢ Hemolytic-uremic syndrome (HUS) ➢ Thrombotic thrombocytopenic purpura

Diagnosis

- **Stool culture** is required for confirmation of *Shigella* infection.
- **Sigmoidoscopy** shows red and swollen mucosa covered by mucopus on the surface. The submucous veins are obscured.
- Enzyme immunoassay used for detecting Shiga toxins in stools.
- PCR for *Shigella* DNA in stools.

Management

- Fluid and **electrolyte** deficits should be corrected by oral rehydration therapy or, if diarrhea is severe, by intravenous replacement of water and electrolyte loss.
- **Antibiotic therapy:** Infections caused by *S. dysenteriae* and *S. flexneri* should be given ciprofloxacin (500 mg twice daily for 3 days). Second-line agents include azithromycin and ceftriaxone.
- **Antidiarrheal medication** should be avoided. Codeine or loperamide may be given to control diarrhea in adults without dysentery.

Amebiasis

Q. Discuss the etiology, pathogenesis, clinical features, diagnosis, investigations, complications, and treatment of amebic dysentery/intestinal amebiasis.

Etiology

- Amebiasis is an **infection caused by protozoan *Entamoeba histolytica***
- *E. histolytica* has three distinct stages:
    1. **Trophozoite stage:** Amebic trophozoites are seen in the stools of patients with acute symptoms.
    2. **Precyst stage:** In the colon, the trophozoite develops into a cyst through an intermediate form termed the precyst.
    3. **Cyst stage: Amebic cysts are the infecting stage** and are found only in stools. They are spherical and have thick chitin walls, and usually four nuclei.
- **Source of infection: Humans** are the only known reservoir for *E. histolytica.* It is reproduced in the colon of infected individual and passes in the feces.
- **Mode of infection:** It is **acquired by fecal-oral route** through ingestion of materials contaminated with human feces containing *E. histolytica.* Pathogenesis of amebiasis is depicted in **Figure 4.6**.
- **Incubation period:** About 2–6 weeks.

Amebic Colitis

Q. Write a short note on amebic colitis/intestinal amebiasis.

Amebic colitis can present in two forms: Amebic dysentery and nondysenteric amebic colitis.

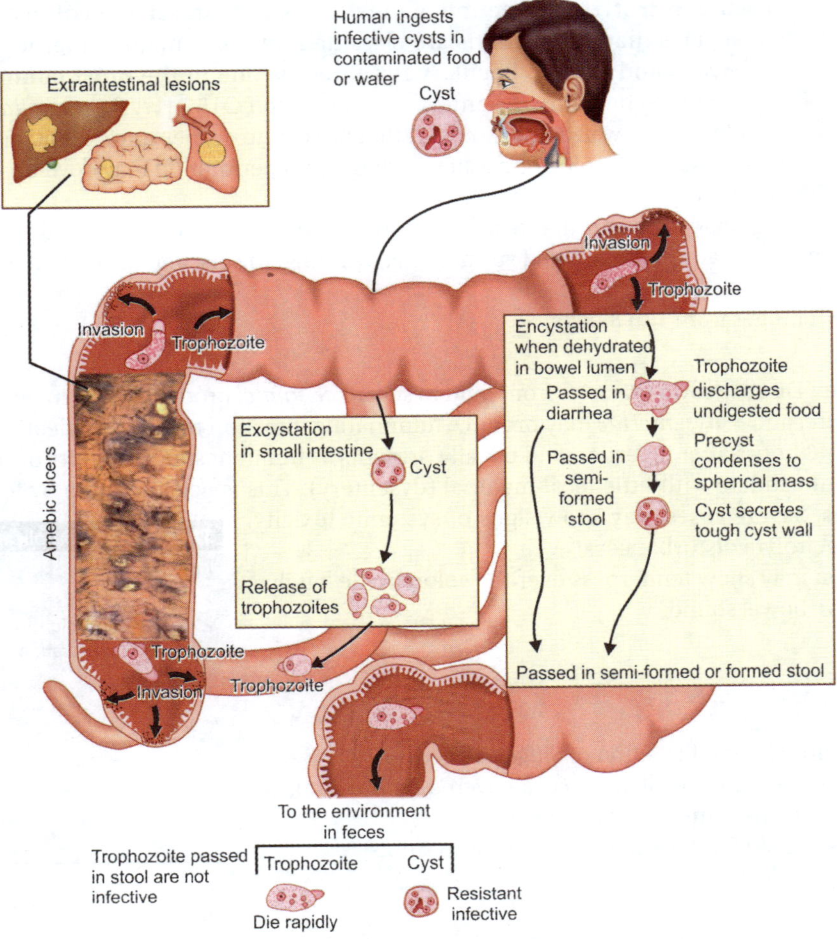

FIG. 4.6: Pathogenesis of amebiasis.

Amebic Dysentery

Pathogenesis

- The amebic cysts are passed in the stool of infected individuals and the **cysts can contaminate water, food, or fingers.** These cysts are tetra-nucleated and can remain viable for weeks to months. However, these are destroyed in temperature below 5°C or above 40°C.
- Amebic dysentery results from ingestion (fecal-oral transmission) of *E. histolytica* cysts. **Amebic cysts colonize the epithelial surface of the terminal ileum and** undergo further nuclear division, and release trophozoites. The trophozoites are carried to the large intestine and may colonize any part of the large intestine, but **most frequently in the cecum and ascending colon causing amebic colitis.** They produce the characteristic "flask-shaped" amebic ulcers with a narrow neck and broad base. These patients pass both cysts and trophozoites in the stool.
- Most often, the amebic infection remains subclinical. However, antibody response usually occurs even without local invasion. These asymptomatic patients should be treated to prevent transmission of infection to others and development of amebic colitis at a later period.
- **Ameboma** is a common complication of amebic dysentery. It is a localized granuloma which presents as a palpable mass in the rectum or causes a filling defect in the colon on radiography.
- **Trophozoite may penetrate blood vessels and reach the liver through** portal vein. In the liver they multiply and produce amebic liver **abscesses** in about 40% of patients with amebic dysentery. The liquid contents of this abscess have a characteristic pinkish color, which may later change to chocolate-brown (like anchovy sauce).
- They can also travel to lungs and brain.

Clinical features of intestinal amebiasis (amebic dysentery)

Q. Write short essay on the clinical features and treatment of intestinal amebiasis.

- It may produce **dysentery of varying severity.** It presents with intermittent diarrhea consisting of **foul smelling** (offensive), **loose, and watery stools** that may contain **mucus and blood.** Sometimes diarrhea alternate with constipation.

- **Other symptoms include abdominal pain**/cramp (especially right lower quadrant which may simulate acute appendicitis), flatulence, and weight loss. Sometimes it is accompanied by systemic symptoms, such as headache, fever, nausea, and anorexia. Less commonly, it may present as acute amebic dysentery, resembling bacillary dysentery or acute ulcerative colitis.
- **Physical examination:** There may be tenderness over the cecum (amebic typhlitis), ascending colon and over the left iliac fossa **(amebic point or Manson–Barr point)** and tender hepatomegaly.

Complications

See **Table 4.13**.

TABLE 4.13: Complications of amebiasis.

Intestinal complications	*Extraintestinal complications*
➢ Massive hemorrhage ➢ Ameboma ➢ Perforation and peritonitis ➢ Toxic megacolon in fulminant cases ➢ Postdysenteric colitis ➢ Rectovaginal fistula ➢ Chronic infection with stricture formation	➢ Amebic liver abscess ➢ Pleuropulmonary amebiasis ➢ Hepaticobronchial fistula ➢ Amebic pericarditis ➢ Cutaneous amebiasis

Diagnosis

- **Microscopic examination of stool:** Presence of motile trophozoites containing red blood cells (hematophagous trophozoites) in fresh sample of stool will confirm the diagnosis. If a fresh stool sample cannot be examined immediately, it should be preserved with a fixative such as polyvinyl alcohol or kept cool (4°C). Presence of amebic cysts alone does not imply disease.
- **Sigmoidoscopy** and barium enema may show the characteristic "flask-shaped" ulcers with normal surrounding mucosa. The aspirated material or scrapings from the ulcer or biopsy of the ulcer may show the trophozoites. Colonic exudate obtained by sigmoidoscopy may microscopically show trophozoites.
- **Serologic tests:** Indirect hemagglutination test, ELISA or counter immunoelectrophoresis can detect antibodies in the blood. They are more useful in extraintestinal amebiasis.
- Amebic fluorescent antibody test is positive in about 90% of patients with liver abscess and in 60–70% with active colitis.
- Detection of *E. histolytica* antigen or DNA in a stool sample.

Diagnosis of amebic liver abscess: It is often suspected on clinical grounds.

Nondysenteric Amebic Colitis

- Usually presents as recurrent bouts of diarrhea with or without mucus, but without any visible blood.
- **Stools examination** shows *E. histolytica* cysts or nonhematophagous trophozoite (trophozoites with no ingested RBCs).

Q. Write short note on uses of metronidazole.

Box 4.6 lists the uses of metronidazole.

Box 4.6: Uses of metronidazole.

- Amebiasis
- Giardiasis
- *Trichomonas vaginalis*
- Anerobic bacterial infections
- Pseudomembranous enterocolitis
- Ulcerative gingivitis
- *Helicobacter pylori* gastritis/peptic ulcer

Q. Enumerate the differences between amebic dysentery and bacillary dysentery.

Differences between amebic dysentery and bacillary dysentery are given in **Table 4.14**.

TABLE 4.14: Differences between amebic dysentery and bacillary dysentery.

Features	*Amebic dysentery*	*Bacillary dysentery*
Macroscopic		
Number of motions	6–8 motions/day	Over 10 motions/day
Amount of stool	Relatively copious	Relatively small
Odor	Offensive	No odor
Nature	Blood and mucus mixed with feces	Blood and mucus, no feces
Color	Dark red	Bright red
Reaction	Acidic	Alkaline
Consistency	Not adherent to the container	Adherent to the container
Microscopic		
RBC	In clumps	Discrete or in rouleaux
Pus cells	Few	Numerous
Macrophages and ghost cells	Very few	Numerous
Eosinophils, and pyknotic bodies	Present	Scarce
Causative agent	Trophozoites of *E. histolytica*	Motile bacteria
Charcot–Leyden crystals	Present	Absent

Brucellosis

Q. Write short essay/note on brucellosis (abortus fever; Malta fever; undulant fever; and Mediterranean fever). Name species that cause brucellosis.

- Brucellosis (Malta fever, undulant fever, Mediterranean fever, and Rock fever of Gibraltar) is a zoonotic disease.
- Brucellosis is an infection caused by one of the four species of *Brucella: Brucella melitensis* (goats, sheep, and camels), *Brucella abortus* (cattle), *Brucella suis* (pigs), and *Brucella canis* (dogs). *Brucella* is a gram-negative organism.
- Natural reservoir of brucellosis is animals.

Mode of Infection

- **Ingestion:** Infected animals may excrete *Brucella* in their milk, and human infection is acquired by ingesting contaminated dairy products (especially unpasteurized raw milk) and uncooked meat.

- **Direct infection:** Animal urine, feces, vaginal discharge, and uterine products may act as sources of infection and they may enter humans through abraded skin.
- **Inhalation of infectious aerosols**
  - Pens, tables, and slaughter houses
  - Conjunctival splashes and injection
- **Person-to-person transmission is very rare,** particularly mother-to-child.

Clinical Features

Q. Write short essay on clinical features and treatment of brucellosis.

Brucellosis involves many organ systems and has a very insidious onset with varying clinical signs. The most common sign in all patients is an intermittent/irregular fever with variable duration, which is termed as *undulant fever.*

Acute brucellosis (<2 months)

- Incubation period of acute brucellosis is 1–3 weeks.
- Acute onset in nearly 50% cases and presents with fever, malaise, headache, chills, fatigue, weakness, backache, generalized myalgia, and night sweats. Patients also have anorexia, lose weight, cough, and arthralgias.
- **Fever:** It is classically high swinging **undulant** pattern with rigors, although continuous and intermittent patterns may be seen.
- **Physical findings** are nonspecific and include splenomegaly (20% of cases may lead to hypersplenism and thrombocytopenia), lymphadenopathy (15% cases) and hepatomegaly (10% cases), sacroiliitis, and arthritis.
- A few may develop localized brucellosis in the form of osteomyelitis, splenic abscess, epididymo-orchitis, pneumonia, meningoencephalitis pleural effusion, and endocarditis.

Subacute brucellosis (2–12 months)

Features are similar to acute form, but less severe.

Chronic brucellosis (>12 months)

- This is characterized by low-grade fever easy fatigability, myalgia, arthralgia, occasional bouts of fever and neuropsychiatric manifestations (e.g., depression).
- Splenomegaly is usually observed.
- Bone and joint complications are the most common complications and include uveitis, sacroiliitis, spondylitis, peripheral arthritis, osteomyelitis, and bursitis.

Diagnosis

- **Culture:** Definitive diagnosis depends on the isolation of the *Brucella.*
- **Serological tests** may also aid diagnosis and are of greater value in chronic disease. In ***Brucella* agglutination test,** a fourfold or greater rise in titer of agglutination antibody (IgM) is highly suggestive of brucellosis. Raised serum IgG level indicates current or recent infection; a negative test excludes chronic brucellosis.
- **Other tests** include ultrasound and CT, bone radiographs, radionuclide scans, and species-specific PCR tests.

Treatment

- ***Regimen A:*** Doxycycline 100 mg PO BID for 6 weeks + streptomycin 1 g IM qd (means one a day) for the first 14–21 days
- ***Regimen B:*** Doxycycline 100 mg PO BID + rifampin 600–900 mg (15 mg/kg) PO qd for 6 weeks

Prevention and Control

- Careful attention to hygiene when handling infected animals, eradication of infection in animals, and pasteurization of milk.
- No vaccine is available for humans.

Cholera

Q. Write a short essay/note on cholera and cholera sicca.

- Cholera is an acute illness caused by the curved, flagellated, halophilic gram-negative bacillus, *Vibrio cholerae.*
- *Vibrio cholerae* colonizes in the small intestine. It causes explosive, severe watery diarrhea with rapid depletion of extracellular fluid and electrolytes.
- *Vibrio cholerae:* It is killed by temperatures of 100°C in a few seconds but can survive in ice for up to 6 weeks. The **major pathogenic strain** has a **somatic antigen (O1)** and has **two biotypes: classical and El Tor. New classical toxigenic strain, serotype O139** (Bengal serogroup) is still major cause of cholera in our country.

Mode of Transmission

By the feco-oral route: Infection spreads via the stools or vomitus of symptomatic patients. Contaminated drinking water is the major source of the dissemination, although contaminated foodstuffs (shellfish and food contaminated by flies), and hands of contact carriers may contribute in epidemics.

Incubation period is about 12–48 hours.

Pathogenesis

- In the small intestine *Vibrio cholerae* proliferates and produces a powerful **exotoxin.** The exotoxin causes massive secretion of isotonic fluid into the intestinal lumen.
- Cholera toxin also releases serotonin (5HT, 5 hydroxy tryptamine) from enterochromaffin cells in the gut. This activates a neural secretory reflex in the enteric nervous system.
- *V. cholerae* also produces other toxins (zona occludens toxin, ZOT, and accessory cholera toxin, ACT) and are responsible for pathogenesis of cholera.
- Severe depletion of extracellular fluid produces hypotension, metabolic acidosis, and hypokalemia.
- In severe cases, massive fluid loss may lead to hypovolemic shock and acute tubular necrosis resulting in renal failure.

Clinical Features

- Majority with cholera may have a mild illness that cannot be distinguished clinically from diarrhea due to other infective causes. Severe cases, present abruptly with severe, painless, watery diarrhea without pain or colic, followed by vomiting (vomiting may be absent).
- **Rice-water stool:** Following the evacuation of normal gut fecal contents, characteristic "rice water" stool is passed, consisting of clear fluid with flecks of mucus.
- **Loss of fluid and electrolytes:** Leading to intense dehydration with muscular cramps. The features of hypovolemic shock include cold, clammy and wrinkled ("washerwomen" skin) skin with loss of skin turgor, tachycardia, hypotension, and peripheral cyanosis. Features of dehydration include sunken eyes, hollow cheeks, and a diminished urine output. The blood pressure drops and the pulse becomes rapid and thready. Death from acute circulatory failure may occur unless fluid and electrolytes are promptly replaced. Rapid improvement occurs with proper treatment.
- **Cholera sicca:** Occasionally, a very **severe form of the cholera** occurs with **accumulation of fluid into the dilated bowel.** This **kills the patient before typical gastrointestinal symptoms** appear. It is called as cholera sicca!

Diagnosis

- **Clinical diagnosis** can be easily made during an epidemic. Otherwise, the diagnosis requires bacteriological confirmation.
- **Stool examination: "Hanging drop" preparation** of the freshly passed stool shows the characteristic rapidly motile (shooting star motility) *V. cholerae* (this is not diagnostic, as *Campylobacter jejuni* may give a similar appearance).
- **Culture** of the stool or a rectal swab can isolate and identify the *V. cholerae* and also establish antibiotic sensitivity.

Treatment/Management

Q. Write a short essay/note on treatment of cholera.

1. **Appropriate and effective rehydration therapy:** Maintenance of circulation by replacement of water and electrolytes is the mainstay of treatment.
   - **Intravenous therapy** is required if there is severe dehydration. Ringer's lactate is the best fluid for intravenous replacement and should contain sodium chloride 5 g/L, potassium chloride 1 g/L and sodium bicarbonate (4 g/L) ("Dhaka solution"). Initial fluid deficit should be replaced within 3–4 hours. Patients with severe cholera may need 200–300 mL/kg of isotonic fluids in the initial 24 hours. It should be continued till the patient is hemodynamically stable and vomiting subsides.
   - **Oral rehydration:** Once the vomiting stops and the patient is hemodynamically stable, fluid should be given orally up to 500 mL hourly. *Oral rehydration solutions (ORS)* are based on the observation that glucose (and other carbohydrates) increases absorption of sodium and water in the small intestine, even in the presence of secretory loss due to toxins.
   - Oral rehydration solutions with resistant starch, based on either rice or cereal, shorten the duration of diarrhea and improves prognosis.
   - Total fluid needed may exceed 50 L over a period of 2–5 days. Accurate assessment can be made by the use of a "cholera cot", which has a reinforced hole under the patient's buttocks, beneath which a graded bucket is placed.
2. **Antibiotics:** 3 days treatment with tetracycline 500 mg 6 hourly, a single dose of doxycycline 300 mg or ciprofloxacin 1 g in adults or cotrimoxazole one tablet daily reduces the duration or excretion of *V. cholerae.* It also reduces the total volume of fluid required for replacement. Other alternative drugs include erythromycin and furazolidone.
3. In children, zinc supplementation may reduce the severity of diarrhea.

Prognosis is good with adequate treatment and there is gradual return to normal of clinical and biochemical parameters within 1–3 days.

Prophylaxis

- **Vaccination:** It is recommended by the WHO during potential or actual outbreak situations.
  - Parenteral vaccination with a killed suspension (WC-rBS) of *V. cholerae* has some protective role.
  - Both live attenuated and whole cell killed vaccine (both oral) are available. Oral vaccines containing killed *V. cholerae* and the B subunit of cholera toxin are of limited efficacy.
- **Chemoprophylaxis** by tetracycline 500 mg twice a day for 3 days. Mass single-dose vaccination along with tetracycline is also advised.

Leptospirosis

Q. Write short essay on the etiology, clinical features, complications, investigations/laboratory diagnosis, complications, and treatment of leptospirosis.

Q. Write a short note on leptospirosis.

Leptospirosis is a globally important zoonotic disease caused by the spirochaete *Leptospira interrogans*.

Synonyms: Autumn fever, seven-day fever, canefield fever, swamp fever, Weil's disease, rice-field fever, and swineherd's disease.

Etiology

- *Leptospira* consists of two species: (1) pathogenic *Leptospira interrogans* (now designated *L. interrogans* sensu lato) and (2) saprophytic/free-living *Leptospira biflexia* (now designated *L. biflexia* sensu lato).
- Leptospirosis is the term used for an infection with any of the subtypes or subgroups of *Leptospira interrogans*.

Epidemiology

Leptospirosis is the most widespread important zoonosis in the world.

Source of Infection

Leptospirosis is ubiquitous in wildlife and in many domestic animals. Reservoirs of organisms include **rodents** (most frequent), foxes, skunks, dogs, and domestic livestock. Many animals shed the organism into the urine in massive numbers for long period but infection is asymptomatic in these animals. Outbreaks of leptospirosis may occur with flooding.

Mode of Transmission

- **Direct contact:** Human infection occur either by direct contact with urine or tissue of an infected animal. Transmission may occur through cuts, abraded skin, and mucous membranes (nasopharynx, oral mucosa, conjunctiva, and vagina). Prolonged immersion in contaminated water favors invasion, as the spirochete can survive in fresh water for months and for up to 24 hours in sea water.
- **Ingestion** of contaminated water, soil or vegetation.

Incubation period is usually 1–2 weeks (7–14 days) but ranges from 1 to 30 days.

Pathogenesis (Fig. 4.7)

Typically illness has two phases (biphasic illness)

1. **Leptospiremic** (initial/first) **phase** is named so because leptospirae are present in the blood and CSF during this phase. After entry of the organisms into the human, they proliferate and disseminate through blood into all organs (leptospiremic phase). The organisms can survive in the nonimmune host. They evade complement-mediated killing, resist ingestion and killing by neutrophils, monocytes and macrophages.
2. **Immune** (second) **phase:** During the immune phase, the antibodies appear and leptospirae disappear from the blood. However, the organism persists in various organs including liver, lung, kidney, heart, and brain.

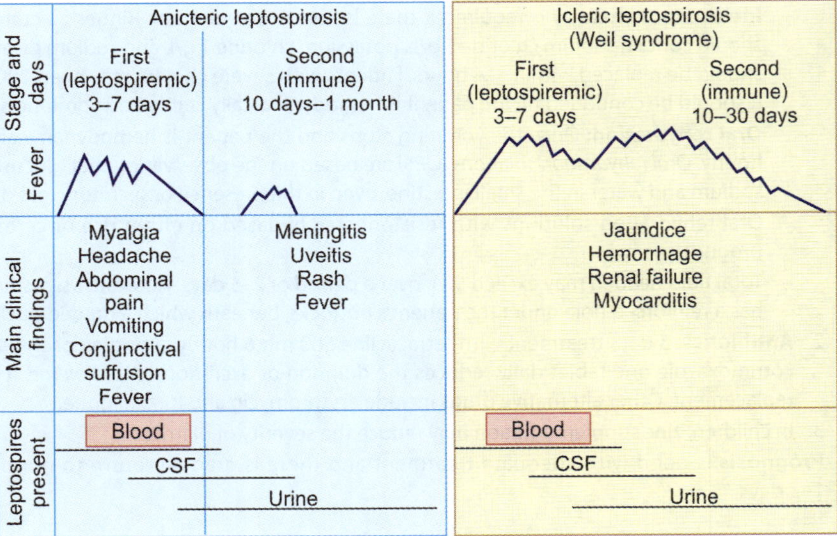

FIG. 4.7: Pathogenesis of leptospirosis.

Clinical Features

Q. Write a short note on the signs and symptoms of Weil's disease.

Most patients with mild leptospirosis are asymptomatic and do not seek medical attention.

1. ***Leptospiremic phase:*** It lasts for up to a week. It produces a nonspecific illness and commonly encountered symptoms include:
   - **Fever:** Usually high-grade with chills and rigors. May be accompanied by malaise and weakness.
   - **Severe headache:** Retro-orbital or occipital.
   - **Myalgia:** Muscle pain occurs in most patients and is severe. The muscles of the thighs and lumbar areas (calf and back) show severe tenderness and may show cutaneous hyperesthesia (causalgia).
   - **Conjunctival suffusion/congestion (Fig. 4.8)** is very helpful and notable sign for detecting the disease. It is characterized by pericorneal reddening or hyperemia (redness without exudate) without conjunctivitis.

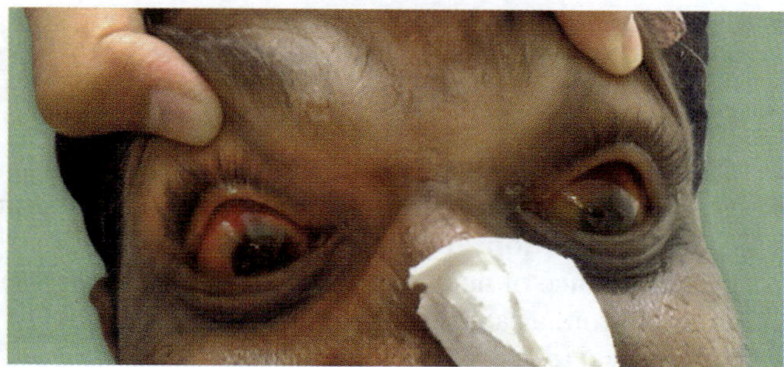

FIG. 4.8: Conjunctival suffusion and jaundice in leptospirosis.

   Other less common features include anorexia, nausea, vomiting, abdominal pain, cough, pharyngitis, uveitis lymphadenopathy, hepatosplenomegaly, and skin rashes.

2. ***Immune (second) phase***
   - In many patients, the first (leptospiremic) phase is followed by a period of apparent recovery, after which the symptoms worsen again for another 2–5 days (immune phase).
   - During the second phase, meningitis, and iridocyclitis are more common.
   - **Meningitis:** Presence of headache, fever, and neck stiffness may suggest meningitis. The CSF is usually show normal number of cells in the first 7 days of illness, although the organisms may be seen. With the onset of antibodies (during immune phase) in the serum aseptic meningitis develops in about 90% of patients, with abnormalities in CSF (refer investigations below).
   - **Other manifestations** which are less frequent include change in the level of consciousness, encephalitis, cranial nerve palsies, and acute dilatation of the gallbladder with cholecystitis.

Weil's Syndrome

Q. Write a short note on Weil's syndrome.

Weil's syndrome is not a specific subgroup of leptospirosis, but indicates severe leptospirosis. It can develop during the second (immune) phase of leptospirosis or as a progressive illness.

Components of Weil's Syndrome

It is dramatic life-threatening event, characterized by:

1. **Jaundice:** The first manifestation of severe leptospirosis is usually jaundice. It develops between fifth and ninth days. Jaundice is deep and is not due to hepatocellular damage, but probably due to cholestasis or sepsis. Hepatic dysfunction such as acute hepatitis and sometimes fulminant may develop.
2. **Renal failure:** Primarily due to impaired renal perfusion and acute tubular necrosis. It presents as oliguria or anuria (acute renal failure) with the presence of albumin, blood, and casts in the urine.
3. **Hemorrhagic manifestations** are common, and include purpura, petechiae appearing on oral, vaginal or conjunctival mucosa, and large areas of bruising. In severe cases, there may be epistaxis, hemoptysis, hematemesis and melena (due to gastrointestinal bleeding), hemorrhage into adrenal glands, pleural, pericardial or subarachnoid spaces (subarachnoid hemorrhage). Thrombocytopenia is common cause of hemorrhagic manifestation.
4. **Pulmonary syndrome:** Adult respiratory distress syndrome (ARDS), pulmonary hemorrhage, pneumonia, and effusion.
5. **CNS:** Meningoencephalitis, subarachnoid hemorrhage, and seizures.
6. **Other features:** DIC, hemolytic anemia, myocarditis and arrhythmias, and multiple organ dysfunction syndrome (MODS).

Investigations

- **Urine examination:**
  - During early part of the illness shows microscopic hematuria, pyuria, and proteinuria.
  - **Demonstration of organism:** The tightly coiled spirochete may be visualized in the urine by phase contrast or dark-field microscopy.
- **Blood:**
  - **Total leukocyte count** may vary, but polymorphonuclear leukocytosis (neutrophilia of more than 70%) with shift to left is very frequent.

- **Anemia** may develop due to intravascular hemolysis, azotemia, and blood loss caused by hemorrhage.
- **Thrombocytopenia** in severe infection.
- **Elevated markers of inflammation:** Raised **erythrocyte sedimentation rate** and C-reactive protein level.
- Raised **blood urea nitrogen (BUN) and hyperkalemia** occur with renal failure.
- **Coagulation studies** may show a prolonged prothrombin time which is reversible with vitamin K administration.
- **Creatinine phosphokinase (CPK)** are elevated in 50% of patients during the first week of illness. This helps in differentiating leptospirosis from viral hepatitis.
- **Liver function tests** show raised AST and ALT (up to five times normal), conjugated hyperbilirubinemia and raised alkaline phosphatase. Marked elevations of bilirubin and mild elevated transaminases level are characteristically found in Weil's syndrome.

- **Chest radiograph** may reveal patchy bronchopneumonia and a small pleural effusion.
- **Electrocardiographic abnormalities** include bradycardia, low voltage, and nonspecific ST-T wave changes.
- **CSF examination:** It may be abnormal in up to 90% of patients. Cell counts are increased (but $<500/\text{mm}^3$) with predominance of neutrophils. Protein levels may be normal or raised and glucose level is normal. In severe jaundice, xanthochromia can be seen.
- **Serological tests:**
  - **IgM antibodies** may be detected in blood by microscopic agglutination test (MAT), during the immune (second) phase of illness. IgM ELISA and immunofluorescent techniques are easy to perform and rapid immunochromatographic tests are specific but are of moderate sensitivity in the first week of disease.
  - **Demonstration of leptospiral antigen** by radioimmunoassay or ELISA.
- **Culture:** Diagnosis can be confirmed by culture (on Fletcher's medium) of the blood or CSF during the first week (leptospiremic phase) of illness or of the urine from the second week onwards. It may take several weeks.
- **Detection of leptospiral DNA** by PCR in blood during early symptomatic disease and in urine from the eighth day of illness.

Modified Faine's Criteria (Table 4.15) includes clinical, epidemiological, and laboratory criteria. A score of more than 26 indicates current leptospirosis.

Treatment

Antibiotic therapy: Leptospirosis is highly susceptible to a broad range of antibiotics. Early antibiotic therapy may prevent the development of major organ system failure or lessen its severity, but it should be given irrespective of the stage of the infection.

- **Mild disease:** Oral treatment with following for 7 days effective when started within 4 days of onset of symptoms.
  - Doxycycline (100 mg orally twice daily) or
  - Ampicillin (750 mg four times daily)
  - Amoxicillin (500 mg four times daily)
  - Azithromycin (500 mg once daily)
- **Severe leptospirosis** should be treated with intravenous penicillin as soon as the diagnosis is considered.
  - Intravenous penicillin (1.5 million units intravenous 6 hourly) or
  - Ceftriaxone 1 g twice a day IV
  - Cefotaxime 1 g IV four times a day
- **Treatment of complications/general care of the patient**
  - Blood product transfusion for hemorrhage, anemia and thrombocytopenia
  - ARDS may require mechanical ventilation. Renal failure may require dialysis. Intravenous corticosteroid is useful for the vasculitic nature of severe leptospirosis, particularly in the setting of pulmonary hemorrhage.

TABLE 4.15: Modified Faine's criteria 2012 for the diagnosis of leptospirosis.

Part A: Clinical data	***Score***
➤ Headache	2
➤ Fever	2
➤ Fever >39°C	2
➤ Conjunctival suffusion	4
➤ Meningism	4
➤ Myalgia	4
➤ Conjunctival suffusion + meningism + myalgia	10
➤ Jaundice	1
➤ Albuminuria/nitrogen retention	2
➤ Hemoptysis/dyspnea	2
Part B: Epidemiological factors	
➤ Rainfall	5
➤ Contact with contaminated environment	4
➤ Animal contact	1
Part C: Bacteriological and Laboratory Findings	
Isolation of Leptospira in culture—Diagnosis certain	
PCR	25
Positive serology	
➤ ELISA IgM positive	15
➤ SAT positive	15
➤ Other rapid tests	15
➤ MAT—single positive in high titer	15
➤ MAT—rising titer/seroconversion (paired sera)	25

Melioidosis

Q. Write short note on melioidosis.

Melioidosis (Whitmore disease) is caused by *Burkholderia pseudomallei; which is* an aerobic, gram-negative motile bacillus, with "safety pin" appearance. It is an opportunistic pathogen found in water and moist soil and produces exotoxin.

Mode of Transmission

- **Contact with contaminated soil or water:** It is the most common route of acquiring the disease.
- **Other routes** include aspiration or ingestion of contaminated water and inhalation of dust from soil. Transmission between infected animals and/or infected people is very rare. Person-to-person transmission may rarely occur through sexual contact with an individual with prostatic infection.

Incubation period varies from 2 days to months to many years. *B. pseudomallei* can survive in phagocytic cells. Hence, melioidosis can result after a latent period.

Risk factors: Immunosuppressive events or chronic diseases, such as diabetes, chronic alcohol use, chronic renal disease, and chronic lung disease.

Clinical Features

- Most infections are asymptomatic.
- **Acute pulmonary infection:** It is the most common form which resembles tuberculosis with presentations of lobar or multilobar pneumonia, necrotizing lesions, and pleural effusions.
- **Focal infection:** Melioidosis can be limited to a focal infection. Localized lesions may occur in the skin (as a result of infected wounds) or various internal organs (as a result of septicemic spread). Many times focal infections become chronic conditions, such as lymphadenopathy, parotitis, cystitis, osteomyelitis, prostatitis, spondylitis, and septic arthritis.
- **Severe systemic form:** It manifests as severe septicemic form. This can be nondisseminated (only involving one organ) or disseminated. Rarely melioidosis can produce encephalomyelitis.

Diagnosis

- It is **difficult** and has been called the great imitator (especially tuberculosis) because there are no pathognomonic lesions. Any organ can be affected and the lesions have no distinguishing characteristics.
- **Isolation of the organism** from blood, sputum, tissues or wound exudates by culture can help to diagnose the disease.
- **Serological tests** for titers may also be used for diagnosis. Serological tests available include agglutination tests, indirect hemagglutination, complement fixation, immunofluorescence, and enzyme assays. Improved methods for rapid diagnosis are being evaluated.

Treatment of melioidosis

- **Systemic antibiotics:** Initial intensive therapy with one of the following regimens:
  - Ceftazidime (2 g IV every 6 hours)
  - Meropenem (1 g IV every 8 hours)
  - Imipenem (1 g IV every 6 hours)

Addition of TMP-SMX (trimethoprim sulfamethoxazole) twice daily during the intensive phase and to be continued for 2–3 months.

- **Surgical drainage of skin wounds** can be effective for localized infection.
- **Long-term treatment** and **multiple drugs** will be necessary for chronic and severe cases. Relapses, as soon as 6 months after treatment, are common.

Rickettsial Diseases

- Rickettsiae are obligate intracellular gram negative parasites.
- Most are zoonoses spread to humans by arthropods (except Q fever).
  Rickettsiae replicate within the cytoplasm of endothelial cells and smooth muscle cells of capillaries, arterioles, and small arteries causing necrotizing vasculitis.
- Most are febrile infections with a characteristic rash.
- An ***eschar*** is the characteristic lesion that develops at the site of inoculation.
- Among the major group of rickettsioses, the commonly reported diseases in India are: (1) *Scrub typhus,* (2) *Murine (endemic) typhus,* (3) *Indian tick typhus, and* (4) *Q fever* **(Table 4.16).**

Box 4.7 lists the investigations in rickettsial disease.

Treatment of rickettsial diseases

- Tetracycline is the drug of choice
- Doxycycline 100 mg BID PO × 7–15 days
- Chloramphenicol 500 mg qid PO × 7–15 days
- IV Chloramphenicol 150 mg/kg per day for 5 days
- *Coxiella* endocarditis: Combination therapy
  - Tetracycline + Cotrimoxazole
  - Tetracycline + Rifampicin

Box 4.7: Investigations in rickettsial disease.

- Polymerase chain reaction (PCR)
- Serological tests
  - **Indirect fluorescent antibody (IFA) test** (Titer ≥1: 200)
  - **Complement fixation test**
  - **Weil Felix test**
    - IgM ELISA test: Highly specific test

TABLE 4.16: Examples of rickettsial diseases and their features.

Diseases	*Rickettsial agent*	*Insect vector*	*Mammalian reservoir*	*Clinical features*
Typhus Group				
Epidemic typhus	*R. prowazekii*	Louse	Human	Fever/chills, myalgia, headache, rash (no eschar) all over body except palm, sole, and face
Murine typhus (endemic typhus)	*R. typhi*	Flea	Rodents	Fever, myalgia, headache, rash (no eschar), trunk, extremities, and milder form of illness
Scrub typhus	*R. tsutsugamushi*	Mite	Rodents	Fever, headache, **rash with eschar*** cigarette burn sign **(Figs. 4.9A to C)**, and lymphadenopathy
Spotted Fever Group				
Indian tick typhus	*R. conorii*	Tick	Rodent and dog	Fever, headache, and **rash with eschar**—first appear on wrist and ankle

Contd...

Contd...

Rocky Mountain spotted fever	*R. rickettsii*	Tick	Rodents and dogs	Fever, headache, and rash (no eschar)—first appear on wrist and ankle, palms, and soles involved, systemic complications—respiratory, cardiovascular, central nervous, renal, and hepatic system
Rickettsial pox	*R. akari*	Mite	Mice	Mild illness, fever, headache, vesicular rash with eschar, lymphadenopathy, and resemblance to chickenpox
Others				
Q fever	*C. burnetii*	Nil	Cattle, sheep, goats	Fever, headache, fatigue, pneumonia, endocarditis, and no rash
Trench fever	*Rochalimaea/ Bartonella quintana*	Louse	Human	Fever, splenomegaly, bone pains, and maculopapular rash

*In scrub typhus, the eschar begins as a small papule, then enlarges, undergoes central necrosis, and eventually acquires a blackened crust with an erythematous halo that resembles a cigarette burn. The eschar resembling **"cigarette burn mark"** is seen in 95% of cases and is most important diagnostic clue of scrub typhus.

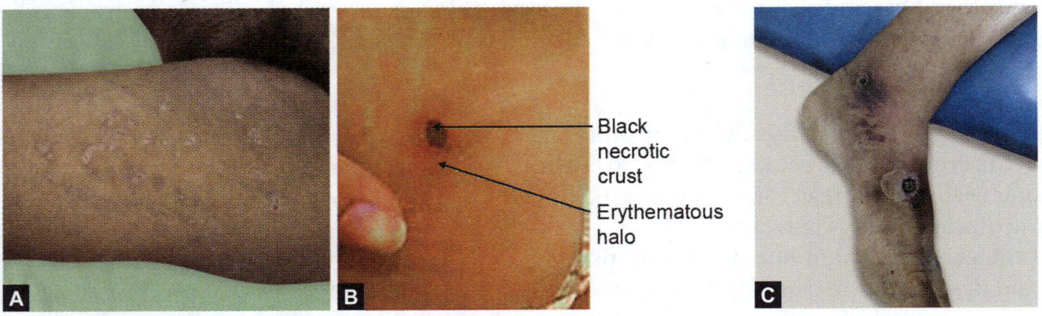

FIGS. 4.9A TO C: (A) Multiple eschar with rash in typhus; (B) Cigarette-burn sign—eschar in typhus; (C) Eschar with rash.

VIRAL INFECTIONS

Measles (Rubella)

Q. Discuss the etiology, clinical features, complications, and prevention of measles (rubella).

- Measles virus, the cause of measles is an RNA virus of the genus *Morbillivirus* in the family *Paramyxoviridae*.
- Measles is highly contagious; approximately 90% of susceptible household contacts acquire the disease.
- Maximal dissemination of virus occurs by droplet spray during the prodromal period (catarrhal stage).

Clinical Features

Measles has three clinical stages

1. **Incubation stage**
   - This stage lasts for about 6–21 days to the first prodromal symptoms and another 2–4 days to the appearance of the rash.
   - **Period of infectivity** is from *4 days before and 2 days after* the onset of rash. Patients with compromised immunity can shed virus for the entire duration of illness.
2. **Prodromal stage with an enanthem (Koplik spots)** and mild symptoms
   - Usually lasts 3–5 days and is characterized by low-grade to moderate **fever, dry cough, coryza,** and **conjunctivitis.**

Q. Write short note on Koplik's spot.

Koplik spots (Fig. 4.10A): Pathognomonic sign of measles are grayish white dots, usually as small as grains of sand, that have slight, reddish areolae; occasionally they are hemorrhagic.
   - Usually tends to occur opposite the lower molars but can spread irregularly over the rest of the buccal mucosa.
   - Rarely, they are found within the midportion of the lower lip, on the palate, described as "grains of salt on a red background" and on the lacrimal caruncle.
   - They appear usually within 12–18 hours and disappear rapidly.
   - Koplik's spots begin to slough when the exanthem appears.
   - The conjunctival inflammation and photophobia may suggest measles before Koplik spots appear. In particular, a **transverse line of conjunctival inflammation,** sharply demarcated **along the eyelid margin,** may be of diagnostic assistance in the prodromal stage.
3. **Final stage with a maculopapular rash (exanthem) (Fig. 4.10B) accompanied by high fever.**
   - Usually starts as faint macules on the upper lateral parts of the neck, behind the ears along the hairline, posterior parts of the cheek.
   - Individual lesions become increasingly maculopapular as the rash spreads rapidly over the entire face, neck, upper arms, and upper part of the chest within approximately the first 24 hours.

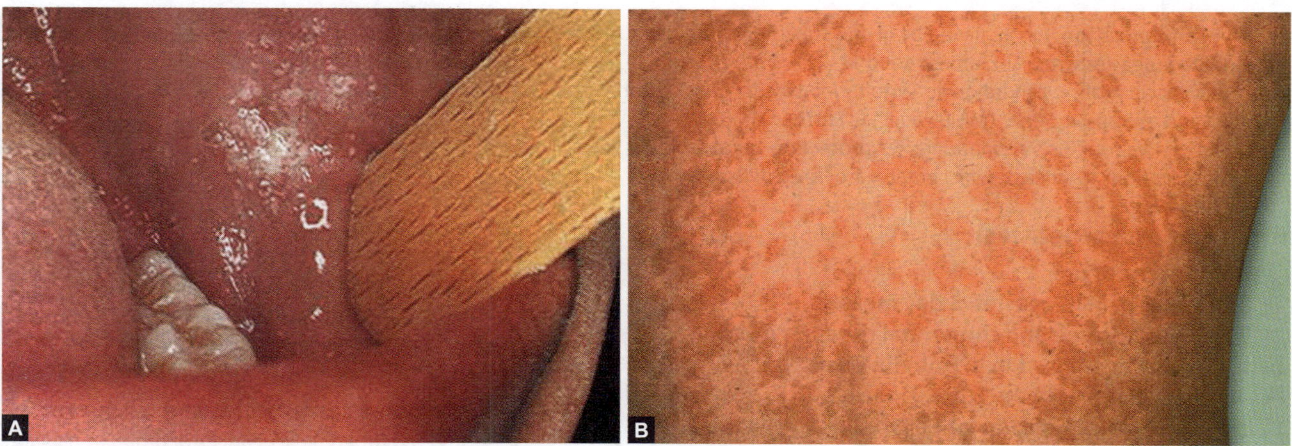

FIGS. 4.10A AND B: (A) Koplik spots—pathognomonic of measles which appears as grayish white dots on the buccal mucosa; (B) maculopapular rashes in measles.

- During the succeeding 24 hours, the rash spreads over the back, abdomen, entire arm, and thighs.
- As it finally reaches the feet on the second to third day, it begins to fade on the face. Associated lymphadenopathy, conjunctivitis, and pharyngitis.
- In hemorrhagic measles **(black measles),** bleeding may occur from the mouth, nose or bowel.
- **Complete absence of rash (modified measles) is rare** except:
  - In patients who have received immunoglobulin (Ig) during the incubation period.
  - In some patients with HIV infection.
  - Occasionally in infants younger than 9 months of age who have appreciable levels of maternal antibody.

Diagnosis

- Diagnosis is usually apparent from the characteristic clinical picture; laboratory confirmation is rarely needed.
- Testing for measles IgM antibodies is recommended in some situations. Measles IgM is detectable for 1 month alter illness, but sensitivity of IgM assays may be limited in the first 72 hours of the rash illness.

Complication (Table 4.17)

They are more common in older children and adults.

Treatment

There is **no specific antiviral therapy** and it is entirely **supportive.**

- **Antipyretics** (acetaminophen or ibuprofen) for fever
- **Bed rest**
- **Maintenance of an adequate fluid intake**
- **Vitamin A supplementation:** Recommended by the American Academy of Pediatrics for children:
  - From 6 months to 2 years of age who are hospitalized for measles and its complications.
  - Older than 6 months of age with measles and immunodeficiency.
  - Recommended regimen as a single dose of:
    - 100,000 IU orally for children 6 months to 1 year
    - 200,000 IU for children 1 year and above
    - Children with ophthalmologic evidence of vitamin A deficiency should be given additional doses the next day and 4 weeks later.
- **Treatment of secondary bacterial infections:** Prompt identification and treatment of secondary bacterial infections (with appropriate antibiotics).
- **Measles encephalitis:** Aerosolized and IV ribavirin may be useful.

Prevention

- **Passive immunization** with intramuscular injection of human normal immune globulin (0.25 mL/kg; maximum: 15 mL) is effective for prevention and attenuation of measles within 6 days of exposure. Indications for passive immunization are mentioned in **Table 4.18**.

TABLE 4.17: Complications of measles.
Due to virus replication
➢ Acute laryngotracheobronchitis (croup) in young children
➢ Giant-cell pneumonitis in immunocompromised children
Due to secondary bacterial infections
Common
➢ Otitis media
➢ Bronchitis
➢ Bronchopneumonia
➢ Gastroenteritis
Others
➢ Noma/cancrum oris
➢ Gangrenous stomatitis
➢ Diarrhea due to undernutrition
Less common
➢ Transient hepatitis
➢ Myocarditis
➢ Conjunctivitis
➢ Keratitis
➢ Corneal ulcers
Postinfectious: Rare CNS complications
➢ Early: Postmeasles encephalomyelitis
➢ Late: Measles inclusion body encephalitis (MIBE) and subacute sclerosing panencephalitis (SSPE)
Others
➢ Guillain–Barré syndrome
➢ Hemiplegia
➢ Cerebral thrombophlebitis
➢ Retrobulbar neuritis
➢ Exacerbate underlying *Mycobacterium tuberculosis*
➢ Measles pneumonia in HIV-infected patients is often fatal

- **Active immunization:** It is achieved by giving subcutaneous injection live attenuated measles virus. All children aged 12–15 months should be given measles vaccination. It can be given simultaneously in combination with rubella and mumps vaccines (MMR vaccine). Further MMR dose is given at the age of 4 years. This vaccination offer protection for at least 15 years. Contraindications for measles vaccination are listed in **Box 4.8**.

TABLE 4.18: Indications for passive immunization.

- Prophylaxis for susceptible household and nosocomial contacts younger than 1 year of age
- Immunodeficient patients (including HIV infected persons previously immunized with live attenuated measles vaccine)
- Pregnant females
- If measles is diagnosed in a household member, to be given to all unimmunized children in the household
- Debilitated children, especially those with a malignant disease
- Patients with active tuberculosis

Box 4.8: Contraindications for measles vaccine.

- Pregnant women
- Children with primary immunodeficiency
- Untreated tuberculosis, cancer, or organ transplantation
- Those receiving long-term immunosuppressive therapy
- Severely immunocompromised HIV-infected children

Rubella (German Measles)

Q. Write short note on:
- **Rubella (German measles, 3 day measles)**
- **Rubella syndrome and congenital rubella syndrome**

Rubella is infection caused by a **Rubella virus** which is an enveloped RNA virus and member of the Togaviridae family. The name is derived from the Latin, meaning ***little red.***

- **Mode of spread via respiratory droplet infection:** Maximum infectivity from up to 10 days before the onset to 2 weeks after the onset of the rash.
- After an incubation period of 14–21 days, the primary symptom of rubella virus infection is the appearance of a rash (exanthema) on the face which spreads to the trunk and limbs and usually fades after three days.
- The skin manifestations are called **"blueberry muffin** lesions".

Clinical Features

Depends on age of the patient and divided into acquired and congenital rubella. Symptoms are mild or absent in children under 5 years.

1. **Acquired rubella**
   - **Prodromal or catarrhal phase:** Characterized by malaise, fever, headache, and mild conjunctivitis. Lymphadenopathy (particularly suboccipital and postauricular and posterior cervical lymph nodes) may be observed during the second week after exposure. **Forchheimer spots** (small petechial lesions on the soft palate) are suggestive but not diagnostic. Splenomegaly may be found.
   - **Eruptive or exanthematous phase:** Occurs within 7 days of the initial symptoms. Characterized by **pinkish red, macular rashes** first appear behind the ears and on the forehead and then spread downwards to the trunk and limbs. These rashes usually last for 2–3 days. May be associated with polyarthritis and generalized lymphadenopathy which may persist for 2 weeks.

   Complications are rare. These include secondary bacterial infection of lung, arthralgia (commoner in females), hemorrhagic manifestations due to thrombocytopenia and postinfectious encephalitis.
2. **Congenital rubella syndrome:** It is the most serious consequence of rubella virus infection of mother during first trimester pregnancy. **Box 4.9** lists the classical triad of congenital rubella syndrome.
   - **Mode of spread:** From the transplacental transmission of the virus from an infected mother to the fetus.
   - **Consequences (Table 4.19)**: The complications of rubella infection of the mother include miscarriage, fetal death, premature delivery or live birth with congenital defects. Infants infected with rubella virus in utero may have many defects. Most common are related to the eyes, ears, and heart. This combination of severe birth defects is known as congenital rubella syndrome.
     - **First trimester infections** lead to abnormalities in 85% of cases and greater damage to organs.
     - **Second trimester infections** lead to defects in 16%. > 20 weeks of pregnancy fetal defects are uncommon.
3. **Expanded rubella syndrome** additionally includes the following manifestations:
   - Hepatosplenomegaly
   - Thrombocytopenic purpura
   - Intrauterine growth retardation
   - Myocarditis
   - Interstitial pneumonia
   - Humoral and cellular immunodeficiency

Box 4.9: Classical triad of congenital rubella syndrome.

- Cataract
- Cardiac abnormalities
- Deafness

TABLE 4.19: Congenital malformations associated with rubella syndrome.
Congenital heart diseases: Patent ductus arteriosus, ventricular septal defect, and pulmonary stenosis
Eye diseases: Corneal clouding, cataracts, chorioretinitis, microphthalmia, and blindness
CNS: Mental retardation and microcephaly
Deafness
Others: Hepatosplenomegaly, myocarditis, interstitial pneumonia, and metaphyseal bone lesions

Diagnosis

Diagnosis is clinically made. However, laboratory diagnosis is needed especially in pregnancy.

- Detection of rubella specific IgM by ELISA in serum, confirmed by demonstration of IgG seroconversion (or a rising titer of IgG) in a serum taken 14 days later.
- Detection of viral genome in throat swabs (or oral fluid), urine and the products of conception (in the case of intrauterine infection).

Treatment

- No specific therapy is available.
- Symptom based treatment is given for various manifestations, such as fever and arthralgia.

Prevention

- **Passive immunization:** Human immunoglobulin can reduce the symptoms but does not prevent the teratogenic effects.
- **Active immunization:** Active immunization is by giving live attenuated rubella vaccine.
  - Aim of vaccination: To reduce the frequency of infection and thereby decrease the chance of exposure to infection by susceptible pregnant females.
  - **Indications:** Should be given to all children at the age of 15 months along with mumps and measles vaccine (MMR vaccine). A second dose is given to young females between the age of 11–13 years and all seronegative females of child-bearing age.
  - **Contraindications:**
    - Contraindicated during pregnancy or if there is a likelihood of pregnancy within 3 months of immunization. It is because of likely risk of vaccine-virus induced fetal damage.
- Patients with immune deficiency diseases or those on immunosuppressive drugs.

Mumps

Q. Write short essay/note on mumps and its prevention.

- Mumps is an acute systemic viral infection caused by paramyxovirus (RNA virus) and is characterized by swelling of the parotid glands.
- **Mode of spread:** The virus is transmitted by the respiratory route (1) by droplet infection, (2) by direct contact or (3) through saliva and fomites. Humans are the only natural hosts of the mumps virus. The peak infectivity is 2–3 days before the onset of the parotitis and for 3 days afterwards.
- **Incubation period** is about 15–20 days (average 18 days).

Clinical Features

Q. Write short essay/note on clinical manifestations of mumps.

Primarily affects school-aged children and young adults (peaks at 5–9 years of age) and is uncommon before 2 years of age.

- **Prodromal symptoms:** Nonspecific and includes malaise, low-grade fever, myalgia, anorexia, headache, anorexia, and tenderness at the angle of the jaw.
- **Parotid gland enlargement:** Prodromal symptoms are followed by severe pain over the parotid glands due to parotitis. Parotitis produces either unilateral or bilateral parotid swelling (75% of cases). It is accompanied by obliteration of the space between the earlobe and the angle of the mandible. The chief complaints at this stage are difficulty in eating, swallowing and talking. Submandibular gland involvement is less frequent.

Diagnosis

- On the basis of the clinical features. In atypical cases diagnosis is confirmed by following investigations:
- **Serological test:** Demonstration of a mumps-specific IgM response in a blood or oral fluid during infection is diagnostic.
- **Demonstration virus:** Culture of virus or identification by genome (PCR) or antigen detection assays, from saliva, throat swab, urine and CSF.

Complications of Mumps (Table 4.20)

Q. Write short essay/note on complications of mumps.

Treatment

- Mumps is generally a benign and self-resolving illness.
- Treatment is symptom-based and supportive. Adequate nutrition and mouth care. Analgesics to relieve pain.

Prevention

MMR vaccine: To be given at the age of 15 months.

TABLE 4.20: Complications of mumps.

➤ Epididymo-orchitis (30%) in adults can lead to infertility
➤ Oophoritis
➤ Mumps pancreatitis
➤ Mumps meningitis (5–10%) and encephalitis. CSF reveals a lymphocytic pleocytosis
➤ Mumps myocarditis
➤ Others: Mastitis, hepatitis, polyarthritis, transient hearing loss, labyrinthitis, and electrocardiographic abnormalities
➤ Abortion (if infection occurs in the first trimester of pregnancy)
➤ Thrombocytopenic purpura

Herpes Viruses Infecting Humans

Q. Write short note on common herpes viruses infecting humans. Enumerate the diseases caused by them.

Herpes viruses are double-stranded DNA viruses. The various diseases caused by them are listed in **Table 4.21**.

TABLE 4.21: Disease caused by various herpes viruses in human beings.

Virus	*Diseases*
Herpes simplex	
➢ Type 1	Herpes labialis (herpes febrilis/cold sore—**Fig. 4.11A**), keratoconjunctivitis, dendritic corneal ulcer, pulp space infections (whitlows), encephalitis with temporal lobe involvement, genital herpes (40%), pneumonitis, tracheobronchitis, ulcerative stomatitis, and esophagitis
➢ Type 2	Genital herpes (60%) and neonatal infections
Cytomegalovirus	Congenital infections (intrauterine growth retardation), perinatal infections, infections in the immunocompromised patients (pneumonitis and retinitis)
Epstein–Barr virus (EBV)	Infectious mononucleosis, Burkitt's lymphoma, nasopharyngeal carcinoma, and hairy leukoplakia in AIDS patients
Varicella-zoster virus	Chickenpox and herpes-zoster (shingles)
Human herpes virus 6	Exanthem subitum (sixth disease) and roseola subitum-slapped cheek appearance **(Fig. 4.11B)**
Human herpes virus 7	Exanthem subitum (sixth disease)
Human herpes virus 8	Kaposi's sarcoma and multicentric Castleman's disease

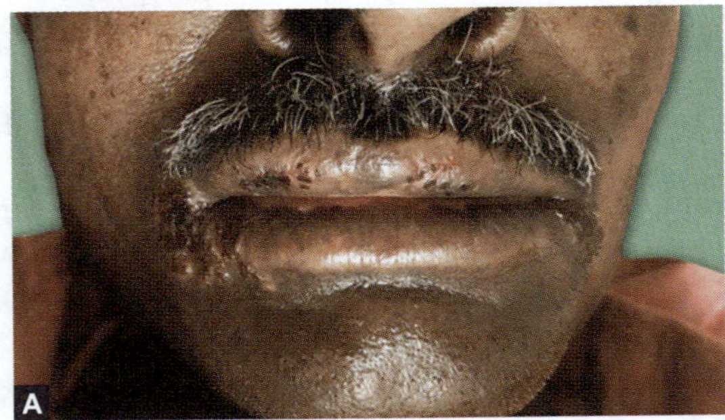
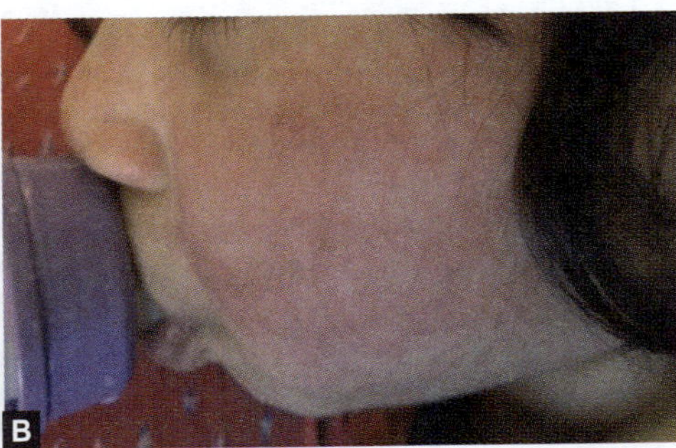

FIGS. 4.11A AND B: (A) Herpes labialis/febrilis caused by herpes simplex type 1 virus; (B) Roseola subitum-slapped cheek appearance in human herpes virus 6 infection.

Infectious Mononucleosis (Glandular Fever)

Q. Write short essay/note on etiology, clinical features, investigations, complications, and treatment of infectious mononucleosis (glandular fever).

Etiology

- Caused by Epstein–Barr virus (EBV). It is a herpes virus that infects and replicates in B lymphocytes in the submucosal lymphoid tissue of nasopharynx and oropharynx.
- **Age:** Peak incidence in 14–16 years for females and 16–18 years for males. Subclinical infection is very common.
- **Mode of transmission** is largely through saliva (e.g., kissing hence the nickname kissing disease).
- **Incubation period:** 7–10 days.

Clinical Features

- Usually presents with nonspecific prodromal symptoms followed by the classical triad of (1) fever, (2) severe pharyngitis, and tonsillitis, and (3) lymphadenopathy (particularly posterior cervical lymph node enlargement but sometimes generalized) and hepatosplenomegaly.
  Other features: Petechial rashes on palate and maculopapular skin rash, the latter develops in 90% of patients who have received ampicillin or amoxicillin (inappropriately) for the sore throat.
- **Gianotti–Crosti syndrome:** A symmetrical rash on the cheeks with, multiple erythematous papules, which may coalesce into plaques, and persists for 15–50 days.

Investigations

- **Peripheral blood smear:** In >90% of, two-thirds are **lymphocytes, 20–40% atypical lymphocytes.** The atypical lymphocytes are large with larger eccentric and folded nuclei with a lower nuclear-to-cytoplasm ratio.

- **Liver function tests: Raised liver enzymes**
- **Serological tests**
  - **Demonstration of heterophile antibodies:** The following tests will be useful for demonstration of heterophile antibodies.
- **Paul Bunnell test** is characteristically positive: Sheep red blood cells agglutinate in the presence of heterophile antibodies.
- **Monospot test** is a sensitive slide test: Horse red cells agglutinate on exposure to heterophile antibodies.
  - **Demonstration specific antibodies against EBV antigens:** These are demonstrated by ELISA.
- **Antibody** against viral capsid antigens (anti-VCA): These antibodies are initially of IgM type and later of IgG type (which persists for life).
- Antibodies to Epstein–Barr nuclear antigen (EBNA): This can be demonstrated by polymerase chain reaction (PCR).

Complications of EBV Infection

See **Table 4.22**.

EBV-associated Oncogenesis

See **Table 4.23**.

Treatment

- Infectious mononucleosis is usually a **self-limiting disease** and **majority requires no specific treatment** and recovery rapidly.
- **Symptomatic treatment** includes rest, acetaminophen, etc.
- Corticosteroids are indicated when there are neurological complications (e.g., meningitis, encephalitis, severe hemolysis, marked thrombocytopenia, and marked tonsillar enlargement causing respiratory obstruction.

TABLE 4.22: Complications of EBV infection.

- Chronic fatigue syndrome.
- Hematological complications:
  - Hemolytic anemia and thrombocytopenia
  - Aplastic anemia, thrombotic thrombocytopenic purpura of hemolytic-uremic syndrome, and disseminated intravascular coagulation (DIC)
- Glomerulonephritis, interstitial nephritis, hepatitis, myocarditis, and pericarditis
- Splenic rupture
- Cardiac: Myocarditis and pericarditis
- Hepatic: Reyes syndrome
- Skin: Ampicillin associated rash (Jarisch–Herxheimer reaction) and oral hairy leukoplakia
- Neurologic complications, e.g., meningitis, encephalitis, transverse myelitis, and Guillain–Barré (GB) syndrome
- Airway obstruction due to marked enlargement tonsils/severe pharyngeal edema

TABLE 4.23: EBV-associated oncogenesis.

Benign EBV-associated proliferations

- Oral hairy leukoplakia, primarily in adults with AIDS
- Lymphoid interstitial pneumonitis, in children with AIDS

Malignant EBV-associated proliferations

- Nasopharyngeal carcinoma
- Burkitt's lymphoma
- Hodgkin disease
- Lymphoproliferative disorders
- Leiomyosarcoma in immunodeficient including AIDS

Chickenpox (Varicella)

Q. Discuss the clinical features, complications, and management of chickenpox.

- Chickenpox is caused by ubiquitous and extremely contagious primary infection with varicella-zoster virus (also called as human herpes virus 3). It is usually a benign illness of childhood (5–9 years of age).
- Varicella zoster virus (VZV) is a dermotropic and neurotropic virus and is a member of the family *Herpesviridae*.
- It causes two distinct clinical entities: Varicella (chickenpox) and herpes zoster (shingles). Primary infection is chickenpox and usually occurs in childhood. The virus remains latent; which reactivate later in life giving rise to herpes zoster.

Mode of Transmission

- By droplet infection from the upper respiratory tract.
- Direct contact with discharge from ruptured lesions on the skin.

Humans are the only reservoirs of VZV. Chickenpox is contagious till pustules disappear.

- **Incubation period** is about 10–21 days.

Clinical Features

- **Distribution of skin lesions:** Chickenpox presents with characteristic rash on the second day of illness that first appears on the trunk followed by the face **(Fig. 4.12A)**, and finally on the limbs. Maximum lesions are found on the trunk and minimum on the periphery of the limbs (centripetal distribution).
- **Appearance of skin lesions:**
  - Rash appear first as **small pink macules** and **progress to papules, vesicles (Fig. 4.12B), and pustules within 24 hours.** Finally these lesions dry up and form scabs.
  - New lesions develop in crops every 2–4 days and each crop is associated with fever. Thus, lesions at all stages of development are seen in any area at the same time.
  - Infectivity lasts from up to 4 days before the lesions appear till the last vesicles crust over.
  - In immunocompromised patients the skin lesions are hemorrhagic and are numerous. Dissemination to other organs is quite common.
- Enanthem is rash/small spots on the mucous membranes **(Fig. 4.12C)** may also be seen.

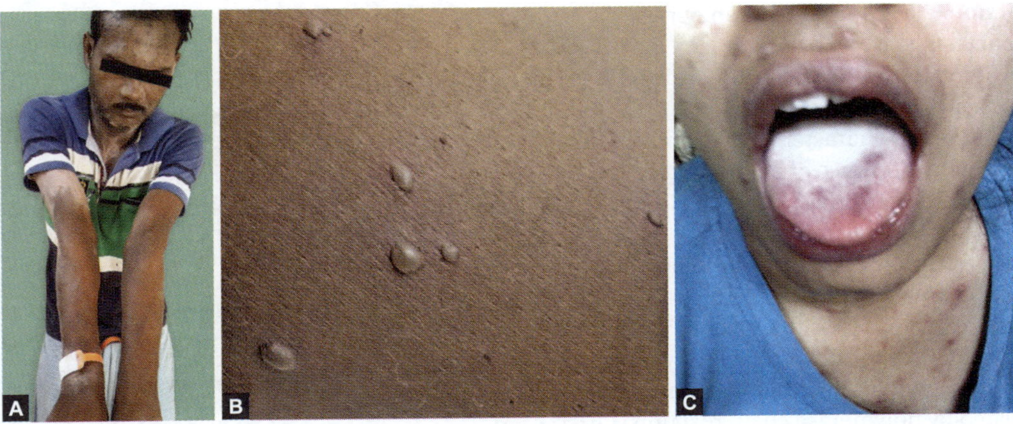

FIGS. 4.12A TO C: Lesions in chickenpox. (A) Involvement of face and body; (B) Vesicles; (C) Chickenpox exanthema (widespread) and enanthem (rash/small spots on the mucous membranes).

Complications of Chickenpox

See **Table 4.24**.

TABLE 4.24: Complications of chickenpox.

➢ Secondary bacterial infection of skin lesions ➢ CNS (rare) – Cerebellar ataxia – Encephalitis – Aseptic meningitis – Transverse myelitis – Guillain–Barré syndrome ➢ Varicella pneumonia (interstitial)	➢ Myocarditis ➢ Acute glomerulonephritis ➢ Corneal lesions ➢ Arthritis, osteomyelitis ➢ Bleeding diatheses ➢ Hepatitis ➢ Reye's syndrome with aspirin use ➢ Perinatal varicella ➢ Congenital varicella (extremely uncommon)

Q. Write short note on complications of chickenpox/varicella.

Diagnosis

- Mainly clinical, by recognition of the skin rash.
- If needed, it may be confirmed by:
  - Detection of antigen (direct immunofluorescence) or DNA (PCR) of fluid aspirated from vesicles.
  - Serology is used to identify seronegative individuals at risk of infection.
  - Isolation of virus by culture of vesicular fluid.
  - Tzanck smear: Prepared by scraping of the base of the vesicular lesion. It shows multinucleated giant cells and epithelial cells with eosinophilic intranuclear inclusion bodies. Its sensitivity is low (60%).

Q. Write short note on treatment of chickenpox/varicella.

Management

- No treatment is needed in majority of patients.
- Medical management of immunologically normal patient is by prevention of avoidable complications. These include good hygiene (daily bathing), meticulous skin care (to avoid secondary bacterial infection).
- Avoid aspirin use in children to prevent Reye's syndrome.
- Symptomatic treatment for itching/pruritus includes antihistamines and local calamine lotion.
- Secondary bacterial infection is managed with local antiseptic or systemic antibiotics (e.g., cloxacillin).

Antiviral Therapy

- Not required for uncomplicated primary VZV infection in children.
- **Drugs used:** Antiviral drugs that are used include acyclovir (15 mg/kg by mouth five times daily), valacyclovir (1 g three times daily) or famciclovir (250 mg three times daily) and famciclovir (500 mg TID) for 5–7 days.
- **Indications:** Though in healthy children, antiviral drugs may reduce the duration of disease when administered within 24 hours of symptoms. However, they are usually not recommended but are indicated in the following cases:
  - For uncomplicated chickenpox when the patient presents within 24–48 hours of onset of vesicles.
  - All patients with complications.
  - Immunocompromised patients and pregnant women, regardless of duration of vesicles. More severe disease in immunocompromised patients requires initial parenteral therapy. Immunocompromised patients may shed virus for a prolonged period and may require prolonged treatment.

Prevention

Three methods for the prevention of VZV infections are:

1. **Live attenuated vaccine:** It is given to prevent chickenpox in immunocompetent children and adults who are at a high risk of infection. It is contraindicated in pregnant or immunocompromised patients.

2. **Passive prophylaxis using zoster immune globulin (ZIG) or varicella-zoster immune globulin (VZIG):**
   - It may be given to individuals who are susceptible, those patients having high risk of severe disease or complication of chickenpox (e.g., immunocompromised, steroid treated or pregnant women with history of significant exposure). It should be given within 96 hours of exposure.
   - It is given prophylactically to newborn infants, infant whose mother develops chickenpox within 5 days before or within 48 hours after delivery.
3. **Antiviral therapy:** As prophylaxis to individuals at high risk and not eligible for vaccine or after 96 hours of exposure. They significantly reduce the severity of disease if not completely preventive.

Shingles (Herpes Zoster)

Q. Write short essay on clinical features, diagnosis, and management of herpes zoster.

Initial infection with VZV produces chickenpox. After this initial infection, VZV persists in latent form in the dorsal root ganglion of sensory nerves or cranial nerve ganglia. Shingles arises from the reactivation of his latent virus later in life.

Clinical Features

- **Age:** It may occur at any age but most common in the elderly.
- **Skin lesions:** The onset of the skin rash is usually preceded (3–4 days before discrete vesicles occur in the skin) by severe pain **(burning discomfort)** in the affected dermatome. Though **rash is similar to chickenpox,** classically they are unilateral and restricted to a sensory nerve (i.e., dermatomal) distribution **(Fig. 4.13A)**. This is associated with a brief dissemination of virus causing viremia and can produce distant satellite "chickenpox" lesions. Virus is from freshly formed vesicles may also cause chickenpox in susceptible contacts. Chickenpox may be contracted from a patient suffering from shingles but not vice versa. Occasionally, paresthesia may develop without rash ("zoster sine herpete").
- **Dermatome involved:** Most commonly involves **thoracic dermatomes or ophthalmic division of the trigeminal nerve** (vesicles may develop on the cornea and can produce corneal ulceration leading to blindness). Bowel and bladder dysfunction may develop with sacral nerve root involvement. Occasionally it may cause cranial nerve palsy, myelitis or encephalitis.

Complications of Shingles (Herpes Zoster)

Q. Write short note on complications of herpes zoster.

- **Herpes zoster ophthalmicus,** leading to loss of vision
- **Ramsay Hunt syndrome (Fig. 4.13B):** It develops due to geniculate ganglion involvement and characterized by involvement of cranial nerves (V and VII). A triad of (1) ipsilateral facial paralysis/palsy (ipsilateral loss of taste and buccal ulceration), (2) ear pain, and (3) vesicles/rashes in the external auditory canal and auricle is seen. It may be mistaken for Bell's palsy.
- **Postherpetic neuralgia is seen in** 10–15% of people with shingles. It results in troublesome persistent pain for 1–6 months or longer, following healing of the skin rash. It is more common in elderly patients.
- **Granulomatous cerebral angiitis** is a cerebrovascular complication. It leads to a stroke-like syndrome in patients with shingles, especially in an ophthalmic distribution.

Q. Write short note on drugs used for the treatment of herpes zoster.

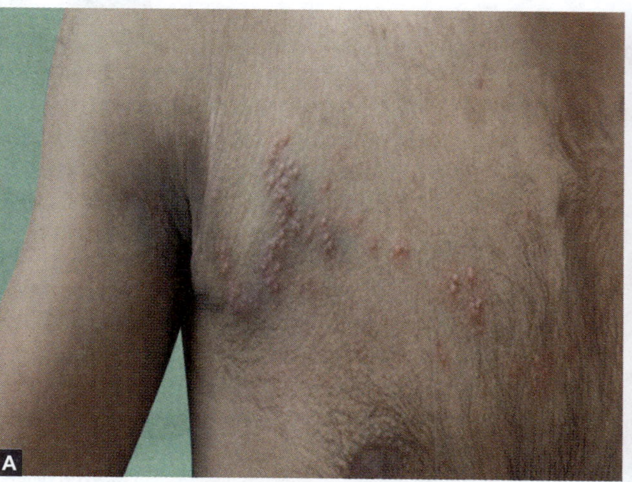

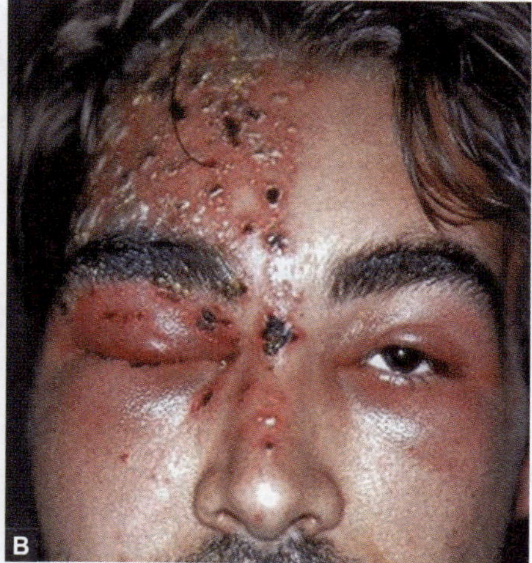

FIGS. 4.13A AND B: (A) Herpes zoster—dermatomal involvement; (B) Ramsay Hunt syndrome.

Management
- **Early therapy with acyclovir or related agents** reduce both early- and late-onset pain, especially in patients above 65 years.
- **Postherpetic neuralgia: Analgesics** along **with amitriptyline** 25–100 mg daily or gabapentin (start with 300 mg daily and slowly increasing to 300 mg twice daily or more). **Capsaicin cream** (0.075%) may be of some help.

Human Papillomaviruses

Q. Write short note on human papillomavirus.

Human papillomavirus (HPV) is a nonenveloped, double-stranded DNA virus with strong tropism for stratified squamous epithelial cells of skin and mucous membranes.

Types of HPV

- **High-risk types** cause dysplastic lesions and invasive carcinoma in the cervix (e.g., HPV-16 and HPV-18).
- **Low-risk types** are responsible for condylomata acuminata (genital wart) and low-grade cervical lesions (e.g., HPV-6 and HPV-11).

Mode of Infection

- Direct contact: Usually mode of infection via direct contact with skin or mucous membrane lesion.
- Sexual contact: Anogenital HPV are usually transmitted sexually. Most important risk factor is number of sexual partners.
- Autoinoculation
- **Incubation period** for genital HPV varies from weeks to months.

Lesions/Diseases Caused by HPV (Table 4.25)

Majority of HPV infections are subclinical and about 80% resolves spontaneously within 12 months.

TABLE 4.25: Lesions/diseases caused by HPV.

Verrucae plantaris ➢ Sites: hands (verrucae palmaris) and feet (verrucae plantaris) ➢ Color: Skin colored ➢ Nature: Flat or dome-shaped papules, surface rough and hyperkeratotic ➢ Usually asymptomatic	**Anogenital malignancies:** Caused by high-risk HPV ➢ Intraepithelial neoplasms: Cervix, vulva, vagina, anus, and penis ➢ Penile carcinoma ➢ Cervical carcinoma: Squamous cell carcinoma
Verrucae plana ➢ Sites: Mainly face, hands or distal forearms ➢ Nature: Flat, reddish or skin-colored papules	**Oral lesions:** Asymptomatic or cause papilloma **Head and neck cancers:** Sites: Oropharynx, tonsils, base of tongue, and soft palate
Condyloma acuminatum ➢ Cause: Low risk HPV ➢ Sites: External **(Fig. 4.14)** or internal genitalia, perianal, the anal canal, and perineum ➢ Nature: Multiple, flat or raised exophytic papillomas, may be with pedicle or broad based, usually self-limited	**Periungual warts** Site: At nail fold; often painful **Skin cancers** (squamous cell carcinoma and basal cell carcinoma) ➢ HPV may act synergistically with ultraviolet light ➢ Usually not caused by high-risk HPV

Diagnosis

- On clinical presentation and appearance.
- **Biopsy:** Necessary to confirm dysplasia or carcinoma.
- **Acetic acid test:** HPV infections can be visualized after application of 3–5% acetic acid with a cotton swab. HPV-positive lesions appear white within 5 minutes.
- **Endoscopic examination (colposcopy and proctoscopy):** To visualize condyloma, dysplasia, and carcinomas.
- **Molecular methods:** To detect HPV viral DNA (e.g., hybrid capture two DNA test).
- PCR to detect HPV viral DNA.

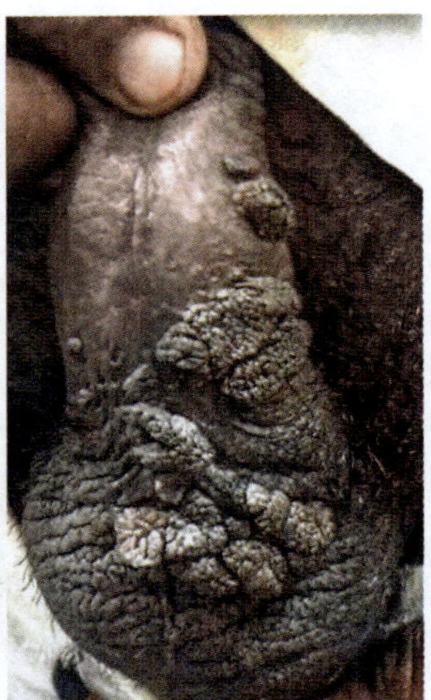

FIG. 4.14: Condyloma acuminatum on the external genitalia of male.

Treatment/Therapy

No specific antiviral treatment available

- **Verrucae**
  - **Keratolysis:** Mechanical removal with a sharp knife and application of salicylic acid: lactic acid: collodion (1:1:4). Vaseline is applied to the surrounding normal skin to prevent its corrosion by chemicals.
  - **Cryotherapy:** Liquid nitrogen is used to freeze warts.
- **Anogenital warts**
  - **Podophyllotoxin:** Application causes death of infected cells. It is applied by patient himself at home twice/day for 3 consecutive days in cycles of several weeks. Serious systemic side effects can develop if it is applied to large areas and absorbed systemically. It is contraindicated during pregnancy.

- **Imiquimod:** Induces the production of antiviral cytokines (e.g., interferon and tumor necrosis factor-α). A 5% cream to be applied thrice weekly for up to 4 months.
- **Ablation:** Either by surgery, laser, and electrocauterization.
- **Cryotherapy** by using liquid nitrogen.
- **Trichloroacetic acid:** Topical application of 50–90% trichloroacetic acid produces coagulation of cell protein and cell death.
- **5-Fluorouracil** can be applied as cream.

HPV Vaccines

- HPV vaccines induce high titers of antibodies which can neutralize infectious viruses. They can prevent about 70% of cervical dysplasias (which can progress to cancer if not treated).
- Types of HPV vaccines: Quadrivalent vaccine and bivalent vaccine.

TABLE 4.26: Examples of diseases caused by arthropod-borne.

Family	Common diseases	Family	Common diseases
Arenaviridae	➢ Lymphocytic choriomeningitis ➢ Lassa fever ➢ Arenaviruses	Flaviviridae	**Mosquito-borne:** ➢ Japanese encephalitis ➢ West Nile encephalitis ➢ Saint Louis encephalitis ➢ Yellow fever ➢ Dengue fever **Tick borne:** Kyasanur forest disease (KFD) **Direct contact:** Ebola disease
Bunyaviridae	➢ California encephalitis ➢ Rift Valley fever ➢ Sandfly fever ➢ Crimean–Congo hemorrhagic fever ➢ Hanta virus—hemorrhagic fever with renal/cardio-pulmonary syndrome	Togaviridae	➢ Chikungunya disease ➢ Sindbis disease ➢ Eastern equine encephalitis ➢ Western equine encephalitis ➢ Venezuelan encephalitis

Arthropod-Borne Viruses (Arboviruses)

Q. Write short essay/note on:

- **Classification of arboviruses**
- **Major clinical syndromes caused by arboviruses**

Arthropod-borne viruses are called as arboviruses. Diseases caused by arboviruses are listed in **Table 4.26** and manifestations of a few diseases are listed in **Table 4.27**.

TABLE 4.27: A few diseases caused by arbovirus and their manifestation.

	Flu-like syndrome	Encephalitis	Hepatitis	Hemorrhage	Shock
Dengue	+		+	+	+
Yellow fever	+		+	+	+
Saint Louis encephalitis	+	+			
West Nile encephalitis	+	+			
Venezuelan encephalitis	+	+			
Western equine encephalitis	+	+			
Eastern equine encephalitis	+	+			
Japanese encephalitis	+	+			

+ = Present; – = Absent

Dengue

Q. Describe classic dengue (break bone fever), dengue hemorrhagic fever (DHF), and dengue shock syndrome (DSS).

Q. Write short essay on the clinical features, diagnosis, and management of dengue hemorrhagic fever.

Dengue is the most rapidly spreading febrile illness caused by flavivirus and transmitted by mosquitoes. It is the most common arthropod-borne viral infection in humans in the world.

Source of Infection

Humans suffering from dengue are main amplifying host of the virus and infective during the first 3 days of the illness (the viremic stage). About 2 weeks after feeding (day time) on an infected individual, mosquitoes become infective and remain so for life. Dengue is usually endemic.

Mode of Transmission

All are transmitted by the daytime *Aedes* mosquito biting. *Aedes aegypti* is the most common mosquito involved in transmission which breeds in stagnant water (e.g., collections of water in containers, water-based air coolers, and tire dumps).
Incubation period: 4–10 days following the mosquito bite.

Classification of Dengue

WHO (2008) classification of dengue

WHO (2008) classifies dengue into nonsevere dengue (with and without warning signs) and severe dengue, the criteria for the same is presented in **Figure 4.13**. Even nonsevere dengue patients without warning signs may develop severe dengue. **WHO (2016) has revised the** classification and is presented in **Table 4.28** and **Figure 4.15**.

*Consequences of dengue virus infection are presented in **Flowchart 4.1**. Presently, expanded dengue has been defined and its features are presented in **Flowchart 4.2**.*

TABLE 4.28: WHO classification of dengue infections and grading of severity of DHF (2016).

DF/DHF	*Grade*	*Signs and symptoms*	*Laboratory*
DF		Fever with two of the following: ➢ Headache ➢ Retro-orbital pain ➢ Myalgia ➢ Arthralgia/bone pain ➢ Rash ➢ Hemorrhagic manifestations ➢ No evidence of plasma leakage	➢ Leukopenia (WBC <5,000 cells/mm³) ➢ Thrombocytopenia (platelet count <150,000 cells/mm³) ➢ Rising hematocrit (Hct) (5–10%) ➢ No evidence of plasma loss
DHF	I	Fever and hemorrhagic manifestation (positive tourniquet test) and evidence of plasma leakage	Thrombocytopenia <100,000 cells/mm³; Hct rise >20%
DHF	II	As in Grade I plus spontaneous bleeding	Thrombocytopenia <100,000 cells/mm³; Hct rise >20%
DHF*	III	As in Grade I or II plus circulatory failure (weak pulse, narrow pulse pressure (≤20 mm Hg), hypotension, restlessness)	Thrombocytopenia <100,000 cells/mm³; Hct rise ≥20%
DHF*	IV	As in Grade III plus profound shock with undetectable BP and pulse	Thrombocytopenia <100,000 cells/mm³; Hct rise ≥20%

Source: WHO. (1997). Dengue haemorrhagic fever: diagnosis, treatment, prevention and control. [online] Available from http://www.who.int/csr/resources/publications/dengue/Denguepublication/en/. [Last accessed December 2020].

(DHF: dengue hemorrhagic fever; Hct: hematocrit)

* DHF III and IV are DSS = Dengue shock syndrome.

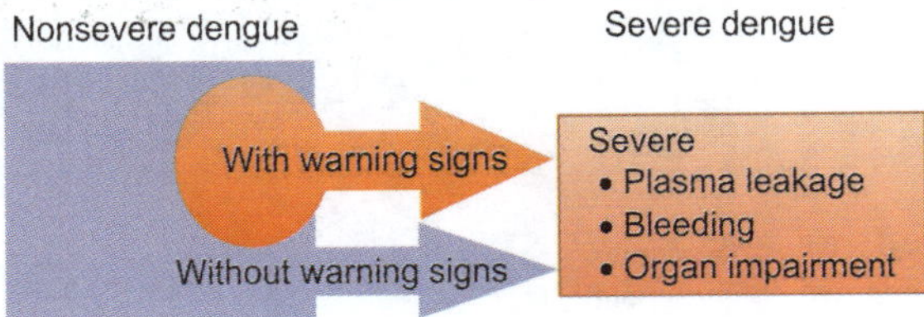

Criteria for nonsevere dengue		Criteria for severe dengue
Without warning signs	With warning signs	
Probable dengue • Live in/travel to endemic area • Fever and two of the following criteria: - Nausea, vomiting - Rash - Aches and pains - Tourniquet test positive - Leukopenia - Any warning sign **Laboratory—confirmed dengue** (important when no sign of plasma leakage)	**Warning signs** (requires strict observation and medical intervention) • Abdominal pain or tenderness • Persistent vomiting • Clinical fluid accumulation • Mucosal bleed • Lethargy, restlessness • Liver enlargement >2 cm • Laboratory: Increase in hematocrit concurrent with rapid decrease in platelet count	• **Severe plasma leakage** leading to - Shock (DSS) - Fluid accumulation with respiratory distress • **Severe bleeding** as evaluated by clinician • **Severe organ involvement** - Liver: AST or ALT ≥1000 - CNS: Impaired consciousness - Heart and other organs

FIG. 4.15: WHO (2008) classification and levels of severity in dengue case.

FLOWCHART 4.1: Manifestations of dengue infection.

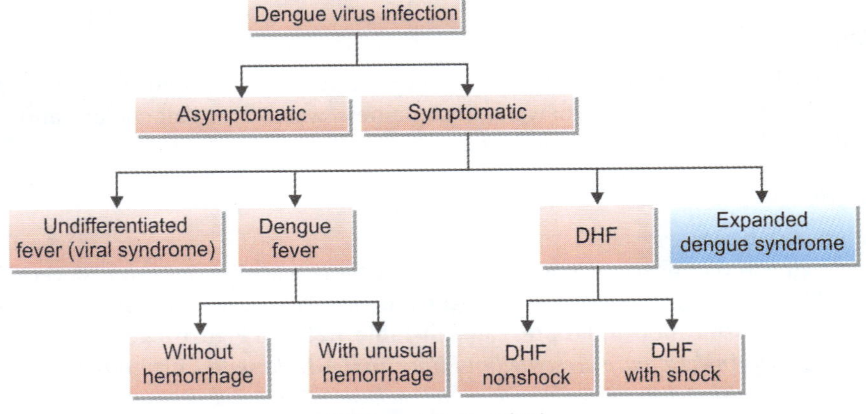

(DHF: dengue hemorrhagic fever)

FLOWCHART 4.2: Expanded dengue syndrome.

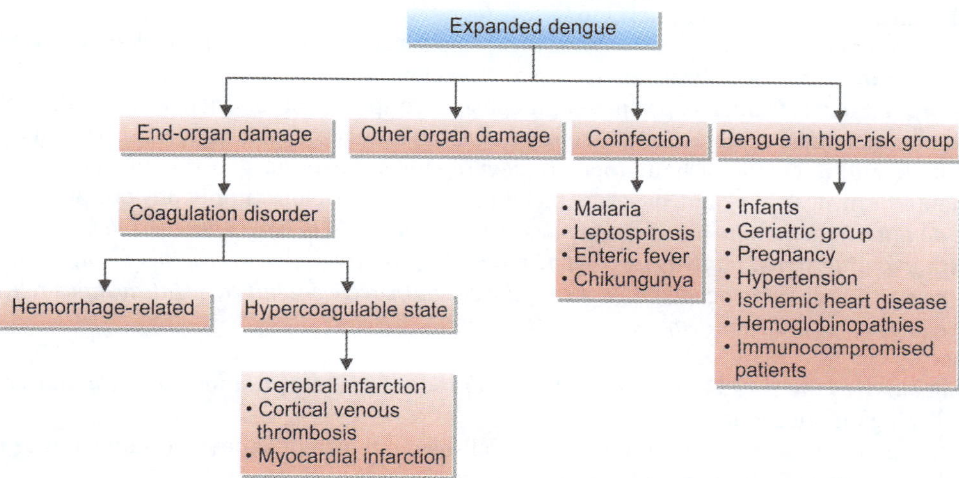

Pathogenesis of Severe Dengue

- Severe dengue is characterized by plasma leakage, hemoconcentration, bleeding, and organ impairment.
- **Plasma leakage:** The cause of plasma leakage probably due to functional endothelial cell activation/dysfunction. The endothelial cell dysfunction in turn may be mediated by activation of infected monocytes and T cells, the complement system and mediators, monokines, cytokines, and soluble receptors.
- **Bleeding**: It may due to thrombocytopenia and associated platelet dysfunction or disseminated intravascular coagulation. Thrombocytopenia may be due to increased destruction or consumption (peripheral sequestration and consumption).

Clinical Features

Dengue is a systemic and dynamic disease. It has a wide clinical spectrum and includes both severe and nonsevere clinical manifestations. Asymptomatic infections are common (especially in children), but it is more severe in infants and the elderly.

Phases of Dengue

After the incubation period, dengue begins abruptly and is followed by the three phases: (1) febrile, (2) critical, and (3) recovery.

1. **Febrile phase**
   - Characterized by the abrupt onset of **high-grade fever** and this phase last for 2–7 days. Fever may be continuous or saddle-back (see below).
   - It often accompanied by **facial flushing, skin erythema, generalized body ache ("break-bone fever"), myalgia, arthralgia, malaise, headache retrobulbar pain** (worsens on eye movements), **severe backache** (which is a prominent symptom), **anorexia, nausea, and vomiting.** Some may have sore throat (pharyngitis), upper respiratory tract symptoms, and conjunctival suffusion. In children, high fever may produce febrile convulsions/seizures.
   - **Saddle-back fever:** In few cases fever subsides and other symptoms disappear after 3–4 days. This remission may last for 2 days and then the fever returns together with others symptoms but milder. This biphasic or "saddle-back" pattern is considered characteristic of dengue.
   - **Mild hemorrhagic manifestations,** such as petechiae and mucosal membrane bleeding (e.g., nose and gums) may be found.
   - Liver is often enlarged and tender.

   Laboratory findings
   - The earliest laboratory abnormality which has a high probability of dengue is a **progressive decrease in total white cell count.**
   - **Tourniquet test (Hess test)**
     - Sphygmomanometer (blood pressure) cuff is tied to the upper arm above the elbow and mark a circle of 5 cm diameter on the flexor aspect of forearm.
     - The cuff is inflated to 80 mm for 5 minutes.
     - Measure the number of petechiae present in the circle (already marked). A test is considered positive when 20 or more petechiae appear in the circle.
2. **Critical phase**
   - Around the time of falling (defervescence = the period of abatement of fever) of fever (usually on days 3–7 of illness), an **increase in capillary permeability** along with **increase of hematocrit** levels may occur. This marks beginning of critical phase.

- **Consequences of plasma leakage are:**
  - **Pleural effusion** and **ascites** may develop.
  - **Shock** occurs when there is a critical volume of plasma leakage and is often preceded by warning signs.
  - **Body temperature** may be **subnormal** when shock occurs.
  - **Organ impairment:** If shock is prolonged, it causes hypoperfusion of organs and leads to progressive organ impairment, metabolic acidosis, and disseminated intravascular coagulation (DIC). This in turn leads to severe hemorrhage and decrease of hematocrit in severe shock. Severe organ impairment (i.e., severe hepatitis, encephalitis or myocarditis) and/or severe bleeding may also develop without obvious plasma leakage or shock.
- ***Nonsevere dengue:*** *Patients who improve after defervescence are said to have nonsevere dengue.*
- ***Dengue with warning signs:*** *Patients who deteriorate will manifest with warning signs and are said to have dengue with warning signs. Cases of dengue with warning signs usually recover with early intravenous rehydration. However, some cases will progress to severe dengue.*

3. **Recovery phase**
   - If the patient survives the 24–48 hour critical phase, a **gradual reabsorption of extravascular compartment fluid** takes place during the subsequent 48–72 hours.
   - It is characterized by **improvement** in the general well-being, return of appetite, disappearance of gastrointestinal symptoms, stabilization of hemodynamic status, and diuresis.
   - **Other features:** Some patients may develop a rash of "isles of white in the sea of red", and some may complain of generalized pruritus (particularly on hands and feet).
   - **Findings**
     - Bradycardia and electrocardiographic changes are common.
     - **Hematocrit** stabilizes or may be low due to the dilutional effect of reabsorbed extracellular fluid (which leaked due to increased vascular permeability).
     - **White blood cell count:** Usually begins to rise soon after defervescence.
     - **Platelet count** recovery is later than that of white blood cell count.
   - **Consequences of excessive intravenous fluids:** If excessive intravenous fluids are administered, massive pleural effusion and ascites may develop leading **to respiratory distress.** During any phase (critical and/or recovery phases), excessive fluid therapy may cause **pulmonary edema** or **congestive heart failure.**
   - The various clinical problems during the different phases of dengue are presented in **Table 4.29**.

TABLE 4.29: Clinical problems during the different phases of dengue.

Phase	*Clinical problems*
Febrile	Dehydration; high fever may cause febrile seizures in young children
Critical	Shock from plasma leakage; severe bleeding; and organ impairment
Recovery	Hypervolemia (only with excessive intravenous fluid therapy)

Severe Dengue

Q. Write short note/essay on dengue shock syndrome.

According to WHO, severe dengue **(Fig. 4.15)** is defined by one or more of the following:
1. Plasma leakage that may lead to shock (dengue shock) and/or fluid accumulation, with or without respiratory distress
2. Severe bleeding
3. Severe organ impairment

Mechanism of severe dengue

Dengue shock

- **Time of occurrence:** Usually develops around defervescence on day **4 or 5 (range 3–7 days) of illness.** It is preceded by the warning signs.
- **Mechanism of shock:** In dengue, **progression of increased vascular permeability** (due to endothelial dysfunction) leads to worsening of **hypovolemia** and results in shock.
- **Consequences:** Initially compensatory mechanisms try to correct the process, but once they fail it goes into the decompensatory phase and organ dysfunction sets in.
  - Severe dengue may be associated with coagulation abnormalities, but they are not sufficient to cause major bleeding. When major **bleeding** develops, it is always associated with profound shock, **hypotension, thrombocytopenia, hypoxia, and acidosis.** They can lead to multiple organ failure and advanced **disseminated intravascular coagulation.**
- Most deaths occur in patients with profound shock complicated by fluid overload. Complications of dengue are listed in **Box 4.10.**

Box 4.10: Complications of dengue.

- Dengue hemorrhagic fever, disseminated intravascular coagulation (DIC), hemophagocytic lymphohistiocytosis (HLH)
- Dengue shock syndrome, polyserositis acalculous cholecystitis, and acute pancreatitis
- Cerebral hemorrhage or edema, cranial nerve palsies, rhabdomyolysis, and hemolytic uremic syndrome
- Hepatitis, encephalitis, myocarditis, aseptic meningitis, GB syndrome, cortical venous thrombosis, pericarditis, atrial fibrillation, heart blocks, and cardiomyopathy
- Vertical transmission (if infection occurs within 5 weeks of delivery).

Diagnosis

Q. Write short note on diagnosis of dengue fever.

- **Blood:** Increasing hemoglobin and hematocrit, leukopenia, thrombocytopenia, and raised live enzymes (AST or ALT).
- **Isolation of** dengue **virus** from the blood (within first 5 days of onset of symptoms) by tissue culture.
- **Detection of dengue virus RNA** by molecular methods like RT-PCR or nucleic acid sequence base amplification (NASBA) during the first few days of illness is diagnostic.
- **Detection of serum NS1 antigen** by enzyme-linked immunosorbent assay (ELISA) is highly specific but **less sensitive** than PCR. It is positive early in the course of illness.
- **Detection of virus specific IgM antibodies** or of rising IgG titers in sequential serum samples (start after 5 days of onset).
- **In severe dengue:** Chest radiograph to look for pleural effusion, and ultrasound abdomen for ascites.

Q. Write short essay on management of dengue fever.

Stepwise Approach to the Management of Dengue

At the first levels of care a stepwise approach should be applied as mentioned in **Table 4.30.**

Step I: Overall assessment

See **Table 4.31**.

Step II: Diagnosis, assessment of disease phase and severity

On the basis of step I determine
- Whether the disease is likely to be dengue
- If dengue, which phase (febrile, critical or recovery)
- Whether there are warning signs
- Hydration and hemodynamic status of the patient
- Whether the patient requires admission.

Step III: Management

Treatment of group A patients (Can be managed at home)

Criteria for group A
- Patients who are able to tolerate adequate volumes of oral fluids and pass urine at least once every 6 hours.
- Do not have any of the warning signs, particularly when fever subsides.

Strategies to be followed:
- Daily review of patients for disease progression (decreasing white blood cell count, defervescence, and warning signs).
- **Treatment plan:**
  - **Fluid intake:** Encourage intake oral rehydration solution (ORS), fruit juice, and other fluids containing electrolytes and sugar to replace losses from fever and vomiting.
  - **Control of fever:** Paracetamol for high fever and if patient is uncomfortable. Tepid sponge if fever is still high. Avoid use of NSAIDs (may aggravate gastritis or bleeding) and aspirin (may develop Reye's syndrome).
  - **To be brought to hospital immediately** if no clinical improvement or bleeding manifestations develop.

TABLE 4.30: A stepwise approach to the management of dengue (WHO).

Step I. Overall assessment
Step II. Diagnosis, assessment of disease phase and severity
Step III. Management ➢ Management decisions: Depending on the clinical manifestations and other circumstances, patients may: – be sent home (Group A); – be referred for in-hospital management (Group B); – require emergency treatment and urgent referral (Group C).

TABLE 4.31: Step I—overall assessment.

History	***Physical examination***
➢ Date of onset of fever/illness ➢ Quantity of oral intake ➢ Assessment for warning signs ➢ Diarrhea ➢ Change in mental state, seizure, and dizziness ➢ Urine output (frequency, volume, and time of last voiding) ➢ Other important relevant histories including coexisting conditions	➢ Mental state ➢ Hydration status ➢ Hemodynamic status ➢ Tachypnea, acidotic breathing, and pleural effusion ➢ Abdominal tenderness, hepatomegaly, and ascites ➢ Rash and bleeding manifestations ➢ Tourniquet test (Hess test)
Investigations	
➢ Complete blood count. ➢ Hematocrit in early febrile phase, establishes baseline, the patient's own hematocrit. ➢ Rapid decrease of white blood cell count makes dengue very likely. ➢ Rapid decrease in platelet count along with a rising hematocrit compared to the baseline is suggestive of progress to the plasma leakage/critical phase of disease. ➢ Other tests include liver function tests (LFT), blood glucose, serum electrolytes, urea and creatinine, bicarbonate or lactate, cardiac enzymes, ECG, and urine specific gravity. A low serum albumin, high ferritin, and a raised CRP (C-reactive protein) are indicative of progress to severe dengue. Laboratory tests are performed to confirm the diagnosis. However, it is not necessary for the acute management of dengue.	

Treatment of group B patients

Patients may require hospital management for close observation, particularly as they approach the critical phase.

Criteria for group B patients: These include patients with:
- Warning signs
- Coexisting conditions (e.g., pregnancy, infancy, old age, obesity, diabetes mellitus, renal failure, and chronic hemolytic diseases) that may make dengue or its management more complicated.
- Certain social circumstances (such as living alone or living far from a health facility without reliable means of transport).

Treatment plan: Obtain the reference **hematocrit** before the start of fluid therapy.

Intravenous fluid:
- **Give only isotonic solutions** such as normal (0.9%) saline or Ringer's lactate.
- Start with 5–7 mL/kg/hour for 1–2 hours, then reduce to 3–5 mL/kg/hour for 2–4 hours, and then reduce to 2–3 mL/kg/hour or less according to the clinical response.

- **Reassess clinical status** and **repeat hematocrit.**
- If hematocrit remains the same or rises only minimally, continue with the same rate (2–3 mL/kg/hour) for another 2–4 hours.
- If vital signs are worsening and hematocrit is rising rapidly, increase rate to 5–10 mL/kg/hour for 1–2 hours.
- Reassess clinical status, repeat hematocrit and review fluid infusion rates accordingly.
- Monitor hematocrit, platelet count, creatinine, electrolytes, and liver function tests.

Treatment of group C patients

Criteria for group C patients: These patients require emergency treatment and urgent referral when they are in the critical phase of disease or have severe dengue. The criteria include patients with **severe:**

- Plasma leakage leading to dengue shock and/or fluid accumulation with respiratory distress.
- Hemorrhages
- Organ impairment (hepatic damage, renal impairment, cardiomyopathy, encephalopathy or encephalitis)

Treatment plan: All patients with severe dengue should be admitted to a hospital with intensive care facilities and blood transfusion.

Intravenous fluid: Judicious intravenous fluid resuscitation is the essential and usually sole intervention required.

- **Replacement of plasma losses** should be immediate and rapid with isotonic crystalloid solution or, in the case of hypotensive shock by colloid solutions. If possible, obtain hematocrit levels before and after fluid resuscitation.

Treatment of shock

- Start intravenous fluid resuscitation with isotonic crystalloid solutions at 5–10 mL/kg/hour over 1 hour. Then reassess the patient's condition (vital signs, capillary refill time, hematocrit, and urine output).
- If no improvement or shock worsens, fluid infusion rate can be increased. Vasopressors and inotropes need to be added.

Treatment of hemorrhagic complications

- Avoid intramuscular injections.
- NSAIDs, antiplatelet agents, and anticoagulants to be withheld temporarily.
- Platelets transfusion if platelet count drops below 10,000/mm^3 or patient develops bleeding manifestations.
- If coagulopathy present, transfuse plasma. Pack red cell transfusion if hemoglobin drops below 8 g%. Steroids indicated if hemophagocytosis is diagnosed.

Management of complications appropriately prevention of dengue infections

Prevention or reduction of dengue virus transmission depends on control of the mosquito vectors or interruption of human-vector contact.

- **Control of the mosquito vectors**
- **Interruption of human-vector contact**
- Currently, no vaccine or antiviral drug against dengue viral infections is available.

Chikungunya

Q. Write short essay/note on chikungunya.

- Chikungunya is a viral fever caused by an *Alphavirus*.
- It is usually not fatal. However during 2005–2006 outbreak occurred in India, where more than 200 deaths were reported mainly related to CNS involvement and fulminant hepatitis.
- Chikungunya (in Swahili of African dialect) means "that bends up". It was used in reference to the stooped posture developed due to the arthritic symptoms of the disease.

Mode of spread: By bites from *Aedes aegypti* mosquitoes.

Source of infection: Humans are the major reservoir of chikungunya virus.

Incubation period: 2–12 days.

Epidemiology: Observed in Tamil Nadu, Karnataka, Kerala, Andhra Pradesh, Rajasthan, Gujarat, and Madhya Pradesh. Significant numbers of cases have been reported from northern India including Delhi.

Clinical Features

Symptoms

- **Fever** (often severe): The fever usually lasts for 2–5 days and may be followed by an afebrile phase and then reappearance of fever **(saddleback pattern).**
- **Maculopapular rash:** Skin involvement is more common in children and occurs about 40–50% of cases. It may appear at the beginning or several days (day 2 or 3 of the disease) of the illness. It is usually a pruritic maculopapular rash predominating on the trunk and limbs.
- **Arthralgia or arthritis:** Adults are more prone to migratory polyarthritis, which produces early morning pain and swelling, most often in the small joints of the ankles, feet, hands, and wrists. However, larger joints may also be affected. Arthritis may persist for months and may become chronic (6 months to several years) in patients who are positive for human leukocyte antigen (HLA)-B27.

- **Other symptoms:** Constitutional symptoms and signs, such as abdominal pain, headache (last for a variable period), anorexia, nausea, conjunctival injection, and slight photophobia. Occasionally, bleeding from skin (petechiae), and epistaxis may occur. Arthritis and skin pigmentation may persist for months to years after convalescence.

Diagnosis

- **Blood:** Leukopenia and thrombocytopenia may occur but is uncommon.
- **Raised aspartate aminotransferases** and **C-reactive protein** may be found.
- **Demonstrating antibodies** using ELISA method for diagnosis.
- Molecular methods include **RT-PCR** to detect structural genes of virus in the blood sample.

Treatment

- **Symptomatic:** No specific treatment available. For arthralgias and arthritis **NSAIDs** (e.g., ibuprofen, diclofenac or naproxen) may be used. Rest is important to reduce morbidity.
- **Hydroxychloroquine** (200 mg once or twice a day) may be given to patients with prolonged joint pains.

Japanese Encephalitis

Q. Write short note on Japanese encephalitis.

- Japanese encephalitis is a mosquito borne encephalitis caused by a *Flavivirus*.
- **Mode of transmission:** It is a viral infection transmitted by infected *Culex tritaeniorhynchus* mosquitoes.
- **Source of infection:** It is a zoonotic disease maintaining Japanese encephalitis virus in nature through pig-mosquito-pig and bird-mosquito-bird cycles. *C. tritaeniorhynchus* feeds mainly on the infected pigs and birds (e.g., herons and sparrows) and transmits the disease. Humans are accidental hosts.
- **Incubation period:** 5–15 days after the mosquito bite.
- **Epidemiology:** It is endemic in Bihar, Uttar Pradesh, Assam, Andhra Pradesh, Karnataka, Tamil Nadu, West Bengal, and Odisha states of India. It is most frequent in the rice growing countries (where irrigated rice fields are present).

Clinical Features

Age group: In endemic regions, the infection occurs in children between 3 and 15 years of age because of high background immunity in older individuals.

Presenting Features

- **Prodromal period:** Following incubation period, the illness starts with fever, severe rigors, headache, malaise nausea, diarrhea, vomiting, cough, and myalgia that last for 1–6 days. Weight loss is prominent.
- **Acute encephalitic stage:** During this stage, fever is high, there is neck rigidity, and neurological signs such as irritability, altered consciousness/behavior, hemiparesis, and convulsions develop. Mental deterioration occurs over a period of 3–4 days and may terminate in coma.
- **Residual neurological defects features**, such as cognitive and speech impairment, emotional liability, cranial nerve palsies (e.g., ocular palsies and deafness), hemiplegia, quadriplegia, and Parkinsonian presentation (extrapyramidal signs in the form of rigidity, dystonia, choreoathetosis, and coarse tremors) occur in about 70% of patients who have had central nervous system (CNS) involvement.
  Mortality ranges from 7% to 40% and is higher in children.

Diagnosis

- **Blood:** Leukocytosis with neutrophilia
- **Cerebrospinal fluid (CSF) examination:**
  - It shows **raised pressure** and cell count. During early stages, neutrophils may predominate but a lymphocytic pleocytosis is typical. CSF **protein is moderately raised** in about 50% of case.
  - **Virus isolation** from CSF
  - **Detection of viral antigens** in CSF by indirect immunofluorescence assay (IFA).
- **Serological tests:** Detect antibodies to viral antigens. The various tests include virus neutralization test, hemagglutination inhibition, and complement fixation. **Antibody detection** in serum and CSF by immunoglobulin M (IgM) capture ELISA is a rapid diagnostic test.
- **EEG:** Persistent abnormalities are common (particularly in children).
- **Imaging studies** by CT scan may show low-density areas in the temporal lobes. MRI scan is more sensitive in detecting early abnormalities.

Treatment

Treatment is supportive/symptomatic and includes management of fever, raised intracranial tension and convulsions.

Prevention

- **Control of the mosquito vectors**
- **Interruption of human-vector contact**
- Vaccines: These include vaccines containing purified formalin-inactivated virus derived from mouse brain (requires three doses on 0, 7, and 14 days) and cell-culture derived live attenuated.

SMALLPOX (VARIOLA)

Q. Write short essay on the clinical features, treatment, and prophylaxis of smallpox.

- It is a severe disease with high mortality caused by variola virus that belongs to the *Orthopoxvirus* genus.
- Smallpox was eradicated worldwide by a global vaccination program and the last case was reported in 1977. In 1980, World Health Organization (WHO) declared world free of smallpox.
- Interest in smallpox has re-emerged because of its potential as a bioweapon. Deliberate introduction of the smallpox virus through aerosolization can produce an epidemic in a few days.

Mode of transmission: Virus spreads through the respiratory or oropharyngeal mucosa. The virus is present in contaminated aerosols, lesional tissue, body fluids, or fomites. It may also spread through contact with lesions (which contains numerous viable virions).

Incubation period: 12–17 days. During incubation period, the virus proliferate within the lymph nodes and subsequently disseminate and seed the other lymphoid tissues throughout the body.

Clinical Features

Prodromal period: It develops abruptly with high fever, headache, backache, prostration, and malaise.

Skin Lesions (Described in Table 4.32)

- **Contagious period:** The disease is most contagious during the period from the development of the rash up to the 10th day. However, the patient remains contagious till scabs fall off.
  - Within 2–3 weeks, the skin lesions develop into scabs that detach. Sometimes, it may lead to scar formation or become hypopigmented.
  - **Uncommon presentations** are flat and hemorrhagic types of lesions.
    - Smallpox: Characterized by soft, flat, confluent, or semiconfluent lesions.
    - Hemorrhagic smallpox: Characterized by widespread hemorrhages into skin and mucous membranes with a very high case-fatality rate.

Vaccination can modify course of disease with milder rash and lower mortality.

Cause of death: May be due to disseminated intravascular coagulation (DIC), hypotension, and multiorgan failure.

TABLE 4.32: Differences between smallpox and chickenpox.

Features	*Smallpox*	*Chickenpox*
Stages of skin rash	All rashes of the same stage	Rash in different stages occur simultaneously
Involvement of palms and soles	Affected	Not affected
Axilla	Free	Affected
Rash prominent on	Extensor surfaces and bony prominences	Mostly on flexor surfaces
Location of rash	Deep seated	Superficial
Type of skin lesion	Vesicles—multilocular and umbilicated	Unilocular—dew drop appearance Pleomorphic rashes
Distribution of rash	Centrifugal	Centripetal
Relation to fever	Fever 2–4 days prior to rash	Fever at the time of rash
Mortality	2–10%	Very few

Treatment

Symptomatic and there is no effective postexposure therapy.

Prophylaxis by Vaccine

- **It is a live attenuated vaccine that employs another virus of *Orthopoxvirus* genus called vaccinia.**
- Vaccination can prevent or reduce the severity of infection if given within 4 days of exposure. However, most countries do not have adequate stock of vaccine.

Differences between smallpox and chickenpox are presented in **Table 4.32**.

RABIES

Q. Describe etiology, clinical features, and treatment of rabies. Add a note on postexposure prophylaxis.

Rabies is caused by a rhabdovirus (genotype 1, single stranded RNA virus of the *Lyssavirus* genus). The virus has a **marked affinity for central nervous tissue and the salivary glands** of a wide range of mammals. Established infection is invariably fatal.

Mode of infection: By **saliva** usually through the **bites or licks** of an infected animal on abrasions or on intact mucous membranes. Other forms of transmission (aerosolized exposure in bat infested caves, postorgan transplant) are rare.

Source of infection: Humans are usually infected from dogs/fox (rarely cats) and bats.

Incubation period in humans: Varies from few weeks to several months. Unusually average is 1–3 months. In general, severe bites (especially on the head or neck) are associated with shorter incubation periods than those elsewhere.

Clinical Features

- **Clinical varieties:** There are two distinct clinical varieties of rabies in humans: (1) Furious rabies (the classic variety) and (2) dumb rabies (the paralytic variety).

- The only characteristic feature in the initial prodromal period is **the pain and tingling** (paresthesia) **at the site of the bite.** There may be fever, malaise, and headache.
- After a prodromal period of 1–10 days, marked anxiety, agitation or depressive features, hallucinations, and paralysis may develop. It may be accompanied by spitting, biting and mania, with lucid intervals in which the patient is markedly anxious.
- **Hyperexcitability** is the hallmark and is precipitated by auditory or visual stimuli. The characteristic **"hydrophobia" (fear of water)** develops in 50% of patients. In hydrophobia, though the patient is thirsty, attempts at drinking (or eating) provoke violent/severe contractions of the diaphragm and other inspiratory (pharyngeal) muscles. **Aerophobia (fear of air) is pathognomonic** of rabies.
- Cranial nerve lesions and autonomic instability are common.
- **Examination:** It shows hyperreflexia, spasticity, and features of sympathetic overactivity (pupillary dilatation and diaphoresis).
- Patient develops **convulsions, respiratory paralysis, and cardiac arrhythmias.** Death usually occurs within 10–14 days of the onset of symptoms.

Dumb rabies presents with a symmetrical ascending paralysis similar to Guillain–Barré syndrome. It commonly develops after bites from rabid bats.

Investigations/Diagnosis

- Diagnosis is usually made on clinical grounds.
- **Skin punch biopsy:** To detect antigen with an immunofluorescent antibody test on frozen section.
- **Reverse transcription polymerase chain reaction (RTPCR):** Isolation of viral RNA
- **Isolation of viruses:** From saliva or the presence of antibodies in blood or CSF
- **Corneal smear test:** It is unreliable.
- **Classic Negri bodies:** They can be demonstrated at postmortem in 90% of patients with rabies. These are eosinophilic, cytoplasmic, ovoid bodies, 2–10 nm in diameter, found in large numbers in the neurons of the hippocampus and the cerebellum.
- **Diagnosis on the biting animal:** By using RTPCR, immunofluorescence assay (IFA) or tissue culture of the brain

Q. Write a short essay/note on treatment of rabies.

Treatment/Management

Established Disease

- Once the CNS disease is established, treatment is symptomatic, as death is virtually inevitable. Only a few patients with established rabies survive.
- **Intensive care:** The patient should be isolated in a quiet, darkened room. Patients who received some postexposure prophylaxis should be given intensive care facilities to control cardiac and respiratory failure and nutritional support. Only palliative treatment can be given once symptoms have appeared.
- **Heavy sedation:** The patient should be heavily sedated with diazepam/morphine, supplemented by chlorpromazine if needed. Sedation should be done liberally in patients who are excitable. Nutrition and fluids should be given intravenously or through a gastrostomy.
- Milwaukee protocol using antivirals (ribavirin and amantadine) along with ketamine and midazolam infusion has been tried.

Prevention

Pre-exposure prophylaxis

- High-risk individuals: Pre-exposure prophylaxis is indicated to individuals with a high-risk of contracting rabies. These include laboratory workers (who work with rabies virus), animal handlers (who handle potentially infected animals professionally), veterinarians, and those who live at special risk in rabies-endemic areas.
- **Method:**
  - **Three doses** on days **0, 7, and 28** (1.0 mL) of **human diploid (HDCV) or chick embryo cell vaccine** given by deep subcutaneous or intramuscular route.
  - A **reinforcing dose after 12 months** and additional reinforcing doses are given every 3–5 years (depending on the risk of exposure).

Q. Write a short note on postexposure prophylaxis of rabies.

Postexposure prophylaxis

Category	*Type of contact*	*Type of exposure*	*Recommended post-exposure prophylaxis*
I	Touching or feeding of animals Licks on intact skin	None	None, if reliable case history is available
II	Nibbling of uncovered skin, minor scratches or abrasion without bleeding	Minor	➢ Wound management ➢ Antirabies vaccine
III	Single or multiple transdermal bites or scratches, licks on broken skin, contamination of mucous membrane with saliva (i.e., licks)	Severe	➢ Wound management ➢ Rabies immunoglobulin ➢ Antirabies vaccine

- **Treatment of the wound:** The wounds should be thoroughly and carefully cleaned with a quaternary ammonium detergent or soap and water. Excise the damaged tissues, the wound left unsutured and open.
- Rabies can be prevented, if treatment is started within a day or two of bite. For maximum protection, hyperimmune serum and vaccine are needed.
- **Human rabies immunoglobulin** should be **given immediately** at dose is 20 IU/kg body weight; **half is injected/infiltrated around the bite wound and** other **half is given intramuscularly** at a different site from the vaccine. Hyperimmune animal serum can be given but hypersensitivity reactions (including anaphylaxis) are common.
- **Vaccine:**
  - **Essen schedule:**
    - Five dose intramuscular regimen—the course for postexposure prophylaxis should consist of intramuscular administration of five injections on days 0, 3, 7, 14, and 28.
    - The sixth injection (D90) should be considered as optional and should be given to those individuals who are immunologically deficient, or at the extremes of age and on steroid therapy.
    - Day 0 indicates date of first injection.
  - **Updated Thai Red cross Schedule**
    - This involves injection of 0.1 mL of reconstituted vaccine per ID site and on two such ID sites per visit (one on each deltoid area, an inch above the insertion of deltoid muscle) on days 0, 3, 7, and 28
  - **Human diploid cell strain vaccine (HDCV)** is the safest vaccine, free of complications.

    Intradermal (ID) regimen—administration of a fraction of intramuscular dose of certain rabies vaccine on multiple sites in the layers of dermis of skin thereby reducing the cost of active immunization.

The treatment may be modified if animal involved (dog or cat) remains healthy throughout the observation period of 10 days by converting postexposure prophylaxis to pre-exposure vaccination by skipping the vaccine dose on day 14 and administering it on day 28.

EBOLA VIRUS DISEASE

Q. Write short note on the clinical features and management of Ebola virus.

Ebola virus disease (EVD), earlier known as **Ebola hemorrhagic fever**, is a severe, often **fatal illness** in humans. EVD outbreaks have a very high fatality rate of around 90%. EVD outbreaks occurred primarily in remote villages in Central and West Africa, near tropical rainforests.

Source of infection: Ebola virus is introduced into the human population through close contact with the blood, secretions, organs, or other bodily fluids of infected animals. Humans recovered from the disease can transmit the virus through semen for up to 7 weeks after recovery from illness.

Mode of Transmission

The natural host of the Ebola virus is the fruit bats of the Pteropodidae family.

Spread of infection: The virus spreads in the **human population through human-to-human transmission**, with infection resulting from **direct contact (through broken skin or mucous membranes) with the blood, secretions, organs or other bodily fluids of infected people**, and **indirect contact with environments contaminated with such fluids.**

Clinical Features

Acute EVD is characterized by **sudden onset of high grade fever**, associated with **severe weakness, muscle pain, headache, vomiting, diarrhea, and skin rash.**

Complications include acute renal failure, hemorrhagic manifestations, DIC, hepatitis, and multiple organ dysfunction syndrome (MODS).

Diagnosis is clinical and serological tests available.

Treatment: Symptomatic and supportive. Isolation is of paramount importance.
- Handling of dead bodies, animal carcases needs to be emphasized.
- No vaccine available

SWINE FLU

Q. Write short note on Swine Flu.

- **Swine influenza virus (SIV)** refers to influenza cases that are caused by orthomyxovirus endemic to pig populations. SIV strains have been classified either as influenza virus C or one of the various subtypes of the genus influenza virus A.
- In late March and early April 2009, cases of human infection with swine influenza A (H1N1) viruses were first reported in Southern California and near San Antonio, Texas.
- **Swine influenza is a respiratory disease of pigs** caused by type A influenza virus that regularly causes outbreaks of influenza in pigs that cause high levels of illness but low death rates in pigs. Swine influenza viruses may circulate among swine throughout the year, but most outbreaks occur during the late fall and winter months similar to outbreaks in humans. The classical swine flu virus (an influenza type A H1N1 virus) was first isolated from a pig in 1930.
- The disease originally was nicknamed swine flu because the virus that causes the disease originally jumped to humans from the live pigs in which it evolved. The virus is a "reassortant"—a mix of genes from swine, bird, and human flu viruses.

Source of Infection

- Droplets from cough or sneeze of an infected individual
- Object contaminated by the cough or touch of an infected person

Infected individual shed the virus from the day prior to illness onset until resolution of fever. Hence infected individuals should be considered to be contagious up to 7 days from the onset of illness.

Signs and Symptoms (Table 4.33)

Patients aged above 65, children below 5 years, pregnant women (especially during the third trimester) and those with underlying medical conditions (e.g., asthma, diabetes, obesity, and heart disease), or those with weakened immune system (e.g., on immunosuppressive medications or infected with HIV) are at **high risk of serious complications**.

The Center for Disease Control and Prevention (CDC) criteria for suspected H1N1 influenza are listed in **Table 4.34**.

TABLE 4.33: Signs and symptoms of swine flu.

Signs	*Symptoms*
➤ High grade fever ➤ Unusual tiredness ➤ Headache ➤ Running nose ➤ Sore throat	➤ Shortness of breath or cough ➤ Loss of appetite ➤ Aching muscles ➤ Diarrhea or vomiting

TABLE 4.34: The CDC criteria for suspected H1N1 influenza.

- ➤ Onset of acute febrile respiratory illness within 7 days of close contact with a person who has a confirmed case of H1N1 influenza A virus infection.
- ➤ Onset of acute febrile respiratory illness within 7 days of travel to a community (within the United States or internationally) where one or more H1N1 influenza A cases have been confirmed.
- ➤ Acute febrile respiratory illness in a person who resides in a community where at least one H1N1 influenza case has been confirmed.

Complications: Adult respiratory distress syndrome (ARDS) and multiple organ dysfunction syndrome (MODS)

Diagnosis

A **confirmed case** of novel influenza A (H1N1) virus infection is defined as a person with an influenza-like illness with laboratory confirmed novel influenza A (H1N1) virus infection by one or more of the following tests:

1. Real-time RT-PCR
2. Viral culture from swabs (nasal, oral, and secretions of respiratory tract) can be used for virus isolation.

Treatment

Mainly supportive and consists of bed rest, increased fluid consumption, cough suppressants, and antipyretics and analgesics (e.g., acetaminophen and nonsteroidal anti-inflammatory drugs) for fever and myalgia.

- **Severe cases** may need **intravenous hydration and other supportive measures.**

Antiviral Agents

- They may also be considered **for treatment or prophylaxis.**
- **Neuraminidase inhibitors:** They **inhibit neuraminidase** which is a glycoprotein on the surface of influenza virus that destroys an infected cell's receptor for viral hemagglutinin. By inhibiting viral **neuraminidase, neuraminidase inhibitor agents decrease the release of viruses** from **infected cells** and, thus, **decrease the spread of virus**. Drugs include oseltamivir and zanamivir. Both are effective against both influenza A or B.
  1. **Oseltamivir (Tamiflu)**
     - Must be administered within 48 hours of symptom onset to provide optimal treatment.
     - **Adult dose**
       - **Treatment for acute illness:** 75 mg PO BID for 5 days
       - **Prophylaxis:** 75 mg PO qd (please refer to duration of prophylaxis specific for postexposure)
  2. **Zanamivir (Relenza)**
     - It is in powder form for inhalation via the Diskhaler oral inhalation device.
     - **Adult dose**
       - **Treatment for acute illness:** 10 mg inhaled orally BID for 5 days
       - **Prophylaxis of household contact:** 10 mg inhaled orally qd for 10 days (initiate within 36 hours)
       - **Prophylaxis for community outbreak:** 10 mg inhaled orally qd for 28 days (initiate within 5 days of outbreak)

Other antiviral agents (e.g., amantadine and rimantadine) are not recommended because of recent resistance to other influenza strains.

- **Vaccination:** Yearly vaccination with season specific strain vaccine before the annual flu season is recommended. Two types of vaccination are available namely intranasal and intramuscular. Monovalent/trivalent vaccines are available.

ZIKA VIRUS

Q. Write short note on Zika virus.

- Zika virus (ZIKV) is an arbovirus, belongs to the *Flavivirus* genus.
- It is enveloped and icosahedral with a nonsegmented, single-stranded, positive-sense RNA genome. It was first identified in Zika forest of Uganda in 1947.

Mode of Spread

- Zika virus is transmitted by ***Aedes* mosquito** species, such as *A. aegypti*, the extrinsic incubation period in mosquitoes is about 10 days. Rarely, mother to child transmission and one case of sexual transmission have been reported.

- The vertebrate hosts of the disease are monkeys and humans. The virus infects dendritic cells near the site of inoculation, and later spreads to lymph nodes and produces viremia.

Incubation period: 10 days.

Clinical Features

- It produces symptoms similar to a mild form of dengue fever with mild headaches, maculopapular rash, fever, malaise, conjunctivitis, and arthralgia. Within 2–4 days, the rash started fading, and fever resolved within 3 days.
- **Neurological complications:** Guillain–Barré syndrome and other neurologic complications
- Congenital infection leads to microcephaly, chorioretinal atrophy, hydranencephaly, intrauterine growth restriction (IUGR), and hydrops fetalis. In January 2016, the US Centers for Disease Control and Prevention (CDC) issued travel guidance on affected countries, including the use of enhanced precautions, and guidelines for pregnant women including considering postponing travel to affected areas. Most dangerous time is during first trimester of pregnancy and damage to the brain of fetus.

Diagnosis

- **Sample to be tested:** Blood saliva and urine
- **PCR:** Useful in the first 3–5 days after the onset of symptoms. It directly detects the virus or specific viral antigens in the clinical specimen.
- **Serology test:** Detects the presence of antibodies and useful only after 5 days.

Treatment

Only symptomatic. No specific antiviral drugs or vaccines are available.

Prevention and Control

- Avoid travel to areas with an active infection
- Control of mosquito

MOLLUSCUM CONTAGIOSUM

Q. Write short note on molluscum contagiosum.

It is caused by a **DNA poxvirus** called the **molluscum contagiosum virus** (MCV). MCV has no nonhuman-animal reservoir (infecting only humans) **(Fig. 4.16)**.

Types: Four types of MCV named MCV-1 to 4; MCV-1 is the most prevalent and MCV-2 is seen usually in adults.

Mode of transmission: The virus spreads from person to person by touching of the affected skin. The virus also spreads by touching a surface with the virus on it, such as a towel, clothing, or toys.

Age group: Children and young adults are infected and also commonly seen in HIV patients.

Appearance of lesions: Lesions begin as small (3–6 mm) papules that are smooth, flesh-colored domes with a central dimple (umbilication). Inside the papule is a white, curd-like core that can be easily expressed. Occasionally, they may be complicated by secondary bacterial infections.

- **Site of lesions:**
  - It can occur anywhere on the skin and mucous membranes, but are usually grouped in one or two areas. Occasionally, they may be widely disseminated.
  - Common sites: Head, eyelids, trunk, and genitalia (predominant site in adults).

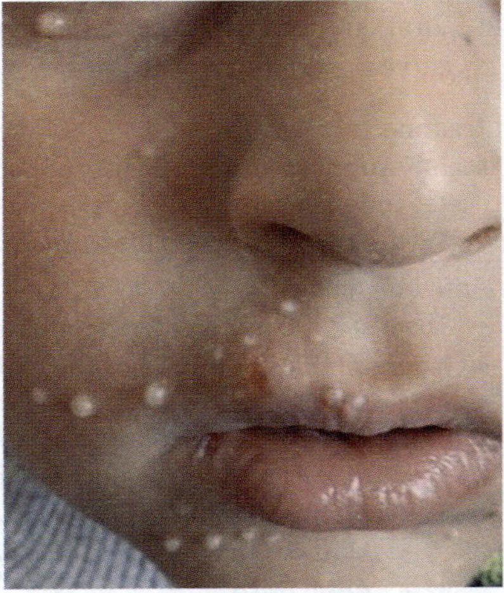

FIG. 4.16: Molluscum contagiosum.

Treatment: Imiquimod and retinoids have been used. Cryosurgery, curettage have also been used in the treatment.

NIPAH VIRUS ENCEPHALITIS

Q. Write a short note on *Nipah virus* encephalitis.

Etiology

It is caused by **a RNA virus** of the family Paramyxoviridae, genus *Henipavirus* first identified in 1999 outbreak, has caused annual outbreaks in Bangladesh, Malaysia, and India. Recent Indian outbreak has occurred in north Kerala in May 2018 has claimed lives.

Transmission

The *Nipah virus* is a zoonotic virus, which means it spreads to humans from either air or through saliva. The fruit bats are the primary carriers of *Nipah virus*. The virus is usually transferred through fluids from the bat. Close contacts with infected pigs and cattle can transmit the disease.

Clinical Features

- The incubation period ranges from 5 to 14 days. The illness presents with high grade fever and headache, followed by drowsiness, disorientation, and mental confusion. This can progress to encephalitis with brainstem dysfunction and coma within 24–48 hours.

- Other neurological signs include seizures, myoclonus, meningismus, autonomic dysfunction, and cerebellar involvement. One-third of patients develop pulmonary signs (ARDS), gastrointestinal, and renal involvement is seen in 5% of cases.

Investigations

- Thrombocytopenia, leukopenia, and elevated transaminases are seen in majority of patients.
- Diffuse bilateral lung infiltrates with basal atelectasis are seen in many cases.
- CSF shows lymphocytic pleocytosis.
- Serum/CSF immunoglobulin (Ig) M capture enzyme immunoassay (EIA) for detection of Nipah IgM antibodies and an indirect EIA for Nipah IgG antibodies are done for the specific diagnosis.

Treatment and Prognosis
- Treatment is supportive only.
- The disease has a fatality rate of around 40%.

Prevention
- Stay away from pigs, bats, or domestic animals in endemic areas.
- Do not drink raw date, palm sap.
- Avoid fruits that have fallen from trees on the ground.

FUNGAL INFECTIONS

Candidiasis (Moniliasis)

Q. Write short note on candidiasis (moniliasis).

Infection of skin or mucous membranes (e.g., oral cavity and vagina) by *Candida* is known moniliasis.

- **Most *Candida* infections occur when the normal commensal flora breach the skin or mucosal barriers.** *Candida* **resides normally in the skin, mouth, gastrointestinal tract, and vagina**. *Candida* species usually live as benign commensals and do not cause disease in healthy individuals. *Candida* species (usually *C. albicans)* are the most common cause of human fungal infections. *Candidas* are small asexual fungi.
- *Candida* species are the most common nosocomial pathogens. *Candida albicans* is the most common cause of candidiasis. Candidiasis may be superficial (noninvasive) or invasive (disseminate). Invasive candidiasis can also be due to nonalbicans *candida* species (e.g., *C. glabrata*) and some of these are resistant to fluconazole.

Lesions/Conditions Caused Due to Candida

- **Oral thrush:** It is characterized by white adherent, painless, discrete, or confluent patches in the mouth. Conditions that predispose to oral *candida* infection include use of broad-spectrum antibiotics, xerostomia, immune dysfunction (e.g., diabetes, immunosuppressive therapy, HIV infection, etc.) or the presence of removable prostheses and lichen planus.
- **Vulvovaginal candidiasis:** More common in diabetics. It presents with pruritus, pain, and vaginal discharge which is usually thin but may appear as whitish "curds" in severe cases.
- **Cutaneous candidiasis:** It may present as intertriginous infection (in the skin folds), paronychia (painful swelling at the nail-skin interface) balanitis (infection of the glans penis), pruritus ani (infection surrounding the anus), vulval candidiasis (in diabetic females), and scrotal candidiasis.
- **Chronic mucocutaneous candidiasis:** It is a heterogeneous infection of the hair, nails, skin, and mucous membranes which persists in spite of intermittent therapy. The onset is usually in infancy or within the first two decades of life. It may be mild and limited to a specific area of the skin or nails or may be severe form (*Candida* granuloma). It occurs in immunocompromised patients with leukemias, lymphomas and AIDS.
- **Deeply invasive *candida* infections:** It may or may not be due to hematogenous spread.
  - **Esophageal candidiasis:** Deep esophageal infection may result from penetration by organisms from superficial esophageal erosions. It present as a dysphagia and retrosternal pain.
  - **Candidiasis of the urinary tract:** It presents with hematogenous renal abscess and bladder thrush. Kidney infection may develop from catheter.
- **Hematogenous dissemination** of *candida* (invasive candidiasis or candidemia): *Candida* may enter into the intravascular compartment either from the gastrointestinal tract or, less often, from the skin through the site of an indwelling intravascular catheter. Then it may spread hematogenously to deep organs, such as brain, chorioretina, heart, and kidneys. It presents with retinal abscesses (extending into vitreous), pulmonary candidiasis, endocarditis, chronic meningitis, and arthritis.

Diagnosis

- **Visualization of hyphae or pseudohyphae** on wet mount (saline and 10% KOH) preparation or in scrapings from infected lesions under microscope.

- Tissue secretions stained with Gram's stain, periodic acid-Schiff stain, or methenamine silver stain may show candida in association with inflammation.
- In invasive disease from blood cultures.

Treatment (Table 4.35): Depends on the site and severity of infection.

TABLE 4.35: Treatment of candidiasis.

Disease	*Treatment*
Cutaneous	Topical azole or topical nystatin
Vulvovaginal	Oral fluconazole (150 mg) or azole cream/suppository or nystatin suppository
Thrush	Clotrimazole troches or nystatin or fluconazole
Esophageal	Fluconazole tablets (100–200 mg/day) or itraconazole solution (200 mg/day) or caspofungin, micafungin, or amphotericin B therapy should be extended for 3 weeks or 2 weeks after the symptoms subside, whichever is longer
Disseminated candidiasis	Ketoconazole 200–400 mg/day, fluconazole 200 mg/day or itraconazole 100 mg per day for 2 weeks
Severe disseminated candidiasis	Intravenous fluconazole (6 mg/kg/day) or amphotericin B Echinocandins (include caspofungin, micafungin and anidulafungin)

Superficial Mycoses

Q. Write short note on superficial mycoses and dermatophytes.

Superficial mycoses are fungal infections of the outermost keratinized (cornfield) layers of the skin or hair shaft resulting in essentially no pathological changes.

Superficial mycoses along with their etiologic agent are as follows:
- **Pityriasis versicolor:** *Malassezia furfur*
- **Black piedra:** *Piedraia hortae*
- **White piedra:** *Trichosporon beigelii*

Tinea nigra: *Exophiala werneckii*

Pityriasis Versicolor

Etiology: *Malassezia furfur (Pityrosporum orbiculare)* which is a lipophilic yeast.
- Normal flora of the superficial epidermis and clusters around the openings of hair follicles.
- Saprophytic on normal skin of trunk, head, neck and **appears in highest numbers in areas with increased sebaceous activity.** Causes superficial chronic infection of stratum corneum.

Predisposing factors: Malnutrition, burns, corticosteroid therapy, immunosuppression, depressed cellular immunity, excess heat, and humidity. It is associated with increased sweating.

Clinical presentation
- Most common in **adolescent and young adult males.**
- **Multiple small, asymptomatic, red to fawn-colored, circular, macules, patches, or follicular papules**. It is hypopigmented. There may be tan to dark brown macules and patches.
- **Most common site: Back, underarm, upper arm, chest, neck,** and occasionally on face.
- Microscopy of skin scrapings shows "spaghetti and meatballs" hyphae. Lesions fluoresce greenish yellow in Wood's light.

Treatment: Topical selenium sulfide or 2% ketoconazole shampoo (apply and remove after 30–60 minutes and repeat daily for 7 days) or a topical imidazole cream (twice daily for 10 days). Oral ketoconazole or oral itraconazole (100 mg twice daily for 1 week) in resistant cases. Altered pigmentation persists for months even after successful treatment.

Dermatophytes

- Cutaneous fungi are called dermatophytes which are keratinophilic fungi—**they possess keratinase** allowing them to **utilize keratin as a nutrient** and energy source.
- They **infect the keratinized** (horny) **outer layer** of the scalp, glabrous skin, and nails causing tinea or ringworm by secreting keratinase—which degrades keratin with varied clinical manifestations and are caused by species of the fungal genera *Trichophyton, Epidermophyton, and Microsporum* (in order of commonality).
- **Lesions on skin** and sometimes nails have a **characteristic circular pattern** that was mistaken by ancient physicians as being a worm down in the tissue.
- These lesions are still today called ringworm infections even though the etiology is known to be a fungus rather than a worm.

Clinical manifestations of ringworm infections are called different names on basis of location of infection sites (**Table 4.36**).

TABLE 4.36: Terminology for ringworm infections and location of infection.

Terminology	*Location of ringworm infection*
Tinea capitis	Head, scalp, eyebrows, and eyelashes
Tinea favosa	Scalp (crusty hair)
Tinea corporis	Body (smooth skin) (**Fig. 4.17A**)
Tinea cruris	Groin (jock itch) (**Fig. 4.17B**)
Tinea unguium	Nails
Tinea barbae	Beard
Tinea manuum	Hand (**Fig. 4.17C**)
Tinea pedis	Foot (athlete's foot)

Kerion

- Inflammatory reaction of tinea capitis caused by *Microsporum canis* or *Trichophyton mentagrophytes.*
- Presents as boggy indurated swellings with crusting and loose hairs.

- Hair follicles may discharge pus.
- In extensive lesions, fever, pain, and regional lymphadenopathy are present.
- Kerion may be followed by scarring and alopecia in areas of inflammation and suppuration.

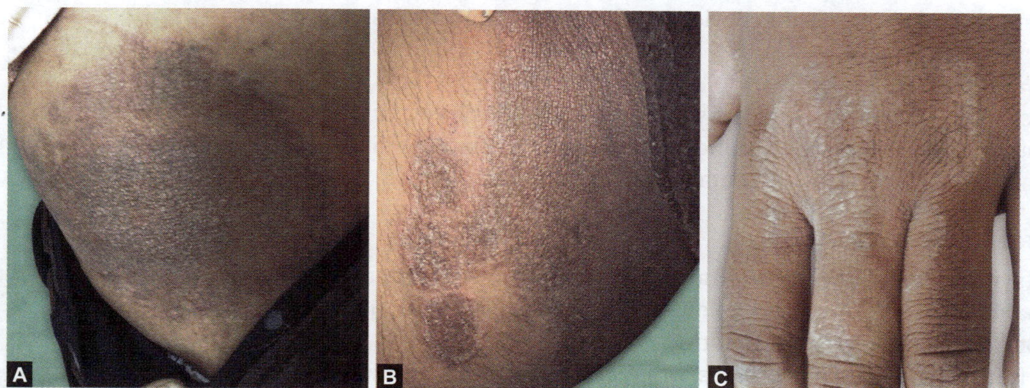

FIGS. 4.17A TO C: (A) Tinea corporis; (B) Tinea cruris; (C) Tinea manuum.

Favus

- Caused by *Trichophyton schoenleinii*
- Characterized by the presence of yellowish, cup-shaped crusts known as scutula. Each scutulum develops round a hair, which pierces it centrally. The scutula have a distinctive mousy odor.
- Cicatricial alopecia is usually found in long-standing cases.

Treatment of Mycoses
- **Topical:** Miconazole, clotrimazole, econazole, and terbinafine
- **Oral:** Griseofulvin, ketoconazole, itraconazole, and terbinafine

OPPORTUNISTIC MYCOSES

Q. Write short essay/note on opportunistic mycoses.

- Occurs in humans with a compromised immune system.
- Causative agents are normal resident flora that becomes pathogenic only when the host's immune defenses are altered, as in immunosuppressive therapy, in a chronic disease (e.g., diabetes mellitus), or during steroid or antibacterial therapy that upsets the balance of bacterial flora in the body.

Etiology

See **Table 4.37**.

TABLE 4.37: Common causative agents responsible for opportunistic mycoses.

• *Candida* species	• *Penicillium* species
• *Cryptococcus neoformans*	• *Fusarium* species
• *Aspergillus* species	• *Alternaria* species
• *Zygomycosis*	
• Rhizopus, mucor, and absidia	

Aspergillosis

- *Aspergillus* species are **ubiquitous saprophytes** in nature.
- In nature >300 species of *Aspergillus* exist, few are important as human pathogens. These include ***(1) A. fumigatus, (2) A. niger, (3) A. flavus, (4) A. terreus, and (5) A. nidulans.***

Clinical Syndromes

The *Aspergillus* species can cause a variety of clinical syndromes:
- **Pulmonary aspergillosis:** These include allergic asthma, bronchopulmonary aspergillosis, and aspergilloma.
- **Invasive aspergillosis**
- **Superficial infections:** Sinusitis, mycotic keratitis, and otomycosis

Treatment: Invasive aspergillosis is treated with intravenous amphotericin B, voriconazole.

Mucormycosis

- It represents a group of **life-threatening infections** caused by fungi of the order Mucorales.
- ***Rhizopus oryzae*** **(in the family Mucoraceae) is by far the most common** cause of infection.

Risk Factors

- **Impaired immune system:** Mucormycosis typically **causes infection primarily in patients with diabetes or defects in phagocytic function** (e.g., associated with prolonged neutropenia or glucocorticoid treatment), solid organ or hematopoietic stem cell transplantation (HSCT), or malignancy. Post COVID-19, lots of cases have been reported.

- **Elevated levels of free iron:** Supports fungal growth in serum and tissues. Hence patients with raised levels of free iron also have increased risk. In iron-overloaded patients with end-stage renal failure, treatment with deferoxamine (iron chelator for the human host) predisposes to the development of rapidly fatal disseminated mucormycosis. Deferoxamine serves as a fungal siderophore, directly delivering iron to the mucorales.

Clinical Categories

Mucormycosis can be divided into at least six clinical categories based on clinical presentation and the involvement of a particular anatomic site. These are (1) rhinocerebral (most common in diabetics), (2) pulmonary (in patients undergoing hematopoietic stem cell transplant), (3) cutaneous, (4) gastrointestinal, (5) disseminated, and (6) miscellaneous.

Rhinocerebral Mucormycosis

- The **initial symptoms** of rhinocerebral mucormycosis are **nonspecific** and include **eye or facial pain** and **facial numbness** followed by the onset of **conjunctival suffusion, blurring of vision**, and soft tissue swelling.
- Fever may be absent in up to half of cases, while **white blood cell counts are typically elevated** as long as the patient has functioning bone marrow.
- If untreated, infection usually spreads from the ethmoid sinus to the orbit, resulting in compromise of extraocular muscle function and **proptosis**, typically with **chemosis**. Onset of signs and symptoms in the contralateral eye, with resulting bilateral proptosis, chemosis, vision loss, and ophthalmoplegia, is ominous and suggests the development of cavernous sinus thrombosis.
- Upon visual inspection, infected tissue may appear to be normal during the earliest stages of fungal spread and then progresses through an erythematous phase, with or without edema, before the onset of a violaceous appearance and finally the development of a black necrotic eschar **(Fig. 4.18)**.

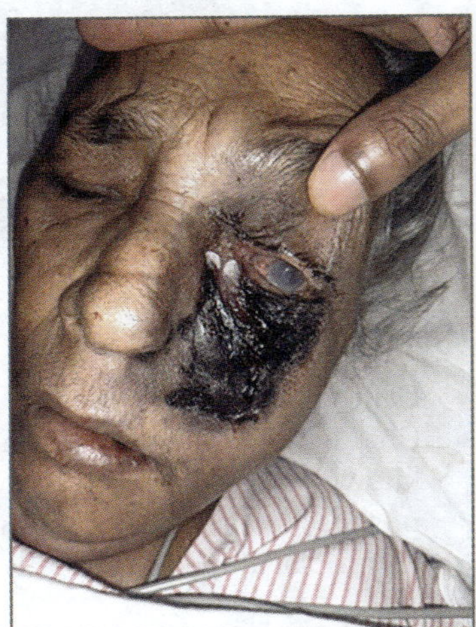

FIG. 4.18: Rhinocerebral mucormycosis.

Definitive Diagnosis

- Diagnosis requires a positive culture from a sterile site (e.g., a needle aspirate, a tissue biopsy specimen, or pleural fluid). A probable diagnosis of mucormycosis can be done by culture from a nonsterile site (e.g., sputum or bronchoalveolar lavage).
- Biopsy with histopathologic evidence of invasive mucormycosis is the most sensitive and specific modality for definitive diagnosis. Biopsy reveals characteristic wide (6–30 μm), thick-walled, ribbon-like, aseptate hyphal elements that branch at right angles.

Treatment: Surgical debridement plus
- Amphotericin B deoxycholate: 1 mg/kg per day
- Liposomal AmB (LAmB): 5–10 mg/kg per day. However, dose escalation of LAmB to 10 mg/kg per day for CNS mucormycosis may be considered in light of the limited penetration of polyenes into the brain.
- Amphotericin B lipid complex (ABLC): 5–7.5 mg/kg
- Posaconazole or isavuconazole is used as step-down therapy for patients who have responded to amphotericin B

Mycetoma

Q. Write short note on mycetoma. Write short note on actinomycosis.

- Mycetoma is a **chronic suppurative infection** of the **deep soft tissues and bones**.
- **Most common site** is the **limbs** but can also occur in the abdominal or chest wall or head.

Etiology

Caused by either (1) **aerobic or anaerobic branching gram-positive bacilli**, ***Actinomycetales*** (actinomycetoma—60%), or (2) by **true fungi, Eumycetes** (eumycetoma—40%).

1. **Actinomycetomas** are caused by **bacteria** such as *Actinomadura, Nocardia,* and *Streptomyces* species.
2. **Eumycetes:** Many **fungi** cause eumycetomas. Most common are *Madurella mycetomatis, M. grisea, Leptosphaeria senegalensis* and *Scedosporium apiospermum*.

Colored grains: Both the above groups characteristically produce colored grains; the color depends on the causative organism. Examples include black grains by eumycetoma, red and yellow grains by actinomycetoma, and white grains by either of them. The disease develops mostly in the tropics and subtropics.

Mode of infection: It is acquired **by inoculation** (e.g., from a thorn) and most commonly affects the foot (**Madura foot**).

Clinical Features

- It begins as a **painless swelling** at the **implantation site**. It becomes chronic and progressively, grows and **spreads within the soft tissues**, and extends into the underlying **bone**. There is usually little pain without fever or lymphadenopathy.
- **Discharging sinuses (Fig. 4.19):** Nodules develop under the epidermis and rupture, producing sinuses through which grains (fungal colonies) may be discharged. Sinuses heal with scarring, while fresh sinuses appear at other places. It can cause progressive disability.
- Deeper soft tissue and bone involvement are less rapid and extensive in eumycetoma than actinomycetoma.

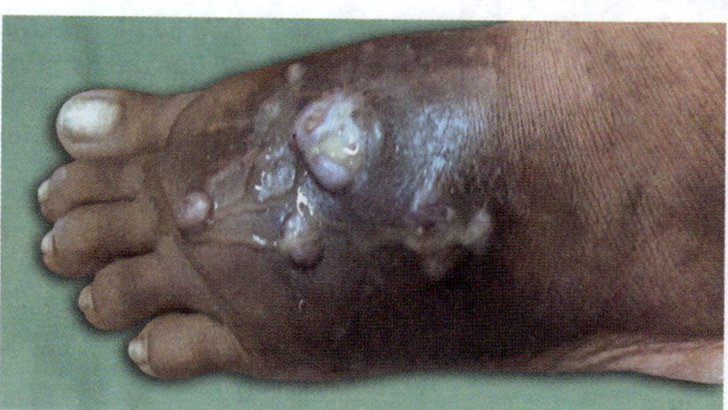

FIG. 4.19: Mycetoma.

Diagnoses/Investigations

- Demonstration *of fungal grains in pus, and/or causative agent by histopathological examination of tissue*
- **Culture and sensitivity** are needed for identification species and susceptibility testing.
- **Serological tests:** Not available.

Management
- **Actinomycetoma:** Treated with prolonged antibiotic combinations. Usual combination is streptomycin and dapsone, with dapsone replaced by cotrimoxazole in cases with intolerance or refractory cases. Other combination includes cotrimoxazole plus amikacin, with rifampicin added in refractory cases and to prevent recurrence.
- **Eumycetoma:** Usually treated with a combination of surgery and antifungal therapy. Most commonly used antifungal drugs are itraconazole and ketoconazole (both 200–400 mg/day). Other drugs include terbinafine monotherapy, voriconazole, and posaconazole. Amphotericin B is usually not effective. Therapy is continued for 6–12 months or longer. In extensive and severe cases, amputation may be needed.

Nocardiosis

- Nocardiosis is a gram-positive bacterial infection caused by aerobic actinomycetes of the genus *Nocardia* found in the soil.
- **Mode of infection:** It is an uncommon infection which occurs most frequently by **direct traumatic inoculation** or occasionally via inhalation or ingestion.

Clinical Features

- **Localized cutaneous infection:** It causes localized cutaneous ulcers or nodules, most frequently in the lower limbs. In tropical countries, chronic destructive infection can produce actinomycetoma, involving soft tissues and bone.
- **Systemic *Nocardia* infection:** Occurs mostly in immunocompromised individuals and results in suppurative disease with lung and brain abscesses.

Microscopic appearance: *Nocardia* species appear as long, filamentous, and branching gram-positive rods. They are weakly acid-fast. They can be cultured but need prolonged incubation.

Treatment

It depends on the result of culture and sensitivity.
- **Systemic infection:** Needs combinations of ceftriaxone, meropenem, amikacin, and cotrimoxazole. They are to be given for 6–12 months or longer. Abscesses are drained surgically wherever possible.
- **Localized cutaneous infection:** Usually treated with a single drug for 1–3 months.

Actinomyces israelii

- *Actinomyces israelii* can produce deep infection in the head and neck, and suppurating disease in the pelvis associated with intrauterine contraceptive devices (IUCDs).
- **Treatment:** Penicillin or doxycycline.

PROTOZOAL INFECTIONS

Malaria

Q. Draw a neat labeled diagram of life cycle of the malarial parasite. Discuss the etiology, epidemiology, clinical features, complications, investigations, and management of malaria.

Q. Discuss the clinical features, diagnosis, and management of *P. falciparum* malaria (both uncomplicated and complicated *P. falciform* malaria).

- Malaria is a **protozoan disease** caused by ***Plasmodium***. Human malaria is usually caused by one of four species of the genus *Plasmodium* namely (1) ***P. falciparum*, (2) *P. vivax*, (3) *P. ovale*, and (4) *P. malariae***. Occasionally, a species of malaria usually found in primates namely ***P. knowlesi*** (simian parasite) can affect man.
- ***Plasmodium falciparum* causes the most severe form** of malaria than the other *Plasmodium* species. *P. vivax* is the most common cause of malaria in India.

Mode of transmission: By the **bite of female anopheles mosquitoes**. Malaria can also be transmitted through contaminated blood transfusions.

A comparison of the developmental characteristics of various species of *Plasmodium* is presented in **Table 4.38.**

TABLE 4.38: Developmental characteristics of various species of *Plasmodium*.

Features	*P. falciparum*	*P. vivax*	*P. ovale*	*P. malariae*
Duration of erythrocytic cycle	48 hours	48 hours	48 hours	72 hours
Type of red cells parasitized	All	Reticulocytes	Reticulocytes	Mature erythrocytes
Relapse	No	Yes	Yes	No
Drug resistance	Yes	+/–	No	No

Life Cycle of the Malarial Parasite (Fig. 4.20) and Pathogenesis

Q. Write short essay on life cycle of malarial parasite.

The life cycle of *Plasmodium* species is simple because it involves only humans and mosquitoes. However, the development of the parasite is complex, because it passes through several morphologically distinct forms. Malarial parasites pass its life cycle in two different hosts namely: (1) human (intermediate host) and (2) female anopheles mosquito (definitive host).

Human Cycle (Fig. 4.20)

Human cycle (infection) starts with the introduction of infectious *sporozoite* by the bite of infected female anopheles mosquito. The *sporozoite* is found in the salivary glands of mosquitoes. During mosquito bite, the mosquito takes a blood meal and sporozoites are released into the human's blood. The different stages of human cycle are:

Pre-erythrocytic (Primary exoerythrocytic) stage

Sporozoites cannot directly enter erythrocyte to start its erythrocyte stage, but undergoes development inside liver cells. The infection of the liver and development of sporozoites into merozoites are referred to as the pre-erythrocytic (exoerythrocytic)

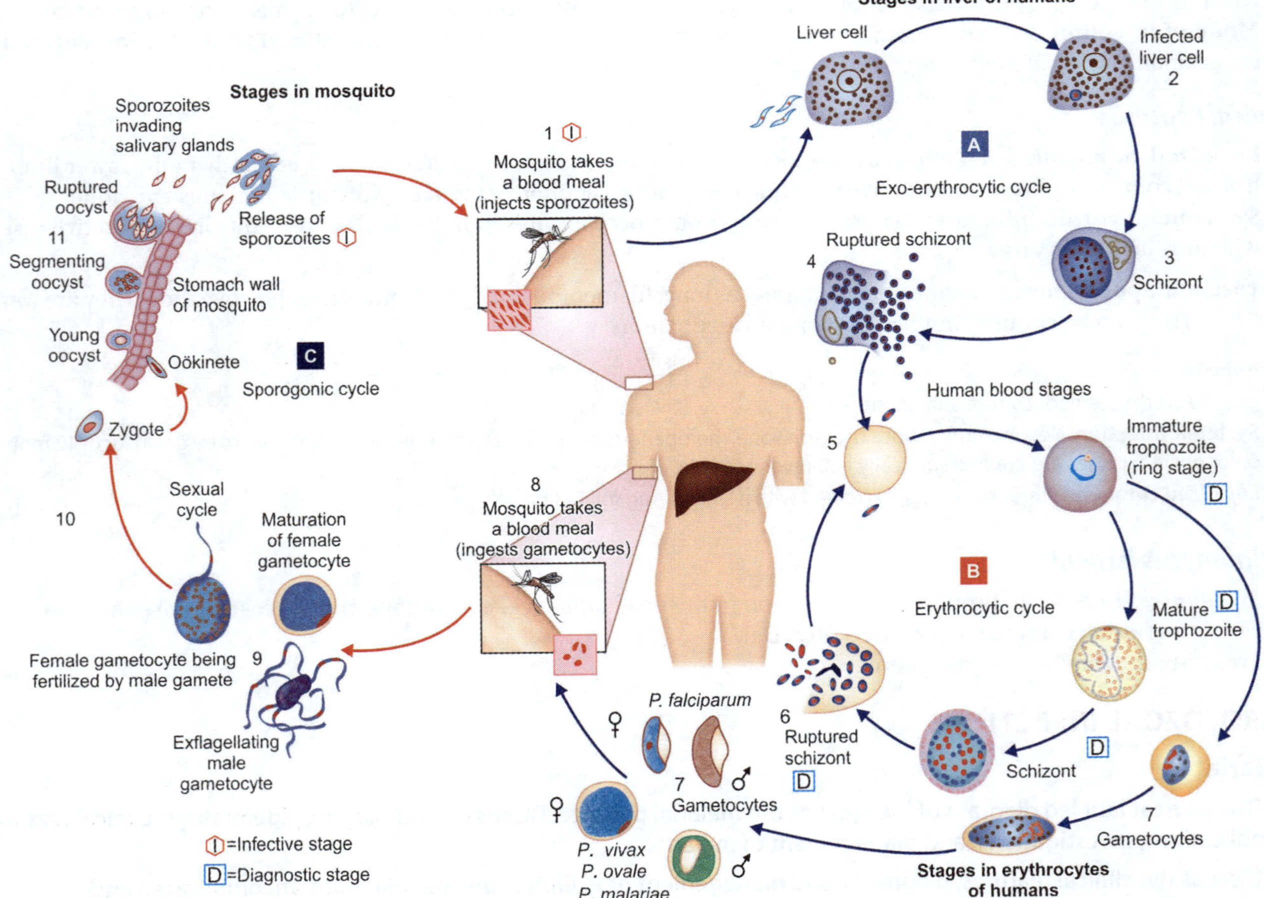

FIG. 4.20: Life cycle of malarial parasites (refer text for description).

stage. Within minutes of entry of sporozoites into the human blood (those which are not destroyed by the immune response), they are carried via the bloodstream and are rapidly (within 30 minutes) taken up by the liver. They enter liver cells and these malaria parasites multiply by asexual reproduction (intrahepatic schizogony), releasing about 30,000 *merozoites* (asexual, haploid forms) when each infected liver cells ruptures. This stage is asymptomatic and during this phase, the parasites are not found in the peripheral blood. The infected hepatocytes rupture and release merozoites into the bloodstream.

- During *P. falciparum* infection, rupture of swollen liver cells usually occurs within 8–12 weeks. *P. falciparum* and *P. malariae* have no persistent exoerythrocytic phase but a new outbreak of fever may result from multiplication of parasites in red cells which have not been eliminated by treatment and immune processes.
- In contrast, *P. vivax* and *P. ovale* releases merozoites into the bloodstream weeks to months after initial infection.

Hypnozoite (latent) stage

The pre-erythrocytic phase disappears completely in *P. falciparum*, whereas a few parasites persist in the liver cells as dormant forms in *P. vivax* and *P. ovale*. The resting phase of parasite (latent phase) is called as hypnozoite. These hypnozoites are capable of developing into merozoites months or years later, causing **relapsing malarial infection.** Thus, the first attack of clinical malaria may develop long after the individual has left the endemic area.

Erythrocytic stage

Once merozoites are released from the liver into the blood stream, they rapidly invade erythrocyte by penetration of the membrane. Within the red cells (erythrocytic stage), asexual division occurs.

- **Asexual forms:** In the red cells parasite develop through the stages of asexual forms changing from *merozoite* to *trophozoite,* to *schizont* and finally appearing as 8–24 new *merozoites.* These asexual forms of parasite can be demonstrated in the thick blood smears.
  - *Ring form*: It is the first stage of the parasite in the red cell and is characterized by the presence of a single chromatin mass (ring form).
  - *Trophozoite:* During this, the parasite assumes an irregular or amoeboid shape.
  - *Schizont:* It is the next stage the parasite has consumed two-thirds of the RBC's hemoglobin and has grown to occupy most of the cell. It shows multiple chromatin masses, each of which develops into a merozoite. Rupture of the schizont releases merozoites into the blood. This causes fever and the periodicity of fever depends on the species of parasite.
  - *Merozoites:* Rupture of the red cell containing merozoites releases the merozoites into the bloodstream. These merozoites are capable of invading additional new erythrocyte and repeating the cycle. The characteristic clinical features of malaria such as paroxysmal fever, chills, and rigors develop during the release of these merozoites into the blood.

  Each cycle of the above process is called erythrocytic schizogony. The periodicity of such cycle takes about 48 h in *P. falciparum, P. vivax,* and *P. ovale* and about 72 hours in *P. malariae. P. vivax,* and *P. ovale* mainly attack reticulocytes and young erythrocytes, whereas *P. malariae* tends to attack old erythrocytes; *P. falciparum* will parasitize any stage of erythrocyte.
- **Sexual forms:** Most malaria parasites within the red cells develop into daughter merozoites. A few merozoites within erythrocytes develop not into trophozoites but undergo a different pathway of development into sexual forms called gametocytes (male and female *gametocytes*). These gametocytes are not released from the red cells until taken up by a feeding mosquito to complete the life cycle. These gametocytes are ingested by the mosquito during a blood meal when mosquito bites the infected human.

Mosquito cycle

A female anopheles mosquito during its blood meal from an infected patient ingests both sexual and asexual forms of parasite, but it is only the mature sexual forms (gametocytes) capable of development.

- The male and female gametocytes of malarial parasite fuse inside the mid-gut (stomach) of the mosquito to form a **zygote**.
- The zygote matures to form an ookinete, which penetrates the gut wall and form an **oocyst**.
- The oocyst matures and forms numerous **sporozoites**. These sporozoites have special predilection toward the **salivary glands** and reach maximum concentration in the salivary ducts of mosquito. The mosquito at this stage is capable of transmitting malarial infection.
- During the blood meal these sporozoites are **inoculated into the new human host**, thus completing the life cycle of *Plasmodium.*

Protection Against Malaria

- Red blood cells containing hemoglobin F, C, or S impair growth of *P. falciparum* parasite. Patients with hemoglobin S especially heterozygotes (AS) are protected against the lethal complications of malaria.
- Attachment of merozoites to red blood cells is mediated via a specific erythrocyte surface receptor. In *P. vivax,* this receptor is related to the Duffy blood group antigen (Fy^a or Fy^b). Thus, an individual who is Duffy-negative (as most of the West African population) will be resistant to infection by *P. vivax.*

Clinical Features

Malaria is a very common cause of fever in tropical countries. The first symptoms of malaria are nonspecific.

P. vivax and *P. ovale* malaria

- **Incubation period** for *P. vivax* is 12–17 days, and for *P. ovale* is 15–18 days.
- **Prodromal symptoms** include headache, fatigue, abdominal discomfort, and muscle aches. These are more severe with *P. malariae* infections.
- **Fever:** The most common symptom of these "benign" malarias is paroxysms of fever. Fever starts with a rigor. The febrile paroxysm synchronizes with erythrocytic stage of the parasite.
  - **Tertian fever:** In *P. vivax* and *P. ovale* malaria infections, the fever recurs every third day (tertian) interval (with 48 hours cycle between spikes).
- ***P. vivax*:** Patients suffering from *P. vivax* malaria may develop **anemia, thrombocytopenia and mild jaundice** with tender hepatosplenomegaly. **Splenic rupture is more common**. Occasionally, *P. vivax* malaria presently develops complications similar to those of *P. falciparum* malaria.
- ***P. ovale*:** The acute symptoms of *P. ovale* may be as severe as those of *P. vivax* infection, but **anemia is less severe** and the risk of **splenic rupture is less common**.
- ***P. vivax* and *P. ovale*:** They have a persistent hepatic cycle and a few parasites persist in the liver cells as dormant forms. This may give rise to relapses.

P. malariae malaria

- **Incubation period: 18–40 days**
- **Prodromal symptoms** include headache, fatigue, abdominal discomfort, and muscle aches and may be more severe than *P. vivax*.
- **Fever:** The febrile paroxysm synchronizes with erythrocytic stage of the parasite.
  - **Quartan fever:** In *P. malariae* infections, the fever recurs every fourth day (quartan) interval (72 hours interval between spikes).
- It is associated with gross splenomegaly, but **splenic rupture is less common** and **anemia is less severe**. Chronic *P. malariae* infections cause **glomerulonephritis and nephrotic syndrome**. *P. malariae* does not relapse, but a persisting undetectable parasitemia may produce repeated exacerbations and the risk of **splenic rupture is less common**.

P. falciparum malaria (malignant tertian or subtertian malaria)

Q. Write short essay on falciparum malaria.

- It is the **most dangerous** type of malarias and patients may be either "**killed or cured**."
- **Incubation period:** 7–14 days (mean 12 days)
- **Prodromal symptoms:** Onset is often insidious, with malaise, headache, myalgia, anorexia, and vomiting.
- **Fever:** Patients develop mild fever having no particular pattern and may last for several days before the onset of the classical "malarial paroxysms."
  - A high irregularly spiking unremitting fever or daily **(quotidian)** paroxysm is more commonly seen in falciparum malaria but usually due to mixed infection (falciparum + vivax).
- **Physical findings:** Patient is often anemic and jaundiced with moderate tender hepatosplenomegaly.
- **Neurological complications** can manifest as acute headache, irritability, agitation, seizures, psychosis, and impaired consciousness.

Box 4.11 lists the jaundice in malaria.

Box 4.11: Jaundice in malaria.

Causes: Jaundice may be due to severe hemolysis and hepatic involvement (malarial hepatopathy) by malaria.

- **Hemolysis:** The malarial parasite, especially *P. falciparum* infects a large number of RBCs. These are destroyed in the spleen and result in hemolytic anemia. It produces elevation of serum bilirubin (dominant unconjugated fraction) level without any significant elevation of the liver enzymes.
- **Malarial hepatitis (malarial hepatopathy):** This term is used to describe dysfunction of liver cells in severe and complicated malaria. However, inflammation of the liver parenchyma is never observed.

Severe Manifestations and Complications of Falciparum Malaria

Q. Write short essay on:
- Complications of malaria
- Complications of falciparum malaria.

- WHO defines complicated falciparum malaria as one of the features shown in the **Table 4.39** along with presence of asexual forms of *P. falciparum* in the peripheral smear. Acute renal failure, acute respiratory distress syndrome, and jaundice are uncommon in children.
- At highest risk of complications from malaria are nonimmune people, and children and pregnant females who live in endemic regions.

TABLE 4.39: Criteria for severe and complicated malaria.

Severe malaria is defined as one or more of the above occurring in the absence of an identified alternative cause and in the presence of *P. falciparum* or *P. knowlesi parasitemia*.

Manifestation	***Features***
World Health Organization criteria from 1990	
Cerebral malaria	Unarousable coma not attributable to any other cause, with a Glasgow Coma Scale score ≤9; coma should persist for at least 30 minutes after a generalized convulsion
Severe anemia	Hematocrit <15% or hemoglobin ≤5 g/dL the presence of parasite count >10,000/μL
Renal failure	Urine output <400 mL/24 hours in adults (<12 mL/kg/24 hours in children) and a serum creatinine >265 μmol/L (>3.0 mg/dL) despite adequate volume repletion
Metabolic (lactic) acidosis	Metabolic acidosis is defined by an arterial blood pH of <7.35 with a plasma bicarbonate concentration of <22 mmol/L; hyperlactatemia is defined as a plasma lactate concentration of 2–5 mmol/L and lactic acidosis is characterized by a pH <7.25 and a plasma lactate >5 mmol/L.
Pulmonary edema or acute respiratory distress syndrome (ARDS)	Breathlessness, bilateral crackles, and other features of pulmonary edema. The acute lung injury score is calculated on the basis of radiographic densities, severity of hypoxemia, and positive end-expiratory pressure
Hypoglycemia	Whole blood glucose concentration of <2.2 mmol/L (<40 mg/dL)
Hypotension and shock (algid malaria)	Systolic blood pressure <50 mm Hg in children 1–5 years or <70 mm Hg in patients ≥5 years; cold and clammy skin or a core-skin temperature difference >10°C
Abnormal bleeding and/or disseminated intravascular coagulation	Spontaneous bleeding from the gums, nose, gastrointestinal tract, retinal hemorrhages, and/or laboratory evidence of disseminated intravascular coagulation
Repeated generalized convulsions	≥3 generalized seizures within 24 hours
Hemoglobinuria	Macroscopic black, brown, or red urine; not associated with effects of oxidant drugs or enzyme defects (like G6PD deficiency)
Added World Health Organization criteria from 2000	
Impaired consciousness	Various levels of impairment may indicate severe infection although not falling into the definition of cerebral malaria. These patients are generally arousable.
Prostration	Extreme weakness, needs support
Hyperparasitemia	5% parasitized erythrocytes or >250,000 parasites/μL (in nonimmune individuals)
Hyperpyrexia	Core body temperature above 40°C
Jaundice (hyperbilirubinemia)	Plasma or serum bilirubin >50 mmol/L (3 mg/dL)
Other (not included in WHO)	
Severe thrombocytopenia	Platelet counts <10,000/cumm
Fluid and electrolyte disturbances	Dehydration, postural hypotension, clinical evidence of hypovolemia
Vomiting of oral drugs	Patients with persistent vomiting may have to be admitted for parenteral therapy
Complicating or associated infections	Aspiration bronchopneumonia, septicemia, urinary tract infection, etc.
Malarial retinopathy	In children dying with cerebral malaria, malarial retinopathy was found to be a better indicator of malarial coma. Similar retinopathy in an adult has also been reported

Cerebral malaria

Q. Write short essay on clinical features and treatment of cerebral malaria.

Q. Write long essay on cerebral malaria-etiopathogenesis, clinical features, and management.

Definition: Cerebral malaria is defined as diffuse encephalopathy in a patient with falciparum malaria which is not attributable to any other cause.

Features: Cerebral malaria manifests as diffuse symmetric encephalopathy.

Neurological

- **Convulsions:** Usually, generalized and often repeated. They occur in both children (50%) and adults (10%) but are more common in children.
- Most common neurological signs in adults are those of a symmetrical upper motor neuron lesion. The abdominal reflexes and cremasteric reflexes are absent.
- Mild neck stiffness may be seen, however, neck rigidity and photophobia and signs of raised intracranial tension are absent. Retinal hemorrhages occur in about 15% of cases, exudates are rare.
- Motor abnormalities like decerebrate rigidity, decorticate rigidity, and opisthotonus occur.
- Fixed jaw closure and tooth grinding (bruxism) are common.
- Neuropsychiatric manifestations, cerebellar signs, extrapyramidal syndromes, and multiple cranial nerve involvement are common in Indian patients.
- **Residual neurological sequelae:** They develop in about 5% of adults and 10% of children. These include hemiplegia, cerebral palsy, cortical blindness, deafness, aphasia, and ataxia. They are more frequent in patients with prolonged deep coma, repeated convulsions, those with hypoglycemia and severe anemia.

Ophthalmological

- **Eyes** may be divergent and a pout reflex may be elicited by stroking the sides of the mouth. The corneal reflexes are preserved (except in deep coma). Transient abnormalities of eye movement (especially dysconjugate gaze) may be found.
- **Ophthalmoscopy:** Retinal hemorrhages may occur and indicate a poor prognosis. Papilledema is rare.

Bad prognostic signs

- Include prolonged impaired consciousness, respiratory failure, renal failure, jaundice, and hypoglycemia.
- The CSF pressure is usually normal. The fluid is clear with <10 cells/μL, CSF lactic acid and protein levels are elevated.
- Cerebral malaria carries a mortality of around 20% in adults and 15% in children. Residual deficits are unusual in adults (<3%). **Box 4.12** lists the causes of neurological manifestations in malaria other than hyperparasitemia.

Box 4.12: Causes of neurological manifestations in malaria other than hyperparasitemia.

- **High-grade fever**
- **Antimalarial drugs** like chloroquine, quinine, mefloquine, and halofantrine.
- **Hypoglycemia,** either due to severe malaria or due to drugs like quinine.
- **Hyponatremia,** most often in the elderly.
- **Severe anemia** and hypoxemia can also cause cerebral dysfunction, particularly in children.

Anemia (Box 4.13)

Box 4.13: Causes of anemia in malaria.

- Hemolysis of:
  - infected red cells
  - noninfected red cells (black water fever)
- Dyserythropoiesis
- Splenomegaly causing
  - Erythrocyte sequestration
  - Hemodilution
- Depletion of folate stores
- Hemorrhage secondary to thrombocytopenia/DIC
- Iron deficiency secondary to RBC breakdown

Renal failure

- Acute kidney injury is common in severe falciparum malaria and usually occurs in adults. It causes progressive oliguria eventually resulting in anuria. It is accompanied by progressive increase serum creatinine and urea levels. It is usually reversible.
- Caused by renal cortical vasoconstriction and resultant hypoperfusion, sequestration, and resultant acute tubular necrosis due to microvascular obstruction and due to massive intravascular hemolysis in black water fever.
- Dehydration and hypovolemia can lead to renal hypoperfusion, but this is reversible with adequate rehydration.

Hypoglycemia

Hypoglycemia is an important and common complication of severe falciparum malaria. It is particularly problematic occurs in three groups of patients:

1. Children with severe disease
2. Patients treated with quinine or quinidine
3. Pregnant women (either on admission or following quinine treatment)

Mechanism: In malaria, hypoglycemia develops due to various mechanisms (**Box 4.14**).

Box 4.14: Causes of hypoglycemia in malaria.

- Failure to hepatic gluconeogenesis
- Increased consumption of glucose by host and malaria parasite.
- Treatment with quinine or quinidine. Both these drugs strongly stimulate pancreas to secrete insulin. This produces hyperinsulinemia resulting in hypoglycemia.

Fluid, electrolyte, and acid-base disturbances

- **Hypovolemia:** Characterized by low jugular venous pressure, postural hypotension, oliguria, and high urine specific gravity. This may be associated with signs of dehydration.
- **Acidotic breathing:** It may develop in severely ill patients in shock, hypoglycemia, hyperparasitemia, and renal failure.
- **Lactic acidosis:** It is a common complication and associated with raised lactic acid levels both in blood and CSF.

Noncardiogenic pulmonary edema

- It is a serious complication of severe falciparum malaria in adults. It carries a high mortality rate (>80%). It can also develop in otherwise uncomplicated vivax malaria, where recovery is usual.
- It may develop several days after antimalarial therapy and at a time when the patient's general condition is improving.
- Noncardiogenic pulmonary edema is associated with hyperparasitemia, renal failure, pregnancy, hypoglycemia, and lactic acidosis. It is aggravated by vigorous administration of IV fluid.

Circulatory collapse ("Algid malaria")

- **Algid malaria** or hypotension due to peripheral circulatory failure may develop suddenly in severe malaria or it may be the presenting feature in some cases of malaria, with a systolic blood pressure <80 mm Hg in the supine position [<50 mm Hg in children], a cold, clammy, cyanotic skin, constricted peripheral veins, and rapid feeble pulse.
- This clinical picture is often associated with a complicating gram-negative septicemia and possible sites of associated infection should be sought in such patients, e.g., lung, urinary tract (especially if there is an indwelling catheter), meninges (meningitis), intravenous injection sites, intravenous lines, etc.
- Circulatory collapse is also observed in patients with pulmonary edema, metabolic acidosis, massive gastrointestinal hemorrhage, dehydration, and hypovolemia.

- Blood and urine culture should be done. Soon after collection of the specimen for culture, broad-spectrum antibiotics should be started.

Malarial hemoglobinuria (Black water fever)

- Malaria hemoglobinuria is uncommon, and is usually associated with hyperparasitemia and/or severe disease. It may or may not be accompanied by renal failure.
  Patients with glucose-6-phosphate dehydrogenase (G6PD) deficiency and other erythrocyte enzyme deficiencies may develop vascular hemolysis and hemoglobinuria when treated with oxidant drugs such as primaquine.
- **Black water fever** typically occurs in nonimmune patients with chronic falciparum malaria, taking antimalarials (especially quinine and primaquine) irregularly. It occurs more commonly in patients with G6PD deficiency.
  - The hemolysis can occur so rapidly that the hemoglobin may drop significantly within a few hours and it may recur periodically at intervals of hours or days. Patient presents with headache, nausea, vomiting, and severe pain in the loins and prostration. Fever up to 39.4°C with a rigor is also seen. Urine is dark red to almost black.
- **Bacterial coinfection**—gram negative septicemia (*Salmonella*) is common in endemic areas.

Box 4.15 lists the chronic complications of malaria.

Box 4.15: Chronic complications of malaria.

- Tropical splenomegaly syndrome
- Quartan malarial nephropathy
- Burkitt's lymphoma

Investigations and Diagnosis

Q. Write short essay on laboratory tests in the diagnosis of malaria.

Malaria should be considered in the differential diagnosis of febrile illness.

Microscopic demonstration of parasite

- **Peripheral smear examination (Fig. 4.21):** The diagnosis of malaria depends on the demonstration of asexual forms of the parasite in stained peripheral-blood smears. Both thin and thick smears should be examined whenever malaria is suspected. Smears are stained by one of the Romanowsky stains (e.g., Wright's, Field's, Leishman's, or Giemsa).
- **Bone marrow aspirate:** Sometimes parasites cannot be detected in peripheral blood smears, even in patient with severe malarial infections. This may be due to partial antimalarials treatment or by sequestration of parasitized cells in deep vascular beds. In these, circumstances examination of smears of bone marrow aspirate reveals parasites or malaria pigment.

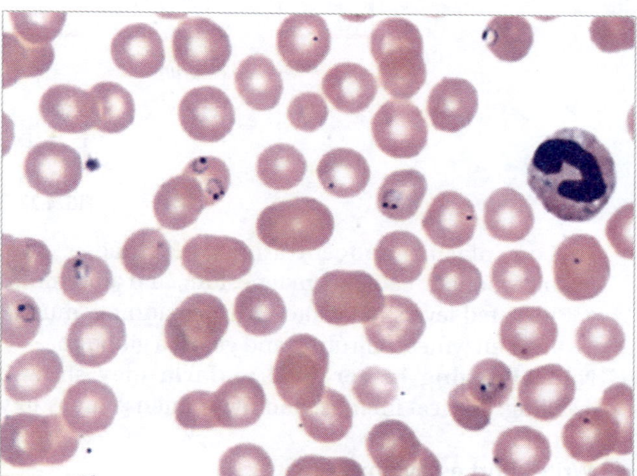

FIG. 4.21: Peripheral smear showing ring forms of malaria.

- **Alternative microscopic methods** have been tried, including faster methods of preparation, dark-field microscopy, and stains like *benzothiocarboxypurine, acridine orange, and Rhodamine-123.*
- **Quantitative buffy coat analysis (QBC) (Fig. 4.22):** It is an alternative and probably more sensitive test than the peripheral smear for detecting the malarial parasite. In this test, the centrifuged buffy coat is stained with a fluorochrome (e.g., acridine orange) that "lights up" (microtube concentration methods with acridine orange staining) malarial parasites. The buffy coat smear is viewed under fluorescence microscopy **(Fig. 4.23)**.

Immunodiagnosis

Serological techniques: They can detect malarial antibodies, but these tests are not specific and are not done routinely. The tests include immunofluorescent assay (IFA) and enzyme-linked immunosorbent assay (ELISA).

Table 4.40 shows comparison of rapid diagnostic tests for malaria antigens.

PCR testing

Molecular diagnosis by polymerase chain reaction (PCR) amplification of parasite nucleic acid (for parasite messenger RNA or DNA) is more sensitive than microscopy or rapid diagnostic tests.

Other laboratory findings

- **Blood:**
  - Normochromic normocytic anemia, thrombocytopenia.
  - Total leukocyte count is low to normal, but neutrophil leukocytosis may be observed in severe infections.
- **Acute-phase protein:** Erythrocyte sedimentation rate (ESR), plasma viscosity, and levels of C-reactive protein are high.
- **Coagulation study:** In severe infections, prothrombin time and partial thromboplastin time may be prolonged and antithrombin III levels are decreased.
- **Other findings in severe malaria:** In complicated malaria there may be metabolic acidosis and:

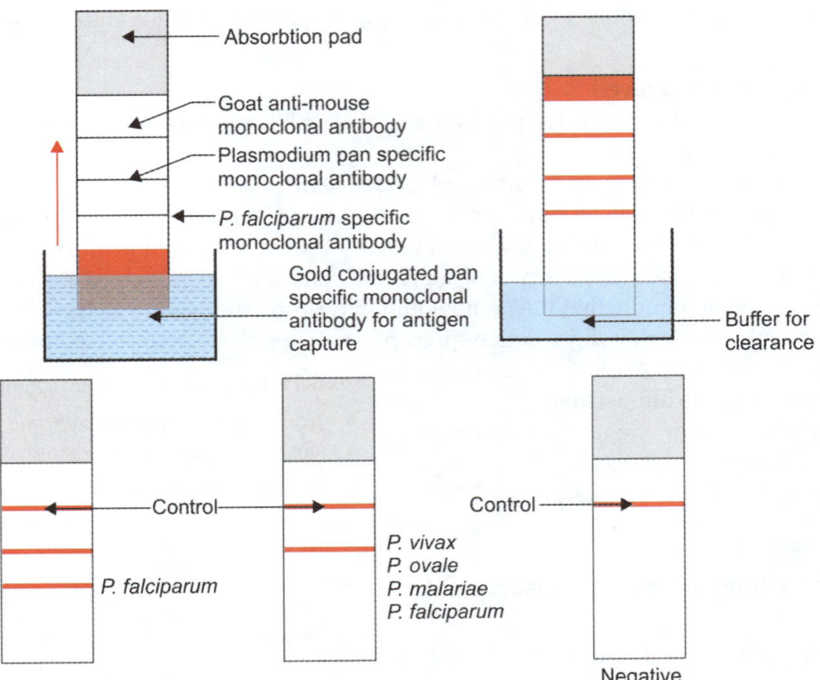

FIG. 4.22: QBC analysis for malaria.

- Low plasma concentrations of glucose, sodium, bicarbonate, calcium, magnesium, and albumin
- Elevated levels of lactate, BUN, creatinine, muscle and liver enzymes, bilirubin, and gamma globulin

- **Neuroimaging in cerebral malaria** may show brain swelling, cortical infarcts, and hyperintense areas in white matter.

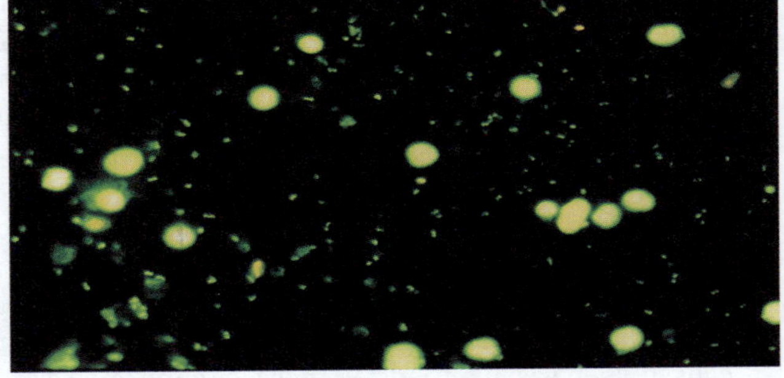

FIG. 4.23: Malarial parasite under fluorescent microscopy.

Q. Write short essay on:
- **Treatment of uncomplicated falciparum malaria**
- **Drugs used in resistant malaria/drug resistant malaria. Drugs for resistant falciparum malaria.**
- **Radical treatment of malaria**
- **Name antimalarial drugs**

TABLE 4.40: Comparison of rapid diagnostic tests for malaria antigens.

	PfHRP2 tests	*PfHRP2 and PMA test*	*pLDH test*
Target antigen	Histidine-rich protein 2 of *P. falciparum*, water soluble protein expressed on RBC membrane	Pan-specific *Plasmodium* aldolase, parasite glycolytic enzyme produced by all species and PfHRP2	Parasite lactate dehydrogenase, parasite glycolytic enzyme produced by all species
Capability	Detects *P. falciparum* only	Can detect all four species	Can detect all four species
Detection limit	>40–100 parasites/μL	Higher for *P. vivax* and other nonfalciparum species	>100–200 parasites/μL for *P. falciparum* and *P. vivax*; may be higher for *P. malariae* and *P. ovale*
Cross-reactivity with autoantibodies	Reported, high (up to 83% with rheumatoid factor)	Not known	Reported low (3.3% with rheumatoid factor)
Indication of viability of parasites	No	No	Positive test indicates presence of viable parasitemia

Management/Treatment

Aims of treatment are presented in **Table 4.41**.

TABLE 4.41: Aims of treatment.

Aims	*Causation*	*Therapy*	*Drugs*
To alleviate symptoms	Symptoms are caused by blood forms of the parasite	Blood schizonticidal drugs	Chloroquine, quinine, and artemisinin combinations
To prevent relapses	Relapses are due to hypnozoites of *P. vivax/P. ovale*	Tissue schizonticidal drugs	Primaquine
To prevent spread	Spread is through the gametocytes	Gametocytocidal drugs	Primaquine for *P. falciparum*, chloroquine for all other

To **counter the threat of resistance of *P. falciparum*** to monotherapies, and to improve treatment outcome, **combinations of antimalarials are now recommended** by WHO for the treatment of falciparum malaria. **Two or more blood schizontocidal drugs** with independent modes of action and thus unrelated biochemical targets in the parasite are used and at present artemisinin-based combination therapy (ACT) is the recommended treatments for uncomplicated falciparum malaria **(Fig. 4.24).**

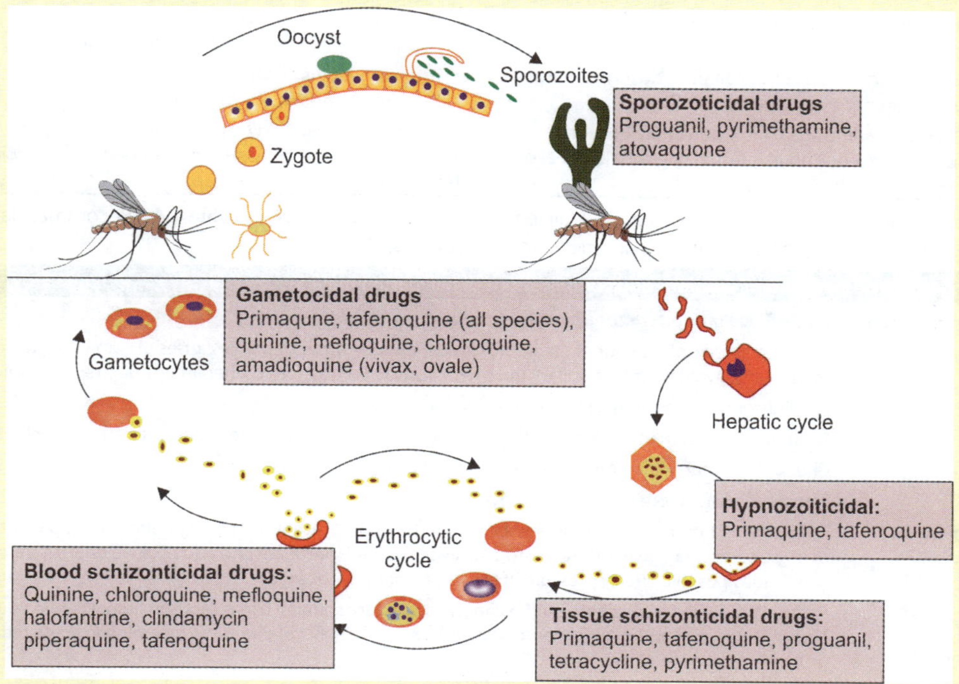

FIG. 4.24: Antimalarial drugs.

- **Artemisinin-based combination therapy (ACT)**
  - Artemisinin and its derivatives (artesunate, artemether, artemotil, and dihydroartemisinin) **produce rapid clearance of parasitemia** and rapid resolution of symptoms. They reduce parasite numbers by a factor of approximately 10,000 in each asexual cycle, which is more than other current antimalarials (which reduce parasite numbers 100- to 1000-fold per cycle). Artemisinin and its derivatives are eliminated rapidly.
  - When given in combination with rapidly eliminated compounds (tetracyclines and clindamycin), a 7-day course of treatment with an artemisinin compound is required; but when given in combination with slowly eliminated antimalarials, shorter courses of treatment (3 days) are effective.
- **Nonartemisinin-based combinations (non-ACTs)** include sulfadoxine—pyrimethamine with chloroquine (SP + CQ) or amodiaquine (SP + AQ). However, the prevailing high levels of resistance have compromised the efficacy of these combinations. There is no convincing evidence that SP + CQ provides any additional benefit over SP, so this combination is not recommended.
  - The ACT used in the national program in India is artesunate + sulfadoxine + pyrimethamine. It is given as:
    - 200 mg artesunate along with sulfadoxine 1,500 mg and pyrimethamine 75 mg on day 1.
    - 200 mg artesunate on days 2 and 3.
  - Another option is to use quinine 600 mg salt three times daily for 5 days orally, followed by a single dose of sulfadoxine 1.5 g combined with pyrimethamine 75 mg.
  - Artemisinin based combinations can be given in second and third trimester of pregnancy. Recommended treatment in first trimester of pregnancy is quinine.
  - If sulfonamide sensitivity is suspected, quinine may be followed by tetracycline 250 m 6 hourly for 7 days.
- Other drugs for treating chloroquine resistant *P. falciparum* are mefloquine (15 mg/kg followed by 10 mg/kg after 8 hours; generally given as ACT) and halofantrine. Recently, dihydroartemisinin (4 mg/kg/day) + piperaquine (18 mg/kg/day) combination for 3 days has been available.
- Summary of treatment of malaria is presented in **Table 4.42**.

TABLE 4.42: Summary of treatment of malaria.

Type of infection	*Suppressive treatment*	*Radical treatment*
P. vivax and *P. ovale*	Chloroquine 25 mg of salt/kg over 36–48 hours	Primaquine 0.25 mg/kg for 14 days
P. malariae and *P. knowlesi*	Chloroquine 25 mg of salt/kg over 36–48 hours	None
P. falciparum	Treatment depends on severity and sensitivity artesunate + pyrimethamine-sulfadoxine or other ACTs, OR quinine plus tetracycline	Primaquine 0.75 mg/kg in single dose as gametocytocidal
Mixed (*P. vivax* + *P. falciparum*)	ACT as for *P. falciparum*	Primaquine as for *P. vivax*

Radical cure of malaria due to *P. vivax* and *P. ovale*.

Primaquine is given at a dose of 15 mg daily for 14 days. It destroys the hypnozoite phase in the liver.

Table 4.43 outlines the treatment of severe malaria.

TABLE 4.43: Treatment of severe malaria.

First drug	*Follow-on treatment (full course of any ACT)*
Artesunate 2.4 mg/kg body weight (bw) IV or IM on admission; then at 12 hours and 24 hours, then once a day for at least 24 hours, followed by full course of ACT OR	➢ Artesunate plus sulfadoxine-pyrimethamine ➢ Artesunate plus amodiaquine ➢ Artesunate plus clindamycin or doxycycline
Artemether 3.2 mg/kg bw IM given on admission then 1.6 mg/kg bw per day for at least 24 hours, followed by full course of ACT	➢ Artemether plus lumefantrine ➢ Dihydroartemisinin + piperaquine
Quinine, 20 mg salt/kg bw on admission (IV infusion or divided IM injection), then 10 mg/kg bw every 8 hour; infusion rate should not exceed 5 mg salt/kg bw per hour; course for 3 days	Doxycycline 100 mg BID (2.2 mg/kg BID for <45 kg) for 7 days OR clindamycin 20 mg base/kg/day divided in three doses for 7 days in pregnancy

Management of severe manifestations and complications of falciparum malaria are presented in **Table 4.44.** Recommendations for treatment of uncomplicated *P. falciparum* malaria in pregnancy are mentioned in **Table 4.45.**

TABLE 4.44: Management of severe manifestations and complications of falciparum malaria.

Manifestation/complication	*Immediate management (in addition to antimalarial treatment)*
Coma (cerebral malaria)	Maintain airway, place patient on his or her side, exclude other treatable causes of coma (e.g., hypoglycemia, bacterial meningitis); avoid harmful ancillary treatment such as corticosteroids, heparin, and adrenaline; intubate if necessary
Hyperpyrexia	Administer tepid sponging, fanning, cooling blanket, and antipyretic drugs
Convulsions	Maintain airways; treat promptly with intravenous or rectal diazepam or intramuscular paraldehyde
Hypoglycemia	Check blood glucose, correct hypoglycemia and maintain with glucose-containing infusion
Severe anemia	Transfuse with screened fresh whole blood
Acute pulmonary edema	Over-enthusiastic rehydration should be avoided so as to prevent pulmonary edema. Prop patient up at an angle of 45°, give oxygen, give a diuretic, stop intravenous fluids, intubate and add positive end-expiratory pressure/ continuous positive airway pressure in life-threatening hypoxemia
Acute renal failure	Exclude prerenal causes, check fluid balance, and urinary sodium; if in established renal failure add hemofiltration or hemodialysis, or if unavailable, peritoneal dialysis. The benefits of diuretics/dopamine in acute renal failure are not proven
Spontaneous bleeding and coagulopathy	Transfuse with screened fresh whole blood (cryoprecipitate, fresh frozen plasma, and platelets if available); give vitamin K injection
Metabolic acidosis	Exclude or treat hypoglycemia, hypovolemia, and septicemia. If severe add hemofiltration or hemodialysis
Shock	Suspect septicemia, take blood for cultures; give parenteral antimicrobials, correct hemodynamic disturbances
Hyperparasitemia	Treat with artemisinins, intravenously or orally

TABLE 4.45: Recommendations for treatment of uncomplicated *P. falciparum* malaria in pregnancy.

First trimester	Quinine + clindamycin for 7 days. ACT should be used if it is the only effective treatment available
Second and third trimesters	ACT known to be effective in the country/region or artesunate + clindamycin to be given for 7 days or quinine + clindamycin to be given for 7 days

Chemoprophylaxis of malaria is presented in **Box 4.16.**

Box 4.16: Chemoprophylaxis of malaria.

- For short-term chemoprophylaxis (<6 weeks), doxycycline in a dose of 100 mg daily. It should be started 2 days before travel and continued for 4 weeks after leaving the malarious area.
- For long-term chemoprophylaxis (>6 weeks), mefloquine in a dose of 5 mg/kg (up to 250 mg) weekly. It should be administered 2 weeks before, during and 4 weeks after leaving the area.

Q. List the uses of chloroquine.

Uses of chloroquine are listed in **Box 4.17**.

Box 4.17: Uses of chloroquine.

- Drug of choice for clinical cure and suppressive prophylaxis of all types of malaria, except that caused by resistant *P. falciparum*
- Extraintestinal amebiasis
- Rheumatoid arthritis, SLE, and chikungunya
- Discoid lupus erythematosus
- Lepra reactions
- Photogenic reactions
- Infectious mononucleosis (symptomatic relief)

Tropical Splenomegaly Syndrome (TSS)

Q. Write short essay/note on tropical splenomegaly syndrome (TSS).

Tropical splenomegaly syndrome or big spleen disease, also known as **hyper-reactive malarial splenomegaly** is massive enlargement of the spleen resulting from abnormal immune response to repeated attacks of malaria. It is seen among residents of endemic areas of malaria.

It is one of the chronic complications of malaria.

Etiopathogenesis

- Chronic or repeated malarial infections produce hypergammaglobulinemia; normocytic normochromic anemia; and massive splenomegaly.

- Tropical splenomegaly syndrome is characterized by the production of cytotoxic IgM antibodies to CD8+ T lymphocytes, antibodies to CD5+ T lymphocytes, and an increase in the ratio of CD4+ to CD8+ T cells. These result in continuous IgM production by B cell and the formation of cryoglobulins (IgM aggregates and immune complexes). This stimulates reticuloendothelial hyperplasia and leads to splenomegaly.

Clinical Features

- Anemia and some degree of pancytopenia are usually found.
- There is increased vulnerability to respiratory and skin infections and many may die due to overwhelming sepsis.
- Physical examination shows massive splenomegaly, hepatomegaly and occasionally low-grade fever.
- The disease generally runs a benign course. Portal hypertension does not develop and the condition is reversible with antimalarial treatment. Some may evolve into malignant lymphoproliferative disorder (e.g., CLL).

Diagnosis of TSS

- **Antimalarial antibodies:** High levels of antimalarial antibodies are found in blood. IgM levels are markedly elevated (up to 20 times).
- There is increase in the serum levels of polyclonal IgM with cryoglobulinemia, reduced C3 and the rheumatoid factor may be positive.
- **Liver biopsy:**
  - Light microscopy of liver shows sinusoidal lymphocytosis and Kupffer cell hyperplasia.
  - **Immunofluorescence microscopy** shows IgM aggregates phagocytosed by RE cells.
- **Peripheral blood:** The peripheral smear shows normocytic normochromic anemia with increased reticulocyte count. Leukopenia and thrombocytopenia may also be seen due to hypersplenism. **Malarial parasites are not found** in the peripheral blood.

Treatment of Tropical Splenomegaly Syndrome

- Chloroquine weekly or proguanil daily has been found to be useful. These drugs may have to be continued for long periods, possibly for life.
- Severe anemia may require blood transfusion.
- Splenectomy may do more harm than good and it may be beneficial in only patients with splenic lymphoma.
- Splenic irradiation or antimitotic therapy is not beneficial and may be even dangerous.

Malaria Vaccines

Q. Write short note on malarial vaccines.

Vaccine Types

The candidate malaria vaccines target the different phases of the parasite's life cycle.

- **The pre-erythrocytic vaccines** target sporozoites or schizont infected liver cells, and are aimed at preventing infection by stopping the progression of hepatic stage. Even a single sporozoite escaping vaccine-induced immunity may cause a fully pathogenic blood stage infection, as was found during the clinical trials of the latest antisporozoite RTS, S vaccine.
- **The erythrocytic stage** vaccines are aimed at reducing parasite multiplication and growth in order to protect against clinical disease, particularly severe disease. These vaccines are designed to induce antibody responses against the targets on the asexual blood stage of the parasite such as merozoite surface proteins (such as MSP-1) or those contained in specialized organelles associated with invasion (such as AMA-1). But, the very short duration during which merozoites stay outside the red cells (about 2 minutes), the high degree of polymorphic variability, and the use of alternative invasion pathways by *P. falciparum*.
- **Transmission-blocking vaccines** are aimed at reducing malaria transmission by interrupting the parasite life-cycle in the mosquito by inducing antibodies that prevent either fertilization of the gametes in the mosquito gut or the further development of the zygote into sporozoites. These vaccines do not protect the immunized individual but rather provide herd benefit. **Antidisease vaccination**, by preventing the parasite surface protein parasite-derived *Plasmodium falciparum* erythrocyte membrane protein 1 (PfEMP1) from interacting with various vascular endothelial cell-surface receptors, may block the sequestration of parasite-infected erythrocytes and prevents the serious complications such as cerebral malaria or placental malaria.
  All these vaccines are in clinical trial stages. RTS, S is the most recently developed recombinant vaccine. It consists of the *P. falciparum* circumsporozoite protein from the pre-erythrocytic stage has been approved to vaccinate children aged 6 weeks to 17 months outside the European Union.

- **Recrudescence of malaria**
  - Exacerbation of persistent undetectable parasitemia, due to survival of erythrocytic forms, no exoerythrocytic cycle (P.f. and P.m.)
- **Relapse**
  - Reactivation of hypnozoites forms of parasite in liver, separate from previous infection with same species (P.v. and P.o.)
- **Recurrence or reinfection**
  - Exoerythrocytic forms infect erythrocytes, separate from previous infection (all species)
  - Cannot always differentiate recrudescence from reinfection

Leishmaniasis

Q. Write short note on leishmaniasis.

Leishmaniasis is a group of diseases caused by unicellular, flagellate, and intracellular protozoa of the genus *Leishmania*, which are transmitted by the bite of the **female phlebotomine sandfly**.

Clinical Syndromes

Visceral Leishmaniasis (Kala-azar)

Q. Write short note on kala-azar or visceral leishmaniasis.

Visceral leishmaniasis (kala-azar) is a generalized visceral infection caused by the protozoon Leishmania donovani complex (comprising *L. donovani, L. infantum,* and *L. chagasi*).

Epidemiology

Mode of transmission: Sandfly of the Genera *Phlebotomus.*

- **Endemic:**
  - Kala-azar is endemic in several countries. More than 90% of visceral leishmaniases are found in India, Bangladesh, Southern Sudan, Nepal, and Brazil.
  - In India, it is endemic in the states of Bihar, West Bengal, Eastern parts of Uttar Pradesh, and parts of Odisha.
- **Sporadic** *cases have been reported from several other parts of* India.

Life cycle of Leishmania (Fig. 4.25)

Leishmania occurs in two forms: (1) extracellular, flagellate promastigote form in the sandfly vector and (2) intracellular, nonflagellate amastigote form in humans.

Incubation period: Usually 1–6 months, but may be several years.

Clinical features of kala-azar

- **Age group:** In India, adults and children are equally affected whereas elsewhere it is mainly seen in small children and infants (except in adults with HIV coinfection).
- **Organs involved:** It primarily affects the host's reticuloendothelial system. In visceral leishmaniasis, monocytes and macrophages of the spleen, liver, bone marrow, and lymph nodes are primarily affected.
- **Onset:** Great majority of individuals infected remain asymptomatic and onset in others may be abrupt.

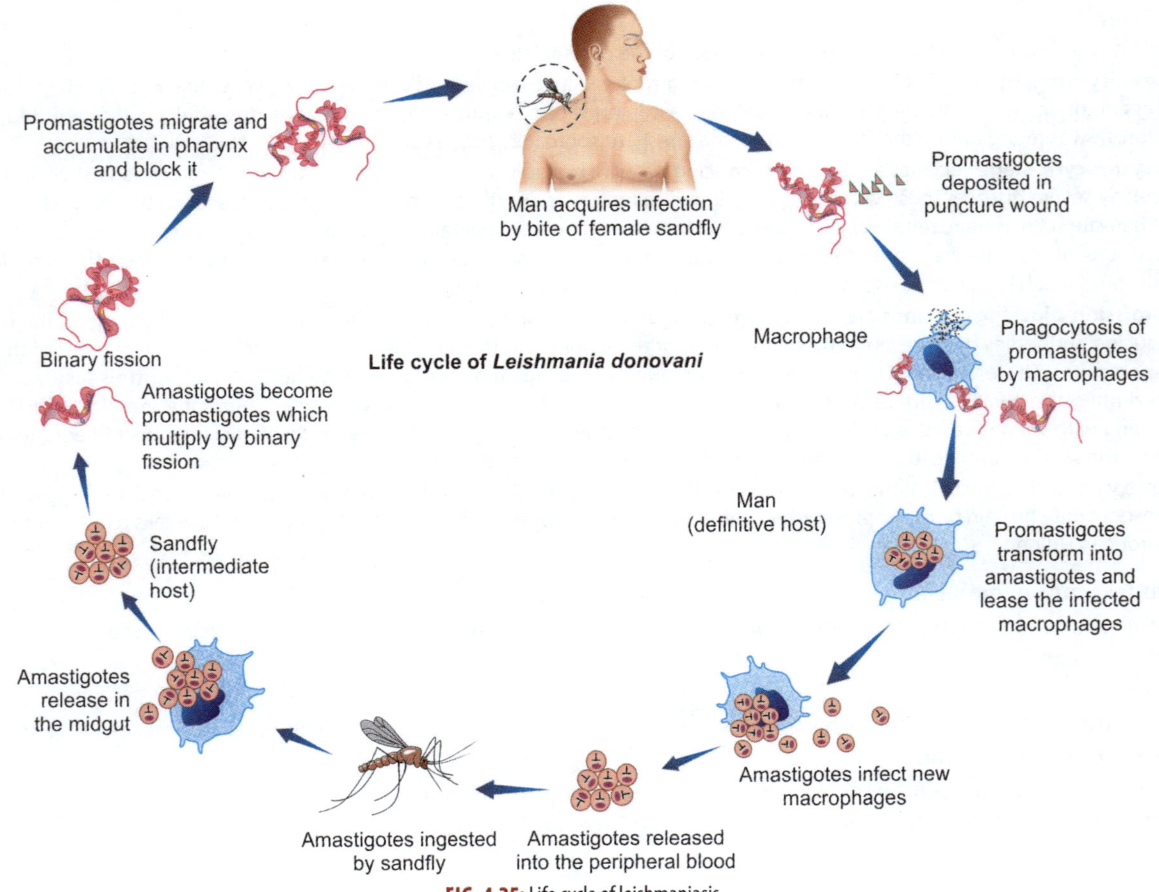

FIG. 4.25: Life cycle of leishmaniasis.

- **Fever:** It is the first sign of infection. Few patients present with a low-grade fever, whereas others present with a high-grade, usually accompanied by rigor and chills. The fever is intermittent showing a double rise of temperature in 24 hours ("camel hump fever"). The intensity of fever decreases over time, and patients may be afebrile for intervening periods ranging from weeks to months. This is followed by a relapse of fever which is often less intense.

Physical findings

- **Massive splenomegaly and hepatomegaly:** Splenomegaly develops in the first few weeks and becomes massive as the disease progresses. Moderate hepatomegaly develops later.
- **Lymphadenopathy:** It is common in patients in Africa, the Mediterranean, and South America. In India, it is more common in patients from West Bengal.
- **Blackish discoloration of the skin:** Disease derived its name; kala-azar is derived from the Hindi word for "black fever." Generalized blackish pigmentation with rough skin is prominent over face is an observed in advanced stage of disease and now it is rare.
- **Anemia:** Moderate to severe anemia develops rapidly, and can produce congestive cardiac failure and associated clinical features.
- **Bleeding manifestations:** Thrombocytopenia, often associated with hepatic dysfunction, may cause bleeding from the retina, gastrointestinal tract, and nose.

Cause of death: Death usually occurs within a year and is either due to bacterial infection or uncontrolled bleeding.

Complications

- **Hypoalbuminemia:** May develop in advanced stage and may manifest as pedal edema, ascites, and anasarca (gross generalized edema and swelling).
- **Immunosuppression:** As the disease advances, severe immunosuppression may lead to secondary infections. These include tuberculosis, pneumonia, malaria, severe amebic or bacillary dysentery, gastroenteritis, herpes zoster, and chickenpox. Skin infections (e.g., boils, cellulitis, scabies, and cancrum oris) are common.

Investigations

Direct evidences

- **Demonstration of amastigotes (Leishman–Donovan bodies):** It can be demonstrated in stained smears of aspirates of bone marrow (50–70% cases), spleen (70–90% cases), liver, lymph nodes, or buffy coat of peripheral blood. Demonstration of LD bodies in splenic smears is the most useful for the diagnosis (98% sensitivity); however, there is a risk of serious hemorrhage in inexperienced hands. It is the gold standard for the diagnosis of visceral leishmaniasis (VL).
- **Culture:** The aspirated material can be cultured in the Novy-MacNeal-Nicolle (NNN) medium for the organism.

Indirect evidences

- **Blood:** Pancytopenia is a common feature (i.e., anemia, granulocytopenia, and thrombocytopenia).
- **Biochemical findings:**
  - Low serum albumin (hypoalbuminemia) and **polyclonal hypergammaglobulinemia** (high serum globulin), chiefly IgG followed by IgM in advanced cases.
  - Liver function test: Mildly elevated bilirubin, AST/ALT and alkaline phosphatase may be seen.
- **Serological/immunodiagnostic tests:**
  - These are less invasive and are useful in community surveillance studies.
  - **Leishmanin (Montenegro) skin test:** Intradermal injection of killed culture of promastigotes produces a delayed-type hypersensitivity and is positive only in patients with cured kala-azar.
  - **Napier's aldehyde** (formal gel) **test and Chopra's antimony test:** These are nonspecific test and should not be employed for the diagnosis of VL. They are used for demonstration of increased immunoglobulins.
  - **Detection of specific antibody:** Various tests such as complement fixation test, indirect hemagglutination test, indirect fluorescent antibody test, and countercurrent immunoglobulins have poor sensitivity and specificity.
- **Antigen detection** by reverse western blotting, dot-enzyme immunoassay (EIA) and latex agglutination test.
- **PCR:** To detect DNA and identify species.

Post-Kala-azar Dermal Leishmaniasis (PKDL)

Time of occurrence: In India, Sudan, and other East African countries, 2–50% of patients develop skin lesions due to local parasitic infection concurrent with or after apparent recovery or cure of visceral leishmaniasis.

Clinical features

Skin lesions may be of three types namely: hypopigmented macules, papules, or nodules and can occur in varying combinations:

- Hypopigmented macules: Earliest lesions and usually found on the trunk and extremities.
- Erythematous patches: These have butterfly distribution on the face.
- Yellowish pink nodules: They are generally found on the skin and rarely on mucus membrane of tongue and eye.

Diagnosis: Demonstration of parasite in the slit smear or by culture of the dermal tissue.

Treatment

Q. Drugs used to treat kala-azar.

General considerations: Blood transfusions to correct severe anemia and treatment of intercurrent bacterial infections with antibiotics.

Pentavalent Antimonial Compounds

- Pentavalent antimonial compounds (sodium stibogluconate and meglumine antimoniate) were the first drugs to be used for the treatment of leishmaniasis and still remain the **mainstay of treatment.** The dose is 20 mg/kg either intravenously or intramuscularly for 40 days. However, many patients may fail to respond due to parasitic resistance.
- **Side effects:** Include arthralgia, myalgia, abdominal pain, raised liver enzymes, pancreatitis (in immunosuppressed patients), ECG changes (T wave inversion and reduced amplitude), and rarely death due to cardiotoxicity.
- For PKDL treatment for 3–4 months is necessary.

Amphotericin B

Q. Write short note on amphotericin B and its side effects.

Amphotericin B deoxycholate is currently used as a primary drug of choice in Bihar, India. In other parts of the world, it is used as a second-line drug when patient is unresponsive to initial antimonial treatment.

- **Dose:** 0.75–1.00 mg/kg given once daily or on alternate days for a total of 15–20 infusion. It has a cure rate of almost 100%.
- **Side effects: Infusion-related side effects** include high fever with chills, thrombophlebitis, diarrhea, and vomiting are common. Other side effects include hypokalemia and renal or hepatic toxicity and thrombocytopenia.
- **Lipid formulations of amphotericin B:** Some of above side effects of amphotericin B deoxycholate can be reduced by using lipid-preparations B lipid complex and amphotericin B colloidal dispersion. In India, liposomal amphotericin B is administered at a total dose of 10 or 15 mg/kg, administered in a single dose or as multiple doses over several days. It may be combined with 7–14 days of oral miltefosine.

Miltefosine

- Miltefosine is an alkyl phospholipid administered orally has shown excellent results. It is the first highly effective, oral drug for treating visceral leishmaniasis.
- **Dose:** 50 mg once a day if weight is <25 kg, and 50 mg twice a day if weight is >25 kg. Duration of treatment is 28 days.
- **Side effects** include vomiting and diarrhea, and occasionally, reversible hepatotoxicity and nephrotoxicity.

Pentamidine

Pentamidine isethionate was used. Dose of 3–4 mg/kg on alternate days for 5–25 weeks was recommended as a second-line drug to treat antimony resistant cases. However, it is abandoned because of its reduced effectiveness and serious side effects (e.g., hypoglycemia, hypotension and induction of diabetes mellitus).

Other Drugs

- Paromomycin (aminosidine): It is antibiotic with antileishmanial action and is highly effective and safe drug. It is given intramuscularly at dose of 11 mg of base/kg daily for 21 days.
- ***Azoles: ketoconazole, fluconazole, and itraconazole***
  - These oral antifungal agents have variable efficacy in leishmaniasis treatment.

Toxoplasmosis

Q. Discuss the etiology, clinical manifestations, diagnosis, and management of toxoplasmosis.

Toxoplasmosis is caused by the intracellular protozoan parasite *Toxoplasma gondii.*

Life Cycle of Toxoplasma gondii

Man is the intermediate host and cat is the definitive host.

Mode of Transmission

- Humans infection occurs via ingestion of:
  - Oocyst discharged in the feces of infected reservoir animal (cat), contaminated salads, vegetables, and water.
  - Raw or undercooked meats containing tissue cysts (bradyzoites). Sheep, pigs, and rabbits are the most common meat sources.
- Transplacental infection from mother to fetus may also occur.

Clinical Manifestations

Q. Write short note on clinical features of toxoplasmosis.

Infection in immunocompetent host

- **Asymptomatic:** Most acute toxoplasmosis is subclinical and goes unnoticed.
- **Painless lymphadenopathy:** In symptomatic patients, it is the most common presenting feature. It may be local or generalized and cervical lymphadenopathy is most common.

- **Other features:**
  - Systemic symptoms are not observed in most patients. If present, these include fever, malaise, fatigue, myalgia, sore throat, and headache.
  - Uncommon features are skin rash and confusion.
  - Rarely: Myocarditis, encephalitis, pneumonia, hepatitis, and polymyositis.
- **Completely resolution occurs within a few weeks to months.**
- **Ocular infection:**
  - Most often ocular involvement (chorioretinitis) is observed in congenital infection
  - Examination shows gray white foci of retinal necrosis with adjacent choroiditis, vasculitis, hemorrhage, and vitreitis. Anterior uveitis may also be seen.

Infection in immunocompromised host

- **In immunocompromised patients, toxoplasmosis is usually due to reactivation of latent infection.**
- **Central nervous system:**
  - It is the most common system affected.
  - Manifestations include encephalopathy, meningoencephalitis, seizures, headache, and focal neurological deficits.
- Pneumonia and ocular involvement may also occur.

Congenital toxoplasmosis

Q. Write short note on congenital toxoplasmosis.

Transmission

Acute toxoplasmosis is mostly subclinical and develops in 0.3–1% of pregnant women.

Clinical manifestations

- Congenital toxoplasmosis may be asymptomatic, but can produce serious disease.
- **CNS:** Manifestations include hydrocephalus, microcephaly, encephalitis, convulsions, tremors, paralysis, and mental retardation. Cerebrospinal fluid may be xanthochromic with raised protein and mononuclear cells. Skull radiograph may show patches of calcification in the brain.
- **Ophthalmic manifestations:** Microphthalmus, nystagmus, chorioretinitis (common), and blindness.
- Other features: Hepatomegaly, jaundice, thrombocytopenia, and purpura may be seen.

Investigations

- **Blood:** Mild lymphocytosis, raised ESR, and mild increase in liver enzymes.
- **Serodiagnosis:** Presence of significant levels of *Toxoplasma* specific IgM antibody indicates acute infection and absence of IgM antibodies virtually rules out acute infection. However, in immunocompromised patients most of the time toxoplasmosis is due to reactivation and there is no rise in IgM antibody. Hence, IgG antibodies are used for presumptive diagnosis.
  - **Sabin–Feldman methylene blue dye test:** A dye test positive with a titer of 1:128 is diagnostic of active toxoplasmosis.
  - **Indirect fluorescent antibody test**
  - **Fluorescent stain for toxoplasma (Goldman's test):** It is useful for detection of parasites in smears and biopsy specimens.
  - **ELISA test.**
- **PCR for toxoplasma DNA** in ocular secretions and amniotic fluid
- **Microscopic examination** of smear or biopsy material (from a lymph node or muscle) shows the parasite.
- **Inoculation** of suspected material into laboratory-bred mice, guinea pigs may show characteristic histological changes.
  These include any of the three infectious stages: tachyzoites in groups, bradyzoites (tissue cysts), or sporozoites within oocyst.
- **Investigations in toxoplasma encephalitis:**
  - **CSF** may be normal or show mild increase in cells and protein
  - **Serum:** IgG antibodies to toxoplasma
  - **Radiological:** CT scan of head may show multiple contrast-enhancing lesions. However, MRI **(Fig. 4.26)** is more sensitive than CT scan in identifying the lesions. Single-photon emission computed tomography (SPECT) helps in differentiating CNS lymphoma from toxoplasmic encephalitis.

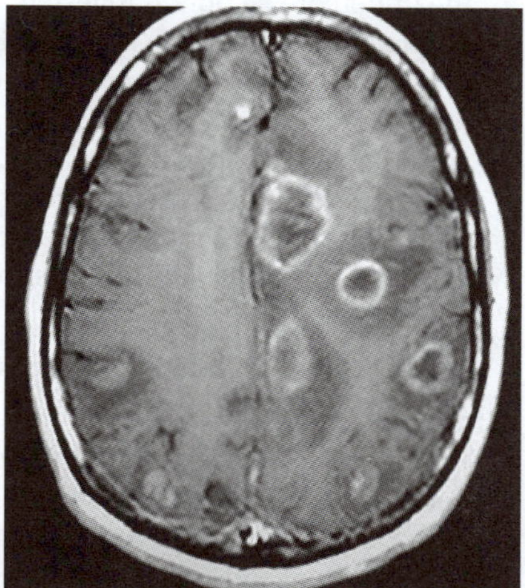

FIG. 4.26: MRI brain showing ring enhancing lesions in toxoplasmosis.

Management

- Acquired uncomplicated toxoplasmosis in an immunocompetent individual is self-limiting and does not require treatment.
- Treatment for severe (especially eye involvement) or progressive disease and for infection in immunocompromised patients:

- Combination of **sulfadiazine 2–4 g daily (1 g 6 hourly) and pyrimethamine** in a single loading dose 25 mg daily both for 4–6 weeks, along with folinic acid/leucovorin. Steroids are added to the above regime for ocular toxoplasmosis.
- If the patient is sensitive to sulfonamides, clindamycin, atovaquone, or azithromycin can be used.

- **Toxoplasmosis in pregnant women:**
  - If a seronegative women acquire toxoplasmosis during pregnancy (especially during first trimester), or seroconverts during pregnancy, there is a greater risk of transmitting the infection to fetus giving rise to an infant with congenital toxoplasmosis. Such pregnancies should be terminated.
  - The aim of management of pregnant women with toxoplasmosis is to reduce the risk of fetal complications.
  - The recommended treatment for a pregnant woman with an established recent infection is spiramycin (3 g daily in divided doses) until term. However, whether it has any significant effect on the frequency or severity of fetal damage is not well established. Infected infants should be treated from birth.

INFECTIONS CAUSED BY HELMINTHS

Cestodes (Tapeworms)

Cestodes (tapeworms) are ribbon-shaped worms which vary from a few millimeters to several meters in length.

Life Cycle (Fig. 4.27)

The tapeworm passes its life cycle in two hosts:

- **Definitive host:** Human is the definitive host and harbors the adult worm.
- **Intermediate host:** It may be pig or cattle depending on type of tapeworm and they harbor larval forms.

Taenia solium

Q. Write a short note on *Taenia solium* and cysticercosis.

Taenia solium, the pork tapeworm, inhabits the intestinal lumen of humans (only definitive host). Adult worms are found only in human. Pigs are the usual intermediate hosts.

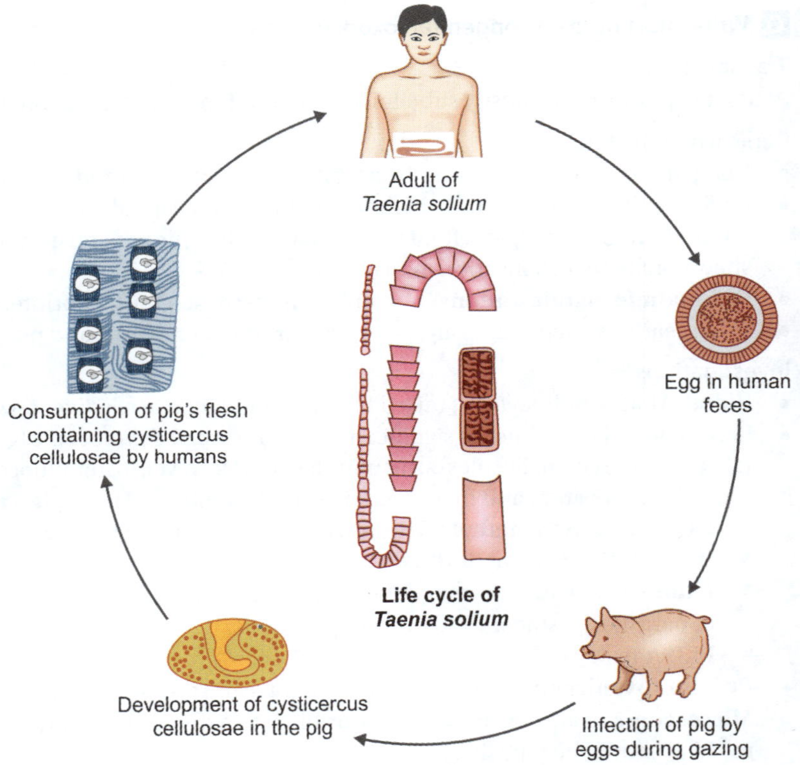

Disease in Humans

Taenia solium causes

- **Intestinal infection:** If cysticerci present in the undercooked pork is ingested.
- **Cysticercosis** (systemic infection from larval migration): If ova present in contaminated food and water are ingested. Feco-oral autoinfection can occur but is rare.

Patients with tapeworms usually do not develop cysticercosis and patients with cysticercosis do not usually harbor tapeworms.

FIG. 4.27: Life cycle of *Taenia solium*.

Cysticercosis

It is the condition in which human tissue is invaded by the larval form of *Taenia solium*.

Mode of infection

- Human cysticercosis results from **ingestion of ova/eggs of *Taenia solium*** which have **contaminated water or vegetable**.
- **Feco-oral autoinfection:** Human harboring adult worm may autoinfect himself either due to unhygienic personal habits.
- **Reversal of peristaltic movements of the intestine** whereby gravid segments are thrown back to the stomach which releases thousands of eggs into the stomach.
- The common sites of cysticerci are subcutaneous tissue, skeletal muscle, brain, and eyes.

Clinical features

Q. Write short note on neurocysticercosis.

Intestinal infection: Presence of adult tapeworm in the intestine usually do not produce symptoms. It is usually discovered when proglottids are found in feces or on underclothing.

Cysticercosis: They are usually range from 10 to 1,000.

- **Superficially placed cysts:** Those in subcutaneous tissues and muscles cause few or no symptoms. They produce palpable or visible nodule (pea-like ovoid bodies) under the skin or mucosa. Eventually, they die and undergo dystrophic calcification. The dead larvae may cause marked tissue response resulting in muscular pain, weakness, fever, and eosinophilia.
- **Neurocysticercosis** results from cysts in the brain. Heavy brain infections may present with meningoencephalitis, epilepsy, personality changes, staggering gait, space-occupying lesion, stroke (due to inflammatory changes in the wall of intracranial arteries located in the vicinity of cysticerci), or hydrocephalus. The cerebral signs usually occur after 5–20 years when the larvae die.

Diagnosis

- **Stool examination:** Eggs and proglottids in stool
- **Radiological investigations:**
  - **Radiographs** of involved soft tissue (buttocks and thigh) may show calcified cysts (*cigar-shaped/rice grain calcification*) in muscles (**Figs. 4.28A to C**).
  - **CT scan** of the brain may show calcified cysticerci, small hypodense lesions (ring or disk-like enhancing lesion) or small hypodense lesions with central bright spot. CT scan is more sensitive than MRI for identifying calcified cysts.
  - **MRI scan:** It is better for identifying cystic lesions, enhancement, and cysticercosis in the ventricles.
- **Serological test:** Specific enzyme-linked immunoelectrodiffusion transfer blot (EITB) using lentil-lectin purified glycoproteins is highly sensitive and specific. IFA and ELISA test are also useful.
- **Histological examination** of the excised subcutaneous nodule or the lesion will show cysticerci.

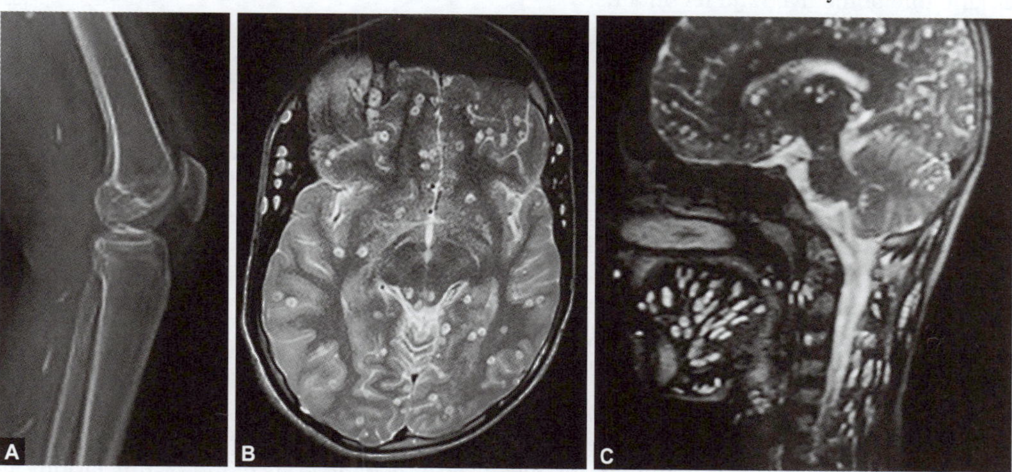

FIGS. 4.28A TO C: X-ray thigh and shows cigar-shaped/rice grain calcification due to calcified cysts of tapeworm in muscles. MRI brain and soft tissue skull showing multiple enhancing lesions (starry sky appearance).

Q. Write short note on:
- **Drug treatment of tapeworm.**
- **Treatment of neurocysticercosis.**

Treatment

Intestinal Infection

For the adult worm in the intestine: Niclosamide (2 g as a single dose), praziquantel (5 mg/kg), or albendazole.

Neurocysticercosis

- **Albendazole:** 15 mg/kg/day for 2–4 weeks is the drug of choice for parenchymal neurocysticercosis.
- An alternative drug is **praziquantel** (PZQ) in the dose of 50 mg/kg in three divided doses daily for 10 days. Single day course is effective in patients with a single cyst or low cyst burdens, but is less efficacious in those with heavier cyst burdens.
- **Corticosteroids:** Successful treatment is accompanied by increased local inflammation. Hence, **prednisolone** is given in the dose of 10 mg 8 hourly for 14 days, starting 1 day before, during and after the course of anthelminthic (albendazole or PZQ).
- **Antiepileptic drugs** should be administered for epilepsy until the reaction in the brain has subsided.
- **Operative intervention** may be necessary for internal hydrocephalus.

Echinococcus granulosus (Taenia Echinococcus) and Hydatid Disease

Q. Write short note on hydatid disease.

Life cycle of *Echinococcus granulosus* (Fig. 4.29)

- **Definitive host:** Dog, wolf, fox, and jackal are the definitive host.
- **Intermediate host:** Human, sheep, pig, cattle, goat, etc., are intermediate host.

Hydatid Disease

Hydatid cyst is the larval stage of *E. granulosus* producing tissue infection of humans or other intermediate hosts (sheep, cattle, camels, and other animals from contaminated water).

Mode of infection: Human is infected accidentally by ingestion of eggs while handling a dog or drinking contaminated water. Canines (especially dogs) are the definitive hosts for *E. granulosus*.

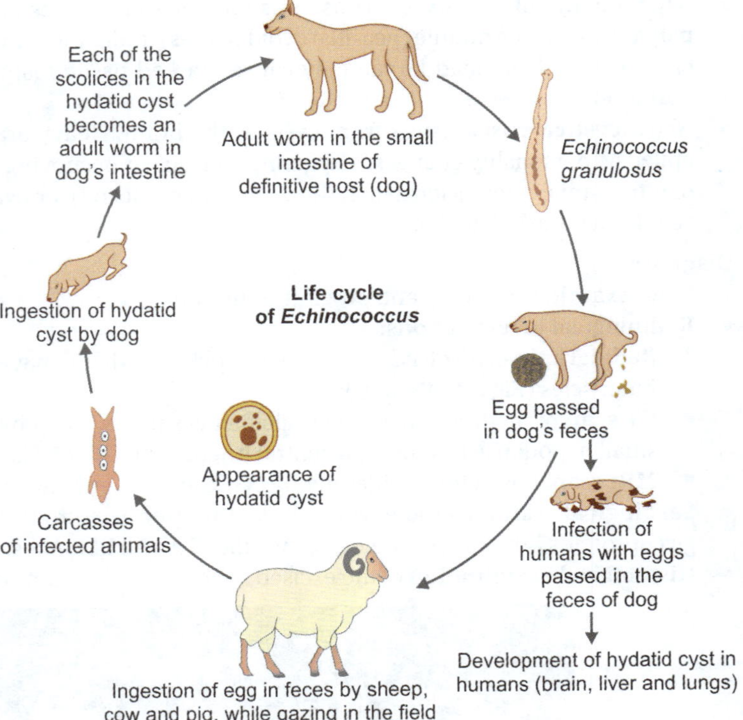

FIG. 4.29: Life cycle of Echinococcus granulosus.

Clinical features

- Humans may ingest the eggs while handling a dog or contaminated water. Usually, hydatid cyst is acquired in childhood and is diagnosed after a latent period of 5–20 years. It may cause pressure symptoms and vary, depending on the site of the cyst (organ or tissue involved).
- **Liver:** In about 75% of the patients, hydatid disease involves the right lobe of the liver and it contains a single cyst. The lesions in liver often present as palpable masses or abdominal pain.
  - Obstruction of bile duct may produce obstructive jaundice.
  - Intrabiliary extrusion of calcified hepatic cysts can cause recurrent cholecystitis.
- **Rupture of a hydatid cysts:** It may occur into the bile duct, peritoneal cavity, lung, pleura, or bronchus. It may cause fever, pruritus, urticarial rash, or an anaphylactoid reaction which may be fatal.
- **Pulmonary** hydatid cyst may rupture producing cough, chest pain, or hemoptysis.
- Hydatid cyst in **central nervous system** may produce epilepsy or blindness.
- Other organs involved: Rarely bone, heart, kidneys, spleen, ovary and thyroid.

Gross appearance of hydatid cyst is shown in **Figure 4.30A**.

Diagnosis

- **Radiological:**
  - **X-ray:** Routine chest radiographs is helpful in the diagnosis of hydatid cysts of lung. Lung lesions appear as round, irregular masses of uniform density. The "meniscus sign" or "crescent sign" is due to the presence of air between the pericyst and the laminated membrane. The "water lily sign" is due to an endocyst floating in a partially fluid-filled cyst. Occasionally, a chest X-ray may show smooth rim of calcified hepatic cyst.
  - **CT scan (Fig. 4.30B), ultrasonography and MRI** can identify the hydatid cysts by showing scolices and daughter cysts.
- **Casoni's skin test** is performed by intradermal injection of 0.2 mL of fresh sterile hydatid fluid. Positive test produces immediate hypersensitivity reaction (not routinely available).

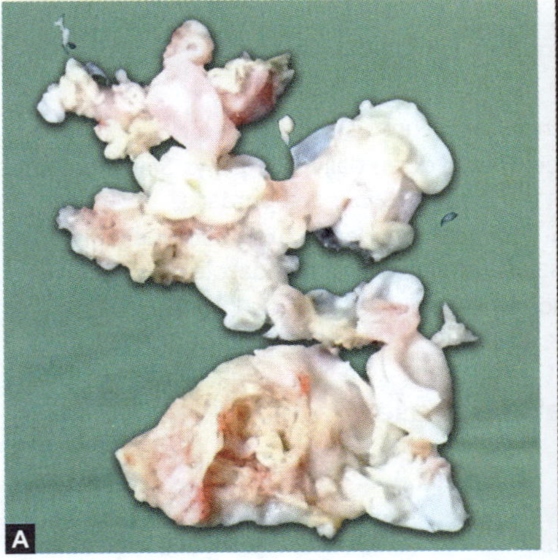

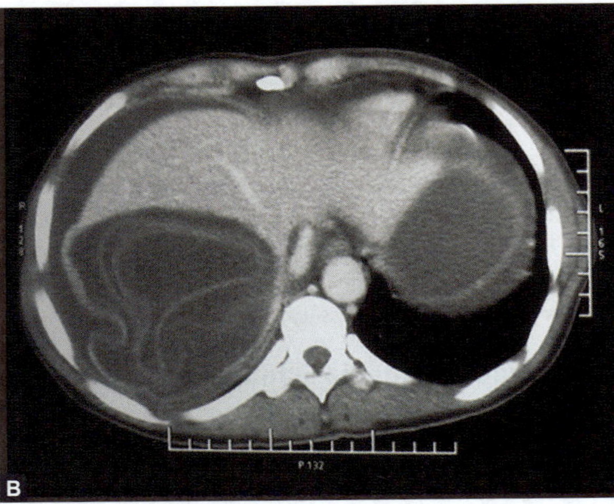

FIGS. 4.30A AND B: (A) Gross appearance of hydatid cyst; (B) hydatid cyst on CT abdomen.

- **Serological test:**
    - Precipitin reaction, complement fixation, immunofluorescent tests, and ELISA are positive in 70–90% of patients.
    - IHAT, ELISA using specific echinococcal antigens

Q. Write short note on medical management of hydatid disease.

Management/Treatment

- Surgical excision of the cysts wherever possible is the treatment of choice. Great care is needed to avoid spillage of fluid and cavities are sterilized with 0.5% silver nitrate or 2.7% sodium chloride.
- In inoperable cases, "high-dose" albendazole (7.5 mg/kg/twice daily or 400 mg twice daily) is given for 1–3 months. In selected cases, the drug can combined with percutaneous puncture, aspiration, injection of scolicidal agent, and re-aspiration (PAIR)
- Praziquantel (20 mg/kg twice daily for 14 days) kills protoscolices and is useful perioperatively.

Enterobius vermicularis (Threadworm/Pinworm)

Q. Write a short note on enterobiasis, pinworm infection, and threadworm infection.

Enterobiasis is an intestinal infection of humans caused by *Enterobius vermicularis* (threadworm).

Mode of Infection

Humans are usually infected by the ingestion of eggs by direct transfer of eggs from the anus to the mouth by way of contaminated fingers or through contaminated food or water. Retroinfection occurs when the eggs hatch in the perianal region and the larvae migrate back into the bowel lumen.

Clinical Features

Q. Write a short note on clinical features of *Enterobius vermicularis*.

- **Perianal itching (pruritus ani):** It is the most common symptom, especially at night. This is due to the gravid female worm which migrates to anal region at night and lays ova around perianal region causing intense itching at night. The ova are carried to the mouth on the fingers and so reinfection or human-to-human infection is common (autoinfection). The adult worms may be seen moving on the buttocks or in the stool.
- **In females:** Migration of adult worm into the female genitalia. It may result in vaginal discharge, salpingitis, and endometritis.
- **Other symptoms** include irritability, insomnia, and enuresis.

Investigations and Diagnoses

Q. Write a short note on laboratory features of pinworm infestations.

- **Direct visualizing the worms** in the perineal and perianal region
- **Stool examination** for eggs may be positive in only 5–10% cases.
    - **Cellophane tape test:** This test is performed by touching the adhesive surface of cellophane tape to the perianal area of skin several times in the morning and removing. It is then examined for eggs on a glass slide under the microscope. Sensitivity of test is about 90%.

Treatment/Management

- **Pyrantel pamoate** given in a single oral dose of 11 mg/kg is the treatment of choice.
- **Other drugs:** A single oral dose of **mebendazole** (100 mg), **albendazole** (400 mg), or piperazine (4 g).
- **Recurring infections:** If infection constantly recurs in a family, each family member should be given mebendazole 100 mg twice daily for 3 days. This should be repeated after 2 weeks (for also to control autoreinfection). During this period all night clothes and bed linens are laundered. Finger nails must be trimmed and hands are washed before meals.

Ascaris lumbricoides (Roundworm)

Q. Write short note on ascariasis or roundworm infection.

Ascariasis is an infection of humans caused by nematode *Ascaris lumbricoides*.

Clinical Features

Q. Write short note on complications of roundworm infestations.

- Infection is usually asymptomatic.
- Heavy infections are associated with nausea, vomiting, abdominal discomfort, anorexia, and malnutrition (fat, protein, carbohydrate, and vitamins) especially in children. However, serious morbidity and mortality are rare in ascariasis.
- The adult worm may be vomited or passed in the stool.

- **Mechanical effects:** The large size of the adult worm and its tendency to aggregate can form bolus of adult worms. It may produce volvulus, intussusception or obstruction of the small intestine (most common in the terminal ileum), hemorrhagic infarction, and perforation.
- **Ectopic ascariasis:**
  - They may occasionally migrate and invade the appendix (causing acute appendicitis), or the bile duct (causing biliary obstruction, suppurative cholangitis, and liver abscess) and pancreatic ducts (pancreatitis).
  - **Pulmonary:** Larval migration through the lungs may produce **pulmonary eosinophilia,** ascaris bronchopneumonia (characterized by fever, cough, dyspnea, wheeze, eosinophilic leukocytosis, and migratory pulmonary infiltrates), eosinophilic granulomas, bronchial asthma, and urticaria.

Investigations and Diagnoses

- Stool examination: Microscopically shows typical ova in the feces and occasionally adult worms are expelled from the mouth or the anus.
- Radiographic study: Barium examination may demonstrate the worms.
- Blood shows eosinophilia.

Management/Treatment

- **Intestinal ascariasis:** A single dose of albendazole (400 mg), pyrantel pamoate (11 mg/kg; maximum 1 g), ivermectin (150–200 µg/kg) or mebendazole (100 mg twice daily for 3 days). The older drug, piperazine citrate is highly effective and less expensive, but slightly more toxic.
- **Obstruction** due to ascariasis adult worms should be treated with nasogastric suction, piperazine citrate, and intravenous fluids. Very rarely, surgical or endoscopic intervention may be needed for intestinal or biliary obstruction.
- **Ascaris bronchopneumonia** is treated symptomatically.

Trichuris trichiura (Whipworm)

Q. Write a short note on trichuriasis/whipworm infection.

Trichuriasis is an intestinal infection of humans caused by *Trichuris trichiura* (whipworm).

Clinical Features

- Infection is usually asymptomatic, but mucosal damage at the attachment of worm in the intestine can produce petechiae. This may cause loss of 0.005 mL blood/worm/day by the patient and cause anemia.
- Occasionally intense infections in children may cause severe mucosal damage leading to colonic ulceration, persistent diarrhea/dysentery, growth retardation, or rectal prolapse.

Treatment: Mebendazole in the dose of 100 mg twice daily for 3 days or albendazole 400 mg once daily for 3 days in the treatment of choice. Heavy infections may need repetitions of dose.

Ancylostomiasis (Hookworm)

Q. Discuss the etiopathogenesis, clinical features, and management and prevention of hookworm disease.

- Ancylostomiasis is a symptomatic infection caused by parasitization with human hookworms *Ancylostoma duodenale* or *Necator americanus.*
- Hookworm infection is one of the major causes of **anemia** in the tropics and subtropics.
- *Ancylostoma duodenale* or old-world hookworm is found in East Asia, Africa, China, Japan, India, and the Pacific Islands.

Necator americanus or new-world hookworm is found in South and Central America and the Caribbean.

Mode of Infection

It occurs through skin by filariform larvae when human walks bare-foot on the focally contaminated soil.

Clinical Features

- **Lesion in skin: Allergic dermatitis**/itching dermatitis ("ground itch dermatitis") develops at the site of entry of the infective filariform larvae. The lesions are usually on the feet, particularly between the toes.
- **Pulmonary manifestations:** The passage of larvae through the lungs in a heavy infection produces cough with blood-stained sputum, fever. There may be bronchitis, patchy pulmonary consolidation/bronchopneumonia, and eosinophilia.
- **Gastrointestinal manifestations:** Light infections (especially in well-nourished individuals) are often asymptomatic. When the worms have reached the small intestine, heavier worm loads may produce epigastric pain, nausea, and vomiting resembling peptic ulcer disease. Other symptoms include abdominal distension, pica, and small frequent loose stools.

- **Pathological effects:** Chronic heavy infection, particularly on a background of malnourishment, may cause:
  - **Iron deficiency anemia** due to chronic intestinal blood loss.
  - **Hypoproteinemia/hypoalbuminemia**
  - **Retarded physical, mental, and sexual development** may occur in older children with heavy infection in children.

Investigations and Diagnoses

- **Stool examination:**
  - **Microscopic examination** of **stool shows** the characteristic **eggs/ovum**. The eggs of both *Ancylostoma duodenale* and *Necator americanus* are 60–70 µm in length and bounded by an ovoid transparent hyaline membrane.
  - **Occult blood:** The stools rarely show gross blood, but tests for occult blood are **usually positive**.
- **Blood:**
  - **Peripheral blood smear:** Characteristically shows **microcytic hypochromic anemia.** There may be **eosinophilia** (as high as 70–80%) in some cases.
  - **Hemoglobin** level is usually **low**.
- **Hypoalbuminemia** is common in severe disease.

Q. Write short essay/note on:
- **Treatment of ancylostomiasis**
- **Mention the drugs used in ancylostoma infestation.**

Treatment/Management
- **Drugs:** A single dose of albendazole in the dose of 400 mg is the treatment of choice. Other drugs include mebendazole (100 mg twice daily for 3 days) and pyrantel pamoate (single oral dose of 11 mg/kg). Eradication of infestation should be confirmed by follow-up stool examination 2 weeks after discontinuation of treatment.
- Improvement of nutrition with a high-protein diet.
- **Anemia:** Mild anemia usually responds to oral iron therapy. Severe anemia is often associated with anasarca, and heart failure. This should be treated carefully, if required with blood transfusions.

Cutaneous Larva Migrans (Creeping Eruption)

Q. Write short note on cutaneous larva migrans (creeping eruption).

- **Definition:** Cutaneous larva migrans (CLM) is a creeping eruptions in the skin caused by the filariform larvae which aimlessly wander through the skin for weeks or months producing a reddish itch papule along the path of travel of the larvae (termed "larva migrans").
- **Cause:** Cutaneous larva migrans is particularly observed with nonhuman hookworms namely *Ancylostoma braziliense* and *A. caninum.*
  - ***Strongyloides stercoralis*** may produce creeping eruptions and its filariform larvae moves rapidly in short line; hence it is termed **larva currens** (reflecting fast movement of strongyloides larva) (**Fig. 4.31**).
- **Sites affected:** The main sites affected in cutaneous larva migrans are the dorsum and sole of the feet, buttocks, pelvic waist, legs, and shoulders. Infestation is usually self-limited. It can persist for a few days to months, but rarely for years.
- **Loeffler's syndrome** (transient migratory pulmonary infiltrates, peripheral blood eosinophilia, and sputum eosinophilia) is found in many cases of cutaneous larva migrans.

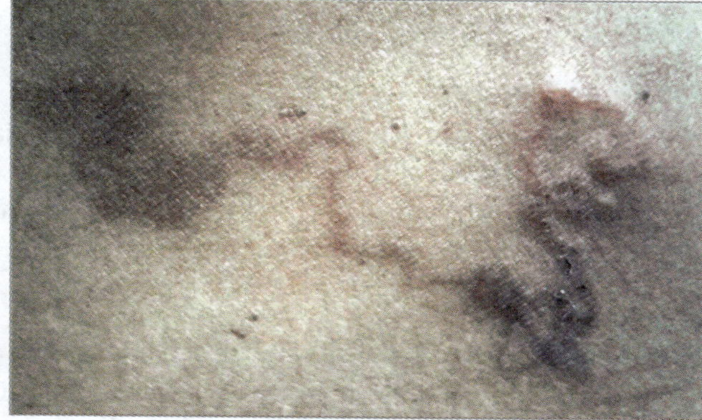

FIG. 4.31: Cutaneous larva migrans.

Clinical Features

There are usually no systemic symptoms and diagnosis is purely made on clinical grounds. Skin shows multiple, clearly defined, intensely pruritic, linear, and serpiginous tracts.

Treatment
- **Ivermectin:** It is the drug of choice and given as a single dose in the dose of 150–200 µg/kg.
- Alternative drug is **albendazole** (200 mg twice a day for 5–7 days).
- Antihistamines may be given for intense itching.

Strongyloidiasis

Q. Discuss clinical features, diagnosis, and treatment of strongyloidiasis.

- Strongyloidiasis is an intestinal infection of humans caused by *Strongyloides stercoralis*.
- The adult worm of *Strongyloides stercoralis* is small and measures 2 mm in length. It is found in many parts of the tropics and subtropics. It lives in the small intestine namely upper part of jejunum.

Clinical Features

- **Skin lesions:** Larval migration through skin may produce itchy rashes at the site of entry. Autoinfection may produce migratory linear weal around the buttocks and lower abdomen (cutaneous larva currens). The classic triad of symptoms is (1) abdominal pain, (2) diarrhea, and (3) urticaria.
- **Pulmonary lesions:** Larval migration through lungs may produce cough, dyspnea, hemoptysis, and bronchospasm.
- **Intestinal lesions:** Adult worms in the intestine may cause abdominal pain, bloating diarrhea, steatorrhea (malabsorption), and weight loss. In heavy infections, damage to the small intestinal mucosa can cause even perforation.
- **Systemic infection:** Systemic strongyloidiasis (the *Strongyloides* hyperinfection syndrome), with dissemination of larvae throughout the body. It may occur in immunocompromised states (e.g., HIV infection and corticosteroid therapy). This may produce diarrhea, severe, generalized abdominal pain, abdominal distension, pneumonia, meningoencephalitis, shock, and death. Gram-negative sepsis may develop.

Diagnosis

- Stool examination: Motile larvae (at least three samples) may be observed on microscopic examination of stool, especially after a period of incubation. Larvae may also be cultured from stool.
- Blood: Eosinophilia may be found in some patients.
- Duodenal/jejunal aspirate may show larvae.
- Serological tests: ELISA for antibody to *S. stercoralis*.
- In patients with disseminated infection: Stool examination, ELISA, and sputum and blood examination for larvae.

Q. Write short note on management of strongyloidiasis.

Treatment

- **Ivermectin** (200 μg/kg/day) for 2 days is the drug of choice.
- **Albendazole:** It is an alternative drug but is less effective drug. It is given orally at a dose of 400 mg twice daily for 7 days.
- **Disseminated systemic infections:** Both ivermectin and albendazole should be given and may be continued for 7 days or till the parasites are cleared.

Filariasis

Q. Discuss the clinical features, diagnosis, and treatment of filariasis.

Conditions included under filariasis are listed in **Box 4.18**.

Box 4.18: Conditions included under filariasis.

- Lymphatic filariasis: Caused by *Wuchereria bancrofti* and *Brugia malayi.*
- Onchocerciasis (river blindness): Caused by *Onchocerca volvulus*
- Loiasis: Caused by *Loa loa*

Lymphatic Filariasis

Q. Write short essay on lymphatic filariasis and bancroftian filariasis and their clinical manifestations and management.

Clinical outcome of lymphatic filariasis may range from subclinical infection to hydrocele and elephantiasis. Life cycle of filariasis is presented in **Figure 4.32**.

Clinical Features

Q. Write short essay on clinical features of filariasis.

Acute filarial lymphangitis: It presents with fever, with chills and sweats, headache, and muscle pain. On examination there will be **pain, tenderness, and erythema along the course of inflamed lymphatic vessels**. The whole episode may last for few days, but it may recur several times in a year. Temporary edema becomes more persistent and regional lymph nodes (e.g., inguinal) are enlarged painful and tender. Inflammation of the **spermatic cord (funiculitis), epididymis (epididymitis), and testis (orchitis)** is common.

- **Chronic stage of the disease:** It is characterized by development of permanent lymphedema ("**elephantiasis**") of legs (**Fig. 4.33**), scrotal edema, **chylous ascites, chylous pleural effusion, and chyluria**. Progressive enlargement of lymphedema may produce coarsening, corrugation, fissuring and bacterial infection of the skin, and subcutaneous tissue. This results in irreversible "elephantiasis." The scrotum may become very large in size because of hydrocele. Chyluria and chylous effusions appear as milky and opalescent which on standing shows fat globules on the top of chylous fluid.
- **Tropical pulmonary eosinophilia.**

Q. Write short essay on laboratory findings in filariasis.

- In the early stages of lymphangitis diagnosis can be made on clinical grounds, and peripheral blood eosinophilia. Microfilariae are not seen in the peripheral blood during early infestation.
- **Peripheral blood:**
  - **Eosinophilia:** Host immune response to the parasite produces massive eosinophilia.
  - **Demonstration of microfilariae:** In the peripheral blood at night.

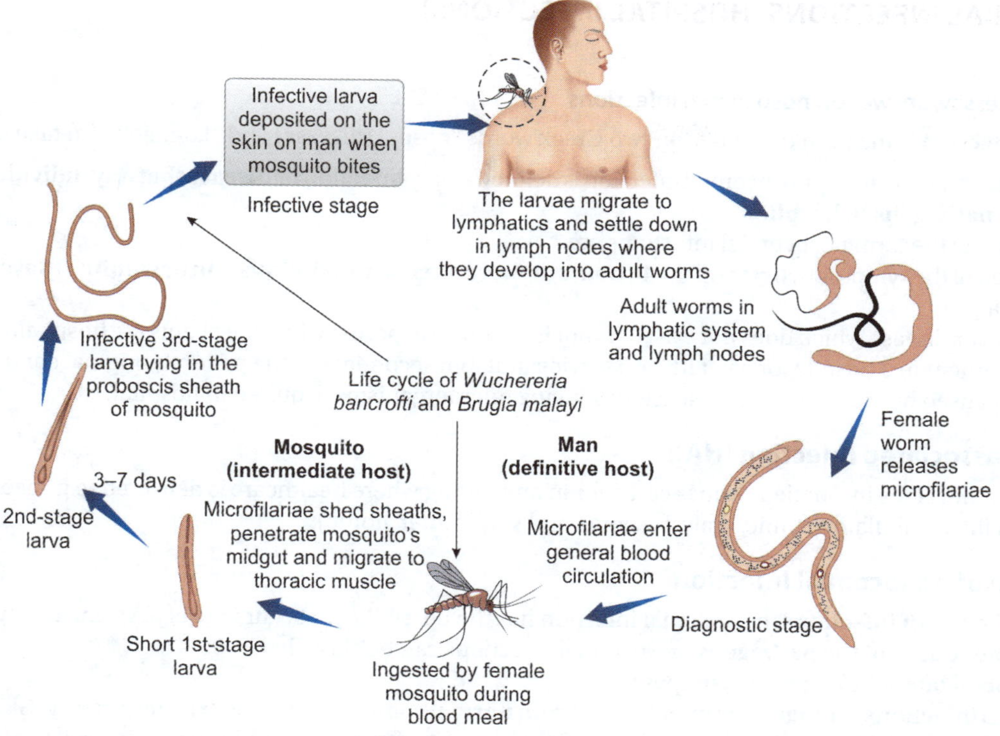

FIG. 4.32: Life cycle of filariasis.

- **Demonstration of microfilariae in other fluids:** Microfilariae can be demonstrated in the hydrocele fluid and may occasionally show an adult worm.
- **Diethylcarbamazine (DEC) provocation test:** In this test, administration of 100 mg DEC usually produces positive blood specimens within 30–60 minutes.
- **Radiology:** Calcified filariae may be demonstrable by radiography.
- **Serological tests:**
  - **Antigen detection and antibody detection in the blood:** By ELISA or immunochromatic method.
- **PCR** for DNA detection.
- **Radionuclide lymphoscintigraphy:** It is used to detect widespread lymphatic abnormalities.
- **Tropical pulmonary eosinophilia:** Serology is strongly positive and IgE levels are markedly raised but circulating microfilariae are not found. The chest X-ray shows miliary changes or mottled opacities. Lung function tests show a restrictive picture.

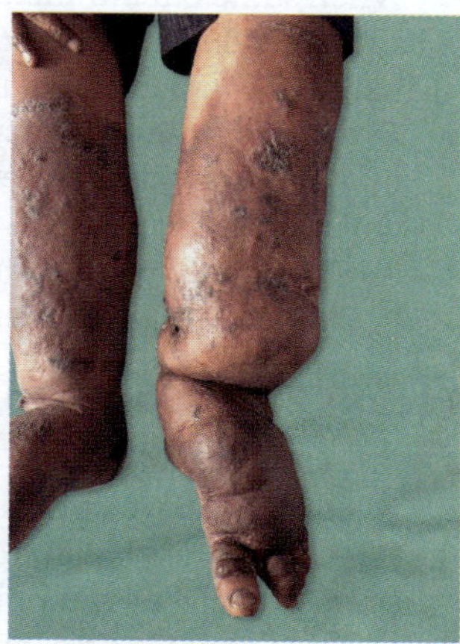

FIG. 4.33: Lymphatic filariasis.

Treatment

- **Aim of treatment:** Reversing and halting the disease progression.
- **Diethylcarbamazine (DEC)** in the dose of 6 mg/kg in three divided doses for 12–21 days kills both microfilariae and adult worms.
  - **Adverse effects:** Due to the host response to dying microfilariae. The intensity of reaction directly proportional to the microfilarial load. The main symptoms include fever, headache, nausea, vomiting, arthralgia, and prostration. They usually develop within 24–36 hours of the first dose of DEC. Antihistamines or corticosteroids may be needed to control these allergic reactions.
- **Ivermectin** kills only microfilariae, but not the adult worms.
- Combined albendazole (400 mg) and ivermectin (200 µg/kg) in a single dose, with or without DEC (300 mg), are also highly effective.
- **Doxycycline 200 mg per day for 4 weeks** plus ivermectin as a single dose (200 µg/kg provides additional benefit by eliminating the bacteria. This interrupts the parasite embryogenesis.
- **Surgery** may be of useful in the treatment established elephantiasis.

Chronic lymphatic pathology

- **Prevention of secondary infection:** Advised to take meticulous care of skin in lymphedematous limbs to prevent secondary bacterial and fungal infections.
- **Control of lymphedema:** Tight bandaging, massage and bed rest with elevation of the affected limb to control the lymphedema.
- **Prevention of further damage:** Prompt diagnosis and antibiotic therapy of bacterial cellulitis to prevent further lymphatic damage and worsening of existing elephantiasis.
- **Surgery:** Plastic surgery may be required in established elephantiasis. Hydroceles and chyluria can be repaired by surgery.

NOSOCOMIAL INFECTIONS (HOSPITAL INFECTIONS)

Introduction

Q. Write short essay/answer on nosocomial infections.

Nosocomial infection is the term derived from two Greek words "nosos" (disease) and "komeion" (to take care of).

Definition: In its broad meaning, nosocomial infection is defined as any **infection or disease that any individual suffers from the invasion of pathogens in hospital.**

Requisites for using the term nosocomial infections are:

- Manifestation of the symptoms, **first appear 48 hours or more after hospital admission or within 30 days after discharge** from hospital**.**
- Any infection or disease which does not exist or is not in incubation period when the clients are hospitalized. They are the result of treatment in a hospital or a healthcare service unit, but secondary to the patient's original condition.
- Infection is caused by the invasion of disease-producing microorganisms acquired in hospital.

Health Care-associated Infection (HAI)

An infection that develops in a patient who is cared for in any setting where healthcare is delivered (e.g., acute care hospital, chronic care facility, ambulatory clinic, dialysis center, and surgicenter, home).

Classification of Nosocomial Infection

According to the site of infections, nosocomial infection has the possibility to occur in every system and every site.

According to the source of the pathogens, nosocomial infections can be classified into:

- **Reactivation of latent infection:** TB, herpes viruses.
- **Endogenous infections (autogenous infections): From normal** commensals of the skin, respiratory, GI, and GU tract are common. It can occur when part of the individual's flora becomes altered and results in an overgrowth of microorganism. When sufficient numbers of microorganisms normally found in one body cavity or lining are transferred to another body site, an endogenous infection develops. For example, transmission of enterococci, normally found in fecal material, from hands to the skin is a cause of wound infections.
- **Exogenous infections (cross infections):** They are due to the invasion of causative microorganisms from the source other than the individual's themselves, such as from hospital personnel, the other individuals, various objects, and hospital environment.
  - **Inanimate environment:** *Aspergillus* from hospital construction, *Legionella* from contaminated water.
  - **Animate environment:** Hospital staff, visitors, other patients, and cross transmission are common.

Factors Predisposing to Hospital Infection

1. Pre-existing condition
2. Need for invasive devices
3. Effect of surgery [(skin wound, tissue trauma, opening colonized viscus, immobilization, and implants of foreign material (joint prostheses, arterial graft)]
4. Effect of antibiotic treatment (colonization by resistant bacteria and fungi)
5. Effect of immunosuppressive treatment (corticosteroids, cancer chemotherapy, radiotherapy, and transplant immunosuppression)
6. Exposure to healthcare workers and other patients, who may transmit pathogens.
7. Exposure to pathogens in the hospital environment

Epidemiology: It develops in **~10%** of patients admitted to hospital.

Etiology: *Staphylococcus aureus, Enterobacteria, Pseudomonas aeruginosa, Acinetobacter* species, coagulase-negative *Staphylococci, Enterococci,* and *Candida* are the most frequent pathogens.

Mechanisms of Transmission

- **Contact:** Direct (person-person), indirect (transmission through an intermediate object-contaminated instruments)
- **Airborne:** Organisms that have a true airborne phase as pattern of dissemination (TB, Varicella)
- **Common-vehicle:** Common animate vehicle as agent of transmission (ingested food or water, blood products, and IV fluids)
- **Droplet:** Brief passage through the air when the source and patient are in close proximity
- **Arthropod borne**

Main Groups of Nosocomial Infection

See **Box 4.19.**

Q. Write short essay/answer on common types of nosocomial infections.

Box 4.19: Main groups of nosocomial infections.

- Catheter-related infections
- Pneumonia
- Respiratory tract infections other than pneumonia
- Surgical site infections
- Urinary tract infections
- Gastrointestinal infections
- Central nervous system infections

Intravascular Catheter-related Infections

- Localized: Peripheral thrombophlebitis, abscess
- Systemic: Bacteremia, sepsis, endocarditis, and metastatic infection.

Microbiology: Coagulase-negative staphylococci (*S. epidermidis*), *S. aureus*, *Candida* species, *Enterococcus* species, and gram-negative rods.

Clinical features

- Local signs of inflammation at the site of entry: Redness, tenderness, swelling, slight purulent exudate—prominent in peripheral lines, less in central lines.
- Systemic signs: Fever, rigors, and no other source of fever
- Clinical improvement after catheter removal
- Elevated inflammatory markers, typical pathogens in blood culture.

Management of Catheter/Line-related Sepsis

- Two blood cultures, one from catheter, one from peripheral to differentiate colonization *versus* catheter-related bacteremia
- Catheter removal, culture of the tip—semiquantitative >15 CFU = infection (insertion of a new catheter not immediately)
- Antibiotics, if symptoms did not resolve after removal, guided by culture results.
- Long-time catheters (Broviac, Hickman)—catheter treatment, antibiotic locks

Prevention and Control

- Choice of catheter and insertion site
- Aseptic and atraumatic insertion (skin disinfection and barrier precautions), fixation to the skin
- TPN—total parenteral nutrition (all-in-one bags) prepared in the pharmacy under sterile precautions
- Minimize opening of the IV set for additive drugs, every opening strictly aseptic
- Maintaining adequate hygiene and dressing of the insertion site and regular review of insertion site
- Replacing giving set and catheter at appropriate intervals
  - Giving set every 72 hours, if lipid emulsions or blood products—24 hours
  - Catheter—peripheral 48 hour, central 7 days, tunneled line much longer
  - Removal of catheter if no longer necessary

Hospital-acquired, Nosocomial Pneumonia (discussed in Chapter 6)

Prevention

- Pulmonary toilet
- Change position second hourly: Elevate head to 30–45°
- Deep breathing, incentive spirometry
- Frequent suctioning
- Bronchoscopy to remove mucous plugging

Other Respiratory Tract Infections

Tracheobronchitis, sinusitis—frequent in mechanically ventilated patients' risk factor for development of nosocomial pneumonia and sepsis.

Urinary Tract Infections (UTI)—Urinary Catheter-related Infections

Source of uropathogens

- **Endogenous:** Most common
  - Catheter insertion
  - Retrograde movement up the urethra (70–80%)
  - Patient's own enteric flora (*E. coli*)
- **Exogenous:**
  - Cross contamination of drainage systems
  - May cause clusters of UTI's.

Etiology: Gram-negatives (*E. coli, Klebsiella pneumoniae, Pseudomonas*, and *Proteus* species), enterococci, and *Candida* species.

Risk factors: Length of catheterization (5%/day), opened drainage system, diabetes, female sex, and age above 50 years. Colonization is often asymptomatic, but there is a risk of ascending infection—pyelonephritis, bacteremia, and sepsis.

Diagnosis:

- **Pyuria: >5 leukocytes per high-power field**
- **Urine** culture: Significant bacteriuria ≥10^5 CFU/mL.

Treatment

- Catheter removal or change
- Antibiotics in symptomatic UTI

Prevention

- Avoid catheter when possible and discontinue ASAP—***MOST IMPORTANT***
- Aseptic insertion by trained healthcare workers
- Maintain closed system of drainage
- Ensure dependent drainage
- Minimize manipulation of the system
- Silver coated catheters
- Maintenance of good patient hygiene
- Replacing catheter at appropriate intervals
- ICU-bacteriological screening—urine culture at appropriate intervals

Surgical Site Infections (SSI)

Infections in the site of surgery and related bacteremias

CDC classification

- **Superficial SSI:** Skin and subcutaneous tissue involved
- **Deep SSI:** Deep soft tissue, fascia, and muscles
- **Organ SSI:** Organs and cavities.

Microbiology: *S. aureus*, coagulase-negative staphylococci, enterococci, *E. coli, Pseudomonas,* and *Enterobacter.*

Antibiotic Prophylaxis

Antibiotics: Bactericidal, effective against considered pathogens, with respect to local resistance, not beta-lactamases inducers. Short course of prophylaxis—first dose IV at induction of anesthesia, second dose if surgery >3 hours.

Prevention of SSI

- **Preoperative:**
  - Minimizing the preoperative hospital stay
  - Cutting better than shaving of surgical site
  - Antibiotic prophylaxis, if indicated
  - Surgical team clothing and washing
  - Skin decolonization
- Chlorhexidine
- Intranasal mupirocin for *S. aureus* carriers
- **Intraoperative:**
  - Regardful (tissue-saving) operation technique
  - Bleeding control
  - Excision of foreign bodies and devitalized tissue
  - Isolation of incised bowel
  - Minimizing of surgical staff and their movement
- **Postoperative:** Aseptic care of the site, sterile covering

Gastrointestinal Infections

Antibiotic-associated colitis

Precipitated by previous antibiotic treatment, mainly lincosamides, ampicillin, and cephalosporins.

Clostridium difficile toxin A (enterotoxin) and toxin B (cytotoxin)

Transmission via spores may cause hospital epidemics.

- **Postantibiotic diarrhea, simple colitis**
- **Pseudomembranous colitis**
- **Toxic megacolon**

Diagnosis:

- **Clinical:** Diarrhea, fever, abdominal pains, vomiting, and related to antibiotic treatment.
- **Laboratory:** *C. difficile* toxin detection—ELISA, antigen detection—latex agglutination (stool culture on selective agar, cytotoxicity test on tissue culture = gold standard, rarely available).
- **Colonoscopy:** Typical morphology with pseudomembranes, typical histology in biopsy specimens.

Treatment

- Stop precipitating antibiotic
- Rehydration, diet
- Antibiotic: Per oral. Metronidazole 3–4 × 500 mg p.o. or vancomycin 4 × 125–250 mg treat at least 7 days
- Probiotic drugs, colestipol, and rifaximin have been tried.
- Toxic megacolon—colectomy

Central Nervous System Infections

CSF shunt-related, rare occurrence, mostly *Staphylococcus aureus* and *Pseudomonas*, often serious course (nosocomial ventriculitis) and high mortality.

Strategies to Reduce Nosocomial Infection

Q. Write short essay/answer on measures to minimize nosocomial infection.

- Modify host: Risk factors such as age, underlying disease are difficult to change.
- Reduce patient exposure to pathogens.
- Reduce the number and virulence of nosocomial pathogens.

Exposure Reduction

- Use of aseptic technique during patient care
- Regular handwashing
- Proper isolation of patients known or suspected of harboring infectious diseases

Handwashing frequently is the single most important measure to prevent nosocomial infections.

SEPSIS

Q. Discuss management of a patient with septic shock.

Systemic Inflammatory Response Syndrome (SIRS)

- SIRS is the body's response to a clinical insult (e.g., infection, inflammation, stress, trauma, and burns)
- Must have at least two of the following:
  - Temperature >38.5°C or <36°C
  - Heart rate >90 beats/min
  - Respiratory rate >20 breaths/min or $PaCO_2$ <32 mm Hg WBC >12,000 cells/mm³, <4,000 cells/mm³, or >10% immature (band) forms

Q. Write short note on sepsis/SIRS/MODS/Septic shock.

Sepsis: SIRS + suspected or confirmed infection (documented via cultures or visualized via physical exam/imaging). Latest definition of sepsis—*Sepsis is defined as life-threatening organ dysfunction caused by the dysregulated host response to infection.* (Sepsis = suspected infection PLUS q SOFA = 2) q SOFA-3 criteria: Hypotension-systolic BP <100 mm Hg, altered mental status-GCS <13, respiratory rate >22.

A continuum of severity describing the host systemic inflammatory response (**Fig. 4.34**).

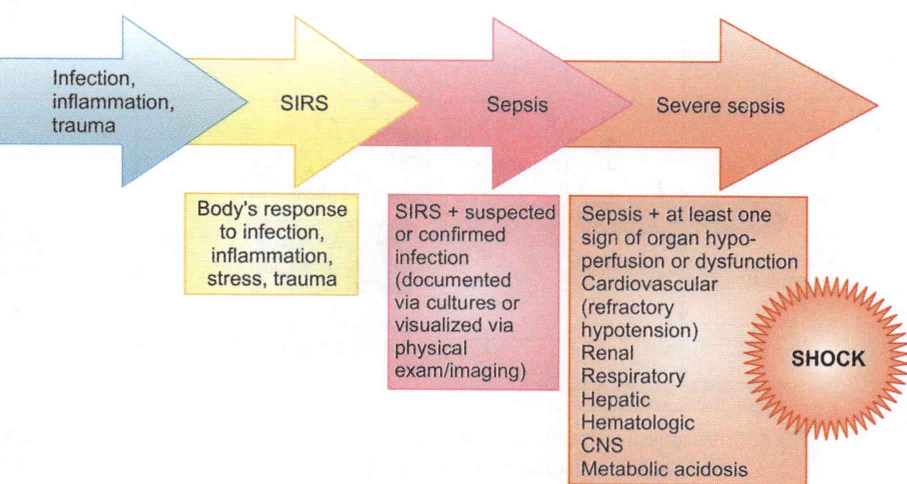

FIG. 4.34: Continuum of severity of sepsis.
(SIRS: systemic inflammatory response syndrome; CNS: central nervous system)

Severe sepsis

All three must be met within 6 hours:

- Documentation of a **suspected source** of infection
- Two or more manifestations of **SIRS** criteria:
  - Temperature >38.3°C/101 F or <36°C/96.8°F
  - Heart rate >90
  - Respiratory rate >20
  - WBC >12 or <4 or >10% bands
- **Organ dysfunction**, evidenced by any one of the following:
  - SBP <90 or MAP <65, or a SBP decrease of more than 40 patients
  - Cr >2.0 or urine output <0.5 cc/kg/ hour for 2 hours
  - Bilirubin >2 mg/dL (32.4 mol/L)
- Or if a provider documents severe sepsis, r/o sepsis, possible sepsis, or septic shock

Septic shock

- There must be documentation of septic shock present and
- **Tissue hypoperfusion** persisting in the hour after crystalloid fluid administration, evidenced by:
  - SBP <90
  - MAP <65
  - Decrease in SBP by >40 points from the patients baseline
  - Lactate ≥4
- Or if the criteria are not met, but there is provider documentation of septic shock or suspected septic shock

Multiple organ dysfunction syndrome (MODS)

- Altered organ function in an acutely ill patient
- Homeostasis cannot be maintained without intervention

Etiology of Sepsis

Septic shock may be caused by **gram-positive** (most common) **or gram-negative bacteria, fungi**, and, very rarely, protozoa or Rickettsiae. The common gram-positive bacteria include ***Staphylococcus aureus*, enterococci, *Streptococcus pneumoniae*,** and gram-negative bacilli which are resistant to usual antibiotics.

Management of Sepsis

Surviving Sepsis Campaign

- Step 1: Identify sepsis
- Step 2: Categorize sepsis
- Step 3: Initiate treatment

TABLE 4.46: Risk factors for sepsis.

Genetic polymorphism	Intrinsic factors
➢ Cytokine responses ➢ Coagulation ➢ Mannose binding proteins	➢ Age ➢ Nutrition ➢ Comorbidities ➢ Vaccination ➢ Immunosuppression
Procedures	**Community factors**
➢ Urinary catheters ➢ Intravenous cannula ➢ Wound dressings	➢ Contacts ➢ Disease outbreaks ➢ Specific exposure
Surgery	**Hospital factors**
➢ Wounds ➢ Emergency versus elective ➢ Dirty versus clean ➢ Prosthetic material	➢ Duration of stay in hospital ➢ Where in hospital (e.g., intensive care unit) ➢ Outbreaks ➢ Local antimicrobial resistance rates

Risk factors for sepsis are listed in **Table 4.46** and pathogenesis of septic shock is illustrated in **Figure 4.35**.

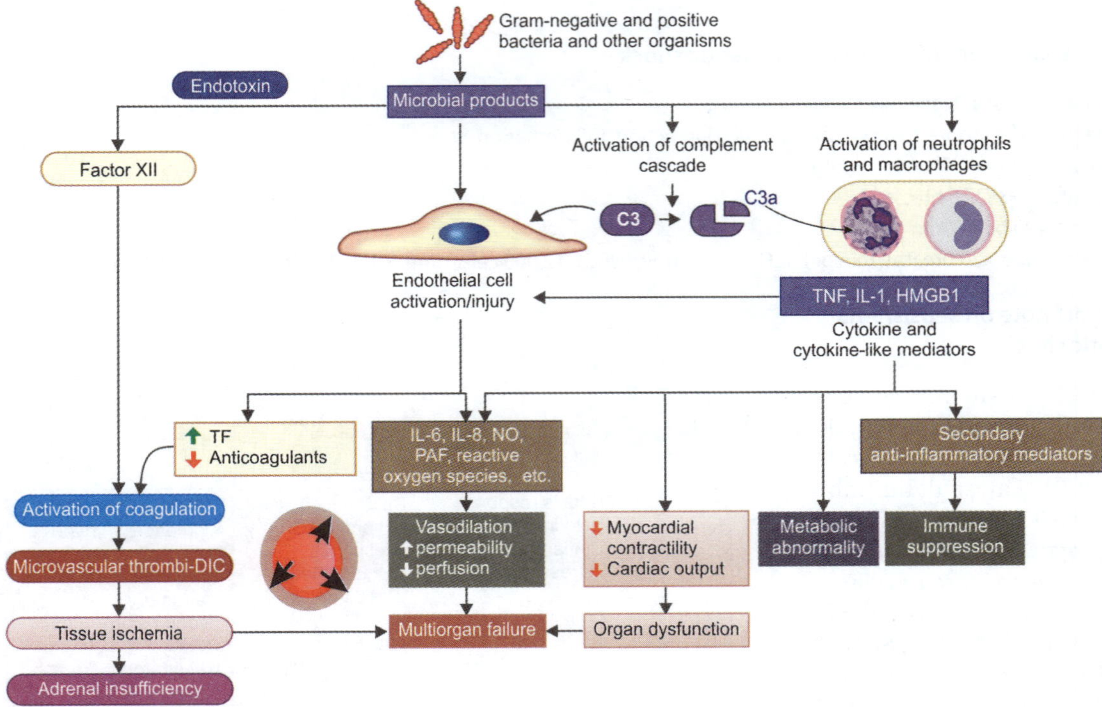

FIG. 4.35: Pathogenesis of septic shock. Microbial products initiate endothelial cell activation/injury activates endothelial cells, complement activation, activation of neutrophils and macrophages, factor XII. These initiating events lead to end-stage multiorgan failure.
(DIC: disseminated intravascular coagulation; HMGB1: high mobility group box 1 protein; NO: nitric oxide; PAF: platelet activating factor; TF: tissue factor)

Identifying acute organ dysfunction as a marker of severe sepsis is presented in **Table 4.47**.

Box 4.20 lists the principles of sepsis management.

- **Initial resuscitation:** Volume resuscitation with normal saline 30 mL/kg over first 30 minutes → if mean arterial pressure <70 mm Hg start inotropes (discussed later).
- **Diagnosis**
  - **Blood culture:** Before the initiation of antimicrobial therapy, at least two blood cultures should be obtained: (1) at least one drawn percutaneously and (2) at least one drawn through each vascular access device if inserted longer than 48 hours.
  - **Other cultures** such as urine, cerebrospinal fluid, wounds, respiratory secretions, or other body fluids should be obtained as per the clinical situation.
  - **Other diagnostic studies** such as imaging and sampling should be performed promptly to determine the source and causative organism of the infection.
- **Antibiotic therapy**
  - **Start intravenous antibiotic therapy** within the **first hour** of recognition of severe sepsis after obtaining appropriate cultures.
  - Empirical choice of antimicrobials should include one or more drugs with activity against likely pathogens, both bacterial or fungal.
    - Penetrate presumed source of infection
    - Guided by susceptibility patterns in the community and hospital
    - Continue broad spectrum therapy until the causative organism and its susceptibilities are defined.
- **Source control:** Evaluate patients for focus of infection amenable to source control measures (**Table 4.48**)
- **Fluid therapy**
  - Crystalloids: **Always use first**!
  - Colloids: FFP if coagulopathy, RBCs if HCT <30, especially, if risk of CAD. Avoid albumin (increase ECF and is costly).
- **Vasopressors**
  - Initiate vasopressor therapy if appropriate fluid challenge fails to restore adequate blood pressure and organ perfusion.
  - Either norepinephrine or dopamine is first-line agents to correct hypotension in septic shock.

TABLE 4.47: Identifying acute organ dysfunction as a marker of severe sepsis.

Cardiovascular	*Respiratory*	*CNS*
Tachycardia	Tachypnea	Altered consciousness
Hypotension	PaO_2 <70 mm Hg	Confusion
	SaO_2 <90%	Psychosis
	PaO_2/FiO_2 ≤300	
Renal	***Hematological***	***Liver***
Oliguria	↓ Platelets	Jaundice
Anuria	↑ PT/APTT	↑ Liver enzymes
↑ Creatinine	↓ Protein C ↑ D-dimer	↓ Albumin ↑ PT

Box 4.20: Principles of sepsis management.

- **Recognize sepsis early** and determine **severity**.
- Organ dysfunction is determined by Sequential Organ Failure Assessment Score (SOFA) which include paO_2, bilirubin, creatinine, and platelet count.
- **Early antibiotics** are critical to resolution of shock.
- **Resuscitate** severe sepsis and septic shock as soon as possible.
- **Early goal directed therapy**

- **Norepinephrine** is more potent and may be more effective than dopamine at reversing hypotension in septic shock patients.
- Dopamine may be particularly useful in patients with compromised systolic function but causes more tachycardia and may be more arrhythmogenic.

- **Inotropic therapy**
  - In **patients with low cardiac output** despite of adequate fluid resuscitation, **dobutamine** can be used to increase cardiac output.
  - Should be combined with vasopressor therapy in the presence of hypotension.
- **Steroids**
  - In patients with septic shock who require vasopressor therapy to maintain blood pressure intravenous corticosteroids are recommended.
  - Administer intravenous hydrocortisone 200–300 mg/day for 7 days in three or four divided doses or by continuous infusion.
- **Recombinant human activated protein C (rhaPC) [drotrecogin alfa (activated)]:** It is recommended in patients at a high risk of death
  - APACHE II (Acute Physiology and Chronic Health Evaluation II) score >25, or
  - Sepsis-induced multiple organ failure, or
  - Septic shock, or
  - Sepsis induced acute respiratory distress syndrome

  Patients should have no absolute or relative contraindication related to bleeding risk that outweighs the potential benefit of rhAPC.
- **Blood product administration:** Red blood transfusion should be given only when hemoglobin decreases to <7 g/dL. Target hemoglobin of 7–9 g/dL.
- **Mechanical ventilation**
  - Sepsis-induced acute lung injury (ALI)/adult respiratory distress syndrome (ARDS)
  - High tidal volumes, >6 mL/kg, coupled with high plateau pressures, >30 cm H_2O, should be avoided. A minimum amount of positive end expiratory pressure should be set to prevent lung collapse at end-expiration.
- **Sedation, analgesia, and neuromuscular blockade in sepsis**
  - The use of protocols and daily interruption/lightening of continuous sedative infusion have shown to reduce the duration of mechanical ventilation and length of stay.
- **Glucose control:** Following initial stabilization of patients with severe sepsis, blood glucose to <150 mg/dL. Glycemic control strategy must include a nutrition protocol with the preferential use of the enteral route.
- **Renal replacement:** Continuous veno-venous hemofiltration and intermittent hemodialysis are considered equivalent in acute renal failure. Continuous hemofiltration offers easier management of fluid balance in hemodynamically unstable septic patients.
- **Bicarbonate therapy:** Bicarbonate is not recommended for improving hemodynamics or reducing vasopressor requirements or for the treatment of hypoperfusion induced lactic academia with pH >7.15.
- **Deep vein thrombosis prophylaxis:** DVT prophylaxis with either low-dose unfractionated heparin or low molecular weight heparin should be used in severe sepsis patients.
- **Stress ulcer prophylaxis:** Stress ulcer prophylaxis should be given to all patients with severe sepsis. H_2 receptor blockers are more efficacious than sucralfate and are the preferred agents. Proton pump inhibitors compared to H_2 blockers have not been assessed.

TABLE 4.48: Measures to control source of infection.

Drainage	
Intra-abdominal abscess Thoracic empyema	Septic arthritis Pyelonephritis, cholangitis
Debridement	
Necrotizing fasciitis Infected pancreatic necrosis	Mediastinitis Intestinal infarction
Device removal	
Infected vascular catheter Urinary catheter	Colonized endotracheal tube
Definitive control	
Sigmoid resection for diverticulitis Amputation for clostridial myonecrosis	Cholecystectomy for gangrenous cholecystitis
qSOFA-Quick SOFA	
Respiratory rate >22/min, altered mentation, SBP <100 mm Hg	Any two positive-poor prognosis

"Surviving sepsis campaign (SSC)": International Guidelines for management of sepsis and septic shock (**Table 4.49**).

TABLE 4.49: Surviving sepsis campaign bundles.

To be completed within 3 hours:
➢ Measure lactate level ➢ Obtain blood cultures prior to administration of antibiotics ➢ Administer broad spectrum antibiotics ➢ Administer 30 mL/kg crystalloid for hypotension or lactate ≥4 mmol/L.
To be completed within 6 hours:
➢ Apply vasopressors (for hypotension that does not respond to initial fluid resuscitation to maintain a mean arterial pressure (MAP) ≥65 mg Hg ➢ In the event of persistent arterial hypotension despite volume resuscitation (septic shock) or initial lactate ≥4 mmol/L (36 mg/dL): – Measure central venous pressure (CVP)* – Measure central venous oxygen saturation ($Scvo_2$)* ➢ Remeasure lactate if initial lactate was elevated*

*Tragets for quantitative resuscitation included in the guidelines are CVP of ≥8 mm Hg, $Scvo_2$ of ≥70%, and normalization of lactate.
SSC (2018) created sets of "sepsis bundles" that clearly outline steps practitioners should take within the first hour ("time zero" or "time of presentation").

Q. Discuss key elements in first hour sepsis bundles.

The five key elements of hours-1 bundle

1. Measure lactate level. Remeasure if initial lactate is >2 mmol/L.
2. Obtain blood culture prior to administration of antibiotics.
3. Administer broad-spectrum antibiotics.
4. Begin rapid administration of 30 mL/kg crystalloid for hypotension or lactate ≥4 mmol/L
5. Apply vasopressors if patient is hypotensive during or after fluid resuscitation to maintain MAP >65 mm Hg.

ANTI-INFECTIVE THERAPY

Antimicrobial Combination Therapy

Limit combination therapy to special situations

- **Synergistic killing,** e.g., β-lactam plus aminoglycoside for endocarditis

- **Mixed infections or severe infections of unknown cause,** e.g., limb infections in diabetic patients
- **To prevent the emergence of resistance,** e.g., *M. tuberculosis*
- Initial empiric therapy

Multidrug Therapy

Tuberculosis, infective endocarditis, malaria, HIV, and leprosy

Antibiotic Chemoprophylaxis

- **Infective endocarditis:** Amoxicillin + gentamicin
- **Splenectomy:** Penicillin
- **Rheumatic fever:** Penicillin
- **Tuberculosis:** INH
- **Meningitis:** Meningococcal and *H. influenzae:* Rifampicin

Beta-lactam antibiotics

Q. Write a short essay/note on β-lactam antibiotics.

Q. Mention four β-lactam antibiotics with dosage.

Q. Mention cephalosporins and name drugs belonging to third generations.

These antibiotics have a β-lactam ring structure and their bactericidal (lysis of bacteria) action is due to their inhibition enzymes involved in cell wall formation in the bacteria [penicillin binding proteins (PBP)].

Types of beta-lactam antibiotics (Flowchart 4.3)

FLOWCHART 4.3: Classification of beta-lactam antibiotics.

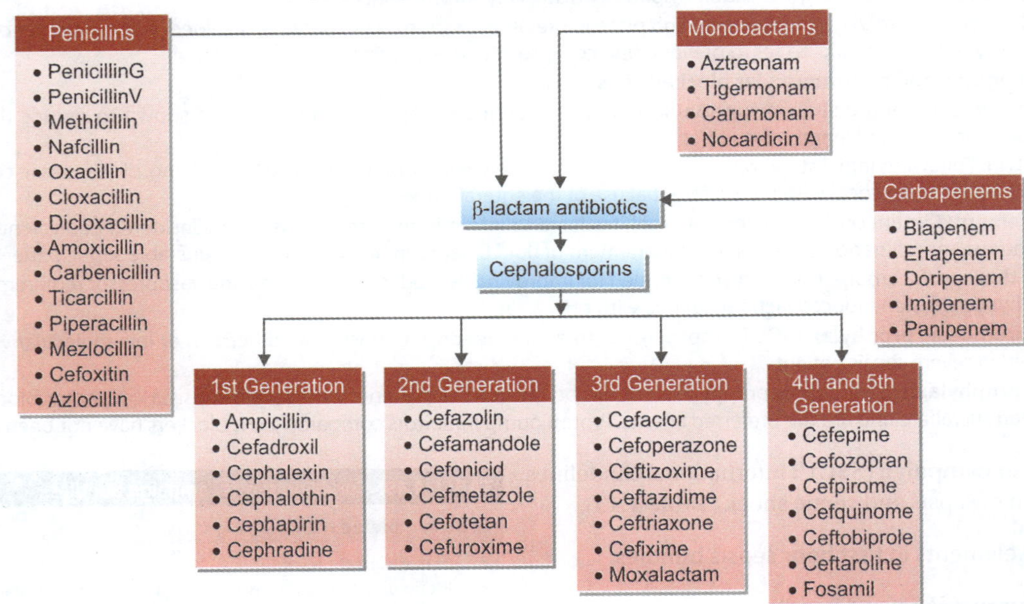

Adverse effects of beta-lactam antibiotics (Box 4.21)

Box 4.21: Adverse effects of beta-lactam antibiotics.

- Generalized allergy to penicillin
- Gastrointestinal upset and diarrhea
- Mild reversible hepatitis
- Leukopenia, thrombocytopenia and coagulation deficiencies, and interstitial nephritis and potentiation of aminoglycoside-mediated renal damage
- Thrombophlebitis with parenteral β-lactams

Drug Resistance

Antibiotic resistance is a challenging and growing problem. The most important mechanism of drug resistance is destruction of drugs by beta-lactamase enzymes.

β-lactamases

Q. Write a short essay/note on β-lactamases.

- β-lactam antibiotics have a β-lactam ring structure. They exert a bactericidal action by inhibiting enzymes involved in cell wall synthesis [penicillin binding proteins (PBP)].
- β-lactamases are bacterial enzymes produced by many gram-positive and gram-negative bacteria. Theses enzymes can inactivate β-lactam antibacterials by hydrolysis of β-lactam ring structure and results in infective compounds.

Production of β-lactamases by these bacteria is the most important factor that contributes to β-lactam antibiotic resistance.

- Many serine-active β-lactamases inhibitors (e.g., clavulanic acid, sulbactam, and tazobactam) in combination with β-lactam antibiotics are used to reduce drug resistance by bacteria containing β-lactamases.

Extended-Spectrum β-Lactamases (ESBL)

Several isolates of *Enterobacteriaceae* and *Pseudomonas* have been identified which produce newer β-lactamases. These enzymes include (1) plasmid-mediated cephamycinases, (2) extended-spectrum β-lactamases (ESBLs), and (3) carbapenem-hydrolyzing enzymes or carbapenemases.

Major Sources of Lactamases (Table 4.50)

- Most commonly β-lactamases are produced by *Klebsiella* species, *Escherichia coli* but can occur in other GNB (gram-negative bacilli), including *Enterobacter*, *Proteus*, *Salmonella*, and *Citrobacter* species, *Morganella morganii*, *Shigella dysenteriae*, *Serratia marcescens*, *Pseudomonas aeruginosa*, and *Burkholderia cepacia*.
- Mutant, plasmid-mediated β-lactamases enzymes are derived from amino acid substitutions in native β-lactamases (particularly TEM-1, TEM-2, and SHV-1).
  Typically associated with multidrug resistance (fluoroquinolones, cotrimoxazole, and aminoglycosides).

TABLE 4.50: Major sources of β-lactamases.

Types of β-lactamases	*Major sources*
TEM, SHV	*Escherichia coli, Klebsiella pneumoniae*
Cefotaxime hydrolyzing (CTX-M)	*Salmonella typhimurium, E. coli, K. pneumoniae*
Oxacillin hydrolyzing (OXA)	*Pseudomonas aeruginosa*
PER-1	*P. aeruginosa, A. baumannii, and S. typhimurium*
PER-2	*Salmonella typhimurium*
VEB-1	*E. coli, P. aeruginosa*

Actions

- β-lactamases are able to hydrolyze all penicillins, cephalosporins (except cephamycins), and monobactams. These are associated with **multidrug resistance** (fluoroquinolones, cotrimoxazole, and aminoglycosides).
- The ESBLs are a group of enzymes capable of hydrolyzing and cause resistance to the oxyiminocephalosporins (cefotaxime, ceftazidime, ceftriaxone, cefuroxime, and cefepime) and monobactams (aztreonam), but not the cephamycins (cefoxitin and cefotetan) or carbapenems (imipenem, meropenem, doripenem, and ertapenem).

Risk factors: Predisposing to infection or colonization with ESBL-producing pathogens is presented in **Table 4.51**.

Treatment recommendations for infections with ESBL producers (Table 4.52)

TABLE 4.51: Risk factors predisposing to infection or colonization with ESBL-producing pathogens.

Critically ill patients/severely debilitated individuals
- Prolonged stay in hospital or ICU unit
- Invasive procedures: e.g., indwelling catheter, central venous catheter, tracheostomy, endotracheal, or nasogastric tube
- Stay in long-term care facility
- Decubitus ulcer
- Total dependence on healthcare workers

Prior antibiotic use in last 3 months
- Exposure to 2nd, 3rd cephalosporins, aztreonam, penicillin, and quinolones
- Delay in appropriate antibiotic therapy

TABLE 4.52: Treatment recommendations for infections with ESBL producers.

- **No treatment needed** for colonization with ESBL producers
- **Imipenem or meropenem**
  - Bloodstream infection
  - Ventilator-associated pneumonia
  - Any producers that appear to have reduced susceptibility to ertapenem
- **Ertapenem or doripenem**
  - Complicated infections of urinary tract
  - Diabetic food infections
  - Intra-abdominal infections
- **Quinolones:** Infections in patients with risk for allergy to carbapenems, if isolates are susceptible
- **Nitrofurantoin or fosfomycin:** Uncomplicated infection of lower urinary tract
- **Tigecycline, colistin, or polymyxin b**
  - Isolates resistant to all other antibiotic options
  - Patients allergic to β-lactams

Carbapenem-Resistant Enterobacteriaceae

Klebsiella pneumoniae Carbapenemase (KPC)

Clonal outbreaks in New York, Israel, Greece, Colombia, Brazil, China, and Canada (Montreal)

Q. Write a short essay/note on New Delhi Metallo-β-lactamase (NDM-1).

NDM-1 (New Delhi Metallo-β-lactamase)

- It is a novel metallo-β-lactamase (MBL) coded by a novel gene bla (NDM-1) in *Enterobacteriaceae*.
- First, it was reported in a Swedish male diabetic, who returned to Sweden after having treatment for gluteal abscess in December 2007 at a hospital in New Delhi. Since the immediate previous treatment was in New Delhi it was named as NDM-1.
- Subsequently, Enterobacteriaceae family containing this genetic element was detected in various regions of India, Pakistan, Bangladesh, Britain, and many other countries.
- Metallo-β-lactamase (MBL) enzymes mediate resistance to almost β-lactam agents (except monobactams, e.g., aztreonam) including carbapenems.
- Organism carrying this gene has multidrug resistance and is susceptible only to tigecycline and colistin.

MISCELLANEOUS

Amikacin

Q. Write short note on amikacin.

- It is a **semisynthetic derivative of kanamycin** and has pharmacokinetics, dose, and toxicity.
- Outstanding feature: Amikacin has the **wide spectrum of activity and effective against many organisms that are resistant to other aminoglycosides**. However, it is effective in relatively higher dose against *Pseudomonas*, *Proteus*, and *Staphylococci*.
- **Indications:** The range of conditions in which amikacin can be used is as same as for gentamicin. It is **reserved for hospital acquired gram-negative bacterial infections where gentamicin/tobramycin resistance is high**. It is effective against tuberculosis, but rarely used for its treatment.
- **Toxicity:** It causes more hearing loss than vestibular disturbance, nephrotoxicity, and neurotoxicity.
- **Dose:** 15 mg/kg/day in 1–3 doses; urinary tract infections 7.5 mg/kg/day. Best given as single daily infusion (minimizes the toxicity).

Indications of Doxycycline

Q. Write short note on indications of doxycycline.

Doxycycline is a tetracycline antibiotic. It is indicated for many different bacterial infections, such as acne, urinary tract infections, intestinal infections, eye infections, gonorrhea, chlamydia, etc.

Cephalosporins

Q. Write short note on cephalosporins.

Cephalosporins are group of semisynthetic antibiotics derived from cephalosporin-C obtained from a fungus *Cephalosporium*. They are chemically related to penicillins.

- First generation cephalosporins: Cephalexin, cephradine, and cefadroxil
- Second generation cephalosporins: Cefuroxime, cefuroxime axetil, and cefaclor
- Third generation cephalosporins: Cefotaxime, ceftizoxime, ceftriaxone, ceftazidime, cefoperazone, cefixime, cefpodoxime, cefdinir, ceftibuten, and cefetamet pivoxil
- Fourth generation cephalosporins: Cefepime and cefpirome

Side Effects of Tetracycline, Chloramphenicol, and Quinolones

See **Table 4.53**.

Q. Write short note on side effects of tetracycline, chloramphenicol, and quinolones.

TABLE 4.53: Side effects of tetracycline, chloramphenicol, quinolones, and lithium.

Drug	*Side effects*
Tetracycline	➢ *Dose related:* Epigastric pain, nausea, vomiting, diarrhea, fatty liver, renal damage, phototoxicity, brown discoloration of teeth, antianabolic effect, increased intracranial pressure, and vestibular toxicity ➢ Hypersensitivity ➢ Superinfection
Chloramphenicol	Bone marrow depression, hypersensitivity reactions, nausea, vomiting, diarrhea, superinfection, and gray baby syndrome
Quinolones/ fluoroquinolones	➢ *GIT:* Nausea, anorexia, vomiting, and bad taste ➢ *CNS:* Dizziness, headache, restlessness, anxiety, insomnia, and tremor ➢ *Skin:* Hypersensitivity, rash, and pruritus ➢ Tendonitis and tendon rupture

Side Effects of Sulfonamides

See **Box 4.22**.

Q. Write short note on side effects of sulfonamides.

Box 4.22: Side effects of sulfonamides.

- Nausea, vomiting, and epigastric pain
- Crystalluria
- Hypersensitivity reactions
- Hepatitis
- Contact sensitization with topical use
- Hemolysis in persons with G6PD deficiency
- Precipitation of kernicterus in premature newborn

Classification of Antifungal Drugs (Table 4.54)

Q. Write short note on antifungal drugs.

TABLE 4.54: Classification of antifungal drugs.

Type of drug	*Examples*
1. Antibiotic – Polyenes – Heterocyclic benzofuran	➢ Amphotericin B (AMB), nystatin, hamycin, and natamycin ➢ Griseofulvin
2. Antimetabolite	Flucytosine
3. Azoles – Imidazoles (topical) – Triazoles (systemic)	➢ Clotrimazole, econazole, miconazole, and oxiconazole (systemic, ketoconazole) ➢ Fluconazole, itraconazole, voriconazole
4. Echinocandin: Impairs β 1,3 glucan synthesis	Caspofungin, micafungin, and anidulafungin
5. Other topical agents	Tolnaftate, undecylenic acid, benzoic acid, quiniodochlor, ciclopirox olamine, butenafine, and sodium thiosulfate
6. Allylamine	Terbinafine

Ketoconazole

Q. Write short note on ketoconazole.

Ketoconazole is antifungal drug belonging to the azole group. It inhibits enzymes involved in steroid hormone biosynthesis and prevents the growth of the fungus. Ketoconazole is available for oral administration (causes severe hepatitis and it has been discontinued in many countries) and for topical application (e.g., for the treatment of tinea, cutaneous candidiasis).

Antiviral Agents

See **Table 4.54**.

Ivermectin

Q. Write short note on ivermectin.

It is an extremely potent semisynthetic derivative of the antinematodal principle obtained from *Streptomyces avermitilis.*

Indications

- Drug of choice for single dose treatment of onchocerciasis and strongyloidiasis
- Bancroftian and brugian filariasis
- Cutaneous larva migrans and ascariasis
- Scabies and head lice

Indications for Intravenous Gamma Globulin (Box 4.23 and Table 4.55)

Q. Write short note on indications for intravenous gammaglobulin.

Box 4.23: Indications for intravenous gamma globulin.

Transplantation
- Allogeneic bone marrow transplantation
- Kidney transplantation with a high antibody recipient or with an ABO incompatible donor
- Hematopoietic stem cell transplantation in patients older than 20 years

Immunodeficiency
- Common variable immunodeficiency (CVID)
- Primary immunodeficiency disorders associated with defects in humoral immunity

Others
- Chronic inflammatory demyelinating polyneuropathy (CIDP)
- Chronic lymphocytic leukemia
- Immune-mediated thrombocytopenia
- Kawasaki disease

Pediatric HIV type 1 infection

TABLE 4.55: Antiviral agents.

Category	*Drugs*
Anti-influenza agents	Amantadine, oseltamivir, peramivir, rimantadine, and zanamivir
Antiherpes virus agents	Acyclovir, cidofovir, docosanol, famciclovir, foscarnet, fomivirsen, ganciclovir, idoxuridine, penciclovir, trifluridine, tromantadine, valaciclovir, valganciclovir, and vidarabine
Antiretroviral agents	➢ **NRTIs:** Zidovudine, didanosine, stavudine, zalcitabine, lamivudine, abacavir, and tenofovir ➢ **NNRTIs:** Nevirapine, efavirenz, and delavirdine ➢ **PIs:** Saquinavir, indinavir, atazanavir, ritonavir, nelfinavir, amprenavir, lopinavir, and tipranavir ➢ **New aRT:** Maraviroc and enfuvirtide
Other antiviral agents	Fomivirsen, enfuvirtide, imiquimod, interferon, ribavirin, and viramidine

Commonly used Immunoglobulins

- Human immunoglobulins:
  - Human normal immunoglobulins: Hepatitis A, measles, rabies, tetanus, and mumps
  - Human specific immunoglobulins: Hepatitis B, varicella, and diphtheria
- Non-human (antisera): Bacterial (e.g., diphtheria, tetanus, gas gangrene, and botulism) and viral (e.g., rabies)

Infections Associated with Skin Rash (Table 4.56 and Box 4.24)

Q. Write short note on infections associated with skin rash.

TABLE 4.56: Infections associated with skin rash.

Macular/maculopapular: Measles, rubella, enterovirus, Epstein–Barr virus, cytomegalovirus, human immunodeficiency virus (HIV), dengue, typhoid, secondary syphilis, and Rickettsiae spotted fevers
Erythematous: Scarlet fever, Lyme disease, toxic shock syndrome (*Staphylococcus* and *Streptococcus*), human parvovirus B19 **Vesicular:** Chickenpox (varicella zoster virus), shingles (varicella zoster virus), and herpes simplex virus
Petechial/hemorrhagic: Meningococcal septicemia, any septicemia with disseminated intravascular coagulation (DIC), Rickettsiae and viruses (*Flavivirus*, *Bunyavirus*, *Arenavirus*, and *Filovirus*)
Urticarial: *Strongyloides*, *Schistosoma*, and cutaneous larva migrans
Others: Tick typhus (eschar), primary syphilis (chancre), anthrax (ulcerating papule), and ulcers associated with other STDs'

Box 4.24: Mnemonic: Very Sick Person Must Take Double Eggs.

- Varicella (Chicken pox): 1st day (rash is often 1st sign in children)
- Scarlet fever: 2nd day
- Pox (Small pox): 3rd day
- Measles (Rubella or 14 day measles): 4th day (*Remember*: Koplik spots appear in pre-eruptive phase on 2nd day of fever)
- Typhus: 5th day
- Dengue: 6th day
- Enteric fever: 7th day

CHAPTER

5

HIV Infection and AIDS

GLOBAL HIV AND AIDS STATISTICS

- There were approximately 38 million people across the globe with human immunodeficiency virus/acquired immunodeficiency syndrome (HIV/AIDS) in 2019.
- An estimated 1.7 million individuals worldwide acquired HIV in 2019, marking a 23% decline in new HIV infections since 2010. 75.7 million people have become infected with HIV since the start of the epidemic (end 2019).
- As of the end of June 2020, 26.0 million people were accessing antiretroviral therapy (ART).
- India has the third largest HIV epidemic in the world. India had 2.35 million people living with HIV. Of this 1.345 million were receiving ART. There were 69,220 new HIV infections and 58,960 AIDS related deaths reported in India in 2019.
- The **90–90–90 targets** by UN AIDS envision that, by 2020, 90% of people living with HIV will know their HIV status, 90% of people who know their HIV-positive status will be accessing treatment, and 90% of people on treatment will have suppressed viral loads. In India, 79% of people living with HIV knew their status, 56% of people living with HIV were on treatment and viral load data is not available.

CHARACTERISTIC FEATURES OF HUMAN IMMUNODEFICIENCY VIRUS

- The human immunodeficiency virus (HIV) causes acquired immunodeficiency syndrome (AIDS)
- Former names of the virus include: human T-cell lymphotropic virus (HTLV-III), lymphadenopathy-associated virus (LAV), and AIDS-associated retrovirus (ARV).
- Discovered independently by Dr Luc Montagnier, Dr Anthony Gallo, and Dr Jay Levy in 1983–84.
- It is an ribonucleic acid (RNA) virus belonging to the *Lentivirus* **genus** of the **Retroviridae family**
- HIV occurs in two genetically different but related main forms—HIV-1 and HIV-2.
  - **HIV-1:**
    - Most common type
    - Four distinct groups of HIV-1, each arising from a different zoonotic transmission event. These include:
      - Group M ("Major")—Majority.
        - Has nine distinct subtypes/clades [A-D, F-H, J-K] and
        - More than 90 known circulating recombinant forms (CRFs)
          - CRF01_AE: Is common in southeast Asia
          - CRF02_AG: Is common in west and central Africa.
      - Group O ("Outlier")—in West Africa
      - Group N ("nonmajor and nonoutlier")—in Cameroon
      - Group P—in Cameroon

        Group P was transmitted from a gorilla, while group M, N, and O were transmitted from a chimpanzee.
  - **HIV-2**:
    - Endemic in West Africa; Prevalence is also higher in France, Spain, Portugal, Brazil, Angola, Mozambique, and parts of India
    - Coinfection with HIV-1 and HIV-2 can occur
    - HIV-2 is inherently **resistant** to non-nucleoside reverse transcriptase inhibitors (**NNRTIs**).

STRUCTURE OF HIV (FIG. 5.1)

- Each mature virion comprises of:
  - Electron-dense and cone-shaped **core**
  - Membrane-associated **matrix protein**
  - **Lipid bilayer envelope** with **surface glycoproteins**, gp120 and gp41.
- About 90–120 nm in diameter
- Spherical in shape
- **Viral core:**
  - **Major capsid protein p24**:
    - Most abundant viral antigen
    - Can be detected early in infection before the development of antibodies
    - Antibodies against p24 antigen are also important serologic markers of infection.

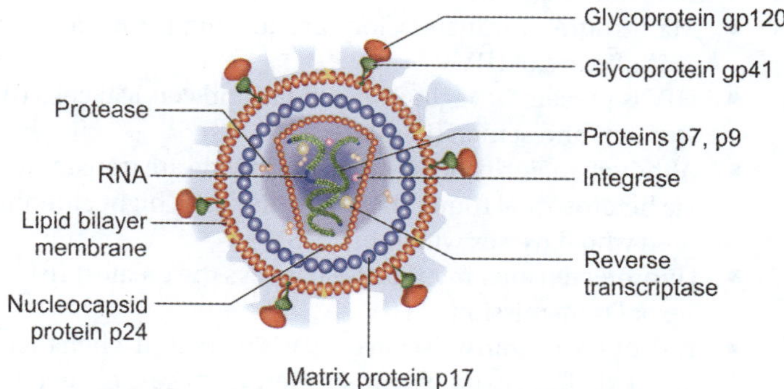

FIG. 5.1: Diagrammatic representation of structure of the human immunodeficiency virus (HIV)-1 virion.

  - **Nucleocapsid protein p7/p9**
  - **Diploid genome**: Two **single-stranded**, positive-sense RNA molecules
  - Three **viral enzymes**:
    - **Reverse transcriptase** [RNA-dependent deoxyribonucleic acid (DNA) polymerase]: Synthesizes DNA by using the genome RNA as a template
    - **Integrase**: Integrates the viral DNA into the host cell DNA
    - **Protease**: Cleaves the various viral precursor proteins.
- Membrane associated matrix protein: **p17**
  - Surrounds the viral core
- Lipid envelope
  - Lipid bilayer is derived from the host cell membrane
  - Two envelope proteins, gp120 and gp41, are embedded in it
    - **gp120:**
      - Projects from the surface as knob-like spikes
      - Interacts with the CD4 receptor and a chemokine receptor (CCR5 or CXCR4) and helps in attachment
    - **gp41:** Mediates the fusion of the viral envelope with the host cell membrane at the time of infection and facilitates entry.
- HIV genome consists of:
  - *Structural genes*:
    - **gag**—encodes the structural proteins—p24, p7, and p17
    - **pol**—codes for reverse transcriptase, integrase, and protease
    - **env**—codes for envelope glycoproteins gp120 and gp41.
  - *Six regulatory genes*
    - Required for replication
      - **tat**—activation of transcription of viral genes
      - **rev**—transport of unspliced messenger RNAs (mRNAs) from nucleus to cytoplasm.
    - Accessory genes—not required for replication
      - **nef**—decreases CD4 proteins and class I MHC proteins on surface of infected cells
      - **vif**—enhances viral infectivity
      - **vpr**—facilitates entry of viral core from cytoplasm into nucleus in nondividing cells
      - **vpu**—enhances virus assembly and release. Note that HIV-2 encodes Vpx instead of Vpu.

TRANSMISSION OF HIV

Q. List the modes modes of transmission of HIV infection and high-risk groups.

- Transmission of HIV occurs when there is an exchange of blood or body fluids containing the virus or virus-infected cells.
- The risk of contracting HIV after exposure depends on:
  - Exposure route
  - The integrity of the exposed site
  - Type and volume of fluid
  - Viral load.
- Exposure route and percentage of transmission of HIV is presented in **Table 5.1**.

Major routes of transmission include:

TABLE 5.1: Exposure route and percentage of transmission of HIV.

Exposure route	*HIV transmission*
Blood transfusion	90–95%
Perinatal	15–30%
Sexual intercourse:	
➢ Vaginal	0.08%–0.19%
➢ Anal	0.5%–3.38% for receptive anal intercourse; 0.06%–0.16% for insertive anal intercourse
➢ Oral	0.005–0.01%
Injecting drugs use	0.63–2.14%
Needle stick exposure	0.13%
Mucous membrane splash to eye and oronasal	0.09%

- **Sexual transmission:**
  - Main route of transmission, accounting for more than 75% of cases of HIV.
  - HIV is present in vaginal secretions and cervical cells (in women) and semen (in men).
  - Although majority of the cases worldwide are transmitted via heterosexual route, HIV transmission is higher among men who have sex with men (MSM).
  - Unprotected anal intercourse conveys the greatest risk of sexual transmission of HIV.
  - Risk of sexual transmission of HIV is increased when there is coexisting sexually transmitted diseases, especially those associated with genital ulceration (e.g., syphilis, chancroid, and herpes).
  - Other risk factors include vaginal/rectal laceration, menstruation, and uncircumcised male partner. Risk of HIV acquisition is decreased with circumcision in heterosexual men. *Male circumcision decreases the risk of female-to-male sexual transmission of HIV by 50% to 60%.*
- **Parenteral transmission:**
  - Intravenous drug users (IDU):
    - Transmission occurs by sharing of needles, and syringes contaminated with HIV-containing blood.
    - Risk factors that determine transmission in this subgroup includes the duration of IDU, frequency of needle sharing, number of needle-sharing partners, number of injections, and prevalence of HIV infection among the users.
  - Transfusion of blood or blood components**:**
    - Recipients of blood transfusion of HIV-infected whole blood or components (e.g., platelets and plasma) was one of the modes of transmission prior to 1985.
    - Screening of donor blood and plasma for antibodies to HIV-1 and HIV-2, as well as determination of the presence of HIV nucleic acid has reduced the risk of this mode of transmission.
    - However, since a recently infected individual may be antibody-negative (window-period), there is a small risk (1 in 1.4–1.8 million units) of acquiring AIDS through transfusion of blood.
    - Note that the likelihood of a person becoming infected with HIV after receiving a single-donor blood product from an HIV-positive patient approaches 100% due to the large volume of transfusion.
  - Hemophiliacs:
    - Mainly those who received large amounts factor VIII and factor IX concentrates before 1985.
    - Increasing use of recombinant-clotting factors has eliminated this mode of transmission.
  - Splash of body fluids on mucosa (e.g., nose, mouth and eyes)
  - Spread through organ transplantation from HIV-infected donors has been reported.
- **Perinatal transmission (mother-to-infant transmission):**
  - Major mode of transmission of AIDS in children.
  - Can occur during gestation (in utero), at the time of delivery (intrapartum), or postpartum through breastfeeding
    - In utero vertical transmission from mother to fetus: **Transplacental spread**
      - Mechanism: Microtransfusions of maternal blood containing the virus to the fetus across the placenta; facilitated by the disruption in the integrity of the placenta
      - Genital tract infections and chorioamnionitis can increase in utero HIV transmission.
    - Intrapartum spread:
      - Due to contact of infant mucosal membranes with infected maternal blood and cervicovaginal fluids during the birth process
      - Microtransfusions across the placenta during labor contractions also contribute to the increased risk of transmission
      - Prolonged rupture of membranes, greater than 4 hours, is associated with increased risk of transmission.
    - Postpartum:
      - Via breastfeeding
      - More likely due to HIV-infected cells within breast milk than cell-free virus
      - The portal of entry is likely to be via intestinal or tonsillar tissues, with breaches in epithelial integrity facilitating transmission.
- **Transmission of HIV infection to healthcare workers**:
  - Via percutaneous, mucous membrane, and cutaneous exposure to blood-contaminated body fluids
  - Percutaneous injury, usually by a needle-stick injury, is the most common mechanism of occupational HIV transmission

- The risk of transmission of HIV to healthcare workers increases when:
    - The device causing the injury is visibly contaminated with blood
    - The device was used for insertion into an artery or a vein
    - The device caused a deep injury or
    - The source patient died within 2 months after the exposure.
- Routes by which HIV is not transmitted are mentioned in **Box 5.1**.

Box 5.1: Routes by which HIV is not transmitted.

- Casual nonsexual contact
- By vectors such as mosquitoes
- Respiratory droplet spread

Note: Saliva, sweat, urine, stool, vomitus, and tears are not considered infectious fluids

The Role of Viral Load in Transmission of HIV

- Viral load is the strongest predictor of transmission
- Higher the plasma viral load, the more likely HIV transmission will occur
- **"Undetectable equals Untransmittable (U = U)"** concept—negligible risk of sexual transmission of HIV when the HIV-infected sex partner has persistently suppressed viral replication on ART.

PATHOGENESIS OF HIV INFECTION AND AIDS

- The interaction between HIV and the host immune system is the basis of the pathogenesis of HIV disease.
- From the site of initial mucosal exposure, virus enters the blood or tissues of an individual.
- HIV is transported by dendritic cells from mucosal surfaces to regional lymph nodes where it establishes a permanent infection.
    - Note that HIV has selective affinity for host cells bearing the CD4 receptor, such as $CD4^+$ T cells (T-helper lymphocytes) which are present in the mucosal lymphoid tissue (largest reservoir of T cells and where majority of memory cells are lodged), monocytes/macrophages, dendritic cells, and microglial cells in the central nervous system.
- This is followed by viremia and dissemination to lymphoid organs, which are the main sites of viral replication.
- As a result, plasma levels of HIV-1 peak within 2 weeks of infection, and patients develop the acute retroviral syndrome. This is associated with significant declines in peripheral $CD4^+$ T-cell counts.
- Within several weeks, there is development of an HIV-specific immune response.
    - This involves both a **humoral immune response**, with the development of antibodies to various antigens, as well a **cell-mediated immune response**.
    - The cell-mediated immune response involves the expansion of HIV-specific CD8 cytotoxic T lymphocytes, resulting in a **CD8 lymphocytosis** and **reversal of the usual CD4:CD8 ratio**.
    - CD8 cytotoxic T lymphocytes kill CD4 cells that are actively replicating the virus, but **not latently infected CD4 cells**.
    - Despite this robust immune response, HIV escapes destruction, because the highly conserved gp120 and gp41 regions needed for viral attachment and entry are protected by highly variable glycoprotein loops that vary over time as a result of mutations caused by the error-prone reverse transcription process.
- The initial peak of viremia in primary infection settles to a plateau phase of persistent chronic viremia.
- With time, there is gradual reduction of the $CD4^+$ T-helper lymphocyte population.
- This makes the patient susceptible to opportunistic diseases.
- This is summarized in **Figure 5.2**.

LIFE CYCLE OF HIV

Q. Discuss the life cycle of HIV.

Life cycle of HIV consists of the following steps **(Fig. 5.3)**:

1. **Attachment**
    - Binding of **gp120** to **CD4 receptor** and one of the coreceptors (**CCR5 or CXCR4**)
    - During initial infection, CCR5 is used but subsequently the virus can adapt to use CXCR4
    - Individuals who are homozygous for the CCR5 delta 32 mutation do not express CCR5 on CD4 cells and are immune to HIV infection.
2. **Fusion**
    - Fusion of the virus with the host cell membrane
    - This involves the use of **gp41**
3. **Uncoating**
    - Uncoating of the viral genomic RNA.
4. **Reverse transcription**
    - Viral RNA is converted to DNA by the enzyme reverse transcriptase
    - This is an error-prone process and multiple mutations may arise, resulting in considerable viral genetic heterogeneity.
5. **Nuclear import**
    - The preintegration complex is transported into the nucleus.

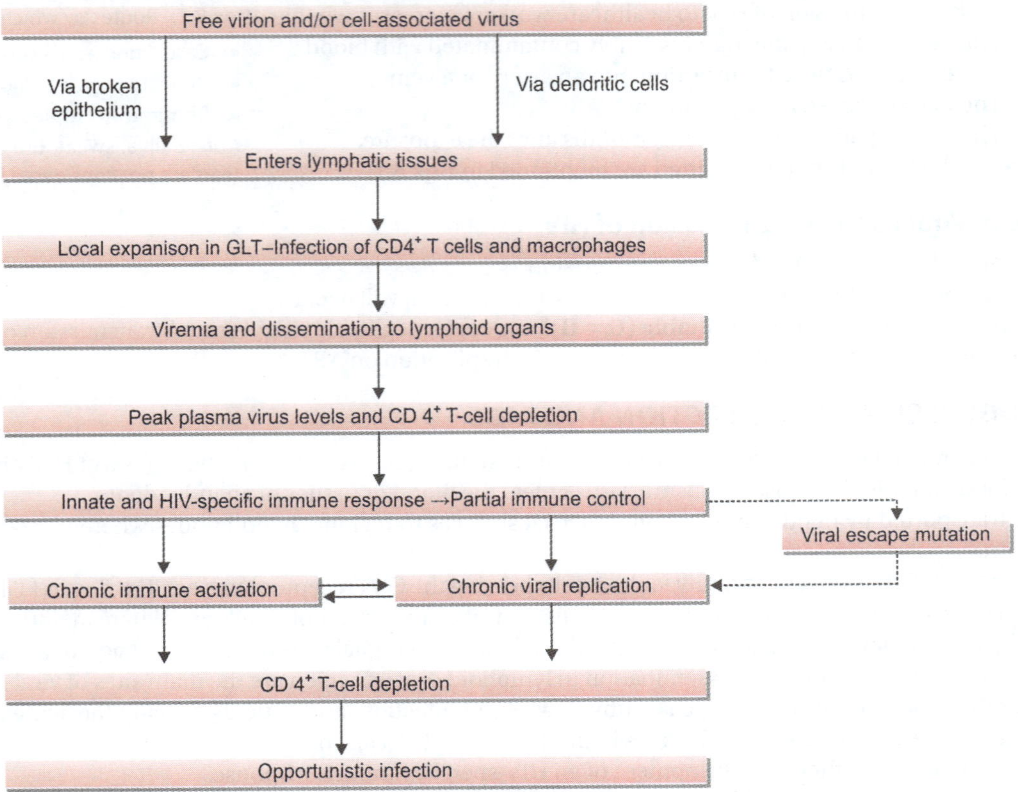

FIG. 5.2: Pathogenesis of HIV infection.

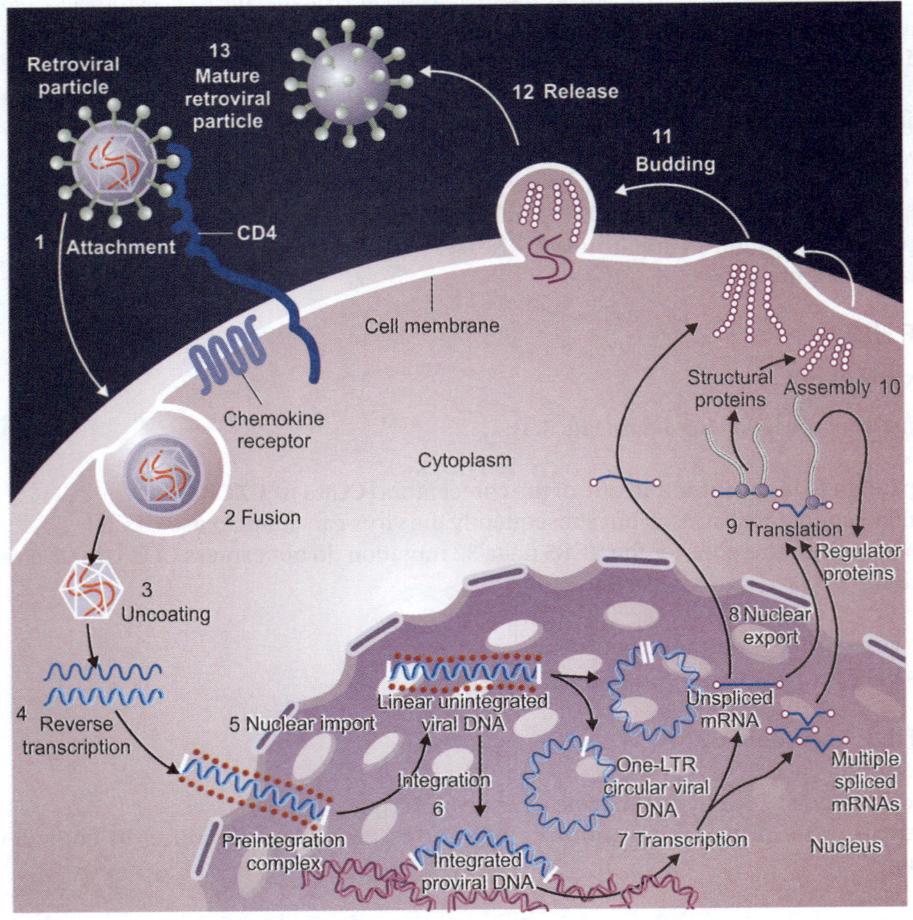

FIG. 5.3: Various molecular steps involved in the life cycle of HIV.

6. **Integration**
   - The enzyme integrase catalyzes the integration of the proviral DNA into the host genome
   - The integrated proviral DNA persists for the life of the cell
   - After the integration of the proviral DNA, there may be a latent infection or productive replication.
   - Latent infection:
     - During this, the provirus remains silent for months or years.
     - This cannot be eliminated by current antiretroviral therapy, which only acts on actively replicating cells.
   - Productive HIV replication: The virus goes through the below described phases.
7. **Transcription:** Proviral DNA is transcribed to yield messenger RNA (mRNA).
8. **Nuclear export:** Export of viral mRNA from the nucleus.
9. **Translation:** Viral structural proteins are synthesized.
10. **Assembly:** Association with the matrix protein Gag and assembly of the virus particle.
11. **Budding:** The immature particle bud from the cell surface, incorporating the host cell membrane into the viral envelope.
12. **Release:** The virus particle is released from the host cell.
13. **Maturation**
    - The enzyme protease mediates maturation to an infectious virus particle
    - This mature virion then infects other CD4 cells and the process is repeated.

NATURAL HISTORY OF HIV INFECTION (FIG. 5.4)

Q. Discuss the natural history of HIV infection.

Q. Discuss acute HIV syndrome.

The clinical picture of HIV infection can be divided into three stages:

1. Acute infection
2. Latent stage
3. Immunodeficiency stage.

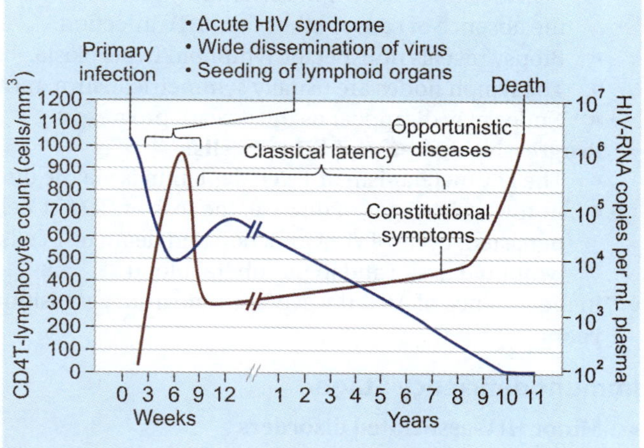

FIG. 5.4: HIV disease progression.

Acute Phase

- There is an **initial infection with HIV** through sexual/parenteral/perinatal transmission.
- This is followed by a **window period**.
  - About 2–6 weeks immediately following infection
  - This period is silent both clinically and serologically
- This is followed by **acute HIV syndrome**
  - Nonspecific flu-like illness
  - Symptoms include fever, sore throat, lymphadenopathy, maculopapular rash, diarrhea, malaise, mucosal ulcers, arthralgia, myalgia, weight loss, and hepatosplenomegaly
  - Patients may also present with neurologic symptoms, such as meningitis, encephalitis, peripheral neuropathy, and myelopathy
  - Opportunistic infections have also been reported at this stage, due to the presence of high level viremia combined with reduced numbers of $CD4^+$ T cells
  - However, may be asymptomatic in up to 60% of the patients
- During this period, uncontrolled viral replication occurs and results in high viral loads. The patient is also unaware of his HIV status. Thus, the patient is highly infectious.
- CD4 cell count can drop transiently.
- Presence of a prolonged symptomatic illness (>14 days) during early infection appears to correlate with more rapid progression to AIDS
- **Early diagnosis** at this stage may be achieved by
  - **HIV RNA** by polymerase chain reaction (PCR)
  - **p24 antigen** positivity.
- **Seroconversion**, i.e., the appearance of HIV-specific antibodies occurs **2 weeks—3 months** after the development of symptoms.
- **Establishment of the viral set point:**
  - By approximately 6 months of infection, plasma viremia reaches a steady-state level, known as the viral set point.
  - The viral set point level is closely associated with the rate of disease progression in the absence of ART, i.e., higher viral set point results in faster progression to AIDS.

- **Fiebig staging,** typically used for research purposes, can be used to characterize viral and immunologic dynamics following HIV transmission **(Table 5.2)**.

TABLE 5.2: Fiebig stages of early HIV infection.

Fiebig stage	*Cumulative duration (days)*	*HIV-RNA*	*p24 antigen*	*Immunoassay*	*Western blot*
1	5	+	–	–	–
2	10	+	+	–	–
3	14	+	+	+	–
4	19	+	+/–	+	Indeterminate
5	88	+	+/–	+	+ (p31 band negative)
6	Open-ended	+	+/–	+	+ (p31 band positive)

Clinical Latency Period

- It is predominantly characterized by **asymptomatic infection**
  - HIV reproduces at relatively lower levels during this phase, with relative **stability of the viral load.**
  - Although CD4⁺ T-cell destruction is ongoing, their levels are sufficiently high enough such that the patient may remain asymptomatic and without any opportunistic infection.
- **Persistent generalized lymphadenopathy (PGL):**
  - Development of persistent generalized lymphadenopathy (PGL) is common.
  - PGL is defined as lymphadenopathy greater than **1 cm** at **2 or more extrainguinal sites** for more than **3 months** in the absence of causes other than HIV infection.
  - Biopsy reveals nonspecific lymphoid hyperplasia.
  - The lymph nodes are usually symmetrical, firm, mobile, and nontender.
  - Nodes may disappear as the disease progresses.
- **Progressive decrease of CD4⁺ T cells:**
  - The key mechanism of T-cell depletion is via the direct killing of T cells by the virus.
  - In the early stages of disease, the loss of CD4⁺ T cells may be replaced by new T cells. Over the years, however, the persistent cycle of viral infection and death of T cells leads to a steady decrease in the number of CD4⁺ T cells, both in lymphoid tissue and in peripheral blood.
- In the absence of ART, the average time from acquisition of HIV to a CD4 cell count <200 cells/μL is approximately **8–10 years.**

Immunodeficiency Stage

- **Minor HIV-associated disorders**
  - Increasing signs and symptoms due to worsening immunity
  - Includes diseases in CDC category B or WHO stage 2 and 3 (See below)
- **AIDS**
  - It is final phase of HIV infection
  - AIDS is defined as a CD4 cell count <200 cells/**μ**L or the presence of any AIDS-defining condition (*See* **Table 5.5**) regardless of the CD4 cell count.
  - This stage is characterized by numerous opportunistic infections and malignancies.
  - Without treatment, individuals with AIDS have a life expectancy of 1–3 years.

PATTERNS OF HIV PROGRESSION

- **Noncontroller:** HIV-infected individuals with plasma **HIV-RNA >10,000 copies/mL without ART**.
- **Rapid progressors**: HIV infected with CD4⁺ T-cell counts of **<300 cells/μL within 3 years** after the last HIV-seronegative test.
- **Slow progressors**: Seropositive **asymptomatic** individuals infected for **8 or more years** with a CD4⁺ T-cell count **above 500 cells/μL** in the **absence of ART**.
- **Long-term nonprogressors**: **Asymptomatic** and **ART-naive** for **10 years** during follow-up with all CD4⁺ cell counts **above 500 cells/μL** during this period.
- **Elite controllers** are HIV-infected individuals who have viral loads **below 50 copies/mL without ART** and maintain normal CD4⁺ counts.
- **Viremic controller**: Infected with HIV and maintaining **viral loads of <2,000 RNA copies/mL without ART.**

HIV CLINICAL STAGING AND CLASSIFICATION (TABLE 5.3)

Q. Write short essay/note on clinical staging and classification of HIV.

- Two clinical staging systems, namely the World Health Organization (WHO) and the Centers for Disease Control (CDC), are in use and are listed below **(Tables 5.3 and 5.4)**.
- Note that the World Health Organization clinical stage is used in low- and middle-income countries while the CDC clinical categories are used in high-income countries.

TABLE 5.3: WHO clinical staging classification of HIV infection.

Primary HIV infection ➤ Asymptomatic ➤ Acute retroviral syndrome **Clinical stage I** ➤ Asymptomatic ➤ Persistent generalized lymphadenopathy **Clinical stage 2** ➤ Unexplained moderate weight loss (<10% of body weight) ➤ Recurrent upper respiratory tract infections (sinusitis, tonsillitis, otitis media, and pharyngitis) ➤ Herpes zoster ➤ Angular cheilitis ➤ Recurrent oral ulceration ➤ Papular pruritic eruptions ➤ Seborrheic dermatitis ➤ Fungal nail infections **Clinical stage 3** ➤ Unexplained severe weight loss (>10% of body weight) ➤ Unexplained chronic diarrhea for longer than one month ➤ Unexplained persistent fever (above 37.5°C for >1 month) ➤ Persistent oral candidiasis ➤ Oral hairy leukoplakia ➤ Pulmonary tuberculosis ➤ Severe bacterial infections (e.g., bacteremia, meningitis, pneumonia, empyema, bone or joint infection) ➤ Acute necrotizing ulcerative stomatitis, gingivitis or periodontitis ➤ Unexplained anemia (<8 g/dL), neutropenia (<500/µL) or HIV-associated immune thrombocytopenia (<50,000/µL) for >1 month	**Clinical stage 4** ➤ Pneumocystis pneumonia ➤ Tuberculosis—extrapulmonary ➤ Pneumonia, recurrent bacterial ➤ Disseminated nontuberculous mycobacterial infection ➤ Candidiasis of esophagus, trachea, bronchi or lungs ➤ Disseminated coccidioidomycosis or histoplasmosis ➤ CNS toxoplasmosis ➤ Cryptococcosis—extrapulmonary (including meningitis) ➤ Progressive multifocal leukoencephalopathy ➤ HIV encephalopathy ➤ Cryptosporidiosis, chronic (>1 month) ➤ Isosporiasis, chronic (>1 month) ➤ Chronic herpes simplex (>1 month) infection ➤ Cytomegalovirus disease (outside liver, spleen, and nodes) ➤ Recurrent nontyphoidal salmonella bacteremia ➤ Leishmaniasis, atypical disseminated ➤ Lymphoma (cerebral or B-cell non-Hodgkin's) ➤ Kaposi's sarcoma ➤ Cervical carcinoma—invasive ➤ Symptomatic HIV-associated nephropathy ➤ Symptomatic HIV-associated cardiomyopathy

TABLE 5.4: CDC clinical staging classification of HIV infection.

Category A	***Category B***	***Category C***
➤ Asymptomatic ➤ Primary HIV infection ➤ Persistent generalized lymphadenopathy	Constitutional symptoms: Fever (38.5°C) or diarrhea for >1 month ➤ Oropharyngeal candidiasis ➤ Oral hairy leukoplakia ➤ Herpes zoster: Involving two separate episodes or more than one dermatome ➤ Persistent vulvovaginal candidiasis ➤ Pelvic inflammatory disease, especially tubo-ovarian abscess ➤ Cervical dysplasia (moderate or severe)/cervical carcinoma in situ ➤ Bacillary angiomatosis ➤ Listeriosis ➤ Idiopathic thrombocytopenic purpura ➤ Peripheral neuropathy	Same as WHO stage 4, with the following modifications: ➤ Pulmonary tuberculosis included ➤ Recurrent salmonella septicemia
Note: Based on the absolute $CD4^+$ counts, the stages may be further classified as follows:		
$CD4^+$ count >500: **A1** $CD4^+$ count >200–499: **A2** $CD4^+$ count <200: **A3**	$CD4^+$ count >500: **B1** $CD4^+$ count >200–499: **B2** $CD4^+$ count <200: **B3**	$CD4^+$ count >500: **C1** $CD4^+$ count >200–499: **C2** $CD4^+$ count <200: **C3**

IMPORTANT INFECTIONS AND PRESENTING PROBLEMS IN AIDS (TABLE 5.5)

TABLE 5.5: AIDS-defining conditions.

Organ system	***AIDS-defining conditions***
Respiratory	Pulmonary tuberculosis ➤ *Pneumocystis jirovecii* pneumonia ➤ Recurrent bacterial pneumonia (>2 episodes in 12 months) ➤ Candidiasis of bronchi, trachea or lungs

Contd...

Contd...

Neurology	➢ Cerebral toxoplasmosis ➢ Cryptococcal meningitis ➢ Progressive multifocal leukoencephalopathy ➢ HIV-related encephalopathy
Ophthalmology	Cytomegalovirus retinitis
Dermatology	Kaposi sarcoma
Gastroenterology	➢ Persistent cryptosporidial diarrhea ➢ Persistent isosporiasis (>1 month's duration) ➢ Esophageal candidiasis
Oncology and hematology	➢ Cervical cancer (invasive) ➢ Non-Hodgkin lymphoma ➢ Primary CNS lymphoma ➢ Burkitt lymphoma
Other	Recurrent salmonella bacteremia ➢ Cryptococcosis ➢ Coccidioidomycosis (disseminated or extrapulmonary) ➢ Histoplasmosis ➢ *Mycobacterium avium* complex (MAC) ➢ Mycobacterial infection (all species) ➢ Herpes simplex bronchitis, pneumonitis or esophagitis, or persistent ulcers for >1 month ➢ HIV wasting syndrome

Q. List of important opportunistic infections in AIDS.

Q. Write short essay/note on AIDS-defining diseases and opportunistic infections in HIV.

Relation between $CD4^+$ cell count and common illness in HIV patients is presented in **Table 5.6** and in **Figure 5.5**.

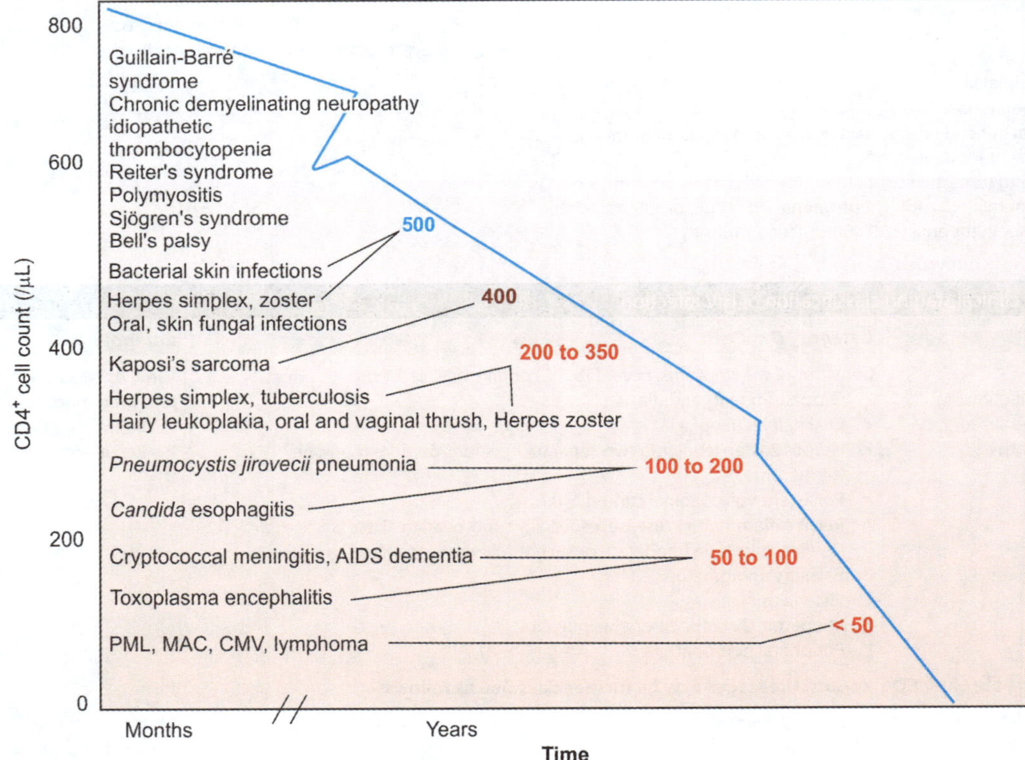

FIG. 5.5: Relation between $CD4^+$ cell count and common illness in HIV patients.

(CMV: cytomegalovirus infection; MAC: mycobacterium avium complex; PML: progressive multifocal leukoencephalopathy)

TABLE 5.6: Features of HIV infection with declining CD4 count.

Absolute CD4 count	***Opportunistic infection/Malignancy***
>400	➢ Bacterial skin infections ➢ Herpes zoster ➢ HIV-associated ITP

Contd...

Contd...

<400	➢ Oral hairy leukoplakia ➢ Oral and vaginal candidiasis ➢ Tuberculosis ➢ Kaposi sarcoma
<200	➢ *Pneumocystis carinii* pneumonia ➢ Esophageal candidiasis ➢ Mucocutaneous herpes simplex ➢ Cryptosporidial/microsporidial diarrhea ➢ Miliary/extrapulmonary tuberculosis ➢ HIV-associated wasting ➢ Peripheral neuropathy ➢ HIV-associated nephropathy
<100	➢ Toxoplasmosis ➢ Cryptococcosis ➢ Non-Hodgkin lymphoma ➢ HIV-associated dementia
<50	➢ Cytomegalovirus ➢ *Mycobacterium avium* complex (MAC) ➢ CNS lymphoma ➢ Progressive multifocal leukoencephalopathy

HIV AND ORGAN SYSTEM INVOLVEMENT

Respiratory System

Q. Enumerate upper/lower respiratory tract infections and pulmonary complications in AIDS (Table 5.7).

Q. Write short essay/note on *Pneumocystis jirovecii* pneumonia (PJP), its treatment, and prophylaxis.

TABLE 5.7: Pulmonary manifestations of HIV.

Etiology and CD4 level	***Organisms (if applicable)***	***Signs and symptoms***	***Laboratory***	***Radiology***	***Initial treatment***	***Prophylaxis***
Sinusitis CD4 level—All	Encapsulated organisms—*Haemophilus influenzae* and *Streptococcus pneumoniae* Lower CD4—mucormycosis	Fever Nasal congestion Headache	Leukocytosis Neutrophilia	CT/MRI—sinusitis—most commonly maxillary sinusitis	Antimicrobial therapy Aggressive local debridement + systemic amphotericin B for mucormycosis	-
Bacterial pneumonia CD4 ~ 300/mcL	*S. pneumonia* *H. influenzae* *Staphylococcus aureus* *Pseudomonas aeruginosa*	Rapid onset of fever, dyspnea, cough, and sputum production	Leukocytosis Neutrophilia Sputum culture Blood cultures often positive	Lobar or diffuse infiltrate	Amoxicillin–clavulanate or ceftriaxone	Immunization: PCV followed by booster immunization with 23PPV
Pneumocystis jirovecii pneumonia—**most common cause**, accounting for 25% of cases of pneumonia in patients with HIV infection CD4 <200	*Pneumocystis jirovecii*	Subacute fever Dyspnea Nonproductive cough Retrosternal chest pain worse on inspiration Auscultation is usually normal Hypoxia on exertion (6-minute walk test) More hypoxia than expected from chest radiographic findings Extrapulmonary involvement may occur rarely	Hypoxemia Increased (A-a) gradient Elevated LDH PFT: Restrictive pattern with reduced diffusion capacity **Diagnosis:** BAL/induced sputum/transbronchial biopsy Silver stain, PCR or immunofluorescence detects *Pneumocystis jirovecii*. Methenamine silver stains the cyst wall Giemsa stains the wall of the trophozoites and sporozoites	CXR: Normal or bilateral perihilar diffuse symmetric interstitial pattern (**Fig 5.6**) CT—patchy ground glass opacities	TMP-SMX, 5 mg/kg (of TMP component) Q8h × 21 days or Clindamycin 600 mg Q8h plus Primaquine 15–30 mg OD × 21 days Other agents that can be used: Dapsone 100 mg Q24h + TMP-SMX 5 mg/kg Q8h × 21 days Atovaquone 750 mg BID × 21 days Pentamidine 4 mg/kg/day × 21 days If pO_2 < 70 mm Hg or (A-a gradient) >35 mm Hg, then add: Prednisone, 40 mg BD × 5 days, then 40 mg OD × 5 days, then 20 mg OD × 11 days	PCP prophylaxis with TMP-SMX for CD4 <200 or CD 4% <15% Continue prophylaxis until CD4 count > 200 × 3 months Other agents that can be used: Pentamidine, Atovaquone, Dapsone + pyrimethamine

Contd...

Contd...

Tuberculosis CD4—Any count	*Mycobacterium tuberculosis*	Patients with **high CD4 count:** Weight loss, fever, cough, night sweats, and lymphadenopathy **Lower CD4 counts:** Disseminated disease	Positive sputum AFB smear Positive sputum and blood cultures; BAL if no productive cough; Typical histopathology of lymph nodes	*CD4 > 200/μL*-Apical, cavitary or nodular lesions *CD4 < 200/μL*—Normal, or middle or lower lobe consolidation, miliary pattern, lymphadenopathy Pleural effusions	2 HRZE 4 HRE Initiation of ART may be associated with TB-IRIS	Latent TB: Isoniazid ± Rifampicin
Atypical mycobacterial infections CD4 <50	*Mycobacterium avium* or *Mycobacterium intracellulare*—MAC Others— *Mycobacterium bovis*	Disseminated disease with fever, weight loss, and night sweats Abdominal pain, diarrhea, lymphadenopathy, and splenomegaly	2 consecutive sputum samples positive for MAC Blood culture, culture of involved tissue Bone marrow biopsy show mycobacteria Anemia Elevated ALP	CXR—Bilateral lower lobe infiltrates suggestive of military spread Alveolar or nodular infiltrates and hilar Mediastinal lymphadenopathy	Clarithromycin, 500 mg PO BD and ethambutol, 15 mg/kg PO OD, and rifabutin, 300 mg/kg PO OD (addition may improve survival and decrease risk of macrolide resistance)	MAC Prophylaxis: CD4 <50 Azithromycin 1,200 mg once weekly or clarithromycin 500 mg twice daily
Rhodococcus equi	*Rhodococcus equi*—gram-positive, pleomorphic, acid-fast nonspore forming bacillus	Fever Cough with expectoration	Cultures: Blood/ sputum/BAL/ pleural fluid/lung tissue	X-ray—cavitary lesions and consolidation	Combination of two of the following: Levofloxacin 750 mg OD Rifampicin 600 mg OD Azithromycin 250 mg OD Duration: 2 months	Secondary prophylaxis until CD4 > 200: Azithromycin 250 mg OD + Levofloxacin 750 mg OD
Fungal infections	Pulmonary cryptococcal disease CD4 < 100	Fever, cough, dyspnea, and hemoptysis Concomitant CNS infection		Focal or diffuse interstitial infiltrate Lobar disease Cavitary disease Pleural effusions Hilar/mediastinal adenopathy	Amphotericin B, 0.7 mg/kg IV OD × 2 weeks and flucytosine, 25 mg/kg IV Q6h × 2 weeks then fluconazole, 400 mg/d PO × 8–10 weeks	Prophylaxis for prior documented disease: Fluconazole 200 mg/d
	Histoplasmosis CD4 < 150	Disseminated disease or cough, dyspnea	Urine Histoplasma antigen	Diffuse interstitial infiltrate or diffuse small nodules	Liposomal amphotericin B 3 mg/kg/d × 1–2 weeks followed by itraconazole 200 mg TID × 3 days, then 200 mg BD for at least 12 months	Prophylaxis if prior documented disease or CD4 < 150 and high risk Itraconazole 200 mg PO daily
	Coccidioides immitis—CD4 count <250/μL	Fever, weight loss, and cough	Enzyme immunoassay for coccidioides—IgM and IgG	CXR—extensive, diffuse reticulonodular infiltrates. Nodules, cavities, pleural effusions, and hilar adenopathy may also be seen	Mild disease: Fluconazole 400 mg OD × 3–12 months Or Itraconazole 200 mg BD × 3–12 months Severe disease: Liposomal amphotericin B 3–5 mg/kg IV daily	Secondary prophylaxis until CD4 > 250/μL Fluconazole 400 mg OD or Itraconazole 200 mg BD
Kaposi sarcoma CD4 < 400	HHV8	Usually associated with skin or mucosal lesions	Typical lesions seen on bronchoscopy	Nodular infiltrates with perihilar location	Treatment for HIV; rarely requires radiotherapy or chemotherapy	-
Lymphoid Interstitial pneumonia CD4 < 200 Note: (Other ILD–NSIP)	EBV	Transitory fever and dyspnea	Transbronchial biopsy/open lung biopsy—interstitial infiltrates of lymphocytes and plasma cells in a perivascular and peribronchial distribution	Reticulonodular infiltrates	Possibly steroids	-

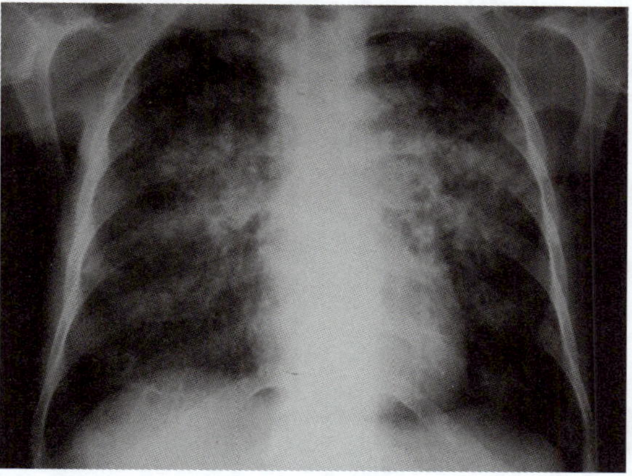

FIG. 5.6: Chest X-ray of pneumocystis pneumonia showing bilateral perihilar infiltrates.

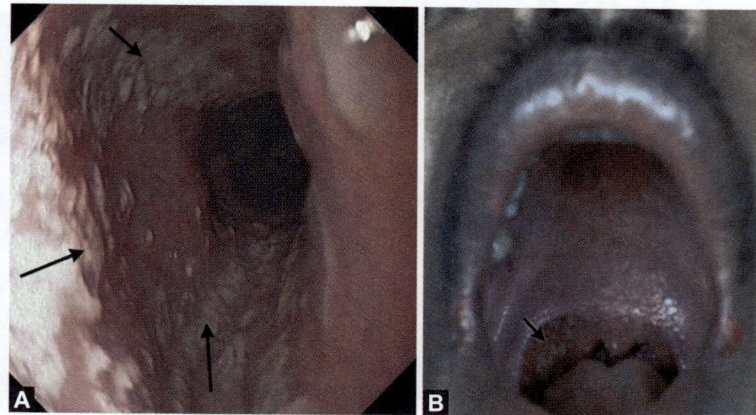

FIGS. 5.7A AND B: (A) Esophageal candidiasis; (B) Oral candidiasis in patient with AIDS.

GASTROINTESTINAL DISEASE

Q. Write short essay/note on gastrointestinal manifestations of AIDS.

Q. List the causes of esophagitis in HIV (Table 5.8).

TABLE 5.8: Esophagitis in HIV.

Etiology and CD4 level	*Clinical features*	*Diagnosis*	*Treatment*	*Comments*
Candida *Candida albicans*—most common CD4 <200 (**Figs. 5.7A and B**)	➢ Dysphagia ➢ Odynophagia **Other risk factors:** ➢ Acute HIV infection ➢ Use of broad-spectrum antibiotics ➢ Corticosteroids ➢ Diabetes mellitus ➢ Hematological or solid organ malignancy and use of antineoplastic agents	➢ Upper endoscopy—hyperemia ➢ Yellow-white mucosal plaques When this is removed, it reveals a friable mucosa Biopsy and culture	Fluconazole 200–400 mg OD × 14–21 days—DOC Other azoles (itraconazole, ketoconazole, posaconazole, voriconazole) and echinocandins (caspofungin, micafungin, anidulafungin) are also effective	When presentation is highly suggestive of *Candida esophagitis*, antifungal therapy can be attempted prior to biopsy Refractory candidiasis: Mucosal candidiasis that fails to resolve despite 7–14 days of daily fluconazole (≥200 mg daily)
Herpes virus Predominantly HSV 1 CD4 <200	➢ Dysphagia ➢ Odynophagia ➢ Nausea ➢ Fever ➢ Epigastric pain	➢ Upper endoscopy: Multiple small superficial ulcers with/without vesicles in the distal part of the esophagus ➢ Biopsy and culture: Diagnostic	Acyclovir 400 mg five times a day × 14–21 days Alternatives: Famciclovir, valacyclovir	May be found in association with candida esophagitis
CMV CD4 <50	➢ Dysphagia ➢ Odynophagia ➢ Nausea ➢ Fever ➢ Epigastric pain	➢ Upper endoscopy: Unique or multiple large, shallow ulcers in the middle or distal esophagus ➢ Histopathology: Large intranuclear "owl-eye" inclusions ➢ Positive immunohistochemical or direct fluorescent staining for CMV	IV ganciclovir 5 mg/kg IV Q12h followed by oral valganciclovir 900 mg PO Q12h, once clinical improvement. Duration of therapy: 3–6 weeks	Culture is neither sensitive nor specific
Other causes of esophagitis: ➢ *Mycobacterium* ➢ Kaposi sarcoma ➢ In patients with well controlled HIV infection with CD4 counts > 200 cells/μL—present mainly with reflux symptoms – Gastroesophageal reflux disease (GERD) – Barrett's esophagus – Gastric ulcers – Inflammatory gastropathy – *Helicobacter pylori* infection				

DIARRHEA IN PATIENTS WITH HIV

Q. List the causes and management of diarrhea in a HIV patient.

- Diarrhea is an important cause of morbidity in patients with HIV and is a predictor of increased mortality.
- Some of the important causes of diarrhea in patients with HIV are described in **Table 5.9**.
- History and physical examination should determine:
  - Small bowel diarrhea versus colonic diarrhea
  - Duration of symptoms

- Other abdominal or constitutional symptoms:
  - Fever
  - Weight loss
  - Hepatosplenomegaly
- Status of HIV disease, including CD4 count
- Medication history and recent changes in medications
- Exposures: Travel, exposure to antibiotics.

- Investigations include
  - For all patients:
    - Stool culture for enteric pathogens
    - Stool for ova and parasites × 3
    - Stool for *Clostridium difficile* toxin.
  - For patients with suspicion of colitis
    - Colonoscopy and biopsy
  - For patient with no suspicion of colitis
    - Upper gastrointestinal (GI) endoscopy and biopsy
  - For patients with diarrhea and concomitant significant abdominal pain
    - Abdominal computed tomography (CT) using oral and intravenous contrast
      - Imaging may show evidence of:
        - Colitis—CMV, herpes simplex virus (HSV), and *Clostridium difficile*
        - Abdominal adenopathy or hepatosplenomegaly—MAC, tuberculosis, histoplasmosis, and lymphoma
        - Biliary tract disease

Treatment:

- Treatment of the underlying cause **(Table 5.9)**
- Empiric therapy is not recommended
- Substitution of an alternative medicine: If a particular antiretroviral medication is the culprit (e.g., ritonavir)
- If chronic diarrhea continues without a diagnosis, symptomatic therapy with an antimotility drug (e.g., loperamide or diphenoxylate with atropine can be attempted.
- **Crofelemer:**
  - 125 mg orally twice daily
  - Blocks chloride secretion and accompanying high-volume water loss in diarrhea
  - Approved by Food and Drug Administration (FDA) for noninfectious diarrhea in HIV-infected patients receiving antiretroviral therapy

TABLE 5.9: Diarrhea in patients with HIV.

Etiology and CD4 level	*Clinical features*	*Investigation*	*Treatment*
Protozoa			
Cryptosporidia CD4 <200	➢ Diarrhea ➢ Crampy abdominal pain ➢ Nausea ➢ Vomiting ➢ Biliary tract disease: ➢ cholecystitis ± cholangitis ± pancreatitis	➢ Stool examination: Oocytes stain with acid fast dyes ➢ Biopsy of small intestine	Nitazoxanide 2,000 mg/day × 14–28 days
Cyclospora spp. CD4 <200	➢ Watery diarrhea ➢ Anorexia and weight loss ➢ Abdominal cramps ➢ Low-grade fever	Stool examination: Modified acid-fast stain: Oocysts appear light pink to deep purple Stool PCR assays	TMP/SMX DS Q12h × 3–4 weeks Alternative: Ciprofloxacin
Cystoisospora belli (Isospora belli) CD4 <200	➢ Nonbloody crampy diarrhea ➢ Malabsorption	Stool examination: Stool stains with large, acid-fast structures Stool PCR assays	TMP/SMX DS Q12h × 3–4 weeks Note: Three weekly regimen of TMP-SMX—prevents recurrence
Microsporidia CD4 <200	➢ Abdominal pain, malabsorption, diarrhea, and cholangitis	Stool examination: Light microscopy: **Modified trichrome stain** Electron microscopic examination of stool specimen, intestinal aspirate or intestinal biopsy specimen required for species identification	Albendazole 400 mg bid × 14–28 days
Cytomegalovirus CD4 <50	➢ Diarrhea ➢ Abdominal pain ➢ Weight loss ➢ Anorexia ➢ Non bloody diarrhea ➢ Monitor for CMV retinitis	➢ Endoscopy ➢ Biopsy—intranuclear and cytoplasmic inclusion bodies	IV ganciclovir 5 mg/kg IV Q12h followed by oral valganciclovir 900 mg PO Q12h, once clinical improvement. Duration of therapy: 3–6 weeks Alternative: Foscarnet and cidofovir

Contd...

Contd...

HSV	Perirectal ulcers and erosions	CECT abdomen: Colitis	Acyclovir 400 mg five times a day × 14–21 days Alternatives: Famciclovir and valacyclovir
Bacteria			
Salmonella, Shigella, and *Campylobacter* spp.	➢ MSM ➢ Fever ➢ Anorexia and fatigue ➢ Diarrhea—may be bloody	➢ Blood and stool culture ➢ Stool fecal leukocytes may be present	Fluoroquinolone (e.g., ciprofloxacin) Erythromycin for campylobacter Duration: 10–14 days
Clostridium difficile	➢ Fever and diarrhea	➢ *C. difficile* toxin ➢ Colitis on contrast CT	Vancomycin and metronidazole
SIBO	➢ Diarrhea ➢ Weight loss ➢ Flatulence and abdominal discomfort	➢ Positive lactulose breath test ➢ Bacterial concentration of >10^3 CFU/mL in jejunal aspirate culture	Metronidazole and ciprofloxacin
Mycobacterium tuberculosis	➢ Chronic diarrhea alternating with constipation ➢ Abdominal distension ➢ Intestinal colic ➢ Fever, weight loss, and night sweats	➢ Abdominal lymphadenopathy or hepatosplenomegaly on imaging ➢ Endoscopy + biopsy	HRZE Duration: 6 months
Mycobacterium avium complex	➢ Diarrhea ➢ Fever, weight loss, and abdominal pain ➢ Lymphadenopathy ➢ Hepatosplenomegaly	➢ Abdominal lymphadenopathy or hepatosplenomegaly on imaging ➢ Blood culture ➢ Anemia ➢ Elevated ALP	Clarithromycin, 500 mg PO BD and Ethambutol, 15 mg/kg PO OD and Rifabutin, 300 mg/kg PO OD
Fungi			
Histoplasmosis	➢ Fever ➢ Diarrhea	Histoplasma antigen—urine and blood culture	Amphotericin B, then itraconazole Duration: 28 days
Coccidioidomycosis	➢ Fever ➢ Diarrhea ➢ Peritonitis with *Coccidioides immitis*	Serology for coccidioidomycosis Culture	Amphotericin B, then fluconazole Duration: 28 days
Other			
HIV enteropathy CD4 <200	➢ Diarrhea > 1 month ➢ Malabsorption ➢ Weight loss ➢ **Diagnosis of exclusion**	Biopsy of small bowel—low grade mucosal atrophy with a decrease in mitotic figures Decreased or absent small bowel lactase	ART
Other causes of diarrhea			

- Infectious:
  - Protozoal:
    - *Entamoeba histolytica*
    - *Leishmania donovani*
    - *Blastocystis hominis*
  - Viral:
    - Adenovirus
    - Rotavirus
    - Norwalk
- Gut neoplasms/tumor invasion:
  - Lymphoma
  - Kaposi's sarcoma
- Pancreatic insufficiency:
  - Infectious pancreatitis:
    - Cytomegalovirus
    - Mycobacterium avium complex
  - Drug-induced pancreatitis:
    - Didanosine
    - Pentamidine

HEPATOBILIARY MANIFESTATIONS OF HIV

Q. Add a note on hepatobiliary manifestations in HIV (Table 5.10).

TABLE 5.10: Hepatobiliary manifestations in HIV.

Etiology	*Clinical features*	*Investigations*	*Treatment*
Liver			
Hepatitis B and hepatitis C	➢ May be asymptomatic ➢ Fatigue, nausea, vomiting, and RUQ pain	Transaminitis Serologies and PCR for viremia	HBV: Antivirals (e.g., TAF and lamivudine) HCV: Direct-acting antiviral combination therapy
MAC	➢ Fever; weight loss; abdominal pain ➢ Anemia ➢ Hepatosplenomegaly ➢ Lymphadenopathy	➢ Elevated serum ALP and LDH ➢ Isolation of MAC from cultures of blood, lymph node, or bone marrow ➢ Histopathologic findings on a liver biopsy specimen showing granulomas with positive acid-fast bacilli stains ➢ Mycobacterial growth from culture of liver tissue obtained by biopsy	Clarithromycin, 500 mg PO BD and ethambutol, 15 mg/kg PO OD, and rifabutin, 300 mg/kg PO OD

Contd...

Contd...

Biliary			
Cholangiopathy (infectious)	➢ Advanced disease ➢ Epigastric pain, nausea, anorexia, and weight loss	Elevated alkaline phosphatase ERCP: Segmental stenosis without gallstones	ART

Others

- Infection:
  - *Mycobacterium tuberculosis*
  - Hepatitis A and E
  - *Pneumocystis jiroveci*
  - *Cryptococcus* spp.
  - Peliosis hepatis—*Bartonella henselae*
  - CMV and microsporidia—can cause both hepatitis and cholangitis
- NAFLD/NASH
- Neoplasms
  - Lymphoma
  - Kaposi sarcoma
  - HCC
- Drugs
  - Atazanavir—indirect hyperbilirubinemia
  - Sulfonamides

MUCOCUTANEOUS MANIFESTATIONS OF HIV/AIDS (TABLE 5.11 AND FIGS. 5.8A TO F)

Q. List the mucocutaneous manifestations of HIV/AIDS.

TABLE 5.11: Mucocutaneous manifestations of HIV/AIDS.

Etiology	*Clinical features*	*Diagnosis*	*Treatment*
Acute HIV infection	Reddish maculopapular lesions on the trunk, face, palms, and soles	➢ HIV RNA levels ➢ P24 antigenemia ➢ Standard screening test may be negative	ART
Oral leukoplakia	Whitish plaques on the lateral aspect of the tongue	➢ Clinical	No treatment
Oral candidiasis **(Fig. 5.7B)**	Creamy white patches overlying inflamed mucosa	➢ Clinical ➢ KOH mount ➢ Culture	Fluconazole 100–200 mg Q24h × 7–14 days
Acute condylomata **(Fig. 5.8A)**	Wart-like papules in the anogenital area	➢ Clinical ➢ Biopsy and typing of HPV	Curettage Podophyllin electrocoagulation, or laser
Molluscum contagiosum (virus pox) **(Fig. 5.8B)**	Umbilicated papules	➢ Clinical ➢ Biopsy	Curettage or electrocoagulation
Herpes simplex virus **(Figs. 5.8C and D)**	➢ Painful vesicles or ulcers that can become very large ➢ Lesions are primarily perianal, vulvar, or peribuccal	Inspection, culture, and immunofluorescence	Valacyclovir, or famciclovir; possibly IV acyclovir
Herpes zoster **(Fig. 5.8E)**	➢ Vesicles on a red surface ➢ Dermatomal distribution ➢ Chronic and disseminated forms are possible in advanced immunodeficiency	➢ Clinical ➢ Can be confirmed by culture and immunofluorescence	Acyclovir Other: Valacyclovir and famciclovir
Kaposi sarcoma (HHV8) **(Fig. 5.8F)**	➢ Macules, papules, or nodules of purple to dark blue color ➢ Edema and ulcers are possible	➢ Clinical ➢ Biopsy, if diagnosis uncertain	ART Local treatment; cryotherapy, radiotherapy, and systemic chemotherapy
Bacillary angiomatosis (*Bartonella henselae*)	Red-to-violet papule or nodule	➢ Biopsy ➢ Culture—difficult	Antibiotics (macrolides, quinolones, and tetracyclines)
Seborrheic dermatitis CD4 <400	➢ Red and squamous plaques on face and trunk ➢ More diffuse in patients with CD4 <200 ➢ May be a cutaneous manifestation of IRIS	➢ Clinical ➢ Biopsy, if diagnosis uncertain	➢ Topical antifungals ➢ Topical anti-inflammatory agents
Prurigo nodularis	Isolated, very itchy squamous papules	Histology	➢ Symptomatic treatment ➢ UV irradiation

Other

- Infectious:
  - Secondary syphilis—papules and nodules
  - Cryptococcosis—papules and nodules
  - Histoplasmosis—mucocutaneous ulcers, papules, and nodules
  - Tinea corporis
  - Norwegian scabies
  - Onychomycosis
- Drug induced
  - Drug rashes: Including toxic epidermal necrolysis, Stevens–Johnson syndrome, and drug reaction with eosinophilia and systemic symptoms (DRESS) syndrome— sulfonamides and non-nucleoside reverse transcriptase inhibitors (NNRTIs)
  - Zidovudine: Blue-black discoloration of nails due to
  - Emtricitabine: Hyperpigmentation of palms and soles
- Other
  - Pruritic papular eruption (itchy red bump disease)—most common skin manifestation of HIV in sub-Saharan Africa
  - Psoriasis—exacerbated by HIV

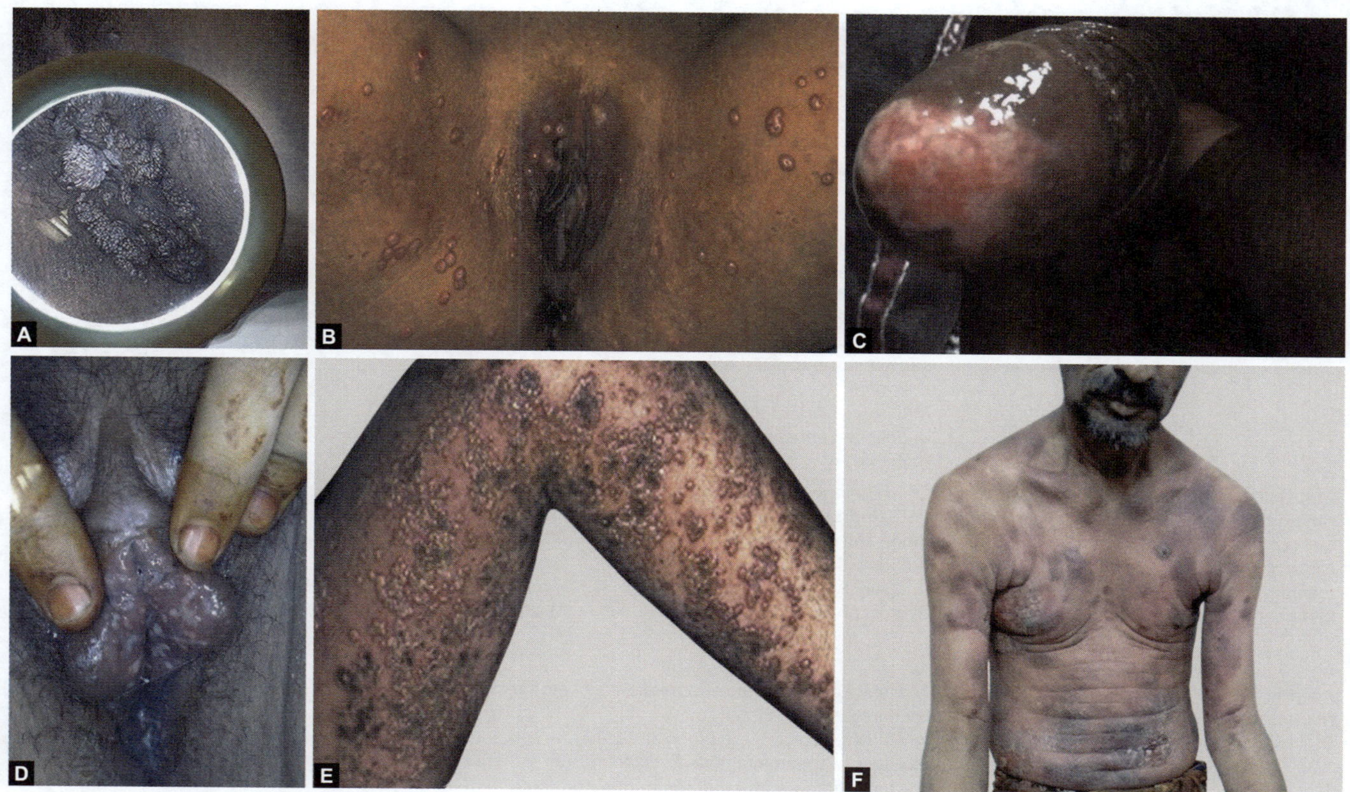

FIGS. 5.8A TO F: (A) Genital warts; (B) Molluscum contagiosum; (C) Genital herpes (male); (D) Genital herpes (female); (E) Herpes zoster on lower limb; (F) Kaposi's sarcoma.

NEUROLOGICAL MANIFESTATIONS OF AIDS (TABLE 5.12)

Q. Discuss the neurological manifestations of AIDS.

Q. Discuss the clinical features and management of cryptococcal meningitis.

TABLE 5.12: Neurological manifestations in patients with HIV/AIDS.

Diagnosis and CD4 level	*Symptoms and signs*	*Investigations*	*Treatment*	*Prophylaxis*
CNS toxoplasmosis— Reactivation of residual *Toxoplasma gondii* cysts from past infection CD4 count <200	Focal deficit, headache, fever, and seizures *Toxoplasma chorioretinitis*— eye pain, decreased visual acuity, raised yellow-white cottony lesions in a nonvascular distribution, "headlight in a fog" appearance **(Fig. 5.9)**	Sabin–Feldman dye test: IgG antitoxoplasma antibodies; CSF—PCR positive in untreated cases *Imaging:* Contrast CT/MRI: **(Fig. 5.10)** Multiple corticomedullary ring-enhancing lesions; edema; "concentric target" sign PET scan—hypodense lesions Definite diagnosis: Brain biopsy; rarely needed	Sulfadiazine 1.5 g + pyrimethamine 200 mg stat followed by 75 mg Q24h + folinic acid 10–25 mg Q24h Duration: Minimum 6 weeks after resolution of signs/symptoms, followed by secondary prophylaxis Alternative: ➢ Pyrimethamine + folinic acid + one of: ➢ Atovaquone ➢ Clarithromycin ➢ Azithromycin ➢ Dapsone ➢ TMP-SMX	Primary prophylaxis: If CD4 <100—TMP-SMX-DS Q24h; Can discontinue if CD4 >200 × 3 months Secondary prophylaxis: Sulfadiazine 2–4 g in two to four doses/day + pyrimethamine 25–50 mg Q24h + folinic acid 10–25 mg Q24h Can discontinue if CD4 >200 × 6 months
CNS tuberculosis— TB meningitis Tuberculoma	Focal deficits, including cranial nerve palsy Meningeal signs Seizures Coma Fundus—choroid tubercles may be seen	CSF—"Cob-web" coagulum, lymphocyte predominant; high protein (100–800 mg/dL), low glucose AFB culture—gold standard NAAT may be positive *Imaging:* Tuberculoma: Lesions are similar toxoplasmosis, except that edema is less marked and single lesions occur more commonly TB meningitis: Meningeal enhancement, Obstructive hydrocephalus—requires neurosurgical intervention *Other:* Spinal arachnoiditis CXR—may reveal evidence of TB	2 HRZE followed by 7 HRE Total duration: 9–12 months Adjunctive corticosteroids: Dexamethasone –0.4 mg/kg/d × 1 week followed by 0.3 mg/kg/d × 1 week followed by 0.2 mg/kg/d × 1 week followed by 0.1 mg/kg/d × 1 week, then tapered and stopped over 3–4 weeks	Latent TB: Isoniazid ± rifampicin

Contd...

Contd...

Primary CNS lymphoma— High-grade B-cell lymphomas associated with EBV infection CD4 count <50	Slow onset of reduced consciousness and headache Focal deficits Seizures Neuropsychiatric symptoms	CSF PCR always positive for EBV; Cytology is seldom positive *Imaging:* Contrast CT/MRI: Variable number of lesions; periventricular contrast enhancement; Lesions are positive in PET scan Stereotactic biopsy	ART High-dose methotrexate-based chemotherapy Radiotherapy Poor prognosis	-
Progressive multifocal leuko-encephalopathy CD4 count <100	Progressive decline in superior cerebral functions Visual defects Focal neurological deficits Seizures	CSF usually positive for JC (John Cunningham) virus *Imaging:* CECT—reduced density of white substance; no contrast enhancement or edema; MRI—increased T2 signal without gadolinium enhancement **(Fig. 5.11)** Brain biopsy	No specific treatment; ART	-
Cryptococcal meningitis— Most common cause of meningitis in AIDS CD4 count <200	Fever and headache Meningeal signs	LP—high opening pressure CSF—India ink stain **(Fig. 5.12)** Blood and CSF positive for cryptococcal antigen; Imaging: Features of raised ICT/ hydrocephalus	Induction: Liposomal amphotericin B 3–4 mg/kg IV Q24h + Flucytosine 25 mg/kg Q6h Consolidation: Fluconazole 400 mg Q24 h × 10 weeks Management of elevated CSF pressure: ➤ Therapeutic lumbar punctures ➤ VP shunt/lumbar drains	Secondary prophylaxis (maintenance therapy)—fluconazole 200 mg PO daily for at least 1 year and until the CD4 count exceeds 100 cells/µL for 3 months
Aseptic meningitis CD4 count > 200	Headache, neck stiffness, photophobia, nausea during primary HIV infection Self-limited illness that subsides spontaneously after several week	Moderate or no immunosuppression; moderate rise in CSF cell count HIV-1 RNA: detectable in blood and CSF HIV-1 p24 antigen might be detected in the blood HIV-1 conventional serology is still negative. Repeat serology testing after 6 weeks is usually positive Imaging is often normal	No specific treatment	-
CMV encephalitis CD4 <50	Behavioral disturbance, cognitive impairment, reduced level of consciousness, lethargy, cranial nerve palsies, nystagmus, myelitis, and polyradiculopathy	CSF PCR is positive CECT/MRI: Periventricular contrast enhancement	Ganciclovir 5 mg/kg IV Q24h Or Valganciclovir 900 mg Q12h Or Foscarnet 90 mg/kg IV Q12h Or Cidofovir 5 mg/kg IV once weekly Duration: Till CMV PCR is undetectable in CSF and serum	Secondary prophylaxis (maintenance therapy): Valganciclovir 900 mg Q24h. Discontinue once CD4 >100 for 6 months
CMV retinitis (*See* **Fig. 5.13**) Most common cause of blindness in AIDS patients with CD4 <50	Decreased visual acuity, floaters, flashing lights (photopsias), and blind spots (scotoma) Retinal hemorrhages with a whitish, granular appearance to the retina "Pizza pie" appearances/ "frosted branch angiitis" appearance	Vitreous fluid PCR for CMV	Immediate sight threatening lesions: Intravitreal ganciclovir (2 mg/ injection) or foscarnet (2.4 mg/ injection) 1–4 doses over 7–10 days + valganciclovir 900 mg Q12h × 14–21 days; then 900 mg Q24h Peripheral lesions: Valganciclovir 900 mg Q12h × 14–21 days; then 900 mg Q24h	Post-treatment suppression: (Secondary prophylaxis) Valganciclovir 900 mg Q24h. Discontinue once CD4 >100 for 6 months
HIV-associated neurocognitive disorders (HAND) Includes Asymptomatic neurocognitive impairment Mild neurocognitive disorder HIV-associated dementia (HIV encephalopathy) CD4 <200	Cognitive defects—Subcortical dementia Memory deficit, impaired executive function, poor attention and concentration Judgment is relatively intact Behavioral and mood changes Motor dysfunction—bradykinesia, loss of coordination and gait imbalance Clinical staging: **Frascati criteria**	Rise in HIV in the CSF; moderate rise in CSF cells and proteins CECT: Cortical or subcortical atrophy; MRI shows enhanced T2 signal	Intensify antiretroviral treatment	-

Contd...

Contd...

Other:

- Encephalitis:
  - Herpes zoster encephalitis
  - Varicella zoster encephalitis
- Focal lesion:
  - Brain abscess
  - Cryptococcoma
- Cerebrovascular disorders
  - Cerebral hemorrhage secondary to vasculitis/thrombocytopenia
  - Nonbacterial endocarditis
- Meningitis
  - Syphilitic
  - Herpes zoster
  - Acute and chronic lymphocytic meningitis
- Eye involvement
  - HIV retinopathy: Microangiopathy that causes cotton-wool spots
  - Varicella zoster virus: Rapidly progressive outer retinal necrosis
  - Herpes zoster: Ocular pain, conjunctival infection and corneal opacification
- Spinal cord
  - Vacuolar myelopathy (similar to subacute combined degeneration of cord)
  - Pure sensory ataxia—due to posterior column involvement
  - Herpes simplex or zoster myelitis
- Peripheral nerve and root
  - Acute inflammatory demyelinating polyradiculopathy—similar to Guillain–Barré (GB) syndrome
  - Distal sensory neuropathy—most common
  - Sensorimotor demyelinating polyneuropathy
  - CMV lumbar polyradiculopathy
  - Herpes zoster
  - Mononeuritis multiplex
  - Leprosy
- Neuromuscular junction and muscle
  - Myasthenia gravis
  - Polymyositis
  - Zidovudine induced myopathy—red ragged fiber on biopsy

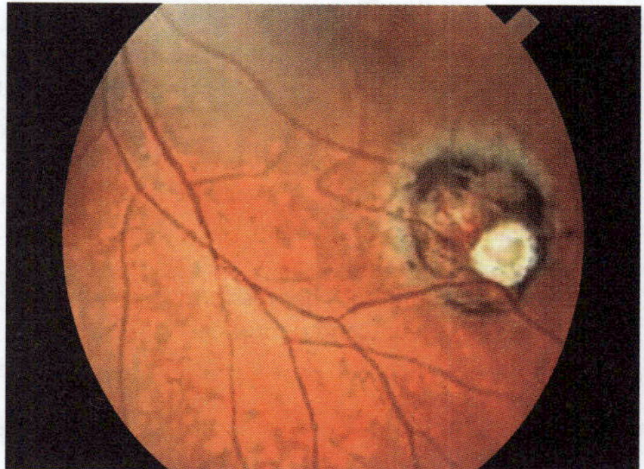

FIG. 5.9: Toxoplasma chorioretinitis.

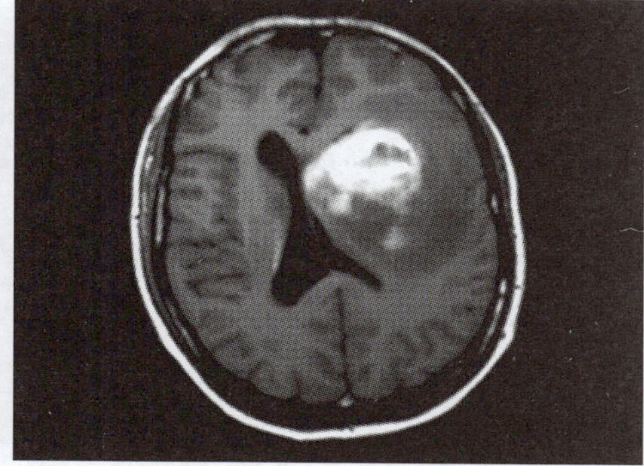

FIG. 5.10: MRI of cerebral toxoplasmosis.

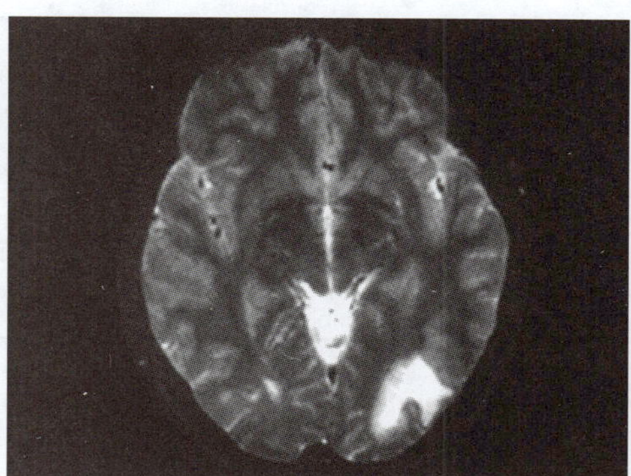

FIG. 5.11: MRI of progressive multifocal leukoencephalopathy (PMLE).

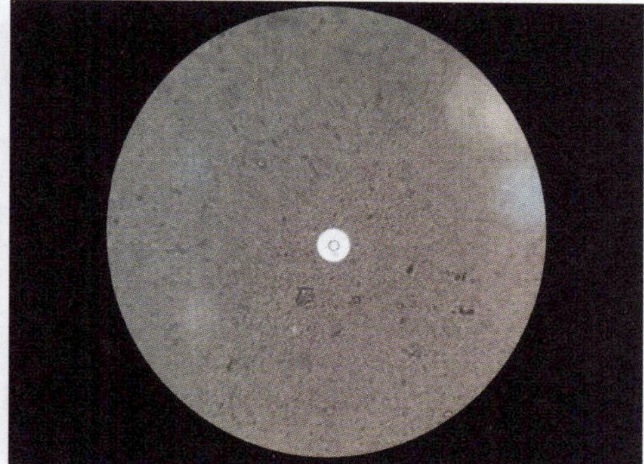

FIG. 5.12: CSF Indian ink showing *Cryptococcus*.

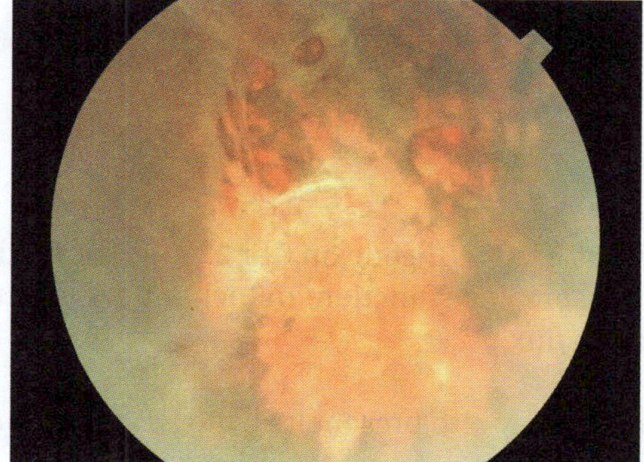

FIG. 5.13: Fundoscopic appearance of CMV retinitis.

CARDIOVASCULAR MANIFESTATIONS OF HIV (TABLE 5.13)

Q. Enumerate the cardiovascular manifestations seen in HIV/AIDS.

TABLE 5.13: Cardiovascular manifestations of HIV.

Disease	*Possible causes/Mechanism*	*Diagnosis*	*Treatment*
Accelerated atherosclerosis and coronary artery disease	Atherogenesis with virus-infected macrophages, Chronic inflammation Endothelial dysfunction Glucose intolerance Dyslipidemia—higher levels of triglycerides, lower levels of HDL cholesterol Protease inhibitors Smoking	ECG Stress testing echocardiography lipid profile CT angiography calcium scoring	Lifestyle modifications: Smoking cessation, low-fat diet and aerobic exercise Antiplatelet Statins Blood pressure control Percutaneous coronary intervention Coronary artery bypass surgery
Cardiomyopathy	HIV-induced cardiomyopathy: Biopsy shows some features of myocarditis Side effects of IFN-α or nucleoside analogue therapy Kaposi sarcoma, cryptococcosis, Chagas disease, and toxoplasmosis	Echocardiogram	Treat the cause: IVIG for HIV-induced cardiomyopathy Stopping IFN-α or nucleoside analog therapy Diuretics, ACE inhibitors, and beta blockers
Primary pulmonary hypertension	Plexogenic pulmonary arteriopathy	ECG, echocardiography, right-heart catheterization	Anticoagulation, vasodilators, prostacyclin analogs Endothelin antagonists PDE-5 inhibitors
Pericardial effusion	Bacteria: *Mycobacterium*, *Staphylococcus*, *Streptococcus*, *Proteus*, *Klebsiella*, *Enterococcus*, *Listeria*, *Nocardia*, viral pathogens: HIV, HSV, CMV, and adenovirus, echovirus Other pathogens: *Cryptococcus*, Toxoplasma, and Histoplasma Malignancy: Kaposi sarcoma and lymphoma Hypothyroidism Immunodeficiency Uremia	Pericardial rub on examination Echocardiography Fluid analysis for Gram-stain, culture, and cytology ECG—low voltage/PR depression Associated pleural and peritoneal fluid analysis Pericardial biopsy	Treat the cause Intensify antiretroviral therapy Pericardiocentesis
Infective endocarditis	Autoimmune Bacteria: *Staphylococcus aureus* or *Staphylococcus epidermidis*, *Streptococcus*, HACEK organisms Fungal: *Aspergillus fumigatus*, *Candida*, and *Cryptococcus neoformans*	Blood cultures and echocardiography	Intravenous antibiotics and valve replacements
Malignancy	Kaposi sarcoma, non-Hodgkin lymphoma, and leiomyosarcoma	Echocardiography and biopsy	Chemotherapy

Others:

- LV systolic dysfunction
- LV diastolic dysfunction
- RV dysfunction
- Nonbacterial thrombotic endocarditis
- Vasculitis
- Autonomic dysfunction
- Arrhythmias: Pentamidine (for PCP) and electrolyte abnormalities
- Cardiovascular collapse and hypotension: Rapid IV administration of pentamidine
- Lipodystrophy: Protease inhibitors

DISEASES OF KIDNEY AND GENITOURINARY SYSTEM IN HIV

Q. Write a short note on HIVAN.

HIV-associated nephropathy

- Classic glomerulopathy of HIV
- Etiopathogenesis:
  - Infection of kidney epithelial cells by HIV and the expression of HIV genes within infected kidney cells
    - Higher viral loads, lower CD4 count—favor infection
    - HIV genes, especially Nef and Vpr are specifically involved
  - Host factors
    - Africans > Europeans, Asians
    - Single nucleotide polymorphisms in *APOL1* gene on Chr 22 → associated with increased risk
    - Proposed mechanism: Endolysosomal dysfunction, mitochondrial dysfunction, and activation of stress kinases due to altered transcellular cation flux
  - Clinical features:
    - Advanced HIV infection—usually; may also present in acute HIV infection
    - Proteinuria—usually nephrotic range
    - Edema

- Rapid decline in renal function
- Hematuria and hypertension may also be seen
- Diagnosis:
  - Urinalysis, including quantification of proteinuria
  - Urea, creatinine, electrolytes, and random blood sugar (RBS)
  - USG abdomen—**increased kidney size**, increased echogenicity
  - Kidney biopsy
    - Pathology:
      - Characterized by the collapsing form of FSGS
      - Light microscopy →
        - Glomeruli: Proliferation and dysregulation of podocytes, glomerular collapse, and pseudocrescent formation
        - Dilated tubules
        - Interstitial inflammation
      - Electron microscopy: Tubuloreticular inclusions

Treatment:
- ART
- ACE-inhibitor/ARB for proteinuria
- Routine CKD care—Target BP: 130/80, management of anemia, mineral-bone disease, avoiding nephrotoxic drug, hemodialysis, and renal transplant
- Renal transplant—Risk of recurrence of HIVAN present

Other renal and genitourinary manifestations in patients with HIV (Tables 5.14 and 5.15):

TABLE 5.14: Kidney diseases associated with HIV/AIDS or its treatment.

	Entity	*Comments*
Glomerular	HIV-associated nephropathy (HIVAN)	See above for detailed discussion
	HIV-associated immune complex kidney disease (HIVICK)	HIVICK can present with various forms, such as post-infectious glomerulonephritis, membranous nephropathy, and a lupus-like pattern.
	Thrombotic microangiopathy	Lower CD4 cell counts, higher viral burden, and AIDS
	Membranoproliferative glomerulonephritis, with or without cryoglobulin-associated vasculitis	Associated with hepatitis C; enfuvirtide
	Membranous nephropathy	Associated with hepatitis B
Tubular	Acute kidney injury	Aminoglycosides, cidofovir, and foscarnet
	Proximal tubule injury (Fanconi syndrome)	Tenofovir disoproxil fumarate, adefovir, cidofovir, and didanosine
	Diabetes insipidus	Amphotericin, tenofovir disoproxil fumarate, didanosine, and abacavir
	Chronic tubular injury	Amphotericin, cidofovir, adefovir, and tenofovir disoproxil fumarate
	Crystal nephropathy	Indinavir, atazanavir, sulfadiazine, ciprofloxacin, and intravenous acyclovir
Interstitial	Interstitial nephritis	Allergy to β-lactam, sulfa drugs, ciprofloxacin, and rifampicin May be associated with immune reconstitution inflammatory syndrome

Other:
TMP-SMX may compete for tubular secretion with creatinine, leading to an increase in the serum creatinine level

TABLE 5.15: Genitourinary manifestations, including sexually transmitted infections.

Condition	*Clinical features*	*Diagnosis*	*Treatment*
Syphilis	Condylomata lata (secondary syphilis)—most common presentation Atypical presentation in HIV: "Lues maligna": ulcerating lesion of the skin due to a necrotizing vasculitis Unexplained fever Nephrotic syndrome Neurosyphilis—asymptomatic/acute meningitis/ neuroretinitis/deafness/stroke	Dark-field examination of appropriate specimens Note: VDRL test ➢ May be false-positive due to polyclonal B cell activation ➢ Development of a new positive VDRL may be delayed in patients with new infections Anti-FTA (anti-fluorescent treponemal antibody) test: May be negative due to immunodeficiency	Benzathine penicillin G Similar to that in HIV-negative patients Patients may develop Jarisch–Herxheimer reaction on initiation of therapy
Vulvovaginal candidiasis	Vulvulus infection: Morbilliform rash that may extend to the thighs, pruritus Vaginal infection: White discharge, plaques, and erythematous vaginal wall Dyspareunia and dysuria	10% KOH mount: pseudohyphal elements	Mild disease: Topical therapy Mod-severe disease: Fluconazole 150 mg OD Q72 hours × two to three doses
HSV	See "mucocutaneous manifestations"		

Other:
- Genitourinary tract infections: Similar to non-HIV/AIDS patients
- Vaginitis:
  - Trichomonas
  - Mixed bacteria

HEMATOLOGICAL MANIFESTATIONS OF HIV

Q. List the hematological manifestations of HIV.

- Hematological manifestations in patients with HIV include
  - **Anemia (Table 5.16)**
  - **Leukopenia**
    - Causes:
      - Decrease in endogenous granulocytic colony-stimulating factor
      - Medications: Zidovudine, TMP-SMX, and ganciclovir

Management
- ART
- Stop offending agents
- G-CSF and GM-CSF: In patients who have profound neutropenia despite removal of the offending agent

  - **Thrombocytopenia**
    - Any stage of HIV infection; however, it is more commonly seen with advanced disease
    - Mechanisms:
      - Immune thrombocytopenia: Development of cross-reactive antibodies between the HIV envelope glycoprotein gp120 and the platelet glycoprotein IIb/IIIa; seen in early-stage HIV
      - Direct infection of megakaryocytes: In late-stage HIV
      - Drug-induced immune thrombocytopenia: TMP-SMX, and rifampicin
      - HCV infection: Due to direct effects on platelet production or hypersplenism

Management
- Virologic suppression with ART
- For those individuals who do not respond to this, corticosteroids, IVIG, or anti-D immune globulin (Rh-positive patient who has not undergone splenectomy) have been used.
- Surgical splenectomy and splenic irradiation—for refractory cases
- Eltrombopag and romiplostim—recently being tried for refractory HIV-related thrombocytopenia

  - **Thrombotic microangiopathy (Table 5.16)**

TABLE 5.16: Causes of anemia in patients with HIV.

Etiology	*Evaluation*	*Treatment*
Uncontrolled HIV infection	HIV viral load	Antiretroviral therapy
Nutritional	B_{12}, folate, iron studies	Supplementation
	Iron deficiency: Endoscopy	Treatment of underlying condition
Medication related	Zidovudine, TMP-SMX, chemotherapy Hemolysis: Dapsone, primaquine, ribavirin	Change medication where possible Support with erythropoiesis-stimulating agents
Chronic inflammation	Exclude other causes Serum iron: reduced Ferritin: Elevated TIBC: Reduced	Erythropoiesis-stimulating agents
Hemolytic anemia 1. Autoimmune 2. Medication-related	LDH, reticulocyte count, haptoglobin, indirect bilirubin Coombs test Dapsone, primaquine (G6PD deficiency)	Corticosteroids for autoimmune hemolytic anemia Discontinue dapsone, primaquine Reduce ribavirin dose
Thrombotic microangiopathy ➢ Thrombotic thrombocytopenic purpura and atypical hemolytic uremic syndrome	Fever, thrombocytopenia, hemolytic anemia, neurologic abnormalities, renal abnormalities Peripheral smear for schistocytes ADAMTS13 level	Plasmapheresis for TTP Eculizumab for atypical HUS
Parvovirus B19	Parvovirus B19 PCR Bone marrow biopsy (pronormoblasts)	Intravenous immune globulin
Bone marrow infiltration	Histoplasma urine/blood antigen Blood culture for MAC LDH for lymphoma Bone marrow biopsy if noninvasive tests are unrevealing	Treatment of underlying etiology

AIDS AND MALIGNANCY

Q. Discuss common cancers in HIV/AIDS (Table 5.17).

TABLE 5.17: Cancers in HIV.

Cancer	Etiology	Clinical features	Investigation	Management
AIDS-defining cancers				
Kaposi's sarcoma	Kaposi sarcoma associated herpes virus (HHV-8)	Skin—Macules, papules, or nodules of purple to dark blue color; Edema and ulcers are possible Pulmonary Kaposi sarcoma—dyspnea, cough, hemoptysis, bilateral lower lobe infiltrates on chest X-ray, pleural effusion Other organs involved—Lymph nodes, GI tract, biliary tract	Clinical Biopsy, if diagnosis uncertain: Proliferation of spindle cells and endothelial cells, extravasation of RBCs, hemosiderin-laden macrophages	ART Cutaneous lesions: ➢ Radiation, ➢ Cryotherapy or ➢ Intralesional vinblastine Extensive disease: ➢ Initial therapy ➢ Interferon α ($CD4^+$ count >150/μL) ➢ Liposomal daunorubicin ➢ Subsequent therapy ➢ Liposomal doxorubicin ➢ Paclitaxel Combination chemotherapy with low-dose doxorubicin, bleomycin, and vinblastine (ABV) Targeted radiation
Non-Hodgkin's lymphoma	EBV	B-type symptoms: Fever, night sweats, or weight loss Lymphadenopathy Extranodal disease—in up to 80% CNS is the most common extranodal site: Headache, cranial nerve palsy, seizures Other sites: GI tract: Dysphagia, abdominal pain Bone marrow: Pancytopenia Lung: Mass lesion, multiple nodules, or an interstitial infiltrate Involvement of liver	MRI or CECT brain: Limited number (one to three) of 3- to 5-cm contrast-enhancing lesions, leptomeningeal enhancement CSF analysis: for staging CT or MRI of the chest/abdomen Biopsy	Combination chemotherapy Palliative radiation therapy
Invasive cervical cancer	HPV Tobacco	Per vaginal bleeding Postcoital spotting Cervical ulceration Bladder and rectal dysfunction, pain, and fistula	Biopsy	Surgery/radiation therapy + chemotherapy
Non-AIDS-defining cancers: ➢ Oral cavity and pharyngeal cancer ➢ Lung cancer ➢ Hepatocellular carcinoma—associated with HBV and HCV ➢ Anal cancer ➢ Penile cancer ➢ Vulval cancer ➢ Multiple myeloma ➢ Leukemia ➢ Melanoma			**NOTE: Lymphoproliferative disorders strongly associated with HIV** ➢ Diffuse large B cell lymphoma—most common lymphoma in patients with HIV; may have CNS involvement ➢ Burkitt's lymphoma ➢ Primary CNS lymphoma ➢ Primary effusion lymphoma ➢ Plasmablastic lymphoma ➢ KSHV(HHV-8) associated multicentric Castleman disease ➢ Classic Hodgkin's lymphoma	

INVESTIGATIONS IN PATIENTS WITH HIV/AIDS

Q. Write short note on laboratory tests for the diagnosis HIV infection.

Indications for Testing

- Symptoms of HIV infection
- Possible HIV exposure
- Individuals who seek screening/treatment for sexually transmitted infections
- Patients with tuberculosis and hepatitis B/C
- Patients who are considering pre-exposure antiretroviral prophylaxis as an HIV prevention strategy
- High-risk groups
  - MSM
  - Commercial sex workers
  - Injection-drug users
  - Sex partners of persons who are HIV-infected, bisexual, or inject drugs
- Routine screening in pregnant women
- In areas of high and extremely high prevalence: All patients not previously diagnosed with HIV who register with a general practice or undergo blood testing for any reason.

Goals of Testing

1. Confirmation of the diagnosis
2. Assess degree of immunosuppression
3. To prepare for treatment
4. To evaluate for coinfections and prior exposures
5. To monitor response to treatment and evaluate for side effects
6. Screening/preventive care

Confirmation of Diagnosis (Fig. 5.14)

- CDC 2014 recommends a three-3 step algorithm for diagnosis of HIV involving two immunoassays and a confirmatory nucleic acid amplification test
- Step 1: Screen with fourth generation **HIV-1/HIV-2/p24 antigen-antibody combination assay**.
  - If negative: Chances of an established HIV-1 or HIV-2 infection are low. No further testing is required.
  - If positive, proceed to step 2
- Step 2: Test the samples with **HIV-1/HIV-2 antibody differentiation assay**
  - If HIV-1 reactive and HIV-2 nonreactive: HIV-1 antibodies detected
  - If HIV-1 nonreactive and HIV-2 reactive: HIV-2 antibodies detected
  - If HIV-1 reactive and HIV-2 reactive: HIV antibodies detected
  - If HIV-1 nonreactive or indeterminate and HIV-2 nonreactive: proceed to step 3
- Step 3: Specimens with screening test positive and negative/indeterminate test on HIV-1/HIV-2 antibody differentiation assay test should be confirmed by **HIV-1 nucleic acid amplification test (NAAT). (HIV-1-RNA testing)**
  - If HIV-1 NAT is positive: Acute HIV-1 infection
  - If HIV-1 NAT is negative: Negative for HIV-1 infection
- Inconsistent or conflicting results should be investigated with follow-up testing on a newly collected specimen
- **Note: Western blot no longer recommended as a confirmatory diagnostic test by CDC**
- **Note: Alternate algorithm, used in some centers, but not recommended by CDC:**
- Step 1: Screening test with HIV-1/2 enzyme immunoassay (EIA) (third-generation assay)
  - If nonreactive: HIV-negative; retest after 3–6 months if clinically indicated
  - If reactive, proceed to step 2

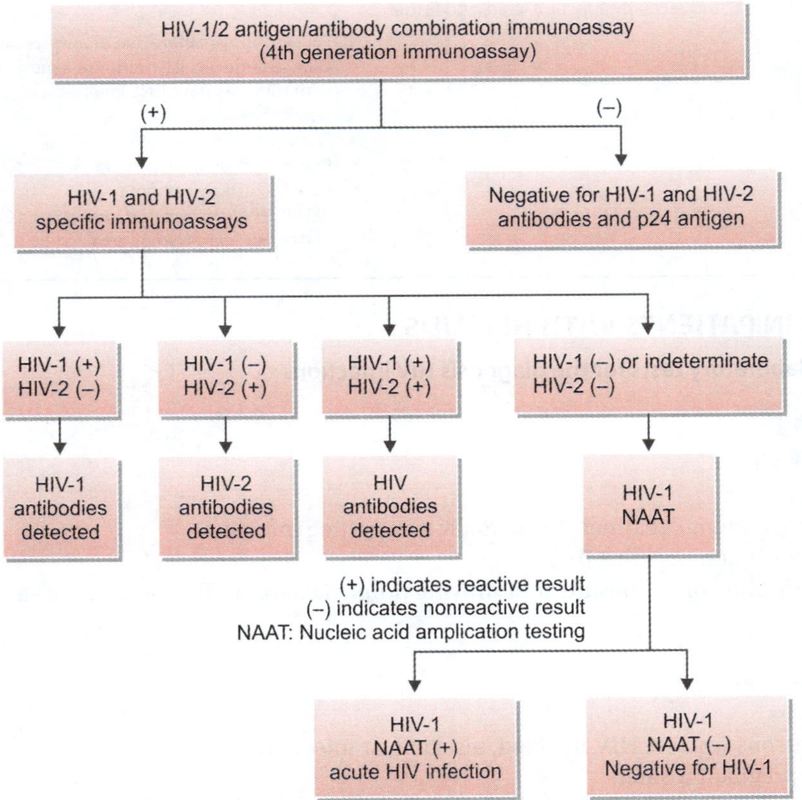

FIG. 5.14: Recommended laboratory HIV testing algorithm.

- Step 2: HIV-1 Western blot
  - If positive, report as HIV-1 positive
  - If inconclusive or nonreactive, proceed to step 3
- Step 3: HIV-2 enzyme immunoassay
  - If Western blot nonreactive and HIV-2 EIA nonreactive: HIV-negative
  - If Western blot inconclusive and HIV-2 EIA nonreactive: Inconclusive and request follow-up specimen after 4–6 weeks
  - If HIV-2 EIA reactive: proceed to step 4
- Step 4: HIV-2 supplemental test
  - If supplemental test is inconclusive or negative: Follow-up specimen
  - If supplemental test is positive: HIV-2 positive

Sequence of appearance of laboratory markers of HIV-1 infection (Table 5.18 and Fig. 5.15)

TABLE 5.18: Sequence of appearance of laboratory markers of HIV-1 infection.

Test	*Target of detection*	*Approximate time to positivity (days)*
Enzyme-linked immunoassay		
First generation	IgG antibody	35–45
Second generation	IgG antibody	25–35
Third generation	IgM and IgG antibody	20–30
Fourth generation	IgM and IgG antibody and p24 antigen	15–20
Western blot		
Western blot	IgM and IgG antibody	35–50 (indeterminate)
		45–60 (positive)
HIV viral load test		
Sensitivity cutoff 50 copies/mL	RNA	10–15
Ultrasensitive cutoff 1–5 copies/mL	RNA	5

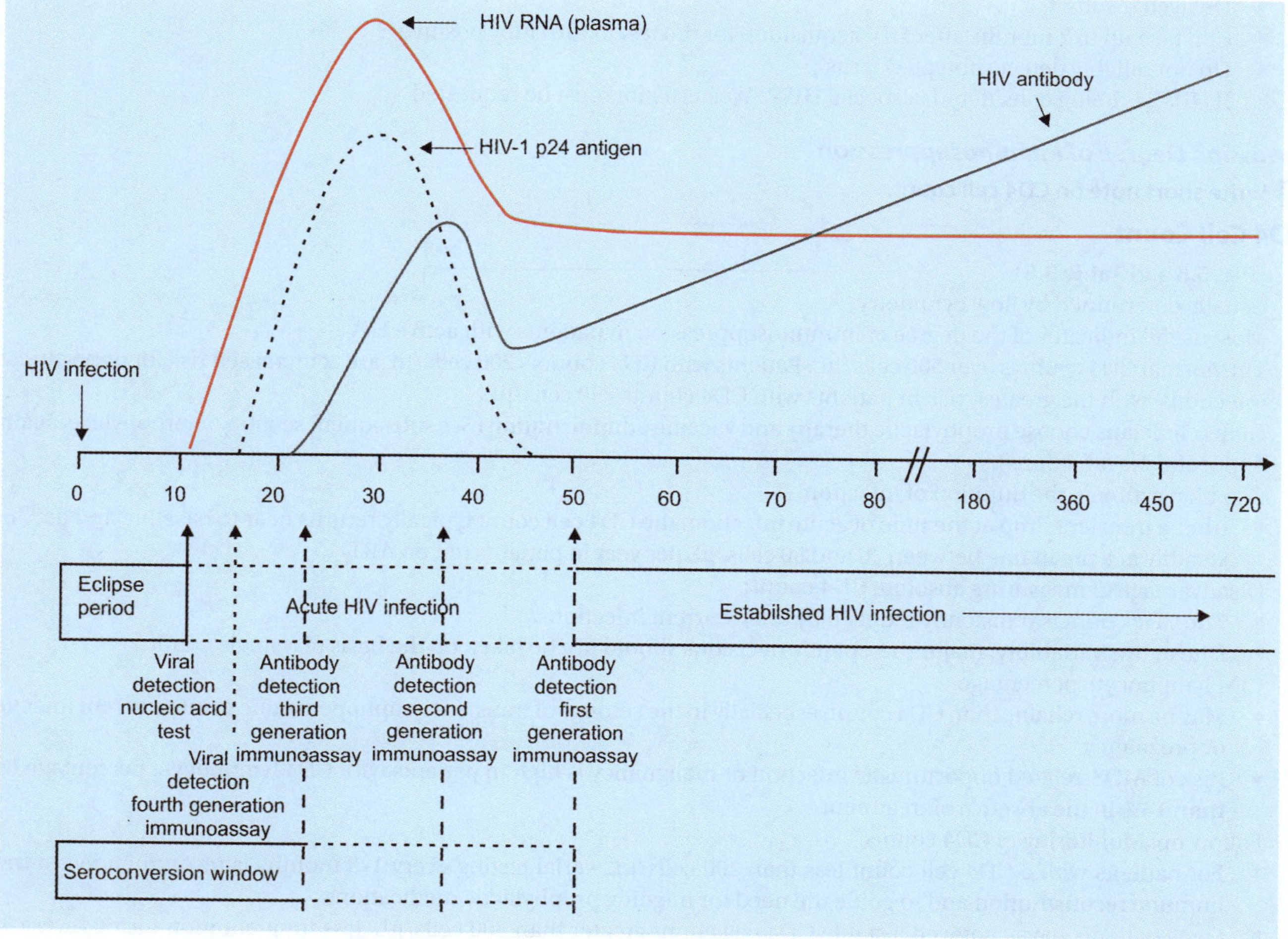

FIG. 5.15: Sequence of appearance of laboratory markers of HIV-1 infection.

Q. Write short note on Western blot testing in HIV.

Western blot (Fig. 5.16)

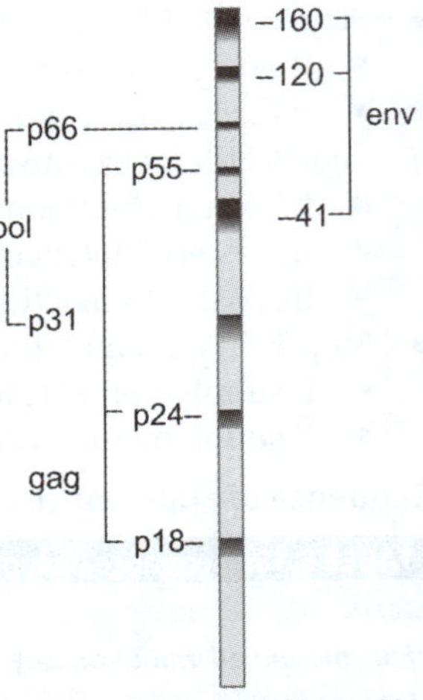

FIG. 5.16: Positive HIV-1 Western blot.

- Previously used confirmatory test
- Procedure:
  - Virions are electrophoresed in a polyacrylamide gel
  - The antigens get separated on the basis of molecular weight
  - This is then transferred onto nitrocellulose and then incubated with patient's serum
  - Antibodies to each component can be detected as discrete bands on the Western blot
- Results:
  - Negative Western blot: No bands are present at molecular weights corresponding to HIV gene products
  - Positive Western blot: If antibodies exist to two of the three HIV proteins, i.e., p24, gp41, and gp120/160
  - Indeterminate: If the results do not fall into the positive or negative categories. May be due to:

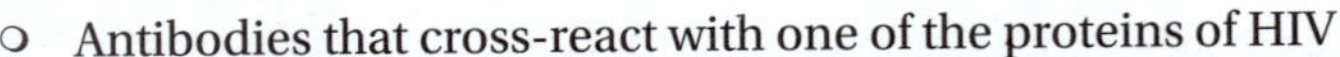

    - Antibodies that cross-react with one of the proteins of HIV
    - Individual is infected with HIV and is in the process of developing an antibody response
    - In both scenarios, the Western blot should be repeated after 1 month to determine if the indeterminate pattern is a pattern in evolution
- Time to positivity:
  - 35–50 days—indeterminate
  - 45–60 days—positive
- Disadvantages:
  - High cost
  - Delayed results
  - Can take up to 2 months after HIV acquisition for the test to turn fully positive
  - Do not reliably detect subtype O virus
  - If HIV-2 is being considered, a special HIV-2 Western blot must be requested

Assessing Degree of Immunosuppression

Q. Write short note on CD4 cell count.

CD4 Cell Count

(*See* **Fig. 5.5** and **Table 5.6**)

- Usually determined by flow cytometry
- Most useful indicator of the degree of immunosuppression in patients with active HIV
- The normal CD4 count is over 500 cells/μL. Patients with CD4 counts <200 cells/μL are at increased risk for opportunistic infections, with the greatest risk in patients with CD4 counts <50 cells/μL.
- Helps clinicians choose prophylactic therapy and vaccine administration (*See* subsequent section on prophylaxis against opportunistic infections).
- Can help estimate the duration of infection:
  - After a transient drop at the time of acute infection, the CD4 cell count typically returns near to baseline and declines steadily at a mean rate between 20 and 50 cells/μL per year in patients not on ART.
- Disadvantage of measuring absolute CD4 count:
  - The CD4 count is transiently reduced by inter-current infections.
  - Due to this variability, major therapeutic decisions should not be taken on the basis of a single count.
- CD4 lymphocyte percentage:
  - May be more reliable than CD4 count, especially in the settings of transient lymphopenia due to intercurrent infection or pregnancy.
  - Risk of AIDS-related opportunistic infection or malignancy is high in patients with CD4 lymphocyte percentage **less than 14%** in the absence of treatment.
- Follow up: Monitoring of CD4 counts
  - For patients with a CD4 cell count less than 200 cells/μL, serial testing every 1–3 months is recommended to track immune reconstitution and to guide the need for ongoing prophylactic medications
  - Once patients have achieved a stable CD4 cell count greater than 300 cells/μL, less frequent monitoring (every 3–6 months) is done. (Note: Some do not recommend routine monitoring)
  - Mild variation in the CD4 cell count does not warrant changes in ART as long viral suppression is maintained.

To Prepare for Treatment

- To characterize the health status of the patient—"safety laboratory tests"
  - Complete blood count: May show anemia, leukopenia, and/or thrombocytopenia
  - Urea, creatinine, electrolytes, and urinalysis: Presence of chronic kidney disease or proteinuria alters the choice of ART. Renal function must be monitored while on therapy, especially for patients on regimens that include tenofovir disoproxil fumarate (TDF) or tenofovir alafenamide (TAF)
  - Liver function tests: May be deranged in viral hepatitis coinfection. LFTs should be monitored on therapy to look for drug-induced liver injury
  - Pregnancy testing: Pregnancy may alter the choice of ART
- Human immunodeficiency virus resistance testing:
  - Timing:
    - At the time of diagnosis
    - When changing antiretroviral regimens
    - When patient has suboptimal viral response
  - Genotypic resistance testing is preferred over phenotypic resistance testing
  - Standard genotypic resistance testing involves testing for mutations in reverse transcriptase and protease genes
  - Resistance testing for integrase inhibitors (integrase strand transfer inhibitor, INSTI) is only recommended if INSTI resistance is a concern
  - Testing may not be successful in patients with HIV RNA levels <500–1,000 copies/mL
  - ART initiation should not be delayed while awaiting resistance testing results in patients with acute or recent HIV infection or pregnancy
- **HLA B*5701**: Presence is associated with a high risk for hypersensitivity to **abacavir**
- Glucose-6-phosphate dehydrogenase deficiency: Before starting the patient on dapsone, primaquine, or sulfonamides
- CCR5/CXCR4 tropism assay: For patients who are being considered for treatment with maraviroc (not routinely used)

To Evaluate for Coinfections and Prior Exposures

- Testing for sexually transmitted infections:
  - Nucleic acid amplification tests from vaginal and cervical swabs—for gonorrhea and chlamydia
  - VDRL/RPR, followed by confirmatory treponemal test—syphilis
- Hepatitis B and C testing
- Testing for latent TB: Tuberculin skin test (TST) or interferon-γ release assay (IGRA)
- Toxoplasma IgG: Seropositive patients are at risk of reactivation disease if severely immunosuppressed (CD4 counts <100), and need primary prophylaxis until they respond to ART
- *Cryptococcus* antigen if CD4 ≤100 cells/μL
- Other investigations: As per clinical presentation

To Monitor Response to Treatment and Evaluate for Side Effects

- **Viral load:**
  - Pretreatment viral load = patient's "baseline."
  - Viral load declines rapidly after initiation of ART
  - Repeat a viral load 4–6 weeks after initiation of therapy and then every 1–3 months until viral suppression is achieved
  - Once patients are stable on therapy, the viral load should be monitored every 6 months, or more frequently after any change in regimen
- **CD 4 count**: *See* section on CD4 counts.
- **Safety laboratory tests:**
  - All patients should be monitored with complete blood count, RFT and electrolytes, and LFTs to track abnormalities due to HIV infection and assess for medication side effects
  - About 4–6 weeks after treatment initiation or change in ART
  - Every 6 months, if stable on therapy
  - Urinalysis should also be obtained for patients on tenofovir-based therapy

Screening/Preventive Care

- Cervical cancer screening:
  - Rationale: Risk of abnormal cervical cytology secondary to human papilloma virus (HPV) infection is 10 times higher in HIV-infected women as compared to the general population
  - Timing: Cervical pap smears every 1–3 years. More intensive follow-up if abnormal results are identified

- Anal cancer screening:
  - Rationale: HIV-infected individuals who practice receptive anal intercourse are at increased risk for HPV-related anal dysplasia
  - Timing: Anal pap smears every 1–3 years
- HbA1c:
  - Rationale: Increased prevalence of diabetes in patients with HIV.
  - Timing: At entry to care and repeated yearly in patients at high risk for diabetes
- Lipid panel:
  - Rationale: Cardiovascular disease is now becoming the leading cause of morbidity and mortality, due to increased inflammation and immune activation
  - Timing: At entry to care and repeated yearly
- Bone density (DEXA) scan:
  - Rationale: HIV and its treatment (especially tenofovir-containing regimens) reduce bone density
  - Timing: All patients should undergo evaluation of bone density at age 50 years.

MANAGEMENT OF A PATIENTS WITH HIV/AIDS

Q. List indications for starting antiretroviral therapy.

Indications of Antiretroviral therapy

Treatment is recommended for all HIV-positive patients irrespective of the CD4 count

- Conditions favoring early initiation of therapy:
  - Acute or recent HIV infection
  - AIDS-defining conditions
  - Pregnancy
  - HIV-associated nephropathy
  - Lower CD4 counts (<200 cells/μL)
  - CD4 decline >100 cells/μL/year
  - HIV RNA >100,000 copies/mL
  - Hepatitis B coinfection and hepatitis C coinfection
- In patients with an AIDS-defining condition or an opportunistic infection: ART should be initiated within 2 weeks of starting treatment for intercurrent conditions.
  - Exceptions:
    - Cryptococcal meningitis: ART should be initiated 5 weeks after starting treatment for cryptococcal infection, as earlier initiation increases the risk of death
    - Tuberculosis: ART should be initiated 2–8 weeks after starting ATTs (except if the CD4 count is < 50 cells/μL). This is because earlier initiation increases the risk of IRIS. See section on HIV-TB co-infection.

Advantages of initiating antiretroviral therapy:

- Reduction in overall mortality
- Reduction in cardiovascular and renal morbidity
- Decreased risk of opportunistic infections and malignancies
- Decreased risk of transmitting HIV to others

Principles of antiretroviral therapy:

- **Goals of treatment**: Reduction of plasma viral load to **less than 50 copies/mL.**
  - Other goals:
    - Improve the CD4 count to over 200 cells/L
    - Improve the quantity and quality of life
    - Reduce transmission of HIV
- **"Hit hard and hit early"** approach: All patients should be treated with combination of preferably three antiretroviral drugs as soon as possible.
- **"First chance = Best chance"**:
  - The choice of medications during the first treatment course determines remaining options when a different treatment regimen becomes necessary.
  - Chances for success are better initially; later on, alternatives are limited by development of resistant mutants.
- Use of fixed dose combinations: Antiretroviral therapy is complex because of various drug interactions and adverse effects. Hence, initial therapy with **single pill fixed-dose combinations** has become the standard of care.

- **Antiretroviral resistance**:
  - HIV resistance occurs due to the high rate of HIV replication, as well as the error-prone nature of antiretroviral drugs
  - Antiretroviral drugs differ in their ability to select for resistant mutations.
  - Some drugs (e.g., emtricitabine, lamivudine, and efavirenz) have a low genetic barrier to resistance, rapidly selecting for a single mutation conferring high-level resistance.
  - On the other hand, drugs, such as PIs and some NRTIs (e.g., zidovudine) select for resistance mutations slowly, and multiple resistant mutations often need to accumulate before the drug's efficacy is lost.
- **Treatment adherence** is key.
  - Current antiretroviral regimens do not eradicate HIV
  - Viral rebound occurs rapidly after treatment discontinuation, followed by CD4 decline, with potential for disease progression
- Therapy should be **regularly monitored**.

Categories of anti-retroviral drugs (Table 5.19)

Q. Discuss and describe the principles of cART, the classes of antiretrovirals used, adverse reactions and interactions.

Q. Write a note on integrase inhibitors.

Q. Write a note on protease inhibitors.

Q. Write a note on HIV entry inhibitors.

Q. Write a note on ibalizumab.

TABLE 5.19: Important antiretroviral therapy agents (alphabetical order within class).

Medication and adult dose (normal renal function)	***Common side effects***	***Comments***
Nucleoside reverse transcriptase inhibitors (NRTIs): Mechanism: Competitive inhibition of HIV-1 reverse transcriptase (*See* **Fig. 5.17**) Need to be phosphorylated intracellularly for activity to occur		
Abacavir 300 mg PO BID	Fever and rash	HLA B*5701 testing prior to initiation May be used in pregnancy Avoid alcohol Avoid abacavir in patients with/at risk for cardiovascular disease
Didanosine 400 mg PO OD	Peripheral neuropathy, pancreatitis and hepatitis	Bimonthly neurologic questionnaire for neuropathy, potassium, bilirubin, amylase, and triglycerides should be done Avoid concurrent use of stavudine, zalcitabine, isoniazid, ribavirin, or allopurinol
Emtricitabine 200 mg PO OD	Skin discoloration in palms/soles Hepatotoxicity in HBV-co-infected patients who discontinue drug	Avoid concurrent lamivudine
Lamivudine 150 mg PO BID or 300 mg PO OD	Rash and peripheral neuropathy Flare of hepatitis in HBV-coinfected patients who discontinue drug	Do not administer with emtricitabine or zalcitabine
Stavudine 40 mg PO BID	Peripheral neuropathy, pancreatitis, hepatitis, lipoatrophy, rapidly progressive ascending neuromuscular weakness (rare)	Monthly neurologic questionnaire for neuropathy, amylase should be done Avoid zidovudine, didanosine, zalcitabine, and isoniazid
Zidovudine (AZT) 300 mg PO BID	Anemia, neutropenia, nausea, headache, lactic acidosis, hepatic steatosis, myopathy (red ragged fibers), nail pigmentation, lipoatrophy, and hyperglycemia	CBC should be done 4–8 weeks after starting AZT Monitor RBS and LFTs
Others: ➢ Zalcitabine		
Nucleotide reverse transcriptase inhibitors (NRTI): Mechanism: Competitive inhibition of HIV-1 reverse transcriptase **(Fig. 5.17)** Need to be phosphorylated intracellularly for activity to occur		
Tenofovir disoproxil fumarate (TDF) 300 mg PO OD	Renal dysfunction, proteinuria, glycosuria (Fanconi syndrome), hypophosphatemia, and bone resorption Flare of hepatitis in HBV-coinfected patients who discontinue drug	Monitor: Creatinine at baseline, at 2–8 weeks, every 3–6 months; urinalysis and urine glucose and protein at baseline and repeated as clinically indicated; consider bone densitometry Avoid atazanavir, didanosine, and probenecid

Contd...

Contd...

Tenofovir alafenamide (TAF) 25 mg PO OD	Nephrotoxicity (less than TDF) Osteoporosis Hepatoxicity Flare of hepatitis in HBV-coinfected patients who discontinue drug	Often combined with emtricitabine 200 mg PO OD Avoid in severe renal insufficiency Avoid inducers of p-glycoprotein (rifampicin, rifabutin, phenytoin, and phenobarbital) Monitor: Creatinine at baseline, at 2–8 weeks, then every 3–6 months; Urinalysis and urine glucose and protein at baseline and repeated as clinically indicated HBsAg, liver enzymes at baseline at 2–8 weeks, every 3–6 months, continue for months after discontinuation Bone densitometry—patients > 50 years of age
Non-nucleoside reverse transcriptase inhibitors (NNRTIs): Mechanism: Noncompetitive inhibitors of reverse transcriptase **(Fig. 5.17)**		
Efavirenz 600 mg OD at night	Rash Deranged LFTs and lipid profile Drowsiness Psychiatric manifestations: Abnormal dreams, depression, and dysphoria	Avoid elvitegravir/cobicistat, etravirine, and indinavir
Nevirapine 200 mg PO OD × 2 weeks, then 200 mg PO BID or 400 mg extended-release OD	Rash, Hepatotoxicity	Contraindicated with moderate or severe hepatic impairment Avoid atazanavir, dolutegravir, and elvitegravir/cobicistat
Others: ➢ Etravirine ➢ Rilpivirine		
Protease inhibitors (PIs): Mechanism: Bind to HIV proteases. This blocks the proteolytic activities of the enzyme, resulting in the inability to form mature, and infectious virions **(Fig. 5.17)**		
Atazanavir 400 mg PO OD Alternate—see comments	PR prolongation Transaminase elevations Nausea and vomiting Hyperglycemia Renal stones	Atazanavir/ritonavir: Atazanavir 300 mg with ritonavir 100 mg OD (given with efavirenz) Atazanavir/cobicistat: Atazanavir 300 mg with cobicistat 150 mg PO OD Avoid in severe hepatic insufficiency
Darunavir Dose—see comments	Diarrhea Headache Skin rash Hepatotoxicity Hyperlipidemia Hyperglycemia	Avoid in patients with sulfa allergy Darunavir/cobicistat: Darunavir 800 mg and cobicistat 150 mg PO OD Darunavir/ritonavir: **For PI-naïve patients:** Darunavir 800 mg and ritonavir 100 mg PO OD **PI-experienced patients:** Darunavir 600 mg and ritonavir 100 mg PO BID
Indinavir 800 mg PO TID	Abdominal pain Nausea Hyperbilirubinemia Fan shaped/Star-burst renal calculi	Avoid efavirenz and etravirine
Lopinavir/ritonavir 400 mg/100 mg PO BD	Skin rash Dyslipidemia Hyperglycemia Elevated transaminases Diarrhea Fatigue	Separate dosing from didanosine by 1 hour Avoid darunavir and elvitegravir/cobicistat Avoid disulfiram and metronidazole with oral solution
Ritonavir 600 mg PO BD or In lower doses for boosting other PIs (e.g., 100 mg PO OD or BD)	Abdominal pain Hyperglycemia Fat redistribution Lipid abnormalities Hepatitis	Not currently used as a single agent because of the high pill burden and the high rate of GI adverse effects and lipid abnormalities. Mainly used for boosting or enhancing the pharmacokinetic profile of other PIs
Others: ➢ Amprenavir ➢ Fosamprenavir ➢ Nelfinavir ➢ Saquinavir ➢ Tipranavir/ritonavir		
Note: ➢ **Cobicistat:** – CYP3A4 inhibitor without antiretroviral activity – Used as a boosting agent. – Increases plasma drug concentrations, half-life and maximum plasma concentrations, thus improving the potency of the antiviral agent. – This allows lower and less frequent dosing of the parent drug, thus reducing the burden of pills. – May falsely increase serum creatinine		

Contd...

Contd...

INSTI—integrase strand transfer inhibitor (Integrase Inhibitors): ➢ Mechanism: Blocks the integrase enzyme and prevents the incorporation of viral DNA into the host chromosome (*See* **Fig. 5.17**)		
Bictegravir 50 mg orally daily	Diarrhea, nausea, and headache	Used in antiretroviral combination with tenofovir alafenamide 25 mg and emtricitabine 200 mg OD
Dolutegravir Treatment-naïve or integrase-naïve patients: 50 mg PO OD *See* comments	Hypersensitivity, insomnia, fatigue, and headache	When administered with efavirenz, fosamprenavir/ritonavir, tipranavir/ritonavir, or rifampicin: 50 mg PO BD When administered to integrase-experienced patients with suspected integrase resistance: 50 mg PO BDAvoid carbamazepine, dofetilide, nevirapine, phenobarbital, and phenytoin
Elvitegravir *See* comments	Diarrhea, rash, and increased liver enzymes	Treatment-naïve: 150 mg OD with cobicistat 150 mg, emtricitabine 200 mg, and tenofovir Treatment-experienced: 150 mg OD, with a protease inhibitor Avoid efavirenz and nevirapine
Raltegravir 400 mg PO BD	Diarrhea, nausea, headache, muscle weakness, rhabdomyolysis, and elevated CPK	Use with caution in patients who are at an increased risk of rhabdomyolysis or myopathy
Others: ➢ Cabotegravir (injectable)		
Entry inhibitors (fusion inhibitors): ➢ Mechanism: Binds to gp41 and prevents the conformational changes necessary for the fusion of the viral and cellular membrane		
Enfuvirtide 90 mg subcutaneously Q12h	Injection site pain and allergic reaction Increased rate of bacterial pneumonia	Indication: ART-experienced patients with HIV replication despite ongoing antiretroviral therapy It does not inhibit HIV-2
Entry inhibitors (CCR5 inhibitors): ➢ Mechanism: Selectively binds to the human CCR5 receptor on the cell membrane, and blocks the interaction of the HIV gp120 and the CCR5 receptor for CCR5-tropic HIV ➢ However, it does not block the viral entry of CXCR4-tropic HIV or HIV that uses both CCR5 and CXCR4 for cell entry		
Maraviroc 150 mg PO BD or 300 mg PO BD	Cough, fever, and rash Hepatotoxicity Musculoskeletal symptoms	Do not administer in patients with severe renal dysfunction Viral tropism testing should be done before initiation of maraviroc Cannot be used for CXCR4-tropic HIV or HIV that uses both CCR5 and CXCR4 for cell entry
Entry inhibitors (postattachment inhibitors)		
Ibalizumab Single loading dose of 2,000 mg followed by a maintenance dose of 800 mg every 2 weeks IV	Rash, diarrhea, and nausea	Humanized monoclonal antibody In combination with other antiretroviral agents in patients with multidrug-resistant HIV-1

Q. What antiretroviral regimen to choose for initial therapy?

- Factors to consider when selecting an ART regimen include
  - Patient-specific factors
    - Pretreatment viral load and CD4 count
    - Results of HIV genotypic drug resistance testing
    - HLA-B*5701 status if considering abacavir
    - Patient preferences and adherence potential
    - Comorbid conditions and coinfections
    - Pregnancy or child-bearing potential
  - Drug-specific factors
    - Genetic barrier to drug resistance
    - Adverse effects
    - Drug-drug interactions
    - Convenience: Pill burden, dosing frequency, and food requirements
    - Cost and access
- Preferred regimens, as per DHHS and WHO are mentioned in **Tables 5.20** and **5.21**, respectively.

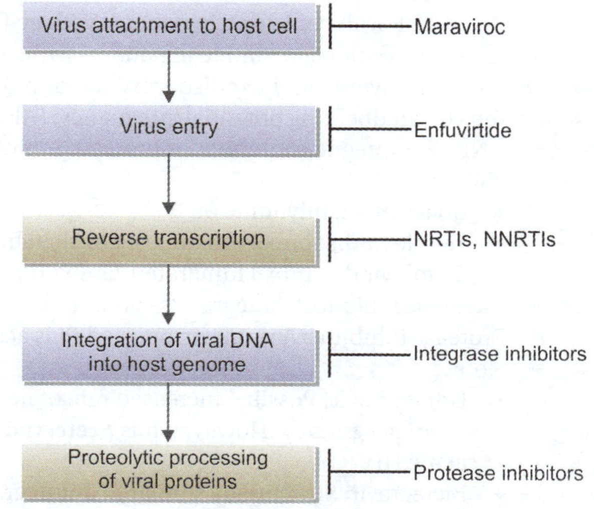

FIG. 5.17: Site of action of antiretroviral therapy (ART).

Special considerations (DHHS 2019)

- *Cardiovascular disease:*
  - If a patient requires a PI: Atazanavir is preferred over other boosted PIs
  - Avoid abacavir in patients with/at risk for cardiovascular disease

TABLE 5.20: Preferred regimens—United States Department of Health and Human Services (DHHS) (Dec 2019).

INSTI + 2 NRTIs preferred: ➢ Bictegravir-emtricitabine-tenofovir alafenamide ➢ Dolutegravir + tenofovir alafenamide-emtricitabine ➢ Dolutegravir-abacavir-lamivudine Note: Tenofovir alafenamide-emtricitabine is the preferred NRTI combination
Alternative regimens
INSTI-based regimens ➢ Elvitegravir/cobicistat-emtricitabine-tenofovir alafenamide ➢ Raltegravir plus tenofovir alafenamide-emtricitabine
PI-based regimens ➢ Atazanavir (boosted with ritonavir or cobicistat) plus tenofovir alafenamide-emtricitabine ➢ Darunavir (boosted with ritonavir or cobicistat) plus tenofovir alafenamide-emtricitabine
NNRTI-based regimens ➢ Doravirine plus tenofovir alafenamide-emtricitabine ➢ Efavirenz plus tenofovir alafenamide-emtricitabine ➢ Efavirenz-emtricitabine-tenofovir disoproxil fumarate
When tenofovir (TAF or TDF) and abacavir cannot be used ➢ Darunavir (boosted with ritonavir or cobicistat) plus dolutegravir ➢ Darunavir (boosted with ritonavir or cobicistat) plus lamivudine ➢ Dolutegravir-lamivudine

TABLE 5.21: World Health Organization (WHO) 2016 recommendations.

For adults and adolescents	
Preferred first-line regimen	1. Tenofovir disoproxil fumarate plus lamivudine (or emtricitabine) plus efavirenz
Alternative first-line regimen	1. Zidovudine plus lamivudine plus efavirenz (or nevirapine) 2. Tenofovir disoproxil fumarate plus lamivudine (or emtricitabine) plus dolutegravir 3. Tenofovir disoproxil fumarate plus lamivudine (or emtricitabine) plus low-dose efavirenz (400 mg/day) 4. Tenofovir disoproxil fumarate plus lamivudine (or emtricitabine) plus nevirapine
For pregnant or breastfeeding women	
Preferred first-line regimen	1. Tenofovir disoproxil fumarate plus lamivudine (or emtricitabine) plus efavirenz
Alternative first-line regimen	1. Zidovudine plus lamivudine plus efavirenz (or nevirapine) 2. Tenofovir disoproxil fumarate plus lamivudine (or emtricitabine) plus nevirapine

- *Hepatitis B coinfection:*
  - Tenofovir (tenofovir alafenamide or tenofovir disoproxil fumarate)-emtricitabine is the preferred NRTI combination for patients with HIV/HBV coinfection
  - Emtricitabine and lamivudine should not be used as monotherapy for the treatment of HBV
- *Kidney disease:*
  - Avoid tenofovir disoproxil fumarate in patients with an eGFR <60 mL/min/1.73 m^2
  - Avoid TDF with cobicistat, in patients with eGFR <70 mL/min/1.73 m^2
  - Avoid tenofovir alafenamide in patients with acute kidney injury or eGFR <30 mL/min/1.73 m^2
- *Osteoporosis:* Avoid tenofovir disoproxil fumarate
- Persons of childbearing potential/pregnancy: (Also see section on HIV-pregnancy below)
  - 2 NRTIs + integrase inhibitor or protease inhibitors preferred
  - NRTIs:
    - Abacavir + lamivudine or
    - Tenofovir disoproxil fumarate + emtricitabine or
    - Tenofovir disoproxil fumarate + lamivudine
  - Integrase inhibitor: Raltegravir is preferred
  - Protease inhibitor: A ritonavir-boosted PI is acceptable
  - Note:
    - Dolutegravir: Possible increased rate of neural tube defects when used at the time of conception; hence **avoid in early pregnancy**. However, it is **preferred** in women presenting **late in pregnancy**, with high viral load or with acute HIV
    - Bictegravir: Structurally similar to dolutegravir
    - Elvitegravir/cobicistat/emtricitabine/tenofovir and other cobicistat-boosted regimens: Decreased drug levels during pregnancy
  - Also *see* World Health Organization (WHO) 2016 Recommendations **(Table 5.21)**
- Baseline resistance testing not available:
  - Regimen containing dolutegravir, bictegravir, or pharmacologically boosted darunavir should be initiated.

Predictors of long-term virologic success in HIV therapy

- Low baseline viral load
- High baseline CD4 count
- Rapid reduction of viral load to undetectable levels
- Patient adherence to prescribed therapy

Changing ART regimen

- Treatment failure
- Adverse events
- Drug interactions
- Pregnancy
- Cost

TREATMENT FAILURE IN HIV

Q. Discuss treatment failure in HIV.

Important definitions:

- **Virologic failure**
  - Inability to achieve or maintain suppression of viral replication to **HIV-1 RNA levels <200 copies/mL**
  - May be either
    - **Incomplete virologic response:** Two consecutive plasma HIV RNA levels ≥200 copies/mL after 24 weeks on ART in patients without previous documented virologic suppression on regimen
    - **Virologic rebound:** Confirmed detectable HIV RNA levels ≥200 copies/mL after achieving virologic suppression.
- **Note: 2010 WHO definitions of clinical, immunological, and virological failure (for adults and adolescents)**
  - **Virologic failure:**
    - Plasma viral load >1,000 copies/mL based on two consecutive viral load measurements after 3 months
  - **Clinical failure**
    - New or recurrent clinical event indicating severe immunodeficiency after 6 months of effective treatment
    - Clinical event refers to WHO clinical stage 4 conditions and some WHO clinical stage 3 conditions, such as pulmonary TB and severe bacterial infections
    - The condition must be differentiated from IRIS occurring after initiating ART
  - **Immunological failure**
    - CD4 count ≤ baseline or
    - Persistent CD4 levels <100 cells/μL.

Risk factors for treatment failure:

- HIV-related factors
  - Transmitted or acquired drug resistance
  - Prior treatment failure
  - Innate resistance to antiretroviral drugs
  - Higher pretreatment HIV RNA level
- Patient and regimen-related factors
  - Poor adherence
  - Drug side effects and toxicities
  - Variable absorption
  - Drug interactions
  - Low genetic barrier to resistance
  - Previous exposure to suboptimal regimens
  - Prescription errors

Management of treatment failure

New antiretroviral regimen should contain at least two, and preferably three, fully active drugs based on

- Patient's treatment history
- Drug resistance testing

Table 5.22 outlines the treatment strategies for management of treatment failure with first-line ARTs.

TABLE 5.22: Treatment in cases of failure of first-line regimen.

	Failing NNRTI plus NRTI regimen	*Failing boosted PI plus NRTI regimen*	*Failing an INSTI plus NRTI regimen*
Likely mechanism	➢ Failure is often due to viral resistance to the NNRTI ➢ NRTI mutations may also be present	➢ Failure is often due to poor adherence, drug-drug interactions, or drug-food interactions ➢ Most patients have either no resistance or resistance to emtricitabine or lamivudine	➢ Resistance to emtricitabine, lamivudine ➢ Possible resistance to the INSTI
Treatment options	➢ Boosted PI plus 2 NRTIs ➢ Dolutegravir plus 2 NRTIs ➢ INSTI plus boosted PI, such as – Raltegravir plus Lopinavir/ritonavir – Dolutegravir plus boosted PI	➢ Continuation of regimen with adherence support and viral monitoring if regimen is well tolerated and there are no concerns of drug interactions ➢ Different boosted PI plus 2 NRTIs ➢ Different boosted PI plus INSTI ➢ INSTI plus 2 NRTIs	➢ In absence of INSTI resistance: – Boosted PI plus 2 NRTIs – Dolutegravir plus 2 NRTIs – Boosted PI plus INSTI ➢ In patients with resistance to raltegravir and elvitegravir, but susceptibility to dolutegravir, options include – Boosted PI plus 2 NRTIs – Twice-daily dolutegravir plus 2 active NRTIs – Twice-daily dolutegravir plus boosted PI

HIV RESISTANCE

Q. Add a note on HIV resistance.

- Important cause of treatment failure in HIV
- Factors favoring drug resistance:
  - Drug related
    - Differing genetic barrier to resistance
      - Emtricitabine, lamivudine, and efavirenz have a low genetic barrier to resistance
      - PIs and some NRTIs (e.g., zidovudine) select for resistance mutations slowly, and multiple resistant mutations often need to accumulate before the drug's efficacy is lost
    - Cross-resistance within drug classes
    - Potency of the drug: Low potency leads to subtherapeutic suppression of viral load, favoring resistance
  - Virus related
    - High rate of HIV-1 replication
    - Error-prone nature of reverse transcriptase
- This leads to mutations which:
  - Alter the coreceptor used for entry into the host cell
  - Increase the removal of a bound drug
  - Change the conformation of a viral enzyme, thus, preventing drug binding
  - Increase the efficiency of a viral enzyme, thus, overcoming drug-based inhibition of that enzyme
- Transmitted drug resistance:
  - Occurs when primary HIV infection is caused by a drug resistance mutation-bearing virus
  - Hence, HIV resistance testing is advised at the time of patient's initial diagnosis
- Acquired drug resistance:
  - Seen in patients with virological failure
- HIV resistance testing has been described earlier

Treatment is as described in the above sections, taking into consideration patient's treatment history and results of drug resistance testing.

SPECIAL CONSIDERATIONS IN PATIENTS WITH HIV

HIV-TB Coinfection

Q. Add a note on HIV-TB coinfection.

Q. Add a note on latent TB infection in patients with HIV.

Active Tuberculosis in Patients with HIV

- TB is the leading cause of death in patients with HIV. Most common opportunistic infection and can occur at any CD4 level.
- HIV infection is the most important risk factor for TB. Patients have an increased risk of acquiring new TB disease as well as have an increased risk of developing active TB from reactivated latent infection.
- Clinical manifestations of TB in patients with HIV varies based on the degree of immunosuppression and sites of TB.

- Pulmonary TB is the most common presentation **(Fig. 5.18A)**
- Extrapulmonary TB is more common in patients with HIV than patients without HIV.
  - In patients with extrapulmonary TB, common presentations include genitourinary tuberculosis, central nervous system TB **(Fig. 5.18B)**, abdominal TB, TB lymphadenitis **(Fig. 5.18C)**, cutaneous TB **(Fig. 5.18D)**, and pleural TB
- Tuberculosis progresses more rapidly, with a subacute or even acute presentation in those with advanced immunosuppression. The diagnosis therefore needs to be made and therapy commenced promptly.

- Diagnosis of tuberculosis (TB) in patients with HIV
  - Sputum smears:
    - Negative in more than half of patients
    - This is mainly due to the absence of pulmonary cavities
  - Nucleic acid amplification testing
    - Use of NAAT in patients with HIV is recommended
    - Advantages include rapid results, increased sensitivity as compared to smear microscopy, and distinction between tuberculosis and nontuberculous mycobacterial infections.
  - Radiologic presentation of chest X-ray varies with state of immunodeficiency.
    - In patients with CD4 T-cell count >350 cells/μL, presentation is similar to that of non-HIV patients, and includes upper lobe infiltrates, cavitation, and pleural disease.
    - In patients with lower CD4 counts, cavitation is less common.
    - They present more often with lower or middle lobe infiltrates, interstitial nodules, miliary infiltrates, mediastinal lymphadenopathy, pleural effusion or sometimes, a normal X-ray.

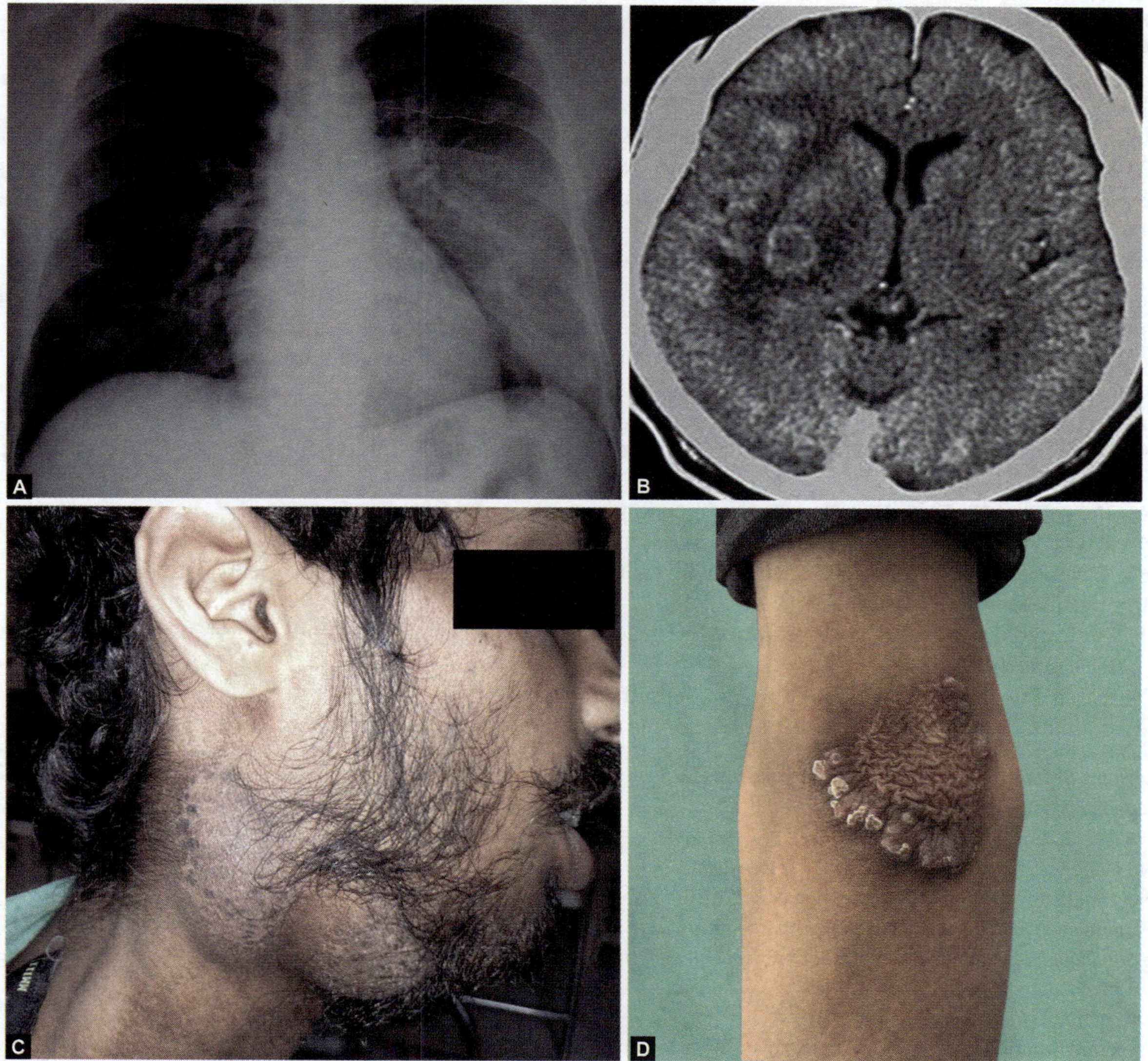

FIGS. 5.18A TO D: (A) Chest X-ray showing tuberculosis involving left lower lobe; (B) CT head showing space occupying lesion—tuberculoma; (C) Matted cervical lymph nodes due to tuberculosis; (D) Cutaneous tuberculosis—lupus vulgaris in a HIV patient.

- Testing of extrapulmonary tuberculosis depends on the site of the disease,
  - For example, for patients with suspected TB lymphadenitis, needle aspiration or biopsy for histopathology, acid fast bacilli, smear, and culture
  - Other samples, depending on the involvement, may include pleural fluid, pericardial fluid, ascites, or cerebrospinal fluid (CSF).

Management of tuberculosis (TB) in patients with HIV

- Recommendations for antituberculosis treatment regimens in adults with HIV infection follow the same principles as for adults without HIV infection
  - Initiation phase: 2 months of isoniazid, rifampin (or rifabutin), pyrazinamide, and ethambutol
  - Continuation phase: 4 months of isoniazid, rifampin (or rifabutin), and ethambutol daily for drug-susceptible TB (longer duration for CNS TB/TB involving the bone/more severe disease)
  - Corticosteroids are recommended for patients with CNS or pericardial disease
- All patients should be given antiretroviral therapy (ART)
  - The preferred cotreatment regimen includes rifampin-based TB therapy plus 2 NRTIs + efavirenz
  - Alternative regimens include:
    - 2 NRTIs plus raltegravir 400–800 mg twice daily with standard rifampin dosing or
    - 2 NRTIs plus ritonavir-boosted protease inhibitor with rifabutin-based TB therapy.
- Recommendations for timing of ART vary by CD4 T-cell count and clinical disease.
  - CD4 T-cell count <50 cells/μL: ART should be started within 2 weeks of starting ATT
  - CD4 T-cell count ≥50 cells/μL and severe clinical disease: ART should be started within 2–4 weeks of starting ATT
  - For patients with CD4 T-cell count ≥50 cells/μL and not severe clinical disease: ART can be delayed beyond 2–4 weeks of starting TB therapy, but should be started within 8–12 weeks.
- TB-IRIS in patients with HIV
  - Patients with HIV infection and TB are at risk of developing immune reconstitution inflammatory syndrome (IRIS) with worsening of signs and symptoms after beginning antiretroviral therapy.
  - Risk of IRIS is higher in those who start ART within 2 weeks of starting ATT compared to those who start at 8–12 weeks of starting ATT.
  - Most IRIS is self-limited and can be managed with anti-inflammatory agents
  - Corticosteroids may rarely be needed to control symptoms.

Latent Tuberculosis in Patients with HIV

- Patients with HIV may often be detected to have latent tuberculosis infection (LTBI), i.e., presence of a *Mycobacterium tuberculosis*-specific immune response in the absence of clinical and radiological disease.
- Guidelines recommend that all persons with HIV should undergo testing for latent tuberculosis infection (LTBI)
  - Options for testing include
  - Tuberculin skin test (TST):
    - Assesses for a delayed hypersensitivity response to an intradermally injected *Mycobacterium tuberculosis* purified protein derivative (PPD)
    - It is read at 48–72 hours following the injection
    - For HIV-positive patients: Positive TST is defined as **induration ≥5 mm**
    - Advanced HIV infection is associated with reduced TST reactivity and decreased sensitivity of the test.
  - Interferon-gamma release assays (IGRAs):
    - Preferred if patient has received prior BCG vaccination, or if patients are unlikely to return after 48–72 hours for TST reporting.
  - Note that a negative TST or IGRA does not definitively exclude a diagnosis of TB
  - All patients with a positive testing for LTBI should undergo testing for active tuberculosis.

Management of latent TB in HIV [TB prophylaxis in HIV]

- Indications:
  - Positive diagnostic test for LTBI,
  - No evidence of active tuberculosis (TB) disease and
  - No prior history of treatment for active or latent TB
  - Patient is a close contact of persons with infectious pulmonary TB, regardless of LTBI status.
- Rule out active TB prior to initiating treatment for LTBI, as treatment of active disease with regimens to treat LTBI can lead to development of drug-resistant TB
- Recommended treatment regimens:
  - Preferred regimen is isoniazid (INH) and pyridoxine for 9 months as either:
    - INH 300 mg orally once daily plus pyridoxine 25–50 mg orally once daily
    - INH 900 mg orally twice weekly by directly observed therapy (DOT) plus pyridoxine 25–50 mg orally once daily.

- Alternative regimens include:
  - Rifampin 600 mg/day orally for 4 months
  - Rifabutin for 4 months, with dose adjusted based on concomitant antiretroviral therapy (ART)
  - Rifapentine plus isoniazid plus pyridoxine for 12 weeks (for patients having ART regimens containing efavirenz or raltegravir)
- ART should be given in addition to LTBI treatment to reduce the risk of TB disease
- Treatment for LTBI reduces the risk of developing active TB by about 60%.

Immune Reconstitution Inflammatory Syndrome (IRIS)

Q. What do you mean by IRIS? List the types and management.

Treatment of HIV infection with combination antiretroviral therapy (ART) results in a rapid improvement in cell immunity. However, restoring the immune response may also lead to a paradoxical worsening of the existing opportunistic disease or to unmasking a new infection. This is referred to as immune reconstitution inflammatory syndrome (IRIS).

- Usually develops within the first 3 months of ART but occasionally develops later.
- Risk factors: Lower CD4 cell counts and high HIV viral load at the time of initiation of ART.
- Types:
  - **Paradoxical IRIS:**
    - Worsening or atypical manifestation (or both) of an established opportunistic infection after ART is initiated
    - Due to the immune response against residual antigens of the pathogen or the dying organism.
  - **Unmasking IRIS:**
    - Disease that occurs for the first time after ART is commenced
    - Due to an immune response against a subclinical infection by an opportunistic pathogen or a missed diagnosis of an opportunistic infection
    - Manifests with accelerated or exaggerated inflammatory presentations of the infection.
  - Immune reconstitution disease (IRD): Patients with HIV infection who are receiving ART also have an increased susceptibility to some autoimmune diseases, such as Graves' disease, and sarcoidosis. This is also referred to as a type of IRIS by some authors.
- Examples and features of immune reconstitution inflammatory syndrome are given in **Table 5.23**
- Fever is the most common clinical manifestation
- Diagnosis: Most or all of the following features should be present
  - Presence of AIDS with a low pretreatment CD4 count (<200 cells/μL)
    - Note: Exception: IRIS secondary to preexisting TB may occur in patients with CD4 counts >200 cells/μL
  - A positive virologic and immunological response to ART
  - The presence of clinical manifestations consistent with an inflammatory condition
  - A temporal association between ART initiation and the onset of clinical features of illness

TABLE 5.23: Examples of IRIS.

IRIS	***Features***
TB-IRIS: *Mycobacterium tuberculosis*—most common pathogen involved in IRIS	Paradoxical exacerbation of TB: Fever, enlargement of lymph nodes, worsening radiographic pulmonary infiltrates, pleural effusion, features of TB meningitis/tuberculoma, and hepatitis
Nontuberculous mycobacteria (NTM) IRIS	Worsening lymphadenitis, pulmonary and abdominal disease
Bacille Calmette–Guérin (BCG)—IRIS	Necrotizing regional lymphadenitis
Leprosy-associated IRIS: *Mycobacterium leprae*	Type 1 lepra reaction
C-IRIS: *Cryptococcus neoformans*	Meningitis and lymphadenitis
Pneumocystosis-associated IRIS: *Pneumocystis jiroveci*	Paradoxical exacerbation of pneumonitis
CMV retinitis after ART or immune recovery uveitis	Acute retinitis after commencing ART Uveitis
Progressive multifocal leukoencephalopathy-IRIS: JC polyomavirus	Multifocal leukoencephalopathy with inflammatory features
Kaposi sarcoma-IRIS: Human herpesvirus 8	Rapid progression of existing and/or new KS lesions
Hepatitis B or C virus associated IRIS	Hepatitis flare and/or liver enzyme elevation May mimic drug-induced liver injury (DILI)
Varicella-zoster virus associated IRIS	Dermatomal or multi-dermatomal zoster Rarely, myelitis
Herpes simplex virus associated IRIS	Herpes lesions with exaggerated inflammation Myelitis or encephalitis (rare)
Inflammatory molluscum contagiosum: Molluscum contagiosum virus	Inflamed molluscum lesions
Inflammatory seborrheic dermatitis: *Malassezia* spp.	Abnormally inflamed seborrheic dermatitis

- Absence of evidence of bacterial superinfection, drug-resistant infection, adverse drug reactions, reduced drug levels or patient noncompliance.

Management:

- **Continue antiretroviral therapy.** Temporary discontinuation of ART should be considered only in patients with life-threatening disease when all other measures have failed
- Unmasking IRIS: Treat the underlying opportunistic infection
- Paradoxical IRIS: Continue treatment of underlying opportunistic infection
- Anti-inflammatory therapy: Reserved for patients with severe inflammation, particularly when it is life-threatening, or causing significant symptoms
  - NSAIDs
  - Glucocorticoids—e.g., prednisone 1.5 mg/kg/day for 2 weeks, then 0.75 mg/kg/day for 2 weeks.

- Prevention:
  - Delay initiation of ART to 5 weeks after starting treatment for cryptococcal infection
  - Delay initiation of ART 2–8 weeks after starting ATTs in cases of tuberculosis. See section on HIV-TB coinfection.

HIV and Pregnancy

Q. Write a note on pregnancy considerations in patients with HIV.

- Mother-to-child transmission (MTCT) accounts for >90% of HIV infection in children.
- Screening:
  - All pregnant women should be screened for HIV infection at entry to antenatal care
  - Testing should be repeated in the third trimester for women at high risk
- Antiretroviral therapy:
  - Start ARTs as early as possible for all pregnant women with HIV infection regardless of CD4 T-cell count or viral load. ART should be continued even after delivery
  - Starting antiretroviral therapy early in pregnancy is associated with decreased viral loads at time of delivery
  - 2 NRTIs + integrase inhibitor or protease inhibitors preferred
    - NRTIs:
      - Abacavir + lamivudine or
      - Tenofovir disoproxil fumarate + emtricitabine or
      - Tenofovir disoproxil fumarate + lamivudine
    - Integrase inhibitor: Raltegravir is preferred
    - Protease inhibitor: A ritonavir-boosted PI is acceptable
  - Note:
    - Dolutegravir: Possible increased rate of neural tube defects when used at the time of conception; hence avoid in early pregnancy. However, it is preferred in women presenting late in pregnancy, with high viral load or with acute HIV
    - Bictegravir: Structurally similar to dolutegravir
    - Elvitegravir/cobicistat/emtricitabine/tenofovir and other cobicistat-boosted regimens: Decreased drug levels during pregnancy
  - World Health Organization (WHO) recommendations. *The antiretroviral drugs dolutegravir and emtricitabine/tenofovir alafenamide fumarate (DTG + FTC/TAF) may comprise the safest and most effective HIV treatment regimen currently available during pregnancy (March 2020)*
    - Preferred first-line regimen: Tenofovir disoproxil fumarate + lamivudine (or emtricitabine) + efavirenz
    - Alternative first-line regimen
      - Zidovudine + lamivudine + efavirenz (or nevirapine)
      - Tenofovir disoproxil fumarate + lamivudine (or emtricitabine) + nevirapine
- Labor and delivery considerations:
  - Mode of delivery:
    - Cesarean delivery at 38 weeks of gestation is recommended for women with viral loads >1,000 copies/mL or unknown viral loads near time of delivery.
    - Scheduled cesarean delivery is not routinely recommended in women with HIV RNA levels ≤1,000 copies/mL
    - Avoid invasive labor procedures, such as an artificial rupture of membranes in the setting of viremia, the use of fetal scalp electrodes, and the use of forceps or vacuum extractor when possible. This is to reduce fetal exposure to bodily fluids.
  - Role of IV zidovudine
    - For women with HIV viral loads >1,000 copies/mL, start zidovudine 2 mg/kg IV over 1 hour at labor onset and then 1 mg/kg/hour IV until delivery.

- For women with HIV infection receiving combination ART during pregnancy and HIV RNA ≤1,000 copies/mL near delivery, intrapartum zidovudine is not required.

- Following delivery:
  - Give postpartum antiretroviral drugs to all **HIV-exposed infants** to reduce perinatal transmission
    - Antiretroviral regimens (at gestational age-appropriate doses) should be given preferably within 6–12 hours of birth
    - **Antiretroviral prophylaxis**
      - To prevent HIV infection in infants with **low risk of transmission**
      - Options:
        - Single drug regimen: Zidovudine alone for 4 weeks for infants born to mother on regular ART with viral load <50 copies/mL
        - Two-drug regimen: Zidovudine for 6 weeks plus three doses of nevirapine during first week of life for infants at higher risk of transmission but in whom presumptive HIV therapy is not needed.
    - **Presumptive HIV therapy:**
      - For infants with **higher risk of HIV acquisition**, such as those born to mothers who
        - Did not have antepartum or intrapartum antiretroviral drugs
        - Only had intrapartum antiretroviral drugs
        - Had antepartum antiretroviral drugs but did not achieve viral suppression near delivery
        - Acquired HIV infection during pregnancy or breastfeeding.
      - Options include
        - Zidovudine for 6 weeks plus emtricitabine and nevirapine for 2–6 weeks
        - Zidovudine for 6 weeks plus emtricitabine and raltegravir for 2–6 weeks
    - **HIV therapy:**
      - To newborns with confirmed infection
      - Administration of three-drug regimen at treatment doses.
- Breastfeeding recommendations:
  - Breastfeeding is not recommended in resource-rich settings due to the availability of safe alternatives
  - However, in resource-limited situations, breastfeeding may be acceptable till safe and adequate diet can be provided.
- Other concerns:
  - Prevention of secondary transmission to partner
  - Family planning
  - Prophylaxis against opportunistic infection: Similar to nonpregnant adults.

TREATMENT OF OPPORTUNISTIC INFECTIONS

It is described in previous sections.

PREVENTION OF OPPORTUNISTIC INFECTIONS (TABLE 5.24)

Q. Enumerate the indications and discuss prophylactic drugs used to prevent HIV-related opportunistic infections.

TABLE 5.24: Prophylaxis for prevention of opportunistic infections (decreasing order of CD4 count).

Condition	*Indications*	*When to stop*	*Therapeutic options*
Mycobacterium tuberculosis (drug sensitive)	➢ Tuberculin skin test >5 mm or ➢ Positive IFN-γ release assay or ➢ Prior positive test without treatment or ➢ Close contact with case of active pulmonary TB (Note: All CD4 counts)	See next column	➢ Isoniazid 300 mg PO + pyridoxine 25 mg PO OD × 9 months OR ➢ Isoniazid 900 mg PO twice weekly + Pyridoxine 25 mg PO daily × 9 months Alternative: ➢ Rifampin 600 mg PO qd × 4 months ➢ Rifabutin for 4 months, with dose adjusted based on concomitant antiretroviral therapy (ART) ➢ Rifapentine plus isoniazid plus pyridoxine for 12 weeks (for patients having ART regimens containing efavirenz or raltegravir)
Coccidiodomycosis	➢ Positive serology and CD4 count <250/μL (endemic area) ➢ Prior documented disease	CD4 count ≥250/μL for 6 months (if it was started for the first indication)	Fluconazole 400 mg PO OD
Pneumocystis jirovecii pneumonia	➢ CD4 count <200/μL ➢ Oropharyngeal candidiasis ➢ Prior episode of PCP	➢ If CD4 count >200/μL for ≥3 months	➢ TMP-SMX-DS 1 tablet PO OD Alternative options: ➢ Atovaquone 1,500 mg PO OD ➢ Dapsone 100 mg PO OD or 50 mg PO BID ➢ Dapsone 50 mg PO OD + pyrimethamine 50 mg PO weekly + folinic acid 25 mg PO weekly ➢ Aerosolized pentamidine 300 mg via Respirgard II nebulizer monthly

Contd...

Contd...

Toxoplasma	➤ Prior toxoplasmic encephalitis and CD4 count <200/μL ➤ Toxoplasma IgG antibody positive and CD4 count <100/μL	➤ If CD4 count >200/μL for ≥3 months	Sulfadiazine 2,000–4,000 mg in two to four divided doses daily PO + pyrimethamine 25–50 mg PO OD + leucovorin 25 mg PO OD Alternate ➤ TMP-SMX 1 DS PO OD or ➤ Clindamycin 600 mg PO TID + Pyrimethamine 25–50 mg PO OD + Leucovorin 25 mg PO OD ➤ Atovaquone 750–1,500 mg PO BID ± pyrimethamine 25 mg PO OD + leucovorin 10 mg PO OD
Histoplasmosis	➤ CD4 count <150 μL and high risk (endemic area or occupational exposure) ➤ Prior documented disease	➤ After 1 year, if CD4 count >150/μL and patient on cART for ≥6 months	➤ Itraconazole 200 mg PO BID or ➤ Fluconazole 400 mg PO OD
Cryptococcus	➤ Prior documented disease	➤ If CD4 count >100/μL, no evidence of active fungal infection, and HIV viral load <500 copies/mL for >3 months	➤ Fluconazole 200 mg PO OD or ➤ Itraconazole 200 mg PO OD
CMV	➤ Prior end-organ disease	➤ If CD4 count >100/μL for 6 months and no evidence of active CMV disease ➤ Restart if prior retinitis and CD4 count <100/μL	➤ Valganciclovir 900 mg bid P Alternative ➤ Cidofovir 5 mg/kg every alternate week IV + Probenecid or ➤ Foscarnet 90–120 (mg/kg)/day IV
MAC	➤ CD4 count <50/μL	If CD4 count >100/μL for ≥6 months	➤ Azithromycin 1,200 mg weekly PO or 600 mg twice weekly PO or ➤ Clarithromycin 500 mg bid PO or ➤ Rifabutin
	➤ Prior documented disseminated disease		➤ Clarithromycin 500 mg PO BID + Ethambutol 15 (mg/kg)/day PO or ➤ Azithromycin 500–600 mg PO OD + ethambutol 15 (mg/kg)/day PO

VACCINATION IN PATIENTS WITH HIV

Q. List the vaccine that should be given to patients with HIV (Table 5.25).

Considerations with vaccination:

- Poor immune response
  - Patients with CD4 count <200 cells/μL, develop poor immune responses to immunization. Thus, it is preferable to wait until the CD4 count increases to >200 cells/μL on ART prior to immunization.
- Live vaccines:
  - Vaccination with live organisms is contraindicated in patients with severe immune suppression, as this may result in disease from the attenuated organisms.
  - Live attenuated vaccines should not be given to patients with CD4 counts of <200 cells/μL, and should be used with caution in those with CD4 counts of <350 cells/μL.

TABLE 5.25: Vaccination in patients with HIV.

Given routinely	*Given if indicated for travel*	*Avoid if CD4⁺ cells <200*	*Avoid*
➤ Tetanus/diphtheria (or Tdap) ➤ Hepatitis A (at-risk patients) ➤ Hepatitis B ➤ Pneumococcal ➤ Hib ➤ Meningococcal ➤ Influenza, yearly ➤ Human papillomavirus (females <40 years)	➤ Typhoid Vi ➤ Polio and IPV ➤ Rabies ➤ Japanese encephalitis ➤ Tick-borne encephalitis	➤ Yellow fever ➤ Measles, mumps, and rubella ➤ Varicella-zoster virus (VZV)	➤ BCG ➤ Oral polio ➤ Oral typhoid

POSTEXPOSURE PROPHYLAXIS FOR HIV

Q. Discuss and describe the principles and regimens used in postexposure prophylaxis for HIV.

Q. Write a short note on postexposure prophylaxis for hepatitis B.

- **What is considered an exposure:**
  - Exposure is defined as contact between blood, tissue, or body fluids (semen, vaginal secretions, breast milk, amniotic fluid, CSF, and pleural/peritoneal/pericardial/synovial fluid) from a source patient and blood, broken skin, or mucosa of exposed patient.
  - Note that contact of a potentially infectious fluid/substance with intact or unbroken skin is not considered a possible exposure.
- **Types of exposure:**
  - Occupational exposures: Healthcare worker
    - Percutaneous exposure: Needlesticks with hollow bore or solid bore needles
      - Visible contamination of needle with blood, insertion of the needle into an artery or a vein, deep injury caused by the device-associated with increased risk of transmission
    - Mucosal exposures: Splashing of blood or body fluids from source into eyes, nose, or mouth of the exposed person
  - Nonoccupational exposures:
    - Sexual exposures (including victims of rape)
    - Injection drug use
    - Biting: Has a theoretical risk of transmission, especially if source patient's saliva contains blood
- **Risk of transmission:**
  - Risk based on source patient:
    - Highest risk: Those with HIV infection and high viral load
    - Risk increases if source is member of group with high risk for HIV acquisition: Men who have sex with men (MSM), injection drug user, commercial sex worker, person from country with ≥1% HIV seroprevalence, and sexual partner of a member of above groups
  - Risk of acquiring HIV by exposure type: *See* **Table 5.1**
    - Blood transfusion (very rare): Highest rate of transmission
- **Patient evaluation:**
  - **Exposed patient:**
    - HIV testing at time of exposure or within 3 days of exposure to determine baseline HIV status
      - Fourth generation HIV-1/HIV-2/p24 antigen-antibody combination assay
      - Positive result on Ag/Ab test must be followed by further antibody testing and/or RNA testing to determine whether patient has acute or chronic infection
    - Baseline testing to assess for undiagnosed conditions prior to starting PEP include complete blood count, renal function tests and electrolytes, liver function tests, hepatitis B and C serology, and pregnancy test for women
    - For sexual exposures, screen for gonorrhea and chlamydia using nucleic acid amplification testing and syphilis using VDRL/RPR.
  - **Source patient:**
    - If HIV status unknown, test for HIV infection
    - If source patient known to be HIV-positive
    - Results of any previous resistance testing and treatment history should be obtained
    - Viral load should be determined, as should HIV drug resistance testing, if status unknown
    - Also test source patient for coinfections including hepatitis B and C.

Treatment

- Decontamination:
  - Wash the area with soap and water.
  - Avoid squeezing or milking the wound.
  - Do not use caustic agents (e.g., bleach).
- Indications for PEP:
  - PEP should be provided following exposure of nonintact skin or mucous membranes to potentially infected body fluid from source that is HIV-positive or has unknown HIV status.
- Exposures for which PEP **not** indicated:
  - Preexisting HIV infection in exposed patient based on baseline blood tests
  - Consistent pre-exposure prophylaxis use by exposed patient
  - Chronic ongoing exposure
  - Exposure to intact skin
  - Exposure to noninfectious bodily materials such as feces, urine, saliva, and sweat
  - Exposure to bodily fluids from a person known to be HIV-negative (unless person at high risk for recent infection within previous 3 months)
  - Certain types of close contact in the absence of blood or ulcers: Kissing, mouth-to-mouth CPR, human bites without visible blood, and exposure to solid bore needles or sharps without recent contact with blood.

- When to start:
  - Start antiretroviral PEP as soon as possible after an exposure
  - Initiation of PEP ≥72 hours after exposure generally not recommended.
- What drugs to give:
  - Three-drug regimen recommended—two NRTIs plus a third drug [preferably an integrase strand transfer inhibitor (INSTI), or a ritonavir-boosted protease inhibitor (PI)]
  - **Preferred** regimen (NACO June 2021):
    - Tenofovir 300 mg **plus** Lamuvidine 300 mg PO OD **plus** Dolutegravir 50 mg orally once daily or raltegravir 400 mg orally twice daily
  - **Alternative regimen** (NACO June 2021):
    - Tenofovir **plus** emtricitabine (or lamivudine) **plus**
    - Third drug:
      - Lopinavir/ritonavir or atazanavir/ritonavir preferred
      - Raltegravir, darunavir/ritonavir, or efavirenz alternative options
    - Antiretroviral agents generally **not recommended** in PEP:
      - Abacavir: Need for early initiation of PEP does not allow time for testing for HLA-B*5701 allele)
      - Didanosine: Rrisk of mitochondrial toxicity
      - Nelfinavir
      - Tipranavir
    - Medications **contraindicated** as PEP:
      - Nevirapine: Risk of fatal hepatotoxicity (rare)
      - Efavirenz for pregnant women
      - Tenofovir for persons with estimated creatinine clearance <60 mL/min
  - Duration of therapy:
    - **28-day course** after exposure
    - If patient tests positive for HIV at baseline, refer for evaluation and treatment of new diagnosis of HIV infection
    - If source patient confirmed HIV-negative, PEP regimen may be discontinued
  - Other management:
    - Treatment of other blood-borne or sexually transmitted infections (hepatitis B, hepatitis C, gonorrhea, and chlamydia)
- Monitoring
  - Monitor for adverse effects of the antiretroviral drugs.
  - Complete blood counts, urea, creatinine, electrolytes, and liver function tests 2 weeks after initiating PEP
  - Repeat testing for HIV, hepatitis B, and hepatitis C infections: At 6 weeks, 12 weeks, and 6 months postexposure.

Postexposure Prophylaxis for Hepatitis B Infection

- PEP for hepatitis B infection is summarized in **Table 5.26**
- Note: Average rate of transmission for hepatitis B virus and hepatitis C virus
  - HBV—
    - If source patient is positive for both HBsAg and HBeAg—37–62%;
    - If source patient is positive for HBsAg but is HBeAg negative—23–37%
  - HCV—1.8%.

TABLE 5.26: Recommended PEP for hepatitis B virus after occupational exposure in healthcare personnel (CDC-2018).

	Source patient	
Exposed patient	***HBsAg (hepatitis B surface antigen) positive or unknown***	***HBsAg negative***
Unvaccinated/incompletely vaccinated or refused vaccination	HBIG (hepatitis B immunoglobulin) × 1; Complete vaccination (0, 1, and 6 months)	No Need for HBIG Complete vaccination (0, 1, and 6 months)
Previously vaccinated (complete series) with Documented complete response (i.e., protective anti-HBs titers)	No treatment	No treatment
Previously vaccinated, known nonresponder (anti-HBs titers <10 mIU/mL, i.e., not protective)	HBIG (hepatitis B immunoglobulin) × 2 Separated by 1 month (No need for revaccination)	No treatment
Previously vaccinated, response unknown	HBIG × 1 Initiate revaccination	No need for HBIG Test for anti-HBs titers. Revaccinate if anti-HBs titers are not protective (anti-HBs titers <10 mIU/mL)

PRE-EXPOSURE PROPHYLAXIS IN HIV

Q. Discuss pre-exposure prophylaxis in HIV.

Pre-exposure prophylaxis (PrEP) refers to the use of antiretroviral agents by HIV-uninfected but at-risk individuals in order to prevent the acquisition of HIV infection.

- **Indications:**
  - HIV-negative patients or patients with indeterminant testing and no signs or symptoms of acute HIV infection in prior 4 weeks and
  - In the following populations:
    - Sexually active adult men who have sex with men (MSM) at substantial risk for acquiring HIV
    - Heterosexually active adult men and women at substantial risk for acquiring HIV
    - Adult injection drug users at substantial risk for acquiring HIV.
- **Evaluation before starting PrEP:**
  - Exclude acute or chronic HIV infection before starting PrEP
    - Patients with positive testing are not eligible for PrEP and should be initiated on HIV treatment
    - Patients with negative or indeterminant test who have signs or symptoms of acute HIV in prior 4 weeks should be advised confirmatory HIV or viral load testing
  - **Baseline renal function:**
    - PrEP is not recommended for patients with a eGFR <30 mL/minute/1.73 m^2.
    - Individuals with an eGFR <60 mL/min/1.73 m^2 are not candidates for PrEP with TDF-FTC.
  - Pregnancy testing
  - Screening for other infections: Hepatitis B, hepatitis C, and other sexually transmitted infections
  - DEXA scan in patients with, or at high risk for, osteoporosis.
- **PrEP options:**
  - Preferred regimen:
    - 2 NRTIs: Tenofovir disoproxil fumarate plus emtricitabine (TDF/FTC).
  - Alternative:
    - Tenofovir alafenamide plus emtricitabine (TAF/FTC) PO OD
    - Preferred for MSM and transgender women with bone and renal issues (eGFR <60 mL/min/1,73 m^2) who are not eligible for TDF-FTC
    - Note: TAF/FTC should **not** be used for those whose main risk for HIV is receptive vaginal sex and those with eGFR <30 mL/minute/1.73 m^2.
  - Duration of therapy for the above regimen:
    - As long as the risk of infection persists
    - PrEP should be continued for one month after the last high-risk exposure
    - However, not more than a 90-day supply should be prescribed
    - Prescription may be renewed only after HIV testing confirms that patient remains HIV uninfected.
  - Alternative regimen:
    - On demand dosing (also known as event-based dosing or "2-1-1" PrEP) **(Fig. 5.19)**:
      - PrEP is taken only when sex is anticipated
      - Has been shown to be effective for MSM having anal sex
      - **Not recommended** in transgender women and heterosexual males and females
      - Should **not** be used in patients with chronic hepatitis B virus infection.
- Patient monitoring:
  - Frequency of follow-up:
    - At 1 month and 3 months after starting treatment, and then every 3 months thereafter
    - More frequent follow-up for:
      - Patients who have been exposed to and/or have symptoms of a sexually transmitted infection (STI)
      - Patients with evidence of renal dysfunction.
  - Tests to be done include 3 monthly HIV testing with a fourth-generation antigen/antibody test, screening for STIs, creatinine, and urinalysis, pregnancy testing, and hepatitis C virus screening every 6 to 12 months.

HIV VACCINE

Q. Add a short note on HIV-vaccine.

- **Need:** In spite of the remarkable achievements in development of antiretroviral therapies and recent advances in new prevention technologies, the rate of new HIV infections continues to outpace efforts on prevention and control.
- **Challenges:**
  - HIV mutates rapidly; HIV mutates in one day as much as influenza viruses do in a year
  - Can be transmitted by cell-free or cell-associated virus

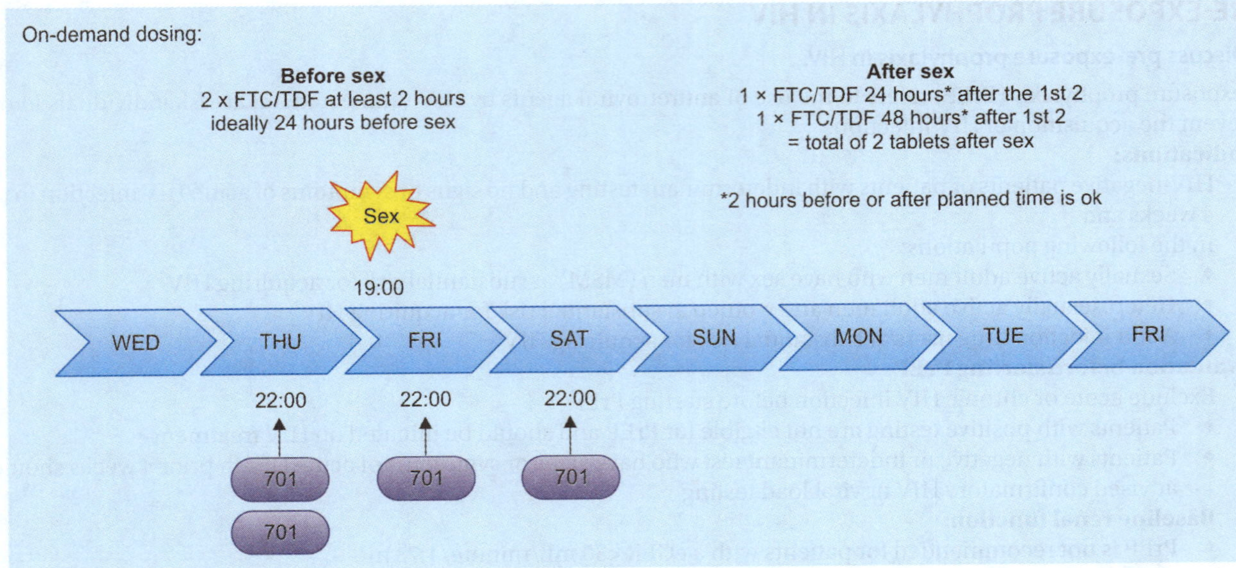

FIG. 5.19: On demand dosing regimen for PrEP.

- HIV provirus integrates itself into the genome of the target cell and remains in a latent form, unexposed to the immune system
- The virus has developed multiple mechanisms to evade the body's defenses.
  - Targets the cells (CD4) that coordinate the immune response to viral infections.
  - Broadly neutralizing antibodies usually appear between 2 and 4 years but by that time the antibodies cannot save them because they are overwhelmed by the mutating virus.

- **Vaccines:**
  - Currently, there is no safe and effective vaccine that is approved for the prevention of HIV infection
  - More than 50 HIV-1 vaccine candidates have been studied since 1987
  - Some of the important vaccine trials are described in **Table 5.27**
  - Research on broadly neutralizing antibodies against certain epitopes on the HIV envelope are underway.

TABLE 5.27: Important HIV-1 vaccines (phase IIb and III efficacy studies).

Vaccine	*Phase*	*Year*	*Results*
Using soluble gp120			
AIDSVAX B/E: 2 recombinant gp120 antigens from subtype B strain and 1 from circulating recombinant forms (CRF01_AE), in alum	III	1999–2003	No protection
AIDSVAX B/B: Recombinant gp120 antigens from two Subtype B isolates, in alum	III	1998–2003	No protection
RV 144 vaccine (Thai trial): Canarypox vector prime + recombinant gp120 boost, in alum	III	2003–2006	31.2% protection
Others:			
HVTN502: Merck adenovirus type-5 vaccine containing HIV gag, pol and nef genes	IIb	2004–2007	Halted because of early transient increased infection in subjects who received the vaccine
HVTN503: Adenovirus type-5 subtype B based vaccine- containing HIV gag, pol, and *nef* genes	IIb	2007–2008	No effect, late increased HIV infection in few male subjects who received the vaccine
HVTN 505: DNA prime followed by recombinant adenovirus type 5 boost (included envelope antigens from HIV-1 subtypes A, B, and C)	IIb	2009–2017	No protection
HVTN 507: Bivalent mosaic antigen delivered by an adenovirus 26 vector and boosted with an alum adjuvanted subtype C gp140 protein	IIb	2017—ongoing	

Mississippi Baby

The "Mississippi baby" was born to an HIV-positive mother who had not received any treatment during pregnancy. Doctors began treating the child by the time she was 30 hours old, but the family stopped antiretroviral therapy at 18 months. She remained off the drugs for the next 27 months with no signs of the virus in her blood. She was monitored closely. However, at 4 years of age, the CD4 cells dropped and in a few weeks the HIV virus levels were detectable. She is presently on treatment.

Berlin Patient

Timothy Ray Brown had HIV for 12 years before he became the first person in the world to be cured of the infection following a stem cell transplant in 2007. The stem cell donor had a specific genetic mutation called CCR5 Delta 32 that protects a person against HIV infection. After the stem cell transplant, Brown was able to stop all antiretroviral treatment and the HIV has not returned till now.

CHAPTER

6

Respiratory System

INTRODUCTION, BASIC APPROACH, SYMPTOMATOLOGY, AND INVESTIGATIONS

Q. Write short note on the normal arterial blood gas (ABG) levels.

Table 6.1 depicts normal arterial blood gas levels.

TABLE 6.1: Normal arterial blood gas (ABG) levels.

Parameter	Value
Arterial oxygen tension (PaO_2)	90–104 mm Hg
Arterial carbon dioxide ($PaCO_2$)	35–45 mm Hg
Arterial oxygen saturation (SaO_2)	95–99%
Arterial blood pH (pH)	7.35–7.45 units
Arterial bicarbonate (HCO_3)	22–30 mEq/L
Base excess (BE)	0 ± 2 mmol/L

HYPERCAPNIA

Q. Write short essay/note on hypercapnic encephalopathy [carbon dioxide (CO_2) narcosis].

Definition

- **Hypercapnia** is defined as a raised **arterial carbon dioxide** ($PaCO_2$) **of 45 mm Hg** (6 kPa) at rest.
- **Hypercapnic encephalopathy:** When **$PaCO_2$ exceeds 90 mm Hg** (12 kPa), severe hypercapnia causes confusion, progressive drowsiness, and CO_2 narcosis.

Causes of Hypercapnia (Table 6.2)

Usually results from **alveolar hypoventilation**.

TABLE 6.2: Causes of hypercapnia.

Central depression of respiratory drive: ➢ Brain-stem lesions ➢ Central sleep apnea, obesity hypoventilation ➢ *Sedatives*: Morphine	**Reduced alveolar ventilation due to pathology within the lungs:** ➢ Chronic bronchitis ➢ Emphysema
Neuromuscular: ➢ Peripheral neuropathy, GB syndrome, poliomyelitis ➢ Myasthenia gravis ➢ Myopathies	**Reduced chest wall** (including diaphragmatic) **movements:** ➢ Trauma ➢ Kyphoscoliosis and pectus excavatum ➢ Ankylosing spondylitis

(GB: Guillain–Barré syndrome)

Clinical Features

- **Headache:** Severe generalized or bilateral frontal or occipital headache (especially **severe on waking up**)
- **Depresses the level of consciousness:**
  - In mild cases, it produces intermittent drowsiness, indifference or inattention, reduction of psychomotor activity, and forgetfulness.
  - In severe cases, it causes mental dullness, drowsiness, confusion, seizures, stupor, and coma. If left untreated, acute hypercapnic respiratory failure can cause death.

Signs

See **Box 6.1**.

Box 6.1: Signs of hypercapnia.

- Asterixis
- Altered sensorium
- Flushed warm extremities
- Bounding peripheral pulses
- Fasciculations
- Papilledema

Investigations

- **Arterial blood gas (ABG) study:** For confirmation of hypercapnia
- **Other relevant investigations** depending on the underlying cause.

Precaution

In chronic hypercapnia [e.g., chronic obstructive pulmonary disease (COPD)], oxygen should be administered in a controlled manner (about 2 L/minute) and morphine and other sedatives should be avoided.

Treatment

- Mechanical ventilation with intermittent positive-pressure respirator. Noninvasive ventilation (NIV) may be sufficient in patients with mild symptoms. BiLevel positive airway pressure (BiPAP): 8–12 cmH_2O (inspiratory pressure) and 3–5 cmH_2O (expiratory pressure)
- Maintenance of acid–base and electrolyte balance
- Treatment of the underlying cause. Respiratory stimulants (doxapram, medroxyprogesterone, and acetazolamide) are used with variable benefits.

HYPOXEMIA

Q. Write short note on hypoxemia.

Definition

Hypoxemia is defined as **arterial oxygen tension (PaO_2) of less than 80 mmHg** (10.6 kPa) in a young healthy adult. As the age advances, the normal arterial oxygen tension (PaO_2) falls gradually.

Causes of Hypoxemia (Table 6.3)

Hypoxemia is rare due to reduced diffusion.

TABLE 6.3: Causes of hypoxemia.

Ventilation-perfusion mismatch in the lung: ➤ Chronic bronchitis ➤ Emphysema ➤ Acute asthma ➤ Pulmonary embolism ➤ Interstitial lung diseases	**Hypoventilation:** ➤ **Central depression of respiratory drive:** Brainstem lesions and central sleep apnea ➤ **Peripheral neuromuscular disease:** Myasthenia gravis peripheral, neuropathy, myasthenia gravis, and myopathies ➤ Malfunctioning of mechanical ventilators
Right-to-left shunts: ➤ Congenital cyanotic heart diseases ➤ Pulmonary collapse/atelectasis ➤ Consolidation, e.g., pneumonia	**Decreased inspired oxygen concentration:** ➤ High altitudes ➤ Malfunctioning of mechanical ventilators

Clinical Features

- **Acute hypoxemia:** It closely resembles acute alcoholism and is characterized by impaired judgment and motor incoordination. On examination, patient has tachypnea, cyanosis, cold peripheries, thready pulse, and hypotension.
- **Chronic hypoxemia:** On long standing, it presents with fatigue, drowsiness, inattentiveness, apathy, delayed reaction time, and reduced work capacity.
- **Consequences:** Centers in the brainstem gets affected and death may occur due to respiratory failure.

Treatment

Treat the underlying cause or mechanism.

Investigations

- **Arterial blood gas (ABG) study:** For confirmation of hypoxemia
- **Calculate the alveolar-arterial O_2 (PAO_2-PaO_2) gradient:** To differentiate various causes of hypoxemia.

CLUBBING

Q. Define clubbing. Enumerate the causes and give the mechanism of clubbing. Enumerate cardiac causes.

Definition

Clubbing (also called Hippocrates fingers) is defined as a selective bulbous enlargement of the distal segment of a digit (fingers and toes) due to an increase in connective tissue especially on the dorsal aspect resulting in loss of the onychonychial angle **(Figs. 6.1A and B).**

Mechanisms

Some of hypotheses are:

- **Role of platelets:** Megakaryocytes from the bone marrow normally break up to the platelets in the pulmonary capillaries. Whenever there are shunts or abnormal circulation (e.g., neoplasm), these megakaryocytes bypass the pulmonary capillaries and reach the systemic circulation. These megakaryocytes preferably lodge in the tips of the digits and locally release platelet-derived growth factor (PDGF) and vascular endothelial growth factor (VEGF). These growth factors along with other mediators increase endothelial permeability and activate and cause proliferation of connective tissue cells (e.g., fibroblasts).
- **Humoral:** Unknown humoral substances dilate vessels in the fingertip (e.g., acromegaly).

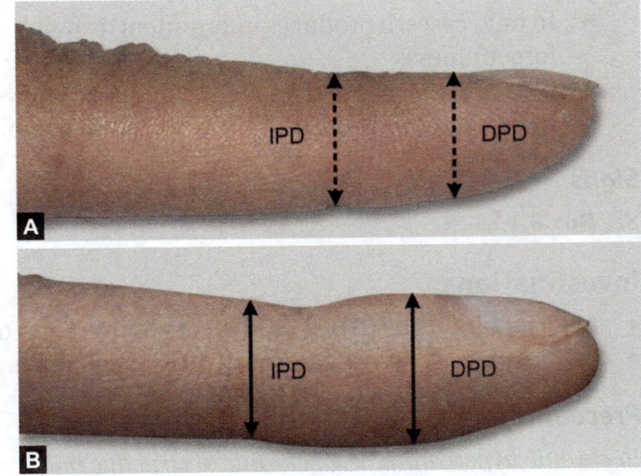

FIGS. 6.1A AND B: (A) Normal finger; (B) Clubbing of finger.
(IPD: interphalangeal distance; DPD: distal phalangeal distance)

- **Persistent hypoxia:** It causes opening of deep arteriovenous fistula in fingers (e.g., tetralogy of Fallot).
- **Reduced ferritin** in systemic circulation: It causes dilation of arteriovenous anastomoses.
- **Vagal theory:** Persistent vagal stimulation causes vasodilation and clubbing (e.g., lung carcinoma).
- **Toxic:** Subacute bacterial endocarditis (SABE).
- **Metabolic:** Thyrotoxicosis.

Grades of Clubbing (Table 6.4)

The process of clubbing usually takes years but in few conditions (e.g., lung abscess and empyema), it may develop quite fast.

TABLE 6.4: Grades of clubbing.

Grade	Features
1	Increased fluctuation due to softening of the nail bed (increased ballotability)
2	Loss of the normal (<165°) onychodermal angle (Lovibond angle), between the nail bed and the nail fold (cuticle)
3	Thickening of the whole distal (end part of the) finger (resembling a parrot beak or drumstick)
4	Hypertrophic osteoarthropathy (pain and tenderness at distal end of long bones due to subperiosteal new bone formation

Causes (Table 6.5)

Clubbing may be hereditary, idiopathic, or acquired and associated with a variety of disorders. Various methods of eliciting clubbing are listed in **Box 6.2**.

Phalangeal depth ratio: It is defined by the ratio of digit's depth measured at the junction between skin and nail (nail bed) and at the distal interphalangeal joint. Normally, the depth at distal interphalangeal joint is more than the depth at nail bed. In clubbing fingers, there is reversal of this ratio. A phalangeal depth ratio of over 1 indicates clubbing. It can be measured by a caliper or a digital photograph.

Pseudoclubbing: It is **increase in longitudinal curvature of the nail with loss of nail and nail plate material.** It is characterized clinically by asymmetrical involvement of fingers and radiographically by resorption of the terminal tufts (acroosteolysis). There is no overgrowth of connective tissue as observed in clubbing.

Causes of pseudoclubbing: (1) Subungual tumor or cyst and (2) subperiosteal bone resorption (e.g., scleroderma, thyroid acropachy, vinyl chloride poisoning, acromegaly, hyperparathyroidism, leprosy, chronic renal failure, acrometastasis, etc.)

TABLE 6.5: Causes of clubbing.

Respiratory: ➢ *Neoplasms:* Bronchogenic carcinoma (especially squamous cell carcinoma), metastasis to lung, mesothelioma ➢ *Suppurative lung disease:* Bronchiectasis, lung abscess, cystic fibrosis, empyema ➢ Asbestosis (with mesothelioma) ➢ Sarcoidosis ➢ Cystic fibrosis ➢ Pulmonary AV fistula ➢ Interstitial lung diseases **Cardiovascular:** ➢ Infective endocarditis ➢ Cyanotic congenial heart diseases, atrial myxoma, and Eisenmenger's syndrome **Gastrointestinal:** ➢ Inflammatory bowel disease (ulcerative colitis and Crohn's disease) ➢ Primary biliary cirrhosis ➢ Hepatoma	**Miscellaneous:** ➢ Hereditary, idiopathic (pachydermoperiostosis or Touraine–Solente–Gole syndrome) ➢ Unidigital clubbing occurs in repeated trauma **Unilateral clubbing:** ➢ Hemiplegia (long standing) ➢ Vascular disease – *Aneurysm:* Subclavian artery, brachiocephalic trunk – Pre-subclavian coarctation of aorta (left-sided clubbing) – Pancoast tumor – Unilateral erythromelalgia – AV fistula used for hemodialysis – Infected arterial graft

Primary hypertrophic osteoarthropathy (PHO) is a rare hereditary disorder with digital clubbing, subperiosteal new bone formation, and arthropathy. It is associated with mutations in the 15-hydroxyprostaglandin dehydrogenase (15-PGDH).

Box 6.2: Various methods of eliciting the signs of clubbing.

1. Lovibond's profile sign (**Fig. 6.2A**)
2. Curth's modified profile sign (**Fig. 6.2B**)
3. Fluctuation test
4. Schamroth's window test (**Fig. 6.2C**)
5. Phalangeal depth ratio

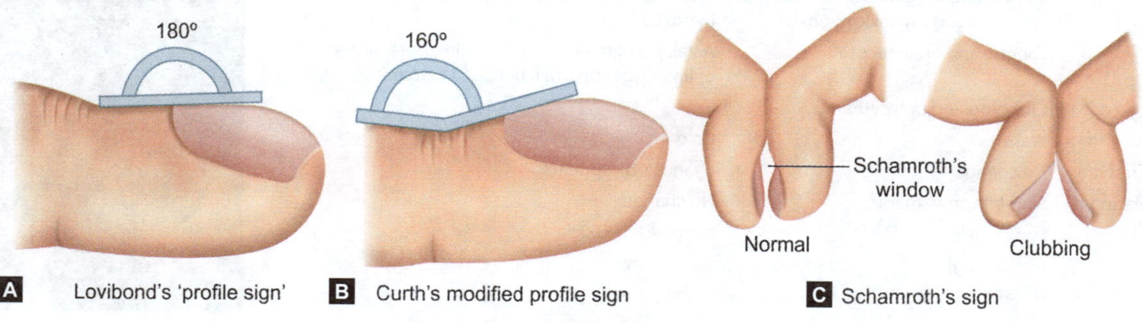

FIGS. 6.2A TO C: Various signs of clubbing.

ABNORMALITIES IN NAILS DUE TO SYSTEMIC DISEASES (TABLE 6.6)

Q. Write short note/essay on abnormalities in nails due to systemic diseases.

TABLE 6.6: Abnormalities in nails due to systemic diseases.

Abnormality and description	*Associated systemic disease*
SHAPE OR GROWTH CHANGE	
➤ **Clubbing**	➤ Discussed above (**Table 6.5**)
➤ **Koilonychia:** Spoon-shaped nails (transverse and longitudinal concavity)	➤ Iron deficiency anemia, rarely in hemochromatosis, Raynaud's disease, SLE, hypothyroidism, or hyperthyroidism
➤ **Pitting:** Punctate depressions in nails	➤ Psoriasis, Reiter's syndrome, pemphigus, lichen planus, alopecia areata, and rheumatoid arthritis
➤ **Onycholysis:** Distal nail plate separated from nail bed and white discoloration of the affected part of the nail	➤ Psoriasis, local infection, hyperthyroidism, sarcoidosis, trauma, amyloidosis, connective tissue disorders, and pellagra
➤ **Beau's lines:** Transverse linear depressions over nails, move distally with the growth of nail	➤ Any severe systemic illness that disrupts nail growth, Raynaud's disease, pemphigus, and trauma
➤ **Onychomadesis:** Proximal separation of nail plate from nail bed	➤ Trauma, drug sensitivity, poor nutrition, pemphigus vulgaris, and Kawasaki disease
➤ **Yellow nails:** Nail has a "heaped-up" or thickened appearance, yellow in color, with obliteration of lunula	➤ Lymphedema, pleural effusion, immunodeficiency, bronchiectasis, sinusitis, rheumatoid arthritis, nephrotic syndrome, thyroiditis, tuberculosis, and Raynaud's disease
COLOR CHANGE	
➤ **Terry's (white) nails:** Most of the nail plate turns white with obliteration of lunula, uniformly affects all nails	➤ Liver failure, cirrhosis, diabetes mellitus, CHF, hyperthyroidism, and malnutrition
➤ **Half-and-half nails (Lindsay's nails):** Proximal portion of nail bed is white because of nail-bed edema (half-brown and half-white appearance)	➤ Renal failure, HIV infection, and Crohn's disease
➤ **Azure lunula (blue nails)**	➤ Hepatolenticular degeneration (Wilson's disease), silver poisoning, and quinacrine therapy
➤ **Mees' lines:** Transverse white bands affecting multiple nails, move distally with nail growth	➤ Arsenic poisoning, Hodgkin's lymphoma, CHF, leprosy, malaria, chemotherapy
➤ **Muehrcke's lines:** Pairs of transverse white lines that disappear on applying pressure, do not move with growth of nail	➤ Specific for hypoalbuminemia of any cause
➤ **Dark longitudinal streaks**	➤ Melanoma, benign nevus, chemical staining, and normal variant in darkly pigmented people
➤ **Splinter hemorrhage:** Longitudinal, thin, reddish lines occurring beneath the nail plate	➤ Subacute bacterial endocarditis, SLE, rheumatoid arthritis, peptic ulcer disease, malignancies, oral contraceptive use, pregnancy, psoriasis, and trauma
➤ **Telangiectasia:** Irregular, twisted, and dilated vessels at the distal portion of cuticle covering the nail bed	➤ Rheumatoid arthritis, SLE, dermatomyositis, and scleroderma
➤ **Longitudinal striations**	➤ Alopecia areata, vitiligo, atopic dermatitis, and psoriasis

CYANOSIS (FIG. 6.3)

Definition: Bluish discoloration of the skin and mucous membrane. It results from an increased concentration of reduced hemoglobin/**deoxyhemoglobin (>5 g/dL)** or abnormal hemoglobin derivatives (e.g., methemoglobin, sulfhemoglobin, etc.) in the capillary blood perfusing the area. Cyanosis is normally detected when the oxygen saturation (SaO_2) is <85%.

Types of Cyanosis (Table 6.7)

TABLE 6.7: Types of cyanosis and difference between them.

Features	*Central cyanosis*	*Peripheral cyanosis*
Mechanism	Inadequate oxygenation of systemic arterial blood (hypoxic hypoxia)	Sluggish peripheral circulation (stagnant hypoxia)
Sites to look	Tongue and oral mucosa	Acral: Tip of the nose, ear lobules, outer aspect of lips, finger tips, nail bed, and extremities
Associations	Clubbing and polycythemia	
Extremities	Warm	Cold
Warming extremities	No change	Cyanosis disappears
Oxygen inhalation	Slight improvement	No change
ABG PaO_2	Low: <85%	Normal: 85–100%
Pulse volume	May be high	Usually low
Dyspnea	Usually present	Usually absent
Exercise	Worsens	May improve

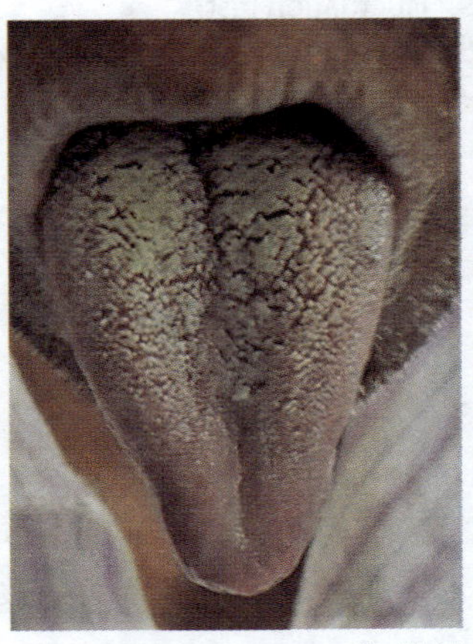

FIG. 6.3: Cyanosis characterized by bluish discoloration of mucous membrane of tongue.

Causes of Cyanosis

Central Cyanosis

- **Cardiac:**
  - Congenital cyanotic heart diseases (*Remember 5 'T's and 2 'E's*): Transposition of great arteries, tetralogy of Fallot, truncus arteriosus, tricuspid valve abnormalities, total anomalous pulmonary venous return (TAPVR), Eisenmenger's syndrome (cyanosis tardive), and Ebstein's anomaly.
  - Acute pulmonary edema (due to left-sided heart failure)
- **Pulmonary:** Acute severe asthma, chronic obstructive pulmonary disease (COPD), cor pulmonale, respiratory failure, respiratory depression, lobar and bronchopneumonia, tension pneumothorax, acute laryngeal edema, and acute pulmonary embolism
- **High altitude** (due to low partial pressure of oxygen)
- **Polycythemia**
- **Enterogenous or pigment cyanosis:** Methemoglobinemia and sulfhemoglobinemia

Peripheral Cyanosis

- **Low-cardiac output:** Congestive heart failure
- **Local vasoconstriction:** Cold, frostbite, Raynaud's phenomenon, and shock
- **Arterial obstruction:** Peripheral vascular diseases (atherosclerosis and Buerger's disease)
- **Venous obstruction:** Superior vena caval syndrome
- **Hyperviscosity syndrome:** Multiple myeloma, polycythemia, and macroglobulinemia
- **Others:** Cryoglobulinemia and mitral stenosis.

Mixed Cyanosis

- All causes of central cyanosis may also cause peripheral cyanosis
- Cardiogenic shock with pulmonary edema
- Congestive cardiac failure due to left-sided heart failure
- Polycythemia (rarely).

Differential cyanosis: Cyanosis only in lower limbs seen in PDA with reversal of shunt

Cyanosis only in upper limbs (reverse differential cyanosis): Coarctation of aorta (ductal type) with transposition of great arteries

Cyanosis in left upper limb and both lower limbs: PDA with reversal of shunt and preductal coarctation of aorta

Intermittent cyanosis: Ebstein's anomaly

Cyclical cyanosis: Bilateral choanal atresia

Orthocyanosis: Development of cyanosis only in upright position due to hypoxia occurring in erect posture. It is seen in pulmonary arteriovenous malformation.

Cyanosis absent despite of sufficient reduced hemoglobin: In severe anemia, carbon monoxide poisoning.

Hyperoxia test (cardiac vs. pulmonary cyanosis): After giving 100% oxygen for 10 minutes, a repeat ABG is done and if PaO_2 is <150 mm Hg then the cause is cardiac and if the PaO_2 improves to >200 mm Hg, the cause is respiratory.

Pseudocyanosis: Caused by metals (gold, silver, mercury, and arsenic) and drugs (minocycline, phenothiazines, chloroquine, and amiodarone)

RESPIRATORY (PULMONARY) FUNCTION TESTS (TABLE 6.8)

Q. Write short note on pulmonary function tests and give their clinical significance.

Q. Write short note on FEV_1 (forced expiratory volume in 1 second).

Abbreviations used in pulmonary function tests are presented in **Table 6.9**.

TABLE 6.8: Pulmonary function test (PFT).

PFT tracings have:
- **Four lung volumes:** Tidal volume, inspiratory reserve volume, expiratory reserve volume, and residual volume
- **Five capacities:** Inspiratory capacity, expiratory capacity, vital capacity, functional residual capacity, and total lung capacity
- Flow–volume curves
- Blood gases and pulse oximetry
- Transfer factor (diffusion)
- Exercise tests
- Exhaled nitric oxide

TABLE 6.9: Abbreviations used in pulmonary function tests.

Abbreviations	*Explanation*
FVC (forced vital capacity)	Volume of air expired with a maximal effort after deep inspiration
FEV_1 (forced expiratory volume in 1 second)	Volume of air expired in the first second after deep inspiration
VC (vital capacity)	Maximum amount of air that can be expelled from the lungs after the deepest possible breath TLC minus RV or maximum volume of air exhaled from maximal inspiratory level (60–70 mL/kg) (3,100–4,800 mL). VC decreases with age

Contd...

Contd...

PEF (peak expiratory flow)	Volume of forcibly expired air during the first 10 seconds after deep inspiration
TLC (total lung capacity)	Sum of all volume compartments or volume of air in lungs after maximum inspiration (4–6 L)
FRC (functional residual capacity)	Sum of RV and ERV or the volume of air in the lungs at end-expiratory tidal position (30–35 mL/kg) (2,300–3,300 mL) measured with multiple-breath closed-circuit helium dilution, multiple-breath open-circuit nitrogen washout, or body plethysmography. It cannot be measured by spirometry
RV (residual volume)	Volume of air remaining in lungs after maximum exhalation (20–25 mL/kg) (1,700–2,100 mL), indirectly measured (FRC-ERV), it cannot be measured by spirometry. RV increases with age
IRV (inspiratory reserve volume)	Maximum volume of air inhaled from the end-inspiratory tidal position (1,900–3,300 mL)
ERV (expiratory reserve volume)	Maximum volume of air that can be exhaled from resting end-expiratory tidal position (700–1,000 mL)
TV (tidal volume)	Volume of air inhaled or exhaled with each breath during quiet breathing (6–8 mL/kg)
IC (inspiratory capacity)	Sum of IRV and TV or the maximum volume of air that can be inhaled from the end-expiratory tidal position (2,400–3,800 mL)
EC (expiratory capacity)	TV + ERV
DLCO (diffusing capacity of lung for carbon monoxide)	Also known as transfer factor, DLCO measures the transfer of inhaled gases into the pulmonary capillaries

Measurement of Airway Obstruction (Fig. 6.4)

Ventilatory Capacity

Ventilatory capacity includes **FEV$_1$** (volume of air expired in the first second after deep inspiration) and **FVC** (volume of air expired with a maximal effort after deep inspiration) and **PEF** (peak expiratory flow rate).

Normally, FEV$_1$/FVC ratio is around 75%.

Patterns of Abnormalities

- **Obstructive ventilatory defect:** It is characterized by narrowing of airways during expiration (e.g., bronchial asthma, chronic bronchitis, and emphysema). These disorders show **markedly reduced FEV$_1$, reduced or normal VC, and reduced FEV$_1$/VC.** In airflow limitation, the FEV$_1$ is reduced as a percentage of FVC. With increasing airflow limitation, FEV falls proportionately more than FVC, so the FEV$_1$/FVC ratio is reduced.
  - **Reversibility of airflow limitation:** When FEV$_1$ is disproportionately reduced, resulting in FEV$_1$/FVC ratio of less than 70%, spirometry should be repeated following inhaled short-acting β_2-adrenoceptor agonists (e.g., salbutamol). A large improvement in FEV$_1$ (over 400 mL) is seen in bronchial asthma and to some extent in chronic bronchitis.
- **Restrictive ventilatory defect:** In restrictive lung disease, **FEV$_1$ and FVC are reduced proportionately and the FEV$_1$/FVC ratio may be normal** or may even increase because of enhanced elastic recoil. This pattern is seen in interstitial inflammation and/or fibrosis that lead to progressive loss of lung volume.

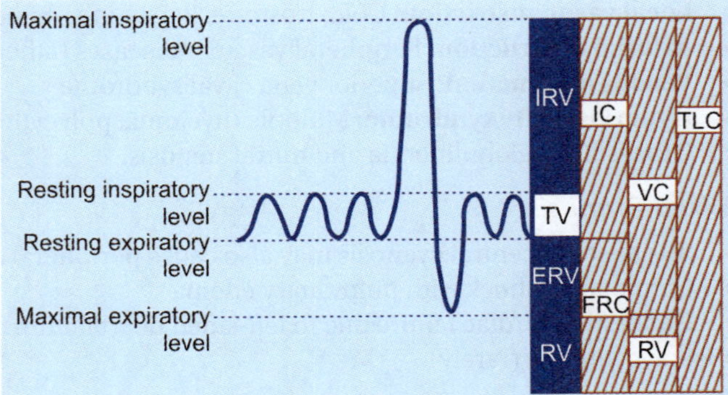

FIG. 6.4: Diagrammatic representation of various lung volume measurements. (TLC: total lung capacity; VC: vital capacity; RV: residual volume; IC: inspiratory capacity; FRC: functional residual capacity; IRV: inspiratory reserve volume; TV: tidal volume; ERV: expiratory reserve volume; RV: residual volume)

Peak Expiratory Flow Rate (PEFR)

Peak flow meters are cheap and simpler than spirometer. Patient is asked to take a full inspiration to total lung capacity and then blow out forcefully into the peak flow meter. PEFR measures the volume of forcibly expired air during the first 10 seconds after deep inspiration. Reduced values are found in airflow obstruction and are not useful in assessing restrictive ventilatory defect. It is mainly useful for diagnosis, to monitor exacerbations and response, and for treatment in asthma.

Lung Volumes

Lung volumes include total lung capacity (TLC) and residual volume (RV). Both can be measured by spirometry.

Total lung capacity (TLC) is the total amount of air in the lungs after taking the deepest breath possible.

Vital capacity (VC) is the maximum amount of air that can be expelled from the lungs after the deepest possible breath and is recorded separately. Patient is asked to make a full but unhurried ("relaxed") exhalation into the spirometer.

Residual volume (RV) is the volume of air in the lungs at the end of full expiration. It is calculated by subtracting the VC (vital capacity) from the TLC (total lung capacity).

Interpretation

- In obstructive lung disease, both TLC and RV are increased.
- In restrictive lung diseases (due to parenchymal lung disease), both TLC and RV are reduced.
- In extraparenchymal diseases with restriction during both inspiration and expiration (ankylosing spondylitis and kyphoscoliosis), RV is increased while TLC is reduced.

Flow–volume Loops (Table 6.10 and Fig. 6.5)

Flow-volume loops measure flow rates against expired volume and show the site of airflow limitation (obstruction) within the lung. At the start of expiration from TLC, maximum resistance is from the large airways. This affects the flow rate for the first 25% of the curve. As air is exhaled, lung volume reduces, and the flow rate depends on the resistance offered by smaller airways.

TABLE 6.10: Flow–volume loops in various disorders.

Disease states	*FVC*	*FEV_1*	*FEV_1/FVC*
Obstructive	Normal	Reduced	Reduced
Stiff lungs	Reduced	Reduced	Normal
Respiratory muscle weakness	Reduced	Reduced	Normal

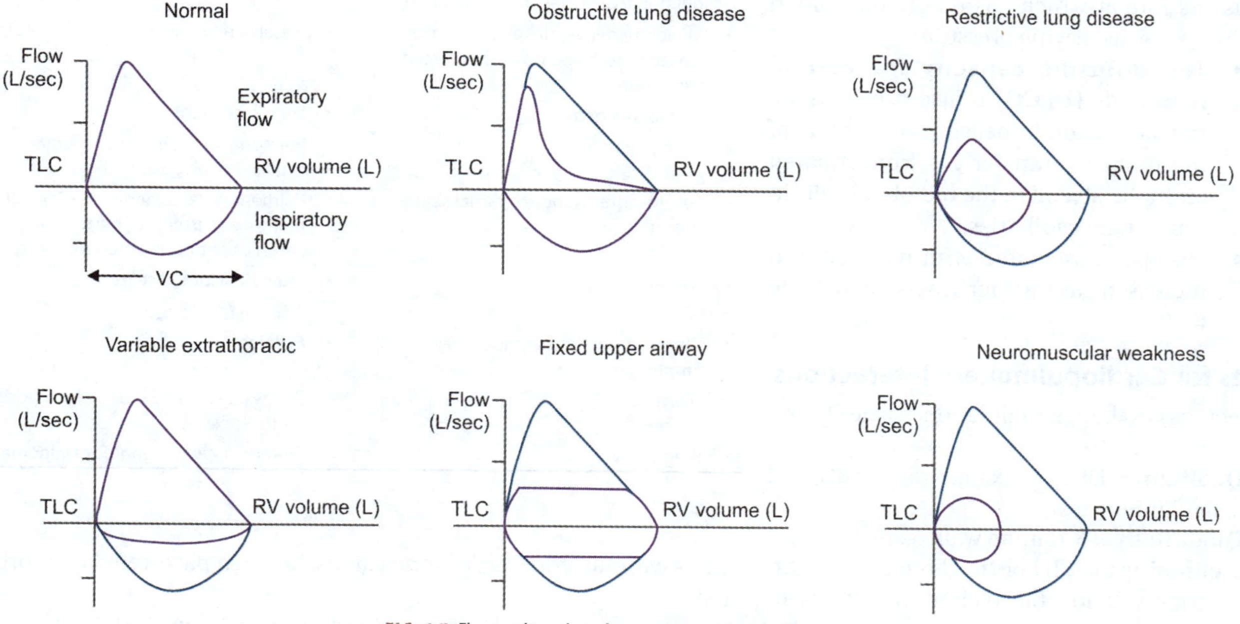

FIG. 6.5: Flow–volume loop for common respiratory diseases.

- **FEV_1** is the volume exhaled during the first second of the FVC maneuver. **It is decreased in both obstructive and restrictive lung disorders.**
- FEF 25–75% is the mean expiratory flow during the middle half of the FVC maneuver; it reflects flow through the small (<2 mm in diameter) airways.
- Interpretation of percent predicted: Normal (>79%), mild obstruction (60–79%), moderate obstruction (40–59%), severe obstruction (<40%).
- **FEV_1/FVC** is the ratio of FEV_1 to FVC × 100 (expressed as a percent); it is an important value because a reduction of this ratio from expected values is specific for obstructive rather than restrictive diseases. Normal value (FEV_1/FVC) is 75–85%, <70% of predicted value in mild obstruction, <60% of predicted value in moderate obstruction, and <50% of predicted value in severe obstruction.

Spirometry interpretation: Obstructive versus restrictive defect (**Table 6.11**)

TABLE 6.11: Spirometry interpretation—obstructive versus restrictive defect.

Obstructive disorders	*Restrictive disorders*
Limitation of expiratory airflow as airways cannot empty as rapidly compared to normal (e.g., narrowed airways from bronchospasm, inflammation, etc.)	Characterized by reduced lung volumes/decreased lung compliance
➢ FVC normal or ↓	➢ FVC ↓ (significantly decreased)
➢ FEV_1 ↓ (significantly decreased)	➢ FEV_1 ↓
➢ FEF 25–75% ↓	➢ FEF 25–75% normal to ↓
➢ FEV_1/FVC ↓ (<0.7)	➢ FEV_1/FVC normal to ↑ (>0.7)
➢ TLC normal or ↑	➢ TLC ↓
Examples: Asthma, emphysema, and cystic fibrosis	Examples: Interstitial fibrosis, scoliosis, obesity, lung resection, neuromuscular diseases, and cystic fibrosis

Arterial blood gases (ABG) and oximetry (*Refer* Table 6.1)

These tests include measurement of: (i) hydrogen ion (H^+) concentration, (ii) PaO_2 and $PaCO_2$, and (iii) oxygen saturation and bicarbonate concentration (derived from the above values) in an arterial blood. These are performed by automatic analyzers.

Uses: (1) To assess the degree and type of respiratory failure and (2) for measuring acid-based status.

Tests for Gas Exchange Function

a. Alveolar-arterial O_2 tension gradient:

- Sensitive indicator of detecting regional V/Q inequality
- It is the difference between the amount of the oxygen in the alveoli [i.e., the alveolar oxygen tension (PaO_2)] and the amount of oxygen dissolved in the plasma (PaO_2).

b. **Dyspnea differentiation index (DDI):**
- To differentiate dyspnea due to respiratory/cardiac diseases

$$DDI = \frac{PEFR \times PaCO_2}{1000}$$

- DDI—lower in respiratory pathology

c. **Diffusing capacity of lung (DL):** Defined as the rate at which gas enters into blood divided by its driving pressure.
- The **diffusing capacity for carbon monoxide (DLCO)** is also known as the transfer factor. It measures the ability of the lungs to transfer gas from inhaled air in the alveoli to the red blood cells in pulmonary capillaries.
- Diseases associated with reduced and increased gas transfer are listed in **Table 6.12**.

TABLE 6.12: Diseases associated with reduced and increased diffusing capacity for carbon monoxide (DLCO).

Increased DLCO [blood flow is in excess of ventilation (a low VQ—SHUNT—"wasted blood")]	*Reduced DLCO [ventilation is in excess of blood flow (a high VQ—DEAD SPACE—"wasted air")]*
➢ Exercise (due to recruitment of capillaries)	➢ Postexercise
➢ Supine position (due to increased pulmonary capillary blood volume)	➢ Standing
➢ Müller maneuver (inspiration against closed mouth and nose after forced expiration)	➢ Valsalva maneuver
➢ Pulmonary hemorrhage	➢ Lung resection
➢ Polycythemia	➢ Pulmonary emphysema (affecting capillary or alveolar bed)
➢ Left-to-right shunt (e.g., atrial septal defect)	➢ Pulmonary vascular disease, including pulmonary arterial hypertension and chronic venous thromboembolism
➢ Obesity	➢ Interstitial lung diseases
➢ Asthma	➢ Anemia
➢ Chronic bronchitis without major emphysema	➢ Evening
➢ Morning	➢ Drugs (e.g., amiodarone, bleomycin, methotrexate)
➢ Pregnancy	➢ Pulmonary lymphangitic carcinomatosis

Tests for Cardiopulmonary Interactions

Reflects gas exchange, ventilation, tissue O_2, and CO_2

- **Qualitative:** History, examination, ABG, and stair climbing test
- **Quantitative:** 6-minute walk test

Stair climbing test: If able to climb three flights of stairs without stopping/dyspnea at his/her own pace-reduced morbidity and mortality. If not able to climb two flights, high-risk.

6-minute walk test: Gold standard. Cardiopulmonary reserve is measured by estimating maximum O_2 uptake (VO_2 maximum) during exercise. Modified, if patient cannot walk—bicycle/arm exercises. If patient is able to walk for >2,000 feet during 6-minute period, VO_2 maximum >15 mL/kg/min, if 1,080 feet in 1 min, VO_2 of 12 mL/kg/min. Simultaneously, oximetry is done and if SpO_2 falls >4%, high-risk.

Exhaled Nitric Oxide

- Nitric oxide is produced by the bronchial epithelium. Its production increases in asthma and other diseases associated with inflammation of airway.
- Measurement of exhaled NO may be helpful in asthma that is difficult to control. Measuring **fractional exhaled nitric oxide** (FeNO) helps to identify patients who are likely to benefit from treatment with corticosteroids. FeNO also predicts the likelihood of steroid responsiveness more consistently than spirometry, bronchodilator response, peak flow variation, or airway hyper-responsiveness to methacholine. A FeNO greater than 50 ppb in adults or greater than 35 ppb in children suggests eosinophilic airway inflammation.

BRONCHIAL ASTHMA

Q. Define and classify bronchial asthma. Discuss the etiology, pathophysiology, clinical features, investigations, diagnosis, complications, and management/treatment of bronchial asthma.

Definition

Asthma is a **chronic inflammatory disorder** of the airways (bronchial tree) in which **breathing is periodically rendered difficult** by **widespread narrowing of the bronchi** (reversible bronchoconstriction).

It is **clinically characterized by recurrent episodes** (paroxysms) **of wheezing, breathlessness** (dyspnea)**, tightness of the chest, and cough.**

Global Initiative for Asthma (GINA)—2015 Definition of Asthma

"Asthma is a heterogeneous disease, usually characterized by chronic airway inflammation. It is defined by the history of respiratory symptoms such as wheeze, shortness of breath, chest tightness, and cough that vary over time and in intensity, together with variable expiratory airflow limitation." *These episodes are usually associated with widespread but variable airflow obstruction that is often reversible either spontaneously or with treatment.*

Characteristics of Asthma

1. **Airflow narrowing:** It is due to combination of muscle edema and viscid bronchial secretion. It is generally reversible spontaneously or with treatment.
2. **Airway hyper-reactivity (AHR)/bronchial hyper-responsiveness (BHR):** It is characterized by increased tendency for airway (tracheobronchial tree) narrowing in response to triggers (stimuli) that have little or no effect in normal individuals.
3. **Bronchial inflammation:** Inflammation of the bronchial walls by T lymphocytes, mast cells, eosinophils with associated plasma exudation, edema, smooth muscle hypertrophy, mucus plugging, and epithelial damage.

Classification (Flowchart 6.1)

FLOWCHART 6.1: Classification of asthma.

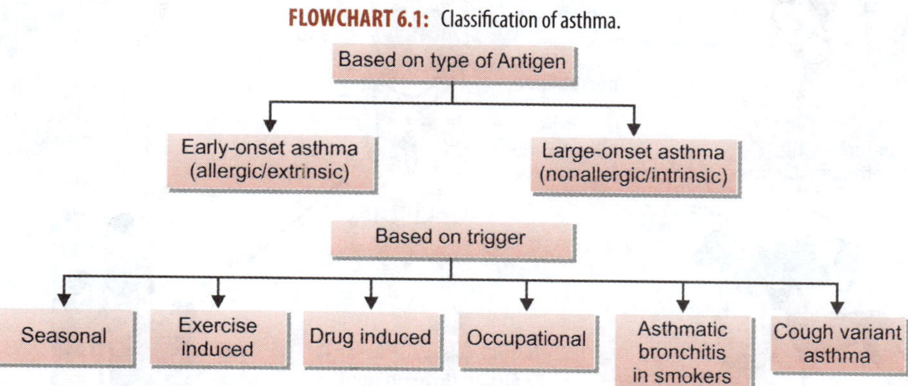

Q. How will you differentiate early-onset (atopic) asthma from late-onset (non-atopic) asthma?

Differentiating features of early-onset asthma and late-onset asthma are presented in **Table 6.13**.

TABLE 6.13: Differentiating features of early-onset asthma and late-onset asthma.

Features	*Early-onset (atopic) asthma*	*Late-onset (nonatopic) asthma*
Onset	Early age (usually begins in childhood)	Late age
Individuals	Atopic individuals	Nonatopic individuals
Role of external allergens	Have strong role	No role
Family history	Positive history of asthma or allergic diseases (e.g., eczema, urticaria, or hay fever)	Less common or absent
Triggering events	Environmental allergens (e.g., dusts, pollens, animal dander, and foods)	Respiratory infections due to viruses (e.g., rhinovirus and parainfluenza virus) Inhaled air pollutants (e.g., smoke and fumes)
Serum level of IgE	Increased	Normal
Skin hypersensitivity test to common inhalant allergens	Positive	Negative
Response to provocation tests	Positive	Negative

Risk Factors and Triggers (Table 6.14)

Risk Factors (Fig. 6.6)

Endogenous factors

- **Genetic predisposition:** Major etiological factor in atopic asthma is genetic predisposition to **type I hypersensitivity (atopy) reaction** and exposure to environmental trigger. One of the **susceptibility loci is on the chromosome 5 (5q)** → several genes involved in regulation of IgE synthesis and mast cell and eosinophil growth and differentiation.
- **Atopy:** Atopic individuals tend to **have higher serum IgE levels**, and a positive family history of allergy is found in 50% of atopic individuals. Patients with asthma commonly suffer from other atopic diseases (e.g., allergic rhinitis and atopic dermatitis/eczema).
- **Airway hyper-responsiveness:** It is an abnormality in which there is an **excessive tendency for airways to contract** (bronchoconstrictor) too easily in response to multiple inhaled triggers that usually do not have any effect on normal individuals
- **Gender and age:** More common in boys than girls and, after puberty, women slightly more commonly than men. Most cases **begin before the age of 25 years**.

Environmental factors

Hygiene hypothesis proposes that individuals with **lack of infections in early childhood** are more prone to asthma than children brought up on farms who are exposed to a high level of endotoxin. Intestinal parasite infection may

TABLE 6.14: Risk factors and triggers involved in asthma.

Risk factors	
Endogenous factors ➢ Genetic predisposition ➢ Atopy ➢ Airway hyper-responsiveness ➢ Gender and age ➢ Ethnicity ➢ Obesity ➢ Early viral infections	**Environmental factors** ➢ Allergens (indoor/outdoor) ➢ Occupational sensitizers ➢ Respiratory infections
Triggers	
➢ Inhaled allergens ➢ Upper respiratory tract viral infections ➢ Air pollution (e.g. sulfur dioxide, irritant gases) ➢ Passive smoking (tobacco smoke)	➢ Drugs (β-blockers and aspirin) ➢ *Physical factors:* Exercise, cold air, and hyperventilation ➢ Emotional stress ➢ Irritants (household sprays paint fumes)

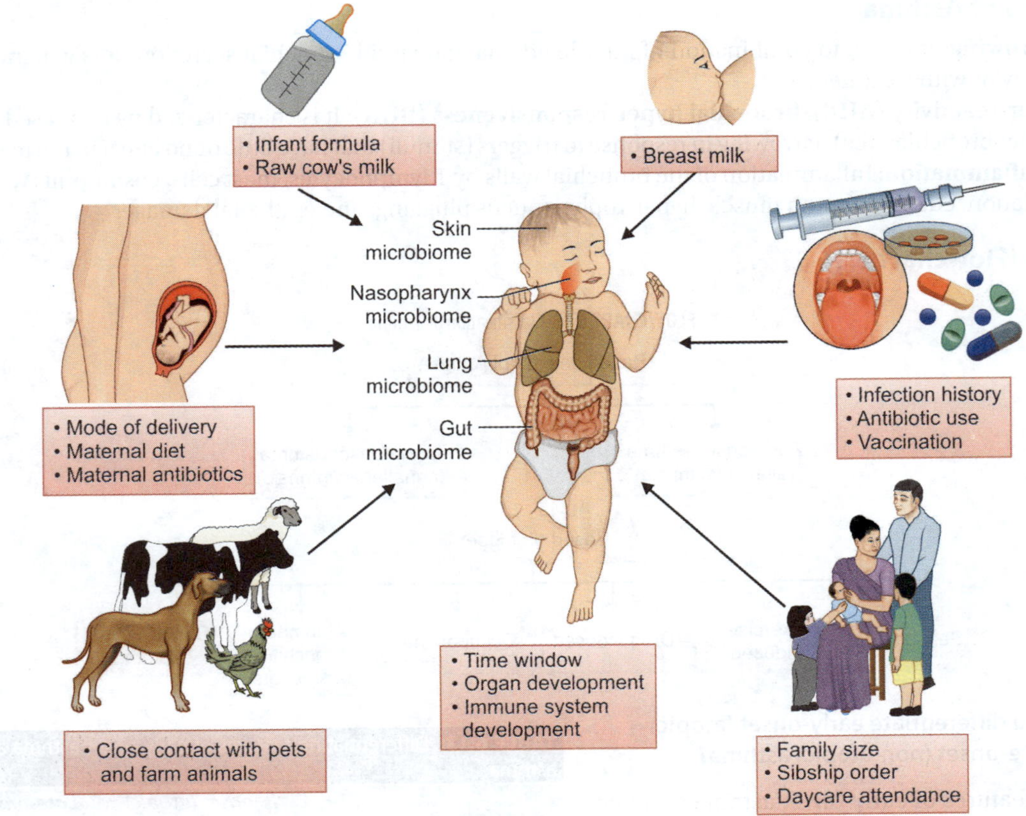

FIG. 6.6: Risk factors for asthma.

also be associated with a decreased risk of asthma. Conversely, early childhood in a "dirtier" environment (exposure to inhaled and ingested products of microorganisms) may allow the immune system to avoid developing allergic responses.

Pathogenesis (Pathophysiology) of Asthma

A. Airway Inflammation

- **Inflammation** is chronic and involves many cell types and inflammatory mediators **(Fig. 6.7)**.
- **Strong T_H2 response: Genetic predisposition** with susceptibility genes makes individuals prone to develop **strong T_H2** (type of T lymphocytes) **reactions against environmental antigens** (allergens).
- **T_H2 cells secrete cytokines,** which promote allergic inflammation and **stimulate B-cells to produce IgE.**

Cells involved in the inflammatory response

Important cells involved in asthma are—**mast cells, eosinophils, dendritic cells (macrophages), and lymphocytes.**

1. Mast cells:
   - **Early reaction** is characterized by **bronchoconstriction, increased mucus production,** and **vasodilation with increased vascular permeability** (causes edema).
   - **Late phase reaction:** It is characterized by **inflammation and airway remodeling.**
2. Eosinophils:
   - **Mediators released from eosinophils:** LTC_4 and basic proteins such as major basic protein (MBP), eosinophil cationic protein (ECP), and eosinophils peroxidase (EPX). They are toxic to epithelial cells.
   - Corticosteroid rapidly decreases the number and reduces the activation of eosinophils.

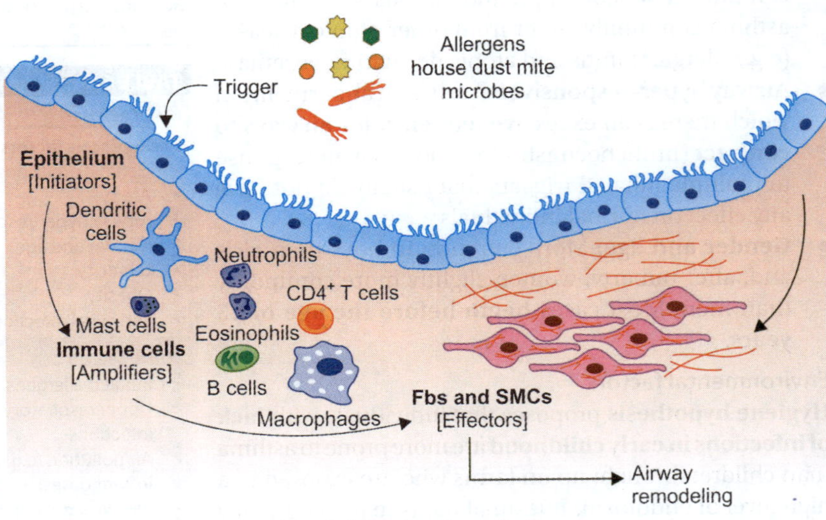

FIG. 6.7: Cells and mediators of asthma.

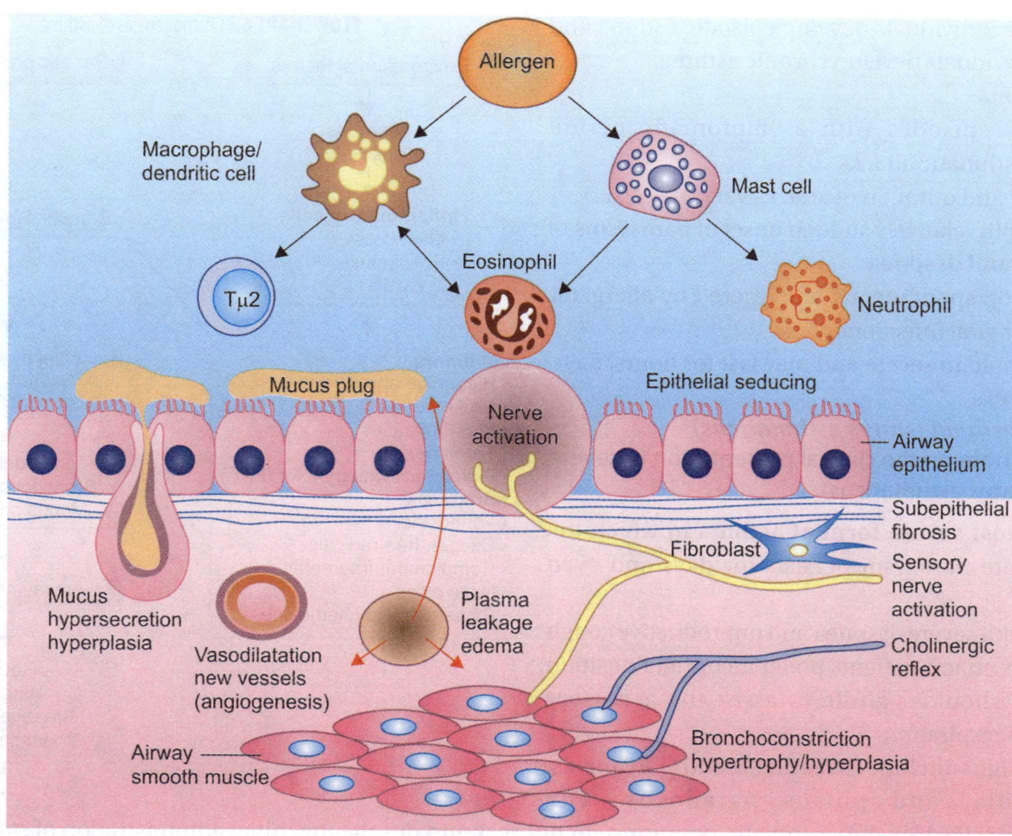

FIG. 6.8: Pathogenesis of asthma.

- Sputum eosinophilia is of diagnostic help and is a biomarker of response to therapy.

3. Dendritic cells and lymphocytes

They release prostaglandin, thromboxane, LTC_4, LTB_4, and platelet-activating factor (PAF).

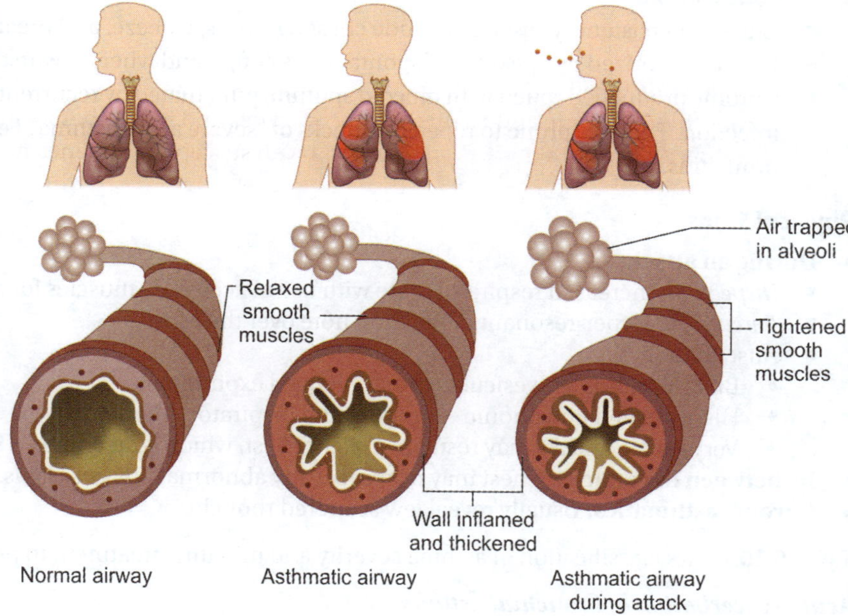

FIG. 6.9: Pathology of asthma.

B. Airway Remodeling

Airway remodeling is the **group of structural** and **functional changes in the bronchial wall due to repeated bouts of inflammation** observed in chronic asthma.

- An **increase in size and number** (hypertrophy/hyperplasia) of the **submucosal glands**
- **Hypertrophy and/or hyperplasia of the bronchial wall smooth muscle**
- **Increased vascularity**
- **Deposition of subepithelial collagen** accompanied by fibrosis and thickening of the basement membrane.

Pathogenesis of asthma is summarized in **Figure 6.8** and **Flowchart 6.2.**

Clinical Features

Q. Write a short note on the clinical presentation of severe acute asthma (status asthmaticus).

- Clinical features are divided into three headings—namely (1) episodic, (2) severe acute (status asthmaticus), and (3) chronic asthma.

- Usually, atopic individuals develop episodic asthma and nonatopic individuals develop chronic asthma.

1. ***Episodic asthma***
   - Occurs as episodes with asymptomatic period between asthmatic attacks
   - Frequency and duration of attacks vary
   - Presents with relatively sudden onset of paroxysms of **wheezing and dyspnea**
   - May develop spontaneous or triggered by allergens, exercise, or viral infections
   - It may be mild to severe and may last for hours, days, or even weeks
2. ***Severe acute asthma (status asthmaticus)***

Q. Write a short note on the clinical presentation of severe acute asthma (status asthmaticus).

   - It is the **most severe form of asthma** in which the severe acute paroxysm persists for days and even weeks.
   - Presents with severe dyspnea and unproductive cough
   - During this attack, patients prefer an upright position fixing the shoulder girdle to assist the accessory muscles of respiration.
   - Physical signs include sweating, central cyanosis, tachycardia, and pulsus paradoxus. The **bronchoconstriction** and asthmatic symptoms **do not respond** despite the initial administration of standard **acute asthma therapy**.
   - It may cause **severe airflow obstruction leading to severe cyanosis and even death**.

FLOWCHART 6.2: Pathogenesis of asthma.

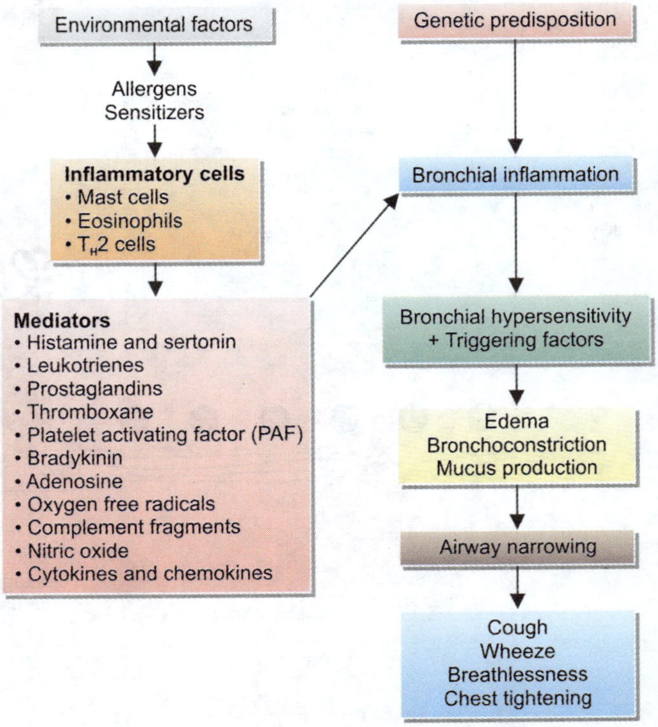

Environmental factors
Allergens
Sensitizers
Inflammatory cells
• Mast cells
• Eosinophils
• T_H2 cells
Mediators
• Histamine and sertonin
• Leukotrienes
• Prostaglandins
• Thromboxane
• Platelet activating factor (PAF)
• Bradykinin
• Adenosine
• Oxygen free radicals
• Complement fragments
• Nitric oxide
• Cytokines and chemokines
Genetic predisposition
Bronchial inflammation
Bronchial hypersensitivity + Triggering factors
Edema
Bronchoconstriction
Mucus production
Airway narrowing
Cough
Wheeze
Breathlessness
Chest tightening

3. ***Chronic asthma***
   - Chronic persistent symptoms include chest tightness, wheeze, and breathlessness on exertion.
   - It is characterized by episodes of spontaneous cough and wheeze, worst during the night.
   - Chronic productive cough with mucoid sputum, punctuated by recurrent attacks of purulent expectoration from frank infection. They are prone to repeated attacks of "severe acute asthma". Features sometimes resemble those of chronic bronchitis.

Physical Signs

- **During an attack:**
  - *Inspection:* Increased respiratory rate with use of accessory muscles for respiration
  - *Percussion:* Hyper-resonant percussion note over the lungs
  - Auscultation
    - Breath sounds are vesicular with prolonged expiration.
    - High-pitched polyphonic expiratory and inspiratory rhonchi
    - Very severe attacks may result in a silent chest, which is an ominous sign.
- **In-between the attacks:** Chest may not reveal any abnormal physical signs.
- **Chronic asthmatics:** Usually reveal few scattered rhonchi.

Table 6.15 shows classification of asthma severity and initiating treatment in persons ≥12 years of age.

Acute exacerbation of bronchial asthma

- Loss of control of any class or variant of asthma
- It is again classified as:
  - *Mild*: The patient is dyspneic, but can complete a sentence in one breath.
  - *Moderate*: The patient is more dyspneic and cannot complete a sentence in one breath.
  - *Severe (severe acute asthma)*: The patient is severely dyspneic, talks in words and may be restless, even unconscious.

Various Causes of Wheeze

See **Box 6.3**.

TABLE 6.15: Classification of asthma severity and initiating treatment in persons ≥12 years of age.

		Classification of Asthma Severity (≥12 years of age)			
			Persistent		
Components of Severity		***Intermittent***	***Mild***	***Moderate***	***Severe***
Impairment Normal FEV_1/FVC: 8–19 years: 85% 20–39 years: 80% 40–59 years: 75% 60–80 years: 70%	Symptoms	≤2 days/week	>2 days/week but not daily	Daily	Throughout the day
	Nighttime awakenings	≤2×/month	3–4×/month	>1/week but not nightly	Often 7×/week
	Short-acting $beta_2$-agonist use for symptom control	≤2 days/week	>2 days/week but not daily, and not more than 1× on any day	Daily	Several times per day
	Interference with normal activity	None	Minor limitation	Some limitation	Extremely limited
	Lung function	➢ Normal FEV_1 between exacerbations ➢ FEV_1 >80% predicted ➢ FEV_1/FVC normal	➢ FEV_1 >80% predicted ➢ FEV_1/FVC normal	➢ FEV_1 >60% but <80% predicted ➢ FEV_1/FVC reduced 5%	➢ FEV_1 <60% predicted ➢ FEV_1/FVC reduced >5%
Risk	Exacerbations requiring oral systemic corticosteroids	0–1/year	← ≥2/years → ← Consider severity and interval since last exacerbation → Frequency and severity may fluctuate over time for patients in any severity category Relative annual risk of exacerbations may be related to FEV_1		
Recommended step for initiating treatment		Step 1	Step 2	Step 3	Step 4 or 5
				and consider short course of oral systemic corticosteroids	
		In 2–6 weeks, evaluate level of asthma control that is achieved and adjust therapy accordingly			

BRITTLE ASTHMA

- Chaotic variations in lung function despite taking appropriate therapy.
- Type 1: Persistent pattern of variability and may require oral corticosteroids, or continuous infusion of β2 agonists.
- Type 2: Has a normal or near-normal lung function but precipitous, unpredictable falls in lung function that may result in death.
- Does not respond well to corticosteroids and does not reverse well with inhaled bronchodilators.

Box 6.3: Various causes (differential diagnosis) of wheeze.

- Bronchial asthma
- Cardiac asthma
- Chronic obstructive lung disease (COPD)
- Recurrent pulmonary emboli
- Systemic vasculitis, including Churg–Strauss syndrome and polyarteritis nodosa
- Carcinoid tumors
- *Others:* Eosinophilic pneumonia, GERD, foreign body aspiration, mediastinal mass, tracheomalacia, and vocal cord dysfunction

Investigations

The diagnosis is mainly clinical and based on a characteristic history. There is no single satisfactory diagnostic test for asthma.

1. ***Lung function tests***

   Pulmonary function tests useful in asthma are FEV_1, VC, and PEFR.
   - **Spirometry:** It is useful, especially in assessing reversibility. Simple spirometry is useful in confirming the airflow limitation with a reduced FEV_1, FEV_1/FVC ratio, and PEF. Asthma can be diagnosed if there **is greater than 15% improvement in FEV_1 or PEFR following the inhalation of a bronchodilator**.
   - **Peak expiratory flow rate (PEFR):** It is useful in demonstrating the variable airflow limitation. PEFR measurements to be done on waking, prior to taking a bronchodilator and before bed after a bronchodilator. The diurnal variation in PEFR of more than 20% (the lowest values typically being recorded in the morning) is considered diagnostic. It also provides good measure of disease severity.
   - *DLCO:* Increased in asthma

   Exercise tests: It is used in the diagnosis of asthma in children. The child is asked to run for 6 minutes on a treadmill (heart rate should be above 160 beats per minute). A negative test does not rule out asthma.

   Airway responsiveness (AHR): AHR is sensitive but nonspecific. **Histamine or methacholine bronchial provocation test:**
   - To detect the presence of airway hyper-responsiveness (a feature of asthma)
   - Useful in patients whom cough is the only/main symptom and is useful in the differential diagnosis of chronic cough.
   - Contraindicated in individuals who have poor lung function (FEV < 1.5 L) or a history of "brittle" asthma.

   Indirect challenge tests are release of endogenous mediators that cause the contraction of airway smooth muscle. These include exercise eucapnic voluntary hyperpnea (EVH), ultrasonically nebulizer hypertonic saline, and dry powder mannitol.

2. ***Imaging***
   - **Chest X-ray:**
     - Usually normal between attacks without any diagnostic features

- During an acute episode or in chronic severe disease, there may be hyperinflated lungs (overinflation).
- It may be helpful in excluding complications such as pneumothorax, lobar collapse (if mucus occludes large bronchus), or in detecting the pulmonary infiltrates associated with allergic bronchopulmonary aspergillosis.

- **High-resolution computed tomography (CT):** It may show areas of bronchiectasis (complication) and thickening of the bronchial walls, but these changes are not diagnostic of asthma.

3. ***Measurement of Allergic Status***
   - **Skin prick tests (SPT):** SPT is performed by intradermal injections of common allergens (house dust mite, cat fur, and grass pollen) and checking the development of a wheal and flare reaction. They are positive in allergic asthma and negative in intrinsic asthma.
   - **Elevated serum IgE levels:** Measurement of total and allergen-specific IgE in serum may be seen.
4. ***Blood and Sputum Tests***
   - Patients with asthma may show increased numbers of eosinophils (eosinophilia) in peripheral blood (>0.4×10^9/L), but sputum eosinophils are a more specific diagnostic finding. Sputum examination may reveal Curschmann's spirals, Creola bodies, and Charcot–Leyden crystals.
   - **Serum periostin** is also a marker of Th2-associated airway inflammation and a better predictor of airway eosinophilia than blood eosinophil counts or FENO.
5. ***Fractional exhaled Nitric Oxide (FENO)***
   It is used as a noninvasive test to measure airway inflammation and as an index of efficacy of corticosteroid response in children (demonstration of insufficient response to anti-inflammatory therapy).
6. ***Trial of Corticosteroids***
   Patients with severe airflow limitation should be given a formal trial of corticosteroids. Prednisolone 30 mg orally/day is given for 2 weeks with lung function measured before and immediately after the course. A substantial improvement in FEV (>15%) confirms the presence of a reversible airflow obstruction and indicates that the administration of inhaled steroids will be beneficial to the patient.
7. ***Arterial blood gas analysis***
   - Hypoxia and hypocarbia during acute attack
   - Hypercarbia during sever acute asthma

TABLE 6.16: Differential diagnosis of asthma.

Disease	*Features*
Chronic obstructive pulmonary disease (COPD)	➢ History of smoking ➢ Less reversible airflow obstruction ➢ Reduced DLCO (diffusing capacity of lung for carbon monoxide)
Bronchiectasis	➢ May be secondary to many disorders ➢ Copious purulent sputum ➢ Computed tomography usually diagnostic
Reactive airways viral syndrome	Transient, usually resolves after several weeks
Rhinosinusitis	➢ Nasal congestion and postnasal drip ➢ Common comorbid illness accompanying asthma
Gastroesophageal reflux disease	Common comorbid illness accompanying asthma
Congestive heart failure	➢ Exertional dyspnea ➢ Moist basilar rales, S_3 gallop, orthopnea, and pink frothy/blood-tinged sputum ➢ Echocardiography is helpful
Laryngeal dysfunction	➢ Stridor ➢ May coexist with asthma
Upper airway obstruction	➢ May exhibit stridor ➢ Flow–volume loop is helpful ➢ Endoscopy diagnostic
Recurrent episodes of bronchospasm	Carcinoid tumors and recurrent pulmonary emboli, Churg–Strauss syndrome

Differential Diagnosis of Asthma (Table 6.16)

Q. Give the differential diagnosis of a 45-year-old male presenting with acute breathlessness.

Differences between bronchial asthma and cardiac asthma are present in **Table 6.17**.

TABLE 6.17: Differences between bronchial asthma and cardiac asthma.

Features	*Bronchial Asthma*	*Cardiac Asthma*
Pathology	Bronchospasm	Pulmonary edema
Age	Young	Elderly (above 50–60 years)
Sex/gender	Both genders	Mostly male
Past history	Of eczema, urticaria (allergy) susceptibility to cold, allergy to pollen, groundnuts, and eggs	No history of allergy, history of left ventricular failure, and right ventricular failure
Family history	Other family members may have similar disease	Hypertension may run in families
Personal history	Highly sensitive individual	Nil
Onset	Acute, usually in early hours of morning or late hours of night	Acute, usually at midnight (very specific) 2–3 hours after sleep
Symptoms		
Dyspnea	Expiratory dyspnea	Both expiratory and inspiratory dyspnea
Expectoration	Scanty and mucoid sputum	Profuse and frothy sputum
Palpitation	Absent	Present
On examination		
Respiratory system	Expiratory wheeze present	Basal crepitations present
Cyanosis	Present during acute severe asthma	Cyanosis present
Pulse rate	May be high	Very high (may be pulsus alternans)
Blood pressure	Normal or slightly more systolic	BP usually high
Heart sounds	Heart sounds are distant	S3, Gallop rhythm may be present

Q. Write short essay/note on:
- **The drugs used in the treatment of chronic bronchial asthma.**
- **Management of acute severe asthma.**
- **List the drugs used for prophylaxis against asthma.**
- **Status asthmaticus.**
- **Long-term complications of asthma.**

Management

Management is discussed under following headings namely:

Avoid Identified Aggravating Factors/Allergens
- This is important in the management of occupational asthma and atopic asthma.
- Avoid causative allergens such as pets, moulds, and certain foodstuffs particularly in childhood.
- If it is due to single allergen, it is easy to reduce or avoid the exposure. However, when multiple allergens are responsible, avoidance is difficult.

Control of Risk Factors Causing Exacerbation

The rapid identification and removal of extrinsic causes of asthma and risk factors that exacerbate asthma should be done.
- Active and passive smoking should be avoided.
- Control, if there is associated rhinitis and GERD (gastroesophageal reflux disease)
- Control obesity
- Individuals intolerant to aspirin should avoid NSAIDs.
- Avoid inadequate use of inhaled corticosteroids.
- Avoid overuse of inhaled short-acting b-agonists (e.g., more than one canister of 200 doses/month).
- Follow proper inhalation techniques.

Desensitization or Immunotherapy

Desensitization is performed by repeated subcutaneous injections of gradually increasing doses of the extracts of allergen(s). However, its benefit is doubtful. GINA, 2017 recommends adding **SLIT (sublingual immunotherapy)** in adult HDM (house dust mite)-sensitive patients with allergic rhinitis who have exacerbations despite ICS treatment, provided FEV-1 is 70% predicted. **Subcutaneous immunotherapy (SCIT)** is also practiced.

Drug Therapy (Table 6.18)

Drug therapy is used to control or suppress clinical manifestations.

The drugs useful in asthma can be divided into bronchodilators (rapidly relieve of symptoms through relaxation of airway smooth muscle), and controllers (inhibit the underlying inflammatory process).

Bronchodilators

1. ***β_2-adrenoreceptor agonists***
   - **β-adrenoreceptor:** There are two types of β-adrenoreceptor namely, β_1 and β_2-adrenoreceptors. β_1-adrenoreceptors are expressed in the heart and β_2-adrenoreceptors are widely expressed in the airways (in bronchial smooth muscles).
   - **β_2-adrenoreceptors agonists** (β_2-agonists) can be divided into **short-acting β_2-agonists** (SABAs) (e.g., salbutamol, levosalbutamol, and terbutaline) and **long-acting β_2-agonists** (LABAs) (e.g., bambuterol, salmeterol, and formoterol).
     - **Catecholamines:** Catecholamines used are adrenaline, isoprenaline, and isoetharine.
       Adrenaline: Most commonly used agent in this group. However, it is not a β_2-selective and produces significant undesirable cardiovascular side effects. The usual dose is 0.3–0.5 mL of a 1:1000 solution administered subcutaneously. It may be repeated thrice at an interval of 20 minutes. They are useful in children.
     - **Salbutamol,** levosalbutamol, **terbutaline, and fenoterol:** These drugs are highly selective for β_2-adrenoreceptors and act predominantly on the respiratory tract.

TABLE 6.18: Drugs useful in asthma.

Relievers	***Controllers***
➢ Short-acting inhaled beta2-agonist bronchodilators (SABA) ➢ Low-dose ICS-formoterol ➢ Short-acting anticholinergics	➢ Inhaled corticosteroids (ICS) ➢ ICS and long-acting beta-2 agonist (LABA), bronchodilator combinations (ICS-LABA) ➢ Leukotriene modifiers ➢ Chromones
Add-on controller medications	
➢ **Long-acting anticholinergic** (at Step 4 or 5 with a history of exacerbations despite ICS ± LABA) - Tiotropium ➢ **Anti-IgE** (with severe allergic asthma uncontrolled on high dose ICS-LABA) - Omalizumab ➢ **Anti-IL5 and anti-IL5R** (severe eosinophilic asthma uncontrolled on high-dose ICS-LABA) - Mepolizumab and reslizumab - Benralizumab ➢ **Anti-IL4R** (severe eosinophilic asthma uncontrolled on high-dose ICS-LABA, or requiring maintenance OCS) - Dupilumab ➢ **Systemic corticosteroids:** - Prednisolone - Hydrocortisone - Methylprednisolone	

- **Powerful and rapidly but short-acting** bronchodilators that relax bronchial smooth muscles
- **Routes of administration:** They are active by inhalation, oral, intravenous, subcutaneous route of administration, but the **preferred route is inhalation**. Inhalation is extremely effective, since, it rapidly decreases airflow obstruction. Intravenous administration has no advantages over inhalation. Other routes of administration are preferably avoided and reserved for selected indications.
- **Dose:**
  - *Salbutamol:* 2–4 mg thrice a day orally or two puffs of 100 μg each as required.
  - *Terbutaline:* 2.5–5 mg thrice a day or two puffs of 100 μg each as required.
  - *Levosalbutamol:* Two puffs of 50 μg each as required.
- **Side effects:** Main untoward effects are tremor and palpitation. Prolonged use of β_2-adrenoreceptor agonists are preferably avoided because they worsen bronchial hyper-responsiveness. Tachycardia, which is less with levosalbutamol compared to salbutamol

- **Bambuterol:** It is a long-acting β_2-adrenoreceptor agonist, which is converted into terbutaline in the body.
  - **Dose:** 10–20 mg once a day, orally
  - **Side effects:** More than with inhaled β-agonists and includes tachycardia, palpitations, and tremors
- **Salmeterol and formoterol:** They are highly selective, potent, and long-acting β_2-adrenoreceptor agonist. They are given once or twice a day by inhalation (either as aerosol or dry powder).
  - *Uses:* Routinely used in place of short-acting β_2-stimulants when the patient requires regular β_2-stimulant therapy. Not to be used as monotherapy but to be used as add-on therapy along with ICS (inhaled corticosteroids) when the response to ICs is suboptimal
  - Salmeterol has a slow onset of action whereas formoterol has a rapid action. Hence, formoterol is suitable for immediate control of symptoms as well.
  - **Dose:**
    - *Salmeterol:* Two puffs of 25 μg each two to three times a day.
    - *Formoterol:* Two puffs of 6 μg each one to three times a day.

Q. Write a short note on action of methylxanthines.

2. **Methylxanthines**

They are of little value as monotherapy but they are beneficial as add-on therapy in patients not controlled with inhaled corticosteroids (ICS). Methylxanthines as an add-on therapy are less effective than long-acting inhaled β_2-agonists.

a. **Theophylline:**
- Theophylline is a medium-potency bronchodilator.
- **Actions:** (i) It improves the movement of airway mucus, (ii) improves diaphragm contractility, and (iii) reduces the release of mediators.
- **Route of administration:** Intravenous, oral, or as suppository. Therapeutic plasma concentrations of theophylline range from 10 to 20 μg/mL. However, the dose required to achieve this concentration varies from patient to patient.
- **Type of preparation:**
  - Acute attacks are treated with short-acting theophylline preparations.
  - For maintenance therapy, long-acting theophylline preparations are used. They are given once or twice a day. Single daily dose in the evening controls nocturnal asthma.
- **Dose:** Usual dose is 100–200 mg (of plain preparation) three times/day, and 300 mg twice/day or 450–600 mg once/day for sustained-release preparation.
- **Side effects:** Nervousness, nausea, vomiting, anorexia, and headache. When plasma levels exceed 30 μg/mL, seizures and cardiac arrhythmias can occur.
- **Precautions:** Theophylline (and aminophylline) clearance is decreased in elderly, liver disease, congestive heart failure, and with concurrent use of erythromycin, allopurinol, and cimetidine. Its clearance is increased with concurrent use of phenobarbitone and phenytoin, and in smokers.

Q. Write short essay/note on adverse effects of and precautions in using aminophylline.

b. **Aminophylline:**
- Aminophylline is a bronchodilator that is effective when given orally, intravenously, and as a suppository. The preferred route of administration is intravenous and may have some role in the management of status asthmaticus (severe acute asthma).
- **Mechanism of action:** Bronchodilator effect is by inhibition of phosphodiesterases in airway smooth-muscle cells, which increase cyclic AMP.
- **Dose:** Loading dose of 5 mg/kg is given slowly intravenously over 20 minutes. This is followed by a maintenance dose of 0.5 mg/kg/h delivered as a continuous intravenous infusion. Patients are already on theophylline; loading dose is preferably withheld or in extreme cases, it is given in a reduced amount at 0.5 mg/kg.
- Rapid infusion of the bolus can lead to sudden death due to cardiac arrhythmias.

c. **Doxophylline (doxofylline):**
- **Mechanism of action:** Bronchodilator effect is by inhibition of phosphodiesterases in airway smooth-muscle cells, which increase cyclic AMP. It has a better safety profile than theophylline. It also inhibits PAF-induced bronchoconstriction and subsequent production of thromboxane A_2.
- **Dose:** 400 mg twice a day.

3. **Anticholinergics:**
- **Antimuscarinic bronchodilators:** They are less effective than β2-agonists in asthma therapy, but may be used as an additional bronchodilator in patients with asthma that is not controlled by inhaled corticosteroids (ICS) and LABA combinations. They may be useful during asthma exacerbations, but are less useful in stable asthma, for example, ipratropium and tiotropium.

Controller Therapies

Q. Write short essay/note on inhaled corticosteroid therapy.

1. **Inhaled corticosteroids (ICS):**
- Inhaled corticosteroids are the most effective controllers for asthma.
- **Mechanism of action:** Corticosteroids are not bronchodilators, but they are the most effective anti-inflammatory agents used in asthma, which reduce number of inflammatory cells as well as their activation in the airways. They decrease bronchial hyper-responsiveness and relieve or prevent airflow obstruction. They also reverse $β_2$-receptor downregulation produced by long-term use of $β_2$-agonists.
- **Uses:** These are beneficial in treating asthma of any severity and age. They are now given as first line of therapy for persistent asthma.
- **Dose:** These are usually given twice daily. Higher doses may be necessary in severe cases.
  - **Beclomethasone dipropionate (200 μg), budesonide (200 μg), or fluticasone (125 μg) is given twice daily as aerosols or dry powder form.**
  - **Ciclesonide is given in a dose of 80–160 μg once a day. Others include flunisolide and mometasone.**
- **Advantages:**
  - **Rapid improvement** of the **symptoms** and **lung function** (within several days).
    - They are effective in preventing asthma symptoms, exercise-induced asthma (EIA), and nocturnal exacerbations and they also prevent severe exacerbations.
    - Early treatment with ICS can prevent irreversible changes in airway function that develops in chronic asthma.
  - **Reduces airway responsiveness** (AHR)
  - Reduces the number of courses of oral corticosteroid therapy (OCS)
- **Side effects:**
  - **Local:** Hoarseness (dysphonia/husky voice) and oropharyngeal candidiasis. These side effects can be minimized by the use of a spacing device along with the metered-dose inhaler and gargling with water after use.
  - **Systemic:** Relatively free from systemic side effects at conventional doses. Long-term use may result in osteoporosis, skin thinning, and adrenal suppression.

2. **Systemic corticosteroids:**

a. **Oral corticosteroids and steroid-sparing agents:**
- **Oral corticosteroids (OCS):** Oral corticosteroids are necessary in patients controlled by inhaled corticosteroids (ICS).
- **Dose:** It should be kept as low as possible to minimize side effects. Prednisolone is started as a single morning dose of 40–60 mg orally/day. Thereafter, the dose is reduced by half every 6 hours. Methylprednisolone is given in a dose of 40–125 mg every 6 hours.
- **Steroid-sparing agents:** Some patients may require continuing treatment with oral corticosteroids. Various immunomodulatory treatments can be used in these patients with severe asthma who have serious side effects with this therapy. Treatment of these patients with low doses of methotrexate (15 mg weekly) can reduce the dose of oral steroids needed to control the disease. Ciclosporin also improves lung function in few steroid-dependent asthmatics.

b. **Parenteral corticosteroids:**
- Corticosteroids are used intravenously (hydrocortisone or methylprednisolone) for the treatment of acute severe asthma.
- **Dose:**
  - Hydrocortisone: Loading dose of 4 mg/kg intravenously followed by 2–3 mg/kg every 6 hours
  - Methylprednisolone: 40–125 mg every 6 hours.
  - Indications for corticosteroids in bronchial asthma
- Acute asthma which does not respond to or even worsen despite bronchodilator therapy
- Severe acute asthma (status asthmaticus).

Corticosteroid-resistant Asthma

- Complete resistance to corticosteroids:
  - <1/1,000 patients
  - Failure to respond to a high dose of oral prednisone/prednisolone (40 mg OD over 2 weeks), ideally with a 2-week run-in with matched placebo
- Corticosteroid-dependant asthma:
  - More common
  - Reduced responsiveness to steroids
  - Control of asthma requires oral corticosteroids

  Mechanisms:
  - Excess of transcription factor AP-1
  - Increase in the alternately spliced form of GR-β
  - Abnormal pattern of histone acetylation in response to corticosteroids
  - Reduction in histone deacetylase activity, as in COPD.

3. **Cromones (anti-inflammatory drugs):**
   - Cromones are not bronchodilators. They inhibit the degranulation of mast cells, thereby preventing release of mediators from these cells.
   - Cromones are not beneficial in the long-term control of asthma due to their short duration of action.
   - Only used as a prophylactic treatment of asthma. For example, **sodium cromoglycate, cromolyn, nedocromil, and ketotifen**
   - **Sodium cromoglycate:** It is useful in children with atopic asthma and in few cases of nonatopic asthma. Sodium cromoglycate is administered as an inhalation. Therapy is started between the attacks or in periods of relative remission. If there is no response within 4–6 weeks, the drug can be discontinued.
   - **Nedocromil sodium:** It is given as an inhalation at a dose of 4 mg, two to four times daily.
   - **Ketotifen** is not a chromone. It is an antihistaminic that inhibits release of mediators. It is useful in the prophylactic treatment of asthma at a dose of 1–2 mg twice daily, orally. The main side effects are drowsiness and weight gain.
4. **Anticholinergics:**

   Q. Write short note/essay on tiotropium/ipratropium bromide uses and side effects.
   - Anticholinergics such as atropine sulfate and atropine methyl nitrate were previously used, but they are presently not used because of their systemic side effects.
   - Currently used anticholinergics are **ipratropium bromide and tiotropium.** These are nonadsorbable quaternary ammonium compounds with minimal side effects. These are administered as aerosol or in dry powder form. Ipratropium is also given as nebulization solution.
   - **Uses:** They are useful in two situations:
     1. Patients with coexistenting heart disease, in whom methylxanthines and β_2-adrenoreceptor agonists cause significant tachycardia.
     2. In refractory cases, bronchodilator action of β_2-adrenoreceptor agonists is enhanced by the addition of ipratropium bromide or tiotropium.
   - **Dose:**
     - *Ipratropium:* Two puffs of 20 µg each, four times/day
     - *Tiotropium:* Two puffs of 9 µg each, once a day
     - *Ipratropium:* 250–500 µg nebulization; may be repeated, if necessary
   - **Side effects:** Dryness of mouth and bitter taste
5. **Leukotriene modifiers:**
   - These include leukotriene receptor antagonists—**LTRAs** (montelukast, zafirlukast, and pranlukast) and 5-lipoxygenase inhibitors (Zileuton).
   - **Uses:** Used as add-on therapy.
     - In patients who do not respond to the conventional agents
     - In patients who require high doses of inhaled steroids (ICS). They can be used as a second choice to inhaled corticosteroids in mild persistent asthma.
   - **Dose:**
     - *Zafirlukast:* 20 mg BID
     - *Montelukast:* 10 mg once a day in the evening
   - **Side effects:** Uncommon and include headache, abdominal pain, skin rashes, angioedema, pulmonary eosinophilia, and arthralgia. Zileuton may cause liver damage.

Anti-IgE—Monoclonal Antibodies

- **Omalizumab,** recombinant humanized monoclonal antibody against IgE, that neutralizes/chelates free circulating IgE without binding to cell-bound IgE. It prevents the binding of circulating IgE to receptors on mast cells and basophils, and decreases release of mediators. Thus, it inhibits IgE-mediated reactions. Monoclonal antibodies (**mepolizumab and**

reslizumab) against interleukin-5 (IL-5), a potent chemoattractant for eosinophils, are indicated for the treatment of severe eosinophilic asthma poorly controlled with conventional therapy.
  - Useful in patients with allergic asthma
  - *Disadvantage:* Treatment is very expensive. Patients should be given a 3–4-month trial of therapy to show objective benefit.
  - *Administration:* Given as a subcutaneous injection once every 2–4 weeks, depending on total serum IgE level and body weight
  - *Side effects:* No significant side effects, very rarely can produce anaphylaxis
- **Anti-TNF therapy** (infliximab or etanercept)—may be beneficial in severe corticosteroid refractory asthma.
- **Methotrexate and cyclosporine** have shown glucocorticoid-sparing effects.
- **Macrolide** antibiotics have both antimicrobial and anti-inflammatory actions raising the possibility of benefit in severe asthma.

Anti-IL-5 therapy

Interleukin (IL)-5 is a proeosinophilic cytokine that is potent and reduces exacerbations in patients with severe asthma who have blood eosinophil counts of 150/μL or greater.
- Mepolizumab and reslizumab are anti-IL-5 monoclonal antibodies
- Benralizumab is an anti-IL-5 receptor alpha antibody

Dosage:
- Mepolizumab is administered subcutaneously, 100 mg every 4 weeks
- Reslizumab is administered 3 mg/kg by intravenous infusion
- Benralizumab is given subcutaneously, 30 mg every 4 weeks first three doses, and then 30 mg every 8 weeks

Anti-IL-4 receptor alpha subunit antibody:

Dupilumab is a fully human monoclonal antibody that binds to the alpha subunit of the IL-4 receptor.

Dose: An initial dose of 400 mg (two 200 mg subcutaneous injections), followed by 200 mg given every other week.

Miscellaneous

Proton pump inhibitor (PPI) may be used in patients with symptomatic gastroesophageal reflux disease and suboptimally controlled asthma.

Bronchial Thermoplasty

- This is invasive procedure for severe asthma. In this therapy, controlled thermal energy is delivered to the airway wall during a series of bronchoscopies. It results in a prolonged reduction in airway smooth muscle mass. But, patient still needs to use their asthma-maintenance medications after the procedure.
- **Risks:** Lung collapse, bleeding, and additional breathing problems, mostly related to the bronchoscope.
- **Benefits:** Patient may use rescue inhalers less often and are able to engage strenuous physical activity than before.

General Measures in Asthmatics

- Avoid:
  - Opiates, sedatives, and tranquilizers in acutely ill patients with asthma
  - β-blockers and parasympathetic agonists in asthmatics
- Expectorants and mucolytic agents have no significant role in the management of bronchial asthma.

Assessment of Asthma Control (Table 6.19)

- Features, which suggest that asthma is under control, are listed in **Box 6.4**.
- Complications of asthma are mentioned in **Box 6.5**.

TABLE 6.19: Assessment of asthma control.

Characteristics	*Controlled asthma*	*Partly controlled asthma*	*Uncontrolled asthma*
Daytime symptoms more than twice/week	No	Any 1 or 2 characteristics present	Any 3 or more characteristics partly controlled asthma
Limitation of activities due to asthma	No		
Nocturnal symptoms/awakening due to asthma	No		
Need for reliever/rescue medicine more than twice/week	No		

Box 6.4: Features of controlled asthma.

- Daytime symptoms develop two times or less/week
- No limitation of daily activities including exercise
- No awakening in the night due to symptoms
- Need for short-acting β-agonists twice or less/week
- No exacerbations

Box 6.5: Complications of asthma.

- Pneumonia
- Collapse of part or all of the lung
- Respiratory failure
- Status asthmaticus

Global Initiative for Asthma (GINA) Severity Grades (Refer Table 6.21)

Severe asthma:

- It is an asthma, which requires treatment with high-dose inhaled corticosteroids and long-acting β_2-agonist and/or leukotriene receptor antagonists for the previous year or systemic corticosteroids for ≥50% of the previous year to prevent from becoming uncontrolled asthma
- Asthma which remains uncontrolled despite this therapy

Stepwise Management of Chronic Asthma (Table 6.20 and Fig. 6.10)

Q. Write short essay/note on step care management of bronchial asthma.

All asthmatics should be educated regarding self-monitoring and correct use of inhalers.

TABLE 6.20: Stepwise management of asthma.

Step	*Management*
Reliever	➤ Low dose ICS + formoterol ➤ Short-acting inhaled β2-agonist as required (required in all steps)
Step 1: (only for intermittent/less frequent symptoms)	➤ ICS+ formoterol ➤ Short-acting inhaled β_2-agonist as required
Step 2: Daily symptoms	**Regular inhaled preventer therapy:** ➤ Low-dose inhaled corticosteroids up to 800 µg daily + formoterol ➤ Leukotriene receptor antagonists (LTRA), (if patient develops side effects to inhaled corticosteroids) and SLIT (sublingual immunotherapy)
Step 3: Severe symptoms	**Inhaled corticosteroids and long-acting inhaled β2-agonist:** ➤ Continue low-dose inhaled corticosteroids plus long-acting β_2-agonist, or ➤ Medium- or high-dose inhaled corticosteroids, or ➤ Low-dose inhaled corticosteroids plus leukotriene receptor antagonists (LTRA), or ➤ Low-dose inhaled corticosteroids plus sustained-release oral theophylline
Step 4: Severe symptoms uncontrolled with high-dose inhaled corticosteroids	**High-dose inhaled corticosteroid and regular bronchodilators:** ➤ Medium- or high-dose inhaled corticosteroids (up to 2,000 µg daily) plus long-acting β_2-agonist ➤ May add leukotriene receptor antagonists (LTRA)
Step 5: Severe symptoms deteriorating	**Regular oral corticosteroids:** ➤ Add oral corticosteroids (prednisolone 40 mg daily) ➤ Consider anti-IgE treatment (omalizumab) ➤ Anti-IL5/anti-IL4 therapy

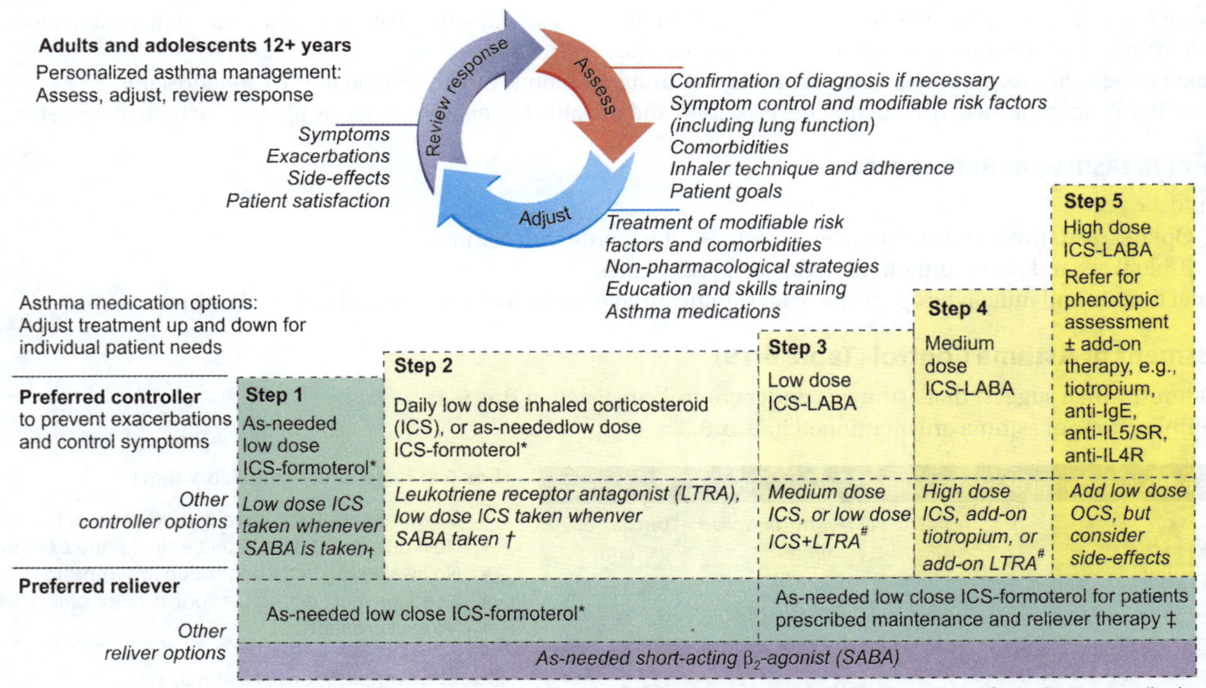

FIG. 6.10: Stepwise management of asthma in adults.
(LABA: long-acting inhaled β_2-agonist; LTRA: leukotriene receptor antagonists; SR: sustained release)

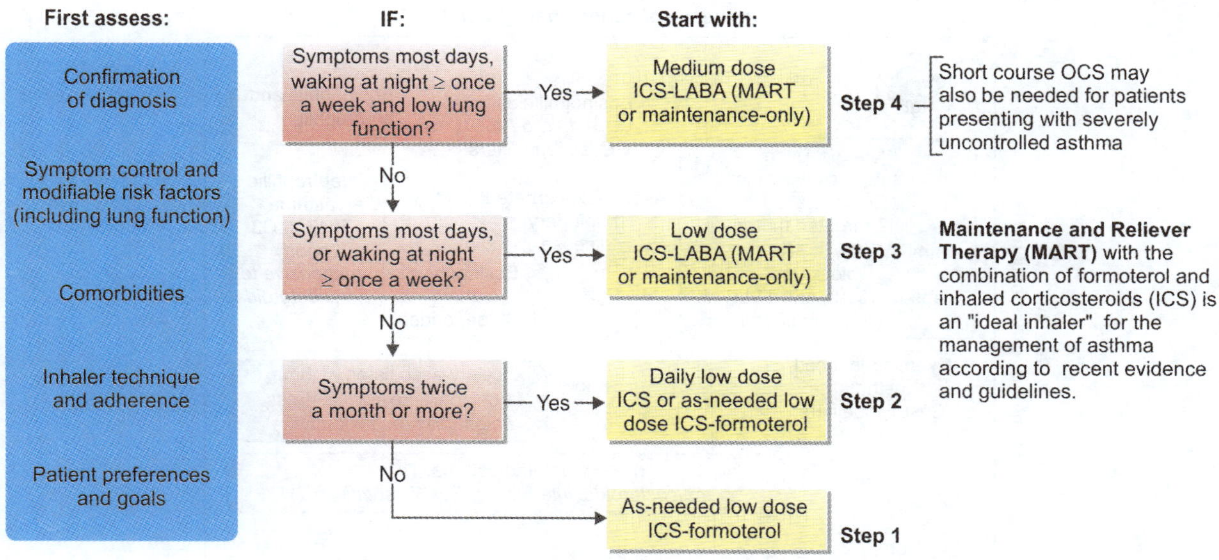

FIG. 6.11: Suggested initial controller treatment in adults and adolescents with a diagnosis of asthma.

Step-down Therapy

Once asthma is controlled, the dose of inhaled (or oral) corticosteroid should be reduced to the lowest dose at which effective control of asthma is maintained.

Suggested initial controller therapy is given in **Figure 6.11**.

Difficult-to-Treat Asthma

Asthma that is uncontrolled despite GINA step 4 or 5 treatment or that requires such treatment to maintain good symptom control and reduce the risk of exacerbations.

Contributory factors may include:
- Incorrect diagnosis
- Incorrect inhaler technique
- Poor adherence
- Comorbidities

Severe asthma is a subset of difficult-to-treat asthma.

It means asthma that is uncontrolled despite adherence with maximal optimized therapy and treatment of contributory factors or that worsens when high-dose treatment is decreased.

It is sometimes called "severe refractory asthma", since it is relatively refractory to high-dose inhaled therapy.

However, with the advent of biologic therapies, the word "refractory" is no longer appropriate.

Phenotypes, endotypes, and biomarkers in severe asthma are shown in **Flowchart 6.3**.

FLOWCHART 6.3: Phenotypes, endotypes, and biomarkers in severe asthma.

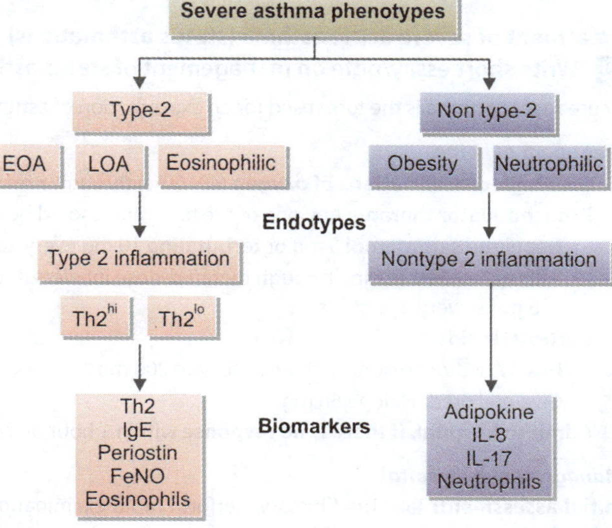

Asthma Phenotype

- The asthma phenotypes differ in terms of genetic susceptibility, environmental risk factors, age of onset, clinical presentation, prognosis, and response to therapies; therefore, asthma is seen as a syndrome rather than a single disease.
- Asthma is divided into **phenotypes:** type 2 inflammation and non-type 2 inflammation. **Type 2 phenotype:** early onset asthma (EOA), late-onset asthma (LOA), and eosinophilic asthma; biomarkers: Th2 cytokines, IgE, periostin, FeNO (fraction of nitric oxide expired), and eosinophilia. **Non-type 2 phenotypes:** asthma associated with obesity and neutrophilic asthma; biomarkers: adipokine, IL-8 or IL-17, and neutrophilia.

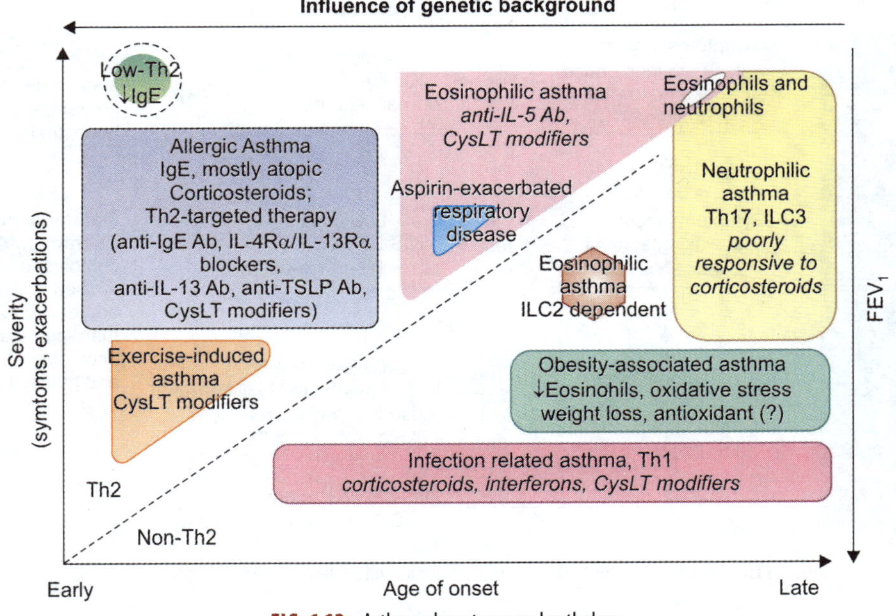

FIG. 6.12: Asthma phenotypes and pathology.

New phenotype/endotype-based therapy to treat severe asthma

Asthma phenotype	*Characterized by difficult-to-treat asthma plus*	*Targeted treatment*
Allergic asthma (IgE)	Total serum IgE = 30–700 IU/mL and demonstrated IgE-mediated hypersensitivity to a perennial allergen	Add anti-IgE biologic ➢ Omalizumab
Eosinophilic	Blood eosinophils >300 cells/uL and 2 or more exacerbations requiring OCS in past year or ≥150 cells/uL and 3 or more exacerbations requiring OCS in past year	Add anti-IL-5 biologic ➢ Mepolizumab ➢ Reslizumab ➢ Benralizumab Add anti-IL-4/IL-13 biologic ➢ Dupilumab
Neutrophilic	Sputum neutrophils in patients who do not respond to high-dose corticosteroids and do not have other type 2 markers	Consider adding a macrolide antibiotic
Airway smooth muscle (ASM) hypertrophy	Patient who does not qualify for other targeted therapies and/or has tried and failed targeted therapies for which he/she might be eligible and obstruction by bronchodilator reversibility	Consider bronchial thermoplasty, an outpatient medical procedure, in addition to regular treatment

Treatment of severe acute asthma (status asthmaticus)

Q. Write short essay/note on management of status asthmaticus.

Acute severe asthma is the term used for an exacerbation of asthma that has not been controlled by the use of standard medication.

Treatment at home

- **Give high concentrations of oxygen** (40–60%) through a mask, if available
- **Bronchodilator therapy:** Any one of the following should be given.
  - Nebulized **salbutamol** 5 mg or **terbutaline** 10 mg every 20 minutes for 3 doses
  - Salbutamol/terbutaline through metered-dose inhalers (four to eight puffs with a spacer every 20 minutes for 3 doses), followed by 4–8 puffs every 2–4 hours
- **Corticosteroids:**
  - Give IV hydrocortisone sodium succinate 200 mg
  - Give oral prednisolone 60 mg
- **Admit to hospital, if there is no response** within 1 hour or if patient becomes drowsy.

Management in hospital

Initial assessment: Take brief history, perform rapid examination of the patient, and assess the severity (**Table 6.21**). Administer high concentration of oxygen (40–60%).

Management algorithm of acute asthma

See **Flowchart 6.4**.

TABLE 6.21: Assessment of severity of asthma.

	Mild	***Moderate***	***Severe***	***Respiratory arrest imminent***
Breathless	Walking Lying down possible	Taking Sitting preferred	At rest Hunched forward	
Talking in	Sentences	Phrases	Words	
Alertness	Possibly agitated	Usually agitated	Usually agitated	Drowsy or confused
Respiratory rate	Increased	Increased	Often >30/min	
Accessory muscles/ suprasternal retractions	Usually not	Usually	Usually	Paradoxical thoracoabdominal movement
Wheeze	Moderate	Loud	Usually loud	Absent
Pulse/min	<100	100–120	>120	Bradycardia
Pulsus paradoxus	Absent	May be present	Often present	Possibly absent due to muscle fatigue
PEF after bronchodilator	>80%	Approximately 60–80%	<60%	

Adapted from: O'Byme P; GINA Executive Committee. Global strategy for asthma management and prevention. National Institutes of Health. 2004. Publication No. 02-3659.

FLOWCHART 6.4: Management algorithm of acute asthma.

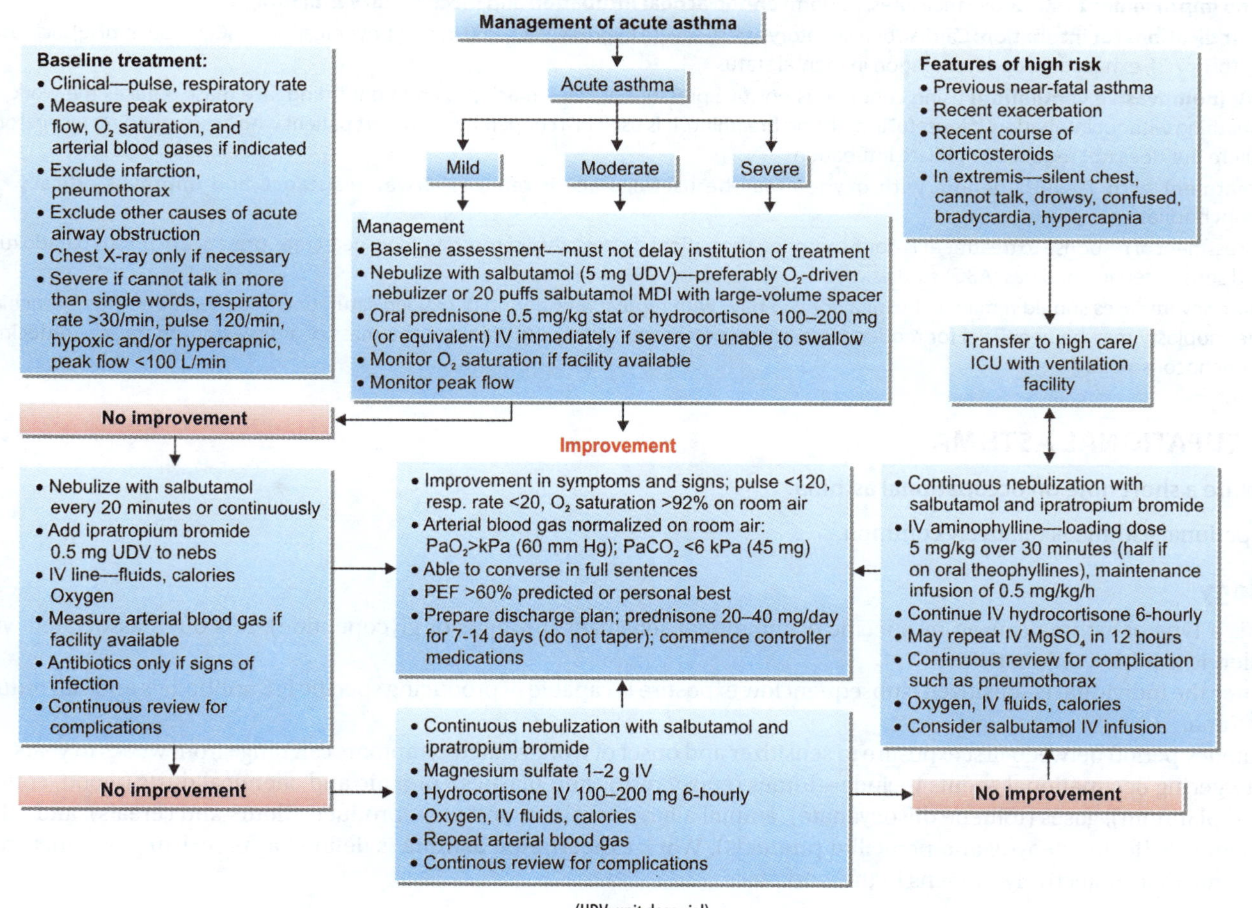

(UDV: unit dose vial)

Exacerbations of asthma

Q. Write short essay on management of acute severe asthma.

Precipitating factors of exacerbations: Viral infections (most common), others include moulds, pollens, and air pollution.

Treatment of mild-to-moderate exacerbation

- β_2-agonists (via inhaler or nebulizer) every 20 minutes for 3 doses (as mentioned above)
- Oral corticosteroids, if there is no immediate response
- Patient is reassessed every hour.

Treatment of severe exacerbation

- Give **high concentration of oxygen** (40–60%)
- **Bronchodilators:**
  - Administer **nebulized (in oxygen) salbutamol** (5 mg) or terbutaline (10 mg) or levosalbutamol (1.25–2.5 mg) immediately and may be repeated after a few minutes, if there is no response.
  - **β_2-agonist (subcutaneously or intravenously)** are indicated in patients with excessive cough, too weak to inspire adequately or moribund.
  - **Terbutaline** is administered subcutaneously (0.25–0.5 mg) or intravenously (0.1–10 µg/kg/min).
  - **Epinephrine (adrenaline)** may be administered in children and young adults. Adult dose is 0.2–0.5 mg as 1:1,000 solution subcutaneously every 20 minutes
  - **Add nebulized ipratropium bromide** 0.5 mg to nebulized salbutamol 5 mg/terbutaline 10 mg to those patients who do not respond within 15–30 minutes. It can be repeated every 20 minutes for 3 doses.
  - **Aminophylline** can be given intravenously to those patients who do not respond to nebulized bronchodilators. Give a loading dose of 5 mg/kg/h as an infusion.
- **Corticosteroids:** In severely ill patients, **hydrocortisone sodium succinate 100 mg** is administered intravenously at presentation and then repeated 4–6 hourly for 24 hours.
- **Antibiotics** are indicated only if there is respiratory infection.
- Role of magnesium sulfate either intravenously or by nebulization is not clear.
- **If no improvement** with above measures, perform **endotracheal intubation** and **mechanical ventilation.**
  - **Indications for intubation:** Cardiac or respiratory arrest, severe hypoxia (PaO_2 <60 mmHg), hypercapnia ($PaCO_2$ > 50 mmHg), acidosis (pH <7.3), exhaustion, or deterioration in mental status
- **NIV (noninvasive ventilation)** using continuous positive pressure of BiPAP machines and tight fitting face mask reduces the work of breathing without intubation. It is useful in assisting breathing. It is used in a cooperative and alert patient who has impending respiratory failure but does not require immediate intubation.
- Treatment with 70–80% helium with oxygen may be useful, since it reduces airway resistance and improves efficacy of bronchodilators.
- Assessment of response to treatment is done by noting the patient distress, respiratory rate, FEV_1, heart rate, presence of pulsus paradoxus, and serial arterial blood gas (ABG) studies.
- More severe cases should remain in hospital for 2–5 days with regular monitoring of oxygen saturation and peak flow rates. Bronchial thermoplasty may be beneficial for moderate-to-severe persistent asthma. This reduces the mass of airway smooth muscle, reducing bronchoconstriction.

OCCUPATIONAL ASTHMA

Q. Write a short note on occupational asthma.

Occupational asthma is relatively common.

Etiology

- It is a type of asthma caused by specific occupational sensitizer (proteins or glycopeptide). It is often associated with allergic rhinitis/conjunctivitis.
- Once the individual is sensitized, subsequent low exposure is capable of producing specific IgE antibodies and can induce asthma.
- Latency period between first exposure to sensitizer and onset of work-related symptoms can range from weeks to years.
- Triggering occupational agents include—fumes (epoxy resins and plastics), organic and chemical dusts (wood, cotton, and platinum), gases (toluene diisocyanate), animal allergens, plants and plant products (flours and cereals), and other chemicals (formaldehyde and penicillin products). **Work-exacerbated asthma** is defined as preexisting or concurrent asthma that subjectively worsens in the workplace.

Management

- Primary prevention (e.g., avoiding sensitizer agent)
- Secondary prevention (e.g., medical surveillance program)
- Tertiary prevention (e.g., appropriate treatment), i.e., treatment as per asthma severity

HYPERSENSITIVITY PNEUMONITIS (EXTRINSIC ALLERGIC ALVEOLITIS)

Q. Discuss the clinical features, diagnosis, and management of hypersensitivity pneumonitis (extrinsic allergic alveolitis).

Q. Write short note on farmer's lung.

Definition

Hypersensitivity pneumonitis (HP) or extrinsic allergic alveolitis is an immune-mediated lung disease that occurs secondary to inhalational exposure to a variety of antigens leading to a widespread diffuse inflammatory reaction in the alveoli and small airways (bronchioles).

Pathogenesis

It is an immune-mediated condition that develops in response to inhaled antigens that are small enough to deposit in distal airways and alveoli. It involves T_H1 and T_H17 lymphocyte subsets. Examples of hypersensitivity pneumonitis are presented in **Table 6.22**.

TABLE 6.22: Examples of hypersensitivity pneumonitis.

Disease	*Sources of antigen*	*Antigen*
Farming/Food processing		
Farmer's lung	Grain, moldy hay	Thermophilic actinomycetes, fungus
Bagassosis	Sugarcane	Thermophilic actinomycetes
Mushroom worker's lung	Mushroom	Thermophilic actinomycetes; mushroom spores
Coffee worker's lung	Coffee beans	Coffee bean dust
Malt worker's lung	Mouldy barley	*Aspergillus* species (clavatus)
Miller's lung	Infested wheat flour	Sitophilus granarius (wheat weevil)
Tobacco grower's lung	Tobacco	*Aspergillus* species
Birds and other animals		
Bird fancier's lung	Avian droppings (most often from pigeons and parakeets)	Protein in avian excreta, feathers
Other occupational and environmental exposures		
Humidifier fever and air-conditioner lung	Humidifiers and air conditioners (contaminated water)	*Bacillus subtilis, Aureobasidium pullulans, Candida albicans*, ameba, thermophilic actinomycetes
Woodworker's lung	Wood dust	*Alternaria* species

Clinical Features

It depends on type, intensity, and duration of exposure to offending antigen. Most of them present following months or years of continuous or intermittent inhalation of offending agent.

Clinical forms: It can present as acute, subacute, or chronic form. Most patients (80–95%) are nonsmokers.

1. **Acute form:**
   - *Onset:* Usually manifests 4–8 hours following exposure to the causative antigen and is often intense in nature.
   - *Symptoms:* Fevers, chills, cough, and malaise accompanied by dyspnea
   - *Resolution:* Symptoms resolve within hours to days, if there is no further exposure to the causative antigen.
2. **Subacute form:** Onset of respiratory (cough, dyspnea, and cyanosis) and systemic symptoms is more gradual lasting for weeks or months.
3. **Chronic form:**
   - Presents with an even more gradual onset of symptoms than subacute form with progressive dyspnea, cough, fatigue, weight loss, and clubbing of the fingers.
   - It usually occurs in patients with continuous low-dose exposure to the causative antigen.
   - Clinically cannot be distinguished from pulmonary fibrosis due to other causes.

Complications

Long-standing disease leads to diffuse pulmonary interstitial fibrosis, pulmonary hypertension resulting in cor pulmonale.

Investigations

- **Chest X-ray:** Findings are nonspecific. It may show diffuse micronodular shadowing with the subsequent development of streaky shadows, particularly in the upper zones. Very advanced cases produce honeycomb lung.
- **High-resolution computed tomography (HRCT):** It shows reticular and nodular changes with ground-glass opacity.
- **Blood:** Raised ESR and neutrophilia (especially in acute form). Eosinophil counts and IgE levels are usually normal.
- **Lung function tests:** These show a restrictive ventilatory defect with normal FEV_1:FVC ratio. Diffusion capacity for carbon monoxide may be significantly impaired in chronic cases.
- **Precipitating antibodies** in the serum against offending agent indicates the evidence of exposure, but not disease.
- **Bronchoscopy with bronchoalveolar lavage (BAL):** Although not a specific, BAL shows increased T-lymphocytes and granulocytes. Most often, CD4:CD8 ratio <1 (normal is about 0.9–2.5). In sarcoidosis, it is usually above 3.5.
- **Lung biopsy:** May show chronic inflammatory cells, ill-defined noncaseating granulomas, and fibrosis in late stages.
- **Provocation test:** If about 4–10 hours after exposure to the inhaled antigen, there is respiratory or systemic findings (e.g., fever and leukocytosis); reduced diffusing capacity, diminished VC (vital capacity), or both; increased radiographic abnormalities; worsening alveolar–arterial oxygen pressure suggests a positive response.

Treatment

- **Prevention:** It should be the aim and can be achieved by identification and avoidance of the offending antigen.
- **Corticosteroids:** Because acute form is usually a self-limited disease, treatment is not necessary. However, corticosteroid has some role in subacute and chronic forms. Prednisolone in large doses (1 mg/kg/day) orally for 1–2 weeks, followed by gradual tapering over the next 4–6 weeks. It may achieve regression during the early stages but not those with established fibrosis.
- **Oxygen therapy** in severely hypoxemic individuals. Symptomatic bronchodilator therapy

DRUG-INDUCED ASTHMA

Drugs Implicated

- Most commonly due to **aspirin (aspirin-induced asthma—**AIA) **followed by ibuprofen, indomethacin, naproxen, phenylbutazone, and mefenamic acid.** About 10% of asthma patients are aspirin sensitive.
- **Drugs that can cause bronchospasm:** Adenosine, prostaglandin analogs, BBs (beta-blockers), cholinergic drugs, streptomycin, pentazocine, and penicillin
- **Nonpharmaceutical agents:** Tartrazine (coloring agent), sulfating agents (preservatives in food/medicines)

Mechanism: Decreased production of prostaglandin E_2 (PGE_2) and enhanced production of leukotriene B_4 (LTB_4).

Associations: Nasal polyps, vasomotor rhinitis, and hyperplastic rhinosinusitis **(Samter's triad)**

Aspirin-induced asthma (AIA): About 1% of asthmatics worsen with aspirin and other COX inhibitors. Mechanism is due to polymorphism of cis-leukotriene synthase.

Two distinct forms:

1. **Cutaneous form:** Associated with urticaria and angioedema
2. **Respiratory form:** Resulting in rhinoconjunctivitis and bronchospasm

Diagnosis: Bronchial challenge with aspirin

Drug treatment of AIA

Treat the underlying asthma and the strict avoidance of aspirin and cross-reacting NSAIDs. Acetaminophen and selective COX-2 inhibitors are safe.

EXERCISE-INDUCED ASTHMA

- Transient airway narrowing associated with exercise, which can occur in patients with or without chronic asthma.
- **Thermal pathway:** Exercise → heat loss → rapid airway rewarming → congestion of vascular bed → airway obstruction
- **Osmotic pathway:** Exercise → water loss → hyperosmolar environment → cell shrinking → mediator release, vascular leak, and bronchospasm

Prevention/treatment of exercise-induced asthma

- Prevention of episode by the inhalation of 2 metered doses of salbutamol or terbutaline a few minutes before exercise. However, regular use may lead to loss of their effect.
- Regular use of sodium cromoglycate or leukotriene modifiers is often needed. Additional use of inhaled b2-adrenoreceptor agonists may be necessary before exercise.
- Single dose short-acting β2 agonist, sodium cromoglycate, or nedocromil sodium immediately before exercise should be used.
- Inhaled corticosteroid twice daily for 8–12 weeks reduces severity.
- If abnormal, spirometry and persistent symptom-inhaled corticosteroid with long-acting β2 agonist
- Leukotriene receptor antagonist may be used

CHRONIC OBSTRUCTIVE PULMONARY DISEASE (COPD)

Q. Write short essay/note on COPD (chronic obstructive pulmonary disease), COLD (chronic obstructive lung disease), or COAD (chronic obstructive airway disease).

Introduction

Chronic obstructive pulmonary disease is also known as chronic obstructive lung disease (COLD), chronic obstructive airway disease (COAD), chronic airflow limitation (CAL), and chronic obstructive respiratory disease (CORD).

Definition

- COPD is a **preventable and treatable pulmonary disease** associated **with** some **significant extrapulmonary effects** that may contribute to the severity in individual patients.
- Pulmonary disease is characterized by **airflow limitation,** which is **not fully reversible.**
- The airflow limitation is usually progressive and associated with an abnormal inflammatory response of the lung to various noxious particles or gases.

Conditions included under COPD: Disease is considered COPD, only if chronic airflow obstruction occurs.

- **Emphysema:** An anatomically defined condition characterized by abnormal and permanent enlargement of the airspaces distal to the terminal bronchioles. It is accompanied by destruction of the airspace walls, without obvious fibrosis (i.e., there is no fibrosis visible to the naked eye).
- **Chronic bronchitis:** It is defined as a chronic productive cough for 3 months in each of two successive years in a patient in whom other causes of chronic cough (e.g., bronchiectasis) have been excluded.
- **Small airways disease:** A condition in which small bronchioles are narrowed.

Pathogenesis

- **Major physiologic change** in the COPD is **airflow limitation**. It can develop due to both small airway obstruction and emphysema. The small airways may become narrowed by cells (hyperplasia and accumulation), mucus, and fibrosis.

- Activation of transforming growth factor-β (TGF-β) contributes to airway fibrosis, whereas absence of TGF-β may produce parenchymal inflammation and emphysema. The mechanism involved in emphysema is better understood than small airway obstruction.

Chronic Bronchitis

Q. Define chronic bronchitis. Describe the etiology, pathology, clinical features, investigations, course, prognosis, treatment, and complications of chronic bronchitis.

Q. Discuss the etiology, pathology, clinical features, investigations, course, prognosis, treatment, and complications of chronic obstructive pulmonary disease.

Incidence

- **Age and gender:** Occurs during **middle and late adult life**. It is more common in **males than in females.**
- It is more common **in smokers than in nonsmokers**. Also more often it develops in urban than in rural dwellers.

Types of Chronic Bronchitis: (1) Simple chronic bronchitis; (2) chronic mucopurulent bronchitis; (3) chronic asthmatic bronchitis; and (4) chronic obstructive bronchitis.

Etiology

Risk Factors

See **Table 6.23.**

TABLE 6.23: Risk factor for chronic obstructive pulmonary disease (COPD).

Environmental:
➢ Tobacco smoke
➢ Indoor air pollution. Cooking with biomass fuels
➢ Toxic industrial inhalants: Occupational dust exposure (e.g., coal dust, silica, and cadmium)
➢ Respiratory infections: Recurrent infection; HIV infection (associated with emphysema), previous tuberculosis
➢ Low-birth weight and bronchopulmonary dysplasia
➢ Lung growth: Childhood infections or maternal smoking may affect growth of lung during childhood
➢ Low socioeconomic status and antioxidant deficiency
➢ Cannabis smoking
Host factors:
➢ Genetic factors: α1-antiproteinase deficiency TGF β-1 polymorphism, *SERPINE2* gene expression
➢ Airway hyper-reactivity

Q. Write short note on risk factors of chronic obstructive pulmonary disease.

Smoking and COPD

- **Cigarette smoking:** It is the most important risk factor for the development of COPD. The risk of developing COPD relates to both the amount and the duration of smoking. However, only about 15–20% of smokers develop clinically significant COPD. This suggests that genetic predisposition and environmental factors play a role in the pathogenesis.
- **Second-hand smoke:** Environmental tobacco smoke that is inhaled involuntarily or passively by someone who is not smoking
- **Environmental tobacco smoke** is generated from the **side stream** (the burning end) of a cigarette, pipe or cigar or from the exhaled **mainstream** (the smoke puffed out by smokers) of cigarettes, pipes, and cigars.
- **Abnormalities due to smoking:** Cigarette smoking is associated with a variety of abnormalities of the respiratory system that predisposes to the development of chronic bronchitis. These include:
  - Sluggishness of movement of cilia
  - Bronchoconstriction due to constriction of smooth muscle
  - Hypertrophy and hyperplasia of mucus secreting glands. **The ratio of the thickness of the mucous gland layer to** the **thickness of the bronchial wall** between the base of the surface epithelium and the inner limit of the cartilage plates is called **Reid index**. It is useful for detecting the increase in the size and number of the mucus glands. Reid index (normally 0.44 ± 0.094) is increased in chronic bronchitis (>0.51). There is a direct correlation between the value of Reid index and the volume of daily sputum production by the patient.
  - Release of proteolytic enzymes from polymorphonuclear leukocytes and release of inflammatory mediators in lungs
  - Inhibits the function of alveolar macrophages
  - Adverse effect on surfactant and favors overdistension of the lungs

Pathogenesis (Flowchart 6.5)

Major physiologic change in COPD is airflow limitation. It can result from both small airway obstruction and emphysema.

- Irritants cause inflammation → infiltration by CD8 + T-lymphocytes, macrophages, and neutrophils.
- **Hypersecretion of mucus:**
  - **Hyperplasia/hypertrophy of the submucosal glands** in **large airways (trachea and bronchi):** Develops as response to inhaled **environmental irritants** and **proteases released from neutrophils** (e.g., elastase and cathepsin). This leads to **hypersecretion of mucus**.
  - **Marked increase of goblet cells in small airways (small bronchi and bronchioles): They produce excessive mucus** → Mucus plugging of bronchial lumen → inflammation and fibrosis of bronchial wall → **leads to airway obstruction**.

Clinical Features

History: Most common three symptoms in COPD are impressive history of cough, sputum production, and exertional dyspnea (breathlessness).

1. **Cough:** Initially, the cough is present only in the winter seasons (often referred as "winter cough" or "smoker's cough"), especially in the mornings ("morning cough"). Later, cough increases in frequency, severity, and duration.
2. **Sputum:** Usually **scanty, mucoid** and more in the mornings. It may be occasionally blood stained (hemoptysis) or frankly purulent ("mucopurulent relapse").
3. **Breathlessness:** It is **relatively insidious in onset** and is due to airflow obstruction. It is aggravated by infection, excessive smoking, and adverse atmospheric conditions. Breathlessness severity can be assessed by the modified MRC dyspnea scale (**Table 6.24**).

Other symptoms: Fever during mucopurulent relapses, wheezing, and tightness in the chest.

FLOWCHART 6.5: Pathogenesis of chronic obstructive pulmonary disease.

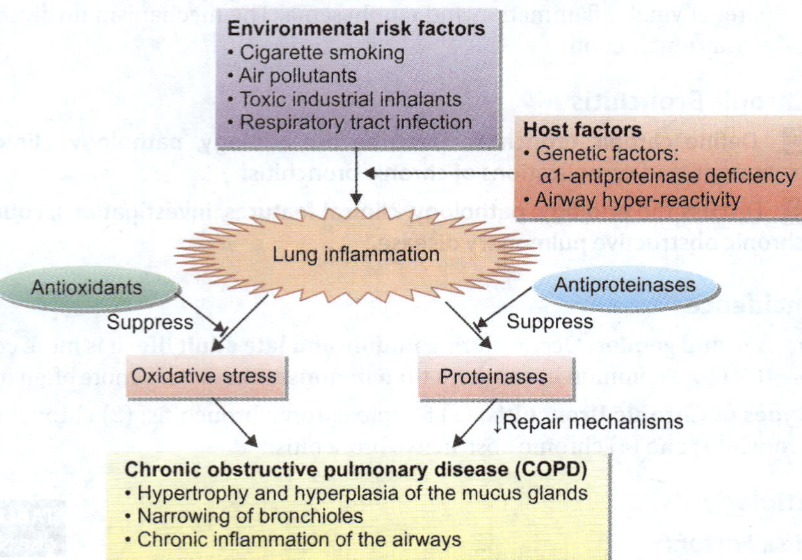

TABLE 6.24: Modified Medical Research Council (mMRC) scale for dyspnea.

Grade	Features
0	No breathless except on strenuous exercise
1	Breathless when hurrying on the level or walking up a slight hill
2	Walks slower than people of same age on the level ground because of breathlessness or has to stop for breath while walking at his own pace on the level ground
3	Stops for breath after walking 100 meters or after a few minutes on the level ground
4	Too breathless to leave the house or gets breathless while dressing or undressing

Physical Signs

- Patient is usually overweight.
- In the early stages, patients are entirely normal on physical examination. At rest, there is no respiratory distress, respiratory rate is normal and accessory muscles of respiration are not acting.
- **Auscultation:** (i) Vesicular breath sounds with prolonged expiration; (ii) inspiratory and expiratory rhonchi; (iii) crepitations that either disappear or change in location and intensity after coughing; and (iv) forced expiratory time >4 seconds.

Associated comorbidities in COPD (Table 6.25): Although COPD affects the lungs, it is associated with comorbidities probably a part of a generalized systemic inflammatory process.

TABLE 6.25: Common comorbidities in chronic obstructive pulmonary disease (COPD).

Cardiovascular disorders:
- Pulmonary hypertension
- Right heart failure and cor pulmonale
- *Vascular disease:* Coronary artery disease, cerebrovascular disease, and peripheral vascular disease
- Systemic hypertension

Nutritional disorders: Cachexia

Musculoskeletal disorders:
- Muscle dysfunction
- Osteoporosis

Cancer: Lung cancer

Other: Sleep disorders, sexual dysfunction, diabetes, depression, anxiety, anemia, osteoporosis, peptic ulcer, and glaucoma

Investigations

Q. Write short note on pulmonary function tests in chronic obstructive airway disease.

- **Radiological examination:**
  - **Chest X-ray:** May assist in the classification of the type of COPD. There are no reliable radiographic signs that indicate the severity of airflow limitation.
    - **Features of emphysema:** Presence of bullae, paucity of parenchymal markings, or hyperlucency
    - **Features of hyperinflation:** Increased lung volumes and flattening of the diaphragm
    - **Chronic bronchitis:** No characteristic abnormality
    - Essential **to identify complications** such as cardiac failure, other complications of smoking (e.g., lung cancer)
  - **High-resolution CT scans (HRCT):** Useful in detection, characterization, and quantification of emphysema
- **Pulmonary function tests (Table 6.26):** In patients with diffuse obstructive disorders, pulmonary function tests show decreased maximal airflow rates during forced expiration, usually expressed as the forced expiratory volume at 1 second (FEV_1) over the forced ventilatory capacity (FVC).

TABLE 6.26: Pulmonary function tests findings in chronic obstructive pulmonary disease (COPD).

- Reduced: FEV_1, FVC, FEV_1: FVC ratio, and PEF
- Increased: TLC, RV, RV, and TLC
- Gas transfer factor for carbon monoxide (diffusion) is reduced

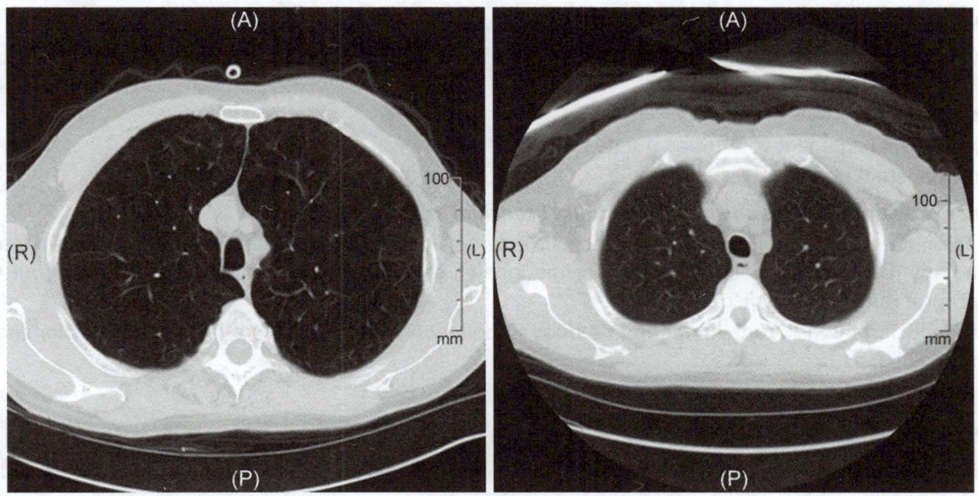

FIG. 6.13: COPD vs normal CT scan.

- **Arterial blood gases (ABG) study:** To demonstrate resting or exertional hypoxemia. It is important in the evaluation of patients with exacerbation.
- **Measurement of lung volumes:** It assesses hyperinflation and is usually performed by using the helium dilution technique.
- **Exercise testing:** Six-minute walk test used to assess exercise tolerance, response to bronchodilator therapy, disability and effectiveness of pulmonary rehabilitation.
- Blood:
  - **Hemoglobin** level and **PCV** may be elevated due to persistent hypoxemia (secondary polycythemia). In patients with normal kidney function, an elevated serum bicarbonate may indirectly identify chronic hypercapnia.
  - **α_1-antiproteinase:** It should be assayed in younger patients with predominantly basal emphysema
- **Electrocardiography:** Often normal. In advanced cases, it may show features of right atrial and ventricular hypertrophy (tall P waves-P-Pulmonary; right bundle branch block; RSR pattern in V_1)

BODE index:
- It is a multidimensional prognostic index. It takes into account several indicators of COPD prognosis **[body mass index (BMI), obstructive ventilatory defect severity, dyspnea severity, and exercise capacity]**.
- The components are derived from measures of the body mass index (weight in kg/height m2), FEV_1 percent predicted, the modified Medical Research Council dyspnea, and 6-minute walk test.
- A BODE score greater than 7 is associated with a 30% 2-year mortality
- A score of 5 to 6 is associated with 15%, 2-year mortality.
- If score is less than 5, the 2-year mortality is less than 10%.

Complications of COPD

Q. Write short note on complications of chronic bronchitis/emphysema.

- **Mucopurulent relapses:** It may develop due to secondary bacterial infection by *Streptococcus pneumoniae, Haemophilus influenzae, or Moraxella catarrhalis.* It presents with fever and increased production of purulent sputum.
- **Carbon dioxide narcosis:** Persistent retention of CO_2 (hypercarbia: high $PaCO_2$) manifests as clouding of consciousness, altered behavior, drowsiness, headache, and papilledema.
- **Respiratory failure:**
  - *Type 1 respiratory failure (low PaO_2 normal $PaCO_2$):* In mild-to-moderate COPD
  - *Type II respiratory failure:* Acute or chronic in severe COPD
- **Secondary polycythemia:** Due to hypoxemia which stimulates erythropoiesis
- **Pulmonary hypertension and right ventricular failure (cor pulmonale)**
- **Pneumonia**
- **Tuberculosis**
- **Lung cancer**
- **Pneumothorax (emphysema)**
- **Deep vein thrombosis**
- **Pulmonary embolism**

Pathogenesis of Complications (Flowchart 6.6)

Management

General measures:

- Regular exercises and management of nutritional status
- Weight loss, if the patient is obese.

Reducing exposure to noxious particles and gases that cause bronchial irritation:

- **Smoking cessation:** Complete smoking cessation and this may be aided by bupropion (a noradrenergic antidepressant) nicotine replacement therapy (by gum, transdermal patch lozenge inhaler, or nasal spray) or varenicline [partial agonist of the nicotinic acetylcholine receptor (nAChR) subtype α-4β_2].
- **Reduce smoke:** Reducing the risk from indoor and outdoor air pollution. Reduce exposure to smoke from biomass fuel, particularly among women and children.
- **Avoid:** Dusty and smoke-laden atmospheres.

Drug therapy (Table 6.27)

Used both for short-term management of exacerbations and for long-term relief of symptoms. However, none of the medications for COPD reduce the rate of decline of lung functions.

- **Bronchodilators:** They are central to the management of breathlessness.
  - β_2**-Adrenergic agonists:** The inhaled route is preferred.
    - *Mild disease:* Short-acting agents namely salbutamol 200 µg or terbutaline 500 µg 6 hourly
    - *Moderate-to-severe disease:* Long-acting agents such as salmeterol 50 µg twice daily or formoterol (12-µg powder inhaled twice daily) or indacaterol (150–300 µg daily) achieve bronchodilation and also reduce the incidence of infective exacerbations. LABAs include salmeterol, formoterol, arformoterol, indacaterol, vilanterol, and olodaterol; all are beta-2 selective.
  - **Antimuscarinic (anticholinergic) drugs:** More prolonged and greater bronchodilatation is achieved by adding ipratropium bromide (40–80 µg 6 hourly) or tiotropium bromide (18 µg once a day) or oxitropium (200 µg twice daily) in severe disease.
  - Oral long-acting theophylline or doxophylline may be beneficial in selected cases. Umeclidinium, aclidinium, and glycopyrronium are newer long-acting anticholinergic drugs available.
- **Phosphodiesterase type 4 inhibitors:** Roflumilast is an inhibitor with anti-inflammatory properties. It may be used as an adjunct to bronchodilators. Weight loss is a significant side effect.

FLOWCHART 6.6: Pathogenesis of complications of chronic bronchitis.

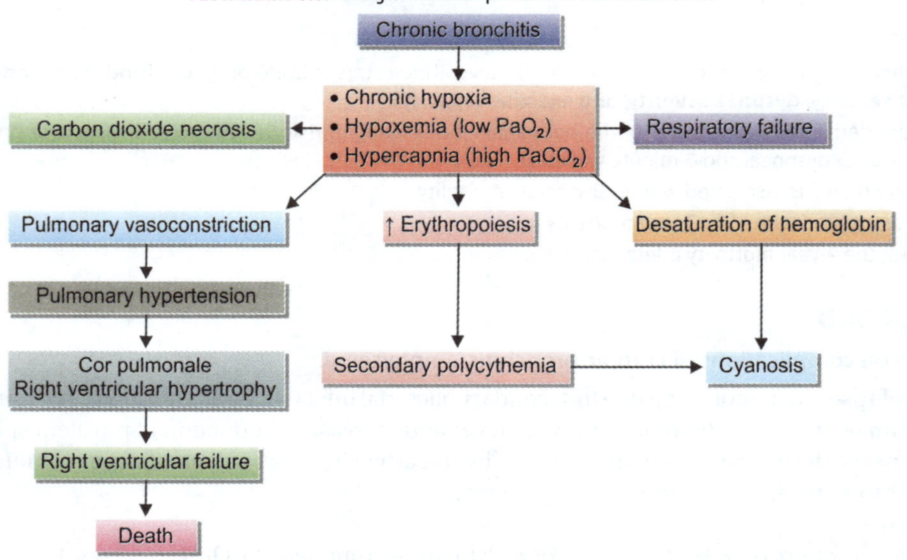

TABLE 6.27: Drug therapy in chronic bronchitis.

➤ **Beta2-agonists:** – Short-acting beta2-agonists (SABA) – Long-acting beta2-agonists (LABA)	➤ **Methylxanthines** ➤ **Inhaled corticosteroids (ICS)** ➤ **Combination long-acting beta$_2$-agonists + corticosteroids in one inhaler**
➤ **Anticholinergics/muscarinic antagonists:** – Short-acting anticholinergics (SAMA) – Long-acting anticholinergics (LAMA)	➤ **Systemic corticosteroids** ➤ **Phosphodiesterase-4 inhibitors**
➤ **Combination short-acting beta$_2$-agonists + anticholinergic in one inhaler**	➤ **Acebrophylline:** An airway mucoregulator and anti-inflammatory agent

- **Corticosteroids:**
  - Inhaled corticosteroids (ICS) reduce the frequency and severity of exacerbations, and are used in moderately severe COPD. These include beclomethasone, budesonide, fluticasone, ciclesonide, flunisolide, and beclametasone.
  - Oral corticosteroids are useful during exacerbations and should be avoided as a maintenance therapy because it may lead to osteoporosis and impaired skeletal muscle function.

Respiratory infections:

- **Treatment of infection:** Bacterial infection precipitates exacerbations. Azithromycin (has both anti-inflammatory and antimicrobial properties) administered daily to subjects with a history of exacerbation in the past 6 months may reduce the exacerbation. If patient develops purulent (yellow or green) sputum, oral tetracycline or ampicillin 250 mg 6 hourly or cotrimoxazole 960 mg 12 hourly for 10 days should be given. If there is no response, sputum culture and sensitivity is done and the antibiotic is changed accordingly.
- **Prevention of infection:** Patients with COPD should receive **vaccination with polyvalent pneumococcal and influenza vaccines**.

Symptomatic measures:

- **Antimucolytic agents:** They reduce viscosity of sputum and can reduce the number of acute exacerbations and total number of days of disability. Mucolytic agents including bromhexine, N-acetylcysteine carbocisteine, ambroxol, and erdosteine can be tried.
- **Antitussives:** Regular use of antitussives to control cough in stable COPD is not recommended.
- Chest physiotherapy

Pulmonary rehabilitation:

- It is an individually designed treatment program consisting of education and cardiovascular conditioning (reverse muscular and cardiovascular dysfunction).
- Program includes breathing technique, chest physiotherapy, postural drainage, activities of daily living (work simplification, energy conservation), and exercise conditioning (upper and lower extremity).

Oxygen Therapy

Q. Write short note on oxygen therapy in chronic obstructive pulmonary disease (COPD).

Long-term domiciliary oxygen therapy (LTOT)

- **Aim of therapy:** To increase the PaO_2 to at least 8 kPa (60 mm Hg) or SaO_2 to at least 90%. It is administered through nasal cannulae for at least 15 hours per day at a low dose (2 L/min)
- **Indications:** In COPD patient with exertional hypoxemia or nocturnal hypoxemia
- Daytime PaO_2 ≤55 mm Hg at rest or oxygen saturation ≤ 88% with or without hypercapnia during a period of clinical stability OR
- Daytime PaO_2 between 56 and 59 mmHg or oxygen saturation > 88% in the presence of secondary polycythemia, nocturnal hypoxemia, peripheral edema, or evidence of pulmonary hypertension
- **Benefits:** LTOT has significant benefits and reduces mortality rates in selected patients. It decreases pulmonary hypertension and prolongs life in hypoxemic COPD patients with right heart failure. It also reduces polycythemia, pulmonary artery pressures, dyspnea, and hypoxemia during sleep and reduces nocturnal arrhythmias.

Pharmacologic therapy in COPD depending on severity (GOLD 2020) is presented in **Figures 6.14A to C.**

Treatment of pulmonary hypertension
By long-term oxygen therapy, sildenafil, bosentan, and synthetic prostacyclin (epoprostenol)

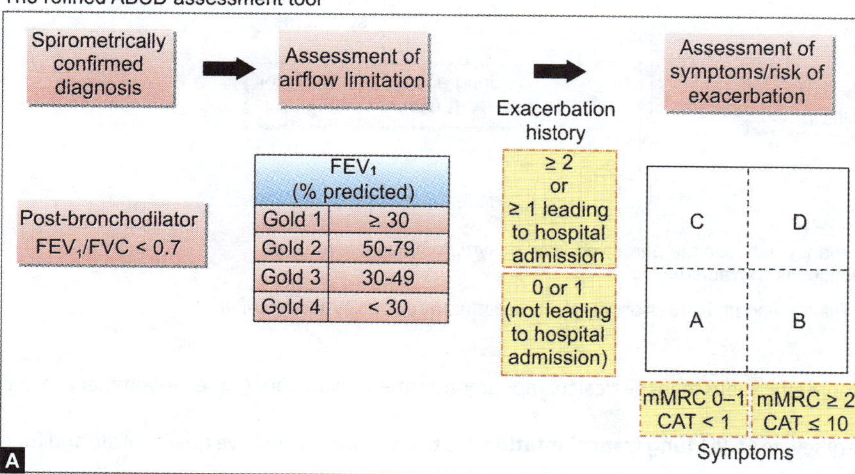

Example: Consider two patients-both patients with FEV_1 <30% of predicted, CAT scores of 18 and one with no exacerbations in the past year and the other with three exacerbations in the past year. Both would have been labeled Gold D in the prior classification scheme. However, with the new proposed scheme, the subject with 3 exacerbations in the past year would be labeled Gold grade 4, group D; the other subject with no exacerbations would be labeled Gold grade 4, group B

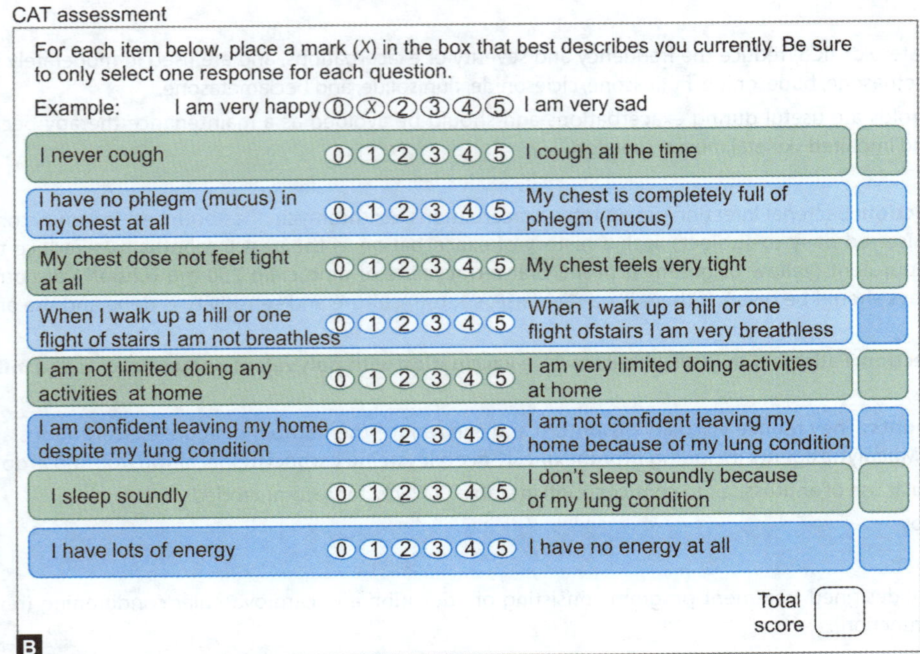

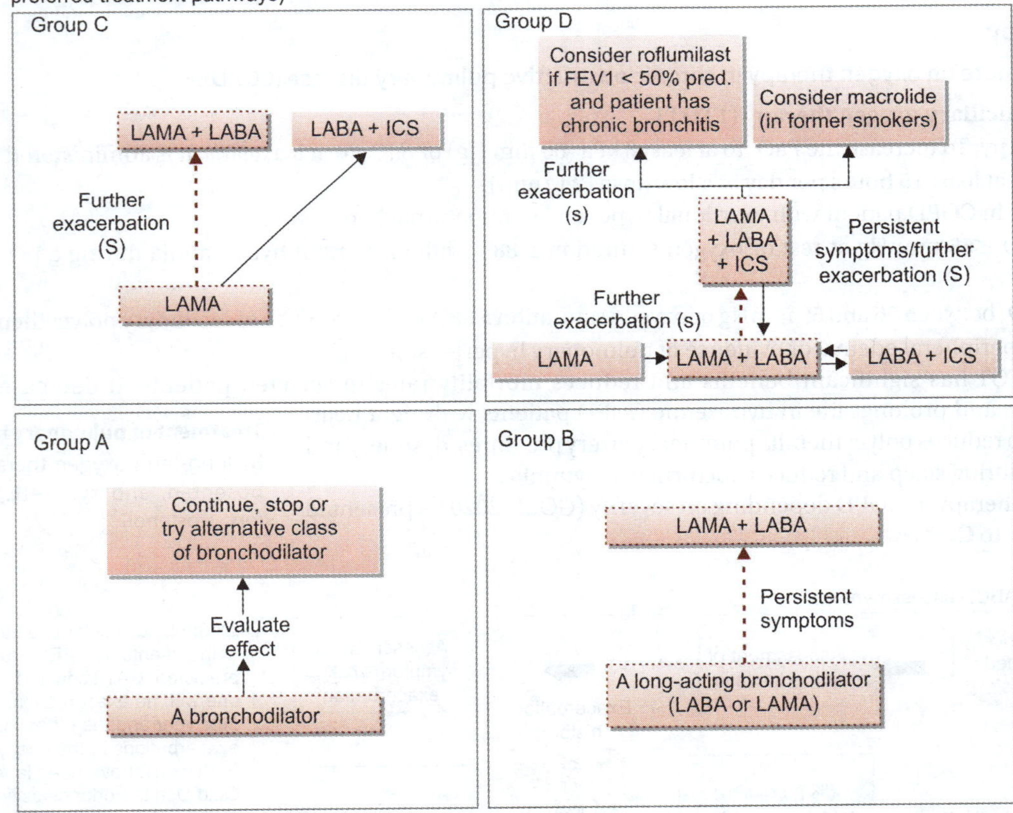

FIGS. 6.14A TO C: Pharmacotherapy based on severity of chronic obstructive pulmonary disease (COPD).

Surgical treatments

Lung volume reduction surgery (LVRS) is more efficacious than medical therapy among patients with upper-lobe predominant emphysema and low-exercise capacity.

In appropriately selected patients with very severe COPD, **lung transplantation** has been shown to improve quality of life and functional capacity.

Criteria and classification of acute COPD exacerbation are shown in **Box 6.6.**

Acute Exacerbations of COPD

- **Definition:** "An event in the natural course of COPD characterized by a change in patient's baseline dyspnea, cough, and/or sputum that is beyond normal day-to-day variations. It is acute in onset and may warrant a change in regular medication in a patient with underlying COPD."
- **Causes of exacerbation:** (1) Infection of the tracheobronchial tree and (2) air pollution. In about one-third of cases, no cause can be identified.
- **Trigging factors:** Infections by bacteria, viruses, or a change in air quality.

Box 6.6: Criteria and classification of acute COPD exacerbation.

Major criteria
- Increase in sputum volume
- Increase in sputum (generally yellow and green)
- Worsening of baseline dyspnea

Additional criteria
- Upper respiratory infection in past 5 days
- Fever of no apparent cause
- Increase in wheezing and cough
- Increase in respiration rate or heart rate 20% above baseline
- Various nonspecific signs and symptoms may accompany these findings, such as fatigue, insomnia, depression, and confusion

Degree of exacerbation
- Mild exacerbation = 1 major criterion + 1 or more additional criteria
- Moderate exacerbation = 2 major criteria
- Severe exacerbation = all 3 major criteria

Q. Write short note/essay on management of a case of acute exacerbation of chronic bronchitis.

Treatment of Severe Acute Exacerbations

Oxygen
- Adequate oxygenation (i.e., to achieve an oxygen saturation of 88–92%) must be assured.
- **Method of administration:** By nasal catheter or through a facemask equipped to control the inspired oxygen fraction. Venturi masks are preferred because they permit a precise fraction of inspired oxygen (FiO_2).

Bronchodilators

Nebulized short-acting β2-agonists (salbutamol 2.5 mg every 20 minutes for initial 1–2 hours) and/or anticholinergic agent (ipratropium bromide 0.5 mg) should be given. Intravenous aminophylline may be added, if the patient fails to respond to the above treatment.

Antibiotics
- **Indications:** Patients with: (1) increase in sputum purulence, sputum volume, or (2) breathlessness (dyspnea), or (3) those requiring mechanical ventilation.
- **Most common organisms during exacerbations:** S. *pneumoniae, H influenzae,* and *M. catarrhalis.* Risk factors for *P. aeruginosa* infection include recent hospitalization, frequent antibiotics use and severe exacerbation.
- **Antibiotics used:**
  - **Outpatient:** Doxycycline, cotrimoxazole, or amoxicillin–clavulanate can be given. Patients older than 65 years are treated with newer fluoroquinolones (levofloxacin, gemifloxacin, and moxifloxacin).
  - **Hospitalized patients:** Intravenous antibiotics (azithromycin or fluoroquinolone or a third-generation cephalosporin-like ceftriaxone or cefotaxime)
  - **Severe exacerbations:** Third-generation cephalosporin plus a fluoroquinolone or an aminoglycoside

Corticosteroids

Intravenous or oral corticosteroids shorten the recovery time and improve lung functions (FEV_1) and hypoxemia.

Diuretics

These are given to patients with gross right ventricular failure.

Respiratory stimulants

These may be used when there is no response to the conventional agents. Doxapram in the dose of 1.5–4 mg/minute as infusion is the most often used agent. Other respiratory stimulants are almitrine, nikethamide, medroxyprogesterone, and acetazolamide.

Mechanical Ventilatory Support
- **Noninvasive positive airway pressure ventilation (NIPPV)**
  - NIPPV is by using tight-fitting facemask to deliver BiPAP.
- **Invasive (conventional) ventilation**
  - It is administered via an endotracheal tube.

Management of associated co-morbidities

It is necessary to manage co-morbidities because they are responsible for mortality and hospitalization.

GOLD staging for severity of COPD and management (Fig. 6.15)

It is used for both chronic bronchitis and emphysema.

EMPHYSEMA

The word "emphysema" literally means inflation or distension with air. Emphysema can be classified depending on the organ or structure involved as:

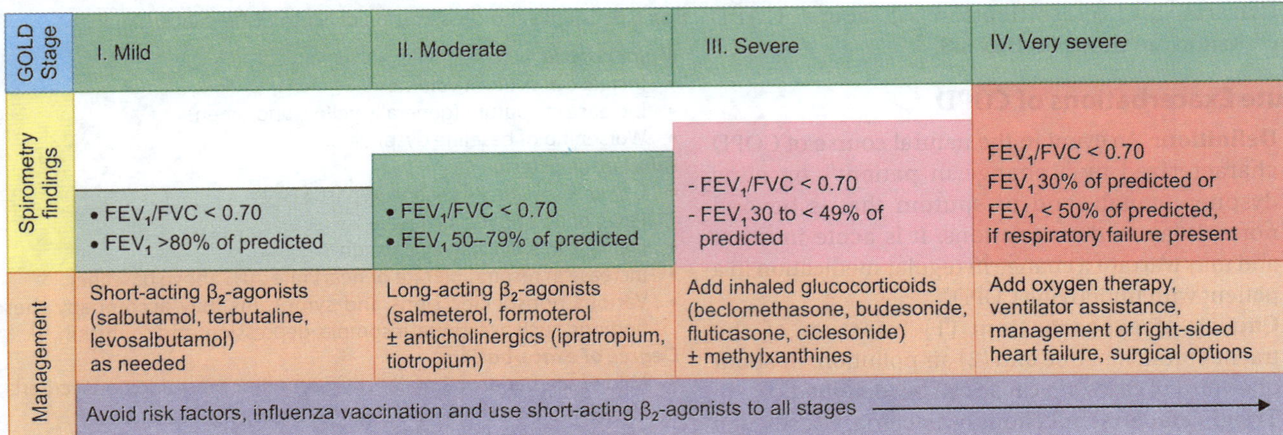

FIG. 6.15: GOLD staging for severity of chronic obstructive pulmonary disease (COPD) and management.

- **Pulmonary emphysema**
- **Compensatory emphysema/hyperinflation:**
  - It is characterized by **dilation of alveoli without destruction of septal walls.** It develops as a compensatory response to loss of extensive lung substance elsewhere (e.g., removal of a diseased lung or lobe).
- **Mediastinal emphysema (Fig. 6.16):**
  - It occurs as a result of entry of air rapidly into the mediastinum following rupture of overdistended alveoli as in severe bronchial asthma, rupture of emphysematous bulla (during coughing) and rupture of esophagus.
  - Severe mediastinal emphysema can lead to cardiac tamponade.
  - *Auscultation:* It may reveal a crunching sound (mediastinal crunch).
- **Subcutaneous emphysema (Fig. 6.16):**
  - It is characterized by the **entry of air into** subcutaneous tissue.
  - *Causes:* Penetrating chest injuries, fracture of ribs of intercostals tube introduction.
  - On palpation, it produces a characteristic crepitation or crackling sensation.
  - *Treatment:* Not needed because the air will get absorbed slowly. In severe cases, subcutaneous incisions may be necessary to relieve pressure.

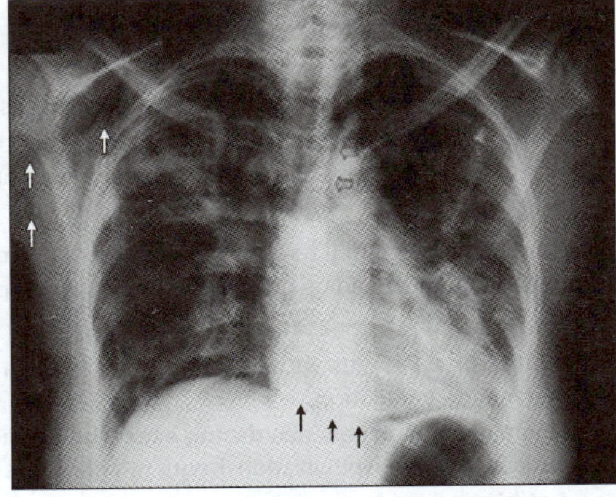

FIG. 6.16: Chest X-ray shows subcutaneous (white arrows) and mediastinal emphysema (black arrows).

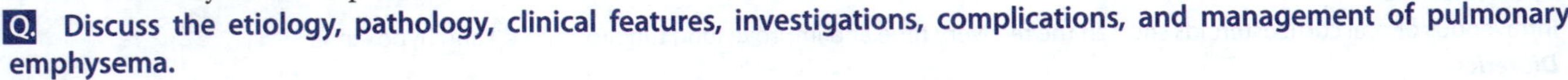

Q. Discuss the etiology, pathology, clinical features, investigations, complications, and management of pulmonary emphysema.

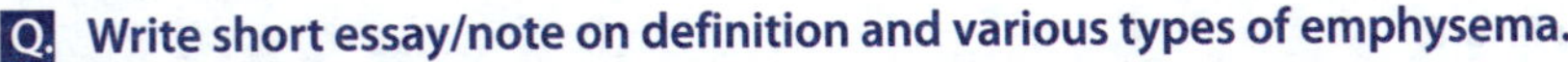

Q. Write short essay/note on definition and various types of emphysema.

Definition: Emphysema (pulmonary) is a **chronic lung disease** characterized by abnormal **irreversible** (permanent) **dilatation of the airspaces distal to the terminal bronchiole.** This is associated with destruction of their walls but without obvious fibrosis.

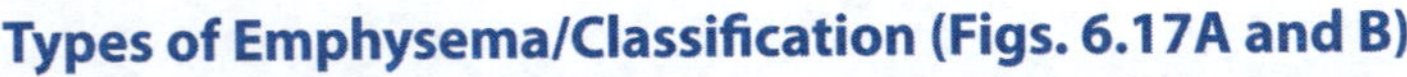

Types of Emphysema/Classification (Figs. 6.17A and B)

Emphysema is **classified according to its anatomic distribution** (location of the lesions) within the lobule into **four major types:** (1) centriacinar, (2) panacinar, (3) paraseptal, and (4) irregular.

1. **Centriacinar (centrilobular) emphysema:**
   - Dilatation **involves the central or proximal parts of the acini** (formed by respiratory bronchioles), whereas distal alveoli are spared.
   - Common and severe in the **upper lobes**, especially in the **apical segments**
   - **Association:** It occurs in **heavy smokers** and in association with **chronic bronchitis** and **coal workers' pneumoconiosis.**
2. **Panacinar (panlobular) emphysema:**
   - All the airspaces beyond terminal bronchiole are more or less uniformly/equally dilated.
   - **Site:** More common in the lower lobes, and is usually most severe at the bases.
   - It is associated with α_1**-antitrypsin (**α_1**-AT) deficiency**

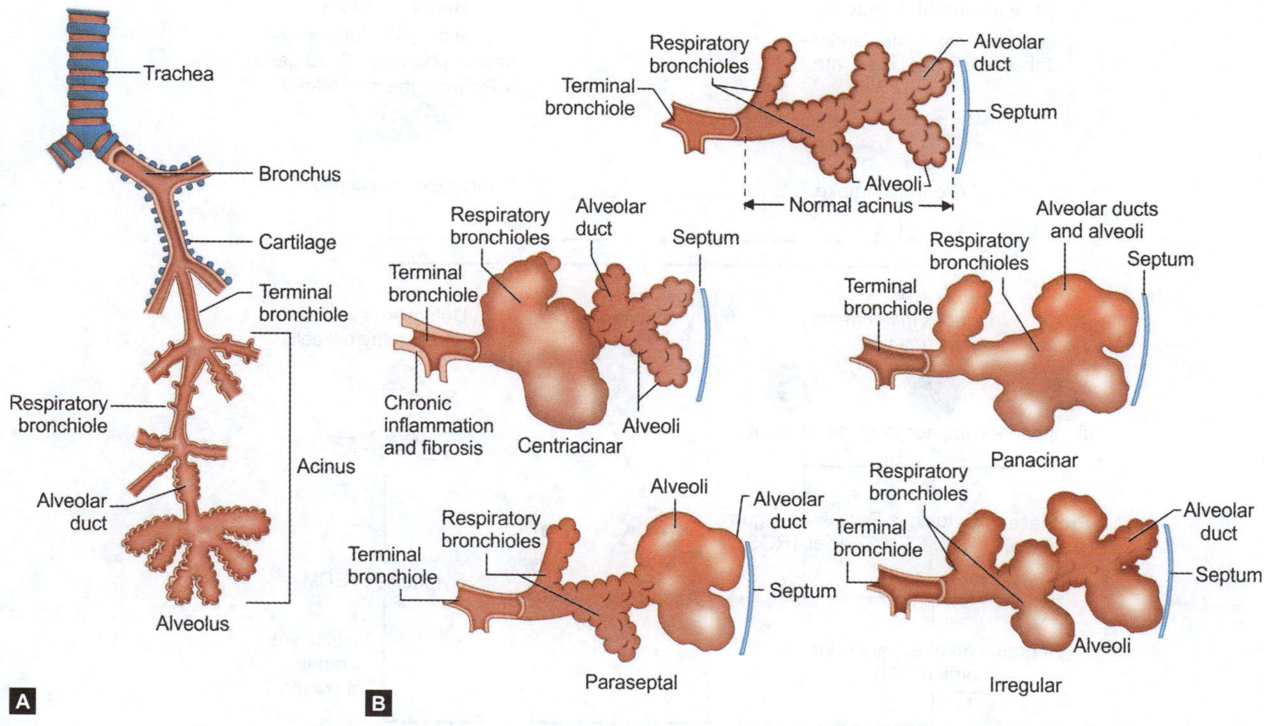

FIGS. 6.17A AND B: (A) Normal components of respiratory tree; (B) Types of emphysema.

3. **Distal acinar (paraseptal) emphysema:**
   - Dilatation affects the distal airspace at the periphery of the lobule and the proximal portion is normal.
   - It is found near the pleura. **Dilated spaces of more than 1 cm in size** are known as **bullae,** which may rupture and cause spontaneous pneumothorax.
   - It occurs **adjacent to areas of fibrosis, scarring, or atelectasis.**
4. **Irregular (scar or cicatricial) emphysema:**
   - Acinus is irregularly involved and may be asymptomatic.
   - It is most common form of emphysema.
   - **It occurs near the scar** and is commonly found **around old healed inflammatory process such as tuberculous scars.**

Etiology and Pathogenesis (Fig. 6.18)

Q. Write short essay/note on etiological factors for emphysema.

The **major event** in emphysema is **destruction of alveolar wall.**

- **Mechanism that checks the destruction of alveolar wall:** These include: (1) **Anti-elastases** (e.g., α_1-antitrypsin) and (2) **antioxidants**. If these two mechanisms are defective → results in (1) **protease–antiprotease imbalance** (e.g., α_1-antitrypsin deficiency) and (2) **imbalance between oxidants and antioxidants.**
  - **Unchecked inflammation and proteolysis:** It develops due to deficiency of the above protective mechanism.
- **Genetic factors:**

Q. Write short note on α1-antitrypsin deficiency.

Deficiency of α_1-antitrypsin: It is inherited as **autosomal recessive**, which exhibits polymorphism → tendency to develop emphysema. **α_1-antitrypsin is a major inhibitor of proteases** (particularly elastase). It is normally present in serum, tissue fluids, and macrophages and a balance is maintained between protease and antiproteases. During inflammation, protease (proteolytic enzyme) is secreted by neutrophils and digests the connective tissue of the lung. α_1-antitrypsin is a protease inhibitor (antiprotease), preventing this proteolytic digestion. Hence, a deficiency or absence of α_1-antitrypsin results in the proteolytic destruction of lung. These patients develop severe panacinar emphysema.

Clinical Features

Manifestations appear late, until, at least one-third of the functioning pulmonary parenchyma is damaged.

- **Dyspnea** is the most striking feature that begins insidiously and steadily progresses, ultimately ending in breathlessness on trivial exertion and even at rest.
- **Cough and expectoration** of scanty mucoid sputum
- **Weight loss,** weakness, anorexia, and lethargy are common with advanced disease.

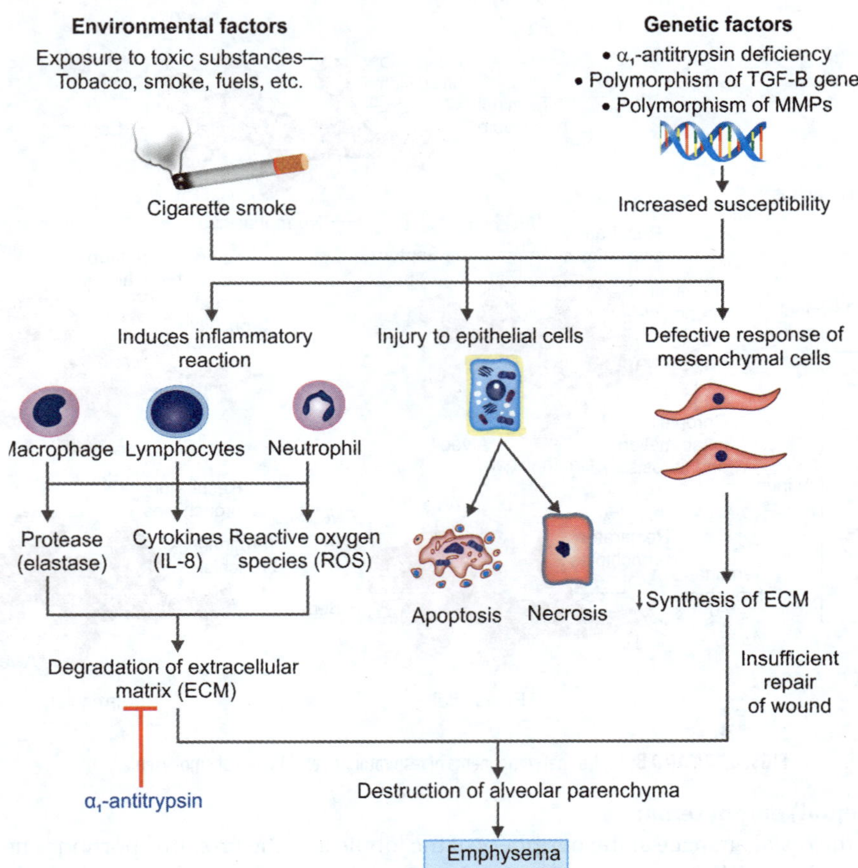

FIG. 6.18: Pathogenesis of emphysema. Exposure to environmental toxins (e.g., cigarette smoke) causes inflammatory reaction, cell death, and proteolysis of extracellular matrix (ECM). α1-antitrypsin (α1-AT) deficiency also results in increased degradation of ECM.
(IL-8: interleukin-8; TNF: tumor necrosis factor; TGF: transforming growth factor)

Physical Findings

General: Body build is asthenic, short, and thick neck; neck veins may appear distend during expiration and collapse during inspiration. Patient leans forward, extending the arms to brace himself during sitting posture.

Respiratory

- **Inspection:**
  - Patient appears **distressed** and **tachypneic**, **hypertrophy of accessory muscles of respiration** (sternomastoid and scalene muscles), length of the trachea above the suprasternal notch is reduced, and apical impulse is invisible or feeble.
  - **During inspiration: Exaggerated tracheal descent** (Campbell's sign), excavation of the suprasternal and supraclavicular fossae, and **indrawing of the costal margins**
  - **Expiration: Prolonged through pursed lips** (purse-lip breathing) and beginning of expiration with a **grunting sound**.
  - **Chest:** Cylindrical or barrel like (**barrel-shaped chest**), anteroposterior diameter of the chest is markedly increased. Whole chest is in a fixed state of full inspiration. Ribs are placed more horizontally and widely. Chest expansion diminished symmetrically. Thoracic kyphosis is exaggerated and the subcostal angle is widened.
  - **Dahl sign:** Above the knee, patches of hyperpigmentation or bruising are caused by constant "tenting" position of hands or elbows.
  - **Hoover's sign:** Briefly, during inspiration, a paradoxical medial movement of the chest. The "subcostal angle" is the angle between the xiphoid process and the right or left costal margin. Normally during inhalation, the chest expands laterally, increasing this angle. When the diaphragms are flattened (as in COPD), inhalation paradoxically causes the angle to decrease.
  - **Harrison's sulcus:** This is a horizontal grove where the diaphragm attaches to the ribs; it is associated with chronic asthma, COPD, and rickets.
- **Percussion:** Hyper-resonant percussion note over the lungs, reduced cardiac dullness, and liver dullness are pushed down or absent. Tidal percussion is negative.
- **Auscultation:** Diminished intensity of the breath sound; breath sounds are vesicular with prolonged expiration. Scattered, faint, high-pitched, and end-expiratory rhonchi may be audible.

Investigations

- **Chest X-ray (Fig. 6.19):**
    - **PA view:** Features include low set, flat diaphragm, translucent lung field, long and narrow heart ("tubular heart"), loss of peripheral vascular markings, prominent pulmonary artery shadows at the hilum and bullae.
    - **Lateral view:** Large retrosternal translucency
- **Computed tomography:** Can identify emphysema with certainty
- **Pulmonary function tests (Table 6.28)**
- **Arterial blood gas studies:** Slightly reduced PaO_2 and normal or mildly elevated $PaCO_2$.

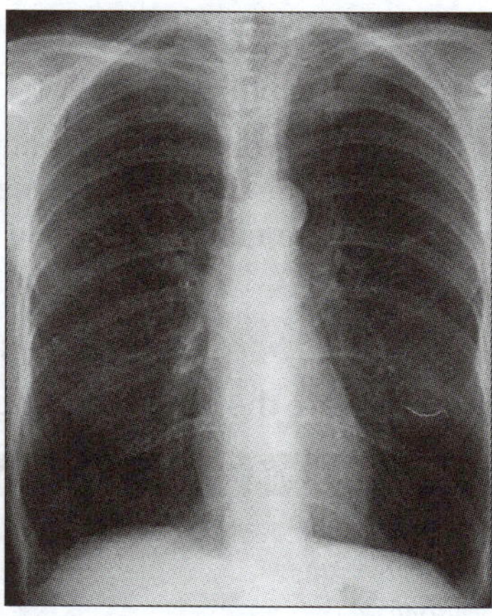

FIG. 6.19: Chest X-ray of emphysema. Posteroanterior (PA) view showing low set, flat diaphragm, translucent lung field, long and narrow heart ("tubular heart"), loss of peripheral vascular markings, and prominent pulmonary artery shadows at the hilum.

Complications

Emphysema progresses steadily and gradually.

Q. Write short note on pulmonary bullae.

1. **Pulmonary bullae:**
    - They represent inflated thin-walled spaces produced due to the rupture of alveolar walls.
    - May be single or multiple, small or large, and resembles an amulet
    - Usually located in the subpleural region along the anterior borders of lungs
    - *Complications:* A subpleural bulla may rupture producing spontaneous pneumothorax. Large bullae can interfere with pulmonary ventilation.

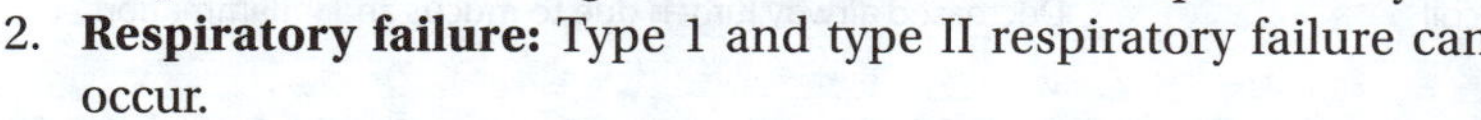

2. **Respiratory failure:** Type 1 and type II respiratory failure can occur.
3. **Pulmonary hypertension and right heart failure (cor pulmonale):** These are late complications and right ventricular failure in emphysema is usually a terminal event.

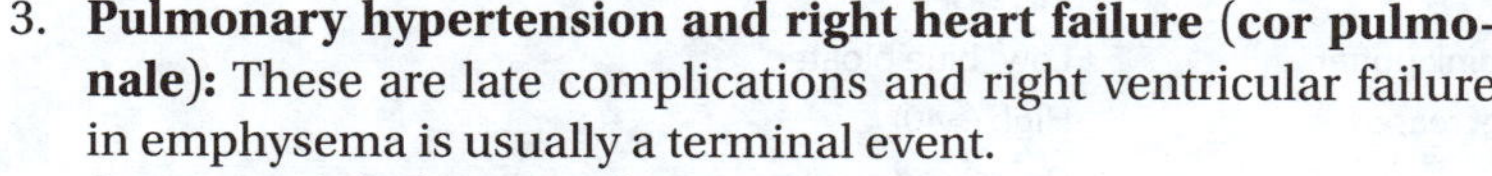

4. **Severe weight loss:** Leading to emaciation

TABLE 6.28: Pulmonary function test findings in emphysema.

Reduced	Increased
Reduced: FEV_1, FVC, FEV_1:FVC ratio, and PEF	**Increased:** TLC, RV, and RV:TLC
GAS transfer factor for carbon monoxide (diffusion) is reduced	

Treatment: Treatment similar as described for COPD

- No specific treatment for established case of emphysema. Bronchodilators and steroids may be helpful in few patients.
- **Prevention of progression:** Cessation of smoking and avoidance of occupational exposure
- **Treatment of aggravating factors and complications:** Treatment of infections, respiratory failure, and right heart failure
- **Physiotherapy**
- **Surgical therapy: Ablation of giant bullae,** lung volume reduction surgery reduced hyperinflation of one or both lungs and/or laser resection
- **Heart and lung transplantation:** In young patients with severe emphysema due to α_1-antitrypsin deficiency

Blue Bloaters (Fig. 6.20A)

Q. What are blue bloaters?

It is a distinctive clinical pattern seen in chronic bronchitis, the characteristics of which are:

- Marked/heavy cyanosis ("blue") and peripheral edema ("bloated") and secondary polycythemia
- Current evidence demonstrates that most patients have elements of both bronchitis and emphysema and by physical examination cannot reliably differentiate "blue bloaters" from "pink puffers".

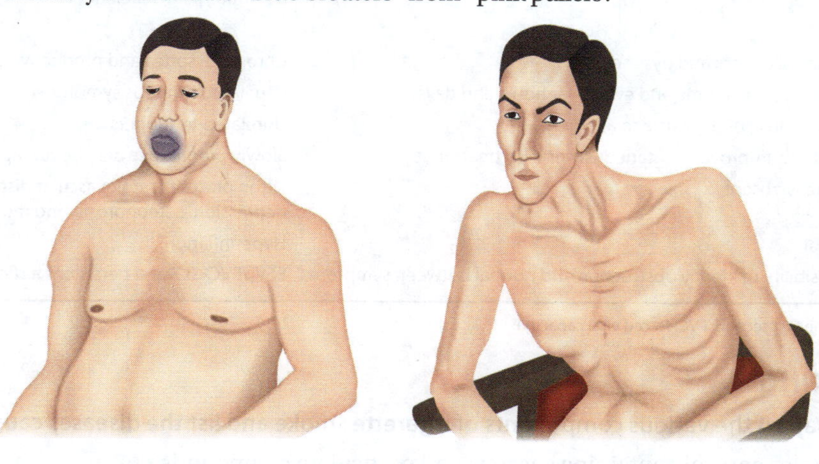

FIGS. 6.20A AND B: (A) Blue bloater (in chronic bronchitis); (B) Pink puffer (in emphysema).

Pink Puffers (Fig. 6.20B)

Q. What are pink puffers?

- It is a distinctive clinical pattern seen in emphysema of lung.
- Patients are thin and noncyanotic at rest (hence "pink").
- They have marked dyspnea ("puffer") and have prominent use of accessory muscle. They develop steadily progressive dyspnea.

Differences between Emphysema and Chronic Bronchitis (Table 6.29)

Q. What are the differentiating features of emphysema and chronic bronchitis?

TABLE 6.29: Differences between emphysema and chronic bronchitis.

Feature	*Emphysema*	*Chronic bronchitis*
Clinical features		
Dyspnea	Severe	Mild to moderate
Cough	Develops after dyspnea starts	Frequent, develops before dyspnea starts
Sputum—amount and nature	Scanty and mucoid	Copious and purulent
Frequency of mucopurulent relapses	Less	More
Cyanosis	Absent	Present
Pulmonary hypertension	Late and mild	Early and severe
Right ventricular failure and respiratory failure	Late and often terminal	Repeated episodes
Mechanism of airway obstruction	Loss of elastic recoil	Decreased airway lumen due to mucus and inflammation
Investigations		
Hematocrit (PCV)	Normal	Increased
PaO_2	Normal to low "pink puffer"	Low "blue bloater"
$PaCO_2$	Normal mildly increased	High (>40)
FEV_1	Decreased	Decreased
Diffusing capacity	Reduced	Normal
Chest X-ray	Features of hyperinflation, bullae, and tubular heart	Increased bronchovascular markings and cardiomegaly
Elastic recoil	Decreased	Normal
Airway resistance	Normal to slightly increased	Increased
Cor pulmonale	Late and mild	Early and marked
Prognosis	Good	Poor

(FEV_1: forced expiratory volume in the first second; $PaCO_2$: partial pressure of carbon dioxide; PaO_2: partial pressure of oxygen)

Differentiating Features of Asthma and Chronic Obstructive Pulmonary Disease (Table 6.30)

Q. What are the differentiating features of asthma and chronic obstructive pulmonary disease?

TABLE 6.30: Differentiating features of asthma and chronic obstructive pulmonary disease (COPD).

Characteristics	*Bronchial asthma*	*COPD*
Age of onset	Usually children and young adults	Usually older individuals
Risk factors	Family history of allergy, exposure to allergens, and occupational sensitizers	Smoking, atmospheric pollution, occupational exposure, and α1-antitrypsin deficiency
Respiratory symptoms		
Main symptoms	Wheezing, cough, and dyspnea	Chronic dyspnea and productive cough
Nature of symptoms	Vary from time to time and even over hours and days	Usually continuous symptoms
Triggers	Exercise, dust, or exposure to allergens	Unrelated to triggers
Recovery of symptoms	Symptoms improve spontaneously or with treatment	Slowly progressive despite therapy
Comorbidities	Generally absent	Often present (cardiovascular diseases, metabolic syndrome, depression, osteoporosis, and muscle wasting)
Chest X-ray	Normal	Hyperinflation
Spirometry	Reversibility of airway obstruction and normal between symptoms	$FEV_1/FVC<0.7$ and persistent airflow limitation

(FEV_1: forced expiratory volume in the first second; FVC: forced vital capacity)

CIGARETTE SMOKING

Q. Write short note/essay on the various components of cigarette smoke and list the diseases caused by smoking.

Cigarette smoke is a complex aerosol containing gaseous and particulate compounds.

Components of cigarette smoke: It consists of mainstream smoke and sidestream smoke.

1. *Mainstream smoke*: It is produced by inhalation of air through cigarette. It is the primary source of smoke exposure in smokers.
2. *Sidestream smoke:* It is produced from emitting of smoke between cigarette puffs and is the main source of environmental smoke or second hand smoke.

Chemical constituents of cigarette smoke: It contains about 2,000–4,000 chemical substances and more than 60 carcinogens. About 95% of the weight of the mainstream smoke is derived from 400 gaseous compounds and about 5% of the weight is made up of about 3,500 particulate components.

Tobacco addiction is due to nicotine present in cigarette smoke and is the total particulate matter responsible for carcinogenesis.

- **Carcinogens:** Tar, polycyclic aromatic hydrocarbons, benzo[a]pyrene, and nitrosamine
- Others:
  - Nicotine causes ganglionic stimulation and depression; tumor promotion
  - Phenol causes tumor promotion; mucosal irritation
  - Carbon monoxide impairs oxygen transport and utilization
  - Formaldehyde produces toxicity to cilia; mucosal irritation
  - Nitrogen oxides produces toxicity to cilia; mucosal irritation

Diseases caused by smoking are listed in **Table 6.31**.

TABLE 6.31: Diseases caused by smoking.

System	*Diseases produced*
General	Cancers of lung, oropharynx, esophagus, stomach, pancreas, bladder, kidney, cervix, colon, and acute myeloid leukemia
Respiratory	COPD, chronic cough, and infections
Cardiovascular	Coronary artery disease, cerebrovascular disease, peripheral artery disease, and abdominal aortic aneurysm
Reproductive	Miscarriage, prematurity, low-birth weight, ectopic pregnancy, SIDS (sudden infant death syndrome)
Gastrointestinal	Gastro-esophageal acid reflux, peptic ulcer, and Crohn's diseases
Others	Poor oral and skin health, cataract, fire-related injuries, osteoporosis, and macular degeneration

(COPD: chronic obstructive pulmonary disease)

Asthma COPD Overlap Syndrome (ACOS)

Major Criteria for ACOS:

- It is characterized by persistent airflow limitation with several features usually associated with asthma and several features usually associated with COPD.
- History or evidence of atopy (e.g., hay fever and elevated total IgE)
- Age 40 years or more
- Smoking >10 pack-years, post-bronchodilator FEV_1 <80% predicted and FEV_1/FVC <70%

  A ≥15% increase in FEV_1 or ≥12% and ≥200 mL increase in FEV_1 post-bronchodilator treatment with albuterol would be a minor criterion.

PULMONARY TUBERCULOSIS

MYCOBACTERIA

Classification

Q. Write short note on classification of mycobacteria and give an account of disease produced by them.

Mycobacteria are classified into three groups:

1. ***Mycobacterium tuberculosis* complex** (*M. tuberculosis, M. bovis, and M. africanum*)
2. ***Mycobacterium leprae***
3. **Atypical mycobacteria** or **nontuberculous mycobacteria** (NTM) or **mycobacteria other than tuberculosis (MOTT)**

Q. Write short note on mycobacteria other than tuberculosis (MOTT)/nontuberculous mycobacteria (NTM).

- MOTT or NTM are ubiquitous in the environment. They occur in soil and water and are **not usually pathogenic** due to their lack of virulence. Therefore, their isolation from a site that is not normally sterile (e.g., sputum, skin, or urine) does not constitute proof of disease. Groups of atypical *Mycobacterium* are listed in **Table 6.32**.
- **Patients with NTM lung disease** often **have predisposing disease of the lung** (e.g., COPD, bronchiectasis, cystic fibrosis, pneumoconiosis, etc.).

- ***Mycobacterium avium* intracellulare:**
  - Also known as MAC (*Mycobacterium avium* complex)
  - Most common nontuberculous mycobacterial infection associated with AIDS
  - Symptoms include fever, swollen lymph nodes, diarrhea, fatigue, weight loss, and shortness of breath.
  - May develop into pulmonary MAC
- ***Mycobacterium marinum*** causes infections of skin and swimming pool granuloma.
- ***Mycobacterium ulcerans*** cause skin infections.
- ***Mycobacterium kansasii*** causes lung disease.

TABLE 6.32: Groups of atypical *Mycobacterium*.

Slow growing:
- **Group I** photochromogens (P): Pigment producers in the presence of light, e.g., *Mycobacterium kansasii, M. marinum, and Mycobacterium simiae*
- **Group II** scotochromogens (S): Pigment producers in the absence of light, e.g., *Mycobacterium scrofulaceum, Mycobacterium szulgai, and Mycobacterium gordonae*
- **Group III** non-photochromogens (N): Do not produce any pigment, e.g., *Mycobacterium malmoense, Mycobacterium xenopi, and M. avium* intracellulare

Fast growing:
- **Group IV** fast growers (3–5 days), e.g. *Mycobacterium fortuitum, Mycobacterium chelonae, and Mycobacterium abscessus*

Therapeutic options in atypical mycobacterial infections (Table 6.33)

TABLE 6.33: Therapeutic options in atypical mycobacterial infections.

Atypical mycobacteria	*Therapeutic options*
MAC (Mycobacterium avium complex)	Clarithromycin or azithromycin + ethambutol + rifampin
M. xenopi	Rifampin + ethambutol + INH
M. kansasii	Rifampin + ethambutol should be treated for at least 18 months
M. malmoense	Rifampin or ethambutol
M. marinum	Rifampin or clarithromycin + ethambutol 2–3 months. Often resistant to isoniazid. Treatment with other antibiotics should be for at least 2 months
Rapid growers	Doxycycline, amikacin, imipenem, quinolones, sulfonamides, cefoxitin, and clarithromycin
Mycobacterium chelonae	Clarithromycin in combination with another agent, sometimes surgical excision is the best approach

Characteristics of Mycobacteria

Q. Write short note on acid–fast bacilli.

- It is an aerobic, slender, and rod-shaped bacterium. It measures 2–10 µm in length.
- It has a high-lipid content in the cell wall, which makes it difficult to stain, but **once stained resists decolorization by acids and alcohol**. Hence, it is termed as acid-fast bacilli (AFB), because once stained by carbol fuchsin (present in **Ziehl–Neelsen stain**), it is not decolorized by acid and alcohol. Acid-fast organisms and structures are listed in **Table 6.34**.

TABLE 6.34: Acid-fast organisms and structures.

Acid-fast organism	*Other acid-fast structures*
➤ *Mycobacteria*	➤ Head of human sperm
➤ *Nocardia*	➤ Embryophore of *T. saginata*
➤ *Isospora*	➤ Hooklets of *E. granulosus*
➤ *Cryptospora*	➤ Keratin
➤ *Microsporidia*	
➤ *Rhodococcus*	
➤ *Legionella*	

TUBERCULOSIS

Tuberculosis (also called Koch's disease) is a **communicable, chronic granulomatous disease** caused by ***Mycobacterium tuberculosis***.

Tuberculosis (TB) is caused by four main mycobacterial species collectively termed *Mycobacterium tuberculosis complex (MTb)*: (1) *Mycobacterium tuberculosis* (reservoir human), (2) *Mycobacterium bovis* (reservoir cattle), (3) *Mycobacterium africanum, and* (4) *Mycobacterium microti. These* are obligate aerobes and facultative intracellular pathogens, which usually infect mononuclear phagocytes.

- **Majority of tuberculosis are due to *Mycobacterium tuberculosis* hominis** (human strain). The source of infection is patients suffering from active open case of tuberculosis.
- **Oropharyngeal and intestinal tuberculosis can be due to drinking milk contaminated by *M. bovis*** (bovine strain) from infected cows. Routine pasteurization has almost eliminated this source of infection.
- ***M. avium and intracellulare* are nonpathogenic to normal individuals. They cause infection in patients suffering from AIDS.**

Epidemiology

- Tuberculosis is common in India. High incidence of tuberculosis is observed with poverty, overcrowding, and chronic debilitating illness.
- In 2019, 1.4 million people died from TB, including nearly 208,000 people who were coinfected with HIV.
- In 2019, 87% of new TB cases occurred in the 30 high TB burden countries. Eight countries accounted for two-thirds of the new TB cases: India, Indonesia, China, Philippines, Pakistan, Nigeria, Bangladesh, and South Africa.
- **Diseases associated with increased risk** of tuberculosis include diabetes mellitus, Hodgkin lymphoma, malnutrition, immunosuppression, alcoholism, chronic lung disease (e.g., silicosis), and chronic renal failure. Alcohol use disorder and tobacco smoking increase the risk of TB disease by a factor of 3.3 and 1.6, respectively.
- **HIV is the most important risk factor.** People who are infected with HIV are 18 times more likely to develop active TB.
- A global total of 206,030 people with multidrug- or rifampicin-resistant TB (MDR/RR-TB) were detected and notified in 2019, a 10% increase from 186,883 in 2018. About half of the global burden of MDR-TB is in 3 countries—India, China, and the Russian Federation.

Determinants of Virulence

- **Three genes:** (1) 1 kagG—encodes catalase, (2) rpo V-signs factor (initiates transcription of many enzymes), and (3) erp—encodes a protein required for multiplication.
- *NRAMP-1* gene: ***NRAMP1* is a transmembrane protein** (a product of *NRAMP1* gene), which **inhibits microbial growth** and it determines the susceptibility to tuberculosis. In individuals with **polymorphisms in the *NRAMP1* (n**atural **r**esistance-**a**ssociated **m**acrophage **p**rotein 1**) gene, tuberculosis may progress due to the absence of an effective immune response**.

Mode of Transmission

- **Inhalation:** It is the **most common mode** of transmission. **Source of organisms is an active open case of tuberculosis to a susceptible individual.** Infection spreads by inhalation of respiratory droplet from other infected patients.

- **Ingestion:** Tuberculosis may be transmitted by drinking nonpasteurized milk from infected cows contaminated with *M. bovis*. It causes oropharyngeal and intestinal tuberculosis. Nowadays, the ingestion mode of transmission occurs when a patient with open case of tuberculosis swallows the infected sputum resulting in tuberculosis of intestine.
- **Inoculation:** It **is extremely rare** and may develop during postmortem examination through cuts resulting from handling tuberculous infected organs.

Primary Tuberculosis

Q. Discuss the pathogenesis, pathology, clinical manifestations, and diagnosis of primary pulmonary tuberculosis.

Q. Write short essay/note on primary complex of Ranke and Ghon complex/features of primary tuberculosis.

Initial infection that occurs on first exposure to the organism (*Mycobacterium tuberculosis*) **in an unsensitized** (previously unexposed tuberculin-negative) **individual** is known as primary tuberculosis. First infection of the lung caused by the tubercle bacillus is termed as primary pulmonary tuberculosis.

Primary infection usually occurs during childhood. Many patients give a history of contact with a case of active pulmonary tuberculosis. About 5% of newly infected people develop clinically significant disease. Source of the organism is always exogenous.

Sites of Primary Tuberculosis

Lung, intestine, tonsil, and skin (very rare)

Primary tuberculosis of lung

It is the **most common site** of primary tuberculosis. Primary pulmonary tuberculosis develops when the bacillus is inhaled and lodged in the alveoli of the lung.

Ghon lesion/focus

Following inhalation, tubercle bacilli reach distal airspaces.

- **Site of deposit:** Lower part of the upper lobe or upper part of the lower lobe near the pleural surface (subpleural) is the usual sites of deposit.
- **Ghon focus:** About 2–4 weeks after the infection, a circumscribed **gray-white area of** about **1- to 1.5-cm develops in the lung** is known as the Ghon focus → the center of which undergoes caseous necrosis.
- **Regional lymphadenitis:** Tubercle bacilli (free or within macrophages) are carried along the lymphatics to the regional draining nodes → which often show caseous necrosis.

Ghon complex

It is the combination of subpleural parenchymal lung lesion (**Ghon focus**) and **regional lymph node** involvement.

Fate of Ghon complex

- **Healing:** In **majority** (about 95%), cell-mediated immunity controls the infection and primary tuberculosis **heals.**
  - The **hallmark of healing is fibrosis.** Ghon complex may undergo progressive fibrosis and calcification. It is radiologically detected as a small calcified nodule **(Ranke complex)** in caseous material and very rarely undergoes ossification.
  - In the majority of individuals infected by *Mycobacterium,* the immune system contains the infection and the patient develops cell-mediated immune memory to the bacteria. This is termed as **latent tuberculosis.**
- **Spread:** Lymphatic and hematogenous spread to other organs or parts of the body occurs during the first few weeks.
  - **Progressive pulmonary tuberculosis:** In few patients, primary lesion in the lung may progress from the beginning (progressive pulmonary tuberculosis or progressive primary pulmonary tuberculosis).
  - **Bronchial spread:** Tuberculous lymph node may rupture/ulcerate through the bronchial wall and discharge caseous material into the bronchial lumen. This results in spread of infection to the related lobe or segment through bronchi.
  - **Hematogenous spread:** In some patients, the tubercle bacilli may enter the blood and produce tuberculous lesions in different parts of the body. The hematogenous spread can be of two types:
    - **Acute form:** It is more likely to occur in infants or young children and results in **miliary tuberculosis** or tuberculous meningitis.
    - **Chronic form:** It is characterized by tuberculosis in the lungs, bones, joints, liver, and kidneys. These lesions may develop months or even years after primary infection. The infection in these secondary foci may remain dormant for years.
  - **Lymphatic spread:** In some cases, the infection may be carried by lymphatics from mediastinal lymph nodes to pleura or pericardium resulting in tuberculous pleurisy with effusion or tuberculous pericarditis with effusion.

Other Sites of Primary Tuberculosis

- **Intestine:** Primary focus always involves the small intestine (usually ileal region) and is associated with mesenteric lymphadenitis.

- **Tonsils:** Primary focus in the pharynx and tonsil with cervical lymph node enlargement
- **Skin:** Primary focus in the skin associated with regional lymphadenopathy

Bronchial Complications

- **Middle lobe syndrome:** Enlarged mediastinal lymph nodes of primary complex may compress a bronchus causing collapse of the lung. Compression of middle lobe bronchus may lead to collapse-consolidation and bronchiectatic changes. This may be present later as the **"middle lobe syndrome or Brock's syndrome"**.
- An unusual phenomenon in primary tuberculosis is obstruction of bronchus by lymph nodes referred to as **epituberculosis** resulting in some clinical signs, e.g., localized wheeze or bronchial breathing.
- **Obstructive emphysema:** Rarely, the compression of bronchus may result in a valve action with air trapping. This leads to obstructive emphysema.
- **Broncholith:** Calcification in a Ghon focus or regional lymph node may be extruded into a bronchus leading to "broncholith" or present as hemoptysis.

Clinical Features: Pulmonary Disease

Primary pulmonary TB

Symptoms:

- Majority are asymptomatic.
- A few patients may present with self-limiting febrile illness, which may lasts no more than 7–14 days. It occurs at the time of tuberculin conversion.
- Clinical disease only occurs, if there is progressive infection. If the infection is severe or the host resistance is low, child may present with reduced appetite and failure to gain weight. Slight dry cough may be occasionally present.

Physical signs:

- Majority of patients do not reveal any abnormal physical signs.
- **General features:** If the lesion is severe or extensive, signs of general debility may be present. Child is thin, pale, and fretful with less glossy hair and less elastic skin.
- **Respiratory system:** Usually no abnormal physical signs detected in the chest. Sometimes, few crepitations may be heard over lung parenchyma involved by the primary complex. More extensive physical signs in the chest may be produced when there are complications. Rarely, pleural effusion can be seen.
- **Erythema nodosum:** It may accompany primary pulmonary tuberculosis. They are bluish-red, raised, and tender; skin lesions are commonly seen on the shins and less commonly on the thighs. In few, it may be associated with fever and polyarthralgia.

Diagnosis

- **History of contact:** With a case of active tuberculosis
- **Tuberculin test:** It is very valuable in children. A positive test in a previously nonsensitized/immunized child strongly indicates the disease. A negative test makes the diagnosis of tuberculosis very unlikely.
- **Chest radiograph:** Primary complex may appear as a peripheral parenchymal lung lesion and an enlarged hilar lymph node.
  - **In children:** Enlargement of (e.g., hilar) lymph node of the primary complex is more prominent than the pulmonary component.
  - **In adults:** Pulmonary component (peripheral parenchymal lesion) of the complex is more obvious than the lymph node component.
- **Bacteriological examination:**
  - Sputum examination—for AFB is preferable
  - Alternatively, three laryngeal swabs or fasting gastric washings can be examined
  - Detection of the tubercle bacilli either in the direct smear or culture confirms the diagnosis.

Postprimary (Secondary) Tuberculosis

Q. Describe the etiology, pathogenesis, pathology, clinical features, complications, and diagnosis of postprimary tuberculosis/secondary tuberculosis.

(Synonyms: Postprimary tuberculosis or reactivation tuberculosis)

- **Tuberculosis** developing **in a previously sensitized** individual (by earlier exposure) is known as secondary tuberculosis.
- It may develop shortly or after many years following primary tuberculosis, when resistance host is reduced.

Source of Infection

- **Endogenous:** Most common source is **reactivation of a latent infection.**
  - Direct progression of a primary tuberculous lesion

- Reactivation of a dormant primary lesion
- Hematogenous spread to the lungs
- **Exogenous:** Rarely exogenous new infection (reinfection)

Any location may be involved in secondary tuberculosis, but lungs are by far the most common site.

Morphology

Gross

- **Site:** In the lungs, postprimary (secondary) tuberculosis usually involves the **apex of the upper lobes** of one or both lungs, **within 1 to 2 cm of the apical pleura**. It commonly involves apical and posterior segments of the upper lobe or apical segment of the lower lobe. This predilection may be due to good ventilation, decreased blood and lymphatic supply of these regions in the erect posture, and the oxygen tension that favors survival of the strictly aerobic tubercle bacilli.
- **Appearance: Initially small focus** (less than **2 cm in diameter) of consolidation**, sharply circumscribed, firm, and **gray-white to yellow** in color. The central caseated liquefied material of a tuberculous primary lesion may be discharged into a bronchus and forms a tuberculous cavity in the lung.
- Regional lymph node involvement is not as prominent as that seen in primary tuberculosis.

Fate of Secondary Tuberculosis (Fig. 6.21)

Healing: In immunocompetent individuals, localized and apical focus may **heal with fibrosis and calcification but** rarely ossification.

Progress: It may occur along several different pathways.

- **Progressive pulmonary tuberculosis:** It occurs mainly in the elderly and immunosuppressed. Apical lesion may expand into surrounding lung and may erode into bronchi and vessels.
  - **Erosion into bronchi:** It leads to release of the central area of caseous necrosis → resulting in a ragged, irregular **apical cavity** surrounded by fibrous tissue. This produces an **important source of infection**, because when the patient coughs, sputum contains bacteria.
  - **Erosion of blood vessels:** It may result in hemoptysis.
- **Spread of infection:** If the treatment is inadequate or if host defenses are impaired, the infection may spread via: (1) airways, (2) lymphatics, or (3) blood vessels.
  - **Local/direct spread:** Tuberculosis can directly spread to the surrounding tissue. In the lung, local spread to the pleura may result in serous **pleural effusions**, **tuberculous empyema**, or **obliterative fibrous pleuritis**.

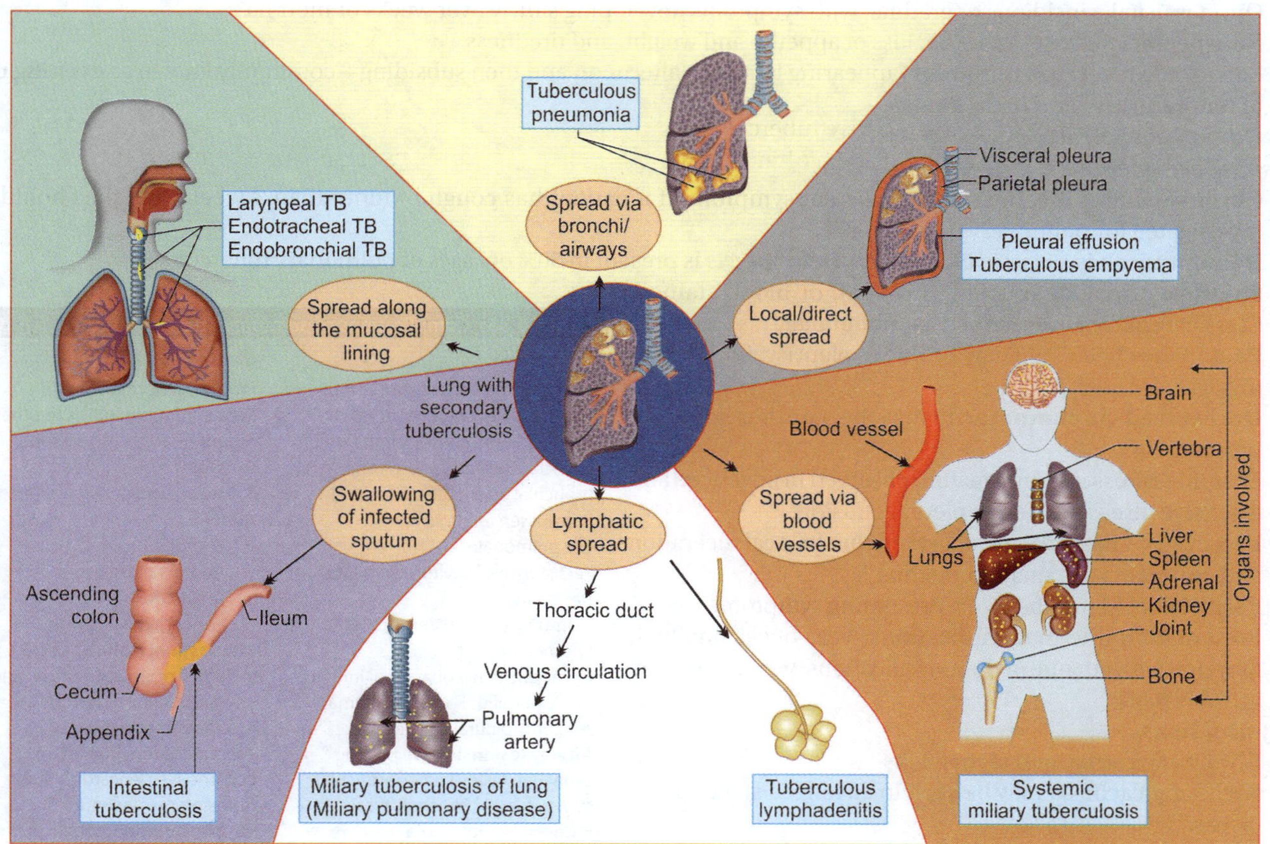

FIG. 6.21: Progress and complications of secondary tuberculosis (TB) of lung.

- **Spread through bronchi/airways:** It may produce tuberculous pneumonia.
- **Spread along mucosal lining:** Spread through lymphatic channels or along the mucosal lining from mycobacteria present in the expectorated infectious material may lead to **endobronchial, endotracheal,** and **laryngeal tuberculosis.** In the past, intestinal tuberculosis was due to drinking of contaminated unpasteurized milk. However, this is rare following pasteurization of milk. Nowadays, it is caused by the **swallowing of coughed-up infective material** in patients with open case of advanced pulmonary tuberculosis. It **mainly develops in the ileum.**
- **Lymphatic spread:** Spread through lymphatic channels mainly reach regional lymph nodes. It may also cause disseminated disease.
  Miliary pulmonary disease: It is the disseminated form of tuberculosis. If the dissemination is only limited to the lungs, it is termed as miliary pulmonary disease.
  Lymphadenitis: It is most frequent presentation of extrapulmonary tuberculosis and usually occurs in the cervical region ("scrofula").

- **Spread via blood vessels**
  Systemic miliary tuberculosis occurs when tubercle bacilli disseminate through the systemic arterial system. Miliary tuberculosis most commonly involves liver, bone marrow, spleen, adrenals, meninges, kidneys, fallopian tubes, and epididymis. Tuberculosis can involve any organ *except nail, hair, and enamel.*
  Isolated organ tuberculosis: Dissemination of tubercle bacilli through blood may seed any organ or tissue → resulting in isolated organ tuberculosis. Commonly involved organs are:
  - Meninges (tuberculous meningitis)
  - Kidneys (renal tuberculosis)
  - Adrenals
  - *Bones (osteomyelitis):* When it involves the vertebrae, the disease is referred to as **Pott's disease**. Paraspinal "cold" abscesses may track along tissue planes and present as an abdominal or pelvic mass.
  - Fallopian tubes (salpingitis)/orchitis.

Clinical Features

Q. Write short note on clinical features of fibrocavitary tuberculosis.

Symptoms of pulmonary tuberculosis:

- Localized secondary tuberculosis may remain asymptomatic.
- Many patients are symptom free, and may be detected on routine radiography.
- Onset is usually insidious or gradual, with symptoms developing slowly over weeks or months.
- **Nonspecific:** Malaise, anorexia, loss of appetite and weight, and tiredness
- **Low-grade fever:** It is **remittent** (appearing late each afternoon and then subsiding—commonly known as **evening rise of temperature**) and **night sweats.**
- *Others:* Amenorrhea

Respiratory symptoms:

- **Chronic cough:** It is the most consistent symptom. If a patient has cough of more than 3 weeks, he/she should be investigated for pulmonary tuberculosis.
- **Hemoptysis:** It is a classical symptom. **Hemoptysis** is present in 50% of cases of pulmonary tuberculosis.
- **Sputum:** It may be mucoid, purulent, or blood stained. Classical sputum is described as "**nummular**".
- **Pain in the chest:** Pain may be due to pleurisy, intercostals myalgia, or cough fracture.
- **Unresolved pneumonia:** It may be another mode of presentation.
- **Breathlessness** may be a feature observed in advanced and extensive disease or due to pleural effusion.
- Localized wheeze may be observed due to local ulceration and narrowing of a major bronchus.
- Recurrent cold may be also a presenting symptom.
- Presentation due to complications: Very occasionally, it may present with one of the complications, which are given in **Table 6.35**.

Physical signs:

- Fever, tachycardia, and tachypnea
- Pallor and cachexia may be seen in advanced stages of the disease.
- Clubbing of finger is unusual.

TABLE 6.35: Complications of pulmonary tuberculosis.

Pulmonary	*Nonpulmonary*
Exudative pleural effusion/empyema Spontaneous pneumothorax Massive hemoptysis pulmonary or bronchial arteritis and thrombosis, bronchial artery dilatation, and Rasmussen aneurysm) Cor pulmonale Persistence of cavities even after treatment Pulmonary fibrosis/emphysema *Infection of cavities:* ➢ Atypical mycobacterial infection ➢ Aspergillus → aspergilloma ➢ Lung/pleural calcification **Airway lesions:** These include bronchiectasis, tracheobronchial stenosis, and broncholithiasis Bronchopleural fistula Bronchogenic carcinoma	Empyema necessitans Spread of tuberculosis to other organs (especially Addison's) Laryngitis *Following swallowing of infected sputum:* ➢ Enteritis ➢ Anorectal disease ➢ Amyloidosis ➢ Poncet's polyarthritis **Mediastinal lesions:** These include lymph node calcification and extranodal extension, esophagomediastinal or esophagobronchial fistula, constrictive pericarditis, and fibrosing mediastinitis Venous thromboembolism

Chest:

- Often, there are no abnormal signs detected.
- **Fine crepitations:** Most common sign is fine crepitations in the upper part (apices) of one or both lungs. They are better heard particularly on taking a deep breath after coughing **(post-tussive crepitations)**.
- Classical physical signs of consolidation (dullness to percussion), cavitation, fibrosis, bronchiectasis, pleural effusion, or pneumothorax may be present.
- **Cavernous bronchial breathing** with **post-tussive suction** may be heard, if there is a superficial collapsible cavity.
- There may be bronchial breathing in the upper part and localized wheeze due to local tuberculous bronchitis or pressure by a lymph node on a bronchus may be heard. Chronic tuberculosis, when accompanied with fibrosis, may show evidence of volume loss and mediastinal shift.

Extrapulmonary manifestations depend on the organ/system involved.

Conditions/diseases that favor reactivation/reinfection of tuberculosis are presented in **Table 6.36**.

TABLE 6.36: Condition/diseases that favor reactivation/reinfection of tuberculosis.

➢ Immunosuppression: HIV, anti-tumor necrosis factor (TNF) therapy, high-dose corticosteroids, and cytotoxic agents ➢ Malnutrition ➢ Diabetes mellitus ➢ Hemophilia ➢ Chronic kidney disease	➢ Silicosis ➢ Malignancies (e.g., lymphoma and leukemia) ➢ Gastrointestinal disease associated with malnutrition (gastrectomy, jejunoileal bypass, cancer of the pancreas, and malabsorption) ➢ Deficiency of vitamin D or A

Investigations

Q. Write short note on diagnosis and investigations of pulmonary tuberculosis.

Presence of an unexplained cough for more than 2–3 weeks, particularly in regions where TB is prevalent, or typical chest X-ray changes, should prompt for further investigation.

Blood examination:

- *Anemia:* Moderate degree
- *White cell count:* Usually normal or below normal
- *ESR:* Usually raised
- *Other findings:*
  - *Serum electrolytes*: Hyponatremia and hyperkalemia may be observed in severe disease.
  - *Liver function tests:* Occasionally may be impaired.

Radiological examination:

For practical purposes, a normal chest radiograph excludes the diagnosis of pulmonary tuberculosis (**Fig. 6.22**).

Radiological Features of Pulmonary Tuberculosis (Table 6.37)

Q. Write short note on the radiological features of pulmonary tuberculosis.

For all practical purposes, a normal chest radiograph excludes the diagnosis of pulmonary tuberculosis.

- *Radiological findings*: It shows ill-defined opacification in one or both of the upper lobes. As the disease progresses features of consolidation, collapse and cavitation develop to varying degrees (**Fig. 6.23**). It is often difficult

TABLE 6.37: Radiological features of tuberculosis of lung.

Radiological shadows that strongly suggest tuberculosis	*Radiological shadows that may be due to tuberculosis*
➢ Patchy or nodular shadows in the upper zone (on one or both sides) ➢ Cavitation (especially if more than one) ➢ Calcified lesion ➢ Pleural effusion/thickening	➢ Oval or round single shadow (tuberculoma) ➢ Hilar and mediastinal shadows (due to enlarged lymph nodes) ➢ Diffuse small nodular shadows (miliary tuberculosis)

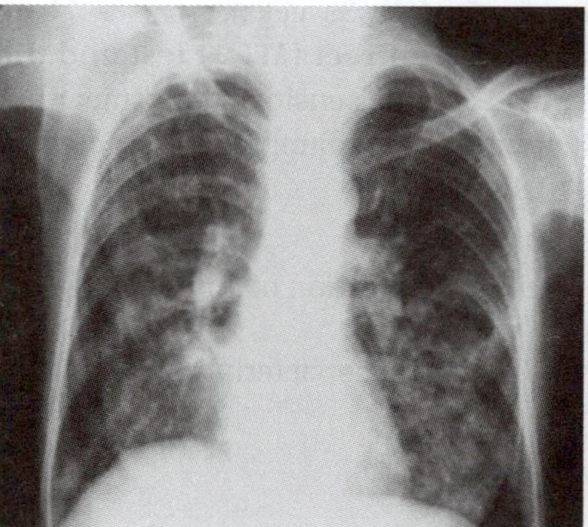
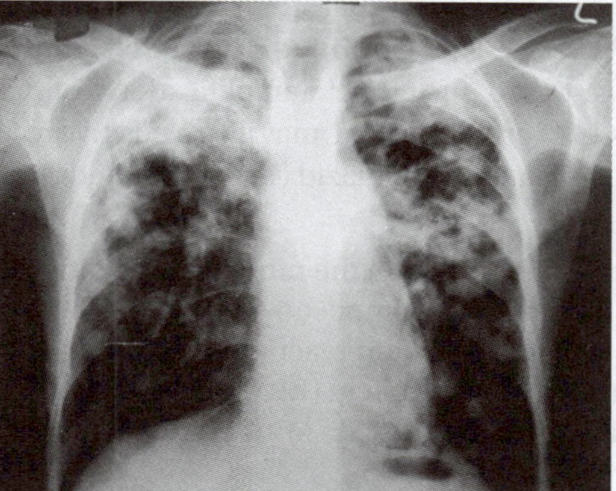

FIG. 6.22: Chest X-rays of tuberculosis showing bilateral infiltrates and thin-walled cavities.

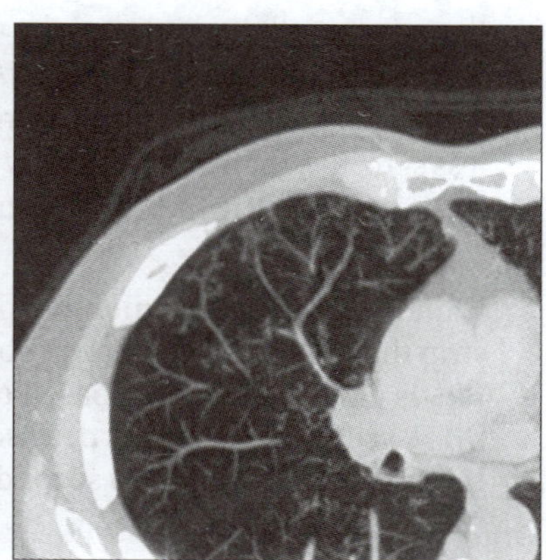

FIG. 6.23: Tree in bud appearance of tuberculosis on computed tomography (CT).

to distinguish between active from quiescent form of tuberculosis on radiological criteria alone, but the presence of a miliary pattern or cavitation favors active disease.

- In extensive disease, collapse may cause significant displacement of the trachea and mediastinum. Occasionally, a caseous lymph node may drain into an adjoining bronchus, resulting in tuberculous pneumonia.
- *CT chest:* It may be useful in evaluating parenchymal and lymph node lesions. It may show **tree in bud appearance** (**Fig. 6.23**).
- ^{18}F-FDG PET scans and ^{11}C-choline PET scans may be done in few selected patients.

Sputum examination

- *Direct microscopic examination of sputum:* It remains the most important first step investigation in pulmonary TB. Earlier, three specimens of sputum should be examined and if two of these smears are positive, diagnosis of TB is certain.
- *Revised WHO definition of a new sputum smear-positive case of pulmonary tuberculosis*: Presence of at least one acid-fast bacillus in at least one sputum sample in countries with a well-functioning external quality-assurance system. Presently, WHO recommends that the number of sputum specimens to be examined for screening of tuberculosis cases can be **reduced from three to two,** in places (i) where a well-functioning external quality-assurance system exists, (ii) where the workload is very high, and (iii) human resources are scarce.
- *Stain*: Rapid identification of the presence of tubercle bacilli by immediate stains is essential and should be done within 24 hours. The most effective stains are the Ziehl–Neelsen and rhodamine–auramine. Auramine–rhodamine staining is more sensitive (though less specific) than Ziehl–Neelsen.
- Grading of smears (RNTCP)

Bacilli observed	*Report*	*Grade*
10 or more AFB/OIF	Positive	3+
1-10 AFB/OIF	Positive	2+
10-99 bacilli/100 OIF	Positive	1+
1-9 AFB/100 OIF	Doubtful (repeat)	Scanty
No AFB/100 OIF	Negative	0

Culture of sputum

- A **positive sputum smear is sufficient for the presumptive diagnosis of TB** but definitive diagnosis requires culture of tubercle bacillus. Smear-negative sputum should also be cultured.
- **Culture medias:** It may be—
  - Liquid/broth culture (Middlebrook 7H12) or the nonradiometric mycobacteria growth indicator tube (MGIT): Faster growth (1–3 weeks) occurs in liquid media. *The BACTEC radiometric growth detection method detects mycobacterial growth by measuring the liberation of $^{14}CO_2$, following metabolism of ^{14}C-labeled substrate present in the medium. The growth can be detected in 4–8 days.*
  - Solid media (Löwenstein–Jensen slopes): MTB grows slowly and may take between 4 and 6 weeks.
- **Drug sensitivity testing:** It should be done in selected cases. It is important in patients with a previous history of TB, treatment failure or chronic disease, and in those who are resident in or have visited an area of high prevalence of resistance, or who are HIV-positive. Using liquid culture in the presence of antimycobacterial drugs (usually first line therapy initially) establishes the drug sensitivity for that strain and usually takes approximately 3 weeks).
- **Nucleic acid amplification (NAA) tests:** The **Amplified *Mycobacterium tuberculosis* direct (MTD) test and the GeneXpert MTB/RIF test**. Cartridge-based nucleic acid amplification test (CBNAAT) is more sensitive than smear but less sensitive than culture, as few as 1–10 organisms/mL may give a positive result. Resistance to rifampin can be detected by Xpert MTB/RIF or MTBDRplus, resistance to isoniazid can be detected by MTBDR plus.

Line probe assay (LPA)

- Immobilization of the multiple probes of interest on the nitrocellulose strip followed by application of amplicons to the strip that determines which probe hybridizes the amplicon.
- LPA is a rapid technique based on polymerase chain reaction (PCR) that is used to detect Mycobacterium tuberculosis (MTB) complex as well as drug sensitivity to rifampicin (RPM) and isoniazid (INH)
- It can detect resistance to second line drugs too.

Other investigations

- Laryngeal swab, early morning gastric lavage, and bronchoalveolar lavage samples can be used for detecting AFB.
- **Tuberculin test:** It is used for diagnosis but is less valuable. However, this test may be negative in patients with active tuberculosis associated with malnutrition or other diseases. It may be positive in patients without active tuberculosis. Strongly positive test favors tuberculosis, whereas a negative test does not exclude tuberculosis.

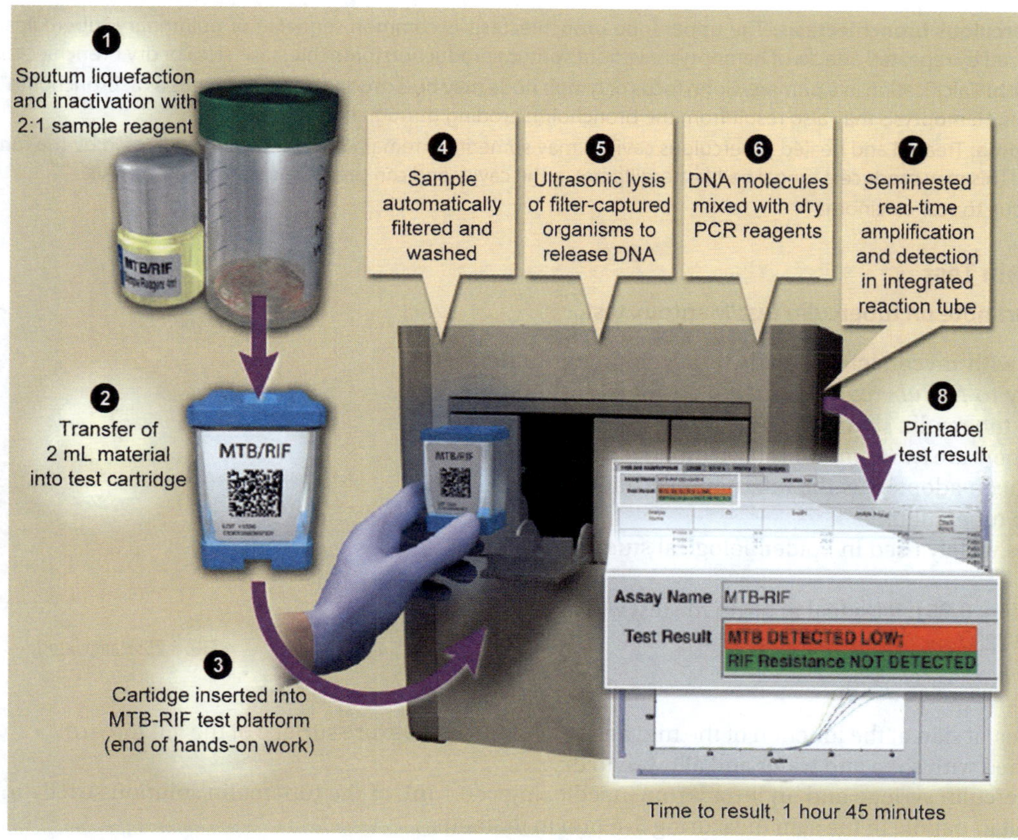

FIG. 6.24: Process of CBNAAT.

Q. Write short note on newer methods of diagnosis of tuberculosis.

- **Interferon gamma release assays (IGRAs):**
  - IGRAs are *in-vitro* tests of cellular immunity. These assays measure cell-mediated immune response by quantifying interferon gamma (IFNγ) released by T cells in response to stimulation by *Mycobacterium tuberculosis*-specific antigens. These specific antigens include early secretory antigenic target-6 (ESAT-6) and culture filtrate protein-10 (CFP10).
  - The test does not differentiate between active and latent infection. This test requires high cost and trained personnel.
- **Other methods of diagnosis:**
  - **MGIT (mycobacteria growth indicator tube)** method: In this method, growth is detected by a nonradioactive detection system using fluorochromes for detection and drug screening.
  - Identification by mycolic acids using high-pressure liquid chromatography
  - *ELISA testing for IgM and IgA:* It is commonly used but has low specificity.
  - Mycobacterial-specific phages (reporter phages) to detect luciferase gene. It can be used to detect drug-resistant isolates.

Causes of Hemoptysis in Pulmonary Tuberculosis

Q. List the causes of hemoptysis in pulmonary tuberculosis.

- **Hemoptysis from a pulmonary cavity**
  - **Rasmussen's aneurysm:** Blood vessels traversing a tuberculous cavity can undergo changes due to inflammatory and necrosis. Over a period of time, these vessels may develop aneurysmal dilatation (Rasmussen's aneurysm). These aneurysms may rupture resulting in hemoptysis.
  - **Allergic response of vessel:** Occasionally, intense allergic response to antigens of tubercle bacilli can damage the walls of the blood vessels in and around the tuberculous cavities leading to hemoptysis.
- **Hemoptysis from endobronchial tuberculosis:**
  - **Tuberculosis of endobronchial region** may be surrounded by vessels with small aneurysmal dilatation. Rupture of these aneurysms can produce hemoptysis.
  - Occasionally, sloughing of the part of the granuloma may result in hemoptysis.
- **Hemoptysis as a sequel of pulmonary tuberculosis:**
  - **Open-healed cavities:** A tuberculous cavity may persist as a sequelae following chemotherapy, which are designated as "open-healed cavities"/INH cysts. The aneurysmal dilations of vessels may also persist in these open-healed cavities, which can rupture producing hemoptysis.

- **Post-tuberculous bronchiectasis:** The upper lobe bronchiectasis is common sequelae of pulmonary tuberculosis. This may be characterized by repeated attacks of hemoptysis without sputum production (bronchiectasis sicca or dry bronchiectasis).
- **Broncholith:** Calcification in a primary/Gohn focus or lymph node may be extruded into a bronchus as a "broncholith" and can cause hemoptysis. Hemoptysis may also result from the broncholith eroding through blood vessels.
- **Aspergilloma:** Treated and healed tuberculous cavities may sometimes remain open and can be infected by the fungus *Aspergillus fumigatus*. This may produce a fungal ball (aspergilloma) in the cavity and can present as severe hemoptysis.

- Hemoptysis due to scar carcinoma

Tuberculin Skin Test

Q. Write a short note on tuberculin test/Mantoux test.

First infection with mycobacteria leads to development of delayed hypersensitivity to *M. tuberculosis* antigens (tuberculin) and this is detected by the tuberculin skin test.

Tuberculins: There are two commonly used tuberculins in present use:

1. PPD-S has been adopted as the international standard for PPD of mammalian tuberculin.
2. PPD-RT23 is widely used in epidemiological studies through- out the world.

Mantoux test (Fig. 6.25): It is ideal to begin the test with 5 IU PPD-S or 1 or 2 IU PPD-RT23.

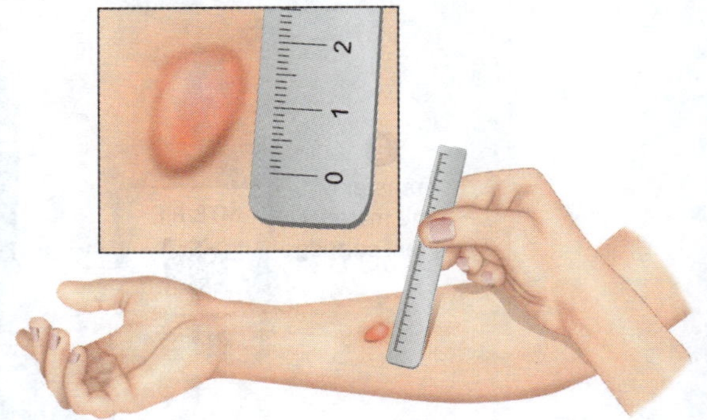

FIG. 6.25: Mantoux test.

Method

- Select an area of skin at the junction of the mid and upper thirds of flexure surface of the left forearm.
- Skin is cleaned with soap and water and allowed to dry.
- Using a tuberculin syringe and an intradermal needle, inject 0.1 mL of the tuberculin solution strictly intradermally. It should result in papule in the skin measuring 5–6 mm in diameter.

Reading and Interpreting the Result

- The test is read after 48–72 hours.
- If a reaction has taken place, there will be an area of erythema (redness) and an area of induration (thickening) of the skin. Measure the diameter of induration across the transverse axis of the arm. The reaction is considered positive, if an area of **induration** of the skin **of 10-mm diameter or more** at the site of injection of PPD. The amount of erythema (redness) present is not important. Induration ≥5 mm is considered as positive in patients with HIV infection (or risk factors for HIV infection, but unknown status), recent close contact to person with known active TB, patients with chest X-ray consistent with prior TB, patients with organ transplants, and other immunosuppressed patient.

Significance

- **Positive tuberculin test: Indicates T-cell-mediated immunity** to mycobacterial antigens. A strongly positive test is particularly valuable in children, especially very young children and favors the diagnosis of tuberculosis.
- **False-negative reactions:** If the diameter of induration is below 10 mm, the test is considered negative. But, a negative test does not exclude tuberculosis. It is seen in certain viral infections, sarcoidosis, malnutrition, Hodgkin lymphoma, immunosuppression, and overwhelming active tuberculous disease, HIV infection, measles, chickenpox, glandular fever (infectious mononucleosis), cancer, corticosteroids, and similar drugs.
- **False-positive reactions:** It is seen in infection by **atypical mycobacteria** or prior **vaccination with BCG** (*Bacillus Calmette–Guerin*) or lymphoma. Most infants immunized with BCG at birth have a negative tuberculin test by 1–2 years. In infants immunized after 1 year, the tuberculin reaction often remains positive for some years. It may also be positive in NTM infections.

Latent Tuberculosis

Q. Describe latent tuberculosis infection (LTBI).

- In the majority of individuals infected by *Mycobacterium tuberculosis*, the immune system contains the infection and the patient develops cell-mediated immune memory to the bacteria. These individuals do not currently have active tuberculosis disease. This is termed latent tuberculosis.
- Individuals with latent tuberculosis are at risk of progression to active tuberculosis. About 5–10% is the lifetime risk of progression. The increased risk of progression from latent tuberculosis to active tuberculosis is during the first 2 years after infection. Groups of individuals at high-risk of tuberculosis infection are listed in **Table 6.38**.

Groups at increased risk of progression to active tuberculosis are listed in **Table 6.39**.

Screening for Latent Tuberculosis

- Tuberculin skin test
- T-cell IGRAs

Prophylaxis (to Prevent Development of Active Tuberculosis)

Refer Tuberculosis Prophylaxis.

ANTITUBERCULOUS DRUGS (ATDS)

Q. Write short note on the terms "bactericidal action" and "sterilizing action" in relation to antituberculous drugs.

- **Bactericidal action:** It is the capacity of antituberculous drugs to rapidly kill large number of actively metabolizing bacilli. Most of the antituberculous drugs (except thiacetazone and PAS) are bactericidal. Isoniazid is the most potent bactericidal. Ethambutol is bacteriostatic at low doses and bactericidal at high doses.
- **Sterilizing action:** It is the capacity of antituberculous drugs to kill special populations of slowly or intermittently metabolizing semi-dormant bacilli (so-called "persisters"), e.g., rifampicin and pyrazinamide.

Q. Write short essay/note on:

- **Management of pulmonary tuberculosis, antituberculous drugs, and their dosages in adults.**
- **List the first- and second-line antituberculous drugs. Explain the rationale for using a multidrug regime.**
- **Bactericidal drugs used in the treatment of tuberculosis.**

Classification of Antituberculous Drugs

See **Table 6.40.**

TABLE 6.38: Groups of individuals at high-risk of tuberculosis infection.

- Employees working at long-term care facilities, hospitals, and medical laboratories
- Individuals having close contact with patients with active tuberculosis
- Residents and employees of congregate living facilities (e.g., prison and jails, nursing homes, hospitals, and homeless shelters)

TABLE 6.39: Groups at increased risk of progression to active tuberculosis.

- Children younger than 5 years of age
- History of tuberculosis infection:
  - Individuals infected with *Mycobacterium tuberculosis* within the past 2 years
  - Past history of untreated or inadequately treated tuberculosis
- Associated conditions:
  - Individuals with HIV infection
  - Silicosis
  - IV drug users
  - Immunocompromised conditions
  - Long-term use of corticosteroids or other immunosuppressants (including anti-TNF-α)
  - Chronic renal failure
  - Diabetes mellitus
  - Malignancy

TABLE 6.40: Classification of antitubercular drugs.

First-line antituberculous drugs	
Isoniazid (H)	Ethambutol (E)
Rifampin (R)	Streptomycin (S)
Pyrazinamide (Z)	
Second-line antitubercular drugs	
Thiacetazone (Tzn)	Newer antitubercular drugs
Para-aminosalicylic acid (PAS)	Ciprofloxacin
Ethionamide (Etm)	Ofloxacin
Cycloserine (Cys)	Moxifloxacin
Kanamycin (Kmc)	Clarithromycin
Amikacin (Am)	Azithromycin
Capreomycin (Cpr)	Rifabutin

First-line Antituberculous Drugs

Q. Write short note on:

- **First-line antituberculous drugs.**
- **Modes of action of first-line drugs.**

1. **Isoniazid (INH):** It is primarily tuberculocidal drug.

   Mechanism of action: Inhibition of mycolic acid cell wall synthesis via O_2-dependent pathways (e.g., catalase-peroxidase reaction). Bactericidal against rapidly multiplying and bacteriostatic against resting bacilli. **Active against both extracellular and intracellular organisms.** Resistance occurs spontaneously in 1 in 10^5 bacilli.

   Pharmacokinetics:
   - Excreted in urine: Decrease dose, if creatinine clearance <30 mL/min
   - Slow versus rapid acetylators ($t_{1/2}$)

   Q. Write short note on toxic effects of INH.

   Adverse effects:

   a. **Peripheral neuropathy:** More common is slow acetylators, diabetic, alcoholics, and malnourished patients
      - Prevention: Pyridoxine 10 mg/day
      - INH neurotoxicity is treated by pyridoxine 100 mg/day. Convulsions should be treated by IV pyridoxine 100 mg.
      - *Other TB-related drugs that cause peripheral neuropathy: Pyridoxine, ethambutol, and cycloserine*

   b. **Hepatitis:**
      - *Increased risk*: Age >35 years, alcohol abuse, rapid acetylators, co-administration of rifampin, pyrazinamide, HIV infection, chronic hepatitis B, pregnant females, and immediate postpartum (3 months).
      - Dose related and is reversible on stopping the drug.

   c. **Others:** Idiosyncratic reactions, SLE, gynecomastia acne, rash, anemia psychosis, memory impairment, and optic neuritis (atrophy).

2. **Rifampicin:**

   Semisynthetic derivative of rifamycin B obtained from *Streptomyces mediterranei.*

Mechanism of action: Inhibition DNA-dependent RNA synthesis. **Bactericidal against both extracellular and intercellular organisms.**

Adverse effects: Patients have discolored (orange) body secretions, hepatitis, thrombocytopenic purpura, respiratory syndrome, shock, renal failure (azotemia). Minor effects are:

- **Cutaneous (red man) syndrome:** Flushing, pruritus, rash (especially face and scalp). Exfoliative dermatitis is more frequent in HIV-positive TB patients.
- Influenza-like (Flu) syndrome
- **Abdominal syndrome:** Pseudomembranous colitis (especially rifabutin)

Newer rifampicin-related antitubercular agents

Q. Write short essay/note on newer rifampicin-related antitubercular agents.

Rifabutin:

- **Actions:** It is related to rifampin. It is active against rifampicin-resistant *M. tuberculosis*; more active than rifampicin against *M. avium* intracellulare complex/NTM; longer t½; extent of absorption remains unchanged with food; recommended instead of rifampicin in patients HIV patients.
- Dose: It is recommended for tuberculosis in HIV-infected patients who are on protease inhibitors. Dose is 150 mg/day.
- Adverse effects: GI distress, rash, myalgias and insomnia, flu-like syndrome, anterior uveitis, leukopenia, skin discoloration, and hepatitis. Patients also have discolored (orange) body secretions.

Rifapentine:

- **Features:** It is lipophilic and has longer duration of action. Mycobacteria resistant to rifampicin are also resistant to this drug. It may be used in the treatment of pulmonary tuberculosis in place of rifampicin. Higher likelihood of relapse, but lower risk of adverse effects and less frequent administration than with rifampicin
- Dose: 600 mg once or twice a week
- Side effects: Similar to rifampicin

Q. Write short essay/note on uses of rifampin.

Uses of rifampin are listed in **Box 6.7**.

Box 6.7: Uses of rifampin.

- Tuberculosis
- Leprosy
- Prophylaxis of *meningococcal* and *H. influenza* meningitis and carrier state
- Second or third choice of drug for MRSA, diphtheroids, and *Legionella* infections
- Combination of doxycycline and rifampin as first line drugs in Brucellosis

3. **Pyrazinamide:**
   - Chemically similar to INH
   - **Mechanism of action:** Inhibition of mycolic acid cell wall synthesis and resembles INH. Bactericidal to slowly metabolizing bacilli in phagosome/granuloma. Most effective in acidic pH (<6.0)
   - **Adverse effects:**
     - Hepatotoxicity: Dose dependent
     - Arthralgias and polyarthralgias (especially shoulders) are common. Arthralgias are not related to the serum uric acid level.
     - Hyperuricemia is common due to inhibition of uric acid secretion by kidney. Development of new-onset gout is rare, but pre-existing gout may be exacerbated.
4. **Ethambutol:**

Q. Write short essay/note on ethambutol.

- **Mechanism of action** (MOA): It inhibits arabinose (arabinosyltransferase) involved in arabinogalactan synthesis. Bacteriostatic
- Excreted in urine (dose reduction required for patients with creatinine clearance <50 mL/min)

Adverse effects:

a. **Retrobulbar neuritis:** Dose-dependent. Usually occurs after many months of treatment. Manifests with reduced visual acuity, central scotoma, disturbance of *red-green* discrimination (loss of ability to see green). Permanent blindness may develop, if not discontinued.

b. Others: Hyperuricemia and peripheral sensory neuropathy.

5. **Streptomycin:**
   - It is an aminoglycoside, bactericidal antibiotic derived from *Streptomyces griseus.*

Adverse effects

a. **Ototoxicity, cochlear and vestibular damage, deafness, and neuromuscular blockage:** Dosage should be reduced, if headache, vomiting, vertigo, and tinnitus occur. Avoid in young children.

b. **Renal damage-nephrotoxicity** (nonoliguric renal failure): Dosage must be reduced to half immediately, if (1) urinary output falls, (2) if albuminuria occurs, or (3) if tubular casts are detected in the urine.

c. **Others:** Rare and include hemolytic anemia, aplastic anemia, agranulocytosis, thrombocytopenia, and lupoid reactions

Mode of Action of First-line Antituberculous Drugs

In a tuberculous lesion (particularly in a cavitary lesion), mycobacteria exist in several foci (**Table 6.41**).

Second-line Antituberculous Drugs

Q. Write short note on second-line antituberculous drugs.

TABLE 6.41: Tuberculous foci and the drugs acting on them.	
Tuberculous foci	***Drugs acting on them***
Extracellular, in alkaline medium	Streptomycin
Rapidly metabolizing mycobacteria (in a cavity)	Rifampicin
Less actively multiplying bacilli in acidic and closed lesions	Isoniazid
Dormant bacilli (that cause a relapse)	Pyrazinamide

- **Ethionamide:** It is structurally related to INH and acts by inhibiting mycolic acid synthesis. It is effective against bacilli, resistant to other drugs, and is effective in infections due to atypical mycobacteria. It is effective against both intracellular and extracellular organisms.
- **Cycloserine:** It is mainly bacteriostatic and acts by inhibiting the synthesis of the bacterial cell wall. It is effective against bacilli resistant to INH or streptomycin and against atypical mycobacteria. Antitubercular activity is less than that of these two drugs.
- **Fluoroquinolones:** Ciprofloxacin, ofloxacin, levofloxacin, moxifloxacin, and gatifloxacin are active against *M. tuberculosis*, even in cases resistant to other drugs. Given orally or IV. It is useful in treating infections resistant to standard drugs and in relapse cases.
- **Capreomycin:** It is bactericidal and its mechanism of action, pharmacokinetics, and adverse reactions are similar to those of streptomycin. Administer with caution in presence of renal impairment.
- **Kanamycin and amikacin:** Both are bactericidal and are active against bacilli resistant to streptomycin, INH, and cycloserine.
- **Macrolides:** Newer macrolides, azithromycin and clarithromycin, also have action against tubercular bacilli. They are used to treat typical mycobacterial infection as well as in relapse cases.

Newer Antituberculous Drugs

- **β-lactams** (imipenem, amoxicillin-clavulanic acid), linezolid, clofazimine, clarithromycin, dapsone, and metronidazole have been used rarely for the treatment of multidrug-resistant (MDR) tuberculosis. However, their roles are not well established.
- **Bedaquiline:** It is a diarylquinoline class of antibiotics that selectively targets the proton pump of ATP synthesis, leading to inadequate ATP synthesis (necessary for bacterial metabolism). It is a new drug used for MDR tuberculosis.
- **Delamanid and pretomanid:** These are nitroimidazole class of antibiotics that inhibit the synthesis of mycolic acids (components of the cell envelope of *M. tuberculosis*). It is still on clinical trials.
- **Sutezolid:** It is oxazolidinone class of antibiotics. It prevents the initiation of protein synthesis by binding to 23s RNA in the 50s ribosomal subunit of bacteria.
- **SQ109**, a 1,2-ethylenediamine: It is an analog of ethambutol.
- **Benzothiazinones:** They inhibit the synthesis of decaprenyl-phospho-arabinose (the precursor of the arabinan) in the mycobacterial cell wall.

Side Effects of the Commonly Used Antituberculous Drugs (Table 6.42)

Q. Write short notes on side effects of the commonly used antituberculous drugs/rifampicin/INH/ethambutol/streptomycin.

TABLE 6.42: Side effects of the commonly used antituberculous drugs.

	Adverse reactions	
Drug (daily dosages)	***Major***	***Less common (rare)***
Isoniazid (H) (5–10 mg/kg)	➤ Hepatitis ➤ Peripheral neuropathy (preventable and treatable with pyridoxine) ➤ Cutaneous hypersensitivity	Giddiness, seizures, optic neuritis, mental symptoms, hemolytic anemia, aplastic anemia, agranulocytosis, lupoid reactions, arthralgia, and gynecomastia
Rifampicin (R) (10 mg/kg)	Febrile reactions ("flu" syndrome; more common with intermittent therapy), hepatitis, cutaneous reactions, and gastrointestinal disturbances	Shortness of breath, shock, hemolytic anemia, interstitial nephritis, and thrombocytopenia
Pyrazinamide (Z) (20 mg/kg)	Anorexia, nausea, flushing, hepatitis, gastrointestinal disturbance, and hyperuricemia	Hepatitis (dose related), vomiting, arthralgia, cutaneous hypersensitivity, and gout
Ethambutol (E) (15 mg/kg)	Retrobulbar neuritis (dose related) and arthralgia	Peripheral neuropathy and rash
Streptomycin (S) and other aminoglycosides (15–20 mg/kg)	8th nerve damage, cutaneous hypersensitivity, giddiness, numbness, and tinnitus	Vertigo, ataxia, deafness, hypokalemia, renal damage, aplastic anemia, and agranulocytosis
Ethionamide (Etm) (10–20 mg/kg)	Anorexia and vomiting	Serious neurologic reactions and hepatitis
Cycloserine (Cys) (10–20 mg/kg)	Headache and somnolence	Psychosis, seizures, and peripheral neuropathy
Quinolones (7.5–15 mg/kg)	GI intolerance and skin rashes	Phototoxicity (with sparfloxacin), dizziness, headache, and insomnia
Thiacetazone (Tzn) (2.5 mg/kg)	Gastrointestinal reactions, cutaneous hypersensitivity, vertigo, and conjunctivitis	Hepatitis, erythema multiforme, exfoliative dermatitis, hemolytic anemia
Para-aminosalicylic acid (PAS) (8–12 g/day)	Gastrointestinal reactions, hepatitis, cutaneous hypersensitivity, and hypokalemia	Acute renal failure, hemolytic anemia, thrombocytopenia, and hypothyroidism

Antituberculous Chemotherapy

Q. Write short essay/note on:
- **Short-course chemotherapy and its advantages.**
- **Discuss regimen of antituberculous chemotherapy.**

Global targets of detecting 70% of infectious cases and curing 85% of those detected. Goals of antituberculous drug therapy are listed in **Box 6.8**.

Short-course Chemotherapy

- Short-course chemotherapy (SCC) is regimens of 6–9-month duration, which are highly effective and widely accepted as the treatment of choice for tuberculosis.
- All the short course regimens have two phases: An initial intensive (bactericidal) phase and a continuation (sterilizing) phase.
  - **Initial phase:** It lasts for 2–3 months and aimed to rapidly kill majority of mycobacteria. The symptoms resolve, sputum becomes negative, and the patient becomes noninfectious.
  - **Continuation phase:** It lasts for 4–6 months during which the remaining bacilli are eliminated so that relapse does not occur.

Advantages of short course of chemotherapy are mentioned in **Box 6.9**.

Box 6.8: Goals of antituberculous therapy.

1. Kill the dividing bacilli
2. Kill the persisting bacilli
3. Prevent emergence of resistance

Box 6.9: Advantages of short-course chemotherapy.

- Easy to take and produces minimal upsets in patients.
- Patient will recover more quickly.
- Sputum becomes negative more quickly. About 85% at 2 months
- Low relapse rate. Even if relapse occurs, the tubercle bacilli remain sensitive and the same treatment can be given repeated.

WHO (2009) Definitions

- **New case:** A patient who has never had been treated for TB or not had anti-TB drugs for less than 1 month. New case may have positive or negative bacteriology and may have tuberculosis at any anatomical site.
- **Previously treated case:** It is defined as a newly registered episode of TB in a patient who has received one month or more of anti-TB drugs in the past. A culture and drug sensitivity test should be done before starting treatment. It is also referred to as "retreatment cases" and forms a heterogeneous group composed of several subcategories:
  - **Relapse:** A patient who has been previously treated for TB and was declared cured and is now been diagnosed bacteriologically positive tuberculous case (either a true relapse or a new episode of TB caused by reinfection).
- **Treatment after failure:** A patient who have been previously treated for TB and whose treatment failed at the end of course of treatment. The sputum smear or culture is positive at 5 months or later during treatment. This includes patients who have a multidrug-resistance strain at any point of time during the treatment.
- **Treatment after loss to follow-up:** Patients have previously been treated for TB and were declared lost to follow-up at the end of their most recent course of treatment (previously known as treatment after default patients) and now have bacteriologically positive tuberculosis.
- **Treatment after default:** A patient who returns to treatment with positive bacteriology, following interruption of treatment for 2 months or more.
- **Other:** All cases, which do not fit the above definitions. It includes patients who are sputum smear-positive at the end of a retreatment regimen (previously defined as chronic cases) and who may be resistant to the first-line drugs.

Categories of Diagnosis and Treatment

Treatment regimen for tuberculosis is presented in **Table 6.43**.

Diagnostic algorithm for pulmonary TB is shown in **Flowchart 6.7**.

Severe Tuberculosis

- **Miliary, disseminated TB** is considered to be severe.
- **Forms of extrapulmonary tuberculosis** (EPTB) classified as severe include: Meningeal, pericardial, peritoneal, bilateral or extensive pleural effusive, spinal, intestinal, and genitourinary.

Less severe: Lymph node, pleural effusion (unilateral), bone (excluding spine), peripheral joint, and skin tuberculosis.

TABLE 6.43: Treatment regimen for tuberculosis—all regimens are daily regimens.

A. DOTS (Directly observed treatment, short course)	***Regimen***
For new TB cases	2 months (HRZE) + 4 months (HRE) **Duration: 6 months**
For previously treated cases: Includes previously treated sputum smear-positive pulmonary TB: ➤ Relapse ➤ Treatment after interruption ➤ Treatment failure	2 months (HRZES) followed by 1 month (HRZE), followed by 5 months (HRE) **Duration: 8 months**
Management of extrapulmonary TB	The CP in both new and previously treated cases may be extended 3–6 months in certain TB such as CNS, skeletal, disseminated TB, and so on based on clinical decision of the treating physicians
B. DOTS PLUS	
1. **MDR TB:** Includes MDR and chronic TB cases (still sputum-positive after supervised retreatment)	6–9 months (KM LVX, ETO CS, Z, and E) followed by 18 months (LVX, ETO, CS, and E) **Duration: 24–27 months**
2. **XDR TB**	6–12 months intensive phase followed by 18 months continuation phase (capreomycin, PAS, moxifloxacin, clofazimine, linezolid, amoxicillin/clavulanate, clarithromycin, thiacetazone) **Duration: 24–30 months**

Note: Since 2017, the thrice weekly regimen has been changed daily regimen.
(H: isoniazid; R: rifampin; Z: pyrazinamide; E: ethambutol; S: streptomycin; KM: kanamycin; LVX: levofloxacin; ETO: ethionamide; CS: Cycloserine; PLHIV: people living with HIV)

FLOWCHART 6.7: Diagnostic algorithm for pulmonary TB.

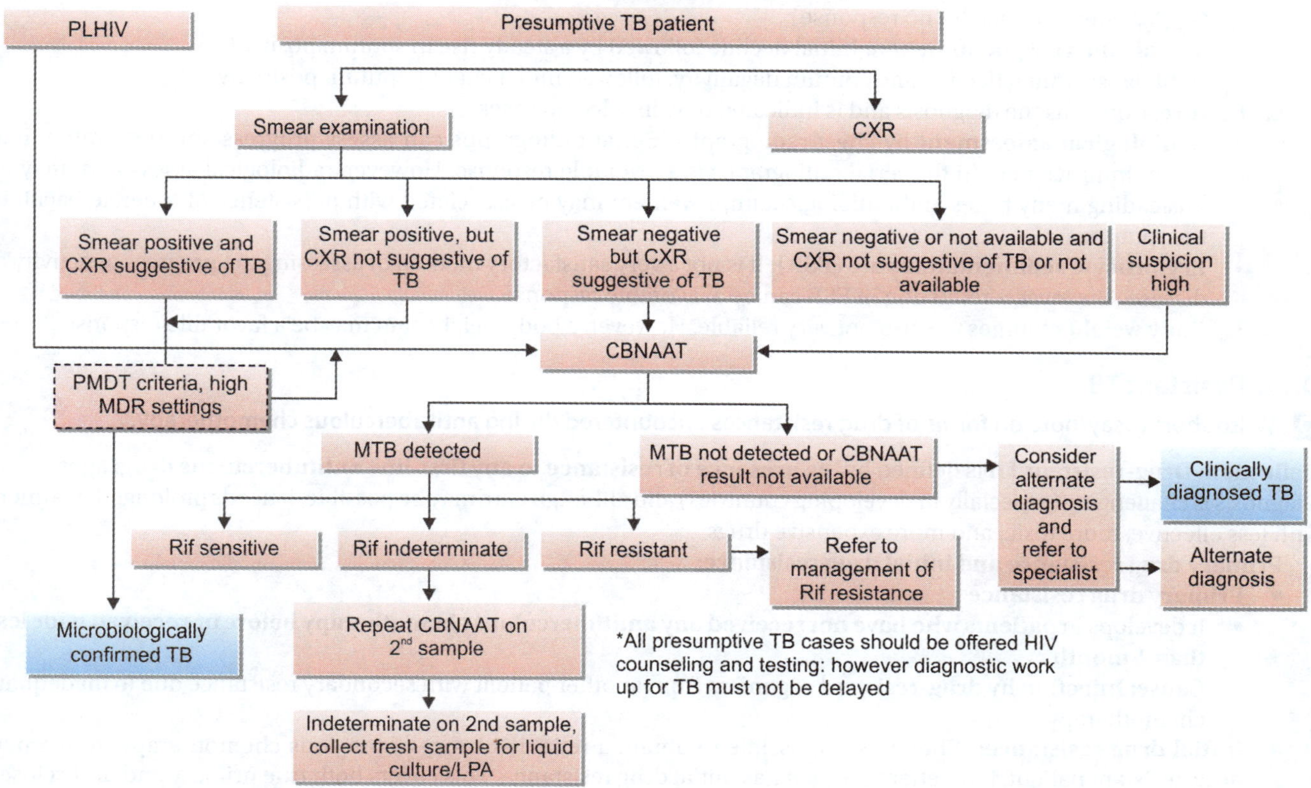

Directly Observed Treatment, Short Course

Q. Write short essay/note on directly observed treatment, short course (DOTS) in tuberculosis.

- Directly observed treatment, short course is an **intermittent method** of administering potent antituberculous regimens to a patient with tuberculosis **under direct supervision.**
- Daily chemotherapy is excellent. However, it is expensive and not possible to supervise therapy and hence compliance rate is low and relapse rate is high.
- **DOTS is a five-point program** (WHO), which can effectively control TB:
  1. Political and administrative support.
  2. Diagnosis in patients attending health facilities is by microscopic examination of sputum.
  3. Good antituberculous drugs are given for short course.
  4. Directly observed treatment, which is easily accessible, acceptable, and accountable.
  5. Systematic monitoring and accountability.

Monitoring the Treatment and Treatment Results

Q. Write short essay/note on monitoring the progress of treatment and the assessment of treatment result.

Main method of monitoring is bacteriological examination. Other methods include radiological assessment, ESR, and body weight changes.

- **Bacteriological examination:** Bacteriological assessment can be made by examining sputum smear and sputum culture.
  a. **Serial sputum smear exminations:** These help to assess the progress and ultimate result.
    - Sputum smear microscopy should be **performed at completion of the intensive phase** of treatment.
    - **New patients:**
      - **If sputum smear is positive at the end of the intensive phase** (2 months), **repeat the sputum smear at the end of the 3rd month.**
      - If the **smear is positive at the end of 3 months,** perform sputum culture and drug susceptibility testing (DST).
    - **Previously treated patients:**
      - If the smear is positive at the end of the intensive phase (3 months), perform sputum culture and DST.
    - **Favorable response:** If sputum bacillary count steadily decreases. In most patients, sputum will be negative in 1 month and almost all in 2 months and all in 3 months. However, sputum culture may be positive for another 1 or 2 months. Finally, both smears and cultures will be negative.

- ♦ **Indications of treatment failure:**
  - Persistence of bacilli (no response)
  - **Fall and rise phenomenon:** Initial decline followed by a steady rise in sputum positivity
  - Relapse: Initial decline and sputum negativity, followed much later by sputum positivity

b. **Culture:** Confirms the diagnosis and is indicated only in selected cases

- ♦ **Radiological assessment** by chest radiographs: Serial radiographs can assess progress and determine final result. Improvement in the serial radiographs is a favorable response. However, radiological assessment may be misleading many times and radiological improvement may be associated with persistence of tubercle bacilli in the sputum.
- ♦ **Erythrocyte sedimentation rate (ESR):** It is not a very satisfactory method of assessing the progress or activity of disease. However, a reduction in ESR can be a favorable response.
- ♦ **Body weight changes** are also not very reliable. However, a body weight gain may be a favorable response.

Drug-Resistant TB

Q. Write short essay/note on forms of drug resistances encountered during antituberculous chemotherapy.

Definition: Drug-resistant TB is defined by the **presence of resistance to any first-line antituberculous drug/agent.** Diagnosis is challenging (especially in developing countries) and although cure may be possible, it needs prolonged treatment with less effective, more toxic, and more expensive drugs.

- **Primary drug resistance and initial drug resistance:**
  - **Primary drug resistance**
    - ♦ It develops in **patients who have not received any antituberculous chemotherapy before or received it for less than 1 month.**
    - ♦ **Cause: Infection by drug-resistant organism** from another patient with secondary resistance due to inadequate chemotherapy.
  - **Initial drug resistance:** When it is impossible to obtain a reliable history of previous chemotherapy from a new drug-resistant patient, it is better to term it has initial drug resistance. This covers both true primary and undisclosed acquired resistance.
- **Secondary or acquired drug resistance: Resistance to one or more antituberculous drugs,** usually due to incorrect chemotherapy.
- **Natural drug resistance:** Mycobacterial strains, which have never been exposed to any antibacterial drug are called "wild strains." Thus, natural drug resistant strain is a wild strain resistant to a particular drug without ever having any contact with it. Thus, neither the patient with naturally resistant bacilli nor his source of infection has had chemotherapy in the past.
- **Transient drug resistance:** A positive culture of bacilli may be resistant to one or more (rarely two) drugs of a regimen during the course of successful chemotherapy. This may be due to resistant organisms for unknown reasons outlived the sensitive part of the bacterial population. Transient resistance does not need any change of treatment, since it does not results in treatment failure.
- **Mono-resistance (MR):** A TB patient whose biological specimen is resistant to one first-line anti-TB drug only.
- **Polyresistance (PDR):** A TB patient whose biological specimen is resistant to more than one first-line anti-TB drug, other than both INH and rifampicin.
- **Rifampicin resistance (RR):** Resistance to rifampicin detected by phenotypic or genotypic methods with or without resistant to other ATD excluding INH. Patient with RR should be managed as if they are in MDR-TB case.

Q. Write short essay on multidrug-resistant (MDR) tuberculosis, its diagnosis, and management.

- **Multiple drug resistance or multidrug-resistant TB:**
  - Multidrug-resistant tuberculosis (MDR-TB) is a form of TB that is **resistance to at least both of INH and rifampicin**, with or without other drug resistance. Hence, a patient should not be classified as multidrug resistant disease, if the patient has an infection with a bacterium susceptible to rifampicin but resistant to many other drugs.
  - MDR-TB can rarely be observed in new cases. It is more common in individuals in re-treatment cases (prior history of TB, particularly if treatment has been inadequate, and those with HIV infection). It is a man-made phenomenon
  - Chronic cases and MDR-TB cases are not synonymous. Chronic patients probably have MDR-TB because they have previously received at least two full courses of treatment with essential antituberculous drugs.
- **Extensive drug-resistance TB (XDR-TB):**
  - Extensively drug resistance TB is a form of TB that is resistant to at least four of the core anti-TB drugs. These drugs include most important (core) anti-TB drugs—(1) isoniazid and (2) rifampicin, and (3) injectable second-line aminoglycoside drugs (amikacin, capreomycin, or kanamycin) + (4) fluoroquinolone (such as ofloxacin or moxifloxacin).
- **Totally drug-resistant TB or (extremely XXDR, TDR):**
  - Totally drug-resistant tuberculosis (TDR-TB) is a form of TB strains that shows in vitro resistance to all first- and second-line drugs tested (isoniazid, rifampicin, streptomycin, ethambutol, pyrazinamide, ethionamide, para-aminosalicylic acid, cycloserine, ofloxacin, amikacin, ciprofloxacin, capreomycin, and kanamycin).

– It was first reported in 2003 from Italy. In early January 2012, twelve cases had been diagnosed in Mumbai and in all cases, the strain of TB was resistant to all first- and second-line antitubercular drugs.

Factors contributing to the emergence of drug-resistant TB are listed in **Table 6.44**.

Q. Write short essay/note on common causes of drug resistance.

Suspicion of Drug Resistant TB

- A close contact of drug resistant TB case
- All retreatment cases
- Extensive disease at start of treatment
- Extrapulmonary TB not responding to standard ATT regime.
- Treatment failures
- No sputum conversion after initial 2 months of ATT
- All HIV patients with TB

TABLE 6.44: Factors contributing to the emergence of drug-resistant tuberculosis (TB).

➤ Drug shortages	➤ Infection due to organisms with primary resistance
➤ Use of poor-quality drugs	➤ Transmission of drug-resistant strains
➤ Inadequate treatment regimen	➤ Prior antituberculosis treatment
➤ Inadequate supervision of therapy	➤ Treatment failure (smear-positive at 5 months)
➤ Poor absorption of drugs	➤ Lack of good laboratory facilities to monitor drug susceptibility
➤ Development of adverse drug reactions	➤ Genetic factors
➤ Inadequate duration of treatment	

Drug Susceptibility Testing (DST)

Q. Write short essay/note on various methods for performing drug susceptibility tests for *M. tuberculosis*.

WHO recommends DST for first-line and second-line anti-TB drugs to detect MDR-TB and XDR-TB, respectively.

Various methods of DST are:

- **Lowenstein Jensen (L-J) culture:** For drug sensitivity testing, it takes 6–8 weeks time.
- **Radiometric methods (BACTEC radiometric method):** Results obtained within 10 days of inoculation.
- **Mycobacteria growth indicator tube (MGIT) system:** Rapid, nonradioactive method.
- **Nitrate reduction assays:** Based on the capacity of *M. tuberculosis* to reduce nitrate to nitrite.
- **Ligase chain reaction (LCR):** Enzyme DNA ligase functions as a link two strands of DNA.
- **Luciferase reporter assay:** Useful for rapid determination of drug resistance.
- **PCR-based sequencing:** Detects mutations responsible for drug resistance.
- **Line probe assays:** Detects drug resistant (particularly rifampicin resistant) bacilli.
- **The Xpert MTB/RIF:** It is a cartridge-based, automated diagnostic test that identifies *Mycobacterium tuberculosis* (MTB) DNA and resistance to rifampicin (RIF) by nucleic acid amplification technique (NAAT). Result is obtained within 2 hours.

Management of Multidrug-resistant Tuberculosis (Flowchart 6.8)

Q. Write short essay/note on multidrug resistant (MDR) tuberculosis, its diagnosis, and its management (drugs used).

FLOWCHART 6.8: Drug-resistant TB—diagnostic algorithm.

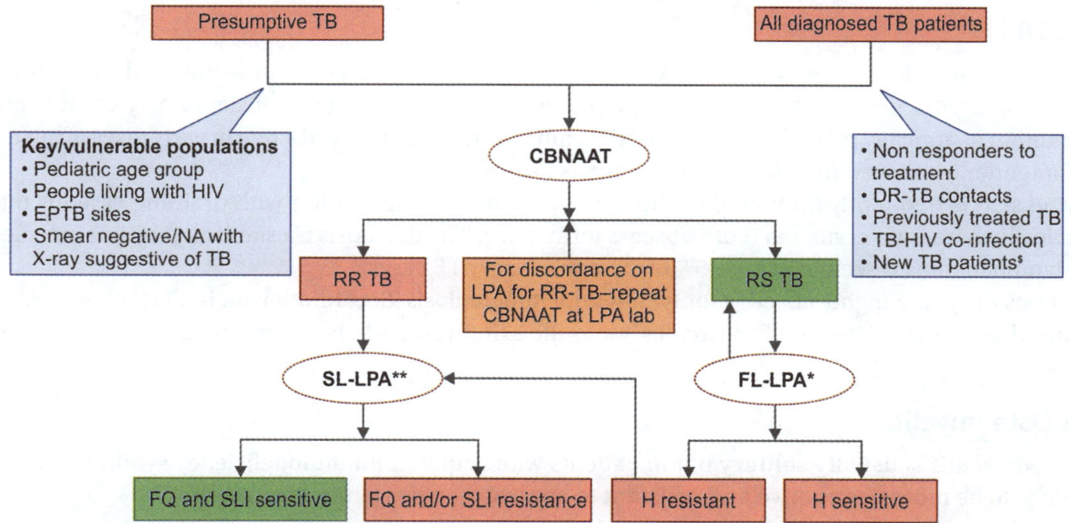

Note: *Offer molecular testing for H mono/poly resistance to TB patients prioritized by risk as per the available lab capacity
**LC DST (Mfx 2.0, Km, Cm, Lzd) will be done only for patients with any resistance on baseline SL-LPA, DST to Z, Cfz, Bdq and Dlm would be considered for policy in future, whenever available, standardized and WHO endorsed.
$States to advance in phased manner as per PMDT scale up plan for universal DST based on lab capacity and policy on use of diagnostics

Q. Write short essay/note on management of multidrug-resistant (MDR) tuberculosis.

Principles for managing a patient with MDR tuberculosis (Table 6.45)

TABLE 6.45: Principles for managing a patient with multidrug-resistant (MDR) tuberculosis.

- DOTS-PLUS strategy is used.
- Use at least 4 reliable drugs.
- Do not use drugs with cross resistance.
- Eliminate drugs that are not safe for the patient.
- Include drugs from Groups 1–5 in a hierarchical order.
- Monitor and manage adverse effects of drugs.
- Never add a single drug to failing regime.

General treatment principles

- Provide 18–24 months' treatment, always with intensive phase of at least 6 months (current WHO guidelines—8 months).
- Provide DOT therapy.
- Warn patients about possible side effects.
- Manage side effects appropriately.
- Perform cultures monthly.

Standard RNTP Guidelines for XDR-TB Management

Intensive phase (6–12 months)	***Continuous phase (18 months)***
Capreomycin (1000 mg)	Moxifloxacin (400 mg)
Moxifloxacin (400 mg)	INH high dose (900 mg)
INH high dose (900 mg)	PAS (12 g)
PAS (12 g)	Clofazimine (200 mg)
Clofazimine (200 mg)	Linezolid (600 mg)
Linezolid (600 mg)	Amoxicillin/clavulanate (875 + 125 mg); 2 tablets in morning and 1 tablet in evening
Amoxicillin/clavulanate (875 + 125 mg); 2 tablets in morning and 1 tablet in evening	

Note: Add pyridoxine (100 mg/day) to ATD regimen

Indications for Treatment with Steroids

Q. Write short essay/note on the indications of corticosteroids use in the management of tuberculosis.

- Severely ill patients, e.g., TB meningitis with decreased consciousness, neurological defects, or spinal block or severe pulmonary TB.
- Severe hypersensitivity reaction to anti-TB drugs.
- To prevent exudation, its organization and stricture formation:
  - TB pericarditis with effusion or constriction
  - Large TB pleural effusion with severe symptoms
  - Meningeal tuberculosis
  - Renal tract TB to prevent ureteric scarring
  - TB laryngitis with life-threatening airway obstruction
- Hypoadrenalism (tuberculosis of adrenal glands)
- Massive lymph node enlargement with pressure effects
- In AIDS patient with severe manifestations of tuberculosis

EXTRAPULMONARY TUBERCULOSIS

Q. Write short essay/note on extrapulmonary tuberculosis.

The term extrapulmonary tuberculosis (EPTB) is used for occurrence of tuberculosis at body sites other than the lung. However, when an extrapulmonary focus is present in a patient with pulmonary tuberculosis, such patients are categorized as pulmonary tuberculosis.

EPTB constitutes 15–20% of all cases of TB immunocompetent patients and in HIV-positive patients, EPTB accounts for more than 50% of all cases of TB.

Sites of EPTB: In order of frequency, these include lymph nodes (mediastinal and/or hilar, cervical), pleura (effusions without radiographic abnormalities in the lungs), genitourinary tract, bones and joints, meninges, peritoneum, and pericardium. However, virtually all organ systems may be affected **except nail, hair and enamel.**

Lymph Node TB

- Most common site for EPTB is lymph node. Extrathoracic nodes are more commonly involved than intrathoracic or mediastinal. Usually, this presents as a firm, painless (nontender) enlargement of a posterior cervical or supraclavicular node (a condition historically referred to as **scrofula**). Lymph nodes are usually discrete in early disease but develop into a matted nontender mass over time. The portal of entry is through the tonsils.
- The overlying skin is frequently indurated or there can be sinus tract formation with draining caseous material, but characteristically there is no erythema (**cold abscess** formation). The diagnosis is established by fine-needle aspiration biopsy. TB lymphadenitis is seen in nearly 35% of extrapulmonary TB cases.
- Antituberculous drugs are highly effective for lymph node tuberculosis. **Scrofuloderma** is a mycobacterial infection of the skin caused by direct extension of tuberculosis into the skin from underlying structures or by contact exposure to tuberculosis.

Tuberculous Osteomyelitis

Tuberculous osteomyelitis is **usually solitary** but in patients with acquired immunodeficiency syndrome, it is frequently multifocal. It tends to be **more destructive and resistant to control** than pyogenic osteomyelitis.

- **Age:** Usually **adolescents or young adults** in developing countries.
- **Source of infection:** Pulmonary or extrapulmonary tuberculosis.
- **Predisposing factors:** Diabetes, elderly, immune compromised states, and general debility.
- **Route of infection:**
  - **Blood-borne:** Usually blood-borne infection, which is from a focus of **active pulmonary or extrapulmonary disease**.
  - **Direct extension:** From lung into a rib and tracheobronchial nodes into adjacent vertebrae.

- **Sites:**
  - **Spine** (thoracic and lumbar vertebrae) commonly known as **Pott's disease.** The **infection breaks through intervertebral disks** to involve multiple vertebrae and **extends down into the soft tissues** forming abscesses (**cold abscess–psoas abscess**).
  - Knees and hips
- **Clinical course:**
  - Low-grade fever with evening rise of temperature
  - Pain on motion and localized tenderness
  - Weight loss
- **Complications:**
  - **Spine**
    - **Destruction of vertebrae:** Causes severe **scoliosis or kyphosis** and neurologic deficits due to spinal cord and nerve compression.
    - **Psoas abscess:** Infection from spine may rupture into the soft tissue anteriorly and pus and necrotic debris may drain along the spinal ligaments and form a **cold abscess, i.e., an abscess lacking acute inflammation. Psoas abscess** is the condition in which infection from lower lumbar vertebrae dissects along the pelvis, and appears as a draining sinus of the skin in the inguinal region. It may be the first manifestation of tuberculous spondylitis.
      - **Tuberculous arthritis**
      - **Sinus tract formation**
      - **Amyloidosis**

Tuberculous Meningitis

Refer **Chapter 15.**

Gastrointestinal Tuberculosis

- TB can affect any part of the bowel.
- Upper gastrointestinal tract involvement is rare.

Intestinal Tuberculosis

Discussed in Chapter 10.

Extrapulmonary sites of tuberculosis and their presentation are summarized in **Table 6.46** and **Figure 6.26**.

TABLE 6.46: Extrapulmonary sites of tuberculosis and their presentation.

Extrapulmonary site	*Presentation*
Pleural	Pleural effusion and pleuritis
Lymph nodes	Tuberculous lymphadenopathy (including mediastinal) nonhealing sinuses
Skeletal system	Tuberculous osteomyelitis, cold abscess, vertebral tuberculosis, and pyarthrosis
Nervous system	Tuberculous meningitis tuberculous arteritis and cerebral tuberculoma
Gastrointestinal	Ulcerations of the tongue, intestinal tuberculosis, and tuberculous peritonitis
Pericardium	Pericardial effusion and tamponade, constrictive pericarditis
Genitourinary	Renal tuberculosis, salpingitis, tubal abscess, and tuberculous epididymitis
Miscellaneous	Addison's disease (tuberculous adrenalitis), skin tuberculosis (Scrofuloderma, Lupus vulgaris, tuberculids), phlyctenular keratoconjunctivitis, choroiditis, iritis, and erythema nodosum

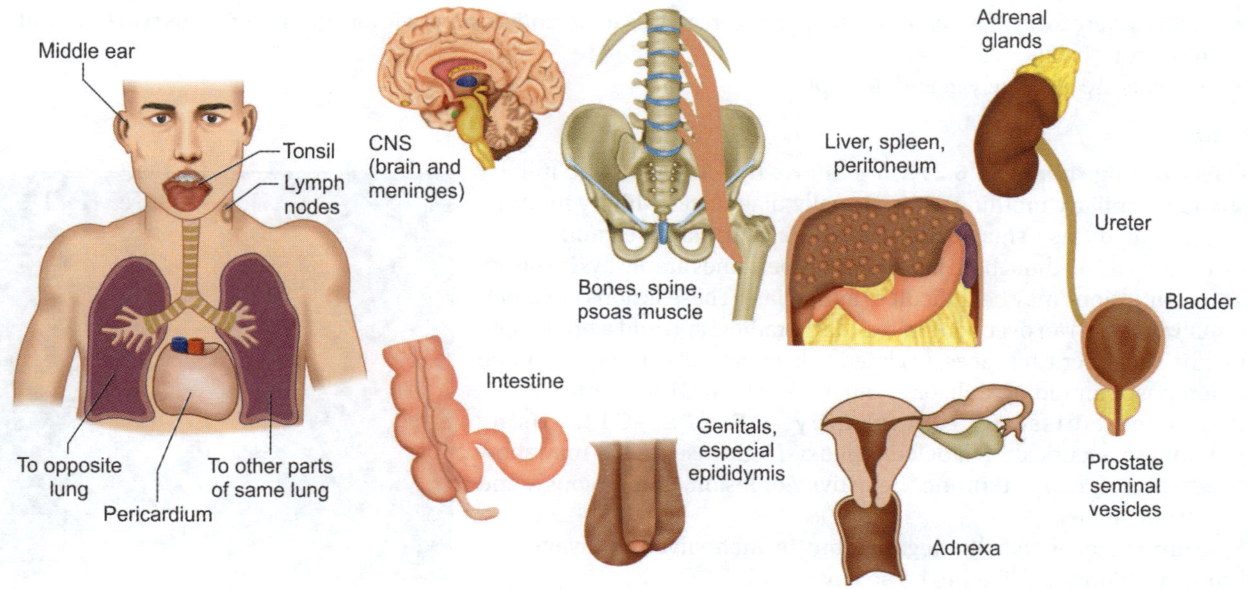

FIG. 6.26: Various extrapulmonary sites of tuberculosis.
(CNS: central nervous system)

Miliary or Disseminated TB

Q. Discuss the pathogenesis, types, clinical features, diagnosis, and management of miliary tuberculosis in adults.

Miliary TB is the disseminated form of tuberculosis. The lesions are usually yellowish granulomas 1–2 mm in diameter. These lesions resemble millet seeds (hence termed miliary).

Route of Spread

Miliary tuberculosis results from widespread hematogenous dissemination of tubercle bacilli. The tubercle bacilli may enter the bloodstream by either hematogenous or lymphatic route.

Types

Q. Write short essay/note on miliary tuberculosis/nonreactive miliary tuberculosis/disseminated nonreactive tuberculosis.

Clinically, the miliary TB patients may be divided into three different types: (1) Classical (acute) miliary tuberculosis, (2) cryptic (obscure) miliary tuberculosis, and (3) nonreactive miliary tuberculosis.

1. **Classical (acute) miliary tuberculosis:**
   - **Age:** Can occur at any age, but more commonly affects children and young adults.
   - **Onset:** Sudden or gradual. Usually present with insidious onset of fever, malaise, and weight loss over weeks.
   - **Other symptoms:**
     - Systemic symptoms include high-grade fever, drenching night sweats, and progressive pallor.
     - Cough and breathlessness are occasionally present.
   - **Signs:**
     - There may not be any abnormal physical signs in the lungs. Widespread crepitations may be heard late in the disease.
     - Hepatosplenomegaly may be seen.
     - **Choroidal tubercles** on ophthalmoscopy—diagnostic
2. **Cryptic (obscure) miliary tuberculosis**

   Q. Write short essay/note on cryptic miliary tuberculosis.
   - **Age:** Usually in the elderly
   - **Symptoms:**
     - Prolonged low-grade pyrexia common presenting manifestation
     - Lassitude, weight loss, and general debility
   - **Signs:**
     - Hepatosplenomegaly may occur
     - Chest is usually normal
     - Choroidal tubercles are rare
3. **Nonreactive miliary tuberculosis:**
   - Rare, usually develops in elderly with disease reactivation
   - Acute severe form of tuberculous septicemia, resulting in necrotic lesions without granulomatous reaction containing numerous bacilli.
   - Patients are extremely ill and die rapidly.

Diagnosis

- **Chest radiograph (Fig. 6.27):** If it shows the characteristic miliary shadows (miliary mottling), it is virtually diagnostic. Miliary mottling appears as diffuse small shadows of 1–2 mm diameter and evenly distributed throughout both lung fields. Upper zones are always involved. The early lesions may be difficult to appreciate. These lesions are better visualized by (1) an over penetrated (dark) radiograph and a bright light behind the outer rib spaces, (2) lateral chest film, (3) underpenetrated anteroposterior radiograph, or (4) high-resolution CT of chest.
- **Positron emission tomography CT (PET-CT):** Using radiopharmaceutical ^{18}F labeled 2-deoxy-D-glucose (FDG) may show "hot" spots. It can determine the activity of lesion, guide biopsy, and detect occult foci.
- **Sputum** smear is usually negative but bronchoalveolar lavage and bronchial biopsy are likely to be positive.

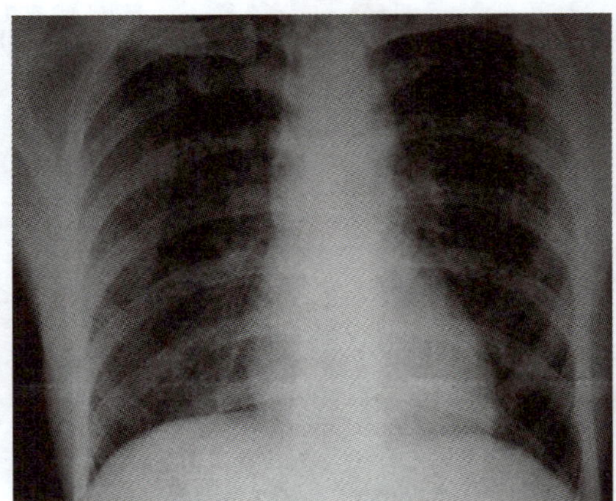

FIG. 6.27: Chest X-ray showing miliary mottling.

- **Culture:** Confirmation of diagnosis should be done by culture of sputum, urine, or bone marrow.
- **Hematological abnormalities:** These include anemia, leukopenia, neutrophilic leukocytosis, and leukemoid reaction. Rarely DIC can develop.
- Elevation of alkaline phosphatase and other liver enzymes may be observed in patient with severe liver involvement.
- Hyponatremia may develop in about 50% cases.
- **Bone marrow biopsy:** May show miliary tubercles/bacilli on histology. Part of the specimen should be sent for culture for tubercle bacilli.
- **Liver biopsy:** May show miliary tubercles.
- **Tuberculin test:** Only of limited value in miliary tuberculosis.

Q. Write short essay/note on management of miliary tuberculosis.

Management

- **Acute and cryptic miliary tuberculosis:** Standard antituberculous chemotherapy. In severely ill patients, prednisolone is given along with chemotherapy. It reduces life-threatening toxicity and gives time for antituberculous drugs to act.
- **If the diagnosis is not proved** (e.g., cryptic miliary tuberculosis): Therapeutic trial of antituberculous chemotherapy.

Tuberculous Pleural Effusion

Q. Discuss the etiology, pathogenesis, clinical features, investigations, complications, and management of tuberculous pleural effusion.

Q. Write short note on tuberculous pleural effusion and its laboratory diagnosis.

- **Age group:** Tuberculous pleural effusion usually occurs in **younger individuals**.
- Underlying pulmonary tuberculosis: **Only one-third** of patients show simultaneous pulmonary tuberculosis.

Pathogenesis

Involvement of pleura by *M. tuberculosis* may occur by various routes namely via lymphatics, bloodstream, or by direct extension.

- **Isolated pleural effusion** usually due to **recent primary infection**. The collection of fluid in the pleural space represents a hypersensitivity response to mycobacterial antigens.
- Pleural disease may also develop from contiguous parenchymal spread from **postprimary/secondary tuberculosis of lung**.
- **Rupture of subpleural caseous focus** into the pleural cavity. This produces delayed hypersensitivity reaction to tuberculous protein. It causes increased permeability of pleural capillaries, mild lymphatic block by fibrosis. Cultures of the pleural fluid from most of these patients with tuberculous pleural effusions are negative (because it is a hypersensitivity response).
- **Sequelae:** If left untreated, the pleura may become thick and fibrotic (pleural fibrosis) and pleural adhesions may develop. Pleural adhesion causes restrictive ventilator dysfunction. Early treatment is necessary to prevent these sequelae.

Clinical Features, Investigations, and Management

Refer Section on pleural effusion later.

Pleural fluid analysis

Q. Write a note on pleural fluid findings in tuberculous pleural effusion.

- **Color:** Fluid is usually straw/amber colored, but sometimes hemorrhagic.
- **Exudative in nature:** Characteristically fluid is an exudate, with a high protein content (>3 g/dL) >50% of that in serum (usually 4–6 g/dL) a normal to low glucose concentration, a pH of ~7.3 (occasionally <7.2) and raised white blood cells (usually 500–6,000/μL).
- **Cells: Predominant lymphocytosis**. Neutrophils may predominate in the early stage (less than 2 weeks), but lymphocytosis is the typical finding later. Mesothelial cells are usually rare or absent. If the pleural fluid shows more than 10% eosinophils, diagnosis of tuberculous effusion is unlikely unless the patient has a pneumothorax or had previously undergone thoracocentesis.
- **Smear for AFB:** Smears prepared from the centrifuged deposit may rarely show the tubercle bacilli (<10% of immunocompetent cases).
- **Culture for *M. tuberculosis*:** Positive in approximately 25–50% of patients and are more common among postprimary/secondary cases.
- **Determination of the pleural concentration of adenosine deaminase (ADA):** It is a useful screening test, and TB can be excluded if the value is very low.

Q. Write short note on adenosine deaminase (ADA).

- It is a T-lymphocyte enzyme.
- In majority of cases, the levels of **ADA in the pleural fluid are elevated** (>40 IU/L) and is probably due to increased activity of T lymphocytes (CD4+) in the pleural fluid.
- Other causes with high ADA include rheumatoid arthritis, lymphoma, chronic lymphatic leukemia, empyema, and mesothelioma. However, because the incidence of tuberculosis far exceeds than any other cause of a lymphocytic pleural effusion (like in India), high ADA level has a predictive value.
- Specificity of raised levels of ADA in diagnosing tuberculous effusion is nearly 0.83 and the reported sensitivity is 77–100%. Specificity increases when pleural fluid lymphocytes/polymorph ratio greater than 3.
- ADA is not useful in HIV patients with TB.
- There are two isoenzymes of ADA namely ADA1 and ADA2. ADA1 isoenzyme is found in all cells and they are high in lymphocytes and monocytes. ADA2 isoenzyme is present only in monocytes. In **tuberculous pleural effusion, ADA2 isoenzyme** is mainly responsible for high ADA concentration.

Interferon-gamma (INF-γ): Produced by lymphocytes specifically sensitized to PPD. Its level above 140 pg/mL is suggestive of TB and is elevated irrespective of immune status. It is more expensive than ADA.

Other tests on pleural fluid: These include raised LDH, raised lysozymes, marked elevation in the levels of soluble interleukin-2 (IL-2) receptors, and PCR for DNA of *M. tuberculosis*. Nucleic acid amplification technology has low sensitivity.

Pleural biopsy: Closed pleural biopsy shows noncaseating granulomas in 80% of patients. It should be stained with Z-N stain and cultured for mycobacteria. Diagnostic yield increases to 90% with pleural biopsy and biopsy cultures for AFB.

Management
- **Therapeutic aspiration of pleural fluid:** May be required in patients with severe symptoms.
- **Antituberculous chemotherapy**
- **Corticosteroids:** May reduce the symptoms of toxemia. However, they do not reduce the incidence of pleural fibrosis. Prednisolone is administered in the dose of 0.75 mg/kg/day for up to 4 weeks with gradual reduction over an additional 2–4 weeks.

BCG Vaccination

Q. Write short essay/note on BCG vaccination (Bacillus Calmette–Guerin vaccine).

BCG (Bacillus Calmette-Guerin) is a freeze-dried, live attenuated (lost its virulence) vaccine derived from *M. bovis*. In India, Danish strain 1331 is being used for BCG vaccine production.
Procedure: 0.1 mL of the reconstituted vaccine is injected intradermally at the junction of the upper and middle thirds of the left upper arm.
Contraindications: Generalized eczema and hypogammaglobulinemia, and immunodeficiency resulting from treatment with antimetabolites, irradiation or systemic corticosteroids.
Advantages: BCG vaccination reduces the risk of miliary/disseminated tuberculosis (TB) and tuberculous meningitis in children. Its efficacy in adults is very variable.
Complications: Secondary infection with local abscess formation, enlargement of regional lymph nodes, cold abscess of draining lymph nodes, local lupoid reactions (rare), erythema nodosum, urticaria, and disseminated BCG infection (rare).

Tuberculosis Chemoprophylaxis—Isoniazid Preventive Therapy

Q. Write a short note on tuberculosis chemoprophylaxis.

- Purpose: To prevent progression of latent tuberculous infection to active disease.
- **Types:**
    - **Primary or infection prophylaxis:** Drug is given to individuals who have not been infected in order to prevent development of disease (e.g., breastfed infants of sputum-positive mother).
    - **Secondary or disease prophylaxis:** Drug is given to prevent development of disease in individuals already infected.

Drugs Used

- **Isoniazid** (H) at the dose of 5 mg/kg/day (not exceeding 300 mg/day) for 6–12 months is used for chemoprophylaxis.
- Alternate option:
    - Isoniazid plus rifampicin (10 mg/kg daily) for 3 months or
    - Isoniazid in the dose of 5 mg/kg (adults 900 mg) plus rifampicin at a dose of 10 mg/kg twice weekly for 3 months.
- **Precaution:** Exclude active TB by history, physical examination, chest radiograph and, if necessary, by other tests before starting chemoprophylaxis.

Indications

- Close contacts of open case of TB who show recent Mantoux conversion.
- Close contacts children aged 5 years or below with strongly positive Mantoux and a TB patient in the family.
- Breastfed neonates/infants of sputum-positive mothers.
- Newly infected patients as shown by recent change in tuberculin test from negative to positive.
- Patients with old inactive disease who are assessed to have received inadequate treatment.
- Certain diseases in which TB is more likely to develop. These include HIV infection, leukemia, Hodgkin's disease, prolonged treatment with prednisolone, severe diabetes mellitus, and patients on anti-malignancy drugs. In India, if tuberculin test is ≥10 mm. [WHO recommends that people living with HIV (PLHIV) who are unlikely to have active TB should receive at least 6 months of isoniazid preventive therapy (IPT) as part of a comprehensive package of HIV care)].

Risks

- **Isoniazid resistance** can occur especially when preventive therapy with isoniazid is inadvertently given to individuals with subclinical or unrecognized TB.
- Hepatotoxicity.

SUPPURATIVE LUNG DISEASE

Bronchiectasis

Q. Define bronchiectasis. Describe the etiopathogenesis, classification, clinical features, investigations, complications, and management of bronchiectasis.

Definition: Bronchiectasis is defined as an **irreversible** (permanent), **abnormal dilation of the cartilage-containing airways bronchi or bronchioles.**

Classification

A. **According to the shape of the bronchial dilation (Figs. 6.28A to C)** based on the bronchographic appearance (Reid's classification)
   - **Tubular (cylindrical):** Characterized by smooth dilation of the bronchi. It is the most common form.
   - **Varicose (bulbous):** In which the bronchi are dilated with multiple indentations.
   - **Cystic (saccular/balloon appearance):** In which dilated bronchi terminate in blind ending sacs.

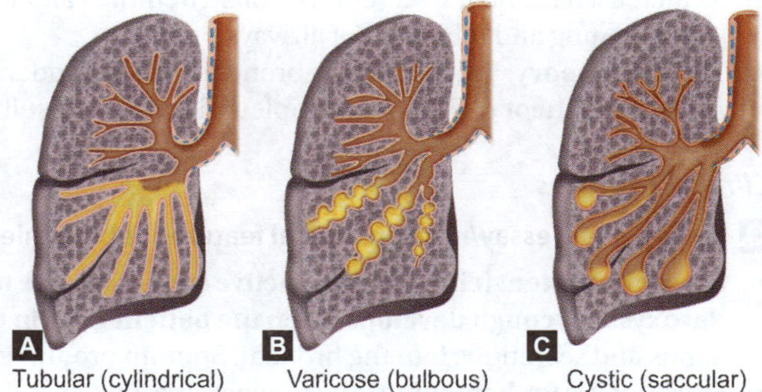

FIGS. 6.28A TO C: Morphological types of bronchiectasis: (A) Cylindrical type; (B) Varicose (bulbous) type; (C) Saccular.

B. **According to the extent of involvement**
   - **Diffuse (generalized) bronchiectasis: Characterized by** widespread bronchiectatic changes throughout the lung. It is **usually bilateral** and commonly affects the **lower lobes. Left lobe is more commonly involved than the right**. It is most severe in the distal bronchi and bronchioles.
   - **Focal (localized) bronchiectasis:** Bronchiectatic change is **restricted to a** localized area of the lung **(single segment of the lung)** and usually occurs in association with obstruction of the airway (parenchymal tumor or aspiration of foreign bodies).

C. **According to the underlying disease/mechanism**
   - Congenital/acquired
   - Cystic fibrosis (CF) associated and noncystic fibrosis bronchiectasis
   - Associated with post fibrosis: Traction bronchiectasis
   - Without much expectorant: Dry bronchiectasis.

Etiology

Q. Write a short essay/note on causes of bronchiectasis.

The dilatation of bronchi and bronchioles is caused by **destruction of the muscle and elastic tissue of bronchial wall**. It represents a secondary disorder as the end stage of many unrelated disorders. It may be divided into obstructive and nonobstructive (postinflammatory). It may also be divided into congenital and acquired **(Table 6.47)**.

Proximal bronchiectasis: In which, dilatation involves larger airways:

- **Allergic bronchopulmonary aspergillosis (ABPA)**
- **Brock's syndrome/middle lobe syndrome:** Primary TB/foreign body/tumor compressing main bronchus.
- **Lady Windermere syndrome (LWS):** These women have the habit of voluntarily suppressing cough. It results in inability to clear the secretions from the right middle lobe and lingual leading to infection and later bronchiectasis.
- **Congenital syndromes: Kartagener's syndrome, yellow nails syndrome, Chandra-Khetarpal syndrome** (immunodeficiency associated with levocardia, bronchiectasis, and paranasal sinus anomalies), **Young's syndrome, cystic fibrosis, Chédiak-Higashi syndrome.**

TABLE 6.47: Causes of bronchiectasis.

Congenital
- Cystic fibrosis (CF)
- Ciliary dysfunction syndromes
  - Primary ciliary dyskinesia (immotile cilia syndrome), Young's syndrome
  - Kartagener's syndrome (sinusitis and transposition of the viscera)
- Primary hypogammaglobulinemia, alpha-1 antitrypsin deficiency
- Others: Bronchial cysts, cul-de-sacs, bronchomalacia, atopic bronchial asthma, pulmonary sequestration, Mounier–Kuhn syndrome or tracheobronchomegaly, Williams–Campbell syndrome (bronchomalacia)

Acquired: children
- Pneumonia (complicating whooping cough or measles)
- Primary tuberculosis
- Inhaled foreign body

Acquired: adults
- Pulmonary tuberculosis, *Mycobacterium avium complex (MAC)*
- Suppurative pneumonia
- Allergic bronchopulmonary aspergillosis (ABPA) complicating asthma
- Postobstructive bronchiectasis: Partial or total obstruction of the bronchial lumen, e.g., endobronchial tumors or foreign bodies, enlarged hilar lymph nodes or tumor masses and bronchostenosis following endobronchial tuberculosis
- Autoimmune diseases, e.g., rheumatoid arthritis, Sjögren's syndrome, systemic lupus erythematosus, inflammatory bowel disease
- Others: Repeated aspiration of gastric juice, inhalation of toxic gas (ammonia), HIV infection, interstitial lung fibrosis (traction bronchiectasis), radiation fibrosis, sarcoidosis, chronic hypersensitivity pneumonitis, bronchiolitis obliterans after lung transplantation

Pathogenesis

Theories of bronchiectasis

- **Pressure of secretion theory (obstruction):** Secretions cause mechanical obstruction and obstruction **impairs clearing mechanisms** of the lung → results in **accumulation of secretions** distal to the obstruction → **leads to secondary infection** → inflammation → weakens and dilates airway.
- **Infection theory: Chronic persistent** (recurrent) **necrotizing infection** and inflammation in the bronchi or bronchioles → increased bronchial secretion → **obstruction** of airways by secretions → inflammation and fibrosis of the airway walls → weakening and dilatation of airways.
- **Traction theory:** Traction of the bronchi walls secondary to fibrosis/scarring.
- **Atelectasis theory:** Negative intrapleural pressure resulting in collapse and bronchial dilatation.

Clinical Features

Q Write a short essay/note on clinical features of bronchiectasis.

- **Severe persistent (chronic) productive cough: It is the most common symptom.** Cough is chronic, daily, and persistent. **Paroxysm of cough develops when the patient rises in the morning** because the postural changes drain the collections of pus and secretions into the bronchi. Sputum production varies with posture.
- **Sputum:** It is **foul-smelling** (due to anaerobic infections), thick, copious, tenacious, and continuously purulent, sometimes bloody.
- **Hemoptysis:** Streaks of blood is common with exacerbations of infection and is commonly recurrent. Rarely massive hemoptysis occurs. Hemoptysis occurs due to rupture of the thin-walled blood vessels present on the walls of dilated bronchi.
- **Pleuritic (chest) pain:** It may be caused due to infection of pleura, or due to segmental collapse caused by retained secretions.
- **Infective exacerbation:** Increased sputum volume with fever, malaise, and anorexia are precipitated by upper respiratory tract infections.
- **General debility:** In severe/widespread bronchiectasis, the patient presents with difficulty maintaining weight, anorexia, exertional breathlessness/dyspnea, wheezing, and orthopnea.
- **Bronchiectasis sicca/dry bronchiectasis:** Occasionally, the patient is asymptomatic or has nonproductive cough. It is termed bronchiectasis sicca and commonly follows TB of upper lobe. Only manifestation will be hemoptysis.
- Situs inversus is found in 50% cases of ciliary dyskinesia.

Physical findings

General examination: It may reveal anemia, **pandigital clubbing** (7% cases), fever, weight loss, night sweat, weakness, **halitosis** (may accompany purulent sputum) and sinusitis. Signs and symptoms of lung infection, such as fever may not be present.

Respiratory system

- Nasal polyps and signs of chronic sinusitis may be present.

- Signs may be unilateral, but are usually bilateral and basal. In dry bronchiectasis, no abnormal physical signs may be found.
- **Auscultation:** Reveals **crackles** and wheezing. Presence of large amounts of secretion is responsible for the characteristic **"bilateral, coarse, leathery crepitations"** of bronchiectasis which may be palpable (tactile fremitus).

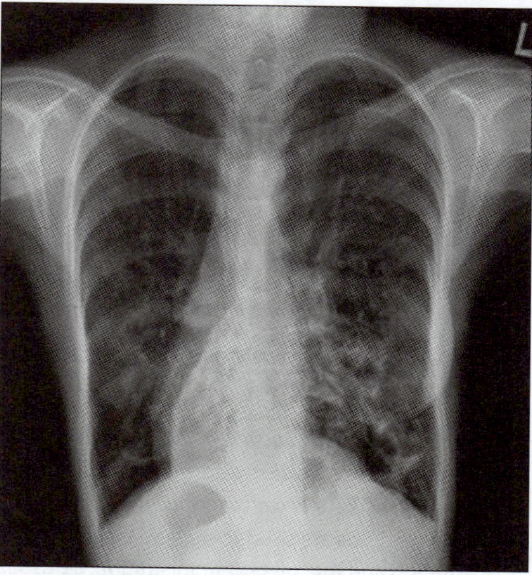

FIG. 6.29: Chest X-ray (CXR) showing bilateral bronchiectasis with dextrocardia with situs inversus.

Investigations

- **Blood:** Anemia, raised ESR and leukocytosis indicating suppuration. ABG studies may show respiratory alkalosis or hypoxemia.
- Sputum examination:
  - If sputum is collected in a conical flask and allowed to stand, it forms three layers (**"three-layered sputum"**), top mucoid layer, middle mucopurulent layer, and purulent layer at the bottom.
  - Stain the sputum by Gram's stain, Ziehl–Neelsen stain for acid-fast bacilli
  - Culture and sensitivity: Culture usually grows organism in the normal nasopharyngeal flora or *Pseudomonas.*
- **Chest radiograph (Fig. 6.29):** It lacks sensitivity. Signs on CXR include the identification of parallel linear densities, tram-track opacities, or ring shadows reflecting thickened and abnormally dilated bronchial walls.
- **Chest computed tomography (CT):** More specific and sensitive, and is the imaging modality of choice for confirmation for bronchiectasis. High-resolution CT **(HRCT) findings (Fig. 6.30)** are:
  - Specific criteria:
    - Thickened, dilated airways (parallel "tram tracks" or as the "signet ring sign"). Internal diameter of the bronchus is minimum 1.5 times more than that of the nearby vessel.
    - Absence of bronchial tapering in the periphery of the chest (presence of tubular structures within 1 cm from the pleural surface)
  - Other findings: Inspissated secretions (e.g., the tree-in-bud pattern) or cysts arising from the bronchial wall (in cystic bronchiectasis).
  - May suggest the etiology of bronchiectasis (e.g., proximal bronchiectasis suggests ABPA).

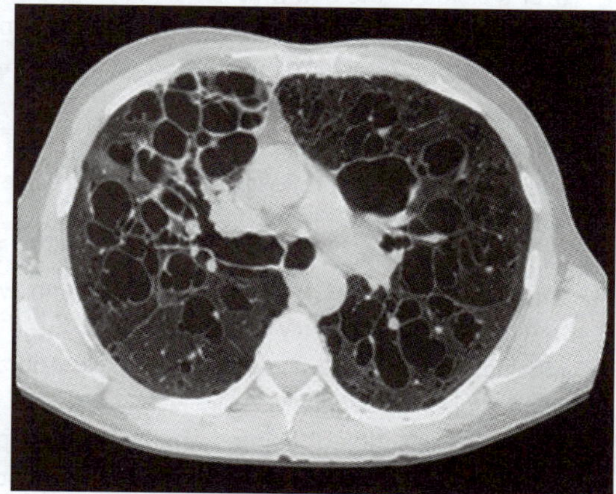

FIG. 6.30: High-resolution CT (HRCT) image of bronchiectasis.

- **Sinus X-rays:** About 30% of patients have rhinosinusitis.
- Bronchoscopy: Does not establish the diagnosis.
  - Indications: (1) to identify the source of secretions, (2) to identify the site of bleeding in patients with hemoptysis, (3) therapeutically to remove secretions, and (4) localized bronchiectasis.
- Bronchography: Rarely indicated.
- **Pulmonary function tests:** It may detect mild to moderate airflow obstruction, but a restrictive pattern evolves with advanced disease.
- Urine examination: In advanced and chronic cases, proteinuria may develop due to renal amyloidosis.
- Electrocardiogram: Usually normal, but right ventricular hypertrophy may be detected when cor pulmonale develops.
- **Sweat electrolytes:** Measurement of sodium and chloride concentrations in sweat is useful in cystic fibrosis.
- **Serum immunoglobulins:** Up to 10% of adults with bronchiectasis have antibody class or subclass deficiency (mainly IgA). Its estimation is also useful when primary hypogammaglobulinemia is suspected.
- **Patients suspected of ciliary dysfunction syndrome:** Assessment of ciliary function may be done by several ways:
  - **Mucociliary clearance (nasal clearance of saccharin):** Measures the time taken for a small pellet of saccharin placed in the anterior chamber of the nose to reach the pharynx, where patient can taste it. Normally, it should be <30 minutes. A prolongation of this time (>60 minutes) is found in patients with ciliary dysfunction.
  - Measurement of ciliary beat frequency: Assessed by using biopsies taken from the nose.
  - Electron microscopy: It can detect structural abnormalities of cilia.
  - Study of the sperms.

Complications of Bronchiectasis (Table 6.48)

TABLE 6.48: Complications of bronchiectasis.

- Hemoptysis
- Pneumonia
- Lung abscess
- Empyema
- Cor pulmonale
- Septicemia
- Meningitis
- Osteomyelitis
- Metastatic abscesses (e.g., brain abscess)
- Generalized edema (100 mL sputum/4–5 g protein)—protein loosing pneumopathy
- Generalized amyloidosis
- Aspergilloma
- Respiratory failure
- Microbial resistance to antibiotics

Q. Write a short essay/note on complications of bronchiectasis.

Management

Goals of treatment of bronchiectasis is presented in **Box 6.10**.

Improvements in secretion clearance and bronchial hygiene

- Bronchial hygiene so as to reduce the microbial load within the airways and minimize the risk of repeated infections.
- Many methods are used to increase secretion clearance in bronchiectasis. These include chest physiotherapy (e.g., postural drainage), hydration and mucolytic administration, aerosolization of bronchodilators, and hyperosmolar agents (e.g., hypertonic saline).
- **Postural drainage:** Postural drainage is valuable and consists of adopting a position in which the affected lobe(s) to be drained is uppermost. Patients must be trained by physiotherapists and this should be performed at least three times daily for 5–10 minutes. Lying over the side of the bed with head and thorax down is effective in most patients. Gentle mechanical chest percussion through hand clapping to the chest helps to dislodge the sputum.
- Bronchoscopic removal of inspissated secretions is rarely necessary.

Antibiotic therapy

Antibiotics for eradication of bacteria

For *Pseudomonas:* Oral ciprofloxacin (500–750 mg twice daily) or ceftazidime by intravenous injection or infusion (1–2 g three times daily) for 7–10 days.

Suppressive antibiotics

- After resolution of an acute infection in patients with recurrences, the use of suppressive antibiotics may minimize the microbial load and reduce the frequency of exacerbations.
- Inhaled antibiotics are safe and effective, e.g., tobramycin, gentamicin

Antibiotics for exacerbation

- Choice of the antibiotic depends on the results of culture and sensitivity of sputum.
- If no specific pathogen is identified and the patient is not seriously ill, oral agents like amoxicillin, ampicillin, cotrimoxazole, tetracycline, one of the fluoroquinolones or a fixed combination of amoxicillin and clavulanic acid are recommended.
- More seriously ill patients with pneumonitis require parenteral antibiotics.
- Duration of therapy: Usually a 7- to 10-day course is sufficient. Few patients may need prolonged therapy for several weeks.

Anti-inflammatory therapy

- Control of the inflammatory response may be of benefit in bronchiectasis.
- Inhaled or oral steroids can reduce the rate of progression of bronchiectasis.
- Macrolide antibiotic: They have immunomodulatory action.

Reversal of airflow obstruction

- Bronchodilators (β-adrenoreceptor agonists, anticholinergics) improve obstruction and help in clearance of secretion. They are useful in patients with demonstrable airflow limitation.
- Inhaled corticosteroids may be useful in some patients.

Surgical treatment

- It can be considered only in refractory cases.
- The procedure involved is excision of bronchiectatic areas. It is usually done in cases where the bronchiectasis is restricted to a single lobe or segment on CT.
- Indications of surgery:
  - Children or young adults with localized lesions who fail to respond to medical treatment.
  - Recurrent hemoptysis
  - Recurrent localized pneumonias
- Lung transplantation is considered in patients with advanced disease and respiratory failure.
- **Treatment of the hemoptysis:** Bed rest and antibiotics. Blood transfusion is given if necessary. Occasionally, fiberoptic bronchoscopy is needed to detect the source of bleeding. If the hemoptysis continues, embolization of bronchial artery is the treatment of choice. Surgical resection may be needed if embolization fails.

Other measures
- General management: Graded exercise, routine deep breathing, and maintenance of good nutrition
- Vaccination
- Promptly treat episodes of sinusitis.
- Treat complicated ABPA with prednisolone and itraconazole.
- Mucolytic dornase (DNase) is recommended in cystic fibrosis-related bronchiectasis. It reduces viscosity of sputum by breaking down DNA released from neutrophils.

Box 6.10: Goals of treatment in bronchiectasis.
- Treatment of the underlying cause/disorder
- Improvements in secretion clearance and bronchial hygiene
- Antibiotics to control active infections
- Anti-inflammatory therapy
- Reversal of airflow obstruction
- Surgery

Management of bronchiectasis is summarized in **Flowchart 6.9**.

FLOWCHART 6.9: Management of bronchiectasis.

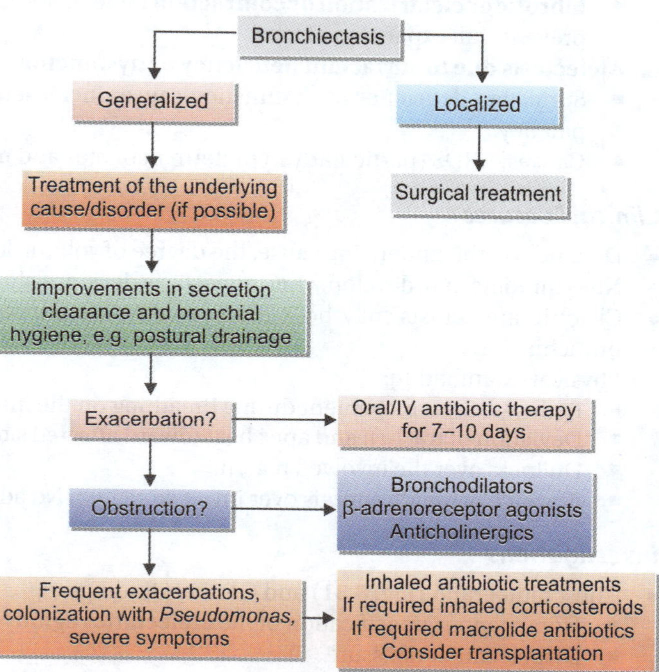

Pseudobronchiectasis

Q. Write a short note on pseudobronchiectasis.

Pseudobronchiectasis (functional bronchiectasis) is characterized by dilated bronchi and is reversible. It is a common in patients with pneumonia of any cause. But re-expansion of the collapsed lung in atelectasis and regeneration of the mucosa in tracheobronchitis leads to reversal of the bronchographic findings. This reversible dilatation of bronchi is termed as pseudobronchiectasis.

Postobstructive Bronchiectasis

Q. Write a short note on postobstructive bronchiectasis.

- It is bronchiectasis that develops distal to a bronchial obstruction.
- **Causes: Partial or total obstruction of the bronchial lumen** due to endobronchial tumors, foreign body aspiration, mucus plugs, enlarged hilar lymph nodes or tumor masses, and bronchostenosis (due to endobronchial TB).

Bronchiectasis Sicca (Dry Bronchiectasis)

Q. Write a short note on bronchiectasis sicca (dry bronchiectasis).

- Usually, bronchiectasis presents with copious sputum.
- **Bronchiectasis sicca** is a condition where bronchiectasis presents with repeated episodes of hemoptysis without sputum production.
- It usually occurs in bronchiectasis of upper lobe following TB.

Atelectasis

Q. Write a short note on atelectasis and signs of lung collapse.

- Atelectasis refers either to **incomplete expansion of the lungs** (neonatal atelectasis) or to the **complete collapse** of previously inflated lung parenchyma.
- It produces areas of relatively airless pulmonary parenchyma.

Classification

Main types are acquired atelectasis:

A. **Obstructive atelectasis (absorption atelectasis)**
   - Most common type
   - **Mechanism:** Complete obstruction (intrabronchial) of an airway causes obstruction of communication between the alveoli and major airways. This leads to absorption of air from the dependent alveoli → diminished lung volume → shifting of the mediastinum toward the atelectatic lung.
   - **Causes:** Due to complete obstruction (intrabronchial) of an airway.
     - Exogenous, e.g., foreign body aspiration, or recurrent aspiration of either gastric or oral contents due to a swallowing disorder
     - Endogenous, e.g., excessive secretions (e.g., mucus plugs) or exudates within smaller bronchi (e.g., in bronchial asthma, chronic bronchitis, bronchiectasis, and postoperative states), bronchial tumors.

B. Nonobstructive atelectasis

- **Compression atelectasis:**
  - Develops due to compression of lung.
  - Causes: It develops from any space-occupying lesion of the thorax (e.g., tumors, cysts, enlarged lymph nodes, and cardiomegaly). It can also occur with chest wall defects (e.g., scoliosis), neuromuscular diseases, and compression by emphysematous bulla.
  - In compression atelectasis, the mediastinum shifts away from the affected lung.
- Relaxation or passive atelectasis
  - Contact between visceral and parietal pleura is lost resulting in passive atelectasis of lung.
  - Causes: Significant volumes of fluid (transudate, exudate or blood) or air (*pneumothorax*) accumulation within the pleural cavity.
- **Fibrotic or cicatrization or contraction atelectasis:** It occurs when focal or generalized pulmonary or pleural fibrosis prevents full expansion of lung.

C. Atelectasis due to surfactant deficiency or dysfunction

- Surfactant deficiency or dysfunction causes increased alveolar surface tension and failure to maintain small airway patency.
- Causes: ARDS (particularly in preterm neonates and meconium aspiration), and pneumonia in elderly.

Clinical Features

- Depends on the underlying cause, the degree of volume loss within the lung, and rate of volume loss.
- No symptoms may develop when atelectasis develops slowly.
- Chronic atelectasis may be a nidus of chronic purulent infection. This may damage bronchial wall leading to bronchiectasis.
- Physical examination:
  - Reduced chest movement during breathing on the involvedregion
  - Deviation of trachea and apex beat toward affected side
  - Dullness over the involved region
  - Absence of breath sounds over involved region. No added sounds.

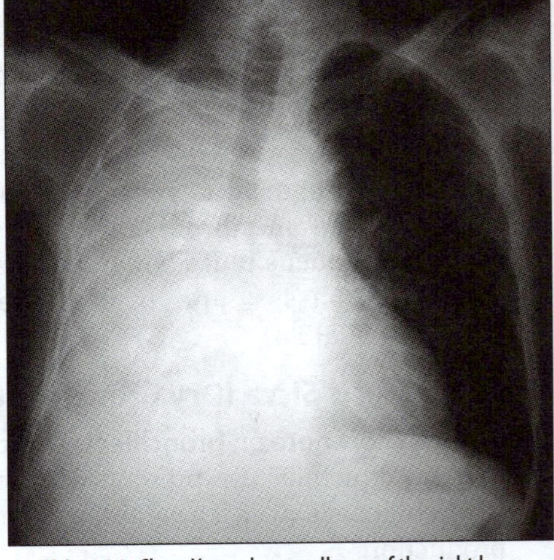

FIG. 6.31: Chest X-ray shows collapse of the right lung.

Investigations

- Chest radiograph **(Fig. 6.31)** and CT chest findings
  - Homogenous opacification of the **atelectatic region**
  - Displacement of fissure
  - Loss of volume and shift of trachea and mediastinum
- Bronchoscopy to identify obstructive lesions and is also useful in removing the mucus plug.
- Arterial blood gas may reveal hypoxemia. Hypocapnia may develop due to tachypnea.

Treatment of collapse

- Emergency bronchoscopy and removal of mucus plug, foreign body
- Treatment of underlying cause

Middle Lobe Bronchiectasis (Middle Lobe Syndrome or Brock's Syndrome)

Q. Write a short note on middle lobe bronchiectasis (middle lobe syndrome or Brock's syndrome).

- It usually develops as a sequel of primary pulmonary TB of lung. It can be also seen with lymphoma and other causes of mediastinal lymphadenopathy.
- It is a type of postobstructive bronchiectasis usually due to obstruction of the middle lobe bronchus by tuberculous lymph nodes.
- This syndrome is characterized by recurrent atelectasis of the right middle lobe in the absence of any endobronchial lesion. Recurrent episodes of atelectasis result in bronchiectasis and fibrosis of right middle lobe.

When a middle-aged woman presents with MAC infection following right middle lobe or lingular lobe bronchiectasis, the patient is diagnosed to have LWS. This appears to be more common in thin females, who have never smoked, and who have no underlying pulmonary disease. Voluntary suppression of cough (hence, fastidious) in these women is hypothesized to cause reduced clearance of secretions from the right middle lobe and lingular segments, which have long and narrow bronchi with acute angulations, thus predisposing the patients to MAC infection.

Ciliary Dysfunction Syndromes or Primary Ciliary Dyskinesia

Q. Enumerate the clinical features, diagnosis, and treatment of ciliary dysfunction syndromes (ciliary dyskinesia syndromes).

Q. Write a short note on primary ciliary dyskinesia (PCD)/Kartagener's syndrome, and Young's syndrome.

- These are a group of genetic disorders characterized by dysfunction of cilia of the respiratory tract epithelium, sperms, and other cells. Dysfunction of cilia causes impairment of mucociliary clearance, left-right body asymmetry, and impaired sperm motility.
- Majority are transmitted as an autosomal recessive disorder.
- **Kartagener or immotile cilia syndrome:** It is an **autosomal recessive** syndrome. It is one of the ciliary dysfunction syndromes with **lack of ciliary function** (due to absence of inner or outer dynein arms of cilia) and causes retention of secretions and recurrent infections. It comprises of recurrent **sinusitis, bronchiectasis, dextrocardia** (with or without situs inversus), and **male infertility** (sperm dysmotility).
- **Young's syndrome:** Patients develop bronchiectasis, sinusitis, and obstructive azoospermia. The cause is not known.

TABLE 6.49: Clinical features of primary ciliary dyskinesia.

System involved	*Clinical features*
Lung	Respiratory distress (in neonates), recurrent infections, and bronchiectasis
Nasal sinus	Chronic sinusitis
Ear	Otitis media, cholesteatoma, hearing loss
Genital tract	Male infertility
Organ laterality	Situs inversus totalis, polysplenia or asplenia
Cardiovascular system	Complex congenital heart disease, vascular anomalies
Central nervous system	Hydrocephalus (rare)

Clinical Features of Primary Ciliary Dyskinesia

See **Table 6.49.**

Diagnosis

- Screening tests
  - Exhaled nasal nitric oxide: Low
  - **Mucociliary clearance (nasal clearance of saccharin):** Tests for ciliary function.
- **Electron microscopy:** It can detect structural abnormalities of respiratory cilia in samples of nasal or airway mucosa. It is characterized by defects in the outer or inner dynein arms of the cilia.
- **Genetic study:** Shows mutation in PCD genes.

Treatment
- No definite treatment.
- Treat bronchiectasis.
- Avoid cough suppressants because cough is the only intact mechanism for mucociliary clearance in these patients.

Suppurative Pneumonias

Q. Write a short essay on suppurative pneumonias and necrotizing pneumonias.

Suppurative pneumonia, aspiration pneumonia, and pulmonary abscess are conditions which have overlap in their etiology and clinical features. Suppurative pneumonia is a type of pneumonic consolidation characterized by destruction of the lung parenchyma by the inflammatory process. Though histologically there is formation of microabscess, the term "lung/pulmonary abscess" is usually used for lesions having a large localized collection of pus, or a cavity lined by chronic inflammatory tissue. The etiological factors are same for both suppurative pneumonia and lung/pulmonary abscess.

Lung Abscess

Q. Define lung abscess. Describe the etiology, clinical features, investigations, diagnosis, complications, and management of lung abscess.

Definition: Lung (pulmonary) abscess is defined as a severe, **local suppurative process within the lung** associated with cavity formation. It is characterized by necrotic area of lung parenchyma containing **pus accompanied by the destruction of lung tissue. Necrotizing pneumonia:** Often used to describe similar pathologic process with multiple small (<2 cm) cavities in contiguous are as of the lung.

Classification

- **Duration of symptoms** prior to diagnosis: acute <1 month, and chronic >1 month
- **Primary or secondary.**

Etiology (Table 6.50)

- Infectious causes: Any pathogen can produce lung abscess.
- Noninfectious causes.

TABLE 6.50: Causes of lung abscess.

A. Infectious causes
1. **Bacteria** – **Usual:** Mouth flora anaerobes, most frequently isolated anaerobes: *Peptostreptococcus, Fusobacterium nucleatum, Prevotella melaninogenica* – **Less common:** *Staphylococcus aureus, Streptococcus pyogenes, Pseudomonas aeruginosa, Klebsiella pneumoniae, Streptococcus pneumoniae*, gram-negative bacilli, such as *Escherichia coli, Haemophilus influenzae type B, Legionella, Nocardia asteroides*. Mixed infections occur when lung abscess develops due to inhalation of foreign material – **Mycobacteria:** *Mycobacterium tuberculosis, M. avium complex, M. kansasii*, other mycobacteria
2. **Fungi:** *Aspergillus spp., Histoplasma capsulatum, Pneumocystis Jirovecii, Coccidioides immitis, Blastocystis hominis, Cryptococcus*
3. **Parasites:** *Entamoeba histolytica, Paragonimus westermani, Strongyloides stercoralis* (postobstructive)
B. Noninfectious causes
1. **Neoplasms:** Primary lung cancer, metastatic carcinoma, lymphoma 2. **Pulmonary infarction:** Due to bland embolus (may be secondarily infected in <5%) 3. **Septic embolism:** Tricuspid endocarditis due to *S. aureus* and others (typically with positive blood cultures), jugular venous septic phlebitis due to ***Fusobacterium necrophorum*** **(Lemierre's syndrome)** 4. **Vasculitis:** Wegener's granulomatosis, rheumatoid lung nodule 5. **Developmental:** Pulmonary sequestration 6. **Airway disease:** Bullae, blebs, or cystic bronchiectasis (usually thin-walled) 7. **Other:** Sarcoidosis, transdiaphragmatic bowel herniation giving appearance of cavity with air fluid level

Pathogenesis

Lung abscess may be **primary or secondary**.

A. **Secondary lung abscess:** Develops as a complication of several conditions.
   - **Complication of necrotizing pneumonia:** The microbes usually associated are: *Staphylococcus aureus, Klebsiella pneumoniae*, and the serotype type 3 *Pneumococcus*.
   - **Pulmonary TB:** Important cause of lung abscess.
   - **Septic embolism:** The source of embolus may be from thrombophlebitis in any part of the systemic venous circulation or from the vegetations of infective bacterial endocarditis on the right side of the heart. The embolus may be trapped in the lung causing multiple pyemic abscesses.
   - **Bronchial obstruction:** By a **bronchial cancer** (primary or secondary) or foreign body (postobstructive pneumonia) → secondary infection
   - Miscellaneous:
     - Direct penetrating trauma to the lungs
     - Spread of infections from a neighboring organ (e.g., suppuration in the esophagus, spine, subphrenic space, or pleural cavity)
     - Spread from an amebic liver abscess
     - Secondary infection of cavitary malignancy, pulmonary infarct.

B. **Primary cryptogenic lung abscesses:** This type of lung abscess has no apparent cause and most of them develop as consequence of **aspiration of infected material**. About 80% of lung abscess is primary (50% of these associated with putrid sputum). Bacteria responsible are usually the mixed anaerobes found in the oropharynx or nasopharynx (aspiration abscess). Predominant organisms found in aspiration abscess include anerobic organisms, streptococci and *Haemophilus influenzae*. Preexisting sources of infection for aspiration are sinusitis, dental sepsis, gingivitis, periodontal infection, etc.
   - **Aspiration of infective material:** Depression of cough reflex favors aspiration from **infected nasal sinuses or tonsils** or periodontitis gingivitis. It may occur during alcoholic stupor, general anesthesia, sleep, epilepsy, coma, head injury or neurological disease-causing loss of consciousness.
   - **Aspiration of gastric contents:** Occurs in achalasia cardia, carcinoma of esophagus, hiatus hernia, and gastroesophageal reflux disease (chemical pneumonitis—Mendelson's syndrome).

   Features of aspiration abscess:
   - **Site and number:** Abscess due to **aspiration** is more common on the **right** lung (because of the more vertical right main bronchus) and is most often **single**.
   - **Segment involved:** Aspiration abscess cavities occur in those bronchopulmonary segments that are most dependent at the time of aspiration.
     - Aspiration in supine position → produces abscess in posterior segment of the upper lobes or superior segments of the lower lobes.
     - Aspiration in the upright position → produces abscess in the basilar segments (bilateral).
   - About one-third of patients develop empyema due to direct extension.
   - Amebic lung abscess typically occurs in right lower lobe due to direct extension of liver abscess through the diaphragm.

Clinical Features

Q. Write short essay on diagnosis of acute lung abscess.

Lung abscess may present either as an acute (symptoms <1 month) or chronic (symptoms >1 month).

- **Acute:**
  - Majority present acutely with dry **cough**, high-grade **fever**, chills, rigors, and pleuritic chest pain.
  - After a few days, when the abscess ruptures into a patent bronchus, the patient suddenly starts expectorating **large amounts of foul-smelling purulent or sanguineous sputum.** The sputum may often be blood-tinged and expectoration **varies with posture.**
- **Chronic:** Lung abscess secondary to aspiration often presents as chronic, insidious in onset with low-grade fever, malaise, weight loss, anorexia, and a deep-seated chest **pain**/discomfort.

Physical findings

General examination: Anemia, fever, **clubbing of the fingers and toes** (may develop rapidly), **halitosis,** and oronasal sepsis.

Respiratory system examination

- **Early stages:** May be normal
- Later:
  - **Signs of consolidation:** Dullness of percussion, increased vocal fremitus and vocal resonance, bronchial breathing, crepitations, and pleural rub.
  - **Signs of cavitation:** Once the abscess opens into a bronchus, signs of cavitation like cavernous or amphoric bronchial breathing and coarse post-tussive crepitations are heard on auscultation.

Investigations

- **Blood:** Normocytic anemia and/or raised inflammatory markers (ESR/CRP), leukocytosis, and raised ESR.
- Sputum:
  - Gram's stain, Ziehl–Neelsen staining for acid-fast bacilli
  - Culture and sensitivity: For aerobic and anaerobic
  - Cytological examination: For malignant cells.
- **Chest radiograph (Fig. 6.32):** It reveals radiolucency in an opaque area of consolidation. The wall of the abscess cavity completely surrounds the radiolucent area. An air-fluid level may be seen in the abscess cavity.
- **CT scan of thorax:** It shows lung abscess.
- **Bronchoscopy:** Indicated (1) to exclude malignancy, (2) to obtain specimens for studies, and (3) for removal of secretions.

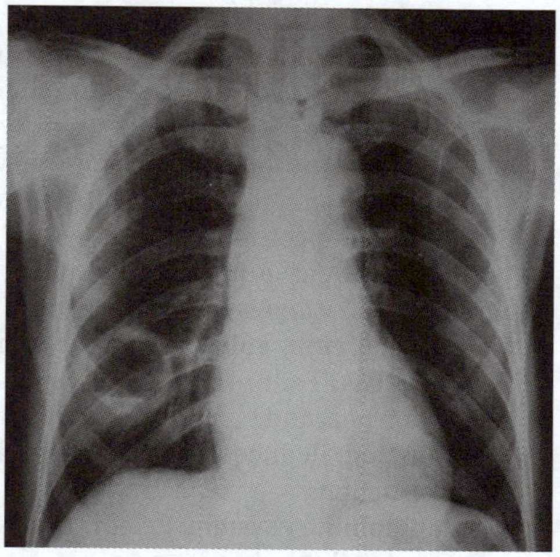

FIG. 6.32: Chest X-ray shows lung abscess in right lower zone.

Complications (Table 6.51)

Q. Write a short essay on management of acute lung abscess/management of lung abscess.

Treatment

- **Postural drainage** (refer bronchiectasis) and chest physiotherapy.
- **Antibiotic therapy:** Choice of drug depends on culture and sensitivity result. Broad guidelines include:
  - **Aspiration abscess:** Antibiotic therapy is similar to that of aspiration pneumonia.
  - **Oral treatment:** Majority respond to oral treatment with ampicillin 500 mg four times daily or cotrimoxazole 960 mg twice daily or clindamycin 300 mg thrice daily.
  - **Anaerobic bacterial infection**, e.g., patients with foul-smelling sputum, oral metronidazole 400 mg 8 hourly should be combined with the above oral treatment. It should not be used alone.
  - **Parenteral antibiotic therapy:** Required in seriously ill patients and consists of beta-lactamase inhibitor (e.g., ampicillin-sulbactam 3 g intravenously every 6 hours) or a carbapenem (e.g., imipenem, meropenem) with clindamycin and metronidazole.
- **Duration of antibiotic therapy:** Usually given for 4–6 weeks. Antibiotic treatment should be continued until the chest radiograph has shown either the resolution of lung abscess or the presence of a small stable lesion. There is a risk of relapse with shorter antibiotic regimen.
- **Large lung abscess:** Aspiration and placement of pigtail catheters may be useful.
- **Resectional surgery:** Indicated in few in cases. These include:
  - Massive hemoptysis
  - Lung abscess associated with symptomatic bronchiectasis
  - Lung abscess associated with localized malignancy
  - Persistent lung abscess cavity.

The surgical procedure is either lobectomy or pneumonectomy. Consider lobectomy/pneumonectomy with large cavities (>8 cm), resistant organisms like *Pseudomonas*, obstructing neoplasm or massive hemorrhage.

TABLE 6.51: Complications of lung abscess.

- Extension of the infection into the pleural cavity: Leading to empyema/pneumothorax/pyopneumothorax/bronchopleural fistula/pleural effusion/pleurocutaneous fistula
- Hemorrhage into the abscess cavity
- Hemoptysis
- Septic emboli may cause metastatic brain abscesses or meningitis
- Secondary amyloidosis (type AA)
- Aspergilloma
- Residual fibrosis and bronchiectasis

Cystic Fibrosis

Q. Write a short note on complications of cystic fibrosis.

Cystic fibrosis is a fatal multisystem genetic disorder because of abnormal ion transport function causing inability to adequately hydrate mucus.

Genetics and Pathogenesis

It is transmitted as an autosomal recessive disorder and characterized by mutation in a gene on the long arm of chromosome 7. This gene codes for a chloride channel known as cystic fibrosis transmembrane conductance regulator (*CFTR*). This influences salt and water movement across epithelial cell membranes.

CFTR protein:

- Normally present in epithelia and functions as cAMP-regulated chloride ion channel and as inhibitor of Na^+ channels.
- Mutation in *CFTR* gene causes intracellular degradation of CFTR. Thus, epithelial membranes are unable to secrete chloride ion in response to cAMP-mediated signals.

Types of epithelia affected:

- **Volume-absorbing epithelia:** Airways and distal intestinal epithelium.
  - In cystic fibrosis, **Na^+ absorption increased and chloride ion secretion is decreased.** This leads to reduced volume of periciliary fluid (with relative dehydration of the airway epithelium), thickening of mucus, adhesion and failure to clear mucus from the airway lumen. Mucus stasis and mucus hypoxia predispose to chronic bacterial infection (favors *Pseudomonas* growth) and ciliary dysfunction. It can lead to bronchiectasis.
- **Salt-absorbing epithelia:** In the sweat duct epithelium, cystic fibrosis is associated with increased sodium and chloride content in sweat. Aquagenic wrinkling of the palms (wrinkling and nodules) that develop after several minutes of immersion in water is quite characteristic.
- **Volume secretary epithelia:** Epithelium of proximal intestine and pancreas
  - **Pancreas:** Failure of Cl-HCO_3 exchanger to secrete Na^+, HCO_3 and water → enzymes retained → steatorrhea, azotorrhea, and pancreatic destruction.
  - **Intestine:** Reduced bicarbonate secretion → low pH in duodenum → thick intestinal mucus → predisposition to obstruction.
  - **Hepatobiliary system:** Retention of biliary secretion, focal biliary cirrhosis, bile duct proliferation, chronic cholecystitis, and cholelithiasis.

Clinical Features

- Most patients present in infancy. Earliest presentation is **meconium ileus**. Pancreatic and intestinal manifestations occur early.
- Pulmonary manifestations occur late. After the neonatal period, maximum morbidity and mortality is due to pulmonary disease.

Respiratory tract

- Upper respiratory tract: Chronic sinusitis, rhinorrhea, and nasal polyps
- Lower respiratory tract:
  - Earliest functional abnormality is small airways disease and earliest symptom is cough. Final expression is bronchiectasis. Earliest and most severe changes in **right upper lobe**.
  - Persistent cough → viscous, purulent sputum. Intermittent exacerbations → increased cough, increased sputum volume, decrements in pulmonary function, weight loss. As exacerbations become more frequent, lung function deteriorates → eventually, respiratory failure.
  - Pathogens: In newly diagnosed patients include *H. influenzae* and *S. aureus* and in established diseases *Pseudomonas aeruginosa* (mucoid form).
  - Chest X-ray: Earliest manifestation is hyperinflation later bronchiectatic changes.
  - Pulmonary function tests: Obstructive pattern with partial bronchodilator response.
  - Complications: Pneumothorax, hemoptysis, clubbing, respiratory failure, cor pulmonale.

Gastrointestinal tract

- Most common is **exocrine pancreatic insufficiency:** Steatorrhea, azotorrhea → consequent malnutrition. Recognized only when secretion of amylase and lipase falls below 90%.
- Endocrine pancreatic insufficiency occurs in 10% much later.
- Others: Intestinal obstruction, appendicitis, recurring acute or chronic pancreatitis.
- Increased incidence of GI malignancy.

Genitourinary tract

- Late onset of puberty in both males and females.
- 95% azoospermic, 20% women infertile, 90% completed pregnancies produce viable infants; breastfeeding normal.
- Retardation of bone age, heatstroke.

Diagnosis

- One or more characteristic clinical features + abnormal sweat chloride ions or nasal bioelectrical response [nasal transepithelial potential difference (TEPD)]. TEPD is the voltage across an epithelium, and is the sum of the membrane potentials for the outer and inner cell membranes. This test measures the salt (sodium and chloride) transport in and out of the cells in the nose in response to different salt solutions. The way nasal cells respond to the changing salt solutions can be used to make a diagnosis of cystic fibrosis.
- Other disorders raised sweat chloride ions: Ectodermal dysplasia, glycogen storage disorders, adrenal sufficiency, mucopolysaccharidoses, acute respiratory disorders (group, epiglottitis, and viral pneumonias), chronic respiratory disorders (alpha-1 antitrypsin deficiency, bronchopulmonary dysplasia).
- Pilocarpine iontophoresis
- Sweat chloride ions >70 mEq/L distinguishing feature

- Nasal TEPD: Increased and on amiloride application → loss of this potential difference and with β-agonist → no response.
- DNA testing (for mutation) not useful because > 1,000 mutations exist.

Treatment
- **Lung disease**
  - Clear secretions: By breathing exercises, flutter valves, chest percussion, and recombinant human DNase
  - Infection: Long courses of culture and sensitivity guided antibiotic therapy; higher doses required; oral/IV/aerosolized
  - Inhaled β-agonists/anticholinergics: Short-term benefit. O_2 and medical management are temporary measures
  - Long-term high-dose NSAID (some patients)
  - The only effective therapy for respiratory failure in cystic fibrosis (CF): Lung transplantation.
- **Gastrointestinal**
  - Pancreatic enzyme replacement (microsphere formulation)
  - Replacement of fat-soluble vitamins
  - Treatment of acute obstruction: Enema of hypertonic radiocontrast material (megalodiatrizoate).
- **Reproductive:** Assisted reproductive technology.

PLEURAL EFFUSION

Normal Composition of Pleural Fluid (Table 6.52)

Q. Discuss the causes/etiology, clinical features, investigations, radiological findings, diagnosis, pleural fluid analysis, complications, and management/treatment of pleural effusion.

TABLE 6.52: Normal composition of pleural fluid.

Feature	*Normal value*
➢ Volume	0.1–0.2 mL/kg
➢ Cells	1,000–5,000/mm^3
– Mesothelial cells	3–70%
– Monocytes	30–70%
– Lymphocytes	2–30%
– Granulocytes	~ 10%
– Eosinophils	0%
➢ Protein	1–2 g/dL
➢ Albumin	50–70%
➢ Glucose	~ plasma level
➢ Lactate dehydrogenase (LDH)	<50% plasma level

Definitions

- **Pleural effusion:** Excessive accumulation of serous fluid within the pleural cavity/space (between parietal pleura and visceral pleura). It can be detected on X-ray when ≥300 mL of fluid is accumulated and clinically, when a minimum of 500 mL is present.
- **Empyema:** Accumulation of purulent fluid (frank pus) within the pleural cavity/space.
- **Hydrothorax:** Passive transudation of fluid into the pleural cavity. It occurs in congestive heart failure, nephrotic syndrome, cirrhosis of liver, severe malnutrition, etc.
- **Hemothorax:** Accumulation of blood within the pleural cavity/space.
- **Chylothorax:** Accumulation of chyle within the pleural cavity/space.

Mechanism of Pleural Effusion

- Increased hydrostatic pressure (e.g., left ventricular failure)
- Decreased oncotic pressure in microcirculation (e.g., hypoalbuminemia)
- Decrease in pleural pressure (e.g., atelectasis)
- Increased permeability of microcirculation (e.g., pneumonia)
- Impaired lymphatic drainage from pleural space (e.g., malignancy)
- Movement of fluid from abdomen to pleural space (e.g., cirrhosis).

Classification and Causes (Table 6.53)

Q. Write a short essay/note on:
- **Causes of pleural effusion.**
- **Causes and diagnosis of exudative pleural effusion.**
- **Causes of transudative pleural effusion.**

TABLE 6.53: Classification and causes of pleural effusion.

Types of effusion	*Causes*	
Transudative effusion	➢ Cardiac failure ➢ Hypoproteinemia (e.g., nephrotic syndrome, cirrhosis of liver, severe malnutrition) ➢ Constrictive pericarditis	➢ Hypothyroidism ➢ Meigs' syndrome (benign ovarian tumors with ascites and pleural effusion) ➢ Peritoneal dialysis
Exudative effusion	➢ Tuberculosis ➢ Bacterial pneumonia ➢ Malignancy ➢ Pulmonary infarction ➢ Autoimmune diseases (e.g., rheumatoid arthritis, systemic lupus erythematosus) ➢ Acute pancreatitis ➢ Postmyocardial infarction syndrome (Dressler's syndrome)	➢ Drug-induced effusion ➢ Benign asbestos-related effusion ➢ Intra-abdominal abscess ➢ Meigs' syndrome (can be transudative as well) ➢ Ruptured amebic liver abscess, chylous pleural effusion ➢ Acute rheumatic fever

Q. Write a short essay/note on causes of left-sided pleural effusion.

Causes of left-sided pleural effusion is listed in **Box 6.11**.

Box 6.11: Causes of left-sided pleural effusion.

- Pancreatitis
- Pericardial inflammation
- Rupture of esophagus
- Left-sided subdiaphragmatic abscess
- Thoracic duct involvement above D_3 level

Clinical Features

- Symptoms (pain on inspiration and coughing) and signs of pleurisy (a pleural rub): They often precede the development of a pleural effusion.
- **Breathlessness:** It may be the only symptom and its severity depends on the size and rate of accumulation of fluid.

Physical Findings in the Chest

Q. Write a short essay/note on signs of pleural effusion.

- **Inspection: Tachypnea.** Shift of trachea to opposite side.
- **Palpation:**
  - **Shift of trachea and mediastinum** (shift of apex beat) to the opposite side
  - **Reduced chest movements** on the affected side, bulging of the intercostal spaces, fullness of the affected chest, and markedly reduced vocal fremitus
  - **Measurements:** Diminished chest expansion, increase in the size of the affected hemithorax and an increase in spinoscapular distance.

Box 6.12: Causes of pleural effusion without trachea/mediastinal shift.

- Minimal effusion
- Loculated effusion
- Bilateral effusion
- Effusion with underlying collapse/fibrosis
- Effusion with fixed mediastinum (malignancy/fibrosis)

- **Percussion:**
  - **Stony dullness** over the fluid. Upper level of the dullness is highest laterally in the axilla, and is lower anteriorly and posteriorly (**Ellis-S-shaped curve**).
  - **Small effusions:** When there is a small effusion, it may be detected as follows:
    - **Left-sided** small pleural effusion may be detected only by the obliteration of Traube's space on percussion.
    - **Right-sided** small effusion may be detectable only by tidal percussion.
  - **Moderate to large effusions:** Percussion reveals a triangular area of dullness or impaired note over the back of chest on the contralateral side or opposite side of the effusion. It may be due to shift of the posterior mediastinum to the opposite side by effusion.
    Causes of pleural effusion without tracheal mediastinal shift are listed in **Box 6.12**.
- **Auscultation:**
  - **Breath sounds: Intensity is markedly diminished** or absent over the fluid.
  - **Vocal resonance: Markedly diminished** over the fluid.
  - **Bronchial breathing or crackles** the level of a pleural effusion
  - Occasional findings: Egophony and enhanced breath sounds can often be appreciated at the superior border of the effusion because of underlying atelectatic lung tissue.

Q. Write a short note on Grocco's sign.

Grocco's sign (Grocco's triangle; paravertebral triangle of dullness): It is a triangular area of paravertebral dullness on the side opposite a pleural effusion. Boundaries of Grocco's triangle are:

- Medial boundary: Midspinal line from the upper level of effusion down to the level of the 10th thoracic vertebra.
- Lower boundary: A horizontal line of about 3–7 cm extending laterally from the 10th thoracic vertebra, along the lower limit of lung resonance.
- Lateral boundary: A curved line connecting the above two lines.

Investigations

Q. Write a short note on radiological findings/X-ray features in pleural effusion.

- **Radiological investigations**
  - 75 mL of pleural fluid: Subpulmonic space without spillover can obliterate the posterior costophrenic sulcus.
  - **Upright chest radiograph**
    - 175 mL is required to obscure the lateral costophrenic sulcus.
    - 500 mL of fluid will obscure the diaphragmatic contour.
    - 1,000 mL of effusion reaches the level of the 4th anterior rib.
    - **Decubitus radiographs and CT scans:** Less than 10 mL (even as little as 2 mL) can be identified.
  - Small effusions are thinner than 1.5 cm, moderate effusions are 1.5–4.5 cm thick, and large effusions exceed 4.5 cm.
  - Effusions thicker than 1 cm are usually large enough for sampling by thoracentesis, since at least 200 mL of liquid is already present.
  - A significant pleural effusion is large enough to produce a pleural fluid strip >10 mm wide on lateral decubitus radiographic views.

Radiological features of pleural effusion in an erect chest film **(Fig. 6.33)** are as follows:

- ♦ **Shift of mediastinum** to the opposite side
- ♦ **Obliteration of costophrenic angle**
- ♦ **Opacity:** Dense uniform opacity in the lower and lateral part on the involved side. Upper border of the opacity is concave upward and is highest laterally.

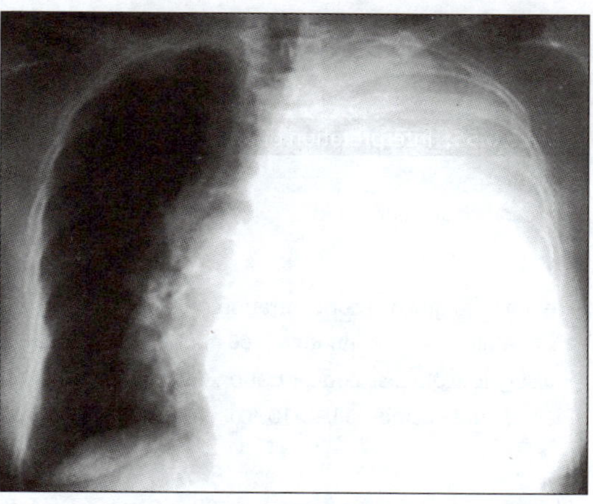

FIG. 6.33: Chest X-ray shows left-sided massive pleural effusion.

- ▪ **Interlobar effusion:** Wider than normal interlobar fissure.
- ▪ **Encysted interlobar effusion:** Round opacity resembling solitary pulmonary nodule (phantom tumor).

- **Ultrasonography**
  - ▪ More accurate than plain chest X-ray for detection of pleural effusion and it can detect as little as 5 mL of effusion.
  - ▪ **Interpretation**
    - ♦ **Transudate versus exudate:** A clear hypoechoic space favors transudate and the presence of moving floating densities suggests an exudate.
    - ♦ Presence of septation favors an evolving empyema or resolving hemothorax.

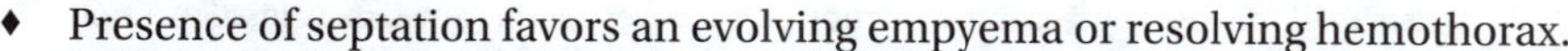

    - ♦ Useful in differentiating loculated pleural effusion from pleural tumor or pleural thickening.
    - ♦ Useful for locating an effusion prior to aspiration and biopsy.
    - ♦ Detection of solid pleural abnormalities may suggest pleural malignancy. However, a CT scanning is indicated where malignancy is suspected.

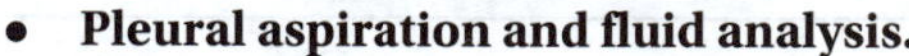

- **Pleural aspiration and fluid analysis.**

Pleural Fluid Analysis

Q. How will you differentiate transudative pleural effusions from exudative pleural effusions?

Q. Write a short essay/note on criteria for distinguishing pleural transudate from exudate.

Q. Write a short essay/note on pleural fluid analysis in a typical pleural effusion.

Differentiation of transudative from exudative effusion **(Table 6.54)**.

TABLE 6.54: Differentiation of transudative from exudative effusion.

Characteristics	*Transudative effusion*	*Exudative effusion*
Cause and mechanism	Noninflammatory process. Ultrafiltrate of plasma, due to increased hydrostatic pressure or decreased serum oncotic pressure with normal vascular permeability	Inflammation process and is rich in proteins due to increased vascular permeability
Appearance	Clear, serous	Cloudy/purulent/hemorrhagic/chylous
Color	Straw yellow	Yellow to red
Specific gravity	<1.018	>1.018
Protein		
➢ Absolute value	Low, <2 g/dL, mainly albumin	High, >2 g/dL
➢ Pleural fluid: serum ratio	<0.5	>0.5
Clot	Absent	Clots spontaneously because of high fibrinogen
Leukocytes		
➢ Total leukocytes	<1,000/mm^3	>1,000/mm^3
➢ Type of cells	>50% lymphocytes or mononuclear cells	>50% lymphocytes (tuberculosis, malignancy)
Differential leukocytes	mesothelial cells	>50% polymorphs (acute inflammation)
➢ Erythrocytes	<500/mm^3	Variable
Bacteria	Absent	Usually present
Lactate dehydrogenase (LDH)		
➢ Absolute value	<200 IU/L	200 IU/L
➢ Pleural fluid LDH: serum LDH ratio	<0.6	>0.6
Glucose	>60 mg/dL (usually same as in blood)	<60 mg/dL (variable)

Interpretation of Pleural Fluid Parameters (Table 6.55)

Light's criteria

TABLE 6.55: Interpretation of pleural fluid parameters.

Parameter	*Interpretation*
Appearance of pleural fluid	Putrid odor (anaerobic empyema), food particles (esophageal rupture), bile-stained (chylothorax/biliary fistula), milky (chylothorax/pseudochylothorax), anchovy sauce-like fluid (ruptured amebic abscess)
Pleural fluid glucose concentration	
➤ Low glucose concentration (<60 mg/dL)	Suggests empyema, malignancy or tuberculosis
➤ Very low glucose concentration (<15 mg/dL)	Empyema, rheumatoid effusions
Pleural fluid eosinophilia (>10% of all cells)	May be observed in resolving infections, pneumothorax, hydropneumothorax, hemothorax and asbestos-related pleural effusion, dantrolene, bromocriptine, nitrofurantoin, paragonimiasis or Churg–Strauss syndrome
Pleural fluid erythrocyte counts >100,000/mm³	Most often in malignancy or pulmonary infarction/embolism, but may result from a traumatic tap
Low pH of pleural fluid <7.2	Complicated parapneumonic effusion, esophageal rupture, rheumatoid pleuritis, tuberculous pleuritis, malignant pleural disease, hemothorax, systemic acidosis, paragonimiasis, lupus pleuritis, urinothorax
Raised pleural fluid amylase	Pancreatic diseases and esophageal rupture. However, routine amylase estimation is not recommended unless the clinical features suggest either of the two diseases
Pleural fluid antinuclear antibody titers or rheumatoid factor	No diagnostic significance and is not indicated in most cases
Mesothelial cells	Absent: Tuberculosis Markedly increased: Pulmonary embolism

Q. Write a short essay/note on Light's criteria for distinguishing pleural transudate from exudate.

- Light's criteria **(Box 6.13)** are used to differentiate exudative from transudative pleural effusion by measuring the lactate dehydrogenase (LDH) and protein levels in the pleural fluid. Exudative pleural effusions must meet at least one of the following criteria, whereas transudative pleural effusions meet none.
- **Precautions:**
  - **Low specificity:** These criteria are highly sensitive for exudative effusions but have lower specificity (i.e., few transudative effusions will be classified as exudative using these criteria).
- In general Light's criteria, occasionally misidentify a transudative effusion as an exudative effusion as in cardiac failure with diuretic therapy

Clinically if a patient should have a transudative effusion, but meets Light's criteria for an exudative effusion, measure serum-pleural fluid albumin gradient, or measure the serum-pleural protein gradient **(Roth's criteria)**
- Serum-effusion albumin gradient of >1.2 g/dL—transudative
- Serum-effusion protein gradient >3.1 g/dL—transudative

Causes of Lymphocytic Pleural Effusion (Table 6.56)

- **Pleural biopsy is indicated in undiagnosed cases.**
- **Other investigations in pleural effusion**
  - **Pleural fluid tumor markers:** Carcinoembryonic antigen (CEA), cancer antigen 125 (CA 125), cancer antigen15-3 (CA 15-3) and cytokeratin 19 fragments (CYFRA). They are not used in routine investigations of pleural effusion.
  - **Blood examination:** Total and differential leukocyte counts, ESR, proteins, sugar, LDH, amylase, rheumatoid factor and antinuclear factor.

Box 6.13: Modified Light's criteria for distinguishing pleural transudate from exudate.

Modified Light's criteria

Pleural fluid is an exudate if one or more of the following criteria are met:

Pleural fluid
- Serum protein ratio >0.5
- Serum LDH ratio >0.6
- LDH >2/3 upper limit of normal serum LDH
- Protein >30 g/L

If only one of the above criteria is met, then calculate the fluid to serum albumin gradient
- If the albumin gradient >12 g/L, consider a transudate

Sensitivity and specificity of tests to distinguish exudative from transudative effusions

	Sensitivity for exudates (%)	*Specificity for exudates (%)*
Light's criteria	98	83
Pleural-fluid cholesterol level >60 mg/dL	54	92
Pleural-fluid cholesterol level >43 mg/dL	75	80
Ratio pleural-fluid cholesterol/serum cholesterol >0.3	89	81
Serum albumin level minus pleural fluid albumin level ≤1.2 g/L	87	92

(LDH: lactate dehydrogenase)

Source: Modified with permission from Light RW. Pleural effusion. Engl J Med. 2002;346:1971-7.

TABLE 6.56: Causes of lymphocytic pleural effusion.

Malignancy ➤ Primary lung cancers ➤ Secondaries	Long-standing congestive cardiac failure
Tuberculosis	Effusion associated with rheumatoid arthritis
Lymphoma	Chylothorax, uremic pleuritis

- **Sputum examination:** For tubercle bacilli and malignant cells.
- Mantoux test
- **Repeat radiograph:** When effusion is massive, a repeat radiograph after removal of a large volume of fluid may reveal an underlying parenchymal lesion.
- Biopsy or fine-needle aspiration of scalene lymph nodes
- Bronchoscopy and biopsy
- Thoracoscopy and biopsy.

Management of pleural effusion

- **Treat the underlying cause** (e.g., heart failure, pneumonia, pulmonary embolism or subphrenic abscess).
- **Therapeutic aspiration:** It may be necessary to relieve breathlessness/dyspnea. At one sitting not >1 L should be removed because it is associated with a small risk of re-expansion pulmonary edema. If there is rapid re-accumulation of fluid insertion of chest tube is necessary.
- **Drainage:** If the fluid is purulent (empyema).
- **Pleurodesis:** For malignant effusion.

Approach to the Diagnosis of Pleural Effusions

See **Flowchart 6.10.**

Re-expansion Pulmonary Edema

Q. Write a short essay/note on re-expansion pulmonary edema.

- It occurs in small number of patients when the lung undergoes rapid inflation of lung (e.g., evacuation of >1 L of air/fluid) after a prolonged period of collapse (usually >3 days) from either pleural effusion or pneumothorax.
- Edema usually involves the entire re-expanded lung. Occasionally, it may involve a single lobe or the contralateral lung, or bilateral.

Mechanism: Exact mechanism is not known. Following may be implicated in its development.

- **Reactive oxygen species:** Ventilation and reperfusion of a previously collapsed lung may cause an inflammatory response, with generation of reactive oxygen species and superoxide radicals, which leads to increased capillary permeability.
- **Increase pulmonary hydrostatic pressure:** It may be due to increased venous return.
- **Pressure-induced mechanical disruption** of alveolar capillaries
- Reduced levels of functional surfactant
- Increased pressure across the capillary-alveolar membrane due to bronchial obstruction
- Alteration of lymphatic clearance.

Clinical Features

- **Onset:** Symptoms usually develop within 24 hours (majority within 1–2 hours after lung re-expansion).
- **Symptoms:** Chest discomfort, persistent severe cough, dyspnea and frothy sputum.
- **Signs:** Tachypnea, tachycardia, and crackles on the affected side of the lung.
- **Chest radiograph:** Features of pulmonary edema.
- Mortality rate is about 20%.

FLOWCHART 6.10: Approach to the diagnosis of pleural effusions.

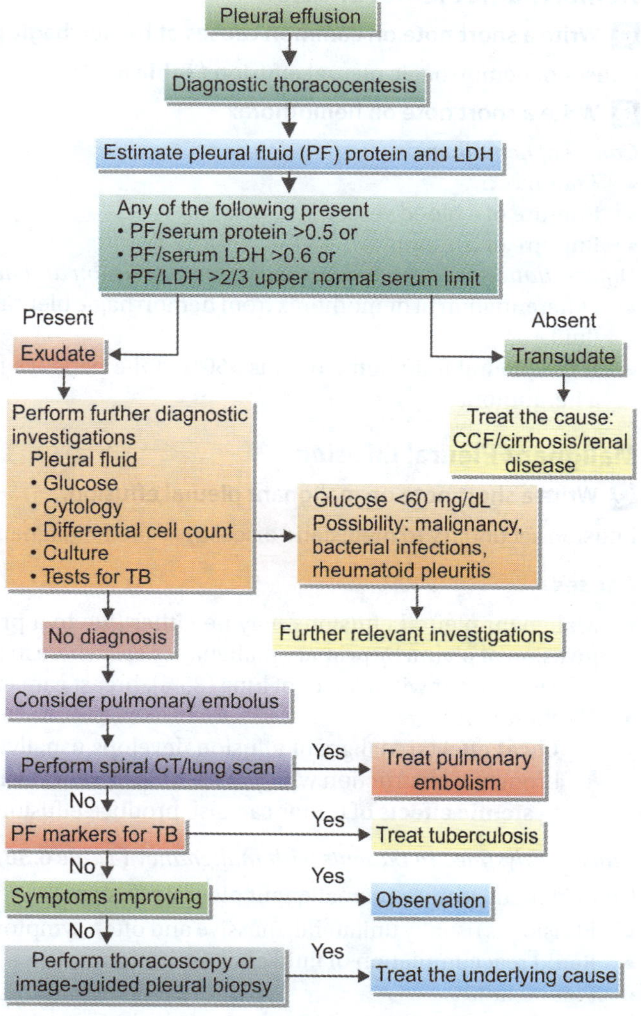

Treatment

- **Supportive treatment:** Most patients recover completely within 5–7 days with supportive treatment (includes oxygen administration in mild cases to mechanical ventilation in severe cases). Patient is advised to lie on unaffected side.
- Others: Use of diuretics, bronchodilators, prostaglandin analogs (e.g., misoprostol), ibuprofen, and steroids is controversial.

Prevention of Re-expansion Pulmonary Edema

- Restricting the drainage of pleural fluid to <1 L.
- Use of low negative pressure (< –20 cm H_2O) during tube thoracostomy.
- Large volumes of fluid can be drained safely if pleural pressures are monitored. If the patient complains of vague chest pressure during thoracentesis, it suggests a sudden drop in intrapleural pressure, and the thoracentesis should be stopped.

Subpulmonic Effusion

Q. Write a short essay/note on subpulmonic effusion. How will you diagnose it?

- It is a small pleural effusion which is seen underneath the lung. Its detection is extremely difficult.
  - Left-sided subpulmonic effusion may show obliteration of Traube's semilunar space of tympany.
  - Right-sided subpulmonic effusion may be suspected with an abnormal tidal percussion.
- Chest radiograph:
  - Posteroanterior view in the erect posture
    - Mild elevation of hemidiaphragm
    - Lateral displacement and slight flattering of the dome of the diaphragm
    - Wide density between the gastric air shadow and upper border of the diaphragm in left-sided subpulmonic effusion
  - Lateral decubitus view with the affected side down: Pleural fluid layering out along the lateral chest wall
- **Ultrasonography:** Reveals subpulmonic effusion with more certainty.

Hemorrhagic Pleural Effusion

Q. Write a short note on common causes of hemorrhagic pleural effusion.

Causes of hemorrhagic pleural effusion **(Table 6.57)**

TABLE 6.57: Causes of hemorrhagic pleural effusion.

➢ Malignancy	➢ Tuberculosis (very rare)
➢ Pulmonary infarction	➢ Postcardiac injury effusion
➢ Asbestos-related pleural effusion	

Q. Write a short note on hemothorax.

Causes of hemothorax

- Trauma
- Rupture of a blood vessel
- Rupture of a tumor

Differentiation between hemorrhagic pleural effusion and hemothorax:

- Differentiation of hemothorax from hemorrhagic pleural effusions can be done by performing a hematocrit on the pleural fluid.
- If the pleural fluid hematocrit is >50% of the patient's peripheral blood hematocrit, it is considered to be diagnostic of a hemothorax.

Malignant Pleural Effusion

Q. Write a short note on malignant pleural effusion.

Effusion secondary to metastatic disease is called malignant pleural effusion.

Causes

- Malignant pleural effusions may be either due to a primary malignancy of pleura (e.g., mesothelioma) or secondary invasion of pleura by primary malignancy elsewhere in the body (more common). Most common malignancy-associated effusions occur with cancer of lung (35%), breast cancers (25%), and lymphomas (10%).
- **Mechanism:**
  - **Local effects:** Malignant effusion develops usually due to the local effects of the tumor, e.g., lymphatic obstruction, bronchial obstruction with pneumonia or atelectasis.
  - **Systemic effects** of tumor can also produce effusion.

Causes of dyspnea in patients with malignancy ***(Table 6.58)***

TABLE 6.58: Causes of dyspnea in patients with malignancy.

➢ Pleural effusion	➢ Underlying lung disease
➢ Direct effects of a tumor on the lung	➢ Pulmonary vascular disease (e.g., pulmonary emboli)
➢ Airway obstruction	➢ Lymphangitis carcinomatosis
➢ Chest wall invasion	➢ Radiation pneumonitis
➢ Pericardial disease	➢ Cardiac compromise

Characteristic features of malignant pleural effusion:

- Effusion is usually unilateral, massive and often symptomatic.
- Rapid reaccumulation of fluid after aspiration
- Pleural fluid
  - Often hemorrhagic, with a high erythrocyte count (>100,000/mm^3)
  - Shows the characteristics of an exudates such as high protein content (>3.0 g/dL), high LDH levels (>200 IU/L), low glucose levels (<60 mg/dL), and a total leukocyte count exceeding 1,000/mm^3
  - Predominant cells are lymphocytes (>50%).
  - Cytological examination may show malignant cells.
- Closed pleural biopsy: It may reveal malignant tumor (in about 40% of cases).

Treatment

- Asymptomatic effusions: Do not require any treatment.
- Mildly symptomatic effusions: Treated by repeated aspirations.
- Severely symptomatic and recurrent effusions: Treated by pleurodesis. This consists of instillation of tetracycline hydrochloride or talcum powder (more effective) or inactivated Corynebacterium parvum into the pleural cavity. It produces a severe inflammatory reaction in the pleura, followed by extensive pleural adhesions. Other treatment modalities include thoracotomy with pleurectomy or pleural abrasion.

Parapneumonic Effusion (Synpneumonic Effusion)

Q. Write a short note on parapneumonic effusion (synpneumonic effusion).

Parapneumonic effusion is a pleural effusion developing as a complicating pneumonia or lung abscess or bronchiectasis.

Synpneumonic effusion is used to describe a sterile parapneumonic effusion in general.

Empyema refers to a grossly purulent pleural effusion.

- More frequently associated with bacterial pneumonias (especially gram-negative and pneumococcal). Effusion in these cases is large and consists of predominant polymorphonuclear leukocytes.
- Less frequent with viral pneumonias and this effusion is small and predominant shows lymphocytes.

Clinical Presentation

- **Acute illness:** Aerobic bacterial pneumonia with pleural effusion presents with an acute illness with fever, chest pain. sputum, and leukocytosis.
- **Subacute illness:** Anaerobic infections present with a subacute illness with weight loss, leukocytosis, mild anemia, and predisposing factor that has resulted in aspiration pneumonia.

Categories of Parapneumonic Effusion (Table 6.59)

TABLE 6.59: Parapneumonic pleural effusion and empyema: Light's classification and corresponding treatment.

Category	*Type*	*Characteristics*	*Treatment*
1.	Nonsignificant	<1 cm thick on an ipsilateral decubitus view. Thoracocentesis not required	Antibiotic
2.	Typical parapneumonic	>1 cm thick, glucose >40 mg/dL pH > 7.20, negative Gram's stain and culture	Antibiotic + consider therapeutic thoracentesis
3.	Borderline complicated	pH 7–7.20 or LDH >1,000 Negative Gram's stain and culture	Antibiotic + pleural drainage tube + consider fibrinolytics
4.	Simple complicated	pH <7.0, positive Gram's stain or culture. Not loculated, no pus	Antibiotic + pleural drainage tube + fibrinolytics
5.	Complex complicated	pH <7.0, positive Gram's stain or culture. Multiloculated	Antibiotics + pleural drainage tube + fibrinolytics + consider VAT
6.	Simple empyema	Frank pus. Single loculation or free-flowing fluid	Antibiotics + pleural drainage tube + fibrinolytics + consider VAT
7.	Complex empyema	Frank pus. Multiple loculations. Often requires decortication	Antibiotics + pleural drainage tube + fibrinolytics + VAT + other surgical procedures if VAT fails

(LDH: lactate dehydrogenase; VAT: video-assisted thoracoscopy)

Investigations

Presence of pleural fluid can be demonstrated with a lateral decubitus radiograph, computed tomography (CT) of the chest, or ultrasound.

Treatment

- When there is **mild** parapneumonic effusion, patient may be **observed** and a repeat tap is done if it persists or increases.
- If the free fluid separates the lung from the chest wall by >1 cm, a **therapeutic thoracentesis** should be done.
- Indications for **more invasive procedure,** i.e., intercostal tube drainage are as following:
  - Loculated pleural fluid
  - Pleural fluid pH <7.20
  - Pleural fluid glucose <3.3 mmol/L (<60 mg/dL)
  - Positive Gram's stain or culture of the pleural fluid
  - Presence of gross pus in the pleural space.
- If there is recurrence after the initial therapeutic thoracentesis and if any of above factors is present, a repeat thoracentesis should be done.

- If the fluid cannot be completely removed with the therapeutic thoracentesis, insert a chest tube and instill a fibrinolytic agent (e.g., tissue plasminogen activator 10 mg) and deoxyribonuclease (5 mg) or performing a thoracoscopy and release the adhesions.
- **Intrapleural thrombolytic agents:** Most effective in the early fibrinolytic stage (e.g., streptokinase, streptodornase, urokinase, and tPA).
  - **Indications:** (1) Occluded small-bore catheter, (2) multiloculated pleural space, and (3) as a trial before committing the patient to surgery.
- **Decortication** is performed when the above measures are not effective.
- **Treatment of underlying cause.**

Chylous Pleural Effusion (Chylothorax)

Q. Write a short note on chylous pleural effusion (chylothorax)/causes of milky pleural fluid.

- **Definition:** It is the accumulation of chyle in the pleural cavity.
- **Mechanism:** A chylothorax results from leakage of chyle from the thoracic duct into the pleural space.
- **Causes:** Most common cause is trauma (most frequently during thoracic surgery). It may also result from lymphomas, lung cancer with mediastinal spread, mediastinal fibrosis, and tumors.
- **Presentation:** Dyspnea and a large pleural effusion on chest X-ray.
- **Pleural fluid findings:**
  - Appears milky and shows the characteristics of exudates **(Fig. 6.34).**
  - Total triglyceride level is >110 mg/dL. The cholesterol level is very low. Sudan III staining shows fat globules.
  - Occasionally, empyema can be so turbid to be confused with chyle. Centrifugation of fluid leaves a clear supernatant fluid in empyema compared to persistence of milky appearance in chylous effusion. In starved patients, chyle may not be milky in appearance.
- If the trauma is not the cause of chylothorax, a contrast-enhanced CT scan of mediastinal and a lymphangiogram should be performed.

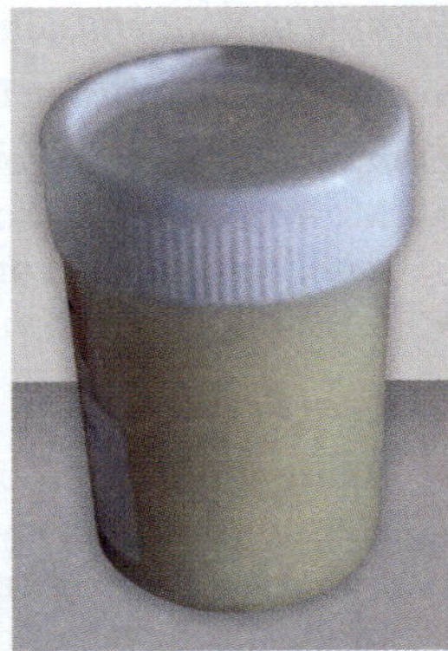

FIG. 6.34: Gross appearance of pleural aspirate in chylothorax.

Treatment

Treatment of choice is insertion of a chest tube and use of octreotide. Long-term tube drainage may result in malnutrition and immune deficiency. Therefore, if patient does not respond, a pleuroperitoneal shunt may be tried. Alternatively, ligation of the thoracic duct and percutaneous transabdominal thoracic duct blockage may be useful.

Pseudochylous Pleural Effusion (Pseudochylothorax)

Q. Write a short essay/note on pseudochylous pleural effusion (pseudochylothorax).

- Rare condition in which the pleural fluid appearance is similar to that of chylous effusion (milky).
- **Causes:** Long-standing benign pleural effusion (e.g., tuberculous effusion, rheumatoid effusion, etc.).
- **Pleural fluid:** Appears milky. Cholesterol level of the fluid is very high (>200 mg/dL) which is responsible for the milky appearance of fluid. Cholesterol crystals can be demonstrated and Sudan III staining does not show fat globules.
- **Differences between pseudochylous thorax and chylothorax (Table 6.60).**

TABLE 6.60: Differences between pseudochylous thorax and chylothorax.

Feature	*Pseudochylothorax*	*Chylothorax*
Triglycerides	<0.56 mol/L (50 mg/dL)	>1.24 mmol/L (110 mg/dL)
Cholesterol	>5.18 mmol/L (200 mg/dL)	<5.18 mmol/L (200 mg/dL)
Cholesterol crystals	Often present	Absent
Chylomicrons	Absent	Present
Etiology	Tuberculosis, rheumatoid arthritis, poorly treated empyema	Neoplasm (lymphoma, metastatic carcinoma), trauma (operative, penetrating injuries), miscellaneous (tuberculosis, sarcoidosis, cirrhosis, lymphangioleiomyomatosis, obstruction of central veins, amyloidosis)

Pleural Effusions in HIV Infection

- A pleural effusion is seen in 7–27% of patients with HIV.
- Leading causes are: Kaposi sarcoma, parapneumonic effusion, TB, lymphoma, *Pneumocystis jirovecii* pneumonia.

Empyema Thoracis

Q. Discuss the etiology, clinical features, investigations, complications, and management of empyema thoracis.

Definition

- Empyema thoracis is defined as collection of pus in the pleural space/cavity. It may be as thin as serous fluid or so thick that it is impossible to aspirate, even with a wide-bore needle. Microscopically, it shows numerous neutrophil leukocytes.

- It usually involves whole pleural space/cavity and unilateral. If only a part of the pleural space is involved, it is termed encysted or loculated empyema.

Etiology

- **Spread of infection from neighboring structures:** For example, bacterial pneumonias, bronchiectasis, lung abscess, rupture of subphrenic abscess through the diaphragm, esophageal perforation, and infection of hemothorax following trauma or surgery.
- **From distant source:** For example, bacteremia.
- **Direct infection from external source:** For example, penetrating chest injury, chest tube placement, and thoracic surgery.
  Common organisms: *Pneumococcus, Streptococcus, Staphylococcus, Pseudomonas, Mycobacterium tuberculosis, H. influenzae*, and anaerobes.

Clinical Features (Table 6.61)

Q. Write a short answer on:
- **Clinical features of empyema.**
- **Physical sign of right-sided empyema.**

TABLE 6.61: Clinical features of empyema.

Systemic features
➢ High-grade, remittent fever
➢ Chills, rigors, sweating, malaise, and weight loss
Respiratory symptoms
Pleuritic chest pain, breathlessness, and dry cough. Copious, purulent sputum develops when the empyema ruptures into a bronchus (bronchopleural fistula)
Physical examination
Clinical signs of pleural effusion plus intercostals tenderness, digital clubbing, and edema of the chest wall

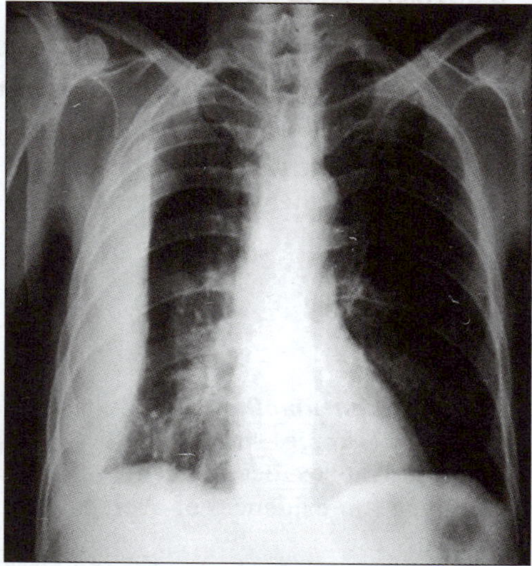

FIG. 6.35: Chest X-ray of loculated effusion—"D" sign.

Investigations

- **Blood:** Polymorphonuclear leukocytosis, high CRP (C-reactive protein).
- **Chest X-ray:** Findings may be similar to those of pleural effusion. However, pleural adhesions may produce a "D"-shaped shadow against the inside of the chest wall **(Fig. 6.35)**. If air is present along with pus (pyopneumothorax), a horizontal "fluid level" mark is detected at the air/liquid interface.
- **Ultrasound:** It shows the position of the fluid, the extent of pleural thickening and whether fluid is collected as a single locule or multiloculated.
- **CT:** It gives information regarding the pleura, underlying lung parenchyma, and patency of the major bronchi. Ultrasound or CT is used to detect the optimal site for aspiration.
- **Aspiration of empyema (Table 6.62)**

TABLE 6.62: Characteristic features of aspirated pus from empyema.

Consistency	Vary from very thin to very thick
Microscopy	Numerous polymorphonuclear leukocytes
Gram's stain	May show positive organism
Culture and sensitivity	To identify the causative organism
Tubercle bacilli	May be found, if it is due to *M. tuberculosis*

TABLE 6.63: Complications of empyema.

➢ **Empyema necessitans** is the formation of a subcutaneous abscess or sinus that develops when the pus track through the chest wall	➢ Pleural fibrosis ➢ Secondary amyloidosis
➢ **Bronchopleural fistula and pyopneumothorax** due to rupture of pus into a bronchus	➢ Metastatic brain abscess

Complications

See **Table 6.63.**

Q. Write a short essay/note on the management on nontuberculous empyema.

Management of Empyema Thoracis

A. Nontuberculous empyema

Acute

- Antibiotics: It should be given depending on the culture and sensitivity report.
- **Drainage of pus:** The pus in the pleural cavity should be drained.
  - **Aspiration:** In early and small empyema with thin fluid, daily aspiration of the fluid with a wide-bore needle is attempted.
  - **Tube drainage** is necessary in most cases.
  - **Limited thoracotomy:** If tube drainage fails or pus is thick or loculated, limited thoracotomy is performed. It involves resection of a small segment of the rib, clearing the empyema cavity breaking down any adhesions and introducing a wide-bore tube (for prolonged drainage).
  - Intrapleural administration of fibrinolytic agents (e.g., streptokinase) is of no benefit.

Chronic

- **Surgery:**
  - Surgical "decortication" of the lung may be necessary when there is gross thickening of the visceral pleura which is preventing re-expansion of the lung in chronic empyema. It involves stripping of the whole grossly thickened visceral pleura in order to allow the lung to re-expand.
  - Surgery is also required if a bronchopleural fistula develops.

B. Tuberculous empyema

- **Antituberculous chemotherapy**
- **Repeated aspiration:** Through a wide-bore needle or tube drainage.
- Rarely, surgical treatment may be required.

PNEUMOTHORAX

Q. Describe the types, etiology, clinical features, investigations, and management of pneumothorax.

Q. Describe etiology, clinical features, investigations, and treatment of tension pneumothorax.

- **Definition:** Presence of air/gas in the pleural cavity/space is known as pneumothorax.
- Pneumothorax may be localized (if there is a prior disease-causing adhesion of visceral pleura to parietal pleura), or generalized (if there are no pleural adhesions).

Classification

See **Flowchart 6.11**

FLOWCHART 6.11: Classification of pneumothorax.

- Classification of pneumothorax
  - Spontaneous
    - Open
    - Closed
    - Tension
    - Primary
    - Secondary
  - Traumatic
    - Iatrogenic
      - Causes
        - Transthoracic needle aspiration
        - Subclavian vessel puncture
        - Thoracocentesis
        - Pleural biopsy
        - Mechanical ventilation
    - Noniatrogenic
      - Causes
        - Penetrating trauma
        - Blunt trauma

Etiology

Spontaneous pneumothorax

- **Primary (simple) spontaneous pneumothorax** occurs in the absence (no evidence) of overt lung disease.
  - It occurs in individual without any underlying lung disease or any trauma.
  - Age: Commonly occurs between the age group of 20–40 years.
  - Risk factors: Smoking, tall stature, and the presence of apical subpleural blebs, mostly familial.
  - About 50% of patients will have a recurrence. Both lungs are affected with equal frequency
- **Secondary spontaneous pneumothorax** occurs in the presence of an underlying lung disease.
  - **Causes:** Most common causes are **COPD** (chronic bronchitis and emphysema) **and** cavitary active pulmonary **TB. It occurs** due to rupture of emphysematous bullae and subpleural TB focus. Other causes include bronchial asthma, suppurative diseases of lung and pleura, cystic fibrosis, and *P. jirovecii* pneumonia.

Traumatic pneumothorax results from penetrating or nonpenetrating injuries to the chest.

- **Iatrogenic:** Following diagnostic or therapeutic interventions. These include transthoracic and transbronchial needle aspiration/biopsy (24%), subclavian vessel puncture (22%), thoracocentesis (22%), pleural biopsy (8%), and mechanical ventilation (7%).
- **Noniatrogenic:** Blunt and penetrating injuries to the chest wall, bronchi, lung or esophagus.

Clinical Features

Q. Write a short note on clinical features of acute pneumothorax.

- A small pneumothorax may be asymptomatic without any abnormal physical signs in the chest.
- Most common symptoms are **sudden onset unilateral pleuritic chest pain** and **breathlessness** (dyspnea).
- **Severity depends on:** (1) extent of lung collapse and (2) amount of preexisting lung disease.
- **Tension pneumothorax:** Distressed with rapid labored respiration, cyanosis, marked tachycardia, and profuse diaphoresis.

Physical Signs

General examination: Patient will be cyanosed, tachypneic, peripheral pulses may be feeble and hypotension may be present.

Respiratory system

- Inspection and palpation
  - **Accessory muscles of respiration in action, trachea and mediastinal** (apex beat) **shift to the opposite side.**
  - **On the affected side:** Fullness of the chest, diminished chest movements, increase in the size and diminished expansion of the hemithorax, increased spinoscapular distance, and markedly diminished vocal fremitus. Subcutaneous emphysema may be present.
- **Percussion:** Hyper-resonant note over the affected hemithorax.
- Auscultation
  - **On the affected side:** Markedly diminished/absent of breath sounds and vocal resonance, absence of adventitious sounds. Open pneumothorax with a bronchopleural fistula, there may be amphoric bronchial breathing.

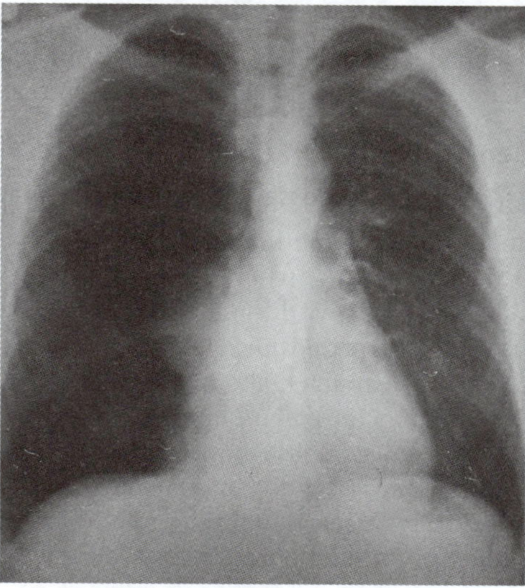

FIG. 6.36: Chest X-ray shows right-sided pneumothorax.

Investigations

Radiological findings on chest radiograph **(Fig. 6.36): Standard erect chest X-ray in inspiration** is recommended for the initial diagnosis of pneumothorax rather than expiratory films. Following features are observed:

- Sharply defined edge of the deflated lung.
- Complete translucency and absence of bronchovascular markings (no lung markings) in the area between the edge of the lung and chest wall. A clear **visceral pleural line/collapsed lung margin** can be seen.
- Mediastinal shift/displacement to the opposite side.
  It may also reveal the presence or absence of pleural fluid, complicating empyema or underlying lung lesion. CT is used in difficult cases.
  CT scanning is done if accurate size estimates are required.
- Recommended only in difficult cases such as patients in whom the lungs are obscured by overlying surgical emphysema.
- To differentiate a pneumothorax from suspected bulla in complex cystic lung disease.
  USG signs of pneumothorax: (1) loss of lung sliding, (2) loss of comet tails, (3) loss of seashore sign (M mode), and (4) stratosphere sign or barcode sign (M mode).

Types of Spontaneous Pneumothorax (Figs. 6.37A to C)

There are three types namely: (1) closed spontaneous pneumothorax, (2) open spontaneous pneumothorax, and (3) tension (valvular) pneumothorax. Differences between closed, open, and tension pneumothorax are listed in **Table 6.64.**

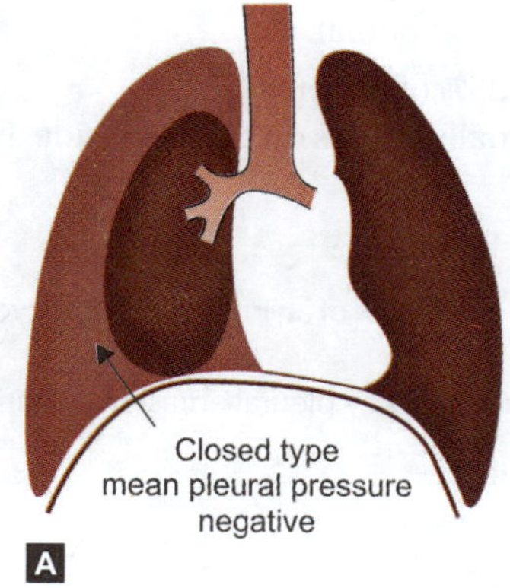

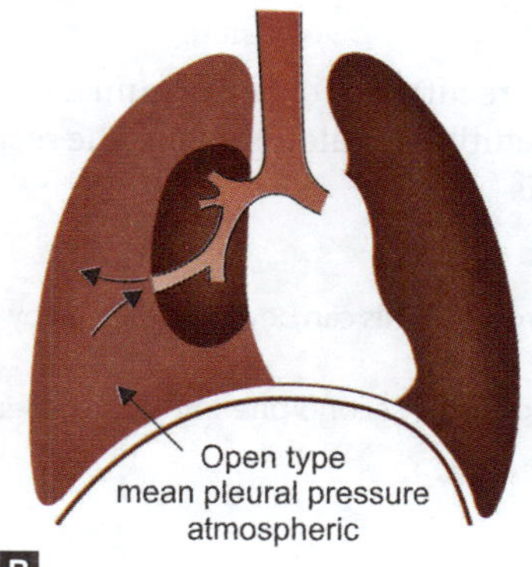

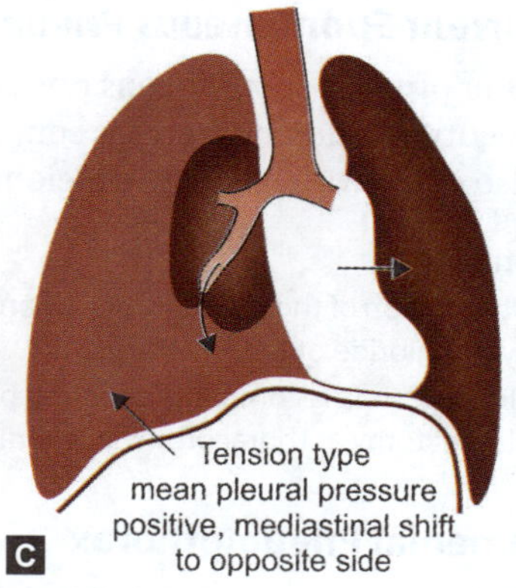

FIGS. 6.37A TO C: Types of spontaneous pneumothorax. (A) Closed type; (B) Open type; (C) Tension (valvular) type.

Closed Spontaneous Pneumothorax

Pneumothorax where the communication between pleural space and the lung seals off and does not reopen. The mean pleural pressure remains negative and air can neither enter nor leave the pleural cavity/space. The trapped air is slowly and spontaneously reabsorbed and the lung re-expands completely in 2–4 weeks. Infection of the pleural cavity is uncommon.

Clinical features: Trivial breathlessness that gradually abates over a few days.

TABLE 6.64: Types of spontaneous pneumothorax (Figs. 6.37A to C).

Closed pneumothorax	*Open pneumothorax*	*Tension pneumothorax*
The pleural tear is **sealed**	The pleural tear is **open**	The pleural tear acts as a **ball and valve** mechanism
The pleural cavity pressure is less than the atmospheric pressure	The pleural cavity pressure is equal to the atmospheric pressure	The pleural cavity pressure is more than the atmospheric pressure

Open Spontaneous Pneumothorax

- Pneumothorax where the communication between bronchus and pleura does not seal off and remains patent and air continues to pass freely between the bronchial tree and pleural space. It results in a bronchopleural fistula.
- Free flow of air through the bronchopleural fistula results in intrapleural pressure (normally negative) same as that of atmospheric pressure throughout the respiratory cycle. This prevents the re-expansion of the collapsed lung. Development of bronchopleural fistula facilitates the spread of infection into the pleural space causing empyema.
- Open pneumothorax usually develops secondary to rupture of an emphysematous bulla, a small pleural bleb, a tuberculous cavity or a lung abscess into the pleural cavity/space.

Clinical features: Presents with breathlessness that does not improve. If there is infection of pleural space, fever and systemic features are observed. The physical signs are those of hydropneumothorax (air and fluid in the pleural space).

Tension (Valvular) Pneumothorax

Q. Write a short essay/note on clinical features and signs of tension pneumothorax.

In tension pneumothorax, the pressure in the pleural space is positive throughout the respiratory cycle.

- Pneumothorax where communication between pleura and lung persists. This is due to formation of a valvular mechanism (one-way valve through) in which air is sucked into the pleural space during inspiration (coughing, sneezing and straining) but not expelled during expiration. Large quantity of air gets "trapped" in the pleural space/cavity and raises the intrapleural pressure much higher than the atmospheric pressure.
- The high intrapleural pressure causes compression of the underlying lung, shifts the mediastinum to the opposite side with consequent compression of the opposite lung also. It also decreases venous return to the heart by compressing the vena cava resulting in reduced cardiac output.

Clinical features: Rapidly progressive breathlessness, central cyanosis, rapid thread pulse, and signs of peripheral circulatory failure. Signs of pneumothorax are present.

Treatment

- Tension pneumothorax should be treated as an acute medical emergency.
- Emergency treatment: Insertion of a large-bore needle into the pleural space through the second anterior intercostal space. The diagnosis is confirmed, if large amounts of air escape through the inserted needle. The needle should be left in place till a thoracostomy tube can be inserted. Cover the open end of the needle with a glove finger. Other methods:
  - Insertion of wide-bore plastic cannula. The opposite end is attached to long rubber tubing, the end of which is placed underwater in a bottle.
  - Introduction of an intercostals catheter connected to a water-seal drainage system.
  - If above methods cannot be performed, simple stab on chest wall to release pressure.

Recurrent Spontaneous Pneumothorax

- After primary spontaneous pneumothorax, recurrence occurs within a year in about 25% of patients.
- Recurrent pneumothorax is common with emphysematous bullae. The recurrence usually occurs on the same side. It can also occur with lymphangioleiomyomatosis (LAM).

Treatment

- Obliteration of the pleural space by artificial pleurodesis. This can be accomplished by intrapleural instillation of an irritant like tetracycline hydrochloride of talc powder.
- Pleurodesis is recommended for all patients following a second pneumothorax. Pleurodesis is achieved by pleural abrasion or parietal pleurectomy at thoracotomy or thoracoscopy.

Catamenial Pneumothorax

Q. Write a short note on catamenial pneumothorax.

- Rare condition occurring in females above the age of 25–30 years.
- It presents with repeated attacks of spontaneous pneumothorax usually on the right side, in association with menstruation. Attacks usually occur within 2 days before or after the onset of menstruation. Hemoptysis may also develop. Most frequently associated with endometriosis of thorax.

Treatment

Ovulation-suppressing drugs, surgical exploration, and pleurodesis.

Clicking Pneumothorax

Q. Write a short note clicking pneumothorax.

In clicking pneumothorax, a small left-sided pneumothorax gets localized in front of the pericardium. This produces alteration of the heart sounds so that the sound becomes loud and resonant ("clicking").

Complications of Pneumothorax

Q. Write a short note on causes of pyopneumothorax.

- **Pyopneumothorax:** It is caused by aspiration or intercostal chest tube insertion (iatrogenic). It may also result from necrotic pneumonia, lung abscess, or caseous pneumonia. Its causes are listed in **Box 6.14**.
- Hydropneumothorax
- **Hemopneumothorax:** Bleeding in pleural space and commonly caused due to rupture of vessels in adhesions. When lung re-expands, bleeding will stop. If bleeding persists, surgical ligation may be required.
- Mediastinal and subcutaneous emphysema

Box 6.14: Causes of pyopneumothorax.

- Complication of pneumothorax
- Thoracocentesis
- Trauma to thorax
- Bronchopleural fistula
- Esophagopleural fistula

Q. Write a short note on management of acute pneumothorax.

Treatment of pneumothorax

- **Goals:** (1) To promote lung expansion, (2) to eliminate the pathogenesis, and (3) to decrease recurrence of pneumothorax.
- **Treatment options according to** (1) classification of pneumothorax, (2) pathogenesis, (3) pneumothorax frequency, (4) the extension of lung collapse, (5) severity of disease, and (6) complication and concomitant underlying diseases.

1. **Primary spontaneous pneumothorax (PSP): Observation:** Small, closed, mildly symptomatic spontaneous pneumothoraces do not require hospital admission. Patient is asked to return to hospital in the event of developing breathlessness.
2. **Secondary spontaneous pneumothorax (SSP):**
   - **Hospitalization and observation:** Small SSP of <1 cm depth or isolated apical pneumothoraces in asymptomatic patients, supplemental high flow (10 L/min) oxygen inhalation of high concentration oxygen may reduce the total pressure of gases in pleural capillaries by reducing the partial pressure of nitrogen. This should increase the pressure gradient between the pleural capillaries and the pleural cavity. Thereby increasing absorption of air from the pleural cavity. The rate of resolution/reabsorption of spontaneous pneumothoraces is 1.25–1.8% of volume of hemithorax/24 hours.

   Active intervention: All other cases will require active intervention (aspiration or chest drain insertion).
   - **Simple aspiration**
     - Recommended as first-line treatment for all PSP requiring intervention.
     - Less likely to succeed in secondary pneumothoraces and in such cases, it is only recommended as an initial treatment in small (<2 cm) pneumothoraces in minimally breathless patients under the age of 50 years.
   - **Repeated and catheter aspiration:** It is reasonable for primary pneumothorax when the first aspiration has been unsuccessful. A volume of <2.5 L has been aspirated on the first attempt.
   - **Intercostal tube and underwater seal drainage:** Suction to an intercostal tube should not be applied directly after tube insertion. But can be added after 48 hours for persistent air leak or failure of a pneumothorax to re-expand. High volume, low pressure (–10 to –20 cm H_2O) suction systems are recommended.
   - **Chemical pleurodesis**

   Q. Write a short note on indications for pleurodesis.
     - Goals: (1) to prevent pneumothorax recurrence and (2) to produce inflammation of pleura and adhesions.
     - **Indications:** Persistent air leak and repeated pneumothorax, bilateral pneumothoraces, those complicated with bullae, occupations where pneumothorax should not occur (e.g., drivers, pilots).
     - Sclerosing agents: **Tetracycline, minocycline, doxycycline, talc, and erythromycin.**
     - The instillation of sclerosing agents into the pleural space should lead to an aseptic inflammation with dense adhesions.
   - Other types pleurodesis:
     - Biological pleurodesis using ***Corynebacterium parvum.***
     - Physical pleurodesis **mechanical abrasions.**

Surgical treatment

- Indication: No response to medical treatment, persistence of air leak, hemopneumothorax, bilateral pneumothoraces, recurrent pneumothorax, tension pneumothorax failed to drain, thicken pleura making lung unable to re-expansion, and multiple blebs or bullae.
- **Open thoracotomy and pleurectomy** remain the procedure with the lowest recurrence rate for difficult or recurrent pneumothorax.
- Minimally invasive procedures, thoracoscopy (VATS), pleural abrasion, and surgical talc pleurodesis are all effective alternative strategies.

Hydropneumothorax

Q. Write a short note on the physical signs of hydropneumothorax.

Similar findings as pneumothorax except the following findings:

- **Percussion note** is **hyper-resonant over the upper air-containing part** and **stony dull over the lower fluid-containing part.**

- **Straight line dullness. Shifting dullness** can be elicited.
- **Amphoric bronchial breathing** in case of bronchopleural fistula.
- **Coin-test** is positive over the upper air-containing part.
- **Succussion splash** can be elicited on the affected side.

PNEUMONIA

Q. Describe the etiology, classification, investigations, complications, indications of hospitalization, and treatment of pneumonia.

Definition: Pneumonia is as an acute respiratory illness, defined as inflammation with exudative solidification of the lung parenchyma. It causes the alveoli to be filled with inflammatory exudates and usually results in consolidation (solidification) of lung.

- **Pathological definition:** Infection of the alveoli, distal airway, and interstitium of the lung. Characterized by increased weight, replacement of the normal sponginess by the consolidation. Alveoli filled by the WBC, RBC, and fibrin.
- **Clinical definition:** Constellation of symptoms and signs (fever, chills, cough, pleural chest pain, sputum, bronchial breathing, egophony, crackles, wheeze, and pleural friction rub) with at least one opacity on chest X-ray PA view.

TABLE 6.65: Classification of pneumonia.

1. Classification depending on the anatomic distribution
   - Lobar pneumonia
   - Bronchopneumonia
   - Interstitial pneumonia
2. Etiological classification
   - Primary
   - Secondary
   - Suppurative
3. Clinical setting in which the infection occurs (if no pathogen can be isolated)
   - Community-acquired acute pneumonia
   - Community-acquired atypical pneumonia
   - Nosocomial pneumonia or hospital-acquired pneumonia
   - Pneumonia in immunocompromised host
   - Health care-associated pneumonia

Classification of Pneumonia

Pneumonias can be classified in different ways **(Table 6.65)**.

1. ***Classification depending on the anatomic distribution***
   a. **Lobar pneumonias (alveolar or air space pneumonia):** The organism causes inflammatory exudates involving many contiguous alveoli (e.g., pneumococcal pneumonia). This radiologically appears as nonsegmental consolidation.
   b. **Bronchopneumonia:** Inflammation involving conducting airways, especially terminal and respiratory bronchioles, and the surrounding alveoli (e.g., staphylococcal pneumonia).
   c. **Interstitial pneumonia:** The inflammation is confined to interalveolar septa. X-ray chest gives a reticular pattern (e.g., *Mycoplasma pneumoniae, P. jirovecii*, and viruses).
2. ***Etiological classification***
   a. **Primary pneumonia:** It is caused by a specific pathogenic organism and there is no preexisting abnormality of the respiratory system. The causative organisms are listed in **Table 6.66**.

TABLE 6.66: List of organisms causing primary pneumonia.

Common	*Less common*
➤ *Streptococcus pneumoniae* (most common) ➤ *Haemophilus influenzae* ➤ *Moraxella catarrhalis* ➤ *Staphylococcus aureus* ➤ *Legionella pneumophila* ➤ *Mycoplasma pneumoniae*	➤ *Enterobacteriaceae (Klebsiella pneumoniae)* and *Pseudomonas* spp. ➤ *Streptococcus pyogenes* ➤ *Pseudomonas aeruginosa* ➤ *Coxiella burnetii* (Q fever) ➤ *Chlamydia* spp. *(C. pneumoniae, C. psittaci, and C. trachomatis)* ➤ Viruses: Respiratory syncytial virus, H1N1 influenza virus, seasonal influenza virus, parainfluenza virus, and human metapneumovirus (children); influenza A and B (adults); adenovirus (military recruits) coronavirus producing severe acute respiratory syndrome (SARS) ➤ *Actinomyces israelii*

Q. Write a short essay on list the bacteria causing pneumonia.

   b. **Secondary pneumonia (including aspiration pneumonia):** (discussed earlier)
   c. **Suppurative pneumonia (necrotizing pneumonia):** (discussed earlier)
3. **Clinical setting in which the infection occurs (if no pathogen can be isolated):** Pneumonia is classified by the setting in which the person has contracted their infection.
   a. **Community setting or community-acquired pneumonia (CAP):** It is defined as an acute pulmonary infection in a patient who is not hospitalized or living in a long-term care facility 14 days or more before presentation and does not meet the criteria for health care-associated pneumonia (HCAP). This category includes both immunocompetent and immunocompromised patients as causative agents are almost similar in both the conditions.
   b. **Nosocomial pneumonia or hospital acquired pneumonia**
      - **Definition:** Hospital-acquired pneumonias (HAPs)are pulmonary infections acquired in the course of a hospital stay (development of pneumonia after >48 hours of hospitalization).
      - Most of this pneumonia occurs outside intensive care units. However, the highest risk is observed in patients on mechanical ventilation [ventilator-associated pneumonia (VAP)]
      - **Etiology:** Predisposing factors include severe underlying disease, immunosuppression, prolonged antibiotic therapy, patients on mechanical ventilation or invasive access devices such as intravascular catheters. The HAPs are serious and may be life-threatening. The various causative organisms causing HAP are shown in **Table 6.67**.

TABLE 6.67: Various etiological agents causing hospital-acquired pneumonia.

Gram-negative rods, Enterobacteriaceae (*Klebsiella* spp., *Serratia marcescens, Escherichia coli*) and *Pseudomonas* spp.
Staphylococcus aureus (penicillin and usually methicillin-resistant

c. **Pneumonia in immune compromised host**: This is a type of pneumonia found in patient whose immune system is compromised, through either genetic defect, immunosuppressive medication, or acquired immunodeficiency such as HIV infection and malignancies.
   - It may be caused by classical organisms, atypical organisms, *M. tuberculosis* or *P. jirovecii*.
   - Usually, symptoms are more than the signs.

d. **Health care-associated pneumonia**
   - **Definition:** Hospital-acquired pneumonias are pulmonary infections acquired in the course of a hospital stay. It occurs:
     - Within 90 days of a 2-day or longer hospitalization. In a nursing home or long-term care residence.
     - Within 30 days of receiving intravenous antibacterial therapy, chemotherapy, or wound care or after a hospital or hemodialysis clinic visit; or in any patient in contact with a multidrug-resistant pathogen.
   - Features of HCAP more closely resemble nosocomial pneumonia and may require treatment accordingly.

Noninfective Pneumonias

- **Lipid/Lipoid pneumonia:**
  - Aspiration of fatty/oily material into lungs.
  - Decreasing order of severity of manifestations: Mineral oil > animal oil > vegetable oil (because vegetable oil to some extent, animal oils can be hydrolyzed in the body).
  - Liquid paraffin causes the most cases of lipoid pneumonia.
  - Chronic persistence of the oil in the lung can produce fibrosis/paraffinomas (paraffin granulomas).
- **Radiation pneumonitis**
  - Dose >25 Gy. Risk depends on radiation dose and volume of lung irradiated.
  - Early phase: Cough, fever, chest X-ray infiltrate.
  - Late phase (3–6 weeks): Dyspnea
  - Lung fibrosis: With excessive dose/large lung volume irradiation.
  - Treatment: Glucocorticoids improve symptoms, but have no ultimate effect on the development of fibrosis.
  - Recall pneumonitis: Pneumonitis due to chemotherapy, within the distribution of a previous radiotherapy field (the radiation sensitizes the lung tissue to the toxic effects of chemotherapy).
- **Chemical pneumonitis**
  - If aspirated fluid: pH <2.5 and volume >0.3 mL/kg result in chemical pneumonia (Mendelson's syndrome)—ARDS/secondary bacterial infection.
  - If gastric pH alkaline: Colonization of gastric mucosa by enteric gram-negative bacilli—pneumonitis.
  - Poor orodental hygiene with gross aspiration and lung abscess.
  - Pathogenesis: Most common mechanism by which pathogenic organisms reach the lower respiratory tract through microaspiration.
  - Others: Hematogenous/inhalation (droplet nuclei/aerosols)/contiguous spread.

Community-acquired Pneumonia

Q. Write an essay on community-acquired pneumonia—its definition, etiology/causative organisms, clinical features, investigations, diagnosis, complications, and treatment/management.

Q. Write an essay on streptococcal pneumonia—its etiopathogenesis, clinical features, complications, and management.

Q. Write a short essay on etiology/organisms causing community-acquired pneumonia.

- Community-acquired pneumonia affects all ages, but is commoner at extremes of age.
- Most cases are spread by droplet infection.
- CAP may occur in previously healthy individuals. However, several factors may impair the effectiveness of local defenses and predispose to CAP **(Table 6.68)**.

TABLE 6.68: Predisposing conditions for community-acquired pneumonia.

- Extremes of age
- Upper respiratory tract infections
- Comorbidities: For example, congestive heart failure, diabetes, chronic kidney disease, recent influenza infection, and malnutrition
- Cigarette smoking
- Alcohol
- Corticosteroid therapy
- Congenital or acquired immune deficiencies, e.g., HIV
- Decreased or absent splenic function, e.g., sickle cell disease or postsplenectomy (risk for infection with encapsulated bacteria)
- Other respiratory conditions: Cystic fibrosis, bronchiectasis, COPD, obstructing lesion (endoluminal cancer, inhaled foreign body)
- Indoor air pollution

- Pneumonia can be classified either according to the organism responsible for infection or anatomical distribution of infection.
- *Streptococcus pneumoniae (Pneumococcus)* is the most common cause. Viral infections are important causes of CAP in children.

- Depending upon the anatomical distribution of infection, it may be classified as lobar pneumonia (localized with the whole of one or more lobes affected) or bronchopneumonia (diffuse in which lobules of the lung are mainly affected, often due to infection centered on the bronchi and bronchioles).
- Potential causative agents in CAP: Bacteria, fungi, viruses, and protozoa.
- Causative agent and salient features of community-acquired acute pneumonia are presented in **Table 6.69**.

TABLE 6.69: Causative agent and salient features of community-acquired acute pneumonia.

Microorganism	*Features*
Streptococcus pneumoniae or Pneumococcus	Most common cause
Haemophilus influenzae	Most common bacterial cause in COPD
Moraxella catarrhalis	Elderly
Staphylococcus aureus	Secondary bacterial pneumonia following viral respiratory illnesses
Enterobacteriaceae (Klebsiella pneumoniae)	In debilitated and malnourished people
Pseudomonas aeruginosa	Common in patients with neutropenia
Legionella pneumophila	Organ transplant recipients

Q. Write a short essay on etiology/organisms causing community-acquired pneumonia.

Types of Presentations of Community-acquired Pneumonia

Two types of presentations of CAP are presented in **Table 6.70**.

TABLE 6.70: Types of presentations of community-acquired pneumonia (CAP).

Classical	*Atypical*
➢ Sudden onset of CAP ➢ High-fever, shaking chills ➢ Pleuritic chest pain, sudden onset of breathlessness ➢ Productive cough ➢ Rusty sputum, blood tinge ➢ Poor general condition ➢ High mortality up to 20% in patients with bacteremia ➢ Cause: *S. pneumoniae*	➢ Gradual and insidious onset ➢ Low-grade fever ➢ Dry cough, no blood tinge ➢ Low mortality 1–2%; except in cases of legionellosis ➢ Cause: *Mycoplasma, Chlamydia, Legionella,* rickettsiae, viruses ➢ Systemic manifestations present

Clinical Features of Community-acquired Pneumonia

- The clinical features vary according to the immune status of the patient and the infecting agent.
- **Systemic features:** Pneumonia (especially lobar pneumonia), usually presents as an acute illness. Sudden onset of fever, rigors, shivering, and malaise are predominant symptoms and delirium may be present. The appetite is lost and there may be headache. Fever can be as high as 39.5–40°C. Swinging fevers often indicates empyema.
- **Pulmonary symptoms**
  - **Cough:** First, it is characteristically short, painful and dry. Later, it is productive with expectoration of mucopurulent sputum. Characteristically rusty sputum may be seen in patients with *S. pneumoniae* (pneumococcal pneumonia) and the occasional hemoptysis can occur.
  - **Chest pain:** It is commonly pleuritic chest pain and may be a presenting feature. It is due to inflammation of the pleura. A pleural rub may be heard. Occasionally, pain may be referred to the shoulder or anterior abdominal wall. Upper abdominal tenderness is sometimes apparent in patients.
  - **Breathlessness:** The alveoli become filled inflammatory exudate impairs gas exchange producing breathlessness.
  - **Other features:** CAP can present with confusion or nonspecific symptoms in the elderly. When symptoms have been present for several weeks or have failed to respond to standard antibiotics, the possibility of TB should always be considered.
- **Extrapulmonary features (Table 6.71):** They are more common in certain infections and sometimes give a clinical clue to the etiology.

TABLE 6.71: Extrapulmonary features of community-acquired pneumonia.

Extrapulmonary symptoms	*Infectious agent*
Myalgia, arthralgia, and malaise	*Legionella* and *Mycoplasma*
Myocarditis and pericarditis	Mycoplasma pneumoniae
Headache, abdominal pain, diarrhea, and vomiting	Legionella pneumoniae
Labial herpes simplex reactivation	Pneumococcal pneumonia
Skin rashes: Erythema multiforme and erythema nodosum	Mycoplasma pneumoniae

Examination

- **Fever:** About 80% are febrile, although this finding is frequently absent in older patients. This is a helpful diagnostic clue if present.
- Respiratory and pulse rate may be raised and the blood pressure low and this may be the most sensitive sign in the elderly.
- **Tachycardia** is common. However, relative bradycardia is a characteristic feature of Legionnaires' pneumonia. There may be delirium.
- Oxygen saturation on air may be low, and the patient cyanosed and distressed.
- **Chest examination:**
  - Chest signs vary, depending on the phase of the inflammatory response.
  - During consolidation phase: Lung is typically dull to percussion and, as conduction of sound is enhanced, auscultation reveals tubular bronchial breath sounds over areas of consolidated lung bronchophony and whispering pectoriloquy. Coarse crackles are heard throughout on auscultation, due to consolidation of the lung parenchyma.

Investigations in Community-acquired Pneumonia (Table 6.72)

TABLE 6.72: Investigations in community-acquired pneumonia (CAP).

Investigation	*Significance*
Complete blood count	
➢ Very high (>20 × 10^9/L) or low (<4 × 10^9/L) WBC count	➢ Marker of severity. In viral and atypical pneumonias, total leukocyte count is often <5,000/mm^3
➢ Neutrophilic leukocytosis >15 × 10^9/L	➢ Suggests bacterial pneumonia
➢ Hemolytic anemia	➢ Occasionally complicates *Mycoplasma*
Urea and electrolytes	
➢ Urea >7 mmol/L (~20 mg/dL)	➢ Marker of severity
➢ Hyponatremia	➢ Marker of severity may occur in patients with Legionnaires' disease
Liver function tests	
➢ Abnormal transaminitis, raised bilirubin	➢ When basal pneumonia inflames liver, or in atypical pneumonia
➢ Hypoalbuminemia	➢ Marker of severity
Erythrocyte sedimentation rate/ C-reactive protein	➢ Nonspecifically elevated
Blood culture	➢ Bacteremia is a marker of severity. Causative organism may be grown (e.g., pneumococcal pneumonia). However, blood cultures are recommended only in hospitalized patients
Serological and antigen detection tests	➢ Pneumococcal antigens can be detected in the serum or urine in pneumococcal pneumonia ➢ Acute and convalescent titers for *Mycoplasma*, *Chlamydia*, *Legionella*, and viral infections
Cold agglutinins	Positive in 50% of patients with *Mycoplasma*
Arterial blood gases	Measure when SaO_2 <93% or when severe clinical features to assess ventilatory failure or acidosis
HIV testing	Since pneumonia is a common in previously undiagnosed HIV infection, a test should be offered to all patients with pneumonia
Sputum: It can be distinguished from saliva by microscopic examination. Sputum contains alveolar macrophages	Gram's stain, culture, antimicrobial sensitivity testing and Ziehl–Neelsen staining
Oropharynx swab	PCR for *Mycoplasma pneumoniae* and other atypical pathogens
Urine	Pneumococcal and/or *Legionella* antigen. Hematuria may occur in patients with Legionnaires' disease
Chest X-ray	Essential for the confirmation of diagnoses, follow-up and detection of complications like parapneumonic effusion and empyema
➢ Lobar pneumonia	➢ Patchy opacification evolves into homogeneous consolidation of affected lobe ➢ Air bronchogram (air-filled bronchi appear lucent against consolidated lung tissue) may be present
➢ Bronchopneumonia	Patchy and segmental shadowing
➢ Complications	Parapneumonic effusion, intrapulmonary abscess or empyema
➢ *Staphylococcus aureus*	Multilobar shadowing, cavitation, pneumatoceles, and abscesses
➢ *Mycoplasma*	Usually, one lobe is involved but infection can be bilateral and extensive
➢ *Legionella*	There is lobar and then multilobar shadowing, with the occasional small pleural effusion. Cavitation is rare
Aspiration	➢ Percutaneous transtracheal aspiration of secretions ➢ Percutaneous transthoracic needle aspiration, preferable under CT guidance
Fiberoptic bronchoscopy with BAL and brushings	Gram's stain, AFB stain, culture, and cytology
Biopsy	A transbronchial biopsy of the lung tissue for culture and histopathology may be done in selected cases. Diagnostic open-lung biopsy, which carries a high-risk, is reserved for selected patients
Pleural fluid	Aspirate and culture when present in more than trivial amounts, preferably with ultrasound guidance

Q. Write a short essay on radiological findings in pneumonias.

Complications of Pneumonia

Q. Write a short essay on complications of pneumonia.

General Complications (Box 6.15)

Box 6.15: General complications of pneumonia.

- Respiratory failure ARDS
- **Bacteremic dissemination** (bacteremia): It **can cause:**
  - Endocarditis (heart valves)
  - Pericarditis (pericardium)
  - Meningitis (meninges)
  - Suppurative arthritis (joint)
  - Metastatic abscesses in kidneys or spleen
  - Sepsis—multisystem failure

Local complications

- Lung abscess
- **Organization:** Delayed and incomplete resolution can cause **ingrowth of granulation tissue into the alveolar exudate.** The intra-alveolar plugs of granulation tissue are known as organizing pneumonia. Gradually, **increased alveolar fibrosis leads to a shrunken and firm lobe and is called as cornification.**
- **Spread of infection to the pleural cavity:** It may result in:
  - Pleuritis

- **Parapneumonic pleural effusion**
- **Pyothorax:** Which may lead to fibrothorax.
- **Pneumothorax**, especially in *S. pneumoniae* due to pneumatocele rupture.

Management Guidelines for CAP

- Rational use of microbiology laboratory.
- Pathogen-directed antimicrobial therapy whenever possible.
- Prompt initiation of antibiotic therapy.
- Decision to hospitalize based on prognostic criteria CURB 65

Severity: The need to hospitalize (severity) a patient is commonly assessed by CURB 65 or the CRB 65 score **(Table 6.73).** The CRB 65 score is used in the community where the serum urea level is not usually available. Other severity score available is Pneumonia Severity Index (PSI), which combines several clinical and laboratory features, and comorbid conditions.

General Management (Treatment) of Pneumonia

- Check the airway, breathing, and circulation. The most important aspects are: oxygenation, fluid balance, and antibiotic therapy.
- **Oxygen:** Oxygen is indicated in all patients with tachypnea, hypoxemia, hypotension or acidosis. The aim is to maintain saturations between 94 and 98%. In patients with known COPD, high concentrations (35% or more), preferably humidified oxygen should be used to maintain a saturation between 88 and 92%. If hypoxia continues or patient develops increasing hypercapnia, ventilate the patient mechanically.
- **Intravenous fluids:** These are required in patients with severe illness, older patients and those who are vomiting. Treat shock (hypotensive showing any evidence of volume depletion) with intravenous fluids initially. Otherwise, an adequate oral intake of fluid is enough.

New Treatment Paradigm

- **Hit Hard Early with Antibiotics → De-escalate.**
  1. ***Antibiotics:*** Administer antibiotics as soon the diagnosis of CAP is established preferably within 4 hours of presentation in hospital and treatment should not be delayed while investigations are awaited. Prompt administration of antibiotics improves the outcome. Empiric regimens **(Table 6.74)**
     Duration of therapy: Minimum of 5 days (usually 7–10 days). Afebrile for at least 48–72 hours. Duration is 10–14 days for patients with *Mycoplasma* and *Chlamydia pneumoniae*. Patients initially treated with intravenous antibiotics can be switched to oral agents when they become febrile. Longer duration of therapy is needed if initial therapy was not active against the identified pathogen or complicated by extrapulmonary infection.
  2. ***Mild analgesics for pleuritic pain***: Pleural pain may prevent the patient from breathing normally and coughing efficiently resulting in sputum retention, atelectasis or secondary infection. Hence, it is relieved by simple analgesia such as paracetamol, codeine or NSAIDs.

TABLE 6.73: CURB 65 rule.

Confusion: New mental confusion
Urea >7 mmol/L (>20 mg/dL)
Respiratory rate >30 breaths/minute
Blood pressure: Diastolic BP <60 mm Hg or systolic blood pressure <90 mm Hg
Age ≥**65** years of age (1 point for each)
Group 1: 0 or 1 of the above—mortality low—1.5%. Likely suitable for treatment at home
Group 2: 2 of the above—mortality—9.2%. Hospitalization for treatment
Group 3: 3 or more of the above—mortality—22%. Likely requires admission to ICU

TABLE 6.74: Empiric regimens for pneumonia.

Setting	*Therapeutic options*
Ambulatory, not requiring hospitalization, age under 60 years	Oral macrolide (erythromycin or azithromycin)
Ambulatory, not requiring hospitalization, comorbidity or age over 60 years	Oral β-lactam/β-lactamase inhibitor + macrolide **or** oral antipneumococcal fluoroquinolone
Requiring hospitalization	β-lactam (cefoperazone or ceftriaxone) + macrolide or antipneumococcal fluoroquinolone
Aspiration pneumonia requiring hospitalization	β-lactam/β-lactamase inhibitor alone (ampicillin/sulbactam, piperacillin/tazobactam)

Antibiotic treatment for community-acquired pneumonia has been shown in **Table 6.75**.

Unresolved/Slow-resolving Pneumonia

- Patient is considered to have responded if: (1) fever declines within 72 hours, (2) temperature normalizes within 5 days, and (3) respiratory signs (tachypnea) return to normal. The expected time course for resolution is controversial.
  - In 1975, Hendin defined slowly resolving as **pulmonary consolidation persisting >21 days.**
  - In 1991, Kirtland and Winterbauer defined slowly-resolving CAP in immunocompetent patients based upon radiographic criteria. **>50% clearing by 2 weeks** or > **complete clearing at 4 weeks.**

TABLE 6.75: Antibiotic treatment for community-acquired pneumonia (CAP).

Antibiotic	*Dosage, route, frequency, and duration*
Doxycycline	100–200 mg PO/IV BID for 7–10 days
Azithromycin	500 mg OD IV—3 days + 500 mg OD PO for 7–10 days
Clarithromycin	250–500 mg BID PO for 7–14 days
Telithromycin	800 mg PO OD for 7–10 days
Levofloxacin	750 mg PO/IV OD for 5 days
Gatifloxacin	400 mg PO or IV OD for 5–7 days
Moxifloxacin	400 mg PO or IV OD for 5–7 days
Gemifloxacin	320 mg PO OD for 5–7 days
Amoxiclav	2 g of amoxicillin + 125 mg of clavulanic acid PO BID for 7–10 days
Ceftriaxone	2 g IV BID for 5–7 days
Ertapenem	1 g OD IV or IM for 7–14 days

(PO: per oral; IV: intravenous; IM: intramuscular; OD: once daily; BID: twice daily)

- **Nonresolving pneumonia** is defined as a clinical syndrome in which focal infiltrates begin with some clinical association of acute pulmonary infection and despite a minimum of 10 days of antibiotic therapy patients either do not improve or worsen or radiographic opacities fail to resolve within 12 weeks.
- **Progressive pneumonia:** Increase in radiographic abnormalities and clinical deterioration during first 72 hours of treatment.
- Causes of unresolved/slow-resolving pneumonia have been shown in **Table 6.76**.

Recurrent pneumonia: Many conditions cause recurrent pneumonias **(Table 6.77)**.

TABLE 6.76: Causes of unresolved/slow-resolving pneumonia.

Incorrect microbiological diagnosis (e.g., tuberculosis instead of classical organisms) or incomplete antimicrobial treatment	➢ Underlying antibiotic resistance ➢ Inadequate dose/duration ➢ Nonadherence ➢ Malabsorption
Complication of CAP (community-acquired pneumonia)	➢ Parapneumonic pleural effusion (exudative), empyema, lung abscess
Underlying neoplastic lesion or other lung disease	➢ Bronchial obstruction causing partial or complete obstruction, bronchoalveolar cell carcinoma, bronchiectasis
Alternative diagnosis	➢ Pulmonary thromboembolic disease, cryptogenic organizing pneumonia, eosinophilic pneumonia, pulmonary hemorrhage
Host factors	➢ Age especially >50 years ➢ Comorbid illness: Diabetes, COPD (chronic obstructive pulmonary disease) ➢ Others, e.g., alcoholism, immunosuppressive/cytotoxic therapy
Superinfection	➢ Fungi, *Mycobacterium tuberculosis*
Defects in defense	➢ For example, impaired cough (sedatives, neuromuscular illness, stroke), impaired mucociliary transport (chronic bronchitis), immune deficiency states—primary and secondary (B-cell and T-cell)

TABLE 6.77: Conditions causing recurrent pneumonias.

➢ Bronchial obstruction (e.g., foreign body, bronchial stenosis, compression of bronchus, endobronchial lesions)
➢ Bronchiectasis
➢ Immunocompromised state
➢ Sequestration of lung
➢ Ciliary dyskinesia
➢ Multiple myeloma and other lymphoreticular malignancies

Prevention of Further Episodes of Pneumonia

- **Cessation smoking**
- **Influenza vaccine** (Flu shot—October through February): It offers 90% protection and reduces mortality by 80%.
- Pneumococcal vaccine (Pneumonia shot): It protects against 23 types of Pneumococci. About 70% of individuals have pneumococci in the respiratory tract. Vaccination reduces mortality.

Pneumococcal Pneumonia (Lobar Pneumonia)

Q. Discuss the etiology, clinical features, investigations, diagnosis, complications, and treatment/management of pneumococcal pneumonia (lobar pneumonia/*S. pneumoniae*).

Definition: Lobar pneumonia is characterized by **diffuse inflammation** affecting the **part or entire lobe, usually the lower lobes.**

Etiology

- Causative organism: Most common form of pneumonia and is caused by *S. pneumoniae* (e.g., *Pneumococcus*, a gram-positive, lancet-shaped *Diplococcus*).
- Mode of infection: By droplet infection.

Risk factors for pneumococcal pneumonia

- **Age:** Younger than 2 years or older than 65 years.
- Strongest independent risk factor for invasive pneumococcal disease: Cigarette smoking
- **Strongest independent risk factor for CAP: Alcoholism**
  (ALPS: Alcoholism, leukopenia, pneumococcal sepsis: Mortality rate 80%)
- Poverty and overcrowding
- **Lowered systemic resistance of the host:** It may be due to:
  - **Chronic diseases:** Diabetes mellitus, severe liver disease, and chronic lung disease
  - **Immunological deficiency:** Defects in innate immunity and humoral immunodeficiency (complement or immunoglobulin), defects in cell-mediated immunity (congenital and acquired), HIV infection.
  - Treatment with immunosuppressive agents
  - **Leukopenia**
  - Asplenia or hyposplenia
- Impaired local defense mechanisms
  - **Loss or suppression of the cough reflex:** For example, **coma**, **anesthesia**, **drugs**, **chest pain**, or neuromuscular disorders. It may lead to aspiration of gastric contents into the lung.
  - **Damage or injury to the mucociliary apparatus:** It may be due to **cigarette smoke, viral diseases, inhalation of hot or corrosive gases**, or genetic defects of ciliary function (e.g., the immotile cilia syndrome).
  - **Accumulation of secretions:** Cystic fibrosis and bronchial obstruction.

- **Interference with the phagocytic or bactericidal action of alveolar macrophages:** It may be due to alcohol intoxication, tobacco smoke, anoxia, or oxygen intoxication.
- Antecedent influenza
- Pulmonary congestion and edema.

Clinical Features

- **Sudden onset of high fever**, **chills** and rigors, **coughs**, and vomiting. Fever is usually high grade (39–40°C). Convulsions may occur in children.
- Cough is initially short, painful and dry, but soon becomes productive with **mucopurulent sputum.** Rust-colored sputum (**"rusty" sputum**) is characteristic but occasionally may be frankly blood stained.
- Nonspecific symptoms include loss of appetite, headache, and pains in the body and limbs
- Localized pleuritic chest pain develops at an early stage due to fibrinosuppurative pleuritis. It may be referred to the shoulder or abdominal wall. It may be companied by pleural friction rub. Breathing is rapid and shallow due to pleuritic pain.
- Other features are tachycardia, hot and dry skin, herpes labialis, and flushed face.

Physical signs in the chest

Q. Write a short note on signs of consolidation

- First 2 days: The physical signs are minimal and include diminished respiratory movements, slight impairment of percussion note, and pleural rub. In early stages, numerous finecrepitations are audible.
- After 2 days: Frank signs of consolidation appear **(Box 6.16)**.

Box 6.16: Signs of consolidation.

- Diminished respiratory movements
- Dull percussion note
- No mediastinal shift
- Markedly increased vocal fremitus and vocal resonance
- High-pitched tubular bronchial breathing
- Bronchophony, egophony and whispering pectoriloquy may be present
- During resolution coarse crepitations
- If parapneumonic effusion develops, additional signs of pleural effusion

Investigations

- **Blood**
  - Severe neutrophil leukocytosis
  - Blood culture may show *S. pneumoniae.*
- **Sputum**
  - Gram's staining of the sputum may show pneumococci which appear as gram-positive, lancet-shaped diplococci.
  - Sputum culture may show *S. pneumoniae.*
  - Assays on sputum are based on detecting nucleic acids for pneumococci.
- **Serological tests:** They can detect pneumococcal antigen in serum, urine, and sputum. Detection of C-polysaccharide (part of pneumococcal cell wall) in urine by an immunochromatography assay is quite sensitive. Urinary antigen remains positive for weeks after onset of severe pneumococcal pneumonia. However, it is often negative in mild pneumococcal pneumonia.
- **Chest radiograph (Figs. 6.38A and B)**
  - Involved lobe or segment appears homogeneous radiopaque with air bronchograms.
  - Associated parapneumonic effusion or empyema can also be detected.
- **Others:** In rare instances, fiberoptic, bronchoscopic aspiration or transthoracic needle aspiration may be necessary.

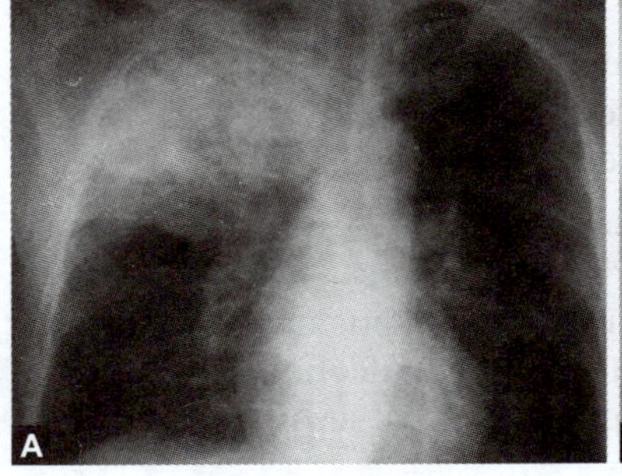

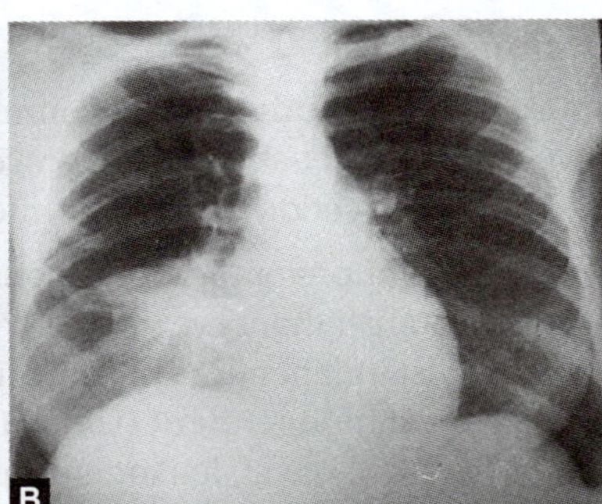

FIGS. 6.38A AND B: Chest X-ray. (A) Shows right upper lobe pneumonia; (B) Shows right middle lobe pneumonia.

Complications (Table 6.78)

Q. Write a short essay on complications of lobar pneumonia.

TABLE 6.78: Complications of lobar pneumonia.

Pulmonary ➢ Delayed/incomplete resolution ➢ Spread to other lobes (rare)	**Cardiovascular** ➢ Acute circulatory failure ➢ Acute pericarditis ➢ Endocarditis (rare)
Pleural: Spread of infection to the pleural cavity: ➢ Sterile pleural effusion ➢ Empyema ➢ Pyothorax	**Neurological** ➢ Mental confusion ➢ Meningism ➢ Meningitis (rare)

Treatment

General measures

- Administration of oxygen in high concentration to all hypoxemic patients.
- Treatment of pleuritic pain with mild analgesics like paracetamol and NSAIDs. However, few may require pethidine 50–100 mg or morphine 10–15 mg intramuscularly or intravenously.

Antibiotic therapy (Discussed earlier)

Vaccine: Two types:

1. Pneumococcal polysaccharide vaccine (PPV): Consists of 23 most common capsular serotypes that produce invasive pneumococcal disease. However, it has poor protection in individuals at greatest risk for severe pneumococcal disease namely elderly, immunocompromised, and infants younger than 2 years.
2. Polysaccharide-protein conjugate pneumococcal vaccine (pneumococcal conjugate vaccine—PCV): It targets seven serotypes responsible for most of pneumococcal infections in children. Hence, it is used mainly in children younger than 2 years.

Indications for vaccination

Refer **Table 6.79.**

TABLE 6.79: Indications for vaccination.

- Age 65 years
- Patients with risk factors: Congestive heart failure, asthma, COPD, diabetes mellitus, chronic liver disease, and alcoholism
- Splenectomized patients including patients with sickle cell anemia
- Persons living in long-term care facilities
- Immunocompromised persons

Staphylococcal Pneumonia

Q. Write a short essay/note on staphylococcal pneumonia.

- It produces bronchopneumonia that is characterized by **widespread** focal/**patchy areas** of **acute suppurative inflammation**.
- They are centered on bronchioles and bronchi with subsequent spread to surrounding alveoli. The involved alveoli show consolidation.
- **Causative agent:** *S. aureus*. Methicillin-resistant *S. aureus* (MRSA) is an important pathogen in nosocomial pneumonia. Recently, community-acquired MRSA (CA-MRSA) infections (skin and soft tissue infections, and necrotizing pneumonia) developing in previously healthy persons have emerged as a serious clinical condition.
- **Predisposing factors:** Common following influenza, in debilitated patients in hospital, and patient with cystic fibrosis.
- **Characteristic features:**
  - Abscess formation is very common. These abscesses are multiple and often bilateral.
  - Abscesses may rupture into pleura leading to pneumothorax or pyopneumothorax.
- Chest radiograph shows bronchopneumonia. It is often bilateral, with multiple thin-walled cyst-like lesions (pneumatoceles).
- Sputum smear shows gram-positive *S. aureus* in clumps.

Treatment

- Drug of choice is penicillin.
- Methicillin-sensitive *S. aureus*: Oxacillin or flucloxacillin.
- Methicillin-resistant *S. aureus*: Vancomycin and teicoplanin.
- Ceftaroline and ceftobiprole, new 5th-generation cephalosporins.
- Drugs used in treatment of resistant *Staphylococcus* (discussed in Chapter 4).

Complications

Toxic shock syndrome (TSS).

Klebsiella Pneumoniae (Friedlander's Pneumonia)

Q. Write a short note on diagnosis and treatment of *Klebsiella pneumoniae* (Friedlander's pneumonia).

- **Causative agent:** *K. pneumoniae* (Friedlander's bacillus).
- **Predisposing factors:** Common in alcoholics and diabetics.
- **Characteristics:**
  - Severe illness with a high-mortality rate.
  - Massive consolidation of one or more lobes. The **upper lobes are** most often affected.
  - Abscess formation and pleural effusion are common.

Investigations

- Sputum:
  - It may be viscid, jelly-like and blood stained **(red-current-jelly sputum)**. Sometimes it may be purulent or rusty.
  - Sputum smear shows gram-negative *K. pneumoniae. K. pneumoniae* can be cultures from the sputum.
- Chest radiograph:
  - It shows air space pneumonia, usually in one of the upper lobes, with abscess formation and pleural effusion.
  - **Bulging interlobar fissure** is a characteristic finding.

Treatment: Antibiotic therapy

- Gentamicin, ceftazidime or ciprofloxacin for 2–3 weeks.
- Severe cases: Piperacillin + tazobactam or meropenem.
- Extended-spectrum β-lactamases (ESBL) producing organisms: Meropenem (or imipenem + cilastatin), amikacin, and tigecycline. Polymyxin B for highly resistant strains.

Atypical Pneumonias

Q. Discuss the etiology (organisms causing atypical pneumonias), clinical features, investigations, and treatment of atypical pneumonias.

- Causes: ***M. pneumoniae, L. pneumophila,*** *Coxiella pneumoniae, C. burnetii,* viruses (influenza, adenovirus, RSV, measles, VZV, and CMV).
- Evolve much more slowly than bacterial pneumonias.
- Symptoms > signs
- They tend to have a slower onset, often with more prominent extrapulmonary symptoms and complications.
- Suspicion of atypical pathogens as the cause of pneumonia should be thought if patient has three or more of the parameters listed in **Table 6.80**.

TABLE 6.80: Parameters that favor the diagnosis of atypical pneumonias.

➢ Age 60 years
➢ Absence of any underlying comorbid condition
➢ Paroxysmal cough
➢ No expectoration
➢ Few clinical signs on examination of chest
If total WBC count 10,000/mm3 is added to the above five parameters, then presence of four features indicates a strong likelihood of atypical pneumonia.

Mycoplasma Pneumoniae

Q. Discuss the clinical features, laboratory diagnosis, and treatment of pneumonias caused by *M. pneumoniae*.

Cause: *M. pneumoniae* which lacks cell wall. It is most often associated with atypical pneumonia.

Clinical Presentation

- Onset is insidious ranging from several days to a week.
- Constitutional symptoms include headache exacerbated by cough, sore throat, malaise, and myalgias. Cough is dry, paroxysmal, and worse at night.
- Clinical course is usually mild and self-limited.

Complications

- **Pulmonary complications:** Pleural effusion, empyema, pneumothorax, and respiratory distress syndrome.
- Infection is severe in sickle cell disease and other HbS-related hemoglobinopathies (functional asplenia). Especially prone to digital necrosis in patients with high titer of cold antibodies.
- **Extrapulmonary complications:**
  - Ear pain: Bullous myringitis
  - Erythema multiforme: Target/iris lesion, Stevens–Johnson (SJ) syndrome
  - Digital necrosis (especially in patients with sickle cell disease)
  - Neurological: Encephalitis, cerebellar ataxia, GBS (Guillain–Barré syndrome), transverse myelitis, peripheral neuropathy.
  - Hematological: Hemolytic anemia and coagulopathy
    - *M. pneumoniae* evokes immunoglobulin M (IgM) antibodies which agglutinate human RBCs at 4°C.
  - Others: Myocarditis, pericarditis, and pancreatitis.

Laboratory Findings and Diagnosis

- Mild leukocytosis can be found.
- Fourfold increase in antibody titers.
- Cold agglutinins are nonspecific but helpful in diagnosis.

Treatment of *Mycoplasma pneumoniae infection*: Macrolides (azithromycin) is the drug of choice, followed by doxycycline and fluoroquinolones.

Chlamydia Pneumoniae

- **Cause:** *Chlamydophila (Chlamydia) pneumoniae* which is an obligate intracellular organism. Another species of *Chlamydophila*, i.e., *Chlamydia psittaci* can also cause pneumonia. It usually infects birds but occasionally infects humans (psittacosis).
- **Mode of transmission:** Through respiratory secretions.
- **Incubation period:** Several weeks.
- **Predisposing factor:** Old age with comorbid diseases.
- **Clinical presentation:** Sore throat, headache, low-grade fever, and cough that can persist for months.
- **Chest radiographs:** Show less-extensive infiltrates than those with other causes of pneumonia.

Treatment: Doxycycline is the drug of choice.

Legionella Pneumonia or Legionnaires' Disease

Q. Write a short essay/note on Legionella pneumonia (Legionnaires' disease).

- ***Pontiac fever:*** Acute self-limiting febrile illness.
- Legionnaires' disease: Pneumonia.
- Most common species causing human infections: *L. pneumophila*
- Most common serogroup causing CAP: 1.
- Most common serogroup causing nosocomial pneumonia: 6
- **Mode of transmission:** Through water droplets originated from infected **humidifier cooling systems,** and from stagnant water in cisterns and shower heads.

Clinical Features

- Fever, chills, and cough with scanty mucoid sputum. Gastrointestinal symptoms like nausea, abdominal pain, and diarrhea are common. **Mental confusion or delirium** may also develop.
- Uncommon features: Myocarditis, pericarditis and prosthetic valve endocarditis, glomerulonephritis, pancreatitis, and peritonitis.

Investigations

- **Chest X-ray:** Shows parenchymal lesions progressing from patchy to lobar consolidation. Pleural effusion may be observed in more than one-third patients. Complete clearing of lung infiltrates may take 1–4 months.
- **Blood:** Relative lymphopenia, very high ESR, hyponatremia, proteinuria, and microscopic hematuria.
- **Culture:** Definitive and most sensitive method, requires 3–5 days.
- **Gram's stain:** Many PMNs, no organisms-suggestive (usual picture with all atypical pneumonias).
- **False +ve AFB stain:** *Legionella micdadei* also known as Pittsburgh pneumonia agent.
- **Direct fluorescent antibody (DFA) test:** Sensitive and specific.
- **Antibody:** Fourfold rise in titer from acute to convalescent stage is diagnostic. Serology has only epidemiologic significance.
- Urinary antigen: Second to culture in terms of both sensitive and specificity.

Treatment: With any one of the following antibacterials: azithromycin, erythromycin, clarithromycin, telithromycin, doxycycline or an extended-spectrum fluoroquinolone for 7-10 days.

Prognosis: Among the atypical pneumonia, Legionnaires' disease presents with most severe clinical course and can progress more severely if the infection is not treated appropriately and early.

Q. Give a short essay/note on antibiotics used in atypical pneumonias.

Actinomycosis

Q. Write a short note/essay on actinomycosis.

- **Cause:** *Actinomyces israelii,* an anaerobic organism present in the oral cavity as a commensal. When local defenses are impaired, it can produce disease.
- Forms:
  - **Oral-cervicofacial actinomycosis:** Present as soft tissue swelling, abscess, and discharging sinuses.
  - **Abdominal actinomycosis:** Presents with discharging sinuses, abdominal mass or abscess.
  - **Pulmonary actinomycosis:** Causes widespread suppurative pneumonia, empyema (often bilateral), and persistent discharging chest wall sinuses.
- Pus obtained from the sinuses show **"sulfur grains".**

Treatment: Antibiotic therapy with benzylpenicillin 18–24 million units intravenously (four divided doses) for 4–6 weeks. This is followed by oral penicillin for 6–12 months.

Acute Bronchopneumonia

Q. Write a short note on acute bronchopneumonia.

- **Bronchopneumonia** is characterized by **patchy** (scattered solid foci) **area of consolidation in the same or several lobes** of the lung.
- It is a type of secondary pneumonia, invariable proceded by bronchial infection. Common in patients with chronicbronchitis.
- Bronchopneumonia is characterized by **widespread** focal/**patchy areas** of **acute suppurative inflammation**. They are **centered on bronchioles and bronchi** with subsequent spread to surrounding alveoli. The involved alveoli show **consolidation**. The **consolidated areas are larger and more numerous in lower lobes** (because of the tendency of secretions to gravitate into the lower lobes) and **frequently bilateral**.

- **Predisposing factors:**
  - In children: As a complication of **measles or whooping cough.**
  - In adults: As a complication of **acute bronchitis or influenza**.
  - In elderly or debilitated patients: As **hypostatic pneumonia.**
- Viral pneumonias and "atypical" pneumonias may also present as bronchopneumonia.

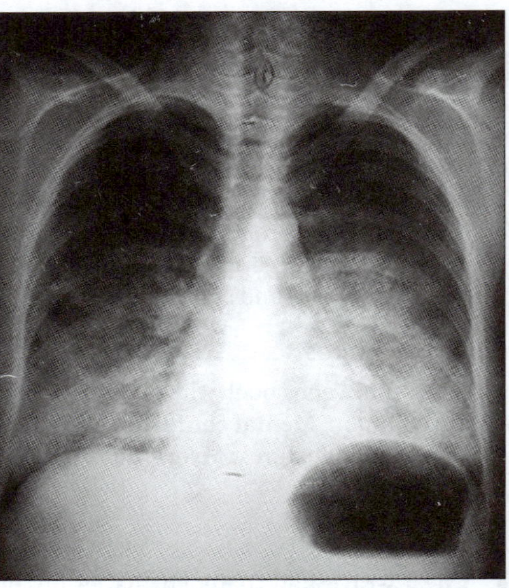

FIG. 6.39: Chest X-ray of bronchopneumonia.

Clinical Features

- High fever, severe cough with purulent expectoration, breathlessness, tachypnea, tachycardia, and central cyanosis.
- **Physical signs in the chest:** Early-stage signs of acute bronchitis, later-stage numerous crepitations.
- **Investigations:**
  - Chest X-ray: Bilateral mottled opacities, predominantly in the lower zones **(Fig. 6.39)**.
  - Blood: Neutrophilic leukocytosis common.

Treatment: Antibiotic therapy.
- Mild cases: Ampicillin or cotrimoxazole given orally is effective.
- Serious cases: Third-generation cephalosporin along with a macrolide.

Aspiration Pneumonia

Q. Write a short note on aspiration pneumonia.

- It develops due to abnormal entry of fluid, particulate exogenous substances or endogenous secretions into the lower airways.
- Types: (1) Chemical aspiration pneumonia and (2) bacterial aspiration pneumonia.

Predisposing Factors

- Acute aspiration of gastric contents into the lungs: Reduced consciousness, as a complication of anesthesia.
- Mechanical disruption of the glottis closure or cardiac sphincter due to tracheostomy, endotracheal intubation, bronchoscopy, upper endoscopy, and nasogastric feeding.
- Disorders of the upper gastrointestinal tract: Esophageal disease, surgery involving the upper airways or esophagus, and gastric reflux.
- Dysphagia from neurologic deficits.
- Miscellaneous conditions: Protracted vomiting, large volume tube feedings, and feeding gastrostomy.

Chemical Aspiration Pneumonia

- Develops due to the aspiration of substances that are toxic to the lower airways, independent of bacterial infection.
- Chemical pneumonitis associated with the aspiration of gastric acid as a complication of anesthesia particularly during pregnancy **(Mendelson's syndrome).** It can produce an extremely severe and sometimes fatal illness because of the intense destructiveness of gastric acid.

Clinical Features

- Abrupt onset of low-grade fever and dyspnea.
- Physical examination reveals cyanosis and diffuse crepitations.
- Chest radiograph: Infiltrates involving dependent pulmonary segments that usually develop within 2 hours of aspiration.

Treatment
- **Tracheal suction:** To clear fluids and particulate matter.
- **Support of respiration:** Mechanical ventilation may be needed.
- **Corticosteroids:** Use controversial.
- **Antibiotics:** In acute events.

Bacterial Aspiration Pneumonia

- Most common type of aspiration pneumonia caused by bacteria that normally reside in the upper airways or stomach.
- **Predisposing factors:** Hospitalized patients with depressed gag reflex, impaired swallowing, or nasogastric or endotracheal tube. Elderly individuals and patients with impaired consciousness (e.g., drug, alcohol, stroke).

Clinical Features

- Highly variable and depend upon the bacteria involved and status of the host.
- Most cases are due to anaerobic bacteria that normally reside in the gingival crevices.
- **Usual features** of pneumonia such as cough, fever, purulent sputum, and dyspnea. The process evolves over a period of several days or weeks instead of hours in usual pneumonia.
- **Other features:** Weight loss and anemia.
- **Oral examination:** May reveal periodontal disease.

Diagnosis

- **Sputum:** Putrid discharge is considered as diagnostic of anaerobic infection.
- **Chest radiograph:** Involvement of dependent pulmonary segments by aspiration. Lower lobes are involved when aspiration occurs in upright position and the superior segments of the lower lobes or posterior segment of the upper lobes when aspiration occurs in recumbent position.

Treatment

- Penicillin. However, about 25% of cases are caused by penicillinase-producing anaerobic bacteria.
- Clindamycin (600 mg 8 hourly IV followed by 300 mg 6 hourly orally) is the drug of choice for anaerobic infections above the diaphragm (e.g., pulmonary infections).
- Other drugs include amoxicillin-clavulanate or newer fluoroquinolones (levofloxacin and gemifloxacin).
- Metronidazole alone should not be used as a monotherapy because of failure rate of about 50%.

Hospital-acquired Pneumonia (Nosocomial Pneumonia)

Q. Write a short essay on hospital-acquired pneumonia (nosocomial pneumonia) and its management.

- Hospital-acquired pneumonia or nosocomial pneumonia is a new episode of pneumonia developing in hospital in a patient who is beyond 2 days (>48 hours) of their initial admission to hospital, which was not incubating at the time of admission. Most common resistant organism causing HAP is *S. aureus.*
- Second most common (urinary infection being first) hospital-acquired infection (HAI) and the leading cause of HAI-associated death. The HAPs are serious and may be life-threatening.
- Ventilator-associated pneumonia: It is a subcategory of nosocomial pneumonia that occurs in patients who have been on ventilator support for any reason. Pneumonia is termed as VAP if it occurs after 48 hours after endotracheal intubation for mechanical ventilation, but within 72 hours of start of ventilation. Most common mechanism of nosocomial pneumonia is aspiration and most common organism is *S. aureus.* The most common multidrug-resistant gram-negative bacilli (MDR-GNB) causing HAP/VAP: *P. aeruginosa.*
- Early-onset HAP and VAP: Occurring within the first 4 days of hospitalization, usually carry a better prognosis, and are more likely to be caused by antibiotic-sensitive bacteria.
- Late-onset HAP and VAP (5 days or more) are more likely to be caused by MDR pathogens, and are associated with increased patient mortality and morbidity.

Criteria

- At least two of three clinical features (fever >38°C, leukocytosis or leukopenia, and purulent secretions), a positive culture of sputum or tracheal aspirate, and a new lung infiltrate.
- *When fever, leukocytosis, purulent sputum, and a positive culture of a sputum or tracheal aspirate are present without a new lung infiltrate, the diagnosis of nosocomial tracheobronchitis should be considered.*

Etiology (Table 6.81)

The organisms causing hospital-acquired pneumonias are different from those causing CAP.

TABLE 6.81: Various etiological agents causing hospital-acquired pneumonia.

- **Early onset:** (within 4 days of hospitalization): *S. aureus*, EGNB, *S. pneumoniae* and *H. influenzae*
- **Late onset:** *S. aureus, Pseudomonas, Enterobacter, Klebsiella, Acinetobacter*

Risk factors for nosocomial pneumonia: Severe underlying diseases, malnutrition, uremia, alcoholism, cigarette smoking, immunosuppression, increasing age, nasogastric tube (lesser risk with orogastric tube), endotracheal tube, decreased level of consciousness, prior AMA use, decreased gastric acidity, and upper abdominal surgery.

Risk factors for VAP: Reintubation, supine positioning, enteral nutrition, heavy sedation, paralytic agents, H_2 antagonists, and antacids.

Clinical Features

The diagnosis should be considered in any hospitalized or ventilated patient who develops:

- Purulent sputum (or endotracheal secretions)

- New infiltrate on chest radiograph
- Unexplained increase in oxygen requirement
- Core temperature of more than 38.3°C
- Leukocytosis or leukopenia

Investigations

- Patients with hospital-acquired pneumonia should have blood cultures, and microbiological confirmation should be sought whenever possible. Vigorous attempts must be made to obtain respiratory secretions for identification of the organism and determining its sensitivity to antibiotics. In mechanically ventilated patients, bronchoscopy-directed protected brush specimens, bronchoalveolar lavage (BAL) or endotracheal aspirates may be obtained.
- Full blood count (FBC), urea and electrolytes (U&E), erythrocyte sedimentation rate (ESR) and C-reactive protein (CRP), and arterial blood gas analysis and a chest X-ray are performed.

Management/Treatment

- The principles of management are similar to those for CAP.These include adequate oxygenation, appropriate fluid balance, and antibiotics.
- In early-onset HAP:
  - Patients who have not received previous antibiotics can be treated with co-amoxiclav or cefuroxime.
  - If the patient has received a course of recent antibiotics are treated with piperacillin/tazobactam or a third-generation cephalosporin
- In late-onset HAP:
  - The choice of antibiotics must cover the gram-negative bacteria, *S. aureus* (including MRSA) and anaerobes.
  - Antipseudomonal cover by a carbapenem (meropenem) or a third-generation cephalosporin combined with an aminoglycoside.
  - MRSA cover may be provided by glycopeptides (vancomycin or linezolid).
- *Acinetobacter baumannii* is usually sensitive to carbapenems but resistant cases may require prolonged administration of nebulized colistin.

Prevention of Ventilator-associated Pneumonia

See **Table 6.82.**

TABLE 6.82: Prevention of ventilator-associated pneumonia.

➤ Good hygiene: Rigorous handwashing by caregivers and sterility of any equipment used
➤ Minimize the risk of aspiration
➤ Semirecumbent positioning of the patient to prevent aspiration
➤ Avoidance of gastric distention
➤ Continuous subglottic suctioning
➤ Adequate nutritional support
➤ Early removal of endotracheal and nasogastric tubes
➤ Oral antiseptic (chlorhexidine 2%) may be used to decontaminate the upper airway.
➤ Use of sucralfate (for stress-ulcer prophylaxis)
➤ Avoidance of prophylactic antibiotic

Influenza

Q. Discuss the etiology, clinical features, investigations, complications, and management of influenza.

Definition

Influenza is an acute systemic viral infection caused by influenza viruses that primarily affects the upper and/or lower respiratory tract.

Etiology

The influenza virus is a spherical or filamentous enveloped RNA virus.

Influenza A Virus

- It is responsible for pandemics and epidemics.
- **Antigenic variation and influenza outbreaks and pandemics:** The most extensive and severe outbreaks of influenza are due to influenza A viruses. This may be because H and N antigens of these viruses undergo periodic antigenic variation. Immunity following viral infection is type-specific and of short duration.
- **Antigenic/genetic shift:** Major antigenic variations (switch in the hemagglutinin or neuraminidase antigen generates. New influenza A subtypes) are called antigenic/genetic shift. Antigenic shift results in a virus of different antigenic character to which most or all of the population is susceptible and is the basis for influenza pandemics. For example, an antigenic shift involving both the hemagglutinin and the neuraminidase occurred in 1957 resulting in severe pandemic. It was due to shift of predominant influenza A virus subtype from H1N1 to H2N2.
- **Antigenic/genetic drifts:** These are due to minor antigenic variations. Minor antigenic variation periodically involve the hemagglutinin or the neuraminidase component or both. Antigenic drift results in viruses that are different enough from preceding strains and enables the virus to evade previously acquired immunity and contributes to yearly seasonal epidemics. Influenza viruses also infect other species (e.g., birds and pigs) and these animal strains may infect humans and spread from person to person.

Clinical features

- Incubation period: 1–3 days
- **Clinical manifestations:** Influenza is respiratory illness characterized by systemic symptoms such as sudden onset of headache, fever, chills, myalgia, nausea, vomiting and malaise. The respiratory signs and symptoms include harsh unproductive cough, and sore throat
- **Physical findings:** Usually minimal in uncomplicated cases. Pharynx may be unremarkable despite a severe sore throat and chest is usually clear.
- In uncomplicated cases, the symptoms usually subside within 3–5 days.

Investigations

- Blood: Leukopenia
- Throat swab or nasopharyngeal aspirate or sputum: Virus may be detected in throat swabs or nasopharyngeal aspirate or sputum.
- Reverse-transcriptase polymerase chain reaction (RT-PCR): Most sensitive and specific technique for detection of influenza viruses.
- Rapid influenza diagnostic tests (RIDTs): Detect influenza virus antigens by immunologic or enzymatic techniques.

Complications

- **Pulmonary complications:** Primary influenza viral pneumonia, secondary bacterial pneumonia (most often due to superinfection with *S. pneumoniae, S. Aureus*, or other bacteria), mixed viral and bacterial pneumonia, exacerbation of underlying asthma and COPD.
- **Extrapulmonary complications:**
  - Myositis, myocarditis, pericarditis, worsening of underlying congestive heart failure and coronary artery disease
  - Neurological complications: Reye's syndrome in children, encephalitis, or transverse myelitis
  - Postinfluenzal asthenia and depression

Management

- Bed rest till fever subsides
- Paracetamol 0.5–1 g every 4–6 hourly.
- Avoid aspirin, particularly in adolescents and children, because of its association with Reye's syndrome.
- **Specific antiviral therapy—administration of neuraminidase inhibitor:** Oral oseltamivir (75 mg twice daily) or inhaled zanamivir (10 mg twice daily) for 5 days reduces the severity of symptoms and duration of illness if given within 48 hours of symptom onset of both influenza A and B. Amantadine (100 mg twice a day) and rimantadine (100 mg twice a day) which are useful only for influenza A.
- Specific treatment of complications

Prevention

Vaccination

- **Indications:** Annual seasonal vaccination is advised to elderly, individuals with chronic medical illnesses (which increases the risk of the complications of influenza), such as chronic cardiopulmonary diseases or immunocompromised or renal disease and their healthcare workers. Specific vaccination gives about 70% protection.
- **Types of vaccine:** Two types of vaccines against seasonal influenza are available, namely inactivated (killed-injectable) and live attenuated vaccines (nasal spray). Both vaccines contain three strains of influenza: an H3N2 virus, an H1N1 (seasonal) virus, and an influenza B virus. Vaccine composition is changed yearly to cover the "predicted" seasonal strains, but vaccination may fail when a new pandemic strain of virus emerges.

Chemoprophylaxis: Antiviral drugs may be used as chemoprophylaxis against influenza. However, they may lead to development of resistance.

Chemoprophylaxis with oseltamivir or zanamivir are helpful against influenza A and B; amantadine and rimantadine are useful for influenza A.

Swine Flu (H1N1 Influenza)

Refer **Chapter 4.**

Avian Influenza

Q. Write short essay on avian influenza.

- Avian influenza is caused by **avian influenza A viruses** and is primary public health concern of the 21st century.
- Avian influenza A viruses caused sporadic avian influenza and small outbreaks in humans, usually after **direct contact with birds** (most commonly poultry). There is no sustained person-to-person transmission.

Clinical Features

- **History of exposure** to infected birds.
- **Incubation period:** Usually 2–5 days after exposure (longer than with human influenza infection).
- **Symptoms:** Fever (at least 100.4°F), cough and myalgia. Watery diarrhea is fairly common. Usually complicated by viral pneumonia causing increasing respiratory distress and cyanosis. Ventilatory support is often necessary and mortality rate may be as high as 50%.

Investigations

- **Blood:** Leukopenia
- **Liver function tests:** Raised hepatic aminotransferase, lactate dehydrogenase, and creatine kinase
- **Chest X-ray:** Infiltrates seen 7 days after the onset of fever.
- Diagnosis:
  - Isolation of virus or detection of H5-specific RNA. Pharyngeal swabs are preferred than nasal swabs, because of greater titers in the throat and lower respiratory tract.
  - Reverse transcriptase polymerase chain reaction assays are more sensitive than commercial rapid antigen tests.

Prevention: Whenever there is an outbreak of avian influenza, avoid live animal markets and poultry farms.

Treatment

Drug treatment: Same as H1N1 influenza (*refer* **Chapter 4)**

Non-pharmacologic approaches

- Influenza surveillance: For early warning, travel restrictions, quarantine, use of N 95 particulate respiratory masks, and communication networking.
- Proper poultry handling and personal hygiene (such as handwashing) and minimizing contact with birds during an outbreak.

Severe Acute Respiratory Syndrome

Q. Write a short essay/note on severe acute respiratory syndrome and its laboratory findings.

An extraordinary outbreak of the coronavirus-associated disease known as severe acute respiratory syndrome (SARS) was described for the first time in 2002-2003 from Southern China and quickly spread to several countries within less than a year. A death rate of nearly 10% was reported. Though, presently it has not been reported from any country, there is possibility of either human or animal reservoirs of the virus and this may lead to return of SARS.

Etiology

SARS is caused by a previously unknown novel coronavirus (SARS-CoV). It is not closely related to any of the previously described coronaviruses.

Mode of spread: By close person-to-person contact via droplet transmission, or fomite.

Clinical Features

- **Incubation period:** 2–7 days (range 1–14 days).
- **Symptoms:** Begins as a systemic disease with persistent fever, chills/rigor, malaise, headache, and myalgias followed by nonproductive/dry cough and dyspnea within 1–2 days. About 25% have diarrhea and about 20% develop ARDS over a period of 3 weeks.
- Older individuals may present with decrease in general well-being, poor feeding, fall without the typical febrile response.

Laboratory Findings

Blood

- Lymphopenia due to the destruction of both $CD4^+$ and $CD8^+$ T-cells. Thrombocytopenia may occur as the disease progresses.
- Raised serum levels of aminotransferases, creatine kinase, and lactate dehydrogenase
- Laboratory features of low-grade disseminated intravascular coagulation (DIC): Thrombocytopenia, prolonged activated partial thromboplastin time and raised D-dimer.

Chest X-ray

- Most frequently peripheral and lower zone or interstitial infiltrates show patchy areas of consolidation. There will no cavitation, hilar lymphadenopathy, or pleural effusion.
- Patchy areas may progress to diffuse involvement.
- Spontaneous pneumomediastinum may occur in few.
- Chest X-ray may be normal in about 25%.

Diagnosis

- **Detection of SARS-CoV:** A rapid diagnosis of SARS-CoV infection by reverse transcription PCR (RT-PCR). The samples use includes:
  - **During early phase:** Respiratory tract (e.g., nasopharyngeal aspirate) samples and plasma
  - **During later phase:** Urine and stool specimen
- Quantitative measurement of SARS-CoV RNA in blood with RT-PCR technique
- Viral culture of respiratory tract samples

Treatment
- No specific therapy
- **Supportive care:** It is the mainstay in therapy and includes maintenance of fluid and electrolyte balance, oxygenation and, if necessary ventilation with proper protection of healthcare workers.
- High-dose methylprednisolone (0.5 g daily) is given if pneumonia or hypoxemia develops. However, its benefit remains to be established.

Middle East Respiratory Syndrome

Q. Write short note on Middle East respiratory syndrome.

- Caused by novel coronavirus, namely Middle East respiratory syndrome (MERS)-CoV
- Most cases have been reported in Arab Peninsula and neighboring countries with more than 70% from Saudi Arabia.
- **Mode of transmission:** Human-to-human transmission can occur although spread may not be efficient. Unlike SARS coronavirus, MERS-CoV does not preferentially infect healthcare workers.

Source of infection: Camels are major reservoir host for MERS-CoV and an animal source of infection in humans.

Incubation period: 2–14 days (mean 5.2 days)
- The virus causes more severe disease in individuals who are old, with weakened immune systems, with chronic diseases (e.g., cancer, chronic lung disease, and diabetes).

Clinical features: Typical MERS symptoms include fever, cough, and shortness of breath. Pneumonia is common, but not always present. Gastrointestinal symptoms, including diarrhea, have also been reported.
- About 36% of reported patients with MERS died mostly due to ARDS. Renal failure also can develop.
- Investigations: Leukopenia, thrombocytopenia, raised elevated liver enzymes, LDH, and creatinine kinase.

Treatment
Neither vaccine nor specific treatment is currently available. Treatment is supportive and based on the patient's clinical condition.

DIFFUSE PARENCHYMAL LUNG DISEASE/INTERSTITIAL LUNG DISEASE

Q. Discuss the etiology and approach to diffuse parenchymal lung disease/interstitial lung diseases.

Definition: Diffuse parenchymal lung diseases [DPLD, also referred to as **interstitial lung diseases (**ILDs)] are a **heterogeneous group of conditions affecting the parenchyma of** lung and alveoli.

- **Diffuse:** Refers to the nonspecific **radiological patterns**
- **Lung parenchyma** includes the alveoli, the alveolar epithelium, the capillary endothelium, the spaces between those structures (interstitium) as well as the perivascular and lymphatic tissues.
- ILD-A misnomer
  - Pathophysiologic processes are not restricted to the interstitium.
  - All of the several cellular and soluble constituents that make up the gas exchange units and others
  - Bronchiolar lumen
  - Terminal bronchioles
  - Pulmonary parenchyma beyond the gas exchange units
  - Pleura
  - Lymphatic
  - Lymph nodes
- **Interstitium of the lung:** It is defined as continuum of loose connective tissue throughout the lung and composed of three subdivisions:
  1. **Bronchovascular** (axial), surrounding the bronchi, arteries, and veins from the lung root to the level of the respiratory bronchiole.
  2. **Parenchymal** (acinar), situated between the alveolar and capillary basement membranes

3. **Subpleural**, situated beneath the pleura, as well as in the interlobular septae
   - Interstitium of the lung is not normally visible radiographically. It becomes visible only when its volume increases.
   - They are noninfectious and nonmalignant and usually chronic diseases that diffusely involve the lungs.
   - Diffuse parenchymal lung diseases can progress fibrosis in the interstitium (interstitial pulmonary fibrosis) of the lung.

Etiology (Table 6.83)

Q. Write short essay/note on causes/etiology of interstitial lung disease.

Many diseases can produce interstitial lung disease. Based on the major underlying histopathology, ILDs can be divided into two groups: (1) those associated with predominant inflammation and fibrosis and (2) those with a predominantly granulomatous reaction in interstitial or vascular.

TABLE 6.83: Major causes of interstitial lung disease (ILD)/diffuse parenchymal lung diseases (DPLD).

ILD/DPLD due to known causes	*ILD/DPLD due to unknown causes*
Nongranulomatous interstitial inflammation (predominant inflammation and fibrosis)	
➢ Drugs: Antibiotics, gold, amiodarone, D-penicillamine, nitrofurantoin, Chemotherapeutic (e.g., busulfan, bleomycin, methotrexate, CCNU) ➢ Asbestos ➢ Fumes and gases ➢ Radiation ➢ Aspiration pneumonitis ➢ Residual of acute respiratory distress syndrome ➢ Smoking related: Pulmonary Langerhans cell histiocytosis, respiratory bronchiolitis interstitial lung disease and desquamative interstitial pneumonia ➢ Acute eosinophilic pneumonia	➢ Idiopathic interstitial pneumonias (IIPs) ➢ Idiopathic pulmonary fibrosis ➢ Pulmonary autoimmune rheumatic diseases (e.g., systemic lupus erythematosus, rheumatoid arthritis) ➢ Pulmonary alveolar proteinosis ➢ Eosinophilic pneumonias ➢ Lymphangioleiomyomatosis (LAM) ➢ Diffuse pulmonary hemorrhage ➢ Goodpasture syndrome ➢ Idiopathic pulmonary hemosiderosis ➢ Lymphocytic interstitial pneumonia (seen in HIV)
Granulomatous interstitial inflammation	
➢ Hypersensitivity pneumonitis (organic dusts) ➢ Inorganic dusts: For example, silicosis, berylliosis	➢ Sarcoidosis ➢ Pulmonary Langerhans cell histiocytosis ➢ Granulomatous lung disease with vasculitis (e.g., Wegener, Churg–Strauss)

Flowchart 6.12 shows classification of ILD and **Flowchart 6.13** shows classification of DLPD.

FLOWCHART 6.12: ILD classification.

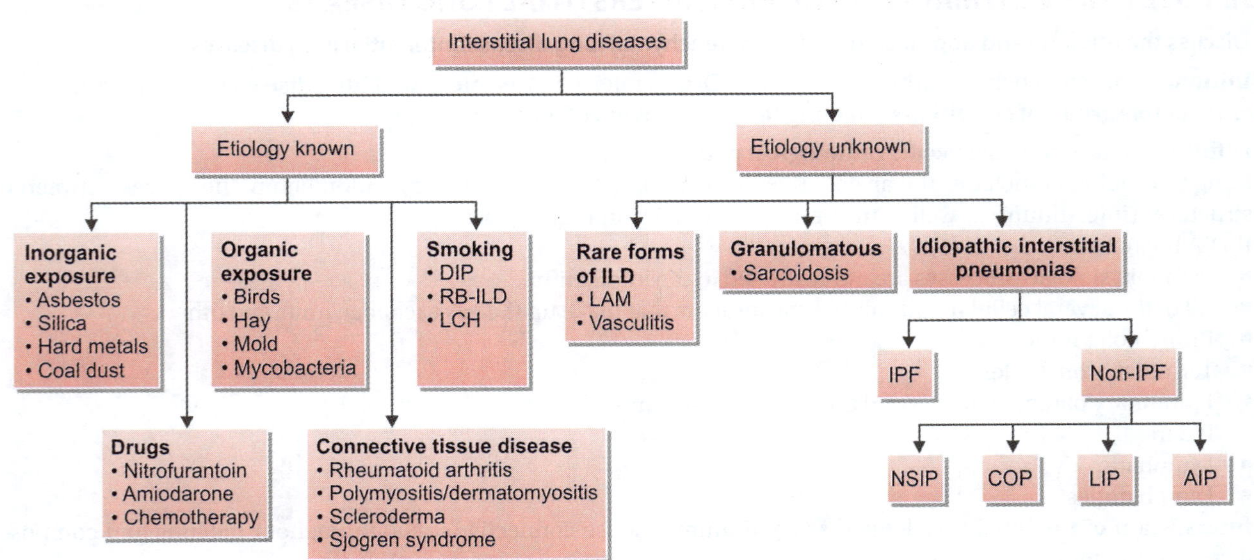

FLOWCHART 6.13: Classification of DLPD.

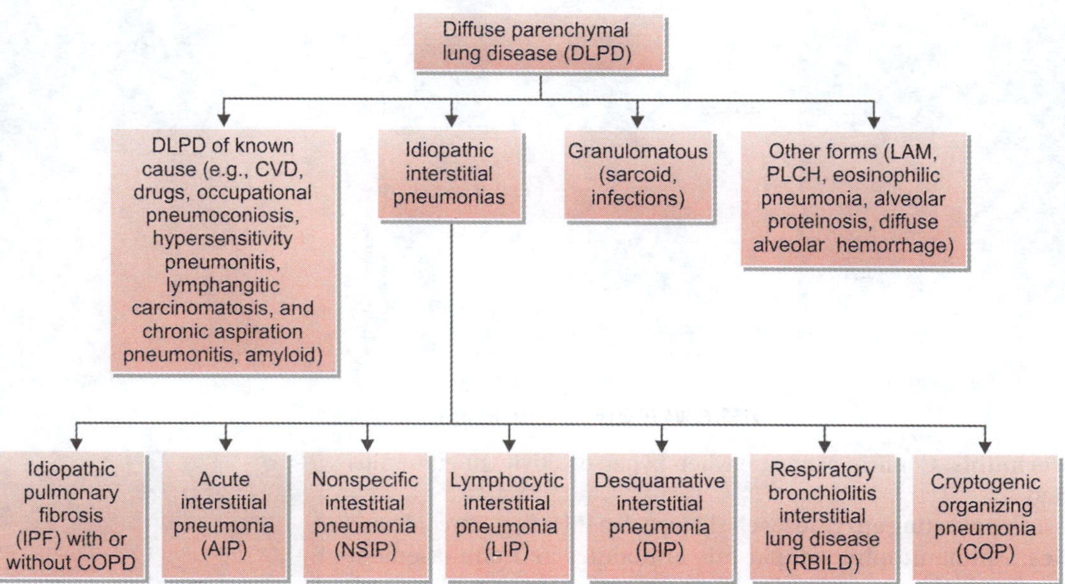

Pathogenesis

See **Flowchart 6.14.**

FLOWCHART 6.14: Pathogenesis of pulmonary fibrosis

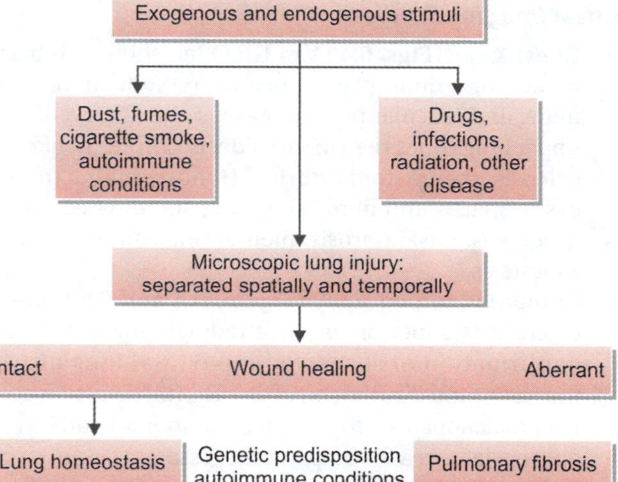

Clinical Features

Q. Write short essay/note on clinical features of diffuse parenchymal lung disease/interstitial lung diseases.

Depending on the duration of illness and clinical presentation, ILDs are divided into acute, subacute, and chronic.

- **Acute presentation** (days to weeks)
  - This presentation is **uncommon** but may develop with drugs, acute idiopathic interstitial pneumonia and hypersensitivity pneumonitis.
  - **Chief symptoms** are cough, dyspnea, and occasionally fever.
  - **Chest X-ray** shows diffuse alveolar opacities which can be confused with "atypical" pneumonia.
- **Subacute presentation** (weeks to months)
  - **Symptoms:** Gradually increasing cough and dyspnea over weeks to months
  - This type of presentation can occur especially with sarcoidosis, and drug-induced ILDs
- Chronic presentation (months to years)
  - Most common presentation in which symptoms are present for months to years.
  - **Common symptoms:** Shortness of breath, dry cough, fatigue, weakness, loss of appetite and weight.

Physical Examination

- Clubbing
- Cyanosis
- Crackles or "velcro rales" are present on chest examination in most forms of ILD
- Scattered late inspiratory high-pitched rhonchi, so-called inspiratory squeaks
- Decreased chest expansion
- Evidence of Pulmonary hypertension/cor pulmonale
- Signs of underlying cause

Investigations

Laboratory Investigation

- **Blood:** Total leukocyte count, ESR, renal and liver functions, antinuclear antibodies, rheumatoid factor and circulating immune complexes.

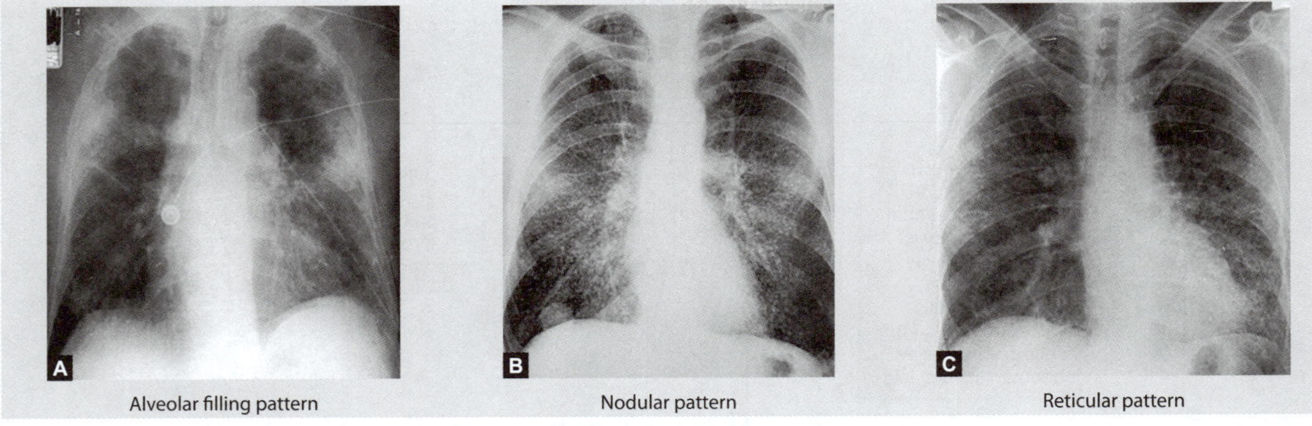

FIGS. 6.40A TO C: Chest X-ray showing patterns of ILD/DPLD.

- **Serum precipitins:** Confirm exposure when hypersensitivity pneumonitis is suspected.
- **Angiotensin-converting enzyme levels:** Elevated in ILDs (e.g., sarcoidosis).
- **Antibodies:** Antineutrophil cytoplasmic antibodies and antibasement membrane antibodies are useful if vasculitis is suspected (e.g., Wegener's granulomatosis, Goodpasture syndrome).

Chest Imaging Studies

- **Chest X-ray (Figs. 6.40A to C):** Often shows a bibasilar reticular or linear pattern or ground-glass appearance. Nodular or mixed pattern of alveolar filling and reticular pattern may also be observed. Nodular opacities in the upper lung zones seen in sarcoidosis, chronic hypersensitivity pneumonitis, silicosis, rheumatoid arthritis. Honeycombing (due to small thick-walled cystic spaces and fibrosis) in long-standing conditions. It indicates poor prognosis. Basal fibrosis, pleural thickening and pleural plaques suggest asbestosis.
- **Computed tomography (Figs. 6.41A and B):** High-resolution CT (HRCT) of chest is superior to chest radiography for (i) early detection and confirmation of suspected interstitial lung disease, (ii) demonstrates the extent and distribution of disease, (iii) detection of coexisting disease (e.g., lymphadenopathy, emphysema, carcinoma) and (iv) to determine the most appropriate area for biopsy (if necessary).
- **Pulmonary function tests:** These show following findings:

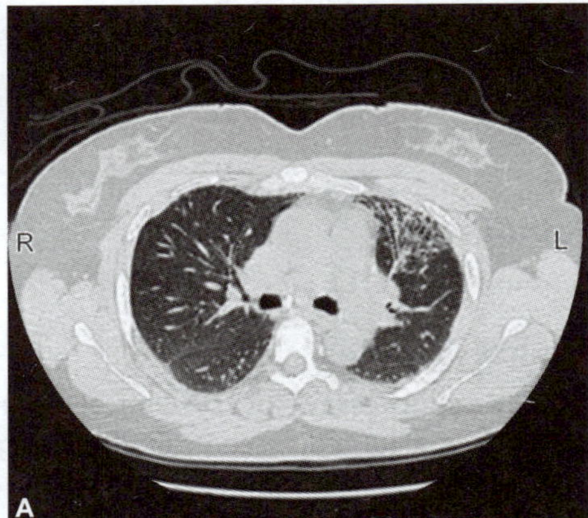

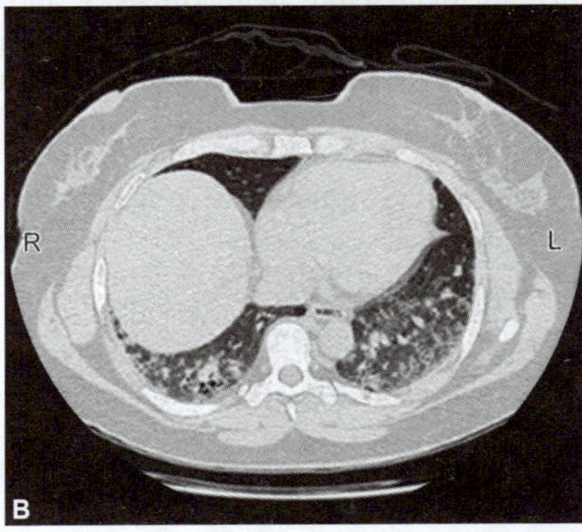

FIGS. 6.41A AND B: CT sections showing patterns of ILD/DPLD.

Q. Write short note on pulmonary function tests in interstitial lung disease.

- Restrictive ventilatory defect in the presence of reduced lung volumes and impaired gas transfer.
- Restrictive defect is characterized by reduced FVC, reduced FEV_1, normal or elevated FEV_1: FVC ratio, total lung capacity, reduced diffusion capacity.
- Obstructive pattern is seen in sarcoidosis, hypersensitivity pneumonitis, Lymphangioleiomyomatosis, tuberous sclerosis, and neurofibromatosis.
  - **Exercise tests:** Help in the evaluation of severity of the disease. The 6-minute walk test records oxygen saturation before, during, and after exercise and measures the total distance walked.
- **Arterial blood gas:** It may reveal hypoxemia and respiratory alkalosis. Hypercapnia is rare and may develop in the end-stage. Increased alveolar-arterial oxygen gradient $[P(A-a)O_2]$
- **Fiberoptic bronchoscopy and bronchoalveolar lavage (BAL):** In selected cases (e.g., sarcoidosis, hypersensitivity pneumonitis, cancer) cellular analysis of BAL may be useful in narrowing the differential diagnosis. Transbronchial biopsy may aid in diagnosis.
  - Sarcoidosis and hypersensitivity pneumonitis: It shows T-cell lymphocytosis (increased CD4 cells in sarcoidosis and CD8 cells in hypersensitivity pneumonitis).
  - Idiopathic pulmonary fibrosis (IPF): It shows predominant neutrophils and eosinophils.

- Pulmonary alveolar proteinosis: It is milky and microscopically contains foamy macrophages with PAS-positive material.

- Diffuse pulmonary hemorrhage: It shows RBCs and hemosiderin-laden macrophages.
- **Biopsy: Open or video-assisted lung biopsy is used for confirmation of diagnosis and assessment of activity.**

Treatment

Major Goals

- Treat the underlying cause if possible.
- Permanent removal of the offending agent if known.
- General
  - Oxygen therapy: For patients with documented hypoxia, SpO_2<89%,–PaO_2<55 mm Hg. Improves exercise tolerance
  - Adequate nutrition and immunizations (pneumococcal, influenza)
  - Pulmonary rehabilitation: Treatment of pulmonary hypertension, single lung transplantation
  - Early identification and aggressive suppression of the acute and chronic inflammatory process, thereby reducing further damage to the lung.

Drugs

- **Corticosteroids** are the mainstay for the suppression of the inflammation present in ILD, though they are not effective in majority, particularly those with significant fibrosis. Prednisone in the dose is 0.5–1 mg/kg once daily for 4–12 weeks. If the patient improves, it is then tapered to maintenance dose of 0.25–0.5 mg/kg level for an additional 4–12 weeks.
- **N-Acetylcysteine:** 600 mg thrice daily. It has been found promising in the management of DPLD.
- **Other immunosuppressants:** If the patient does not respond to steroids, another immunosuppressant, such as cyclophosphamide or azathioprine (1–2 mg/kg lean body weight per day) mycophenolate mofetil, rituximab with/ without glucocorticoids may be tried.
- **Other drugs:** Include colchicine, cyclosporine.
- **Pirfenidone** is an antifibrotic drug used for idiopathic pulmonary fibrosis (IPF). Mechanism of action is via the downregulation of the production of growth factors and procollagens I and II leading to decrease in fibroblast proliferation.
- **Nintedanib,** an oral tyrosine kinase inhibitor has been shown to slow down disease progression in 2 randomized placebo-controlled trials by reducing annual decline in forced vital capacity (FVC).

Idiopathic Interstitial Pneumonias

Idiopathic interstitial pneumonias (IIPs) are characterized by diffuse inflammation and fibrosis in the lung parenchyma in which the etiology is not known. They form a major subgroup of interstitial lung diseases or diffuse parenchymal lung diseases. The lung parenchyma shows varying combinations of fibrosis and inflammation.

Classification of idiopathic interstitial pneumonias (ATS/ERS joint consensus statement-2002). Based on mainly histological patterns/in order of relative frequency is presented in **Table 6.84**.

TABLE 6.84: Classification of idiopathic interstitial pneumonias based mainly on histological patterns/in order of relative frequency.

- Idiopathic pulmonary fibrosis (IPF)/usual interstitial pneumonia (UIP)
- Nonspecific interstitial pneumonia (NSIP)
- Cryptogenic organizing pneumonia (COP)/bronchiolitis obliterans organizing pneumonia (BOOP)
- Acute interstitial pneumonia (AIP)/(Hamman–Rich syndrome) rapidly fatal
  - Respiratory bronchiolitis-associated interstitial lung disease (RBILD)
  - Desquamative interstitial pneumonia (DIP)
  - Lymphoid interstitial pneumonia (LIP)

Idiopathic Pulmonary Fibrosis

Q. Write short essay/note on clinical features, investigations, and treatment of idiopathic pulmonary fibrosis.

Also known as usual interstitial pneumonia (UIP) and was previously called as cryptogenic fibrosing alveolitis (CFA).

Definition: It is a progressive fibrosing interstitial pneumonia of unknown cause.

Contributory factors: Cigarette smoking, chronic aspiration, antidepressants, infections (e.g., Epstein–Barr virus), exposure to occupational dusts (e.g., wood and metal dusts) and chronic gastroesophageal reflux.

Clinical features and investigations are discussed under ILD.

Diagnostic criteria are as are shown in **Table 6.85**.

TABLE 6.85: Diagnostic criteria idiopathic pulmonary fibrosis.

Major criteria	*Minor criteria*
1. Exclusion of other known causes of interstitial lung disease	1. Age >50 years
2. Abnormal pulmonary function with restriction and/or decreased diffusing capacity	2. Insidious onset of otherwise unexplained dyspnoe
3. Bibasilar reticular abnormalities on HRCT scans	3. Duration of illness >3 months
4. BAL or TBB not pointing to another disease	4. Bibasilar, inspiratory crackles on auscultation

Treatment

- Refer to treatment of "interstitial lung disease" as discussed above.
- Corticosteroids: Response is poor.

OCCUPATIONAL LUNG DISEASES

Q. Write short essay/note on common occupational lung diseases and their etiology/common causes of pneumoconiosis.

- Exposure to dusts, gases, vapors, and fumes at work can cause many types of lung disease. It is difficult to distinguish occupational and environmental lung diseases from those of nonenvironmental origin.
- **Pneumoconioses** are defined as **lung diseases produced by organic as well as inorganic particulates and chemical fumes and vapors**. However, sometimes the term occupational lung diseases and pneumoconiosis are used interchangeably.
- **Common** pneumoconiosis is due to inorganic (mineral) dusts. Occupational exposure and associated lung diseases are listed in **Table 6.86**.

TABLE 6.86: Occupational exposure and associated lung diseases.

Occupational exposure	*Disease associated with chronic exposure*
Diseases due to inorganic (mineral) dusts: Common pneumoconiosis	
➤ Coal	Coal-worker's pneumoconiosis (CWP)
➤ Silica	CWP
➤ Asbestos	Silicosis
➤ Beryllium	Asbestos-related diseases
➤ Iron oxide	Berylliosis
➤ Tin dioxide	Siderosis
	Stannosis
Diseases due to organic dusts	
➤ Cotton, flax or hemp dust	Byssinosis
➤ Moldy hay, grain, straw	Farmer's lung
➤ Mold malting	Malt worker's lung
➤ Contaminated bagasse (sugar cane)	Bagassosis
Diseases due to gases and fumes	
➤ Irritant gases, isocyanates cadmium	Occupational asthma, bronchitis, ARDS
➤ Platinum salts	Occupational asthma
Diseases due to biological substances	
➤ Proteolytic enzymes, allergens from animals and insects (excreta), contaminated grain dust	Occupational asthma, bronchitis
Diseases due to chemicals and radioactive substances	
➤ Polycyclic hydrocarbons, radon	Bronchial carcinoma

Coal-workers' Pneumoconiosis

Q. Write a short essay/note on coal-worker's pneumoconiosis.

Definition: Coal-workers' pneumoconiosis (CWP) is the **parenchymal lung disease caused by prolonged inhalation of carbon particles** (coal mine dust).

- Coal-worker's pneumoconiosis develops in coal miners with a prolonged history of inhalation of coal dust. The coal mine dust particles about 2–5 μm in diameter are retained in the small airways and alveoli of the lung. The incidence of the disease depends on the total dust exposure, and availability of ventilation and dust suppression. The risk of this disease is reduced due to improved ventilation and working conditions.
- Incidence is more in anthracite coal miners compared to bituminous miners.

Classification: Based on the size and extent of radiographic nodularity, CWP is subdivided into:

- Simple coal-worker's pneumoconiosis (SCWP)
- Progressive massive fibrosis (PMF).

Simple Coal-worker's Pneumoconiosis

- Simple coal-worker's pneumoconiosis (SCWP) refers to the deposition of coal dust in the lung and produces small radiographic (micronodular) shadows/nodules on the chest X-ray in an otherwise asymptomatic individual. It is the most common type of pneumoconiosis.
- It develops after prolonged exposure (15–20 years) to coal dust.
- SCWP does not impair lung function and does not progress if the miner leaves the industry/exposure ceases.
- Grading of simple coal-workers pneumoconiosis: Depending on the chest X-ray appearance, simple CWP is divided into three categories **(Table 6.87)**.
- Simple pneumoconiosis (categories 2 and 3) can progress to progressive massive fibrosis (PMF).

TABLE 6.87: Grading of simple coal-worker's pneumoconiosis.

Category	*Chest X-ray appearance*
1	Few small round opacities
2	Numerous small round opacities but normal lung markings still visible
3	Very numerous small round opacities and normal lung markings partly or totally obscured

Progressive Massive Fibrosis

Q. Write a short essay/note on progressive massive fibrosis.

- Progressive massive fibrosis (PMF) progresses even after the miner leaves the industry/exposure ceases.
- Chest X-ray: Characterized by single or multiple round fibrotic nodules/masses several centimeters in diameter (>1 cm in size to large dense masses), invariably in the upper lobes. Sometimes, these nodules show central necrotic cavities.
- Lung function tests: Mixed restrictive and obstructive ventilatory defect with loss of lung volume, irreversible airflow limitation and reduced gas transfer.
- Clinical features: Progressive breathlessness/dyspnea and cough with blackish sputum **(melanoptysis)**.
- Complications: Respiratory failure, right ventricular failure, and Caplan's syndrome.

Caplan's Syndrome

Q. Write a short essay/note on Caplan's syndrome (rheumatoid pneumoconiosis).

- Caplan's syndrome is the combination of pneumoconiotic nodules with seropositive rheumatoid arthritis.
- Pneumoconiotic nodules are round, fibrotic and measure 0.5–5 cm diameter and are found mainly in the periphery of the lung fields.
- Rheumatoid factor is positive and pathological features are similar to a rheumatoid nodule.
- This syndrome can also seen in pneumoconiosis (e.g., silicosis) other than CWP.

Asbestos-related Lung and Pleural Diseases

Q. Write a short essay/note on the asbestos-related diseases of lungs and pleura.

- **Asbestos types:** Asbestos has the unique property of occurring naturally as a fiber. It is remarkably resistant to heat, acid, and alkali. Major types are: **chrysotile** (white asbestos), **crocidolite (blue asbestos) and amosite (brown asbestos)**. All of these types **are fibrogenic** and have the potential to cause asbestos-related diseases. It is widely used for roofing, insulation and fireproofing.
- **Occupational exposure:** It is highest with workers involved in the production of asbestos products (mining, milling, and **manufacturing), shipyard** and construction industries. Exposure can also occur in automobile and railroad workers and those involved in thermal and electrical wire insulation.

Asbestos-related Diseases

1. Asbestosis (progressive pulmonary fibrosis)—highest dose is required to cause asbestosis.
2. Benign localized pleural fibrous plaques—calcification of parietal pleura more pronounced on the diaphragm and mediastinum.
3. Benign pleural effusions
4. Carcinoma of lung
5. Malignant mesotheliomas of pleura and mesothelioma of peritoneum (rare)
6. Laryngeal carcinomas

Asbestosis

- **Definition:** Asbestosis is defined as interstitial fibrosis of the lung caused by exposure to **asbestos dust**. It does not include asbestos-induced pleural diseases and carcinoma of lung that are found in asbestos-exposed workers.
- **Duration of exposure:** Development of asbestosis is directly related to the intensity and duration of exposure. It develops after moderate-to-severe exposure for at least 10 years.
- **Clinical features:** Progressive exertional breathlessness, finger clubbing, and late-inspiratory crepitations/crackles over the lower zones of lung.
- **Investigations:**
  - Radiography:
    - Chest radiographic hallmark of asbestosis is presence of irregular or linear opacities in the lower lung fields. An indistinct heart border or a "ground-glass" appearance in the lung fields may be observed.
    - HRCT: May show subpleural curvilinear lines 5–10 mm in length which appear to be parallel to the pleural surface. Plain chest X-ray may not show pleural disease; however, CT can demonstrate pleural disease in more than 90% cases. Honeycomb lung may also be seen.
  - **Pulmonary function tests:** Restrictive pattern with a decreased both lung volumes and diffusing capacity.
  - **Lung biopsy:** May show asbestos bodies and fibrosis.
- **Complications:** Respiratory failure, right ventricular failure, and bronchial carcinoma

Lung Cancer

- Most common cancer associated with asbestos exposure. Minimum latent period ranges from 15 to 20 years between first exposure and development of cancer.
- Histological, it may be squamous cell carcinoma or adenocarcinoma.

Mesothelioma

- Mesothelioma is a primary malignant tumor of mesothelial lining of pleura and/or peritoneum and both can develop with asbestos exposure and is most commonly caused by blue asbestos.
- In contrast to lung cancer, development of mesothelioma has no association with smoking.
- Relatively short period of exposure (even 1–2 years) that occurred more than 20–40 years ago is associated with development of mesothelium.

- **Clinical presentation:** Persistent chest pain (due to involvement of chest wall), breathlessness (due to pleural effusion), and usually unilateral hemorrhagic pleural effusion. As the tumor advances, it encases the underlying lung, may invade into the lung parenchyma, the mediastinum, and the pericardium.
- Diagnosis is confirmed by video-assisted thoracoscopic biopsy of pleura.
- Mesothelioma is almost invariably fatal.

Silicosis

Q. Write a short essay/note on silicosis.

Definition: Silicosis is a **parenchymal lung disease** associated with **inhalation of crystalline silicon dioxide** (silica).

- Occupational exposure: High-risk occupations include mining, stone cutting, sand blasting, and quarrying (e.g., granite), pottery and ceramics industry, foundry work, boiler scaling, glass and cement manufacturing, etc.
- Silica is highly fibrogenic and causes the development of hard nodules that coalesce as the disease advances. Pulmonary fibrosis depends on dose and develops after many years of exposure.
- **Associated risk:** Silicosis is associated with increased risk of tuberculosis (silicotuberculosis), lung cancer and COPD. The increased risk is lifelong even if exposure ceases. Chemoprophylaxis using INH for 9 months is recommended if latent tuberculosis is diagnosed with a positive tuberculin test. Other diseases that can develop in silicosis include chronic renal insufficiency and autoimmune diseases (e.g., scleroderma, rheumatoid arthritis, and Wegener's granulomatosis).
  Forms of silicosis (silica-induced lung disease): Chronic, acute, or accelerated
- **Chronic or simple silicosis**
  - Most common form of silicosis. It occurs after many decades (10 to 20 years) of exposure to relatively low levels of silica.
  - Clinically characterized by gradually progressive dyspnea and dry cough. It is often compatible with normal life.
  - **Radiological features:** Variable and similar to those of coal-worker's pneumoconiosis. It may show multiple well-circumscribed 3–5 mm-nodular opacities mainly in the mid- and upper zones. As the diseases progresses, extensive fibrosis develops and resembles PMF. The involvement of hilar lymph nodes by chronic silicosis is characteristic (but is uncommon and non-specific), with a tendency toward peripheral calcification, which produces the so-called **egg-shell calcification.**
  - **Pulmonary function tests:** Mixed pattern of obstruction and restriction with a reduced diffusion capacity.
  - No specific treatment
- **Acute silicosis**
  - It occurs after intense exposure (very high concentration of dust) to very fine crystalline silica dust over a few months (about less than 10 months of exposure) and is usually rapidly fatal within years.
  - Characterized by pulmonary edema, interstitial inflammation, and accumulation of proteinaceous fluid rich in surfactant within the alveoli.
  - Chest radiograph: May show miliary infiltration or areas of consolidation. HRCT chest may show pattern known as "crazy paving".
- **Accelerated silicosis**
  - It occurs after a few years (typically 5–10 years) of exposure to silica.
  - More aggressive course associated with rapidly progressive features of dyspnea and pulmonary fibrosis.
  - Involves mainly middle and lower zones of the lungs as compared to chronic silicosis.

PULMONARY FIBROSIS

A wide variety of lung disorders heals by producing fibrous tissue and results in fibrosis of the lung.

Types of Pulmonary Fibrosis

Q. Write a short essay/note on types of pulmonary fibrosis and causes of interstitial fibrosis.

1. **Replacement fibrosis:** In this, the damaged lung parenchyma (e.g., suppuration and infarction) replaced by fibrous tissue.
   - **Common causes:** Pulmonary tuberculosis, bronchiectasis, lung abscess, pulmonary infarcts, and necrotizing pneumonias
2. **Focal fibrosis:** In focal fibrosis, the extent of fibrosis varies from small nodular lesions to extensive areas.
   - **Common causes:** Coal-worker's pneumoconiosis (CWP), asbestosis, and silicosis
3. **Interstitial fibrosis:** In this, fibrosis is diffuse and represents the end result of interstitial lung diseases.
   - **Common causes** of interstitial lung disease (*refer* **Table 6.83**).

Clinical Features of Replacement Fibrosis

History of cough with/without expectoration and dyspnea. Sputum may be blood-tinged.

Physical findings in the chest

- Inspection and palpation:
  - **Features on the affected side:** Shifting of the trachea and mediastinum toward the affected side. Drooping of the shoulder, flattening, hollowing, and crowding of the ribs, diminished movements of the chest wall and scoliosis of the spine. The hemithorax is smaller, its expansion and spinoscapular distance are diminished and spinoacromial distance is increased. Vocal fremitus is usually decreased.
  - Chest expansion is reduced.
- **Percussion: On the affected side,** there is impaired note.
- Auscultation:
  - When fibrosis is extensive, the intensity of breath sound is reduced and vesicular in character with prolonged expiration.
  - Vocal resonance is reduced. Crepitations are heard.
  - Sometimes if trachea or major bronchus is pulled up due to fibrosis, tubular bronchial breathing can be heard.

Fibrothorax

- **Causes of fibrothorax:** Empyema, pleural effusion, traumatic hemothorax, tuberculosis, benign asbestos pleural effusion, connective and collagen vascular disorders, uremia, paragonimiasis, and drug-induced (e.g., ergot alkaloids, bromocriptine, **pergoline**, methysergide, and methotrexate).
- **Clinical features** of fibrothorax: (1) marked limitation of chest movements, (2) mediastinal shift to same side, trachea may be central or shifted to affected side, (3) decrease in size of hemothorax, and (4) crowding of ribs.

Radiological findings on the affected side: Shift of the mediastinum toward the affected side. Smaller hemithorax than the other unaffected hemithorax. Crowding of the ribs, pulling of hilum upward, raised diaphragm (tenting), and lung fields show fibrous bands.

Management/treatment of replacement fibrosis
- **Symptomatic measures:** For example, breathing exercises, expectorants
- **Treatment of infections:** Antibiotics
- **Treatment of the underlying disease/cause:** For example, tuberculosis
- **Surgery:** Resection in selected cases.

Primary Bronchial Tumors

Q. Write a short essay/note on classification of primary bronchial tumors.

Classification of primary tumors of the lung **(Table 6.88)**.

TABLE 6.88: Classification of tumors of the lung.

Benign tumors (5%)	*Malignant tumors (95%)*
Benign epithelial tumors ➤ Papillomas ➤ Adenomas **Mesenchymal tumors** ➤ Chondroma ➤ Lipoma **Miscellaneous tumors** ➤ Pulmonary hamartoma ➤ Sclerosing hemangioma	**Nonsmall-cell carcinoma** (75%) ➤ Squamous or epidermoid carcinoma ➤ Large-cell carcinoma ➤ Adenocarcinoma – Bronchioloalveolar cell carcinoma (presently termed adenocarcinoma in situ) **Small-cell carcinoma** (oat cell carcinoma) (25%) **Adenosquamous carcinoma/Sarcomatoid carcinoma** **Salivary gland tumor:** Mucoepidermoid carcinoma, adenoid cystic carcinoma **Carcinoid tumor:** Typical carcinoid, atypical carcinoid

LUNG CANCER (BRONCHIAL CARCINOMA)

Q. Discuss the etiology/risk factors, clinical features, investigations, diagnosis, metastatic and nonmetastatic complications, and management of bronchial carcinoma (bronchogenic carcinoma, lung cancer).

- Carcinoma of the lung is the **most common cause of cancer death**. This is mainly due to the carcinogenic effects of **cigarette smoke.**
- In the past, the term bronchogenic carcinoma was used for primary lung cancer, to indicate the origin from the bronchi. Now it is known that about 5% of primary lung cancers do not arise from bronchus. Hence, the term lung cancer is used.
- Bronchial carcinoma is the most common primary malignant tumor of the lung and arises from the bronchial epithelium or mucous glands.

Incidence

- **Age and gender:** Mostly found between **50 and 80 years** of age. More common in males, but there is a recent increase in females due to increased smoking among females.
- More in urban than rural dwellers and more in smokers than nonsmokers.

Etiology

- **Cigarette (tobacco) smoking**
  - There is strong evidence that tobacco smoking is the most important cause of cancer of lung. Smoking also multiplies the risk of other carcinogenic influences, such as asbestos and uranium. The **strongest association** of smoking is with **squamous-cell and small-cell carcinomas**. The risk of cancer is directly proportional to the amount of daily smoking,

tendency to inhale and duration of smoking habit. Compared to nonsmokers, the smokers have 10 times and heavy smokers (more than 40 cigarettes per day for several years) are at 60 times more risk of lung cancer. Females are more susceptible to tobacco carcinogens than males. Cessation of smoking for 10 years reduces risk but not to the level in nonsmokers. However, only 11% of heavy smokers develop lung cancer, which indicates that genetic factors are involved. **Pipe and cigar smokers have lower incidence than cigarette smokers**. Bidi smoking may be associated with more risk of lung cancer than cigarette smoking. Secondhand smoke exposure (passive smoking) is also a risk factor. Adenocarcinoma is usually not related to smoking.

- More than 60% of new lung cancers occur in nonsmokers (smoked <100 cigarettes per lifetime) or former smoker (smoked 100 cigarettes per lifetime, quit 1 year), 1 in 5 women and 1 in 12 men diagnosed with lung cancer have never smoked.
- **Major carcinogens in tobacco smoke** include both initiators and promoters (such as phenol derivatives). These include **polycyclic aromatic hydrocarbons (e.g.,** Benzo[*a*]pyrene, dibenzanthracene) and **radioactive elements and other contaminants** (e.g., arsenic, nickel, cadmium, molds, and vinyl chloride).
- **Environmental tobacco smoke = Mainstream smoke + Sidestream smoke**
  Mainstream smoke refers to the smoke inhaled by smoking directly while sidestream smoke refers to the smoke emitted by the burning cigarette. Both contain carcinogens.
- **In Indians** with lung cancer, history of active tobacco smoking was found in 87% of males and 85% of females. History of passive tobacco exposure is found in 3%. Thus, 90% of all cases in India resulted from tobacco exposure.
- The relative risk of developing lung cancer is: 2.64 for beedi smokers, 2.23 for cigarette smokers and 2.45 as the overall relative risk (RR).
- **Lung cancer in never smokers:**
  - Definition: <100 cigarettes in lifetime. It accounts for 25% of lung cancers and is distinctly associated with: female cases, east Asian populations, positive family history, adenocarcinoma type, *EGFR* mutation, and better prognosis.

- **Industrial and occupational hazards**
  - **Ionizing radiation:** High dose of ionizing radiation is carcinogenic (uranium mining—oat-cell carcinoma is the most common type).
  - **Uranium:** It is weakly radioactive and uranium miners (both nonsmokers and smokers) have higher incidence of lung cancer than in the general population.
  - **Asbestos:** Exposure increases the risk and risk increases when associated with smoking. It develops after a latent period of about 10 to 30 years. In insulation and shipyard workers, risk of lung cancer increases after 10 years of exposure, and with concurrent smoking, the risk increases to 90-fold.
  - **Other carcinogens:** Chloromethyl, ethers, and mustard gas (squamous and undifferentiated are the most common types), chromium, nickel, vinyl chloride, polyaromatic hydrocarbons, cadmium, formaldehyde and dioxin.
- **Atmospheric pollution:** The risk of **lung cancers is higher in urban areas** than rural areas, suggesting role of air pollution. Major air pollutants include polycyclic hydrocarbons from fossil fuels and motor vehicle exhaust, especially diesel smoke. Studies from China have shown coal burning at home is a significant risk factor for development of lung cancer in nonsmoking females. Coal smoke contains potential carcinogens SO_2, CO, TSP, B (a) P, radon, thorn.
- **Diet: Vitamin A deficiency** *leads to squamous metaplasia *increased **susceptibility to cancer**. Folate, carotenoid-rich fruits and vegetables, vitamin E and beta-carotene are associated with reduced risk of lung cancer.
- **Idiopathic pulmonary fibrosis:** It is associated with increased risk of lung cancer.
- **Prior lung diseases such as** chronic bronchitis, emphysema, and **tuberculosis**
- **Genetic predisposition:** Genetic polymorphisms involving cytochrome *P-450* gene CYP1A1*increased capacity to metabolize procarcinogens present in the cigarette smoke *increased risk of lung cancer.
  - First-degree relatives of lung cancer probands have a two-to-three fold excess risk of lung cancer and other cancers, many of which are not smoking-related.
  - Individuals with inherited mutations in *RB* (retinoblastoma) and *p53* (Li–Fraumeni syndrome) genes may develop lung cancer.
- A rare germline mutation (T790M) involving the epidermal growth factor receptor (EGFR) may be linked to lung cancer susceptibility in nonsmokers.

Examples of the oncogenes and tumor suppressor genes involved in lung cancer are presented in **Table 6.89**.

TABLE 6.89: Examples of the oncogenes and tumor suppressor genes involved in lung cancer.

Histology	*Oncogene*	*Tumor-suppressor genes*
Adenocarcinoma	*EGFR, KRAS, ALK*	*TP53, CDKN2A/B(p16, p14), LKB1*
Squamous-cell carcinoma	*EGFR, PIK3CA, IGF-1R*	*TP53, TP63*
Small-cell carcinoma	*MYC, BCL-2*	*TP53, RB1, FHIT*
Large-cell carcinoma	(not well studied)	

Pathology

Clinical subgroups of lung cancer (Table 6.90): Lung carcinomas can be divided into two clinical subgroups on the basis of likelihood of metastases and response to therapies.

- Small-cell lung cancer (SCLC) and nonsmall-cell lung cancer (NSCLC) (includes adenocarcinoma, squamous-cell carcinoma and large-cell carcinoma) account for approximately 90% of all epithelial lung cancers.
- Among women and young adults (<60 years), adenocarcinoma tends to be the most common form of lung cancer.
- Neuroendocrine tumors of the lung arise from Kulchitsky cells of the bronchial mucosa and consist of typical carcinoid, atypical carcinoid, and small-cell lung cancer.

TABLE 6.90: Clinical subgroups of lung cancer.

Small-cell lung carcinomas (SCLC)—highly metastatic, high response to chemotherapy	***Nonsmall-cell lung carcinomas (NSCLC)—less metastatic, less responsive***
Small-cell (oat-cell) carcinoma	➢ Squamous (epidermoid) carcinoma ➢ Adenocarcinoma (including bronchioloalveolar carcinoma) ➢ Large-cell carcinoma

Lung Cancer in India

- Nonsmall-cell lung cancer constitutes 75–80% of lung cancers. More than 70% of them are detected in stages III and IV. Thus, curative surgery cannot be done in these cases. In many Western countries, adenocarcinoma has become the most common lung cancer. However, in India, squamous-cell carcinoma is still the most common carcinoma in both males and females.
- Small-cell lung carcinoma constitutes 20% of all lung cancers. It is detected at an extensive stage in 70% of patients at the time of diagnosis.

Site: Depending on the site, the lung cancers are divided into:

- **Central (hilar):** Lung cancers arise in and around the **hilus** of the lung are the **most common**. About 75% arise from first, second, and third-order bronchi. Squamous-cell and small-cell carcinomas are generally centrally placed.
- **Peripheral:** Lung cancers may also arise in the periphery of the lung from the alveolar septal cells or terminal bronchioles. They are **usually adenocarcinomas, including bronchioloalveolar type**.

Bronchioloalveolar carcinoma (BAC) is a subtype of adenocarcinoma that grows along the alveoli without invasion. It can present with profuse, mucoid sputum (bronchorrhea).

TABLE 6.91: Manifestations due to the location of the primary tumor.

Due to a central or endobronchial growth	***Due to a peripheral growth***
➢ Cough ➢ Hemoptysis ➢ Wheeze and stridor ➢ Breathlessness/dyspnea ➢ Postobstructive pneumonitis presenting with fever and productive cough	➢ Chest pain from pleural or chest-wall involvement ➢ Dyspnea on a restrictive basis ➢ Symptoms of lung abscess due to cavitation of tumor

Clinical Features

More than 50% of patients present with locally advanced or metastatic disease at the time of diagnosis. Majority patients present with signs, symptoms, or laboratory abnormalities that may be due to the (i) primary lesion, (ii) local tumor growth, (iii) invasion or obstruction of adjacent structures, (iv) metastatic tumor, or (v) as a paraneoplastic syndrome. Clinical manifestations of bronchial carcinoma can be studied under the following headings:

1. Manifestations due to the location of the primary tumor/growth **(Table 6.91).**
2. **Manifestations due to the regional spread of tumor in the thorax (Table 6.92).**
3. **Manifestations of extrathoracic metastasis (Table 6.93).**

TABLE 6.92: Manifestations of lung cancer due to regional spread of tumor in the thorax.

Pathological basis	***Local effects***
➢ Obstruction of airway by tumor	Pneumonia, abscess, atelectasis, focal emphysema
➢ Tracheal obstruction	Stridor (a harsh inspiratory noise) and dyspnea
➢ Local spread into pleura	Pleuritis and malignant effusion
➢ Local spread to pericardium	Pericarditis, effusion, tamponade
➢ Compression of SVC by tumor	Superior vena cava syndrome
Invasion of structure	**Its effects**
➢ Recurrent laryngeal nerve	Hoarseness of voice and "bovine" cough
➢ Phrenic nerve	Diaphragm paralysis and dyspnea
➢ Sympathetic ganglia	Horner syndrome
➢ Esophagus	Dysphagia
➢ Chest wall (direct extension)	Destruction of rib producing rib pain, pathological fractures and intercostal neuralgia
➢ Superior sulcus tumor (destruction of the T1 and C8 roots in the lower part of the brachial plexus by an apical lung tumor)	Pancoast's syndrome (pain in the inner aspect of the arm, sometimes with small muscle wasting in the hand)
➢ Lymphatic obstruction	Pleural effusion
➢ Vascular obstruction	Superior vena cava (SVC) syndrome
➢ Pericardial and cardiac extension	Pericardial effusion, cardiac tamponade, arrhythmias or cardiac failure

Paraneoplastic Syndromes (Table 6.94)

Q. Write short essay/note on:
- **Paraneoplastic syndromes/manifestations associated with bronchogenic carcinoma.**
- **Mention the nonmetastatic manifestations/complications of bronchial carcinoma.**

- Paraneoplastic syndromes are symptom complexes in cancer patients which are not directly related to mass effects or invasion or metastasis or by the secretion of hormones indigenous to the tissue of origin.

TABLE 6.93: Manifestations of extrathoracic metastasis.

Site of metastasis	Manifestations
Adrenal glands (~50%)	Usually asymptomatic, Addison's disease
Liver (30–50%)	Anorexia, nausea, biliary obstruction, weight loss, right upper quadrant pain, and pain
Brain (20%)	Headache, vomiting, focal neurologic deficits, epileptic seizures confusion, and raised intracranial pressure
Bone (20%)	Bony pain, pathologic fractures or raised alkaline phosphatase
Bone marrow	Cytopenias or leukoerythroblastosis
Lymph node	Lymphadenopathy—commonly to mediastinal, cervical, supraclavicular region (scalene node), and even axillary or intra-abdominal nodes
Epidural and bone metastases	Spinal cord compression (if spine is involved) syndromes

TABLE 6.94: Paraneoplastic syndromes in lung cancer.

System involved	Manifestations
Systemic	➢ Anorexia, cachexia, weight loss, fever
Endocrine	➢ Syndrome of inappropriate secretion of antidiuretic hormone causing hyponatremia (small-cell carcinoma) ➢ Ectopic ACTH secretion resulting in hypokalemia, rather than full-blown Cushing's syndrome (small-cell carcinoma) ➢ Hypercalcemia due to ectopic production of parathyroid hormone or parathyroid hormone-related peptide (squamous-cell carcinoma) ➢ Carcinoid syndrome, acromegaly, hypoglycemia, hyperthyroidism ➢ Gynecomastia
Skeletal	➢ Clubbing of fingers (usually NSCLC) nonsmall-cell carcinoma ➢ Hypertrophic pulmonary osteoarthropathy (usually adenocarcinoma)—HPOA
Neuromyopathic	➢ Polyneuropathy ➢ Myelopathy encephalomyelitis, opsoclonus-myoclonus, limbic encephalitis ➢ Cerebellar degeneration ➢ Myasthenia (Lambert–Eaton syndrome) and retinal blindness (small-cell carcinoma)
Hematological	➢ Migratory venous thrombophlebitis (Trousseau's syndrome) ➢ Marantic endocarditis ➢ Disseminated intravascular coagulation (DIC) ➢ Anemia, granulocytosis, leukoerythroblastosis
Cutaneous	➢ Dermatomyositis ➢ Acanthosis nigricans
Renal	➢ Nephrotic syndrome ➢ Glomerulonephritis

- Lung cancer may occasionally be associated with paraneoplastic syndromes. They are summarized in **Table 6.94**.
- Paraneoplastic syndromes manifest due to the peptide hormones secreted by the tumor and may be in the first manifestations of lung cancers. They are often relieved by successful treatment of the primary lung cancer. They are common with small-cell carcinoma.

Lamber–Eaton Myasthenic Syndrome (LMS)

- Autoimmune disorders of neuromuscular junction due to anti-voltage-gated calcium channel antibodies.
- Proximal muscle weakness, usually in lower extremities
- Occasionally autonomic dysfunction and rarely cranial nerve symptoms
- Frequently depressed deep tendon reflexes
- In contrast to patients with myasthenia gravis, strength improves with serial effort.

Treatment of LMS
- Chemotherapy is the initial treatment of choice.
- 3, 4–diaminopyridine: It increases duration of presynaptic action potential by blocking potassium efflux, prolonging the activation of VGCC and increasing calcium entry into nerve terminals.

Differential Diagnosis of Large Bronchus Obstruction (Table 6.95)

Investigations

Main aims of investigation: (1) to confirm the diagnosis, (2) establish the histological cell type, (3) to stage the extent of the disease and (4) to assess fitness to undergo treatment.

- Imaging:
  - **Chest X-ray**
  - Plain chest radiographs may show evidence of lung cancer or nonspecific appearances **(Table 6.96)**.
  - **Evidence of lung cancer:** A normal finding does not rule out the presence of an underlying tumor. Tumor is visible if greater than 1 cm diameter.
- **Computed tomography (CT) of chest and abdomen:** It is important for diagnosis and staging of carcinoma. Used—
  - To know the tumor size and extent of disease [pleural extension, to detect occult abdominal disease (e.g., liver and adrenals)].
  - To evaluate mediastinal or hilar lymph-node involvement. If nodal involvement is observed, it should be confirmed by histopathology.

TABLE 6.95: Causes of large bronchus obstruction.

Common
➤ Neoplasm (bronchial carcinoma or adenoma)
➤ Enlargement of tracheobronchial lymph nodes (malignant or tuberculous)
➤ Inhaled foreign bodies (more common in the right lung)
➤ Bronchial casts or plugs composed of inspissated mucus or blood clot (especially, asthma, cystic fibrosis, hemoptysis, and debility)
➤ Collections of mucus or retained mucus in the bronchi as a result of ineffective expectoration (especially, postoperative following abdominal surgery)
Rare
➤ Aneurysm of aorta
➤ Giant left atrium
➤ Pericardial effusion
➤ Congenital bronchial atresia
➤ Bronchial stricture (e.g., following tuberculosis or bronchial surgery/lung transplant)

TABLE 6.96: Common radiological presentations of bronchial carcinoma.

Findings	Interpretation
Unilateral enlargement at hilum	Central tumor or enlargement of hilar lymph node or a peripheral tumor in the apical segment of the lower lobe
Peripheral lung opacity with/without cavitation, solitary pulmonary nodule	Usually irregular but well circumscribed, and may contain irregular cavitation (squamous-cell carcinoma may cavitate)
Collapse of the whole lung, lobe or segment	Endoluminal (tumor within the bronchus) tumor or compression of the main bronchus by enlarged lymph glands may produce occlusion leading to complete collapse
Broadening of mediastinum, enlarged cardiac shadow, elevation of a hemidiaphragm	Paratracheal lymphadenopathy (widening of the upper mediastinum). Malignant pericardial effusion (enlargement of the cardiac shadow). Raised hemidiaphragm (phrenic nerve palsy). Mediastinal widening due to mediastinal invasion
Pleural effusion	Usually indicates tumor invasion of pleural cavity/space distal to a bronchial carcinoma. Usually, effusion is unilateral and large and may mask an underlying mass or pleural tumor (D/D mesothelioma)
Destruction of rib (osteolytic lesions)	Direct extension of tumor or bloodborne metastasis
Single mass/diffuse, multinodular lesion/fluffy	Bronchoalveolar carcinoma

- To plan biopsy procedures: Used for guided biopsy of suspected lesions to know whether a tumor is accessible by bronchoscopy or percutaneous CT-guided biopsy.
- To assess the response to treatment

- **Cytological examination:** Specimens that may be obtained for examining for malignant cells include: sputum, bronchial brushings and washings, percutaneous (CT-guided) needle-aspiration biopsy from a peripheral tumor and fine-needle aspiration of lymph node, skin, or liver in patients with metastasis.
- **Fiberoptic bronchoscopy:**
    - It permits visualization and biopsy of an intrabronchial tumor.
    - Useful for collecting bronchial washings from the suspicious segments for cytological study.
    - It helps in assessment of operability and the proximity of central tumors to the main carina
- **Percutaneous aspiration and biopsy:** Peripheral lung tumors cannot be seen by fiberoptic bronchoscopy. Hence, samples are obtained by aspiration or biopsy through the chest wall under CT guidance.
    - Diagnosis of lung cancer rests on the morphologic or cytological features correlated with clinical and radiographic findings.
- Uses of **immunohistochemistry:**
    - To verify neuroendocrine differentiation within a tumor, with markers, such as neuron-specific enolase (NSE), CD56 or neural cell adhesion molecule (NCAM), synaptophysin, chromogranin, and Leu7.
    - Helps in differentiating primary from metastatic adenocarcinomas. For example, thyroid transcription factor 1 (TTF-1) is positive in more than 70% of pulmonary adenocarcinomas and is a reliable indicator of primary lung cancer, provided a thyroid primary has been excluded.
    - To narrow the differential diagnosis: For example, cytokeratins 7 and 20.
- **Investigations for staging to guide treatment:**
    - Fine-needle aspiration: (1) Endoscopic ultrasound-guided fine-needle aspiration (FNA) of tumor or lymph node, (2) endobronchial ultrasound-guided fine-needle aspiration, and (3) endoscopic ultrasound via the esophagus
    - Scalene node biopsy, mediastinoscopy, pleural aspiration, and biopsy and barium swallow
    - Ultrasonography examination of liver and adrenal glands.
    - **If metastasis is suspected:** Bone scans, bone marrow trephine biopsies, and brain CT.
    - **Positron emission tomography (PET) imaging /CT:** It helps in detecting intrathoracic tumor, assessing the extent of mediastinal nodal involvement and detection of distant metastases. PET images combined with CT are better than CT or PET alone.
- **Other investigations:** Complete blood count for the detection of anemia, and biochemistry for liver involvement, hypercalcemia, and hyponatremia.
- **Molecular testing for guiding treatment:** Test for *EGFR* mutations and ALK fusion

Staging

- **Staging of nonsmall-cell carcinoma (Table 6.97)**: Staged into stages I to IV depending on the size and location of primary tumor, involvement of lymph nodes, and distant metastasis (TNM International Staging System).
- **Staging of small-cell carcinoma:** It is staged into limited-stage and extensive-stage disease depending on whether the tumor can be encompassed within a tolerable radiation therapy port.

TABLE 6.97: TNM staging of nonsmall-cell carcinoma.

TNM	Description
Tx	Main tumor cannot be assesses, or cancer cells seen on sputum cytology or bronchial washing but no tumor can be found
T1	Tumor ≤3 cm in diameter; surrounded by lung or pleura; does not invade main bronchus
T1a	Tumor 2 cm or less in greatest dimension
T1b	Tumor >2 cm but ≤3 cm
T2	Tumor >3 cm in diameter; may invade pleura; may extend into main bronchus bur remains 2 cm or more distal to carina
T2a	Tumor >3 cm but ≤5 cm
T2b	Tumor >5 cm but ≤7 cm
T3	Tumor >7 cm, invasion of chest wall, diaphragm, pleura or pericardium; main bronchus <2 cm distal to carina; atelectasis of entire lung
T4	Invasion of mediastinum, heart, great vessels, trachea, esophagus, vertebral body or carina; separate tumor nodules; malignant pleural effusion
N0	No nodal metastasis
N1	Involvement of ipsilateral peribronchial or hilar nodes and intrapulmonary nodes
N2	Involvement of ipsilateral mediastinal or subcarinal nodes
N3	Involvement of contralateral nodes or any supraclavicular nodes
M0	No distant metastasis
M1	Distant metastasis

Staging of the Small-cell and Nonsmall-cell Carcinomas (Table 6.98)

Q. Discuss the staging, diagnosis and treatment of small cell carcinoma.

- **Assessing fitness for treatment:** Before radical treatment, an assessment of fitness for treatment should be done. These include:
  - Evaluation of performance (Karnofsky performance status: Eastern cooperative Oncology Group Performance Status).
  - Full lung function test: Specifically FEV_1 and diffusion capacity
  - Tests for any cardiovascular disease if there is evidence of disease (e.g., cardiopulmonary exercise testing, stress echo or occasionally preoperative angiography).

Treatment

1. **Nonsmall-cell carcinoma**

   a. **Surgical treatment**: Surgical resection of the tumor is done in early stage (1A, 1B, IIA, IIB and selected IIIA) of non-small cell lung cancer.
   - **Postoperative chemotherapy** (adjuvant therapy): Where surgical staging of resected lung cancer has lymph node involvement, patients need adjuvant chemotherapy.
   - **Preoperative chemotherapy** (neoadjuvant chemotherapy: May improve survival in stage IIIB patients and can effectively "down-stage" disease. Commonly used drugs are carboplatin, pacilitaxel ± bevacizumab (an antiangiogenesis drug).

   Contraindications to surgical resection
   - Stage IIIB or IV
   - Extensive invasion into surrounding structures: Involvement of vena cava, atrium, recurrent laryngeal or phrenic nerve and contralateral lymph nodes. Others include SVC obstruction, malignant effusion, and pericardial tamponade
   - Medically unfit: Poor cardiac or pulmonary status, predicted postoperative FEV1% <40%, predicted postoperative DLCO% <40% and exercise studies for marginal candidates

   b. **Radiotherapy**

   Radiotherapy for cure: Radiotherapy is much less effective than surgical therapy. In selected cases with adequate lung function and early stage NSCLC, high-dose radiotherapy or continuous hyperfractionated accelerated regimens (CHART) is a good alternative to surgical resection. It is the treatment of choice if surgery is contraindicated due to comorbidities.

   Radiation treatment for symptoms: Radiation can be used as palliative for distressing symptoms/complications in lung cancer. Indications for palliative radiotherapy are: bone and chest wall pain from metastases or direct invasion, recurrent hemoptysis and occluded trachea, bronchi and superior vena cava obstruction.

   Stereotactic ablative radiotherapy (SABR) is able to deliver large doses of radiation with a high precision of 1–2 mm to small lesions of <1 cm3 using an external 3D coordinated system that is linked with movements during the respiratory cycle reserved for people with early stage cancer who have been unable/unwilling to undergo surgical resection due to medical comorbidities.

   Percutaneous radiofrequency ablation (RFA) for early stage peripherally based lung tumors or metastases in medically inoperable patients.

   c. **Chemotherapy**

   Adjuvant chemotherapy with radiotherapy improves response rate and extends median survival.
   - **Older drugs:** Drug regimen, namely cisplatin/carboplatin + 1 other (Paclitaxel/Docetaxel/Gemcitabine). Common side effects are nausea and vomiting and are best treated with 5-HT3 receptor antagonists.

- **Newer targeted agents** against epidermal growth factor receptors and tyrosine kinases in NSCLC (in particular adenocarcinoma) in selected patients. Can also be used where intravenous chemotherapy produces severe toxicity or as second-line chemotherapy.
  - *EGFR* mutation-positive NSCLC: Erlotinib, afatanib, and gefitinib
  - Crizotinib for *ALK/ROS-1* mutation-positive NSCLC
  - Osimertinib for *EGFR T790M* mutation-positive NSCLC.
  - Immune checkpoint inhibitors: Pembrolizumab, nivolumab, and atezolizumab which act through the programmed death-ligand 1/2 (PD-L1 and PD-L2)
  - Tirapazamine, thalidomide, vandetanib
  - Antiangiogenesis (e.g., bevacizumab)
  - Nintedanib with docetaxel
  - Vinorelbine + Carboplatin or Cisplatin

Treatment of nonsmall-cell lung cancer is summarized in **Table 6.99**.

2. **Small-cell carcinoma**

General treatment plan for small-cell carcinoma **(Table 6.100)**

- If the patient responds to treatment plan, prophylactic radiotherapy to brain is advised. High-dose radiotherapy to the entire brain is also advised to patients with documented brain metastasis.
- **Chemotherapeutic regimens for small-cell carcinoma**
  - Commonly used combination Cisplatin/carboplatin + etoposide, ifosfamide, irinotecan plus cisplatin, carboplatin and etoposide with/without vincristine.

Laser therapy and tracheobronchial stents

- In selected patients with inoperable lung cancer, palliation of symptoms due to tracheobronchial narrowing from intraluminal tumor or extrinsic compression can be achieved by bronchoscopic laser treatment.
- It helps to clear tumor tissue and allow reaeration of collapsed lung. It is useful mainly when the tumor is the main bronchi.
- In case of extrinsic compression by malignant nodes, endobronchial stents can be used to maintain airway patency.

TABLE 6.98: Staging of carcinomas of lung.

Stages of nonsmall-cell carcinoma based on TNM classification	
Occult carcinoma	TX, N0, M0
IA	T1a,bNOMO
IB	T2aNOMO
IIA	T2bN0M0; T1a, bN1M0; T2aN1M0
IIB	T2bN1M0; T3N0M0
IIIA	T1a, b, T2a, b, N2M0; T3N1, N2M0; T4N0, N1M0
IIIB	T4N2M0; any T N3M0
IV	Any T any NM1
Stage of small-cell carcinoma	***Description***
Limited stage	➤ 30–40% of small cell lung cancers ➤ Confined to the hemithorax, mediastinum, and ipsilateral supraclavicular lymph node ➤ Within the confines of radiation port
Extensive stage	➤ 60–70% of small cell lung cancers ➤ Any distant spread

TABLE 6.99: Treatment of nonsmall-cell lung cancer.

Stage IA: ➤ Lobectomy is treatment of choice. T1N0, lobectomy has 70% 5-year recurrence-free survival ➤ If inoperable: – 30% cure rate with XRT alone – Stereotactic radiosurgery (CyberKnife) – Radiofrequency ablation
Stage 1B: ➤ Lobectomy ➤ Adjuvant chemotherapy adds a 4–12% survival benefit. Best in tumors >4 cm
Stage II: ➤ Lobectomy is treatment of choice ➤ Adjuvant chemotherapy now standard ➤ Consider adjuvant XRT to mediastinum
Stage III: ➤ Combination chemotherapy with XRT is the treatment of choice. ➤ Surgery has yet to be established consistently as benefit in randomized trials. ➤ Neoadjuvant therapy followed by surgical resection is option in IIIA.
Stage IV: ➤ Chemotherapy

TABLE 6.100: General plan of treatment small-cell carcinoma.

Stage	***Status of patient***	***Treatment***
Limited stage	With good performance status of patient	Chemotherapy + radiotherapy
	With poor performance status of patient	Modified chemotherapy and/or palliative radiotherapy
Extensive stage	With good performance status of patient	Chemotherapy ± local radiotherapy
	With poor performance status of patient	Modified chemotherapy and/or palliative radiotherapy

TABLE 6.101: Neurological manifestations of bronchial carcinoma.

Regional effects	***Remote effects (paraneoplastic)***
➤ Nerve paralysis – Recurrent laryngeal nerve – Phrenic nerve ➤ Intercostal neuralgia ➤ Horner's syndrome ➤ Pancoast's syndrome	➤ Polyneuropathy ➤ Myelopathy ➤ Polymyositis and dermatomyositis ➤ Eaton–Lambert syndrome ➤ Cerebellar degeneration ➤ Cortical degeneration ➤ Limbic encephalitis
Metastatic effects: Brain and spine	

Flowchart 6.15 shows treatment of small cell lung cancer.

FLOWCHART 6.15: Small cell lung cancer: treatment.

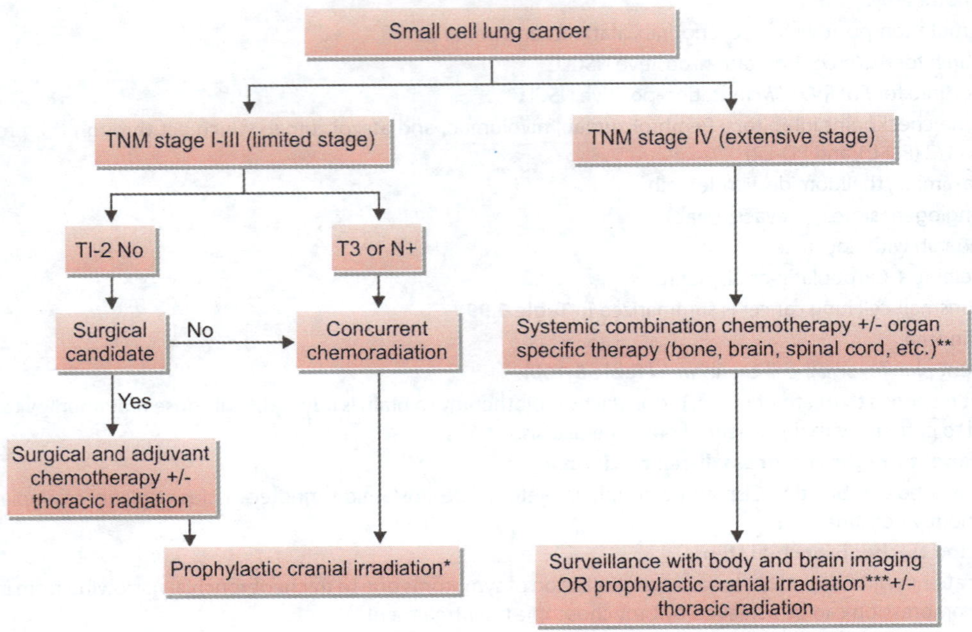

Neurological Manifestations of Bronchial Carcinoma (Table 6.101)

Q. Write short note on the neurological manifestations of bronchial carcinoma.

Hypertrophic Osteoarthropathy (Hypertrophic Pulmonary Osteoarthropathy)

Q. Write short note on pulmonary hypertrophic osteoarthropathy (hypertrophic pulmonary osteoarthropathy).

- Hypertrophic osteoarthropathy (HOA) is characterized by clubbing of digits and in more advanced stages, by periosteal new-bone formation and synovial effusions.
- Clubbing is almost always found in HOA but can occur as an isolated manifestation.
- Primary HOA is also called Pierre-Marie-Bamberger syndrome.

Clinical features

- **Sites involved:** Most common are the distal parts of the long bones of wrists (radius and ulna) and ankles (tibia and fibula).
- **Symptoms:** Pain and swelling of the wrists and ankles, to a lesser extent in knees and shin. Pain is aggravated by dependency and relieved by elevation of the affected limb.
- **Physical examination:** Digital clubbing, swollen and tender joints, and pitting edema of the anterior aspect of shin.
- **Investigations**
  - **X-ray (Fig. 6.42):** Periosteal thickening and subperiosteal new bone formation along the shaft of distal ends of long bones. The ends of distal phalanges may show osseous resorption.
  - **Radionuclide studies of bones:** It shows pericortical linear uptake along the cortical margins of long bones. These changes may be detected even before any radiographic changes.

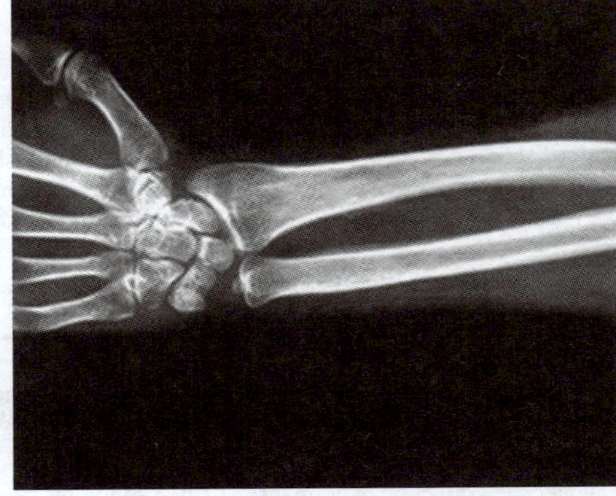

FIG. 6.42: X-ray of the wrist showing subperiosteal new bone formation—HPOA.

Treatment

- Identify and treat the associated disease.
- Vagotomy or percutaneous blocking of the vagus nerve: It may give relief in few patients.
- Analgesics: Aspirin or other nonsteroidal anti-inflammatory drugs.

Pancoast's Syndrome (Pancoast's Tumor; Superior Sulcus Tumor Syndrome)

Q. Write short essay/note on clinical features of Pancoast (superior pulmonary sulcus) tumor.

Q. Write short note on Horner's syndrome.

- Pancoast's tumor also known as Pancoast-Tobias tumor or superior sulcus tumor.
- Pancoast's **tumor is a tumor at the apex of lung which** may invade the **neural structures around the first rib, subclavian vessels,** and the **cervical sympathetic plexus. Chest X-ray appearance is shown in Figure 6.43.**
- Local extension of the tumor can involve the eighth cervical (C_8) and first thoracic (T_1) nerves.
- **Features of Pancoast's syndrome:**
  - Shoulder pain which radiates in the distribution of ulnar nerve of the arm (i.e., along the C_8, T_1 distribution).
  - Wasting of the small muscles of the hand from due to C_8, T_1 nerve involvement.
  - Pain and tenderness over the first and second ribs and radiological evidence of rib destruction due to local invasion by tumor.
  - **Horner's syndrome** (enophthalmos, ptosis, miosis, and anhidrosis) on the same side as the tumor due to involvement of the sympathetic pathway as it passes through the T_1 root.
- **Investigations:** CT scan, fine-needle aspiration, and MRI.

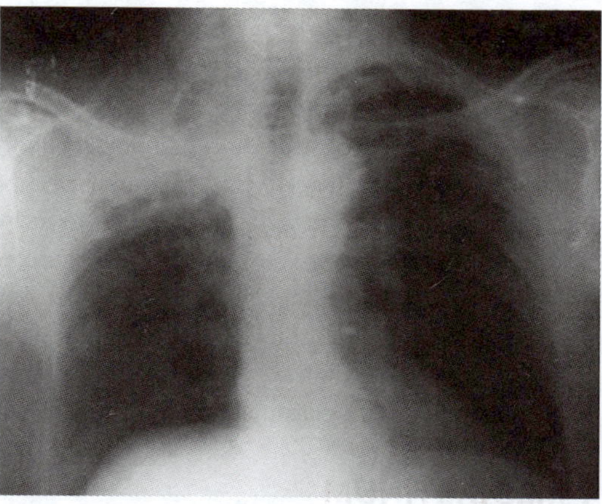

FIG. 6.43: X-ray showing mass lesion in the right upper zone with erosion of ribs—Pancoast's tumor.

TABLE 6.102: Causes of superior vena cava obstruction.

Neoplastic	*Non-neoplastic*
➢ Primary – Bronchial carcinoma (75%) – Lymphomas (20%) – Thymoma – Parathyroid tumor ➢ Metastatic tumors	➢ Tuberculosis ➢ Fibrosing mediastinitis ➢ Retrosternal goiter ➢ Central venous catheter causing thrombosis ➢ Aortic arch aneurysm

Treatment: Combined chemoradiotherapy and surgery. Preoperative radiotherapy along with chemotherapy (cisplatin and etoposide) is given followed by en-bloc resection of the tumor.

Superior Vena Cava Syndrome

Q. Write short essay/note on:
- **Causes, clinical features, and management of superior vena cava (SVC) syndrome.**
- **Superior vena cava obstruction.**

It develops due to the obstruction of SVC secondary to compression and/or invasion by tumors or other lesions in the superior mediastinum **(Table 6.102).**

Bronchial carcinoma and lymphoma are the most common causes and others are very rare causes of SVC obstruction.

Clinical Features

- Due to involvement of other structures of mediastinum (*refer* to mediastinal tumors)
- Due to involvement of SVC: Headache, visual disturbances change in the state of consciousness and orthopnea.
- **Physical signs:**
  - Distended, **nonpulsatile neck veins,** dilated veins on the upper thorax and upper limbs
  - Conjunctival edema, suffusion, and subconjunctival hemorrhage
- **Features based on location of SVC obstruction**.
  - **Preazygos or supra-azygos***:* Obstruction to the return of blood above the entry of azygos vein into the SVC produces distension of veins and edema of the face, neck, and upper extremities.
  - **Postazygos or infra-azygos:** Obstruction below the entry of azygos vein into the SVC causes retrograde flow of blood through the azygos via collaterals to the inferior vena cava. This leads to the symptoms and signs of preazygos disease and dilation of the veins over the abdomen. This is usually more severe and poorly tolerated than preazygos obstruction.

Investigation and diagnosis

- Based on **clinical features.**
- **Chest radiograph:** Widening of the superior mediastinum (mostly on the right side). Pleural effusion may be found in about 25% patients.
- **CT of the chest:** Most useful
- **Invasive procedures:** Bronchoscopy, percutaneous needle biopsy, mediastinoscopy, and thoracoscopy

Treatment

- Diuretics, head elevation and oxygen for temporary symptomatic relief in few patients.
- If there is tracheal obstruction: Emergency radiotherapy
- Radiotherapy (elective): It is the treatment of choice for nonsmall-cell tumors of lung and metastatic tumors producing SVC syndrome.
- Chemotherapy: For example, small-cell carcinoma of lung or lymphoma.
- Seriously-ill patients may be given empiric corticosteroids and cyclophosphamide intravenously for temporary relief.
- Endovascular stent placement

MEDIASTINUM

Q. Define mediastinum. What are its various compartments?

Mediastinum is the region of the thoracic cavity located between the pleural cavities (sacs) in the chest. It extends anteroposteriorly from the sternum to the spine (paravertebral gutter and ribs) and sagittally from the thoracic inlet (above) to the diaphragm (below) and laterally mediastinal pleura. It has numerous organs and structures which make it a veritable Pandora's box, within which congenital cysts, benign tumors, and primary and malignant neoplasms may develop.

TABLE 6.103: Various compartments of mediastinum and their normal contents.

Compartment	Normal contents
Superior mediastinum	➤ Trachea, upper esophagus, thymus gland, thoracic duct, lymph nodes ➤ Vessels: Superior vena cava (SVC), arch of aorta and its branches ➤ Nerves: Phrenic nerve, vagus nerve, left recurrent laryngeal nerve
Anterior mediastinum	➤ Thymus gland ➤ Anterior mediastinal lymph nodes, internal mammary artery and vein ➤ Adipose tissue
Posterior mediastinum	➤ Esophagus, lymph nodes ➤ Vessels: Descending aorta, azygos vein ➤ Thoracic duct, sympathetic chain
Middle mediastinum	➤ Heart, ascending aorta, arch of aorta, vena cavae, brachiocephalic arteries and veins, pulmonary arteries and veins ➤ Trachea, main bronchi, hilar lymph nodes ➤ Phrenic nerves

Compartments

Mediastinum is divided into four compartments based on the lateral chest radiograph **(Table 6.103)**.

Common Mediastinal Tumors, Cysts, and Masses (Figs. 6.44A and B)

Q. Write short essay/note on causes of mediastinal mass.

Clinical Features

Q. Write short essay/note on clinical features, investigations, and management of mediastinal tumors.

- **Age group:** Germ-cell tumors and lymphoma/leukemias are more common between 20 and 40 years of age.
- Clinical features are due to the compression and/or invasion (infiltration) of the structures of mediastinum **(Table 6.104)**. Benign tumors cause compression without invasion, whereas malignant tumors compress and invade the vital structures of mediastinum.

Investigations

- **Cytological examination of sputum** for malignant cells.
- **α-fetoprotein and β-human chorionic gonadotropin levels:** Elevated in nonseminomatous germ-cell tumors of anterior or superior mediastinum in male.

Superior:
- Thymoma and thymic cyst
- Malignant lymphoma
- Thyroid lesions
- Parathyroid adenoma

Posterior:
- Neurogenic tumors
- Most common mass of the posterior compartment schwannoma, neurofibroma malignant peripheral nerve sheath tumor (MPNST) neuroblastoma, ganglioneuroma, ganglioneuroblastoma

Meningoceles

Thoracic spine lesions:
- Pott's disease

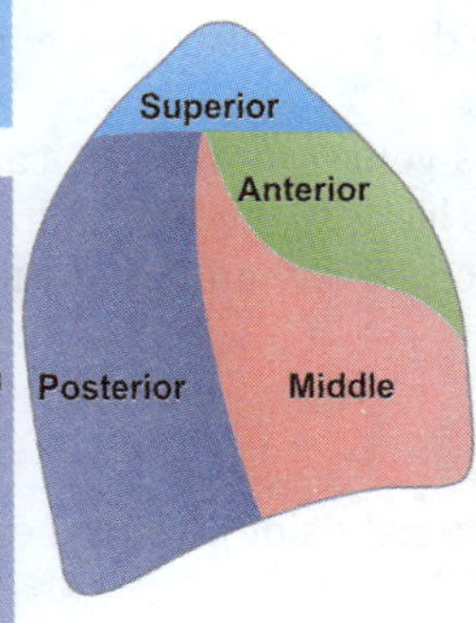

Anterior
- **Thymus:** Thymoma, thymic cyst, thymic hyperplasia, thymic carcinoma
- **Lymphoma:** Hodgkin's lymphoma, lymphoblastic lymphoma, mediastinal DLBCL
- **Germ cell tumors:** Teratoma, seminoma, nonseminomatous tumors
- **Thyroid** (intrathoracic)
- **Others:** Parathyroid adenoma, hemangioma, lipoma, liposarcoma, hemangioma, fibroma, fibrosarcoma, paraganglioma

Foramen of Morgagni hernia

Middle
- **Lymphadenopathy:** Most common mass of the middle compartment Lymphoma, metastatic lung cancer, metastatic breast cancer, sarcoidosis
- **Cysts:** Bronchogenic, pericardial, esophageal duplication

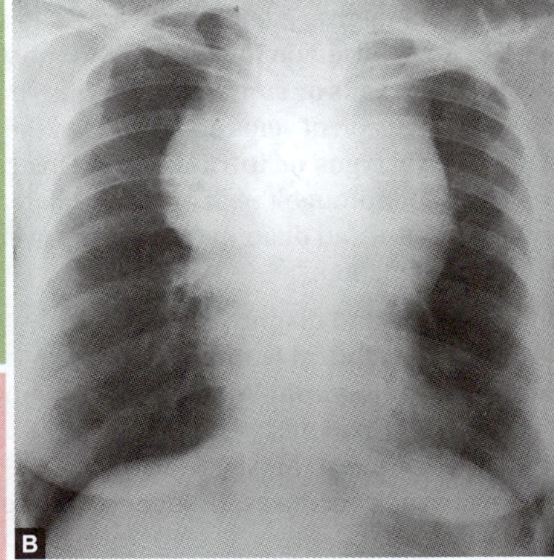

FIGS. 6.44A AND B: (A) Location of most common lesions of mediastinum. (B) Superior and anterior mediastinal mass—thymoma.

- **Radiological investigations:**
  - **Plain radiograph of chest:**
- **Benign tumor** appears as a sharply circumscribed opacity in the mediastinum which may encroach on one or both lung fields.
- **Malignant tumor** appears as a lesion with ill-defined margins and often causes a generalized widening of the mediastinal shadow.
  - **Fluoroscopic examination:** For diaphragm analysis
  - **Barium swallow:** For identifying esophageal involvement
  - CT scan of thorax
  - **Magnetic resonance imaging (MRI):** Useful for evaluating cystic lesions
  - Positron emission tomography (PET)
- **Bronchoscopy** if there is suspicion of lung cancer.
- **Mediastinoscopy:** To remove lymph node from anterior mediastinum.
- **Exploratory thoracotomy:** For removal of part or entire tumor for histopathological examination.

TABLE 6.104: Structures involved and clinical features of malignant mediastinal invasion.

Structure	Clinical features
Trachea and main bronchi:	Stridor, breathlessness, cough, collapse of lung
Esophagus:	Dysphagia, esophageal displacement or obstruction on barium swallow examination
Phrenic nerve:	Diaphragmatic paralysis and dyspnea
Left recurrent laryngeal nerve:	Paralysis of left vocal cord producing hoarseness and 'bovine' cough
Sympathetic trunk:	Horner's syndrome
Superior vena cava (SVC):	SVC syndrome: Nonpulsatile distension of neck veins, subconjunctival edema, and edema and cyanosis of head, neck, hands and arms. Dilated anastomotic veins on chest wall.
Pericardium:	Pericarditis and/or pericardial effusion, cardiac tamponade

Management
- Benign mediastinal tumors: Surgical removal.
- SVC obstruction: Refer to SVC syndrome.
- Lung cancer with lymph nodal metastases: Radiotherapy and/or chemotherapy.
- Treatments of lymphomas and leukemias.

Solitary Pulmonary Nodule

- Criteria: A single discrete pulmonary opacity surrounded by normal lung tissue. Not associated with adenopathy or atelectasis.
- Size and nature: Solitary pulmonary nodule must be 3 cm or less in diameter. Lesions larger than 3 cm are almost always malignant. Malignant nodules have a tumor doubling time between 30 and 300 days, whereas benign nodules, it is either less than 30 days or more than 300 days.
- Prompt diagnosis and resection are usually advisable. Chest X-ray appearance of solitary pulmonary nodule is shown in **Figure 6.45.**
- Differential diagnosis of solitary pulmonary nodules **(Table 6.105)**.

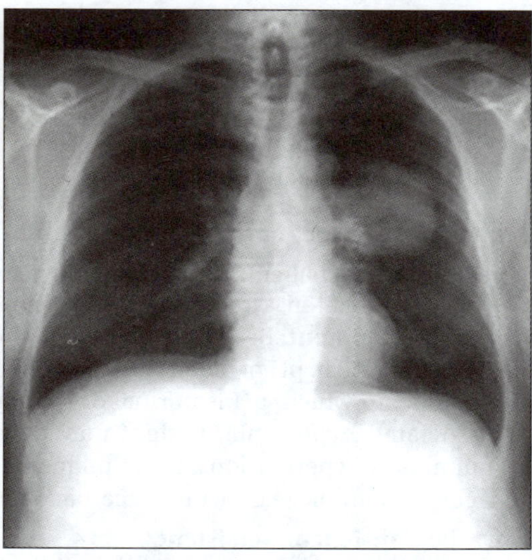

FIG. 6.45: Chest X-ray of solitary pulmonary nodule.

RESPIRATORY FAILURE

Q. Define respiratory failure. Describe in detail the causes and management of various types of respiratory failures.

Q. Discuss the role of oxygen therapy in chronic type II respiratory failure complicating chronic bronchitis.

Q. Write short essay/note on:
- **Acute respiratory failure**
- **Clinical features of type I and type II respiratory failure.**

Definition

- Respiratory failure is the term used when pulmonary gas exchange fails to maintain normal arterial oxygen and carbon dioxide levels.
- Respiratory failure is a syndrome of inadequate gas exchange due to dysfunction of one or more essential components of the respiratory system:
  - Chest wall (including pleura and diaphragm)
  - Airways
  - Alveolar-capillary units
  - Pulmonary circulation
  - Nerves
  - CNS or brainstem

TABLE 6.105: Differential diagnosis of solitary pulmonary nodules.

Malignant tumors	Noninfectious granulomas
➢ Bronchogenic carcinoma (adenocarcinoma, large cell, squamous, small cell) ➢ Carcinoid ➢ Pulmonary lymphoma	➢ Rheumatoid arthritis ➢ Wegener's granulomatosis ➢ Sarcoidosis ➢ Paraffinoma
Benign tumors	**Others**
➢ Hamartoma ➢ enoma ➢ Lipoma	➢ Miscellaneous ➢ Bronchiolitis obliterans organizing pneumonia (BOOP) ➢ Abscess
Infectious granulomas	**Pseudotumor**
➢ Tuberculosis ➢ Histoplasmosis ➢ Coccidioidomycosis	➢ Spherical pneumonia ➢ Pulmonary infarction ➢ Arteriovenous malformation ➢ Bronchogenic cyst ➢ Amyloidoma

- **Criteria:** Respiratory failure is present when **PaO_2 is 60 mm Hg (8.0 kPa) and/or $PaCO_2$ is 50 mm Hg (6.5 kPa).**
- **Features of respiratory failure:** (1) breathlessness at rest, (2) central cyanosis, (3) raised respiratory rate and (4) drowsiness, confusion, or unconsciousness. In such patients, arterial blood gas analysis to be done.

Classification

It can be classified in different ways: (1) type I, II, III and IV, (2) acute and chronic type I respiratory failure; acute and chronic type II respiratory failure, and (3) type I (hypoxemic) respiratory failure and type II (hypercapnic) respiratory failure.

Type I or Hypoxemic (PaO_2<60 at sea level): Failure of Oxygen Exchange

Increased shunt fraction (Q_S/Q_T)
- Due to alveolar flooding
- Hypoxemia refractory to supplemental oxygen

Type II or Hypercapnic ($PaCO_2$>45): Failure to Exchange or Remove Carbon Dioxide

- Decreased alveolar minute ventilation (V_A)
- Often accompanied by hypoxemia that corrects with supplemental oxygen.

Type III Respiratory Failure: Perioperative Respiratory Failure

- Increased atelectasis due to low functional residual capacity (FRC) in the setting of abnormal abdominal wall mechanics.
- Often results in type I or type II respiratory failure.
- Can be ameliorated by anesthetic or operative technique, posture, incentive spirometry, postoperative analgesia, and attempts to lower intra-abdominal pressure.

Type IV Respiratory Failure: Shock

Type IV describes patients who are intubated and ventilated in the process of resuscitation for shock.

Goal of ventilation is to stabilize gas exchange and to unload the respiratory muscles, lowering their oxygen consumption.

Rate of development: Respiratory failure may be
- Acute: In which, pH of blood may drop to below 7.2.
- Chronic: In which, pH is normal or slightly reduced and bicarbonate is elevated due to renal compensation. Due to associated hypoxemia, patient may develop polycythemia, pulmonary hypertension and cor pulmonale.
- Acute on chronic (e.g., acute exacerbation of advanced COPD)

It may be **transient or persistent**.

Various mechanisms of producing respiratory failure are listed in **Table 6.106**.

- **Hypoventilation:** It may be due to (1) low tidal volume, (2) increased dead space, or (3) reduced respiratory rate.
  In hypoventilation $PaCO_2$ increases, PaO_2 decreases, and alveolar arterial oxygen gradient is normal.
- **Ventilation–perfusion (V/Q) mismatch:** It is the **most common cause of hypoxemia** and administration of 100% O_2 will markedly improve hypoxemia. There is elevation of alveolar–arterial oxygen gradient.
- **Shunt:** If there is a shunt, deoxygenated blood bypasses ventilated alveoli and mixes with oxygenated blood and produces hypoxemia. In these patients, hypoxemia will persist even if patient is given 100% oxygen. Hypercapnia will not develop when shunt fraction is more than 60%. There is elevation of alveolar–arterial oxygen gradient.
- **Diffusion abnormality** is an uncommon cause of hypoxemia.

TABLE 6.106: Mechanisms of producing respiratory failure.

Decreased inspired oxygen concentration
➢ High altitude: Acute mountain sickness, chronic mountain sickness
Hypoventilation
➢ Diminished ventilatory drive, e.g., drug overdose, primary alveolar hypoventilation, stroke
➢ Impaired neuromuscular transmission, e.g., Guillain–Barre syndrome, myasthenia gravis, phrenic nerve injury, spinal cord lesion, amyotrophic lateral sclerosis
➢ Weakness of muscle, e.g., myasthenia gravis, muscular dystrophies, electrolyte disturbances
➢ Disorders of chest wall, e.g., kyphoscoliosis, ankylosing spondylitis, severe obesity
➢ Disorders of pleura, e.g., pneumothorax, pleural effusion
➢ Parenchymal lung disease
➢ Airway obstruction, e.g., COPD, acute severe asthma, foreign body, vocal cord palsy
Ventilation–perfusion (V/Q) mismatch
➢ Interstitial lung disease
➢ Obstructive airway disease, e.g., chronic bronchitis, emphysema, bronchiectasis, bronchial asthma
➢ Alveolar diseases, e.g., pneumonia, acute respiratory distress syndrome (ARDS)
➢ Pulmonary vascular diseases, e.g., pulmonary embolism, pulmonary hypertension
➢ Decreased cardiac output
Shunt
➢ Intracardiac right to left shunts, e.g., tetralogy of Fallot.
➢ Intrapulmonary shunts, e.g., pulmonary arteriovenous shunts, alveolar collapse, pneumonia, pulmonary edema, pulmonary hemorrhage
Diffusion abnormality
➢ Interstitial lung disease, ARDS, interstitial pneumonias

Acute Type I and Chronic Type I Respiratory Failure

Q. Write short essay/note on the causes of acute type I respiratory failure.

Acute type I respiratory failure usually develops abruptly, often in patients with previously normal lungs. Common causes of acute and chronic type I failure are listed in **Table 6.107**.

Acute Type II and Chronic Type II Respiratory Failure

Common causes of acute and chronic type II failure are listed in **Table 6.108**.

Q. Write short essay/note on management of type I and type II respiratory failure.

Management of Respiratory Failure

Flowchart 6.16 shows an approach to identify the mechanism of respiratory failure.

1. **Secure airway by:**
   - Endotracheal intubation or tracheostomy
   - Invasive mechanical ventilation
   - Noninvasive ventilation
2. **Supplemental oxygen as needed**
3. **Treat underlying condition.**
   - **Infection:** Antimicrobials and source control
   - **Airway obstruction:** Bronchodilators, glucocorticoids
   - **Improve cardiac function:** Positive airway pressure, diuretics, vasodilators, morphine, inotropy, and revascularization.
4. Respiratory stimulants, such as *doxapram hydrochloride, nikethamide, progesterone, modafinil, acetazolamide* can increase or maintain ventilation for a short time, at most 24 hours. However, its role is controversial.

Flowchart 6.17 shows step-by-step approach to respiratory failure.

TABLE 6.107: Causes of acute and chronic type I respiratory failure.

Acute type I respiratory failure	*Chronic type I respiratory failure*
➢ Pneumonia ➢ Pulmonary edema ➢ Acute asthma ➢ Pulmonary embolism ➢ Acute respiratory distress syndrome (ARDS) ➢ Pneumothorax	➢ Diseases with widespread pulmonary fibrosis ➢ Chronic pulmonary edema ➢ Chronic disorders of chest wall or neuromuscular diseases ➢ Chronic pulmonary thromboembolism

TABLE 6.108: Causes of acute and chronic type II respiratory failure.

Acute type II respiratory failure
➢ **Respiratory depressant drugs**, e.g., diazepam, opiates, alcohol ➢ **Severe obstruction to the airflow,** e.g., severe acute asthma, laryngeal and tracheal obstruction, acute exacerbation of chronic obstructive pulmonary disease (COPD) ➢ **Disorders of respiratory muscles,** e.g., acute polymyositis ➢ **Injuries to chest,** e.g., tension pneumothorax, massive hemothorax, and flail chest ➢ **Brainstem damage,** e.g., stroke, encephalitis, trauma **Disorders of spinal cord, nerves, and neuromuscular transmission**, e.g., spinal trauma, transverse myelitis, acute GB syndrome, poliomyelitis, myasthenia gravis, and botulism
Chronic type II respiratory failure
➢ COPD (most common) ➢ Chest wall abnormalities, e.g., marked kyphoscoliosis, marked obesity ➢ Amyotrophic lateral sclerosis, muscular dystrophy ➢ Central hypoventilation

SLEEP APNEA/HYPOPNEA SYNDROME

Q. Write short note on sleep apnea syndromes.

- Sleep apnea is defined as an intermittent recurrent reduction or cessation of breathing (upper airway obstruction) during sleep.
- **Apnea:** Defined by the American Academy of Sleep Medicine (AASM) as the cessation of airflow for at least 10 seconds.
- **Hypopnea:** Defined as a recognizable transient reduction (but not complete cessation) of breathing for 10 seconds or longer, a decrease of greater than 50% in the amplitude of a validated measure of breathing, or a reduction in amplitude of less than 50% associated with oxygen desaturation of 4% or more.
- **Respiratory effort-related arousal** (RERA): It is an event characterized by increasing respiratory effort for 10 seconds or longer leading to an arousal from sleep. It does not fulfil the criteria for a hypopnea or apnea.

Types of sleep apnea: (1) Obstructive sleep apnea (OSA), (2) central sleep apnea, and (3) mixed sleep apnea (combination of factors).

- **Obstructive** sleep apnea is characterized by continued thoracoabdominal effort in the setting of partial or complete air flow cessation.
- **Central** sleep apnea is characterized by the lack of thoracoabdominal effort in the setting of partial or complete airflow cessation.
- **Mixed** sleep apnea has both obstructive and central features. They generally begin without thoracoabdominal effort and end with several thoracoabdominal efforts in breathing.

FLOWCHART 6.16: Approach to identify the mechanism of respiratory failure.

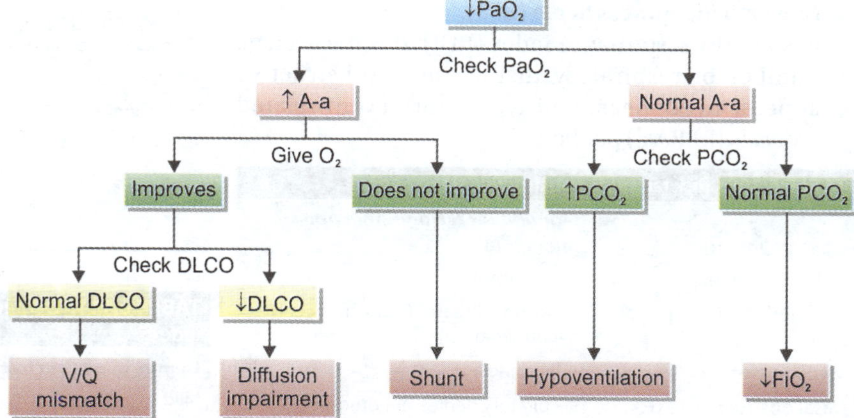

(A-a: alveolar–arterial gradient; DLCO: diffusing capacity of the lungs for carbon monoxide; FiO_2: fraction of inspired oxygen; O_2: oxygen; PaO_2: partial pressure of oxygen; $PaCO_2$: partial pressure of carbon dioxide; Q: perfusion, the blood that reaches the alveoli V: ventilation is the air that reaches the alveoli; V/Q: ventilation/perfusion ratio)

Obstructive Sleep Apnea

Risk Factors

Refer **Table 6.109**.

Clinical Features (Table 6.110)

Pickwickian syndrome (obesity-hypoventilation syndrome): It is characterized by morbid obesity (body mass index greater than 40 kg/m²), chronic sleep-induced central hypoventilation with hypercapnia ($PaCO_2$ greater than 45 mm Hg) during wakefulness. Awake resting hypoxemia, hypersomnolence, signs of cor pulmonale (right-sided heart failure and lower extremity edema), and nocturnal hypoventilation.

FLOWCHART 6.17: Step-by-step approach to respiratory failure.

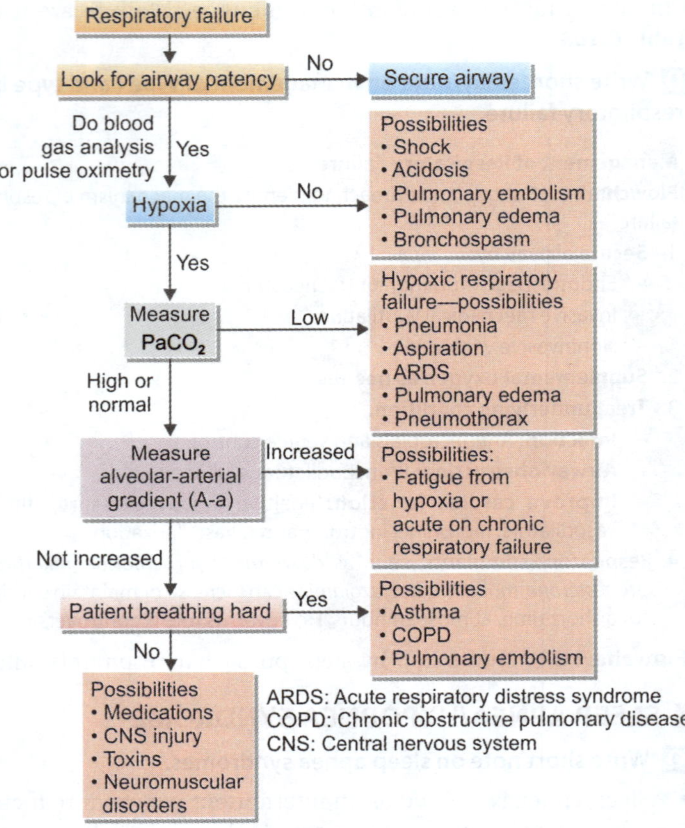

Physical Examination

- Obesity: Body mass index (BMI) greater than 30 kg/m²
- Large neck circumference: Greater than 17 inches in men and 15 inches in women
- Abnormal (increased) Mallampati score
- Narrowing of the lateral airway walls
- Other risk factors mentioned in **Table 6.109** may be found.

Diagnosis

- Diagnosis can be made on the basis of history and pulse oximetry demonstration of at least a 10 mm Hg increment in $PaCO_2$ during sleep.
- Polysomnography
  - Sleep stages are recorded via an EEG, electro-oculogram, and chin electromyogram (EMG).
  - Heart rhythm is monitored with a single-lead ECG.
  - Leg movements are recorded via an anterior tibialis EMG.
  - Breathing is monitored, including airflow at the nose and mouth (using both a thermal sensors and a nasal pressure transducer), effort (using inductance plethysmography), and oxygen saturation.
  - The breathing pattern is analyzed for the presence of apnea and hypopneas
  - Apnea-hypopnea index (AHI): AHI is defined as the average number of episodes of apnea and hypopnea per hour.

  Diagnosis of sleep apnea is confirmed if AHI ≥5 **(Table 6.111)**.
- Excessive daytime sleepiness (EDS) assessed by **Epworth Sleepiness Scale** (ESS).
- Respiratory disturbance index (RDI): It is the average number of respiratory disturbances (obstructive apneas, hypopneas, and respiratory event-related arousals [RERAs]) per hour.

TABLE 6.109: Risk factors for obstructive sleep apnea.

Obesity (major)	*Mandibular retrognathia and micrognathia*
Male sex (major)	Family history
Enlarged tonsils (especially in children)	Endocrine diseases (e.g., acromegaly, hypothyroidism)
Menopause	Advancing age
Nasal obstruction (e.g., nasal deformities, rhinitis, polyps, adenoids), smoking	Respiratory depressant drugs (e.g., alcohol, sedatives, strong analgesics)

TABLE 6.110: Clinical features of obstructive sleep apnea.

Nocturnal features	*Daytime features*
➢ Snoring, usually loud, habitual ➢ Witnessed apnea, which often interrupt the snoring and end with a snort ➢ Nocturnal gasping and choking sensations ➢ Nocturia ➢ Insomnia ➢ Restless sleep	➢ Nonrestorative sleep (i.e. waking up as tired as when they went to bed) ➢ Morning headache, dry or sore throat ➢ Excessive daytime sleepiness (EDS) ➢ Daytime fatigue/tiredness ➢ Cognitive deficits; memory and intellectual impairment (short-term memory, concentration) and impaired work performance ➢ Decreased vigilance ➢ Morning confusion ➢ Personality and mood changes, including depression, anxiety and irritability

TABLE 6.111: Degree of obstructive sleep apnea and apnea hypopnea index.

Degree of obstructive sleep apnea	*Apnea–hypopnea index (AHI)*
Mild	5–15
Moderate	16–30
Severe	>30

Treatment

- Mild apnea: Wider variety of options
- Moderate-to-severe apnea: Should be treated with nasal continuous positive airway pressure (CPAP).
  1. Conservative nonsurgical treatment
     - Weight reduction in obese individuals
     - Avoidance of alcohol for 4–6 hours prior to bedtime.
     - Sleeping on one's side rather than on the stomach or back.
  2. **Nasal CPAP therapy**
     - Most effective for OSA. Increases the caliber of the airway in the retropalatal and retroglossal regions. It increases the lateral dimensions of the upper airways and thins the lateral pharyngeal walls. Maintains upper airways patency during sleep, preventing the soft tissues from collapsing.
     - **Indications:** (1) Patients with an apnea–hypopnea index (AHI) greater than 15 regardless of symptomatology. (2) For patients with an AHI of 5–14.9, if the patient has one of the following: excessive daytime sleepiness (EDS), hypertension, or cardiovascular disease.
  3. **Other modalities:** BiPAP therapy and oral appliance therapy.
  4. **Surgery for obstructive sleep apnea,** e.g., nasal surgery (septoplasty, sinus surgery, and others), tonsillectomy ± adenoidectomy, uvulopalatopharyngoplasty (UPPP).
  5. **Pharmacotherapy:**
     - Many drugs (e.g., mirtazapine, protriptyline, theophylline, naloxone, doxapram, oxymetazoline nasal application, inhaled nasal corticosteroids, and acetazolamide) have been tried without much benefit in OSA.
     - Modafinil is used in patients who have residual daytime sleepiness despite optimal use of CPAP.
     - Selective serotonin reuptake inhibitor agents such as paroxetine and fluoxetine have been shown to increase genioglossus muscle activity and decrease REM sleep (apneas are more common in REM).

Central Sleep Apnea

- It occurs without obstruction of the airway.
- *Causes:* Congenital central sleep apnea (Ondine's curse) and a many neurological lesions.
- *Mechanisms:* Primary central alveolar hypoventilation syndrome.
- Etiology not known. Probably due to high chemoresponsiveness of the respiratory system. Apnea is terminated with an abrupt, large breath.
- Daytime somnolence is less common.
  - *Others:* High altitude, stroke, neurodegenerative diseases (e.g., Parkinson's disease), left ventricular failure with Cheyne-Stokes breathing.

Treatment

- Administration of oxygen during sleep.
- Nasal CPAP.
- Noninvasive positive-pressure ventilation (bilevel nasal positive pressure).
- Acetazolamide and theophylline may be tried though effect is modest.
- Treatment of underlying cause: β-blockers in congestive heart failure.

TABLE 6.112: Therapeutic indications for oxygen therapy.

➢ Pulmonary edema	➢ Respiratory paralysis
➢ Acute attack of bronchial asthma	➢ Anaerobic infections
➢ Chronic obstructive pulmonary disease (COPD)	➢ High altitude
➢ Acute respiratory distress syndrome (ARDS)	➢ Prevents development of severe pulmonary hypertension

Oxygen Therapy

Q. Write short essay/note on different types of oxygen therapy.

Therapeutic Indications for Oxygen Therapy (Table 6.112)

Q. Write short essay/note on common therapeutic indications of oxygen therapy in clinical practice.

Hazards of Oxygen Therapy

- CO_2 narcosis
- Pulmonary complications: Irritation of respiratory tract, pulmonary edema, ARDS, consolidation, reduction in lung compliance → fibrosis.
- In premature infants and neonates: Retrolental fibroplasias, blindness, bronchopulmonary dysplasia
- Idiopathic epilepsy

Technique of Administration

- Fraction of inspired oxygen (FiO_2) while inhaling 100% oxygen depends upon rate of oxygen flow and minute ventilation of patient. Merits and demerits of various techniques of oxygen administration are presented in **Table 6.113**.
- Oxygen delivery system can be divided into:
  - Low-flow systems
  - High-flow systems

Hyperbaric Oxygen Therapy

Hyperbaric oxygen (HBO) exposure (breathing oxygen at increased ambient pressure), usually 2–3 atmospheres absolute (ATA) causes an increase in PaO_2.

Indication for HBOT

- Poisoning: Carbon monoxide
- Infections: Clostridial myonecrosis
- Acute ischemia: Crush injury
- Chronic ischemia: Radiation necrosis
- Ischemic ulcers: Diabetic ulcers

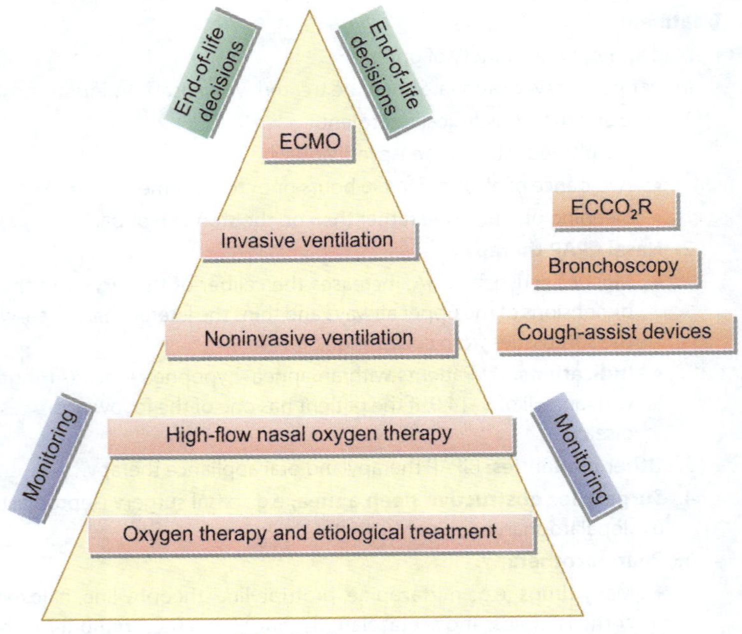

FIG. 6.46: Types of oxygen therapy.

NONINVASIVE POSITIVE PRESSURE VENTILATION (NPPV)

- Delivers respiratory support with positive airway pressure via a sealed facemask, nasal mask, or helmet device.
- NPPV includes continuous positive airway pressure (CPAP) and bilevel positive airway pressure (BiPAP) ventilation. NPPV can be delivered by home devices or ventilators.
  - CPAP: Delivers continuous positive airway pressure throughout the respiratory cycle and prevents alveolar collapse during expiration.
  - CPAP is often used in the treatment of obstructive sleep apnea and pulmonary edema.
  - BiPAP: Delivers two different airway pressures during inspiration and expiration to decrease the work of breathing. BiPAP is often used for COPD exacerbations, weaning, and neuromuscular weakness
  - Benefits of NPPV:
    - NPPV decreases the need for mechanical ventilation in appropriately selected patients, especially in patients with neuromuscular disease, COPD, pulmonary edema, and postoperative respiratory insufficiency.
- Disadvantages of NPPV: NPPV is generally safe but can cause skin damage, eye irritation, claustrophobia, and aerophagia and be difficult to tolerate for some patients. Use should be limited to patients who are conscious, are cooperative, able to protect their airway, and are hemodynamically stable.

TABLE 6.113: Merits and demerits of various techniques of oxygen administration.

Merits	*Demerits*
Nasal catheter, nasal cannula (simple plastic tubing + prongs)	
➢ Easy to fix ➢ Keep hands free ➢ Not much interference with further airway care ➢ Useful in both spontaneous breathing and apneic	➢ Mucosal irritation (uncomfortable) ➢ Gastric dilatation (especially with high flows) - Exact FiO_2 delivered is unknown because it is influenced by peak inspiratory flow demand
Simple face mask	
➢ Simple ➢ Lightweight ➢ Delivers oxygen at FiO_2 of 35–55% using flows of 5–12 L/min	➢ Need to remove when speak, eat, drink, vomiting, expectoration of secretions ➢ Drying/irritation of eyes ➢ Uncomfortable when facial burns/trauma ➢ Application problem when *Ryle's tube* in situ
Partial rebreathing mask (polymask)	
➢ FiO_2 delivered >0.60 is delivered in moderate-to-severe hypoxia ➢ Exhaled oxygen from anatomic dead space is conserved	➢ Insufficient flow rate may lead to rebreathing of CO_2 ➢ Claustrophobia ➢ Drying and irritation of eyes
Nonrebreathing mask	
➢ Use a reservoir bag to achieve higher oxygen concentrations (up to 80%). ➢ Flow rates are generally at least 8–15 L/min	➢ Air dilution (if not fitting properly) ➢ Rebreathing (if O_2 flow is inadequate) ➢ Interfere with further airway care ➢ Uncomfortable (sweating, spitting)
Venturi masks: Allow the precise administration of oxygen via a Venturi facemask. Usual FiO_2 values delivered are 24%, 28%, 31%, 35%, 40%, and 50%.	
Heated humidified high-flow nasal cannula (HFNC): ➢ Delivers heated and humidified oxygen at high flows and concentrations such that it flushes out a significant amount of nonoxygenated air from the upper airway. ➢ The system can be titrated up to 60 L/min and 100% FiO_2 and may provide a small amount of PEEP at high-flow rates.	

Mechanical Ventilation

Q. Write short essay on noninvasive ventilation.

Types of mechanical ventilation: (1) Invasive and (2) noninvasive. Indications for mechanical ventilation are mentioned in **Box 6.17**.

Box 6.17: Indications of mechanical ventilation.

- Apnea with respiratory arrest
- Acute lung injury
- Respiratory rate >35 breaths per minute
- Vital capacity <15 mL/kg
- PO_2 <60 at FiO_2 0.6
- Respiratory muscle fatigue
- Obtundation or coma
- Bradypnea
- PCO_2 of >50 mm Hg with pH <7.25

General Principles of Ventilation

- Endotracheal tube should be inserted to an average depth of 23 cm in men and 21 cm in women (measured at the incisor).
- Pressure in the cuff generally should not exceed 25 mm Hg.
- Tracheostomy should be done if anticipating ventilator setting for more than 3 days.
- Routine suctioning is not recommended because it may be associated with complications (e.g., desaturation, arrhythmias, bronchospasm, severe coughing, and introduction of secretions into the lower respiratory tract).

Modes of ventilatory support: Controlled mode ventilation (CMV), assist control mode ventilation (ACMV), synchronized intermittent mandatory ventilation (SIMV), and continuous positive airway pressure/positive end-expiratory pressure (CPAP/PEEP).

- **Controlled mode ventilation**
  - Used for initiation of the ventilation
  - No patient contribution
  - All variables are independent (FiO_2, TV, RR, I/E).
- **Assist control mode ventilation**
  - Inspiratory cycle is initiated either by the patient or if patient effort is not present, then by a timer signal present within the ventilator.
  - Also commonly used for initiation
  - Synchronization of ventilator cycle with patient's inspiratory effort.
  - Drawbacks: Respiratory alkalosis, myoclonus and seizures
- **Synchronized intermittent mandatory ventilation (SIMV)**
  - Patient is allowed to breathe spontaneously without ventilator assist in between the ventilator breaths.
  - Ventilator breath is delivered in synchrony.
  - Mandatory are the number of present breaths
  - Intermediate mode
  - Helpful in weaning
- **Continuous positive airway pressure (CPAP)**
  - Not a true mode of ventilation
  - All ventilation occurs because of patients spontaneous efforts ventilator just gives fresh gas to the breathing circuit with operator-depended positive pressure.
  - Used to access the extubation potential in the patient who requires very little ventilator support or inpatient with intact respiratory system function who require an ET tube for airway protection.

Weaning

- Arterial pH: 7.35–7.40
- SO_2 >90% with FiO_2 0.5
- PEEP <5 mm Hg
- Intact cough reflex (assessed during suctioning)
- Weaning index: RR/TV <105
- Patient off inotropes

Complications of Ventilation

- **Pulmonary:** Barotrauma (>50 mm Hg), interstitial emphysema, pneumomediastinum, subcutaneous emphysema, pneumothorax, **ventilator-associated pneumonia (VAP)**, tracheal stenosis.
- **Hypotension:** Resulting from elevated intrathoracic pressure and decreased venous return and it is responds to volume repletion.
- **Gastrointestinal:** Stress ulcers and cholestasis.
  - Neuromuscular weakness
  - Pressure sores
  - Raised intracranial pressure
  - Sinusitis, oral ulcers

Extracorporeal Membrane Oxygenation

Extracorporeal membrane oxygenation (ECMO) is a type of mechanical cardiopulmonary support that is used to support patients with cardiac failure or both cardiac and respiratory failure, despite optimal conventional care, by removing blood from the venous system, oxygenating it, and returning it to either the venous (venous-venous [VV] ECMO) or arterial (veno-arterial [VA] ECMO) system.

- Veno-venous ECMO: Used to support patients with respiratory failure
- Veno-arterial ECMO: Used to support patients with cardiac failure or both cardiac and respiratory failure.

Extracorporeal Carbon Dioxide Removal

$ECCO_2R$ therapy is a useful and effective supportive treatment for adults in the ICU with both ARDS and AE-COPD.

Indications

- Acute severe heart or lung failure with high mortality risk, despite optimal conventional therapy.
- Hypoxic respiratory failure, with a partial pressure of arterial oxygen (PaO_2)/fraction of inspired oxygen (FiO_2) < 150 mm Hg with FiO_2 >0.9 and Murray score of 2–3.
- ARDS
- Severe cardiac failure of any cause
- Primary allograft failure following heart or lung transplantation
- As a bridge to either cardiac or lung transplantation or placement of a ventricular-assist device.

Contraindications

Most contraindications are relative:

- Conditions incompatible with normal life if the patient recovers
- Preexisting conditions which affect the quality of life (CNS status, end-stage malignancy, risk of systemic bleeding with anticoagulation).

Complications

- Bleeding due to anticoagulants used is seen in around 50% of patients and can be life threatening.
- Systemic thromboembolism due to clots formed in the circuit
- Heparin-induced thrombocytopenia, canula-related problems, and neurological dysfunction have also been reported.

Acute Lung Injury and the Acute Respiratory Distress Syndrome

Q. Describe acute respiratory distress syndrome (ARDS), noncardiogenic pulmonary edema, and acute lung injury (ALI).

Definition: Acute respiratory distress syndrome (ARDS) is a sudden and progressive form of acute respiratory failure in which the alveolar capillary membrane becomes damaged and more permeable to intravascular fluid resulting in severe dyspnea, hypoxemia, and diffuse pulmonary infiltrates.

The Berlin definition of ARDS **(Table 6.114)**: An acute, diffuse, inflammatory lung injury that leads to increased pulmonary vascular permeability, increased lung weight, and a loss of aerated tissue.

ARDS and ALI are serious diseases characterized by damage to alveolar epithelium and pulmonary capillary endothelium. Alveoli become filled with edema fluid of high-protein content and inflammatory cells.

Etiology of ARDS and ALI (Table 6.115)

ARDS may develop due to diffuse lung injury from many medical and surgical disorders. The lung injury may be direct (e.g., toxic inhalation) or indirect (e.g., in septicemia).

TABLE 6.114: The Berlin definition of acute respiratory distress syndrome (ARDS).

The Berlin definition of acute respiratory distress syndrome (ARDS)	
Timing	Within 1 week of a known clinical insult/new/ worsening respiratory symptoms
Chest X-ray	Bilateral opacities—not fully explained by effusions, lobar/lung collapse or nodules
Origin of edema	➢ Respiratory failure not fully explained by cardiac failure or fluid overload ➢ Need objective assessment (e.g., echocardiography) to exclude hydrostatic edema If no risk factor is present.
Oxygenation	
Mild	200 mm Hg <PaO2/FiO_2 ≤300 mm Hg with PEEP or CPAP >5 cm H_2O
Moderate	100 mm Hg <PaO2/FiO_2 ≤200 mm Hg with PEEP >5 cm H_2O
Severe	PaO_2/FiO_2 ≤100 mm Hg with PEEP >5 cm H_2O

TABLE 6.115: Disorders commonly associated with ARDS.

Direct lung injury	
Pulmonary infections	Pneumonia (viral, bacterial, fungal *Pneumocystis jirovecii, Mycoplasma)*
Aspiration	Aspiration of gastric contents (vomitus)
Inhalation of toxic gas	Ammonia, chlorine, nitrogen dioxide, ozone, oxygen, smoke
Blunt chest trauma	Pulmonary contusion
Near drowning	
Indirect lung injury	
Systemic disorders	Shock, septicemia, uremia, eclampsia
Severe trauma	Multiple bone fractures (fat embolism), flail chest, head trauma, burns
Blood	Multiple transfusions
Drug overdose	
➢ Narcotic overdose	Heroin, methadone, morphine, dextropropoxyphene
➢ Nonnarcotic drugs	Barbiturates, thiazides, nitrofurantoin
Others	Acute pancreatitis, cardiopulmonary bypass, trauma, Goodpasture's syndrome, SLE

FLOWCHART 6.18: Pathophysiology of acute respiratory distress syndrome (ARDS).

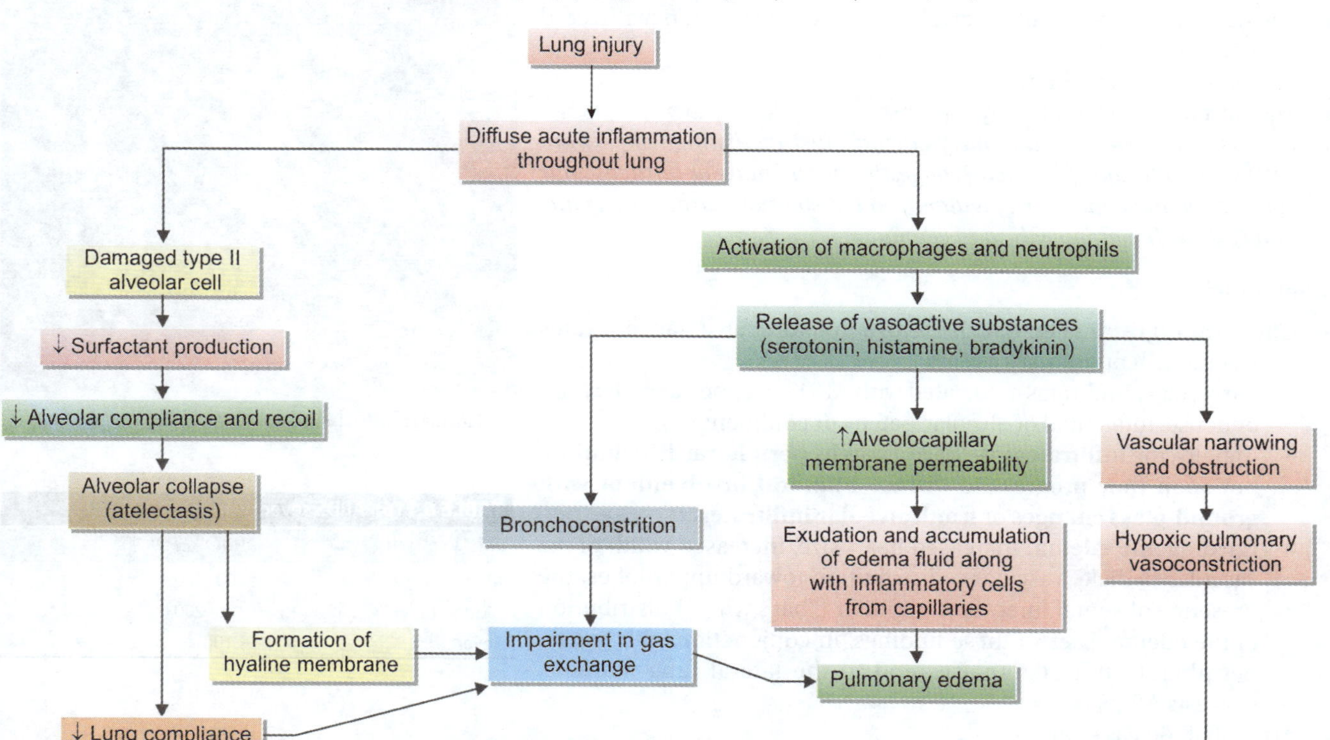

Pathophysiology (Flowchart 6.18)

Natural history of ARDS can be divided into three: Exudative, proliferative, and fibrotic.

1. **Exudative phase (1–7 days):** Diffuse acute inflammation (e.g., neutrophils) occurs throughout the lungs, involving both endothelial and epithelial surfaces. Activated neutrophils are sequestered into the lungs and increase the capillary permeability as well as damages type I and II alveolar cells. The leaked proteins aggregate in the air spaces with cellular debris and dysfunctional pulmonary surfactant to form the characteristic hyaline membranes. Activated macrophages and neutrophils release cytokines and chemokines which progressively recruit more inflammatory cells and amplify the inflammatory response. There is loss of surfactant and impaired surfactant production as a secondary event. The net effect is alveolar collapse (most marked independent regions of the lung) and results in hypoxemia due to ventilation-perfusion mismatch and increased pulmonary shunt.
2. **Proliferative phase (3–7 days):** Resolution often starts at this phase along with the initiation of repair process. The alveolar exudate undergoes organization and neutrophils disappear with appearance of lymphocytes. Type II pneumocytes starts proliferating. Connective tissue and other structural elements in the lungs proliferate in response to the initial injury, including development of fibroblasts. The terms “stiff lung” and “shock lung” frequently used to characterize this stage.
3. **Fibrotic phase (>10–14 days):** It occurs in some cases and is characterized by proliferation of fibroblasts resulting in interstitial fibrosis. Lung function may continue to improve for as long as 6–12 months after onset of respiratory failure, depending on the precipitating condition and severity of the initial injury.

Results

- Hypoxemia (V/Q mismatch, impaired hypoxic pulmonary vasoconstriction)
- Increase in dependent densities (surfactant dysfunction, alveolar instabilities)
- Decreased compliance (surfactant dysfunction, decreased lung volume, fibrosis)
- Collapse/consolidation (increased compression of dependent lung)
- Increased minute ventilation (increased in alveolar dead space)
- Increased work of breathing—WOB (increased elastase, increased minute volume requirement)
- Pulmonary hypertension (vasoconstriction, microvascular thrombi, fibrosis, PEEP (positive end expiratory pressure).

Clinical Features

- Development of **acute dyspnea and hypoxemia within hours to days** of an inciting event.
- **Tachypnea, tachycardia,** cyanosis and the need for a high-fraction of inspired oxygen (FiO_2) to maintain oxygen saturation.

- Febrile or hypothermic
- Sepsis—hypotension and peripheral vasoconstriction with cold extremities.
- Bilateral rales/crepitations
- Manifestations of the underlying cause.
- *Because cardiogenic pulmonary edema must be distinguished from ARDS, carefully look for signs of congestive heart failure or intravascular volume overload, including jugular venous distension, cardiac murmurs and gallops, hepatomegaly, and edema.*

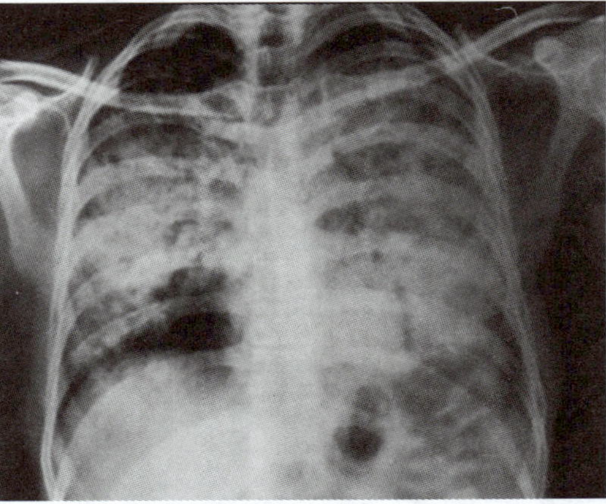

FIG. 6.47: Bilateral alveolar shadows in ARDS on chest X-ray.

Investigations

- **Chest radiograph (Fig. 6.47):** Diffuse, bilateral alveolar infiltrates consistent with pulmonary edema
  - Early stage: Infiltrates associated with ARDS **may be variable:** Mild or dense, interstitial or alveolar, patchy or confluent.
  - Initially, the **infiltrates** may have a **patchy peripheral distribution**, but soon they progress to **diffuse bilateral involvement with ground-glass changes** or **frank alveolar infiltrates.**
  - **Cardiogenic edema:** Increased heart size, increased width of the vascular pedicle, vascular redistribution toward upper lobes, the presence of septal lines, or a perihilar ("bat's wing") distribution of the edema. Lack of these findings, in conjunction with patchy peripheral infiltrates that extend to the lateral lung margins, suggests ARDS.

TABLE 6.116: ARDS severity and PaO_2/FiO_2.

ARDS severity	*PaO_2/FiO_2*
Mild	200–300
Moderate	100–200
Severe	<100

- Arterial blood gas analysis:
  - PaO_2/FiO_2 ratio and severity **(Table 6.116)**
  - In addition to hypoxemia, arterial blood gases often initially show a respiratory alkalosis.
  - However, in ARDS occurring in the context of sepsis, a metabolic acidosis with or without respiratory compensation may be present.
  - As the condition progresses and the work of breathing increases, the partial pressure of carbon dioxide (PCO_2) begins to rise and respiratory alkalosis gives way to respiratory acidosis.
- To exclude cardiogenic pulmonary edema
  - Echocardiogram: Left ventricular ejection fraction, wall motion, and valvular abnormalities
  - Plasma B-type natriuretic peptide (BNP) value.
- CT scan: Diffuse consolidation with air bronchograms, bullae, pleural effusions, pneumomediastinum and pneumothorax. Later may show lung cysts.

Management

Goals of management of patients with ARDS

- Treatment of respiratory system abnormalities
- Diagnose and treat the precipitating/initiating cause of ARDS. Support or treat other organ system dysfunction or failure.
- Maintain oxygenation.
- General critical care, adequate early nutritional support, prophylaxis against deep vein thrombosis (DVT) and gastrointestinal (GI) bleeding.

Maintaining adequate oxygenation

- Positive end-expiratory pressure (PEEP) is employed.
- When utilized in sufficient amounts, PEEP allows FiO_2 to be lowered from high potentially toxic concentrations.
- **Lung-protective mechanical ventilation**
  - Mechanical ventilation using limited tidal volumes
  - The goals of lung-protective ventilation are to avoid injury due to overexpansion of alveoli during inspiration ("volutrauma") and injury due to repetitive opening and closing of alveoli during inspiration and expiration ("atelectatrauma").
- **Low tidal volume ventilation (LTVV)**
  - Set initial tidal volume to 8 mL/kg IBW.
  - Reduce tidal volume to 7 mL/kg IBW then 6 mL/kg IBW over the next 1–3 hours.
  - Set respiratory rate to <35 bpm to match baseline minute ventilation.
- **Permissive hypercapnia** is defined as clinician-allowed hypercapnia during assisted ventilation, despite an ability to achieve a level of minute ventilation sufficient to maintain a normal.

Fluid management

- Primary ARDS due to aspiration, pneumonia, or inhalational injury, usually can be treated with fluid restriction.
- Secondary ARDS due to remote infection or inflammation requires initial fluid and potential vasoactive drug therapy.

Prone positioning ventilation

About two-thirds of patients with ARDS improve their oxygenation after being placed in a prone position.

Adjuncts to lung protective mechanical ventilation

Inhaled nitric oxide, inhaled prostacyclin, tracheal gas insufflation, extracorporeal membrane oxygenation (ECMO) or extracorporeal CO_2 removal ($ECCO_2R$)

Corticosteroids

Corticosteroids have little or no role in acute phase of ALI or ARDS. However, the role of corticosteroids in later phases of ALI or ARDS has been controversial.

Experimental therapies

- Surfactant replacement therapy: Improves oxygenation but no improvement in mortality.
- Ketoconazole: Antifungal that inhibits thromboxane synthase and 5-lipooxygenase

Future nonventilatory therapeutic options

- Gene therapy for ALI/ARDS
- Mesenchymal stem cells (MSC)

SARCOIDOSIS

Q. Discuss the clinical features, investigations, and management of sarcoidosis.

Definition: Sarcoidosis is a multisystem disorder of unknown etiology characterized by noncaseating granuloma which mainly affects lung but can also affect any other organs.

Etiology

- Etiology of sarcoidosis **remains unknown**, but several lines of evidence suggest that it is a disease of disordered immune regulation in genetically predisposed individual.
- Factors that play a role in its pathogenesis are: (1) **Environmental agents** (infectious and noninfectious), (2) **genetic** (e.g., HLA-A1 and HLA-B8), and (3) **immunological** (cell-mediated immune response).
- The granuloma is the pathologic hallmark of sarcoidosis. The sarcoid granulomas develop as an exaggerated cell-mediated immune response to an unidentified environmental antigen. Infectious or noninfectious agent in a genetically susceptible individual. Probable infectious inciting agent includes: mycobacteria (both *Mycobacterium tuberculosis* and nontuberculous mycobacteria), *Propionibacterium acnes, Borrelia burgdorferi*, viruses, fungi, spirochetes, and *Rickettsia*.

Pathology

- **Noncaseating granulomas** are composed of an **aggregate of epithelioid cells and lymphocytes** (mainly CD4+ T-cell).
- Epithelioid cells are modified macrophages and characteristically have abundant eosinophilic cytoplasm and vesicular nuclei. Schumann bodies and stellate inclusion as asteroid bodies enclosed within giant cells are formed in approximately 60% of granulomas.
- **Organs involved:** Sarcoidosis can affect every organ of the body. **It most commonly** affects the **lung** and the **lymph nodes** in the **mediastinum and hilar regions**. Other organs commonly affected are the liver, spleen, skin, parotid glands, and eye.

Clinical Features

- **Age and gender:** It occurs mainly in 3rd or 4th decade of life. More predominant in women.
- **More prevalent** in Swedes, Danes, and US blacks.
- **Systems involved:** Pulmonary (90%), lymph nodes (70%), hepatic (50–80%), cardiac (30%), cutaneous (25%), and ocular (20%)

Manifestations of Sarcoidosis

- **Asymptomatic form** (30–45%): It is usually detected incidentally on a routine chest X-ray (~30%) or abnormal liver function tests.
- Acute or subacute form (10–15%)
- Chronic form (40–60%).

Pulmonary manifestations

- First site of involvement. Begins with alveolitis involving small bronchi and small blood vessels. Alveolitis either clear-up spontaneously or lead to granuloma or fibrosis.
- Other features: Interstitial lung diseases, atelectasis, cavitation, unilateral pleural effusion, pulmonary nodules, miliary mottling, lymphadenopathy.

- Most patients have pulmonary manifestations, and most presenting with incidental findings on CXR as an interstitial disease.
- Symptoms include dry cough, dyspnea, and chest discomfort.
- Unpredictable course.

Extrapulmonary Involvement

1. Lymph nodes: Lymph nodes are involved in almost all cases (mainly hilar and mediastinal nodes), but any nodes may be involved. Involved nodes are characteristically enlarged, discrete, and sometimes calcified.
   - **Typical:**
     - Bilateral hilar and right paratracheal lymph nodes
     - Middle mediastinal lymph node (**50%** of cases).
     - Left paratracheal, aortopulmonary, and subcarinal lymph nodes
     1-2-3 sign present in **95%** of cases. This is called **Garland triad**.
   - **Atypical:**
     - Unilateral hilar lymph node
     - Anterior or posterior mediastinal lymph nodes
     - Lymph node calcification (amorphous, punctate, popcorn or egg-shell calcification).
   - Tonsil may be affected in about quarter to one third of the cases.
2. Skin (33%): Erythema nodosum, plaques, maculopapular eruptions, subcutaneous nodules, lupus pernio, keloid, infiltration of previous scars by granuloma
3. Eyes (25%): Anterior uveitis, iridocyclitis, retinitis, phlyctenular conjunctivitis, lacrimal gland involvement—keratoconjunctivitis sicca (dry eyes).
4. Salivary glands: Parotid gland enlargement.

Q. Write short note on Heerfordt–Waldenström syndrome.

- **Heerfordt's syndrome**/uveoparotid fever/Heerfordt–Mylius syndrome/Waldenström's uveoparotitis is a rare manifestation of sarcoidosis. It is characterized by uveitis, swelling of the parotid gland, chronic fever, and facial nerve palsy (in some cases).

5. Heart: Cardiac arrhythmias, heart block, sudden death, and CHF
6. Liver and spleen: Granulomatous liver disease, hepatosplenomegaly, Budd–Chiari syndrome.
7. Nervous system: Cranial nerve palsy, pachymeningitis, space-occupying lesion, diabetes insipidus due to hypothalamic involvement, mononeuritis multiplex, peripheral neuropathy
8. Kidneys: Nephrocalcinosis, hypercalciuria, and renal stones
9. Musculoskeletal
   - Arthropathies, osteoporosis, phalangeal bone cysts, polymyositis, chronic myopathy
   - Endocrine
   - Diabetes insipidus, anterior pituitary dysfunction, Addison's syndrome.
10. Lupus pernio
    - It is a specific complex involvement of skin around nose, eye and cheeks.
    - These chilblains-like lesions often cause is figuration by eroding the cartilage and bone, especially around the nose.
    - It is diagnostic for chronic form of sarcoidosis and is associated with more sever pulmonary disease.
    - Associated with poor prognosis of sarcoidosis.

Q. Write short note on Löfgren's syndrome.

Löfgren's syndrome: It is an acute triad of erythema nodosum, joint pains, and radiographic evidence of bilateral hilar adenopathy. It is often seen in young women and resolves over 6 months to 2 years with NSAIDs.

Investigations

Q. Write short note on radiological/X-ray findings in sarcoidosis.

- Radiological investigations
  - **Classic radiographic patterns of pulmonary sarcoidosis (Table 6.117):** The chest X-ray is the most commonly used tool to assess the lung involvement in sarcoidosis. According to the pattern of involvement on X-ray findings, sarcoidosis is classified into four stages.
  - **Computed tomography of the chest (contrast-enhanced):** Helps in better delineation of the hilar and mediastinal lymph nodes.

TABLE 6.117: Staging of pulmonary sarcoidosis according to radiographic patterns and corresponding clinical features.

Stage	*X-ray finding*	*Clinical features*
I	Bilateral hilar lymphadenopathy (BHL) without any parenchymal abnormalities (50% cases)	Often asymptomatic, but may be associated with erythema nodosum and arthralgia. Majority resolve spontaneously within 1 year
II	BHL with diffuse pulmonary infiltrates (30% cases)	May present with breathlessness or cough. Majority resolve spontaneously
III	Diffuse pulmonary infiltrates without BHL (10% cases)	Disease is less likely to resolve spontaneously
IV	Evidence of diffuse pulmonary fibrosis	Can progress to ventilatory failure, pulmonary hypertension and cor pulmonale

- **HRCT:** Characteristic appearance is presence of reticulonodular opacities that follow a perilymphatic distribution, centered on bronchovascular bundles and the subpleural areas. Confluence of many interstitial granulomas can produce large, irregular, mass-like opacities (alveolar sarcoid). Small satellite nodules are usually found at the periphery of these large nodules termed the "galaxy sign" (a collection of stars). Honeycombing is not common.
- **Gallium 67 scan:** Shows diffuse uptake
- **PET scan:** Using radiolabeled fluorodeoxyglucose is more useful than gallium-67 scan to detect areas of granulomatous disease in the chest and other sites and select potential area for biopsy.
- **MRI:** May be useful in the assessment of extrapulmonary sites (e.g., brain, heart, and bone).

- **Complete blood count:** There may be a mild normochromic, normocytic anemia, lymphocytopenia (characteristic), eosinophilia, raised ESR, hyperglobulinemia, elevated serum alkaline phosphatase.
- **Serum biochemistry:** Serum calcium is often raised (hypercalcemia due to increased production of 1,25-dihydroxyvitamin D by the granuloma) and there is hypergammaglobulinemia.
- **Serum angiotensin-converting enzyme (ACE) level** is elevated in more than 75% of patients with untreated sarcoidosis. Elevated levels are not of diagnostic value because it may also be elevated in lymphoma, pulmonary tuberculosis, asbestosis, and silicosis. However, it is useful in assessing disease activity and response to treatment.
- **Mantoux test:** Skin sensitivity to tuberculin is reduced or absent. So, Mantoux test is a useful screening test and a strongly positive reaction virtually rules out sarcoidosis.
- **Lung function tests:** They show atypical restrictive lung defect in patients with pulmonary infiltration or fibrosis. There is a decrease in TLC, FEV, and FVC, and gas transfer. Lung function is usually normal in patients with extrapulmonary disease or those with only hilar lymphadenopathy on chest X-ray.
- **Bronchoscopy:** May show a "cobblestone" appearance of the mucosa.
- **Bronchial and transbronchial biopsy:** Most useful investigation. It usually shows noncaseating granulomas composed of epithelioid cells and multinucleate giant cells.
- **Bronchoalveolar lavage (BAL):** Shows increased proportion of lymphocytes, mostly activated Th1 (subset of Cd4+ cells) cells. BAL fluid also shows an increased CD4:CD8 T-cell ratio.
- **Kveim (or Kveim-Siltzbach) test:** It involves intradermal injection of 0.1 mL of an antigen obtained from sarcoidosis spleen extract. Development of small nodule at the injection site indicates the test as positive. The nodule is biopsied at 4–6 weeks and shows typical noncaseating epithelioid granuloma. However, this test is obsolete now.
- Mediastinoscopic biopsy of mediastinal or hilar lymph nodes.
- Exercise tests: May show oxygen desaturation.
- Bone marrow examination may show granulomas in about 30% cases

Differential diagnosis of bilateral hilar lymphadenopathy **(Table 6.118)**

Various causes of granuloma are listed in **Table 6.119**.

TABLE 6.118: Differential diagnosis of bilateral hilar lymphadenopathy.

1. **Lymphoma**	Involvement of only the hilar lymph nodes is rare
2. **Pulmonary tuberculosis**	Symmetrical enlargement of hilar lymph nodes is rare
3. **Carcinoma of the bronchus**	Malignant spread to the contralateral hilar lymph nodes is rarely symmetrical

TABLE 6.119: Causes of granulomas.

Infectious diseases	*Noninfectious diseases*
➢ Mycobacterial infections ➢ *Mycobacterium tuberculosis* ➢ Nontuberculous mycobacteria (NTM) ➢ Fungal infections: *Histoplasma, Cryptococcus, Coccidioides, Blastomyces, Pneumocystis jirovecii, Aspergillus* ➢ Other infections: Brucella, Chlamydia, Cat scratch disease	➢ Sarcoidosis, lymphoma, chronic beryllium disease, hypersensitivity pneumonitis, Wegener's granulomatosis, Churg–Strauss syndrome, talc granulomatosis, rheumatoid nodule, foreign body

Treatment

Treatment should be based on symptoms or presence of organ or life-threatening disease.

Minimal or no symptoms

- No treatment is required when there is only hilar lymph adenopathy.
- Persisting infiltration found on the chest X-ray with normal lung function tests requires careful monitoring.

Symptomatic single organ disease

Symptoms limited to only one organ: Topical steroid therapy is preferable.

Symptomatic multiple organ disease

Multiorgan or disease too extensive for topical therapy requires systemic therapy and are usually immunosuppressive including glucocorticoids, cytotoxics, or biologics.

- **Glucocorticoids:** Remain the drugs of choice and given immediately in the presence of hypercalcemia, pulmonary impairment, renal impairment and uveitis. Prednisolone is given 20–40 mg/day for 6 weeks, followed by a maintenance dose of 7.5–10 mg daily for 6–12 months.
- **Steroid-sparing agents:** In patients with severe disease, methotrexate (10–20 mg/week), azathioprine (50–150 mg/day) and the use of specific tumor necrosis factor (TNF)-α inhibitors is useful in patients developing toxicity with glucocorticoids. Chloroquine, hydroxychloroquine, and low-dose thalidomide may be useful for skin, bone, and joint involvement.
- Selected patients may be considered for single lung transplantation.

Bronchopulmonary Aspergillosis

Q. Write short essay/note on bronchopulmonary aspergillosis and classify bronchopulmonary aspergillosis.

Bronchopulmonary aspergillosis is the term used for the bronchopulmonary diseases caused by fungus *Aspergillus* species, the most common being *Aspergillus fumigates*. Others fungus in *Aspergillus* species include *A. clavatus, A. niger, A. flavus* and *A. terreus.*

Classification of Bronchopulmonary Aspergillosis (Table 6.120)

Q. Write short note on classification of bronchopulmonary aspergillosis.

TABLE 6.120: Classification of bronchopulmonary aspergillosis.

- Allergic bronchopulmonary aspergillosis (ABPA-asthmatic pulmonary eosinophilia)
- Extrinsic allergic alveolitis (*Aspergillus clavatus*) (hypersensitivity pneumonitis)
- Intracavitary aspergilloma
- Invasive pulmonary aspergillosis
- Chronic and subacute pulmonary aspergillosis

Allergic Bronchopulmonary Aspergillosis (ABPA-Asthmatic Pulmonary Eosinophilia)

Q. Discuss the clinical features, diagnostic criteria and management of allergic bronchopulmonary aspergillosis (ABPA-asthmatic pulmonary eosinophilia).

Allergic bronchopulmonary aspergillosis (ABPA) occurs due to hypersensitivity reaction against germinating fungal spores in the wall of the airway. Usually hypersensitivity reactions are seen to *A. fumigatus* and rare cases are due to other Aspergilli and other fungi.

- It can complicate bronchial asthma or cystic fibrosis.
- It is one of the causes of pulmonary eosinophilia.

Pathogenesis

Exact pathogenesis of ABPA is not known but probably occurs as a result of a hypersensitivity reaction to germinating fungal spores in the airway wall. Thus, it may be due to *Aspergillus*-specific IgE-mediated type I hypersensitivity reactions or specific IgG-mediated type III hypersensitivity reactions and abnormal T-lymphocyte cellular immune response.

Clinical features

- Fever, breathlessness, coughing up of thick sputum casts and worsening of asthmatic symptoms.
- Aspergillus may grow in the walls of proximal bronchi and may produce **proximal bronchiectasis.** It may cause repeated episodes of eosinophilic pneumonia which manifest as wheeze, cough, fever, and expectoration with sputum-containing fungal mycelia.

Investigations

- Radiological signs on chest X-ray:
  - Radiographically show infiltrates which may be mistaken for pneumonia. Segmental or lobar collapse on chest X-rays in patients where asthma symptoms are stable, suggestive of ABPA.
  - Repeated pneumonic episodes may show fleeting shadows of infiltrates on chest radiographs. Other findings include transient area of opacification (due to mucoid impaction of the airways), band-like opacities with rounded distal margin (gloved-finger appearance), and "ringsing" and "tramlines" (due to thickened and inflamed bronchi). Eventually, it may result in central bronchiectasis and progressive pulmonary fibrosis.
- Other relevant investigations and diagnostic features of allergic bronchopulmonary aspergillosis are mentioned in **Table 6.121**.

TABLE 6.121: Diagnostic features of allergic bronchopulmonary aspergillosis.

Rosenberg-Patterson criteria	
Major criteria (ARTEPICS)	***Minor criteria***
A = Asthma (bronchial) **R** = Roentgenographic fleeting pulmonary opacities **T** = Skin test positive (immediate wheal- and-flare response) for *Aspergillus* (type I) **E** = Eosinophilia in peripheral blood (>1,000/mm³) **P** = Precipitating antibodies (IgG) in serum **I** = IgE in serum elevated (>1,000 IU/mL) **C** = Central/proximal bronchiectasis (inner two thirds of chest CT field) **S** = Serum *A. fumigatus*-specific IgG and IgE (more than twice the value of pooled serum samples from patients with asthma who have *Aspergillus* hypersensitivity)	➤ Sputum - Fungal hyphae of *A. fumigates* and eosinophils on microscopic examination of sputum - Expectoration of brownish black mucus plugs in sputum - Culture of *A. fumigatus* from sputum ➤ Delayed skin reaction to *Aspergillus* antigen (type III). ➤ Presence of 6 of 8 major criteria makes diagnosis almost certain

Management

- Corticosteroids: Oral prednisolone 30 mg daily for 7–10 days causes rapid clearing of the pulmonary infiltrate. Prednisolone should be gradually tapered to a maintenance dose of 5–10 mg/day for long term. Asthma responds to inhaled corticosteroids.
- Antifungal agents: Oral itraconazole Dose: 200 mg bid for 16 weeks, then once a day for 16 weeks, or voriconazole should be used in patients on high doses of steroids. It reduces exacerbations and requirement of steroids.
- Humanized monoclonal antibody against IgE: Omalizumab is undertrial.
- Bronchoscopic extraction of the casts: If there is persistent lobar collapse, bronchoscopic (usually under general anesthesia) removal of impacted mucus and casts may result in reinflation of the collapsed lobe.

Aspergilloma

Q. Discuss the etiology, clinical features, diagnosis, and management of intracavitary aspergilloma (fungal ball).

Aspergilloma is the growth of *Aspergillus* fungus within previously damaged lung tissue and forms a ball of fungus (mycelium) within lung cavities. Most commonly the fungal ball is produced by *Aspergillus fumigatus* and rarely by other fungi (e.g., Zygomycetes and Fusarium).

Etiology

- An intracavitary aspergilloma may develop in any area of damaged lung with abnormal cavity. Inhaled *Aspergillus* may reach and germinate in this cavity forming "aspergilloma."
- **Causes of cavitation associated with Aspergillum:** Colonization and proliferation of fungus in a preexisting lung cavity.
  - **Common cause:** Tuberculosis cavity occurs most often in the upper lobes.
  - **Less common causes:** Lung abscess, sarcoidosis, histoplasmosis, blastomycosis, AIDS pneumonia, bronchiectasis, rheumatoid nodules, pulmonary infarction, and lung cancer
- When there are multiple aspergilloma cavities in a diseased area of lung, it is termed as a "complex aspergilloma."
- Aspergilloma (fungus ball) consists of fungal hyphae, inflammatory cells, fibrin, mucous, and tissue debris.

Clinical Features

- Simple aspergilloma is usually asymptomatic.
- Occasionally it may cause recurrent scanty-to-**massive hemoptysis.** The source of hemoptysis is usually bronchial blood vessels. It may be due to local invasion of blood vessels lining the cavity, endotoxins released from the fungus or mechanical irritation of the vessels inside the cavity during rolling of the fungus ball.
- Nonspecific systemic features such as lethargy and weight loss may be present.

Diagnosis

- Chest X-ray: Shows a round cavity with a tumor-like opacity inside. It is distinguished from a carcinoma by the presence of a crescentic air shadow (halo) between the fungal ball and the upper wall of the cavity. If the radiographs are repeated in a different position, the fungal ball occupies the dependent portion of the cavity. **Crescent sign of Monad (Fig. 6.48).**
- HRCT is more sensitive for demonstration of the fungal ball.
- Serum precipitins to *Aspergillus fumigatus* can be detected.
- Sputum:
  - Microscopic examination shows fungal hyphal fragments.
  - Culture usually grows the fungus.
- Positive skin tests (hypersensitivity) to extracts of *Aspergillus fumigatus*.

Management

- No treatment required for asymptomatic patients.
- Antifungal drugs have not been useful and corticosteroids may predispose to invasion.
- **Surgical removal:**
  - Aspergillomas complicated by hemoptysis should be excised surgically in suitable patients.
  - For patient unfit for surgery, palliative procedures such as ultrasound or CT-guided local injection of amphotericin B is given into the cavity and bronchial artery embolization is done to control hemoptysis.

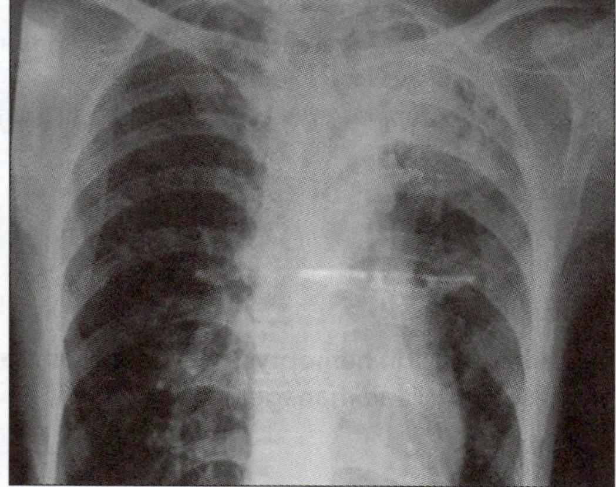

FIG. 6.48: Chest X-ray shows air crescent sign of aspergilloma in the left upper zone.

Invasive Pulmonary Aspergillosis

Q. Discuss the etiology, clinical features, diagnosis, and management of invasive pulmonary aspergillosis.

Invasive pulmonary aspergillosis (IPA) is invasion of previously healthy lung tissue by *Aspergillus fumigates* and usually develops as a complication in patients who are immunocompromised (with profound neutropenia) either by drugs (especially immunosuppressants) and/or disease.

Risk factors for invasive aspergillosis

Refer **Table 6.122**.

Clinical features

Acute IPA (≤1 month): Causes severe necrotizing pneumonia.

They present with fever, cough (sometimes productive), chest discomfort, mild-to-massive hemoptysis, and shortness of breath.

Subacute (1–3 months):

- Local invasion of pulmonary vessels causes thrombosis and infarction.
- Epithelial spread: Involvement of tracheobronchial mucosa produces fungal plaques and ulceration.
- Systemic spread through blood may occur to the brain (causes seizures, ring-enhancing lesions, cerebral infarctions, intracranial hemorrhage, meningitis, and epidural abscess), heart, kidneys, and other organs.

TABLE 6.122: Risk factors for invasive aspergillosis.

- Prolonged neutropenia (<500 cells/mm^3 for >10 days) most common and risk is related to duration and degree
- Solid-organ (particularly lung transplantation) or allogeneic stem cell transplantation
- Prolonged (>3 weeks), high dose corticosteroid therapy
- Leukemia and other hematological malignancies
- Cytotoxic chemotherapy
- Advance AIDS
- Severe COPD
- Critically ill patients on intensive care units
- Chronic granulomatous disease

Diagnosis

- Sputum:
  - Microscopic examination shows fungal hyphal fragments.
  - Culture usually grows the fungus.
- Serum precipitins to *Aspergillus fumigatus* can be detected.
- Chest X-ray: Nonspecific and includes round densities, pleural-based infiltrates (suggestive of pulmonary infarctions) and cavitations.
- HRCT: Very useful for diagnosis particularly in neutropenic patients. Characteristically it shows macronodules (usually ≥1 cm) surrounded by a "halo" (low attenuation due to hemorrhage surrounding the pulmonary nodule) during first 5 days.
- Detection of cell wall components **(galactomannan and β-1, 3-glucan)** in blood or BAL fluid is useful for early confirmation of the diagnosis, and also its serial estimation may be useful in assessing the evolution of infection during treatment.
- PCR to detect *Aspergillus* DNA in BAL fluid and serum.
- Bronchoscopy and BAL transbronchial biopsy is of little value and may produce complications. However, biopsy may be needed for confirmation.

Management

Treatment should not be delayed because IPA has a high mortality rate. It requires aggressive antifungal therapy and immunosuppression should be reduced if possible.

Voriconazole and liposomal amphotericin B allow a safer and more effective treatment of invasive aspergillosis when compared with amphotericin B-deoxycholate.

First-line agents: The treatment of choice is intravenous voriconazole (6 mg/kg every 12 hours for two doses and then 4 mg/kg twice a day). It is better tolerated and more effective than amphotericin B. Antifungal therapy with amphotericin (1.0–1.5 mg/kg/day) with or without flucytosine is equally effective.

Second-line agents: Intravenous echinocandin derivatives such as caspofungin, micafungin, and anidulafungin are used in refractory cases or if the patient cannot tolerate first-line agents.

In less immunosuppressed patients, oral itraconazole (200 mg twice a day) may be given.

Fungal Infections of Lung

Refer **Box 6.18.**

Box 6.18: Fungal infections of the lung.

Endemic fungal pneumonia pathogens in healthy and in immunocompromised individuals

- *Histoplasma capsulatum*
- *Coccidioides immitis*
- *Blastomyces dermatitidis*
- *Paracoccidioides brasiliensis*
- *Sporothrix schenckii*
- *Cryptococcus neoformans*

Opportunistic fungal infections organisms in patients with congenital or acquired defects in the host immune defenses

- *Candida spp.*
- *Aspergillus spp.*
- *Mucor spp.*
- *Cryptococcus neoformans*

HEMOPTYSIS

Q. Write essay on hemoptysis (its definition, causes, clinical features, investigations, and management).

Definition

- Hemoptysis is defined as coughing of blood originating from below the vocal cords.
- Hemoptysis can range from blood-streaking of sputum to the presence of gross blood in the absence of any accompanying sputum.
- Life threatening (or) massive hemoptysis is defined as coughing of blood > 150 mL/time (or) > 600 mL/24 hours.
- Only 5% of hemoptysis is massive but mortality is 80%.
- Clinical definition of massive hemoptysis is any bleeding that result in a threat to life because of airway or hemodynamic compromise due to bleeding.

Causes of Hemoptysis (Tables 6.123 and 6.124)

Q. Write short essay/note on common causes of hemoptysis.

TABLE 6.123: Causes of hemoptysis.

Structure involved	*Common causes*	*Uncommon causes*
Bronchial disease	Bronchial carcinoma, bronchiectasis, acute and chronic bronchitis	Bronchial adenoma, foreign body
Parenchymal disease of lung	Pulmonary tuberculosis (Rasmussen's aneurysm— dilation of a pulmonary artery in a tuberculous cavity), lung abscess, pneumonia (particularly *Klebsiella*), fungal infections (aspergilloma and invasive aspergillosis, pulmonary contusion/laceration(traumatic)	Parasites (e.g., hydatid disease, flukes), trauma, actinomycosis, mycetoma
Vascular diseases of lung	Pulmonary infarction	Goodpasture's syndrome, polyarteritis nodosa, idiopathic, pulmonary hemosiderosis, primary pulmonary hypertension
Cardiovascular disease	Acute left ventricular failure	Mitral stenosis, aortic aneurysm, pulmonary thromboembolism
Hematological disorders		Leukemia, hemophilia, anticoagulants, hemorrhagic diathesis

TABLE 6.124: Causes of massive hemoptysis.

➢ Pulmonary tuberculosis	➢ Cystic fibrosis	➢ Mitral stenosis
➢ Pulmonary infarction	➢ Lung abscess	➢ Pulmonary arteriovenous malformation
➢ Bronchiectasis	➢ Necrotizing pneumonia	
➢ Bronchogenic carcinoma		

Clinical Clues for the Diagnosis of Cause of Hemoptysis (Table 6.125)

TABLE 6.125: Clinical clues for the diagnosis of cause of hemoptysis.

Clinical clues	*Suggested diagnosis*
Anticoagulant use	Medication effect, coagulation disorder
Tobacco use	Acute bronchitis, chronic bronchitis, pneumonia, lung cancer
Dyspnea on exertion, fatigue, orthopnea, paroxysmal nocturnal dyspnea, frothy pink sputum	Congestive heart failure, left ventricular failure, mitral stenosis
Fever, productive cough	Upper respiratory tract infection, acute bronchitis, pneumonia, lung abscess
History of cancer (e.g., breast, colon, or kidney)	Endobronchial metastasis from carcinoma
History of chronic lung disease, recurrent lower respiratory tract infection, cough with copious purulent sputum	Bronchiectasis, lung abscess
Pleuritic chest pain, calf tenderness	Pulmonary embolism or infarction
Toxic symptoms	Tuberculosis
Weight loss	Emphysema, lung cancer, tuberculosis, bronchiectasis, lung abscess
Melena, alcoholism, chronic use of NSAIDs	Gastritis, gastric or peptic ulcer, esophageal varices
Association with menses	Catamenial hemoptysis
Cachexia, clubbing, hoarseness	Lung cancer, small-cell carcinoma
Clubbing	Lung cancer, bronchiectasis, lung abscess
Dullness to percussion, fever, crepitations	Pneumonia

Differences Between True and False Hemoptysis (Table 6.126)

TABLE 6.126: Differences between true and false hemoptysis.

True hemoptysis	*False hemoptysis (Spurious)*
Below vocal cords	Above vocal cords
Persists as blood-tinged sputum	Does not persist
May be mixed with sputum	Not mixed with sputum
History of cardiopulmonary disease	Obvious by ENT examination
Chest X-ray may be abnormal	Normal chest X-ray

Differences Between Hemoptysis and Hematemesis (Table 6.127)

Q. Write short essay/note on differences between hematemesis and hemoptysis.

TABLE 6.127: Differences between hemoptysis and hematemesis.

Hemoptysis	*Hematemesis*
Coughing of blood. Cough precedes hemoptysis	Vomiting of blood. Nausea and vomiting precedes hematemesis
History of cardiopulmonary disease	History of gastrointestinal disease
Bright red in color	Dark brown in color
Sputum remains blood stained after the attack for few days	Usually followed by melena
Mixed with sputum	Mixed with gastric contents
Blood is frothy due to admixture of air	Airless and not frothy
Alkaline	Acidic
Sputum contains hemosiderin-laden macrophages	No
Melena absent	Melena present

Investigations

When a patient comes with massive hemoptysis, initial diagnostic tests **(Table 6.128)** must begin in concert with efforts to stabilize the patient and control the bleeding.

- Other test includes antineutrophil cytoplasmic antibody, antiglomerular basement membrane antibody, and antinuclear antibody.
- Chest X-ray: Posteroanterior and lateral views may provide important diagnostic clues. It may provide evidence of a localized lesion, including tumor (malignant or benign), pneumonia, mycetoma or tuberculosis.

Chest X-ray may be useful in pulmonary thromboembolism, mitral stenosis, primary pulmonary hypertension, pulmonary hemosiderosis, and bronchial adenoma.

- **Computed tomography of the chest:** Useful in delineating lesions that are not seen on a plain chest X-ray and it defines **the lesions better than seen on X**-ray.
  - It is valuable in selected cases to show the presence of lung cavities, solid masses, and mediastinal and hilar lymphadenopathy.
  - Along with fiberoptic bronchoscopy, it gives a greater positive yield of pathology and is useful for excluding malignancy in high-risk patients.
  - Allows application of special imaging techniques, for example, HRCT (1–3 mm thickness section)→ **bronchiectasis** and spiral CT with pulmonary angiography→**pulmonary embolism**.
- **Electrocardiogram:** It may be useful in unsuspected mitral stenosis, pulmonary thromboembolism and pulmonary hypertension.
- **Bronchoscopy:** Most important diagnostic procedure.
- Angiography
- Isotope lung scans: Useful when pulmonary embolism is suspected in a patient with a normal chest radiograph.

TABLE 6.128: Common laboratory tests and their interpretation.

Test	*Diagnostic findings*
Total leukocyte count with differential count	Raised leukocyte count and shift to the left in upper and lower respiratory tract infections
Hemoglobin and hematocrit	Decreased in anemia
Platelet count	Reduced in thrombocytopenia
Prothrombin and partial thromboplastin time	Increased in anticoagulant use, disorders of coagulation
Arterial blood gas	Hypoxia, hypercarbia
D-dimer	Raised in pulmonary embolism
Sputum	
➢ Gram stain, and culture and sensitivity	*Klebsiella pneumoniae*, identify organism in acute exacerbations of chronic bronchitis, bronchiectasis and lung abscess
➢ AFB (Ziehl–Neelsen stain) and culture	Pulmonary tuberculosis
➢ Cytological examination	Neoplasm (bronchial carcinoma)
Tuberculin test	Positive in TB
ESR	↑in infection, autoimmune disorders (e.g., Wegener's syndrome, SLE, Goodpasture's syndrome) and malignancy
Urine microscopy	RBCs and red cell casts in hemorrhagic diathesis and Goodpasture's syndrome

Q. Write short essay/note on:
- **Outline the management of a case of hemoptysis.**
- **Management of massive (potentially lethal) hemoptysis.**

Treatment
- **Medical**
  - Endotracheal tube (single wide bore (or) double lumen)
  - Large-bore IV line for fluids, blood transfusion
  - Avoid cough suppressants (if necessary benzodiazepine)
  - Position of the patient in sitting (or) bleeding side down
  - Supplemental oxygen/mechanical ventilation
  - Vasopressin 0.2–0.4 units/min IV
- **Surgical**
  - Emergency resection for bronchogenic mass
  - Surgical resection for aspergilloma
  - Resection of bronchogenic mass after patient stabilization
- **Endobronchial**
  - Identify: **S**ource, **R**ate and to **S**low (or) **A**rrest bleeding.
  - The rigid bronchoscope is preferred as it enables blood to be aspirated more easily.
  - The fiberoptic bronchoscopy may be used for cold saline lavage, which may sometimes arrest bleeding. The iced saline is instilled in 50–100 mL aliquots followed by suctioning and repeated until there is noticeable improvement.

- Other techniques used to control bleeding include: Topical thrombin or fibrinogen, topical coagulation with laser photocoagulation (Nd:YAG), argon plasma coagulator, endobronchial brachytherapy in high doses (10–12 Gy/h for a total of 500–4,000 Gy), endobronchial cryotherapy.
- A balloon catheter passed through the bronchoscope can be inflated proximally in the bleeding bronchus. This will isolate the source of bleeding from the rest of the lung and the contralateral lung, preventing asphyxiation by blood flooding.

- **Endovascular**
  - In most patients, the bleeding originates from bronchial arteries rather than pulmonary arteries.
  - Transcatheter embolization is effective in immediate control of massive hemoptysis (73–98%).
  - Causes of recurrence: Incomplete embolization of artery, recanalization of previously embolized artery, revascularization through collateral circulation, progression of basic lung disease.

Management of hemoptysis is summarized in **Flowchart 6.19.**

FLOWCHART 6.19: Management of hemoptysis.

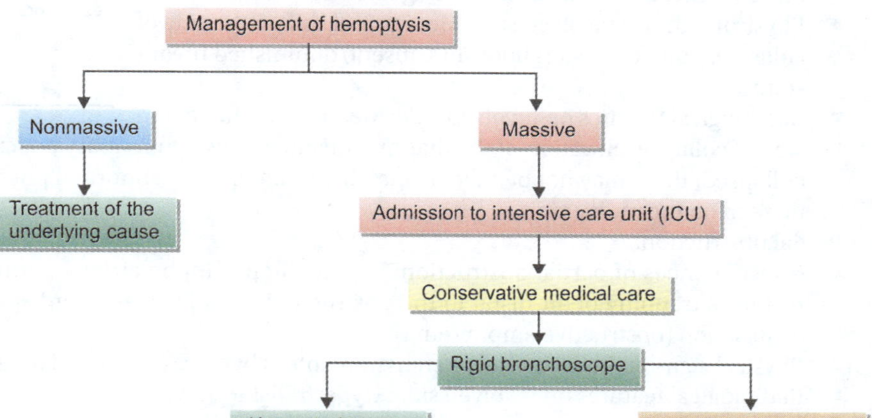

DYSPNEA

Q. Discuss briefly the differential diagnosis of acute-onset dyspnea.

Q. Write short note on respiratory causes of acute breathlessness (dyspnea).

Dyspnea or breathlessness is defined as **subjective experience of breathing discomfort** (i.e., uncomfortable need to breathe). It is a sense of awareness of increased respiratory effort that is unpleasant and recognized by the patient as being inappropriate. Patient often complains of tightness in the chest.

Causes of Dyspnea (Table 6.129)

Acute dyspnea: Dyspnea arising over the course of a few minutes to 24-28 hours is termed acute dyspnea.

TABLE 6.129: Causes of acute and chronic dyspnea.

Acute dyspnea	*Chronic dyspnea*
Cardiovascular system	
Cardiogenic acute pulmonary edema	Chronic heart failure, myocardial ischemia
Respiratory system	
➢ Acute severe bronchial asthma	➢ COPD
➢ Acute exacerbation of COPD	➢ Chronic bronchial asthma
➢ Spontaneous pneumothorax	➢ Bronchial carcinoma
➢ Pneumonia	➢ Interstitial lung disease (e.g., sarcoidosis, fibrosing alveolitis, extrinsic allergic alveolitis, pneumoconiosis)
➢ Acute pulmonary embolism	
➢ ARDS	
➢ Inhaled foreign body (especially in children)	
➢ Lobar collapse	➢ Chronic pulmonary thromboembolism
➢ Laryngeal edema (e.g., anaphylaxis) or obstruction	➢ Lymphatic carcinomatosis
	➢ Large pleural effusion(s)
➢ Metabolic acidosis (e.g., diabetic ketoacidosis, lactic acidosis, uremia, overdose of salicylates, ethylene glycol poisoning)	➢ Severe anemia
	➢ Obesity
➢ Psychogenic hyperventilation (anxiety or panic-related)	➢ Deconditioning

Bronchial Obstruction

Q. Write short note on the causes, clinical presentation, and management of bronchial obstruction.

Causes

See **Table 6.130**.

Clinical Features

Depends on the following:

- Cause of obstruction
- Degree of obstruction: Complete or partial obstruction.
- Presence or absence of secondary infection
- Effect on function of lung.

TABLE 6.130: Causes of bronchial obstruction.

Causes	Disease/lesion
Tumors	Bronchial adenoma or carcinoma
Enlarged tracheobronchial lymph nodes	Malignancy, Hodgkin lymphoma, non-Hodgkin lymphoma, tuberculosis
Inhaled foreign bodies	Common foreign bodies nuts, peas, beans, small pieces of toys, articles of food
Bronchial casts or plugs	Inspissated mucus (in asthma or pulmonary eosinophilia) or blood clots (severe hemoptysis)
Ineffective expectoration	Results in collection of mucus or mucopus in the bronchus
Rarely	Congenital bronchial atresia, post-tuberculous bronchial stricture, aortic aneurysm

Degree of Obstruction

- Complete obstruction:
  - Consequences of complete obstruction: Absorption of air distal to the obstruction, closure of alveolar spaces, collapse and solidification of the affected lung distal to obstruction.
  - Physical signs on involved side: Mediastinal shift to the side of collapse, dull percussion note, and absent/diminished breath sounds.
  - Radiological features on involved side: Mediastinal shift to the side of collapse, elevation of the diaphragm and a dense pulmonary opacity. When only small portion of the lung is collapsed, there may not be mediastinal displacement and abnormal physical signs, but a characteristic opacity will be seen on the radiograph.
- Partial obstruction:
  - Consequences of partial obstruction: Less resistance to the airflow during inspiration than during expiration and results is trapping of air distal to the obstruction. This leads to overdistension of the part of the lung distal to the obstruction (obstructive emphysema).
  - Physical signs on involved side: Percussion note is hyperresonant and breath sounds are diminished.
  - Radiological features on involved side: Hypertranslucency.

Features of Secondary Infection

- Secondary bacterial infection usually develops distal to the obstruction and is usually caused by microorganism of low virulence. Sometimes suppuration can produce lung abscess.
- It may manifest as a recurrent pneumonia in the same segment/lobe of the involved lung.

Effect on Function of Lung

- Symptoms usually follow if there is obstruction of a main or lobar bronchus.
- Sudden occlusion may produce severe breathlessness and hypoxemia.

Management

- Identify the cause of obstruction: By chest X-ray, bronchoscopy and biopsy.
- Treat the underlying cause.
- Remove foreign bodies, bronchial casts, plugs and secretions by bronchoscopy.

PULMONARY EOSINOPHILIC SYNDROMES

Q. Write short essay/note on:

- **Causes of eosinophilia**
- **Diagnosis, differential diagnosis and management/treatment of tropical pulmonary eosinophilia.**

Heterogenous group of pulmonary disorders characterized by pulmonary parenchymal or peripheral blood eosinophilia

1. ***Loeffler's syndrome (simple pulmonary eosinophilia)***
   - It is a clinical syndrome characterized by:
     - Mild respiratory symptoms
     - Peripheral blood eosinophilia, and
     - Transient, migratory pulmonary infiltrates.
   - Affects all ages
   - **Immune hypersensitivity to *Ascaris lumbricoides*** is the likely cause. Other parasites such as Necator, Ancylostoma, and Dirofilaria, can be associated
   - Chest X-ray: Transient, migratory, nonsegmental interstitial and alveolar infiltrates (often peripheral or pleural based).
   - Pulmonary function tests: Typically reveals mild-to-moderate restrictive ventilatory defect with a reduced diffusing capacity of the lungs for carbon monoxide (DLCO).

2. ***Drug and toxin-induced pulmonary eosinophilic syndromes***
   - Onset: Acute or subacute.
   - Respiratory symptoms: Vary widely in severity.
     - Mild Loeffler's-like illness with dyspnea, cough, and fever
     - Severe fulminant respiratory failure
   - Drugs implicated are acetyl salicylate, nitrofurantoin, bleomycin, methotrexate, minocycline, sulfa drugs, gold salts, INH, etc.
3. ***Idiopathic acute eosinophilic pneumonia***
   - More common in younger men (mean age about 30 years).
   - Occurs commonly in previously healthy persons. Also seen in persons with history of chronic myeloid leukemia (CML), HIV infection, recent commencement of smoking, etc.
   - Diagnostic criteria:
     - Acute onset of febrile respiratory manifestations (≤1 month duration before consultation).
     - Bilateral diffuse infiltrates on chest X-ray.
     - Hypoxemia, with PaO_2 on room air < 60 mm Hg, and/or PaO_2/FiO_2 ≤300 mm Hg, and/or oxygen saturation on room air <90%.
     - Lung eosinophilia, with >25% eosinophils in BAL (or eosinophilic pneumonia at lung biopsy).
     - Absence of infection, or of other known causes of eosinophilic lung disease (especially, exposure to drug known to induce pulmonary eosinophilia).

Treatment
- Initial doses of methyl-prednisolone used in the range from 60 to 125 mg every 6 hours.
- After resolution of respiratory failure, oral prednisolone (in doses of 40–60 mg per day) may be continued for 2–4 weeks with a subsequent slow taper over the next several weeks.
- Idiopathic acute eosinophilic pneumonia (AEP) carries an excellent prognosis.

4. ***Tropical pulmonary eosinophilia***

Q. Write short note on tropical pulmonary eosinophilia, its diagnosis and management.

Tropical pulmonary eosinophilia (TPE) was first described in the early 1940s by Weingarten, in India. It is seen mainly in South and South-east Asia and Africa.

Definition: Tropical pulmonary eosinophilia is an occasional atypical host response (hypersensitivity reaction) of an individual to a mosquito-borne filarial infection by tissue-dwelling human nematode (microfilariae) *Wuchereria bancrofti and Brugia malayi.*

Pathogenesis: When filarial parasites are destroyed, the antigens released initiate an immediate IgE-mediated reaction. There is dense inflammatory reaction with eosinophils which over time, progresses to granuloma formation and fibrosis. In children, marked enlargement of lymph nodes and spleen **(Meyers-Kouwenaar syndrome)** may be evident. In adults, symptoms are predominantly due to lung involvement. Microfilariae are trapped in the pulmonary capillaries and produce symptoms of lung involvement.

Clinical features
- Paroxysmal dry cough, fever, malaise, anorexia, weight loss, dyspnea or wheeze/nocturnal bronchospasm (asthma-like symptoms) and miliary pulmonary infiltrates **(Weingarten syndrome or tropical pulmonary eosinophilia).**
- Tropical pulmonary eosinophilia is a complication seen mainly in India. If untreated, it may progress to chronic interstitial lung disease. Spontaneous resolution over several weeks.
- Other features:
  - Presentation can be similar to status asthmaticus
  - Chest pain, muscle tenderness, pericardial and CNS involvement
  - Rarely, patients remain asymptomatic.
- Chest examination: Coarse crackles and rhonchi.
- Generalized lymphadenopathy and hepatosplenomegaly may be present.

Diagnosis
- **History** of long period of residence in an endemic area.
- Peripheral blood:
  - Absence of microfilariae in the despite repeated examinations.
  - Marked peripheral blood **eosinophilia** in excess of 3,000/mL.
- Chest X-ray—miliary mottling.
- Serological findings
  - High titers of antifilarial antibodies.
  - Elevated levels of total IgE (at least 1,000 units/mL).
- **Therapeutic response to DEC** (6 mg/kg/day for 3 weeks) within 7–10 days of initiating therapy.

Treatment: Diethylcarbamazine in a dose of 2 mg/kg orally three times a day for 14–21 days or for as long as 4 weeks. It is directly filaricidal to both adult worms and microfilariae.

5. ***Chronic eosinophilic pneumonia***
   - Typically subacute presentation.
   - Symptoms present for several months before diagnosis.
   - Common presenting complaints include: Low-grade fevers, drenching night sweats, moderate (10–50 pound) weight loss, cough.
   - History of atopy, allergic rhinitis, or nasal polyps may be found.
   - About 2/3 develop adult-onset asthma: Preceding or concurrent with the occurrence of CEP.
   - No major extrapulmonary manifestations
   - Chest X-ray: Bilateral opacities in upper and mid zone. Photographic negative of pulmonary edema.
   - Corticosteroids are the mainstay of therapy for CEP. Dramatic clinical, radiographic, and physiological improvements.
6. ***Allergic bronchopulmonary aspergillosis*** *(discussed earlier)*
7. ***Churg–Strauss syndrome:*** It is a form of necrotizing vasculitis in several organs, associated with eosinophilic tissue inflammation and extravascular granulomas. It occurs in asthmatics and presents with fever and peripheral hypereosinophilia (discussed on page 714).
8. ***Idiopathic hypereosinophilic syndrome***
   - Several names: Eosinophilic leukemia, Loeffler's fibroblastic endocarditis, disseminated eosinophilic cardiovascular disease.
   - **Clinical features:** Often nonspecific and include:
     - Weakness, fatigue, low-grade fevers, myalgias, cough, angioedema, rash, retinal lesions, and dyspnea.
     - Can affect every organ system.
     - Cough is nocturnal, either nonproductive or productive of small quantities of nonpurulent sputum.
     - Wheezing and dyspnea without evidence of airflow obstruction on spirometry.
     - Pulmonary hypertension, ARDS, and pleural effusions.
     - Progressive chronic heart failure due to eosinophilic myocarditis and endocarditis, intracardiac thrombi and endocardial fibrosis.
     - Encephalopathy with neuropsychiatric dysfunction, thromboembolic events such as hemiparesis. Peripheral neuropathy is extremely common in IHS.
     - Hepatosplenomegaly, lymphadenopathy
   - **Investigations:**
     - Anemia, thrombocytopenia
     - Elevated vitamin B_{12} levels
     - Bone marrow: Universally affected with a striking eosinophilia (up to 25–75% of the differential count).

Treatment
- Glucocorticoids are the first-line therapy in all patients without FIP1L1/PDGFRA mutation.
- Patients with FIP1L1/PDGFRA mutation: Imatinib is the drug of choice with a very good response rate.
- Other drugs include: Hydroxyurea, vincristine, interferons, anti-IL-5 monoclonal antibody (e.g., mepolizumab) and an anti-CD52 antibody (alemtuzumab).

Causes of Calcification in Lung Parenchyma (Box 6.19)

Q. Write short note on causes of calcification in lung parenchyma.

Box 6.19: Calcification in lung parenchyma.

Micronodules

Pulmonary alveolar microlithiasis, occupational lung diseases (e.g., silicosis, coal-worker's pneumoconiosis)

Large nodules or masses
- Granulomatous disease (tuberculosis, histoplasmosis)
- Primary lung cancer (5–10%)
- Metastasis to lung (e.g., osteosarcoma, chondrosarcoma)
- Nonmalignant metastatic calcification in lung (e.g., renal failure, hyperparathyroidism)
- Multiple pulmonary chondroma (e.g., with Carney triad)
- Others: Chickenpox pneumonia, hemosiderosis, pulmonary hemorrhage

Breath Sounds (Fig. 6.49)

Q. Write short note on:
- **Causes of bronchial breathing, tubular and amphoric breathing. Three components of tubular breathing.**
- **Cavernous breathing.**

Normal breath sounds are produced by vibration of vocal cords due to turbulent flow in the larynx. This sound is harsher anteriorly over the upper lobes (particularly on the right).

- **Vesicular breath sounds:** Healthy lungs filter out most of the high-frequency component, and the resulting low-pitched, rustling sounds are called vesicular. Inspiration is longer than expiration and there is no gap in between and rustling in character.

- Conditions with diminished vesicular breath sounds are heard in bronchial asthma, tumors, pleural effusion (small), pleural thickening, collapsed lung with occluded bronchus, and emphysema.
- **Bronchial breath sounds** are produced by the passage of air through the trachea and large bronchi. It is loud and high pitched. Inspiration and expiration are of equal duration, there is a gap between inspiration and expiration, and the quality is guttural or aspirate.
    - Types of bronchial breathing
        - **Tubular:** High pitched and heard in pneumonia with consolidation, partially collapsed lung or lobe and above the level of pleural effusion (relaxation atelectasis)
        - **Cavernous:** Low pitched and heard in thick-walled cavity with communicating bronchus.
        - **Amphoric:** Low pitched with high tone and a metallic quality. It is heard in bronchopleural fistula, rarely over a superficial cavity and tension pneumothorax.
- Bronchovesicular breath sound: This is classically seen in obstructive lung disease where expiration is prolonged; however, there is no gap in between.

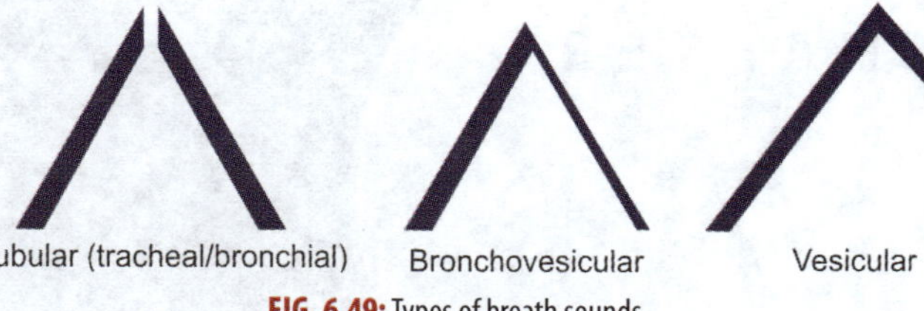

FIG. 6.49: Types of breath sounds.

Indications of Bronchoscopy (Table 6.131)

Q. List the indications for bronchoscopy.

TABLE 6.131: Indications of bronchoscopy.

Diagnostic	*Therapeutic*
➢ Diagnosis of lung cancer ➢ Chest radiographic abnormality (lung tumor or changes suggestive of bronchial obstruction, such as appearance of early volume loss or undoubted collapse, unresolved pneumonia or hemidiaphragmatic paralysis) ➢ Evaluation of hemoptysis ➢ Evaluation of persistent or recurrent cough ➢ Evaluation of paralyzed vocal cord ➢ To obtain positive sputum cytology ➢ Staging of lung cancer ➢ Diagnosis of diffuse lung disease ➢ Identification of infecting agents	➢ Insertion of an endotracheal tube for general anesthesia in patients in whom extension of neck may be dangerous (atlantoaxial subluxation) ➢ Tamponade of endobronchial bleeding, either with end of bronchoscope itself or by using a Fogarty ➢ Removal of foreign bodies ➢ Aspiration of secretions in acute inflammatory lobar atelectasis where physiotherapy has proved unsuccessful in achieving this end ➢ Relief of tracheobronchial narrowing by laser treatment ➢ Treatment of lung cancer by placement of stents or delivery of endobronchial radiotherapy (brachytherapy)

Bronchoalveolar Lavage

Q. Write a short note on bronchoalveolar lavage.

Bronchoalveolar lavage (BAL) is a diagnostic procedure used to recover cellular and noncellular components of the epithelial lining fluid from the alveolar and bronchial air spaces.

Common findings on BAL

Increased neutrophils (>5%) (Normal <3%)	Idiopathic pulmonary fibrosis (IPF), acute respiratory distress syndrome (ARDS), infections, connective tissue disorders, pneumoconiosis
Eosinophilia (Normal <1–2%)	>25%: suggesting eosinophilic lung diseases such as acute eosinophilic pneumonia, chronic eosinophilic pneumonia, and Churg–Strauss syndrome
Lymphocytosis (Normal <15%)	>50%: Hypersensitivity pneumonitis ➢ When greater than or equal to 15% lymphocytes are present, CD4/CD8 ratios can be assessed. - Elevated CD4/CD8: Hypersensitivity pneumonitis (chronic or smoker), sarcoidosis, berylliosis, asbestosis, Crohn disease, connective tissue disorders - Normal CD4/CD8: Tuberculosis, malignancies - Low CD4/CD8: Acute hypersensitivity pneumonitis, silicosis, drug-induced lung disease, HIV infection, BOOP (COP)
Alveolar macrophages (normal >80%)	Decreased in sarcoidosis (to less than 50%)
RBCs	Alveolar hemorrhage
Diagnosis of infection	*Mycobacterium tuberculosis, Aspergillus. Pneumocystis carinii, Toxoplasma gondii Strongyloides stercoralis, Legionella pneumophila, Cryptococcus neoformans, Histoplasma capsulatum, Mycoplasma pneumoniae,* Influenza A and B viruses, respiratory syncytial virus
Diagnosis of malignancy	
Progressively darkening aliquots of bloody BAL fluid is highly suggestive of diffuse alveolar hemorrhage	
Pulmonary alveolar microlithiasis—Calcospherites can be demonstrated in BAL fluid	

CHAPTER

7

Cardiology

INTRODUCTION AND SYMPTOMATOLOGY

Chest Pain

Q. Write a short essay on the differential diagnosis of chest pain. List the noncardiac causes of chest pain.

Chest pain is a common symptom of cardiac disease. It can be due to noncardiac causes, such as anxiety or diseases involving the respiratory, musculoskeletal, or gastrointestinal systems.

Common Causes of Chest Pain (Fig. 7.1)

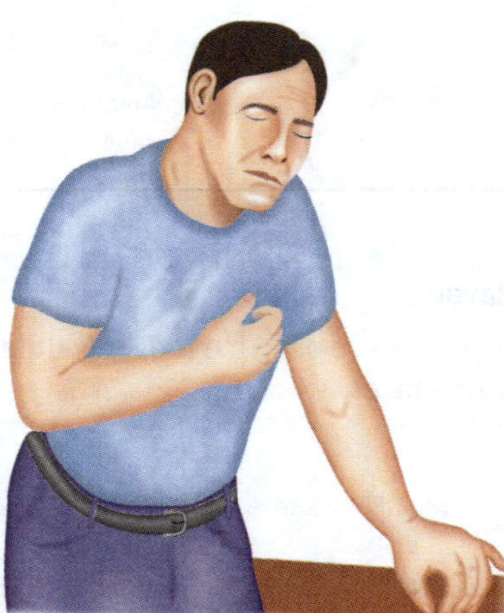

FIG. 7.1: Causes of chest pain.

Differential Diagnosis of Chest Pain (Table 7.1)

TABLE 7.1: Differential diagnosis of chest pain.

Potentially life-threatening causes	*Common non-life-threatening causes*
➢ Acute coronary syndromes: Acute myocardial infarction (MI), ST-segment elevation MI, non-ST-segment elevation MI ➢ Unstable angina ➢ Pulmonary embolism ➢ Aortic dissection ➢ Myocarditis ➢ Tension pneumothorax ➢ Acute chest syndrome/crisis in sickle cell anemia ➢ Pericarditis ➢ Boerhaave's syndrome (perforated esophagus) ➢ Gastrointestinal: Perforated peptic ulcer, acute pancreatitis, acute cholecystitis	➢ Gastrointestinal: – Biliary colic – Gastroesophageal reflux disease – Peptic ulcer disease ➢ Pulmonary: – Pneumonia – Pleuritis ➢ Musculoskeletal pain: Costochondritis (Tietze's syndrome), intercostal myalgia/neuralgia, fracture of the ribs (cough, trauma), secondaries in the ribs, Bornholm disease ➢ Thoracic radiculopathy: Texidor's twinge (precordial catch syndrome) ➢ Emotional: Anxiety ➢ Neural: Shingles/herpes zoster

Differential Features of Ischemic Cardiac and Noncardiac Pain (Table 7.2)

TABLE 7.2: Differential features of ischemic cardiac and noncardiac pain.

Features	*Ischemic cardiac pain*	*Noncardiac pain*
Site	Central, diffuse	Peripheral, localized
Character of pain	Tight, squeezing, dull, constricting, choking or 'heavy'	Sharp, stabbing, catching
Precipitation/provocation	Exertion, emotion	Spontaneous, not related to exertion
Radiation	Jaw/neck/shoulder	Usually no radiation
Relieving factors	Rest (in less than 5 minutes), nitrates	Not relieved by rest or by nitrates
Associated features	Breathlessness, diaphoresis	Depends on the cause

Differentiating Features

Differentiating features of the common causes of chest pain are shown in **Table 7.3.**

TABLE 7.3: Differentiating features of the common causes of chest pain.

Disease	*Description*	*Location*	*Radiation*	*Associations*
Acute coronary syndromes	Crushing, tightening, squeezing, or pressure like	Retrosternal, left anterior chest or epigastric	Right (R) or left (L) shoulder, R or L arm/hand/jaw	Dyspnea, diaphoresis, nausea
Pulmonary embolism	Heaviness, tightness	Whole chest (massive) or focal chest (segmental)	None	Dyspnea, unstable vital signs, feeling of impending doom if massive or just tachycardia, tachypnea if segmental
Aortic dissection	Ripping, tearing	Midline, substernal	Interscapular area of back	Secondary arterial branch occlusion (paraplegia)
Pericarditis/cardiac tamponade	Sharp, constant or pleuritic	Substernal	None	Fever, dyspnea, pericardial friction rub
Pneumothorax	Sudden, sharp, lancinating, pleuritic	One side of chest	Shoulder, back	Dyspnea
Perforated esophagus	Sudden, sharp, after forceful vomiting	Substernal	Back	Dyspnea, diaphoresis, signs of sepsis

Palpitations

Q. Discuss the approach to a patient with palpitations.

- Palpitation is the term used to describe an uncomfortable increased awareness of one's own heartbeat or the sensation of slow, rapid, or irregular heart rhythms.
- Palpitations do not always indicate the presence of arrhythmia and conversely, an arrhythmia can occur without palpitations. Palpitations are usually noted when the patient is quietly resting.
- Palpitation can be either intermittent or sustained and either regular or irregular. **A change in the rate, rhythm, or force of contraction can produce palpitations**.

Causes of Palpitations

See **Table 7.4**.

TABLE 7.4: Causes of palpitations.

Cardiac causes: ➢ **Cardiac arrhythmias:** – Premature atrial and ventricular contractions – Supraventricular and ventricular arrhythmias ➢ **Structural heart diseases:** – Atrial myxoma, valvular heart disease – Congenital heart disease, cardiomyopathy – Mitral valve prolapse, pacemaker	**Drug-induced:** ➢ Alcohol (use or withdrawal) ➢ Atropine ➢ Amphetamines ➢ Caffeine, nicotine ➢ Cocaine ➢ Beta agonists, theophylline
Psychosomatic disorders: Generalized anxiety, major depression, and panic disorder	**Endocrine:** Hyperthyroidism, hypoglycemia, and pheochromocytoma
High output states: Anemia, beriberi, fever, pregnancy, and thyrotoxicosis	**Miscellaneous and idiopathic:** Emotional stress, hyperventilation, premenstrual syndrome, and strenuous physical activity

Evaluation of Palpitation (Box 7.1)

Box 7.1: Evaluation of palpitation.

- Detect and identify any underlying arrhythmia
- Determine presence of any organic heart disease
- Determine any precipitating cause

Clinical presentation

- **Duration and frequency of palpitations:**
  - Duration may be either short-lasting or persistent
  - Note onset and offset of palpitations
  - Frequency: It may occur daily, weekly, monthly, or yearly.
- **Types of palpitations:** They are classified according to the rate, rhythm, and intensity of heartbeat as follows:
  - **Extrasystolic palpitations:** Due to ectopic beats, usually produce feelings of 'missing/skipping a beat' and/or a 'sinking of the heart' interspersed with

periods during which the heart beats normally. Patients report that the heart seems to stop and then start again. It can often be seen in even in young individuals, usually without any disease of the heart, and generally benign.
  - **Tachycardiac palpitations** is the rapid fluctuation like "beating wings" in the chest. It may be regular (e.g., in atrioventricular tachycardia, atrial flutter, or ventricular tachycardia) or irregular or arrhythmic (e.g., in atrial fibrillation).
  - **Anxiety-related palpitations** are perceived as a form of anxiety. They begin and end gradually.
- **Associated symptoms and circumstances:**
  - Palpitations developing after sudden changes in posture are usually due to intolerance to orthostatic or to episodes of atrioventricular nodal re-entrant tachycardia.
  - Occurrence of syncope or other symptoms, such as severe fatigue, dyspnea, or angina, in addition to palpitations, is more common with structural heart disease.
  - Hypersecretion of natriuretic hormone results in polyuria/postpalpitation diuresis in atrial fibrillation.
  - Palpitations associated with anxiety or during panic attacks are usually due to sinus tachycardia secondary to the mental disturbance.
  - Palpitations may be produced by an increase in the sympathetic drive during physical exercise.
- **Typical description:**
  - **Flip-flopping in the chest:** Palpitations are sensed as the heart seeming to stop and then start again, producing a pounding or flip-flopping sensation. This type of palpitation is generally caused by supraventricular or ventricular premature contractions.
  - **Rapid fluttering in the chest:** It is due to a sustained ventricular or supraventricular arrhythmia, including sinus tachycardia.
  - **Pounding in the neck:** An irregular pounding feeling in the neck is caused by atrioventricular dissociation, with independent contraction of the atria and ventricles, resulting in occasional atrial contraction against a closed tricuspid and mitral valve. This produces cannon A waves, which are intermittent increases in the "A" wave of the jugular venous pulse. **Cannon A** waves may be seen with ventricular premature contractions, third-degree or complete heart block, or ventricular tachycardia (VT).

Physical examination

It may help to confirm or refute the presence of an arrhythmia as a cause for palpitations:
- Measurement of the vital signs
- Assessment of the jugular venous pressure and pulse
- Auscultation of the chest and precordium

Investigations

- **Electrocardiogram:**
  - Resting electrocardiogram can be used to diagnose the arrhythmia.
  - If exertion induces the arrhythmia and palpitations, exercise electrocardiography can be used to make the diagnosis.
  - It may reveal bundle branch block (LBBB), short PR interval, delta waves, prolonged QT interval, ischemia, and enlargement of heart chambers, prior myocardial infarction, or other organic diseases of the heart.

If the arrhythmia is not frequent, other methods must be used. These include:
- **Continuous electrocardiographic (Holter) monitoring** or telephonic monitoring.
- **Echocardiography:** To evaluate any structural heart disease and assessment of left ventricular function.
- **Electrophysiology study** is an invasive test of electrical conduction system of heart.
- **Blood tests:** Hemoglobin, serum glucose level, serum electrolytes, and thyroid function tests depending on the clinical findings.

Management of palpitation
- Most of the causes do not have serious arrhythmias or underlying structural heart disease.
- In symptomatic patients, occasional benign atrial or ventricular premature contractions can often be treated by beta-blockers.
- Avoid precipitation factor, such as alcohol, tobacco, or illicit drugs.
- If caused by pharmacologic agents: Consider alternative therapies if appropriate or possible.
- Psychiatric causes: By cognitive therapy or pharmacotherapy.
- Reassurance: After all the serious causes have been excluded.

Dyspnea

Q. Write short note on causes of acute dyspnea.

Definition: "Dyspnea" is a term used to characterize a subjective experience of breathing discomfort that is comprised of qualitatively distinct sensations that vary in intensity. The experience derives from interactions among multiple physiological, psychological, social, and environmental factors, and may induce secondary physiological and behavioral responses.

Causes of Dyspnea

Refer **Table 6.129**.

Mechanisms

- **Chemoreceptors:**
  - **Peripheral:** Carotid and aortic bodies (sensitive to changes pO_2, pCO_2, and H^+)
  - **Central:** Medulla (sensitive only to changes pCO_2, not pO_2, change in pH of CSF).
- **Increased work of breathing:**
  - **Airflow obstruction:** Bronchial asthma, chronic obstructive pulmonary disease (COPD), and tracheal obstruction
  - **Decreased pulmonary compliance:** Pulmonary edema, fibrosis, and allergic alveolitis
  - **Restricted chest expansion:** Ankylosing spondylitis, respiratory paralysis, and kyphoscoliosis.
- **Increased ventilatory drive:**
  - **Increased physiological dead space (V/Q mismatch):** Consolidation, collapse, pleural effusion (PE), and pulmonary edema
  - Hyperventilation due to receptor stimulation
  - **Chemoreceptors:** Acidosis, hypoxia (shock, pneumonia), and hypercapnia
  - **J receptors at alveolo-capillary junction:** Pulmonary edema, pulmonary embolism, and pulmonary congestion (activates Hering-Breuer reflex which terminates inspiratory effort before full inspiration is achieved—rapid and shallow)
  - **Muscle spindles in intercostal muscles:** Tension-length disparity
  - **Central:** Exertion, anxiety, thyrotoxicosis, and pheochromocytoma
- **Impaired respiratory muscle function:** Poliomyelitis, Guillain-Barré syndrome (GBS), and myasthenia gravis.

Orthopnea

Dyspnea develops in recumbent position and is relieved by sitting up or by elevation of the head with pillows.

- Pulmonary congestion during recumbency (cannot be pumped out of LV) seen in congestive heart failure (CHF), COPD, and bronchial asthma.
- Increased venous return
- Diaphragm elevation leading to decreased vital capacity.

Basics: *A normal 70 kg person breathes 12–15/minute with a tidal volume of 600 mL. A normal individual is not aware of respiratory effort until ventilation is doubled, and dyspnea is not experienced until ventilation is tripled.*

Causes of dyspnea in COPD are listed in **Box 7.2**.

Paroxysmal nocturnal dyspnea (PND): Attacks of dyspnea occur at night and awaken the patient from sleep.

- It is due to decreased responsiveness of respiratory center in brain during sleep and pulmonary congestion (due to increased sympathetic activity during REM sleep) 2–3 hours after onset of sleep.
- Takes 10–30 minutes for recovery after upright posture.
- Causes: Specific sign of LV dysfunction and includes ischemic heart disease, aortic valve disease, hypertension, and cardiomyopathy.

Differences between **orthopnea and paroxysmal nocturnal dyspnea** are presented in **Table 7.5**.

Box 7.2: Dyspnea in COPD.

- Hypoxia and hypercapnia: Chemoreceptors
- Increased airway resistance and hyperinflation
- Deconditioning: Reduced threshold at which respiratory muscles produce lactic acidosis

TABLE 7.5: Differences between paroxysmal nocturnal dyspnea and orthopnea.

	Paroxysmal nocturnal dyspnea	*Orthopnea*
Definition	Episode of sudden onset of dyspnea 2–2.5 hours after sleep	Dyspnea in recumbent posture
Timing	Patient wakes up from rapid eye movement (REM) sleep	Occurs soon after lying down
Method of relief	Sits up with legs hanging down, stands up, air hunger, self ventilates to comfort	Gets up, uses more pillows, sleeps in erect posture
Mechanism	Depressed respiratory center. Sympathetic overactivity during REM → catecholamine surge resulting in tachycardia → interstitial pulmonary congestion → respiratory center lags behind → perceived as acute dyspnea. There is sudden transient increase in PCWP	Shifting of venous blood (>400 Ml) into pulmonary circulation, V/Q mismatch, compression of diaphragm, postural diastolic dysfunction. There is a slow sustained rise in pulmonary capillary wedge pressure (PCWP)
Associated symptoms	Angina, perspiration, palpitation, rarely hemoptysis	All the symptoms of congestive cardiac failure (CCF)
Oxygen saturation	Transient hypoxia	Normal
Differential diagnosis	Night mares/panic attacks/nocturnal hypoglycemia/ obstructive sleep apnea (OSA)	COPD/gross obesity/acute asthma/gross ascites

Trepopnea

Aggravation of dyspnea when lying on one side and relieved by lying on opposite side. Its causes are:

- **Unilateral lung disease:** Uninvolved normal lung receives more blood supply due to gravity.
- **Congestive heart failure:** Lying on right side enhances venous return and sympathetic activity.
- **Lung tumor:** Gravity-induced compression of blood vessels or lung.

Platypnea: Dyspnea on sitting or standing and relieved by supine position. Its causes are:

- Venous to arterial shunting (lung bases)
- Intracardiac shunts (ASD, pneumonectomy)
- Intrapulmonary right to left shunt [hepatopulmonary syndrome, pulmonary embolism (PE), COPD]
- Acute respiratory distress syndrome (ARDS)

Bendopnea

A newly described symptom in patients with heart failure, is mediated via a further increase in ventricular filling pressures during bending in subjects whose sitting ventricular filling pressures are already high, particularly in patients with low cardiac index.

A patient sits in a chair, bends at the waist, and touches his/her feet. Bendopnea is considered present if dyspnea occurs within 30s of bending.

Approach to Dyspnea

- **Onset and duration:**
  - **Minutes to hours (rapid onset):** Pneumothorax, acute asthma, PE, pulmonary edema, and foreign body.
  - **Hours to days (gradual onset):** Pneumonia, pleural effusion, anemia, Guillain-Barré syndrome (GBS).
  - **Months to years (slow onset):** Pulmonary tuberculosis (PTB), COPD, carcinoma, and fibrosing alveolitis.
- **Severity of dyspnea (Table 7.6)**
- **Aggravating and relieving factors:**
  - **Improves on weekend/holidays:** Occupational asthma, extrinsic allergic alveolitis
  - **Recumbency/sleep:** Orthopnea/paroxysmal nocturnal dyspnea (PND)

Q. NYHA functional classification of cardiac disability (Table 7.6).

- **Associated symptoms:**
  - **Pleuritic chest pain:** Pneumonia, pulmonary infarction, rib fracture, and pneumothorax
  - **Central nonpleuritic chest pain:** Myocardial infarction, massive pulmonary embolism
  - **Cough or wheeze:** Asthma, pulmonary embolism, and pneumothorax

TABLE 7.6: Severity of dyspnea.

Medical Research Council (MRC) grading of severity of dyspnea	*New York Heart Association (NYHA) classification of severity of heart failure (angina, fatigue, palpitation, or dyspnea)*
1. Not troubled by breathlessness except on strenuous exertion 2. Short of breath when hurrying on level ground or walking up slight hill 3. Walks slower than people of same age or stops after 15 minutes when walking at own pace on level 4. Stops after 100 yards (90 m) or after few minutes in level ground 5. Too breathless to leave house, dress or undress	Class I: No limitation with ordinary physical activity Class II: Mild/slight limitation of ordinary physical activity Class III: Marked limitation of physical activity, symptoms with exertion Class IV: Symptoms at rest. Unable to carry out physical activity without discomfort

Arterial Pulses

Q. Write short essay/note on the clinical value of examination of radial and carotid pulses at bedside.

Definition of arterial pulse: It is a pressure distension wave produced by the contraction and relaxation of the left ventricle against a partially filled aorta which is transmitted to peripheries and is felt against bony prominences.

Peripheral arterial pulses: These include radial, brachial, carotid, femoral, popliteal, posterior tibial, and dorsalis pedis pulses. Right radial pulse is the first pulse to be examined during clinical examination. Normal pulse wave is depicted in **Figure 7.2**.

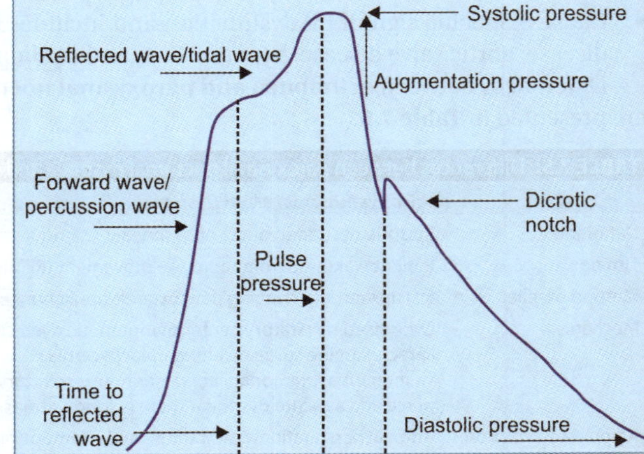

FIG. 7.2: Normal carotid and peripheral pulse wave.

Examination of the Arterial Pulse (Table 7.7)

- The character of the pulse is determined by stroke volume and arterial compliance, and is best assessed by palpating a major artery, such as the carotid or brachial artery.
- **Pulse rate**

TABLE 7.7: Assessment of arterial pulse.

Characteristics	*Best assessed by palpating*
➤ Rate	Radial artery
➤ Rhythm	
➤ Volume	Carotid artery
➤ Character or quality	Carotid artery (except collapsing pulse which is appreciated better at radial artery)
➤ Radiofemoral delay	
➤ Whether felt in all peripheral vessels	
➤ Condition of vessel wall	

TABLE 7.8: Causes of bradycardia and tachycardia.

Bradycardia	*Tachycardia*
Physiological: Athletes, sleep **Pathological:** ➤ Severe hypoxia ➤ Hypothyroidism/myxedema ➤ Hypothermia ➤ Sick sinus syndrome ➤ Vasovagal syncope ➤ Drugs—β-blockers, verapamil, and digoxin ➤ Heart block ➤ Raised intracranial tension	**Physiological:** Infants, children, emotion, exertion, and pregnancy **Pathological:** ➤ Tachyarrhythmias ➤ High output states: Anemia, pyrexia, anxiety, beriberi, thyrotoxicosis, cardiac failure, cardiogenic shock, and drugs (e.g., atropine, nifedipine, salbutamol, terbutaline, nicotine, and caffeine)

- Normal (resting) pulse rate in an adult is between 60 and 100 beats/minute (bpm).
- Should be counted for 1 full minute by palpating the radial artery.
  - **Sinus bradycardia:** Resting pulse rate is less than 60 beats/minute.
  - **Sinus tachycardia:** Resting pulse rate is more than 100 beats/minute.
- Causes of bradycardia and tachycardia are listed in **Table 7.8**.

Pulse deficit (Apex-pulse deficit) is the difference between the heart rate (counted by auscultation) and pulse rate when counted simultaneously for 1 full minute.

Causes: Pulse deficit of more than 10/minute occurs in atrial fibrillation and less than 10/minute may be found with ventricular premature beats or slow/controlled atrial fibrillation (AF).

Rhythm:

- Rhythm is assessed by palpating the radial pulse. The normal rhythm is regular.
- Causes of various types of arterial pulse rhythm abnormalities are listed in **Box 7.3**.

Box 7.3: Causes of various types of arterial pulse rhythm abnormalities.

Regularly irregular:
- Atrial tachyarrhythmias, sinus arrhythmia, and partial AV blocks
- Ventricular bigeminy, trigeminy

Irregularly irregular:
- Atrial or ventricular ectopics
- Atrial fibrillation
- Atrial tachyarrhythmia with AV blocks
- Frequent extrasystoles

Regular with occasional irregularity:
Extrasystoles

Q. What are the causes for irregularly irregular pulse?

- **Ventricular ectopics:** These develop as occasional or repeated irregularities superimposed on a regular pulse rhythm.
  Intermittent heart block also present with occasional beats dropped from an otherwise regular rhythm.
- **Atrial fibrillation:** It develops an irregularly irregular pulse. This irregular pattern persists when the pulse increases in response to exercise. On the contrary pulse irregularity due to ectopic beats usually disappears with exercise.

Pulse volume:

- Pulse volume is best assessed by palpating the carotid artery. However, the **pulse pressure** (i.e., difference between systolic and diastolic blood pressure) provides an accurate measure of pulse volume.
- Pulse volume is normal when pulse pressure is between 30 and 60 mm Hg, low when it is less than 30 mm Hg and large volume when more than 60 mm Hg.

Pulse character or quality:

- Differences between atrial fibrillation and ventricular premature contractions (VPCs) are shown in **Table 7.9A**. Causes of hypokinetic and hyperkinetic pulse are listed in **Table 7.9B**. Various types of pulse quality and its causes are mentioned in **Table 7.10**.
- **Grading of pulse:** Palpation of pulse is done by the fingertips and intensity of the pulse is graded from 0 to 4 +. 0 = pulse not palpable; 1 + = faint, but detectable pulse; 2 + = slightly more diminished pulse than normal; 3 + = normal pulse; and 4 + = bounding pulse.

TABLE 7.9A: Differences between atrial fibrillation and ventricular premature contractions (VPCs).

	Atrial fibrillation	*VPCs*
Apex pulse deficit	Usually >10	Usually <10
JVP "a" wave	Absent	Normal
S1	Variable intensity	Normal
Effect of exercise/ hand grip	Irregularity persists	Pulse becomes regular

TABLE 7.9B: Causes of hypokinetic and hyperkinetic pulse.

Hypokinetic pulse	*Hyperkinetic/bounding pulse*
➤ Congestive cardiac failure ➤ Hypovolemia ➤ Shock ➤ Mitral stenosis ➤ Aortic stenosis ➤ Constrictive pericarditis	**Physiological:** Fever, pregnancy, alcoholism, and exercise **Pathological:** ➤ **High output states:** Anemia, cor pulmonale, cirrhosis liver, beriberi, thyrotoxicosis, AV fistula, and Paget's disease ➤ **Cardiac cause:** Aortic regurgitation, bradycardia, complete heart block, PDA, systolic HTN, rupture of sinus Valsalva into heart chamber, and aortopulmonary window

Q. Write short note on: (1) Corrigan's/water hammer/collapsing pulse and its causes, (2) pulsus paradoxus and its causes, and (3) pulsus alternans.

TABLE 7.10: Various types of pulse quality and its causes.

Types	*Wave forms*	*Causes*
Catacrotic pulse	Percussion (p)—ejection of blood Tidal (t) Dicrotic—elastic recoil of vessel (reflected waves)	Normal
Pulsus parvus et tardus	A low amplitude (parvus) with a slow rising and late peak (tardus)	Severe aortic stenosis (AS)
Anacrotic pulse	Single peak low volume	Severe aortic stenosis
Pulsus bisferiens: Single pulse wave with two peaks in systole	Rapid rising, twice beating and both waves felt in systole	Severe aortic regurgitation (AR), moderate AR + AS, hypertrophic obstructive cardiomyopathy (HOCM)
Pulsus dicroticus	Twice beating. First wave in systole, second wave in diastole. Seen when pulse rate and diastolic pressure are low	Typhoid fever, severe left ventricular failure (LVF), dehydration, and dilated cardiomyopathy endotoxic shock
Watson's water hammer pulse or collapsing pulse	High (large) volume pulse, sharp rise (systolic pressure is high), ill-sustained, sharp fall (diastolic pressure is low), pulse pressure is at least 60 mm Hg	Aortic regurgitation, patent ductus arteriosus (PDA), AP window, rupture of sinus Valsalva, arteriovenous fistula, hyperdynamic circulation states
Pulsus paradoxus: Exaggerated reduction in the strength of pulse during normal respiration	Systolic blood pressure falls more than 10 mm Hg during inspiration (exaggeration of normal phenomenon)	Constrictive pericarditis, acute severe asthma/COPD, cardiac tamponade, tension pneumothorax, massive pulmonary embolism
Absent pulsus paradoxus in an expected disease		If associated ASD, VSD, AR, and pericardial adhesions
Reverse pulsus paradoxus		Positive pressure ventilation, HOCM
Pseudo-pulsus paradoxus		Complete heart bock with AV dissociation
Jerky pulse—Spike and dome		HOCM
Pulsus alternans	Alternating weaker and stronger volume pulses in regular rhythm, doubling rate of Korotkoff sound on lowering cuff pressures	Left ventricular failure
Plateau pulse		Severe AS
Pulsus bigeminus	Pulse wave with normal beat followed by a premature beat and a compensatory pause, occurring in rapid succession, resulting in alteration of the strength of pulse	Digoxin toxicity
Sinus arrhythmia	Increase pulse rate with inspiration and decrease with expiration	Absent sinus arrhythmia in CCF and autonomic neuropathy

Diagrammatic appearances of various arterial waveforms are presented in **Figure 7.3**.

Radiofemoral delay:

- A delayed femoral pulsation compared to right radial pulse occurs in coarctation of aorta.
- Demonstrated by simultaneous palpation of right radial artery and one femoral artery.
  - **Apico-carotid** delay is seen in severe aortic stenosis where there is a delay between apical impulse and the carotid upstroke.

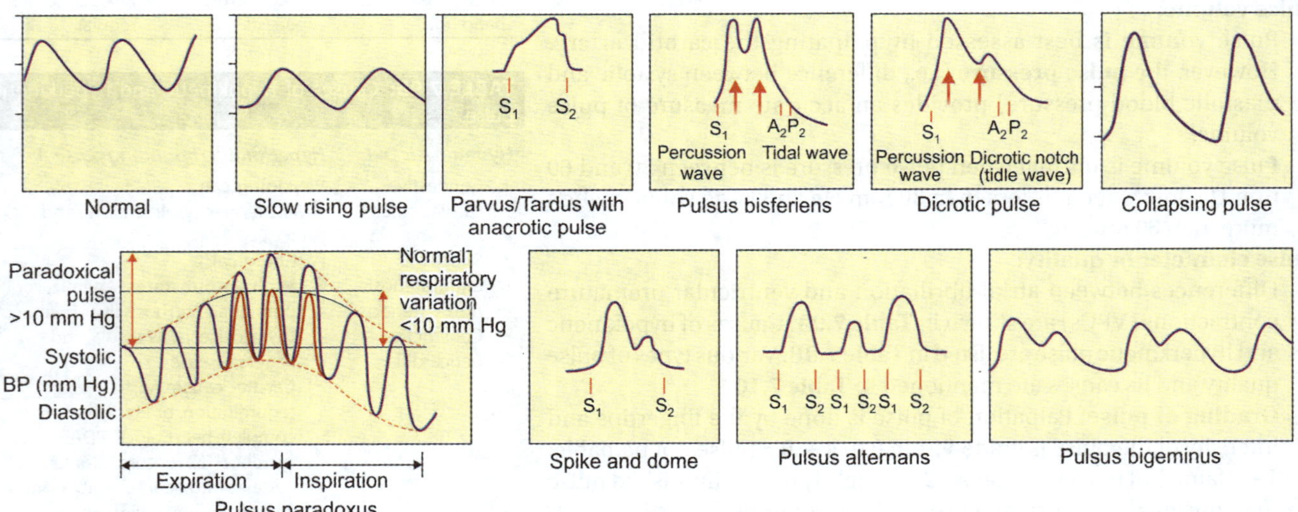

FIG. 7.3: Diagrammatic appearances of various arterial waveforms. A_2, aortic component of the second heart sound; P_2, pulmonary component of the second heart sound; S_1 first heart sound.

Reduced or absent arterial pulses:

- It indicates impaired blood flow.
- Causes: (1) congenital (e.g., coarctation of the aorta), (2) intrinsic disease of artery (e.g., atherosclerosis, thrombosis, arteritis), (3) disorders with vasospasm (e.g., Raynaud's phenomenon), (4) extrinsic compression of blood vessel (e.g., thoracic outlet syndrome, trauma, and neoplasms).

Jugular Venous Pressure

Q. Write short essay/note on jugular venous pulse (JVP) and its clinical significance.

Definition: Jugular venous pulse is defined as the **oscillating top of undulating vertical column of blood in the right internal jugular vein that faithfully reflects the pressure and volumetric changes in the right atrium that varies with all phases of cardiac cycle and respiration**. JVP is the vertical height of oscillating column of blood.

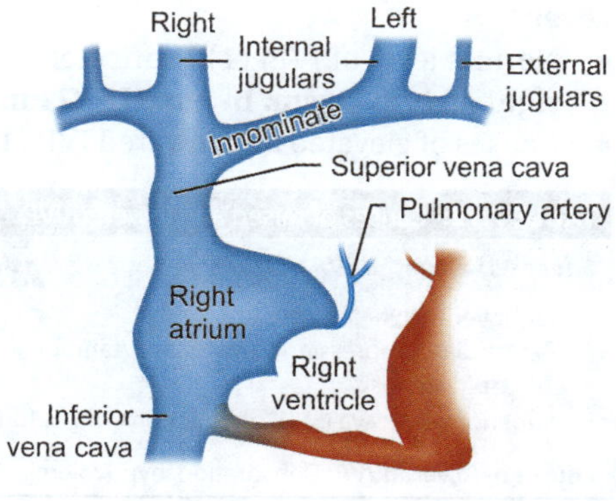

FIG. 7.4: Diagrammatic appearance of anatomic relations of jugular veins and right atrium.

Advantages of Internal Jugular Vein (IJV) vs External Jugular Vein (EJV)

- IJV is **anatomically (Fig. 7.4) closer** to and has a **direct course to right atrium** while EJV does not directly drain into superior vena cava.
- IJV is valveless and pulsations can be seen. EJV has valves and pulsations cannot be seen.
- EJV can become small and barely visible when there is vasoconstriction secondary to hypotension (as in congestive heart failure).
- EJV is superficial and prone to kinking.

Importance of Right Internal Jugular Vein

- Right internal jugular veins extend in an almost straight line to superior vena cava, thus favoring transmission of the hemodynamic changes from the right atrium.
- The left innominate vein is not in a straight line and may be kinked or compressed between aortic arch and sternum, by a dilated aorta, or by an aneurysm.

Technique of Measuring JVP

- **Position:** Semireclining position with 45° angle between the trunk (not the neck) and the bed turn the head slightly toward left shoulder, so that the neck muscles are relaxed **(Fig. 7.5A)**. Tangential light source can be put from opposite side.
  - **Not in sitting position:** Because the upper level of venous column is below the clavicle.
  - **Not in supine position:** Because the whole venous column moves beyond the angle of jaw into the intracranial cavity.
- **Identify jugular venous pulsation:**
  - Assure good lighting (can use tangential beam of light through torch).
  - Look between the two heads of sternocleidomastoid.
  - Note the upper level of pulsation, waveform, and respiratory variation.
  - Do not mistake the carotid pulsations for venous pulsations **(Table 7.11)**.

Q. List the differences between jugular venous pulse from carotid pulse.

- **Measurement of JVP:** Measure the vertical distance (in cm) between the horizontal lines drawn from the upper level of venous pulsation and the sternal angle.
  - This can be done by using two rulers—one placed horizontal to the upper level of pulsation and another taking the vertical distance of that ruler from the sternal angle.

Q. Method of calculation of central venous pressure from jugular venous pressure.

- **Calculate the right atrial pressure (RAP) or central venous pressure (CVP)**

TABLE 7.11: Differences between jugular venous pulsations and carotid pulsations.

Jugular vein	*Carotid artery*
➤ Pulsations not palpable	➤ Pulsations palpable
➤ Pulsations obliterated by pressure above the clavicle	➤ Pulsations not obliterated by pressure above the clavicle
➤ Pulse wave level of reduced during inspiration and increased on expiration	➤ No effects of respiration on pulse
➤ Usually two pulsations per systole (x and y descents)	➤ One pulsation per systole
➤ Prominent descents	➤ Descents not prominent
➤ Pulsations more prominent with abdominal pressure	➤ No effect of abdominal pressure on pulsations
➤ Changes with position	➤ No change with position
➤ More lateral in position in the neck	➤ Medial in the neck
➤ Has a definite upper level	➤ No upper level
➤ More superficial	➤ Deeper in location
➤ Wavy and undulant	➤ Brisk and jerky
➤ Descents are more prominent	➤ Only positive waves

- Normally, the center of right atrium is 5 cm below the sternal angle at any position of the patient. Hence, 5 cm is added to the above value to obtain the RAP.
- Conversion: 1.3 cm of H_2O or blood = 1 mm Hg

Evaluation/Interpretation of JVP (Box 7.4)

Box 7.4: Evaluation of jugular venous pulse (JVP).

(1) Level, (2) waveform, (3) venous hum, (4) respiratory variation in level and wave pattern, (5) abdominojugular reflux, and (6) liver size and pulsations.

Level:

- Normal level of JVP: **(1) From sternal angle <4 cm, (2) from center of right atrium <9 cm. In mm Hg <7 mm Hg.**
- Causes of elevated and lowered JVP **(Table 7.12)**.

TABLE 7.12: Causes of raised and lowered JVP.

Causes of elevated JVP (jugular venous distension)	
➤ Right ventricular failure	➤ Circulatory overload
➤ Pericardial compression (constriction/tamponade): little or no pulsations when severe	➤ Renal failure
➤ Tricuspid stenosis	➤ Excessive fluid administration
➤ Superior vena cava (SVC) obstruction—no pulsations	➤ Atrial septal defect with mitral valve disease
Causes of lowered JVP: Dehydration, hypovolemia	

Q. Write short essay/note on normal wave patterns of JVP and their variations.

Wave pattern (Figs. 7.5A and B)

The normal JVP consists of three ascents or positive waves (a, c and v) and two descents or negative waves (x, x' and y):

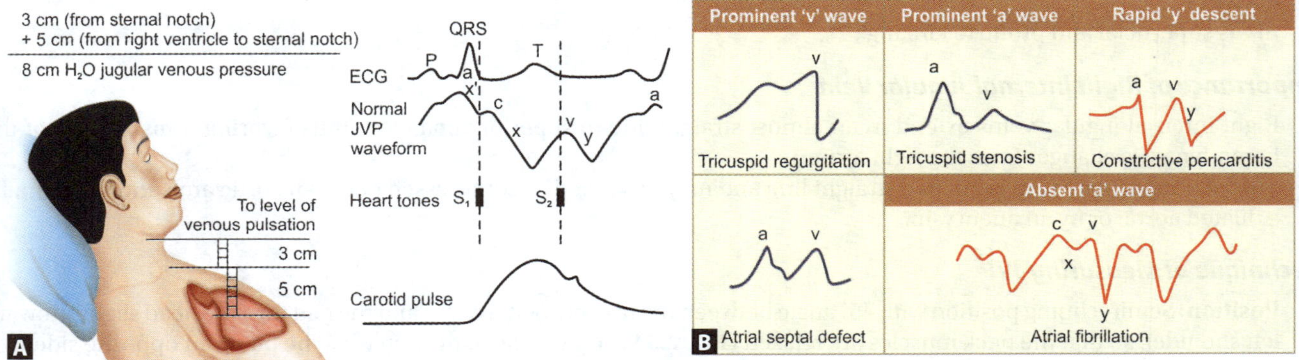

FIGS. 7.5A AND B: (A) Wave patterns in jugular venous pressure (JVP); (B) Abnormalities of JVP.

- **a wave (ascent):** Due to **a**ctive atrial contraction leading to retrograde blood flow into neck veins.
- **x wave (descent):** Due to continued atrial relaxation.
- **c wave:** Due to impact of the **c**arotid artery adjacent to the jugular vein and retrograde transmission of a positive wave in the right atrium. It is produced by the right ventricular systole and the bulging of the tricuspid valve into the right atrium. Not usually seen in humans.
- **x' wave (descent):** Due to descent of floor of right atrium (tricuspid valve) during right ventricular systole and continued atrial relaxation.
- **v wave (ascent):** Due to passive atrial filling (**v**enous filling).
- **y wave (descent):** Due to opening of tricuspid valve and subsequent rapid inflow of blood from right atrium into the right ventricle leading to a sudden fall in right atrial pressure.

Wave patterns in jugular venous pressure are presented in **Figure 7.5A**.

Best way to identify the waves (ascents and descents): Simultaneously auscultate and observe the wave pattern.

- **"a" ascent:** Clinically corresponds to S_1 (though it actually occurs before S_1); sharper and more prominent than "v" wave.
- **"x" descent:** Follows S_1; less prominent than "y" descent.
- **"c" ascent:** Occurs simultaneously with carotid pulse; but never seen normally.
- **"v" ascent:** Coincides with S_2; less prominent than "a" ascent.
- **"y" descent:** Follows S_2; more prominent than "x" ascent.

Note: h wave —between the bottom of "y" descent and beginning of "a" ascent, during the period of diastasis (relatively slow ventricular filling).

Patient with prominent jugular veins is depicted in **Figure 7.6**.

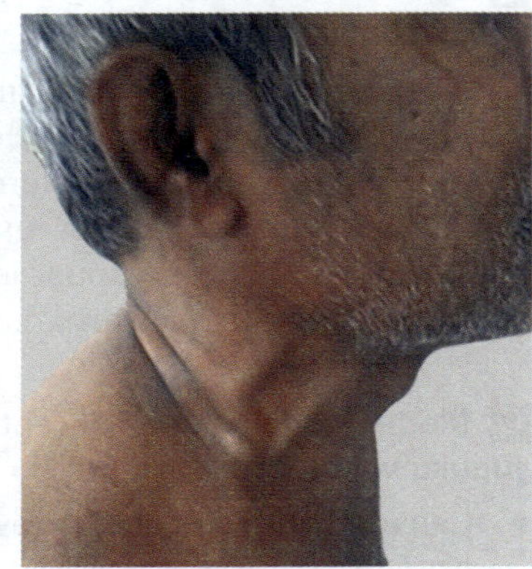

FIG. 7.6: Prominent jugular veins.

Abnormalities of wave patterns of JVP

- **Prominent "a" waves (giant a-wave or Venous Corrigan):** Due to resistance to atrial emptying at:
  - **Tricuspid level:** Tricuspid stenosis, right atrial tumors.
  - **Right ventricular level:** Concentric hypertrophy due to severe pulmonary hypertension, right ventricular cardiomyopathy, severe aortic stenosis, acute pulmonary embolism, and acute tricuspid regurgitation.
- **Cannon waves:** Very prominent "a" waves due to atrial contraction against closed tricuspid valve.
  - **Regular cannon waves:** Junctional rhythm, ventricular tachycardia 1:1 retrograde conduction, and isorhythmic AV dissociation.
  - **Irregular cannon waves:** Complete heart block, ventricular tachycardia, ventricular ectopy, ventricular pacing, and classic AV dissociation.
- Rapid and regular neck pulsations, which are due to prominent and regular A waves, may be seen as a bulging in the neck, sometimes termed as **"frog sign"** and is most typical of re-entrant supraventricular arrhythmias, particularly AVNRT or atrioventricular re-entrant tachycardia due to a pre-excitation syndrome.
- **Absent "a" waves:** Atrial fibrillation (AF), post DC conversion of AF, sinoventricular conduction in hyperkalemia.
- Single wave
  - **"a" and "v" wave merge:** Heart rate >120 beats/minute
  - **Early "v" wave with obliterated "x" wave:** Severe chronic tricuspid regurgitation, acute tricuspid regurgitation
- **Absent "x" wave** (failure of atrial pressure to fall): Atrial fibrillation, severe chronic tricuspid regurgitation, acute tricuspid regurgitation, and constrictive pericarditis.
- **Prominent "x" wave:** Cardiac tamponade
- **Prominent "v" wave:** Right ventricular failure, tricuspid regurgitation, atrial septal defect with/without mitral regurgitation.
- **Diminished "v" wave:** Hypovolemia, venodilators
- **Rapid "y" descent:** Causes of prominent "v" wave, constrictive pericarditis (Friedrich's sign).
- **Slow "y" descent:** Tricuspid stenosis, pericardial tamponade, and tension pneumothorax.
- **c-v wave with prominent "y" descent:** Tricuspid regurgitation (lateral ear lobe pulsations—Lancisi's sign).
- **Steeply rising "h" wave:** Restrictive cardiomyopathy, constrictive pericarditis, and right ventricular infarction.
- **Equal "a" and "v" wave** (M Pattern): Atrial septal defect.

Venous hum (Pontain's murmur)

- Continuous bruit over neck veins (normally noiseless) due to increased velocity of blood flow or decreased viscosity of blood.
- Best heard with the bell of the stethoscope over the right supraclavicular fossa/root of neck, patient in standing position.
- Causes:
  - **Physiological:** Children, pregnancy
  - **Pathological:** Hyperkinetic states, anemia (indicates **chronic compensated severe anemia**), thyrotoxicosis, beriberi, and intracranial AV fistula. Indicates chronic compensated severe anemia.

Respiratory Variation of JVP

- **Normal:** Venous column in IJV rises during expiration and falls during inspiration.
- **Reason:**
  - During inspiration venous return to the right side of the heart increases due to increased negative thoracic pressure. However, this is accommodated by the inspiratory decrease in pulmonary vascular resistance. As a result, pulmonary artery, right ventricle, and right atrial pressures fall in spite of increased venous return.
  - During expiration, due to increased positive intrathoracic pressure, pulmonary circulation is compressed by the thoracic cage resulting in increased pulmonary resistance and pressure.

Kussmaul's Sign

Q. Write short essay/note on Kussmaul's sign.

- Normally, during inspiration there will be decrease in the height of jugular venous pulsation and drop in jugular venous pressure (respirophasic changes).
- Kussmaul's sign is paradoxical rise in JVP during inspiration.
- **Causes:** Constrictive pericarditis, right ventricular infarction, restrictive cardiomyopathy, severe right-sided heart failure, and acute severe asthma. Rarely can be seen in cardiac tamponade, tricuspid stenosis, and severe tricuspid regurgitation.
- **Reason:** Increased venous return in inspiration cannot be accommodated by the heart in the above-mentioned conditions leading to a translation of the venous blood back through the SVC and presents as distended jugular veins even during inspiration.

Abdominojugular/Hepatojugular Reflux

Q. Write a short note on abdominojugular/hepatojugular reflux test and its clinical significance.

- **Technique:** When pressure is applied over the liver by pressing firmly (40 mm Hg) over the abdomen for around 30 seconds, the venous pressure gets exaggerated initially due to increased venous return. Later the myocardium accommodates the

extravenous return and the level falls. Normally within 2–3 cardiac cycles, i.e., within 3 seconds.
- **Normal response:** Upper level of jugular venous pulsation moves upward by less than 3 cm and then falls down within 5 seconds even when the pressure is continued.

Significance
- **Positive test:** Rise in JVP (more than 3 cm) for >10 seconds of firm mid-abdominal compression.
  - **Early cardiac failure:** First sign of right heart failure (RHF).
  - **False positive:** Valsalva (abdominal guarding), fluid overload
- **False negative:** SVC/IVC obstruction, Budd–Chiari syndrome where there is no rise in JVP.
  This test also helps to differentiate venous pulsation from the arterial pulsation.

Square Root Sign

It is found in constrictive pericarditis on **cardiac catheterization** to note pressure tracings. A rapid halt of ventricular filling occurs as the ventricular wall is impeded by the abnormal pericardium causing an abrupt rise in LV pressure **(Fig. 7.7)**. This has been described as the square root sign.

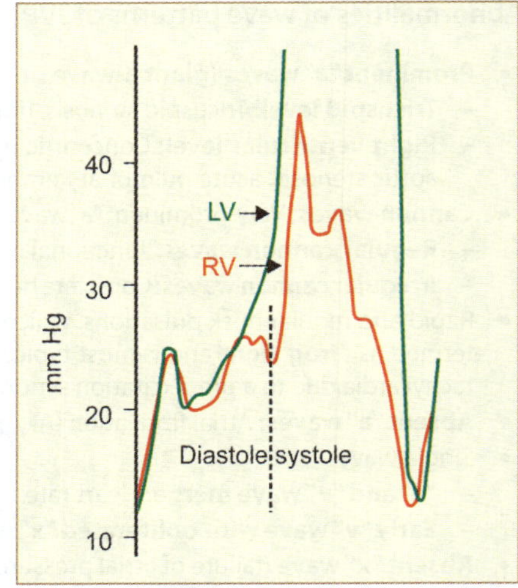

FIG. 7.7: Ventricular pressure curve in constrictive pericarditis.

APICAL IMPULSE

Q. Write a short note on apical impulse.

***Definition*:** It is the outermost and lowermost point of maximum impulse (PMI) in early systole, which imparts a perpendicular gentle thrust to a palpating finger, followed by a slight medial retraction in the late systole.

***Cause of normal apical impulse*:** Anterior and counter clock-wise rotation of LV due to isovolumic contraction during early systole and medical retraction due to clock-wise rotation of the LV during late systole. Characteristics of normal apical impulse are listed in **Box 7.5**.

Box 7.5: Characteristics of normal apical impulse.
- Location: Left 5th ICS at or around half an inch medial to mid-clavicular line and <10 cm from mid-sternal line
- Extent: <2.5 cm in diameter which is one ICS
- Duration: <50% of systole
- Mildly tapping in character

Abnormal Apical Impulse
- **Absent:** Dilated cardiomyopathy, pericardial effusion, behind the rib, dextrocardia, obesity, COPD, left pleural effusion
- **Tapping:** Mitral stenosis (palpable S_1—**closing snap**)
- **Hyperdynamic:** Increased in amplitude, duration is >1/3 to <2/3 of systole, occupies more than one intercostal space. Occurs in LV volume overload [AR (aortic regurgitation), MR (mitral regurgitation), VSD (ventricular septal defect), PDA (patent ductus arteriosus), and high output states]
- **Heaving:** Increase in amplitude, duration is >2/3 of systole and occupies more than one intercostal space. Occurs in LV pressure overload [AS (aortic stenosis), HTN (hypertension), coarctation of aorta]
- **Diffuse:** Occupying more than 1 ICS. Occurs in LV aneurysm, LV dilatation as in AR
- **Double:** Hypertrophic obstructive cardiomyopathy (HOCM), AS with AR, left dyssynergy (LBBB), LV aneurysm
- **Triple or quadruple:** HOCM
- **Retractile:** Severe TR (tricuspid regurgitation)
- **Medial apical retraction:** Left ventricular enlargement
- **Lateral apical retraction:** Right ventricular enlargement

Cheyne–Stokes Breathing

Q. Write short essay on mechanism, causes, consequences, and management of Cheyne–Stokes breathing.

Definition: This is a cyclical pattern of respiration due to impaired responsiveness of the respiratory center to carbon dioxide. It is characterized by gradual increases and decreases in respiration. It has two alternative periods, namely (1) rapid deep respiration called hyperpnea and (2) complete stoppage of respiration called apnea.

Mechanism (Fig. 7.8)

- Spontaneous rhythmic activity of breathing is abolished when there is anoxemia. Consequent apnea causes accumulation of carbon dioxide.
- Hypercapnia stimulates respiratory centers → produces hyperventilation → leads to reduced carbon dioxide → causes depression of the respiratory center → resulting in apnea. The cycle is repeated.

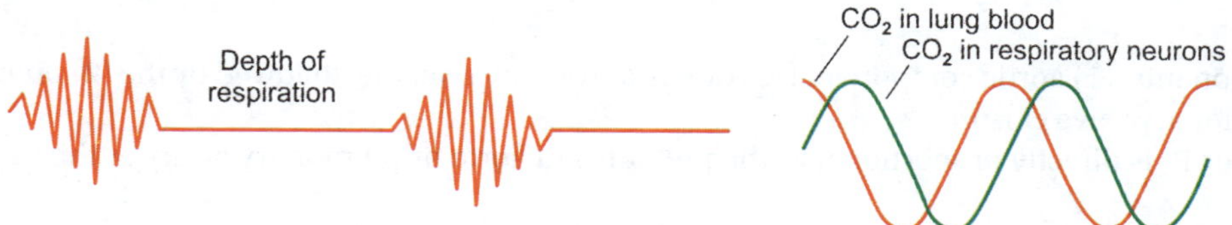

FIG. 7.8: Cheyne–Stokes breathing and levels of carbon dioxide (CO_2).

Conditions Associated with Cheyne–Stokes Breathing

- **Physiological conditions:** During deep sleep, high altitude, and newborn babies
- **Pathological conditions:** Severe heart (left ventricular) failure, uremia, chronic hypoxia, diffuse cerebral atherosclerosis, stroke, head injury and hemorrhage, increased intracranial pressure, severe pneumonia, and narcotic drug (e.g., barbiturates, opiates) poisoning.

HEART SOUNDS

Relative, brief, auditory vibrations of variable intensity, frequency, and quality.

First Heart Sound (S_1)

Q. What is the mechanism of first heart sound? Write short note on the variations in first heart sound.

Mechanism

During systole the atrioventricular (AV), i.e., mitral and tricuspid valves, closes and blood tries to enter the atrium and lead to back bulging of the AV valves into the respective atria. But the taut (stretched or pulled tight) chordae tendineae stop the back bulging and causes the blood to flow forward. This will cause vibration of the valves, blood, and the walls of the ventricles.

Timing

- Just precedes carotid upstroke.
- S_1 will appear to initiate the outward LV thrust of apex beat.

Characteristics

- Medium-to-high frequency but lower pitch than S_2.
- Q-M_1 60 ms, Q-T_1 90 ms, M_1-T_1 30 ms.
- First heart sound has two components: (1) Mitral component (M1) due to mitral valve closure followed by (2) tricuspid component (T_1) due to tricuspid valve closure.
- S_1 is best heard at the apex. It is best heard with the diaphragm of stethoscope.

Intensity

Determined by structural integrity of mitral valve, **position of AV valves at time of ventricular contraction,** integrity of isovolumetric systole, heart rate, P-R interval, and myocardial contractility.

Abnormalities of S_1

Table 7.13 lists the causes of variations in the intensity of first heart sound.

- **Variation in the intensity of first heart sound:** Atrial fibrillation, complete heart block (CHB), ventricular tachycardia, atrial flutter with varying block, atrial tachycardia with varying block, and ventricular ectopics.
- **Splitting of S_1:** Abnormalities in splitting of first heart sound are presented in **Table 7.14**.

TABLE 7.13: Causes of variations in the intensity of first heart sound.

Loud first heart sound (S_1)	*Soft first heart sound (S_1)*
➢ Mitral stenosis (mild to moderate) ➢ Tachycardia ➢ Hyperdynamic circulation: Exercise, anemia, fever, thyrotoxicosis, Paget's disease, pregnancy, beriberi, and increased cardiac output ➢ Short P-R interval ➢ Left atrial myxoma ➢ Tricuspid stenosis ➢ Thin people	➢ Mitral or tricuspid regurgitation ➢ Obesity ➢ Emphysema ➢ Pericardial effusion ➢ Severe calcified mitral stenosis ➢ Left ventricular failure ➢ Shock ➢ Bradycardia ➢ First-degree block ➢ Long P-R interval

TABLE 7.14: Abnormalities in splitting of first heart sound.

Wide splitting of first heart sound	*Reversed splitting of first heart sound*
➢ Ebstein's anomaly T1 delayed ➢ Atrial septal defect (ASD) ➢ Complete right bundle branch block (RBBB) ➢ Left ventricular pacing	➢ Complete left bundle branch block ➢ Severe mitral stenosis ➢ Myxoma of left atrium ➢ Right ventricular pacing ➢ Ectopic beats from right ventricle

Second Heart Sound (S_2)

Q. What is the mechanism of second heart sound? Write short note on the variations in second heart sound.

It is due to the closure of aortic and pulmonary valve.

Characteristics

- It has two components: (1) aortic component (A_2) due to aortic valve closure, followed by the (2) pulmonary component (P_2) due to pulmonary valve closure.
- Loudness of A_2 or P_2 is directly proportional to the pressures in aorta or pulmonary artery at the beginning of diastole, respectively.
- The second heart sound is **medium to high pitched** (higher frequency) because:
  - The semilunar valves are more taut
  - The great elastic coefficient of the taut arteries provides the principle vibrations of the second heart sound.
- P_2 only heard at second left intercostal space. *Loudest sound in pulmonary area is A_2.*
- A_2 is audible at region of right second intercostal space, left parasternal space, and apex.
- Normal splitting:
  - **Splitting during inspiration:** During inspiration, the aortic valve closes early than pulmonary valve and produces a physiological **inspiratory splitting of second heart sound**. Split is audible in second and third intercostal space and amplitude of $A_2 > P_2$.
  - Normally, during expiration both aortic and pulmonary valves close almost simultaneously and produce a **single expiratory second heart sound**.
  - Frequency of both A_2 and P_2 components are same.

Hangout time/interval: The interval between the pressure crossover point and the incisura (the onset of A_2 or P_2) has been termed "hangout time". During inspiration, pulmonary vascular impedance declines with a further increase in the pulmonary hangout time, which is the mechanism for inspiratory splitting of S_2.

Abnormalities of Second Heart Sound (S_2)

- **Absent S_2:** Old age as in calcific aortic stenosis (due to absence of A_2) or chronic emphysema.
- **Single second heart sound (S_2):** May be either due to absent A_2 (e.g., severe aortic stenosis or atresia) or absent P_2 (e.g., severe pulmonary stenosis or atresia) and tetralogy of Fallot.
- **Variation in the intensity S_2 (Table 7.15).**
- **Splitting of S_2:** Physiological splitting of S_2 is normally found in children and young adults during inspiration. Normal interval is A_2-P_2 30 ms and A_2-OS 30–150 ms.
- **Wide split S_2:** It may be variable or fixed **(Table 7.16)**.
- **ASD with variable split S_2:** Sinus venosus type of ASD or ASD with atrial fibrillation.
- **Reversed (paradoxical) splitting S_2:** May be due to early P_2 or delayed A_2 **(Table 7.17)**.

TABLE 7.15: Variations in the intensity of second heart sound.

Aortic component (A_2)		
➢ Loud A_2: Essential hypertension, hyperhemodynamic circulatory states, syphilitic aortic regurgitation, and aortic aneurysm		
➢ Soft A_2: Aortic stenosis and regurgitation		
Pulmonary component (P_2)		
Causes of loud P_2	**Diminished (soft) P_2**	**Absent P_2**
➢ Normal in infants and children ➢ Adults with chest deformity or thin chests ➢ Pulmonary arterial hypertension ➢ Left to right shunts ➢ Hyperkinetic circulatory states	➢ Normal in elderly ➢ Thick chested adults ➢ Pulmonary stenosis ➢ Dysplastic valve	➢ Tetralogy of Fallot ➢ Transposition of great arteries ➢ Truncus arteriosus ➢ Pulmonary atresia ➢ Absent pulmonary valve

TABLE 7.16: Causes of wide split of second heart sound.

Wide split S_2		*Wide fixed split*
➢ **Due to early A_2:** - Mitral regurgitation - Ventricular septal defect - Constrictive pericarditis	➢ **Due to late P_2:** - Right bundle branch block - Ectopic from left ventricle - Left ventricular pacemakers	➢ Atrial septal defect ➢ Severe right ventricular failure ➢ Massive acute pulmonary embolism

TABLE 7.17: Causes of reversed or paradoxical split.

Early P_2	*Delayed A_2*	
➢ Left bundle branch block ➢ Right ventricular pacing ➢ PVCs of right ventricular origin ➢ Wolff–Parkinson–White (WPW) syndrome (type B)	➢ Severe aortic stenosis ➢ Severe systemic hypertension ➢ Acute myocardial infarction ➢ Hypertrophic cardiomyopathy	➢ Severe aortic regurgitation ➢ Large patent ductus arteriosus ➢ Aneurysm of ascending aorta ➢ Poststenotic dilatation in aortic stenosis

- **Pseudo-paradoxical split:** Normally S_2 split in expiration and inspiration. But during inspiration patients with muffled P_2, so that single S_2 will be heard in inspiration.
- **Narrow splitting:** Aging, artifactual muffling of P_2, severe pulmonary arterial hypertension, and murmur obscuration.

Third Heart Sound

Q. Write short note on the significance of third heart sound.

- Third heart sound (S_3) is also called as **protodiastolic sound**/ventricular gallop.
- S_3 is a low-pitched early diastolic sound produced due to rapid ventricular filling immediately after opening of the atrioventricular valves.
- S_3 best heard with the bell of stethoscope at the apex. It coincides with rapid ventricular filling. It occurs 0.12–0.18 seconds after S_2 and has low frequency and low intensity.

Causes of Third Heart Sound (Table 7.18)

- A third heart sound is a normal finding in children, in young adults, and during pregnancy.
- A third heart sound is usually pathological after the age of 40 years. In heart failure S_3 occurs with a tachycardia and S_1 and S_2 are quiet (lub-da-dub).

TABLE 7.18: Causes of third heart sound.

Physiological S_3: Children, young adults under 40 years, athletes, and pregnancy
Pathological: ➢ **Hyperdynamic/high output states:** AV fistula, thyrotoxicosis ➢ **Left-sided S_3** (arising from the left ventricle)**:** Left ventricular failure (most common cause), aortic regurgitation, mitral regurgitation, ischemic heart disease, and hypertrophic cardiomyopathy ➢ **Right-sided S_3** (arising from right ventricle): Right ventricular failure, tricuspid regurgitation, and pulmonary hypertension

Fourth Heart Sound

Q. Write short note on significance of fourth heart sound.

- Fourth heart sound (S_4) is less common and is also called **presystolic/atrial gallop.** It occurs just before the first sound (da-lub-dub). It occurs 0.11 seconds prior to S_1.
- It is soft and low-pitched, best heard with the bell of the stethoscope at the apex.
- It is always pathological and is produced by a rapid (forceful) empting of the atrium into the noncompliant or stiff ventricle. It cannot occur when there is atrial fibrillation.
- Third and a fourth heart sound causes a "triple" or "gallop" rhythm. S_4 may be confused with spilt S_1. Firm pressure by the diaphragm of stethoscope eliminates S_4 but not split S_1.

Box 7.6: Causes of fourth heart sound.

Left sided S_4:
- Systemic hypertension with left ventricular hypertrophy
- Hypertrophic cardiomyopathy
- Ischemic heart disease (especially acute myocardial infarction)
- Acute mitral regurgitation
- Anemia, thyrotoxicosis, and AV fistula

Right sided S_4:
- Right ventricular hypertrophy due to pulmonary hypertension, pulmonary stenosis

Causes of Fourth Heart Sound (Box 7.6)

Summation Gallop

Q. Write short note on summation gallop.

- Summation is the presence of S_1, S_2 merging with S_3 and S_4.
  It occurs when both S_3 and S_4 are present in a patient with tachycardia.
- Shortening of diastole causes joining of the two sounds (S_3 and S_4) and produce a single loud sound.

Pericardial Friction Rub

Q. Write short note on pericardial rub.

- It is the sound produced due to sliding (apposition) of the two inflamed layers (visceral and parietal pericardium) of the pericardium.
- **Phases:** It is triphasic: (1) midsystolic, (2) mid-diastolic, and (3) presystolic.
- **Character:** It is scratchy, grating, leathery, or creaking in character. Its intensity vary over time, and with the position of the patient.
- **Best heard:** With diaphragm of stethoscope on the left sternal boarder (3rd and 4th space) leaning over at the end of expiration. It may be audible over any part of the precordium but is often localized.
- Confused with Hamman's sign in post-open heart surgery (crunch sound from mediastinal air).
- A pleuropericardial rub is a similar sound that occurs in time with the cardiac cycle but is also influenced by respiration and is pleural in origin. Occasionally, a "crunching" noise can be heard caused by air in the pericardium (pneumopericardium).

Cardiac Sounds on Auscultation

Ejection Sound/Click

Usually sharp, high frequency sound audible immediately after S_1. Its causes are listed in **Box 7.7**.

Box 7.7: Causes of ejection sound/click.

- **Aortic valve:** Aortic stenosis, bicuspid aortic valve
- **Pulmonary valve:** Pulmonic stenosis, vary with respirations
- **Prosthetic valves:** Mechanical, not bioprosthetic

Mid-Late Systolic Sounds

- Click, high frequency sound found in mitral valve prolapse.
- Occurs earlier with Valsalva maneuver or squatting to standing.

Early Diastolic Sounds

Q. Write short note on opening snap.

Opening snap of mitral stenosis (MS)

- It is caused by the opening of atrioventricular valve.
- **Characteristics:** High-pitched sound audible at the apex in left lateral decubitus position. 0.04–0.12 sec after A_2 (S_3 occurs 0.12 sec after A_2). Occurs after S_2, before S_3.
- Severe mitral stenosis is associated with short A_2-OS interval and softer OS or absent OS.

Mechanism of Opening Snap (OS)

- Stenotic anterior mitral valve leaflet suddenly bulging download into the left ventricular cavity like a dome, with a snapping sound when the mitral valve is rapidly opened during diastole. So, OS is audible only if anterior mitral leaflet of mitral valve is mobile.
- OS occurs when movement of AMV suddenly stops, at point when LVP drops below that of LAP.

Differences between opening snap second and third heart sound are listed in **Table 7.19**.

TABLE 7.19: Differences between opening snap second and third heart sound.

	Opening snap (OS)	*S_2 (second heart sound)*	*S_3 (third heart sound)*
Area	Just inside apex/entire chest wall	2nd and 3rd left intercostal space	Only apex
Relation to posture	A_2-OS interval widens on standing	A_2-P_2 interval narrows on standing	Disappear of sitting
Intensity on standing	Remain same/intensified	Decreases	–
Relation to respiration	A_2-OS interval constant throughout respiration	Split increase on respiration	None
Intensity on respiration	Same	–	RVS_3 load during inspiration
A_2-OS/A_2-P_2/A_2-S_3 interval	–	A_2-P_2 interval shorter than A_2-OS interval	A_2-S_3 interval is longer than A_2-OS interval
Pitch	High (Best heard with diaphragm)	High	Low (Best heard with bell)

MURMURS

- Sudden deceleration of blood produces heart sounds. Heart murmurs are produced by turbulent flow (Raynold's number >2,000) across an abnormal valve, septal defect or outflow obstruction, or by increased volume or velocity of flow through a normal valve.
- Murmurs may occur in a healthy heart. These "innocent" murmurs occur when stroke volume is increased, e.g., during pregnancy, and in athletes with resting bradycardia or children with fever **(Box 7.8)**.

Box 7.8: Mechanism of murmurs.

- **Blood viscosity:** Increased or decreased blood velocity
- **Valve:** Narrowed or incompetent, organic or relative
- Abnormal connection
- Vibration of loose structure
- Diameter of vessel increased or decreased

Box 7.9: Grading of systolic murmurs (Freeman and Levine).

- Grade 1 = very faint
- Grade 2 = quiet but heard immediately
- Grade 3 = moderately loud
- Grade 4 = loud with thrill
- Grade 5 = heard with stethoscope partly off the chest, thrill present
- Grade 6 = no stethoscope needed, thrill present

Note:

- Thrills are associated with murmurs of grades 4–6
- Diastolic murmurs are only graded till 4

Features to be Observed in Murmur

- **Timing:** By simultaneous palpation of the carotid arterial pulse and note whether systolic, diastolic, and continuous.
- **Shape:** Crescendo (grows louder), decrescendo, crescendo-decrescendo, and plateau
- **Intensity:**
    - Systolic murmurs are graded on a 6 point scale (Levine and Freeman) **(Box 7.9)**
    - Diastolic murmurs are usually not graded but can be described as (1) **very soft** (2) **soft,** and (3) **loud with/without thrill.**
- **Duration**
- Location of maximum intensity depends on the site where the murmur originates.
- **Character** blowing, harsh, rumbling, and musical
- **Pitch** high, medium, low depending on the velocity of the jet
- **Radiation/conduction:**
    - Reflects the intensity of the murmur and the direction of blood flow
    - Mitral regurgitation murmur (PSM) radiates to axilla
    - Aortic stenosis murmur (ESM) conducts to the carotid.
- **Variation** with respiration/position/other maneuvers
- **Best heard** with bell or diaphragm of the stethoscope.

Systolic Murmurs

Q. Write short essay/note on differential diagnosis of ejection systolic murmurs (ESM). List the causes of systolic murmurs.

Ejection Systolic (Mid-systolic) Murmurs

Ejection systolic (mid-systole) murmurs occur when there is ventricular outflow tract obstruction. It begins shortly after the first heart sound (S_1) and ends before the second heart sound with a crescendo-decrescendo or diamond-shaped pattern, reflecting the changing velocity of blood flow.

Various Systolic Murmurs and its Causes (Table 7.20)

Q. Write short note on causes of pansystolic murmur.

Various Diastolic Murmurs and Its Causes (Table 7.21)

Q. Write short note on causes of mid-diastolic murmurs.

TABLE 7.20: Various systolic murmurs and its causes.

Early systolic murmurs: ➢ VSD (small muscular VSD/large VSD with pulmonary hypertension) ➢ Acute severe MR ➢ Acute severe TR	**Late systolic murmurs:** ➢ Mitral valve prolapse ➢ Tricuspid valve prolapse ➢ Papillary muscle dysfunction
Mid-systolic/ejection systolic murmurs: ➢ Aortic stenosis ➢ Pulmonary stenosis ➢ Hypertrophic obstructive cardiomyopathy (HOCM)	**Pansystolic murmurs:** ➢ Mitral regurgitation ➢ Tricuspid regurgitation ➢ Ventricular septal defect ➢ Rare: Early PDA/PDA with Eisenmenger

TABLE 7.21: Various diastolic murmurs and its causes.

Early diastolic murmur:	Mid diastolic murmur:	Late diastolic murmurs/ presystolic murmur:
➢ Aortic regurgitation ➢ Pulmonary regurgitation	➢ Mitral stenosis ➢ Tricuspid stenosis ➢ Carey Coombs murmur of acute rheumatic fever ➢ Austin Flint murmur of chronic aortic regurgitation ➢ Flow MDM ➢ Across mitral valve: MR, AR, VSD, PDA ➢ Across tricuspid valve: ASD, TR, TAPVC (total anomalous pulmonary venous connection) ➢ Atrial myxoma ➢ Ball-valve thrombus ➢ Cor triatriatum ➢ Rytand's murmur of complete heart block	➢ Mitral stenosis ➢ Tricuspid stenosis ➢ Myxoma

Continuous Murmurs

Q. Write short note on the common causes of continuous murmurs of heart.

The continuous murmur is a murmur that begins in systole and continues without interruption, encompassing the second sound, throughout diastole or part of diastole.

Causes of Continuous Murmurs (Table 7.22)

TABLE 7.22: Causes of continuous murmurs.

➢ **Systemic to pulmonary communication:** – Patent ductus arteriosus – Aortopulmonary window – Anomalous origin of left coronary artery from pulmonary artery (ALCAPA) – Tricuspid atresia – Truncus arteriosus – Shunts for TOF surgery: Waterson, Potts, or Blalock-Taussig shunt ➢ **Systemic to right heart connection:** – Coronary AV fistula – Rupture sinus of Valsalva ➢ **Left atrium to right atrium connection:** – Lutembacher syndrome	➢ **Arteriovenous fistula:** – Systemic – Pulmonary ➢ **Normal flow through constricted arteries:** – Coarctation of aorta – Peripheral pulmonary stenosis – Renal artery stenosis ➢ **Increased flow through normal vessels:** – Venous: Cervical venous hum, Cruveilhier-Baumgarten murmur – Arterial: Mammary soufflé, uterine soufflé, thyrotoxicosis, tumors (e.g., hepatocellular carcinoma, renal cell carcinoma)

Systolic-Diastolic Murmur/To-and-Fro Murmur

- The presence of a systolic-diastolic murmur (systolic murmur and diastolic murmur), so called a to-and-fro murmur, is not a continuous murmur.
- It is separating the two murmurs through a small "silence".
- It involves two components: A systolic one, in which the blood flows in one direction, and a diastolic one in which the blood flows in the opposite direction.
- In contrast to true continuous murmur, the blood flows in the same direction in both systole and diastole.
- To-and-fro murmurs are two murmurs that occur through a single channel.
- Causes of systolic-diastolic murmur are presented in **Table 7.23**.

TABLE 7.23: Causes of systolic-diastolic and to-and-fro murmur.

Systolic-diastolic murmur:	To-and-fro murmur:
➢ VSD with AR	➢ AS with AR ➢ Pulmonary hypertension with pulmonary regurgitation

Innocent Murmurs

Q. Write short note on innocent murmurs.

Characteristics: Short, systolic (rarely continuous) soft murmur. Normal heart sounds and no hemodynamic abnormalities.

Examples of innocent murmurs are listed in **Box 7.10**.

Venous hum (jugular venous hum; cervical venous hum, Pontian's murmur).

Named murmurs and its causes are listed in **Table 7.24**.

Box 7.10: Examples of innocent murmurs.

Systolic:
- Vibratory systolic murmur (Still's murmur)
- Pulmonic systolic murmur (pulmonary trunk)
- Mammary soufflé
- Peripheral pulmonic systolic murmur (pulmonary branches)
- Supraclavicular or brachiocephalic systolic murmur
- Aortic systolic murmur
- Still's murmur: Medium frequency, vibratory, originating from leaflets of pulmonary valve

Continuous:
- Venous hum
- Continuous mammary soufflé

TABLE 7.24: Named murmurs.

Name of the murmur	*Cause/lesion*
Carey Coombs murmur: Mid-diastolic murmur	Rheumatic fever
Austin Flint murmur: Mid-late diastolic murmur	Aortic regurgitation
Graham-Steel murmur: High pitched, diastolic murmur	Pulmonary regurgitation
Rytand's murmur: Mid-diastolic atypical murmur	Complete heart block
Dock's murmur: Diastolic murmur	Left anterior descending (LAD) artery stenosis
Mill wheel murmur due to air in RV cavity	Following cardiac catheterization
Still's murmur: Inferior aspect of lower left sternal border, systolic ejection sound, vibratory/musical quality	Subaortic stenosis, small VSD
Gibson's murmur: Continuous machinery murmur	Patent ductus arteriosus (PDA)
Key–Hodgkin murmur: Diastolic murmur	Aortic regurgitation, e.g., syphilitic
Cabot–Locke murmur: Diastolic murmur heard best at the left sternal border	Anemic patients and the murmur resolves with treatment of anemia
Roger's murmur: Loud pansystolic murmur heard maximally at the left sternal border	Small VSD
Pontain's murmur: Cervical venous hum	Severe anemia
Cole-Cecil murmur	AR murmur in left axilla due to higher position of apex
Cruveilhier-Baumgarten murmur	Venous hum diagnostic of portal vein hypertension

Q. Write short note on mammary soufflé.

Mammary soufflé is an innocent systolic or continuous cardiac murmur (probably of arterial origin) heard during late pregnancy or in the early postpartum period. It is to be differentiated from pathologic lesions and is unaffected by the Valsalva maneuver.

Changing Murmurs

Murmurs which change in character or intensity from moment to moment **(Box 7.11)**.

Box 7.11: Changing murmurs.

- Carey Coombs murmur
- Infective endocarditis
- Atrial thrombus
- Atrial myxomas

Dynamic Auscultation

Q. Write short essay/note on dynamic auscultation in cardiac diseases.

This is a technique of altering circulatory dynamics by means of a variety of physiological and pharmacological maneuvers and determining their effects on heart sounds and murmurs.

Q. Write short essay/note on maneuvers useful in differentiating murmurs due to various cardiac diseases.

Interventions most commonly employed are:

- Respiration
- Postural changes
- Valsalva maneuver
- Isometric exercise
- Post-premature ventricular contractions (PVC)
- Vasoactive agents, e.g., amyl nitrite, methoxamine, and phenylephrine.

Various valvular lesions and dynamic auscultation findings are presented in **Table 7.25**.

Usefulness of dynamic auscultation in differential diagnosis of valvular lesions is depicted in **Table 7.26**.

Usefulness of amyl nitrate in differential diagnosis of murmurs is depicted in **Table 7.27**.

TABLE 7.25: Various valvular lesions and dynamic auscultation findings.

Valvular lesion	Features that augmenting/increasing the murmur intensity	Features that decrease/reduce the murmur intensity
Mitral stenosis (MS)	MDM accentuated by: Exercise, squatting, amyl nitrate, isometric hand grip, and left lateral position	Reduced mid-diastolic murmur (MDM), softening of opening snap (OS), and A_2-OS gap widening by: Inspiration, sudden standing
Mitral regurgitation (MR)	Augmentation of the murmur by: Squatting, isometric exercise and left lateral position	Decrease murmur by: Sudden standing, Valsalva, and amyl nitrate
Aortic stenosis (AS)	Murmur increases on: Post PVC beat, squatting and lying flat from standing	Reduces AS murmur by: Valsalva, standing and handgrip
Aortic regurgitation (AR)	Early diastolic murmur (EDM) increases on: Expiration, sitting up and leaning forward, squatting, isometric exercise, and vasopressors	Decreases with: Amyl nitrate and Valsalva
Mitral valve prolapse (MVP)	Murmur and click later, LV volume increase by: Squatting, postectopic, isometric exercise (intensity increases)	Murmur and click earlier (intensity decreases) and left ventricle (LV) volume decrease by: Standing and Valsalva
Hypertrophic obstructive cardiomyopathy (HOCM)	Increase murmur by: Expiration, Valsalva strain, standing, postectopic, and amyl nitrate	Decrease murmur by: Inspiration, sustained handgrip, squatting, and methoxamine

TABLE 7.26: Usefulness of dynamic auscultation in differential diagnosis of valvular lesions.	
Differential diagnosis	
Aortic stenosis (AS) versus hypertrophic obstructive cardiomyopathy (HOCM)	Squatting: Increases in AS, decreases in HOCM
	Valsalva/standing: Decreases in AS, increases in HOCM
Aortic stenosis (AS) versus mitral regurgitation (MR)	Handgrip and phenylephrine: Decreases in AS, increases in MR
	Post-PVC and amyl nitrate: Increases in AS, decreases in MR
Mitral stenosis (MS) versus Austin Flint murmur	Amyl nitrate: Increases in MS, decreases in Austin Flint murmur
Pulmonary stenosis (PS) versus aortic stenosis (AS)	Respiration: Increases with inspiration in PS, increases with expiration in AS
Mitral stenosis (MS) versus tricuspid stenosis (TS)	Respiration: Increases with expiration (MS) and increases with inspiration (TS)
Mitral regurgitation (MR) versus tricuspid regurgitation (TR)	Respiration: Increases with expiration (MR) and increases with inspiration (TR)
Pulmonary stenosis (PS) versus small ventricular septal defect (VSD)	Amyl nitrate: Increases in PS, decreases in VSD
	Phenylephrine: Decreases in PS and increases in VSD
	Respiration: Increases with inspiration in PS, no variation with respiration in VSD
Pulmonary regurgitation (PR) versus aortic regurgitation (AR)	Squatting and sustained handgrip: No change in PR, increased in AR

CONDUCTION SYSTEM OF THE HEART (FIG. 7.9)

Q. Write short essay/note on the conduction system of the heart.

An electrical discharge from the sinoatrial (sinus) node initiates the normal heart beat. It is then sequentially depolarized in the atria followed by ventricles as it passes through specialized conducting tissue.

- **Sinus node (SA node):** It is located in the lateral and epicardial aspect where the superior vena cava joins the right atrium.
  It is a natural pacemaker of the heart and controls the rate and rhythm of the heart (rate of 60–100 beats/minute). It has the fastest inherent discharge.
- **Atrioventricular (AV) node:** The impulse from the SA node spreads through the atrial musculature and down to the atrioventricular (AV) node that is situated above the tricuspid valve. Passage via the AV node is relatively slow, and is responsible for the normal physiological delay in ventricular depolarization. AV node functions as a back-up pacemaker with an intrinsic rate of 40–60 beats/minute.
- **His bundle and Purkinje fibers:** The impulse then travels downward to the bundle of His and through its branches (right bundle branch and left bundle branch) to the Purkinje network of fibers that convey the impulse to the ventricular

TABLE 7.27: Usefulness of amyl nitrate in differential diagnosis of murmurs.	
Valvular lesions	***Amyl nitrate response***
Systolic murmur:	
Aortic stenosis (AS) versus mitral regurgitation (MR)	Increased in AS and decreased in MR
Tricuspid regurgitation (TR) versus mitral regurgitation (MR)	Increased in TR and decreased in MR
Pulmonary stenosis (PS) versus tetralogy of Fallot (TOF)	Increased in PS and decreased in TOF
Pulmonary stenosis (PS) versus ventricular septal defect (VSD)	Increased in PS and decreased in VSD
Diastolic murmur:	
Mitral stenosis (MS) versus Austin Flint murmur	Increased in MS and decreased in Austin Flint murmur
End-diastolic murmur of pulmonary regurgitation (PR) with aortic regurgitation (AR)	Increased in PR and decreased in AR

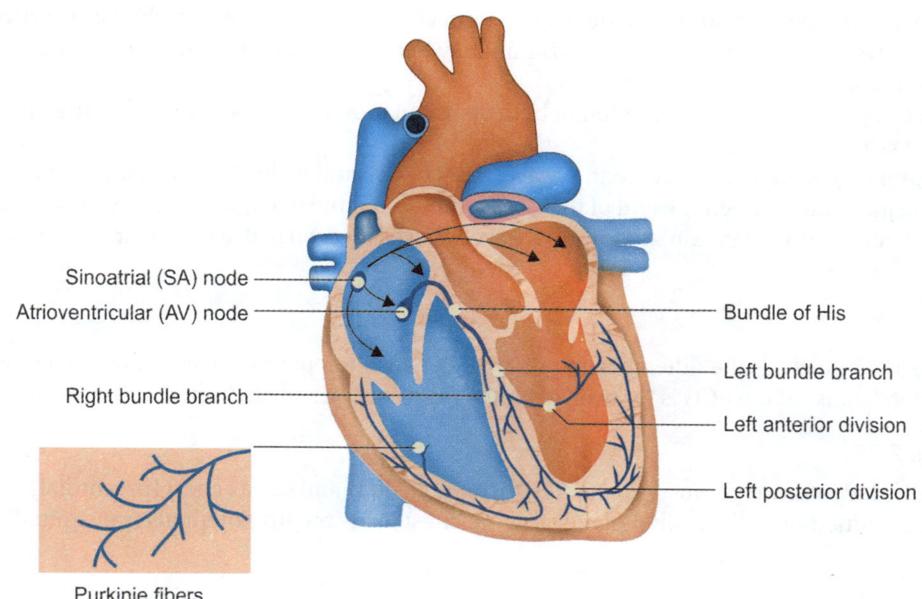

FIG. 7.9: Conduction system of heart.

endocardium and then epicardium. Potential pacemaking properties also exist in the cells of the AV node, bundle of His, and Purkinje fibers. Ventricular cells also act a back-up pacemaker with an intrinsic rate of 20–45 beats/minute.

ELECTROCARDIOGRAM

Q. Write short essay on analysis of an electrocardiogram (ECG).

Sinus Rhythm: Waveforms and Intervals (Fig. 7.10)

Electrocardiogram is the recording of sequential sum of depolarization and repolarization of all myocardial cells. The electrical depolarization of myocardial tissue produces a small dipole current. It can be detected by electrode pairs on the body surface. These signals are amplified and either printed on special graph paper or displayed on a monitor.

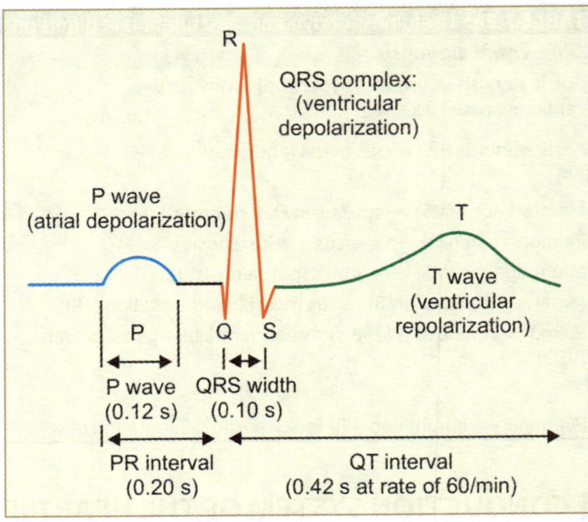

FIG. 7.10: Electrocardiograph showing various components.

- **Depolarization** is the sudden change within myocardium, during which it undergoes a dramatic electrical change. Entire myocardium is depolarized in a coordinated manner.
  - **P wave:** The ECG waveforms are labeled alphabetically beginning with the P wave (represents atrial depolarization).
  - The SA node triggers **atrial depolarization**, producing a beginning P wave.
  - **QRS complex:** Depolarization slowly spreads through the AV node, which produces a depolarization wave which is too small to be detected from the body surface. The bundle of His, bundle branches, and Purkinje system are then activated, initiating ventricular myocardial depolarization. During this, QRS complex is produced that represents the duration of ventricular depolarization. Because of the larger size of the ventricular muscle mass than that of the atria, the QRS complex is larger than the P wave. Normal value is 100–110 ms or less. The QRS complex is subdivided into specific deflections or waves.
    - **Q wave:** If the initial QRS depletion in a particular lead is negative, it is termed a Q wave, indicates septal depolarization.
    - **R wave:** The first positive deflection is termed an R wave.
    - **S wave:** A negative deflection after an R wave is an S wave.
    - **Subsequent positive or negative waves** are labeled R′ (R prime) and S′ (S prime), respectively.
    - Lowercase letters (qrs) are used for waves of relatively small amplitude. An entirely negative QRS complex is termed a QS wave.
  - **PR interval:** It is the interval between the onset of the P wave and the onset of the QRS complex. Normal value is 120–200 ms. It largely reflects the duration of AV nodal conduction between atrial and ventricular depolarization.
- **Repolarization** is the restoration of the electrical polarity of myocardial muscle.
  - Repolarization is a slower process and spreads from the epicardium to the endocardium.
  - Atrial repolarization does not produce a detectable signal (too low in amplitude) whereas ventricular repolarization produces the T wave. However, atrial repolarization may become apparent in conditions, such as acute pericarditis and atrial infarction.
  - **QT interval:** It represents the total duration of both ventricular depolarization and repolarization. It varies inversely with the heart rate.
  - **ST-T-U complex:** It consists of ST segment, T wave, and U wave and is due to ventricular repolarization. The J point represents the junction between the end of the QRS complex and the beginning of the ST segment.
  - **U wave:** Small, rounded, upright wave following T wave. Most easily seen with a slow heart rate. Indicates repolarization of Purkinje fibers.

ECG Leads

The standard 12-lead ECG records the difference in potential between ten physical electrodes placed on the surface of the body. The term twelve "leads" of the ECG is for twelve number of recordings made from pairs or sets of these electrodes.

Type of Leads (Fig. 7.11)

The ECG leads are divided into two groups: (1) six limb (extremity) leads and (2) six chest (precordial) leads. The limb leads record potentials transmitted onto the frontal plane, and the chest leads record potentials transmitted onto the horizontal plane.

Reading 12-lead ECGs

The best way to read 12-lead ECGs is to develop a step-by-step approach **(Box 7.12)**.

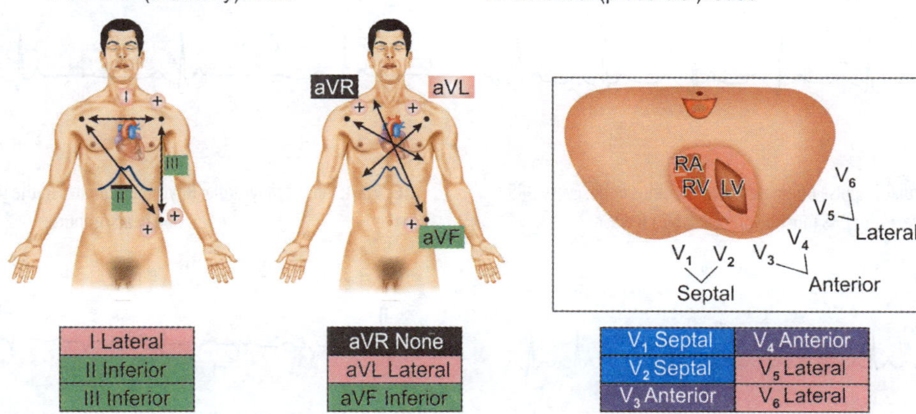

FIG. 7.11: Diagrammatic representation of the connections or directions, net axis of each lead in a 12-lead electrocardiogram.

Step 1: Determining the Heart Rate (Fig. 7.12)

- The ECG is normally recorded at a speed of 25 mm/sec. Each small, square, in the graph is 1 mm and represents 0.04 seconds and big boxes with heavier lines represent 0.20 s (200 ms).
- **Rule of 300/1,500:** For regular rhythms, count the number of "big boxes" between two QRS complexes, and divide this into 300. The heart rate (beats per minute) can also be computed readily from the interbeat [R-number of small (0.04 s) units into 1,500].
- **6-second rule:** For irregular rhythms, ECG records 6 seconds of rhythm per page, count the number of beats present on the ECG, multiply by 10.
- Variations of heart rate and its causes are listed in **Table 7.28.**

Q. Write short note on sinus tachycardia.

Step 2: Determine Regularity (Figs. 7.13 to 7.25)

- Look at the R-R distances (using a caliper or markings on a paper).
- Regular (are they equidistant apart)? Occasionally irregular? Regularly irregular?
- Irregularly irregular-atrial fibrillation.

Step 3: Determining the Axis (Fig. 7.26)

- Normal QRS axis from –30° to +110°, –30° to –90° is referred to as a left axis deviation (LAD), +110° to +180° is referred to as a right axis deviation (RAD) and –180° to –90° is referred as north-west axis/extreme axis/axis in no man's land.
- QRS complex in leads I and aVF determine if they are predominantly positive or negative. The combination should place the axis into one of the 4 quadrants above.
- Various causes of axis deviation are listed in **Table 7.29.**

Box 7.12: Steps in reading ECG.

1. Calculate rate
2. Determine rhythm
3. Determine QRS axis
4. Check individual waves
5. Calculate intervals
6. Assess for hypertrophy
7. Look for evidence of infarction/dyselectrolytemia/drug effects

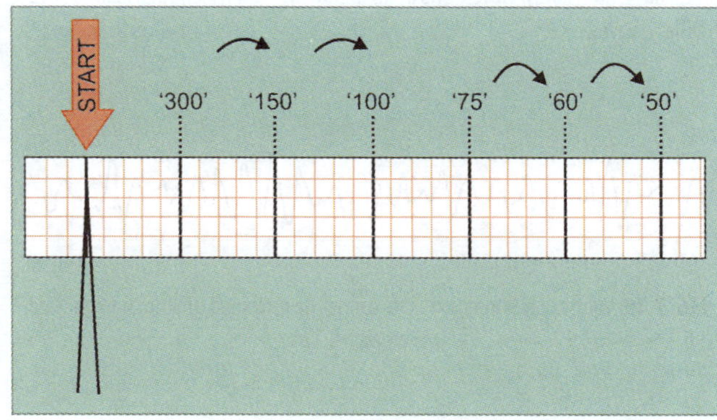

FIG. 7.12: Determination of heart rate by ECG.

TABLE 7.28: Variations of heart rate and its causes.
Normal: 60–99 beats/min (bpm)
Bradycardia <60 bpm: Hypothermia, increased vagal tone (due to vagal stimulation or e.g., drugs), athletes, hypothyroidism, beta blockade, marked intracranial hypertension, obstructive jaundice, uremia, structural SA node disease, or ischemia
Tachycardia >100 bpm: Any cause of adrenergic stimulation (including pain); thyrotoxicosis; hypovolemia; vagolytic drugs (e.g., atropine) anemia, pregnancy; vasodilator drugs, including many hypotensive agents; fever, myocarditis

Step 4: Check Individual Waves

- **Assess P waves (Box 7.13)**
- **Normal:** Always positive in lead I and II, always negative in lead aVR. Commonly biphasic in lead V_1 and best seen in leads II. <2.5 small squares in duration and <2.5 small squares in amplitude.

Step 5: Calculate Intervals

PR interval: Normal is 0.12–0.20 seconds.

- **Long PR interval** may indicate heart block **(Figs. 7.27 to 7.30)**
- **Short PR interval:** Tachycardia and pre-excitation syndromes (e.g., Lown-Ganong-Levine syndrome, Wolff-Parkinson-White syndrome).

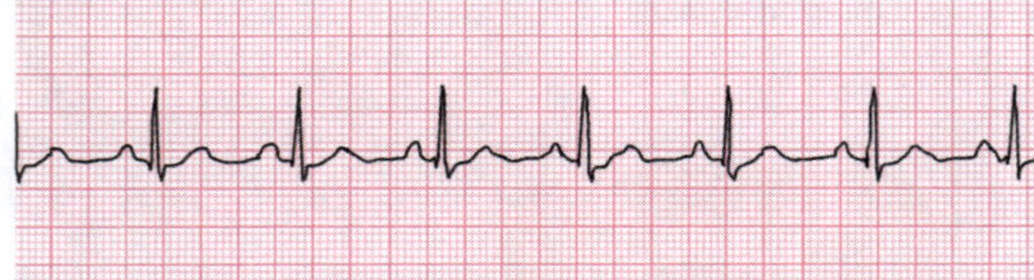

FIG. 7.13: Sinus rhythm: Cardiac impulse originates from the sinus node. Every QRS must be sinus node. Every QRS must be preceded by a P wave.

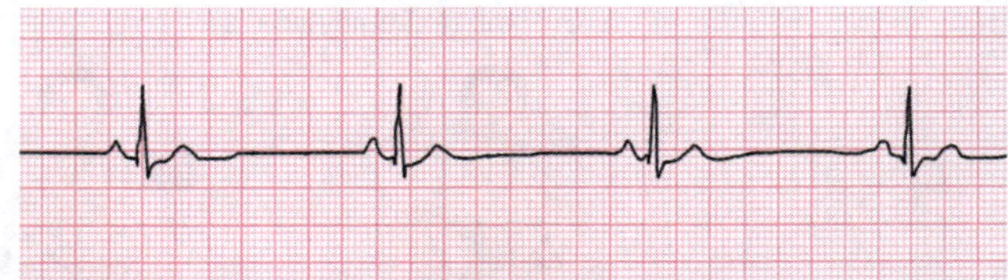

FIG. 7.14: Sinus bradycardia: Rhythm originates in the sinus node. Rate of less than 60 beats/minute.

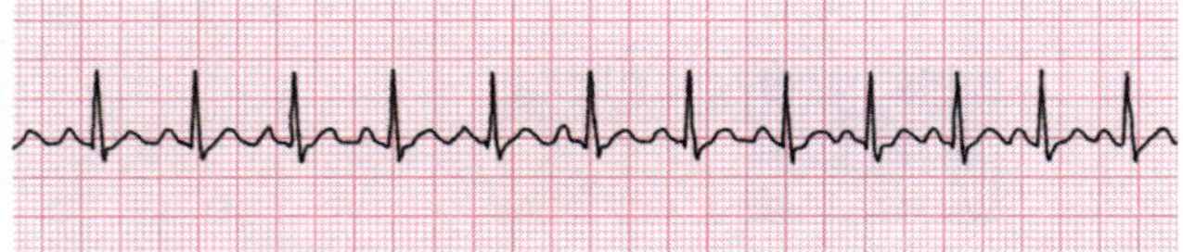

FIG. 7.15: Sinus tachycardia: Rate >100 beats/minute, otherwise, normal.

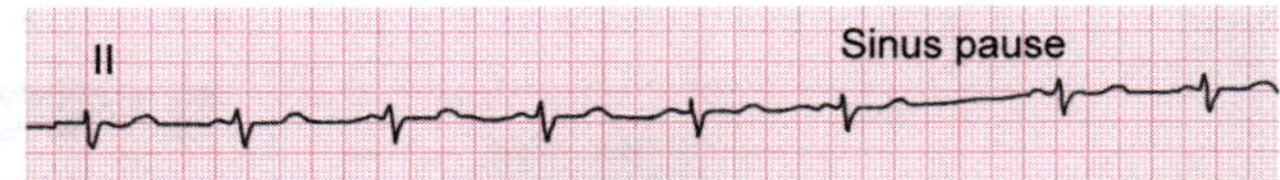

FIG. 7.16: Sinus pause. In disease (e.g., sick sinus syndrome) the SA node can fail in its pacing function. If failure is brief and recovery is prompt, the result is only a missed beat (sinus pause). If recovery is delayed and no other focus assumes pacing function, cardiac arrest follows.

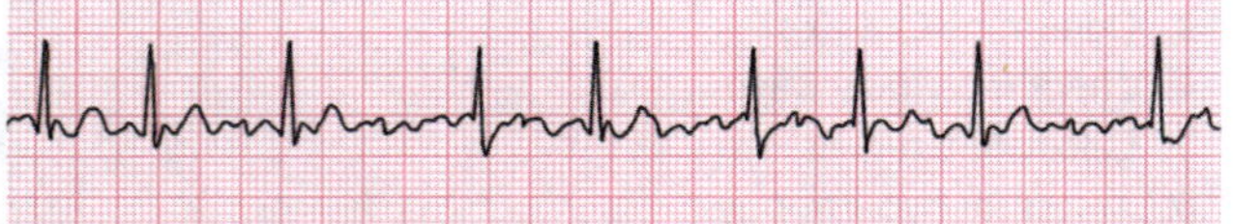

FIG. 7.17: Atrial fibrillation. Rate = ~150 beats/minute, irregularly irregular, baseline irregularity, no visible p waves, QRS occur irregularly with its length usually <0.12 s, fibrillary waves.

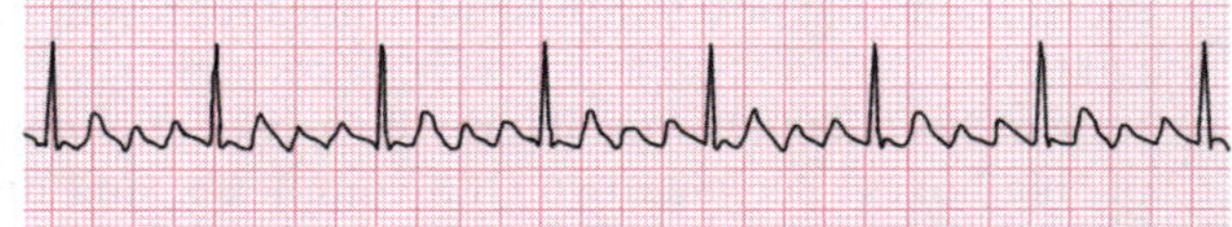

FIG. 7.18: Atrial flutter. Atrial rate = ~300 beats/minute, P waves absent but have flutter waves, ECG baseline adapts "saw- toothed' appearance".

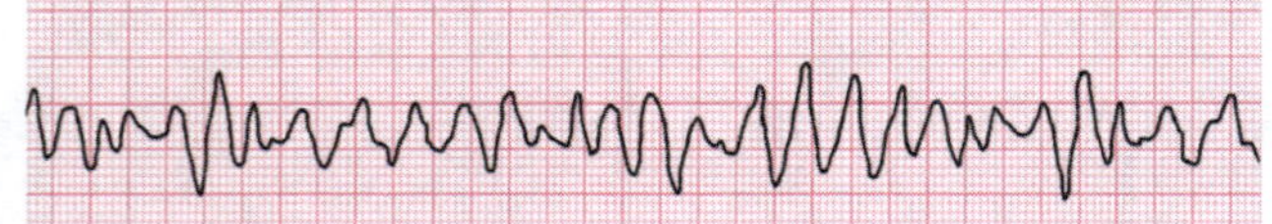

FIG. 7.19: Ventricular fibrillation. Rate cannot be discerned, rhythm unorganized, QRS broad >0.12 s.

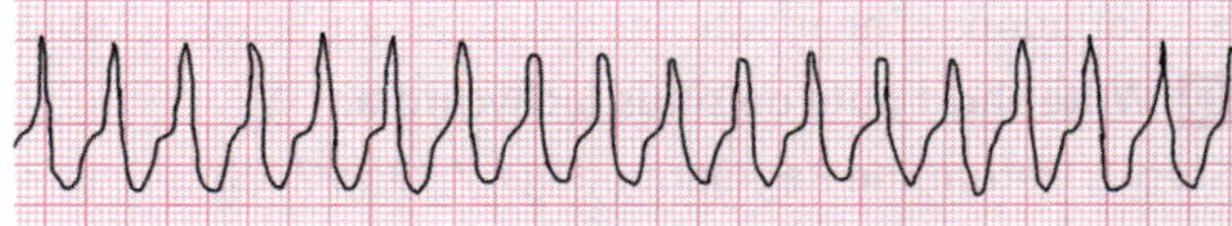

FIG. 7.20: Ventricular tachycardia. Rate = 100–250 beats/minute, broad QRS, regular.

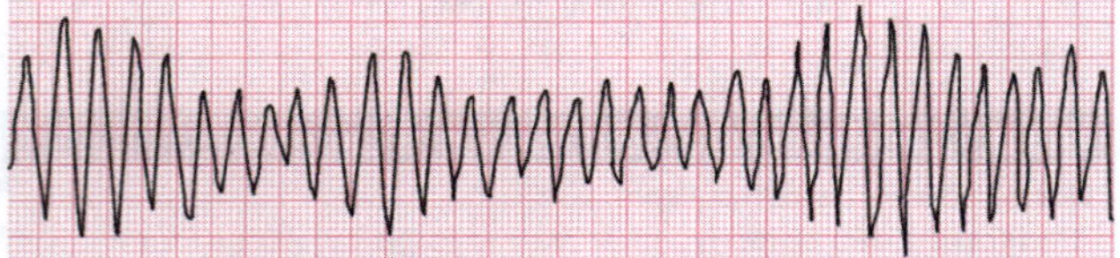

FIG. 7.21: Torsades de pointes (literally means twisting of points) is a distinctive form of polymorphic ventricular tachycardia characterized by a gradual change in the amplitude and twisting of the QRS complexes around the isoelectric lines.

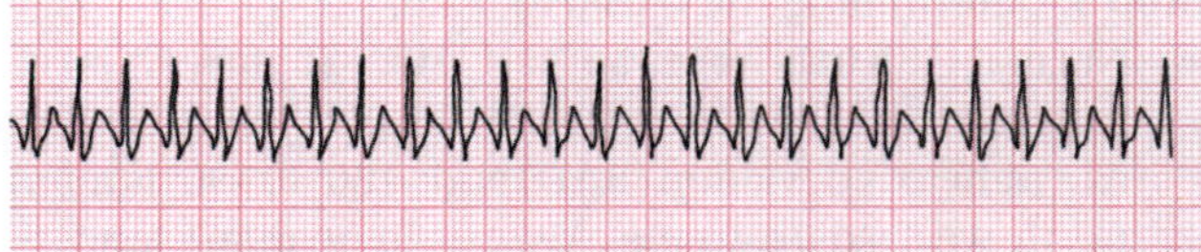

FIG. 7.22: Supraventricular tachycardia. Tachycardiac rhythm originating above the ventricular tissue. Atrial and ventricular rate = 150–250 beats/minute regular rhythm, p is usually not discernable.

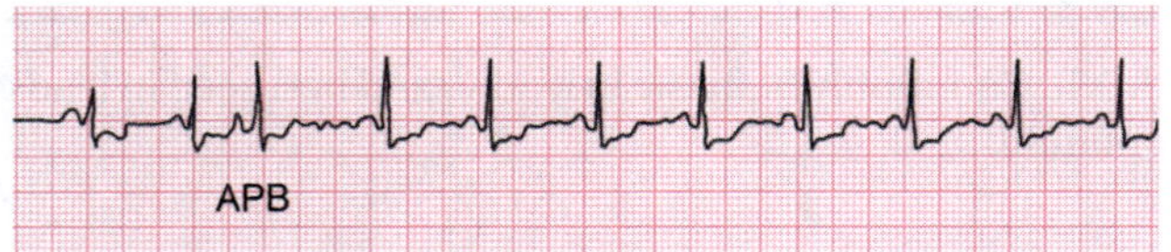

FIG. 7.23: Atrial premature beat (APB). It arises from an irritable focus in one of the atria. It produces different looking P wave, because depolarization vector is abnormal. QRS complex has normal duration and same morphology.

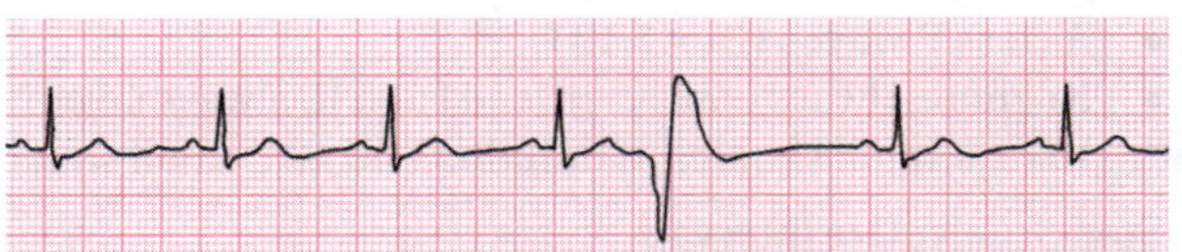

FIG. 7.24: Premature ventricular complexes (PVCs). Occasionally irregular rhythm, broad QRS arising from ventricles no p-wave associated with PVCs. It can be monomorphic/polymorphic.

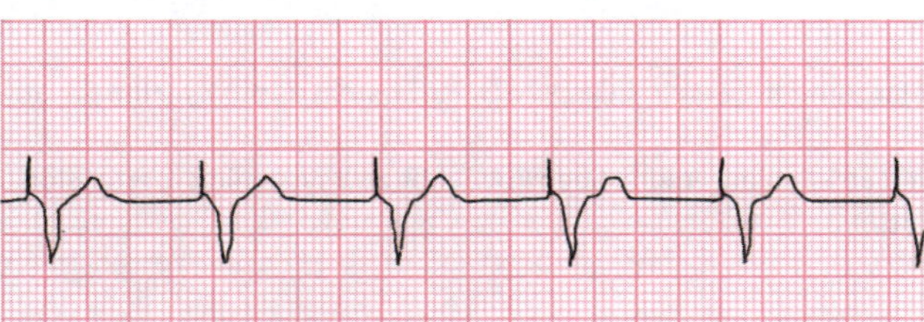

FIG. 7.25: Artificial pacemaker. Sharp, thin spike before each complex, ventricular paced rhythm shows wide ventricular pacemaker spikes.

TABLE 7.29: Causes of axis deviation.

Cardiac axis	*Causes*
Left axis deviation	Left anterior hemiblock, left ventricular hypertrophy, Wolff–Parkinson–White syndrome, inferior MI, ostium primum ASD, and ventricular tachycardia Normal variation in pregnancy, obesity; ascites, and abdominal distention
Right axis deviation	Tall thin adults, right ventricular hypertrophy, COPD, ostium secundum ASD, left posterior hemiblock, Wolff–Parkinson–White syndrome, anterolateral MI
North West	Dextrocardia, severe emphysema, hyperkalemia, lead transposition, artificial cardiac pacing, and ventricular tachycardia

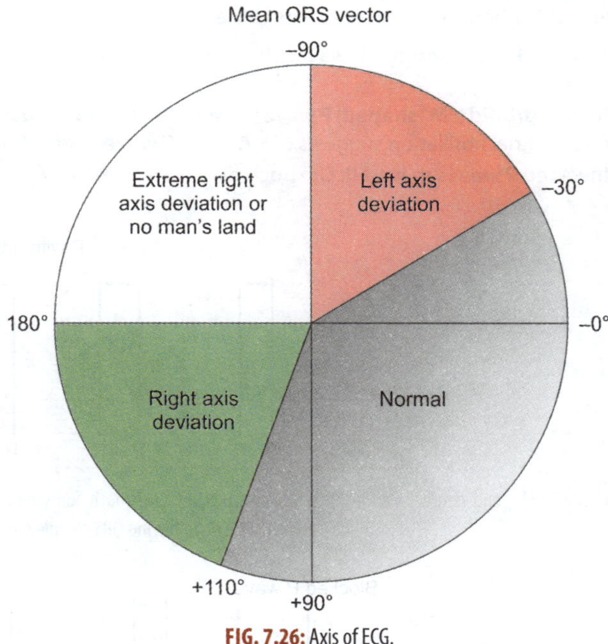

FIG. 7.26: Axis of ECG.

QRS-complex

- **Normal characteristics:** Duration is 0.04–0.11 seconds.
- **Broad/wide QRS** (>0.12s): Ventricular hypertrophy, intraventricular conduction disturbance, bundle branch blocks, aberrant ventricular conduction, ventricular preexcitation, ventricular ectopic or escape pacemaker, and ventricular pacing by cardiac pacemaker
- Height of QRS–Sokolow index (SV2 + RV5) <35 mm (<45 mm for young)
- Increased height: In RV/LV hypertrophy
- **Decreased height:** Low voltage QRS (<5 mV in limb leads/<10 mV in chest leads): Obese patient, restrictive cardiomyopathy, pericardial effusion, hypothyroidism, hypothermia, and myocarditis.

Q Waves

- The normal Q wave in lead I is due to septal depolarization. It is small in amplitude (less than 25% of the succeeding R wave, or less than 3 mm). Its duration is <0.04 sec or one small box. It is seen in L1 and sometimes in V5, V6.
- **Pathological Q wave** of infarction in the respective leads is due to dead muscle. It may also be seen in cardiomyopathies, i.e., hypertrophic (HOCM), infiltrative myocardial disease.
- **Absent Q waves** in V5-6 is most commonly due to LBBB.

Bundle Branch Blocks (Figs. 7.31A and B)

- **Left bundle branch block (LBBB):** Indirect activation causes left ventricle to contract later than the right ventricle.
- **Right bundle branch block (RBBB):** Indirect activation causes right ventricle to contract later than the left ventricle.

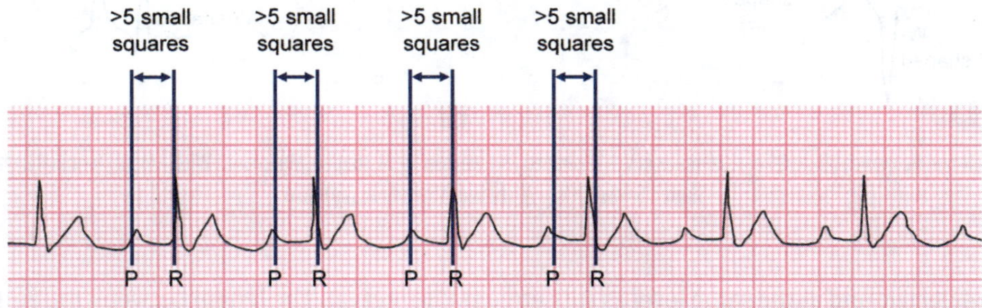

FIG. 7.27: First-degree heart block. P wave precedes QRS complex but P-R intervals prolong (>5 small squares) and remain constant from beat to beat.

Box 7.13: Abnormal P waves and its causes.

Tall (>2.5 mm), pointed P waves (P pulmonale): Suggests right atrial enlargement. Seen in COPD, ASD, TS, Ebstein anomaly (Himalayan P waves)

Notched/bifid ("M" shaped) P wave (P "mitrale") in limb leads: Suggests left atrial enlargement. Seen in MS, MR, and systemic hypertension. Coarse atrial fibrillation suggests LAE **Absent P waves:** Atrial fibrillation/flutter

Inverted P waves in lead II: Dextrocardia

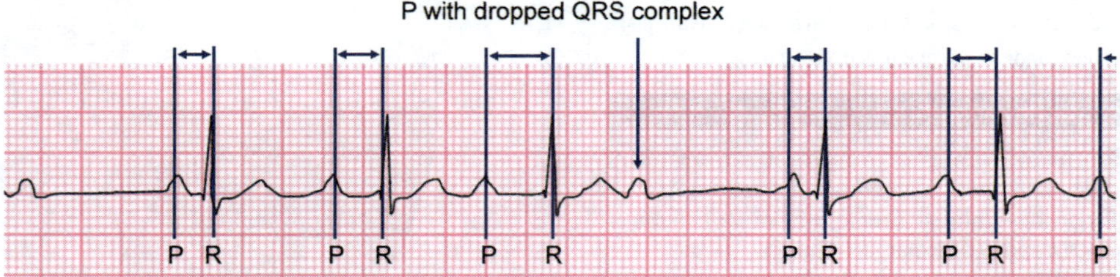

FIG. 7.28: Second-degree heart block—Mobitz type I or Wenckebach. Runs in cycle, first P-R interval is often normal. With successive beat, P-R interval lengthens until there will be a P wave with no following QRS complex. The block is at AV node, often transient, may be asymptomatic.

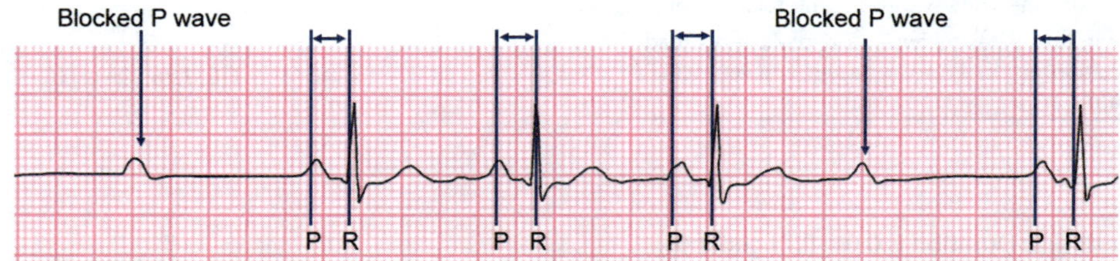

FIG. 7.29: Second-degree heart block—Mobitz type 2. P-R interval is constant, duration is normal/prolonged. Periodically, no conduction between atria and ventricles—producing a p wave with no associated QRS complex (blocked p wave). The block is most often below AV node, at bundle of His or BB, may progress to third-degree heart block.

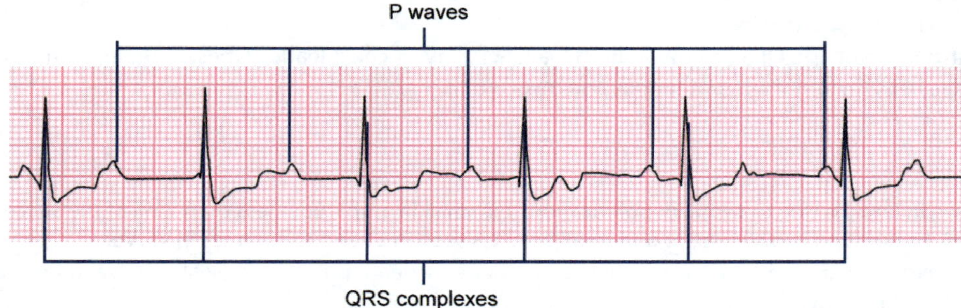

FIG. 7.30: Third-degree heart block (complete heart block). No relationship between P waves and QRS complexes. An accessory pacemaker in the lower chambers will typically activate the ventricles-escape rhythm. Atrial rate = 60–100 beats/minute. Ventricular rate based on site of escape pacemaker. Atrial and ventricular rhythms both are regular.

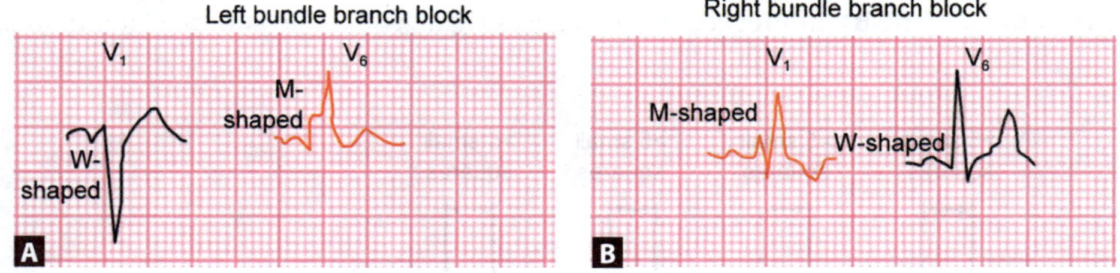

FIGS. 7.31A AND B: (A) Left bundle branch block: QS or rS complex in V_1 - W-shaped RsR' wave in V_6 - M-shaped. Mnemonic: WILLIAM; (B) Terminal R wave (rSR') in V_1 - M-shaped. Slurred S wave in V_6 - W-shaped. Mnemonic: MARROW.

ST Segment

- ST segment is isoelectric and at the same level as subsequent PR-interval. The length between the end of the S wave (end of ventricular depolarization) and the beginning of repolarization. From J point on the end of QRS complex, to inclination of T wave.

- Causes of ST-segment elevation are shown in **Box 7.14** and **Figure 7.32** and causes of ST-segment depression are listed in **Box 7.15**.

T Wave

- Normally, a repolarization directs from epicardium to endocardium = T wave is concordant with QRS complex
- Causes of T wave inversions are listed in **Box 7.16**.
- **Tall T waves** (height more than 2/3 of neighboring QRS): Hyperkalemia (steeple T waves), hyperacute MI.

QT Interval

- It represents the time taken for ventricular depolarization and repolarization. The duration of the QT interval is proportionate to the heart rate. The faster the heart beats, the faster the ventricles repolarize so the shorter the QT interval. Therefore, what is a "normal" QT varies with the heart rate. QT interval should be 0.35–0.45 seconds.
- For each heart rate you need to calculate an adjusted QT interval, called the "corrected QT" (QTc):
- QTc = QT/square root of RR interval—**Bazett's formula**
- **Prolonged QTc** (>440 ms) **(Box 7.17)**: A prolonged QT can be very dangerous. It can predispose an individual to a type of ventricular tachycardia—Torsades de pointes.
- **Short QTc** (<350 ms): Hypercalcemia, digoxin effect.

U Waves

- U wave need not be always seen on an electrocardiogram. It is small, round, and symmetrical and follows the T wave and seen positive in lead II. U waves are due to repolarization of the papillary muscles or Purkinje fibers. It is the same direction as T wave in that lead.
- **Prominent U waves:** These are seen in hypokalemia, hypercalcemia, thyrotoxicosis, or exposure to digitalis, epinephrine, and Class 1A and 3 antiarrhythmics.
- An inverted U wave may represent myocardial ischemia or left ventricular volume overload.

Step 6: Assess for Hypertrophy

Left Ventricular Hypertrophy (LVH)

Q. Write short note on causes of left ventricular hypertrophy and left ventricular dilatation.

- Criteria of LVH:
  - *High QRS voltages in limb leads: Sokolow-Lyon index: S in V_1 or V_2 + R in V_5 or V_6 (whichever is larger) ≥35 mm OR R in aVL ≥11 mm*
  - *Deep symmetric T inversion in V_4, V_5, and V_6*
  - *QRS duration >0.09 sec, associated left axis deviation*
- Romhilt-Estes scoring system is used for diagnosing LVH.
- **Common causes of left ventricular hypertrophy and left ventricular dilatation** are listed in **Table 7.30**.

Ventricular Hypertrophy (RVH)

Criteria of right ventricular hypertrophy and its causes are listed in **Table 7.31**.

Step 7: Look for Evidence of Infarction/Dyselectrolytemia

- **ECG in myocardial infarction (MI):** There are two types of MI—ST-elevation myocardial infarction (STEMI) and non-STEMI (NSTEMI).

Box 7.14: Causes of ST-segment elevation.

- Ischemia
- Early repolarization
- Acute pericarditis: ST elevation in all leads except aVR
- Pulmonary embolism
- Hypothermia
- Hypertrophic cardiomyopathy
- High potassium
- Cerebrovascular accident (CVA)
- Acute sympathetic stress
- Brugada syndrome
- Cardiac aneurysm
- Left ventricular hypertrophy
- Idioventricular rhythm including paced rhythm

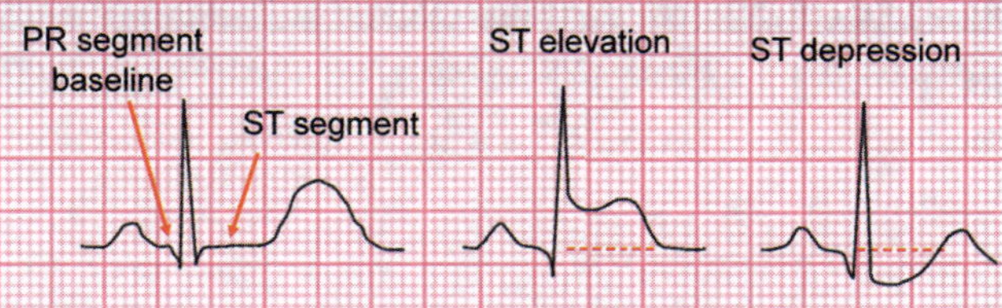

FIG. 7.32: ECG showing ST-segment elevation.

Box 7.15: Causes of ST-segment depression.

- Myocardial ischemia/NSTEMI
- Reciprocal change in STEMI
- Posterior MI
- Digoxin effect (Reverse tick mark/'sagging' morphology, resembling Salvador Dali's moustache)
- Hypokalemia
- Bundle branch block
- Ventricular hypertrophy
- Ventricular pacing

Box 7.16: Causes of T wave inversions.

- CAD/ischemia
- Cardiomyopathies (hypertrophic), myocarditis, pericarditis, and pulmonary embolism
- Valvular disorders
- Raised intracranial tension, CNS bleed, and ventricular hypertrophy
- Bundle branch block
- Pacing

Box 7.17: Causes of prolonged QTc.

- Hypokalemia, hypomagnesemia, and hypocalcemia
- Hypothermia
- Myocardial ischemia
- Raised intracranial pressure
- Congenital long QT syndrome, e.g., Jervell and Lange-Nielsen syndrome, Romano-Ward syndrome
- **Drugs**, e.g., chlorpromazine, haloperidol, quetiapine, quinidine, and procainamide

- **Romhilt-Estes point score system (≥5 points definite LVH)**
  i. Any limb lead R or S ≥20 mm/SV_1 + SV_2 ≥30 mm or RV_5 + RV_6 ≥30 mm—3 points
  ii. ST-T changes with digitalis—1 point, without digitalis—3 points
  iii. LAE—3 points
  iv. Left axis deviation (≤30)—2 points
  v. QRS duration ≥90 ms—1 point
  vi. Delayed intrinsicoid deflection in V_5/V_6 ≥50 ms—1 point

TABLE 7.30: Common causes of left ventricular hypertrophy and dilatation.

Common causes of left ventricular hypertrophy	***Common causes of left ventricular dilatation***
➢ Pressure overload: Systemic hypertension, aortic stenosis, IHD, coarctation of aorta (COA) ➢ Volume overload: Mitral or aortic regurgitation, dilated cardiomyopathy ➢ Both right and left ventricular volume overload: Ventricular septal defect (VSD) ➢ No pressure or volume overload: Hypertrophic cardiomyopathy (HCM) systemic	➢ Aortic regurgitation (AR) ➢ Mitral regurgitation (MR) ➢ VSD ➢ Persistent ductus arteriosus (PDA) ➢ Ischemic heart disease (IHD) ➢ Hyperkinetic circulatory states, e.g., anemia, thyrotoxicosis, and beriberi ➢ Dilated cardiomyopathy

TABLE 7.32: ECG findings depending on the location of myocardial infarct.

Location of MI	***Lead with ST changes***	***Affected coronary artery***
Anterior	V_1, V_2, V_3, V_4	Left anterior descending artery (LAD)
Septum	V_1, V_2	
Left lateral	I, aVL, V_5, V_6	Left circumflex
Inferior	II, III, aVF	Right coronary artery (RCA)
Right atrium	aVR, V_1	
Posterior	Posterior chest leads	
Right ventricle	Right sided leads	

- **STEMI criteria:**
    - ♦ ST elevation in >2 chest leads >2 mm elevation
    - ♦ ST elevation in >2 limb leads >1 mm elevation
    - ♦ Q wave >0.04s (1 small square).

  ECG findings depending on the location of myocardial infarct are presented in **Table 7.32**. Sequential ECG changes in STEMI are presented in **Figures 7.33A to F**.
- **Non-ST-elevation myocardial infarction (NSTEMI):**
    - NSTEMI is also known as subendocardial or non-Q-wave MI. In a patient with acute coronary syndrome (ACS) in which the ECG does not show ST elevation, NSTEMI (subendocardial MI) is suspected if ECG shows T wave inversion (symmetrical, arrowhead) with/without ST depression.
    - An ST depression is more suggestive of myocardial ischemia than infarction.

  Usefulness of electrocardiogram is listed in **Box 7.18**.

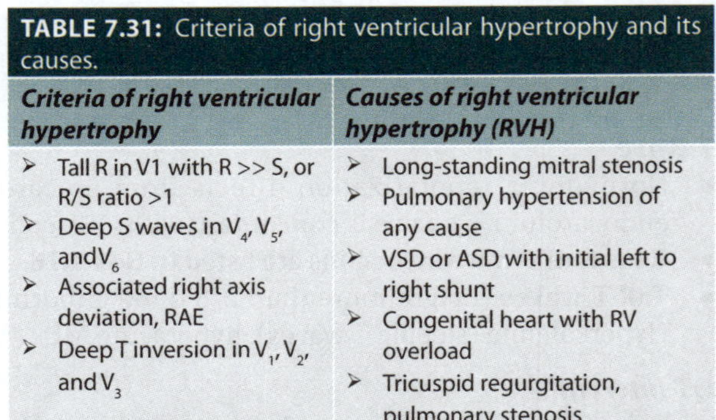

TABLE 7.31: Criteria of right ventricular hypertrophy and its causes.

Criteria of right ventricular hypertrophy	***Causes of right ventricular hypertrophy (RVH)***
➢ Tall R in V1 with R >> S, or R/S ratio >1 ➢ Deep S waves in V_4, V_5, and V_6 ➢ Associated right axis deviation, RAE ➢ Deep T inversion in V_1, V_2, and V_3	➢ Long-standing mitral stenosis ➢ Pulmonary hypertension of any cause ➢ VSD or ASD with initial left to right shunt ➢ Congenital heart with RV overload ➢ Tricuspid regurgitation, pulmonary stenosis

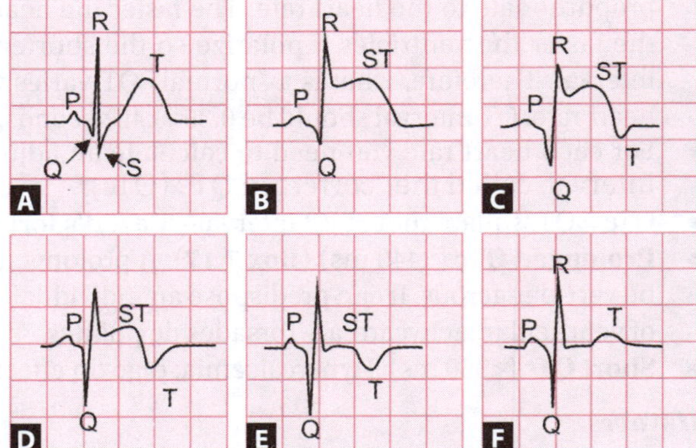

FIGS. 7.33A TO F: Sequential ECG changes in STEMI: (A) Normal ECG; (B) 0 hour: pronounced/hyper acute tall T wave initially, ST elevation (convex type); (C) 1–24 hours: depressed R wave, and pronounced T wave. Pathological Q waves may appear within hours or may take greater than 24 hours—indicating full-thickness MI. Q wave is pathological if it is wider than 40 ms or deeper than a third of the height of the entire QRS complex; (D) Day 1–2: exaggeration of T wave continues for 24 hours; (E) Days later: T wave inverts as the ST elevation begins to resolve. Persistent ST elevation is rare except in the presence of a ventricular aneurysm; (F) Weeks later: ECG returns to normal T wave, but retains pronounced Q wave.

Box 7.18: Usefulness of electrocardiogram.

- Cardiac arrhythmias
- Conduction defects
- Hypertrophy of cardiac chamber (atrium or ventricle)
- Electrolyte abnormalities (hypokalemia, hyperkalemia, hypocalcemia, and hypercalcemia)
- Effects of drugs (digitals)
- Hypothermia
- Pericarditis

ISCHEMIC HEART DISEASE

Q. Discuss the etiology, risk factors, clinical features, investigation, and treatment of ischemic heart disease (IHD).

Definition: Ischemic heart disease is a group of heart diseases in which there is an imbalance between myocardial blood supply and its oxygen demand. IHD is the **leading cause of death** in both males and females.

Etiology

- Coronary arterial occlusion is the main cause of myocardial ischemia.
    - Mostly due to coronary atherosclerosis and its complications. Coronary atherosclerosis narrows one or more of the epicardial coronary arteries → decreases the coronary blood flow in about 90% of cases. Hence, IHD is often known as coronary artery disease (CAD) or coronary heart disease.
- Other rare causes: Emboli, vasculitis, coronary vasospasm, hematologic disorders, such as sickle cell disease, and diminished availability of blood or oxygen (lowered systemic blood pressure as in shock).

Risk Factors for Atherosclerosis

Q. Write short essay/note on:

- **Risk factors for coronary arterial disease**
- **Risk factors for atherosclerosis**

They were identified through several studies most important being the Framingham heart study and atherosclerosis risk in communities study.

Classification of risk factors

The risk factors may be broadly classified as modifiable, nonmodifiable, and additional **(Table 7.33)**.

TABLE 7.33: Risk factors for atherosclerosis.

A. Modifiable major risk factors: Hyperlipidemia, hypertension, cigarette smoking, and diabetes mellitus
B. Nonmodifiable risk factors: Increasing age (men ≥45 years and females ≥55 years), male gender, family history, and genetic abnormalities (e.g., familial hypercholesterolemia)
C. Additional risk factors: Inflammation, raised CRP level, hyperhomocysteinemia, metabolic syndrome, lipoprotein (a), raised procoagulant levels, inadequate physical activity, stressful lifestyle, obesity, and alcohol

Pathogenesis of Atherosclerosis

Q. Discuss pathogenesis of atherosclerosis.

Atherosclerosis is a progressive inflammatory disorder of the arteries characterized by focal deposits of lipids in the intima. It may be clinically silent until they become large enough to reduce tissue perfusion, or until ulceration and disruption of the atheromatous lesion lead to thrombotic occlusion or distal embolization of the vessel.

Early Atherosclerosis

- **Fatty streaks** may be the earliest or precursor lesions of atherosclerosis. Endothelial injury and dysfunction leads to adhesion of leukocyte (mainly monocyte) to endothelium, increased vascular permeability, platelet adhesion, and movement of low-density lipoproteins (LDL) across the endothelium into the intima. This initiates the atheroma formation. Lipid accumulated in the intima is engulfed by the macrophages and form foam cells. This is followed by migration and proliferation of smooth muscle cells into the intima. Lipids accumulate both intracellularly (within macrophages and smooth muscle cells) and extracellularly. This results in formation of atheromatous plaque.
- **Atheromatous plaque (Figs. 7.34A to E):** It consists of three regions: (1) Superficial fibrous cap (formed by fibrous tissue synthesized by smooth muscle cells around the lipid core), (2) lipid-rich necrotic core (formed by lipid-laden foam cells that have undergone apoptosis), and (3) shoulder. Some atheromatous plaques bulge into the lumen of the coronary artery and narrow its lumen. This may limit the blood flow, particularly during increased myocardial demand leading to ischemic symptoms. Depending on the structure of plaque, they can be divided into stable and vulnerable (unstable) plaques:
    - **Stable plaques:** They have dense collagenous and thick fibrous caps with minimal inflammation and negligible underlying atheromatous necrotic core. These are less likely to undergo rupture.
    - **High-risk or vulnerable plaque:** They have core with many foam cells and abundant extracellular lipid (large lipid core). The fibrous cap is thin with few smooth muscle cells or groups of inflammatory cells (high density of macrophages and T lymphocytes) and increased inflammation. These are likely to undergo rupture.

Sequential changes in coronary artery atherosclerosis causing occlusion of lumen in ischemic heart disease are shown in **Figures 7.34A to E.**

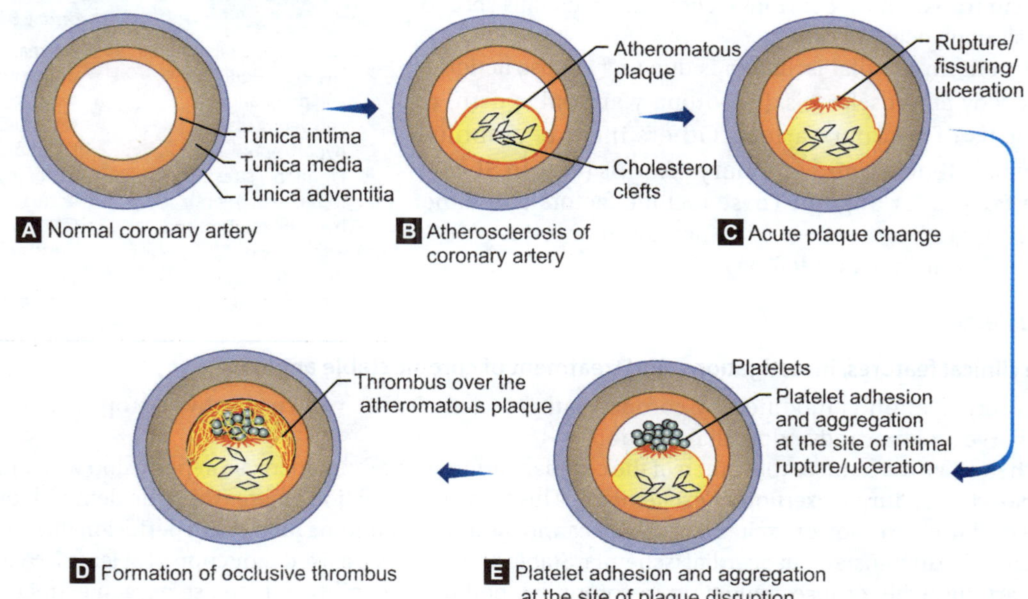

FIGS. 7.34A TO E: Sequential changes in coronary artery atherosclerosis causing occlusion of lumen in ischemic heart disease.

Advanced atherosclerosis/complicated plaques: Atherosclerotic plaques can undergo clinically important changes **(Box 7.19)**.

- **Rupture, ulceration, or erosion:** Plaque protrudes into the lumen and can disturb the blood flow → resulting in turbulent flow of blood → which can damage the endothelium → cause rupture, ulceration, or erosion of the intimal surface of plaques.
- **Hemorrhage into a plaque:** It may occur due to rupture of the fibrous cap of the plaque or of the thin-walled vessels formed due to neovascularization.
- **Thrombosis and embolism:** Ulceration/erosion/rupture of endothelial surface → exposes the blood to highly thrombogenic subendothelial collagen → favors **thrombus formation** → can partially or completely occlude the lumen (depending on the size of the lumen) → lead to ischemia. The thrombus may become organized or fragment to form thromboemboli.
- **Atheroembolism:** Plaque rupture → discharge atherosclerotic debris into the bloodstream → results in atheroemboli.
- **Aneurysm formation:** Atherosclerosis even though an intimal disease may cause pressure or ischemic atrophy of the underlying media. It may also damage the elastic tissue and cause weakening the wall → result in aneurysmal dilation → which may rupture.
- **Calcification:** It may occur in the central necrotic area of the plaque (dystrophic calcification).

Box 7.19: Complications of atheromatous plaque.

- Rupture, ulceration, or erosion
- Hemorrhage into a plaque
- Thrombosis and embolism
- Atheroembolism
- Aneurysm formation
- Calcification

Nonatherosclerotic Causes of ACS

The prevalence of nonobstructive coronary artery disease, defined clinically as luminal stenosis <50%, in patients presenting with myocardial infarction (MI) is estimated to be as high as 30% in women and 11% in men. Important causes include:

- **Spontaneous coronary artery dissection (SCAD):** It accounts for up to 35% of ACS in women aged <50 years, and has a true prevalence as high as 4% of all cases of ACS. Systemic conditions associated with SCAD, include fibromuscular dysplasia, peripartum status, extreme emotion or exercise, and connective tissue diseases, such as Marfan syndrome, Ehlers-Danlos syndrome, and Loeys-Dietz syndrome.
- **Coronary artery embolism**—direct, paradoxical, or iatrogenic
- **Coronary vasospasm** at the epicardial or microvascular level
- **Coronary artery bridging**—a portion of myocardial muscle overlying a segment of an epicardial coronary artery is defined as a myocardial bridge.
- Stress-induced cardiomyopathy/**Takotsubo syndrome (TTS)**

CORONARY ARTERY DISEASE

Q. Discuss etiology, clinical manifestations, investigations, diagnosis, and management of angina pectoris.

Angina Pectoris

Definition: Angina pectoris is a clinical syndrome that presents as **paroxysmal** and **recurrent attacks of substernal or precordial chest discomfort** due to **transient myocardial ischemia**, which falls short of inducing necrosis of myocardial cell.

- **Cause:** Transient myocardial ischemia is due to: (1) obstruction of coronary flow by atherosclerosis, (2) coronary arterial spasm, or (3) thrombosis of coronary artery. Others include embolus, coronary ostial stenosis, and coronary arteritis (e.g., in SLE).
- **Precipitate factors for angina:** These include factors that either increase the oxygen requirement of myocardium or reduce blood supply to the myocardium **(Table 7.34)**.

TABLE 7.34: Factors precipitating angina.

Factors that increase oxygen demand or cardiac work	*Factors that decrease oxygen supply or coronary blood flow*
➤ Exercise and tachycardia ➤ Hypertension, anemia, and pregnancy ➤ Left ventricular hypertrophy ➤ Emotional stress (anger, fright, excitement), hyperthyroidism, and arrhythmias ➤ Aortic stenosis or regurgitation	➤ Decreased oxygenation due to anemia or reduced oxygen saturation ➤ Duration of diastole (coronary blood flow occurs mainly in diastole) ➤ Coronary perfusion pressure (aortic diastolic pressure minus coronary sinus or right atrial diastolic pressure)

Stable Angina Pectoris

Q. Discuss the clinical features, investigations, and treatment of chronic stable angina.

- Coronary autoregulation is modified by coronary atherosclerosis, left ventricular hypertrophy, and alterations in autonomic nerve function and endothelial function.
- Coronary atherosclerosis reduces the lumen of the coronary arteries. It cannot increase in perfusion when the demand for flow is increased (e.g., during exertion or excitement). This leads to a situation where when the demand for blood flow is increased (e.g., during exertion or excitement), there cannot be a corresponding increase in perfusion due to the atheroma.
- Stable angina is due to transient myocardial ischemia. Stable angina shows a fixed reduction of at least 70% in the diameter of coronary arteries which causes reduction in coronary blood flow. Inability to increase oxygen extraction or reduced coronary blood flow, together with increased myocardial demand, leads to angina.

Clinical Features

History

Diagnosis of angina is mainly depends on the clinical history.

Classical or Stable or Exertional Angina Pectoris

It is characterized by:

- **Chest pain:** Constricting discomfort/squeezing/tightening/heaviness/aching in the front of the chest. Pain may radiate to left arm, neck (throat), jaw (chin) or less commonly to right arm, back, and epigastrium. Typical chest pain lasts 2–5 minutes. **Levine's sign** (clenched fist held over the chest) may be positive.
- **Brought on by physical exertion**, such as after meals and in cold, windy weather or by anger or excitement/emotion.
- **Relieved** (usually within minutes) with **rest or sublingual glyceryl trinitrate**. Occasionally, it may disappear with continued exertion ("walking through the pain"). Pain seldom lasts more than 20 minutes.

Typical angina has all the three features mentioned above. Atypical angina has two out of the three, and non-anginal chest pain ***(Table 7.35)*** *one or less of these features. Many patients with angina may have silent episodes of angina, i.e., without any symptoms.*

TABLE 7.35: Differentiating features of chest pain of ischemic and nonischemic origin.

	Favors ischemic origin	*Against ischemic origin*
Character	Constricting, squeezing, burning, and heaviness	Dull ache, knife-like, sharp, jabs, and pleuritic
Location	Substernal, anterior thorax, arms, shoulders, neck, teeth, and interscapular	Left submammary area, left hemithorax
Provoking factors	Exertion, excitement, cold, meals, and stress	Pain after completion of exercise, pain with movement

Types of Angina

- **Stable angina** (described above)
- **Unstable angina**
- **Refractory angina:** Patients with severe coronary disease in whom revascularization is not possible and angina is not controlled by medical therapy.
- **Variant (Prinzmetal's/vasospastic) angina**: Pain occurs without exertion and usually at rest. It is due to spasm of coronary artery and more frequent in women. Characteristically, it is associated with transient ST-segment elevation on the ECG during the pain. Provocation tests (e.g., hyperventilation, cold pressure testing, or ergometrine challenge) may be needed for establishing the diagnosis. Prognosis is usually better than those with fixed, significant obstructive lesions. Usually the response to β-blockers may be poor. Calcium channel blockers are used for the treatment.

Q. Write short note on angina decubitus.

- **Angina decubitus:** Pain develops while lying flat (raises end-diastolic left ventricular volume, myocardial wall tension, and hence oxygen demand).

Q. Write short note on nocturnal angina.

- **Nocturnal angina:** Unusual form of angina that develops in aortic regurgitation especially syphilitic. It is characterized by paroxysmal, nocturnal angina pains accompanied by nightmares, dyspnea, palpitations, skin flushing, profuse sweating, and wide pulse pressure. It does not relieve by sublingual nitroglycerine.

Q. Write short note on microvascular angina.

- **Cardiac syndrome X (microvascular angina):** These patients have angina-like pain, a positive exercise test and angiographically normal coronary arteries. They form a heterogeneous group. It occurs in patients with metabolic syndrome and is more common in women. This type has a good prognosis. Response to nitrates is less reliable and they are difficult to treat. The myocardium shows an abnormal metabolic response to stress, indicating that the myocardial ischemia probably results from abnormal dilator responses of the coronary microvasculature to stress. About 1% die and 0.6% suffer a stroke within 1 year after their first hospital admission.

Others

- **Status anginosus:** Frequent, recurrent, sustained angina refractory to usual treatment.
- **Walk-through angina:** Angina with effort that disappears gradually during activity that is sustained (although usually at reduced intensity) and after which improved exercise tolerance results.
- **Second-wind angina:** A brief rest after an initial attack results in a markedly improved threshold free from angina. A synonym is "warm-up" angina.
- **Caudal angina:** Angina symptoms occurring in the scalp or head via referred pain.
- **Angina equivalents:** Symptoms other than pain or discomfort that are ischemic related and serve as angina surrogates, e.g., dyspnea, diaphoresis, fatigue, or light-headedness.
- **Silent angina:** Objective manifestations of ischemia without symptoms.

Classification of Angina

- Severity of angina is classified by New York Heart Association Classification in class I to class IV (described earlier).
- Canadian Cardiovascular Society functional classification of angina is shown in **Table 7.36**.

Physical Examination

- Usually no abnormal findings in angina. Occasionally a third/ fourth heart sound may be detected during an angina episode, dyskinetic cardiac apex, mitral regurgitation, and even pulmonary edema may be appreciated.
- Physical examination should include a careful search for evidence hyperlipidemia (e.g., xanthelasma, tendon and xanthoma), valve disease (particularly aortic stenosis characterized by slow rising carotid impulse and ejection systolic murmur radiating to the neck), important risk factors (e.g., hypertension and diabetes mellitus), left ventricular dysfunction (cardiomegaly and gallop rhythm), manifestations of arterial disease (carotid bruits and peripheral vascular disease), and unrelated conditions that may exacerbate angina (anemia and thyrotoxicosis), and obesity. Check the blood pressure to identify coexistent hypertension.
- Physical signs of myocardial ischemia: The presence of one or more of these during an attack of pain may be suggestive of myocardial ischemia.

TABLE 7.36: Canadian Cardiovascular Society (CCS) functional classification of angina.

Class	*Features*
I	Ordinary physical activity does not cause angina, such as walking and climbing stairs. Angina with strenuous or rapid or prolonged exertion at work or recreation
II	Slight limitation of ordinary activity. Walking or climbing stairs rapidly, walking uphill, walking or stair climbing after meals, or in cold, or in wind, or under emotional stress, or only during the few hours after awakening. Walking more than two blocks on the level and climbing more than one flight of ordinary stairs at a normal pace and in normal conditions
III	Marked limitation of ordinary physical activity: Walking less than two blocks, climbing less than one flight of stairs
IV	Any physical activity brings on angina; angina at rest

Investigations

Electrocardiography (ECG)

Q. Write a short essay/note on the investigations in a case of suspected angina pectoris.

Resting ECG and ECG in between attacks are normal in most patents (even in patients with severe coronary artery). ECG may show evidence of previous MI and there may be T-wave flattening or inversion in some leads, due to myocardial ischemia or damage. The most convincing ECG evidence of myocardial ischemia is the demonstration of reversible ST-segment depression or elevation, with/without T-wave inversion, during the attack of pain (whether spontaneous or induced by exercise testing, such as treadmill testing or bicycle ergometry).

Exercise ECG: An exercise tolerance test (ETT) is usually done by using a standard treadmill or bicycle ergometer protocol (recording of ECG before, during and after exercise). During this process, patient's ECG, BP, and general condition are monitored.

- **Indications:**
  - Two sets of cardiac enzymes at 4-hour intervals should be normal.
  - No significant abnormality in 12-lead ECG at the time of arrival and pre-exercise.
  - Absence of ischemic chest pain at the time of exercise testing.
- **Contraindications for exercise testing (Box 7.20)**
- Indications for terminating exercise testing of ECG **(Box 7.21)**
- **Interpretation:** Planar or down-sloping ST-segment depression of 1 mm or more indicates ischemia. Up-sloping ST depression is less specific and often found in normal individuals (modified Bruce protocol is followed).
- **Advantages:** Exercise testing is useful means of assessing the severity of coronary disease and identifying high-risk individuals (i.e., post-infarct angina, poor effort tolerance, ischemia at low workload, left main or three-vessel disease, and poor LV function).
  - **Disadvantages:** It may produce false-positive results in the presence of digoxin therapy, left ventricular hypertrophy, bundle branch block, or Wolff–Parkinson–White (WPW) syndrome. The accuracy is lower in women than in men. The test is considered inconclusive (rather than negative) if the patient cannot achieve an adequate level of exercise because of locomotor or other noncardiac problems.

Box 7.20: Contraindications for exercise testing.

Absolute:
- Acute myocardial infarction (within 2 days)
- High-risk unstable angina
- Uncontrolled cardiac arrhythmias causing symptoms or hemodynamic compromise
- Symptomatic severe aortic stenosis
- Uncontrolled symptomatic heart failure
- Acute pulmonary embolus or pulmonary infarction
- Acute pericarditis or myocarditis
- Acute aortic dissection

Relative:
- Left main coronary stenosis
- Moderate stenotic valvular heart disease
- Electrolyte abnormalities
- Severe arterial hypertension
- Bradyarrhythmias or tachyarrhythmias
- Hypertrophic cardiomyopathy and other forms of outflow tract obstruction
- Mental or physical impairment leading to inability to exercise adequately
- High-degree atrioventricular block

Box 7.21: Indications for terminating exercise testing.

- Drop in systolic BP of >10 mm Hg from baseline BP despite an increase in workload, when accompanied by other evidence of ischemia
- Moderate to severe angina
- Increasing nervous system symptoms (e.g., ataxia, dizziness, or near-syncope)
- Signs of poor perfusion (cyanosis or pallor)
- Sustained ventricular tachycardia
- ST elevation (>1.0 mm) in leads without diagnostic Q-waves (other than V_1 or aVR)

Other forms of stress testing

- **Myocardial perfusion scanning:** It is performed using radioactive isotopes. It may be helpful in the (1) evaluation of patients with an equivocal or uninterpretable exercise test and (2) patients who cannot perform exercise. The scintiscans of the myocardium are obtained at rest and during stress (either

TABLE 7.37: Indications for coronary angiography.

➤ Strongly positive stress test	➤ Noninvasive tests have failed to establish the cause of atypical chest pain
➤ Indeterminate stress tests but clinical features of IHD	➤ Previous re-vascularization procedure
➤ Strong suspicion of left main coronary artery or three-vessel disease	➤ Presence of heart failure
➤ Patients with known or possible angina pectoris who have survived cardiac arrest	➤ Nonatherosclerotic cause of ischemia (e.g., coronary arterial anomaly)
➤ Patients considered for revascularization, i.e., a percutaneous coronary intervention (PCI) or coronary artery bypass grafting (CABG)	➤ Frequent readmission for chest pain. Occupation demands a definitive diagnosis
➤ Unable to perform noninvasive tests	➤ Chronic stable angina pectoris with severely symptomatic despite medical therapy

exercise testing or pharmacological stress, such as a controlled infusion of dipyridamole, adenosine or dobutamine), after the administration of an intravenous radioactive isotope, such as thallium (201thallium) or technetium (99technetium sestamibi). The radioactive isotopes are taken up by viable perfused myocardium. If there is a perfusion defect during stress but not at rest, it indicates evidence of reversible myocardial ischemia, whereas a persistent perfusion defect seen during both phases is usually indicative of previous MI.

- **Stress echocardiography:** It is an alternative to myocardial perfusion scanning and has similar predictive accuracy. On transthoracic echocardiography the ischemic segments show reversible defects in contractility during exercise or pharmacological stress, whereas infarcted regions do not contract at rest or during stress.

Coronary arteriography: It gives detailed anatomical information about the extent and nature of coronary artery disease. It is usually done with a view to coronary artery bypass graft surgery or percutaneous coronary intervention (PCI). It is done under local anesthesia and requires specialized radiological equipment, cardiac monitoring, and an experienced team. Indications for coronary angiography are listed in **Table 7.37**.

Newer modalities

These include multiple-slice spiral computed tomographic coronary angiography (CTCA), intravascular ultrasound, magnetic resonance coronary angiography (MRCA), and positron emission tomography (myocardial viability is assessed using glucose metabolism).

Laboratory Tests

- Fasting lipid profile
- Fasting glucose and/or glycated hemoglobin (HbA1c) level if available; additional oral glucose tolerance test (OGTT) if both are inconclusive.
- Complete blood count (CBC) and hematocrit
- Creatinine level with estimation of glomerular filtration rate (GFR)
- Biochemical markers of myocardial injury (Troponin T or I) if clinical evaluation suggests an acute coronary syndrome (ACS).
- Thyroid function tests
- Liver function tests early after beginning statin therapy.

Advice to patients with angina is presented in **Table 7.38**.

TABLE 7.38: Advice to patients with angina.

Stop smoking: **Reduce/maintain ideal body weight exercise:** ➤ Take regular exercise (may promote collateral vessels) but avoid unaccustomed strenuous exercises ➤ Avoid walking or exercise after a heavy meal or in very cold weather ➤ Take sublingual nitrate before any exertion that may induce angina	**ABCDE:** **A** = Aspirin and Antianginal therapy **B** = Beta-blocker and Blood pressure **C** = Cigarette smoking and Cholesterol **D** = Diet and Diabetes **E** = Education and Exercise

Q. Write a short essay/note on:

- **Treatment of angina pectoris.**
- **Management of chronic stable angina.**
- **Drugs used in the treatment of chronic stable angina/antianginal drugs.**
- **Drug treatment of angina pectoris.**

Management of angina pectoris

Management can be discussed under three headings: (A) general measures, (B) drug treatment, and (C) surgical treatment. Goals of treatment of angina pectoris are listed in **Box 7.22**.

Box 7.22: Goals of treatment of angina pectoris.

- Assessment of severity and extent of arterial disease
- Measures to control symptoms
- Identification and control of risk factors (e.g., smoking, hypertension, diabetes, and hyperlipidemia)
- Identification of high-risk patients for treatment and measures to improve life expectancy

General measures

- Careful explanation about the nature of their condition (disease process).
- Evaluate the risk factors and steps to correct them where possible. Advice to be given to the patient is listed in **Table 7.38**.
- Correction of precipitating underlying conditions, e.g., anemia, hyperthyroidism, valvular disease, and arrhythmias should be treated.

TABLE 7.38: Advice to patients with angina.

Stop smoking: **Reduce/maintain ideal body weight exercise:** ➤ Take regular exercise (may promote collateral vessels) but avoid unaccustomed strenuous exercises ➤ Avoid walking or exercise after a heavy meal or in very cold weather ➤ Take sublingual nitrate before any exertion that may induce angina	**ABCDE:** **A** = Aspirin and Antianginal therapy **B** = Beta-blocker and Blood pressure **C** = Cigarette smoking and Cholesterol **D** = Diet and Diabetes **E** = Education and Exercise

- **Management of coexistent conditions:** Identification and treatment of aggravating conditions, such as aortic stenosis, hypertrophic cardiomyopathy, and control of hypertension and diabetes (ACE inhibitors are useful in these patients).
- **Lipid management:** Identify hypercholesterolemia (hyperlipidemia) and treat with diet and drugs (with the goal of reducing LDL <100 mg dL; goal of <70 mg/dL in very high-risk patients).
- Lifestyle modification.

Q. Write short essay/note on lifestyle modifications in cardiovascular disease.

- **Healthy diet:** Increase polyunsaturated fatty acid consumption, mainly from oily fish: **2 to 3 servings of oily fish per week** may help prevent cardiovascular disease (CVD).
- Saturated fatty acids must comprise less than 10% of the total energy intake. Protein with low saturated fats should replace those high in these harmful fats.
- Limit salt intake to less than 5 grams per day.
- Consume 30 to 45 grams of fiber/day (e.g., wholegrain products, fruits, and vegetables). Avoid simple carbohydrates with high glycemic load.
- Consume 200 grams of vegetables and 200 grams of fruits per day.
- Limit consumption of alcoholic beverages.

Antianginal Drug Treatment

Antiangina drugs can be divided into five groups. They are used to relieve or prevent the symptoms of angina. These include: (1) nitrates, (2) β-blockers, (3) calcium antagonists, (4) potassium channel activators, and (5) I_f channel antagonist.

1. Nitrates

Short-acting (glyceryl trinitrate (GTN), nitroglycerine) or long-acting (isosorbide dinitrate, isosorbide mononitrate)

Mechanism of action: Nitrates directly act on smooth muscle in the walls of blood vessels and produce dilatation of arteries and veins. This lowers blood pressure, reduces venous return to heart, and produces dilatation of coronary blood vessels. Nitrates cause reduction in myocardial oxygen demand (lower preload and afterload) as well as an increase in myocardial oxygen supply (coronary vasodilatation) predominantly by perfusing the subendocardial region.

Indications: Prophylaxis and treatment of angina. Prophylactically to use the drug before taking exercise that is liable to produce pain. Prophylactic use of GTN should be encouraged because physical activity promotes the formation of collateral vessels. For predominant nocturnal angina, long-acting nitrates can be given at the end of the day.

Contraindications: Nitrates should not be given along with phosphodiesterase type 5 (PDE-5) inhibitors (e.g., sildenafil, tadalafil, and vardenafil) within the same 24 hours period because it may produce sever hypotension. Other contraindications include obstructive hypertrophic cardiomyopathy, severe aortic stenosis, constrictive pericarditis, mitral stenosis, and closed-angle glaucoma.

- **Glyceryl trinitrate (GTN):**
  - **Preparations:** (1) metered-dose aerosol (400 µg per spray) or (2) as a tablet (300 or 500 µg).
  - **Action:** Sublingual GTN has a short duration of action and will relieve an attack of angina in 2–3 minutes.
- **Isosorbide dinitrate** (10–20 mg 2 to 3 times daily) has prolonged action and is given by mouth. Headache is a common side effect but tends to diminish if the patient perseveres with the treatment. Tolerance can develop with continuous nitrate therapy which can be avoided by a 6–8-hour nitrate-free period. Hence, doses are given in the morning and afternoon.
- **Isosorbide mononitrate** (20–60 mg once or twice daily) can also be given by mouth.

2. β-blockers

Mechanism: These drugs lower oxygen demand of myocardium by reducing heart rate, blood pressure, and myocardial contractility. They inhibit apoptosis by inhibiting beta adrenoceptors, and have antioxidant and antiproliferative properties. They also counteract the direct adverse effects of catecholamines and have antiarrhythmic action. They are useful to control tachycardia, hypertension, and continued angina.

- **Cardioselective β-blockers:** These include slow-release **metoprolol** 50–200 mg daily, **bisoprolol** 5–15 mg daily, and **atenolol** (50–200 mg/day). They have fewer peripheral side effects.
- **Non-selective β-blockers: Propranolol** is started in a small initial dose (20 mg thrice daily) and gradually increased to 80–120 mg three times daily. They may aggravate coronary vasospasm by blocking the coronary artery β2-adrenoceptors.
- **Carvedilol** (3.125–25 mg twice a day) has additional advantage of having antiarrhythmic effects.

3. Calcium channel antagonists (calcium channel blockers)

- **Dihydropyridine calcium antagonists** [e.g., nifedipine, amlodipine (dihydropyridines), felodipine, and nicardipine]. They produce coronary and peripheral arterial dilatation, and negative inotropy. They often cause a reflex tachycardia.
  - **Nifedipine:** It is a powerful coronary and systemic arteriolar dilator. This can cause marked reflex tachycardia. Short-acting nifedipine are not used because it can increase mortality due to myocardial infarction. Long-acting preparations are given usually along with a β-blocker. Dose is 5–20 mg 3 times daily.
  - **Amlodipine:** Dose is 2.5–10 mg daily. Side effects are ankle edema and reflex tachycardia.
- **Non-dihydropyridine calcium antagonists,** e.g., verapamil (phenylalkylamines) and diltiazem (benzothiazepines). They produce coronary and peripheral arterial dilatation and negative inotropy, and also reduce conductivity. Because of its negative inotropic effect, they should be avoided in patients with impaired ventricular function (uncompensated heart failure).
  - **Verapamil:** Dose is 40–80 mg thrice daily. Useful antiarrhythmic properties. Common adverse effect is constipation.
  - **Diltiazem:** 60–120 mg 3 times daily. Similar antiarrhythmic properties to verapamil.
  - β-blockers reduce mortality after myocardial infarction. Hence, it is reasonable to start a β-blocker and then add a calcium channel blocker if needed. However, β-blockers should not be combined with verapamil, because of their synergistic effect on heart rate and myocardial contractility.

4. Second-line antianginal drugs

- Potassium channel activators/openers: **Nicorandil** increases potassium ion conductance by opening ATP-sensitive potassium channels resulting in smooth muscle relaxation causing arterial and venous dilatation. It does not develop tolerance as seen with nitrates. They also provide protection of myocardium during ischemia and prevention of intracellular calcium toxicity. It is given in the dose of 10–30 mg twice daily orally.
- I_f channel antagonist: **Ivabradine** selectively inhibits inward sodium-potassium current [important pacemaking current in the cells sinus (SA) node]. This slows the rate of diastolic depolarization and induces bradycardia ("bradycardic" drug). In contrast to β-blockers and rate-limiting calcium antagonists, it does not have other cardiovascular effects. Thus, it does not affect contractility, AV nodal conduction or hemodynamics. It can be combined with other agents and is safe to use in patients with heart failure. It may produce brightness in visual fields because it also blocks the retinal current and has transient side effect. It is contraindicated in sick sinus syndrome and AV block.
- **Ranolazine:** It inhibits late sodium channels in cardiac cells. It does not affect heart rate and blood pressure. It is the drug of choice in bradycardic and hypertensive patients. It is metabolized by cytochrome P450 3A4. Dose is 500–1,000 mg twice a day. Side effects include constipation, dizziness, and prolongation of QT interval.
- **Trimetazidine:** Dose is 20 mg three times daily. It is associated with greater improvements in time to onset of angina, and the mean weekly number of anginal episodes.
- **Fasudil**: It is an inhibitor of Rho kinase that is involved in the vascular smooth muscle contractile response. It is of benefit in patients with stable and microvascular angina (angina with normal coronary arteries).
- **Allopurinol:** The drug significantly improves endothelium-dependent vasodilation and completely abolishes oxidative stress.
- **Therapeutic angiogenesis** for management of refractory angina using VEGF is under trials.

None of these groups is more effective than another group. It is conventional to start therapy with low-dose aspirin, a statin, sublingual GTN, and a β-blocker. If needed later add a calcium channel antagonist or a long-acting nitrate. The goal is the control of angina with minimum side effects and the simplest possible drug regimen. Indications and contraindications of various antianginal drugs are given in **Table 7.39**.

TABLE 7.39: Indications and contraindications of various antianginal drugs.

Drug	Indication	Contraindication
β-Blockers	➢ Postmyocardial infarction ➢ CHF (compensated) ➢ Ventricular tachycardia ➢ Supraventricular tachycardia (SVT) ➢ Systemic hypertension ➢ Hyperthyroidism	➢ Decompensated HF ➢ Severe bradycardia or AV block ➢ Severe depression ➢ Symptomatic PAD ➢ Raynaud's phenomenon ➢ Severe COPD
DHP-CCB	➢ Systemic hypertension ➢ Raynaud's phenomenon or ➢ Prinzmetal's angina ➢ Severe bradycardia or AV block	Hypotension
Non-DHP-CCB	➢ SVT ➢ Systemic hypertension	➢ Severe bradycardia ➢ Significant AV block ➢ LV dysfunction or HF
Nitrates	LV dysfunction or HF	➢ Severe aortic stenosis ➢ PDE-5 inhibitor use
Ivabradine	Increased resting heart rate	➢ Bradycardia ➢ 2° AV block
Ranolazine	➢ Bradycardia or AV block ➢ Low blood pressure ➢ LV dysfunction ➢ Possible diabetes	➢ Treatment with QT prolonging agents ➢ Moderate or severe hepatic dysfunction
Nicorandil	Refractory angina	➢ Severe aortic stenosis ➢ PDE-5 inhibitor use

(AV: atrioventricular; CCBs: calcium channel blockers; COPD: chronic obstructive pulmonary disease; DHP: dihydropyridine calcium antagonists; LV: left ventricular; PAD: peripheral artery disease; PDE-5 inhibitor: phosphodiesterase type 5 inhibitor)

Q. Write a short essay/note on antiplatelet drugs and its indications.

5. Antiplatelet therapy

Antianginal drugs ameliorate only symptoms but may not reduce mortality. To reduce the risk of adverse events, such as MI, antiplatelet drugs are given.

Aspirin:

- Aspirin inhibits the synthesis of prostaglandins, namely thromboxane A_2, which is a potent vasoconstrictor and platelet activator.
- Dose: Low-dose therapy in the dose of 75–150 mg/day.

P2Y12 antagonists:

- **Clopidogrel**
- It is a thienopyridine which inhibits ADP-dependent activation of the GPIIb/IIIa complex and prevents platelet aggregation.
- It is an equally effective antiplatelet agent that can be used in patients who cannot tolerate aspirin.
- It may have a synergistic effect when combined with aspirin in patients following acute coronary syndrome or implantation of a drug-eluting stent. The benefit of its combination with aspirin was not found chronic stable angina.
- Dose: 75 mg daily
- **Prasugrel and ticagrelor** are new P2Y12 antagonists and have higher platelet inhibition compared to clopidogrel.

6. Statins

Irrespective of the LDL or cholesterol levels. Proprotein convertase subtilisin/kexin type 9 (PCSK9) inhibitors confer a mortality benefit to patients with IHD whose LDL levels remain >70 mg/dL despite high-intensity statins.

Invasive (Surgical) Treatment: Revascularization

Percutaneous Coronary Intervention (PCI)

- Percutaneous coronary interventions include angioplasty [percutaneous transluminal coronary angioplasty (PTCA)] or stent placement in the coronary artery. It is the process to maximize and maintain dilatation of a stenosed coronary artery. A coronary stent is a piece of coated metallic "scaffolding" (fine guidewire) that can be deployed on a balloon. In this process, a small inflatable balloon and metallic coronary stent introduced percutaneously into the arterial circulation via an arterial catheter through the femoral, radial, or brachial artery under radiographic control. It is passed across the coronary stenosis and balloon is inflated to dilate the stenosis. Dilatation can be repeated if symptoms recur.
- **Types of stents:** Two types, namely **(1) bare-metal stents and (2) drug-eluting stents.** The drug-eluting stents are coated stents lined with substances (e.g., sirolimus and paclitaxel) that prevent neointimal hyperplasia and reduce the risk of coronary artery reocclusion. Recent data suggest both types of stents to be equally effective over long-term follow-up.
- **Indications for PCI:**
  - Ideal for single-vessel or two-vessel coronary disease without significant lesions in the proximal left anterior descending artery (LAD), with normal LV function, with high risk on noninvasive testing and a large area of viable myocardium.
  - Undergone prior PCI with either recurrence of stenosis or high risk on noninvasive testing.
  - Failure of medical therapy and with acceptable risk for PCI. Treatment of choice for unstable angina (UA) when rest pain recurs in spite of full medical treatment.
  - Lesion suitable for PCI
  - No diabetes
- **Complications of the procedure:** Bleeding, hematoma, dissection, and pseudoaneurysm from the arterial puncture site. Serious complications are acute myocardial infarction (2%), stroke (0.4%), and death (1%). Long-term complication is restenosis (33% of cases) which is due to a combination of elastic recoil and smooth muscle proliferation (neointimal hyperplasia). It tends to occur within 3 months.

Coronary Artery Bypass Grafting (CABG)

- In CABG, autologous veins (reversed segments of the patient's own saphenous vein) or arteries (internal mammary artery/radial artery/gastroepiploic arteries) are anastomosed to the ascending aorta at one end and to the native coronary arteries distal to the area of occlusion/stenosis at the other end.
- Usually done under cardiopulmonary bypass but, in few cases, it can be done in the beating heart ("off-pump" surgery). Aspirin (75–150 mg daily) and clopidogrel (75 mg daily) both improve graft patency, and one or other should be given indefinitely.
- **Indications:**
  - Significant left main coronary disease.
  - Triple-vessel disease/two blood vessel disease with reduced left ventricular function (left ventricular ejection fraction is <50%).
  - Two-vessel disease with significant proximal left LAD disease and either LVEF <50% or demonstrable ischemic on noninvasive testing.
  - Failure of medical therapy and with acceptable risk for CABG.
  - Diabetes
  - Prior CABG, PCIs (percutaneous coronary interventions) with recurrent rest enosis
  - Abnormal stress test
- **Risks:** Higher risks in elderly, those with poor left ventricular function and those with significant comorbidity, such as renal failure.
- **Minimally invasive operative procedures for bypass grafting (MIDCAB):** Laparoscopic approaches may be useful in patients with previous CABG and those with coexistent medical conditions which would increase the operative risks of "full" CABG).

Novel therapy in angina is summarized in **Box 7.23**.

Flowchart 7.1 shows scheme for the investigation and management of stable angina.

Prognosis

- Critical stenosis (>70%) of coronary arteries and 5 years mortality rate: One artery—2%, two arteries—8%, and three arteries—11%. 50% stenosis of left main coronary artery has a mortality rate of about 15% per year.

Box 7.23: Novel therapy in angina.

Newer drugs:
- Ivabradine: Selectively blocks I_f in a current-dependent fashion in pacemaker cells of the sinoatrial node
- Ranolazine: Partial fatty acid oxidation (pFOX) inhibitor, late sodium current blocker
- Trimetazidine: Inhibitor of partial fatty acid oxidation (pFOX)
- Perhexiline: Inhibits mitochondrial carnitine palmitoyltransferase-1 (CPT-1)
- Etomoxir/Oxfenicine: CPT 1 inhibitor
- Nicorandil: Activation of ATP-sensitive K^+ channels
- Rho kinase inhibition: Fasudil
- Molsidomine and linsidomine act by releasing nitric oxide
- Others: Testosterone, endothelin receptor blockers (bosentan), allopurinol

TMLR: Transmyocardial laser revascularization
EECP: Enhanced external counter pulsation
Chelation therapy: Intravenous EDTA infusions
Spinal cord stimulation, coronary sinus reducing device, apheresis

Other novel agents:
- **Monoclonal antibodies:** Inclacumab is a P-selectin monoclonal antibody, in patients with NSTE–ACS undergoing PCI. It reduces myocardial damage
- **Stem cell therapy:** The use of stem cells derived from bone marrow or myocardium to improve cardiac function has been promising

FLOWCHART 7.1: Scheme for the investigation and management of stable angina.

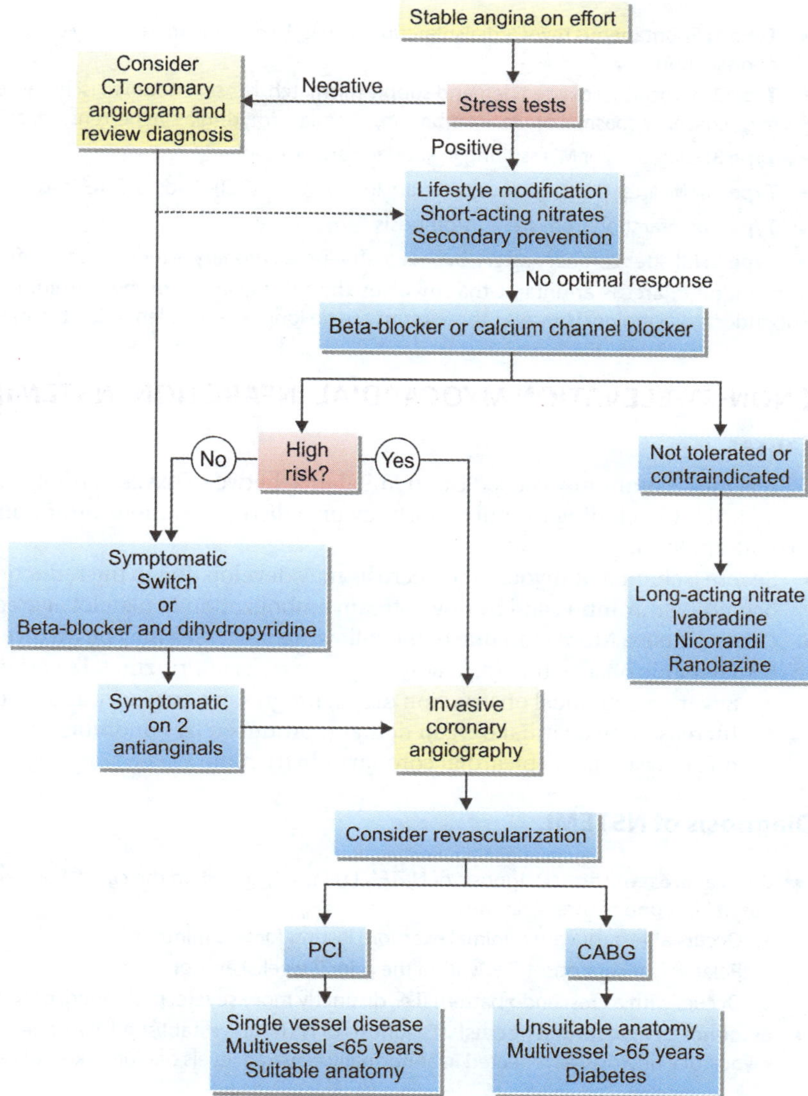

(CABG: coronary artery bypass grafting; PCI: percutaneous coronary intervention)

- Other poor prognostic factors are advanced age (>75 years), diabetes, morbid obesity, accompanying peripheral vascular and or cerebrovascular disease, previous myocardial infraction, high levels of plasma CRP, and evidence of LV dysfunction.

ST-ELEVATION MYOCARDIAL INFARCTION (STEMI)

Q. Discuss the etiology (risk factors), clinical features, investigations, complications, and management of acute coronary syndrome/ACS (ST-elevation myocardial infarction—STEMI)/acute myocardial infarction.

Q. Write short essay/note on risk factors of acute myocardial infarction.

- STEMI is due to the **formation of an occlusive thrombus at the site of rupture of an atheromatous plaque** in a coronary artery. Usually there is minimal prior narrowing of coronary lumen.
- **Other causes:** Coronary spasm, rarely coronary emboli as well as by ostial narrowing due to aortitis, hypercoagulable state and use of cocaine. Congenital anomalies, such as the origin of the left anterior descending coronary artery from the pulmonary artery may cause myocardial ischemia in infancy, but this cause is very rare in adults.
- Limitation of the ability to increase flow to meet increased myocardial demand occurs with 50% coronary stenosis while 80% coronary stenosis causes myocardial ischemia at rest or with minimal stress.

Types of Myocardial Infarction

- **Type 1:** Spontaneous myocardial infarction with ischemia due to a primary coronary event, e.g., plaque erosion/rupture, fissuring or dissection.
- **Type 2:** Myocardial oxygen demand supply mismatch, i.e., secondary to ischemia due to increased oxygen demand or decreased supply (e.g., coronary spasm, coronary embolism, anemia, arrhythmias, hypertension, or hypotension).
- **Type 3:** Diagnosis of MI resulting in sudden cardiac death.
- **Type 4a:** MI after percutaneous coronary intervention (PCI)—post-PCI related.
- **Type 4b:** Infarction from stent thrombosis.
- **Type 5:** MI after coronary artery bypass graft—post-coronary artery bypass graft.

Transmural infarct is an infarct that involves the full thickness of myocardium. Subendocardial infarct is an infarct which involves subendocardial region. However, these terms are no longer used. Silent infarct is infarct without symptoms but with only ECG changes.

NON-ST-ELEVATION MYOCARDIAL INFARCTION (NSTEMI)

Causes

- It is most commonly caused by an imbalance between oxygen supply and oxygen demand. This imbalance results from a partially occluding thrombus forming on a disrupted atherothrombotic coronary plaque or on eroded coronary artery endothelium.
- Severe ischemia or myocardial necrosis may develop due to the reduction of coronary blood flow caused by the partially occluding thrombus and by downstream embolization of platelet aggregates and/or atherosclerotic debris.
- **Other causes:** More than one of the following processes may be involved.
  - Dynamic obstruction (e.g., coronary spasm, as in Prinzmetal's variant angina)
  - Severe mechanical obstruction due to progressive coronary atherosclerosis
  - Increased myocardial oxygen demand produced by conditions, such as fever, tachycardia, and thyrotoxicosis in the presence of fixed epicardial coronary obstruction.

Diagnosis of NSTEMI

- **Clinical presentation:** Diagnosis of NSTEMI is largely based on the clinical presentation. Typically, chest discomfort is severe and has at least one of three features:
  1. Occurs at rest (or with minimal exertion) lasting for >10 minutes.
  2. Relatively recent onset (i.e., within the prior 2 weeks) and/or
  3. Occurs with a crescendo pattern (i.e., distinctly more severe, prolonged, or frequent than previous episodes).
- **Evidence of myocardial necrosis:** Diagnosis of NSTEMI is established, if a patient with the above clinical features shows the evidence of myocardial necrosis, as reflected in abnormally elevated levels of biomarkers of cardiac necrosis.

ACUTE CORONARY SYNDROME

Q. Write short essay on acute coronary syndromes.

Ischemic heart disease (IHD) forms a spectrum of diseases **(Flowchart 7.2)** and consists of stable angina and acute coronary syndromes (includes STEMI, NSTEMI, and unstable angina).

FLOWCHART 7.2: Spectrum of ischemic heart disease.

Ischemic heart disease
- Chronic coronary artery disease (CAD) with stable angina
- Acute coronary syndrome
  - ST-elevation myocardial infarction (STEMI)
  - Non-ST-elevation myocardial infarction (NSTEMI)
  - Unstable angina (UA)

Acute coronary syndrome (ACS) is a term used for spectrum of clinical presentations due to acute myocardial ischemia. It includes:

- ST-elevation myocardial infarction (STEMI) **(Flowchart 7.3)**: Majority of STEMI has Q-wave MI (QwMI).
- **Non-ST-elevation myocardial infarction (NSTEMI):** A small percentage of STEMI and majority of NSTEMI have non-Q-wave MI (NQwMI, previously known as subendocardial infarction). However, the terms Q-wave or non-Q-wave infarctions are not used at present.
- **Unstable angina (UA):** It Includes patients with ACS but with normal ECG, without elevation of cardiac injury markers and no ST elevation in the ECG. Management of unstable angina and NSTEMI is similar.

FLOWCHART 7.3: New classification scheme of acute coronary syndrome.

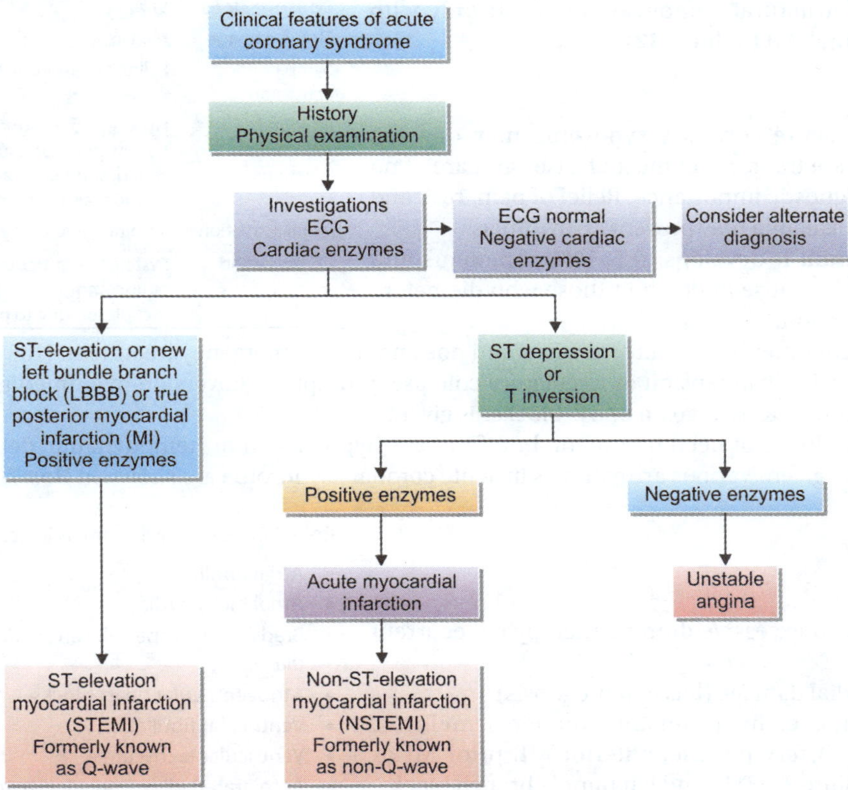

Pathophysiology (Table 7.40)

TABLE 7.40: Pathophysiology of stable angina and acute coronary syndrome.

Stable angina	*Unstable angina*	*NSTEMI*	*STEMI*
➢ Progressive narrowing of coronary lumen ➢ Stable fibrous cap	➢ Progressive narrowing ➢ Acute worsening of coronary lumen due to thrombus formation	➢ Acute worsening of coronary lumen due to thrombus formation ➢ Subocclusive/transient coronary thrombus with myocardial necrosis	➢ Minimal prior narrowing of coronary lumen ➢ Acute rupture of thin fibrous cap ➢ Occlusive thrombus formation ➢ Acute injury pattern ➢ Myocardial necrosis

Clinical Features of Acute Coronary Syndrome

Symptoms

- **Prolonged cardiac pain:** Myocardial ischemia causing chest discomfort is termed angina pectoris. Thus, classic manifestation of ischemia is angina, which is usually described as a heavy chest pressure or squeezing, a burning feeling, or difficulty breathing.
- The discomfort often radiates to the left shoulder, neck, or arm. It typically builds in intensity over a period of a few minutes.
- The pain may begin with exercise or psychological stress, but ACS most commonly occurs without obvious precipitating factors.
- Pain may be absent in patients with prior cardiac, prior stroke, age >75 years, and diabetes mellitus. Painless MI is more common in females compared to males.
- Any patient with severe chest pain that lasts for more than 20 minutes may be suffering from a myocardial infarction. This pain usually does not respond to sublingual GTN.
- **Other features:** Features include anxiety and fear of impending death, nausea and vomiting, breathlessness, and collapse/syncope.

TABLE 7.41: Various signs of acute coronary syndrome and its causes.

Type	*Complication*
Ischemic	Infarct extension, reinfarction, and angina
Mechanical	Cardiogenic shock, cardiac failure, mitral regurgitation, ventricular aneurysm, and cardiac rupture (papillary muscle, ventricular septum, and cardiac wall)
Arrhythmic	Atrial or ventricular arrhythmia, dysfunction of sinus or atrioventricular node
Thromboembolic	Left ventricular mural thrombus, CNS embolus (e.g., stroke) and peripheral embolus
Inflammatory	Pericarditis

Physical Signs (Table 7.41)

Sometimes infarction occurs without any physical signs.

Complications of Acute Coronary Syndrome

Major mechanical and structural complications occur only with significant, often transmural, MI (**Table 7.42**).

TABLE 7.42: Complications of acute myocardial infarction.

Cause of signs	*Sign*
Tissue damage	Mild fever
Sympathetic activation	Pallor, sweating, and tachycardia
Impaired myocardial function	Hypotension, oliguria, cold peripheries, narrow pulse pressure, raised JVP, third heart sound, soft first heart sound, diffuse apical impulse, and basal crepitations in the lung
Vagal activation	Vomiting and bradycardia
Complication	Systolic murmur due to mitral regurgitation or uncommonly due to VSD, pericardial friction rub due to pericarditis

Arrhythmias

- Many patients with acute coronary syndrome may develop arrhythmia and they are transient in most of cases and are of no hemodynamic or prognostic importance. Relief of pain, rest, and the correction of hypokalemia may prevent arrhythmias.
- **Ventricular fibrillation:** It develops in 5–10% of patients and appears to be the major cause of death in those who die before receiving medical attention.
- **Atrial fibrillation** is common but usually transient and does not need emergency treatment. However, if it produces a rapid ventricular rate with hypotension or circulatory collapse, prompt cardioversion by immediate synchronized DC shock is required. In other cases, digoxin or a β-blocker is given.
- **Bradycardia:** Usually does not need treatment, but if there is hypotension or hemodynamic deterioration, atropine (0.6–1.2 mg IV) may be given. Various arrhythmias in acute coronary syndrome are shown in **Box 7.24**.

Box 7.24: Various arrhythmias in acute coronary syndrome.

- Atrial fibrillation
- Atrial tachycardia
- Bradycardia (especially after inferior MI) and tachycardia
- Atrioventricular heart blocks
- Ventricular fibrillation
- Ventricular tachycardia
- Accelerated idioventricular rhythm
- Ventricular ectopic beats

Cardiogenic Shock

- **Causes:**
  - Arrhythmia
  - Hypovolemia due to excessive diuretic therapy or recurrent vomiting
  - Extensive myocardial damage (has bad prognosis)
- **Risk factors:** Older age, hypertension, diabetes mellitus, multivessel coronary artery disease, anterior MI, prior MI or angina, prior heart failure, STEMI, and left bundle branch block.

Left Ventricular Failure

It commonly leads to pulmonary edema.

Mechanical Complications

- **Myocardial rupture:** Part of the necrotic muscle in a fresh infarct can result in tear or cardiac rupture. Most frequent during 3 to 7 days after transmural infarcts.
- **Rupture of the ventricular free wall:** It is most common and result in hemopericardium and cardiac tamponade. It is usually fatal.
- **Rupture of the ventricular septum:** It is less common and can lead to an acute VSD and left-to-right shunt. It usually presents with sudden hemodynamic deterioration and produces a new loud pansystolic murmur radiating to the right sternal border.
- **Rupture of papillary muscle:** It can lead to acute severe mitral regurgitation, which presents with a pansystolic murmur and third heart sound.

Embolism

Thrombus may form on the endocardial surface of freshly infarcted myocardium due to local abnormality in myocardial contractility (causing stasis) and endocardial damage (creating a thrombogenic surface). This can lead to systemic thromboembolism and occasionally causes a stroke. Venous thrombosis and pulmonary embolism may also develop patients on prolonged bed rest, but are now less common with the use of prophylactic anticoagulants and early mobilization.

Ventricular Aneurysm

After acute transmural infarction, the affected ventricular wall may bulge outward during systole resulting ventricular aneurysm. It develops as a late complication of large transmural infarcts.

Pericarditis

- **Early pericarditis:** A transmural myocardial infarct → can involve the pericardium → cause fibrinous or fibrinohemorrhagic pericarditis. Usually, develops on second or third day.
- **Delayed form of pericarditis (postmyocardial infarction syndrome/Dressler syndrome):** It develops 2 to 10 weeks after infarction—probably immunologically mediated reaction to necrotic muscle. It is characterized by fever, pericarditis, and pleurisy. Treatment is with aspirin or other nonsteroidal anti-inflammatory drugs (NSAIDs) or corticosteroids.

Investigations

Q. Write short essay/note on ECG changes in acute myocardial infarction.

Electrocardiogram (ECG)

The 12-lead ECG is central to confirming the diagnosis and should be done and interpreted within 10 minutes of arrival. The initial ECG may be normal or nondiagnostic in about 30% of cases. Repeated ECGs are needed, especially where the diagnosis is uncertain or the patient has recurrent or persistent symptoms.

Changes in ECG: Characteristic changes are observed in leads that "face" the ischemic or infracted area (e.g., anteroseptal, anterolateral, strict anterior, inferior, and posterior wall infarction).

- **STEMI: ST-segment deviation** is the earliest ECG change. With proximal occlusion of a major coronary artery, ST-segment elevation (or new bundle branch block) is observed initially. Later, there is diminution in the size of the R wave and, in transmural (full-thickness) infarction, there is development of a Q wave. Subsequently, the T wave becomes inverted and persists after the ST segment has returned to normal.
- **NSTEMI and unstable angina:** It is due to partial occlusion of a major vessel or complete occlusion of a minor vessel, causing unstable angina or partial-thickness (subendocardial) MI. They usually produce ST-segment depression and T-wave changes. When infarction is present, there may be some loss of R waves in the absence of Q waves.
  Anatomic site of infarct, ECG lead and location of myocardial infarct are discussed earlier.

Plasma Cardiac Biomarkers (Biochemical Markers of Cardiac Injury)

Q. Write a short essay/note on serum markers in acute myocardial infarction.

Unstable angina: There is no detectable rise in cardiac biomarkers or enzymes in unstable angina and the initial diagnosis is made from the clinical history and ECG only.

Myocardial infarction: Causes arise in the plasma concentration of enzymes and proteins that are normally concentrated within cardiac cells. These include creatine kinase (CK), aspartate aminotransferase (AST), lactate dehydrogenase (LDH), myoglobin, and troponins (troponin I and troponin T). These markers leak from the necrotic myocardial cells into the blood circulation.

- **Cardiac creatine kinase (CK):** It is a **nonspecific enzyme marker** and is present in brain, myocardium, and skeletal muscle. It has two isoforms designated "M" and "B". **MB** heterodimers chiefly in cardiac muscle (lesser amounts in skeletal muscle).
  - MB form of creatine kinase (CK-MB) is sensitive but not specific, because it is also raised with skeletal muscle injury.
  - CK-MB levels rise within 4 to 6 hours of the onset of MI, peaks at 12 hours, and returns to normal within 72 hours.
  - Total CK is also raised in diseases of skeletal muscle (e.g., polymyositis and muscular dystrophies), hypothyroidism, and stroke.
- **Lactate dehydrogenase:** It not specific marker. It **starts rising** after **24–48 hours**. It remains **for many days** and **returns to normal in 7–14 days**. An elevated LDH_1 (an isoenzyme of LDH) is a more sensitive indicator of myocardial infarction than total LDH.
- **Myoglobin:** It is an oxygen-carrying respiratory protein found only in skeletal and cardiac muscle. It is an **earliest marker of MI**, the level rises within 1–3 hours, **peaks in about 8–12 hours** and **return to normal in about 24–36 hours**.
- **Cardiac troponins:** These are proteins involved in heart muscle contraction. **Increased plasma levels establish the diagnosis of myocardial infarction.** Cardiac-specific proteins are of two types, namely cardiac **Troponins I (cTnI) and T (cTnT)**. They are **most sensitive and specific markers** of myocardial infarction. Levels begin to **rise at 4–6 hours** and **peak at 48 hours**. The elevated troponin levels may **remain for 7–10 days** after acute MI and therefore, this assay is particular useful in the evaluation of patients who present sufficiently long after their episode of chest pain. Further, about one-third of patients with unstable angina also have elevated cTn, which classifies these groups of patients to non-ST-elevation MI.
- **Aspartate aminotransferase:** Starts to rise by about 12 hours and reaches a peak on the first or second day.
- **Other enzymes:** (1) Ischemia modified albumin, (2) N terminal Pro BNP, (3) suPAR (soluble urokinase-type plasminogen activator receptor), and (4) Glycogen phosphorylase isoenzyme BB.
  Various enzyme levels in acute coronary syndrome are shown in **Figure 7.35** and **Table 7.43**.

Other Blood Tests

- Leukocytosis with a peak on first day.
- Erythrocyte sedimentation rate (ESR): Raised and may remain so for days.
- C-reactive protein: Elevated.
- **Heart-type fatty acid-binding protein (H-FABP)** as a plasma marker for the diagnosis of patients presenting with chest pain suggestive of myocardial infarction, especially in the early hours (within 2 hours) after onset of symptoms. However, their use as a diagnostic tool for MI is limited.

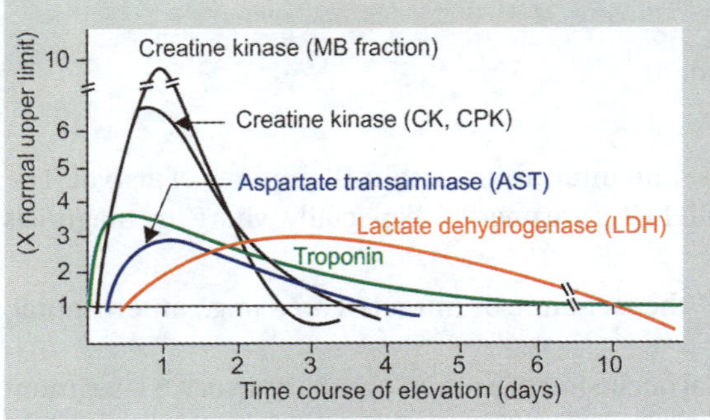

FIG. 7.35: Various enzyme levels following acute myocardial infarction.

TABLE 7.43: Characteristics of plasma biomarkers for acute myocardial infraction (AMI).

Marker protein	Elevation in plasma after AMI (h)	Peak plasma concentration (h)	Normalization of plasma level (days)
Myoglobin	2–3	6–12	1–2
Cardiac troponin I	3–8	12–24	7–10
Cardiac troponin T	3–8	12–24	7–10
Creatine kinase MB	2–6	12–24	2–3

Chest X-ray

- It may show evidence of pulmonary edema that is not evident on clinical examination.
- Heart size is usually normal but there may be cardiomegaly due to previous myocardial damage or pericardial effusion.

Echocardiography

It is useful for assessing ventricular function and for detecting complications (e.g., mural thrombus, cardiac rupture, ventricular septal defect, mitral regurgitation, and pericardial effusion).

Radionuclide Scanning

It helps to detect the site of necrosis and the extent of damage to ventricular function.

Q. Write short essay/note on:
- **Management of a case of acute myocardial infarction in the first 24 hours.**
- **Management of a case of acute myocardial infarction.**

Management

Immediate management: The first 24–48 hours, the patients should be admitted immediately to hospital. During first 24–48 hours the risk for fatal arrhythmia is highest and as a result, there is a significant risk of death or recurrent myocardial ischemia. Patients are best treated in an intensive coronary care unit.

Management of acute myocardial infarction

Initial treatment

Admit in intensive coronary care unit, attach a cardiac monitor, and secure an intravenous line.

- **General treatment ("M O N A C"):**
  - **M**orphine 2–4 mg q 5–10 minute to control chest pain.
  - **O**xygen 4 L/minute: Hypoxemia in uncomplicated MI is usually due to ventilation-perfusion abnormalities and may be exacerbated by CHF. Therefore, oxygen is given to patients suspected of having an acute coronary syndromes and oxygen saturation <90%.
  - **N**TG (nitroglycerine) sublingual or spray, followed by infusion for persistent chest pain
  - **A**spirin 160–325 mg chew and swallow or/and
  - **C**lopidogrel 300 mg oral
- **Confirm diagnosis:** By investigations, namely:
  - Electrocardiogram (ECG)
  - Plasma cardiac biomarkers: Troponin T or I and CK-MB
- **Specific therapy:**
  - Thrombolysis or percutaneous coronary interventions
  - β-blockers unless contraindicated
  - Treat complications (arrhythmias, congestive failure, and shock)

Control of Pain by Analgesics

- Proper control of pain is necessary not only to relieve distress but also to lower adrenergic drive which reduces vascular resistance, BP, infarct size, and susceptibility to ventricular arrhythmias.
- **Intravenous opiates:** Initially, morphine in the dose of 2–4 mg or diamorphine 2.5–5 mg is administered along with antiemetics (metoclopramide 10 mg), and repeated until the patient is comfortable.
- β-blockers, nitroglycerine, and thrombolysis may also help in reducing the pain. Antianginal therapy (*refer* earlier)

Antiplatelet therapy

- **Aspirin:** In acute coronary syndrome, oral aspirin (75–325 mg daily) improves survival and reduce mortality. The first dose (300 mg) should be given orally within the first 12 hours and should be continued indefinitely if there are no side effects.
- **Combination therapies:** Combination of aspirin and an ADP-receptor blocker (clopidogrel, prasugrel or ticagrelor) is recommended in patients with STEMI who are undergoing primary PCI (for up to 12 months) or (clopidogrel) fibrinolysis and in those who have not undergone reperfusion therapy. In acute coronary syndrome, with/without ST-segment elevation, ticagrelor (180 mg, followed by 90 mg twice daily) is found to be more effective than clopidogrel in reducing vascular death, MI or stroke, and other causes of death.
- **Glycoprotein IIb/IIIa receptor antagonists:** These are powerful inhibitors of platelet aggregation and prevent thrombus formation (e.g., **tirofiban, eptifibatide, and abciximab**). Abciximab is a monoclonal antibody which binds tightly and has a long half-life. They are beneficial in patients who undergo PCI, those with recurrent ischemia and those with high risk (e.g., diabetes mellitus and raised troponin concentration).

  Various antiplatelet agents and their dosage are mentioned in **Table 7.44**.

Anticoagulants (antithrombin therapy)

Prophylactic anticoagulants are given to prevent deep vein thrombosis and pulmonary embolism in patients who do not receive fibrinolytic agents. They reduce the risk of thromboembolic complications, and prevent reinfarction in the absence of reperfusion therapy or after successful thrombolysis.

Preparations:

- **Unfractionated heparin:** Given as an initial bolus dose of 60 IU/kg (with a maximum dose of 4,000 units) followed by an initial infusion of 12 IU/kg/hour (maximum 1000 units/hour). The dose is adjusted to attain the activated partial thromboplastin time at 1.5–2 times control. Heparin is given before the completion of infusion of rt-PA or tenecteplase or patients receiving STK.
- **Low-molecular weight heparin:** It is used as an adjunct to thrombolytics. It produces higher reperfusion rate and lower reocclusion rate compared to unfractionated heparin. Dose of 5,000 units is given twice a day subcutaneously.
- **Direct thrombin inhibitors:** These appear better than the unfractionated heparin in patients undergoing PCI. These include hirudin and bivalirudin. Pentasaccharides (subcutaneous fondaparinux 2.5 mg daily) are safe and effective. However, fondaparinux is not used as sole agent and contraindicated if PCI is planned.

  Antithrombin preparations should be continued for at least 48 hours and preferably for 8 days or till discharge or coronary revascularization.

Statins

High-dose statins are recommended in all patients during the first 24 hours of admission for STEMI, irrespective of the patient's cholesterol concentration, if there is no contraindications (e.g., allergy, active liver disease). They are recommended during the early phase of therapy up to at least 4 weeks. Patient on statin therapy presenting with STEMI should continue statin.

Advantages:

- Statins lower cholesterol and has direct effects on endothelial function, oxidative stress, inflammation, thrombosis as well as plaque stabilization. High-dose atorvastatin (40–80 mg) or rosuvastatin (20–40 mg) therapy before emergency percutaneous coronary intervention has following advantages:
  - Reduce periprocedural inflammatory response
  - Reduce myocardial dysfunction
  - Prevent contrast-induced nephropathy.

  Management of acute coronary syndrome is indicated in **Flowchart 7.4**.

TABLE 7.44: Various antiplatelet agents and their dosage.

Oral antiplatelets	
Aspirin	Initial dose of 325 mg nonenteric formulation followed by 75–100 mg/day of an enteric or a nonenteric formulation
Clopidogrel	Loading dose of 300–600 mg followed by 75 mg/day
Prasugrel	Pre-PCI: Loading dose 60 mg followed by 10 mg/day
Ticagrelor	Loading dose of 180 mg followed by 90 mg twice daily
Intravenous antiplatelet therapy	
Abciximab	0.25 mg/kg bolus followed by infusion of 0.125 µg/kg per min (maximum 10 µg/min) for 12–24 hours
Eptifibatide	180 µg/kg bolus followed 10 min later by second bolus of 180 µg with infusion of 2.0 µg/kg per min for 72–96 hours following first bolus
Tirofiban	5 µg/kg per min followed by infusion of 0.15 µg/kg per min for 48–96 hours
Others	**Phosphodiesterase inhibitors**—Cilostazol

Thrombolytic (or Fibrinolytic) Therapy in Acute Coronary Syndrome

Q. Write short essay/note on indications, contraindications, and therapeutic schedule of thrombolytic therapy in acute myocardial infarction.

Indications for Thrombolysis in Acute Myocardial Infarction (Box 7.25)

Fibrinolytic therapy should be initiated within 30 minutes (door-to-needle time or first medical contact-to-needle time).

FLOWCHART 7.4: Management of acute coronary syndrome.

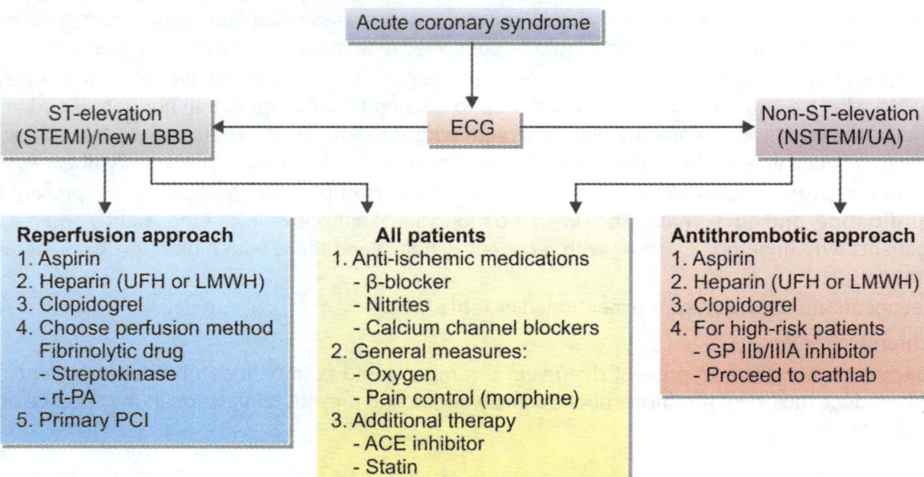

(LMWH: low-molecular-weight heparin; UFH: unfractionated heparin; NSTEMI: non-ST-elevation myocardial infarction; STEMI: ST-elevation myocardial infarction)

Box 7.25: Indications for thrombolysis in acute myocardial infarction.

Thrombolysis: Definitely beneficial
- ST-segment elevation of more than 0.1 mV in two or more contiguous leads, with time to therapy 12 hours or less
- Left bundle branch block (LBBB) obscuring ST-segment analysis and history of acute myocardial infarction for less than 12 hours

Thrombolysis: Some benefit
- ST-segment elevation with time to therapy 12–24 hours

Thrombolysis: Not indicated
- ST-segment depression only (unless leads V_1-V_4 show ST depression related to posterior wall myocardial infarction)
- Time to therapy >24 hours

TABLE 7.45: Various thrombolytic agents and their dosage.

Thrombolytic agent	*Dose*
Alteplase (tissue plasminogen activator-tPA)	15 mg bolus followed by 50 mg intravenously over the first 30 minute, followed by 35 mg over the next 60 minutes
Streptokinase (STK)	1.5 million units (MU) intravenous infusion over 1 hour
Tenecteplase (TNK)	Given as a single weight-based intravenous bolus of 0.53 mg/kg over 10 seconds
Reteplase (rPA)	Double-bolus regimen consisting of a 10 MU bolus given over 2–3 minutes, followed by second 10-MU bolus 30 minutes later

Thrombolytic agents (Table 7.45): These include plasminogen activators, i.e., *streptokinase (STK), urokinase (UK), human tissue plasminogen activator (tPA-alteplase), recombinant plasminogen activator (rPA-reteplase), tenecteplase, anisoylated plasminogen streptokinase activator complex (AP- SAC, anistreplase), and single-chain urokinase plasminogen activator (scu-PA).*

Mechanism of action: Thrombolytic or fibrinolytic agents lyse thrombi/clot to recanalize the occluded vessels (mainly coronary arteries) by the activation of plasminogen to form plasmin. They are curative rather than prophylactic.

- **Fibrin-specific fibrinolytics:** They generate fibrin-specific fibrinolytics at the site of thrombus/clot. Examples include rPA (reteplase), tenecteplase (TNK), and scu-PA. They have lower mortality rate compared with STK and also lack the significant acute side effects of hypotension and allergy caused by STK.
- **Generation plasmin in the systemic circulation:** These agents generate plasmin in systemic circulation producing a systemic lytic state. This leads to a reduction in blood viscosity, and produces strong anticoagulant and antiplatelet effects. Examples include streptokinase (STK) and urokinase (UK). STK use is associated with lower incidence of intracranial hemorrhage, especially in older individuals.
  Thrombolytic therapy is not recommended for patients with NSTEMI and unstable angina.

Signs of Reperfusion

Signs of reperfusion are shown in **Box 7.26**.

Contraindications to Thrombolytic Therapy (Box 7.27)

Complications of Thrombolytic Therapy

- **Hemorrhage:** It is the major complication. The most common site is in the region of puncture sites, genitourinary system, and intracranial hemorrhage (in about 0.5% of patients).
- **Allergic reactions:** These may develop with use of STK and APSAC.
- **Hypotension:** It may develop if STK is infused rapidly.

Thrombolysis in myocardial infarction (TIMI) grading system (Box 7.28): It is a simple qualitative scale to grade the flow in the culprit coronary artery when assessed by angiography.

Rescue PCI should be considered in patients with failure of reperfusion (persistent chest pain and ST-segment elevation >90 minutes) with thrombolytic agents.

Box 7.26: Signs of reperfusion.

- Immediate relief of chest pain
- Reduction of the initial ST-segment elevation by 50% within 60–90 minutes of fibrinolytic therapy
- Onset of reperfusion arrhythmias (e.g., accelerated idioventricular rhythm and frequent ventricular ectopics)
- Early peaking of CK-MB enzyme

Box 7.28: Thrombolysis in myocardial infarction (TIMI) grading system.

- **TIMI 0:** Absence of antegrade flow beyond a coronary occlusion
- **TIMI 1:** Faint antegrade coronary flow beyond the occlusion, although filling of the distal coronary bed is incomplete
- **TIMI 2:** Flow is delayed or sluggish antegrade flow with complete filling of the distal territory
- **TIMI 3:** Flow is normal which fills the distal coronary bed completely

Box 7.27: Contraindications to thrombolytic therapy.

Absolute:

- History of cerebrovascular hemorrhage anytime in life
- History of nonhemorrhagic stroke or other cerebrovascular event within the past 1 year
- Uncontrolled marked hypertension (systolic BP >180 mm Hg, diastolic BP >110 mm Hg). However, STK can be given.
- Suspected aortic dissection
- Active internal bleeding (excluding menses)
- Known intracranial aneurysm/AV malformation/neoplasm (primary or metastatic)
- Intracranial/spinal surgery within last 3 months)

Relative:

- Current use of anticoagulants (INR ≥2)
- Recent (<2 weeks) invasive or surgical procedure, prolonged (>10 min) CPR
- Known bleeding diathesis
- Recent trauma (including traumatic resuscitation)
- Pregnancy
- Hemorrhage ophthalmic condition
- Active peptic ulcer disease
- History of severe hypertension that is currently controlled

Percutaneous Coronary Intervention (PCI)

Percutaneous coronary intervention is the treatment of choice, provided it is performed promptly by a qualified interventional cardiologist in an appropriate facility.

Indications: Patients with STEMI with following features:

- Symptoms of ischemia of less than 12 hours duration.
- Symptoms of ischemia of less than 12 hours duration who have contraindications to fibrinolytic therapy, irrespective of the time delay from first medical contact.
- Cardiogenic shock or acute severe heart failure (HF), irrespective of time delay from MI onset.
- It may be recommended if there is clinical and/or ECG evidence of ongoing ischemia between 12 and 24 hours after symptom onset. **Maximum acceptable delay** for primary PCI from presentation to balloon inflation is 60 minutes if a patient presents within 1 hour of symptom of onset or 90 minutes if a patient present later.

Types of PCI: Types include primary PCI, rescue PCI, and facilitated PCI (described below).

Glycoprotein IIb/IIIa inhibitors (e.g., abciximab and tirofiban) may be used in patients undergoing percutaneous interventions.

Reperfusion Options for STEMI

- **Fibrinolysis:** It is usually preferred in the following situations:
  - Early presentation (≤3 hours from symptom of onset)
  - In patients where primary PCI cannot done because of the following:
    - Catheterization laboratory occupied/unavailable
    - Vascular access difficulties
    - Lack of access to a skilled PCI laboratory
  - Delay to primary PCI:
    - Door-to-balloon time minus door-to-needle time is >1 hour.
    - Door-to-balloon time is >90 minutes.
- **Primary PCI:** In which PCI is used solely in acute MI. It is indicated in cardiogenic shock, and in patients in whom thrombolytic therapy is contraindicated. **It is generally preferred with following conditions:**
  - Skilled PCI laboratory is available with good surgical backup.
    - Door-to-balloon time is ≤90 minutes.
    - Door-to-balloon time minus door-to-needle time is ≤1 hour.
  - High-risk STEMI:
    - Cardiogenic shock
    - Killip class CHF ≥3
  - Contraindications to fibrinolysis including increased risk of bleeding and intracranial hemorrhage.
  - Late presentation (>3 hours after symptom of onset).
    - **Rescue PCI:** It is combination of PCI with thrombolytic therapy and PCI is performed within 12 after failed thrombolysis/fibrinolysis for patients with continuing or recurrent myocardial ischemia.

- **Indications:** STEMI in aged <75 years who received fibrinolytic therapy and have cardiogenic shock, severe congestive heart failure (Killip class III), or hemodynamically compromising ventricular arrhythmias.
- It may be performed in patients with symptoms of persistent ischemia.

- **Facilitated PCI:** In this type PCI is done following initial pharmacological regimen aimed at improving patency of coronary arteries before PCI.
  - The pharmacological regimens include GB IIB/IIIa inhibitors, full-dose or reduced-dose of fibrinolytic therapy, and combination of a GP IIb/IIIa inhibitor, and a reduced-dose fibrinolytic/thrombolytic agent. However, this type of reperfusion may be inferior to thrombolysis alone or primary PCI and is usually not recommended in most patients with STEMI.

Coronary Artery Bypass Grafting

- Recommended in:
  - Failed PCI with persistent pain or hemodynamic instability in patients with coronary anatomy suitable for surgery.
  - Persistent or recurrent ischemia refractory to medical therapy in patients who have coronary anatomy suitable for surgery, and are not candidates for PCI or fibrinolytic therapy.
  - Patients with STEMI at the time of operative repair of mechanical defects.

Management of Complications

- **Ventricular dysfunction:**
  After STEMI ventricular remodeling occurs, ventricular dysfunction can be prevented by ACE inhibitors and nitrates.
  Hemodynamic classification of ventricular dysfunction is shown in **Box 7.29**.
  This classification has prognostic value with highest mortality in class IV patients.
- **Cardiogenic shock:**
  - This results when there is infarction of ≥40% of left ventricle. The patient has systolic BP <90 mm Hg and pulmonary capillary wedge pressure >18 mm Hg.
  - Cardiogenic shock is best managed by invasive means (Primary PCI). Use of intra-aortic balloon pump and IV vasopressors may be beneficial.
- **Right ventricular infarction (discussed later):**
  - Clinically significant right ventricular infarction is rare and occurs in patients with inferior infarction.

Box 7.29: Hemodynamic classification of patients with acute myocardial infarction.

Based on Clinical Examination (Killip's)			
Class I	**Class II**	**Class III**	**Class IV**
Rales and S3 absent	Crackles, S3 Gallop, elevated jugular venous pressure	Frank pulmonary edema	Shock SBP <90 mm Hg
Mortality: 6%	Mortality: 17%	Mortality: 38%	Mortality: 81%
Based on Invasive Monitoring			
Subset I	**Subset II**	**Subset III**	**Subset IV**
Normal hemodynamics PCWP <18 CI >2.2	Pulmonary congestion PCWP >18 CI >2.2	Peripheral hypoperfusion PCWP <18 CI <2.2	Pulmonary congestion and peripheral hypoperfusion PCWP >18 CI <2.2

(CI: cardiac index; PCWP: pulmonary capillary wedge pressure)

Pericarditis

- Common complication in first week of transmural myocardial infarct.
- Radiation of pain to trapezius muscle is helpful in distinguishing it from ischemia.
- Pericardial rub may be present.

Treatment of pericarditis

Aspirin 650 mg qid and **withhold anticoagulants**.

Management of other complications

These include: (1) thromboembolism, (2) left ventricular aneurysm, (3) sinus bradycardia, (4) AV block, and (5) ventricular tachycardia and fibrillation and acute mitral regurgitation, VSR, and tricuspid regurgitation.

Their management is discussed in individual sections.

Aftercare and Rehabilitation

- **Physical activities:** To be restricted for 4–6 weeks because replacement of infarct by fibrous tissue takes 4–6 weeks. Advised gradual mobilization and return to work over 6 weeks. Exercise and sexual activity within the limits.
- **Complications:** Patients who had complications, the regimen depends on the type of complication.
- **Lifestyle and risk factor modification:** Control of risk factors such as obesity by regular exercises, cessation of smoking, lifestyle modifications, and control of plasma lipids by diets and drugs.
- Secondary prevention drug therapy:
  - **Aspirin and clopidogrel:** Low-dose aspirin (75–150 mg daily) unless there is any contraindication. Clopidogrel (75 mg daily) for up to 12 months, particularly after stent implantation. It may be given as an alternative when aspirin is contraindicated, or in combination with aspirin particularly in patients with unstable angina or recurrent cardiac events.
  - **β-blocker:** Oral β-blockers are continued indefinitely (unless any contraindications). Carvedilol, bisoprolol, or metoprolol (extended release) are given to patients with heart failure. Role of β-blockers in the secondary prevention in unstable angina is not known.
  - ACE inhibitor is given early after an acute coronary syndrome. Long-term treatment with an ACE inhibitor (e.g., enalapril 10 mg twice daily or ramipril 2.5–5 mg twice daily) is found to counteract ventricular remodeling, prevent the onset of heart failure, and reduce recurrent MI.
  - **Statin therapy** started in the hospital for all patients with coronary artery disease.
  - **Warfarin** after myocardial infarction is given to patients having a high-risk of systemic thromboembolism due to atrial fibrillation, mural thrombus, congestive heart failure, or previous embolization.
  - **Nitrates:** Short-acting nitrates, for chest pain. Long-acting nitrates are given for relief of symptom when β-blocker alone is unsuccessful or is contraindicated.
  - **Aldosterone antagonist** (e.g., eplerenone) is given early after myocardial infarction to patients who have LVEF ≤40%, despite optimum dose of ACE inhibitors and β-blockers, and have either CHF or diabetes.
- **Device therapy:** Implantable cardiac defibrillators can prevent sudden cardiac death in patients who have severe left ventricular impairment (ejection fraction ≤30%) after MI.

Non-ST-Segment-Elevation Acute Coronary Syndrome (NSTEACS)

Q. Briefly discuss unstable angina and non-ST-elevation myocardial infarction.

- It includes unstable angina (UA) and non-ST-elevation myocardial infarction (NSTEMI).
- Both are caused by coronary artery spasm, progression of the underlying coronary artery disease (CAD), or hemorrhage into a nonoccluding atheromatous plaque with subsequent thrombosis producing coronary obstruction over a period of few hours. The difference between UA and NSTEMI is that the NSTEMI shows an occluding thrombus, which leads to myocardial necrosis and a rise in serum troponins or CKMB.

Non-ST-elevation MI (NSTEMI)

- It usually shows ST depression and T inversion in the ECG along with elevation in serum troponins or CKMB.
- Myocardial function (as shown by ejection fraction) in NSTEMI is less deranged when compared to STEMI. However, in NSTEMI early as well as late reinfarction rates are higher than in STEMI.

Unstable Angina (UA)

Q. Write a short essay/note on unstable angina.

- **Three principal presentations include:**
  - **Rest angina:** Angina occurring at rest and prolonged, usually >20 minutes.
  - **New-onset angina:** New-onset angina of at least CCS Class III severity.
  - **Increasing angina:** Previously diagnosed angina that has become distinctly more frequent, longer in duration, or lower in threshold (i.e., increased by >1 CCS) class to at least CCS Class III severity.

- Normal ECG (no ST elevation), without elevation of cardiac injury markers (normal level of cardiac enzymes).
- Patients with UA have a high risk of developing MI or sudden death when compared to patients with stable angina. Thus, they need aggressive treatment in the hospital.
  Classification of risk categories in NSTEMI/UA and its management are mentioned in **Table 7.46**.

RIGHT VENTRICULAR MYOCARDIAL INFARCTION (RVMI)

- **Right ventricular myocardial infarction** is seen in patients with an acute inferior MI secondary to complete occlusion of the proximal RCA.
- Right ventricular function is very preload dependent, and frequently, hypotension responds to fluid resuscitation.

- The clinical triad of hypotension, elevated jugular venous pressure, and clear lung fields in the setting of STEMI should prompt an evaluation for RV infarct or massive pulmonary embolism.
- One-mm ST elevations in the V_1 or V_4R leads are the most sensitive marker of RV involvement.
- Initial therapy is IV fluids. If hypotension persists, inotropic support with dobutamine and/or IABP may be necessary. Right-sided mechanical support devices are available when pharmacologic support fails.
- Management protocol is same as other ACS. Caution should be exercised while using nitrates and beta blockers.

TABLE 7.46: Risk categories in NSTEMI/UA.

Category	*Management*
High risk (12–30%)	
➢ Prolonged chest pain (>20 minutes or ongoing), plus: ➢ ECG: (1) Transient ST changes, (2) sustained ST depression, and (3) deep Twave inversion (>5 leads) ➢ Biochemical markers: Troponin/CKMB abnormal ➢ Recurrent ischemia ➢ Acute MI in last 4 weeks ➢ Hemodynamic compromise	➢ Aspirin + heparin/ low-molecular-weight heparin (LMWH) ➢ GP IIb/IIIa antagonist ➢ Early percutaneous coronary intervention (PCI)
Intermediate risk (4–8%)	
➢ No high-risk features but ≥1 of: – Ongoing chest pain – Crescendo angina – Borderline positive troponin I (0.4–2.0) – Previous intervention: PCI or CABG – Increased baseline risk (diabetes mellitus, elderly)	➢ Aspirin ± clopidogrel ➢ Ultrafraction heparin (UFH) or LMWH ➢ PCI
Low risk (<2%)	
➢ No high or intermediate features ➢ Chest pain, single episode, exertional ➢ ECG: Normal or nonspecific or unchanged ➢ May include previous history of CAD or risk factors	➢ Aspirin ➢ No heparin ➢ Observe

Prinzmetal's Variant Angina

Q. Write a short essay/note on clinical features and treatment of Prinzmetal's angina (variant angina).

In 1959 Prinzmetal et al. described a syndrome of severe ischemic pain that usually occurs at rest and is associated with **transient ST-segment elevation.**

Etiology

- **Focal spasm of an epicardial coronary artery** is the cause of Prinzmetal's variant angina (PVA) and leads to severe transient myocardial ischemia and occasionally infarction.
- The cause of the spasm is not well defined, but it may be related to hypercontractility of vascular smooth muscle due to adrenergic vasoconstrictors, leukotrienes, or serotonin.

Clinical Features

- Pain occurs without exertion and usually at rest. It is more frequent in women.
- Associated with migraine, Raynaud's phenomenon, and aspirin-induced asthma. Younger patients with history of cigarette smoking.

Investigation

- Characteristically, it is associated with transient ST-segment elevation on the ECG during the pain.
- Coronary angiography is gold standard for diagnosis. Focal spasm commonly accompanied by **stenosis within 1 cm of spasm** is the hallmark (most commonly in right coronary artery).
- Provocation tests (e.g., hyperventilation, cold pressor testing, or ergometrine or intracoronary acetylcholine challenge) may be needed for demonstration of focal spasm and establishing the diagnosis.

Management

- Nitrates and calcium channel blockers are the main therapeutic agents. Aspirin may actually increase the severity of ischemic episodes, possibly as a result of the sensitivity of coronary tone to modest changes in the synthesis of prostacyclin.
- The response to β-blockers is variable but usually poor. Prazosin can be useful.
- Coronary revascularization may be helpful in patients with discrete, flow-limiting, proximal fixed obstructive lesions.

Prognosis

- Many patients pass through an acute, active phase, with frequent episodes of angina and cardiac events during the first 6 months after presentation.
- Prognosis is better in patients with no or mild fixed coronary obstruction than patients with severe, fixed, significant obstructive lesions. Survival at 5 years is excellent (~90–95%).
- Nonfatal MI occurs in up to 20% of patients by 5 years. Patients with PVA who develop serious arrhythmias during spontaneous episodes of pain are at a higher risk for sudden cardiac death. In most patients who survive an infarction or the initial 3- to 6-month period of frequent episodes, there is a tendency for symptoms and cardiac events to diminish over time.

HYPERTENSION

Q. Classify hypertension. Discuss the clinical features, baseline investigations, diagnosis, complications, and management of essential hypertension.

Q. Discuss the causes and investigations of secondary hypertension.

Hypertension is a hemodynamic disorder and about 15% of the general population can be regarded as hypertensives.

Definition: A well-accepted definition of hypertension was suggested by Evans and Rose:

- "Hypertension should be defined in the terms of blood pressure level above which investigation and treatment do good more than harm."
- The following diagnostic criteria has been suggested by the 2017 American College of Cardiology/American Heart Association (ACC/AHA) guidelines; meeting one or more of these criteria using ambulatory blood pressure monitoring (ABPM) to qualify as hypertension.
    - A 24-hour mean of 125/75 mm Hg or above
    - Daytime (awake) mean of 130/80 mm Hg or above
    - Nighttime (asleep) mean of 110/65 mm Hg or above.

Hypertension is defined arbitrarily at levels above generally accepted normal (Joint National Committee—JNC 7/8 recommendations) and is presented in **Table 7.47A**. Other guidelines for classification of hypertension are summarized in **Table 7.47B**.

TABLE 7.47A: Systolic and diastolic values used in the classification of hypertension (JNC 7/8).

Classification	*Systolic BP (mm Hg)*		*Diastolic BP (mm Hg)*
Normal	<120	and	<80
Prehypertension	120–139	or	80–89
Stage 1 hypertension	140–159	or	90–99
Stage 2 hypertension	≥160	or	≥100
Isolated systolic hypertension	>140	and	<90

TABLE 7.47B: Current classification of high blood pressure.

SSP (mm Hg)		*DBP (mm Hg)*	*ESH/ESC 2018*	*AHA/ACC 2017*	*Position of the DHL, 2017*	*NICE 2016*
<120	and	<80	Optimal	Normal	Optimal	Normal
120–129	and	<80	Normal	Elvated	Normal	Normal
130–139	or	80–89	Upper range of normal	Grade I hypertension	Upper range of normal	Upper range of normal
140–159	or	90–99	Grade I hypertension	Grade II hypertension	Grade I hypertension	Grade I hypertension (>135/85 mm hg)*
160–179	or	100–109	Grade II hypertension	Grade II hypertension	Grade II hypertension	Grade II hypertension (≥150/95 mm hg)*
≥180	or	≥110	Grade III hypertension	Grade II hypertension	Grade III hypertension	Severe hypertension*

A comparium of the new definitions of normal blood pressure and the different grades of high blood pressure by the American Heart Association (ANA) and American Colllege of Cardiology (ACC) with the definitions by the European Society of Cardiology (ESC) and European Society of Hypertension (ESH), as well as the most recent position of the German Hypertension League (*Deutsche Hochdruckliga*, DHL) and the National Institute for Hearth and Care Eexellence (NICE) of the United Kingdom.

The lowering of cutoff values led to an increase in the prevalence of hypertension in the USA from 32% to 46%.

*The value refers to further measurements In the outpatient setting or at hone.
(DBP: dastolic blood pressure; SBP: systolic blood pressure)

Classification and Causes (Table 7.48 and Fig. 7.36)

Q. Write short note on the causes of hypertension.

- **Primary or essential hypertension:** It constitutes about 85% of the cases in which it is not possible to define a specific underlying cause. About 70% of these patients give a positive family history.
- **Secondary hypertension:** It constitutes remaining 15% of the cases and is due to a specific disease or abnormality.

Q. Write short essay or note on secondary hypertension and its causes.

Q. Write short note on causes of isolated systolic hypertension.

Essential Hypertension

In about 85–95% of cases, a specific underlying cause of hypertension cannot be identified and such hypertension is termed as essential hypertension. The exact pathogenesis is not known. It has multifactorial etiology and many factors may contribute to its development.

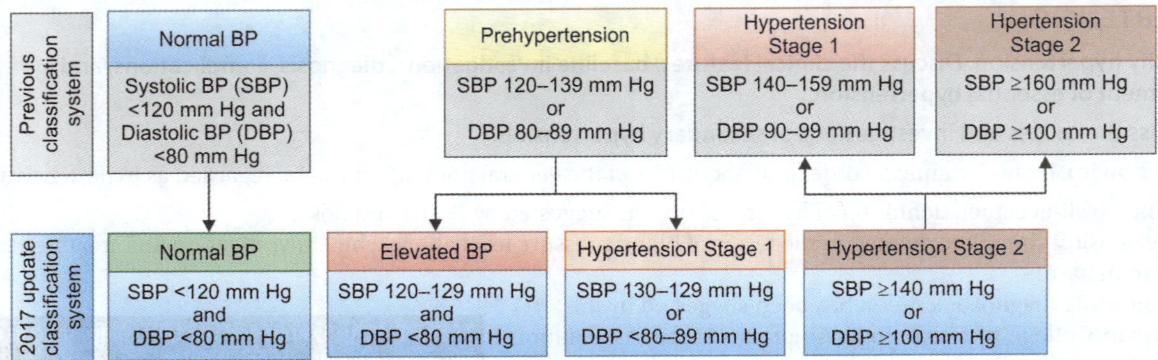

FIG. 7.36: 2017 updated classification of high blood pressure in adults.

Etiology

Q. Write short essay or note on risk factors for hypertension.

Genetic factors: Blood pressure tends to run in families and this may be partly due to environmental influences.

Environmental factors: Several environmental factors may be involved and these include salt intake, obesity, occupation, alcohol intake, family size, and crowding.

- **Obesity:** Higher blood pressures are seen in obese individuals compared to thin individuals. Sleep disordered breathing/obstructive sleep apnea often observed with obesity may be an additional risk factor.
- **Alcohol intake:** There is close relationship between the consumption of alcohol and blood pressure level.
- **Sodium intake:** Higher sodium intakes may be associated with an increase in blood pressure. A high potassium diet can have protective role against the effects of a high sodium intake. *About 60% of hypertensive are salt sensitive. Primary aldosteronism, bilateral renal artery stenosis, renal parenchymal disease, and low-renin essential hypertension are all salt sensitive.*
- **Stress:** Acute pain or stress is associated with raised blood pressure. However, the relationship between chronic stress and blood pressure is not known.

TABLE 7.48: Major causes of hypertension (systolic and diastolic).

Primary/essential hypertension (~85% of case)
Secondary hypertension (~15% of case)
Renal
Renal parenchymal disease (most common cause of secondary hypertension): Acute glomerulonephritis, polycystic kidney disease, chronic nephritis, diabetic nephropathy, and hydronephrosis (obstructive uropathy)
Renal artery stenosis (renovascular hypertension) Renin producing tumors
Endocrine
Adrenal disorders: Cushing's syndrome, primary aldosteronism, primary adrenal hyperplasia, and pheochromocytoma
Others: Hypothyroidism (myxedema), hyperthyroidism (thyrotoxicosis), hypercalcemia, acromegaly, carcinoid, and exogenous hormones
Cardiovascular
Coarctation of aorta, polyarteritis nodosa
Neurologic
Psychogenic, porphyria, lead poisoning, primary dysautonomia (Riley-day syndrome), increased intracranial pressure, and GB syndrome
Obstructive sleep apnea
Preeclampsia/eclampsia
Medications and toxins
High-dose estrogens, alcohol and drugs—oral contraceptives, anabolic steroids, corticosteroids, decongestants, nonsteroidal anti-inflammatory agents (NSAIDs), COX-2 inhibitors, carbenoxolone, sympathomimetics, cyclosporine, sibutramine, bromocriptine, and erythropoietin
Stress
Postoperative, pain, burns, hypoglycemia, alcohol withdrawal, and hypoglycemia
Causes of isolated systolic hypertension: Atherosclerosis, aortic regurgitation, patent ductus arteriosus, thyrotoxicosis, and coarctation of aorta

Humoral Mechanisms

The autonomic nervous system, the renin–angiotensin, natriuretic peptide, and kallikrein kinin system play a role in the physiological regulation of short-term changes in blood pressure. They may also be probably involved in the pathogenesis of essential hypertension.

- *A low-renin, salt-sensitive, essential hypertension* in which patients have renal sodium and water retention has been found.
  Low-renin hypertension is more common in elderly and diabetics. These patients are salt-sensitive and diuretic responsive.
- *Normal renin hypertension* (nonmodulators) is more common in males and postmenopausal females. They are salt sensitive.
- *High-renin hypertension* is characterized by high plasma renin activity and responsiveness to angiotensin II antagonists.
- Low calcium intake has been associated with an increase in blood pressure in epidemiologic studies.
  Insulin resistance is responsible for essential hypertension in majority of the patients.
- **Metabolic syndrome:** It is characterized by hyperinsulinemia, glucose intolerance, reduced levels of HDL cholesterol, hypertriglyceridemia, and central obesity (all related to insulin resistance). Metabolic syndrome is associated with hypertension and is a major risk factor for cardiovascular disease.

Fetal factors

Impaired intrauterine growth resulting in low-birth weight is associated with subsequent development of high blood pressure.

Approach to Newly Diagnosed Hypertension

Q. Discuss the approach to a case of hypertension in the young.

Hypertension is usually asymptomatic and the diagnosis is usually made at routine examination or when a complication arises. A routine BP checkup is necessary every 5 years in adults.

Goals of the initial evaluation with high BP are to:

- Obtain accurate BP measurements
- Identify contributing factors, and risk factors and any underlying cause (secondary hypertension)
- Quantify cardiovascular risk
- Detect any complications (target organ damage)
- Identify comorbidity that may influence the choice of antihypertensive therapy.

These are attained by a careful history, clinical examination, and few simple investigations.

Ambulatory Blood Pressure Monitoring (ABPM)

Q. Write short note on ambulatory blood pressure monitoring.

Ambulatory blood pressure monitoring is the preferred method for confirming the diagnosis of hypertension. High-quality data suggest that ABPM predicts target-organ damage and cardiovascular events better than office blood pressure readings. ABPM records the blood pressure at preset intervals (usually every 15 to 20 minutes during the day and every 30 to 60 minutes during sleep).

Uses of ABPM are listed in **Box 7.30**.

Box 7.30: Uses of ambulatory blood pressure monitoring.

- Confirm white coat and masked hypertension
- Suspected episodic hypertension (e.g., pheochromocytoma)
- Determining therapeutic response (i.e., blood pressure control) in patients who are known to have a substantial white coat effect)
- Hypotensive symptoms while taking antihypertensive medications
- Resistant hypertension
- Autonomic dysfunction

Home and Ambulatory BP Recordings

- A transient rise in BP may occur by exercise, anxiety, discomfort, and unfamiliar surroundings.
- **White coat hypertension:** It is a transient increase in blood pressure in normal individuals when blood pressure is recorded either in a hospital or in a physician's clinic.
- **Isolated ambulatory or masked hypertension:**
  - It is reversal of white coat hypertension in which individuals have normal blood pressure (<140/90 mm Hg) in a hospital or in a physician's clinic but have increased ambulatory or home blood pressure values.
  - These individuals have increased prevalence of organ damage, with an increased prevalence of metabolic risk factors.

- Paradoxical hypertension:
  - It is characterized by a paradoxical increase in blood pressure in patients on antihypertensive agents.
  - This is observed in patients with:
    - Diabetes and hypertension who are on β-blockers, if they develop hypoglycemia. It is due to sympathetic stimulation following hypoglycemia.
    - Bilateral renal artery stenosis who are given ACE inhibitors.
    - Pheochromocytoma who is administered pure β-blockers.

History

- Record family history, lifestyle (exercise, salt intake, and smoking), other risk factors, history of drug intake or alcohol.
- Symptoms of causes of secondary hypertension **(Table 7.49)** or complications such as coronary artery disease (e.g., angina and breathlessness).

Clinical Features

Clinical features of hypertension may be due to hypertension itself and the underlying cause of hypertension. Clinical features due to hypertension per se:

- Majority of patients are asymptomatic and hypertension is usually detected during routine examination.
- Acute hypertension may produce transient headache and polyuria.
- Long-standing hypertension may cause left ventricular hypertrophy and heaving apical impulse, accentuation of the aortic component of the second heart sound (A2), a fourth heart sound (S4), very short early diastolic murmur, and fundal changes (refer complications).

TABLE 7.49: Findings and specific investigations in various secondary hypertension.

Findings	*Disease suspected*	*Specific investigation*
Paroxysmal hypertension, palpitations, headache, and diaphoresis	Pheochromocytoma	Urine VMA, metanephrine, plasma metanephrine
Fatigue, weight gain, menstrual irregularities, and diastolic hypertension	Hypothyroidism	Serum thyroid-stimulating hormone (TSH)
Weight loss, tachycardia, tremors, heat intolerance, and systolic hypertension	Hyperthyroidism	Serum TSH
Depression, muscle weakness, kidney stones, and osteoporosis	Hyperparathyroidism	Serum calcium, parathormone (PTH)
Headaches, fatigue, visual disturbances, enlarged tongue, and enlarged extremities	Acromegaly	Growth hormone (GH)
Weight gain, muscle weakness, striae, obesity, amenorrhea, and moon facies	Cushing's syndrome	Serum cortisol
Obesity, snoring, and daytime somnolence	Obstructive sleep apnea (OSA)	Polysomnography
Enlarged palpable kidneys, family history positive	Autosomal dominant polycystic kidney disease (ADPKD)	Ultrasound abdomen
Proteinuria, elevated serum creatinine, edema, and anemia	Chronic kidney disease (CKD)	Ultrasound
Abdominal/renal bruit	Renovascular cause	MR angiogram
Fatigue, hypokalemia, and hypernatremia	Aldosteronism	Plasma renin to aldosterone ratio, MRI abdomen

Objectives of clinical examination

- Identify any underlying cause of hypertension
- Recognize risk factors that lead to complications
- Abnormal signs to detect complications if already developed.

Nonspecific findings: Optic fundi may be abnormal; there may be evidence of generalized atheroma or specific complications, such as aortic aneurysm or peripheral vascular disease. Findings and specific investigations in various secondary hypertension are mentioned in **Table 7.49**.

Q. Write short note on causes and investigations of secondary hypertension.

Target Organ Damage (Complications of Hypertension)

Q. Write short essay or note on complications of hypertension/target organ damage in systemic arterial hypertension.

Target organ damage in hypertension can be clinically detected.

Central Nervous System Complications

- **Transient ischemic attacks (TIAs):** Carotid atheroma and TIAs are more common in patients with hypertension.
- **Cerebrovascular accidents (strokes)** are a common complication of hypertension and may be due to cerebral hemorrhage or infarction (due to cerebral atherothrombosis).
- **Subarachnoid hemorrhage** is also a complication of hypertension.
- **Hypertensive encephalopathy** is a rare complication characterized by very high blood pressure, neurological manifestations (includes transient disturbances in speech and vision, paresthesias, seizures, disorientation, and loss of consciousness), and papilledema.

TABLE 7.50: Grading of hypertensive retinopathy—Keith-Wagener-Barker classification.

Grade 1: Mild narrowing of the arterioles—"copper wire"
Grade 2: Moderate narrowing—copper wire and AV nicking, changes associated with long-standing essential hypertension
Grade 3: Severe narrowing—silver wire changes, hemorrhage, cotton wool spots, and hard exudates
Grade 4: Grade 3 + papilledema. Grade 3 and 4 highly correlated with progression to end-organ damage and decreased survival

Ophthalmic (Retinal) Complications

Q. Write short essay or note on grades of hypertensive retinopathy.

Hypertensive retinopathy (Table 7.50 and Fig. 7.37).

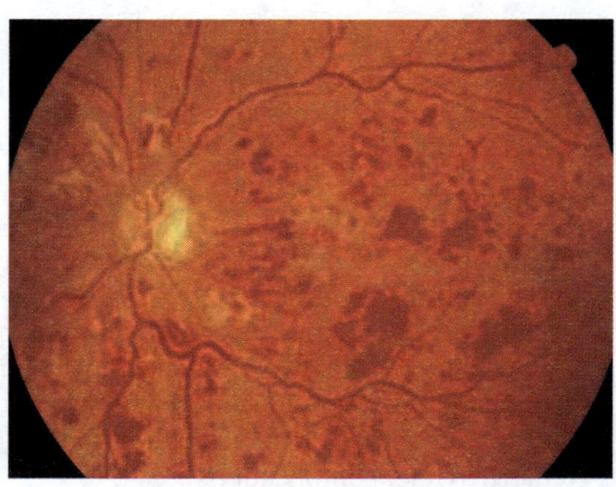

FIG. 7.37: Fundus image of hypertensive retinopathy.

Cardiovascular Complications

- **Coronary artery disease** (angina, myocardial infarction): Increased cardiac mortality and morbidity associated with hypertension are chiefly due to a higher incidence of coronary artery disease. High BP may produce left ventricular hypertrophy with a forceful apex beat and fourth heart sound. ECG or echocardiography is useful in risk assessment.

- **Left ventricular failure and pulmonary edema:** It may develop with severe hypertension.
- **Atrial fibrillation** is common and may be due to diastolic dysfunction caused by left ventricular hypertrophy or the effects of coronary artery disease.

Blood Vessels

Larger arteries show thickening of the internal elastic lamina, hypertrophy of smooth muscle, and deposition of fibrous tissue. Smaller arteries show hyaline arteriosclerosis in the wall, narrowing of the lumen, and aneurysm. **Atherosclerosis** may develop in coronary and cerebral blood vessel. Hypertension is a major risk factor involved in the pathogenesis **of aneurysm of aorta** and dissecting hematoma of aorta **(aortic dissection).**

Renal Complications

Long-standing hypertension may cause to damage the renal vasculature and produce (1) proteinuria, (2) hematuria, and (3) progressive renal failure.

Investigations

Basic investigations in all patients:
- **Urinalysis:** For protein, blood, and glucose.
- **Blood urea and creatinine:** To assess renal function.
- **Serum electrolytes:** For hypokalemia (is usually due to diuretic therapy) and alkalosis in hyperaldosteronism
- **Fasting and postprandial blood glucose:** For hyperglycemia
- **Lipid profile:** Serum total cholesterol and HDL cholesterol
- **Electrocardiogram:** 12-lead ECG for left ventricular hypertrophy and coronary artery disease.

Secondary Investigations in Selected Patients

- **Chest radiograph:** For detecting the cardiac size, evidence of cardiac failure and aortic dilatation, coarctation of the aorta
- **Ambulatory BP recording:** To detect borderline, masked hypertension or "white coat" hypertension
- **Echocardiogram:** To detect or quantify left ventricular hypertrophy and function
- **Renal ultrasound:** To detect renal disease
- **MRI, renal isotope scan, and renal angiography:** To detect or confirm renal artery stenosis
- **Urinary catecholamines:** To detect pheochromocytoma
- **Urinary cortisol and dexamethasone suppression test:** To detect Cushing's syndrome
- **Thyroid function tests:** To detect hypothyroidism or hyperthyroidism
- **Serum calcium and parathyroid hormone level:** To detect hyperparathyroidism
- **Plasma renin activity and aldosterone:** To detect possible primary aldosteronism
- **Growth hormone:** To detect acromegaly

Treatment
- **Objective of antihypertensive therapy:** To reduce the incidence of adverse cardiovascular events (e.g., coronary artery disease), stroke, and heart failure.
- **Target blood pressure:** For most patients, a target is <140 mm Hg systolic blood pressure and ≈85 mm Hg diastolic blood pressure. For patients with diabetes, renal impairment, or established cardiovascular disease the target is <130/80 mm Hg.

Management of hypertension can be studied under three headings.
- General measures
- Antihypertensive drug therapy
- Treatment of underlying cause (in secondary hypertension).

General Measures

Q. Write short essay/note on nonpharmacological treatment of hypertension.

- **Lifestyle modifications:** Recommended for all patients with hypertension and prehypertension. A reduction in systolic blood pressure of 5 mm Hg has been associated with about 10% reduction in mortality caused by stroke and heart disease:
  - Control of obesity: Maintain normal body weight (BMI 20–25 kg/m^2)
  - Diet: Dietary Approaches to Stop Hypertension or **DASH** eating plan.
    - Restrict salt in the diet (<100 mEq sodium or <6 g NaCl or <2.4 g Na/day).
    - Reduce intake of fat and saturated fat.
    - Increase consumption of diet rich in fruit and vegetables (≥5 portions of fresh fruit and vegetables/day), potassium.
    - Limit/reduce alcohol consumption to ≤3 units/day men and ≤2 units/day women.

- Cardiovascular risk reduction: Stop/avoid cigarette smoking and increase intake of oily fish.
- Regular aerobic/physical exercises: Perform ≥30 minute brisk walk most days of the week. Relaxation classes, meditation, and biofeedback.

Q. Write short essay or note on various types of antihypertensive drugs.

Antihypertensive Drug Therapy (Table 7.51)

Q. Write short note on α-adrenergic blockers.

Diuretics

- Indications include heart failure and elderly and systolic hypertension
  - **Thiazide diuretics:**
    - **Adverse drug reactions:** These include impotence, postural hypotension, allergic rashes, bone marrow depression, hypokalemia, hyperuricemia, hypercalcemia, and impaired glucose tolerance/diabetes.
    - Used as first-line agent in elderly patients with systolic hypertension. If blood pressure is not controlled with a thiazide diuretic, add ACE inhibitors, angiotensin receptor blockers, or calcium channel blockers.
    - **Loop diuretics:** Furosemide or others are used if there is renal impairment or when greater sodium excretion is needed or they are used in conjunction with an ACE inhibitor.

β-adrenoreceptor Antagonists (β-blockers)

Q. Write short essay or note on β-blockers, uses, and its side effects.

Uses and contraindications for β-blockers are mentioned in **Table 7.52**. Beta blockers are no longer used as first-line antihypertensive therapy. They may be useful in following situations in:

TABLE 7.51: Various antihypertensive drugs (dose).

Drugs by class	*Properties*	*Initial dose*	*Dosage range (mg)*
β-adrenergic antagonists			
Atenolol	Selective	50 mg PO daily	25–100
Betaxolol	Selective	10 mg PO daily	5–40
Bisoprolol	Selective	5 mg PO daily	2.5–20
Metoprolol	Selective	50 mg PO bid	50–450
Metoprolol XL	Selective	50–100 mg PO daily	50–400
Nebivolol	Selective with vasodilatory properties	5 mg PO daily	5–40
Nadolol	Nonselective	40 mg PO daily	20–240
Propranolol	Nonselective	40 mg PO bid	40–240
Propranolol LA	Nonselective	80 mg PO daily	60–240
Timolol	Nonselective	10 mg PO bid	20–40
Pindolol	ISA	5 mg PO daily	10–60
Labetalol	α- and β-antagonist properties	100 mg PO bid	200–1,200
Carvedilol	α- and β-antagonist properties	6.25 mg PO bid	12.5–50
Carvedilol CR	α- and β-antagonist properties	10 mg PO daily	10–80
Acebutolol	ISA, selective	200 mg PO bid, 400 mg PO daily	200–1,200
Calcium channel antagonists			
Amlodipine	DHP	5 mg PO daily	2.5–10
Diltiazem		30 mg PO qid	90–360
Diltiazem LA		180 mg PO daily	120–540
Diltiazem CD		180 mg PO daily	120–480
Diltiazem XR		180 mg PO daily	120–540
Diltiazem XT		180 mg PO daily	120–480
Isradipine	DHP	2.5 mg PO bid	2.5–10
Nicardipine	DHP	20 mg PO tid	60–120
Nifedipine	DHP	10 mg PO tid	30–120
Nifedipine XL (or CC)	DHP	30 mg PO daily	30–90
Nisoldipine	DHP	20 mg PO daily	20–40
Verapamil		80 mg PO tid	80–480
Verapamil SR		120 mg PO daily	120–480

Contd...

Contd...

Angiotensin-converting enzyme inhibitors			
Benazepril		10 mg PO bid	10–40
Captopril		25 mg PO bid–tid	50–450
Enalapril		5 mg PO daily	2.5–40
Fosinopril		10 mg PO daily	10–40
Lisinopril		10 mg PO daily	5–40
Moexipril		7.5 mg PO daily	7.5–30
Quinapril		10 mg PO daily	5–80
Ramipril		2.5 mg PO daily	1.25–20
Trandolapril		1–2 mg PO daily	1–4
Perindopril		4 mg PO daily	2–16
Angiotensin II receptor blockers			
Azilsartan		40 mg PO daily	40–80
Candesartan		8 mg PO daily	8–32
Eprosartan		600 mg PO daily	600–800
Irbesartan		150 mg PO daily	150–300
Olmesartan		20 mg PO daily	20–40
Losartan		50 mg PO daily	25–100
Telmisartan		40 mg PO daily	20–80
Valsartan		80 mg PO daily	80–320
Direct renin inhibitor			
Aliskiren		150 mg PO daily	150–300
Diuretics			
Chlorthalidone	Thiazide diuretic	25 mg PO daily	12.5–50
Hydrochlorothiazide	Thiazide diuretic	12.5 mg PO daily	12.5–50
Hydroflumethiazide	Thiazide diuretic	50 mg PO daily	50–100
Indapamide	Thiazide diuretic	1.25 mg PO daily	2.5–5
Methyclothiazide	Thiazide diuretic	2.5 mg PO daily	2.5–5
Metolazone	Thiazide diuretic	2.5 mg PO daily	1.25–5
Bumetanide	Loop diuretic	0.5 mg PO daily (or IV)	0.5–5
Ethacrynic acid	Loop diuretic	50 mg PO daily (or IV)	25–100
Furosemide	Loop diuretic	20 mg PO daily (or IV)	20–320
Torsemide	Loop diuretic	5 mg PO daily (or IV)	5–10
Amiloride	Potassium-sparing diuretic	5 mg PO daily	5–10
Triamterene	Potassium-sparing diuretic	50 mg PO bid	50–200
Eplerenone	Aldosterone antagonist	25 mg PO daily	25–100
Spironolactone	Aldosterone antagonist	25 mg PO daily	25–100
α-adrenergic antagonists			
Doxazosin		1 mg PO daily	1–16
Prazosin		1 mg PO bid–tid	1–20
Terazosin		1 mg PO at bedtime	1–20
Centrally acting adrenergic agents			
Clonidine		0.1 mg PO bid	0.1–1.2
Clonidine patch		TTS 1/week (equivalent to 0.1 mg/day release)	0.1–0.3
Guanfacine		1 mg PO daily	1–3
Guanabenz		4 mg PO bid	4–64
Methyldopa		250 mg PO bid–tid	250–2,000
Direct-acting vasodilators			
Hydralazine		10 mg PO qid	50–300
Minoxidil		5 mg PO daily	2.5–100
Miscellaneous			
Reserpine		0.5 mg PO daily	0.01–0.25

- Younger individuals, particularly who have an intolerance or contraindication to ACE inhibitors and angiotensin II receptor antagonists.
- Women of childbearing potential
- Patients with increased sympathetic drive
- Patients having hypertension and other diseases, such as coronary heart disease (postmyocardial infarction or angina) and heart failure.

Nonselective (β1 and β2)

- **Mechanism of action:** Sympatholytic effect, antihypertensive effect, and relief of anxiety, palpitation and angina. Large portion of the drug is destroyed during its passage through liver, e.g.:

TABLE 7.52: Uses and contraindications for β-blockers.

Uses of β-blockers	
➢ Angina pectoris ➢ Cardiac arrhythmias ➢ Acute myocardial infarction and postmyocardial infarction period (to prevent reinfarction) ➢ Dissecting aortic aneurysm ➢ Hypertrophic cardiomyopathy ➢ Fallot's tetralogy (cyanotic spells)	➢ Hypertension ➢ Thyrotoxicosis ➢ Pheochromocytoma ➢ Anxiety with somatic symptoms ➢ Chronic open-angle glaucoma ➢ Portal hypertension ➢ Migraine prophylaxis ➢ Essential tremor
Contraindications of β-blockers	
➢ Chronic obstructive pulmonary disease and asthma ➢ Cardiac failure ➢ Heart block	➢ Peripheral vascular disease ➢ Diabetes mellitus (masks sympathetic signs of hypoglycemia)

INDIVIDUALIZING ANTIHYPERTENSIVE THERAPY

Compelling indications (major improvement in outcome independent of blood pressure)	
Diabetes mellitus	ACE inhibitor or ARB
Heart failure with reduced ejection fraction	ACE inhibitor or ARB, beta blocker, diuretic, and aldosterone antagonist
Postmyocardial infarction	ACE inhibitor or ARB, beta blocker, aldosterone antagonist
Proteinuric chronic kidney disease (nondiabetic)	ACE inhibitor or ARB
Angina pectoris	Beta blocker and calcium channel blocker
Atrial fibrillation/flutter rate control	Beta blocker, nondihydropyridine calcium channel blocker
Previous CVA/TIA	ACE inhibitor ± diuretic
Antihypertensive agents with a favorable effect on symptoms in comorbid conditions	
Benign prostatic hyperplasia	Alpha blocker
Essential tremor	Beta blocker (non cardioselective)
Hyperthyroidism	Beta blocker
Migraine	Beta blocker, calcium channel blocker
Osteoporosis	Thiazide diuretic
Raynaud phenomenon	Dihydropyridine calcium channel blocker
Contraindications	
Angioedema	Do not use an ACE inhibitor
Peripheral vascular disease	Avoid beta blocker
Bronchospasm	Do not use a nonselective beta blocker
Liver disease	Do not use methyldopa
Pregnancy	Do not use an ACE inhibitor, ARB, or renin inhibitor
Second- or third-degree heart block	Do not use a beta blocker, nondihydropyridine calcium channel blocker unless a functioning ventricular pacemaker
Bilateral renal artery stenosis	Avoid ACE inhibitors/ARB/renin inhibitor
Drug classes that may have adverse effects on comorbid conditions	
Depression	Avoid beta blocker, central alpha-2 agonist
Gout	Avoid loop or thiazide diuretic
Hyperkalemia	Avoid aldosterone antagonist, ACE inhibitor, ARB, and renin inhibitor
Hyponatremia	Avoid thiazide diuretic
Renovascular disease	Avoid ACE inhibitor, ARB, or renin inhibitor

- **Dosage:** Started with 40 mg twice a day and gradually increased to 160 mg 6 hourly. Slow-release forms are administered as a single daily dose, e.g., propranolol
- **Side effects:** Gastric disturbances, bronchospasm, bradycardia, cardiac failure, tiredness, bad dreams, hallucinations, cold hands, and muscle weakness.

Cardioselective (β1)

- **Mechanisms of action:** They act more on the cardiac β_1-adrenoceptors than β_2-adrenoceptors that mediate vasodilatation and bronchodilatation. **Examples: Metaprolol and atenolol**
- **Dose:** Metaprolol 50 mg twice daily to 100 mg thrice daily, atenolol 50–100 mg once daily and bisoprolol 5–10 mg daily. Sustained release preparation of metoprolol is given in the dose of 12.5–100 mg once daily.

- **Indications:**
  - Hypertensive with mild airway obstruction (COPD, asthma), peripheral vascular disease, and type 1 diabetes. However, caution is necessary.
  - Ischemic heart disease and supraventricular tachycardia.
- **Side effect:** Similar to propranolol and also cause hyperkalemia.

Combined α- and β-blockers (Labetalol and Carvedilol)

- Sometimes, these combined β- and α-adrenoceptor antagonists are more effective than pure β-blockers.
- **Mechanism of action and side effects:** Similar to propranolol.
- **Dose:** Labetalol 100–200 mg twice daily and carvedilol 6.25–25 mg twice daily. Labetalol can be used as an infusion in the treatment of malignant phase hypertension.

Angiotensin-converting Enzyme (ACE) Inhibitors

Q. Write short essay or note on mechanism of action, indications, and side effects of angiotensin-converting enzyme (ACE) inhibitors.

Q. Write short note on ramipril.

- These include captopril, enalapril (20 mg daily), lisinopril (10–40 mg daily), ramipril (5–10 mg daily), and perindopril.
- **Mechanisms of action:** They inhibit the conversion of angiotensin I to angiotensin II and produce powerful arteriolar and venous dilatation, and inhibit release of aldosterone.
- **Dosage:** Start with a small dose (captopril 6.25 mg and enalapril 2.5 mg) and then gradually increase.
- **Indication:** Used in hypertension, chronic cardiac failure or left ventricular dysfunction, postmyocardial infarction or cardiovascular disease, diabetic nephropathy, and stroke secondary prevention.
- **Contraindication:** Renal failure (creatinine >3 mg/dL) and bilateral renal artery stenosis because they can reduce the filtration pressure in the glomeruli and precipitate renal failure. Electrolytes and creatinine levels should be checked before and 1-2 weeks after starting therapy. Other contraindications include peripheral vascular disease hyperkalemia and pregnancy.
- **Adverse reaction:** First-dose postural hypotension, cough, angioedema, skin rashes, blood dyscrasias, hyperkalemia, renal dysfunction neuropathy, and diarrhea.

Peripheral Vasodilators

- **Mechanism of action:** Peripheral vasodilators act on arteriolar smooth muscles or smooth muscles of venules and produce peripheral arteriolar and venous dilatation.
- Drugs include hydralazine, prazosin (alpha blocker), diazoxide, and sodium nitroprusside.

Angiotensin Receptor Blockers

Q. Write short essay or note on angiotensin receptor blockers and indications.

- **Mechanism of action:** They block the angiotensin II type I receptor and have similar effects to ACE inhibitors. Renin-angiotensin-aldosterone system (RAAS) plays an important role in the regulation of blood pressure.
  - Renin catalyzes cleavage of angiotensinogen and produces angiotensin I.
  - Angiotensin I is converted to angiotensin II by the action of ACE. Angiotensin II is the most active hormone of the renin-angiotensin system. There are two angiotensin II receptors, namely AT1 (most effective) and AT2 (its function is not established).
  - When angiotensin II binds to its AT1 receptor, it produces many effects such as vasoconstriction, cell proliferation, hypertrophy, and aldosterone secretion and provides feedback inhibition of further renin release by the kidney.
  - The angiotensin receptor blockers block the action of angiotensin II by blocking AT1 receptors.
- **Dose:** Losartan 50–100 mg daily, candesartan 2.0–32 mg daily, valsartan 40–320 mg daily, telmisartan 40 mg daily, olmesartan 10–40 mg daily, and irbesartan and azilsartan (40–80 mg daily).
- **Side effects:** These drugs are better tolerated than ACE inhibitors. Side effects include hypotension, drowsiness, and dizziness. These drugs do not cause cough.
- **Indications:** ACE inhibitor intolerant hypertension, <55 years old, hypertension with LVH, heart failure or left ventricular dysfunction, myocardial infarction (to reduce myocardial remodeling), diabetic nephropathy (to slow its progression), and chronic renal disease.

Calcium Channel Blockers (Calcium Antagonists)

Q. Write short essay or note on uses/indications of calcium channel blockers and its side effects.

- They are effective and usually well-tolerated antihypertensive drugs. Various indications of calcium channel blockers are listed in **Table 7.53**.

- **Contraindications:** Unstable angina, heart failure, hypotension, postinfarct patients, severe aortic stenosis, and second- and third-degree AV block.
- **Side effects:** Flushing, palpitations, and fluid retention. The main side effect of verapamil is constipation.

Nifedipine and Verapamil

Dosage: Nifedipine 10–20 mg three to four times daily and verapamil 180–360 mg/day in divided doses. Short-acting nifedipine should be avoided.

TABLE 7.53: Indications of calcium channel blockers.

➢ Angina pectoris/Prinzmetal's angina ➢ Hypertension and hypertensive crisis ➢ Cardiac arrhythmias ➢ Elderly patients with systolic hypertension ➢ Congestive cardiac failure ➢ Valvular diseases (mitral and aortic regurgitation) ➢ Hypertrophic cardiomyopathy	➢ Peripheral vasospastic conditions, e.g., Raynaud's disease, migraine ➢ Pulmonary hypertension ➢ Cor pulmonale (chronic bronchitis with pulmonary hypertension) ➢ Subarachnoid hemorrhage (to prevent vasospasm) ➢ Achalasia cardia ➢ Biliary dyskinesia

Centrally Acting Drugs

Reserpine: It is a mild antihypertensive with central and peripheral action.

It is given in the dose of 0.1–0.5 mg daily. Its side effects include nasal congestion, depression, and Parkinsonism.

α-methyldopa: It is a precursor of dopamine and noradrenaline.

- **Mechanism of action:** Converted to α-methyl noradrenaline which acts on alpha-2 receptors in brain and causes inhibition of adrenergic discharge in adrenal medulla → fall in peripheral vascular resistance and fall in blood pressure.
- **Side effects:** Cognitive impairment, postural hypotension, positive Coombs test, etc. Not used therapeutically now except in hypertension during pregnancy.
- **Dose:** 250–500 mg twice or thrice daily.

Clonidine: Not frequently used because of tolerance and withdrawal hypertension. Side effect is dryness of mouth. Dose: 0.1–1.0 mg daily.

Newer antihypertensive agents are listed in **Table 7.54**.

TABLE 7.54: Newer antihypertensive agents.

Direct renin inhibitor	Aliskiren
Protein kinase C inhibitors	Staurosporine
Calcium channel blocker	Cilnidipine, azelnidipine, and clevidipine
Nonselective β-blocker and weak α-blocker	Bucindolol
Chymase inhibitors	SPF-32629A
Prostacycline analog	Treprostinil
Serotonin receptor antagonist	Ketanserin
Endothelin receptor antagonist	Ambrisentan, sitaxsentan, bosentan, and darusentan
Advanced glycation end product (AGE) crosslink breaker	Alagebrium
Phosphodiesterase type 5 (PDE-5) inhibitor	Sildenafil

Guidelines for Starting Antihypertensive Agents

Refer **Figure 7.38.**

Recommendations in Hypertension Management Suggested by JNC8 (Table 7.55)

Q. Discuss the recommendations in hypertension management suggested by JNC8.

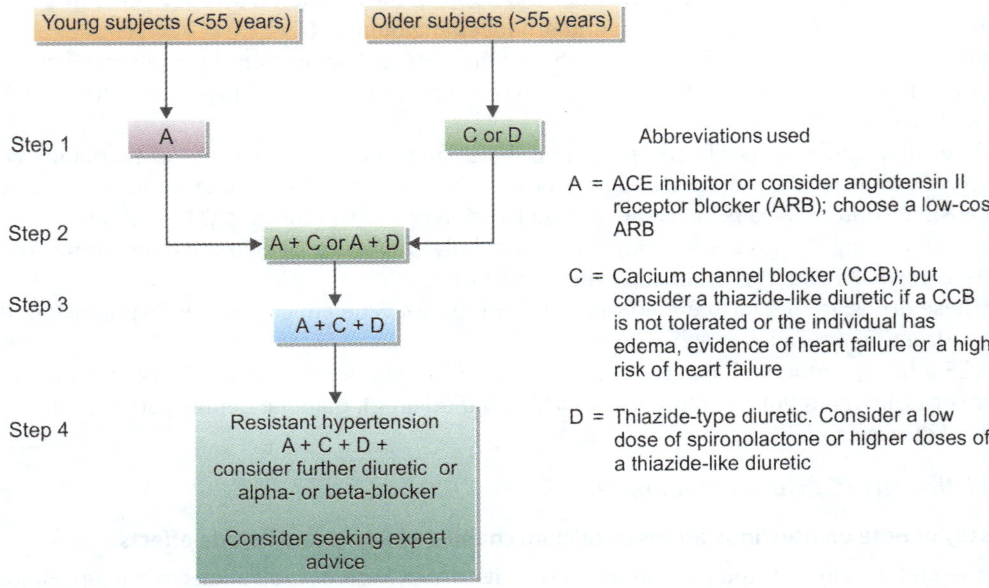

FIG. 7.38: Choosing antihypertensive drug and its combinations for patients newly diagnosed with hypertension.

TABLE 7.55: JNC8 recommendations in hypertension management.	
1.	**Elderly: In the general population aged ≥60 years:** Start drug treatment to reduce BP of ≥150/90 mm Hg **AND** treat patients for blood pressure goal of <150/90 mm Hg
2.	**Diastolic blood pressure:** In general individuals aged <60 years: Initiate drug treatment to reduce diastolic BP of ≥90 mm Hg **AND** treat patients for diastolic BP goal of <90 mm Hg
3.	**Systolic blood pressure:** In general individuals aged <60 years: Initiate drug treatment to reduce systolic BP of ≥140 mm Hg **AND** treat patients for systolic BP goal of <140 mm Hg
4.	**Chronic kidney disease: In the population aged ≥18 years with chronic kidney disease:** Initiate drug treatment to reduce BP of ≥140/90 mm Hg **AND** treat patients for BP goal of <140/90 mm Hg
5.	**Diabetes mellitus: In the population aged ≥18 years with diabetes:** Initiate drug treatment to reduce BP of ≥140/90 mm Hg **AND** treat patients for BP goal of <140/90 mm Hg
6.	**Non-black-first line: In the non-black individuals, including patients with diabetes** recommend antihypertensive treatment with the following: Thiazide-type diuretic, calcium channel blocker (CCB), angiotensin-converting enzyme inhibitor (ACEI), or angiotensin receptor blocker (ARB)
7.	**Black-first line: In the black individuals, including patients with diabetes:** Recommend antihypertensive treatment with: Thiazide-type diuretic **OR** calcium channel blocker (CCB)
8.	**Chronic kidney disease-first line or add on in adults aged ≥18 years with chronic kidney disease and hypertension:** Initial or add-on antihypertensive treatment to improve kidney outcomes with: An ACEI **OR** An ARB
9.	**Do not combine** ACEI and ARB ➢ If BP goal is not reached **within 1 month of treatment** increase the dose of the drug or add second drug and if not reached with 2 drugs, add and titrate a third drug from the above-mentioned class. ➢ If goal BP cannot be reached using only the drugs from class of thiazide-type diuretic, CCB, ACEI, or ARB due to some contraindication or the need to use more than 3 drugs to reach goal BP, antihypertensive drugs from **other classes** can be added

Hypertensive Encephalopathy

Q. Discuss briefly about hypertensive crisis/hypertensive emergencies.

- It is more **generalized** term and is not defined by a specific blood pressure reading.
- It develops in previously hypertensive/normotensive patients.
- It is a clinical syndrome that is associated with acute severe or abrupt elevation of blood pressure. Characterized by severe increase in systolic and/or diastolic blood pressure associated with signs or symptoms of acute end-organ damage.
- No blood pressure threshold for diagnosis. Usually, systolic blood pressure >180–220 mm Hg, diastolic blood pressure >120–130 mm Hg, and mean arterial pressure (MAP) >180 mm Hg
- Increased cerebral blood flow → hyperfiltration → localized or diffuse cerebral edema → cerebral ischemia resulting from arteriolar spasm.
- Severe headache, vomiting, visual disturbances, confusion, focal or generalized seizures.
- Fundoscopy examination (key role): **Papilledema**
- It includes: (1) hypertensive emergency and (2) hypertensive urgency.

Hypertensive Emergencies

Reason includes renovascular disease, pheochromocytoma, nonadherence to antihypertensive medication, hyperaldosteronism, erythropoietin administration, acute glomerular nephropathy, and eclampsia.

Hypertensive Urgency

- Severe elevation in BP >180/120 mm Hg without symptoms or signs of acute target organ involvement.
- Adequate treatment of these conditions, a BP lowering within 24 hours by administration of oral drugs.
- ICU admission is usually not required.

Treatment

Requires an immediate BP reduction in few minutes to hours in an ICU care and brought by IV drugs.

"Malignant" or "Accelerated" Phase Hypertension

Q. Write short essay or a note on accelerated hypertension.

- It is a rare condition that may complicate hypertension of any etiology. It occurs when blood pressure rises rapidly with severe hypertension (diastolic blood pressure >120 mm Hg). Histologically, it is characterized by fibrinoid necrosis in the walls of small arteries and arterioles and intravascular thrombosis.
- **Diagnosis:** Presence of high BP and rapidly progressive end-organ damage, such as retinopathy (grade 3 or 4 with flame-shaped hemorrhages, cotton wool spots, hard exudates, and papilledema), renal dysfunction (e.g., proteinuria and hematuria), and/or cerebral edema and hemorrhage with resultant hypertensive encephalopathy. Left ventricular failure may develop.
- If this is untreated, it may lead to death within months from progressive renal failure, heart failure, aortic dissection, or stroke.

Q. Write short essay or note on treatment of hypertensive crisis (hypertensive emergencies).

Q. Discuss the management of accelerated/malignant hypertension.

Management of Hypertensive Emergencies

- Normalization of BP is usually not recommended.
- Sudden fall in BP may cause acute hypoperfusion of vital organs and results in myocardial ischemia or infarction, hemiplegia, or acute renal failure.
- Older patients with long-lasting hypertension and preclinical organ involvement (LVH, atherosclerosis, and arteriolar remodeling) are at risk of these complications as the lower limit of autoregulation shifted to right.

How fast and how much BP to be lowered to be given importance

- **Goal:** Reduce mean arterial pressure (MAP) by no more than 20–25%, diastolic blood pressure (DBP) to 100–110 mm Hg within few minutes to 2 hours.
- More aggressive and rapid BP reduction needed in acute pulmonary edema and aortic dissection.
- More slow reduction needed for acute cerebrovascular damages with monitoring of neurological status.
- Constant infusion of intravenous agents required (no intermittent IV boluses/oral/sublingual drugs—drastic BP fall).

Various hypertensive emergencies and their treatment are presented in **Table 7.56**.
Drugs used in hypertensive emergencies and their dosage, action, and adverse effects are presented in **Table 7.57**.

Resistant Hypertension

Q. Write short note on resistant hypertension.

Definition: Resistant hypertension is defined as blood pressure above goal (>140/90 mm Hg; >130–139/80–85 mm Hg in patients with diabetes mellitus; >130/80 mm Hg in chronic kidney disease), *despite treatment with ≥3 antihypertensive drugs of different classes, including a diuretic, at optimal doses.*

- Resistant hypertension is observed in about 10–20% of patients with hypertension.
- Almost 50% of these patients experience an adverse cardiovascular event compared with patients with blood pressure controlled by three or fewer antihypertensive agents. Noncompliance to medication is an important cause.
- Diagnosis requires exclusion of both pseudoresistance and reversible or organic causes.

Treatments for Resistant Hypertension

- **Nonpharmacologic intervention:** Reinforce lifestyle changes.
- **Drug intervention:** Look for drug compliance, optimize doses. Add drugs from other classes.
- **Device therapy:** Two techniques:
    1. Percutaneous transluminal radiofrequency sympathetic denervation of the renal arteries.
    2. Carotid baroreflex activation.
- **Medical therapy:** Aldosterone antagonist, angiotensin-converting enzyme (ACE) inhibitors and angiotensin II receptor blockers (ARBs) plus chlorthalidone.
- Percutaneous angioplasty with/without stent placement.
- Surgical revascularization or, nephrectomy in unilateral cases.

TABLE 7.56: Various hypertensive emergencies and their treatment.

Diagnosis	*Suggested drugs*	*Targets*	*Remarks*
Acute aortic dissection	Esmolol/labetalol + nitroprusside would be a better combination	Reduce SBP as rapidly as possible down to 100–110 mm Hg, simultaneously control tachycardia due to the sympathetic activation	Avoid volume depletion Use β-blockers before vasodilators Hydralazine is contraindicated
Acute pulmonary edema	Nitroglycerine infusion, IV enalapril, Nitroprusside infusion, and IV furosemide	Reduce blood pressure by 20–30%	Hypotension may develop with enalaprilat
Acute coronary syndrome	Nitroglycerine infusion β-blockers (metoprolol or labetalol)	Reduce blood pressure by not more than 20–30%	Beware of hypotension in right ventricular infarction Avoid hypotension
Acute renal failure	Labetalol IV, nicardipine infusion, and dialysis	Reduce blood pressure not more than 20–30%	Avoid nitroprusside and ACE inhibitors
Subarachnoid hemorrhage	Labetalol bolus and infusion Esmolol bolus and infusion Nicardipine infusion	Systolic pressure <160 mm Hg or mean arterial pressure <130 mm Hg (to reduce recurrence)	Control of pain will help in BP control
Intracranial bleed	Labetalol and infusion Nitroglycerine infusion Nimodipine, a dihydropyridine calcium blocker is effective	To prevent rebleeding and reduce edema formation. May benefit from gradual 20–25% reduction in BP	Avoid lowering blood pressure by more than 10–15% in 24 hours
Hypertensive encephalopathy	IV sodium nitroprusside is the drug of choice, rapid onset of action. IV labetalol, nicardipine, and hydralazine	Mean BP should be reduced by 20% within first hour	

TABLE 7.57: Drugs used in hypertensive emergencies.

Drug	*Administration*	*Onset*	*Duration of action*	*Dosage*	*Adverse effects and comments*
Fenoldopam	IV infusion	<5 min	30 min	0.1–0.3 µg/kg/min	Tachycardia, nausea, and vomiting
Sodium nitroprusside	IV infusion	Immediate	2–3 min	0.5–10 µg/kg/min (initial dose, 0.25 µg/kg/min for eclampsia and renal insufficiency)	Hypotension, nausea, vomiting, apprehension; risk of thiocyanate and cyanide toxicity is increased in renal and hepatic insufficiency, respectively; levels should be monitored; must shield from light
Diazoxide	IV bolus	15 min	6–12 h	50–100 mg q 5–10 min, up to 600 mg	Hypotension, tachycardia, nausea, vomiting, fluid retention, hyperglycemia; may exacerbate myocardial ischemia, heart failure, or aortic dissection
Labetalol	IV bolus	5–10 min	3–6 h	20–80 mg q 5–10 min, up to 300 mg	Hypotension, heart block, heart failure, bronchospasm, nausea, vomiting, scalp tingling, paradoxical pressor response; may not be effective in patients receiving α- or β-antagonists
	IV infusion			0.5–2 mg/min	
Nitroglycerin	IV infusion	1–2 min	3–5 min	5–250 µg/min	Headache, nausea, and vomiting. Tolerance may develop with prolonged use
Esmolol	IV bolus	1–5 min	10 min	500 µg/kg/min for first 1 min	Hypotension, heart block, heart failure, bronchospasm
	IV infusion			50–300 µg/kg/min	
Phentolamine	IV bolus	1–2 min	3–10 min	5–10 mg q 5–15 min	Hypotension, tachycardia, headache, angina, and paradoxical pressor response
Hydralazine (for treatment of eclampsia)	IV bolus	10–20 min	3–6 h	10–20 mg q 20 min (if no effect after 20 mg, try another agent)	Hypotension, fetal distress, tachycardia, headache, nausea, vomiting, and local thrombophlebitis. Infusion site should be changed after 12 h
Methyldopate (for treatment of eclampsia)	IV bolus	30–60 min	10–16 h	250–500 mg	Hypotension
Nicardipine	IV infusion	1–5 min	3–6 h	5 mg/h, increased by 1.0–2.5 mg/h q 15 min, up to 15 mg/h	Hypotension, headache, tachycardia, nausea, and vomiting
Clevidipine	IV infusion	2–4 min	5–15 min	1–2 mg/h, double dose every 90 seconds up to 16 mg/h	Hypotension, reflex tachycardia
Enalaprilat	IV bolus	5–15 min	1–6 h	0.6255 mg q6h	Hypotension

ACUTE RHEUMATIC FEVER

Q. Define rheumatic fever. Discuss the etiology, risk factors, pathogenesis, clinical features, investigations, diagnosis, complications, and management of rheumatic fever.

Definition: Rheumatic fever (RF) is an **acute, poststreptococcal, immune-mediated, and multisystem inflammatory disease.**

It occurs as a sequel to group A streptococcal pharyngitis.

- Multisystem disease affecting connective tissue particularly of the heart, joints, brain, cutaneous, and subcutaneous tissues.

Phases

There are two major phases:

1. **Acute rheumatic fever (ARF):** It frequently manifests as acute rheumatic carditis.
2. **Chronic rheumatic heart disease (RHD)** is the permanent heart valve damage resulting from one or more attacks of ARF. About 40–60% of patients with ARF will develop RHD. The most common valve affected is the mitral followed by aortic, in that order. However, all four valves can be affected. The deforming fibrotic valvular lesions are the principal/key features of chronic RHD.

Epidemiology and Incidence

- **Age group:** Most common in children between 5 and 15 years. It is rare <3 years of age.
- **Sex:** Both sexes are equally affected. However, certain clinical manifestations, such as mitral stenosis and Sydenham chorea, have a female preponderance after puberty.
- **Socioeconomic conditions:** Rheumatic fever is a worldwide disease and it is prevalent in regions with poor economic conditions, overcrowding, and substandard housing. Incidence and mortality rate of RF and RHD have markedly decreased over the past century, due to improved socioeconomic conditions and rapid diagnosis and treatment of streptococcal pharyngitis. In India, the annual incidence is 0.18 to 0.3 per 1,000 school children.
- **Poor economy and overcrowding:** It is a predisposing factor in developing countries. It is a major cause of death and disability in children and adolescents in socioeconomically deprived regions.

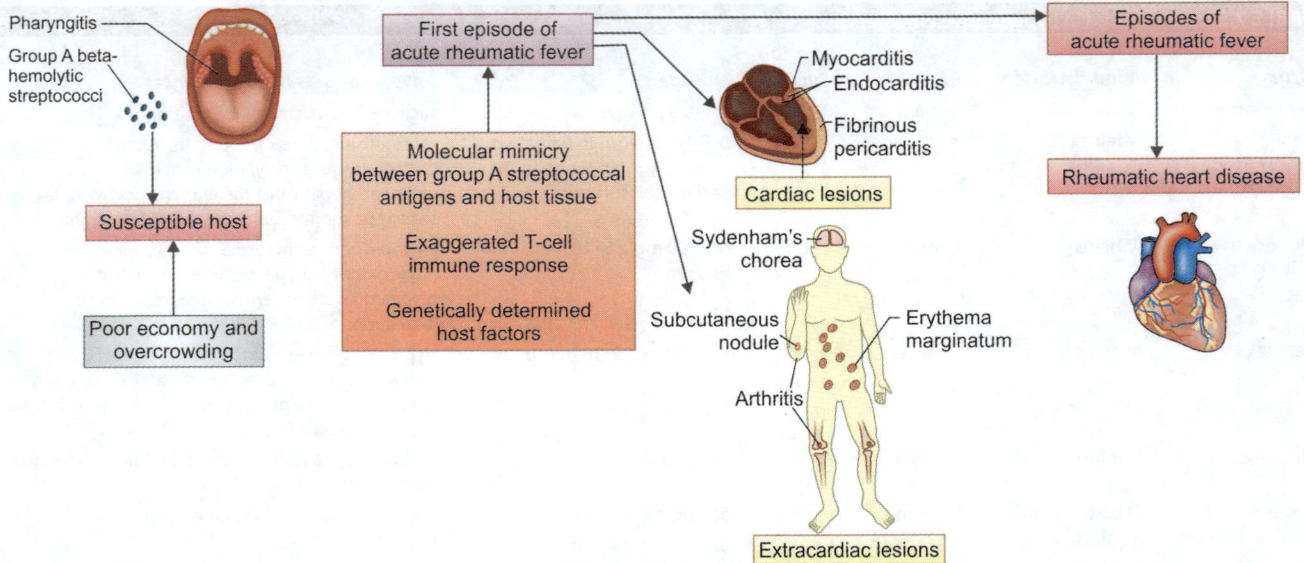

FIG. 7.39: Pathogenesis of rheumatic fever and rheumatic heart disease.

Etiology

- Acute rheumatic fever is a poststreptococcal disease.
- It develops after a latent period of 2 to 6 weeks after an episode of pharyngitis (sore throat) or tonsillitis by group A β-hemolytic streptococci. It occurs most often in children.
- Rheumatogenic potential of various serotypes of group A streptococci varies. M-protein is one of the well-defined determinants of bacterial virulence. M-type 5 is commonly responsible for rheumatic fever and other rheumatogenic serotypes include 1, 3, 6, 14, 18, 19, and 24. M-type 12 is highly prevalent, but usually does cause rheumatic fever.
- Recently virus (coxsackie B-4) has been suggested as causative agent with streptococcus acting as conditioning agent.

Pathogenesis (Fig. 7.39)

Immunologically mediated disease: Exact pathogenesis of rheumatic fever is not known. Streptococcal infection introduces the streptococcal antigens into the body may activate both antibody and T cell-mediated reactions against streptococci.

Molecular Mimicry

- Antibodies may be produced by B-lymphocytes against various antigenic components of the *Streptococcus.*
- These antibodies cross-react with human tissues because of the antigenic similarity between streptococcal components and human connective tissues (molecular mimicry). One of them produced against the M proteins of streptococci seems to cross-react with certain similar self-antigens in the myocardial cells and glycoproteins of the valves in the heart. This may be the mechanism for pancarditis in acute rheumatic fever.
- Immunologically mediated inflammation and damage (autoimmune) to human tissues which have antigenic similarity with streptococcal components—such as heart, joint, and brain connective tissues.

Streptococcal Super Antigens

- Super antigens are glycoproteins synthesized by bacteria and viruses. They can bridge class II major histocompatibility complex molecules to specific T-cell receptors, simulating antigen binding and activation of **$CD4^+$ T-cells**. These T-cells along with antibodies **cross-react with self-proteins in the heart**. These reactions produce cytokines leading to activation of macrophages, which are seen in lesions of rheumatic fever.

Host Factors

- Rheumatic fever occurs in a susceptible host and only 0.3–3% of individuals with acute streptococcal pharyngitis develops rheumatic fever.
- In India, HLA-DR3 is associated more frequently in patients with rheumatic fever and rheumatic fever has low frequency of HLA-DR2.

Clinical Manifestations

Acute rheumatic fever is a multisystem disorder. It usually presents with fever, anorexia, lethargy, and joint pain.

Previous history of sore throat: Only two-thirds of patients remember having any upper respiratory symptoms (episode of streptococcal pharyngitis) in the past 2–3 weeks.

Migrating Polyarthritis

- Migrating polyarthritis is the most common major manifestation. It occurs early when streptococcal antibody titers are high in about 75–90% of patients.
- It is acute, painful, migratory, and asymmetric and is of short duration **(fleeting and flitting).** Usually >5 joints are affected and mainly involves large joints (knees, ankles, wrists, elbows, and shoulders). The joints are involved in quick succession. Small joints and cervical spine are less commonly involved.
- Involved joints show signs of inflammation (red, swollen, and tender) with or without effusion. Pain and swelling develop quickly and subside within 5–7 days. Arthritis does not progress to chronic disease and over a period of time involved joints heal without any residual deformity (licks the joints).
- Excellent response of high-dose aspirin (salicylates) and NSAIDs.
- **Jaccoud's arthritis** is a rare deformity of the metacarpophalangeal joints following repeated attacks of rheumatic fever.
- In children below 5 years, arthritis is usually mild but carditis is more prominent.

Poststreptococcal Reactive Arthritis (PSRA)

- Arthritis developing after an episode of Group A streptococcal pharyngitis without other major criteria of acute rheumatic fever is known as PSRA.
- It develops 10 days after pharyngitis, can involve large joints, small joints or axial skeleton, cumulative and persistent and does not respond to acetylsalicylic acid.
- In contrast, arthritis of rheumatic fever develops 2 to 3 weeks after an episode of Group A streptococcal pharyngitis, migratory and transient, and usually involves only the large joints and responds well to acetylsalicylic acid.
- A small percentage of PSRA patients may subsequently develop valvular heart disease. Hence, patients should be followed up carefully for several months to look for evidence of carditis.

Carditis

Q. Write short essay/note on diagnosis of rheumatic fever.

- Early and most serious manifestation that occurs in 60–70% of patients.
- It manifests as pancarditis involving all three layers of the heart **(endocardium, myocardium, and pericardium).** On microscopic examination, myocardium shows **Aschoff body** that is pathognomonic of rheumatic myocarditis. **Rheumatic endocarditis** may involve valvular (valvular endocarditis) or mural endocardium (mural endocarditis). Rheumatic pericarditis produces pericardial effusion and thick fibrinoserous exudates.
- Carditis leaves a sequelae and permanent damage to the organ (bites the heart).
- Valvular damage is the hallmark of RF. Chronic phase is characterized by fibrosis, calcification, and stenosis of heart valves (fish-mouth valves).
- It is more common in younger children, and may be asymptomatic. It is detected only on echocardiograph.

Manifestations of Carditis

Pancarditis involves the endocardium, myocardium, and pericardium. Incidence of carditis decreases with increasing age. It ranges from 90% at 3 years to around 30% in adolescence.

- **Myocarditis:**
  - Tachycardia: Disproportionate to fever and persists during sleep
  - Features of congestive heart failure: Breathlessness (due to heart failure or pericardial effusion). Cardiac failure may be either caused by dysfunction of myocardium or valvular regurgitation.
  - Physical examination may reveal third heart sound (S_3), fourth heart sound (S_4), or a summation gallop.
  - Arrhythmias, prolongation of PR interval being the most common
- **Endocarditis:** Murmurs are most commonly observed during acute rheumatic fever. It may be new or changed murmurs and include:
  - Apical pansystolic murmur is a high-pitched, blowing-quality murmur of mitral regurgitation that radiates to the left axilla.
    1. Apical soft mid-diastolic murmur (also known as a **Carey Coombs murmur)** is heard during active carditis due to valvulitis with nodules forming on the mitral valve leaflets. It accompanies severe mitral insufficiency.
    2. An early diastolic murmur of aortic regurgitation and is high-pitched, blowing, decrescendo, and heard best along the right upper and mid-left sternal border after deep expiration while the patient is leaning forward.
- **Pericarditis:**
  1. Chest/pericardial pain (due to pericarditis or pancarditis)
  2. Pericardial friction rub and precordial tenderness
  3. Pericardial effusion (uncommon and always small). Rheumatic pericarditis never causes constriction.

Other clinical features of acute rheumatic carditis: These include palpitations, cardiac enlargement (cardiomegaly), and syncope due to conduction defects.

Skin Lesions

Q. Write a short essay/note on skin lesions in acute rheumatic fever.

Subcutaneous Nodules

1. Occur in 9–20% of cases and often associated with carditis.
2. Appears as a small (0.5–2.0 cm), painless, mobile hard nodules beneath skin appears 4 weeks after onset of RF. Thus, it helps to confirm rather than make the diagnosis.
3. Most common along extensor surfaces of joint-knees, elbows, wrists, and also on bony prominences, tendons, dorsum of feet, occipital or cervical spine.
4. Delayed manifestation, disappears: Leaves no residual damage.

Erythema Marginatum

1. Occur in <7% and often associated with chronic carditis and are evanescent.
2. Unique, transient, serpiginous-looking lesions of 1–2 inches in size.
3. Pink/red macules clear centrally, serpiginous spreading edge. More on trunks and limbs, nonitchy and almost never on the face. The resulting red rings or "margins" may coalesce or overlap.
4. Worsens with application of heat.

Chorea (Sydenham's Chorea, Chorea Minor, Saint Vitus Dance)

Others

1. Epistaxis, arthralgia, tender lymph nodes, scarlet fever rash, abdominal pain, tonsillar exudates in older children, etc.
2. Systemic manifestations are rare and include pleurisy, pleural effusion, and pneumonia.

Duration of Attack of Rheumatic Fever

1. **Acute rheumatic fever:** Average duration of an untreated acute attack is about 3 months.
2. **Chronic rheumatic fever:** It is defined as persistence of disease for >6 months. It occurs in <5% of patients and may lead to persisting congestive heart failure.

Laboratory Investigations

Investigations for Evidence of Preceding Streptococcal Infection (Specific)

1. **Isolation of group A streptococci/Throat swab culture:** Group A β-hemolytic streptococci is usually in only 10–25% of cases. It can be done also in family members and contacts. However, serologic tests are usually done to show the evidence of streptococcal infection.
2. **Streptococcal antibody tests (serologic tests):**
   - Serological tests usually confirm a recent group A β-hemolytic streptococcal infection.
   - Raised streptococcal antibody levels are found in the early stages of acute rheumatic fever. However, in two situations their levels may be low:
     - When the interval between the streptococcal pharyngitis and detection of rheumatic fever in >2 months (e.g., chorea)
     - In patients with rheumatic carditis only
   - Common serologic tests:
     - **Antistreptolysin O antibodies** (ASO titers): Rising titers, or levels of >200 U (adults) or >300 U (children). This test is positive in 80% of cases. ASO titers are normal in 20% of adult cases of rheumatic fever and most cases of chorea.
     - Anti-DNase B
     - Antihyaluronidase (AH)
     - Antistreptozyme test (ASTZ) is a very sensitive indicator of recent streptococcal infection and is also helpful in ruling out rheumatic fever. Titers >200 units/mL are considered positive.

   The above four tests when combined together help in conforming the diagnosis in 95% of cases.

Investigations for Evidence of a Systemic Illness (Nonspecific)

- **Acute phase reactants:** These tests confirm the presence of an inflammatory process, but are nonspecific.
  - Erythrocyte sedimentation rate (ESR) is raised.
  - Raised C-reactive protein (CRP) in the blood
- **Other tests confirming an inflammatory reaction:**
  - **Peripheral blood:** Polymorphonuclear leukocytosis and anemia (due to suppression of erythropoiesis)
  - **Serum:** Increase in serum complements, and increase in serum mucoproteins, α_2, and γ globulin levels

Investigations for Evidence of Carditis

- **Chest radiography:** Chest X-ray may show evidences of cardiac failure, cardiomegaly, and pulmonary congestion.
- **Electrocardiogram:** ECG changes commonly include:
  - Most consistent change is a prolongation of the PR interval and T-wave inversion.
  - Other findings are rarely second-degree AV block features of pericarditis and reduction in QRS voltages.
- **Echocardiography:** It can detect myocardial dysfunction, cardiac dilatation, valvular abnormalities, and pericardial effusion.

Diagnosis of Acute Rheumatic Fever

Q. Write a short essay/note on diagnosis of rheumatic fever/revised Duckett Jones criteria for the diagnosis of rheumatic fever.

- Diagnosis of acute rheumatic fever (ARF) is made by the presence of combination of typical clinical features together with evidence of the precipitating group A streptococci (GAS) infection. This uncertainty led Dr T Duckett Jones in 1944 to develop a set of criteria known as Jones Criteria to aid diagnosis.
- **Modified Jones criteria:** Presently diagnosis is based on modified Jones criteria (**Table 7.58**).

Exceptions to Jones Criteria

- Chorea alone, if other causes have been excluded.
- Insidious or late-onset carditis (indolent carditis) with no other explanation.
- Patients with documented RHD or prior rheumatic fever, one major criterion, or of fever, arthralgia or high CRP suggests recurrence.

TABLE 7.58: Revised Jones Criteria for Acute Rheumatic Fever 2015.

Diagnostic categories	***Criteria***
Primary episode of rheumatic fever	**Two major or one major and two minor manifestations plus evidence of preceding group A streptococcal infection**
Recurrent attack of rheumatic fever in a patient without established rheumatic heart disease	
Recurrent attack of rheumatic fever in a patient with established rheumatic heart disease	Two minor manifestations plus evidence of preceding group A streptococcal infection
Rheumatic chorea	Other major manifestations or evidence of group A streptococcal infection not required
Insidious-onset rheumatic carditis	
Chronic valve lesions of rheumatic heart disease (patients presenting for the first time with pure mitral stenosis or mixed mitral valve disease and/or aortic valve disease)	Do not require any other criteria to be diagnosed as having rheumatic heart disease
Major manifestations	***Minor manifestations***
➢ Carditis ➢ Polyarthritis ➢ Chorea ➢ Erythema marginatum ➢ Subcutaneous nodules	➢ Clinical: Fever and polyarthralgias ➢ Laboratory: Elevated erythrocyte sedimentation rate or leukocyte count ➢ Electrocardiogram: Prolonged P-R interval
Supporting evidence of a preceding streptococcal infection within the last 45 days ➢ Elevated or rising antistreptolysin O or other streptococcal antibody ➢ A positive throat culture ➢ Rapid antigen test for group A *Streptococcus* ➢ Recent scarlet fever **Revised Jones criteria, low-risk populations:** Major criteria: carditis (clinical and/or subclinical), arthritis (polyarthritis), chorea, erythema marginatum, and subcutaneous nodules Minor criteria: polyarthralgia, fever (≥38.5° F), sedimentation rate ≥60 mm and/or C-reactive protein (CRP) ≥3.0 mg/dL, and prolonged PR interval (unless carditis is a major criterion) **Revised Jones criteria, moderate- and high-risk populations:** Major criteria: carditis (clinical and/or subclinical), arthritis (monopolyarthritis or polyarthritis, or polyarthralgia), chorea, erythema marginatum, and subcutaneous nodules Minor criteria: fever (≥38.5° F), sedimentation rate ≥30 mm and/or CRP ≥3.0 mg/dL, and prolonged PR interval (unless carditis is a major criterion)	

Q. Write a short essay/note on treatment of rheumatic fever with carditis.

Management of Acute Rheumatic Fever

1. Step I: Primary prevention (eradication of streptococci)
2. Step II: Anti-inflammatory treatment (aspirin and steroids)
3. Step III: Supportive management and management of complications
4. Step IV: Secondary prevention (prevention of recurrent attacks)

Q. Write a short essay/note on prophylaxis of rheumatic fever.

Step I: Primary Prevention (Eradication of Streptococci)

- Primary prevention is accurate diagnosis and treatment of group A β-hemolytic streptococcal pharyngeal infection.
- Antistreptococcal therapy/primary prevention are mentioned in **Table 7.59**.

TABLE 7.59: Antistreptococcal therapy for primary prevention.

Drug	Dose	Mode and duration
Benzathine penicillin G **OR**	600,000 U for patients <27 kg 1,200,000 U for patients >27 kg	Intramuscular once
Penicillin V (phenoxymethylpenicillin) **OR**	Children: 250 mg 2–3 times daily or adolescents and adults: 500 mg 2–3 times daily	Oral for 10 days
Procaine penicillin	Daily 600,000 units	Intramuscular for 10 days
Erythromycin	20–40 mg/kg/day 2–4 times daily (maximum 1 g/day)	Oral for 10 days

Step II: Anti-inflammatory Treatment

- **Arthritis only:**
    - **Aspirin** usually rapidly relieves the symptoms of arthritis within 24 hours and also helps to confirm the diagnosis. Aspirin is given in the dose of **75–100 mg/kg body weight/day** divided into four doses for 6 weeks (attain a body level 20–30 mg/dL). It should be continued till the ESR has fallen. It produces mild toxicity such as nausea, tinnitus, and deafness and serious toxicity as vomiting, tachypnea, and acidosis.
- **Carditis or severe arthritis:**
    - **Corticosteroids** produce more rapid symptomatic relief compared to aspirin. They are indicated in patients with carditis or severe arthritis. However, their long-term use is not found to be beneficial.

Step III: Supportive Management and Management of Complications

Bed rest is important, because it reduces joint pain and cardiac workload.

- **Patients without carditis:** Advice bed rest until temperature and ESR are normal.
- **Patients with carditis:** Bed rest to be continued for 2–6 weeks after the ESR and temperature has returned to normal. Avoid strenuous exercise in patients who had carditis.

Treatment of congestive cardiac failure: Digitalis and diuretics

1. **Treatment of chorea:** Diazepam or haloperidol
2. Rest to joints and supportive splinting

Step IV: Secondary Prevention of Rheumatic Fever (Prevention of Recurrent Attacks)

1. Patients with acute rheumatic fever are susceptible to further attacks of rheumatic fever if another streptococcal infection occurs.
2. Secondary prevention is directed at preventing acute group A β-hemolytic streptococcal (GABHS) pharyngitis in patients at substantial risk of recurrent acute rheumatic fever by long-term prophylaxis. Duration of prophylaxis is controversial and its broad outlines are provided in **Table 7.60**.
3. Regimens for secondary prevention of rheumatic fever are mentioned in **Table 7.61**.

TABLE 7.60: Categories of rheumatic fever and duration of prophylaxis.

Category	Duration
Rheumatic fever without carditis	At least for 5 years or until age 21 years, whichever is longer
Rheumatic fever with carditis but without residual heart disease (no valvular disease)	At least for 10 years or well into adulthood, whichever is longer
Rheumatic fever with carditis and residual heart disease (persistent valvular disease) and postvalve surgery cases	At least 10 years since last episode and at least until age 40 years; sometimes lifelong

TABLE 7.61: Regimens for secondary prevention of rheumatic fever.

Drug	Dose	Route
Penicillin G benzathine **OR**	600,000 U for children, <27 kg and 1.2 million U for children >27 kg, every 3 weeks	Intramuscular
Penicillin V **OR**	250 mg, twice a day	Oral
Sulfadiazine or sulfisoxazole	0.5 g, once a day for patients <60 lb; 1.0 g, once a day for patients >60 lb	Oral
For individuals who are allergic to penicillin and sulfonamide drugs		
Macrolide or azalide (erythromycin and azithromycin)	Variable	Oral

Rheumatic Chorea

Q. Write a short essay/note on clinical features, diagnosis, and treatment of Sydenham's chorea.

It is also known as **Sydenham's chorea, Saint Vitus dance,** St. Johannis chorea, **chorea minor**, or rheumatic chorea.

Definition: Rheumatic chorea is a syndrome characterized by chorea, muscle weakness, and emotional instability.

Etiology

Triggering factor is pharyngeal infection by group A β-hemolytic streptococci.

Clinical Features

Age and gender: Occur in 5–10% of cases, mainly in girls of 1–15 years of age.

Onset of chorea: Rheumatic chorea is a late neurological manifestation of acute rheumatic fever. Usually occurs 3–8 months after the triggering infection by A β-hemolytic streptococci when all the other signs may have disappeared. If there is no previous rheumatic manifestation, the term pure chorea is used.

First sign: Emotional lability, difficulty walking, talking, writing which is observed in 30% of patients with acute rheumatic fever (ARF).

Characterized by spasmodic, brief, purposeless (unintentional), involuntary, jerky movements. Choreiform movements particularly affect the head/face (darting movement of tongue) upper limb hands or feet. Speech may be affected and may be explosive and halting and fidgety. It can be unilateral (hemichorea) or bilateral.

Mild forms may be difficult to diagnose and following signs are helpful in these cases:

- **Milkmaid's grip:** When the patient is asked to squeeze the examiner's fingers, a squeezing and relaxing motion (like milking a cow) occurs. This is described as milkmaid's grip and is due to inability to maintain muscular contraction.
- **Bag-of-worms appearance** is due to asynchronous contractions of the lingual muscles.
- **Jack-in-the-box sign:** When the patient is asked to keep the tongue protruded out, it retracts involuntarily.
- **Pronator sign:** Holding the arms outstretched may elicit "spooning" (hyperextension of the fingers with dorsiflexion of the wrist).

Severe forms: Patients is unable to get up or sit, and has violent continuous jerks that may cause physical injury. Additional features include hypotonia, pendular knee jerks, and mild generalized muscular weakness.

Prognosis

1. Usually benign and spontaneously resolves in 2–3 months. Disappears leaving no residual damage.
2. About 25% of affected patients develop chronic rheumatic valve disease.

Management

1. Rule out other causes of chorea such as systemic lupus erythematosus, Huntington's disease, and Wilson's disease.
2. Rest: Complete mental and physical rest. Keep the patient in a quiet room.
3. Padded side-boards for beds to prevent physical injury.
4. Drugs: Haloperidol or sodium valproate with diazepam. Steroids may be needed in severe cases.
5. Rheumatic fever prophylaxis.

VALVULAR HEART DISEASE

Mitral Valve

It is called so because it resembles the Bishops "miter."

Mitral Valve Apparatus

It consists of different components **(Box 7.31)**. Normal mitral valve is bicuspid (two leaflets), funnel-shaped valve between left atrium and left ventricle with its apex in the left ventricle. The two valve leaflets are attached by (about 120) chordae tendineae to two papillary muscles. Mitral valve orifice is about 4–6 cm^2 (average 5 cm^2).

Box 7.31: Different components of mitral valve apparatus.

- Mitral annulus
- Mitral leaflets: (1) anterior mitral leaflet (AML), and (2) posterior mitral leaflet (PML)
- Subvalvular apparatus: Chordae tendineae and papillary muscles
- Left ventricular wall where the papillary muscle attaches
- Left atrium

MITRAL STENOSIS

Q. Discuss the etiology, pathophysiology, clinical features, investigations, complications, and management of mitral stenosis.

Q. Write a short essay/note on juvenile mitral stenosis and pediatric mitral stenosis.

Mitral stenosis (MS) is a valvular heart disease is characterized by the narrowing of the orifice of the **mitral** valve due to structural abnormality of the **mitral** valve apparatus.

Etiology (Table 7.62) and Pathology

1. Rheumatic fever is the most common cause of mitral stenosis. It develops secondary to previous rheumatic fever due to infection with group A β-hemolytic *Streptococcus.*
2. Mitral stenosis is more common in females.

3. The latent period from the first attack of rheumatic fever and the development of onset of symptoms due to mitral stenosis is usually as short as 1–2 years in India, compared to long in Western countries. This may be due to repeated attacks of severe carditis in India.
4. Clinical manifestation in **juvenile mitral stenosis**/malignant mitral stenosis develops below the age of 19 years and is common in India. Pediatric mitral stenosis manifests below the age of 12 years. Pin-point mitral valve is seen. Atrial fibrillation is rare. Valve calcification is uncommon.

TABLE 7.62: Causes of mitral stenosis (MS).

➢ Rheumatic fever (leading cause) ➢ Congenital mitral stenosis (parachute mitral valve/Shone complex) ➢ Metastatic carcinoid tumor to the lung, or primary bronchial carcinoid ➢ Severe calcification of mitral valve apparatus, e.g., in elderly ➢ Systemic lupus erythematosus ➢ Rheumatoid arthritis (extremely rare) ➢ Endomyocardial fibrosis ➢ Gout ➢ Methysergide treatment	➢ Lutembacher's syndrome (combination of acquired mitral stenosis and an atrial septal defect) ➢ Mucopolysaccharidosis—Hurler syndrome and Hunter syndrome ➢ Whipple's disease ➢ Infective endocarditis with large vegetations **Mimics of MS** ➢ Myxoma ➢ Ball valve thrombus ➢ Cor triatriatum

Rheumatic Mitral Stenosis

In rheumatic MS, chronic inflammation produces:
- Diffuse thickening of the mitral valve leaflets due to fibrosis and/or calcification
- Fusion of commissures and cusp
- Fusion and shortening of the chordae tendineae.

The above morphological changes progress and cause rigidity of mitral valvular cusps which in turn leads to narrowing at the apex of the funnel-shaped ("fish-mouth") mitral valve → severe narrowing (stenotic) of valve orifice and progressive immobility of the valve cusps.

Salient features of mitral stenosis are presented in **Box 7.32**.

Box 7.32: Salient features of mitral stenosis (MS).
- First chamber to fail in MS: Left atrium
- Ventricle to fail in MS: Right ventricle
- Atria that fibrillates in MS: Affects both right and left atria
- Left ventricle in MS: Left ventricular end-diastolic volume (LVEDV) is reduced in 15%, while it is normal in the rest
- The most common complication of MS: Atrial fibrillation (AF)

Pathophysiology and Hemodynamics (Fig. 7.40)

Long latent period: Mitral stenosis clinically manifests after a latent period about 20 years from the first episode of acute rheumatic fever. Its symptoms usually start when the mitral valve surface area reduces to 2.5 cm^2.
- Normally, the mitral valve opens during (left ventricular) diastole and allows the flow of blood from left atrium to the left ventricle. During ventricular diastole, the pressures in the left atrium and the left ventricle are equal.

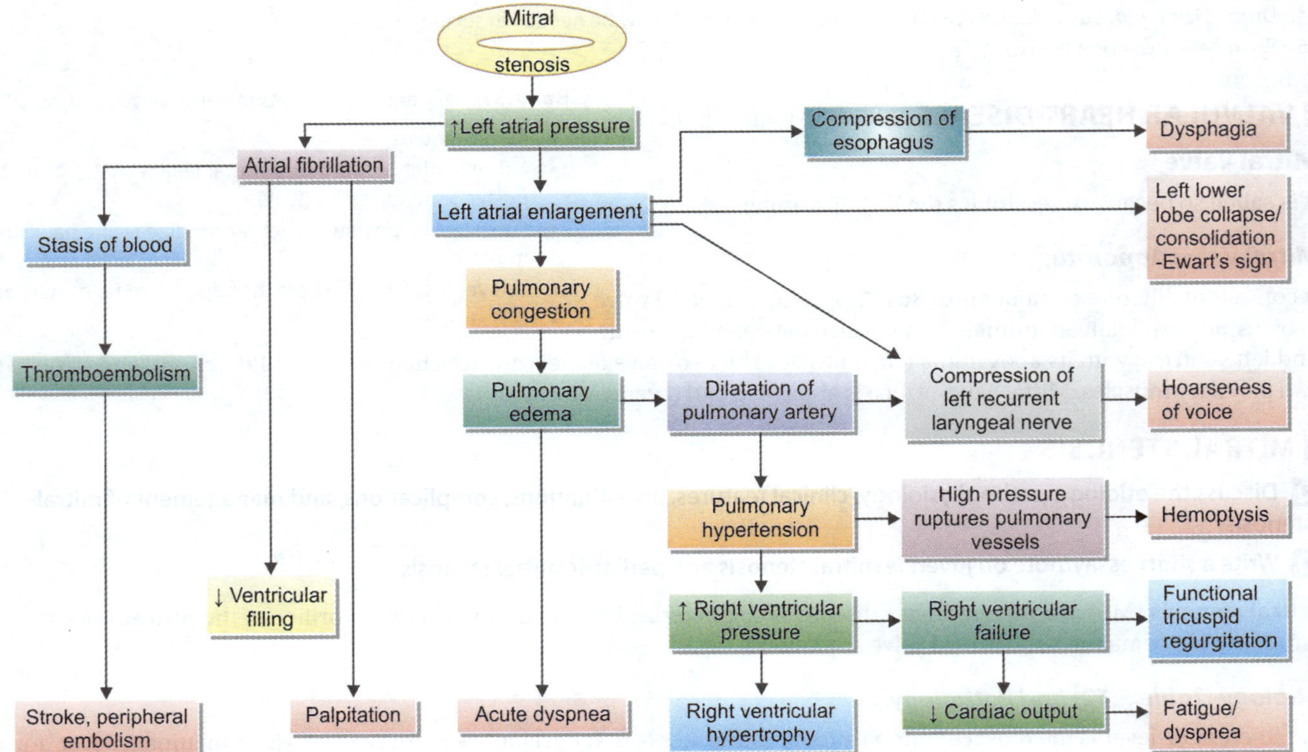

FIG. 7.40: Pathophysiology of mitral stenosis.

- Mitral stenosis obstructs the blood flow from left atrium to left ventricle and raises the pressure in the left atrium (up to 25 mm Hg in severe stenosis). Initially, this **rise in left atrial pressure** may occur only during exercise, but later it is raised even during rest.
- Raised left atrial pressure is reflected back in the pulmonary veins that produce **pulmonary venous hypertension** and subsequently pulmonary arteries which produce **pulmonary arterial hypertension.** The symptoms consist of episodes of paroxysmal nocturnal dyspnea (PND) evident as pulmonary edema and hemoptysis, i.e., **Winter bronchitis.**
- Repeated episodes of PND produce arteriolarization of pulmonary capillaries and veins → pulmonary arterial hypertension. During this period, there may be resolution of symptoms and signs of pulmonary venous hypertension. **Patient develops progressive exertional dyspnea.** Patient feels better in terms of symptoms, although the disease has progressed.
- Pulmonary arterial hypertension (pulmonary hypertension) progressively increases in severity over the next 10–15 years till finally the right ventricle fails (early fourth decade). Types of pulmonary hypertension in MS are presented in **Box 7.33**.
- **Consequences of chronic pulmonary hypertension:**
  - **Hypertrophy of right ventricle:** Which may later undergo dilatation → right ventricular failure
  - **Functional tricuspid regurgitation** due to dilatation tricuspid valve ring secondary to dilatation of right ventricle
  - **Pulmonary valve incompetence** (regurgitation) may develop due to dilatation of pulmonary valve ring
- **Consequences of raised left atrial pressure:** Causes left atrial dilatation and this enlarged left atrium is prone to:
  - Atrial fibrillation
  - Stasis of blood with thrombus formation
  - Detachment of the thrombus resulting in systemic embolism
- Reduced ejection fraction of left ventricle is found one-third of patients due to:
  - Decreased preload due to impaired filing
  - Increased afterload secondary to reflex vasoconstriction (secondary to decreased cardiac output)
- **Severe mitral stenosis:** There is decompensation by tachycardia or high flow. Tachycardia reduces diastolic LV filling time thereby increasing pressure in LA. Hyperkinetic circulatory states increase flow rate across mitral valve leading to increased transmitral gradient leading to increased LA pressure.

Box 7.33: Types of pulmonary hypertension in mitral stenosis (MS).

- **Passive pulmonary hypertension:** Due to passive backward transmission of elevated left atrial pressure by venous and capillary
- **Reactive pulmonary hypertension:** Due to reflex spasm of pulmonary arterioles in response to elevate pulmonary venous and left atrial pressure
- **Obliterative pulmonary hypertension:** Due to chronic hypertension producing fibrosis of pulmonary bed

Clinical Features

Q. Write a short essay/note on clinical features of mitral stenosis.

Symptoms

- **Dyspnea on exertion** is due to pulmonary hypertension and is slowly progressive.
  - Precipitated by severe exertion, excitement, fever, anemia, sexual intercourse, pregnancy, thyrotoxicosis, and atrial fibrillation.
- **Fatigue on exertion:** Due to pulmonary hypertension and low cardiac output. It is slowly progressive.
- **Hemoptysis:**
  - Rupture of bronchial veins or of pulmonary vein or bronchial vein collaterals—pulmonary apoplexy
  - Rupture of pulmonary capillaries during pulmonary edema
  - Pulmonary congestion, embolism, and infarction
  - Winter bronchitis
  - Pulmonary hemosiderosis due to chronic recurrent pulmonary edema
  - Anticoagulant use
- **Chest pain:** Develops in about 15% patients due to (1) right ventricle enlargement, right ventricular hypertrophy, and pulmonary hypertension; (2) coexistent coronary artery disease (CAD); (3) coronary embolism; and (4) angina due to decreased cardiac output.
- Palpitations develop when there are atrial fibrillations (AF), chamber enlargement (right ventricle and pulmonary artery).
- **Systemic thromboembolism:** Paroxysmal AF results in embolism most commonly to the cerebral vessels resulting in stroke, but mesenteric, renal, and peripheral emboli (e.g., ischemic limb) can also develop.
- **Syncope:** PAH, arrhythmias, and ball valve thrombus
- **Hoarseness of voice—La Ortner's syndrome:** Due to compression of the left recurrent laryngeal nerve due to the dilated pulmonary artery or giant left atrium
- Right heart failure
  - **Orthopnea and paroxysmal nocturnal dyspnea:** Due to left atrial failure
  - **Winter bronchitis:** Patients with MS are susceptible to recurrent attacks of bronchitis, especially during the winter.

Physical Signs

General examination

- **Mitral facies** is characterized by cyanotic lips and face, malar flush (dusky pink discoloration over the upper cheeks due to arteriovenous anastomoses and vascular stasis), and mild jaundice. It may develop when MS is very severe with low cardiac output and peripheral vasoconstriction.
- Peripheral edema and ascites when right heart failure develops.
- **Pulse:**
  - Pulse in low volume and peripheral pulse may be absent if embolism develops.
  - Pulse rhythm is irregularly irregular and varying volume in atrial fibrillation.
- **Blood pressure:** May be mildly reduced. Mean of three readings to be taken if atrial fibrillation is present.
- **Jugular veins:**
  - **Jugular venous pressure** is raised when congestive heart failure develops.
  - **Jugular venous pulse:** (1) Prominent a waves (due to vigorous right atrial systole) observed when there is pulmonary hypertension without atrial fibrillation, (2) absence of waves in atrial fibrillation, and (3) prominent V waves (C-V waves) and rapid y descent when there is development of functional tricuspid regurgitation.

Inspection and Palpation of Precordium

- **Apex beat** is not shifted and is tapping character of S_1 at apex (closing snap). Apex beat is shifted when there is coexistent of MS with mitral regurgitation (MR)/aortic stenosis (AS)/systemic hypertension/ischemic heart disease (IHD)/myocarditis.
- **Diastolic thrill** at apex
- **Palpable pulmonary component of second heart sound (P_2)** if there is pulmonary arterial hypertension.
- **Left parasternal heave:** Present when there is right ventricular hypertrophy or left atrial enlargement.
- **Epigastric pulsations** of right ventricular type.
- Precordial bulge in juvenile/malignant MS.

Other findings: Right heart failure is associated with peripheral edema, tender hepatomegaly, and ascites.

Auscultation

Q. Write a short essay/note on auscultatory findings in mitral stenosis.

- **Loud first heart sound:**
  - In mitral stenosis, the forces that open and close the mitral valve increase as left atrial pressure increases. Hence, the first heart sound (S_1) is loud and can be palpable (tapping apex beat) in mitral stenosis.
  - When associated with atrial fibrillation, the intensity of first heart sound varies.
  - A low intensity of the first heart sound in MS may be due to (1) calcification of the mitral valve, (2) congenital MS, and (3) dominant associated mitral/aortic regurgitation.
- **Loud second heart sound:** It is a sign of pulmonary hypertension. The second heart sound is closely split and the pulmonary component of the second heart sound (P_2) is loud.
- **Mitral opening snap:**
  - OS is a sharp, snappy sound heard during early diastole, following the sound of aortic valve closure (A_2) by 0.05–0.12 s.
  - Opening snap (OS) is produced due to the sudden (abrupt) opening of the dome of the stenosed mitral valve with the force of the increased left atrial pressure during diastole. It is the most important auscultatory sign of valvular involvement in MS. Absent OS indicates the calcification of body of the leaflets.
  - The time interval between A_2 and OS is inversely proportional to the severity of the MS.
  - **Best heard:** During expiration, just medial to the cardiac apex with the diaphragm of the stethoscope.
  - **Other conditions with OS:** Mitral regurgitation (10%), tricuspid stenosis, and atrial septal defect
  - **Well's index:** Q-S1 interval minus A_2-OS interval and is expressed in units of 0.01 seconds. More than 2 units indicate MVA <1.2 cm².
- **Murmur of mitral stenosis:**
  - **Mid-diastolic/presystolic murmur:** Turbulent blood flow through stenosed mitral valve produces the characteristic **low pitched, rumbling, mid-diastolic murmur**, and sometimes accompanied by a thrill. Murmur is best heard with the bell of the stethoscope held lightly at the apex with the patient lying on the left side.
    - Duration of the murmur varies and usually depends on the severity of stenosis. In severe MS, the mid-diastolic murmur is long and merges with the presystolic murmur to produce a holodiastolic murmur.
      - **To increase intensity of MDM:** Left lateral position using bell of stethoscope, while holding expiration auscultate after walking (isotonic exercise), and squatting (increased peripheral resistance in these procedures contribute to the increased murmur).
      - In the early phase of mitral stenosis, a **presystolic murmur** may be the only auscultatory abnormality. Mechanism of presystolic murmur: (1) atrial contraction, (2) persistent atrioventricular gradient, and (3) left ventricular contraction in presystole reducing mitral funnel.

- ○ **Presystolic accentuation of the murmur:** Atrial contraction contributes to increased gradient in presystole. Hence, mid-diastolic murmur is accentuated by exercise. In patient with sinus rhythm, the murmur becomes louder during atrial systole and during long R-R interval in atrial fibrillation is termed as **presystolic accentuation.**
- ○ **Absence of presystolic murmur in MS:** Atrial fibrillation, mild MS, prolonged PR interval, bradycardia, and elevated left ventricular dysfunction (LVEDP)
- ○ **Causes of absent mid-diastolic murmur:** Thick chest wall and emphysema, **dampened MS** (severe pulmonary hypertension throttling the left-sided input), low cardiac output, and marked RV enlargement with RV occupying the apex.

- **Systolic murmur:** When **pulmonary hypertension** develops, it will lead to right ventricular hypertrophy and dilatation with secondary tricuspid regurgitation. This produces a systolic murmur and giant "*v* waves" in the venous pulse.
  - ♦ If MS coexists with mitral regurgitation, it produces a loud pansystolic murmur that radiates toward the axilla and is heard at the lower left sternal border. **Functional tricuspid regurgitation** produces a pansystolic murmur. It is accentuated during inspiration (de Carvallo's sign).
- **Murmur of pulmonary regurgitation (Graham Steell murmur):** It is a high-pitched early diastolic decrescendo murmur heard along the left sternal border and indicative of severe pulmonary hypertension.

Diagrammatic representation of timing of heart sounds and murmur in mitral stenosis are shown in **Figure 7.41**.

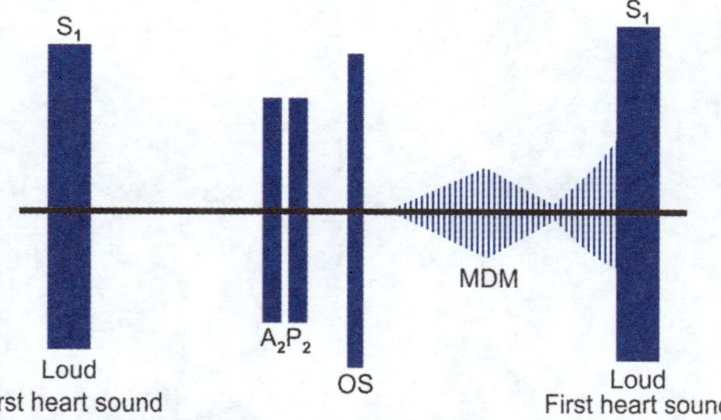

FIG. 7.41: Diagrammatic representation of timing of heart sounds and murmur in mitral stenosis features are loud first heart sound, an opening snap (OS), mid-diastolic murmur (MDM) with presystolic accentuation.

Auscultatory findings in mitral stenosis are listed in **Box 7.34**.

Grades of mitral stenosis and its features are presented in **Table 7.63**.

TABLE 7.63: Grades of mitral stenosis and its features.

Grade of mitral stenosis (valve area in cm²)	*S_2-OS interval in second*	*Signs*
Very mild (2.5 to 2.1)		
Mild (2 to 1.6)	0.08–0.12	Short MDM/or presystolic murmur or murmur may appear with exercise
Moderate (1 to 1.5)	0.06–0.08	MDM + presystolic murmur with a gap between them. Varying degree of MDM in atrial fibrillation
Severe (<1)	0.04–0.06	MDM + presystolic murmur with no gap, presystolic murmur with atrial fibrillation

Note: Normal mitral valve orifice is 4–6 cm²
(MDM: mid-diastolic murmur; OP: opening snap; S_2: second heart sound)

Box 7.34: Auscultatory findings in mitral stenosis.

- Loud S_1
- Loud P_2 and narrow split of S_2 if pulmonary arterial hypertension
- Opening snap
- Mid-diastolic murmur at apex with presystolic accentuation
- Tricuspid regurgitation: Pansystolic murmur
- Pulmonary hypertension: Ejection systolic/ early diastolic (Graham Steell) murmur

Q. Write a short essay/note on grading the severity of mitral stenosis.

Clinical judgment of the severity of mitral stenosis: Following features suggest severe MS:
- Presence of pulmonary hypertension
- More closeness of the opening snap to the second heart sound (short A2-OS interval)
- Lengthy mid-diastolic murmur

Investigations

Radiological features of mitral stenosis (Chest X-ray) (**Figs. 7.42A to D**)

Q. Write a short essay/note on radiological/X-ray chest findings in mitral stenosis.

Due to enlargement of left atrium
- Enlarged left atrial appendage causes filling up of normal concavity between pulmonary artery shadow and the left ventricle.

- **Double atrial shadow:** Border of enlarged left atrium together with right atrial border gives an appearance like atrium within an atrium.
- **Straightening of left heart border:** Mitralization of heart

Due to left atrial appendage enlargement, large pulmonary artery, hypoplastic aorta, under filled left ventricle.

Consequences of left atrial enlargement:

- Pushing of left main bronchus upward causing wide carinal angle (splaying of carina)
- Pushing esophagus backward visible in lateral view of chest X-ray
- Left shift of aorta (Bedford sign)
- Walking man sign (shift of left bronchus forwards) (**Fig. 7.42B**)

Pulmonary venous/capillary hypertension

- **Grade 1:** Cephalization (prominence of veins of upper lobe of lung) of pulmonary vasculature (pulmonary venous pressure ≤20 mm Hg) (inverted moustache sign/antler's horn sign).
- **Grade 2:** Kerley lines (A, B, C) (pulmonary venous pressure 20–25 mm Hg), peribronchial, perivascular cuffing (**Figs. 7.42C and D**)

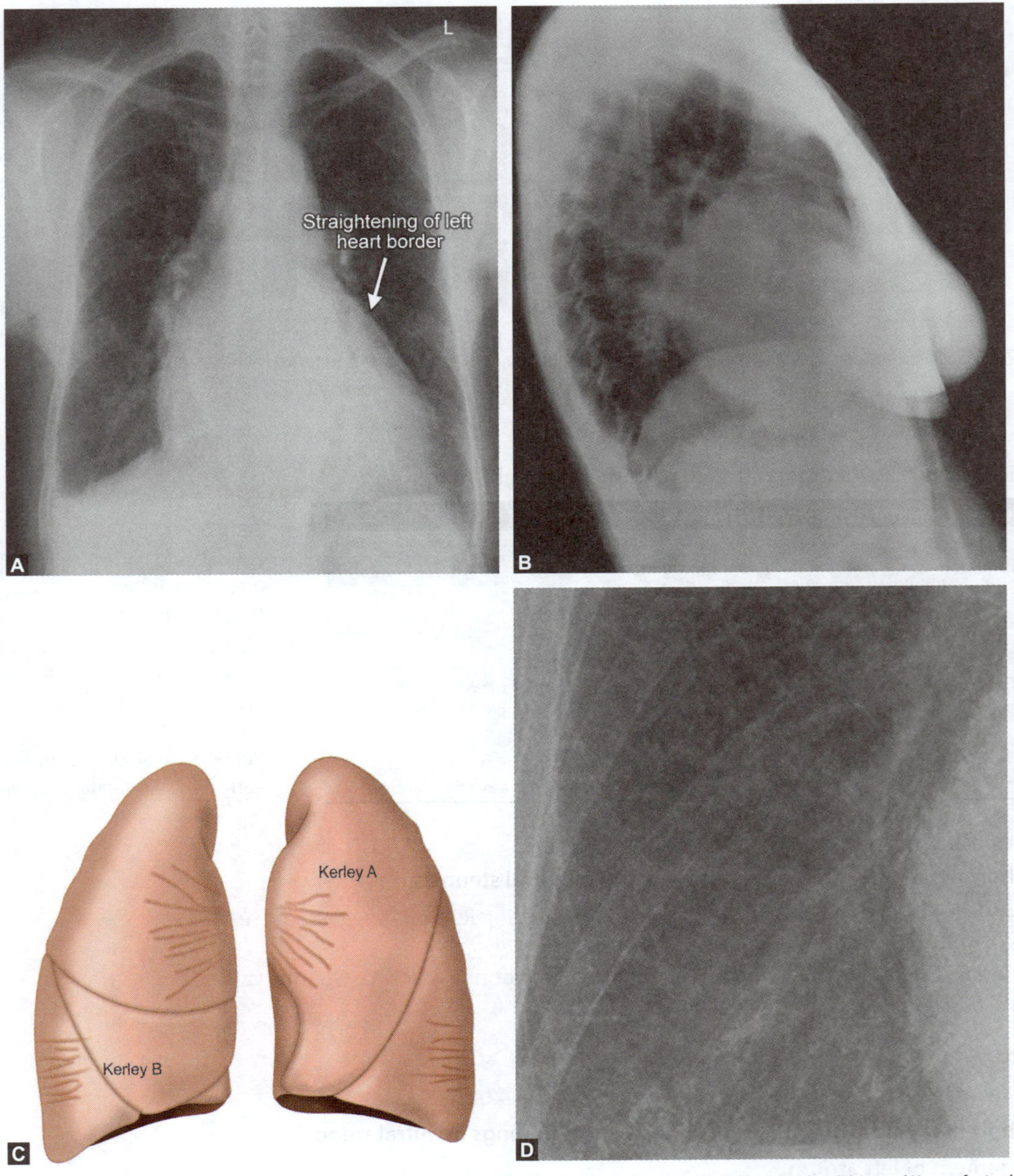

FIGS. 7.42A TO D: (A) X-rays of mitral stenosis showing double atrial shadow and straightening of left heart border; (B) Lateral X-ray of mitral stenosis showing walking man sign; (C) Diagrammatic of Kerley lines; (D) X-ray of Kerley lines.

- Kerley A line: Linear opacities extending from the periphery to hila; they are caused by distension of anastomotic channels between periphery and central lymphatic's
- Kerley B line: Short horizontal lines situated perpendicularly to the pleural surface at the lung base; they represent edema of interlobar septa.
- Kerley C line: Reticular opacities at lung base, representing Kerley B line en face.

- **Grade 3:** Batwing opacities (pulmonary venous pressure >25 mm Hg)

Pulmonary arterial hypertension

Prominent pulmonary outflow tract: Enlarged pulmonary arteries (diameter of right descending pulmonary artery >14 mm in women and >16 mm in men) + pruning of peripheral pulmonary vessels.

Right ventricle

- **Right ventricular hypertrophy:** In presence of cardiomegaly, acute angle is observed between apex of enlarged heart and diaphragm.
- **Sternal contact sign:** Earliest and most sensitive sign in the lateral X-ray is obliteration of Holtzneck's space, i.e., retrosternal space.

Others

- Right atrial enlargement
- Calcification of mitral valve/pericardium/MacCallum patch
- Pulmonary hemosiderosis

Electrocardiogram

It can confirm enlargement of left atrium ("P" mitrale), right ventricular hypertrophy, tall R waves in V_1-V_3, P mitrale, and atrial fibrillation.

Echocardiogram

- It can reveal thickening of mitral valve area, valvular leaflet, thickening and shortening chordae tendineae, fusion of commissures, calcification of leaflets and chordae, and diastolic doming (due to commissural fusion).
- **Wilkins score (4 to 16):** 4 points each for leaflet thickness, leaflet mobility, leaflet calcification, and chordal involvement.

Transesophageal echocardiography (TEE)

To assess mitral regurgitation (MR) severity and to rule out left atrial appendage (LAA) thrombus.

Doppler

Provides definite evaluation of MS. It shows pressure gradient across mitral valve, pulmonary artery pressure, and left ventricular function.

Cardiac catheterization

It is not usually needed. It is used to assess coexisting condition such as coronary artery disease, pulmonary artery pressure, mitral stenosis and regurgitation.

TABLE 7.64: Complications of mitral stenosis.

➢ Atrial fibrillation	➢ Ortner's syndrome	➢ Pulmonary edema
➢ Thrombus formation	➢ Hemoptysis	➢ Pulmonary infarction
➢ Systemic embolization	➢ Dysphagia	➢ Cardiac cirrhosis
➢ Pulmonary hypertension	➢ Lower lobe pneumonia	➢ Pulmonary hemosiderosis
➢ Infective endocarditis	➢ Right heart failure	

Complications of Mitral Stenosis (Table 7.64)

Q. Write a short essay/note on complications of mitral stenosis.

- **Atrial fibrillation (AF):**
  - The most common complication of MS prevalence and incidence varies according to age and roughly parallels the age of the patient (e.g., second decade—10% and sixth decade and beyond—80%).
    - **AF worsens symptoms of MS by:** (1) Decreasing diastolic filling time—leads to increased LA pressure, (2) loss of atrial contribution to LV filling—leads to increased LA pressure, and (3) LA thrombus leading to systemic embolization.
    - **Prognosis:** 5-year survival of AF without MS is 85% and with MS is 64%
    - AF causes decrease in cardiac output by 20% in MS.
- **Systemic embolism:**
  - **Source of emboli:** Left atrial thrombus, vegetations of infective endocarditis (rare)
  - **Factors predisposing to systemic embolism in MS:** Atrial fibrillation, spontaneous echo contrast in left atrium, size of left atrium, age, and low cardiac output.
  - **Clinical features:** Depends on the localization of emboli. Cerebral (strokes, abscess), coronary (leads to chest pain), and renal (leads to hypertension)
    - Leriche syndrome: Claudication of thigh (due to embolism at branching of common iliac artery) + impotence
    - Ball valve or free floating thrombus may produce syncope in specific body position, variability in physical findings, and requires urgent surgery.
- **Infective endocarditis:** May develop infrequently with isolated mitral stenosis.

- **Ortner's syndrome** is a very rare complication of severe pulmonary hypertension secondary to mitral stenosis. It is characterized by paralysis of left recurrent laryngeal nerve due to compression between the enlarged tense pulmonary artery and the aorta at ligamentum arteriosum. It produces hoarseness of voice.
- **Damped MS:** Development of pulmonary hypertension diminishes the cardiac output (throttle effect) and results in temporary symptom-free period (period of illusion). The MDM may not be audible, only OS will be present.

Management

Mild mitral stenosis may not require any treatment other than treatment of attacks of bronchitis.

- **Medical management: MS with** minor symptoms are treated medically.
  - Rheumatic fever prophylaxis to be given. However, infective endocarditis prophylaxis is not necessary.
  - **Indications for anticoagulation:** (1) Atrial fibrillation (persistent or paroxysmal), (2) embolic events, (3) left trial thrombus, (4) left atrial diameter >55 mm, and (5) spontaneous echo contrast.
  - Restrict/decrease sodium intake.
  - **Diuretics:** Early symptom such as mild dyspnea (due to pulmonary congestion) is usually treated with low doses of diuretics.
  - Beta-blockers or non-dihydropyridines (DHP) calcium channel blockers (e.g., verapamil or diltiazem) to reduce heart rate (even in sinus rhythm, more useful in atrial fibrillation)
  - Digoxin if atrial fibrillation with right heart failure. Atrial fibrillation also needs anticoagulation to prevent atrial thrombus and systemic embolization.
- **Surgical management:**

  Four operative measures are available.

  1. **Trans-septal balloon mitral valvotomy (BMV):**
     - Also known as percutaneous balloon valvuloplasty (PBV) is the treatment of choice.
     - **Procedure:** Under local anesthesia, a catheter is passed through the femoral vein into the right atrium. The interatrial septum is punctured and the catheter is passed into the left atrium and across the mitral valve. A balloon is passed over the catheter across the valve, and briefly inflated to split the valve commissures.
     - **Indications:** Pliable mitral valves with little involvement of the subvalvular apparatus and minimal mitral regurgitation.
     - **Contraindications:** Moderate or severe mitral regurgitation, severe calcification, severe subvalvular fibrosis, thrombus in left atrium or ventricle, recent embolism, bleeding disorders, and interatrial septal thickness >3 mm (relative contraindication).
     - **Complications:** Mitral regurgitation may be severe enough to need surgery (2%), mortality (1–2%), cardiac perforation (1%), and cerebral embolism (1%).
  2. **Closed mitral valvotomy (CMV):**
     - **Indication:** Mobile, noncalcified mitral valves without regurgitation
     - **Contraindication:** Left atrial thrombus, mitral valvular calcification, severe subvalvular disease, or moderate or severe mitral regurgitation
     - **Advantages:** Cardiopulmonary bypass is not required and good result is obtained for 10 years or more.
     - **Disadvantage:** The valve cusps may refuse necessitating another operation.
  3. **Open mitral valvotomy (OMV):**
     - It is usually performed and is preferred over closed valvotomy or mitral valve replacement.
     - **Procedure:** Under direct view, the valvular cusps are carefully separated from each other and commissures are incised.
     - **Advantage:** Less chances of traumatic mitral regurgitation, concurrent annuloplasty can be done for mitral regurgitation. Removal of LA thrombus (if present), calcium in leaflets, amputation of LA appendage, and separation of fused chordae can also done along with this surgical procedure.
     - **Disadvantage:** Needs cardiopulmonary bypass.

Q. Write a short essay/note on indications for mitral valve replacement.

  4. **Mitral valve replacement (MVR):**
     - **Indications:**
       - Mitral stenosis associated with mitral regurgitation
       - Severely damaged or severely calcified stenotic valve which cannot be reopened without producing significant mitral regurgitation
       - Moderate or severe mitral stenosis and presence of thrombus in the left atrium even after anticoagulation therapy
     - **Type of prosthesis:** Mechanical prosthesis if age is <65 years and bioprosthesis if age is >65 years.
     - Artificial valves usually work successfully for >20 years and anticoagulants are usually given postoperatively to prevent thrombus formation and its embolization.

MITRAL REGURGITATION

Q. Discuss the etiology, pathophysiology, clinical features, investigations, complications, and management of chronic mitral regurgitation.

- **Management of acute severe mitral regurgitation in pulmonary edema.**

Mitral regurgitation (MR) or mitral insufficiency (MI) or mitral incompetence is a disorder of the heart in which the mitral valve does not close properly.

Etiology (Box 7.35)

Q. Write a short essay/note on causes of acute mitral regurgitation/mitral regurgitation.

Lesion in any one of five components of mitral valve apparatus namely, (1) valve leaflets, (2) the annulus, (3) the chordae tendineae, (4) papillary muscles, or (5) the left ventricle can produce mitral regurgitation (MR).

Mitral regurgitation may be **acute or chronic.**

- **Causes of MR in IE:** Leaflet perforation, vegetations preventing leaflet function, rupture of chordate tendineae, and annular abscess
- **Causes of MR in RHD:** Rigid and retracted leaflet and shortening of chordae tendineae.
- **Causes of MR in CAD:** Regional wall motion abnormalities, ischemia of papillary muscle, and LV failure.

Box 7.35: Causes of mitral regurgitation.

Causes of acute mitral regurgitation:
- **Infective endocarditis, rupture of a papillary muscle** (e.g., acute myocardial infarction and mitral valve prolapse), chest trauma, cardiac surgery, acute rheumatic carditis, and dysfunction of prosthetic valve.

Causes of chronic mitral regurgitation:
- **Damage to valve leaflets: Rheumatic heart disease,** myxomatous degeneration, mitral valve prolapse (MVP), **infective endocarditis**, and SLE.
- **Damage to annulus:** Abscess (IE), **annular calcification**, and dilated cardiomyopathy
- **Damage to chordae tendineae:** Myxomatous degeneration (MVP, Marfan syndrome, Ehlers–Danlos syndrome), infective endocarditis, and acute rheumatic fever
- **Damage to papillary muscles: Coronary artery disease** [ischemia, myocardial infarction, rupture (MI), dilated cardiomyopathy]
- **Damage to left ventricle:** Ischemia and dilated cardiomyopathy

Note: Major causes are highlighted in bold letter

Pathophysiology

- **Acute mitral regurgitation:** During this, the normal compliance of the left atrium does not permit much dilatation and the pressure of left atrium rises. This markedly increases the left atrial pressure and pulmonary venous pressure and cause pulmonary edema. Since part of the stroke volume is regurgitated, the stroke volume increases (to a lesser degree than it does in chronic MR) to maintain the forward cardiac output. This may result in the enlargement of the left ventricle.
- **Chronic mitral regurgitation:** Causes gradual dilatation of left atrium but little increase in left atrial pressure because the regurgitant flow is accommodated by the large left atrium. In longstanding cases, the left ventricle slowly dilates and the left ventricular diastolic and left atrial pressures gradually increase due to chronic volume overload of the left ventricle. MR begets MR.

Clinical Features

Symptoms

- Symptoms depend on the rapidity of development of the mitral regurgitation.
- **Acute mitral regurgitation:** Usually presents dyspnea due to acute pulmonary edema.
- **Chronic mitral regurgitation:** It may be asymptomatic for many years. It may become symptomatic only after the onset of irreversible LV dysfunction.
  - **Palpitation** is the most common symptom due to increased stroke volume or atrial fibrillation.
  - **Dyspnea and orthopnea:** Due to pulmonary venous hypertension and left ventricular failure occur late in the course of mitral regurgitation
  - **Fatigue and lethargy:** Due to reduced cardiac output
  - **Symptoms of right heart failure:** Develop in the late stages and lead to congestive cardiac failure
  - Cardiac cachexia
  - **Thromboembolism:** Less common than in mitral stenosis. However, subacute infective endocarditis is more common.
  - *Other symptoms and complications are similar to mitral stenosis.*

Signs

Pulse: Volume is high and in severe mitral regurgitation, it may be mildly collapsing.

- Irregular rhythm and varying volume if there is atrial fibrillation.

Jugular veins

- **Uncomplicated mitral regurgitation:** Jugular venous pressure (JVP) is normal.
- **With atrial fibrillation:** Disappearance of a waves
- **With pulmonary hypertension:** Prominent a waves
- **With right ventricular failure and functional tricuspid regurgitation:** Jugular venous pressure is raised and very prominent v waves.

Blood pressure: In severe mitral regurgitation: wide pulse pressure. Three recordings are necessary if patient has atrial fibrillation (AF). Pulsus alternans in acute MR.

Inspection and palpation

- Hyperdynamic precordium
- **Apex beat:** Shifted to the left (due to left ventricular dilatation), forceful (feels active and rocking), and diffuse (hyperdynamic) in character due to left ventricular volume overload
- **Cardiomegaly:** In chronic MR. Acute MR does not produce cardiomegaly.
- Systolic thrill (if MI is severe) at the apex
- Left parasternal heave and palpable P_2
- Epigastric pulsations of right ventricular type

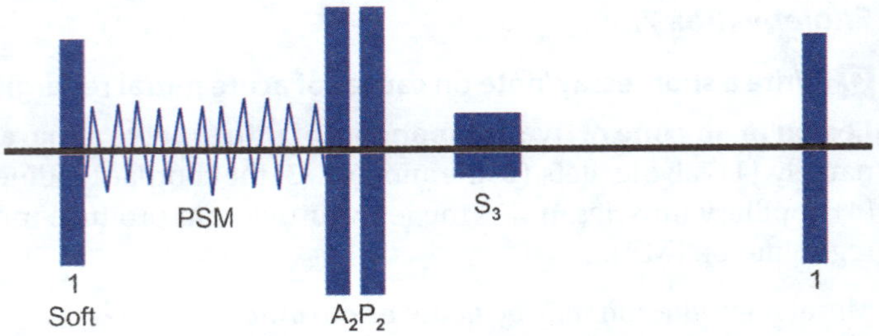

FIG. 7.43: Diagrammatic representation of timing of heart sounds and murmur in mitral regurgitation. Features are normal or soft first heart sound, pansystolic murmur (PSM), extending to the second heart sound (A_2, P_2). A third heart sound (S_3) may develop with severe mitral regurgitation.

Auscultation (Fig. 7.43)

- **Soft first heart sound (S_1):** Because of the incomplete apposition of the mitral valve cusps and partial closure of these valve cusps when ventricular systole begins. It is loud if there is coexistent MS, MVP-MR, or papillary muscle dysfunction MR.
- **Widely split second heart sound (S_2)** is due to aortic valve closure (A1) occurring early but the split is mobile.
- **Pulmonary component (P_2) of S_2** is loud and palpable in pulmonary hypertension and also due to anterior displacement of pulmonary artery caused by dilated LA.
- **Left ventricular third heart sound (S_3):** Indicates severe mitral regurgitation
- S4 is a sign of acute MR as left atrium is not dilated in acute MR.
- Pulmonary ejection sound in pulmonary hypertension

Murmur of mitral regurgitation

- **Apical pansystolic murmur:** The typical features of murmur in mitral regurgitation are:
  - High-pitched, blowing, and usually holosystolic/pansystolic loudest at the apex
  - Plateau-shaped, best heard with diaphragm of stethoscope
  - Commonly radiates widely over the precordium and into the axilla and left interscapular area (if anterior leaflets involved as in rheumatic) or radiating to base (if posterior leaflets involved)
  - It is produced due to the mitral regurgitant jet occurring throughout the whole of systole.
  - It may be accompanied by a thrill.
- Character of murmur depends on the underlying pathology in mitral regurgitation (**Table 7.65**).
- **Severe MR with soft or no murmur (silent MR):** It is observed with left ventricular dilation, acute mitral regurgitation (MR), paraprosthetic MR, COPD, obesity, dampened MR.

TABLE 7.65: Features of murmur depending on the underlying pathology in mitral regurgitation (MR).

Pathology	*Features of murmur*
Giant left atrium (>6 cm)	Radiates to the entire interscapular region
Ruptured chordate tendineae	"Cooling" or "sea gull" quality
Flail mitral leaflet	"Musical" quality and late systolic
Papillary muscle dysfunction	Late systolic
MVP-MR	Mid-systolic
Acute MR	Musical and tapering
Severe MR	Holosystolic murmur with mid-systolic accentuation, i.e., Christmas tree appearance

(MVP: mitral valve prolapse)

- **Dynamic auscultation:**
  - Non-MVP MR murmur is distinguished from MVP murmur by increase with squatting and decrease with standing (opposite with MVP).
  - MR murmur is distinguished from AS/HCM murmur by increase with isometric handgrip (opposite for AS/HCM).
- Short mid-diastolic flow murmur: Sometimes a short, rumbling mid-diastolic murmur may be detected at the apex in severe cases due to an increased flow across the mitral valve. It may follow the third heart sound.
- Other murmurs:
  - Ejection systolic murmur or early diastolic murmur at pulmonary area when there is pulmonary hypertension.
  - Pansystolic murmur at lower left sternal border when there is functional tricuspid regurgitation.
  - Opening snap can be heard in 10% patients with MR.

Signs indicating severity of mitral regurgitation (Box 7.36)

Q. Write a short note on clinical assessment of the severity of mitral regurgitation.

Box 7.36: Signs indicating severity of mitral regurgitation (MR).

Mild MR: Only murmur
Moderate MR: Murmur + thrill and cardiomegaly
Severe MR: Murmur + thrill, cardiomegaly, LV S3, flow mid-diastolic murmur, and pulmonary hypertension

Other signs in MR: These include signs related to:

- Atrial fibrillation/flutter
- Pulmonary venous congestion, e.g., crepitations, pulmonary edema, and effusions
- Pulmonary hypertension and right heart failure
- Left and right heart failure

Signs in acute mitral regurgitation

- Normal apical impulse since there is no ventricular dilatation
- Third and/or fourth heart sound
- An early systolic or pansystolic murmur

Differences between acute and chronic mitral regurgitation are listed in **Table 7.66**.

TABLE 7.66: Differences between acute and chronic mitral regurgitation (MR).

Characters	Acute MR	Chronic MR
Pulse	Alternans	High volume
Atrial fibrillation	Absent	+
Jugular venous pressure (JVP)	Grossly elevated	Mild elevation
Cardiomegaly	Absent	Present
Pulmonary hypertension	Very severe	Variable
S_1	Normal	Soft
S_3	Present	+/-
S_4	Present	Can never be present
Murmur	Late systolic	Pan systolic

TABLE 7.67: Differences between mitral regurgitation (MR) due to mitral valve prolapse and that due to rheumatic heart disease.

Characters	Mitral valve prolapse MR	Rheumatic heart disease MR
Leaflets affected	Any	Posterior
S_1	Loud	Soft
Click	Midsystolic click	No
Murmur	Midsystolic	Holosystolic
Squatting and isometric handgrip	Decrease murmur	Increases murmur
Association	Atrial septal defect (ASD) and polycystic kidney disease	Mitral stenosis

Differences between mitral regurgitation due to mitral valve prolapsed and that due to rheumatic heart disease are listed in **Table 7.67**.

Investigations

- **Electrocardiogram (ECG):** It can reveal:
  - Enlargement/hypertrophy of left atrium (if not in atrial fibrillation)
  - Dilatation and hypertrophy of left ventricle
  - Hypertrophy of both left and right ventricle in pulmonary hypertension
  - Atrial fibrillation
- **Chest X-ray:** May show the following abnormalities: All signs as described for MS:
  - Enlargement of the left atrium (more than in MS) and the left ventricle
  - Pulmonary venous congestion
  - Pulmonary edema: Interstitial edema in acute MR, chronic decompensated MR, or with coexistent MS
  - Annular calcium appears as a C-shaped opacity in posterior third of heart in lateral or RAO (right anterior oblique) view.
- **Echocardiogram:**
  - Shows a dilated left atrium and left ventricle
  - Structural abnormalities of mitral valve, e.g., prolapsed, chordal, or papillary muscle ruptures, if present
  - **Doppler echocardiogram:**
    - Detects and assesses the severity of regurgitation (quantification of regurgitation)
    - Mitral annular calcification between mitral valve apparatus and posterior wall
  - **Transesophageal echocardiography (TEE):** Useful to identify structural valve abnormalities and can be helpful before surgery, especially in MVP. Intraoperative TEE helps in the assessment of the efficacy of valve repair. MVP is defined as >2 mm systolic displacement of mitral leaflet into the left atrium (LA).
- **Cardiac catheterization:** This can show dilated left atrium and left ventricle mitral regurgitation, pulmonary hypertension, and coexisting coronary artery disease (if present).

Complications of mitral regurgitation are listed in **Box 7.37**.

Box 7.37: Complications of mitral regurgitation.

- Progressive heart failure is the most common cause of death.
- **Less frequent:** Sudden death, stroke, and fatal endocarditis
- Atrial fibrillation, infective endocarditis, and left ventricular failure
- Pulmonary hypertension (late) and right ventricular failure (very late)
- Rarely systemic embolism

Management

- Asymptomatic mild mitral regurgitation can be managed conservatively.
- Moderate mitral regurgitation can be treated medically.

Medical Management

- **Acute MR:** Afterload reduction with nitroprusside
- **Chronic MR:** In mitral regurgitation, high afterload may worsen the degree of regurgitation, and hypertension is treated with vasodilators, e.g., ACE inhibitors and nifedipine are used.
- Diuretics
- Treatment of AF: Digoxin and anticoagulants
- Anticoagulation
- Infective endocarditis prophylaxis
- Rheumatic fever prophylaxis

Surgery (Table 7.68 and Box 7.38) Mitral Valve Replacement

TABLE 7.68: European Society of Cardiology (ESC) guidelines for surgical intervention in mitral regurgitation.

Symptomatic patients who present with	*Asymptomatic patients with*
➢ Severe mitral regurgitation ➢ Left ventricular ejection fraction (EF) >30% ➢ End-diastolic dimension (ESD) of under 55 mm	➢ Left ventricular dysfunction ➢ End-systolic dimension >45 mm and/ or ejection fraction of under 60% ➢ New-onset atrial fibrillation and/or pulmonary hypertension

Box 7.38: Conditions in which repair of mitral valve is possible.

- Mitral valve prolapse (MVP)
- Papillary muscle dysfunction
- Leaflet perforation due to infective endocarditis (IE)
- Chordal rupture
- Annular dilation
- Rheumatic mitral regurgitation (MR) in the young

Combined Mitral Stenosis and Mitral Regurgitation

Clinical assessment of the dominance of lesions (**Table 7.69**).

TABLE 7.69: Clinical assessment of the dominance of lesions in the presence of combined mitral stenosis and mitral regurgitation.

Parameter	*Predominant mitral regurgitation*	*Predominant mitral stenosis*
Pulse volume	High	Low
Blood pressure	Wide pulse pressure	Narrow pulse pressure
Cardiomegaly	++	--
S_1	Soft	Loud
LVS3	++	-
Mid-diastolic murmur	Short	Long, loud with presystolic accentuation

MITRAL VALVE PROLAPSE (MVP)

Q. Write a short essay/note on mitral valve prolapse (MVP) or Barlow's syndrome.

- Mitral valve prolapse (MVP) is an abnormal movement of one or both of the mitral valve leaflets >2 mm beyond annular plan into the left atrium during systole with or without mitral regurgitation.
- **Barlow's syndrome:** Involves the posterior leaflet and cusps. **Reads syndrome**/floppy valve syndrome is considered as a variant of Barlow that affects both mitral cusps as well-other valves like aortic valve.
- **Cobb's syndrome** selectively affects the anterior mitral cusp.
- MVP syndrome is also called as **systolic click-murmur syndrome.**
- MVP is one of the more common causes of mild mitral regurgitation.

Pathogenesis

- It is caused by congenital anomalies or degenerative myxomatous changes (e.g., Marfan syndrome and cystic medical necrosis) that are associated with excessive or redundant mitral leaflet tissue. Familial incidence with an autosomal dominant mode of inheritance.
- Prolapse of the cusp occurs in systole → tensing of the chordae → pulling of papillary muscles which sometimes may interfere with blood supply.
- **Conditions associated with MVP:** Atrial septal defect (20%), polycystic kidney disease, chronic rheumatic heart disease, ischemic heart disease, and cardiomyopathies.

Clinical Features

Symptoms

- **Age and gender:** More common in females between 15 and 30 years. But, severe mitral regurgitation caused by prolapsed mitral valve is more common in older males compared to young females.
- May be asymptomatic or present with anxiety neurosis
- Symptoms include atypical chest pain (precordial stabbing), palpitation, syncope or presyncope, and fatigue.
- **Rarely:** Symptoms of left ventricular failure (exertional dyspnea, orthopnea, and paroxysmal nocturnal dyspnea) in patients with mitral regurgitation, sudden death, and transient ischemic attacks.

Signs

- Asthenic built, straight back/pectus excavatum
- **Mid-systolic click:** In mildest forms, the valve is competent but bulges back into the atrium during systole, causing a mid-systolic click to occur >0.14 seconds after S_1 without any murmur.
- **Late systolic murmur:** When there is mitral regurgitation, the click is followed by a late systolic murmur apical murmur (rarely "whooping" or "honking"). Its length increases as the regurgitation becomes more severe. The systolic murmur of mitral valve prolapse increases during standing and Valsalva maneuver, but decreases during squatting and isometric exercise.

Investigations

- **Electrocardiogram (ECG):** Nonspecific ST-T changes or inverted T waves in leads II, III, and aVF
- **Echocardiography:** Used for confirmation of the diagnosis. Color Doppler is used to assess the degree of mitral regurgitation.

Complications

- These include arrhythmias, sudden rupture of the chordate, progressive mitral regurgitation, and infective endocarditis.
- Rare complications include transient cerebral ischemic attacks, embolism, acute severe mitral regurgitation, and sudden death.

Management

- **Medical:**
  - Reassurance for patients without symptoms
  - β-**blockers:** For atypical chest pain
  - **Antiarrhythmic drugs:** For the treatment of arrhythmias
  - **Transient ischemic attacks:** Aspirin, dipyridamole, or anticoagulants
  - No need for infective endocarditis prophylaxis
- **Surgical:** Mitral valve repair or replacement in severe mitral regurgitation

Prognosis: Long-term prognosis is good.

AORTIC STENOSIS

Q. Write a long essay on the classification, causes/etiology, clinical features, investigations, and management of valvular aortic stenosis.

- Aortic stenosis is a chronic progressive disease and characterized by obstruction to the left ventricular stroke volume.
- Normal aortic valve area 3–4 cm^2 without any gradient across it. Critical aortic stenosis develops when an aortic valve area becomes <0.8 cm^2 or a gradient of >50 mm Hg.

Classification and Etiology of Aortic Stenosis (Table 7.70)

TABLE 7.70: Classification and etiology of aortic stenosis.
Valvular aortic stenosis:
➢ **Acquired: Rheumatic aortic stenosis** (young adults, middle-aged, elderly), **calcific aortic valvular disease** (CAVD—in middle aged to elderly), systemic lupus erythematosus (SLE), Fabry disease, chronic kidney disease, Paget's disease of bone, rheumatoid arthritis, infective endocarditis, senile degenerative aortic stenosis (middle-aged to elderly), previous radiation exposure, homozygous familial hypercholesterolemia, and ochronosis
➢ **Congenital:** Congenital aortic stenosis (infants, children, adolescents), bicuspid aortic valve (BAV), calcification and fibrosis of congenitally **bicuspid aortic valve** (young adults to middle-aged)
Subvalvular aortic stenosis:
➢ Membranous diaphragm
➢ Hypertrophic cardiomyopathy
➢ Congenital subvalvular aortic stenosis (infants, children, and adolescents)
Supravalvular aortic stenosis:
➢ Hourglass constriction of aorta
➢ Congenital supravalvular aortic stenosis (infants, children, and adolescents)
➢ Williams syndrome
Williams syndrome: Characterized by Elfin facies, supravalvular aortic stenosis, idiopathic hypercalcemia, mental retardation, and behavioral profile. On examination, the right upper limb blood pressure may be a higher than the left upper limb and the pulse volume on the right arm better than left. This is called *Coandă Effect*
Shone's complex: It is a rare combination of four left-sided congenital cardiac anomalies including parachute mitral valve, supravalvular ring, coarctation of the aorta, and subaortic obstruction

Pathophysiology

- Normal aortic valve area is 2.5–3.5 sq. cm.
- Hemodynamically significant AS occurs when the aortic valve is reduced by 60–75%.
- Critical AS when valve area <0.8 cm^2/gradient >80%.
- Initially, cardiac output is maintained. Pathological hallmark is fixed outflow obstruction to the left ventricle. It limits the increase in cardiac output required during exercise. The coronary blood flow may be inadequate and patients may develop angina even in the absence of concomitant coronary disease. Obstruction to the outflow leads to left ventricular hypertrophy (LVH). Wall stress due to outflow obstruction manifests in two forms.
  - **Development of concentric LVH:** Wall stress is not allowed to rise by development of concentric LVH. This type is more likely in females.
  - **Ventricular dilation and eccentric hypertrophy:** Rise in wall stress and systolic dysfunction are features of this type. This type is more likely in males.
- Later the left ventricle cannot overcome the outflow tract obstruction and pulmonary edema develops. In aortic stenosis, pulmonary arterial hypertension is due to increased LV diastolic pressure.

Clinical Features

Usually, asymptomatic aortic stenosis is moderately severe (aortic orifice reduced to one-third of its normal size). It is commonly diagnosed in asymptomatic patients during routine clinical examination.

Symptoms

Q. Write a short note on symptomatic triad of aortic stenosis.

- **Age of onset of symptoms:** Bicuspid aortic valve between 50 and 70 years, calcific aortic stenosis >70 years, and rheumatic aortic stenosis between 40 and 50 years of age.
- **Symptomatic triad of aortic stenosis:** Three cardinal symptoms are (1) breathlessness (dyspnea), (2) angina, and (3) syncope.
- **Exercise intolerance:** Most common initial presentation. Dyspnea with exertion due to cardiac decompensation or fatigue with exertion due to inadequate rise of cardiac output with exertion.
- **Angina** is typical exertional and is due to mismatch in myocardial oxygen demand-supply ratio, or coexistent coronary artery disease (CAD).
- **Exertional syncope (or presyncope):** Due to failure of cardiac output to rise to meet demand, leading to a fall in BP.
- **Heart failure:** Orthopnea and paroxysmal nocturnal dyspnea (PND).
  - The average survival after the onset of symptoms were 5, 3, and 2 years respectively for angina, syncope, and dyspnea.
- Infective endocarditis
- Embolism
- Gastrointestinal bleed due to angiodysplasias (**Heyde syndrome**), acquired von Willebrand syndrome.

If untreated, the approximate time interval from the onset of symptoms to death is 1.5–2 years for heart failure (dyspnea, PND), 3 years for syncope, and 5 years for angina.

Signs

- **Appearance:** Severe AS produces "Dresden China" look-asthenic appearance with pale skin.
- **Pulse:**
  - Parvus and tardus pulse: Slow rising, late peaking, and low amplitude
  - Pulsus bisferiens if AS is associated aortic regurgitation (AR)
  - Anacrotic pulse and apicocarotid delay in severe AS
  - Coanda effect in supravalvular AS
  - Normal pulse if there is coexistent AR, hypertension (HTN)
- **Blood pressure:**
  - Low systolic and pulse pressures. Systolic decapitation (SBP <120 mm Hg)
  - Normal BP if there is coexistent AR and HTN
- **Carotid shudder:** Thrill in carotids
- **Jugular venous pressure (JVP):** Prominent a waves **(Bernheim effect)**
- **Apex beat:** Thrusting/heaving LV type apex beat due to LV pressure overload. It is not usually displaced because hypertrophy (as opposed to dilatation) does not produce significant cardiomegaly.
- Palpable LV S4

Auscultation (Fig. 7.44)

- S_1 is normal. If loud suspect coexistent MS.
- S_2-A_2: Soft (single S_2) in rheumatic AS, loud in BAV, normal in sub/supravalvular AS. In severe AS, paradoxical (reversed) split of second heart sound A_2 (splitting on expiration)
- Systolic ejection click in bicuspid aortic valve (BAV):
  - **Ejection mid-systolic murmur:** Harsh/rough, radiates to the neck (to carotids arteries) and also the precordium with late peaking in severe AS. Best heard in the base of heart (aortic area). Murmur is likened to a saw cutting wood and especially in older patients may have a musical quality like the "mew" of a seagull. It is diamond-shaped (crescendo decrescendo). The murmur is usually longer in severe AS. The intensity of the murmur should not be correlated with the severity of AS because it is less intense when the cardiac output is reduced. In severe AS, it may not be audible. In calcific AS, high-frequency components radiate to apex producing a long systolic murmur at apex—**Gallavardin phenomenon**/hour-glass conduction due to periodic wake phenomenon. With LV failure, murmur intensity decreases and murmur may disappear.
  - Differences between aortic stenosis and mitral regurgitation presented in **Table 7.71**.

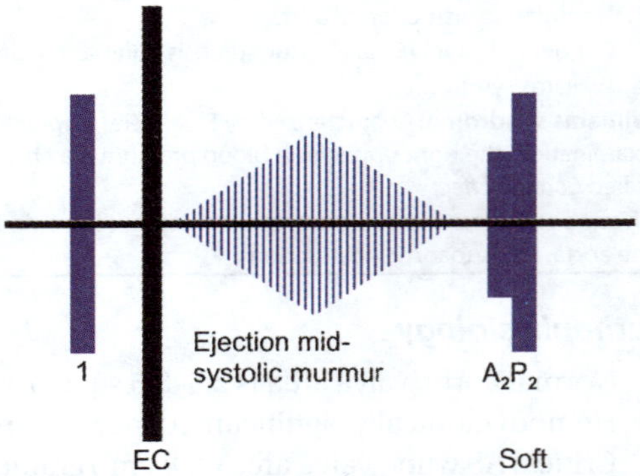

1 EC Ejection mid-systolic murmur A_2P_2 Soft

FIG. 7.44: Diagrammatic representation of timing of heart sounds and murmur in aortic stenosis. Features are diamond-shaped ejection mid-systolic murmur. An ejection click (EC) may be present in young patients with a bicuspid aortic valve. Soft second heart sound (A_2, P_2).

TABLE 7.71: Differences between aortic stenosis and mitral regurgitation.

Features	Aortic stenosis	Mitral regurgitation
Site of systolic murmur	Aortic area + Apex	Apex
Nature of murmur and its relation with A_2	Usually ejection-mid systolic. Stops before A_2	Pan systolic. Continues till A_2
Post-VPC intensity	Increases	No change/decreases
Carotid pulse	Slow rising, low volume	Quick rising high volume

(VPC: ventricular premature contraction)

Severity of aortic stenosis (Box 7.39)

Box 7.39: Signs indicating severity of aortic stenosis.

Mild: Only murmur (early peaking)
Moderate: Low volume pulse, mid-systolic peaking murmur, pulsus parvus et tardus
Severe: Anacrotic pulse, paradoxical split S_2, late peaking murmur, palpable S_4 apicocarotid delay

Investigations

- Chest X-ray:
  - Rounding of apex due to concentric left ventricular hypertrophy with normal heart size or a relatively small heart
  - Prominent dilation of ascending aorta (more prominent if bicuspid aortic valve) due to turbulent blood flow above the stenosed aortic valve causing poststenotic dilatation
  - Calcification of aortic valve (if present)
- Electrocardiogram (ECG):
  - Left ventricular hypertrophy correlation between QRS voltage
  - Atrial fibrillation in 10–15%
  - AV conduction defects and IVCD in 5% of calcific AS due to extension of calcium to conduction system
- Echocardiography:
  - Helps in evaluation of severity and gradient across the aortic valve
  - Dobutamine stress echo:
    - **Severe AS:** Increase in gradient. No change in valve area
    - **Mild AS:** Increase in valve area
    - Also assesses contractile reserve and predicts improvement in LV function after surgery
- **Doppler:** Useful for detecting the severity of stenosis and associated aortic regurgitation
- **Cardiac magnetic resonance and cardiac CT:** They may be required for assessing the presence of aneurysm, dissection, or coarctation of thoracic aorta.
- **Cardiac catheterization** is rarely needed because since all these information can be obtained from noninvasive with echocardiography and CMR. **Coronary angiography is needed before aortic valve surgery and for detecting any associated coronary artery disease.**

Treatment

Asymptomatic patients: Irrespective of the severity of AS, asymptomatic patients have a good immediate prognosis. Hence, should be managed conservatively with regular review for assessment of symptoms and echocardiography.

Medical treatment

- Avoid vigorous physical activity in patients with severe AS.
- **Diuretics** decrease dyspnea but may also reduce cardiac output.
- **ACE inhibitors:** To be used with caution and given only if there is LV failure
- **Avoid beta-blockers:** Because they produce LV failure.
- **Vasodilators for other purposes such as angina:** Be careful in titration as there will be no compensatory increase in cardiac output.
- **Atrial fibrillation:** Cardioversion can be tried.
- Infective endocarditis prophylaxis for those who have undergone valvular replacement
- Rheumatic fever prophylaxis

Surgical treatment

Indications

- **Symptomatic patients:** Symptoms are a good index of severity in aortic stenosis, and all symptomatic patients should undergo aortic valve replacement.
- **Asymptomatic patients:** Surgical intervention for severe aortic stenosis is recommended in patients with:
  - Symptoms during an exercise test or with a fall of blood pressure
  - Left ventricular ejection fraction of <50%
  - Moderate-to-severe aortic stenosis undergoing CABG, surgery of the ascending aorta, or other cardiac valve.

Surgical procedures

- **Balloon dilatation (valvuloplasty)** may be tried in adults (especially elderly) as an alternative to surgery. But results are poor and they should be reserved for patients unfit for surgery or as a "bridge" to surgery (as systolic function will often improve).
- **Aortic valve replacement:** The above procedure causes only temporary relief from the obstruction and aortic valve replacement will be usually needed after few years.
- **Percutaneous valve replacement:** Transcatheter implantation with a balloon expandable stent valve may be done for patients unsuitable for surgical aortic valve replacement.
- **ROSS procedure:** Replacement of deceased aortic valve by pulmonic valve and implantation of homograft instead of native pulmonic valve.
- **Transcatheter aortic valve replacement (TAVR)** and **transcatheter aortic valve implantation (TAVI)** are procedures for select patients with severe symptomatic aortic stenosis.

Aortic Sclerosis

Q. Write a short note on aortic sclerosis.

- Aortic sclerosis is characterized by irregular thickening of the aortic valve leaflets seen on echocardiography but without significant aortic obstruction. It may produce a systolic ejection murmur without any symptoms. Pulse and BP will be normal.
- About 25% patients are above the age 65 years and 40% over 85 years.
- **Risk factors:** Dyslipidemia, diabetes, hypertension, and smoking. Higher prevalence in Paget disease and end-stage renal disease (ESRD)
- There may be coexisting mitral annular calcification. Even if there is no AS, calcific aortic sclerosis increases cardiovascular death and MI by 50%.
- Rate of progression is variable so difficult to predict in an individual patient. The valve area declines 0.1–0.3 cm^2 per year; the systolic pressure gradient across the valve can increase by as much as 10–15 mm Hg per year.

Treatment

- No medical treatment available.
- Rosuvastatin has been shown to decrease progression of less severe AS to severe AS. Other drugs tried include ACE inhibitors.

Bicuspid Aortic Valve (BAV) Disease

Q. Write a short note on bicuspid aortic valve disease.

- Bicuspid aortic valve is the **most common congenital heart disease** found in 1–2% of live births.
- Male-to-female ratio is 3:1.
- Some cases are inherited as autosomal dominant and NOTCH1 gene mutation are found in some cases.
- **Associated conditions:** Other congenital cardiac diseases (e.g., dilatation of proximal ascending aorta secondary to abnormalities of the aortic media), coarctation of aorta, ventricular septal defect (VSD), and atrial septal defect (ASD). Calcification is common in adults with bicuspid aortic valve.
- **Auscultatory findings:** Ejection click best heard at the apex and may be associated murmurs of aortic stenosis or aortic regurgitation.
- **Diagnosis:** By echocardiography

Complications

- **Aortic regurgitation:** About 20% develop severe AR
- **Aortic stenosis:** Due to calcification and severe AS occurs after 50 years of age
- **Infective endocarditis**
- **Ascending aortic dilation:** Due to medial degeneration and is not related to severity of aortic stenosis
- **Aortic dissection:** Risk is increased by five to nine times.

Treatment

- Medical management: Control of hypertension and use of β-blockers.
- Surgical treatment: Aortic valve replacement and may also require aortic root surgery.

Prognosis

Life-expectancy is usually not shortened.

AORTIC REGURGITATION

Q. Discuss the etiology, clinical features, complications, investigations, and treatment of aortic regurgitation.

Aortic regurgitation (AR) is incompetency of the aortic valve which causes backflow (reflux) of blood from the aorta through the aortic valve into the left ventricle during diastole.

Etiology (Box 7.40)

- Aortic regurgitation may be caused by diseases of the aortic valve (e.g., endocarditis) or diseases of the aortic root (e.g., Marfan syndrome) causing dilatation of the aortic root.
- Aortic regurgitation can be acute or chronic.
- **Acute aortic regurgitation** of significant severity leads to sudden increased blood volume in the left ventricle during diastole. The left ventricle does not have sufficient time to dilate in response to the sudden increase in volume. This causes rapid increase in end-diastolic pressure of left ventricle → leading to an increase in pulmonary venous pressure. As pressure increases throughout the pulmonary circulation, the patient develops dyspnea and pulmonary edema. In severe cases, left ventricular failure with cardiogenic shock may develop. Decreased myocardial perfusion may lead to myocardial ischemia.
- **Chronic aortic regurgitation:** Produces increased blood volume in the left ventricle during diastole. To maintain the net cardiac output, the total volume of blood pumped from the left ventricle into the aorta increases, and consequently the left ventricle enlarges. AR begets AR. There is fall in the diastolic blood pressure and decreased coronary perfusion. Myocardial ischemia occurs due to:
  - Increased myocardial oxygen demand due to increased afterload, increased LV ejection time, and increased LV mass
  - Decreased myocardial oxygen supply due to decreased aortic diastolic pressure, decreased diastolic filling time due to increased LV ejection time, and decreased effective stroke volume.

Box 7.40: Causes of aortic regurgitation.

Acute aortic regurgitation:
- Infective endocarditis
- Aortic dissection
- Acute rheumatic fever
- Ruptured sinus of Valsalva aneurysm
- Failure of prosthetic valve
- Trauma

Chronic aortic regurgitation:
- **Congenital:** Bicuspid aortic valve or disproportionate cusps
- **Acquired:**
  - Rheumatic heart disease
  - Infective endocarditis
  - Trauma
  - Aortic dilatation, e.g., aneurysm and dissection
  - Arthritides, e.g., ankylosing spondylitis
  - Rheumatoid arthritis
  - Syphilitic aortitis
  - Hypertension
  - Connective tissue disorders, e.g., Marfan syndrome, Ehlers–Danlos syndrome
  - Osteogenesis imperfecta and methysergide

Clinical Features

Symptoms

- **Age and gender:** About three-fourths of patients with pure or predominant valvular AR are males. Females with primary valvular AR have associated rheumatic mitral valve disease. Chronic AR usually begins during late 50s. Usually, the prevalence and severity of AR increase with age.
- Acute AR:
  - Sudden, severe shortness of breath
  - Chest pain if myocardial perfusion pressure is decreased or an aortic dissection is present
  - Rapidly developing heart failure, pulmonary edema, and cardiogenic shock
- Chronic AR:
  - Relatively asymptomatic for 10–15 years and significant symptoms occur late. Symptoms may not develop until left ventricular failure occurs.
  - Palpitations, especially on lying down, may persist for many years. Sinus tachycardia, during exertion or with emotion, may produce palpitations as well as head pounding.
  - Exertional dyspnea: Usually, the first symptom of diminished cardiac reserve. It depends on the extent of left ventricular dilatation and dysfunction. It is followed by orthopnea, paroxysmal nocturnal dyspnea, and excessive diaphoresis.
  - Angina pectoris: Anginal chest pain develops even in the absence of coronary artery disease (CAD) at rest as well as during exertion. Nocturnal angina may be accompanied by marked diaphoresis. These episodes of angina can be prolonged and usually do not respond satisfactorily to sublingual nitroglycerine. Mechanisms of angina in AR:
    - Associated CAD
    - Low aortic diastolic pressure leading to decreased myocardial perfusion (because coronary flow occurs mainly in diastole)
    - Increased myocardial oxygen demand due to myocardial hypertrophy
- Congestive heart failure
- Sudden cardiac death
- Arrhythmias are not common.

Signs

Q. Write a short essay/note on peripheral signs of aortic regurgitation.

Peripheral signs of aortic regurgitation

Pulses:

- **Peripheral pulses:** Prominent, large-volume (bounding), or collapsing
- **Low-diastolic and increased/wide pulse pressure:** Pulse pressure is the difference between the systolic and diastolic blood pressures. In aortic regurgitation, there is increased/wide pulse pressure. **Table 7.72** shows list of (rare) signs of wide pulse pressure that indicates a hyperdynamic circulation in aortic regurgitation.

Inspection and palpation

- Prominent neck pulsations and thrill in the carotids
- **Apex beat:** Displaced inferiorly and toward the axilla. The point of maximal impulse may be diffuse or hyperdynamic.
- Pre-systolic impulse
- **Diastolic thrill:** May be palpable along the left sternal border in patients with thin-chest (Erb's maneuver)
- **Prominent systolic thrill:** May be palpable in the suprasternal notch and transmitted upward along the carotid arteries

Auscultation

- **First heart sound (S_1):** May be soft
- A_2 component of second heart sound (S_2): Soft in rheumatic aortic regurgitation and loud and **"tambour"** like in syphilitic AR. Narrowly split, single, or paradoxically split second heart sound.
- S_3 gallop, third heart sound (S_3), if left ventricular dysfunction is present.
- Fourth heart sound (S_4) prominent in left ventricular hypertrophy
- Murmurs:
  - **Early-diastolic murmur:** Early-holodiastolic murmur, immediately after A_2, usually as a high-pitched blowing sound that is loudest at the left sternal border, and decrescendo. Best heard in at the end of expiration, in sitting and leaning forward position. The duration of the murmur correlates better with the severity of AR than does the loudness of the murmur.
  - **Cole-Cecil murmur:** It is the term used for the diastolic murmur of AR when well or predominantly heard in the left axilla.

TABLE 7.72: Signs of wide pulse pressure in aortic regurgitation (AR).

Sign	*Feature*
Light house sign/Morton and Mahon sign	Alternate flushing and blanching of forehead
Landolfi's sign	Change in pupillary size in synchronous with cardiac cycle
Becker's sign	Retinal artery pulsations
De Musset's sign	Head nodding with each heart beat/pulse
Müller's sign	Systolic pulsations of uvula
Quincke's sign	Capillary pulsations in the lip or nail bed. Detected by pressing a glass slide on patients lip or nail bed
Corrigan's sign	Dancing carotids
Locomotor brachii	Prominent pulsation of brachial artery
Watson's water hammer pulse/collapsing pulse	Bounding and forcible, rapidly increasing and subsequently collapsing pulse
Pulsus bisferiens	Double peaking in single systole
Pistol shot femorals or Traube sign	Sharp bang heard on auscultation over the femoral arteries in time with each a heart beat
Duroziez's sign	To and fro murmur heard when the femoral artery is auscultated with pressure applied distally
Hill's sign	Popliteal cuff systolic pressure exceeds brachial cuff pressure by >20 mm Hg (Mild AR: 20–40 mm Hg, moderate AR: 40–60 mm Hg, severe AR: > 60 mm Hg)
Drummond sign	Systolic expulsion of air from nose when mouth is closed
Mayan's sign	When arm is raised, diastolic BP drops by >15 mm Hg
Rosenbach's sign	Pulsations of liver
Gerhardt's sign	Pulsations of spleen
Ashrafian sign	Pulsatile pseudoproptosis
Bozzolo sign	Pulsatile nasal mucosa
Palmar click	Pulsating palm
Dennison/Shelley sign	Pulsatile cervix
Lincoln sign	Popliteal pulsation
Sherman sign	Dorsalis pedis prominent pulsation in age of 75 years or more

  - If the murmur is musical (cooing dove murmur), it signifies eversion or perforation of an aortic cusp.
  - **Harvey sign:** When regurgitation is caused by primary valvular disease, the diastolic murmur is heard best along the left sternal border in the 3rd and 4th intercostal space. When murmur is caused mainly by dilation of the ascending aorta, the murmur is more readily audible along the right sternal border.
- A functional systolic flow murmur may also be present because of increased stroke volume, although concurrent AS may also be present.

Q. Write a short note on Austin Flint murmur.

- **Austin Flint murmur:** It may be audible at the cardiac apex in severe AR. It is a low-pitched, mid-diastolic rumbling murmur caused due to:
  - AR jet impinges on anterior mitral leaflet (AML) forces it down and reduces the mitral orifice.
  - Turbulence produced when AR jet meets mitral inflow jet
  - AML fluttering due to AR jet
  - LV endocardial vibrations due to AR jet
- The auscultatory features of AR are intensified by strenuous and sustained handgrip (increases systemic vascular resistance).
- As heart failure develops, peripheral vasoconstriction may occur and arterial diastolic pressure may rise, even though severe AR is present (**Box 7.41**). Thus, pulse pressure can be normal or narrow in severe AR.

Indicators of severity of aortic regurgitation are listed in **Box 7.42**.

Box 7.41: Causes of AR with normal/low pulse pressure.

- Acute AR
- AR with AS or severe MS
- AR with CHF
- AR

(AR: aortic regurgitation; AS: aortic stenosis; CHF: congestive heart failure; MS: mitral stenosis)

Box 7.42: Indicators of severity of aortic regurgitation.

- **Duration of murmur:** If murmur > two-thirds of diastole, murmur becomes holodiastolic and rough in quality
- Bisferiens pulse
- S_3
- Positive Hill's sign >60 mm Hg
- **Cardiomegaly:** Apical impulse displaced down and out
- Austin Flint murmur
- A_2 soft
- Marked peripheral signs

Acute Aortic Regurgitation

- **Clinical presentation:** Sudden in onset with acute left ventricular failure
- Signs:
  - **Pulse pressure:** Normal and near normal systolic and diastolic pressures
  - **S_1:** Soft or absent
  - **P_2:** Normal or increased
  - **S_3:** Usually audible
  - Murmur:
    - Early diastolic murmur is short and functional systolic murmur across aortic valve is less loud.
    - Austin Flint murmur is usually absent.
- Investigations of acute aortic regurgitation:
  - **ECG and chest X-ray:** Do not show evidence of left ventricular enlargement. Chest X-ray may show redistribution of upper lobe vessels due to pulmonary venous hypertension.

Investigations of Chronic Aortic Regurgitation

- **Chest X-ray:** It shows cardiomegaly due to the enlargement/dilatation of the left ventricle in an inferior and leftward direction. The ascending aorta (and the aortic arch or knob) is also severely dilated. Left atrial enlargement is not found unless there is significant left ventricular dysfunction. Calcification of the ascending aortic wall and the aortic valve may be observed in syphilitic aortic regurgitation. Later, it may show features of left heart failure.
- **Electrocardiography (ECG):** It shows the adaptive changes in the left ventricle due to the volume overload. These include: (1) LV hypertrophy: Tall R waves and deeply inverted T waves in the left-sided chest leads, (2) left axis deviation, (3) left atrial enlargement, (4) LV volume overload pattern (prominent Q waves in leads I, aVL, and V_3 to V_6 and relatively small r waves in V_1), and (5) LV conduction defects (typically late in the disease process).
- **Echocardiography:**
  - Aortic valve structure and morphology (e.g., bileaflet versus trileaflet, flail, thickening).
  - Presence of vegetations or nodules (may require transesophageal echocardiography in selected cases)
  - Quantitative measurements of regurgitant volume, fraction and orifice area assessed
  - Fluttering anterior mitral leaflet
  - Regurgitant volume, fraction, and orifice area
  - Associated lesions of the aorta, e.g., dilation, aneurysm, dissection, or ectasia
  - LV structure and function
- Doppler echocardiography: To assess the severity. Transesophageal echocardiography is not usually needed.
- **Cardiac magnetic resonance and cardiac CT:** To assess the thoracic aorta for the aneurysm, dissection or coarctation but are rarely needed. Cardiac MR can quantify regurgitant volume.
- Cardiac catheterization

- **Coronary angiography:** Indicated for the assessment of coronary anatomy prior to aortic valve surgery in patients with risk factors for coronary artery disease
- Other tests:
  - **VDRL and TPHA:** If syphilitic cause is suspected
  - RA factor, ANA, ESR and CRP: To exclude connective tissue disorders.

Q. Write a short essay/note on the management of acute severe aortic regurgitation in pulmonary edema.

Treatment

- Underlying cause of AR-like dissection, endocarditis, syphilis has to be treated.
- **Prophylaxis:** Rheumatic fever prophylaxis is needed if due to rheumatic. Infective endocarditis prophylaxis is not required.
- **Acute severe AR:** Surgical intervention is usually needed, but the patient may be medically supported with **dobutamine** to augment cardiac output and shorten diastole and **sodium nitroprusside** to reduce afterload in hypertensive patients.
- **Chronic severe AR**

Medical treatment

- Vasodilator therapy may be used in selected conditions to reduce afterload in patients with systolic hypertension to reduce wall stress and optimize LV function. In normotensive patients, vasodilator therapy may not be useful because it does not reduce regurgitant volume (preload) significantly.
- The acute administration of sodium nitroprusside, hydralazine, nifedipine, or felodipine reduced PVR and results in an immediate augmentation in forward cardiac output and a reduction in regurgitant volume. Nitroprusside and hydralazine induced acute hemodynamic changes lead to a consistent decrease in end-diastolic volume (EDV) and an increase in ejection fraction (EF).

Surgical treatment

- AR usually requires replacement of the diseased valve with a prosthetic valve, although valve-sparing repair is available like **transcatheter aortic valve replacement/implantation (TAVR/TAVI).**
- Indications for aortic valve surgery (**Box 7.43**)
- **Types of valves:** For patients undergoing AV replacement, careful consideration should be given to the relative risks and benefits of mechanical versus bioprosthetic valves.
  - **Mechanical valves:** More durable but require long-term anticoagulation with warfarin due to increased risk of thrombosis
  - **Bioprosthetic (tissue) valves** carry a greater risk of long-term deterioration (e.g., rapid calcification and degeneration of the valves) and risk of reoperation but avoid the need for long-term warfarin. Thus, they are preferred in the elderly and when anticoagulants must be avoided. They are contraindicated in children and young adults.
- **Aortic root dilation causing AR:** For example, Marfan syndrome. Treated by encircling suture or subcommissural annuloplasty, or aortic graft with prosthetic valve (coronaries need to be reimplanted) or aortic graft alone.

Box 7.43: Indications for aortic valve surgery.

- Patient is symptomatic (dyspnea, NYHA class IIIB, angina) with chronic severe aortic regurgitation
- Patient is asymptomatic, with a resting left ventricular ejection fraction (LVEF) of <55%
- Patient is asymptomatic, with left ventricular (LV) ejection fraction >55% but with left ventricle dilation (LV end-diastolic dimension >70 mm or end-systolic dimension >55 mm)
- Fractional shortening (FS) <0.27
- Acute severe aortic regurgitation, e.g., endocarditis
- If undergoing CABG, surgery of the ascending aorta or other cardiac valve

(CABG: coronary artery bypass grafting; NYHA: New York Heart Association)

Difference between rheumatic and syphilitic aortic regurgitation (Table 7.73)

Q. What are the differences between rheumatic and syphilitic aortic regurgitation?

TABLE 7.73: Differences between aortic regurgitation (AR) of rheumatic and syphilitic etiology.

Feature	*Rheumatic AR*	*Syphilitic AR*
Age group	10–40 years	Older than 40 years
Angina	Less common	More common
Early-diastolic murmur (EDM) best audible at	Erb's area	Aortic area
Character of EDM	Soft, blowing	Cooling dove or seagull
Character of A_2	Soft	Loud and tambour
Association with aortic stenosis or mitral valve disease	May be associated	Not associated
Decompensation	Relatively late	Relatively early
Calcification aorta	Not seen	May be present
Features of underlying cause or etiology	Other features of RHD may be present	Stigmata of syphilis present

(RHD: rheumatic heart disease)

Difference between Acute and Chronic Aortic Regurgitation (Table 7.74)

Q. What are the differences between acute and chronic aortic regurgitation?

Difference between Austin Flint murmurs from the murmur of mitral stenosis (Table 7.75)

Q. What are the differences between Austin Flint murmur and the murmur of mitral stenosis (MS)?

TABLE 7.74: Differences between acute and chronic aortic regurgitation.

Clinical features	*Acute aortic regurgitation*	*Chronic aortic regurgitation*
Congestive cardiac failure	Early and sudden	Late and insidious
Arterial pulse	Low volume Pulsus alternans	High volume, collapsing, water hammer, pulsus bisferiens
Blood pressure	Normal/low	Wide pulse pressure
Contour of peak of pulse	Single	Bisferiens
Left ventricle impulse	Near normal	Laterally displaced
S_1	Soft to absent	Normal
A_2	Soft	N/decreased
S_3	Common	Absent
S_4	Consistently absent	Usually absent
Aortic systolic murmur	Grade 3/less	Grade 3/more
Aortic regurgitant murmur	Short, medium-pitched	Long, high-pitched
Austin Flint murmur	Mid-diastolic	Presystolic, mid-diastolic
Peripheral signs	Absent	Present

TABLE 7.75: Differences between Austin Flint murmur and the murmur of mitral stenosis.

Feature	*Austin Flint murmur*	*Mitral stenosis murmur*
Diastolic thrill at apex	Absent	Present
Wide pulse pressure	Present	Absent
Peripheral signs of AR	++	-
Heart sounds and murmur		
➢ First heart sound (S_1)	-	Loud
➢ P_2	-	Loud
➢ Third heart sound (S_3)	+	-
➢ Opening snap (OS)	-	+
➢ Presystolic accentuation	±	+
➢ Associated EDM at aortic area	++	-
➢ With amyl nitrite	Murmur decreases	No change
Evidence of pulmonary hypertension, RV enlargement and/or hypertrophy	Absent	Present
Evidence of LV enlargement and/or hypertrophy	Present	Absent
Atrial fibrillation	-	May occur

(EDM: early-diastolic murmur; LV: left ventricular; RV: right ventricular)

Tricuspid Stenosis (TS)

Q. Write a short essay/note on tricuspid stenosis (TS).

Tricuspid stenosis is a **narrowing of the tricuspid valve** opening. Uncommon valve lesion that is more common in females than males.

Etiology (Box 7.44)

Box 7.44: Causes of tricuspid stenosis.

- Rheumatic (frequently associated with mitral and/or aortic valve disease)
- **Carcinoid syndrome:** Tricuspid stenosis and regurgitation are found in carcinoid syndrome
- Congenital
- Infective endocarditis
- **Anorectics:** Fenfluramine
- Fabry disease

Pathophysiology

Tricuspid valve stenosis reduces the cardiac output, which is restored to normal when the pressure of right atrium increases—results in systemic venous congestion—hepatomegaly, ascites, and dependent edema.

Clinical Features

Symptoms

- Usually, symptoms are due to associated left-sided rheumatic valve lesions (e.g., mitral stenosis)
- Tricuspid stenosis may produce symptoms of right heart failure: Abdominal pain/hepatic discomfort (due to hepatomegaly), peripheral edema, and ascites
- Little or no dyspnea and fatigue is common.

Signs

- **Jugular venous pressure (JVP):** JVP is raised with prominent a waves (giant a waves) and slowly descent due to the loss of normal rapid right ventricular filling.
- **Mid-diastolic murmur:** Loud first heart sound and a rumbling mid-diastolic murmur (higher-pitched than the murmur of mitral stenosis) with presystolic accentuation, best heard at the lower left sternal border and increases/louder during inspiration **(De Carvallo's sign).**
- **Tricuspid opening snap (OS):** Occasionally heard
- **Right heart failure:** Hepatomegaly with presystolic pulsation felt over the liver, ascites, and peripheral edema

Investigations

- **Chest X-ray:** May show a prominent right atrial bulge
- **ECG:** Enlarged right atrium
- **Echocardiogram:** May reveal thickened and immobile tricuspid valve.

Treatment

- **Medical management:** Diuretic therapy and salt and fluid restriction
- **Surgical treatment:** Tricuspid valve replacement.

Tricuspid Regurgitation

Q. Write a short essay/note on tricuspid regurgitation. What is De Carvallo's sign?

In tricuspid regurgitation, tricuspid valve does not close properly, causing blood to flow backward (leak) into the right atrium.

Etiology

Tricuspid regurgitation is common. Most commonly, it is functional secondary to right ventricular dilatation.

Causes of Tricuspid Regurgitation

- **Primary/organic:** Rheumatic heart disease, endocarditis (IV drug abuse), Ebstein anomaly and carcinoid syndrome
- **Secondary:**
  - **Functional tricuspid regurgitation:** Right ventricular dilatation due to chronic left heart failure
  - Right ventricular infarction, inferior wall infarction
  - Pulmonary hypertension (e.g., cor pulmonale)
  - Cardiomyopathy

Clinical Features

- Symptoms are usually nonspecific. Tiredness due to reduced forward flow.
- Valvular regurgitation increases the right atrial and systemic venous pressure. Patients may develop of right heart failure, i.e., edema, ascites, and hepatomegaly with systolic pulsations due to venous congestion.
- **JVP:** Raised with most prominent "giant" v wave in the jugular venous pulse (a *cv* wave replaces the normal *x* descent)
- Earlobe pulsations **(Lancisi's sign)**
- **Blowing pansystolic murmur:** At the lower-left sternal border that is increased during inspiration and reduced during expiration (**De Carvallo's sign**).
- P_2 may be loud (due to pulmonary hypertension) and RV S_3 is heard.
- **Severe TR:** Right jugular venous thrill and an RV impulse at the left lower sternal border. Long-standing severe TR may lead to RV dysfunction-induced heart failure and atrial fibrillation (AF)
- **Echocardiogram:** It shows dilated right ventricle and thickened valve.

Treatment

- **Functional tricuspid regurgitation** due to right ventricular dilatation usually disappears with treatment of the underlying cause of right ventricular overload. Treatment consists of with diuretic and vasodilator treatment of congestive cardiac failure.
- **Organic tricuspid regurgitation:** TR is usually well tolerated when there is normal pulmonary artery pressure. Severe organic tricuspid regurgitation may require operative repair of the tricuspid valve by annuloplasty or plication or valve repair, or occasionally tricuspid valve replacement. In drug addicts with infective endocarditis of the tricuspid valve, surgical removal of the valve is recommended to eradicate the infection.

Pulmonary Stenosis

Q. Write a short essay/note on pulmonary stenosis.

Pulmonary stenosis (PS) is characterized by obstruction to blood flow from the right ventricle to the pulmonary artery.

Etiology

- **Congenital:** Usually, PS is a congenital lesion. It may be associated with rubella during pregnancy. May be an isolated lesion or associated with a ventricular septal defect (Fallot's tetralogy).
- **Acquired:**
  - Rheumatic (very uncommon)
  - Carcinoid syndrome

Pulmonary stenosis may be classified as valvular, subvalvular (infundibular), or supravalvular.

Clinical Features

Symptoms

- Mild pulmonary stenosis may be asymptomatic.
- Fatigue, syncope, dyspnea, and the symptoms of right heart failure. Angina or syncope indicates severe pulmonary stenosis.

Signs

- **Systolic thrill:** The ejection systolic murmur (described below) is often associated with a thrill. It is best felt when patient sits up, learns forward, and breathes out.
- Right ventricular heave (sustained impulse) and epigastric pulsation may be felt.
- Pulmonary closure sound (P2) is soft and delayed.
- **Wide splitting of second heart sound:** Due to delay in right ventricular ejection
- **Ejection systolic murmur:** It is a principal physical sign. It is best heard on inspiration at the left upper sternum in the second intercostal space. It radiates toward the left shoulder. With progressive severity, the murmur gets harsh/louder longer and peaks later in systole. This murmur is usually preceded by an ejection sound (click).
- **Ejection click:** Mild stenosis is characterized by a systolic ejection click which is often more prominent in expiration. This seemingly paradoxical behavior of the pulmonary ejection click is explained by an inspiratory increase in RV end-diastolic pressure, which opens the valve in late diastole and hence absence of systolic ejection click during inspiratory phase.
- **High-pitched diastolic murmur** after a prominent P_2 may be evident in patients with pulmonary regurgitation secondary to pulmonary hypertension **(Graham Steell murmur).**
- If stenosis is valvular, pulmonary ejection sound/click will be heard.
- **Moderately severe stenosis** is associated with a right ventricular fourth sound and a prominent jugular venous *a* wave.
- **Features of severe pulmonary stenosis:** (1) Loud harsh murmur, (2) inaudible pulmonary closure sound (P_2), (3) increased right ventricular heave, (4) prominent a waves in the jugular pulse, (5) right ventricular hypertrophy in ECG, and (6) chest X-ray shows poststenotic dilatation in the pulmonary artery.

Investigations

- **ECG:** Shows both right ventricular and right atrial hypertrophy
- **Chest X-ray:** Shows a prominent pulmonary artery (extending into the left pulmonary artery branch) owing to poststenotic dilatation
- Doppler echocardiography is the definitive investigation.
- Cardiac catheterization

Treatment

- Mild and even moderate pulmonary valve stenosis and regurgitation do not result in RV overload and may require no specific treatment other than prophylaxis for infective endocarditis.
- Moderately severe and severe pulmonary valve stenosis (resting gradient >50 mm Hg with a normal cardiac output) is currently treated by percutaneous balloon valvotomy or, if this is not available, by surgical valvotomy. Postoperatively pulmonary regurgitation may develop which is benign in nature.

Prognosis

Long-term prognosis is very good.

INFECTIVE ENDOCARDITIS

Q. Discuss the etiology, pathology, clinical features, complications, investigations, management/treatment of subacute bacterial endocarditis (SBE).

Infective endocarditis (IE) is an **infection of the endocardium of heart valves or the mural endocardium.**

Definition

Infective endocarditis is defined as an endovascular infection of cardiovascular structures by microbes. These structures include heart valves, atrial and ventricular endocardium, large intrathoracic vessels, and intracardiac foreign bodies (e.g., prosthetic valves, pacemaker leads, and surgical conduits).

- The causative organism may be bacterium, fungus, chlamydia, or rickettsia. Majority of cases are due to infection by streptococci and staphylococci.
- Consequences of infective endocarditis: Valvular dysfunction, localized or generalized sepsis, and source for embolism.

Classification

- **According to the clinical course:** Acute, subacute, and chronic
- **According to the causative organism:** Bacterial, viral, rickettsial, or fungal

- **According to the nature of valve or device:** Native or prosthetic
- **According to the side affected:** Left-sided or right-sided infective endocarditis
- **According to the side affected and nature of valve/device:** (1) Left-sided infective endocarditis, (2) left-sided prosthetic infective endocarditis, (3) right-sided infective endocarditis, and (4) device-related (permanent pacemaker, implantable cardioverter defibrillator) infective endocarditis.

Differences between acute endocarditis and subacute endocarditis (Table 7.76)

TABLE 7.76: Differences between acute and subacute endocarditis.

Characteristic	*Acute infective endocarditis*	*Subacute infective endocarditis*
Onset	Acute	Insidious
Condition of valve	Infection of normal heart valve as well as damaged valves	Infection of structurally abnormal/deformed valves or at sites where the endothelium is damaged by a high pressure jet of blood
Virulence of organisms	Highly virulent (suppurative) and invasive organisms	Low virulent
Source of infection or portal of entry	Often evident	Common sources of infection are periodontal infections (dental treatment), gastrointestinal tract infections, and urinary tract infections
Lesions	Vegetations are more florid. Affected valve is rapidly destroyed. Abscess (local and metastatic) formation is more common	Less destructive. Formation of vegetations, embolic episodes, mycotic aneurysms, valve regurgitation, splenic and renal infarcts, and immune glomerulonephritis
Clinical features	Of acute infection	Of complications
Course	Fulminant course, death within 6 weeks	Protracted course of weeks
Complications	Acute heart failure or overwhelming sepsis	Infectious complications are uncommon
Causative organisms	➢ *Staphylococcus aureus* ➢ *Pseudomonas* ➢ *Candida* ➢ *Streptococcus pneumoniae* ➢ *Neisseria gonorrhoeae*	*Streptococcus viridans (S. sanguis and S. mitis), Streptococcus milleri, Streptococcus bovis, Enterococcus faecalis, Staphylococcus aureus, HACEK* Group*

(***HACEK:** H = *Haemophilus parainfluenzae, Haemophilus aphrophilus, Haemophilus paraphrophilus, Haemophilus influenzae;* **A** = *Actinobacillus actinomycetemcomitans;* **C** = *Cardiobacterium hominis;* **E** = *Eikenella corrodens;* **K** = *Kingella kingae, Kingella denitrificans*)

Predisposing Factors

- Underlying heart disease:
  - About 72% of patients have a pre-existing structural cardiac abnormality.
  - Congenital isolated aortic valvular stenosis is most often associated with infective endocarditis (IE). Other congenital heart diseases include ventricular septal defect (VSD), tetralogy of Fallot (TOF), idiopathic subaortic stenosis, and atrial septal defect (uncommon).
  - IE commonly involves mitral valve followed by aortic valve and uncommonly tricuspid valve (1%).
  - Major risks for IE are cardiac prosthetic valves and parenteral narcotic drug abuse.
- **Impaired host defense mechanism:** It may occur in diabetes mellitus, malignancies (e.g., leukemias and lymphomas), cytotoxic therapy, and neutropenia.
- **Conditions with bacteremia:** Most important predisposing factors to the development of endocarditis are conditions that lead to bacteremia. Transient bacteremia from any cause may lead to infective endocarditis and include the following surgical procedures from different sources:
  - **Respiratory tract:** Tonsillectomy and/or adenoidectomy, surgical operations (incision or biopsy) involving respiratory mucosa, and any invasive procedure of the respiratory tract used to treat an established infection (e.g., drainage of an abscess or empyema)
  - **Oral cavity:** All dental procedures in which there is handling of gingival tissue or the periapical region of teeth or perforation of the oral mucosa (e.g., dental extractions, suture removal, placement of orthodontic band, root canal treatment).
  - **Gastrointestinal tract:** Procedures done in an established GIT infection
  - **Genitourinary tract:** Procedures performed in an established infection (e.g., cystoscopy during known enterococcal urinary tract infection—UTI)
  - **Skin and musculoskeletal system:** Procedures involving infected tissue.

Common Organisms for Infective Endocarditis (Table 7.77)

Q. Write a short essay/note on common causative agents for infective endocarditis.

More than 75% of infective endocarditis is caused by streptococci or staphylococci.

Postoperative Endocarditis or Prosthetic Valve Endocarditis

- It develops after cardiac surgery and may affect native or prosthetic valves and other prosthetic materials.

TABLE 7.77: Organisms causing infective endocarditis.

Native valves	%	*Narcotic addicts*	%	*Prosthetic valves*	%
Streptococcus viridians	30–40	*Staphylococcus aureus*	50–60	*Staphylococcus epidermidis*	20–30
Staphylococcus aureus	10–30	Streptococci	8–15	*Staphylococcus aureus*	15–20
Staphylococcus epidermidis	1–3	*Staphylococcus epidermidis*	2–5	*Streptococcus viridans*	5–20
Enterococci	5–15	Enterococci	8–10	Enterococci	5–10
Other streptococci	15–20	Other streptococci	10–15	Other streptococci	1–5
Gram -ve bacilli	2–10	Gram -ve bacilli	4–8	Gram -ve bacilli	10–20
Fungi	2–4	Fungi	4–5	Fungi	5–15
Culture-negative	5–10	Culture-negative	5–8	Culture-negative	<5

- Depending on the time of development of endocarditis following surgery, it can be divided into early, intermediate, and late endocarditis.
  - Early (within 60 days of surgery) endocarditis is caused by intraoperative or hospital-acquired infections. The most common organism is a coagulase-negative *Staphylococcus (S. epidermidis)* which is a normal commensal in the skin and followed by fungi *(Candida, Aspergillus).*
  - Late (after 1 year) endocarditis is caused by infection with community-acquired organisms. The causative organism is the same with those causing acute and subacute endocarditis of native valve.
  - Endocarditis developing between 60 days and 1 year is due to a mixture of hospital-acquired episodes caused by less virulent organisms community-acquired episodes. The organisms include *Streptococcus viridans* and Enterococci.
- Types of prosthetic valves:
  - Aortic prosthetic valve is more prone to endocarditis than mitral prosthetic valve.
  - During first 3 months after surgery mechanical heart valves develop endocarditis more frequently than bioprosthetic ones. However, later on the rates of infection for the two valve types are same and are comparable at 5 years.

Right-sided endocarditis: Develops in intravenous drug users and are mainly caused by organisms found on the skin (e.g., *Staphylococcus aureus, Candida).* It usually presents with acute endocarditis and affects mainly tricuspid valve.

Culture-negative Endocarditis (Box 7.45)

- It is defined as endocarditis without etiology following inoculation of at least three independent blood samples in a standard blood culture system with negative cultures after 7 days of incubation and subculturing.
- They constitute 5–10% of cases of endocarditis.

Box 7.45: Causes of culture negative endocarditis.

- It is usually due to prior antibiotic therapy
- Inadequate quantity of blood taken for culture
- Anaerobic infection
- Some may be due to a variety of fastidious organisms that does not grow in normal blood cultures. These include *Coxiella burnetii* (cause of Q fever), *Chlamydia* species, *Bartonella* species (cause trench fever and cat scratch disease), and *Legionella*
- Right-sided endocarditis
- Noninfective endocarditis

Pathogenesis

Mechanism by which virulent organisms infect apparently normal valves is poorly understood.

The probable sequence of events, which occur with the infection of a damaged valve by less-virulent organisms is as follows:

- **Endocardial damage/injury and denudation**
- **Formation of sterile thrombus**
- **Adherence of the microorganisms:** Transient bacteremia → microorganisms gain access to the circulation and adhere and gets deposited to the sterile vegetations (infection of thrombi)
- **Proliferation of microorganisms within vegetations**
- **Formation of emboli:** The vegetation may get detached and form infective emboli → cause spread of infection to visceral organs such as kidney, spleen, and brain. They may result in infarction or abscess. Septic emboli cause arteritis with weakness of arterial wall leading to mycotic aneurysms.
- **Deposition of immune complexes: Antigen and antibody may form immune complexes and can produce** focal glomerulonephritis and microscopic hematuria, diffuse glomerulonephritis, vasculitis of cerebral vessels leading to cerebrovascular accidents, and perisplenitis.

Clinical Features

Q. Write a short essay/note on important signs of infective endocarditis.

- The clinical features of infective endocarditis depend on the causative organism and the presence of predisposing cardiac conditions.
- Endocarditis may be acute or a more insidious "subacute" form. However, there is overlap between the two because the clinical pattern depends not only on the causative organism, but also depends on the site of infection, prior antibiotic therapy, and the presence of a valve or shunt prosthesis.

Subacute Endocarditis (SBE)

Clinical suspicion of subacute endocarditis is necessary when a patient with congenital or valvular heart disease develops certain features. These include:

Evidence of infection

- Vague symptoms such as unusual tiredness, fatigue, lassitude, loss of appetite, loss of weight
- Persistent or intermittent low-grade or high-grade **fever** (84%) with night sweats, chills, and rigors
- **Clubbing (Fig. 7.45A)** in fingers is a late sign and is found only in 10–20% of patients.
- **Splenomegaly:** Spleen is frequently palpable and the liver may also be enlarged.
- Brownish pigmentation of face and limbs

Evidence of new valve lesion (regurgitant)/murmurs or change of murmur

- **New murmur:** Particularly, a diastolic murmur is the diagnostic feature. It is detected in about 15% of patients during initial period. However, most patients develop a murmur during the course of the disease.
- **Changing murmurs:** Apart from integrity of valves, factors such as change in cardiac output, temperature, and hematocrit may be responsible for change of murmurs. However, new regurgitant murmur developing in acute sepsis is almost diagnostic of endocarditis.

Evidence of embolism

- **Cutaneous manifestations:** These include the following:
  - **Purpura and petechiae** (20–40%) (**Fig. 7.45B**), subconjunctival splinter (**Fig. 7.45C**), or subungual splinter hemorrhages due to microthromboemboli
  - **Janeway lesions:** Erythematous, nontender nodules, on palms or soles
  - **Ocular manifestations:** Roth spot (**Fig. 7.45D**) are flame-shaped hemorrhages which may occasionally appear like cotton wool spots.
- **Septic infarcts/abscess:** Spleen (painful splenomegaly), kidney (loin pain, hematuria, and renal failure), brain (convulsions, hemiplegia, aphasia, loss of vision, and cerebellar disturbances), peripheral arteries (claudication, absence of peripheral pulses, and gangrene), or lungs (pulmonary infarction, pleurisy, and pleural effusion due to right-sided endocarditis)
- **Mycotic aneurysms**

Evidence of immunological phenomena

- **Osler nodes (Fig. 7.45E):** Tender, small, painful, swollen, purplish/erythematous subcutaneous papules/nodules in pulp of distal fingers due to hypersensitive angiitis. Cultures are negative and persist for hours to several days.
- **Roth spots (Fig. 7.45F)** are circular retinal hemorrhages with white or pale centers spots composed of fibrin.
- **Focal segmental glomerulonephritis:** Develop due to deposition of antigen-antibody complexes in glomeruli. Grossly, the outer surface of kidney develops a flea-bitten appearance due to patchy hemorrhagic foci involving the glomeruli. Patents develop **microscopic hematuria.**

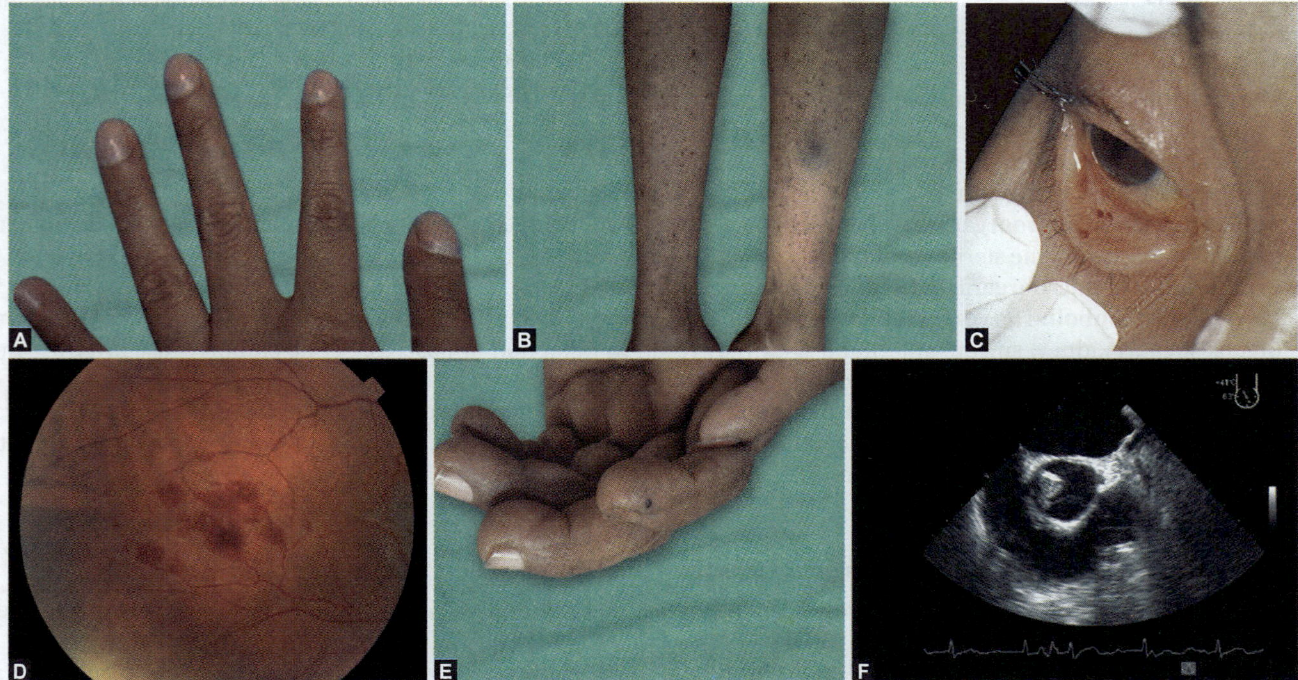

FIGS. 7.45A TO F: Signs of infective endocarditis: (A) Clubbing; (B) Petechiae; (C) Subconjunctival hemorrhage; (D) Roth spots; (E) Osler's nodes; (F) Echocardiography showing vegetation.

Investigations

Aim of investigations: (1) To confirm the diagnosis of infective endocarditis, (2) to identify the causative organism for appropriate therapy, and (3) to assess the patient's response to therapy.

Q. Write a short essay/note on tests for infective endocarditis.

Microbiological Investigations

- ***Blood cultures*** are the crucial investigations in infective endocarditis (1) to identify the causative microorganism, and (2) guide antibiotic therapy. At least three sets of blood samples for cultures should be taken from different venipuncture sites over 24 hours before commencing therapy. Aseptic technique should be followed and the risk of contaminants should be minimized. Blood samples for cultures should not be obtained from an in-dwelling line. Both aerobic and anaerobic cultures are needed.
- ***Serological tests*** are useful if there is suspicion of diagnosis and the cultures are negative. Culture-negative cases may be due to organisms which will not grow in blood cultures such as *Coxiella, Bartonella, Legionella, and Chlamydia.*
- ***Electrocardiogram:*** ECG will help to detect complications such as conduction abnormalities (AV block) and occasionally myocardial infarction due to emboli. PR prolongation/heart block is associated with aortic root abscess.
- ***Chest X-ray:*** It may show evidence of cardiac failure, cardiomegaly, and pulmonary edema in left-sided disease, pulmonary emboli/abscess in right-sided disease.
- ***Echocardiography:*** It plays a key role to identify the presence and size of vegetations (**Fig. 7.45F**), assess valve damage, abscess formation, detect intracardiac complications, and assess cardiac function. However, if vegetations are not detected, the diagnosis of endocarditis cannot be excluded.
    - **Transthoracic echocardiography (TTE):** It is a first-line noninvasive imaging test with sensitivity of 60–75% and high specificity for demonstrating vegetations, valvular dysfunction, ventricular function, and abscesses. Vegetations as small as 2–4 mm can be detected.
    - **Transesophageal echocardiography (TOE):** It is a second-line invasive imaging test with greater sensitivity (>90%) and specificity than TTE. It can detect vegetations even smaller ones (1–1.5 mm), aortic root abscess, and prosthetic valve endocarditis.
- ***Complete blood counts:*** May show normocytic normochromic anemia (reduced hemoglobin) and increased WBC counts and increased or reduced platelets
- ***Urea and creatinine:*** May be increased due to glomerulonephritis
- ***Liver biochemistry:*** Serum alkaline phosphatase may be increased.
- ***Inflammatory markers:*** Increased erythrocyte sedimentation rate (ESR) and C-reactive protein are observed. CRP also helps in monitoring response to therapy; it is reduced in response to therapy and increased with relapse.
- ***Urine:*** Proteinuria and hematuria occur frequently.

Modified Duke Criteria for the Diagnosis of Infective Endocarditis (Table 7.78)

- Diagnosis by these guidelines requires either pathologic or clinical criteria
- *If clinical criteria are used:*
    - *Definite endocarditis, two major, or one major + three minor, or five minor criteria are required for diagnosis*
    - *Possible endocarditis = One major and one minor, or three minor criteria*

Complications

Q. Write a short essay/note on complications of infective endocarditis.

- ***Cardiac complications:*** These are **due to direct valvular damage** and **consequences of local invasion.** The infection may spread locally from valve into the valve ring, adjacent mural endocardium, or chordae tendineae.
    - **Ring abscess:** Vegetations may erode the **underlying myocardium** and produce an **abscess** which is known as ring abscess.
    - **Perforation and rupture:** May involve valve leaflets, aorta, or interventricular septa (depending on the site of infection)
    - **Myocardial abscess** usually due to *S. aureus*
    - **Suppurative pericarditis**
    - **Valvular dysfunction and heart failure:** Stenosis or insufficiency. Heart failure is most common and is due to valvular regurgitation.
    - Prosthetic dehiscence
    - Valvular distortion/destruction chordal rupture
    - Conduction abnormalities
    - Purulent pericarditis

TABLE 7.78: Modified Duke criteria for the diagnosis of infective endocarditis (IE).

Clinical criteria

Major:

Positive blood cultures for IE (one of the following):

Typical microorganisms consistent with IE from two separate blood cultures:

- *Staphylococcus aureus*
- *Viridans Streptococci*
- *Streptococcus gallolyticus* (formerly *S. bovis*), including nutritional variant strains *(Granulicatella* spp and *Abiotrophia defectiva)*
- *HACEK* group: *Haemophilus* spp, *Aggregatibacter* (formerly *Actinobacillus actinomycetes comitans), Cardiobacterium hominis, Eikenella* spp., and *Kingella kingae*
- Community-acquired *Enterococci*, in the absence of a primary focus; **OR**

Persistently positive blood culture:

- For organisms that are typical causes of IE: At least two positive blood cultures from blood samples drawn >12 hours apart
- For organisms that are more commonly skin contaminants: Three or a majority of >4 separate blood cultures (with first and last drawn at least 1 hour apart)

Single positive blood culture for *Coxiella burnetii* or phase I IgG antibody titer >1:800

Evidence of endocardial involvement (one of the following):

Echocardiogram positive for IE:

- Vegetation (oscillating intracardiac mass on a valve or on supporting structures, in the path of regurgitant jets, or on implanted material, in the absence of an alternative anatomic explanation) **OR**
- Abscess **OR**
- New partial dehiscence of prosthetic valve

New valvular regurgitation

Increase in or change in pre-existing murmur not sufficient

Minor:

- Fever >38°C (100.4°F)
- Predisposition: Predisposing heart lesion or intravenous drug use
- Vascular phenomena: Arterial petechiae, subungual/splinter hemorrhages, emboli, septic pulmonary infarcts, mycotic aneurysm, intracranial hemorrhage, conjunctival hemorrhages, and Janeway lesions
- Immunological phenomena: Focal segmental glomerulonephritis, Osler nodes, and Roth spots
- Microbiologic evidence, including a single culture positive but not meeting a major criterion, or for an unusual organism that can cause infective endocarditis

Pathologic criteria

Demonstration of microorganisms by culture or histologic examination in:

- Vegetation
- Embolus from a vegetation
- Intracardiac abscess

Histological confirmation of active endocarditis in vegetation or intracardiac abscess

(****HACEK:*** **H** = *Haemophilus parainfluenzae, Haemophilus aphrophilus, Haemophilus paraphrophilus, Haemophilus influenzae;* **A** = *Actinobacillus actinomycetemcomitans;* **C** = *Cardiobacterium hominis;* **E** = *Eikenella corrodens;* **K** = *Kingella kingae, Kingella denitrificans)*

- ***Renal:*** At least in four forms: (1) prerenal due to low cardiac output, (2) microabscess formation secondary to septic emboli, (3) glomerular dysfunction as a result of circulating immune complexes, and (4) renal failure as a result of antibiotics.
- ***Embolic events*** (discussed under evidence of embolism—subacute endocarditis)
  - Vegetations are usually friable and likely to be break, detach, and cause embolism
  - **Embolic complications** (due to septic emboli): Emboli contain large numbers of virulent organisms → abscesses develop at the sites of arrest of the emboli. Septic emboli from the left side of the heart: They enter systemic circulation and its consequences are:
    - Septic infarcts (e.g., spleen, kidney, or brain)
    - Mycotic aneurysms
    - Small emboli (microthromboemboli) may produce: (1) splinter or subungual hemorrhages, and (2) Janeway lesions
    - Septic emboli from the right side of the heart: They enter pulmonary circulation → lead to pulmonary abscess.
- ***Immunological phenomena:***
  - **Focal segmental glomerulonephritis:** Develop due to deposition of antigen-antibody complexes in glomeruli. Grossly, the outer surface of kidney develops a flea-bitten appearance due to patchy hemorrhagic foci involving the glomeruli.
  - **Osler nodes:** They are small, tender subcutaneous nodules in the pulp of the digits and persist for hours to several days.
  - **Roth spots** are retinal hemorrhages with white or pale centers composed of fibrin.

Q. Write a short essay/note on management of infective endocarditis/subacute infective endocarditis.

Management

Medical treatment

- Blood should be collected for cultures before starting the empirical antibiotic therapy. However, this should not delay therapy in unstable patients.

- If source of infection is identified, it should be removed as soon as possible (e.g., tooth with an apical abscess should be extracted).
- **Empirical treatment regimen:** Penicillins are fundamental to the therapy of bacterial endocarditis. Empirical treatment regimen depends on the mode of presentation, the suspected organism, and whether the patient has a prosthetic valve or penicillin allergy (**Table 7.79**).

TABLE 7.79: Antimicrobial treatment of common causative organisms in infective endocarditis.

Organism	***Antimicrobial treatment with dose and duration***
Infective endocarditis awaiting culture report, no suspicion of staphylococci	Benzylpenicillin IV 1.2 g 4 hourly, 4–6 weeks **PLUS** Gentamicin IV 80 mg 12 hourly, 2–6 weeks
	OR Amoxicillin/clavulanate 12 g/day in four divided doses plus gentamicin 1 mg/kg thrice a day for 4–6 weeks
Suspected staphylococcal endocarditis (IVDU, recent intravascular devices or cardiac surgery, acute infection)	Vancomycin IV 1 g 12 hourly (30 mg/kg/day—(not to exceed 2 g/day) for 6 weeks **PLUS** gentamicin IV 80–120 mg 8 hourly for 1–2 weeks. In prosthetic valve endocarditis, add rifampicin 20 mg/kg/day in two divided doses.
Streptococci highly sensitive to penicillin	Benzylpenicillin IV 1.2 g 4 hourly for 4 weeks **OR** Ceftriaxone IV 2 g once a day for 4 weeks **OR** Benzylpenicillin or ceftriaxone for 2 weeks plus gentamicin 3 mg/kg once a day for 2 weeks Vancomycin 30 mg/kg/day in two divided doses (not to exceed 2 g/day) for 4 weeks in penicillin-sensitive patients
Streptococci less sensitive to penicillin	Benzylpenicillin IV 1.2 g 4 hourly or ceftriaxone IV 2 g for 4–6 weeks and gentamicin 3 mg/kg/day (as single infusion) for at least 2 weeks
Anaerobic streptococci	Benzylpenicillin IV 1.2 g 4 hourly, metronidazole
Staphylococcal endocarditis (methicillin-sensitive)	Cloxacillin 2 g 4 hourly **OR** Cefazolin 2 g 8 hourly, vancomycin 1 g 12 hourly, **OR** Flucloxacillin 2 g 4 hourly **OR** Benzylpenicillin 1.2 g 4 hourly for 4–6 weeks **PLUS** gentamicin 80–120 mg (1mg/kg) three times a day for 3–5 days
Enterococcal endocarditis	Ampicillin/amoxicillin 2 g 4 hourly for 4–6 weeks **OR** vancomycin 1 g twice daily **PLUS** Gentamicin 1 mg/kg three times a day for 6 weeks
Candida	Amphotericin B 1 mg/kg QID 2 weeks' maximum up to 4 weeks. Do not exceed 50 mg/day Flucytosine 150 mg/kg oral for 4 days
Coxiella burnetii	Doxycycline 100 mg twice daily with either hydroxychloroquine 600 mg daily **OR** rifampin (900 mg/day) for 18–24 months
Bartonella	Doxycycline (100 mg PO or IV twice daily) **PLUS** gentamicin (1 mg/kg IV every 8 hours) for 14 days

Prognosis: It is fatal in about 20% patients and higher in those with prosthetic valve endocarditis and those infected with antibiotic-resistant organisms.

Surgical treatment (Box 7.46)

Decisions to carry out surgical intervention in patients with infective endocarditis should take into account the (1) patient specific features such as age, noncardiac morbidities, presence of prosthetic material or cardiac failure, and (2) infective endocarditis features such as causative organism, size of vegetation, presence of perivalvular infection, and systemic embolization.

Cardiac surgery consists of debridement of infected material and valve replacement. Antimicrobial therapy should be started before surgery.

Box 7.46: Indications for surgical treatment in infective endocarditis.

- Endocarditis of prosthetic valve
- Large vegetations
  - Left-sided large vegetation (10 mm) with an episode of embolization
  - Very large (15 mm) and mobile vegetation (high-risk of embolism)
- Progressive cardiac failure due to valvular damage
- Active infection persisting, i.e., fever and evidence of bacteremia for >7–10 days in spite of adequate antibiotic treatment
- Abscess formation, perivalvular involvement, *S. aureus*, and fungal endocarditis

Bacterial Endocarditis Prophylaxis

Q. Write a short essay/note on antibiotic prophylaxis against infective endocarditis during dental procedure/during urogenital surgery.

Q. Write a short essay/note on prophylaxis of infective endocarditis.

Prophylaxis is not needed for routine local anesthetic injections through noninfected tissue, placement of removable prosthodontic or orthodontic appliances, shedding of deciduous teeth, vaginal delivery, and hysterectomy or tattooing, bronchoscopy, laryngoscopy, endotracheal intubation, cystoscopy, colonoscopy, or skin suturing.

Indications

Cardiac lesions: For which antibiotic prophylaxis is advised is listed in **Box 7.47**.

Q. Write a short note on infective endocarditis/subacute infective endocarditis (SBE) prophylaxis.

- **Procedures:** Endocarditis prophylaxis is advised in patient at high or moderate risk for endocarditis. These include following procedures:

- **Dental procedures:** Extraction, periodontal procedures, implant placement, root canal instrumentation, and intraligamentary injections (anesthetic)
- **Respiratory procedure:** Bronchoscopy with rigid bronchoscope operations involving the mucosa
- **Gastrointestinal procedures:** Sclerotherapy of esophageal varices, stricture dilation, ERCP, biliary tract surgery, and surgery involving mucosa
- **Genitourinary procedures:** Urethral dilation, prostate or urethral surgery, or cystoscopy

Antibiotic Regiment for Prophylaxis of Endocarditis in Adults at Moderate- or High-risk

Oral cavity, respiratory tract, or esophageal procedures

- Standard regimen: **Amoxicillin 2.0 g PO 1 hour before procedure**
- Inability to take oral medication: Ampicillin 2.0 g IV or IM within 30 minutes of procedure
- Penicillin allergy:
  - Clarithromycin 500 mg PO 1 hour before procedure
  - Cephalexin or cefadroxil 2.0 g PO 1 hour before procedure
  - Clindamycin 600 mg PO 1 hour before procedure or IV 30 minutes before procedure
- Inability to take oral medication: Cefazolin 1.0 g IV or IM 30 minutes before procedure

Note: For patients at high-risk administer of half-dose 6 hours after the initial dose.

Box 7.47: Infective endocarditis prophylaxis.

High-risk group:
- Prosthetic heart valves
- Prior bacterial endocarditis
- Complex cyanotic congenital heart disease
- Surgically constructed systemic-pulmonary shunts
- Repaired shunts within 6 months
- Valvulopathy after cardiac transplantation

Moderate-risk group:
- Congenital cardiac malformations (other than those listed in other two groups)
- Acquired valvular dysfunction (e.g., rheumatic heart disease)
- Hypertrophic cardiomyopathy
- Mitral valve prolapse with valvular regurgitation, thickened leaflets, or both

Negligible-risk group:
- Isolated secundum atrial septum defect
- Surgical repair of atrial septal defect, ventricular septal defect, or patent ductus arteriosus
- Previous coronary artery bypass graft surgery
- Mitral valve prolapse without valvular regurgitation
- Physiologic, functional, or innocent heart murmurs
- Previous Kawasaki syndrome without valvular dysfunction
- Previous rheumatic fever without valvular dysfunction
- Cardiac pacemakers (intravascular and epicardial) and implanted defibrillators

Genitourinary and Gastrointestinal Tract Procedure

- High-risk patients: Ampicillin 2.0 g IV or IM plus gentamicin 1.5 mg/kg IV or IM within 30 minutes of procedure. Repeat ampicillin, 1.0 g IV or IM or amoxicillin 1.0 g PO 6 hours later
- High-risk penicillin-allergic patients: Vancomycin 1.0 g IV or 1M over 1–2 hours plus gentamicin 1.5 m/kg IV or IM within 30 minutes before procedure, no second dose recommended
- Moderate-risk patients: Amoxicillin 2.0 g PO 1 hour before procedure or ampicillin 2.0 g IV or IM 30 minutes before procedure
- Moderate-risk, penicillin-allergic patients: Vancomycin 1.0 g IV inferred over 1–2 hours and completed within 30 minutes of procedures.

Culture-Negative Infective Endocarditis

Culture-negative infective endocarditis (IE) is defined as endocarditis without etiology following inoculation of three blood samples in a standard blood culture system (e.g., negative cultures after 7 days).

Reasons for culture-negative in infective endocarditis:
- Administration of antimicrobial agents prior to blood culture incubation
- Inadequate microbiological techniques
- Infection with highly fastidious bacteria or nonbacterial pathogens (e.g., fungi)

Noninfective Endocarditis

Q. Write a short essay/note on noninfective endocarditis.

It is characterized by the formation of sterile platelet and fibrin thrombi on cardiac valves and adjacent endocardium.
- It develops in response to trauma, circulating immune complexes, vasculitis, or a hypercoagulable state
- Symptoms are caused due to systemic arterial embolism.
- Diagnosis is by echocardiography and negative blood cultures.

Marantic Endocarditis (Nonbacterial Thrombotic Endocarditis—NBTE)

Etiology

- NBTE is often encountered in a number of conditions. These include debilitated patients with cancer or sepsis, hence previously termed **marantic endocarditis** (root word **marasmus,** relating to malnutrition). It frequently develops

concomitantly with deep venous thrombosis, pulmonary emboli, or underlying systemic hypercoagulable state and advanced malignancy. There is a striking association with mucinous adenocarcinomas, potentially relating to the procoagulant effects of tumor-derived mucin or tissue.
- Other less common causes include systemic lupus erythematosus, antiphospholipid syndrome, rheumatic heart disease, rheumatoid arthritis, and burns.

Vegetations are small, bland, and usually attached to the line of closure of valve leaflets.

Treatment: Consists of systemic anticoagulant therapy and treatment of the underlying malignancy or associated condition.

Libman–Sacks Endocarditis
- Libman–Sacks endocarditis (otherwise known as verrucous endocarditis) is characteristic cardiac manifestation of the autoimmune disease such as systemic lupus erythematosus.
- Pathogenesis: It produced due to circulating immune complexes.
- Endocarditis: It is characterized by small- or medium-sized vegetations on either side of the valve leaflets. They appear mulberry-like clusters of verrucae and consist of accumulations of immune complexes and mononuclear cells.

HEART FAILURE

Q. Define heart failure. Discuss the types, common cause, pathophysiology, clinical features, and management of heart failure.

Q. Describe the etiology, clinical features, and management of chronic heart failure. Mention the factors which will acutely decompensate a patient with chronic stable heart failure.

Q. Discuss the symptoms and signs of heart failure. Outline the rational management.

Q. Describe the etiology, classification, clinical features, diagnosis, and management of congestive cardiac failure (heart failure).

Q. Outline the clinical features, investigations, and treatment of congestive cardiac failure with hypertensive heart disease.

Definition

Heart failure or cardiac failure is the pathophysiological process in which the heart as a pump is unable to meet the metabolic requirements of the tissue for oxygen and substrates despite the venous return to heart is either normal or increased.
- It is a complex syndrome that can result from any structural or functional cardiac disorder. In heart failure, **heart is unable to pump blood at a rate of sufficient to meet the metabolic demands of the tissues** or can do so only at an elevated filling pressure.
- Older term **congestive heart failure** (CHF) should be avoided because not all patients with heart failure have volume overload. Hence, the term heart failure is preferred.
- Heart failure is the **common end stage** of many forms of **chronic heart disease** and most **common reason for hospitalization in adults >65 years of age.**
- Heart failure **usually develops insidiously** from the cumulative effects of chronic work overload (e.g., in valve disease or hypertension) or ischemic heart disease (e.g., following myocardial infarction with heart damage). However, acute hemodynamic stresses, such as fluid overload, sudden valvular dysfunction, or myocardial infarction, can cause sudden heart failure.

Pathophysiology

Q. Write a short essay/note on pathophysiology of heart failure.

- Cardiac output is determined by preload (the volume and pressure of blood in the ventricles at the end of diastole), afterload (the volume and pressure of blood in the ventricles during systole), and myocardial contractility.
- Myocardial contractility (inotropic state): It depends on the adrenergic nervous activity and the levels of circulating catecholamines.

Heart Failure

- In the intact heart, myocardial failure causes reduction of the volume of blood ejected with each heartbeat and an increase in the volume of blood remaining after systole. This increased diastolic volume stretches the myocardial fibers and restores the myocardial contraction. However, the failing myocardium results in myocardial depression (of the ventricles).
- Heart failure is a progressive disorder that is initiated after an index event that either damages the heart muscle (with loss of functioning cardiac myocytes) or disturbs the myocardial ability to generate force (prevents the heart from contracting

normally). The common feature of these events is a decrease in the pumping capacity of the heart. The compensatory mechanisms include tachycardia, increased myocardial contractility, and activation of neurohumoral systems.

If the **heart failure progresses,** the compensatory mechanisms are overwhelmed and **become pathological.** Thus, there is pathological peripheral vasoconstriction and sodium retention. Heart failure is the **common end stage** of many forms of **chronic heart disease.**

Heart failure **usually develops insidiously** from the cumulative effects of chronic work overload (e.g., in valve disease or hypertension) or ischemic heart disease (e.g., following myocardial infarction with heart damage). However, acute hemodynamic stresses, such as fluid overload, sudden valvular dysfunction, or myocardial infarction, can cause sudden heart failure.

Q. Write a short note on ventricular remodeling/cardiac remodeling.

Ventricular remodeling/cardiac remodeling: Refers to the changes in size, shape, structure, and physiology of the heart after injury to the myocardium.

- Left ventricular remodeling is the process by which mechanical, neurohormonal, and possibly genetic factors alter ventricular size, shape, and function.
- Remodeling occurs in several clinical conditions, including myocardial infarction, hypertension, cardiomyopathy, and valvular heart disease.
- It is characterized by *hypertrophy, loss of myocytes, and increased interstitial fibrosis.*

Mechanism of heart failure is depicted in **Flowchart 7.5**.

FLOWCHART 7.5: Mechanism of heart failure.

Left ventricular failure
• Ischemic heart disease
• Valvular heart disease
• Myocarditis
• Restrictive pericarditis

Reduced cardiac output

Right ventricular failure
• Cor pulmonale
• Right-sided valvular heart disease
• Right-sided disease of myocardium
• Pulmonary hypertension

Compensatory mechanisms

Neurohumoral activation

Cardiac compensatory mechanisms

Sympathetic nervous system

Activation of renin-angiotensin-aldosterone mechanism
Vasopressin system
Endothelin system

Tachycardia and increased myocardial contractility

Vasoconstriction

Sodium and water retension

Increased intravascular volume

Increased cardiac workload

Increased blood pressure and cardiac workload

Compensatory hypertrophy and dilatation

Further stress on myocardium

Congestive heart failure

Types of Heart Failure

Q. Write a short note on types of heart failure.

Depending on Output

- **Low-output heart failure:**
  - **Systolic heart failure:** Characterized by decreased cardiac output and decreased left ventricular ejection fraction
  - **Diastolic heart failure:** Characterized by elevated left and right ventricular end-diastolic pressures and may have normal left ventricular ejection fraction

- **High-output heart failure:** Characterized by failure of the heart to maintain sufficient circulation despite an increased cardiac output *(defined as cardiac output >8 L/minute or a cardiac index >3.9 L/minute/m²)*. Examples include cardiac failure associated with hyperthyroidism, anemia, pregnancy, arteriovenous fistulae, beriberi, and Paget's disease.

Diastolic and Systolic Dysfunction

- **Systolic dysfunction:** Systolic heart failure is characterized by an abnormality of **ventricular contraction.** The ejection fraction is usually below 40%. Causes include coronary artery disease, hypertension, and valvular heart disease.
- **Diastolic dysfunction:** Characterized by an impaired **ventricular relaxation** and increased ventricular stiffness resulting in reduced filling (diastolic dysfunction). Causes include hypertension, coronary artery disease, hypertrophic obstructive cardiomyopathy (HOCM), and restrictive cardiomyopathy.

Acute and Chronic Heart Failure

- **Acute heart failure** is characterized by sudden development of heart failure. This suddenly reduces cardiac output and systemic hypotension without peripheral edema. Examples include acute myocardial infarction and rupture of a cardiac valve. Acute left heart failure may develop either de novo or as an acute decompensated episode, on a background of chronic heart failure (acute-on chronic heart failure).
- **Chronic heart failure** is characterized by gradual development of heart failure and systemic arterial pressure is well maintained, but edema develops. Examples include dilated cardiomyopathy and multivalvular disease.
- **Compensated heart failure** is the term used to describe the condition of those with impaired cardiac function, in whom adaptive/compensatory changes have prevented the development of overt heart failure. Severe overt or acute heart failure may be precipitated by minor insult such as an infection or development of atrial fibrillation.

Left-sided, Right-sided, and Biventricular Heart Failure

The left side of the heart consists of the functional unit of the left atrium, left ventricle, and mitral and aortic valves. The right side of the heart consists of the right atrium, right ventricle, and tricuspid and pulmonary valves.

- **Left-sided (left ventricular) heart failure** is characterized by:
  - Reduction in left ventricular output
  - **Increase in left atrial and pulmonary venous pressure:** An acute increase in left atrial pressure produces pulmonary congestion or pulmonary edema (e.g., myocardial infarction). A more gradual increase in left atrial pressure leads to reflex pulmonary vasoconstriction, which prevents the development pulmonary edema (e.g., in mitral stenosis and aortic stenosis). This increases pulmonary vascular resistance and leads to pulmonary hypertension, which in turn can impair the function of right ventricle.
- **Right-sided (right ventricular) heart failure** is characterized by:
  - Reduction in right ventricular output
  - Increase in right atrial and systemic venous pressure
  - Causes of isolated right heart failure, e.g., chronic lung disease (cor pulmonale), multiple pulmonary embolism, and pulmonary valvular stenosis
- **Biventricular heart failure** is characterized by failure of the ventricles of the left and the right heart.
  - Dilated cardiomyopathy or ischemic heart disease, affects both ventricles
  - Disease of the left heart leads to chronic elevation of the left atrial pressure, pulmonary hypertension, and leading to right heart failure.

Forward and Backward Heart Failure

- Forward heart failure is characterized by decreased cardiac output, inadequate perfusion of organs that causes poor tissue perfusion. Reduced renal perfusion activates renin–angiotensin–aldosterone system resulting in excessive absorption of sodium by renal tubules.
- Backward heart failure is characterized by a normal cardiac output, severe salt and water retention, and venous congestion in the pulmonary and systemic circulation.

Causes of heart failure are listed in **Table 7.80**.

Q. Write a short note on causes of heart failure.

In practice, the most common causes of heart failure are ischemic heart disease and hypertensive heart diseases.

Q. Write a short essay/note on factors that precipitate heart failure.

Factors that may precipitate or aggravate heart failure in preexisting heart disease (Box 7.48).
Risk factors for heart failure: Hypertension, diabetes mellitus, use of cardiotoxic substances (e.g., alcohol, tobacco, and cocaine), hyperlipidemia, and coronary artery disease

TABLE 7.80: Causes of heart failure.

Reduced Ejection Fraction (<40% HFrEF)	
➢ **Coronary artery disease:** Myocardial infarction, myocardial ischemia	➢ **Chronic pressure overload:** Hypertension, obstructive valvular disease (e.g., mitral/tricuspid stenosis), and endomyocardial fibrosis
➢ **Chronic volume overload of ventricle:** Regurgitant valvular disease (e.g., mitral/aortic regurgitation), left-to-right shunt (e.g., ventricular septal defect, patent ductus arteriosus, and atrial septal defect)	➢ **Chronic lung disease:** Cor pulmonale, pulmonary vascular disorders
➢ **Nonischemic dilated cardiomyopathy**	➢ Chagas disease
➢ **Toxic/drug-induced damage**	
Preserved ejection fraction (EF >50%)	**Heart failure with mid-range EF (HFmrEF):** EF 41–49%
➢ Pathologic hypertrophy, aging, and restrictive cardiomyopathy	
High-output states	
➢ Metabolic disorders: Thyrotoxicosis	➢ Chronic anemia
➢ Nutritional disorders (beriberi)	

(HFrEF: heart failure with reduced ejection fraction)

Box 7.48: Precipitating factors for heart failure.

- Intercurrent illness, e.g., **infection**
- Supervening heart diseases, e.g., myocardial ischemia or **infarction,** myocarditis, and infective endocarditis
- Cardiac **arrhythmia,** e.g., atrial fibrillation
- Poor compliance with therapy
- Administration of a drug with negative inotropic (β-blocker), disopyramide, or fluid-retaining properties [nonsteroidal anti-inflammatory drugs (NSAIDs) and corticosteroids]
- Pulmonary embolism
- Conditions associated with increased metabolic demand, e.g., **anemia** pregnancy and thyrotoxicosis
- IV fluid overload, e.g., postoperative IV infusion
- Systemic hypertension
- Excess salt intake
- Physical and emotional stress

(IV: intravenous)

TABLE 7.81: Symptoms and signs of heart failure.

Symptoms	*Signs*	
Left ventricular (LV) failure		
Dyspnea: ➢ Exertional dyspnea ➢ Orthopnea ➢ Paroxysmal nocturnal dyspnea ➢ Acute pulmonary edema Cough Fatigue Decreased urine output	Cardiac sign: ➢ Enlargement of LV ➢ Gallop rhythm S_3 ➢ Systolic murmur in apex Pulmonary sign: ➢ Crepitations Pleural effusion	**Think FACES:** **F**atigue, **A**ctivities limited, **C**hest congestion, **E**dema or ankle swelling, and **S**hortness of breath
Right ventricular failure		
Leg swelling Symptom of gastrointestinal—anorexia Symptom of renal origin—oliguria Pain in right hypochondrium Dyspnea	Raised JVP Hepatojugular reflux positive Hepatomegaly Edema Pleural fluid and ascites	

(JVP: jugular venous pressure)

Clinical Manifestations of Heart Failure (Table 7.81)

Q. Write a short essay/note on clinical features (symptoms and signs) of heart failure and acute left ventricular failure.

Symptoms

Dyspnea

- Exertional dyspnea
- Orthopnea, bendopnea
- Paroxysmal nocturnal dyspnea (PND)
- Cardiac asthma is closely related to PND and nocturnal cough. It is characterized by wheezing (secondary to bronchospasm) which is most prominent at night. Acute pulmonary edema represents a severe form of cardiac asthma.
- Acute pulmonary edema
- Cheyne-Stokes respiration.

Nocturia

It is observed during early heart failure. It is because renal perfusion and diuresis is better at night when the patient is supine. Cerebral symptoms includes confusion, difficulty in concentration, impaired memory, headache, insomnia, and anxiety. These symptoms may be produced due to arterial hypoxemia and reduced cerebral perfusion.

Nonspecific symptoms

- Fatigue due to low cardiac output and weakness due to decreased perfusion of skeletal muscles
- Low-grade fever due to reduction of cutaneous blood flow
- Anorexia, nausea, and abdominal fullness/pain due to congestion of liver and portal venous system.

Signs

Dependent/cardiac edema

- **Dependent/cardiac edema:** Due to gravity, fluid accumulates over dependent parts of the body. In ambulant patients, it is found symmetrically in the both legs, particularly in the pretibial region and around the ankles. It is less in the morning and become more toward the evening. In bedridden patients, it is observed in the sacral region.
- **Anasarca:** In advanced heart failure, the fluid accumulating throughout the body and is severe termed as anasarca. Face and upper limbs are usually spared until the terminal stages.

Cyanosis

It is usually observed in lips and nail beds. The extremities appear cold and pale due to reduced blood flow.

Pulse

Pulse volume is reduced and pulsus alternans is a sign of severe heart failure.

Blood pressure

- Reduced pulse pressure is due to reduced stroke volume.
- Occasionally, there may be mild elevation of diastolic blood pressure due to generalized vasoconstriction.
- Hypotension is prominent in acute heart failure.

Jugular venous pressure (JVP)

- JVP is raised because of elevated systemic venous pressure.
- JVP may not be raised at rest during early stages of heart failure. It may be demonstrated:
  - During and immediately after exercise
  - With sustained pressure on the abdomen (positive hepatojugular or abdominojugular reflux).

Third and fourth heart sound

- Presence of a third heart sound in highly suggestive of heart failure
- Triple/quadruple/summation gallop is seen.

Respiratory system

- **Percussion:** Dull percussion notes over the bases of lungs (infrascapular, infra-axillary areas)
- **Auscultation:** Inspiratory crepitations over the bases of lungs. If there is pulmonary edema, coarse crepitations are heard widely over both lung fields associated with expiratory rhonchi.

Liver (congestive hepatomegaly)

- **Hypoglycemia** can develop in long-standing cases due to depletion of glycogen stores in liver and increased production of lactic acid from glucose, induced by hypoxia.
- **Jaundice:** Hyperbilirubinemia of both conjugated and unconjugated type may be a late feature. In acute hepatic congestion, jaundice is severe and liver enzymes are markedly elevated.

Effusion

- **Pleural effusion** develops more commonly on the right side and is due to raised pleural capillary pressure and transudation of fluid into pleural space.
- **Ascites** is due to transudation secondary to raised pressure in the hepatic vein, portal veins, and veins draining the peritoneum.
- **Pericardial effusion:** Rare.

Renal system

- Poor renal perfusion leads to oliguria and prerenal azotemia (uremia). Blood urea is usually raised out of proportion to serum creatinine.
- **Urine:** Specific gravity of urine is high, mild proteinuria is seen, and urinary sodium is low.

Cardiac cachexia

Chronic heart failure is sometimes associated with severe anorexia, marked weight loss (cardiac cachexia), impaired absorption due to gastrointestinal congestion, and skeletal muscle atrophy due to immobility.

Framingham Criteria for Diagnosis of Heart Failure (Table 7.82)

The diagnosis of heart failure should not be made on history and clinical findings alone. It requires evidence of cardiac dysfunction (by investigation) and identification of the underlying cause of heart failure in all cases.

TABLE 7.82: Framingham criteria for diagnosis of heart failure.

Major	*Minor*
➢ Paroxysmal nocturnal dyspnea	➢ Extremity edema
➢ Distension of neck vein	➢ Night cough
➢ Rales	➢ Dyspnea on exertion
➢ Cardiomegaly	➢ Hepatomegaly
➢ Acute pulmonary edema	➢ Pleural effusion
➢ S_3 gallop	➢ Vital capacity reduced by one-third from normal
➢ Increased venous pressure (>16 cm H_2O)	➢ Tachycardia (>120 beats per minute)
➢ Positive hepatojugular reflux	
➢ Weight loss >4.5 kg over 5 days' treatment	

Criteria for diagnosis of heart failure: one major + two minor

Investigations in Heart Failure

- **Chest X-ray:** It may reveal cardiomegaly. Other findings include phantom tumor (fluid in horizontal or oblique fissures of lungs which disappears after treatment with diuretics), bat's wing appearance [hazy opacification spreading from the hilar regions on both sides (**Fig. 7.46**)], and pleural effusion (bilateral or unilateral).
- **Electrocardiography:** It may reveal previous MI, active ischemia, ventricular hypertrophy (e.g., due to hypertension), atria abnormality, arrhythmias, and conduction abnormalities (e.g., arrhythmia).
- **Echocardiography** is very useful to: (1) determine the etiology, (2) detect any unsuspected valvular heart disease (e.g., occult mitral stenosis), (3) identify patients who will benefit from long-term drug therapy (e.g., ACE inhibitors), (4) assess cardiac chamber dimension (size and shape), ejection fraction, valvular functions, cardiomyopathies, and regional wall motion abnormalities, and (5) differentiate between systolic and diastolic heart failure.
- **Stress echocardiography:** It helps in assessing the viability in dysfunctional myocardium. Dobutamine stress identifies contractile reserve in stunned or hibernating myocardium.

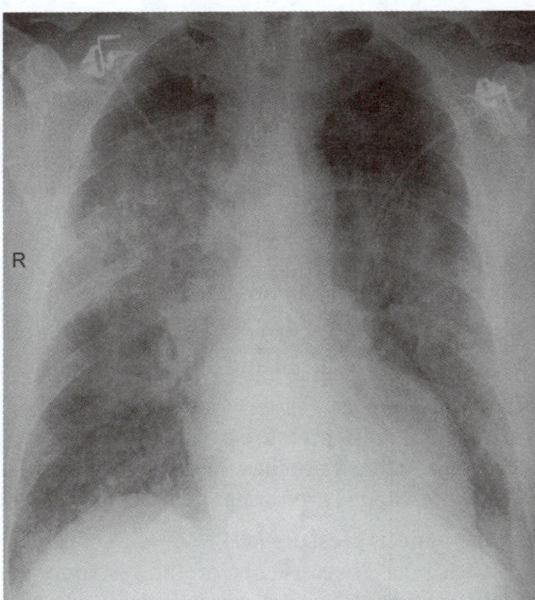

FIG. 7.46: Chest X-ray in heart failure showing bat wing appearance.

- **Nuclear cardiology:** Radionucleotide angiography (RNA) is useful for quantify ventricular ejection fraction, single photon emission computed tomography (SPECT), or positron emission tomography (PET) can reveal myocardial ischemia and viability in dysfunctional myocardium.
- **CMR (cardiac MRI):** It helps to assess the viability in dysfunctional myocardium with the use of dobutamine for contractile reserve or with gadolinium for delayed enhancement ("infarct imaging").
- **Cardiac catheterization:** It is useful in the diagnosis of ischemic heart failure (and suitability for revascularization), measurement of pulmonary artery pressure, left atrial (wedge) pressure, and left ventricular end-diastolic pressure.
- **Cardiac biopsy:** It is useful in the diagnosis of cardiomyopathies (e.g., amyloid) and follow-up of cardiac transplanted patients to assess rejection.
- **Cardiopulmonary exercise testing:** Peak oxygen consumption (VO) is useful in predicting hospital admission and death in heart failure.
- **Ambulatory 24-hour ECG monitoring (Holter):** May be necessary in patients with suspected arrhythmia. It may be useful in severe heart failure or inherited cardiomyopathy to decide the necessity of defibrillator.
- **Brain natriuretic peptide (BNP) or N-terminal portion of proBNF** (NPproBNP) is elevated in heart failure and highly sensitive for the diagnosis of its diagnosis. It is a marker of risk **(>100 pg/mL)** and is useful in the investigation of patients with breathlessness or peripheral edema (to differentiate cardiac from respiratory cause of acute dyspnea).
- **Blood tests:** Full blood count, liver function tests, serum urea, creatinine and electrolytes, cardiac enzymes in acute heart failure, thyroid function may help to establish the nature and severity of the underlying heart disease and detect any complications.
- **Invasive hemodynamic monitoring:** Useful in selected patients with acute heart failure who have persistent symptoms is spite of empiric standard therapies.

Complications in Advanced Heart Failure

- **Renal failure: Cardiorenal syndrome** (poor renal perfusion caused by low cardiac output) may be worsened by therapy [e.g., diuretics, angiotensin-converting enzyme (ACE) inhibitors, and angiotensin receptor blockers].
- **Hypokalemia:** Due to the result of treatment with potassium-losing diuretics or hyperaldosteronism produced by activation of the renin–angiotensin system and impaired aldosterone metabolism due to congestion of liver.
- **Hyperkalemia:** Due to the effects of drugs which promote renal resorption of potassium (e.g., combination of ACE inhibitors or angiotensin receptor blockers, and mineralocorticoid receptor antagonists).
- **Hyponatremia:** May develop in severe heart failure and is a poor prognostic sign. It may be due to diuretics, inappropriate retention of water (due to high ADH secretion), or failure of the cell membrane ion pump.
- **Hepatic dysfunction:** Due to hepatic venous congestion and poor arterial perfusion.
- **Thromboembolism:** Deep vein thrombosis and pulmonary embolism may develop due to the effects of a low cardiac output and immobility. Systemic emboli may develop in patients with atrial fibrillation or flutter, or with intracardiac thrombus complicating conditions such as mitral stenosis, MI, or left ventricular aneurysm.
- **Atrial and ventricular arrhythmias:** Very common and include atrial fibrillation (20%), sudden death (50%) due to a ventricular arrhythmia, ventricular ectopic beats, and nonsustained ventricular tachycardia. They may be due to electrolyte changes (e.g., hypokalemia and hypomagnesemia), the underlying heart disease, and the proarrhythmic effects of sympathetic activation.

Q. Write a short essay on management of congestive heart failure.

Management of Heart Failure

Aim of treatment: (1) Relief of symptoms, (2) prevent and control of disease causing cardiac dysfunction and heart failure, (3) retard disease progression, and (4) improve quality and length of life.

A. ***General Lifestyle Advice/Measures***

- **Education of patients and their relatives:** Explanation of nature of disease, about the causes and treatment of heart failure.
- **Measures to prevent heart failure:** Cessation of smoking and illicit drugs, control of hypertension, diabetes and hypercholesterolemia, and pharmacological treatment following myocardial infarction. Identify and treat any factor that aggravates the heart failure.
- **Treatment of the underlying cause of heart failure (e.g., coronary artery disease):** Wherever possible to prevent progression to heart failure
- **Dietary modifications:** Good general nutrition and maintain desired weight and body mass index. Avoid large meals, foods rich in salt, or added salt. Diet low in fat, rich in fruit and vegetables, and increase fiber. Fluid restriction (limited to 1.5 L) is needed only when heart failure is severe. Alcohol has a negative inotropic effect and should be avoided. Omega-3 polyunsaturated fatty acids reduce mortality and admission.
- **Physical activity, exercise, and emotional rest:**
  - **Physical activity and exercise:** Regular low level endurance exercise (e.g., 20–30 minutes walking three or five times/week at 70–80% of peak heart rate) reverses "deconditioning" of peripheral muscle metabolism and is advisable in patients with compensated heart failure. Avoid strenuous isometric activity.
  - **Bed rest:** Reduces the demands on the heart. Bed rest for a few days is for patients with exacerbations of congestive cardiac failure. However, prolonged bed rest may predispose to deep vein thrombosis. This can be avoided by daily leg exercises, low-dose subcutaneous heparin, and elastic support stockings.

B. ***Drug Therapy/Management***

Function of heart can be improved by increasing contractility, reducing preload or afterload. Drugs that reduce preload are used in patients with high end-diastolic filling pressures and pulmonary or systemic venous congestion. Drugs that reduce afterload or increase myocardial contractility are used in patients with signs and symptoms of a low cardiac output.

- **Diuretic therapy:**
  - In heart failure, diuretics act by increasing the urinary excretion of salt (sodium) and water leading to reduction in blood and plasma volume. Diuretics reduce preload and improves pulmonary and systemic venous congestion. They may also reduce afterload and ventricular volume and increase cardiac efficiency.
  - Loop diuretics (e.g., furosemide 20–40 mg once or twice) and thiazide diuretics (e.g., hydrochlorothiazide 25 mg once or twice, or metolazone 2.5–5 mg OD) are given to patients with fluid overload.
  - In severe heart failure, the combination of a loop and thiazide diuretic may be needed. Regular monitoring of serum electrolytes and renal function is necessary because of risk of hypokalemia and hypomagnesemia.
  - Mineralocorticoid receptor antagonists, such as spironolactone (12.5–25 once or twice), are potassium-sparing diuretics and are beneficial in patients having heart failure with severe left ventricular systolic dysfunction.
- **Angiotensin-converting enzyme inhibitors (ACEI) therapy:**
  - **Mechanism of action:** They prevent the conversion of angiotensin I to angiotensin II. This in turn prevents peripheral vasoconstriction, activation of the sympathetic nervous system, and salt and water retention due to aldosterone release. Thus, they interrupt the vicious circle of neurohumoral activation that is characteristic of moderate and severe heart failure. They also prevent the undesirable activation of the renin-angiotensin system caused by diuretic therapy.
  - **Uses:** ACEIs improve survival in patients in all functional classes (NYHA I - IV) and are given to all patients at risk of developing heart failure. They improve effort tolerance and mortality. They can also improve outcome, prevent the onset of overt heart failure in patients with asymptomatic heart failure following myocardial infarction.
  - **Initiation:** Start low dose; if tolerated then gradual increase in few days to weeks to target dose or maximum tolerable dose with regular blood pressure monitoring. Serum creatinine should be measured concomitantly and potassium-sparing diuretics should be discontinued.
  - **Drugs and dosage:** Captopril (6.25 mg thrice till 50 mg thrice a day), enalapril (2.5 mg twice to 10–20 mg twice a day), lisinopril (2.5–5 mg once to 20–40 mg once a day), and ramipril (1.25–2.5 mg once till 10 mg once a day).
- **Angiotensin II receptor antagonists (ARA)/blockers therapy:**
  - **Indications:** ARAs are indicated as second-line therapy in patients intolerant of ACEI or alternative to ACEI.
  - **Drugs and dosage:** Losartan (25–50 mg once till 50–150 mg once a day), valsartan, and telmisartan. Olmesartan (20–40 mg twice till 160 mg twice).
    - Same initiation and monitoring as ACEI and titration by doubling the dose.
- **Beta-adrenoceptor blocker therapy:**
  - **Indications:** To all patients with current or prior HF and a LVEF ≤40% (HFrEF) in the absence of a contraindication
  - Start low and increase gradually over a 12-week period even during hospitalization.

- Drugs and dosage bisoprolol (1.25–2.5 mg once till 10 mg once), carvedilol (3.125 twice till 50 mg twice), and metoprolol succinate (12.5 once till 200 mg once)

- **Aldosterone receptor antagonists:**
  - **Indications:** NYHA II-IV, EF <35%, no contraindication (GFR >30, creatinine: 2.5 mg/dL male and 2.0 mg/dL female, K<5 mg/dL). They improve survival in patients with heart failure.
  - **Dose:** Spironolactone 12.5–25 mg once till 50 mg daily
  - **Monitoring:** Stop all K+ supplements, check K+, and creatinine 2–3 days after starting then 1 week and every month for 3 months and every 3 months and when clinically indicated.
  - **Side effects:** Increase K+ (10–15%), gynecomastia, or breast pain
- **Digoxin (Cardiac glycoside):**
  - Digoxin is a cardiac glycoside that is used in patients in atrial fibrillation with heart failure. It can be used as add on therapy in symptomatic heart failure patients already receiving ACEI and beta-blockers. No mortality benefit, only decrease in frequency of hospitalizations.
  - No loading required. Usual dose 0.125–0.25 mg daily (low dose 0.125 mg alternate day if >70 years, chronic kidney disease, low lean body mass). Maintain 5–0.9 ng/dL plasma concentration (narrow therapeutic range).
- **Vasodilators and nitrates (Hydralazine Nitrate Combination):**
  - The combination of hydralazine and nitrates reduces afterload and preload. Their use is limited by pharmacological tolerance and hypotension.
  - **Indication:** African-American origin, NYHA III-IV, low EF on ACEI and BB, patients intolerant or contraindication of ACEI or ARA (e.g., in severe renal failure)
  - **Dose:** 37.5 mg hydralazine and 20 mg and isosorbide dinitrate start one tab TID to increase till two tabs TID.
- **Ivabradine:**
  - Ivabradine acts on the inward current if, in the SA node and reduces the heart rate. It reduces hospital admission and mortality rates in patients with heart.
  - It is best given to patients who cannot take β-blockers or in whom the heart rate remains high despite β-blockade. It is not useful in patients with atrial fibrillation.
- **Anticoagulation therapy** is indicated in patients with heart failure who are at risk for thromboembolism. These include patients with atrial fibrillation, valvular heart disease, documented left ventricular thrombus, or a history of embolic stroke.

C. ***Nonpharmacological treatment of heart failure***

Q. Write a short note on implantable cardioverter defibrillator (ICD).

- **Device therapy:**
  - **Implantable cardioverter defibrillator (ICD):** Patients with symptomatic ventricular arrhythmias and heart failure have a very bad prognosis. Irrespective of their response to antiarrhythmic drug therapy, implantation of a cardiac defibrillator improves survival of all these patients. It is indicated in nonischemic or ischemic heart disease (at least 40 days post-MI) with LVEF of <35% with NYHA class II or III symptoms or NYHA 1 with EF <30% on chronic medical therapy, who have reasonable expectation of meaningful survival for >1 year.
  - **Cardiac resynchronization therapy (CRT):**
    - Indicated for patients who have LVEF of 35% or less, sinus rhythm, left bundle-branch block (LBBB) with a QRS duration of 150 ms or greater, and NYHA class II, III, or ambulatory IV symptoms
    - In this, both the LV and RV are paced simultaneously to generate a more coordinated left ventricular contraction and improve cardiac output. It improves symptoms and survival.
- **Coronary revascularization:** Coronary artery disease is the most common cause of heart failure. Patients with angina and left ventricular dysfunction have a higher mortality from surgery (10–20%), but most patients' symptoms and prognosis are improved. Coronary artery bypass surgery or percutaneous coronary intervention may improve function in region of the myocardium that is "hibernating" because of inadequate blood supply. The "hibernating" myocardium can be identified by stress echocardiography and specialized nuclear or MR imaging. Before recommending for surgery factors such as age, symptoms and evidence for reversible myocardial ischemia must be considered.
  - **Hibernating myocardium and myocardial stunning:**
    - **Hibernating myocardium** is the reversible left ventricular dysfunction with decreased myocardial perfusion, which is just sufficient to maintain viability of the heart muscle. It is due to an underlying chronic coronary artery disease. Myocardial hibernation is produced due to repetitive episodes of cardiac stunning which may occur, e.g., with repeated exercise in a patient with coronary artery disease. It responds positively to inotropic stress and indicates the presence of viable heart muscle that may recover after revascularization.
    - **Myocardial stunning** is reversible ventricular dysfunction that persists following an episode of ischemia when the blood flow has returned to normal. This is due to a mismatch between flow and function.

- **Heart (Cardiac) transplantation:**
  - Cardiac transplantation is an established and successful treatment of choice for younger patients with severe intractable heart failure, whose life expectancy is <6 months.
  - **Indications:** Usually, reserved for young patients with severe symptoms despite optimal therapy. Most common indications are coronary artery disease and dilated cardiomyopathy.
  - **Contraindication:** Patients with pulmonary vascular disease due to long-standing left heart failure, complex congenital heart disease (e.g., Eisenmenger's syndrome), or primary pulmonary hypertension
- **Ventricular assist devices (VADs):** There is limited supply of donor organs and VADs take over pumping for the ventricles. Hence, VADs are used as (1) a bridge to cardiac transplantation, (2) potential long-term therapy, and (3) short-term restoration therapy following a potentially reversible insult (e.g., viral myocarditis).

Newer Agents in Heart Failure Management

Q. Discuss newer agents in heart failure management.

- **Nesiritide (recombinant analog of BNP):**
  - **Actions:** (1) Increase natriuresis, diuresis, and cardiac index. (2) Reduce pulmonary capillary wedge pressure, pulmonary artery pressure, pulmonary vascular resistance, and systemic blood pressure in a dose-dependent manner. (3) Reversal of the deleterious neurohormonal response associated with heart failure. (4) Reduce levels of endothelin 1, aldosterone, and norepinephrine.
  - **Advantages:** Does not require ICU admission or invasive monitoring, lower incidence of tachycardia and proarrhythmic effects, and lessen the need for supportive therapies, such as diuretics.
- **Endopeptidase inhibitor (ACE + neutral peptidases),** e.g., omapatrilat
- **Calcium sensitizer:** For example, levosimendan. **Levosimendan** is a novel agent with inotropic properties developed specifically for the management of ADHF (acute decompensated heart failure). It acts by sensitizing troponin C to calcium.
- **Endothelin receptor antagonist:** For example, bosentan and tezosentan. Effective in acute coronary syndromes, acute renal failure, and acute heart failure. Indirectly improve contractility while decreasing pulmonary capillary wedge pressure.
- **Vasopressin antagonists (V2 RA):** For example, tolvaptan, lixivaptan, and conivaptan. It can be used as adjuvant to diuretic in advanced heart failure.
- **Enoximone:** Type 3 phosphodiesterase inhibitor
- **Angiotensin receptor-neprilysin inhibitor:** Sacubitril-valsartan for NYHA class II to IV heart failure with reduced ejection fraction.

Management of heart failure based on symptoms, cardiac output, and pulmonary capillary wedge pressure is depicted in **Figure 7.47**.

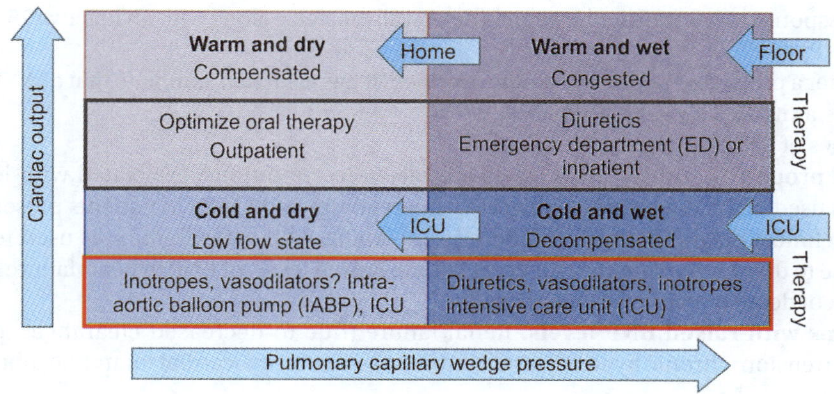

FIG. 7.47: Management of heart failure based on symptoms, cardiac output, and pulmonary capillary wedge pressure.

Refractory Heart Failure

Q. Write a short note on refractory heart failure and its management.

- Optimal "triple therapy" for patients with chronic congestive heart failure (CHF) includes diuretics, digoxin, and either angiotensin-converting enzyme inhibitors or hydralazine plus nitrates.
- Refractory CHF is defined as symptoms of CHF at rest or repeated exacerbations of CHF despite "optimal" triple-drug therapy.

Management: It is managed as end-stage heart failure, i.e., stage D (**Fig. 7.48**). Novel agents and nonpharmacological agents can be tried.

Mechanical circulatory support depending on cause:
Intra-aortic balloon pump (IABP) therapy,
ventricular assist devices (VADs),
Device therapy-permanent,
implantable VAD, transplant/artificial heart

All the measures of Stage A, B and C
temporary intravenous inotropic support

Stage D: End stage disease, refractory symptoms requiring special intervention

Aldosterone receptor antagonists

Depending on the cause revascularization, mitral valve surgery

Device therapy: Cardiac resynchronization therapy (CRT) if there is bundle branch block
Implantable cardioverter defibrillator (ICD)

Dietary restriction of sodium, diuretics and digoxin

ACE inhibitors and beta blockers in all patients. All measures of stage A and B

Stage C: Have symptoms (previous/current) and structural heart damage

Care measures as in Stage A along with ACE inhibitors or ARBs in all patients,
beta blockers in selected patients and spironolactone (if LVEF <40%)
Surgical consultation for coronary artery revascularization and
valve repair/replacement (as appropriate)

Stage B: Asymptomatic but have signs of structural heart damage

Risk factor control: Control of BP and diabetes, weight reduction,
quit smoking, lipid management, atrial fibrillation
ACE inhibitors and ARAs in some patients
Education of patients and their relatives

Stage A: Asymptomatic with no heart damage but have high-risk factors for heart failure

FIG. 7.48: ACC/AHA guidelines (four stages of heart failure and treatment options for systolic heart failure).

Brain Natriuretic Peptide

Q. Write a short essay on brain natriuretic peptide (BNP).

- It is called so because it was first discovered in porcine brain. It is a 32-amino acid peptide predominantly secreted by the left ventricles (as a response to left ventricular stretching or wall tension); along with an inactive 76-amino acid N-terminal fragment (NT-proBNP).
- It is activated only after a prolonged period of volume overload. It has an action similar to that of ANP but greater diagnostic and prognostic value as it has a longer half-life.
- **Utility:** Normal values of BNP: <50 pg/mL or <50 ng/L
  - **Diagnostic and prognostic utility:** BNP levels are raised in conditions associated with left ventricular systolic dysfunction. It is used in the diagnosis of congestive heart failure and useful in patients presenting in the emergency room when the clinical diagnosis of heart failure is uncertain. BNP measurement is used to assess prognosis and monitor response to therapy in patients with heart failure. Raised levels of BNP in heart failure may be associated with an increased risk of death or cardiovascular events.
  - **Other conditions with raised BNP levels:** Renal failure (due to decreased clearance), pulmonary embolism, pulmonary hypertension, chronic hypoxia, atrial fibrillations, acute myocardial infarction, obese patients, and sepsis.

Pulmonary Edema

Q. Describe the clinical features, diagnosis and management of acute pulmonary edema.

Q. Define pulmonary edema. Enumerate the causes of pulmonary edema.

Q. Discuss the etiology, clinical presentation, investigations and management of cardiogenic pulmonary edema. Add a note on the pathophysiology.

Q. Discuss the etiology/causes, clinical features, and management of acute left ventricular failure.

Q. Define pulmonary edema.

Definition

Pulmonary edema is a condition characterized by accumulation of excess fluid in interstitium and alveoli of the lung as a result of an alteration in one or more of starling forces.

Classification and Causes of Pulmonary Edema (Table 7.83)

TABLE 7.83: Various causes of pulmonary edema.

Cardiogenic pulmonary edema (CPE)	*Noncardiogenic pulmonary edema NCPE [other name of NCPE = ARDS (Acute respiratory distress syndrome)]*
Cardiac disorders: Atrial outflow obstruction, LV systolic dysfunction, and LV diastolic dysfunction **Dysrhythmias** **LV hypertrophy and cardiomyopathies** **LV volume overload** **Myocardial infarction** **LV outflow obstruction**	**Direct injury to lung:** Chest trauma, pneumonia, and pulmonary embolism **Indirect injury to lung:** Sepsis, multiple transfusions, cardiopulmonary bypass, pancreatitis, and toxins **Lung injury plus increased hydrostatic pressure:** Neurogenic pulmonary edema, high altitude pulmonary edema, and re-expansion pulmonary edema

(LV: left ventricular)

Q. Write a short essay/note on noncardiac causes of pulmonary edema.

Pulmonary edema can result from hemodynamic disturbances (hemodynamic or cardiogenic pulmonary edema) or from direct increases in capillary permeability (noncardiogenic pulmonary edema due to microvascular injury). Based on underlying cause it can be classified as:

- **Cardiogenic pulmonary edema** is defined as a high pulmonary capillary hydrostatic pressure (as estimated clinically from the pulmonary capillary wedge pressure—PCWP) is responsible for abnormal fluid accumulation in alveoli of the lung.
- **Noncardiogenic pulmonary edema** is caused by various disorders in which factors other than elevated pulmonary capillary pressure are responsible for protein and fluid accumulation in the alveoli.

Stages in Development

- **Interstitial edema:** This is an early stage where edema is limited to interstitium of lung.
- **Alveolar edema:** This occurs later, and characterized by the movement of edema fluid, macromolecules, and red blood cells into the alveoli.

Clinical Features of Acute Pulmonary Edema

Cardiogenic pulmonary edema (CPE)

- **Clinical features of left heart (acute ventricular) failure:** Extreme breathlessness, shortness of breath orthopnea, and paroxysmal nocturnal dyspnea, anxiety, and feelings of drowning. Cough, pink frothy sputum.
- **Physical findings:**
  - Tachypnea and tachycardia
  - Hypertension
  - Cool extremities may indicate low cardiac output
  - Auscultation reveals fine, crepitations, or wheezes
  - **CVS findings:** S_3, accentuation of pulmonic component of S_2, and jugular venous distention
  - Patients with (RV) failure may present with hepatomegaly, sustained hepatojugular reflux, and peripheral edema. Change in mental status, caused by hypoxia or hypercapnia.

Differences between CPE and NCPE

- **CPE:** A history of an acute cardiac event is usually present. Physical examination shows an S_3 gallop, jugular venous distention, and crackles on auscultation.
- **NCPE:** They have a warm periphery, a bounding pulse, and no S_3 gallop or jugular venous distention. Definite differentiation is based on pulmonary capillary wedge pressure (PCWP) measurements. The PCWP is generally >18 mm Hg in CPE and <18 mm Hg in NCPE.

Unusual Type Pulmonary Edema

- **Neurogenic pulmonary edema:** Seen in patients with central nervous system disorders and without apparent preexisting LV dysfunction
- **Re-expansion pulmonary edema:** Develops after removal of air or fluid that has been in pleural space for some time, post-thoracocentesis. Patients may develop hypotension or oliguria resulting from rapid fluid shifts into lung.
- **High altitude pulmonary edema:** Occurs in young individuals who have quickly ascended to altitudes above 2,700 meters (8,000 feet) and who then engage in strenuous physical exercise at that altitude, before they have become acclimatized. Reversible in <48 hours.

Investigations

Same as heart/cardiac failure and ARDS.

Q. Write a short essay/note on treatment of acute pulmonary edema/acute left ventricular failure.

Treatment of Acute Cardiogenic Pulmonary Edema

- **Initial management:** ABCs of resuscitation, i.e., airway, breathing, and circulation
- Medical treatment of CPE focuses on three main goals:
  - Reduction of pulmonary venous return (preload reduction)
  - Reduction of systemic vascular resistance (afterload reduction)
  - Inotropic support
- **Oxygenation:** Oxygen should be administered to all patients to keep oxygen saturation at greater than 90%. Methods of oxygen delivery include the use of a face mask [noninvasive ventilation which includes (BiPAP) and (CPAP)], and intubation and mechanical ventilation. Oxygen corrects hypoxia and positive pressure raises intra-alveolar pressure reducing transudation of fluid.
- **Preload reduction** decreases pulmonary capillary hydrostatic pressure and reduces fluid transudation into the pulmonary interstitium and alveoli. **Nitroglycerin** oral or I/V 10–100 µg/min.
- **Diuretics:** They reduce the circulating blood volume and hasten the relief of pulmonary edema. **Intravenous furosemide** has a venodilator action by which it reduces venous return. This effect occurs within a few minutes while diuresis may take 30 minutes.
- **Morphine sulfate:** Morphine 2–5 mg intravenously slowly, and repeated if necessary, reduces anxiety and reduces venous return.
- **Afterload reduction** increases cardiac output and improves renal perfusion, which allows for diuresis in the patient with fluid overload.
  - **ACE inhibitors:** Enalapril 1.25 mg IV or captopril 25 mg sublingually
  - Angiotensin II receptor blockers
  - Nitroprusside for 3–4 µg/kg/min IV infusion
- **Inotropic agents:** Dobutamine and dopamine
- **Intra-aortic balloon pumping (IABP):**
  - The IABP is inserted percutaneously through the femoral artery to descending aorta using a modified technique. Fluoroscopy may be used for correct positioning of the balloon, and Helium gas is used to inflate the balloon.
  - The IABP decreases afterload as the pump deflates; during diastole the pump inflates to improve coronary blood flow.
- **Ultrafiltration** is a fluid removal procedure that is particularly useful in patients with renal dysfunction and expected diuretic resistance.
- Correction of precipitating causes, e.g., infection or arrhythmias
- Treatment of underlying cause.

CARDIAC ARRHYTHMIAS

Q. Write a short note on definition of cardiac arrhythmias.

Definition

An abnormality (disturbance) of either rate or electrical rhythm of contraction of the heart is called a cardiac arrhythmia.

- Arrhythmias are usually due to structural disease of the heart but may also occur because of abnormal conduction or depolarization in an otherwise healthy heart.

Main Types of Arrhythmia

- **Bradyarrhythmia:** The heart rate is slow and <60/min during the day or <50/min at night.
- **Tachyarrhythmia:** The heart rate is fast and >100/min.

Sinus Arrhythmia

Q. Write a short essay on sinus arrhythmia.

- Sinus arrhythmia is a normal physiological phenomenon and involves cyclic changes in the heart rate during breathing. Normal variation (phasic changes) of the heart rate in relation to breathing (during respiration) may occur due to fluctuations of normal parasympathetic nervous system (autonomic) activity/tone. *During inspiration, parasympathetic tone falls and the heart rate increases, and on expiration, the heart rate decreases.* This variation is normal, especially in children and young adults.
- The nonrespiratory form may occur in diseased hearts and sometimes confused with sinus arrest (also known as "sinus pause").
- Typically, sinus arrhythmia results in predictable irregularities of the pulse.

- **Significance:** It is the most common arrhythmia and is manifestation of normal autonomic nervous activity. Absence of this normal variation in heart rate with breathing (sinus arrhythmia) or with changes in posture may be seen in autonomic neuropathy and cardiac failure.

Treatment is not usually needed unless symptomatic bradycardia is present.

Ectopic Beats (Extrasystoles; Premature Beats)

Q. Write a short essay/note on ectopic beats (extrasystoles; premature beats).

- **Definition:** Ectopic beat is a heartbeat occurring as a result of an impulse originating in an area other than the sinoatrial (SA) node.
- **Classification of ectopic beats** is based on the site of origin of the impulse (ectopic focus).
  - **Supraventricular:** Atrial ectopics, atrial premature beats arising from atrium
  - **Junctional:** Arising from AV junction
  - **Ventricular:** Arising from ventricular muscle
- **Symptoms:** Extra beats, thumping beats, or missed beats
- **Signs:** Irregularity in rhythm, missing of beats, postectopic bounding beat, and cannon waves on JVP.

Supraventricular Ectopics (Atrial Ectopics; Atrial Premature Beats)

Q. Write a short essay/note on supraventricular ectopics (atrial ectopics; atrial premature beats).

- **Atrial premature complexes (APCs)** can be found on 24-hour Holter monitoring in over 60% of normal adults. They are usually asymptomatic and benign.
- **Causes:** Idiopathic in healthy individuals, anxiety, excessive coffee, tea or tobacco, ischemic and valvular heart disease
- **Electrocardiogram (ECG)** shows early abnormal p waves with a morphology that differs from the sinus p waves. It may be inverted if it originates near the AV node. R-R interval preceding and following the ectopic beat is less than twice the basal R-R interval (i.e., pause following the ectopic is not fully compensated).
- Supraventricular ectopics sometimes may precipitate atrial tachycardia, flutter, and fibrillation.

Treatment: Treatment is useful only if they cause palpitations. Treatment of the underlying cause. Trigger for paroxysmal supraventricular tachycardias (e.g., alcohol, tobacco, or adrenergic stimulants) should be identified and eliminated. In their absence, mild sedation or beta-blocker may be tried.

Ventricular Premature Complexes (VPCs)/Ventricular Premature Beats (VPB)/Ventricular Ectopics

Q. Write a short essay/note on ventricular ectopics [ventricular extrasystoles; ventricular premature beats, premature ventricular contractions (PVC)].

- Of adult males, >60% will exhibit VPCs during a 24-hour Holter monitoring.
- In patients with previous MI, if frequent (>10 per hour) or complex VPCs are present, they are associated with increased mortality.
- **Causes:** Idiopathic in healthy individuals, excessive tea, coffee and alcohol, acute myocardial infarction, myocardial ischemia, myocarditis, digitals toxicity, hypokalemia, and mitral valve prolapse

Electrocardiogram

- These premature beats have wide, bizarre QRS complex, >0.12 seconds in duration and usually without a preceding P wave. They arise from an abnormal (ectopic) site in the ventricular myocardium.
- Usually, following a premature beat, there is complete compensatory pause because the AV node or ventricle is refractory to the next sinus impulse.
- The pause is fully compensated so that the sum R-R intervals preceding and following the ectopic QRS equals double the normal sinus R-R interval.
- When a VPC depolarizes the ventricles at a similar time as a conducted atrial beat, a **fusion beat** is observed.
- The term *bigeminy* refers to a normal complex followed by premature complex; *trigeminy* indicates a premature complex that follows two normal beats; a premature complex that occurs after three normal beats is called *quadrigeminy.* Two successive VPCs are known as a couplet, whereas three successive VPCs are called a triplet. Arbitrarily, three or more successive PVCs are termed Salvos/*ventricular tachycardia.* VPCs having different contours are often called multifocal.

Treatment

- In the absence of cardiac disease, isolated asymptomatic VPCs, regardless of configuration and frequency, does not require any treatment.
- Beta-blockers are useful in symptomatic VPCs that occur mainly in the daytime or under stressful situations and in specific settings such as thyrotoxicosis and mitral valve prolapse.
- Implantable cardiac defibrillator (ICD) placement improves prognosis in patients with inducible VT and LV dysfunction.

Tachycardia

Q. Write a short note on tachycardia/narrow-complex and wide-complex tachycardia. Write a note on tachycardia.

Definition: Tachycardia is defined as a heart rate of >100/minute.

Classification

- Depending on origin:
  - **Supraventricular tachycardia** is a tachycardia which utilizes atrial or AV nodal tissue as part of its mechanism (i.e., originating above the bundle of His).
  - **Ventricular tachycardia:** Originates below the level of bundle of His
- Depending on QRS complex:
  - **Narrow-complex** (QRS complex <0.12 seconds) tachycardia: Usually, tachycardia that originates from or above AV node generally produces narrow QRS complexes.
  - **Wide-complex** (QRS >0.12 seconds) tachycardia: Usually, tachycardias that originate below the AV node produce wide QRS complexes.

Supraventricular Tachycardia

Q. What do you understand by the term supraventricular tachycardia? Name various supraventricular tachycardia.

Q. Write a short note on paroxysmal supraventricular tachycardia (PSVT).

- Supraventricular tachycardia (SVT) is an arrhythmia and the term commonly used to describe regular tachycardia (heart rate exceeding 100 beats/minute) that arises from the atrium or the atrioventricular junction. Its conduction is via the His–Purkinje system. Hence, on ECG, the QRS shape during tachycardia is usually similar to that seen in the same patient during baseline rhythm. Various causes of supraventricular tachycardia are presented in **Table 7.84**.
- These are usually associated with a narrow QRS complex and are characterized by a re-entry circuit or automatic focus involving the atria. The term SVT is misleading, as, in many cases, the ventricles also form part of the re-entry circuit, such as in patients with AV re-entrant tachycardia.

TABLE 7.84: Various causes of supraventricular tachycardia (SVT).

Tachycardia	*ECG findings*
Sinus tachycardia	P wave is similar to sinus rhythm preceding QRS
AV nodal re-entry tachycardia (AVNRT) also referred as paroxysmal SVTs	No visible P wave, or inverted P wave immediately before or after QRS complex
AV reciprocating tachycardia (AVRT) complexes	P wave visible between QRS and T wave
Atrial fibrillation	Irregularly irregular RR intervals and no organized atrial activity
Atrial flutter	Visible flutter waves at 300/min (saw tooth appearance) usually with a 2:1 AV conduction
Atrial tachycardia	Organized atrial activity with P wave appearing morphological different from sinus rhythm preceding QRS
Multifocal atrial tachycardia	Multiple P wave morphologies (>3) and irregular RR intervals
Accelerated junctional tachycardia	ECG similar to AVNRT

(ECG: electrocardiogram)

Sinus Tachycardia

Q. Write a short note on sinus tachycardia.

Definition

It is characterized by a heart rate of >100/ minute with normal P waves, P-R interval, and QRS complexes.

- If rate-dependent blocks appear or an accessory path is present, there may be widened QRS complexes.
- Causes: It is usually due to an increase in sympathetic activity associated with exercise, emotion, or pregnancy. Pathological causes include anemia, thyrotoxicosis, anxiety, fever, heart failure, pheochromocytoma, drugs, e.g., β-agonists (bronchodilators) embolism and shock.

Treatment

- Identification and treatment of the underlying cause
- If the tachycardia produces myocardial ischemia, treat with β-blockers.

AV Node Re-entry Tachycardia

AV Node Re-entry Tachycardia (AVNRT) is the most common cause of **paroxysmal supraventricular tachycardia (PSVT).** AVNRT produces a regular tachycardia with a rate of 120–240/min.

Mechanism: AVNRT is due to re-entry in a circuit involving the AV node and there are two functionally and anatomically different right atrial input pathways.

- Superior "fast" pathway has a longer effective refractory period and conducts faster.
- Inferior "slow" pathway characterized by a short effective refractory period and slow conduction

If the atrial impulse occurs early (e.g., an atrial premature beat) when the fast pathway is still refractory, the slow pathway takes over in propagating this atrial impulse to the ventricles. It then travels back through the fast pathway which has already recovered its excitability. Thus, initiating the most common "slow, fast, or typical," AVNRT.

Clinical features

- It is common in women than men (F:M = 2:1).
- It usually occurs suddenly without any structural heart disease or obvious provocation. However, exertion, coffee, tea, and alcohol may aggravate or induce the arrhythmia.
- Episodes/attack may last from a few seconds to many hours and may stop spontaneously or may continue indefinitely until medical intervention.
- During the attack, the patient is usually aware of a rapid, very forceful, regular heartbeat, and may experience chest discomfort, lightheadedness, or breathlessness. Sometimes, polyuria (due to the release of atrial natriuretic peptide) may develop.

ECG: Usually shows a tachycardia at a rate of 140–240/minute with normal regular QRS complexes. Occasionally, the QRS complexes will show typical bundle branch block.

Management

- Treatment is not always required.
- Episode/attack may be terminated in patients without hypotension by **carotid sinus pressure or by the Valsalva maneuver.**
- If these maneuvers are unsuccessful, **adenosine** (3–12 mg rapidly IV in incremental doses until tachycardia stops) or **verapamil** (5 mg IV over 1 min) will restore sinus rhythm in most of the patients. Intravenous β-blocker or flecainide may be helpful.
- Rarely, when there is severe hemodynamic compromise, the tachycardia should be terminated by DC cardioversion.
- Recurrent SVT: Catheter ablation will permanently prevent SVT in >90% of cases.

Atrial Fibrillation

Q. Discuss the etiology, pathophysiology, clinical features, complications, diagnosis, and management of atrial fibrillation.

Definition

- Atrial fibrillation (AF) is an arrhythmia characterized by disorganized atria and produces multiple atrial foci fire impulses at a rate of 350–600/minute. There is no atrial contraction but only fibrillation. The ventricles respond at irregular intervals, usually at a rate of 100–140/minute.
- It is the most common cause of sustained cardiac arrhythmia.

Etiology (Table 7.85)

Any condition that raises the atrial pressure, increases atrial muscle mass, causes atrial fibrosis, or inflammation and infiltration of the atrium, may produce atrial fibrillation. Many genetic (gene defects linked to chromosomes 10, 6, 5, and 4) and systemic causes also may be responsible for atrial fibrillation.

TABLE 7.85: Causes of atrial fibrillation.

Cardiac	*Noncardiac*
➢ Hypertensive heart disease ➢ Valvular heart disease (e.g., rheumatic heart disease) ➢ Ischemic heart disease ➢ Heart failure ➢ Cardiomyopathy ➢ Pericarditis ➢ Congenital heart disease ➢ Postcardiac surgery	➢ Pulmonary: Pneumonia, COPD, pulmonary embolism ➢ Hyperthyroidism/thyrotoxicosis ➢ Excess catecholamine/sympathetic activity ➢ Drugs and alcohol ➢ Significant electrolyte imbalance
Lone atrial fibrillation	**Reversible/transient AF**
➢ Younger patients <60 ➢ No underlying cause ➢ Usually not much symptoms ➢ Normal heart structure ➢ No associated co-morbidities	➢ Acute upper respiratory tract infections (URTI), chest infection AMI, pericarditis, thyrotoxicosis, pulmonary embolism, after CABG, holiday heart syndrome

(AF: atrial fibrillation; AMI: acute myocardial infarction; CABG: coronary artery bypass grafting; COPD: chronic obstructive pulmonary disease)

Mechanisms of Atrial Fibrillation (Fig. 7.49)

- AF is a complex arrhythmia. It is characterized by (1) abnormal automatic firing at a rate of 350–600/minute and (2) the presence of multiple interacting re-entry circuits looping around the atria.
- Episodes of atrial fibrillation are initiated by rapid bursts of depolarizing automatic ectopic beats arising from conducting tissue in the pulmonary veins or from diseased atrial tissue. The atria respond electrically at this rapid rate. Many of them reach the AV node during its refractory period, and hence not conducted.
- AF becomes maintained by continuous, rapid (300–600/min) activation of the atria by multiple re-entrant conduction within the atria or sometimes because of continuous ectopic firing. Re-entry occurs in enlarged atria or in which conduction is slow (occurs in many forms of heart disease).

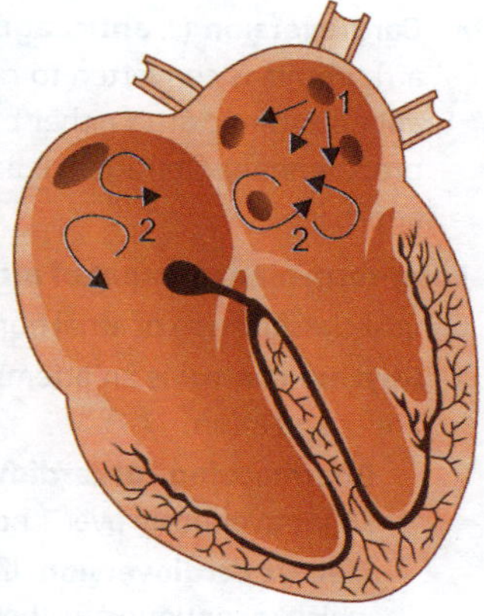

FIG. 7.49: Mechanisms of atrial fibrillation: (1) Ectopic beats, originating from the pulmonary veins usually trigger atrial fibrillation; (2) Re-entry within the atria maintains atrial fibrillation.

Clinical Features

Symptoms

Usual symptoms include palpitations, fatigue, syncope, angina, and symptoms of cardiac failure and thromboembolism.

Cardinal signs

- Irregularly irregular pulse, varying volumes of pulse, pulse deficit (apex pulse deficit)
- Blood pressure: Hypotension, mean of three recordings to be taken
- Absence of a waves on JVP
- Varying intensity of the first heart sound, disappearance of the fourth heart sound, and disappearance of the PSA of the mid-diastolic murmur of mitral stenosis (MS) in a few.

Investigations

Q. Write a short note on ECG changes in atrial fibrillation.

- Electrocardiogram (**Box 7.49**)
- 2D ECHO to look for LA size, thrombus, LV function
- Holter monitoring: For paroxysmal AF
- Exercise stress test: Ischemic heart disease (IHD)
- Catheterization: Before ablation
- Thyroid function tests and serum electrolytes in all patients
- Chest X-ray
- Fasting lipid profile.

Box 7.49: ECG changes in atrial fibrillation.

- No clear P waves
- Fine very irregular, disorganized atrial fibrillatory or F waves, coarse fibrillary waves indicate LAE
- F waves: Several independent re-entrant wavelets within atria, which may be fine or coarse
- Atrial rate: 350–500 bpm
- **Ventricular rate:** Irregularly irregular, conduction of AV node
- **RS complexes:** Rhythm is rapid and irregular, narrow/broad. Broad-BBB, aberrant conduction, and pre-excitation
- Long R-R interval is followed by short R-R intervals. Atrial impulse may find the RBBB still refractory. **Ashman phenomenon** is characterized by wide QRS complexes with a short cycle following long cycle commonly seen in ASD.

(ASD: atrial septal defect; AV: atrioventricular; BBB: bundle branch block; ECG: electrocardiogram; LAE: left atrial enlargement; RBBB: right bundle branch block)

Q. Write a short note on complications of atrial fibrillation.

Complications: Thromboembolism, precipitation/worsening of cardiac failure, syncope, hypotension, angina, precipitation of pulmonary edema in mitral stenosis.

Management/Treatment

Goals of management

- Hemodynamic stabilization
- Heart rate control or restoration of sinus rhythm
  - Minimize symptoms associated with excessive heart rates
  - Prevent tachycardia-associated cardiomyopathy
- Prevention of recurrent AF
- **Reduction of the risk of thromboembolism:** Anticoagulation prevents embolic complications.
- **Treatment of underlying cause:** When atrial fibrillation develops as a complication of acute precipitating event (e.g., alcohol toxicity, chest infection, pulmonary embolism, or hyperthyroidism), the provoking primary disorder/cause should be effectively treated. It will often restore sinus rhythm.

Strategies for the acute management of AF

- **Ventricular rate control** is achieved by drugs which block the AV node.
- **Cardioversion (± anticoagulation): Cardioversion** is a procedure by which an abnormally fast heart rate (tachycardia) or cardiac arrhythmia is converted to normal rhythm using electricity or drugs. Cardioversion is achieved electrically by DC shock or medically antiarrhythmic drug either by intravenous infusion (e.g., flecainide, propafenone, vernakalant, or amiodarone) or orally (flecainide or propafenone). Oral agent is administered to a particular patient who is previously tested in hospital and found to be safe ("pill in pocket" approach).

Long-term management of atrial fibrillation

Clinical classification of atrial fibrillation is presented in **Table 7.86**. Long-term management of persistent atrial fibrillation has two options:

1. **Rhythm control** is an attempt to restore and maintain normal sinus rhythm by antiarrhythmic drugs plus DC cardioversion plus oral anticoagulation.
   - **Pharmacological cardioversion:** By quinidine, ibutilide, flecainide, propafenone, or amiodarone. The dose of amiodarone 5–7 mg/kg intravenously over 1 hour followed by 1.2–1.8 g/24-hour infusion.
   - **Electric cardioversion:** If there is failure of medical cardioversion, electric cardioversion is done after 3 weeks of warfarin therapy which is continued further for another 4 weeks after cardioversion. Anticoagulation is to be given to these patients.
2. **Rate control:** If sinus rhythm cannot be restored, treatment is aimed to control the ventricular rate to <100/minute and to prevent embolic complications. This is achieved by AV nodal slowing agents plus oral anticoagulation.
   - Calcium channel blockers (calcium antagonists):
     - **Verapamil:** 5–10 mg intravenously over 2 minutes. If required repeat in 30 minutes.
     - **Diltiazem:** 10 mg intravenously over 2 minutes. If required repeat same dose in 15 minutes. An infusion at 10–15 mg/hour is started to maintain ventricular rate below 100/minute.

TABLE 7.86: Clinical classification of atrial fibrillation (AF) and choice of treatment.

Terminology	*Clinical features*	*Treatment*
Initial event (first detected episode)	Symptomatic/asymptomatic. Onset unknown	Rhythm/rate control
Paroxysmal (may be vagotonic AF or adrenergic AF)	Intermittent episodes that stop spontaneously (self-termination) within 7 days and most often <48 hours	Rhythm control. Vagotonic AF responds to digitalis, disopyramide while beta-blockers are helpful for adrenergic AF
Persistent	Prolonged, not self-terminating, lasting >7 days which requires termination by electrical or chemical cardioversion	Rhythm/rate control
Permanent ("accepted")	Not spontaneously terminated or terminated but relapsed, no cardioversion attempt	Rate control

Note: Atrial fibrillation may be asymptomatic and the first detected episode should not be considered as the true onset.

- **β-blockers:** Propranolol 1 mg intravenously over 2 minutes. Dose is repeated every 5 minutes up to a maximum of 5 mg.
- **Digoxin:** 0.25–0.5 mg intravenously, then 0.25 mg after 4–6 hours and another after 12 hours. At present less commonly used.
- **Amiodarone:** 150 mg over 10 minutes followed by 1 mg/minute over 6 hours and then 0.5 mg/minutes for next 18 hours. Adverse effects include: hepatic toxicity (hepatitis that can progress to cirrhosis), pulmonary toxicity (cough and dyspnea), thyroid dysfunction (hypothyroidism, hyperthyroidism), sun sensitivity, and ocular symptoms.

Prevention of recurrence

- After restoring the sinus rhythm (either by electric or pharmacological cardioversion), recurrence is prevented by quinidine, amiodarone, or dronedarone (safer than amiodarone).
- When cardioversion is unsuccessful or if atrial fibrillation is likely to recur, following treatment is given:
  - Allow the patient to remain in atrial fibrillation but reduce the ventricular rate by digitals, diltiazem, verapamil, or propranolol.
  - **Chronic anticoagulation**
  - Reduction in stroke risk; by warfarin or antiplatelet agents.

Reduction of the risk (prevention) of thromboembolism (anticoagulation)

One of the complications of atrial fibrillation is embolism. First step is to determine the need for anticoagulation. A scoring system known as **CHA_2DS_2-VASc (Table 7.87)** is used to assess the risk of embolism.

Indications: Atrial fibrillation in patients with rheumatic mitral stenosis or with mechanical prosthetic heart valve. Other indications include:

- Transesophageal echocardiography should be done in patients with atrial fibrillation to exclude an atrial thrombus.
  - If no atrial thrombi: Heparin is given before cardioversion (if conversion to sinus rhythm) and followed by warfarin for 4 weeks.
  - If atrial thrombi present: Warfarin is given for 3 weeks prior to cardioversion and is continued for another 4 weeks after cardioversion.
- If cardioversion is unsuccessful and patient remains in atrial fibrillation, long-term warfarin should be given.

Anticoagulants: With warfarin, the INR should be maintained between 2.0 and 3.0 (2.5 and 3.5 in case of underlying valvular lesion). Newer oral anticoagulants include dabigatran (a direct thrombin inhibitor in the dose of 150 mg BID), apixaban (5 mg BID), and rivaroxaban (20 mg OD).

TABLE 7.87: CHA_2DS_2-VASc stroke risk scoring system for non-valvular atrial fibrillation.

Risk factor	*Score*	
C: Congestive heart failure	1	**0 points: Low-risk** (no prophylaxis required) **1–2 points: Moderate-risk** (oral anticoagulant or aspirin recommended) **≥3 points: High-risk** (oral anticoagulant recommended)
H: Hypertension	1	
A: Age >75 years	2	
D: Diabetes mellitus	1	
S_2: Prior stroke or TIA	2	
V: Vascular disease	1	
A: Age 65–74 years old	1	
Sc: Sex category (female)	1	

(TIA: transient ischemic attack)

Aspirin: In the dose of 325 mg/day may be used as an alternative to warfarin when patient is allergic to warfarin or is contraindicated, patient <75 years of age with no previous stroke or transient ischemic attack without hypertension, diabetes, or heart failure.

Radiofrequency ablation (RF) ablation therapy: Indications are:

- Very symptomatic patients who refuse antiarrhythmic drug therapy
- Young patients where only effective antiarrhythmic drug is amiodarone
- Patients with significant bradycardia for whom antiarrhythmic drug therapy will require pacemaker
- **Surgical procedure for AF** is the "cut-and-sew" maze procedure

Atrial Flutter

Q. Define atrial flutter. Discuss the causes, electrocardiographic features, and management of atrial flutter.

Definition

Atrial flutter is a cardiac arrhythmia usually characterized by an organized, regular, rapid atrial rate between 250 and 350/minute. The ventricles respond to every second, third, or fourth beat (2:1, 3:1, or 4:1 AV block).

Common Causes

- **Cardiac causes:** Organic heart diseases (e.g., ischemic, rheumatic, congenital), pericarditis, following open heart surgery (1st week)
- Acute respiratory failure

ECG: Characteristic saw-toothed flutter waves ("F" waves) between QRS complexes. QRS complexes are regular.

Management

- **Restoration to sinus rhythm:** Treatment of a symptomatic acute paroxysm is direct electrical cardioversion. Atrial flutter of >1–2 days should be treated similar to atrial fibrillation and anticoagulated for 3 weeks prior to cardioversion.
- **Control of ventricular rate:** By using digoxin, β-blockers, or verapamil/diltiazem followed by conversion to sinus rhythm using quinidine, amiodarone, disopyramide, or flecainide
- **Prevention of recurrences:** Recurrent paroxysms can be prevented by class III antiarrhythmic agents (*refer* **Table 7.91**) such as quinidine, amiodarone, disopyramide, or flecainide. Treatment of choice for patients with recurrent atrial flutter is catheter ablation.
- **Prevention of stroke:** Risk of stroke is similar to that of atrial fibrillation and the management is almost identical but anticoagulants may be stopped earlier after successful ablation.

Wolff–Parkinson–White Syndrome (WPW Syndrome)

Q. Write a short essay on Wolff–Parkinson–White (WPW) syndrome.

Wolff–Parkinson–White (WPW) syndrome is an extra electrical (accessory) pathway (Bundle of Kent) between atria and ventricles and causes tachycardia.

Accessory pathways: Extra electrical pathway consists of an abnormal band of rapidly conducting fibers which connects the atria and ventricles. These conducting fibers resemble Purkinje tissue, in that they conduct very rapidly and are rich in sodium channels. Accessory pathways may be of two types.

1. **Concealed accessory pathway:** About 50% of cases, this pathway only conducts in the retrograde direction (from ventricles to atria) and thus does not change the appearance of the ECG in sinus rhythm. It is called as a concealed accessory pathway.
2. **Manifest accessory pathway:** In remaining 50%, the pathway conducts anterograde direction (from atria to ventricles). Thus, AV conduction in sinus rhythm is mediated via both the AV node and the accessory pathway and distorts the QRS complex. Premature ventricular activation via this pathway shortens the PR interval and produces a "slurred" initial deflection of the QRS complex, and is called a delta wave. This manifests as an accessory pathway. Because AV node and accessory pathway have different conduction speeds and refractory periods, a re-entry circuit can develop, producing tachycardia. When this is **associated with symptoms, it is termed as Wolff–Parkinson–White (WPW) syndrome.**

ECG (Fig. 7.50): During tachycardia is indistinguishable from that of AVNRT.

- Short PR interval (<0.12 second)
- Slurred upstroke of the QRS complex (Delta wave)
- Wide QRS complex

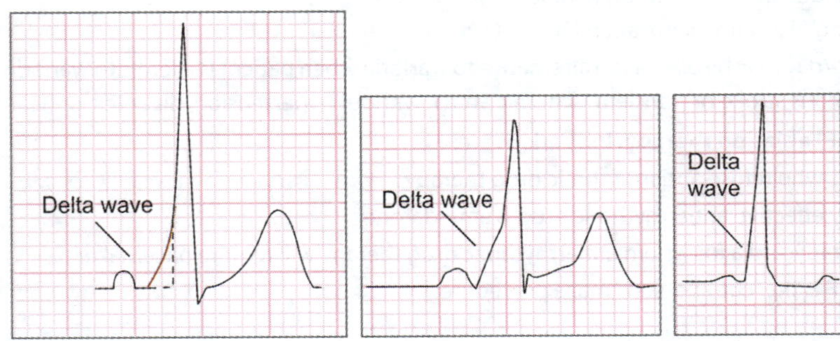

FIG. 7.50: ECG findings in Wolff–Parkinson–White (WPW) syndrome.

Complications: Atrial flutter, atrial fibrillation, supraventricular tachycardia, ventricular tachycardia, ventricular fibrillation, and death

Treatment
- Carotid sinus pressure or intravenous adenosine used for termination of the tachycardia
- Acute episodes of PSVT in Wolff–Parkinson–White (WPW) syndrome are treated similar to that of PSVT.
- Life-threatening atrial fibrillation is treated as an emergency with DC cardioversion.
- In nonlife-threatening atrial fibrillation (AF), lidocaine (3–5 mg/kg) or procainamide (15 mg/kg) administered IV over 15–20 minutes will usually show the ventricular response. Ibutilide can also be used.
- *Avoid IV verapamil and digitalis in WPW and AF,* because they can increase ventricular response (by shortening the refractory period of accessory pathway). Beta-blockers are of no use in controlling ventricular response during AF when conduction proceeds over the bypass tract.
- Catheter ablation of bypass tracts is possible in >90% of the patients and is the treatment of choice in patients with symptomatic arrhythmias. Surgical ablation may be required in an occasional patient in whom catheter ablation fails.

Sick Sinus Syndrome

Q. Write a short essay on sick sinus syndrome.

- It comprises a number of abnormalities namely sinus bradycardia, sinus arrest, combinations of sinoatrial and AV blocks, tachycardia-bradycardia, and supraventricular tachycardia.
- It is characterized by sinus node dysfunction with an atrial rate inappropriate for physiologic requirements.
- **Cause:** Usually due to ischemia, fibrosis, drug-induced, or autonomic dysfunction.

Clinical Features
- Majority are asymptomatic
- Clinical features are due to cerebral hypoperfusion and reduced cardiac output. These include syncope, palpitations, and dizziness. There may be symptoms caused due to worsening of underlying conditions (e.g., congestive heart failure, angina pectoris, and cerebrovascular accident).
- A slow heart rate, fever, left ventricular failure, or pulmonary edema suggest sick sinus syndrome.

Treatment of recurrent symptomatic bradycardia or prolonged pauses by implantation of a permanent pacemaker.

Ventricular Tachycardia (VT)

Q. Write a short essay on ventricular tachycardia.

- **Most common cause of wide complex tachycardia (80%)**
- VT heart rate is 100–200 bpm and if more than rate >220 bpm, it is ventricular fibrillation (VF).
- Major cause of morbidity and mortality in patients with structural heart disease
- Major cause of sudden cardiac death—60% cases on Holter monitoring
- Relatively organized tachyarrhythmias with discrete QRS complexes
- Recurrence is more common in <1 year of onset
- The occurrence of three or more VPC complexes with a rate of >120 bpm in succession is called as VT.

Types of VT
- **Nonsustained VT** is termination of VT by self <30 seconds.
- **Sustained** VT is presence of VT for >30 seconds or hemodynamically unstable but terminated in <30 seconds.
- **Slow VT:** Heart rate >100 or <120 bpm.
- **Pulseless VT:** VT with hemodynamic collapse that requires DC cardioversion
- **Refractory VT:** VT that does not revert to sinus rhythm on medication use or use of three shocks
- **VT storm:** Repeated VT episodes requiring the DC shocks/ICD shocks

Etiology (Table 7.88)
Re-entry is the most common mechanism.

TABLE 7.88: Causes of ventricular tachycardia (VT).

	Reversible causes of VT
➢ Ischemic heart disease: Acute MI, after chronic infarction ➢ Dilated cardiomyopathy ➢ Hypertrophic cardiomyopathy ➢ Post-CABG, post-TOF surgery ➢ Idiopathic ➢ Specific etiology—genetic	➢ Hypoxia ➢ Hyperthyroidism, catecholamines ➢ Electrolyte abnormalities: Hypokalemia, hypomagnesemia, hypocalcemia, and metabolic acidosis ➢ Drugs, alcohol, and starvation

(CABG: coronary artery bypass grafting; MI: myocardial infarction; TOF: tetralogy of Fallot)

Clinical Features (Table 7.89)

TABLE 7.89: Clinical features of ventricular tachycardia.

➢ Asymptomatic	➢ Presyncope
➢ May have palpitations—transient/sustained	➢ Cannon a waves
➢ Chest pain: Angina	➢ Absent pulse
➢ Syncope/dizziness	➢ Hypotension
	➢ Variable S_1

Diagnosis

- ECG: 12 lead with long rhythm strip of lead II
- 24-hour Holter monitoring in case of transient episode
- 2D echo for the etiology
- Routine investigations, serum electrolytes, calcium, magnesium, and ABG

Treatment

- **Prompt restoration of sinus rhythm** followed by prophylactic therapy.
- **Hemodynamically unstable patients: Synchronized DC** cardioversion is the treatment of choice (if systolic BP is below 90 mm Hg).
- **If the patient is stable and arrhythmia is well tolerated:** With preserved left ventricular function **IV procainamide** 50 mg/min. In presence of left ventricular dysfunction, **IV 150 mg amiodarone** given as a bolus, followed by a continuous infusion. **IV lidocaine** can be used but may depress left ventricular function, causing hypotension, or acute heart failure.
- **Correction of electrolyte or acid–base imbalance,** e.g., hypokalemia, hypomagnesemia, acidosis, and hypoxemia
- **Prevention of VT:** Beta-blockers reducing ventricular automaticity and amiodarone can be added if additional control is needed. Do not use class Ic antiarrhythmic drugs in patients with coronary artery disease or heart failure because they depress myocardial function and can be proarrhythmic (increases the possibility of a fatal arrhythmia).
- **Implantable cardiac defibrillator** is the absolute indication in the presence of LVEF <30% and is recommended for patients with high risk of arrhythmic death (e.g., poor left ventricular function, or associated with hemodynamic compromise). Rarely, surgery (e.g., aneurysm resection) or catheter ablation may be required for patients with VT associated with a myocardial infarct scar.

Torsades De Pointes

- A special type of ventricular tachycardia (VT) characterized by **polymorphic QRS complexes that change in amplitude and cycle length,** giving the appearance of oscillations around the baseline. This is associated with QT prolongation.
- **QT prolongation** may result from electrolyte disturbances (particularly hypokalemia and hypomagnesemia), antiarrhythmic drugs (quinidine), phenothiazines, tricyclic agents, and bradyarrhythmias. It may be due to congenital long QT syndrome (Andersen–Tawil syndrome, Romano–Ward syndrome, Jervell and Lange-Nielsen syndrome).
- The electrocardiographic hallmark is polymorphic VT preceded by marked QT prolongation, often in excess of 0.60 second.

Treatment

- Correct electrolyte abnormalities or underlying cause
- Intravenous **magnesium** (8 mmol over 15 minutes, then 72 mmol over 24 hours) should be given in all patients.
- Avoid class IA and class III antiarrhythmic agents.
- Lidocaine does not prolong QT interval. Isoproterenol bridge before temporary pacemaker. Phenytoin 100 mg every 5 minutes maximum dose of 500 mg.
- Temporary pacemaker
- Beta-blockers (BBs) to be used to prevent syncope in patients with congenital QTc prolongation syndrome

Brugada Syndrome

- Named by the Spanish cardiologists, Pedro Brugada and Josep Brugada
- Major cause of **sudden unexpected death syndrome** (SUDS), and is the most common cause of sudden death in young men without known underlying cardiac disease in Thailand and Laos.
- Genetic abnormality of the cardiac **sodium channels,** leading to ventricular tachycardia and/or sudden cardiac death.
- Hereditary: 60% of Brugada patients have a family history of SCD. Mutations of SCN5a genes resulting in diminished inward sodium current in the region of the RV outflow tract epicardium appear responsible for this syndrome.
- The large potential difference between the normal endocardium and rapidly depolarized RV outflow epicardium gives rise to **ST segment elevation in V_1 to V_3** in sinus rhythm and predisposes to local re-entry and life-threatening ventricular arrhythmias in the absence of structural heart disease.
- Arrhythmias frequently occur during sleep. Affects relatively young and predominant in males.

Treatment

- No benefit from beta-blockers
- Implantable cardiac defibrillator (ICD) treatment to manage recurrences. A history of syncope spontaneous ST segment elevation and inducibility of VT with programmed stimulation.

Ventricular Fibrillation

Q. Write a short note/essay on causes, diagnosis, and treatment of ventricular fibrillation.

- It is characterized by very rapid, irregular, and uncoordinated movement of the ventricles with no mechanical effect.
- Patient is pulseless and becomes rapidly unconscious, and respiration ceases (cardiac arrest).
- ECG: Shows shapeless/bizarre, rapid oscillations
- Ventricular fibrillation rarely reverses spontaneously.

Treatment: Electrical defibrillation.

Atrioventricular Blocks

Q. Discuss the causes, clinical features, and management of atrioventricular blocks and AV conduction disturbances.

Heart block or conduction block may develop at any level in the conducting system. Block in either the AV node or the His bundle produces AV block, whereas block lower in the conduction system results in bundle branch block.

Types: Atrioventricular block consists of three forms: (1) first-degree AV block, (2) second-degree AV block, and (3) third-degree (complete) AV block.

First-degree Atrioventricular (AV) Block

- In this type of block, AV conduction is delayed.
- ECG shows simple prolongation of the PR interval to >0.22 seconds. Every atrial depolarization is followed by conduction to the ventricles but occurs with delay. So, all the P waves are conducted and the QRS is normal as the delay is most often in the AV mode.

Second-degree Atrioventricular (AV) Block

In this type of AV block, dropped beats occur because some impulses from the atria fail to conduct to the ventricles.

Types

- **Mobitz type I second-degree AV block** (Wenckebach block phenomenon): It is characterized by progressive slowing of AV conduction until it is totally blocked. ECG shows progressive lengthening of successive PR intervals until a P wave fails to conduct (culminating in a dropped beat).
- **Mobitz type II second-degree AV block:** In this type, the PR interval remains constant but some atrial impulses (P waves) are not conducted. It occurs when a dropped QRS complex is not preceded by progressive PR interval prolongation. The QRS complex is usually wide (>0.12 second).
- **2:1 or 3:1 (advanced) block:** It occurs when every second or third P wave conducts to the ventricles. The block is defined by a ratio in which the first digit represents the total number of P waves, and the second digit represents the number of P waves conducted (i.e., the number of QRS complexes). This form of second-degree block is neither Mobitz I nor II.

Third-degree (Complete) Atrioventricular Block

Q. Write a short essay on complete heart block.

Complete heart block occurs when all the atrial activities fail to conduct (AV conduction fails completely) to ventricles and both the atria and ventricles beat independently (AV dissociation). In this ventricular activity (and the life) is maintained by spontaneous escape rhythm arising in the AV node or bundle of His (narrow QRS complexes) or the distal Purkinje tissues (broad QRS complexes). Distal escape rhythms are slower and less reliable. Causes of complete heart block are listed in **Box 7.50**.

Box 7.50: Causes of heart block.

Congenital

Acquired:

- Myocardial ischemia or infarction
- Idiopathic fibrosis
- Inflammation:
  - Acute (e.g., aortic root abscess in infective endocarditis)
  - Chronic (e.g., sarcoidosis and Chagas disease)
- Trauma (e.g., intracardiac surgery)
- Drugs (e.g., digoxin intoxication and β-blocker)
- Tumors and infections involving the conducting system
- Infections: Rheumatic autoimmune disease and neuromuscular diseases
- Lev's disease
- Lenegre's disease

Clinical features of complete heart block

- Regular (except in congenital complete AV block), high volume slow pulse (25–50/minute) which does not vary with exercise. Usually, there is a compensatory increase in stroke volume and produces a large-volume pulse.
- Irregular cannon waves on JVP in the neck
- Stokes-Adams attacks
- Varying intensity of first heart sound

ECG: Constant P-P and R-R intervals, complete AV dissociation (i.e., the atria and ventricles beat independently) and there is no relation between the P waves and the QRS complexes.

Adams–Stokes Attacks (Stokes–Adams–Morgagni Attacks)

Q. Write a short essay on Adams–Stokes attacks (Stokes–Adams–Morgagni attacks) and their clinical features.

Stokes–Adams attack is characterized by a recurrent episode of sudden loss of consciousness unrelated to posture with or without convulsions due to a disorder of heart rhythm in which there is bradycardia or absent pulse.

Etiology

Episodes of ventricular asystole may complicate intermittent high-grade AV block (Mobitz type II or complete heart block), profound bradycardia, or ventricular standstill. Sinoatrial disease and neurocardiogenic syncope may produce similar symptoms.

Clinical Features

- **Prodrome** preceding the attack may be observed in few patients.
- **Sudden loss of consciousness:** Patient may fall to the ground with sudden loss of consciousness without warning and results in collapse. During the attack, patient is pale with a death-like appearance and deeply unconscious. The pulse is usually very slow or absent. Recovery is rapid and after a few seconds, the patient recovers consciousness with characteristic flush as the heart starts beating again and pulse quickens.
- Occasionally, brief anoxic generalized convulsions/seizures and death may occur if there is prolonged asystole or severe prolonged bradycardia (>10 seconds) causing cerebral hypoxia/ischemia. Prolonged bradycardia may produce cyanosis.
- Usually there are no sequelae, but patients may injure themselves due to the sudden fall.

Treatment of heart block: (1) Removal of offending agent, (2) Injection atropine/injection isoprenaline if symptomatic, and (3) pacemaker insertion.

Therapeutic Procedures

Defibrillation and Cardioversion

Q. Write a short note on defibrillation and cardioversion.

Introduction

- By the passage of sufficiently large electrical current (from an external source) through the heart, it can be completely depolarized. This will interrupt any arrhythmia and produce a short period of asystole and is usually followed by the resumption of normal sinus rhythm.
- **Cardioversion** is a procedure by which an abnormally fast heart rate (tachycardia) or cardiac arrhythmia is converted to a normal rhythm using electricity (defibrillation) or drugs.

Defibrillation

- In this technique, ventricular fibrillation is converted to sinus rhythm by defibrillators which deliver direct current (DC). When the defibrillator is discharged, a high-voltage field electric shock of short duration is delivered to the heart. This electric shock envelopes the heart and depolarizes the myocardium which causes an organized heart rhythm to emerge.
- **Method:** Defibrillators deliver a DC, high-electrical energy, short-duration shock through two large electrodes or paddles coated with conducting jelly or a gel pad. One electrode is positioned over the upper right sternal edge and the other over the cardiac apex. Present-day modern units deliver a biphasic shock. Advantage is that the shock polarity is reversed during mid-shock and this decreases the total shock energy needed to depolarize the heart.

Direct current cardioversion (DCC)

- **Transthoracic electric shock:** It is used to convert sinus rhythm in tachyarrhythmias which do not respond to medical treatment or that are associated with hemodynamic compromise (e.g., hypotension and worsening heart failure).
- **Precautions:**
  - A short-acting general anesthetic or powerful sedation is used in elective cardioversion.
  - Withdraw digitalis therapy at least 36 hours before cardioversion
  - Patients with long-standing (>48 hours) atrial fibrillation or flutter should be anticoagulated adequately for at least 3 weeks before cardioversion to reduce the risk of embolization.
  - Levels of cardiac enzyme may rise after a cardioversion.
- **Difference between defibrillation and cardioversion:** A nonsynchronize shock is used to defibrillate and accidental defibrillation (in patient who do not need it) may itself precipitate ventricular fibrillation. A synchronized shock (i.e., one delivered during the QRS complex) is used for all cardioversions except for very rapid ventricular tachyarrhythmias, such as ventricular flutter or VF.
- **Indications for DCC:** Ventricular fibrillation, sustained ventricular tachycardia, atrial fibrillation/flutter, and supraventricular tachycardia.

Cardiac Pacemakers

Q. Write a short note on types of cardiac pacemakers and its indications.

Temporary pacing

- It involves delivery of an electrical impulse into the heart to initiate depolarization and to trigger cardiac contraction.
- **Indication:** Transient AV block, arrhythmias complicating acute MI or cardiac surgery, to maintain the rhythm in other situations of reversible bradycardia (i.e., due to metabolic disturbance or drug overdose), or as a bridge to permanent pacing

Transvenous pacing: It is done in patients with symptomatic bradycardias. In this procedure under the guidance of cardiac fluoroscopic imaging, a thin (French gauge 5 or 6), bipolar pacing electrode wire is inserted via an internal jugular vein, a femoral vein, or a subclavian vein and is positioned at the apex of the right ventricle. The electrode is connected to an external pacemaker with an adjustable energy output and pacing rate usually about 60–80/minute.

Complications: Pneumothorax, brachial plexus or subclavian artery injury, local infection or septicemia (usually *Staphylococcus, aureus),* and pericarditis.

Transcutaneous pacing is performed in selected patients with asymptomatic bradycardia or conduction abnormalities. It may be lifesaving for patients with cardiac arrest precipitated by bradycardia. This method consists of depolarizing the myocardium by current flow between two large adhesive electrodes positioned anteriorly and posteriorly on the chest wall.

Permanent pacing

Pacing electrodes (leads) can be placed via the subclavian or cephalic veins and are designed to both pace and sense either the ventricles or the atria, or more commonly, both chambers.

Indication for permanent pacing (Table 7.90)

TABLE 7.90: Indication of permanent pacing.
➤ Acquired AV block in adults
– Complete heart block associated with any one of the following:
◆ Symptomatic bradycardia
◆ CHF
◆ Asystole >3 seconds
◆ Escape rate <40 beats per minute
◆ Post-AV junction ablation, myotonic dystrophy
– Second-degree AV block with symptomatic bradycardia
– Atrial fibrillation, atrial flutter, or rare cases of supraventricular tachycardia with complete heart block, bradycardia, or any of the conditions listed under above
➤ After myocardial infarction
– Persistent advanced second-degree AV block or complete heart block with block in His–Purkinje system.
– Transient advance AV block with associated bundle branch block
➤ Bifascicular trifascicular block
– Bifascicular block with intermittent complete heart block associated with symptomatic bradycardia
– Bifascicular or trifascicular block with intermittent type II second-degree AV block without symptoms
➤ Sinus node dysfunction with documented symptomatic bradycardia: The most common indication of pacing
➤ Hypersensitive carotid sinus, recurrent syncope associated with clear, spontaneous events provoked by carotid sinus stimulation

(AV: atrioventricular; CHF: congestive heart failure)

Antiarrhythmic Drugs (Table 7.91)

Q. Write a short essay on antiarrhythmic drugs.

TABLE 7.91: Vaughan Williams classification of antiarrhythmic drugs.

Class	*Mechanism of action*	*Examples*
I. Na^+ channel blocker	Change the slope of phase 0	Ia: Quinidine, disopyramide, procainamide, and moricizine
		Ib: Lidocaine, phenytoin, and mexiletine
		Ic: Flecainide and propafenone
II. β-blocker	↓heart rate and conduction velocity	Propranolol, metoprolol, esmolol, and acebutolol
III. K^+ channel blocker	Action potential duration (APD) or effective refractory period (ERP)	Amiodarone, sotalol, bretylium, and dronedarone
	Delay repolarization	Vernakalant, azimilide, and tedisamil
IV. Ca^{++} channel blocker	Slowing the rate of rise in phase 4 of SA node.	Verapamil and diltiazem
Others		Adenosine, magnesium, and digitalis

Therapy of Various Arrhythmias (Table 7.92)

Amiodarone

Q. Write a short note on amiodarone and its use in clinical practice.

Amiodarone is an unusual iodine containing highly lipophilic long-acting antiarrhythmic drug.

TABLE 7.92: Various types of arrhythmias and their therapy.

Arrhythmias	Acute therapy		Chronic therapy	
	First choice	*Alternatives*	*First choice*	*Alternatives*
Atrial fibrillation/atrial flutter	Esmolol	Verapamil,	Digoxin	Propranolol
Paroxysmal supraventricular tachycardia (PSVT)	Adenosine	Esmolol, diltiazem, and verapamil	Digoxin, verapamil, and propranolol	Propafenone
Ventricular tachycardia (VT)	Lidocaine cardioversion	Procainamide, mexiletine, and amiodarone	Amiodarone, Dofetilide	Mexiletine, propranolol, and propafenone
Torsades de pointes	Pacing	Isoprenaline and magnesium	Propranolol	Pacing
Ventricular fibrillation (VF)	Electrical defibrillation	Lidocaine and amiodarone	Amiodarone	Procainamide and dofetilide
Wolff–Parkinson–White (WPW) syndrome	Cardioversion	Amiodarone, propafenone, and procainamide	Amiodarone and propranolol	Quinidine and propafenone

Indications: Useful in wide range of ventricular and supraventricular arrhythmias.

- Resistant ventricular tachycardia/pulseless VT
- Recurrent ventricular fibrillation
- To maintain sinus rhythm in atrial flutter when other drugs have failed. For patients with heart failure or left ventricular hypertrophy, only amiodarone is recommended.

Duration of action: Long. Hence suitable for long-term prophylactic therapy

Adverse reactions: These are dose-related and increase with duration of therapy. These reactions include fall in blood pressure, bradycardia, and myocardial depression on IV injection and on drug cumulation. Nausea, gastrointestinal upset with oral medication, photosensitization, and bluish skin discoloration pigmentation may develop in about 10% of patients. Pulmonary alveolitis and fibrosis are serious adverse reactions. Cirrhosis occurs uncommonly. Neurologic dysfunction, and hyperthyroidism (1–2%) or hypothyroidism (2–4%) can be seen.

Dose:

- Oral 400–600 mg/day for few weeks, followed by 100–200 mg for maintenance therapy
- Slow IV injection of 100–300 mg (5 mg/kg) over 30–60 minutes

DISEASES OF THE MYOCARDIUM

Myocarditis

Q. Write a short essay/note on acute myocarditis.

- Acute myocarditis is an acute inflammatory disease of the myocardium (heart muscle).
- Myocarditis may present with a wide range of symptoms, ranging from mild dyspnea or chest pain that resolves without specific therapy to cardiogenic shock and death.
- Major long-term sequelae of myocarditis is DCM (dilated cardiomyopathy) with chronic heart failure.
- Three distinct forms of inflammatory cardiomyopathy (myocarditis associated with cardiac dysfunction) are recognized: Idiopathic, autoimmune, and infectious.

Etiology (Table 7.93)

Q. Write a short essay/note on causes of myocarditis.

Clinical Features of Myocarditis

Range from an asymptomatic or present with fatigue, palpitations, chest pain, dyspnea, and fulminant congestive cardiac failure depending on the type of myocarditis.

Classification: Depending on the clinical presentations, myocarditis can be classified into four groups:

1. **Fulminant myocarditis:** Has abrupt onset and follows a viral prodrome (fever, chills, myalgia, and constitutional symptoms) or influenza-like illness, and produces severe acute heart failure or cardiogenic shock. Prognosis is good.
2. **Acute myocarditis:** It presents with heart failure, acute myocardial infarction, or sudden cardiac death. It may progress to dilated cardiomyopathy and chronic heart failure. More common in children/teenagers.

TABLE 7.93: Causes of myocarditis.

Infections: ➤ **Viral:** Most common cause. Coxsackie A and B, influenza, HIV, dengue virus, parvovirus B19, hepatitis C, Epstein–Barr virus ➤ **Bacterial:** Diphtheria, *S. aureus, Mycoplasma pneumoniae* ➤ **Protozoal:** Trypanosomiasis *(Trypanosoma cruzi)*, toxoplasmosis ➤ **Spirochetal:** Lyme disease *(Borrelia burgdorferi)* ➤ **Fungal**
Toxic: ➤ **Direct injury:** Drugs (e.g., cocaine, lithium, and anti-cancer drugs, such as doxorubicin) ➤ **Hypersensitivity reactions** and associated myocarditis: - Drugs: Penicillins and sulfonamides - Lead and carbon monoxide - Others: Bee venom, wasp venom, scorpion venom, and snake venom
Autoimmune conditions: Systemic lupus erythematosus and rheumatoid arthritis
Others: Acute rheumatic fever, chemical agents, radiation, and giant cell myocarditis (thymoma and Crohn's disease)

3. **Chronic active myocarditis:** It is rare and have insidious onset. It is seen in older adults and microscopically shows chronic inflammation of the myocardium.
4. **Chronic persistent myocarditis:** It shows focal myocardial infiltrates and cause chest pain and arrhythmia without causing ventricular dysfunction.

Physical examination may be normal or present with soft muffled heart sounds, a prominent third sound, inappropriate tachycardia, arrhythmias including conduction blocks, signs of congestive heart failure, and pericardial friction rub (associated with pericarditis).

Investigations

- **Chest X-ray:** May show mild cardiac enlargement
- **ECG** changes are common but nonspecific. May show standard T wave abnormalities and arrhythmias. Heart block may develop in diphtheritic myocarditis, Lyme disease, and Chagas disease.
- **Cardiac enzymes:** Biochemical markers of myocardial injury such as troponin I and T, creatine kinase may be raised during the early phases.
- **Echocardiography:** May show left ventricular dysfunction, and global hypokinesia with or without pericardial effusion
- **Cardiac magnetic resonance imaging:** MRI may show myocardial inflammation or infiltration. May show increased myocardial T_2 signal on inversion recovery sequence and delayed contrast enhancement after gadolinium-DTPA infusion.
- **Viral antibody titers:** May be increased
- Endomyocardial biopsy is sometimes useful to confirm the diagnosis and may show acute inflammation. Although controversial, still the current gold-standard test for diagnosis. It should be considered when there is suspicious of giant cell myocarditis, hypersensitivity/eosinophilic myocarditis, and cardiac involvement in a systemic disease.
- **Viral RNA, DNA:** Genome by polymerase chain reaction (PCR) or in situ hybridization.
- **Blood:** Leukocytosis, elevated ESR, or eosinophilia

Complications: Ventricular arrhythmia, heart block, congestive heart failure, acute pericarditis, progression to chronic myocarditis, or chronic dilated cardiomyopathy (e.g., Chagas disease).

Management

- Identify, treat, eliminate, or avoid the underlying cause.
- Prolonged bed rest during the acute phase of the illness and restriction of physical activities for 6 months (till ECG is normal). Because physical activities can induce potentially fatal ventricular arrhythmias.
- Treatment of heart failure with diuretics, ACE inhibitors/all receptor antagonists, β-blockers, spironolactone ± digoxin. Arrhythmias are treated by amiodarone and β-blockers. Digoxin should be used with caution.
- **Antibiotics:** Specific antimicrobial therapy if a causative organism has been identified.
- NSAIDs should not be given in the acute phase but may be given in the late phase.
- Corticosteroids and immunosuppressive agents use is controversial.
- **Immunoglobulin:** High-dose intravenous immunoglobulin appears to hasten the resolution of the left ventricular dysfunction and improved survival.
- Refractory patients may rarely need cardiac transplantation or temporary circulatory support (with a mechanical ventricular assist device).

CARDIOMYOPATHY

Q. Define and classify cardiomyopathy.

Definition

Cardiomyopathies are the heterogeneous group of diseases of the myocardium that affect the mechanical or electrical function of the heart.

- The term cardiomyopathy should be restricted to the conditions which primarily affect the myocardium. It does not include myocardial involvement due to congenital, acquired valvular, hypertensive, and coronary arterial or pericardial abnormalities.
- *Etiology:* They can be genetic/inherited or have infective, toxic causes, or idiopathic.

Classification

Cardiomyopathies may be classified according to a variety of criteria, including the underlying genetic basis of dysfunction. Two fundamental forms of cardiomyopathy **(Box 7.51)** are:

1. *Primary cardiomyopathy:* Consists of heart muscle disease predominantly involving the myocardium and/or of unknown cause.
2. *Secondary cardiomyopathy:* Consists of myocardial disease of unknown cause or cardiomyopathy associated with systemic disease (e.g., chronic alcohol use, amyloidosis).

Box 7.51: Etiologic classification of cardiomyopathy.

Primary cardiomyopathy
- Idiopathic (D, R, H)
- Familial (D, R, H)
- Eosinophilic endomyocardial fibrosis (R)
- Endomyocardial fibrosis (R)

Secondary cardiomyopathy
- *Infective (D):* Viral, bacterial, fungal, protozoal, metazoal, rickettsial, spirochetal myocarditis.
- *Metabolic (D):* Familial storage disease (D, R): Glycogen storage disease, mucopolysaccharidosis, hemochromatosis, Fabry's disease
- *Deficiency (D):* Electrolytes, nutritional
- *Autoimmune disease:* Systemic lupus erythematosus, polyarteritis nodosa, rheumatoid arthritis
- *Infiltrations and granulomas diseases (R, D):* Amyloidosis, sarcoidosis, malignancy
- *Neuromuscular:* Muscular dystrophy, myotonic dystrophy, Friedrich's ataxia (H, D)
- *Sensitivity and toxic reaction (D):* Alcohol, drugs, radiation
- Peripartum heart disease Takotsubo (stress) cardiomyopathy

(D: dilated cardiomyopathy; H: hypertrophic cardiomyopathy; R: restrictive cardiomyopathy)

Clinical Classification of Cardiomyopathy (Fig. 7.51 and Table 7.94)

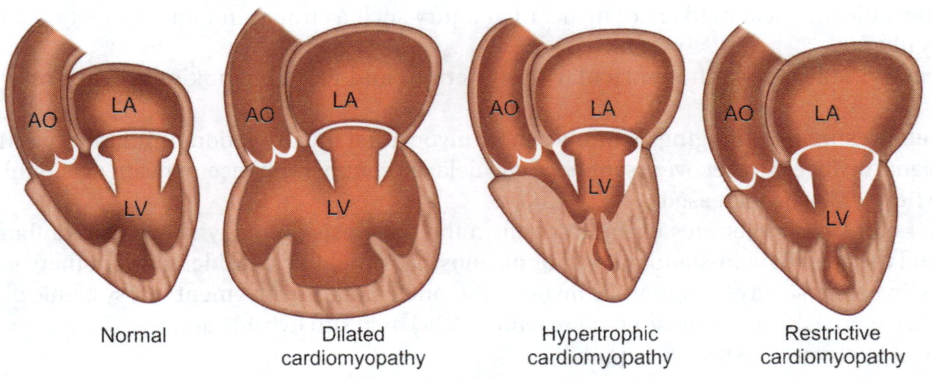

FIG. 7.51: Clinical classification of cardiomyopathy.
(AO: aorta; LA: left atrium; LV: left ventricle)

TABLE 7.94: Salient features of three major clinical types of cardiomyopathies.

Functional type (Left ventricular ejection fraction)	*Abnormality*		
	Structural	*Functional*	*Dysfunction*
Dilated/congestive (<40%)	Dilatation of ventricle	Poor ventricular contraction	Systolic dysfunction
Hypertrophic (50–80%)	Hypertrophy of left ventricle generalized or involves the upper portion of interventricular septum	Impairment of ventricular filling and left ventricular ejection due to outflow tract obstruction	Predominantly diastolic dysfunction
Restrictive/obliterative (45–90%)	Small ventricle with" stiff wall"	Impairment of ventricular filling	Diastolic dysfunction

Dilated (Congestive) Cardiomyopathy (DCM)

Q. Write short essay/note on dilated cardiomyopathy (congestive cardiomyopathy).

- DCM is characterized by dilatation/enlargement of the ventricular chambers and systolic dysfunction (impaired contraction of left and/or right ventricular) with preserved wall thickness.
- Left ventricular mass is increased but thickness of wall is normal or reduced. Dilatation of the valve rings may cause functional incompetence of mitral and tricuspid valves.

- Most common of all cardiomyopathies.
- Responsible for about one in three cases of heart failure and third most common cause of heart failure.

Etiology

- **Familial DCM:** One-fifth to one-third of patients has familial forms of DCM. It is inherited as an autosomal dominant disorder and is associated with more than 20 varieties of single-gene mutations. Most of these mutations involve genes encoding the cytoskeleton of the myocyte (dystrophin, lamin A and C, emerin, and metavinculin). Most of the X-linked inherited skeletal muscular dystrophies (e.g., Becker and Duchenne) are associated with cardiomyopathy.
- **Sporadic DCM:** Causes include:
  - **Myocarditis:** Coxsackie, adenoviruses, HIV, bacteria, fungal, mycobacteria, parasitic (Chagas disease)
  - **Toxins:** Alcohol, chemotherapy (e.g., adriamycin, trastuzumab, cyclophosphamide), metals (cobalt, lead, mercury, arsenic)
  - Autoimmune diseases (SLE, systemic sclerosis, dermatomyositis)
  - **Endocrine:** Diabetes mellitus, thyrotoxicosis, hypothyroidism
  - **Neuromuscular:** Muscular dystrophies, Friedrich's ataxia, myotonic dystrophy

Clinical Features

- It is three times more common in men than women and the peak incidence is in middle age.
- Symptoms may be gradual in onset or may cause sudden cardiac death due to arrhythmias. Thromboembolism, conduction defects and sporadic chest pain may be present.
- Symptoms/signs of heart failure
  - Fatigue and weakness
  - Pulmonary congestion (left heart failure), dyspnea (rest, exertional, nocturnal), orthopnea
  - Systemic congestion (right heart failure), edema, nausea, abdominal pain, nocturia
  - Low cardiac output
  - Hypotension, tachycardia, tachypnea
  - Narrow pulse pressure
  - Elevated jugular venous pressure (JVP)
  - **Arrhythmia:** Atrial fibrillation, conduction delays, complex PVCs, sudden death

Investigations

- **Chest X-ray:** Generalized enlargement of heart, CHF
- **Electrocardiogram:** ECG shows tachycardia, conduction abnormalities (AV block, LBBB), diffuse nonspecific ST segment and T wave changes, arrhythmias (i.e., atrial fibrillation, ventricular premature contractions or ventricular tachycardia)
- **24-hour Holter monitor:** If lightheadedness, palpitation, syncope
- **Echocardiogram, CTI, CMRI:** Show left ventricular dilation with normal or minimally thickened or, thinned walls, global hypokinesia, low EF
- Elevated BNP
- Cardiac catheterization to rule out coronary artery disease
- Myocardial biopsy, rarely necessary.

Treatment

- *Control and conventional management of heart failure:* Salt restriction, fluid restriction, and initiate standard treatment of heart failure. Medical therapy consists of ACE inhibitors, diuretics, digoxin and hydralazine/nitrate combination. L-carnitine, antioxidants and chelating agents have been tried.
- Anticoagulation prophylaxis
- Implantation of a cardiac defibrillator and/or cardiac resynchronization therapy in some patients.
- Cardiac transplantation in certain patients.

Prognosis: Majority particularly >50 years die within 4 years of onset. Spontaneous improvement or stabilization occurs in 25% of cases. Death is due to progressive heart failure, ventricular tachycardia. Sudden cardiac death (SCD) is a constant threat.

Alcoholic Cardiomyopathy

- Individuals who consumes >90 g/day of alcohol for many years.
- Clinical picture resembling idiopathic or familial DCM.
- Partially genetically predetermined (ALDH2).
- Abstention may halt the progression or may even reverse.

Peripartum Cardiomyopathy

- Cardiac dilatation with CHF develops during last trimester or within 6 months of delivery.
- Typically present in multiparous of age >30 years.

- Unknown cause
- Inflammatory myocarditis, immune activation, multiple gestations have been incriminated.
- Symptoms, signs and management are that of IDCM
- Further pregnancy should be discouraged.

Hypertrophic Cardiomyopathy

Q. Write short essay/note on hypertrophic cardiomyopathy (HCM).

- HCM is characterized by left ventricular hypertrophy, typically of a nondilated chamber, without any obvious cause.
- Two significant features are:
  - **Asymmetric myocardial hypertrophy** of the left ventricle with greater hypertrophy of the interventricular septum.
  - A dynamic left ventricular outflow tract pressure gradient, related to narrowing of the sub aortic area which may produce LV outflow tract obstruction.
- It is familial and transmitted as an autosomal dominant trait.

Clinical Features

- *Asymptomatic:* Echocardiographic finding only and family history may be positive.
- *Symptomatic:* Dyspnea in 90%. Other symptoms include effort-related such as angina and breathlessness, arrhythmia, and sudden death.

Signs

- Rapidly rising carotid pulse ("jerky" "spike and dome")/bisferiens pulse (two systolic peaks).
- Double apical impulse
- Reversed pulsus paradoxus on arterial pulse with Bernheim a wave in JVP.
- Harsh ejection systolic murmur best heard at the lower-left sternal border as well as the apex due to left ventricular outflow tract obstruction. This murmur increases during standing and Valsalva maneuver (which reduce ventricular preload) but decreases during squatting and sustained hand grip (which increase afterload), and also by leg rising (which increases preload).
- Pansystolic murmur at mitral area due to mitral regurgitation.

Investigations

- *Electrocardiogram:* Abnormal in 85–90% of cases. Shows left ventricular hypertrophy, abnormal ST-Ts, giant T-wave inversions, abnormal Q' waves, bundle branch block (BBB).
- *Chest X-ray:* Normal or shows mild-to-moderate cardiac enlargement.
- Echocardiography is diagnostic. Increased LV wall thickness ≥15 mm, **systolic anterior motion** (SAM) of the mitral valve and dynamic LV outflow tract obstruction.
- Genetic testing for evaluation of family members.
- Apical nonobstructive cardiac hypertrophy (Yamaguchi syndrome) is a relatively rare form of hypertrophic cardiomyopathy.
- Typical features of apical HCM include giant T-wave negativity on the electrocardiogram, especially in the left precordial leads, a "spade-like" configuration of the left ventricular cavity at end-diastole on left ventriculography.

Treatment

- *Avoid:* Dehydration, digitalis, diuretics, dihydropins, and vasodilators.
- *Drug therapy:* Beta-adrenergic blockers, calcium-channel blockers (verapamil, diltiazem, etc.), disopyramide and antiarrhythmics (amiodarone).
- Implantable cardiac defibrillator (ICD).
- Myectomy (partial surgical resection of septum) may improve outflow tract obstruction.
- Iatrogenic infarction of the basal septum (septal ablation) using a catheter delivered alcohol solution.
- Transplantation.

Prognosis

- Risk of SCD higher in children. Clinical deterioration usually is slow.
- Poor prognosis in males, young age of onset, family history of SCD, history of syncope, exercise induced hypotension (worst).
- Progression to DCM occurs in 10–15%.

Restrictive (Obliterative) Cardiomyopathy

Q. Write short essay/note on restrictive cardiomyopathy (obliterative cardiomyopathy).

- Rare condition in which ventricular filling is impaired because of the stiff ventricles. Hallmark is an abnormal diastolic function.
- It resemblances constrictive pericarditis, and it is important to differentiate because constrictive pericarditis is an operable disease.
- Much less common than DCM or HCM outside the tropics, but frequent cause of death in Africa, India, South and Central America and Asia primarily because of the high incidence of endomyocardial fibrosis in those regions.

Causes

- **Idiopathic**
- **Myocardial:**
  - *Noninfiltrative:* Idiopathic, scleroderma
  - *Infiltrative:* Amyloidosis, sarcoidosis, Gaucher's disease, Hurler disease
  - Storage disease: Hemochromatosis, Fabry disease, glycogen storage diseases
- **Endomyocardial:** Tropical endomyocardial fibrosis, hypereosinophilic syndrome, carcinoid, metastatic malignancies, radiation, anthracycline drugs.

Clinical Features

- Symptoms of right and left heart failure. Exercise intolerance, dyspnea, peripheral edema, ascites, and enlarged tender liver.
- Systemic embolism may develop in about 25% cases.
- Jugular venous pressure may be raised with diastolic collapse and positive Kussmaul's sign.
- Mild cardiac enlargement, the cardiac apex is easily palpable, and a mitral regurgitation murmur may be heard (not found in constrictive pericarditis).
- Heart sounds are soft and third and fourth heart sounds may be heard.

Investigations

- **Electrocardiogram:** Shows nonspecific ST-T wave changes, low voltage, arrhythmias
- **Chest X-ray:** Shows mild cardiomegaly.
- **Doppler echocardiography:** Abnormal mitral inflow pattern, symmetrically thickened LV walls and systolic dysfunction, prominent E wave (rapid diastolic filling), reduced deceleration time (increased left atrial pressure).
- **Cardiac MRI and CT:** Show symmetrically thickening of left ventricle wall, and normal or slightly reduced ventricular volumes and systolic function. These findings are useful in differentiating it from constrictive pericarditis.
- **Cardiac catheterization:** Shows increased ventricular filling pressures with dip-and-plateau pattern.

Treatment

- No satisfactory medical therapy.
- Drug therapy must be used with caution:
  - Diuretics for extremely high-filling pressures.
  - Chronic anticoagulation is often recommended.
  - Vasodilators may decrease filling pressure.
  - Calcium-channel blockers to improve diastolic compliance.
  - Digitalis and other inotropic agents are not indicated.
- Transplantation may be indicated.

Stress Cardiomyopathy

- Stress cardiomyopathy is a clinical syndrome characterized by an acute and transient (<21 days) left ventricular (LV) systolic (and diastolic) dysfunction often related to an emotional or physical stressful event, most often identified in the preceding days (1–5 days).
- First described in Japan in 1990; also called as **Takotsubo cardiomyopathy,** broken heart syndrome, apical ballooning syndrome.
- Prevalence is currently estimated at 1 to 2% of patients with suspected acute coronary syndrome.
- Exact pathophysiology is unknown and most accepted hypothesis is norepinephrine and NPY are stored in the pre-synaptic terminations of the post-ganglionic sympathetic system.
- Risk factors include female sex, menopausal, psychiatric illness, diabetes mellitus , obstructive airway disease, substance abuse disorder.

Clinical Presentation

- Clinical presentation of typical patient with stress cardiomyopathy include postmenopausal woman who presents with acute or subacute onset of chest pain (>75%) and/or shortness of breath (approximately 50%), often with dizziness (>25%) and occasional syncope (5–10%)
- In majority of the cases, the patient has experienced an emotional or physical stress that he/she may not share with the healthcare provider unless asked.
- Physical examination reveals features of acute decompensated left-sided heart failure and a systolic murmur when there is accompanying LV outflow tract obstruction.
- Diagnosis is based on RWMA beyond territory supplied by single coronary artery with reversible in due course and associated with physical/emotional stress.
- Electrocardiogram is abnormal in >95% patients with ischemic ST segment and T wave changes. T wave inversion are usually deep and wide associated with prolonged QTc likely occurring after 24-48 hours of the precipitating factor.

Treatment

- Management is mainly supportive therapy and prevention of complications until recovery. Treatment of heart failure with or without cardiogenic shock is as per guideline directed heart failure management.
- Anticoagulation is considered for apical thrombus (for upto 3 months) or large area of akinesis (until LVEF improves)
- Recurrence is seen in 2–4% of patients and in hospital mortality is seen upto 5% of patients.
- Recovery of LVEF is seen from 48 hours up to 6 weeks.

CONGENITAL HEART DISEASES

Q. Write short note on:
- **Common congenital heart diseases seen in adults.**
- **Enumerate cyanotic heart diseases.**

Congenital heart disease (CHD) is the most common group of structural malformations in children. CHD occurs in 8 per 1000 infants. About 1 in 10 stillborn infants have a cardiac anomaly.

Classification of Congenital Heart Diseases

Classification of congenital heart diseases is summarized in **Table 7.95**.

TABLE 7.95: Classification of congenital heart diseases.

Acyanotic	*Cyanotic*
With (left to right) shunts ➢ Ventricular septal defect ➢ Atrial septal defect ➢ Patent ductus arteriosus	**With (right to left) shunts** ➢ Tetralogy of Fallot ➢ Tricuspid atresia ➢ Ebstein's anomaly ➢ Transposition of great vessels ➢ Truncus arteriosus ➢ Total anomalous pulmonary venous communication
Without shunts (obstructive lesions) ➢ Aortic stenosis ➢ Coarctation of aorta	**Without shunts (obstructive lesions)** Pulmonary stenosis

Acyanotic Congenital Heart Diseases

Persistent Ductus Arteriosus (Patent Ductus Arteriosus)

Q. Write short essay on persistent ductus arteriosus (patent ductus arteriosus).

Etiology

Rubella infection during the first trimester of pregnancy and fetal valproate syndrome is associated with a high incidence of patent ductus arteriosus (PDA). **Patent (persistent) ductus arteriosus** is a congenital anomaly in which the **ductus arteriosus remains open after birth**. This produces a persistent communication between the proximal left pulmonary artery and the descending aorta. Since the pressure in the aorta is higher than that in the pulmonary artery, it produces a continuous arteriovenous left-to-right shunt the volume of which depends on the size of the ductus. About 50% of the left ventricular output is recirculated through the lungs, with a consequent increase in the work of the heart. PDAs may occur as an **isolated anomaly** (about 90%), **or associated with** other abnormalities, such as ventricular septal defect **(VSD), coarctation of the aorta, or pulmonary or aortic valve stenosis.**

Clinical features

Symptoms

- More common in females with female-to-male ratio of about 2:1.
- When the shunt is small, then it may be asymptomatic for years.
- If the shunt is moderate-to-large, there is retardation of growth and development. It produces left heart volume overload. Cardiac failure may develop producing dyspnea. In some cases, it may raise pulmonary artery pressure resulting in pulmonary hypertension and Eisenmenger's syndrome.

Q. Write short essay on differential cyanosis.

Persistent ductus with reversed shunting: When the pulmonary vascular resistance increases, pulmonary artery pressure may rise until it equals or exceeds aortic pressure. Then the shunt through the patent ductus arteriosus may reverse causing Eisenmenger's syndrome. Patients with Eisenmenger's syndrome are cyanotic and may have **differential cyanosis**. It is characterized by cyanosis and clubbing of the toes but not the fingers because the right-to-left ductal shunting is distal to the subclavian arteries.

Signs

Q. Write short essay on cardiac findings in patent ductus arteriosus.

- **Bounding pulse:** Pulses are increased in volume.
- **Apex beat** is shifted down and out and hyperdynamic.
- PDA produces a characteristic **continuous harsh murmur known as "machinery-like"/Gibson's murmur.** It is heard with late systolic accentuation and maximal in the first left intercostal space below the clavicle and frequently accompanied by a continuous thrill at the upper-left sternal edge. However, in a large PDA when pulmonary hypertension develops the murmur becomes softer.
- First heart sound is loud (due to loud mitral component).
- Graham Steell murmur of pulmonary hypertension will be present.

Investigations

- **Chest X-ray** shows enlargement of the pulmonary artery with increased vascular markings (plethoric fields).
- **ECG** is usually normal with smaller ductal shunts. It may demonstrate left atrial enlargement, left ventricular hypertrophy, sinus tachycardia or atrial fibrillation in patients with moderate or large shunts.

- **Echocardiogram and color Doppler** shows PDA and the amount of blood flow through the ductus arteriosus.
- **Magnetic resonance imaging and computed tomography:** It can assess the degree of calcification, which is important, if surgical therapy is considered.

Complications: Cardiac failure, hypertensive pulmonary vascular disease, endarteritis, paradoxical embolism.

Management

- Small ductus arteriosus may predispose to endarteritis and ductus closure should be done unless clinically silent.
- Ductus closure is indicated for any child or adult who is symptomatic from significant left-to-right shunting through the PDA.
- Transcatheter-occluding devices (e.g., coils, buttons and umbrellas) are increasingly used.
- Video-assisted thoracoscopic clip closure.
- Surgical ligation or division of the PDA remains the treatment of choice for the rare very large ductus arteriosus.
- Symptomatic patients with PDA usually improve with a medical regimen of diuretics, digoxin and angiotensin-converting enzyme inhibition, antidysrhythmic medications with anticoagulation may be useful in patients with atrial fibrillation or flutter.
- **Pharmacological treatment in the neonatal period:** In the first week of life, if the ductus is patent; a prostaglandin synthetase inhibitor (e.g., indomethacin or ibuprofen) may be used to induce its closure. However, if there is an impaired lung perfusion (e.g., severe pulmonary stenosis and left-to right shunt through the ductus), the ductus must be kept open with prostaglandin treatment to improve oxygenation.

Coarctation of Aorta

Q. Write short essay on coarctation of aorta.

Coarctation of the aorta (COA) is narrowing of the lumen of the aorta at the region or just distal to the insertion of the ductus arteriosus distal to (just below) the origin of the left subclavian artery.

Etiology: It is congenital heart disease associated with other abnormalities, such as bicuspid aortic valve (80% of cases) and 'berry" aneurysms in the circle of Willis, Turner's syndrome. Other lesions that may be associated include patent ductus arteriosus, ventricular septal defect and patent ductus arteriosus, mitral stenosis or regurgitation.

Types: Two classic forms.

1. **Infantile (preductal) form:** Characterized by tubular hypoplasia of the aortic arch proximal to a patent ductus arteriosus. It produces symptoms in early childhood.
2. **Adult (postductal) form:** Shows narrowing of the aorta, opposite the closed ductus arteriosus (ligamentum arteriosum) distal to the arch vessels.

Clinical features

Symptoms

- It is twice common in men compared to women.
- It may present as cardiac failure in the newborn but often asymptomatic for many years when detected in older children or adults.
- May present with headaches and epistaxis/nosebleeds due to hypertension proximal to the coarctation.
- Occasionally present with weakness or cramps/claudication in the legs and cold legs due to decreased blood flow to the lower part of the body limbs.

Signs

Q. Write short note on radiofemoral delay and Suzman's sign.

- **Pulse:** The femoral pulses and pulses in the lower limbs are weak, delayed (radiofemoral delay) in comparison with the radial pulse. If coarctation is proximal to the left subclavian artery, asynchronous radial pulses in right and left arms are observed. Prominent pulsations in the neck. In severe coarctation, pulses are poor.
- **BP:** It is raised in the upper limbs, but normal/low in the legs (difference >20 mm Hg).
- **Heart sounds and murmurs:**
  - *Ejection systolic murmur (ESM):* Systolic murmur is heard posteriorly, over the spine due to coarctation.
  - Systolic or continuous murmurs over lateral thoracic wall due to collaterals.
  - An ejection click and systolic murmur in the aortic area, if associated with bicuspid aortic valve. Heaving apical impulse.
- **Bruits:** Aortic narrowing causes formation of collaterals mainly in the periscapular, internal mammary and intercostal arteries, and may produce localized bruits.
- **Suzman's sign:** It is characterized by dilated, tortuous, pulsatile arteries around the scapulae and intercostals regions in the back. It is seen better when the patient bends forwards with hands hanging down.
- **Corkscrew**-shaped retinal arteries. Absence of papilledema despite high BP.

Investigations

- **Chest X-ray:** In early childhood, it is often normal. Later, it may show post-stenotic dilatation of aorta and indentation of the descending aorta at the site of the coarctation. This produces an aorta shaped like a **'figure 3'** (due to combination of dilated left subclavian artery above, stenosed, coarcted segment in the middle and dilated poststenotic aorta below in the upper right mediastinum. Tortuous and dilated collaterals may erode the undersurfaces of the ribs producing notching of the under-surfaces of the posterior ribs **("rib notching" or "Dock' sign")** extending from third to ninth ribs. It may be unilateral or bilateral, and found only after 6 years of age.
- **CT, MRI, and CMR scanning** is the best imaging method to accurately demonstrate the coarctation and quantify flow.
- **ECG:** May demonstrate left ventricular hypertrophy.
- **Echocardiography** sometimes shows the coarctation and other associated anomalies. It confirms left ventricular hypertrophy.

Complications: Hypertension, left ventricular/congestive heart failure, infective endocarditis (at the site of coarctation, bicuspid aortic valve or collateral channels), cerebral hemorrhage due to rupture of Berry aneurysm and rupture or dissection of aorta.

Treatment

- If untreated, death may occur due to complications (e.g., left ventricular failure, dissection of the aorta or cerebral hemorrhage).
- Treat hypertension and congestive heart failure. Avoid ACE inhibitors and angiotensin II receptor antagonists because they may lead to inadequate perfusion of lower-body and may precipitate renal failure.
- *Surgical correction:* Intervention is needed if there is a peak–peak gradient across the coarctation of >20 mm Hg and/or proximal hypertension. In neonates surgical repair is required. In older children and adults, balloon dilatation and stenting or surgery is advisable. Recurrence of stenosis may occur as the child grows. A balloon dilatation is preferred for recoarctation (sometimes stenting).

Atrial Septal Defect

Q. Write short essay on atrial septal defect.

An atrial septal defect (ASD) is an abnormal, fixed opening in the atrial septum. It is due to incomplete formation of the atrial septum.

Types of ASD

- **Ostium secundum** defects (**75–85%** of ASDs) are located in the region of the midseptum (fossa ovalis).
- **Ostium primum (atrioventricular septal)** defects (**10–15%**) are located in the lower portion of the atrial septum.
- **Sinus venosus** defects:
  - **Superior sinus venosus type defect (5–10%):** Defects are located in the superior part of the septum near the orifice of the superior vena cava (SVC).
  - **Inferior sinus venosus (IVC) type defect (1%):** Defects are located on the inferior part of the septum near the IVC entry point.
- **Coronary sinus (1%)** septal defect (in which a defect between the coronary sinus and the left atrium allows a left-to-right shunt to occur through an 'unroofed' coronary sinus).

Hemodynamics

In ASD flow of blood is between the left and right atria. Normal RV is more compliant than the LV and initially a large volume of blood shunts through the atrial defect from the left atrium to right atrium and then to right ventricle. This increases right ventricular output and markedly increased pulmonary blood flow through the pulmonary arteries. As a result, there is progressive enlargement of right atrium, right ventricle and pulmonary arteries. Eventually, pulmonary hypertension develops and sometimes reversal of the shunt from right to left (tend to occur later in life).

Clinical Features

Symptoms

- ASDs are often **asymptomatic till adulthood**.
- Two to three times more common in women than in men.
- Symptoms include easy fatigability, recurrent chest infection, exertional dyspnea, palpitations related to arrhythmias (especially atrial fibrillation), platypnea-orthodeoxia-dyspnea with standing, relieved by rest and cardiac failure.
- *After 40 years:* Deterioration due to atrial fibrillation, increased left to right shunt due to hypertension and coronary artery disease (CAD) which decrease left ventricular (LV) compliance.

Signs

- **Pulse:** No variation in rate or volume with Valsalva, irregularly irregular pulse with AF.
- **JVP:** (1) a and v waves have equal height that is reflection of LA waves and (2) a wave becomes taller when pulmonary hypertension develops or associated mitral stenosis (MS).
- Systolic pulsations in second and third left intercostals space due to dilated pulmonary artery.

- Characteristic physical signs due to the volume overload of the right ventricle:
  - ***S_2- wide fixed split:** Wide, fixed splitting of the second heart sound (S_2).*
    - Wide due to (1) increased RV ejection time (delay in right ventricular ejection) and (2) increased pulmonary hangout interval.
    - Fixed because the atrial septal defect equalizes left and right atrial pressures throughout the respiratory cycle.
  - A systolic flow murmur over the pulmonary valve not due to atrial septal defect.
  - Diastolic flow murmur over the tricuspid valve may be heard in children with a large shunt.
- S_1-loud and P_2 is loud (due to increased recoil of the dilated PA and close proximity of dilated PA to chest wall).
- Ventricular heave/parasternal impulse present.

Investigations

- **Chest X-ray (Fig. 7.52):** It shows enlargement of the heart (right atrium, right ventricle) and prominent pulmonary arteries (Jug handle appearance) with pulmonary plethora. Hilar dance on fluoroscopy is characteristic.
- **ECG:** Incomplete right bundle branch block (RBBB due to right ventricular depolarization) and right axis deviation (due to dilatation of the right ventricle). Ostium primum defects may show left axis deviation.
- **Echocardiography:** May show hypertrophy and dilatation of the right heart and pulmonary arteries.
- Subcostal views with 2D and color Doppler demonstrates the ASD and helps in calculation of the left right shunt (QP: QS ratio).
- **CMR and CT** helps to assess for anomalous pulmonary venous drainage.
- **MRI:** Can be used to identify size and location of defect, A major advantage of MRI is the ability to quantify right ventricular size,
- volume, and function along with the ability to identify the systemic and pulmonary venous return.
- **Cardiac catheterization:** In nonrestrictive ASD, pressure gradient between atria is less than 3 mm Hg.

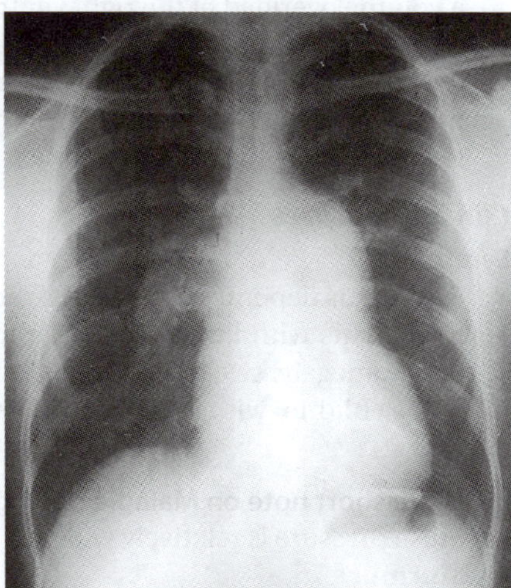

FIG. 7.52: Chest X-ray of atrial septal defect showing jug handle appearance.

Complications: Congestive heart failure (in neonates), paradoxical embolism, atrial fibrillation. Others include pulmonary hypertension (late), Eisenmenger's syndrome (very late), and very rarely infective endocarditis.

Management

- Prompt treatment of respiratory infections.
- Indications for intervention
  - ASD with significant left to right shunting resulting in right atrial/ventricular enlargement irrespective of symptoms.
  - Atrial septal defects in which pulmonary flow is increased 50% above systemic flow (i.e., flow ratio of 1.5:1).
  - Thromboembolic events.
- **Contraindications to surgery:** Severe pulmonary hypertension and shunt reversal.
- **Surgical options available are:**
  - Median sternotomy with direct closure of small to moderate defect.
  - Larger defects closed with autologous pericardium or synthetic patches like polyester polymer (Dacron) or polytetrafluoroethylene (PTFE).
  - Surgical closure of the defect is done in patients above 3 years of age, provided there are no signs of pulmonary hypertension and the pulmonary flow is 50% more than the systemic blood flow (Qp:Qs>1.5/1).
  - A transcatheter septal clamshell device closure may be used for most secundum ASDs (if suitable size).
- Uncorrected ASD does not require antibiotic prophylaxis for endocarditis unless other high-risk conditions are present.

Prognosis: Long-term prognosis thereafter is excellent after surgical intervention.

Patent Foramen Ovale

- It may be found in >25% of adult population and is hemodynamically insignificant.
- Usually asymptomatic but may be associated with paradoxical emboli and increased incidence of embolic stroke.

Ventricular Septal Defect

Q. Write short essay on ventricular septal defect (VSD).

VSD is the most common congenital heart disease (2 per 1,000 live births).

Etiology

- Congenital ventricular septal defect are due to incomplete septation of the ventricles. Embryologically, the interventricular septum has two portions, namely (1) a membranous and (2) a muscular portion (which is further divided into inflow, trabecular and outflow portions). Most congenital ventricular defects are "perimembranous," i.e., at the junction of the membranous and muscular portions. Congenital ventricular septal defect may be isolated or may be associated with other congenital heart disease.

- **Causes of acquired ventricular septal defect:** Ventricular septal rupture as a complication of acute MI, infective endocarditis or rarely from trauma/cardiac catheterization.

Hemodynamic Consequences

- Left ventricular pressure is higher than right ventricle. Therefore, blood flows from left-to-right ventricle and this causes a volume overload of the right ventricle and increased pulmonary blood flow.
- The shunt volume in a VSD depends on the shunt size of the defect and the pulmonary vascular resistance. If the defect is large (at a later stage), large volumes of blood flows through the pulmonary vasculature leading to pulmonary hypertension. When the right ventricular pressure becomes higher than left, the blood starts to shunt from right to left leading to Eisenmenger's complex. It is characterized by cyanosis.

Clinical Features

Symptoms

- Symptoms depend on the size of the defect and severity the shunt.
- In patients with large VSD, symptoms develop soon after birth. It includes dyspnea, repeated pulmonary infection, hepatomegaly, sweating, and failure to thrive. Irreversible pulmonary vascular disease after 1–2 years of age.
- Some children with isolated VSD develop subpulmonic stenosis: Patient not at risk of pulmonary vascular disease.

Signs

Q. Write short note on Maladie de Roger.

- Pulse pressure is relatively wide.
- **Murmur:**
  - Blood flow from the high-pressure left ventricle to the low-pressure right ventricle during systole produces a **pansystolic murmur (PSM)**. It is usually heard best at the left sternal edge (3rd, 4th and 5th intercostal space) and radiates all over the precordium. S_1 and S_2 are masked by a pansystolic murmur.
  - **A small defect usually produces a loud** PSM **murmur** (**Maladie de Roger**) presenting in older children when there is no other hemodynamic disturbance.
  - **Large defect produces a softer murmur**, especially when the right ventricular pressure is raised. This can be detected immediately after birth, while pulmonary vascular resistance is high, or when the shunt is reversed as in Eisenmenger's syndrome.
- Precordium is hyperkinetic with a systolic thrill at left sternal border (LSB).
- Prominent parasternal pulsation, tachypnea and indrawing of the lower ribs on inspiration.
- Mortality—27% by 20 years and 69% by 60 years.

Investigations

- **Chest X-ray:** Shows cardiomegaly proportional to the volume overload. Mainly LV, LA, and RV enlargement. Increased pulmonary blood flow, PAH.
- **Electrocardiogram:** May show right/left or combined ventricular hypertrophy. RBBB is common. **Katz Wachtel sign**, i.e., large equiphasic QRS in V_2-V_4 suggestive of biventricular hypertrophy.
- **Doppler echocardiography** is useful to determine location of VSD, morphology of LV outflow, aortic valve involvement.
- **Cardiac catheterization** to assess pulmonary vascular resistance in complicated VSD.

Complications: These include congestive heart failure, pulmonary hypertension, Eisenmenger's syndrome, right ventricular outflow tract obstruction, infective endocarditis.

Natural History

- Spontaneous closure occurs in about 40% of cases.
- Development of RVOT obstruction/infundibular stenosis (*Gasul's transformation*) may occur in 5% of the defects. Though patient requires surgery, it prevents development of pulmonary vascular obstructive disease.
- Aortic insufficiency develops in approximately 5% of patients. This may either be related to prolapse of an aortic valve cusp into VSD or lack of support to the aortic root.

Management

- **Small VSD:** No medication or surgery needed if asymptomatic. About 75–80% closes by 2 years and it needs observation.
- **Cardiac failure in infancy:** It is initially managed with digoxin and diuretics. If failure persists surgical repair of the defect should be performed.
- **Moderate/large VSD:** Repair by intervention
  - Large hemodynamically significant VSD: L to R shunting with Qp/Qs ≥ 2:1, even if asymptomatic, ideally before 1 year.
  - Growth failure, unresponsive to medical therapy is an indication for surgery.
- Surgical closure is contraindicated in fully developed Eisenmenger's syndrome. These patients may be treated by heart–lung transplantation.

Eisenmenger's Syndrome

Q. Write short essay on Eisenmenger's syndrome.

Eisenmenger syndrome characterized by an untreated congenital cardiac defect with intracardiac communication that leads to pulmonary hypertension, reversal of flow, and cyanosis.

- It develops as a consequence of the reversal of a left-to-right shunt to a right-to-left shunt. It develops in patients with congenital heart disease, such as PDA, VSD, and ASD.
- VSD Eisenmenger is called as Eisenmenger complex.

Clinical Features

Symptoms

Dyspnea, fatigue, dizziness, and syncope.

Signs

- **Central cyanosis and clubbing:** It develops due to the mixing of deoxygenated blood with oxygenated blood. It is generalized in ASD and VSD reversal, whereas it is differential (only lower limbs) in PDA with reversal.
- Signs of pulmonary hypertension and its sequelae (refer 'pulmonary hypertension').
- **Heart sounds:** S_2 is loud with palpable P_2.
  - In ASD with reversal: S_2 fixed but narrowly split
  - In VSD with reversal: S_2 single
  - In PDA with reversal: S_2 mobile but narrowly split
  - Right ventricular S_4 and pulmonary ejection click appear.
- **Murmurs:** The murmurs of the underlying cause (ASD, VSD, PDA) decrease in intensity, duration and finally disappear with the development of Eisenmenger's syndrome. Early diastolic murmur at pulmonary area and pansystolic murmur of TR appear.

Complications: Right heart failure, infective endocarditis, pulmonary infections, severe hemoptysis, secondary polycythemia, pulmonary thrombosis with infarction, brain abscess, cerebral stroke, and ventricular arrhythmias.

Treatment

- Surgical correction of underlying defect (refer treatment of ASD, VSD and PDA).
- Do not advise vasodilator therapy using calcium channel blockers. It causes systemic vasodilatation and increases right-to-left shunt.
- Long-term oxygen inhalation may be useful to relieve symptoms.
- Phlebotomy when hyperviscosity syndrome develops due to polycythemia.
- Heart-lung transplantation is the only curative treatment.
- Relief of symptoms: By drugs such as prostanoids (e.g., epoprostenol, iloprost, treprostinil), endothelin receptor antagonists (e.g., bosentan) and phosphodiesteraase-5 inhibitors (e.g., sildenafil, tadalafil).

CYANOTIC CONGENITAL HEART DISEASES

Tetralogy of Fallot

Q. Write short essay on Fallot's tetralogy or Tetralogy of Fallot (TOF).

It is the most common congenital cyanotic heart disease in adults (75%). It consists of four features **(Fig. 7.53A)**:

1. Ventricular septal defect usually large and similar in aperture to the aortic orifice.
2. Pulmonary stenosis: Right ventricular outflow tract obstruction mostly subvalvular (infundibular) but may be valvular, supravalvular or a combination of these.
3. Overriding of dextroposed aorta
4. Right ventricular hypertrophy

Presence of ASD along with TOF is known as **pentalogy of Fallot.**

Etiology

- It occurs in about 1 in 2,000 births and is the most common cause of cyanosis in infancy after the first year of life.
- It is due to abnormal development of the bulbar septum that separates the ascending aorta from the pulmonary artery.

Pathophysiology

- When RV and LV pressures become identical, there is little or no left to right shunt. Hence, VSD is silent.
- Right ventricle empties into pulmonary artery across pulmonic stenosis producing ejection systolic murmur. Hence, the more severe the pulmonary stenosis, more is the left-to-right shunt and less is the flow into the pulmonary artery and the ejection systolic murmur is shorter.
- When tetralogy causes elevation of right ventricular pressure, right-to-left shunting of cyanotic blood across the ventricular septal defect occurs.
- Congestive failure usually does not develop because right ventricle is effectively decompressed by ventricular septal defect.

Clinical Features

Symptoms

- Symptoms depend on the severity of pulmonary stenosis and may present any time after birth.
- Paroxysmal attacks of dyspnea, anoxic spells, predominantly after waking up. Child cries becomes blue (cyanosis due to increased right sided pressures, resulting in a right to left shunt), lose consciousness and may develop convulsion. Frequency varies from once a few days to many attack every day.

- Squatting is common
- **Fallot's spell ("tet spell"):** It is lethal, unpredictable, episodes in which the child suddenly becomes increasingly cyanosed usually during feeding, crying, fever or exercise and may become apneic and unconscious. This is because of spasm of the subpulmonary muscle (infundibular septum), systemic vasodilatation producing increased right-to-left shunting across VSD and acute increase right ventricular outlet obstruction.
  - Progression of spell may lead to metabolic acidosis which further reduces systemic resistance and increases pulmonary vascular resistance. This can cause sudden death.
  - **Fallot's spell** can be relieved by increasing systemic/peripheral resistance. This diminishes (reduces) right-to-left shunting, increases systemic venous return and increases pulmonary blood flow. Example of postural maneuver that increases peripheral/systemic resistance is sitting posture/squatting (Fallot sign).
- Adults have growth retardation, fatigue and dyspnea on exertion but cyanotic spells are not usual. Secondary polycythemia due to chronic hypoxia and can produce thrombotic strokes.

Signs

- **Combination of cyanosis with a loud ejection systolic murmur:** In the pulmonary area (as for pulmonary stenosis) is the most characteristic feature. The ejection systolic murmur is heard in the second and third left intercostal spaces and is due to pulmonary outflow obstruction. Intensity and duration of ejection systolic murmur is inversely proportional to severity of right ventricular outflow tract obstruction. However, cyanosis may not be seen in the newborn or in patients with only mild right ventricular outflow obstruction ("acyanotic tetralogy of Fallot").
- **Second heart sound:** Pulmonary obstruction results in delayed P_2 and **P_2 become soft or inaudible** (too soft to be heard). Since P_2 is inaudible, hence $S_2 = A_2$ (S_2 is single loud second heart sound).
- Aorta is displaced anteriorly too, A2 becomes loud. Ascending aorta in TOF is large, results in an aortic ejection click.
- Other signs include clubbing, parasternal heave, systolic thrill.

Investigations

- **Chest X-ray (Fig. 7.53B):** Shows an abnormally small pulmonary artery, large right ventricle and a 'boot-shaped' heart ("Coeur en Sabot").
- **ECG:** Shows right ventricular hypertrophy.
- **Echocardiography:** It is diagnostic and highly sensitive. It shows that the aorta is not continuous with the anterior ventricular septum.
- Cardiac catheterization is rarely required.

Treatment

- **Definitive management:** Consists of total correction of the defect by surgical means (relief of the pulmonary stenosis and closure of the ventricular septal defect) in infants and children prior to 5 years of age.
- **Blalock–Taussig shunt:** It is a shunt/anastomosis between a subclavian artery and pulmonary artery on the same side. In babies with severely hypoplastic pulmonary arteries (severe pulmonary stenosis), initially palliation in the form of a Blalock–Taussig shunt may be performed. This increases pulmonary blood flow and pulmonary artery development, and may facilitate later definitive correction.
- **Treatment of cyanotic spells:**
  - Patient is asking to assume squatting (knee-to-chest) position.
  - Oxygen administration
  - Intravenous fluids to increase venous return.
  - Morphine IV in the dose of 0.1 mg/kg reduces the release of catecholamines. This increases the period of right ventricular filling.
  - Propranolol IV in the dose of 0.01 mg/kg followed by oral dose of 3–5 mg/kg/day in divided doses.
- **Antibiotic prophylaxis** for prevention of endocarditis.

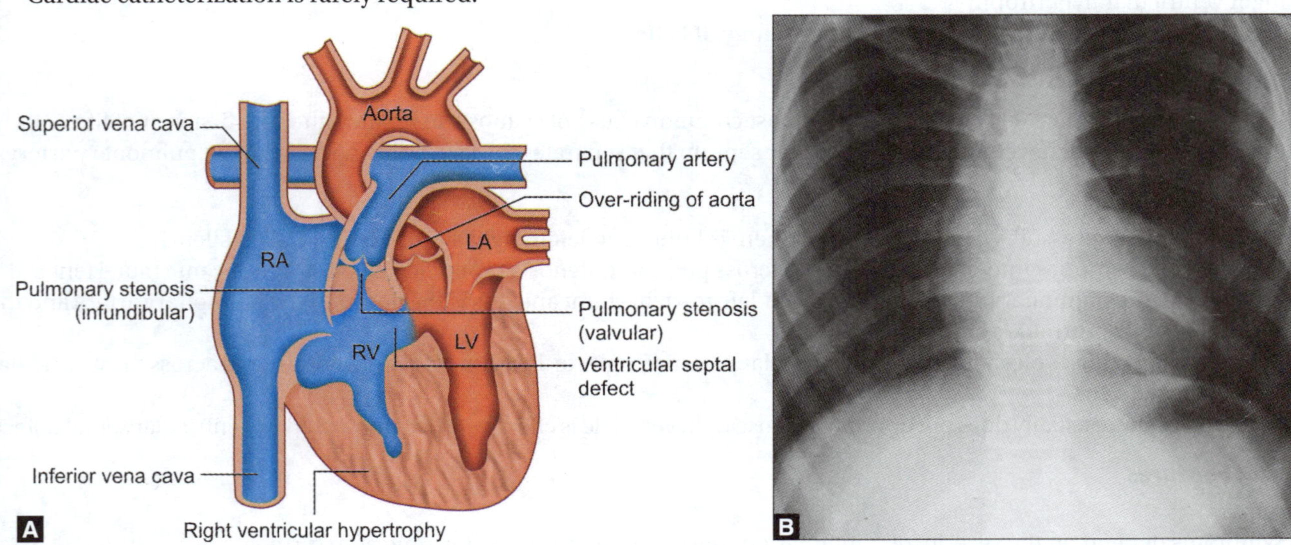

FIGS. 7.53A AND B: (A) Diagrammatic representation of tetralogy of Fallot. Four components are: (1) Ventricular septal defect; (2) subpulmonic stenosis/pulmonary valvular stenosis; (3) aorta overriding the VSD and (4) right ventricular hypertrophy; (B) X-ray shows an abnormally small pulmonary artery, large right ventricle and a 'boot-shaped' heart.
(LA: left atrium; LV: left ventricle; RV: right ventricle; RA: right atrium)

Complications: These include (1) intravascular thrombosis, cerebrovascular accidents and embolism secondary to polycythemia, (2) brain abscess and (3) infective endocarditis.

Ebstein Anomaly

- Ebstein's anomaly is a cyanotic congenital heart disease that is characterized by abnormalities of the tricuspid valve and atrialization of right ventricle. It is associated with maternal lithium consumption.
- **Clinical features:** Patients present with episodic tachyarrhythmia's (associated WPW syndrome) and cyanosis. They are prone to develop paradoxical embolism, brain abscess and sudden cardiac death.
- On examination, there is central cyanosis and clubbing, prominent a waves in JVP and hepatomegaly. On auscultation, patient will have a split first heart sound, split second heart sound, S_3 and S_4. Pansystolic murmur of TR is present.
- ECG reveals right axis deviation, "Himalayan" giant P waves, RBBB, preexcitation pattern. CXR reveals gross cardiomegaly often called as wall to wall heart or the box heart.
- Doppler echocardiography is diagnostic.

Prognosis: After total surgical correction is good (especially if the operation is performed in childhood). About 66% live to 1 year, 49% to 3 years, and 24% to 10 years.

Management
Medical management include treatment of arrhythmias, embolism and nitric oxide. Surgical repair includes tricuspid replacement, selective plication of the atrialized right ventricle and closure of intracardiac shunt (Danielson repair, Carpentier technique).

DISEASES OF THE PERICARDIUM

Acute Pericarditis

Q. Write short essay/note on:
- **Acute pericarditis.**
- **Causes and management of pericarditis.**

Definition: Acute pericarditis is defined as an acute inflammation of the pericardium.

Etiology

Q. Write short note on causes of pericarditis.

Various common causes of pericarditis are listed in **Box 7.52**.

Box 7.52: Common causes of pericarditis.

- Idiopathic
- Infections
  - Viral (Coxsackie A and B, Echovirus, HIV)
  - Pyogenic (*Pneumococcus, Staphylococcus, Legionella*)
  - Tuberculosis: Most common cause in India
  - Fungal (Histoplasmosis, *Candida*)
  - Syphilis, parasitic
- Acute myocardial infarction
- Metastatic neoplasm
- Hypothyroidism
- Radiation therapy (up to 20 years earlier)
- Chronic renal failure
- Connective tissue disorder (RA, SLE)
- Drug reaction (Procainamide, hydralazine)
- Autoimmune following heart surgery and MI (Dressler's syndrome)
- Trauma

(MI, myocardial infarction; SLE, systemic lupus erythematosus)

Classification

- **Depending on the duration:** Pericarditis is classified as acute (<6 weeks), subacute (6 weeks to 6 months) and chronic (>6 months).
- **Depending on the nature of inflammation:** Pericarditis may be associated with pericardial effusion and also may coexist with myocarditis. Depending on the nature of pericardial inflammation, it may be classified as serous, hemorrhagic or purulent pericarditis.
  - *Fibrinous pericarditis:* Fibrinous exudate may heal and form varying degrees of adhesion formation.
  - *Serous pericarditis:* Produces a large effusion of turbid, straw colored fluid with high protein content.
  - Hemorrhagic pericarditis is usually due to malignant disease (e.g., carcinoma of the breast or bronchus, and lymphoma).
  - *Purulent pericarditis:* May develop as a complication of septicemia, by direct spread from an intrathoracic infection, or from a penetrating injury.

Clinical Features

Pericardial pain

- Pericardial inflammation produces characteristic pericardial pain. It is sharp, retrosternal (central) chest pain which radiates to the shoulders and neck. Radiation of pain to trapezius muscle ridges is a feature that favors pericardial pain.
- Pain may be steady and constrictive. Typically aggravated by deep breathing, movement, and a change of position/lying down, coughing exercise and swallowing.
- Typically relieved by sitting up and leaning forward.

Nonspecific symptoms

- Low-grade fever, and malaise. Myocarditis may be associated with pericarditis.
- Large pericardial effusion can compress adjacent bronchi and lung and produce dyspnea (Ewart's sign).

Pericardial friction rub

- Pericardial friction rub is a high-pitched superficial scratching or crunching sound, produced by movement of the inflamed pericardium. It is diagnostic of pericarditis.
- Best heard by applying firm pressure with the diaphragm of stethoscope at the lower left sternal edge at the end of expiration with the patients sitting upright and leaning forward. Usually heard in systole but may also be audible in diastole.
- It has a "to-and-fro," leathery quality. It is usually transitory, repeatedly disappearing and re-appearing.
- **Three phase:** Classical pericardial friction rub has three phases corresponding to movement of heart during three phases of cardiac cycle, namely (1) atrial systole, (2) ventricular systole and (3) ventricular diastole (rapid ventricular filling during early diastole). However, in some it may be heard as only one (monophasic) or two (biphasic) rubs.

Other features

- **Pulsus paradoxus** (paradoxical pulse) is characterized by weakness/disappearance of arterial pulse during inspiration.
- **Cardiac tamponade:** Characterized by the accumulation of pericardial fluid under pressure.
- **Constrictive pericarditis:** Results from scarring and consequent loss of elasticity of the pericardial sac. Typically pericardium is thicker than normal and shows chronic inflammation, sometimes with calcification.
- **Effusive-constrictive pericarditis:** Characterized by constrictive physiology with a coexisting pericardial effusion, usually with tamponade.

Investigations

- **Blood:** Leukocytosis (bacterial pericarditis) or lymphocytosis (viral pericarditis) and raised erythrocyte sedimentation rate (ESR).
- **Cardiac enzymes (CPK-MB, troponin T):** Normal unless associated with myocarditis.
- **Electrocardiogram:** ECG is diagnostic and changes may be found over the affected area, which may be widespread. These are as follows:
  - Widespread **concave upwards (saddle shaped/smiling face) ST elevation** in multiple leads (particularly leads I, II, aVL, aVF, and V1-V3) and reciprocal ST depression in leads aVR and V.
  - **PR segment depression** is a characteristic feature of acute pericarditis.
  - The above changes evolve over time and later followed by resolution of the ST elevation, T wave flattening/inversion (due to myocarditis) and finally T wave normalization.
  - Finally ECG becomes normal.
  - When there pericardial effusion QRS voltage is reduced. Electrical alternans is seen with effusion.

Differential diagnosis

- **Myocardial infarction (Table 7.96):** The early ECG changes observed in pericarditis should be differentiated from the ST elevation observed in myocardial infarction (limited to the infarcted area, e.g., anterior or inferior). Most reliable feature may be the ratio of ST segment elevation (in millimeters) to T-wave amplitude in lead V6; ratio >0.24.
- **Chest X-ray:**
  - May be normal in pericarditis without effusion. Stenciled borders of heart.
  - Rapid increase in the size of the cardiac shadow (cardiomegaly-pear-shaped) may be seen in pericarditis with effusion. (money bag/water-bottle appearance). Oreo cookie sign/epicardial fat pad sign can be seen on lateral X-ray chest.
- **Echocardiography** used for confirmation of the pericardial effusion.
- **CT and cardiac MR** may be useful when there is thickening (>4 mm) or inflammation of pericardium and myocardium.
- **Paracentesis:** Diagnostic paracentesis is performed when there is pericardial effusion.

TABLE 7.96: Differences in ECG changes between acute pericarditis and acute ST-elevation myocardial infarction.

ECG finding	*Acute pericarditis*	*Acute ST-elevation MI*
Shape of ST-segment	Concave upward	Convex upward
Reciprocal ST-segment changes	–	+
Location of ST-segment changes	Diffuse (except aVR and V_1)	Depends on coronary artery affected
Q waves	–	+
Depression of PR-segment	+	–
Concomitant presence of ST and T changes	– (T wave inversion occurs after ST segments have normalized)	+

Q. Write short note on management of pericarditis.

Treatment

- Treatment of the underlying cause (e.g., tuberculosis, uremia, autoimmune disease).
- Bed rest and avoid physical activity.
- **Analgesics:** The pain is usually relieved by oral NSAIDs (high dose aspirin indomethacin or ibuprofen). It also decreases the inflammation in idiopathic or viral pericarditis.

- **Aspirin** in the dose of 600 mg 4 hourly is the drug of choice for patients with a recent myocardial infarction. Ibuprofen 300–800 mg 3 times daily may also be used. They can be given till pain and pericardial effusion disappears and ESR, CRP values return normal. It usually takes 7 to 10 days.
- Indomethacin is a more potent anti-inflammatory drug and can be given in the dose of 25 mg 3 times daily. It should be avoided in elderly patients because it can decrease the coronary blood flow.
- **Colchicine** 0.5 mg twice a day is also effective in combination with NSAIDs.
- **Corticosteroids** (10–30 mg/day for 2–4 weeks) should be reserved for patients with an immune cause or patients who do not respond to NSAIDs. Because their use is associated with an increased rate of recurrence. Colchicine or corticosteroids reduce the symptoms but does not hasten the cure.

- **Purulent pericarditis:** Antimicrobial therapy, pericardiocentesis and surgical drainage (if required).
- **Indications for hospitalization:** Fever (38°C), leukocytosis, large pericardial effusion, lack of response to NSAIDs after 1 week of therapy acute trauma, cardiac tamponade, immunosuppressed state, recurrent pericarditis.

Pericardial Effusion

Q. Write short essay/note on pericardial effusion and its causes.

Definition: Pericardial effusion is an accumulation of fluid within the potential space of the serous pericardial sac.

- Slowly developing pericardial effusions may be asymptomatic. If it develops over a short period, and volume of effusion is large, it may lead to compromisation of ventricular filling leading to embarrassment of the circulation. This is known as cardiac tamponade.
- **Type:** Pericardial effusion may be transudate (hydropericardium), exudate (pyopericardium) or hemopericardium.
- **Etiology:** It commonly develops during an episode of acute pericarditis (*refer* **Box 7.52**).

Clinical Signs

Symptoms commonly reflect the underlying pericarditis. Sometimes, a sensation of retrosternal oppression may be present.

Signs

- Cardiovascular examination is normal except if the effusion is large, apex beat/impulse is not palpable (sometimes palpable medial to the left border of cardiac dullness).
- Increase in cardiac dullness on percussion.
- Heart sounds are faint, soft, distant or muffled.
- A pericardial friction rub due to pericarditis may be audible in the early stages. It becomes quieter as fluid accumulates and pushes the layers of the pericardium apart.
- **Ewart's sign:** Rarely, large effusion may compress the base of the left lung. It produces an area of dullness to percussion and tubular breath sounds on auscultation in the left axilla or left base (below the angle of the left scapula) and termed as Ewart's sign.

Investigations

Q. Write short note on radiological findings in pericardial effusion.

- **Chest X-ray:** Shows increased size of the cardiac silhouette, large globular or pear-shaped heart or water-bottle appearance with sharp outlines and lucent pericardial fat lines. Typically, the pulmonary veins are not distended Oreo cookie sign/ Epicardial fat pad sign.
- **Electrocardiogram:** ECG often shows low voltage QRS complexes (<0.5 mV in limb leads) in the presence of large effusions with sinus tachycardia. Electric alternans characterized by alternation of QRS amplitude or axis between beats) due to a to-and-fro motion of the heart within the fluid-filled pericardial sac may be observed.
- **Echocardiography** is the most useful investigation for demonstrating the pericardial effusion. It is also useful to monitor the size of the effusion and its effect on cardiac function.
- **Cardiac CT or MRI** is advisable if loculated pericardial effusions are suspected (postcardiac surgery).
- **Pericardial aspiration (pericardiocentesis):** It is aspiration of pericardial fluid effusion with aseptic technique under echocardiographic guidance. A needle is inserted medial to the cardiac apex or below the xiphoid process, directed upwards toward the left shoulder. It is indicated for diagnostic purposes (e.g., tuberculous, malignant or purulent effusion) or for the treatment of cardiac tamponade. Complications of pericardiocentesis include arrhythmias, damage to myocardium and coronary vessels, air embolism, and pneumothorax. The pericardial fluid is can be sent for investigations, such as:
    - Cell counts, protein, glucose and LDH to differentiate exudates from transudates, Gram's stains and AFB stain.
    - Cytology for malignant cells
    - Mycobacterium culture
- **Pericardial biopsy** may be advisable if when tuberculosis is suspected and pericardiocentesis is not diagnostic.
- **Other tests:** Depending on the underlying causes, e.g., blood cultures, autoantibody screen.

Treatment

- Treat the underlying cause if possible.
- Anti-inflammatory drugs (aspirin or indomethacin). Most effusions resolve spontaneously, but rapid effusion may produce cardiac tamponade.
- **Therapeutic pericardiocentesis:** Indicated to relieve the pressure and a pigtail catheter drain may be left in temporarily to allow sufficient release of fluid.
- **Pericardial fenestration:** If pericardial effusions accumulate (e.g., malignancy), it may be treated by pericardial fenestration. This procedure consists of creating a window in the pericardium to allow the slow release of fluid into the surrounding tissues. It may be performed either transcutaneously under local anesthetic or by a conventional surgical approach.
- **Intrapericardial instillation of chemotherapeutic agents** may be useful in malignant effusion.

Cardiac Tamponade

Q. Write short essay/note on clinical features, signs and management of pericardial tamponade.

- Cardiac tamponade is the term used for acute heart failure that results from large or rapidly developing pericardial effusion which compresses the heart and impair diastolic filling.
- Minimum amount of pericardial fluid necessary for the development of cardiac tamponade depends on the speed of its accumulation. About 250 mL in rapidly developing effusions and more than 2000 mL in slowly developing effusions.

Etiology: Pericardial effusion (*refer* **Box 7.52**).

Clinical Features

Symptoms

- Due to reduced cardiac output: Dyspnea, orthopnea, substernal chest discomfort radiating to neck and jaw.
- Due to systemic venous congestion: Pain in the right upper quadrant and pedal edema in slowly developing cardiac tamponade (subacute tamponade).

Signs

- Friedreich's sign: Markedly raised jugular venous pressure with sharp rise and *y* descent.
- Pulsus paradoxus or paradoxical pulse: An exaggeration in the normal variation in pulse pressure seen with inspiration. There is drop in systolic blood pressure of ≥10 mm Hg. Pulsus paradoxus is the hallmark of cardiac tamponade.
- *Kussmaul's sign:* Rise in JVP/increased neck vein distension during inspiration.
- *Others:* Reduced cardiac output, hypotension, tachycardia, and oliguria.
- **Beck's triad of hypotension, muffled heart sounds, and elevated jugular venous pressure** remains a useful clue to the presence of severe tamponade.

Investigations

- *Chest X-ray:* Discussed earlier in pericarditis.
- **Electrocardiogram:** May show sinus tachycardia, reduction in QRS voltage, nonspecific ST-T changes and electrical alternans (alternation of QRS complex amplitude or axis between beats).
- **Echocardiography:** A pericardial effusion appears as a lucent separation between parietal and visceral pericardium and shows separation visceral and parietal layers for the entire cardiac cycle.
  - Small effusions are first evident over the posterobasal left ventricle.
  - Early diastolic collapse of the right ventricle and collapse of the right atrium (which occurs during ventricular diastole) are sensitive and specific signs.
  - Right atrial collapse is considered more sensitive.
  - RV collapse more specific for tamponade.

Management

- Emergency pericardiocentesis is necessary.
- If patient is hypotensive, as a temporary measure expansion of blood volume by saline, blood, plasma, and dextran.
- Avoid positive pressure mechanic ventilation in acute tamponade because it reduces cardiac filling further.
- Treatment of underlying cause.

Chronic Constrictive Pericarditis

Q. Write short essay/note on chronic constrictive pericarditis.

- Constrictive pericarditis is an end stage inflammatory process involving pericardium.
- It is characterized by progressive thickening, fibrosis, and calcification of the pericardium and visceral and parietal pericardium usually becomes adherent resulting in obliteration of the pericardial space. In some cases, the constricting process is formed by the visceral pericardium (epicardium) alone.

Pathophysiology: The heart is encased in a solid shell and cannot fill properly. The calcification may extend into the myocardium and may impair myocardial contraction. Following features develop:

- Restricted diastolic filling of the heart by fibrotic pericardium.
- Limitation of venous return to the heart → reduced ventricular filling → inability to maintain adequate preload.
- Filling pressures of the heart tend to become equal in both the ventricles and the atria.
- Systolic function is rarely affected until late in the course of the disease.
- **Preservation of myocardial function in early diastole aids in distinguishing constrictive pericarditis from restrictive cardiomyopathy.**

Etiology (Box 7.53) Clinical Features

The symptoms and signs are due to:

- Reduced ventricular filling which is similar to cardiac tamponade (i.e., Kussmaul's sign, Friedreich's sign, pulsus paradoxus.
- Systemic venous congestion: Symptoms consistent with CCF (especially right-sided heart failure), such as ascites, dependent edema, hepatomegaly and raised JVP.
- Reduced cardiac output: Inability of the heart to increase stroke volume produces fatigue, hypotension, and reflex tachycardia.
- Rapid ventricular filling: **Pericardial knock** (occurs 0.09–0.12 second after A_2) can be heard in early diastole at the lower left sternal border.
- Rarely pulmonary venous congestion causing dyspnea, cough, orthopnea.

Box 7.53: Causes of constrictive pericarditis.

- Idiopathic
- Infectious:
  - **Tuberculosis**
  - Viral especially Coxsackie B
  - Bacterial
  - Fungal
  - Parasitic
  - Postradiotherapy
- Postcardiac surgery
- Post-traumatic
- Neoplastic
- Connective tissue diseases (e.g., rheumatoid arthritis and SLE)
- Toxic/metabolic: Uremia, chylous pericardium, methysergide
- Post-myocardial infarction
- Familial

Investigations

- **ECG:** Rarely normal, nonspecific and highly variable. Atrial arrhythmias are frequent, with atrial fibrillation occurring late in course. Low voltage (<50% cases) and LA enlargement (19–37%).
- **Chest X-ray:** Pulmonary venous congestion and pleural effusions (late in the disease). **Calcified pericardium** is highly suggestive of constrictive pericarditis when present in a patient with constrictive/restrictive physiology.
- **Echocardiography:** Pericardial thickening better seen through transesophageal echo, normal RV and LV chamber size, LA and RA enlargement, abnormal septal and posterior wall motion, paradoxical septal motion, premature opening of the pulmonic valve and dilated IVC without respiratory variation.
- **Magnetic resonance imaging/CT scan** can confirm pericardial thickening. Pericardial thickening >4 mm assists in differentiating constrictive disease from restrictive cardiomyopathy, and thickening >6 mm adds even more specific for constriction. Normal pericardial thickness does not exclude pericardial constriction, and the clinical situation must always be taken in account.
- **Cardiac catheterization:** Ventricular pressure initially decreases rapidly (steep y descent on RA pressure waveform tracings) and then increases abruptly to a level that is sustained until systole (the "dip-and-plateau waveform" or "square root sign" seen on RV or LV pressure waveform tracings).

Treatment

- Pericardiectomy (resection of the pericardium) is the only definitive treatment.
- **Pharmacologic therapy**
  - **Steroids** for subacute constrictive pericarditis (before pericardial fibrosis occurs).
  - **Diuretics** to relieve congestion and optimize clinical volume status (may decrease preload to the point of reducing cardiac output).
  - Treatment of the causative disease (e.g., antituberculosis medication).
  - Avoid beta-blockers and calcium channel blockers (CCBs).

PULMONARY HYPERTENSION

Q. Write short essay/note on pulmonary hypertension.

Definition (WHO)

- Pulmonary hypertension (PH) is defined as an increase in blood pressure in pulmonary circulation (either in the arteries, or both in arteries and veins).
- Normal pressure as measured at right heart catheterization is 14–18 mm Hg at rest and 20–25 mm Hg on exercise. Hemodynamically it is defined as an increase in mean pulmonary arterial pressure to 25 mm Hg at rest.
- Definition may be refined by giving consideration of the pulmonary wedge pressure; the cardiac output and the transpulmonary pressure gradient (mean PAP - mean PWP).

WHO Classifications of Pulmonary Hypertension

WHO classification of pulmonary hypertension has been shown in **Table 7.97**.

Q. Write short essay/note on causes of pulmonary hypertension.

TABLE 7.97: WHO classifications of pulmonary hypertension, 2008 (Dana point).

- **Pulmonary arterial hypertension**
  - Idiopathic pulmonary arterial hypertension (IPAH)
  - Familial: BMPR2, ALK 1, unknown
  - Associated with PAH
    - Connective tissue disease: Scleroderma, SLE, rheumatoid arthritis
    - Congenital heart disease
    - Portal hypertension (5–7% of patients)
    - HIV (0.5% of patients)
    - Drugs/toxins: aminorex, dexfenfluramine, or fenfluramine-containing products, cocaine, methamphetamine
    - Others: Hereditary hemorrhagic telangiectasia, hemoglobinopathies, myeloproliferative disorders, splenectomy
  - Associated with venous/capillary involvement
    - Pulmonary veno-occlusive disease (evidence of pulmonary vascular congestion)
    - Pulmonary capillary hemangiomatosis
  - Persistent pulmonary hypertension (PH) of newborn
- **PH owing to left heart disease:** Systolic dysfunction, diastolic dysfunction and valvular disease.
- **PH secondary to chronic hypoxemia:** Chronic obstructive lung disease, interstitial lung disease, sleep disordered breathing, alveolar hypoventilation disorders, chronic exposure to high altitude, developmental abnormalities
- **Chronic thromboembolic pulmonary hypertension (CTEPH):** Thromboembolic obstruction of proximal or distal pulmonary arteries
- **Miscellaneous (usually extrinsic compression of pulmonary arteries):** Sarcoidosis, histiocytosis X, lymphangiomyomatosis, compression of pulmonary vessels (adenopathy, tumor, fibrosing mediastinitis, thyroid disorders, glycogen storage disease, Gaucher's disease)

Clinical Features

Symptoms: Insidious in onset and is usually diagnosed late. Usual symptoms include exertional breathlessness/dyspnea (60%), fatigue (19%), palpitation and near syncope/syncope (13%), chest pain (7%), palpitations (5%), LE edema (3%), and hoarseness of voice (2%).

Signs: These include:
- Cold extremities, peripheral edema, **cyanosis,** and rarely clubbing
- Raised jugular venous pulse, prominent V wave if tricuspid regurgitation is present
- Left parasternal lift/heave due to right ventricular hypertrophy.
- Large pulsatile liver
- Auscultatory signs in pulmonary hypertension **(Box 7.54)**
- **Signs of underlying cause**, e.g., interstitial lung disease or cardiac, liver, or connective tissue disease.

Box 7.54: Auscultatory signs in pulmonary hypertension.

- Pulmonary ejection sound (ES)
- Abnormal second heart sound (S_2): Loud P_2, narrow splitting
- Right atrial fourth heart sound (S_4)
- Right ventricular third heart sound (S_3)
- Pulmonary ejection systolic murmur (ESM)
- Pulmonary early diastolic murmur (EDM): Graham Steel murmur
- Tricuspid pansystolic murmur (PSM)

Investigations

- **Chest X-ray**
  - Enlargement of the pulmonary artery and its main branches
  - Peripheral "pruning" of vascular shadows
  - Enlarged right atrium, and right ventricle
  - Findings of underlying lung or cardiac pathology
- **Electrocardiogram:** Shows right axis deviation, R/S wave ratio greater than one in lead V1, right bundle branch block (incomplete or complete) and increased P wave amplitude in lead II (due to right atrial enlargement).
- **Echocardiography:** Most useful for detecting pulmonary hypertension and excluding cardiac disease. It shows tricuspid regurgitation, right atrial and ventricular hypertrophy, flattening of interventricular septum, small LV dimension, dilated pulmonary artery, and secondary causes (if any).
- **Transthoracic echocardiography:** Doppler assessment of the tricuspid regurgitant jet is a noninvasive method of determining the pressure of pulmonary artery.
- **Right heart catheterization:** Mean PAP pressure at rest >25 mm Hg, with exercise >30 mm Hg, wedge pressure <15 mm Hg.
- **Other tests**
  - Complete blood counts, prothrombin time, partial thromboplastin time, and liver function tests.
  - Autoantibodies if autoimmune disease is suspected.
  - HIV-ELISA if the patient has risk factors.
  - Arterial blood gas to exclude hypoxia and acidosis as contributors to pulmonary hypertension.
  - Sleep studies if sleep apnea suspected.
  - Pulmonary function tests to establish airflow obstruction or restrictive lung disease.
  - High-resolution computed tomography of chest to exclude occult interstitial lung disease.
  - Helical CT to detect pulmonary thromboembolism.
  - Ventilation-perfusion scanning to differentiate chronic thromboembolism from primary pulmonary hypertension.

Treatment
- Early recognition and treatment of the underlying cause.
- **Medical:** Diuretics mainly to treat edema from right heart failure, digoxin (for atrial tachyarrhythmias), **oxygen** (keep oxygen saturation ≥90%) and anticoagulants (IPAH) to keep INR 2.0–2.5.

- **PAH-specific therapy**
  - **Calcium channel blockers:** Indicated in patients who respond to vasodilators during catheterization. High doses required, e.g., nifedipine 240 mg/day, or amlodipine, 20 mg/day.
  - **Oral endothelin receptor antagonists (ERAs):** For example, bosentan, sitaxsentan, ambrisentan. Liver function be monitored monthly throughout the duration of use.
    - Bosentan initiated at 62.5 mg BD for first month and increased to 125 mg BD.
    - Ambrisentan initiated as 5 mg OD and can be increased to 10 mg daily.
  - **Phosphodiesterase type 5 inhibitors (PDE 5-I):** For example, sildenafil, tadalafil, vardenafil. The most common side effect is headache. Effective dose for sildenafil is 20–80 mg TID and for tadalafil is 40 mg OD.
  - **Prostaglandins:** For example, epoprostenol (prostacyclin), treprostinil, iloprost, prostacyclin 1P receptor antagonist (Selexipag).
  - **Guanylate cyclase stimulant:** For example, riociguat.
- Pneumococcal and influenza vaccination.
- **Surgical therapy**
  - Atrial septostomy (the creation of a right-to-left shunt).
  - Lung transplantation
  - Pulmonary thromboendarterectomy for chronic proximal thromboembolic pulmonary hypertension.

SUDDEN CARDIAC DEATH

Q. Write a short note on sudden cardiac death.

Sudden cardiac arrest (SCA) and SCD refer to the sudden cessation of cardiac activity with hemodynamic collapse.

- **Sudden cardiac death** is defined as an unexpected, nontraumatic, natural death due to cardiac causes occurring in a short period (within 1 hour of symptom onset) in an individual with or without any previously identified heart disease but in whom the time and mode of death are unexpected.
- It has four temporal elements: (1) Prodromes, (2) onset of terminal event, (3) cardiac arrest, and (4) biologic death.
- Bimodal age distribution with one peak between birth and 6 months of age and another after 65 years of age. It is a male preponderance.

Causes

Causes of SCD have been shown in **Box 7.55**.

Treatment

- Identifying individuals at high risk of SCD: Combination of factors more useful, most important parameter is left ventricular ejection fraction (LVEF).
- Pharmacological agents
  - Beta blockers, ACEI, amiodarone
  - Revascularization
  - ICD/CRT.

Box 7.55: Causes of sudden cardiac death.

- **Coronary artery disease:** Coronary atherosclerosis, developmental anomalies, coronary artery embolism, others (e.g., vasculitis, dissection)
- **Myocardial diseases:** Cardiomyopathies, myocarditis and other infiltrative processes, right ventricular dysplasia
- **Valvular diseases:** Mitral valve prolapse, aortic stenosis and other forms of left ventricular outflow obstruction, endocarditis
- **Conduction system abnormalities**: Wolff-Parkinson-White (WPW) syndrome, Brugada syndrome, long QT syndromes

CARDIAC ARREST

Definition: Cardiac arrest is a sudden loss of cardiac pump function which can reversed by a prompt intervention, without which it lead to death.

Causes of Cardiac Arrest

Causes of cardiac arrest have been shown in **Box 7.56**.

Q. Write short note on causes of cardiac arrest.

Diagnosis of cardiac arrest (TRIAD): (1) Loss of **consciousness**, (2) loss of apical and central **pulsations** (carotid, femoral) and (3) apnea**.**

ECG: Three basic patterns

1. Ventricular tachyarrhythmia: Ventricular fibrillation (VF)/sustained type of pulseless ventricular tachycardia.
2. Ventricular asystole or a bradyasystolic rhythm with an extremely slow rate.
3. Pulseless electrical activity (PEA) previously referred to as electromechanical dissociation.

Box 7.56: Causes of cardiac arrest (6 H and 4 T).

- **H**ypoxia
- **H**ypotension
- **H**ypothermia
- **H**ypoglycemia
- Acidosis (**H**$^+$)
- **H**yperkalemia (electrolyte disturbance)
- Cardiac **T**amponade
- **T**ension pneumothorax
- **T**hromboembolism (pulmonary, coronary)
- **T**oxicity (e.g., digoxin, local anesthetics, insecticides)

Q. Write short essay/note on management of cardiac arrest.

Management

Chain of Survival

It refers to the sequence of events that is required to maximize the chances of survival in a patient with cardiac arrest. Survival is most likely if all links in the chain are strong. The chain of survival consists of following links, namely:

- Immediate identification of cardiac arrest and activation of the emergency response system (ERS) by a trained individual.
- Immediate cardiopulmonary resuscitation (CPR) with chest compressions.
- Quick defibrillation.
- Effective advanced life support (ALS).
- Integrated post-cardiac arrest care.

Immediate Identification and Activation of ERS

- Immediate identification of cardiac arrest: Assessment is of crucial importance. It includes: (1) unresponsiveness (check the individual for a response, gently shake shoulders and ask 'are you all right?'), (2) no breathing or no normal breathing (i.e. only gasping) and (3) no pulse felt within 10 seconds.
- Activation of ERS: After activation of the ERS, all rescuers should immediately begin CPR.

Q. Write short essay/note on cardiopulmonary resuscitation (CPR).

- ***CPR***
  - It provides artificial ventilation and perfusion to the vital organs, particularly heart and brain until spontaneous cardiopulmonary function is restored. It consists of both basic life supports (BLS) and advanced life support (ALS). BLS provides adequate oxygen and perfusion to vital organs (brain and heart) until advanced cardiac life support is available **(Table 7.98)**.

TABLE 7.98: Phases of life support and its steps.

Phases	***Steps***
Phase-1: BLS	C = Circulation, A = Airway, B = Breathing
Phase-2: (ALS	D = Drugs, E = ECG, F = Fibrillation
Phase-3: Prolonged life support	Postresuscitation care

BLS consists of maneuver purpose of which is to maintain a low level of circulation until more definitive treatment with advanced life support can be provided.

- **Change from A-B-C to C-A-B:** CPR includes four sequential: **C**irculation, **A**irway and **B**reathing (CAB) and defibrillation. Previously, the sequence used to be **A**irway, **B**reathing and **C**irculation (ABC).
  - **Circulation:** The brain cannot survive for more than 3 minutes without circulation. Hence, start chest compressions immediately for a patient without central pulsations.
    - **Chest compressions (cardiac massage):**
      - Place the patient on a hard surface (wooden board).
      - The palm of one hand is placed in the concavity of the lower half of the sternum 2 fingers above the xiphoid process (avoid xiphisternal junction → fracture and injury). The other hand is placed over the hand on the sternum.
      - **Shoulders** should be positioned directly over the hands with the **elbows** locked straight and arms extended. Use your upper body weight to compress.
      - Sternum must be depressed **at least 5 cm** in adults, and **2–4 cm** in children, **1–2 cm** in infants.
      - **Push hard and push fast.** Must be performed at a rate of 100–120/min.
      - During CPR the ratio of chest compressions to ventilation should be: single rescuer = 30:2 and in the presence of 2 rescuers, **chest compressions must not be interrupted for ventilation.**
      - Chest compressions must be continued for 2 minutes before reassessment of cardiac rhythm (2 minutes = equivalent to 5 cycles 30:2).
    - **Assessment of the adequacy of chest compressions:** Systolic BP = 60–80 mm Hg, diastolic BP (>40 mm Hg) and COP = 30% of normal.
    - **Complications of chest compressions:** Fractures of rib/sternum, rib separation, pneumothorax, hemothorax, contusions of lung, lacerations of liver, fat emboli.
  - **Airway:** Loss of consciousness usually produces obstruction of airway due to loss of the muscle tone in the airway and falling back of the tongue. Hence, **clear the airway. Basic techniques for airway patency:**
    - **Head tilt, chin lift:** Place one hand on the forehead and the other on the chin. The head is tilted upwards to displace the tongue anteriorly.
    - **Jaw thrust method:** In this angles of mandible are grasped with both hands and the mandible is lifted forward.
    - **Finger sweep:** Sweep out foreign body in the mouth by index finger in unconscious patients and **not in a conscious or convulsing patient**.
    - **Heimlich maneuver:** Useful to remove the foreign body in a conscious patient. It is done while the patient is standing up or lying down. In this subdiaphragmatic abdominal thrust elevates the diaphragm and expels a blast of air from the lungs that displaces the foreign body. In infants this is performed by a series of blows on the back and chest thrusts.
  - **Breathing:** Rescue breathing can be mouth-to-mouth breathing or mouth-to-nose breathing (if there is serious injury of the mouth or it cannot be opened). With the airway open (using the head-tilt, chin-lift maneuver), pinch the nostrils shut for mouth-to-mouth breathing and cover the person's mouth with rescuer making a seal.

    - ◆ **Mouth-to-mouth breathing:** With the airway held open, pinch the nostrils closed, take a deep breath and seal your lips over the patients mouth. Blow steadily into the patient's mouth watching the chest rise as if the patient was taking a deep breath. Volume of each rescue breath should produce visible chest rise.
    - ◆ **Mouth-to-nose breathing:** Seal the mouth shut and breathe steadily through the nose.
    - ◆ **Mouth-to-mouth and nose:** It is used in infants and small children.
  - **Assessment of restoration of breathing and circulation:** Contraction of pupil, improved color of the skin, free movement of the chest wall, swallowing attempts and struggling movements.
  - **Indications for termination of BLS:** Pulse and respiration returns, emergency medical help arrives, physician declared patient is deceased, in a nonhealth setting, another indication to stop BLS would be that the rescuer was exhausted and physically unable to continue to perform BLS.
- **ALS:** The purpose is to restore normal cardiac rhythm by defibrillation when the cause is tachyarrhythmia, or to restore cardiac output by correcting other reversible causes of cardiac arrest. It includes:
  - Circulation by cardiac massage.
  - Airway management by equipment.
  - Breathing by advanced techniques.
  - Defibrillation by manual defibrillator.
  - Drugs.

Advanced techniques for airway patency: (1) Face mask, (2) oropharyngeal airway, (3) nasopharyngeal airway, (4) laryngeal mask airway, (5) endotracheal intubation, (6) combitube, (7) cricothyrotomy, (8) tracheostomy.

Advanced breathing: Expired air contains **16% O_2** so supplemental 100% O_2 should be used as soon as possible. Successful breathing is achieved by delivery of a tidal volume of **800–1,200 mL** in adults at a rate of **10–12 breaths/min** in adults. Advanced techniques include:

- **Self-inflating resuscitation bag** (Ambu bag), **(2) Mechanical ventilator or in ICU. Advanced circulation**
- It consists of continuation of chest compression and establishing an intravenous access, attaching a cardiac monitor/defibrillator, assessing the rhythm, defibrillation and administering appropriate drugs for rhythm as well as the condition.
- Continuous chest compression is performed at the rate of 100/minute and ventilation is provided at 8–10 breaths/minute (1 breath/6–8 seconds).

Rhythm in cardiac arrest

It may be (1) shockable rhythm (ventricular tachycardia/ventricular fibrillation) and (2) nonshockable rhythm (asystole and pulseless electrical activity).

- Rhythm checks should be performed done only after 2 minutes of CPR and not immediately following a defibrillation attempt.

Shockable rhythms: Ventricular fibrillation or pulseless ventricular tachycardia (VT).

Defibrillation: Completely depolarize all myocardial cells so SA node can re-establish as pacemaker. Voltage of electricity discharge High from 150 J to 360 J (biphasic) 360 J (monophasic). Continue CPR for 2 minutes and briefly check the monitor for rhythm. If VT/VF persists give second shock and immediately resume CPR and continue for 2 minutes, and repeat this cycle.

Drugs:

- **Adrenaline:** Given as a **vasopressor** α-1 effect (not as an inotrope). **Dose** is **1 mg** (**0.01 mg/kg**) **IV** every **4 minutes** (alternating cycles) while continuing CPR.
  - Given: (1) Immediately in nonshockable rhythm (non-VT/VF), (2) In VF or VT given after the 3rd shock.
  - **Repeated** in alternate cycles (every 4 minutes).
  - Once adrenaline → always adrenaline.
- **Amiodarone: Given** in shockable rhythm **after the 3rd shock**. If unavailable give **lidocaine** 100 mg IV (1–1.5 mg/kg). **Dose is 300 mg IV** bolus (5 mg/kg).
- **Vasopressin (ADH):** 40 IU single dose once.
- **Magnesium: Given** (1) VF/ VT with hypomagnesemia, (2) Torsade de pointes, (3) Digoxin toxicity. **Dose is 2 g IV.**
- **Calcium: Dose is 10 mL of 10%** calcium chloride IV.
  - **Indications:** PEA caused by hyperkalemia, hypocalcemia, hypermagnesemia, and overdose of calcium channel blockers.
  - Calcium solutions and $NaHCO_3$ should not be given simultaneously by the same route.
- **Thrombolytics:** Fibrinolytic therapy is considered when cardiac arrest is caused by proven or suspected **acute pulmonary embolism**. If a fibrinolytic drug is used in these circumstances consider performing CPR for at least 60–90 minutes before termination of resuscitation attempts. Example: Alteplase, tenecteplase (old generation: streptokinase).
- **Sodium bicarbonate:** Used in (1) severe metabolic acidosis (pH < 7.1), (2) life-threatening hyperkalemia, (3) tricyclic antidepressant overdose.
  - Dose: (Half correction) 1/2 base deficit × 1/3 body weight
  - Adverse drug reactions: (1) Increases CO_2 load, (2) inhibits release of O_2 to tissues, (3) impairs myocardial contractility and (4) causes hypernatremia.
- **Atropine:** Its routine use in **pulseless electrical activity** (PEA) and asystole is not useful. **Indicated** in sinus bradycardia or AV block causing hemodynamic instability. **Dose is 0.5 mg IV**. Repeated up to a maximum of 3 mg (*full atropinization*).

Nonshockable rhythms: Pulseless electrical activity (PEA) and asystole.

- PEA is characterized by cardiac electrical activity in the absence of any palpable pulse. They usually have some very weak mechanical myocardial contractions and does not produce a detectable pulse.

- Start CPR. Begin with chest compressions, and continue for 2 minutes before the rhythm check is repeated.
- Give 1 mg adrenaline IV immediately and re-check rhythm after 2 minutes of CPR.
- If PEA or asystole persists, continue CPR and recheck rhythm every 2 minutes. Administer adrenaline every 3–5 minutes. Do not give atropine.
- Check rhythm. If it shows change, check for pulse. If pulse appears, start post-resuscitation care. If there is still no pulse, continue CPR with rhythm check every 2 minutes and adrenaline every 3–5 minutes. If the rhythm develops into VF/VT, defibrillate the patient.

IV fluids: Infuse fluids rapidly if hypovolemia is suspected. Use **normal saline** (0.9% NaCl) or **Ringer's** solution. **Avoid dextrose** which is redistributed away from the intravascular space rapidly and causes hyperglycemia which may worsen neurological outcome after cardiac arrest. Dextrose is indicated only if there is **documented hypoglycemia.**

Postresuscitation care

- Maintain adequate airway and support breathing.
- Continue cardiac monitoring.
- Vasoactive medications (norepinephrine, dobutamine and epinephrine) and IV fluids to support circulation.
- Avoid hyperthermia, hyperglycemia (maintain blood sugar <200 mg/dL).
- Treating the precipitating cause of cardiac arrest.

SYNCOPE

Q. Write short essay/note on cardiac syncope/syncope.

Definition: Syncope is defined as a transient loss of consciousness due to inadequate cerebral blood flow with loss of postural tone.

- It is associated with loss of postural tone, with spontaneous return to baseline neurologic function without any resuscitative efforts.
- **Presyncope** is the term used for lightheadedness in which the individual thinks he/she may black out.
- **Classical vasovagal syncope:** Syncope triggered by emotional or orthostatic stress such as venipuncture (experienced or witnessed), painful or noxious stimuli, fear of bodily injury, prolonged standing, heat exposure, or exertion.

Mechanism: Global hypoperfusion of cerebral cortices or focal hypoperfusion of the reticular activating system.

- About one-third of individuals may develop a syncopal episode during their lifetime.
- Its incidence increases with age (sharp rise at age 70 years).
- Cardiac syncope has a high incidence (about 24%) of subsequent cardiac arrest.

TABLE 7.99: Causes of syncope.

Cardiac causes
➢ **Cardiac arrhythmias:** Ventricular tachycardia, paroxysmal supraventricular tachycardia, long QT syndrome, Brugada syndrome, bradycardia (Mobitz type II or 3rd degree heart block)
➢ **Structural cardiac or cardiopulmonary disease:** Cardiac valvular disease (AS, MS, PS), obstructive cardiomyopathy, atrial myxoma, acute aortic dissection, pericardial disease/tamponade, pulmonary embolus/pulmonary hypertension, acute myocardial infarction/ischemia
Noncardiac causes
➢ **Neurocardiogenic syncope 'vasovagal or vasodepressor syncope':** Classical vasovagal syncope, situational syncope, carotid sinus syncope, glossopharyngeal neuralgia, micturition syncope
➢ **Orthostatic hypotension:** Autonomic failure which may be primary (e.g., pure autonomic failure, multiple system atrophy, Parkinson's disease with autonomic failure) or secondary (e.g., diabetic neuropathy)
➢ **Neurovascular syncope:** Vascular steal syndromes

Causes of Syncope

Causes of syncope have been shown in **Table 7.99**.

Causes of nonsyncopal attacks (Box 7.57): Episodes that may be confused with syncope include disorders without impairment of consciousness and disorders with partial or complete loss of consciousness.

Box 7.57: Causes of nonsyncopal attacks.

- **Seizures.**
- **Metabolic or toxic abnormalities:** Hypoglycemia and encephalitis rarely syncope.
- **Neurologic syncope:** Subarachnoid hemorrhage, transient ischemic attack, complex migraine headache.
- Psychiatric syncope
- **Drug-induced loss of consciousness:** Drugs of abuse and alcohol.

Investigations

- ECG: Factors that suggests arrhythmia-induced syncope are prolonged intervals (QRS, QTc), severe bradycardia, pre-excitation, evidence of myocardial infarction.
- Holter monitoring
- Echocardiography
- Neurological: CT brain and MRI, EEG
- Laboratory evaluation: Full blood count (FBC) and hematocrit, random blood sugar (RBS) test, electrolytes, pregnancy test.
- Head up tilt table test.

COR PULMONALE

Q. Discuss the etiology, pathogenesis, clinical features, investigations, and management of chronic cor pulmonale.

- Cor pulmonale is a Latin word means "pulmonary heart" and is defined as **symptoms and signs of fluid overload secondary to lung disease.**

- Cor pulmonale is a disease of the right ventricle characterized by its hypertrophy and dilation with or without failure secondary to diseases directly affecting the lung parenchyma, pulmonary vasculature, chest bellows or central. This excludes pulmonary alterations produced due to diseases that primarily affect the left side of the heart (e.g., congenital heart diseases).

Types of Cor Pulmonale

Q. Write short essay/note on types and causes of cor pulmonale.

Q. Write short essay/note on acute cor pulmonale.

According to rate of development: Acute or chronic.

- **Acute cor pulmonale** develops due to a sudden increase in right ventricular pressure. It usually follows ***acute massive pulmonary embolism*** that is sufficient enough to obstruct more than 60% of pulmonary circulation. It leads to acute pulmonary hypertension, acute right ventricular dilatation and failure. Other example is acute respiratory distress syndrome.
- **Chronic cor pulmonale:** It can be further divided hypoxic type or vascular obliterans type.
  - **Hypoxic subtype:** Chronic obstructive pulmonary disease (COPD) is the most common disease associated with hypoxic subtype.
  - **Obliterans subtype:** Most common process associated with this subtype is pulmonary thromboembolic disease.

Etiology and Clinical Features (Box 7.58)

Usually the signs and symptoms are minimal except in the advanced stage. Mostly the clinicians focus on the disease producing cor pulmonale rather than on cor pulmonale itself.

Symptoms

Similar to those of right side heart failure: Fatigability, dyspnea on exertion, syncope, chest pain, palpitation, abdominal distension, edema of the lower extremity, exercise-induced peripheral cyanosis and excessive daytime somnolence.

Signs

- Pedal edema
- Accentuated A wave of the jugular venous pulsations and prominent jugular V wave, indicating the presence of tricuspid regurgitation.
- Palpable left parasternal lift.
- Accentuated pulmonic component of the second heart sound, right sided S_4 heart sound, ejection systolic murmur in the pulmonary area. In addition there may be pansystolic murmur of tricuspid regurgitation or early-diastolic murmur of pulmonary regurgitation.
- **Overt right side heart failure:** In a patient with chronic cor pulmonale reveal following signs:
  - Increasing peripheral edema
  - Jugular venous pressure: Raised and hepatojugular reflux positive
  - Tender hepatomegaly and enlargement of heart
  - Right ventricular third heart sound and a gallop rhythm, and right sided fourth heart sound.

Investigations

- **Chest X-ray**
  - Enlarged pulmonary artery and right ventricle, distended azygous or other central vein.
  - In pulmonary embolism Wester mark sign "oligemia of lung lobe or entire lung." Hampton's hump 'wedge-shaped opacity'
  - In COPD anterior-posterior diameter increased, diaphragm flattened, honeycombing and hyperlucency of lung.

Box 7.58: Causes of cor pulmonale.

Diseases of lung: Chronic obstructive pulmonary disease (COPD, e.g., chronic bronchitis and emphysema), pulmonary tuberculosis, interstitial lung disease, high altitude dwelling, cystic fibrosis, pleural fibrosis

Diseases of pulmonary circulation: Recurrent pulmonary thromboembolism, primary pulmonary hypertension, collagen vascular diseases, chronic liver disease

Diseases of thorax: Kyphoscoliosis, neuromuscular diseases, sleep apnea syndrome, obesity

Diseases of respiratory control: Brainstem lesions, central sleep apnea—Ondine's curse.

Management of Chronic Cor Pulmonale

These include (1) general measures, (2) additional measures in cor pulmonale due to COPD and (3) surgical treatment.

- **General measures**
- **Nonpharmacological treatment:**
  - Oxygen therapy.
  - Phlebotomy.
  - Noninvasive positive pressure ventilation (NIPPV).
- **Pharmacological treatment:**
  - Diuretics.
  - Anticoagulation.
  - Vasodilators
- **Treatment to decrease pulmonary hypertension**
  - Treatment of underlying disease.
  - Oxygen therapy is the most important treatment for reducing pulmonary hypertension. The long-term oxygen therapy retards its progression of pulmonary hypertension and oxygen therapy should be started if the arterial oxygen tension is 55 mm Hg or less.
- **Treatment of right heart failure**
  - Restriction of salt intake
  - Digoxin: Role not clear
  - Diuretics
- **Chronic anticoagulation** with Warfarin may benefit patients with cor pulmonale due to thrombo-occlusive pulmonary disease.
- **Surgical treatment**
  - Pulmonary embolectomy: If pulmonary emboli are not resolved.
  - Heart lung transplantation: For primary pulmonary hypertension.

- **Electrocardiogram:** Right axis deviation, P pulmonale (large P wave) in the inferior and anterior leads 'right atrial enlargement', right bundle branch block, right precordial T-wave inversions, delayed intrinsicoid deflection of right precordial leads, RVH, S1 Q3 T3 pattern and QR pattern in lead V1 or V3R.
- Arterial blood gas analysis: Hypoxia, hypercapnia.
- BNP: Used as biomarker for pulmonary hypertension in COPD patients.
- Echocardiography: Hypertrophy and dilatation of right ventricle.
- Others: Contrast-enhanced computed tomography/high-resolution computed tomography (CECT/HRCT) chest, nuclear scan for detecting pulmonary embolism, rarely right heart catheterization.

DISEASES OF VESSELS

Aortic Aneurysms

Q. Write short note on aneurysm of aorta.

Definition of aneurysm: It is an abnormal permanent focal dilatation of a blood vessel/artery to 1.5 times its normal diameter.

Classification of Aortic Aneurysm

Q. Write short note on classification of aortic aneurysms and its common causes.

- **Depending on the gross appearance:** (1) Fusiform aneurysm and (2) saccular aneurysm, (3) cylindrical, and (4) arterial dissection.
- **Depending on the sites/region involved:** (1) Thoracic part of aorta, (2) ascending aorta, (3) arch of aorta, (4) descending aorta, (5) abdominal aorta (commonest site is infrarenal portion).
- **Depending on the etiology:** Atherosclerosis (commonest cause), cystic medial necrosis, syphilis (aneurysm of ascending aorta), rheumatic aortitis, and trauma.

Aortic Dissection

Q. Write short note on aortic dissection.

Definition: Aortic dissection develops when **blood from the aortic lumen enters into the aortic wall** through a breach in the integrity of the aortic wall.

- Blood enters the media, split it into two layers and travels along the layers of the media creating a "false blood-filled lumen" alongside the existing or "true lumen."
- Usually, the false lumen re-enters the true lumen, producing a double-barreled aorta. However, it may rupture into the surrounding structures (e.g., left pleural cavity, pericardium) with fatal consequences.
- Dissection may damage aortic valve and compromise the branches of the aorta.
- Affects males more than females during 5th to 7th decades. Men/Female ratio 2:1 to 5:1. Proximal dissection peak age is 50–55 years and distal dissection peak age is 60–70 years.
- Dissection in younger patients is usually associated with Marfan's syndrome, pregnancy or trauma.

Box 7.59: Predisposing factors for aortic dissection.

- **Systemic hypertension** (~80%)
- **Aortic diseases:** Aortic atherosclerosis, dilatation, nonspecific aneurysm, arteritis, coarctation, bicuspid aortic valve. Previous aortic surgery (e.g., coronary artery bypass grafting (CABG), aortic valve replacement)
- Trauma
  - Direct iatrogenic, e.g., cardiac catheterization, intra-aortic balloon pumping
  - Indirect trauma, e.g., sudden deceleration
- Hereditary connective tissue diseases, e.g., Marfan syndrome, Ehlers-Danlos syndrome
- Chromosomal aberrations: Turner's syndrome, Noonan's syndrome
- Others: Third trimester of pregnancy or first stage of labor, giant cell arteritis, Behçet's disease, and syphilis

Predisposing Factors and Classification

- *Predisposing factors for aortic dissection have been shown in* **Box 7.59** *and classification in* ***Figure 7.54***. **Stanford anatomical classification**
  - **Type A dissections (66%):** Dissection involving either both the ascending and descending aorta or only the ascending aorta (types I and II of the DeBakey classification). It is more common but dangerous.
  - **Type B dissections:** They have dissection limited to descending aorta (usually begin distal to the subclavian artery) and do not involve the ascending part and (DeBakey type III).

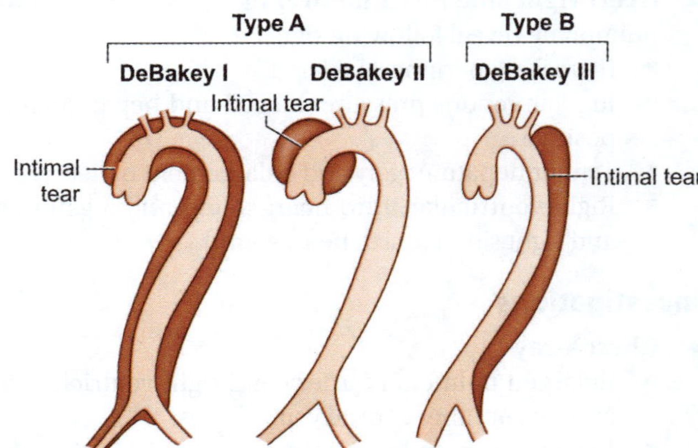

FIG. 7.54: Classification of aortic dissections. Type A (proximal) involves the ascending aorta (DeBakey I and II). Type B (distal or DeBakey III) dissections arise beyond the subclavian artery.

- **DeBakey classification (Fig. 7.54)**
  - Type I: Involves ascending to descending aorta
  - Type II: Limited to ascending or arch of aorta
  - Type III: Involves descending aorta only.
- **According to the timing of diagnosis** from the initial onset of symptoms:
  - **Acute** diagnosis is made <2 weeks of symptoms
  - **Subacute** 2–8 weeks of symptoms
  - **Chronic** >8 weeks of symptoms.

Clinical Features

Symptoms

- Sudden (abrupt) onset of severe, tearing, migratory pain, beginning in the anterior chest, radiating to the back between the scapulae (interscapular area), and moving downward as the dissection progresses. Pain may be misdiagnosed as that of myocardial infarction. Usually anterior chest pain develops when there is involvement of the ascending aorta, pain is intrascapular when descending aorta is involved. Collapse is common.
- **Others:** Syncope, dyspnea, weakness, hypertension or hypotension.

Signs

Asymmetry of pulses and blood pressure: It may produce asymmetry of the brachial, carotid or femoral pulses and blood pressure.

- Signs of aortic regurgitation.
- **Signs of occlusion of branches of aorta:** It may occlude orifices of branches of aorta and cause MI (coronary), stroke (carotid) paraplegia (spinal), mesenteric infarction with an acute abdomen (celiac and superior mesenteric), renal failure (renal) paraplegia (spinal cord) and ischemia of limb (usually leg).
- **Others:** Pulmonary edema, hemopericardium, cardiac tamponade.

Investigations

- **Chest X-ray:** May show widening/broadening of superior mediastinum and distortion of the aortic "knuckle" but these may be absent in 10% of cases. A small left-sided pleural effusion may be found.
- **Electrocardiogram:** ECG may show left ventricular hypertrophy in patients with hypertension (33% of cases). ECG is necessary to rule out any ischemic changes or MI. Rarely changes of acute MI (usually inferior) may be evident.
- **Doppler echocardiography:** It may reveal aortic regurgitation, and dilated aortic root.
- **Transesophageal echocardiography (TEE):** May be useful since it can show images of the first 3–4 cm of the ascending aorta (sensitivity 98–99% and specificity 94–95%).
- **CT and MRI angiography:** Highly (98–100%) specific and sensitive MRI is the gold standard for diagnosis.

Management/Treatment

Mortality rate of acute aortic dissection if untreated is 1–5% /hour and 90% within 3 months. Hence urgent treatment is needed.

- **Goal: Reduction of systolic blood pressure** (100–120) and **diminution of dp/dt** (reflects force of LV ejection) through use of a beta blocker. Therapy is targeted to halt the progression of the dissection. The course of the tear rather than the tear itself leads to compromise of vasculature or rupture.
- **Initial medical management consists of control of pain and antihypertensive treatment**. About 50% of patients are hypertensive and they are given urgent antihypertensive medication to reduce systolic blood pressure to below 120 mm Hg. This may be achieved by
  - Intravenous beta-blockers (e.g., labetalol, metoprolol) and vasodilators (GTN).
  - Intravenous calcium channel blockers (e.g., verapamil or diltiazem) are used if β-blockers are contraindicated.
  - If the above drugs fail to control BP adequately, sodium nitroprusside may be given.
- **Type A dissections need emergency surgery** to replace the ascending aorta (arch replacement) if fit enough, because medical management has a high mortality (50% within 2 weeks).
- Better prognosis with **type B dissections** and have a survival of 89% at 1 month. They are initially treated medically unless they develop complications such as actual or impending external rupture, or vital organ (gut, kidneys) or limb ischemia. In these patients very high morbidity and mortality rate associated with surgery.
- **Surgical therapy:** Percutaneous or minimal access endoluminal repair and involves either "fenestrating" (perforating) the intimal flap or endovascular implantation of a stent graft placed from the femoral artery.

Cause of death: Acute aortic regurgitation, major branch vessel obstruction, aortic rupture (into pericardium, left pleural cavity, or mediastinum).

Marfan's Syndrome

Q. Write short note on Marfan's syndrome and its clinical features.

It is an autosomal dominant disorder of connective tissue characterized by mutations in the *fibrillin* gene on chromosome 15.

Systems Affected

- **Cardiovascular system:** Weakening of the media of the aortic root cause dilatation (**Fig. 7.55D**), regurgitation and dissection. Mitral valve prolapse, mitral regurgitation.
- Skeletal system: Tall stature, arachnodactyly, wrist (**Fig. 7.55A**) and/thumb sign (**Fig. 7.55B**), joint hypermobility, scoliosis, chest deformity, and high arched palate (**Fig. 7.55C**).
- Eyes: Dislocation of the lens (superior and temporal).

Investigations: Chest X-ray (**Fig. 7.55D**), echocardiography, MRI or CT may detect aortic dilatation.

Treatment

β-blockers reduces the rate of aortic dilatation and risk of rupture. Elective replacement of the ascending aorta: in patients with progressive aortic dilatation.

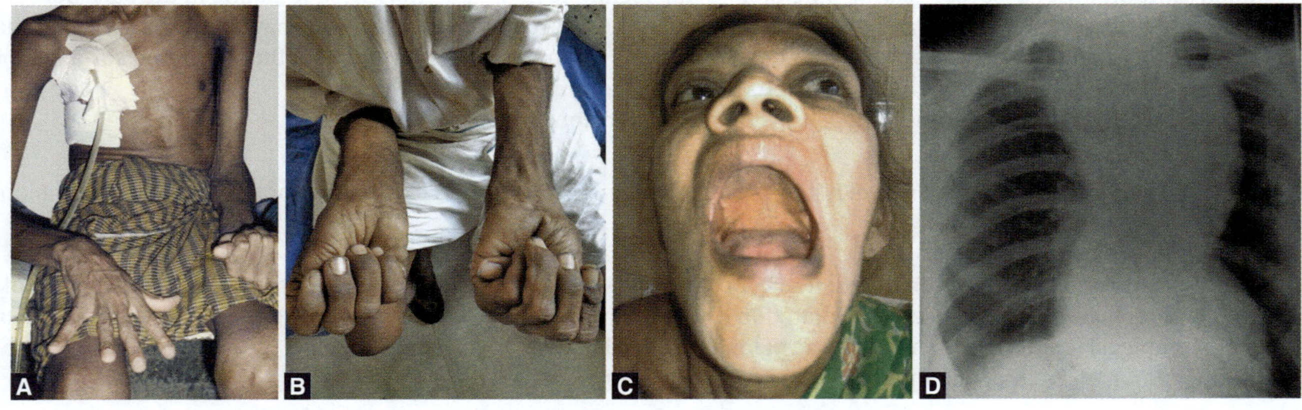

FIGS. 7.55A TO D: Features of Marfan's syndrome: (A) Wrist sign with right pneumothorax on intercostal drainage; (B) Thumb sign; (C) High arched palate; (D) Chest X-ray showing aortic root dilatation.

RAYNAUD'S PHENOMENON AND RAYNAUD'S DISEASE

Q. Write short note on Raynaud's phenomenon, its causes and Raynaud's disease.

- **Raynaud's phenomenon:** Chronic episodic attacks of digital ischemia due to spasm of the digital arteries usually precipitated by exposure to cold or emotional stress and relieved by heat. An underlying disease or cause is present and most commonly connective tissue disease, such as systemic sclerosis. If there is no underlying cause, it is termed **Raynaud's disease** (primary or idiopathic Raynaud's phenomenon).
- Affects 5–10% of population.

Causes of Raynaud's Phenomenon and Clinical Features

Causes of Raynaud's phenomenon have been shown in **Table 7.100**.

- **Characterized by sequential color changes:** White (pallor due to vasospasm), >blue (cyanosis due to deoxygenated blood) > and red (rubor due to reactive hyperemia). Pallor is essential for diagnosis.
- **Age of onset and gender:** Usually less than 40 years of age, but it may occur over this age. F:M = 5:1. However, in secondary cases it depends on the underlying disease, and is not restricted to female sex.
- Raynaud's phenomenon usually involves the hands and less common in the feet. Rarely, involves nose, ear lobe, tongue, etc.
- **Typical attack** is characterized by sudden attack of pallor in one or more digits, followed after a few minutes by cyanosis or/and sometimes by erythema. Attacks are usually precipitated by cold (either local or of the whole body), by pressure or by psychological stimuli. Episodes may occur infrequently or many times each day.
  - **Primary Raynaud's:** Usually bilateral, symmetrical and involves several digits (fingers).
  - **Secondary Raynaud's:** Involves only one or a few digits and asymmetry is not unusual.
- **Severe cases:** Usually seen in secondary type and may be complicated by:
  - Telangiectasias of the nail fold
  - Thinning and ridging of the nail

TABLE 7.100: Causes of Raynaud's phenomenon (Secondary Raynaud's).

Connective tissue disease and vasculitis, e.g., systemic sclerosis, SLE, rheumatoid arthritis, Sjögren's syndrome, Mixed connective tissue disease	Hematological disease, e.g., cryoglobulinemia, cold agglutinins, paroxysmal hemoglobinuria, Waldenström's macroglobulinemia
Obstructive arterial disease, e.g., atherosclerosis, thromboangiitis obliterans (TAO) (Buerger's disease)	**Neurological disease,** e.g., thoracic outlet syndrome (cervical rib), carpal tunnel syndrome
Trauma or vibration: Reflex sympathetic dystrophy, vibration exposure, arteriovenous fistula	**Miscellaneous,** e.g., paraneoplastic syndrome, chronic renal failure, primary pulmonary hypertension
Drugs and toxins, e.g., Ergot, β-blockers, methysergide	

- Atrophy or sclerosis of the fingers (sclerodactyly).
- **Skin necrosis:** Rare in primary Raynaud's phenomenon but not uncommon in secondary Raynaud's phenomenon and may lead to destruction of the digits.

Investigations

- **Blood test**
  - Complete blood count, ESR, urinalysis
  - Patient with ANA, specific antigen like Sm antigen or topoisomerase or centromere or DsDNA to rule out SLE or scleroderma.
- **Chest X-ray:** To look for cervical rib or evidence of ILD.
- **Specific test:** Nail fold capillary microscopy procedure differentiates primary from secondary Raynaud phenomenon. Patients with connective tissue diseases may have enlarged deformed capillary loops surrounded by avascular areas.

Treatment

General measures

- Lifestyle modifications to minimize exposure to cold.
- Patient's education to recognize and terminate attacks promptly by returning to a warmer environment and applying local heat to hands (e.g., by placing their hands in warm water or by using a hair dryer).
- Cessation of smoking because nicotine induces cutaneous vasoconstriction.
- Stress modification and social support to minimize vasoconstriction induced by hyperactivity of sympathetic nervous system.
- Treatment of underlying cause.
- **Drugs:** Calcium channel blockers (e.g., nifedipine, amlodipine), sildenafil, prostaglandin analogues (e.g., ilaprost), bosentan, losartan, topical glyceryl trinitrate.
- **Sympathectomy:** Patients with refractory, disabling attacks or with an acutely ischemic digit that is unresponsive to other measure.

CIRCULATORY FAILURE: SHOCK

Q. Write short note/essay on:

- **Septic shock, SIRS and sepsis (*refer* Chapter 4).**
- **Anaphylactic shock and neurogenic shock.**
- **Management of septic shock.**

Definition

Q. Define acute circulatory failure/shock.

- Shock (acute circulatory failure, low-output state) is defined as a state with impaired cardiac pump, circulatory system, and/or volume that can lead to compromised blood flow to tissues.
- Kumar and Parrillo (1995): Shock is a state in which profound and widespread reduction of effective tissue perfusion leads first to reversible, and then if prolonged, to irreversible cellular injury.

Classification and Causes

Classification and causes of shock have been shown in **Table 7.101**.

Q. Write short note/essay on classification and causes of shock.

Q. Causes of cardiogenic shock.

TABLE 7.101: Classification and causes of shock.

Type of shock and insult	*Causes*	*Physiologic effect*	*Compensation*
Cardiogenic: Heart **fails to pump** blood out	Myocardial infarction (MI), arrhythmia, aortic stenosis, mitral regurgitation, myocarditis, rupture of papillary muscle, right ventricular infarction with excessive diuretic therapy	Decreased cardiac output	Baroreceptor mechanism. Increased systemic vascular resistance Increased heart rate and contractibility
Obstructive: Heart pumps well, but the outflow is obstructed	Extracardiac obstructive causes, such as pericardial effusion, tension pneumothorax, tamponade, acute massive pulmonary embolism		
Hypovolemic: Heart pumps well, but **not enough blood volume** to pump	Hemorrhage, fluid loss (vomiting, diarrhea, burns)		
Distributive: Heart pumps well, but there is **peripheral vasodilation**	Septic, anaphylactic, and neurogenic shock pancreatitis, burns, multi-trauma via activation of the inflammatory response	Reduced systemic vascular resistance	Increased cardiac output. Increased heart rate and contractibility No change in neurogenic shock

Stages of Shock

Stages of shock have been shown in **Table 7.102**.

TABLE 7.102: Stages of shock.

Stage	*Pathophysiology*	*Clinical findings*
Insult (initial stage)	Example: Splenic rupture with blood loss	
Preshock (compensatory stage)	Hemostatic compensation Mean arterial blood pressure (MAP) = Reduced. Decreased cardiac output is compensated by increase in heart rate and systemic vascular resistance	MAP is maintained Heart rate will be increased Extremities will be cool due to vasoconstriction
Shock (progressive stage)	Compensatory mechanisms fail	MAP is reduced. Tachycardia, dyspnea, restlessness
End organ dysfunction (refractory stage)	Cell death and organ failure	Decreased renal function, liver failure, disseminated intravascular coagulopathy, death

Pathogenesis of Various Types of Shock

Pathogenesis of various types of shock has been shown in **Flowchart 7.6**.

FLOWCHART 7.6: Pathogenesis of various types of shock.

Cardiogenic (e.g., myocardial infarction)
Damage to myocardium
↓ Systolic and diastoilc function
Obstructive
↓ Diastolic filling (e.g., tension pneumothorax)
↑ Ventricular after load (e.g., massive pulmonary embolism)
↓ Diastolic function
↓ Systolic function
Hypovolemic (e.g., hemorrhage, fluid loss)
↓ Preload
↓ Diastolic filling
Distributive (e.g., septic shock)
↓ Preload
Myocardial depression
↓ Diastolic filling
↓ Systolic and diastolic function
↓ Cardiac output
↓ Systemic vascular resistence
↓ Systemic vascular resistence
↓ Cardiac output
↓ Mean arterial blood pressure
Shock
Maldistribution of blood flow
Multiple Organ Dysfunction Syndrome (MODS)

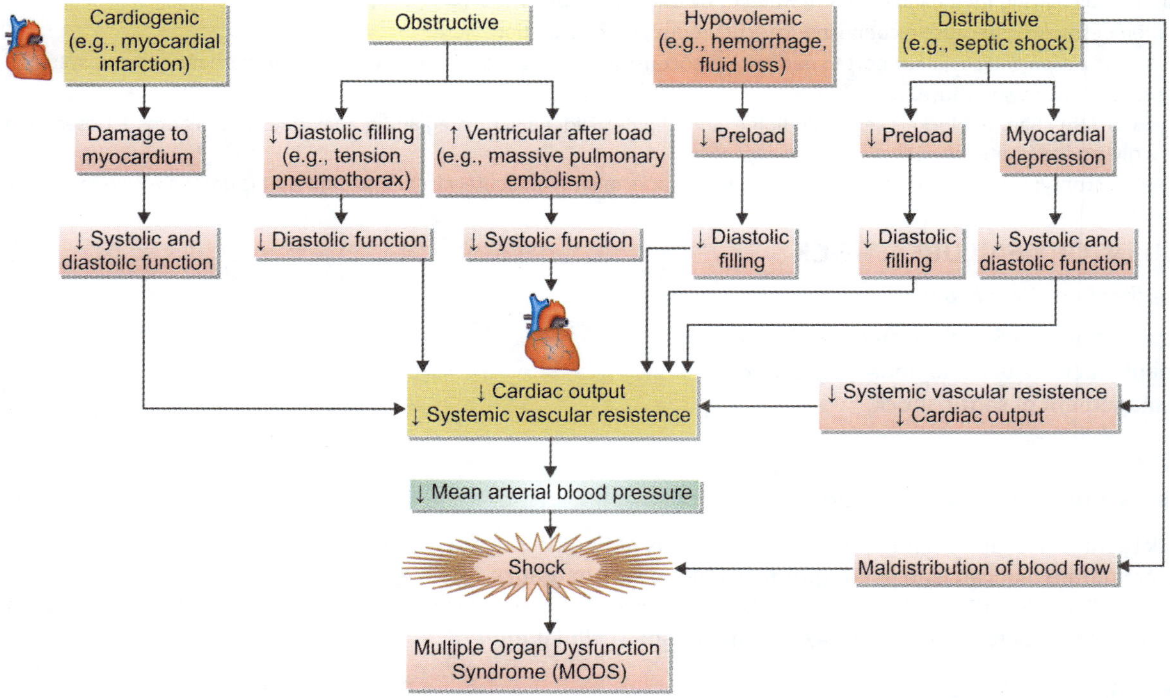

Clinical Features

Clinical features of various types of shock have been shown in **Table 7.103**.

TABLE 7.103: Clinical features of various types of shock.

	Hypovolemic shock	*Distributive shock*	*Cardiogenic shock*	*Obstructive shock*
Heart rate	Increased	Increased (normal in neurogenic shock)	Increased or decreased	Increased
Jugular venous pressure (JVP)	Low	Low	High	High
Blood pressure	Low	Low	Low	Low
Skin	Cold	Warm (cold in severe shock)	Cold	Cold
Capillary refill	Slow	Slow	Slow	Slow

Q. Write short notes on hypovolemic shock.

Types of Shock

- **Neurogenic shock**
  - Neurogenic is the rarest form of shock. Caused by the loss of sympathetic control of resistance vessels resulting in massive dilatation of arterioles and venules.

- A type of distributive shock that results from the loss or suppression of sympathetic tone.
- Causes massive vasodilatation in the venous vasculature → venous return to heart → cardiac output.
- Most common cause is spinal cord injury above T6.

- **Sepsis** (discussed in Chapter 4)
  - **Sepsis syndrome:** SIRS with confirmed infectious process associated with organ failure or hypotension
  - Two phases:
    - **'Warm' shock-early phase:** Hyperdynamic response, vasodilation
    - **"Cold" shock**-late phase: Hypodynamic response
  - Decompensated state
- **Anaphylactic shock** (discussed in Chapter 20)
  - A type of distributive shock that results from widespread systemic allergic reaction to an antigen.
  - Differences between anaphylactic shock and anaphylactoid shock (**Table 7.104**).
  - This hypersensitive reaction is **life-threatening**.
- **Cardiogenic shock.**
  - The impaired ability of the heart to pump blood. Pump failure of the right or left ventricle.
  - Most common cause is left ventricular myocardial infarction (anterior). Occurs when >40% of ventricular mass damage.
  - Mortality rate is 80% or more.

TABLE 7.104: Differences between anaphylactic shock and anaphylactoid shock.

Anaphylactic shock	*Anaphylactoid shock*
➢ Insect envenomation ➢ Antibiotics (beta- lactams, vancomycin, sulfonamides) ➢ Heterologous serum (antitoxin, antisera) ➢ Blood transfusion ➢ Immunoglobulins (esp. IgA deficient) ➢ Egg-based vaccines ➢ Latex	➢ Ionic contrast media ➢ Protamine ➢ Opiates ➢ Polysaccharide volume expanders (dextran, hydroxyethyl starch) ➢ Muscle relaxants ➢ Anesthetics

Q. Write short note/essay on management of shock.

Management of Shock

Goal of management: (1) Treat reversible causes, (2) protect ischemic myocardium, and (3) improve tissue perfusion.

Patient Monitoring

- Initial assessment (ABC)
- Airway:
  - Does patient have mental status to protect airway?
  - Glasgow Coma Scale (GCS) less than "eight" means "intubate"
  - Airway is compromised in anaphylaxis.
- **Breathing:** If patient is conversing with you, airway (A) and breathing (B) are fine, place patient on oxygen.
- **Circulation:** Vitals (heart rate and blood pressure), 2 large bore IV, start fluids (careful if cardiogenic shock), put on continuous monitor.
  - In a trauma, perform ABCDE, not just ABC.
- **Deficit or disability:**
  - Assess for obvious neurologic deficit.
  - Moving all four extremities—Yes/No Pupils-Reaction
  - Glasgow Coma Scale (M6, V5, E4).
- **Exposure:** Remove all clothing on trauma patients.

General Measures

- Optimize oxygen content
  - Hemoglobin: Check if appears pale or anemic, check coagulation status.
  - SaO_2: Just a pulse oximeter tells you the SpO_2. Check SaO_2 on ABG.
- Optimize cardiac output
  - Cardiac output (CO) = Stroke volume (SV) x Heart rate (HR)
  - Stroke volume depends on preload, contractility and afterload
    - Preload: Look at response to fluid bolus.
      - If improves BP could be suggestive of decreased preload (volume) and a reasonable contractility.
      - If no improvement or worsening BP could be suggestive of a contractility problem or excess preload (volume) situation.
      - Look at CVP
    - Contractility
      - Check any history suggestive of ischemic disease or CCF.
      - Check ECHO and ECG.
      - A high systolic pressure could be suggestive of good contractility.
    - Afterload
      - Check ECHO if suggestive of any obstructive features.
      - If peripheries cold could indicate increased vascular resistance.

- If peripheries warm could indicate vasodilation and decreased vascular resistance.
- A low diastolic blood pressure could indicate low vascular resistance.
- A high diastolic blood pressure could indicate increased vascular resistance.

- **Heart rate**
  - If low, 2 possible interventions, namely electric pacing or pharmacological intervention.
  - If high, 2 possible interventions, namely electric cardioversion/defibrillation or pharmacological intervention.

Optimize Blood Pressure

Q. Write short note/essay on sympathomimetic amines and vasopressor agents in shock.

- Vasopressors and inotropes (sympathomimetic amines and vasopressin) **(Table 7.105)**
  - Dobutamine alone is useful to augment cardiac output if arterial pressure is near-normal. Otherwise, a combination of dopamine and dobutamine is preferred initial sympathomimetic agents.
  - Vasopressin
    - Vasopressin constricts vascular smooth muscle directly via V1 receptors, and also increases responsiveness of the vasculature to catecholamines.
    - Vasopressin may also increase blood pressure by inhibition of vascular smooth muscle nitric oxide production.
- **Milrinone** can be used to increase cardiac contractility.
- **Steroids** can be used in specific types as septic shock.

TABLE 7.105: Common sympathomimetic amines used in shock.

Sympathomimetic amine (receptor activated) and dose	*Actions*
Dopamine: (Dopaminergic + α + β_1) ➢ 0.2–1 mg/minute	Vasodilation of renal, mesenteric, cerebral and coronary vessels Increase myocardial contraction, heart rate and cardiac output. Rise in systolic blood pressure
Dobutamine: (β_1) ➢ 2–8 µg/kg/minute	Marked increase in myocardial contraction, minimal increase in heart rate and minimal peripheral vessels vasodilatation
Noradrenaline: (α + β_1) ➢ 2–8 µg/minute	Increased myocardial contraction, heart rate, cardiac output, and rise in blood pressure vasoconstriction in skin, muscle and splanchnic beds. Coronary vasodilation
Adrenaline: (α + β_1+ β_2) ➢ 1–8 µg/kg/minute	Increased myocardial contraction, heart rate and cardiac output. Rise in mean blood pressure vasoconstriction in most except skeletal muscles and coronary arteries. Vasodilatation in skeletal muscles and coronary arteries
Isoproterenol: (β_1+ β_2) ➢ 5–10 µg/minute	Increased myocardial contraction, heart rate cardiac output and rise in systolic blood pressure Vasodilatation mainly in skeletal muscles
Phenylephrine: (α_1) ➢ 30–60 µg/minute	Vasoconstriction

Treatment of Underlying Cause

- **Hypovolemic shock**
  - Rapid replacement of blood, colloid, or crystalloid.
  - Identify source of blood or fluid loss and treat it. Endoscopy/colonoscopy or angiography.

Q. Write short note on management of cardiogenic shock.

Cardiogenic Shock (Box 7.60)

Extracardiac obstructive shock

- Pericardial tamponade: Pericardiocentesis and surgical drainage (if needed).
- Pulmonary embolism
  - Heparin
  - Ventilation/perfusion lung scan
  - Pulmonary angiography
  - Consider: Thrombolytic therapy, embolectomy at surgery.

Septic shock

- Identify site of infection and drain, if possible.
- Antimicrobial agents (key rules).
- ICU monitoring and support with fluids, vasopressors, and inotropic agents.

Box 7.60: Management of cardiogenic shock.

Left ventricular infarction
- Intra-aortic balloon pump (IABP)
- Cardiac angiography
- Revascularization: Angioplasty, coronary bypass

Right ventricular infarction
- Fluid and inotropes with PA catheter monitoring

Mechanical abnormality
- Echocardiography
- Corrective surgery

Management of neurogenic shock

Hypovolemia: Treat with careful fluid replacement for BP<90 mm Hg, UO <30 cc/hr.

- Observe closely for fluid overload
- Vasopressors may be needed.
- Hypothermia: Warming. Avoid large swings in patient's body temperature.
- Treat hypoxia
- Maintain ventilatory support.
- Alpha agonist to augment tone if perfusion still inadequate
  - Dopamine (>10 mg/kg per min)
  - Ephedrine (12.5–25 mg IV every 3–4 hour)
- Treat bradycardia with atropine 0.5–1 mg doses to maximum 3 mg, may need transcutaneous or transvenous pacing temporarily.

PULMONARY EMBOLISM AND VENOUS THROMBOSIS

Pulmonary Embolism (PE)

Q. Discuss the etiology, clinical features, investigations, diagnosis and management of pulmonary thromboembolism and pulmonary infarction.

Definition

- **Pulmonary embolism** (pulmonary thromboembolism—PTE) is defined as an embolism in which emboli occlude pulmonary arterial tree (pulmonary artery or its branches). Pulmonary embolism is the second most common cause of unexpected death in most age groups. It accounts for about 15% of all postoperative deaths. Present in 60–80% of patients with DVT, more than 50% of them are asymptomatic.
- **Pulmonary infarction:** It is ischemic necrosis of lung tissue following embolic occlusion. It develops in less than 10% of cases of pulmonary embolism. They are more common in patients with an underlying cardiac or pulmonary disease.

Source of Emboli

Pulmonary embolism usually results from dislodgement of venous thrombi and the source of these emboli are as follows:
- **Thromboemboli**
  - **Deep leg veins:** Deep venous thromboses (DVTs) are the source in more than 95% of cases of pulmonary emboli. Deep leg veins include popliteal, femoral or iliac veins. Other source of thromboemboli is from pelvic veins, abdominal veins and vena cava.
  - **Other sites:** Rarely, source of emboli may be right atrium or right ventricle.
- **Other nonthrombotic emboli:** They are rare and include septic emboli (from endocarditis involving the tricuspid or pulmonary valves), tumor emboli (especially choriocarcinoma), fat (long bone fractures), air, amniotic fluid emboli, and foreign material during IV drug use.

Causes and Risk Factors

Causes and risk factors (predisposing factors) for venous thrombosis and embolism have been shown in **Table 7.106**.

TABLE 7.106: Risk factors (predisposing factors) for venous thrombosis and embolism.

Primary (genetic)	Secondary (acquired)
➢ **Deficiency of antithrombotic (anticoagulant) factors** (e.g., Antithrombin III deficiency, protein C and S deficiency) ➢ **Increased prothrombotic factors** (e.g., activated protein C (APC) resistance (factor V mutation/factor Va/factor V Leiden)	➢ **Surgery:** Major abdominal/pelvic, hip/knee surgery, postoperative intensive care ➢ **Obstetrics:** Pregnancy, postpartum ➢ **Cardiorespiratory disease:** COPD, congestive cardiac failure ➢ **Lower limb conditions:** Fracture, varicose veins ➢ **Malignancy:** Abdominal/pelvic, advanced/disseminated cancers, concurrent chemotherapy ➢ Antiphospholipid antibody syndrome ➢ **Miscellaneous:** Increasing age, prolonged bed rest, prolonged immobilization, trauma

Q. Write short essay/note on the predisposing causes of pulmonary embolism.

Q. Write short note on Virchow's triad.

Virchow's triad: It consists of three factors that predispose to thrombus formation and includes (1) endothelial injury, (2) altered blood flow and (3) hypercoagulability. These factors favor the adhesion of platelets at the site of endothelial damage. These platelets undergo aggregation and release factors which generate thrombin generation. Venous thrombi form and flourish in the presence of stasis and hypercoagulability.

Pathological Consequences

Embolization: The deep venous thrombi may detach from their site of formation. These emboli pass to the vena cava, right atrium and right ventricle, and finally lodge in the pulmonary arterial circulation. In the lung, they produce acute pulmonary embolism.
- **Acute massive pulmonary embolism:** When emboli lodges in the main pulmonary artery (may result in death). Massive pulmonary embolism shows 60% or more obstruction of the pulmonary circulation. Massive PE accounts for 5–10% of cases.
- **Pulmonary infarction:** It results from embolism to smaller pulmonary arteries. Most (about 75%) small pulmonary emboli do not produce infarcts. However, in the patients with congestive heart failure or chronic lung disease an embolus can cause infarction.
- **Pulmonary hemorrhage:** Obstruction of medium-sized pulmonary arteries by emboli and subsequent rupture of these vessels can result in pulmonary hemorrhage.
- **Pulmonary hypertension:** Multiple recurrent pulmonary emboli → may cause mechanical blockage of the arterial bed → result in chronic pulmonary hypertension → right ventricular failure.

Clinical Features of Pulmonary Embolism and Pulmonary Infarction

- Dyspnea (75–85%), pleuritic chest pain (57–87%), cough (40–53%), hemoptysis, syncope, similar to obstructive lung disease (chronic).
- **Massive pulmonary embolism:** Rarer condition characterized by sudden collapse because of an acute obstruction of the right ventricular outflow tract. Symptoms include collapse/hypotension, unexplained hypoxia, engorged neck veins, and acute right heart failure (acute cor pulmonale).

Physical findings

- Patient may be normal.
- There may be tachypnea (respiratory rate >16/min) in 96% of cases, rales (58%), accentuated second heart sound (53%), tachycardia (heart rate >100/min), fever (temperature >37.8 °C), diaphoresis, S_3 or S_4 gallop.
- Other clinical signs and symptoms suggesting thrombophlebitis, lower extremity edema, cardiac murmur, cyanosis and clinical evidence of DVT may be present.

Wells Scoring System

Wells scoring system for the diagnosis of pulmonary embolism has been shown in **Box 7.61**.

Box 7.61: Wells scoring system for the diagnosis of pulmonary embolism (PE).

Clinically suspected DVT: 3.0 points

- Alternative diagnosis is less likely than PE: 3.0 points
- Tachycardia (heart rate >100): 1.5 points
- Immobilization (≥3d)/surgery in previous four weeks: 1.5 points
- History of DVT or PE: 1.5 points
- Hemoptysis: 1.0 point
- Malignancy (with treatment within six months) or palliative: 1.0 point

Score >4-PE likely. Consider diagnostic imaging and score 4 or less-PE unlikely.

Diagnosis

Q. Write short essay/note on diagnosis of pulmonary embolism.

Pulmonary embolism is the Great Masquerader. Its symptoms and signs are nonspecific and the diagnosis is difficult. Not all leg pain is due to deep vein thrombosis and not all dyspnea is due to pulmonary embolism. Pulmonary embolism should be considered if a patient has pleuritic chest pain, hemoptysis or dyspnea that is out of proportion to the size of pleural effusion.

- **Nonimaging diagnostic modalities**
  Blood tests
  - **Pulmonary infarction:** It results in polymorphonuclear leukocytosis, raised ESR and raised lactate dehydrogenase levels in the serum.
  - **D-dimer assay:** D-dimer is a specific degradation product produced during the breakdown of endogenous fibrin (fibrinolysis) by plasmin. It is best screening test for PE or DVT. Its significance are:
    - **Raised D-dimer:** The quantitative raise in plasma D-dimer [measured by enzyme-linked immunosorbent assay (ELISA)] indicates the presence of DVT or PE or clinically ineffective thrombolysis. The sensitivity of the D-dimer is >80% for DVT (less sensitive than for PE because the size of DVT thrombus is smaller) and >95% for PE. However, raised D-dimer is not specific, because it may be also raised in other conditions (e.g., myocardial infarction, pneumonia, sepsis, cancer, postoperative state and during second or third trimester of pregnancy). It has no role in hospitalized patients because levels are usually raised due to systemic illness. A positive test or normal test in high-risk patients requires further specific diagnostic tests, such as Doppler of legs for deep vein thrombosis, spiral CT pulmonary angiography (CT-PA), perfusion scanning of the lungs and pulmonary angiography.
    - **Normal D-dimer:** If D-dimer is normal, it rules out the diagnosis of embolism (unless patient has a high-risk of PTE clinically).
  - **ECG** is often normal but helps in excluding other differential diagnoses (e.g., acute myocardial infarction and pericarditis). It may show sinus tachycardia, changes of acute pulmonary hypertension and right ventricular strain. Other abnormalities include atrial fibrillation; ECG changes include the **S I Q3T3** sign: an S wave in lead 1, a Q wave in lead III, and an inverted T wave in lead III.
  - **Arterial blood gases:** Show a hypoxemia (reduced PaO_2) and a normal or hypocapnia (low $PaCO_2$) i.e. type I respiratory failure pattern and an increased alveolar–arterial oxygen gradient.
- **Noninvasive Imaging Modalities**
  - **Ultrasound scanning:** For the detection of clots in deep veins, pelvic or iliofemoral veins.
  - **Venous ultrasonography:** Color Doppler ultrasound of the leg veins examines the venous flow dynamics and is the investigation of choice in suspected DVT. Normally, manual compression of calf increases the Doppler flow pattern. Loss of normal respiratory variation is seen when there is occluding DVT or any obstruction within the pelvis.

- Chest X-ray
  - Pulmonary embolism
    - Normal or nearly normal
    - Increased radiolucency in lung zones (due to decreased or absent blood flow)
    - Small infiltrative shadows (due to linear atelectasis)

- Elevated hemidiaphragm
- Difference in the diameter of pulmonary arteries and their main branches on either side.
- Abrupt "cut-off" of a blood vessel
- Enlarged right descending pulmonary artery (Palla's sign).

- Pulmonary infarction
  - May be normal during early stages
  - Parenchymal, peripheral, wedge-shaped (pulmonary infarct) density above the diaphragm (Hampton's hump). Previous infarcts may appear as opaque linear scars.
  - Translucent under perfused distal zone, infiltrative shadow abutting against the pleura (usually appears 12–36 hours later) (Westmark's sign).
  - Abrupt cutoff of a pulmonary artery
  - Blunting of a costophrenic angle (due to a small pleural effusion).

- **Chest CT:** CT of the chest with intravenous contrast is the main imaging test for the diagnosis of PE.
- **Lung scanning:** It is the second line diagnostic test for PE and performed in patients who cannot tolerate intravenous contrast. The perfusion scan defect favors absent or decreased blood flow possibly due to PE whereas a normal perfusion scan excludes significant pulmonary embolism. However, an abnormal perfusion scan may be due to lung pathology (e.g., asthma and chronic obstructive pulmonary disease). In such patients, a ventilation-perfusion scan is needed though it may still give ambiguous results.
- **Magnetic resonance (MR) (contrast-enhanced) imaging:** It is useful mainly in detecting large proximal PE but is not reliable for smaller segmental and subsegmental PE.
- **Echocardiography** is not useful for diagnosis of acute PE, but is very useful for detecting conditions that mimic PE (e.g., acute myocardial infarction, pericardial tamponade, and aortic dissection).
- **Radionuclide ventilation/perfusion scanning ($^{V/Q}$scan):** It uses less radiation and contrast and is a good diagnostic tool. Pulmonary Tc scintigraphy shows under perfused regions indicative of pulmonary infarcts. However, this test should be interpreted in consideration of history, examination and other investigations.

- **Invasive diagnostic modalities**
  - **Pulmonary angiography:** Chest CT with contrast has replaced invasive pulmonary angiography as a diagnostic test. It is performed in patients planned for interventional procedure (e.g., catheter-directed thrombolysis). Features of PE includes visualization of a filling defect in the lumen, abrupt blockage ("cutoff") of vessels, segmental oligemia or avascularity, a prolonged arterial phase with slow filling, and tortuous, tapering peripheral vessels.

Q. Write short essay/note on management of pulmonary embolism.

Management

Supportive measures

- Prompt recognition and treatment.
- Bed rest in acute stage.
- Oxygen should be given to hypoxemic patients to maintain arterial oxygen saturation above 90%.
- Intravenous saline and/or noradrenaline may be necessary to maintain venous pressure in massive embolism.
- Avoid diuretics and vasodilators because they will reduce cardiac output.
- Analgesics: Opiates may be needed to relieve pain and distress.
- External cardiac massage in the moribund patient may dislodge and breaking up a large central embolus.

Anticoagulation

- **Unfractionated heparin:** Initial dose is 5,000–10,000 units IV, followed by maintenance.
- Maintenance: By any one of the three regimens namely (1) continuous intravenous, (2) intermittent intravenous and (3) intermittent subcutaneous.
- Dosage and monitoring of anticoagulant therapy.
  - After initiating heparin therapy, repeat APTT every 6 hour for first 24 hours and then every 24 hours when therapeutic APTT is achieved.
  - Warfarin 5 mg/d can be started on day 1 of therapy; there is no benefit from higher starting doses.
  - Platelet count should be monitored at least every 3 day during initial heparin therapy.
  - Therapeutic APTT should correspond to plasma heparin level of 0.2–0.4 IU/mL.
  - Heparin is usually continued for 5–7 days. Heparin can be stopped after 4–5 d of **warfarin** therapy when INR is in 2.0–3.0 range.
- Novel oral anticoagulants.
  - **Rivaroxaban** is an oral factor Xa inhibitor approved by the FDA in November 2012 for the treatment of DVT or PE. Apixaban was approved for treatment of PE in August 2014.
  - Direct thrombin inhibitors: **Argatroban, ximelagatran.**
- Anticoagulation is maintained for at least 6 months.

Thrombolytic therapy
- Indications: Hemodynamic instability, hypoxia on 100% oxygen, and right ventricular dysfunction by echocardiography.
- Approved thrombolytics for pulmonary embolism
  - Streptokinase: 250,000 IU as loading dose over 30 minutes, followed by 100,000 U/h for 24 hours.
  - Urokinase: 4400 IU/kg as a loading dose over 10 minutes, followed by 4400 IU/kg/h for 12–24 hours.
  - Recombinant tissue-plasminogen activator:100 mg as a continuous peripheral intravenous infusion administered over 2 hour
- **Contraindications**
  - Absolute: Active internal bleeding
  - **Relative:** Recent surgery, bleeding disorder (thrombocytopenia, renal failure, liver failure), hypertension >200 mm Hg systolic or 110 mm Hg diastolic, hypertensive retinopathy with hemorrhages or exudates.

Surgical therapy: Include surgical pulmonary embolectomy, inferior vena caval filters (to prevent recurrent emboli) and venous interruption.
Prophylaxis: To prevent pulmonary embolism (*refer* prophylaxis for venous thrombosis).

VENOUS THROMBOSIS

Q. Discuss the risk factors, clinical features, investigations, diagnosis, and treatment of venous thrombosis [deep venous thrombosis (DVT)].

Venous thrombosis is the formation of thrombus in the venous circulation namely veins or right side of the heart.

Sites of Venous Thrombosis

Most commonly deep or superficial veins of the leg are involved.
- **DVT:**
  - Usually develops in the lower extremity, starting at the larger calf vein level and progressing proximally to involve popliteal, femoral, or iliac veins. In about 80–90% pulmonary embolism, the source is deep vein thrombus. Lower extremity DVTs are found in associated with venous stasis and hypercoagulable states. More prone to embolization into the lungs and produce pulmonary infarction. About 50% of DVTs are asymptomatic and are detected after embolization.
  - **Other systemic veins,** e.g., pelvic veins
  - **Right side of the heart:** Atrium (e.g., in patients with atrial fibrillation and cardiac failure) and right ventricle.
- **Superficial venous thrombi:** They develop in the varicosities involving saphenous veins. It can cause local congestion, swelling (edema), pain, and tenderness. Embolization is very rare.

Risk Factors of Venous Thrombosis (refer Table 7.106)

Clinical Features of Deep Venous Thrombosis

- Often DVT is asymptomatic with minimal symptoms and signs in about 50% of patients. It may present with clinical features of pulmonary embolism.
- Usually unilateral (only one leg) but may be bilateral (both legs), and thrombus may extend proximally into the inferior vena cava. Bilateral DVT develops more commonly associated with underlying malignancy.
- Major presenting features are: Pain in the calf or tenderness, or both, swelling (ankle edema), redness, an increase in temperature (affected calf is warmer) and dilatation or engorgement of the superficial veins.
- **Homan's sign:** Pain in the posterior calf on forced dorsiflexion of the foot while the knee is fully extended. It can be usually demonstrated, but is not diagnostic and may be observed with all lesions of the calf. This test should not be done, because it has the possibility to dislodge the DVT and development of pulmonary embolism.
- **Moses test** is tenderness over calf muscles on squeezing the muscles from side to side. It is also not done because of possibility of pulmonary embolism.
- **Thrombosis in the iliofemoral region:** Severe pain, swelling of the thigh and/or ankle edema.
- **Complete occlusion of a large vein:** Cyanosis of the limb, severe edema, and very rarely lead to venous gangrene.

Diagnosis of DVT

Q. Write short essay/note on Wells probability score.

Wells clinical prediction guide for diagnosis of DVT is presented in **Table 7.107**. It incorporates risk factors, clinical signs, and the presence or absence of alternative diagnoses. *It helps in quantifying the pretest probability of*

TABLE 7.107: Wells probability score.

Clinical parameter	*Score*
Active cancer (ongoing treatment or within 6 months of palliative)	+1
Paralysis or recent plaster immobilization of the lower extremities	+1
Recently bedridden for >3 days or major surgery <4 weeks	+1
Localized tenderness along the distribution of the deep veins	+1
Swelling of entire leg	+1
Calf swelling >3 cm compared to the asymptomatic leg	+1
Pitting edema (greater in the symptomatic leg)	+1
Previously documented DVT	+1
Collateral superficial veins (nonvaricose)	+1
Alternative diagnosis (at least as likely as DVT)	-2

DVT namely high score is 3 or more, a moderate score 1–2 and a low score 0. It groups the patients into high, moderate, or low-risk categories.

Complications

- Pulmonary embolism
- **Post-thrombotic syndrome:** Consists of edema, skin pigmentation, venous eczema/dermatitis, ulceration around the medial malleolus, venous claudication, nocturnal cramping, and lifelong pain in the involved limb.
- **Venous gangrene:** Due to complete obstruction of large veins.

Investigations

- **D-Dimer:** Raised (>500 ng/mL) but is not specific. May be raised in trauma, recent surgery, hemorrhage, cancer, etc. In DVT, it remains raised for 7 days.
    - **Negative D-dimer assay:** Rules out DVT in patients with low-to-moderate risk and a Wells score ≤1. No further investigations needed.
    - **Positive D-dimer assay:** With a moderate-to-high risk of DVT (Wells score ≥2) need diagnostic investigation, e.g., Doppler ultrasonography.
- **B mode venous compression, ultrasonography or Doppler (duplex) ultrasonography:** Compression ultrasound is the imaging investigation of choice and has sensitivity for proximal DVT (of the popliteal vein or above) of 99.5%. Venous thrombosis is associated with failure to compress the vascular lumen.
- **Contrast venography** (phlebography) can reliably detect below knee thromboses, but is now rarely by **venography** with noninvasive.
- **Impedance plethysmography (IPG)** also detects above knee thrombi.
- **Radiofibrinogen scanning** is very accurate in calf vein and lower thigh thrombi.

Treatment of DVT

- Bed rest till the patient is fully anticoagulated.
- **Legs:** Elevation by 15° and physiotherapy.

Prophylaxis

Q. Write short essay/note on prophylaxis of venous thrombosis (deep venous thrombosis-DVT).

- Prophylaxis for DVT and pulmonary embolism is indicated in at high-risk patients **(Box 7.62)**.

Prophylaxis of DVT

- Nonpharmacological measures:
    - Mechanical VTE (antiembolism stockings) thigh or knee length.
    - Foot impulse devices.
    - Physiotherapy
    - Intermittent pneumatic compression devices (thigh or knee length): Compress the calf intermittently (usually once a minute).
- Pharmacological prophylaxis
    - Fondaparinux or low-molecular weight heparin or unfractionated heparin are given before operation or on admission to hospital, continued until the patient is ambulatory.
    - When risk factors are present treatment with warfarin to be given for a prolonged time.

Box 7.62: High-risk factors for deep vein thrombosis and pulmonary thromboembolism.

- **Patients undergoing major surgery**, e.g., abdominal, thoracic or gynecological
- **Fractures:** Involving pelvis or extremities
- **Significant medical comorbidities**, e.g., heart disease, metabolic, endocrine or respiratory diseases pathologies, acute infectious diseases, inflammatory conditions
- **Patients admitted with major medical diseases:**
    - Acute coronary syndrome, acute congestive failure [New York Heart Association (NYHA) classes III, IV]
    - Acute respiratory diseases (respiratory failure with or without mechanical ventilation), chronic respiratory disease (e.g., chronic obstructive pulmonary disease)
    - Active cancer or cancer treatment
    - Inflammatory bowel disease
    - Acute arthritis of lower extremities
    - Sepsis, stroke, paraplegia, obesity
    - Varicose veins with phlebitis

DISORDERS OF BLOOD LIPIDS AND LIPOPROTEINS

Q. Write short essay/note on structure of lipoproteins and their transport in body.

Classes of lipid: Most important are:

- **Cholesterol:** It is composed of hydrocarbon rings.
- **Triglycerides (TG):** These are esters composed of glycerol linked to three long-chain fatty acids.
- **Phospholipids:** Composed of a hydrophobic "tail" consisting of two long-chain fatty acids connected to a hydrophilic head containing a phosphate group by glycerol. Phospholipids are present in cell membranes and constitute important signaling molecules.

Both plasma cholesterol and TG are clinically important because they are major treatable risk factors for atherosclerosis.

Lipoproteins

Lipids are poorly water soluble, but are absorbed from the gastrointestinal tract and transported throughout the body. This is achieved by lipids by forming complexes known as lipoproteins. Lipoproteins are spherical or disc-shaped and composed of:

- **Hydrophobic core:** Consisting of TG and cholesterol ester which is enveloped by a less hydrophobic surface coat (mentioned below).
- **Less hydrophobic surface coat:** Consisting of phospholipids, unesterified cholesterol and special proteins called apolipoproteins. Some apolipoproteins make these lipoproteins to act as enzyme co-factors or cell receptor ligands.

Types of Lipoprotein

- Chylomicrons
- Very low-density lipoprotein (VLDL)
- Intermediate-density lipoprotein (IDL)
- Low-density lipoprotein (LDL): Lipoprotein [Lp(a)] is a type of lipoprotein similar to LDL with the addition of apolipoprotein (a)/Lp(a) links lipid metabolism with blood coagulation.
- High-density lipoprotein (HDL).

VLDL particles containing more cholesterol ester are more atherogenic than LDL particles.

Transport and Storage of Lipids

Transport and storage of lipids have been shown in **Figure 7.56.**

Three main pathways involved in metabolism of lipid are:

1. **Exogenous (dietary) lipid pathway**
   - Dietary lipids are digested and absorbed in the small intestine and form chylomicrons in the epithelial cells of the intestines. Chylomicrons are the largest lipoprotein particle containing TG and cholesterol ester.

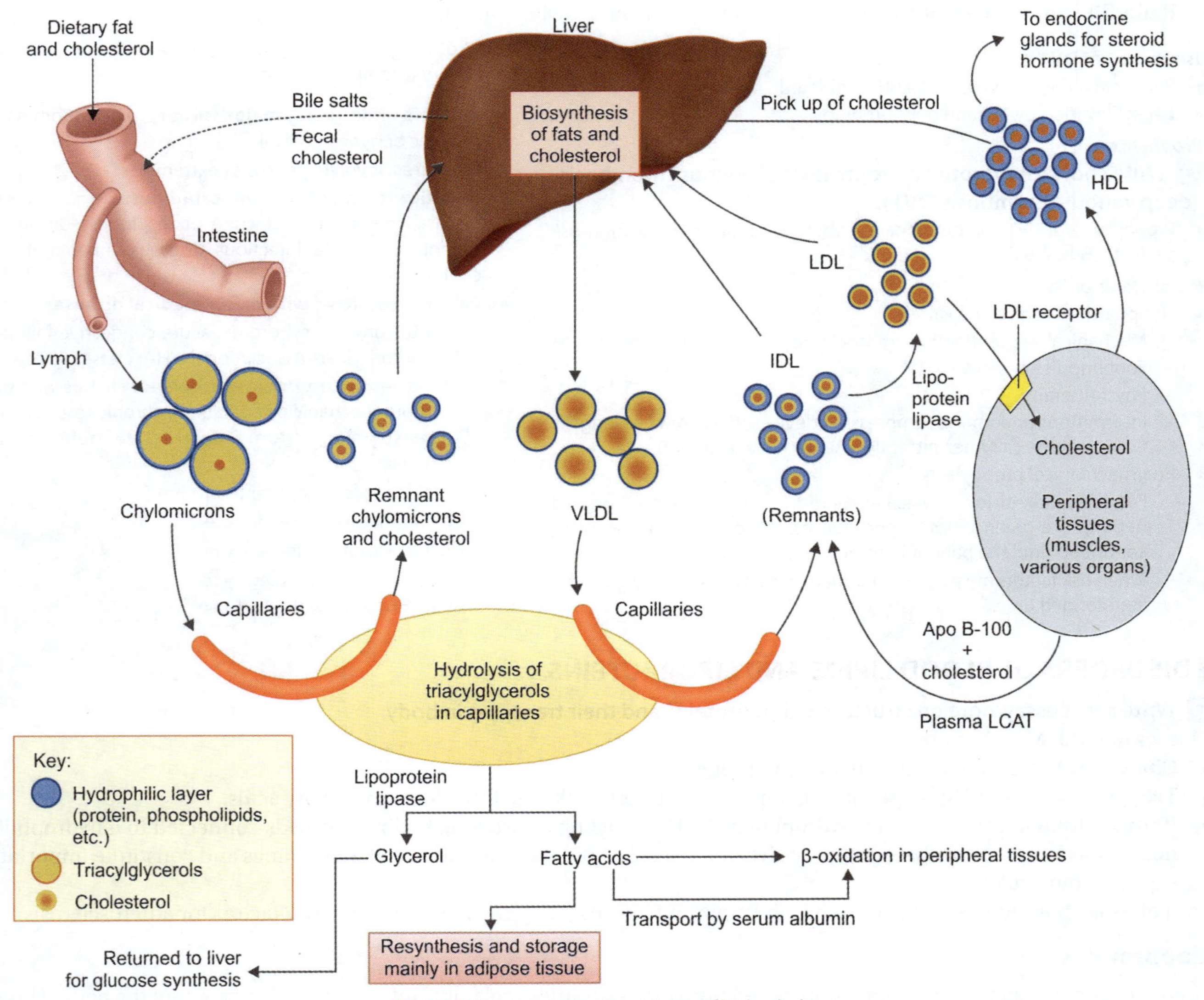

FIG. 7.56: Absorption, transport and storage of lipids in body.
(IDL: intermediate-density lipoproteins; LCAT: lecithin cholesterol acyltransferase; LDL: low-density lipoproteins; VLDL: very low-density lipoproteins)

- Chylomicrons enter the blood circulation and are hydrolyzed by lipoprotein lipase (LPL) located on the endothelium of tissue capillary beds and release fatty acids. These fatty acids are utilized locally for energy production or stored as TG in muscle or fat.

2. **Endogenous pathway**
   - During fasting, the liver is the main source of plasma lipids and constitute endogenous pathway.
   - TGs and cholesterol ester are produced by the liver and these lipids are secreted by the liver into the circulation as very low-density lipoproteins (VLDL). VLDL is also rich in TG but differ from chylomicrons in that they contain full-length Apo B100.
   - VLDL secreted into the circulation undergoes metabolic processing similar to that of chylomicrons. Hydrolysis of VLDL TG by capillary LPL releases fatty acids to tissues (utilized by fat and muscle) and remaining lipid portion of VLDL is converted into 'remnant' particles termed as intermediate-density lipoproteins (IDL).
   - Major part of IDL is taken up and quickly cleared by LDL receptors in the liver. Some of IDL is processed by hepatic lipase, which converts the IDL to LDL by removing TG.
   - LDL is an atherogenic lipoprotein. LDL particles carry the majority of the cholesterol in the blood and are a source of cholesterol for cells and tissues.
   - **Regulation of plasma LDL concentration:** LDL cholesterol is taken up by receptor-mediated endocytosis through the LDL receptor in the peripheral cells or liver.
     - **Controls the rate of cholesterol synthesis:** The supply of cholesterol through this pathway down-regulates further expression of the LDL receptor gene. This in turn decreases the synthesis and activity of the rate-limiting enzyme for cholesterol synthesis, HMGCoA reductase. This negative feedback loop, along with the modulation of cholesterol esterification, controls the intracellular free cholesterol level.
3. **Reverse cholesterol transport**
   - It is the process in which cholesterol is removed from the peripheral tissues and is returned to the liver. This protects against excessive cholesterol accumulation in peripheral tissues.
   - High-density lipoproteins (HDL) are the main lipoprotein along with lipid-poor Apo A1 (derived from the liver, intestine and the outer layer of chylomicrons and VLDL) involved in his reverse cholesterol transport process. HDL is produced and catabolized in the liver and intestines.
   - HDL is able to accept more free cholesterol from atherogenic lipoproteins and peripheral tissues to the liver. A circulating enzyme called lecithin cholesterol acyltransferase (LCAT) esterifies these HDL.

Hyperlipidemia

Q. Write short essay/note on hyperlipidemias, their causes, and management.

Hyperlipidemia is characterized by an abnormality in the lipid profile, consisting of a variety of disorders with raised total cholesterol, LDL or TG, or conversely, lower levels of HDL.

Classification and Causes

- **Primary hyperlipidemia:** It is a genetic disorder of lipid metabolism (e.g., familial hypercholesterolemia). It is characterized by a genetic mutation, which causes impaired clearance of LDL from the circulation due to absence of LDL receptors.
- **Secondary hyperlipidemia:** These are characterized by hyperlipidemia secondary to a disease/disorder other than the genetic defect (**Table 7.108**).

TABLE 7.108: Causes of secondary hyperlipidemia.

Increased LDL cholesterol level	*Increased triglyceride level*	*Decreased HDL cholesterol level*
➤ Diabetes mellitus ➤ Hypothyroidism ➤ Nephrotic syndrome ➤ Obstructive liver disease ➤ Drugs – Anabolic steroids – Progestins – Beta-adrenergic blockers (without intrinsic sympathomimetic action) – Thiazides	➤ Alcoholism ➤ Diabetes mellitus ➤ Hypothyroidism Obesity ➤ Renal insufficiency ➤ Drugs – Beta-adrenergic blockers (without intrinsic sympathomimetic action) – Bile acid binding resins – Estrogens – Ticlopidine	➤ Cigarette smoking ➤ Diabetes mellitus ➤ Hypertriglyceridemia ➤ Menopause ➤ Obesity ➤ Uremia ➤ Anabolic steroids ➤ Beta-adrenergic blockers (without intrinsic sympathomimetic action) ➤ Progestins

(LDL: low-density lipoprotein; HDL: high-density lipoprotein)

Management Strategies

- Lipid profile of an individual should be interpreted along with the risk factors for CAD.
- Coronary heart disease risk based on risk factors other than the LDL level is listed in **Box 7.63**.

Box 7.63: Coronary heart disease risk based on risk factors other than the LDL level.

Positive risk factors
- **Sex:** Male ≥45 years and female ≥55 years or postmenopausal without estrogen replacement therapy
- **Family history of premature coronary heart disease:** Myocardial infarction or sudden death before age 55 in father or other male first-degree relative or before age 65 in mother or other female first-degree relative)
- Current cigarette smoking
- **Hypertension:** Blood pressure ≥140/90 mm Hg or patient is receiving antihypertensive drug therapy
- **HDL cholesterol level** <35 mg per dL (<0.90 mmol per L)
- **Diabetes mellitus**
- **Negative risk factor#:** High HDL cholesterol level (≥60 mg per dL [≥1.60 mmol per L])

(LDL: low-density lipoprotein; HDL: high-density lipoprotein)

#Subtract one positive risk factor if negative risk factor is present.

- **Major modifiable risk factors:** (1) Hypercholesterolemia, (2) smoking, (3) diabetes mellitus and (4) hypertension as per Framingham Risk Score (FRS). It provides the risk of an individual and developing a cardiac event in the next 10 years.
- Emerging risk factors: That may contribute to the risk of CAD include:
  - Apolipoprotein B
  - Lipoprotein (a)
  - C-reactive protein
  - Hyperhomocysteinemia
  - Small, dense LDL particles
- CAD equivalents: These include:
  - Diabetes mellitus
  - Patients with FRS ≥20%
  - In these patients, the goals of treatment are same as those for patients with established CAD.
- LDL cholesterol goals in different categories (**Table 7.109**).

Management

- Therapeutic lifestyle changes.
- **Patients with normal-weight, dyslipidemia [body mass index (BMI) 18.5–24.9 kg/m^2]:** Focus on healthy eating and regular exercise.
- **Overweight and obese patients (BMI ≥25 kg/m^2):** Reduce caloric intake from fats, simple carbohydrate and ≥30 mins physical activity most days.
- Intake of soluble fiber to be increased (10–25 g/day).
- Diet (rich fruits, veg, nuts, whole grains, monounsaturated oils; low red meat, animal fat) reduces LDL 5–15% (ATP III TLC diet).
- **Aerobic exercise:** Running, walking, cycling, swimming enhance weight reduction facilitates achieving optimum lipid levels.

- Therapeutic drug classes, their effect on lipid profile and side effects are presented in **Table 7.110**.
- **Table 7.111** shows drugs to be considered depending on cholesterol level.
  Ezetimibe inhibits the absorption of cholesterol from the diet.
  Omega-3 fatty acid: Useful to reduce TG levels. Dose is 1–2 g/day.
  Newer agents:
- **Torcetrapib** is a cholesteryl ester transfer protein (CETP) inhibitors.

TABLE 7.109: Cardiovascular risk categories and recommendations—2019 ESC/EAS Guidelines for the management of dyslipidemias.

Risk	*Description*	*Recommendation*
Very-high-risk	➤ Documented ASCVD, either clinical or unequivocal on imaging. (previous ACS , stable angina, coronary revascularisation, stroke and TIA, and peripheral arterial disease.) ➤ Unequivocally documented ASCVD on imaging includes those findings that are known to be predictive of clinical events, such as significant plaque on coronary angiography or CT scan or on carotid ultrasound. ➤ DM with target organ damage, ≥3 major risk factors or early onset of T1DM of long duration (>20 years). ➤ Severe CKD (eGFR <30 mL/min/1.73 m^2). ➤ Family history with ASCVD or with another major risk factor. ➤ *A calculated score **≥10%** for 10-year risk of fatal CVD.*	**Target:** An LDL-C reduction of at least 50% from baselined and an LDL-C goal of <1.4 mmol/L (<55 mg/dL) are recommended. **Intervention:** Lifestyle intervention plus drug (if LDL >1.8 mmol/L </70 mg/dL)
High-risk	➤ Markedly elevated single risk factors, in particular TC >8 mmol/L (>310 mg/dL), LDL-C >4.9 mmol/L(>190 mg/dL), or BP ≥180/110 mm Hg. ➤ Patients with FH without other major risk factors. ➤ Patients with DM without target organ damage, with DM duration ≥10 years or another additional risk factors. ➤ Moderate CKD (eGFR 30–59 mL/min/1.73 m^2) ➤ *A calculated score **≥5% and <10%** for10-year risk of fatal CVD*	**Target**: An LDL-C reduction of at least 50% from baselined and an LDL-C goal of <1.8 mmol/L (<70 mg/dL) are recommended. **Intervention:** Lifestyle intervention PLUS drug (if LDL > 2.5 mmol/L < /100 mg/dL)
Moderate-risk	➤ Young patients (T1DM <35 years; T2DM <50 years) with DM duration <10 years, without other risk factors. ➤ *Calculated score **≥1% and <5%** for10-year risk of fatal CVD*	**Target** -an LDL-C goal of <2.6 mmol/L (<100 mg/dL) should be considered **Intervention** -Lifestyle intervention plus drug (if LDL > 4.4 mmol/L < /150 mg/dL)
Low-risk	*Calculated score <**1%**for10-year risk of fatal CVD*	**Target:** An LDL-C goal <3.0 mmol/L (<116 mg/dL) may be considered. **Intervention:** Lifestyle intervention plus drug (if LDL > 4.9 mmol/L < /190 mg/dL)

(CKD: chronic kidney disease; CVD: cardiovascular disease; LDL: low-density lipoprotein; T2DM: type 2 diabetes mellitus)

TABLE 7.110: Drug classes, their effect on lipid profile and side effects.

Drug class	*Total cholesterol levels*	*LDL levels*	*HDL levels*	*Triglycerides*	*Side effects*
Bile acid binding resins	20%	10–20%	3–5%	Neutral	Unpalatability, bloating, constipation, heartburn
Nicotinic acid	25%	10–25%	15–35%	20–50%	Flushing, nausea, glucose intolerance, abnormal liver function test
Fibric acid analogs	15%	5–15%	14–20%	20–50%	Nausea, skin rash
HMG-CoA reductase inhibitors	15–30%	20–60%	5–15%	10–40%	Myositis, myalgia, elevated hepatic transaminases

(LDL: low-density lipoprotein; HDL: high-density lipoprotein)

- **PCSK9 inhibitors**
  - Monoclonal antibodies have been developed that lower LDL-C. They work by inhibiting the Proprotein convertase subtilisin/kexin type 9 (PCSK9) enzyme, which is involved in breaking down the LDL-C receptor.
  - Two PCSK9 inhibitors are approved. **Evolocumab** is dosed at 140 mg subcutaneously every 2 weeks or 420 mg sc every 4 weeks. **Alirocumab** is dosed at 75 or 150 mg every 2 weeks or 300 mg every 4 weeks.

TABLE 7.111: Drugs to be considered depending on cholesterol level.

LDL cholesterol level	*Drugs to be considered*
High LDL-C level only	Statins first, resins or intestinal absorption blocker second, niacin third
High LDL-C and low HDL-C levels	Statins first, niacin second
High LDL-C, low HDL-C, and high triglyceride levels	Niacin and statins first, fibrates second
High triglyceride levels, with/without low HDL-C levels	Fibrates first, niacin second
Low HDL-C levels only	Niacin first, fibrates second

(LDL-C: low density lipoprotein cholesterol; HDL-C: high-density-lipoprotein cholesterol)

ASCVD Risk

ASCVD stands for atherosclerotic cardiovascular disease, defined as a nonfatal myocardial infarction (heart attack), coronary heart disease death, or stroke. It estimates the risk of ASCVD within a 10-year period among patients without pre-existing cardiovascular disease who are between 40 and 79 years of age who have never had one of these events in the past. This risk estimate considers age, sex, race, cholesterol levels, blood pressure, medication use, diabetic status, and smoking status.

Moderate- or high-intensity statin therapy is recommended for
- Individuals with clinical ASCVD
- Individuals with primary elevations of LDL ≥190 mg/dL
- Individuals 40 to 75 years of age with diabetes and an LDL 70 to 189 mg/dL without clinical ASCVD
- Individuals without clinical ASCVD or diabetes who are 40 to 75 years of age with LDL 70 to 189 mg/dL and a 10-year ASCVD risk of 7.5% or higher.

LIPODYSTROPHY

Q. Write a short note on lipodystrophy.

Lipodystrophy is changes in the distribution body fat. Lipoatrophy implies partial or complete decrease of fat. However, the terms lipoatrophy and lipodystrophy are used interchangeably in clinical practice.

Classification of Lipodystrophies

- **Total lipodystrophy:** Two types namely congenital and acquired.
  - **Berardinelli-Seip (congenital):** Autosomal recessive, hypermetabolic state.
  - **Seip-Lawrence (acquired):** Begins <15 years old, often <5 years
- **Partial lipodystrophy**
  - **Kobberling-Dunnigan syndrome:** Inherited form, autosomal dominant
  - **Progressive partial lipodystrophy:** Acquired forms
- **Centrifugal:** One type is seen primarily in infants from Japan. 90% are under 5 years. Centrifugally spreading loss of abdominal fat over 3–8 years with regional lymphadenopathy. Resolves completely after progression stops.
- **Semicircular:** Adult women affected with single or multiple, asymptomatic, symmetric depressions of anterolateral thigh. Often after trauma, resolves in several years.
- **Annular atrophic panniculitis:** 10 cm band of atrophy, bilaterally, around the ankles of children and young adults. Rare.
- **Lipoatrophia annularis:** Bracelet-like constrictions of upper extremities 1–2 cm wide on women following a period of swelling and erythema of extremity. Arthralgias and pain of affected extremity. Persist up to 20 years.
- **Localized lipodystrophy: Secondary** to injection of medications especially insulin.
- **HIV-associated lipodystrophy:**
  - Occurs in effectively treated AIDS patients with reverse transcriptase inhibitors and protease inhibitors.
  - Fat redistribution from face, buccal, buttocks and limbs is lost to neck, upper back and inter abdominal areas.
  - Peripheral lipodystrophy, central fat accumulation and lipomatosis.

Q. Write short note on indications for low-dose aspirin.

Indications for low-dose aspirin (**Box 7.64**).

Box 7.64: Indications for low-dose aspirin.

- Secondary prevention of cardiovascular disease: CAD (coronary artery disease, stroke, post-CABG (coronary artery bypass grafting)
- Primary prevention of ischemic heart disease
- Transient ischemic attacks (TIA)
- Antiphospholipid antibody (APLA) syndrome
- Pre-eclampsia
- Essential thrombocytosis, polycythemia vera
- Venous thromboembolism—prophylaxis

STRAIGHT BACK SYNDROME

Q. Write short essay/note on straight back syndrome (SBS).

- In straight back syndrome, there is loss of normal curvature upper thoracic spinal which reduces the anteroposterior diameter of the chest. This deformity compresses or "pancakes" the heart (cardiomegaly) and great vessels so as to appear enlarged. There is displacement of the heart toward left, resulting in cardiac murmurs.
- **Clinical features:** Chest pain, tracheal compression and mitral valve prolapse (MVP).
- **Chest X-ray:** Lateral chest X-ray reveals significant reduction of distance from the middle of the anterior border T8 to a vertical line connecting T4 and T12. A value less 1.2 cm is diagnostic.
- ECG often shows right bundle branch block.

CARDIAC TUMORS

Myxoma

- Most common type of primary cardiac tumor in adults seen in third to sixth decade of life.
- Most common in females.
- Most are sporadic, but some are familial (autosomal dominant)-10%.
- Most are solitary and located in left atrium arising from inter atrial septum near fossa ovalis.
- Its presentation most commonly mimics that of mitral valve disease.
- "Tumor plop" is a characteristic low-pitched sound which may be audible during early or mid-diastole and is thought to result from the tumor abruptly stopping as it strikes the ventricular wall.
- **Symptoms and signs:** Fever, weight loss, cachexia, malaise arthralgia, rash, clubbing, and Raynaud's phenomenon. Peripheral or pulmonary embolization can develop.
- **Investigations:**
  - Anemia, polycythemia, elevated ESR, thrombocytopenia or thrombocytosis.
  - 2-D echocardiography: Useful screening tool
  - CT and MRI are investigations of choice
- Treatment is surgical excision using cardiopulmonary bypass.

Rhabdomyomas are the commonest cardiac tumor in children.

DIGOXIN

Q. Write short essay/note on digoxin, manifestations of digoxin/digitalis toxicity, and its management.

Digoxin is a purified glycoside derived from *Digitalis lanata* having cardiac inotropic property.

Pharmacological Actions

- Force of myocardial contraction is increased by a direct action of digitalis.
- **Heart rate:** Decreased and bradycardia is more marked in CHF.
- **Electrophysiological properties:**
  - Prolongs the refractory period of V node → slows the ventricular rate.
  - Reflex vasodilation in CHF.

Pharmacokinetics

- Has a good oral absorption.
- Digoxin concentration in the heart is 30 times more than in the plasma.
- The elimination half-life for digoxin is **36–48 hours** in patients with normal or near-normal renal function. This permits once-a-day dosing; near steady-state blood levels are achieved one week after initiation of maintenance therapy.
- About 85% of digoxin is excreted through the kidneys and the remaining 15% through the stool.

Indications

- **Cardiac arrhythmias:** Supraventricular tachycardia, tachyarrhythmias and atrial fibrillation with a fast ventricular rate.
- Heart failure with reduced ejection fraction (HFrEF)
- Heart failure accompanied by atrial fibrillation or flutter with a rapid ventricular rate.

Dosage and Route of Administration

The dosage and route is determined based on the desired action.

- **Rapid digitalizing (loading dose) regimen**
  - **Intravenously:** Initial loading dose of 0.25–0.5 mg followed by 0.25 mg every 6 hour. Careful monitoring of clinical response and toxicity should be performed before each dose.

- **Orally:** Initial loading dose is 0.5–1 mg followed by 0.25 mg 6 hourly. Careful monitoring of clinical response and toxicity before each dose.
- **Slow digitalization:** Maintenance dose (0.125–0.25 mg/day) given from the beginning. Dose may be increased every 2 weeks depending on clinical response, serum levels of the drug, and toxicity.
- As per ACCF/AHA guidelines, a loading dose to initiate digoxin therapy in patients with heart failure is not required.

Digoxin Toxicity and its Management

Digitalis has high toxicity low margin of safety. Definite toxicity defined as nausea/vomiting, with cardiac effects and resolution of side effects on discontinuation. Serum digoxin concentration (SDC) is not a necessary criterion but SDC >2.0 ng/mL helpful.

Manifestations of Digoxin Toxicity

- Extracardiac manifestations
  - Nonspecific but more common
  - **Gastrointestinal (60–80%):** Nausea/vomiting, anorexia, abdominal pain, diarrhea
  - Malaise (30–40%), lethargy, fatigue
  - **Neurological (20–30%):** Dizziness, confusion, headache, visual changes (flashing lights, halos, color disturbances in green-yellow spectrum, blurred vision)
- Cardiac side effects
  - More specific but less common
  - Almost any permutations and combinations of heart block (partial to complete), brady and tachydysrhythmias can be produced.
  - **Classical:** Paroxysmal atrial tachycardia, ventricular bigeminy, bidirectional ventricular tachycardia, nodal and ventricular extrasystoles.
- **ECG changes of digoxin toxicity:** Inverse check mark with proximal ST segment depressed, in leads other than those with tall R waves, with T wave not rising above baseline (Inverted T), with shortened QTc.

Management of Digoxin Toxicity

- Stop digoxin.
- **Blood test:** Urea, electrolytes and plasma digoxin concentration.
- **Correction of hypokalemia:** Intravenous supplementation of no more than 20 mmol/h of potassium. More rapid infusion may cause asystole.
- **Heart blocks:** Atropine and temporary cardiac pacing.
- Malignant ventricular arrhythmias
- Phenytoin (100 mg intravenously, repeated after 5 minutes if required) opposes digitalis binding and may improve atrioventricular conduction by its anticholinergic properties.
- Ultra-short-acting beta blockers, e.g., esmolol.
- Avoid cardioversion wherever possible, due to the risk of precipitating asystole.
- **Digoxin-specific antibody fragments:** Digoxin-specific fab antibody fragments (Digibind) are the most effective but expensive.
- Hence, reserved for treatment of serious toxicity, especially in the presence of malignant cardiac dysrhythmias.

VALSALVA MANEUVER

Q. What is the Valsalva maneuver?

The Valsalva maneuver is a forceful attempted exhalation against a closed glottis.

Method (Fig. 7.57)

- **Instruction:** Take a deep breath, close your mouth and pinch your nose with the thumb and index finger and attempt to breathe out gently, keeping your cheek muscles tight, not allowing the air to escape by keeping the lips pursed.
- **"Standard" or "quantitative:"** Blowing out with an open glottis into a tube of a sphygmomanometer against the pressure of 40 mm Hg.

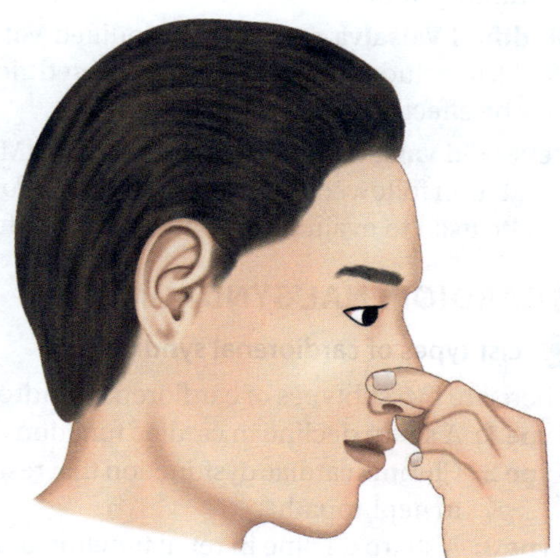

FIG. 7.57: The Valsalva maneuver.

Phases of Valsalva Maneuver

Physiological effects on blood pressure heart rate and phases of Valsalva maneuver are presented in **Table 7.112** and **Figure 7.58.**

Phase 1: The onset of blowing. The pressure within the chest and abdomen increases and presses upon the arteries in the chest, which results in an increase in mean arterial blood pressure. This activates the baroreceptor reflex, which results in an increase in parasympathetic (vagal) activity and hence in a drop in heart rate. The increased intrathoracic pressure also reduces the amount of blood that comes into the right atrium (decreased venous return or preload).

Phase 2: A decrease of venous return results in a lower amount of blood that is ejected from the heart, which results in a decrease of central venous pressure and consequently in a decrease of mean arterial blood pressure. This activates the baroreflex, which results in a decrease of the parasympathetic (vagal) activity and consequent increase of the heart rate,

TABLE 7.112: Various phases of Valsalva maneuver and its associated changes.

Phase	1	2a	2b	3	4
Intrathoracic pressure	Increased	Increased	Increased	Normal	Normal
Mean arterial blood pressure	Increased	Decreased	Increased	Decreased	Increased
Heart rate	Decreased	Increased	Decreased	Increased	Decreased
Sympathetic activity	Decreased	Decreased	Increased	Increased	Increased
Parasympathetic (vagal) activity	Increased	Increased	Decreased	Decreased	Increase

and in an increase in sympathetic activity, which constrict the arteries (an increase of peripheral resistance), which results in a slight rise of the blood pressure at the end of phase 2 (2b).

Phase 3: Relaxation—the end of the maneuver. The intrathoracic pressure decreases, so the intrathoracic arteries widen, which results in a brief drop in blood pressure. At the same time, the venous blood fills the heart.

Phase 4: The heart ejects the blood into the arterial system against increased peripheral resistance (which has developed in phase 2), so the blood pressure rises again (blood pressure overshoot). This activates the baroreflex, which results in a drop in heart rate (bradycardia). Eventually, both the blood pressure and heart rate normalize.

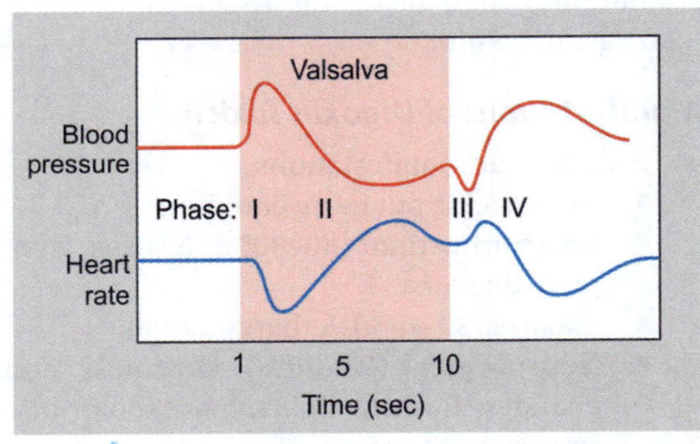

FIG. 7.58: Mean arterial blood pressure and heart rate changes during the Valsalva maneuver.

Uses

- Eustachian tube dysfunction
- Heart murmurs: Valsalva increases murmurs in hypertrophic cardiomyopathy and mitral valve prolapse and decreases them in atrial septal defects and aortic stenosis.
- Congestive heart failure: Valsalva responses lost
- Function of the autonomous nervous system: An abnormal blood pressure response (for example, an absence of the blood pressure rise in phase 4) suggests an abnormality of the sympathetic system.
- An abnormal heart rate response suggests an abnormality of the parasympathetic Valsalva maneuver can be used as a provocative test to check for:
  - Neurogenic orthostatic hypotension
  - Chiari malformation, the Valsalva maneuver (coughing) triggers a headache at the back of the head.
- Diagnosis of inguinal hernia, prolapse of the uterus, bladder or vagina, varicocele and intrinsic sphincter deficiency in stress urinary incontinence system.
- Valsalva maneuver can help: Equalize the pressure between the middle ear and the ambient pressure during scuba diving, driving from a steep hill, elevator descending, parachuting or plane landing or in individuals with Eustachian tube dysfunction.

Modified Valsalva maneuver: Modified Valsalva maneuver is used to terminate an attack of supraventricular tachycardia (SVT); it includes blowing against a closed glottis followed by lying down face up and raising legs with the help of an assistant, may be effective in 19–54% of cases.

Reversed Valsalva—Müller's maneuver: Müller's maneuver is the opposite of the Valsalva maneuver and includes forced exhalation followed by an attempted forceful inhalation with a closed mouth and nose or just with a closed glottis. The test can be used to evaluate weakness of the soft palate and throat walls in individuals with obstructive sleep apnea.

CARDIORENAL SYNDROME

Q. List types of cardiorenal syndrome.

There are five subtypes of cardiorenal syndrome:

Type 1: A sharp decline in cardiac function that results in an acute decrease in renal function, e.g., cardiogenic shock.

Type 2: Chronic cardiac dysfunction that results in a sustained reduction in renal function, e.g., chronic heart failure resulting in nephropathy.

Type 3: A sharp decline in renal function that results in an acute reduction in cardiac function, e.g., acute kidney injury.

Type 4: Chronic decline in kidney function that results in chronic cardiac dysfunction, e.g., chronic kidney disease.

Type 5: Systemic diseases that result in both cardiac and renal dysfunction, e.g., diabetes, hypertension.

CHAPTER

8

Hematology

DISORDERS OF RED BLOOD CELL

INTRODUCTION

Hemoglobin Structure

A hemoglobin molecule is a conjugated protein composed of iron-containing pigment called **heme** and protein **globin**. About 65–70% of hemoglobin is synthesized in normoblasts and 30–35% is synthesized at the reticulocyte stage.

- Each molecule of **heme** consists of protoporphyrin with an iron in ferrous state (Fe^{++}). Heme synthesis occurs mainly in the mitochondria of normoblasts.
- Each **globin** chain is made up of **two pairs of distinct polypeptide** chains (composed of a number of amino acids) bound to a heme molecule.
  - **Hemoglobin A (HbA)** is composed of two α and two β globin chains ($\alpha_2 \beta_2$) and normally represents more than 95% of the hemoglobin in adult red blood cells (RBCs). Fetal hemoglobin is replaced by adult hemoglobin during the first year of life (hemoglobin switching).
  - **Fetal hemoglobin (HbF)** contains two α and two γ globin chains ($\alpha_2 \gamma_2$). It is the major hemoglobin (70–90%) during fetal development and is normally found in low levels in adults.
  - **Hemoglobin A2 ($\alpha_2 \delta_2$)** is normally found at low levels in adults (2%).
  - Normal hemoglobin in the adult are HbA ($\alpha_2 \beta_2$) and HbA_2 ($\alpha_2\delta_2$)
  - Normal hemoglobin in the fetus are HbF ($\alpha_2 \gamma_2$) and Hb-Bart's (γ_4).

Red Cell Indices

- **Mean corpuscular volume (MCV):** It is used for classification and differential diagnosis of anemias.
  - **Normal range: 82–98 fL** (fL stands for femtoliters)

  Microcytic anemia has MCV < 80 fL and macrocytic anemia has MCV >100 fL.
- **Mean corpuscular hemoglobin (MCH):**
  - **Normal range: 27–32 pg**

  MCH < 26 pg is seen in microcytic anemia and MCH > 33 pg is seen in macrocytic anemia.
- **Mean corpuscular hemoglobin concentration (MCHC):** It is a better indicator of hypochromasia than MCH.
  - **Normal range: 31–35 g/dL**

  MCHC < 31 g/dL is seen in hypochromic RBC such as iron deficiency anemia (IDA) and thalassemia. MCHC is increased in hereditary spherocytosis.
- **Red Cell Distribution Width (RDW):**
  - RDW is a quantitative measure of **anisocytosis.**
  - **Normal RDW is 11.5–14.5%.**

  RDW = (Standard deviation + mean cell volume) × 100
  - **Significance:** RDW is used for differentiating anemia due to iron deficiency and thalassemia. Increased in IDA (along with low MCV) and megaloblastic anemia (with high MCV) while in thalassemia trait, RDW is normal with low MCV.

  RBC count: Normal range in males 4.5–5.5 millions/cu mm; females 4–4.5 millions/cu mm

Reticulocyte Count

Reticulocytes are immature, non-nucleated RBCs released from bone marrow. They are demonstrated by using visual method brilliant cresyl blue/new methylene blue stain or by automated method.

Reticulocyte count is expressed as a percentage of RBC count (normal <2.5%). Reticulocyte count reflects the erythropoietic activity of the bone marrow and provides an estimate of red cell production. Increased erythropoiesis results in increased reticulocyte release. The reference range of the corrected reticulocyte percentage in adults is 0.5–1.5%. Causes of increased and reduced reticulocyte count are listed in **Table 8.1**.

TABLE 8.1: Causes of increased and reduced reticulocyte count.

Causes of increased reticulocyte count (reticulocytosis)	*Causes of reduced reticulocyte count*
➤ Hemolytic anemias ➤ Hemolytic crisis ➤ Hemorrhage ➤ Following treatment in iron/folic acid/vitamin B_{12} deficiency anemias. *Highest counts are found on 6th/7th day of treatment and indicate marrow response to iron and 3rd day in response to vitamin B_{12}*	➤ Due to decreased erythropoietic activity ➤ Aplastic anemia ➤ Aplastic crisis due to parvovirus (in hereditary spherocytosis and sickle cell disease) ➤ Pure red cell aplasia ➤ Fanconi anemia ➤ Myelofibrosis

- **Reticulocyte production index (RPI)** is expressed as % and it accounts for premature release of reticulocytes from bone marrow in anemia. It is important in determining if a patient's bone marrow is responding appropriately to the level of anemia.

  Reticulocyte index =

  $$\text{Recticulocyte count} \times \frac{\text{Hematocrit}}{\text{Normal hematocrit for the age}}$$

  Reticulocyte production index (RPI) =

  $$\text{Reticulocyte count} \times \frac{\text{Hematocrit}}{\text{Normal hemoglobin for the age}} \times 0.5$$

Significance: Normal RPI is 1.0–2.0. However, RPI < 2 with anemia indicates decreased RBC production (hypoproliferative anemia) and RPI > 2 with anemia indicates hemolysis or loss of RBCs leading to compensatory production of reticulocytes and is observed in hyperproliferative anemia.

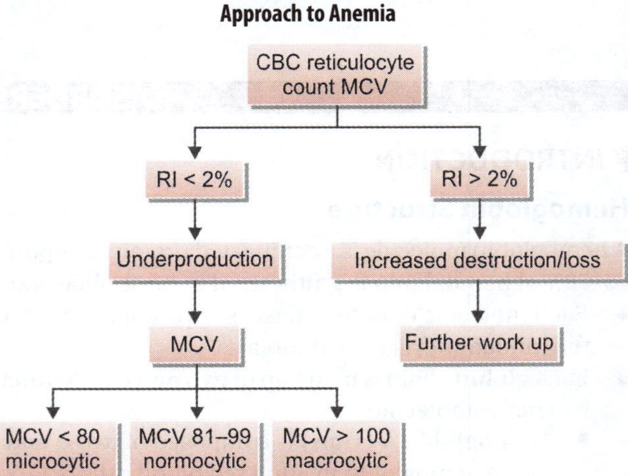

RBC Abnormalities

Various RBC abnormalities are presented in **Figures 8.1 to 8.4**.

Term	Description	Appearance	Condition
Normocyte	• Normal RBC is biconcave, 7.2 µm in diameter		• Normal RBC normochromic • Normocytic anemia
Microcyte	• RBCs smaller than normal and less than 6 µm in diameter		• Iron deficiency anemia • Thalassemia • Sideroblastic anemia
Macrocyte-round	• Larger than normal and more than 9 µm in diameter		• Liver disease • Alcohol abuse • Hypothyroidism • Antifolate drugs
Macroovalocyte	• Larger than normal, more than 9 µm in diameter and also oval		• Megaloblastic anemia due to vitamin B_{12} and folic acid deficiency
Anisocytosis	• Variation in size		• Severe anemia of any type • Iron deficiency anemia • Megaloblastic anemia • Moderate to severe thalassemia • Sideroblastic anemia • Post-transfusion

FIG. 8.1: Variation in size of red blood cells and associated conditions.

Q. Discuss the RBC abnormalities seen on a peripheral blood smear examination.

Q. Define, describe, and classify anemia based on red blood cell size and reticulocyte count.

Term	Description	Appearance	Condition
Normal	• Biconcave, flattened on smear	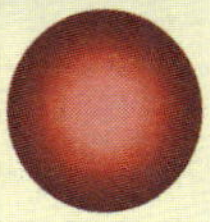	• Normal
Poikilocytosis	• Variation in shape	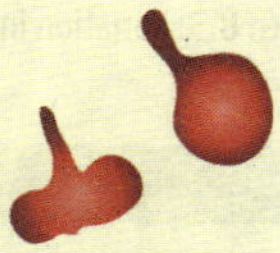	• Severe anemia • Iron deficiency anemia • Thalassemia • Sideroblastic anemia
Spherocytes	• Smaller and stain darker without any central pallor	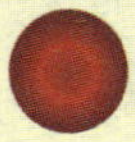	• Hereditary spherocytosis • Immunohemolytic anemia
Target cells or leptocytes	• Only the periphery and the central regions of the cell appear hemoglobinized	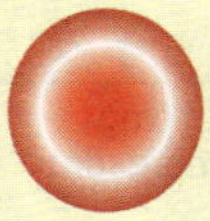	• Thalassemia • Sickle cell anemia • Hemolytic anemia • Postsplenectomy • Liver disease
Sickle cells	• Thin, elongated, slightly curved and have shape of a sickle	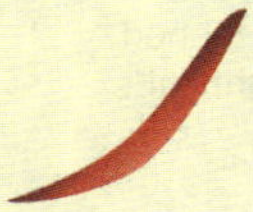	• Sickle cell anemia
Bite cells	• Pairs of spicules	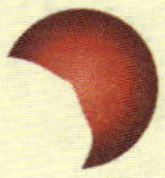	• G6PD deficiency
Schistocytes (Fragmented cells)	• Small, irregular shaped, triangular or spiculated cells	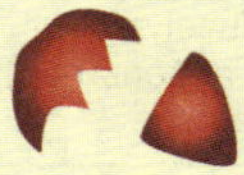	• Microangiopathic hemolytic anemia [e.g. disseminated intravascular coagulation (DIC), thrombotic thrombocytopenic purpura (TTP)]

FIG. 8.2A: Variation in shape of red blood cells and associated conditions.

Term	Description	Appearance	Condition
Acanthocytes/ spur cells	• RBCs with few spicules of uneven (irregular) length and shape	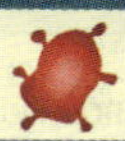	• Abetalipoproteinemia • Liver disease
Echinocyte/ Burr cells	• Very small irregular shrunken cells with pointed projections. Resemblance to the small thorny 'burrs'	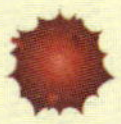	• Uremia • Post-transfusion
Elliptocyte or Ovalocyte	• Oval in shape	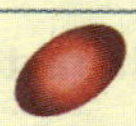	• Hereditary ovalocytosis • Hemolytic anemia
Pencil shaped cells	• Elongated thin cells (exaggerated ovalocytes)	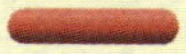	• Iron deficiency anemia
Tear drop and pear-shaped cells	• These abnormal RBCs have a teardrop or pear-like shape	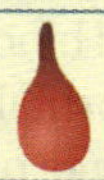	• Myelofibrosis • Marrow infiltration
Stomatocytes	• Red cells with a slit-like area of central pallor	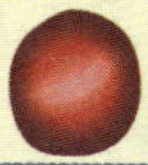	• Hereditary stomatocytosis • Liver disease

FIG. 8.2B: Variation in shape of red blood cells and associated conditions.

Term	Description	Appearance	Condition
Normochromic	Cell with 1/3 central pallor	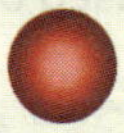	• Normal RBC
Hypochromic	Central pallor more than 1/3	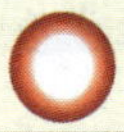	• Iron deficiency anemia • Thalassemia • Sideroblastic anemia
Polychromasia	Cells stained purple and are larger than normal	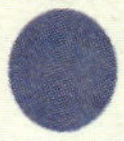	• Hemolytic anemias • Response to therapy in deficiency anemias

FIG. 8.3: Variation in color of red blood cells.

Term	Description	Appearance	Condition
Basophilic stippling (punctate basophilia)	• Red cells contain small, blue black inclusions and represent precipitated ribosomal RNA	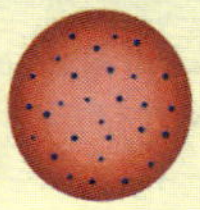	• Lead poisoning • Megaloblastic anemias • Hemolytic anemias like thalassemias • Sideroblastic anemias • Alcoholism • Pyrimidine-5 nucleotidase deficiency
Howell-Jolly bodies	• Small, round, densely staining dark blue particles and represent nuclear remnants	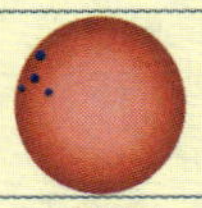	• Megaloblastic anemias • Acute hemolytic anemias • Postsplenectomy state
Cabot rings	• Rings or figure of eight shaped and are probably remnants of the nuclear membrane	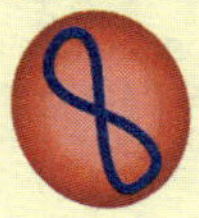	• Hemolytic anemia • Megaloblastic anemia • Leukemia • Rarely after splenectomy
Pappenheimer bodies/ siderotic granules (RBCs with Pappenheimer bodies are called siderocytes)	• Aggregates of ferritin and appear pale blue, but are easily demonstrable with Perl's stain (Prussian blue reaction)	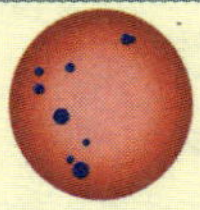	• Sideroblastic anemias • Megaloblastic anemias • Hemolytic anemias • Postsplenectomy
Hemoglobin H inclusions	• Free β chains in red cells. Small, regular, multiple and diffusely distributed (golf ball like appearance). Stained by supravital stains.	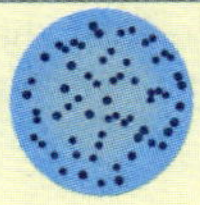	• α-thalassemias
Heinz bodies	• Refractive, single or multiple rounded inclusions of denatured globin detected by supravital stains	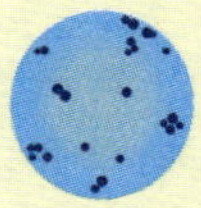	• Intake/exposure to oxidizing drugs or chemicals. • G6PD deficiency • Unstable hemoglobin disease
Hemoglobin C crystals	• Crystallization of hemoglobin C	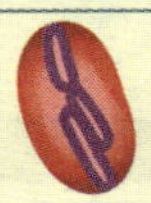	• Splenectomy in homozygous hemoglobin C

FIG. 8.4: Inclusions in red blood cells and associated conditions.

ANEMIA

Q. Describe and discuss the morphological characteristics, etiology, and prevalence of each of the causes of anemia.

Definition

Anemia is defined as **decrease** in circulating red blood cell mass. It is characterized by decrease of **hemoglobin concentration (Hb)/RBC count/hematocrit (PCV)** below normal for the patient's age, sex, and altitude of residence.

Normal adult hemoglobin level is in the range of 13–17 g/dL in males and 12–15 g/dL in females.

Classification of Anemia

Anemia may be classified (1) based on the morphology of red cells (morphological classification) and (2) based on the etiology/cause of anemia.

Morphological and Etiological Classification (Table 8.2)

Q. Write short essay/answer on etiology of anemia.

TABLE 8.2: Morphological classification.

Normocytic normochromic	Microcytic hypochromic	Macrocytic

Etiological classification	
Blood loss	
Acute	**Chronic**
Loss of large volume over short period **Trauma,** postpartum bleeding	Small volume over long period Peptic ulcer, hemorrhoids, carcinoma of colon, hookworms, excessive menstrual loss
Impaired red cell production	
Disturbed Proliferation and Maturation	**Marrow Replacement**
Defective DNA synthesis ➢ Megaloblastic anemias—deficiency or impaired utilization of vitamin B_{12} and folic acid ➢ Anemia of renal failure—deficiency of erythropoietin ➢ Anemia of chronic disease—iron sequestration and relative erythropoietin deficiency ➢ Anemias of endocrine disorders ***Defective hemoglobin synthesis*** ➢ Defective heme synthesis: Iron deficiency, sideroblastic anemia ➢ Defective globin synthesis: Thalassemia	***Primary hematopoietic neoplasms:*** Acute leukemia Myelodysplastic syndromes **Marrow infiltration (myelophthisic anemia)** ***Metastatic neoplasms*** **Disturbed Proliferation and Differentiation of Stem Cells** Aplastic anemia Pure red cell aplasia
Increased red cell destruction (hemolytic anemias)	
Intrinsic (Intracorpuscular)	**Extrinsic (Extracorpuscular)**
Hereditary ➢ Abnormal Membrane: Spherocytosis, elliptocytosis ➢ Enzyme deficiencies: Glucose-6-phosphate dehydrogenase, pyruvate kinase ➢ Disorders of hemoglobin synthesis – Deficient globin synthesis: Thalassemia – Hemoglobinopathies: Sickle cell anemia ***Acquired*** Membrane defects: Paroxysmal nocturnal hemoglobinuria	***Antibody-mediated*** ➢ Iso-hemagglutinins: Transfusion reactions, Rh disease of the newborn ➢ Autoantibodies: Idiopathic, primary, drug-associated, systemic lupus erythematosus ***Mechanical trauma to RBCs:*** ➢ Microangiopathic hemolytic anemia: Disseminated intravascular coagulation ***Infections:*** Malaria

Clinical Features

Q. Discuss the clinical features of anemia. How to approach a case of anemia?

Symptoms

They depend on (1) speed of onset of anemia, (2) severity of anemia, (3) age of the patient, and (4) underlying illness. General clinical features are due to either tissue hypoxia or compensatory mechanisms.

- **Due to tissue hypoxia:**
  - Nonspecific symptoms: Weakness, malaise, lassitude, and easy fatigability
  - Dyspnea on mild exertion, angina, intermittent claudication, transient cerebral ischemia
  - Central nervous system (CNS): Headache, vertigo, tinnitus, dizziness, syncope, irritability, sleep disturbances, and lack of concentration
  - Gastrointestinal tract (GIT): Anorexia, indigestion, nausea, bowel disturbances
  - Female genital tract: Amenorrhea, polymenorrhea.
- **Due to compensatory mechanisms:**
  - Cardiac features: Dyspnea on mild exertion, palpitation, tachycardia, and congestive cardiac failure.

Signs

- Pallor **(Figs. 8.5A and B)** is observed on skin, palms, mucous membranes (oral, vaginal, rectal), nail beds, and palpebral conjunctiva.

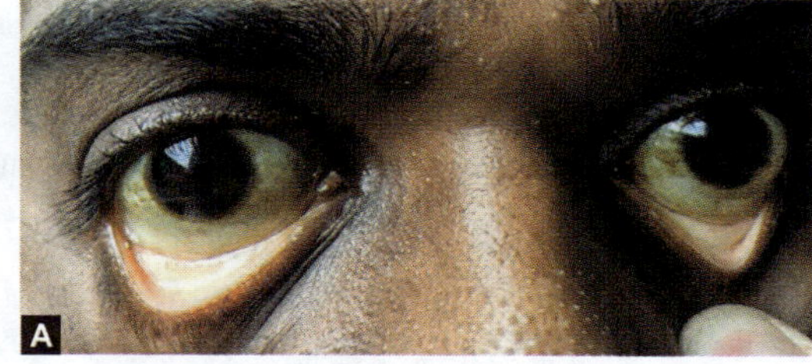

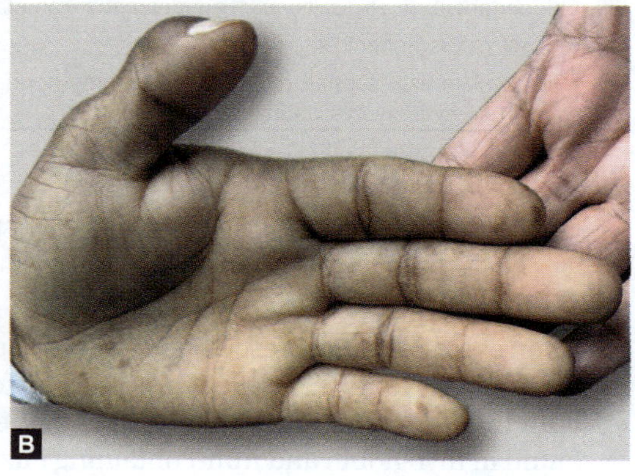

FIGS. 8.5A AND B: (A) Pallor of palpebral conjunctiva; (B) Pale palms with pale creases.

- Pulse: Tachycardia, wide pulse pressure
- Cardiovascular system (CVS): Cervical venous hum, hyperdynamic precordium, ejection systolic murmur (best heard over the pulmonary area), cardiac dilatation and later, signs of cardiac failure
- Ankle edema.

Signs suggesting etiology of anemia (Table 8.3)

TABLE 8.3: Various signs of anemia suggesting the probable etiology.

Sign	*Probable etiology*
Angular cheilitis, blue sclera, koilonychia	Iron deficiency anemia
Glossitis	Iron, vitamin B_{12}, and folate deficiency anemia
Neurological changes (neuropathy, dementia, ataxia), knuckle pigmentation	Vitamin B_{12} deficiency
Jaundice	Hemolytic anemia, megaloblastic anemia
Splenomegaly	Malaria, chronic hemolytic anemia, acute infection, leukemia, lymphoma, portal hypertension, megaloblastic anemia, iron deficiency anemia (rare)
Frontal bossing, dental malocclusion, skin ulcers	Chronic hemolytic anemia (e.g., beta-thalassemia, sickle cell anemia)
Leg ulcers	Sickle cell disease

History in diagnosis of anemias (Table 8.4)

TABLE 8.4: History suggesting the possible etiology of anemia.

Signs and symptoms	*Possible etiology of anemia*
Known normal complete blood cell count in the past	Probably not a hereditary/congenital disorder
Anemia known since childhood	Inherited/congenital hemolytic anemia
Splenectomy, gallstones, and/or jaundice	Chronic hemolytic anemia, liver disease
Family history of splenectomy, gallstones, and/or jaundice	Hereditary hemolytic anemia (RBC enzyme or membrane disorder, thalassemia, or hemoglobinopathy)
Poor or unconventional diet, malnutrition, or severe alcoholism	Bone marrow hypoplasia, folate deficiency
Paresthesias, foot numbness, loss of balance, altered mental status	Cobalamin (vitamin B_{12}) deficiency
Gastrectomy, surgical removal of the ileum, chronic malabsorption disorder	Cobalamin (vitamin B_{12}) deficiency
Chronic gastritis, peptic ulcer disease, chronic use of ASA or NSAIDs, recurrent epistaxis or rectal bleeding, melena, menorrhagia, metrorrhagia, multiple pregnancies, duodenal surgery, gastrectomy	Iron deficiency
Chronic rheumatologic, immunologic, infectious, or neoplastic disease	Anemia of inflammation, autoimmune hemolytic anemia
Decreased urine output	Anemia secondary to renal insufficiency
Dark urine	Hemolytic anemia (intravascular hemolysis)
Recent onset of infections, mucosal and skin bleeding, easy bruising, oral ulcerations	Bone marrow aplasia/hypoplasia, acute leukemia, myelodysplasia, myelophthisis
Occupational/environmental toxin exposure (benzene, ionizing radiation, lead)	Bone marrow aplasia/hypoplasia, acute leukemia, myelodysplasia, lead poisoning
Drug/medication exposure:	
➤ Penicillin, cephalosporin, procainamide, quinidine, quinine, sulfonamide	Drug-induced immune hemolytic anemia
➤ Fava beans, dapsone, naphthalene	Oxidant-induced hemolysis (G6PD deficient)
➤ Cancer chemotherapeutic drugs (recent use)	Bone marrow aplasia/hypoplasia, oxidant damage, fluid retention/dilutional anemia, megaloblastic anemia
➤ Cancer chemotherapeutic drugs (past use)	Bone marrow hypoplasia, myelodysplasia, acute myeloid leukemia
➤ Chloramphenicol, gold salts, sulfonamides, anti-inflammatory drugs	Bone marrow aplasia/hypoplasia
➤ Ethanol, chloramphenicol	Acute reversible bone marrow toxicity
➤ Methotrexate, azathioprine, pyrimethamine, trimethoprim, zidovudine, sulfa drugs, hydroxyurea, antimetabolites	Bone marrow aplasia/hypoplasia, megaloblastic anemia

IRON METABOLISM (FIG. 8.6)

Iron is required for synthesis of normal heme of hemoglobin. Its deficiency leads to decreased erythropoiesis and anemia.

Distribution of Iron

Iron is an essential metal present in the human body. The total body iron content (3–4 g) is divided into functional and storage compartments **(Table 8.5)**. Iron in the body is extensively recycled between the functional and storage pools.

- **Functional:** Approximately 80% (2.5 g) of the functional iron is present in hemoglobin. The remaining functional iron is found in myoglobin and iron-containing enzymes (catalase, cytochromes, and peroxidases).
- **Storage:** The storage pool contains 15–20% (0.5–1.5 g) of total body iron. Free iron is highly toxic because it can result in tissue damage due to its capacity to form free radicals. Therefore, iron is bound to protein and stored in the body in two

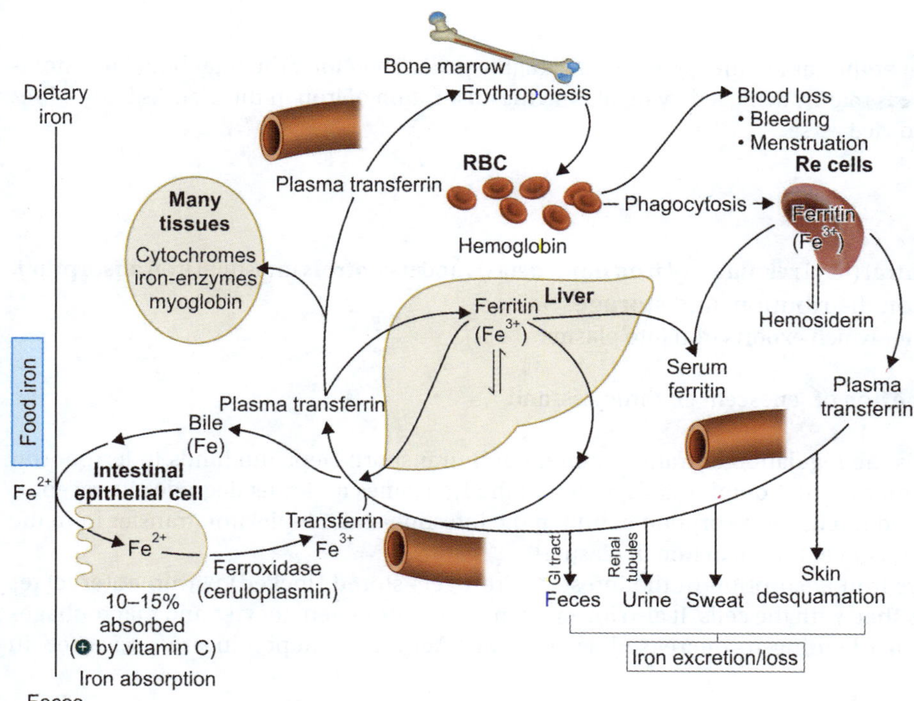

FIG. 8.6: Iron metabolism.

TABLE 8.5: Iron distribution in healthy young adults.

Pool	Grams	%
Functional		
Hemoglobin	2.5	68
Myoglobin	0.15	4
Transferrin (iron-binding blood plasma glycoprotein)	0.003	0.1
Iron-containing enzymes	0.02	0.6
Storage		
Ferritin and hemosiderin in tissue	1.0	27
Ferritin, serum	0.0001	0.004

forms, namely "**ferritin**" and "**hemosiderin**". The storage iron can be readily mobilized whenever there is increase in the requirements of iron, as may occur after blood loss. Two-third of the iron is stored as ferritin and one-third as hemosiderin.

- **Ferritin** (Fe^{3+}) is a protein–iron complex (apoferritin + iron) found in all tissues but particularly in liver, spleen, bone marrow, and skeletal muscles. Very small amounts of ferritin circulate in the serum, the value normally being 15–300 µg/L. **Serum ferritin levels reflect the iron stores** and are a sensitive indicator of the amount of iron in the body. Serum ferritin level is usually below 12 µg/L in iron deficiency and it is very high (as high as 5,000 µg/L may be observed) in conditions associated with iron overload. Ferritin is water-soluble and not visible by light microscopy.
- **Hemosiderin** is an aggregate of iron and protein which is found in the reticuloendothelial cells of bone marrow, spleen, and liver. It is formed when iron is in excess (amorphous iron deposition).

Daily requirements: The recommended dietary allowance 10–15 mg. The daily requirement in **adult males is 5–10 mg/day and in females 20 mg/day.**

Dietary sources: The diet contains iron either in the form of heme contained in animal products and/or nonheme iron in vegetables. Of 10–50 mg in the diet, only 10–15% is normally absorbed.

Iron Absorption

Site of absorption: Iron is absorbed from the **duodenum** and **proximal jejunum**. Iron balance is maintained mainly by regulating the dietary absorption of iron (by the synthesis of apoferritin within mucosal cells).

Transport of Iron

- **Transferrin:** Iron is transported in plasma by the iron transport protein **transferrin**, which is synthesized in the liver. The major function of plasma transferrin is to deliver iron to erythroid precursors for the synthesis of hemoglobin. In normal individuals, transferrin is about 33% saturated with iron, with an average serum iron level of 120 µg/dL in men and 100 µg/dL in women. Thus, the total iron-binding capacity of serum is in the range of 310–340 µg/dL. Unsaturated transferrin protects against infections (iron overload and infection).
- **Lactoferrin:** It binds iron in milk. It has antimicrobial effect (protects newborns from gastrointestinal infections).
- **Haptoglobin:** It binds hemoglobin in the plasma.

Iron Excretion/Loss

Iron metabolism is unique as it is very efficiently utilized and reutilized by the body. There is no physiological regulated mechanism for iron excretion and 1–2 mg/day is lost by shedding of epithelial cells of GI tract, skin epithelial cells (by sweat), and renal tubules and by menstruation, pregnancy, multiple births, lactation, and bleeding.

Regulation of Iron Balance

Iron is essential for cellular metabolism; at the same time, excess of it is highly toxic. Therefore, the total body iron stores must be properly regulated. Iron balance is mainly achieved by regulating the absorption of iron in the diet. As body stores decrease, the absorption of iron rises and vice versa.

Hepcidin

Q. Write short note on role of hepcidin.

It is synthesized in the liver and is the **central** (key) **regulator of iron homeostasis** and it **controls** intestinal iron **absorption,** plasma iron concentrations, tissue iron distribution, and **storage**.

- Ferroportin is the cellular iron exporter which exports iron into plasma
  - from absorptive enterocytes,
  - from macrophages that recycle the iron of senescent erythrocytes, and
  - from hepatocytes that store iron.
- The major mechanism of hepcidin is the regulation of transmembrane iron transport. Hepcidin binds to ferroportin and forms hepcidin–ferroportin complex. This complex is degraded in the lysosomes and thus degrades its receptor ferroportin. By this mechanism, hepcidin reduces resorption of iron in the intestine and inhibits iron transfer from the enterocyte to plasma (thereby reduces concentration of iron in plasma).
- When hepcidin levels rise, it lowers iron absorption in the intestine, iron gets stored (locked) within enterocytes forming mucosal ferritin, and iron is shed with the cells. It also lowers iron release from hepatocytes and macrophages (through degradation of ferroportin) leading to decreased serum iron. Actions of hepcidin are presented in **Figure 8.7**.

Significance of hepcidin

- Increased hepcidin concentration is seen in inflammation (chronic disease anemia)
- Reduced hepcidin production → hereditary hemochromatosis.

Functions of Iron

1. **Heme iron:** Hemoglobin, myoglobin, cytochrome c oxidase, catalase
2. **Nonheme iron:** Fe-S complexes (xanthine oxidase), DNA synthesis (ribonucleotide reductase).

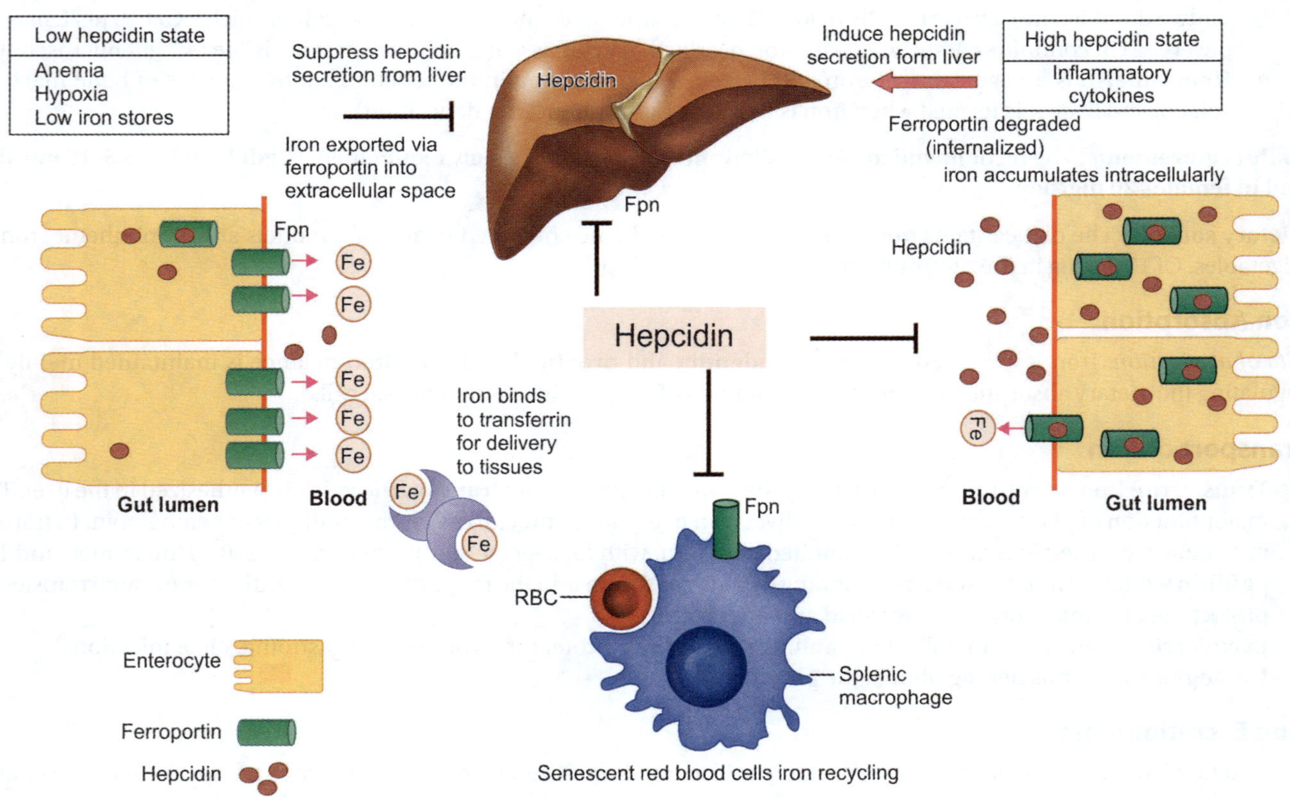

FIG. 8.7: Actions of hepcidin.

IRON DEFICIENCY ANEMIA (IDA)

Q. Discuss the etiology, clinical features, investigations, and management of iron deficiency anemia.

Etiology (Table 8.6)

TABLE 8.6: Causes of iron deficiency anemia.

Decreased iron intake	Increased demand/requirement for iron
➢ Milk-fed infants ➢ Elderly with improper diet, poor dentition ➢ Low socioeconomical sections ➢ Vegetarians (poorly absorbable inorganic iron)	➢ Rapid growth in infancy or adolescents ➢ Pregnancy and lactation
Decreased absorption of iron	**Increased iron loss**
➢ Total/partial gastrectomy ➢ Intestinal absorption is impaired in sprue, other causes of intestinal steatorrhea, and chronic diarrhea ➢ Specific items in the diet, such as phytates of cereals, tannates, carbonates, oxalates, phosphates, and drugs, can impair iron absorption	➢ Chronic blood loss due to bleeding from the: ➢ Gastrointestinal tract (peptic ulcers, gastric or colonic carcinoma, hemorrhoids, hookworm infestation, schistosomiasis, or NSAID) ➢ Urinary tract (renal or bladder tumors) ➢ Genital tract (menorrhagia, uterine cancer)
Iron refractory iron deficiency anemia (IRIDA) is a rare inherited disorder caused by loss-of-function mutations of the *TMPRSS6/matriptase 2* gene.	

- IDA is due to deficiency of iron causing defective **heme synthesis**. Iron deficiency anemia is the most common cause of anemia.
- Daily requirement of iron is 10–15 mg. Children consuming large amounts of cow milk develop IDA because iron from cow milk is poorly absorbed and calcium in the milk inhibits iron absorption.

Stages of Iron Deficiency

- **Stage 1: Negative iron balance** is characterized by decreased bone marrow iron stores.
- **Stage 2: Iron-deficient erythropoiesis**—erythropoiesis is impaired when serum iron falls to <50 mcg/dL (<9 µmol/L) and transferrin saturation to <16%.
- **Stage 3: Iron deficiency anemia**—microcytosis and then hypochromia develop. Eventually iron deficiency affects tissues, resulting in symptoms and signs.

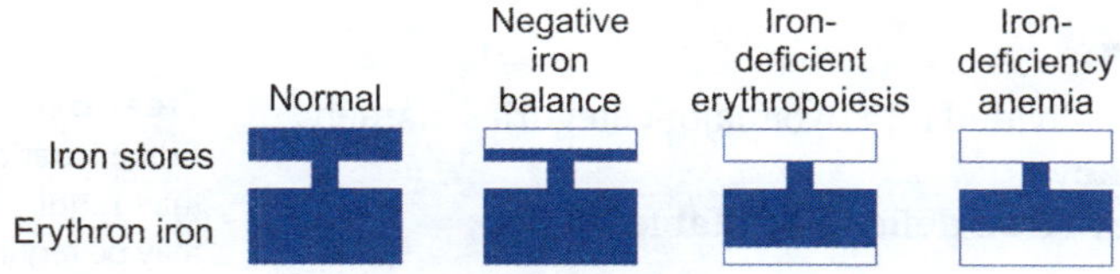

	Normal	Negative iron balance	Iron-deficient erythropoiesis	Iron-deficiency anemia
Iron stores				
Erythron iron				
Marrow iron stores	1–3+	0–1+	0	0
Serum ferritin (µg/L)	50–200	<20	<15	<15
TIBC (µg/dL)	300–360	>360	>360	>400
SI (µg/dL)	50–150	NL	<50	<30
Saturation (%)	30–50	NL	<20	<10
Marrow sideroblasts (%)	40–60	NL	<10	<10
RBC protoporphyrin (µg/dL)	30–50	NL	>100	>200
RBC morphology	NL	NL	NL	Microcytic/ hypochromic

Q. Discuss the clinical manifestations and complications of iron deficiency anemia.

Q. Write short note on Plummer-Vinson syndrome.

Clinical Features

- Clinical features of iron deficiency anemia include the usual symptoms and signs of anemia
- Characteristic signs of advanced iron deficiency include:
  - Cheilosis (fissures at the corners of the mouth)/angular stomatitis
  - **Atrophic glossitis (Fig. 8.8)**
  - Brittle fingernails, platonychia, and ***koilonychia*** (spooning of the fingernails) **(Figs. 8.9A and B)**, brittle hair

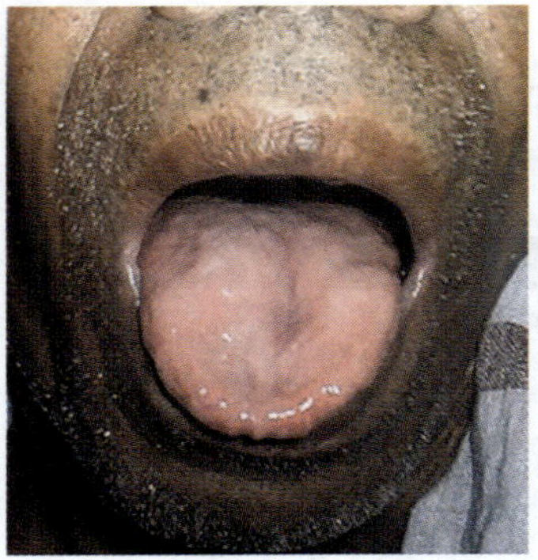

FIG. 8.8: Atrophic glossitis producing bald tongue in iron deficiency anemia. There is also mild cheilosis.

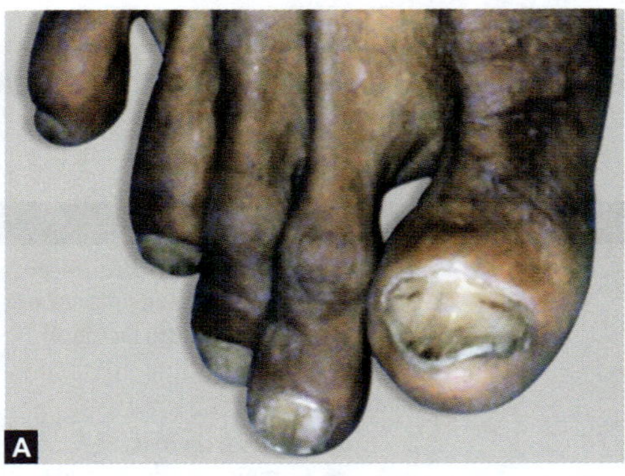

FIGS. 8.9A AND B: Koilonychia (Spooning of the fingernails) in iron deficiency anemia.

- **Blue-tinged sclerae,** alopecia
- **Pica** is the unusual craving for substances which have a "crunching" sound with no nutritional value like clay or chalk. Craving for ice (pagophagia) specific to iron deficiency or less commonly for clay (geophagia) or starch (amylophagia); pagophagia is believed to be the most specific to iron deficiency.

- **Restless leg syndrome** is seen in around 25% of patients with IDA.
- **Beeturia** is a phenomenon in which the urine turns red following ingestion of beets. Beeturia is increased in individuals with iron deficiency (49–80% of individuals with iron deficiency).

- **Plummer-Vinson syndrome or Patterson-Brown-Kelly** or **sideropenic dysphagia** develops in long-standing iron deficiency.
  - Iron deficiency (microcytic hypochromic) anemia
  - Atrophic glossitis
  - Esophageal/post-cricoid webs resulting in dysphagia for solids than liquids. The web can be demonstrated either by endoscopy or by barium swallow.
  - These patients have increased risk of squamous cell carcinoma of pharynx and esophagus.

Diagnosis of Iron Deficiency Anemia

Q. Discuss the investigations/diagnosis of iron deficiency anemia.

Laboratory Investigations

These investigations may be divided into two major categories, namely:

1. **To confirm iron deficiency.**
2. **To determine the cause of iron deficiency (Table 8.7).**

Treatment of Plummer-Vinson syndrome: Administration of iron. Severe obstruction by the web may require dilatation. Regular upper GI endoscopy may be required for the early detection of cancers.

To confirm iron deficiency	*To determine the cause of iron deficiency*
Hemoglobin and hematocrit (PCV): Decreased	Stool: Examine for occult blood and hookworm infestation.
Red cell indices: **MCV**: <80 fL; **MCH:** <25 pg; **MCHC:** <27 g/dL. **RDW: Increased,** >15%. Earliest sign of iron deficiency	
Peripheral smear: Microcytic hypochromic RBCs. Severe anemia—ring/pessary, pencil/cigar-shaped cells with moderate anisocytosis and poikilocytosis **(Fig. 8.10)**	Endoscopy: This includes upper gastrointestinal endoscopy, sigmoidoscopy, and colonoscopy.
Reticulocyte count: Low for degree of anemia	
Bone marrow: Moderate erythroid hyperplasia and micronormoblastic maturation	Urine: Examine for bleeding and for parasites such as schistosomiasis.
Absence of bone marrow iron: "Gold standard" test, demonstrated by negative Prussian blue reaction	
Hepcidin: Decreased. Hepcidin regulates iron concentrations and tissue iron distribution.	Investigations for malabsorption
A response to a therapeutic trial of iron administration may be helpful in confirming the diagnosis of iron deficiency anemia.	

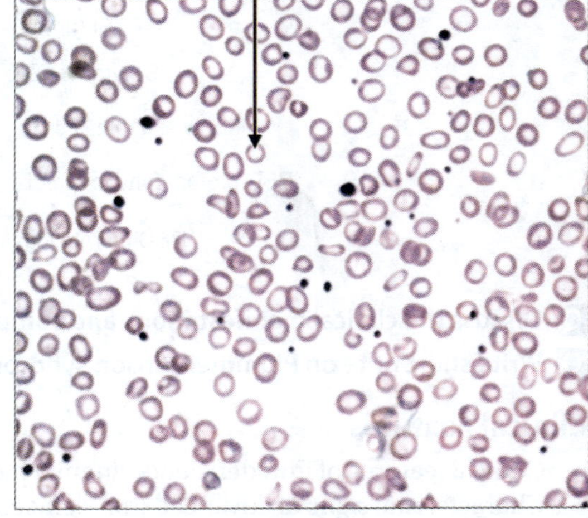

FIG. 8.10: Peripheral blood smear showing microcytic hypochromic red blood cells.

Soluble transferrin receptor (sTfR) and sTfR-ferritin index—reflect overall erythropoiesis, which is increased in iron deficiency. sTfR-ferritin index (sTfR ÷ log[ferritin]).

The sTfR reflects erythropoiesis, while the ferritin reflects the tissue iron stores; thus, a high sTfR-ferritin index (above 2–3) is a sign of iron deficiency due to increased erythropoietic drive and low iron stores. In anemia of chronic disease/anemia of inflammation, sTfR-ferritin index <1.

TABLE 8.7: Serum iron profile in IDA.

	Normal range	*Value in IDA*	*Observation*
Serum ferritin	15–300 µg/L	<15 µg/L	↓
Serum iron	50–150 µg/dL	10–15 µg/dL	↓
Serum transferrin saturation	30–40%	<15%	↓
Total iron-binding capacity (TIBC)	310–340 µg/dL	350-450 µg/dL	↑
Serum transferrin receptor (TFR)	0.57–2.8 µg/L	3.5–7.1 µg/L	↑
Red cell protoporphyrin	30–50 µg/dL	>200 µg/dL	↑

Differential Diagnosis

The microcytic hypochromic anemia does not necessarily mean only iron deficiency. The various causes of microcytic hypochromic anemia are listed in **Box 8.1**.

Complications of severe iron deficiency anemia are listed in **Box 8.2**.

Box 8.1: Differential diagnosis of microcytic hypochromic blood picture.

- Iron deficiency
- Thalassemia: It is an inherited defect in globin chain synthesis. It can be differentiated from iron deficiency by serum iron values, normal or increased serum iron levels, and transferrin saturation. The red blood cell distribution width (RDW) index is generally normal or reduced in thalassemia and elevated in iron deficiency.
- Anemia of chronic disease
- Sideroblastic anemia
- Lead poisoning

Box 8.2: Complications of severe iron deficiency anemia.

- During pregnancy: Poor pregnancy outcomes such as premature births and low birth weight babies
- Heart failure
- Delayed growth and development in infants and children
- Increased susceptibility to infections
- Exacerbates cardiorespiratory problems, especially in the elderly

Q. Discuss the management/treatment of iron deficiency anemia.

Q. Write short note on (1) iron therapy and (2) parenteral iron therapy.

Management

Treatment can be divided into:

- Treatment of underlying cause for iron deficiency. The correct management of iron deficiency is to identify and treat the underlying cause for deficiency.

Oral iron therapy

Most patients can be treated with oral iron preparations.

- **Iron preparations and dose:** Oral iron dose is 6 mg/kg/day. Commonly used and best are ferrous sulfate (200 mg three times daily, a total of 180 mg ferrous iron), ferrous gluconate (300 mg twice daily, only 70 mg ferrous iron), ferrous fumarate (325 mg two or three times daily), and others.
- *Alternate-day dosing appears to result in equivalent or better iron absorption than daily dosing, usually with fewer adverse effects.*
- **Side effects:** Few patients may develop metallic taste, nausea, dyspepsia, constipation, black tarry stools, or diarrhea. These can be reduced by taking iron tablets with food or reducing the dose or by using preparation with less iron (e.g., ferrous gluconate) or a controlled-release preparation or a liquid preparation.
- **Duration of oral iron therapy:**
  - Iron should be given to correct the Hb level to normal range and usually occurs within 4–6 weeks. If it does not occur, it may be due to failure of response to therapy.
  - Once the hemoglobin returns to normal, oral iron therapy should be continued to replace the iron stores. This may take 6 months to 1 year.
  - Patients having iron deficiency due to malabsorption, deficient intake, continuing blood loss, etc., may require long-term iron supplements at a minimum dose.
- **Response to oral iron therapy:** The response appears within 7–10 days of treatment with iron in the form of an increased reticulocyte count (usually not exceeding 10%, normal <2.5%).
- **Causes of failure to respond to oral iron therapy:** It may be due to one or more of the following reasons:
  - **Failure to take the iron tables:** Patients taking iron preparations have gray- or black-colored stools.
  - Continuing hemorrhage/blood loss.
  - **Incorrect/wrong diagnosis:** For example, thalassemia trait.

- Ingestion of drugs which reduce iron absorption: Certain drugs if taken along with oral iron (e.g., H_2-receptor blockers, proton-pump inhibitors, antacids, tetracyclines) may interfere with iron absorption.
- Severe malabsorption.

Parenteral iron therapy

Parenteral iron therapy should be given only after the definite diagnosis of iron deficiency; otherwise it may lead to iron overload and its consequences. Iron stores are replaced much faster with parenteral iron than with oral iron, but the hematological response is not quick.

Indications of parenteral iron therapy:

- Intolerant to oral iron preparation.
- Severe malabsorption.
- Primary blood loss is uncontrollable: When rate of iron (blood) loss exceeds the rate of its absorption.
- Chronic GI tract disease (e.g., inflammatory bowel disease) which may worsen with oral iron.

Calculation of total iron dose required.

Iron dose in mg = Body weight (kg) × 2.3 × (normal Hb—patient's hemoglobin, g/dL) + 500 or 1,000 mg (to provide body iron stores).

Route of administration: Parenteral iron can be given by slow intravenous infusion or by intramuscular injection.

Types of parenteral iron preparations: These include iron-sorbitol, iron-dextran (imferon), and preparations with much lower rates of adverse effects such as iron sucrose or sodium ferric gluconate, ferric carboxymaltose, and iron isomaltoside.

Iron-sorbitol

- It is administered only intramuscularly and never by the intravenous route.
- Dose is 1.5 mg of iron/kg body weight daily, to a dose not exceeding 2.5 g.

Iron-dextran (Imferon)

Low-molecular-weight iron dextran is most commonly used. It may be given either intramuscularly or intravenously (more ideal). Test dose is required before administration to prevent anaphylaxis.

- **Intramuscular:** Dose is 100 mg daily till the total required dose is administered or to a maximum of 2 kg. It should be given deep intramuscularly into the buttocks using a "Z-tract technique."
- **Slow intravenous infusion:** Total dose intravenous infusion is rarely required. If a large dose is to be given (>100 mg), it should be diluted in 5% dextrose in water or 0.9% NaCl solution and infused slowly.

Iron-sucrose

- It has lesser adverse effects and is considered to be the safe intravenous iron preparation.
- It is given as a single dose of 100–200 mg as an intravenous injection or up to 500 mg infused over a period of 3 hours.

Sodium ferric gluconate

- It is the preferred form of parenteral iron owing to the low incidence of adverse reactions.
- It is administered intravenously at a dose of 125 mg over 10 minutes.

Ferric carboxymaltose: A novel iron complex that consists of a ferric hydroxide core stabilized by a carbohydrate shell allows for controlled delivery of iron to target tissues. Administered intravenously, it is effective in the treatment of iron-deficiency anemia, delivering a replenishment dose of up to 1,000 mg of iron during a minimum administration time of ≤15 minutes with least reactions.

Ferumoxytol: It is a superparamagnetic iron oxide nanoparticle coated with a low-molecular-weight (LMW) semisynthetic carbohydrate. It can be given in doses of 17 mL (equivalent to 510 mg of elemental iron).

Iron isomaltoside/ferric derisomaltose can be administered in a single infusion, at a dose of 20 mg/kg, over 15 minutes.

Side effects/toxicity of parenteral iron preparations

- Pain and swelling at the site of injection/infusion
- Anaphylactic reactions: Fever, generalized urticarial rash, lymphadenopathy, splenomegaly, and arthralgias
- Hemochromatosis

Red Cell Transfusion

- **Indication:** It is reserved for patients who have symptoms of anemia, cardiovascular instability, continued and excessive loss of blood loss from any site, and require immediate intervention.
- Transfusions correct the anemia acutely as well as transfused red cells provide a source of iron for reutilization.

MACROCYTIC ANEMIA

Q. Describe the metabolism of vitamin B_{12} and the etiology and pathogenesis of B_{12} deficiency.

Vitamin B_{12} and folic acid are closely related, and both are essential for normal DNA synthesis and nuclear maturation.

Vitamin B_{12} Metabolism

- Vitamin B_{12} is present only in animal proteins and dairy products and not present in vegetables. Therefore, strict vegetarians do not get an adequate quantity of vitamin B_{12}.

- A balanced diet (not rigid vegetarian!) contains significantly large amounts of vitamin B_{12} which accumulates in the body (liver) and is enough for several (about 3) years. Hence, if there is any dietary deficiency or malabsorption of vitamin B_{12}, its clinical manifestations appear only after about 2-4 years.
- Normal daily requirement is about **2–3 µg**.

Absorption, Transport, and Storage (Fig. 8.11)

- Vitamin B_{12} in food is usually in coenzyme form (as deoxyadenosylcobalamin and methylcobalamin) and bound to binding proteins in the diet.
- In the stomach, peptic digestion at low pH is required for release of vitamin B_{12} from binding protein in the food. The released vitamin B_{12} binds with salivary protein called **haptocorrin**, which is secreted in salivary juice.
- These haptocorrin-B_{12} complexes leave stomach along with unbound special protein called **intrinsic factor** (IF), which is produced by gastric (fundus and cardia) parietal (oxyntic) cells.
- As haptocorrin-B_{12} complexes pass into the second part of the duodenum, pancreatic proteases release vitamin B_{12} from haptocorrin. Vitamin B_{12} then associates with the intrinsic factor and forms IF-B_{12} complex.
- This stable IF-vitamin B_{12} complex is transported to the ileum, where it is endocytosed by ileal enterocytes. These ileal enterocytes express a receptor on their surfaces for the intrinsic factor. These receptors are called **cubilin**.
- In the ileal epithelium, vitamin B_{12} combines with a major carrier protein, **transcobalamin II**, and is actively transported into the mucosal cells and then into the blood.
- Transcobalamin II-vitamin B_{12} complex delivers vitamin B_{12} to the liver and other cells of the body, particularly rapidly proliferating cells in the bone marrow and mucosal lining of the gastrointestinal tract.

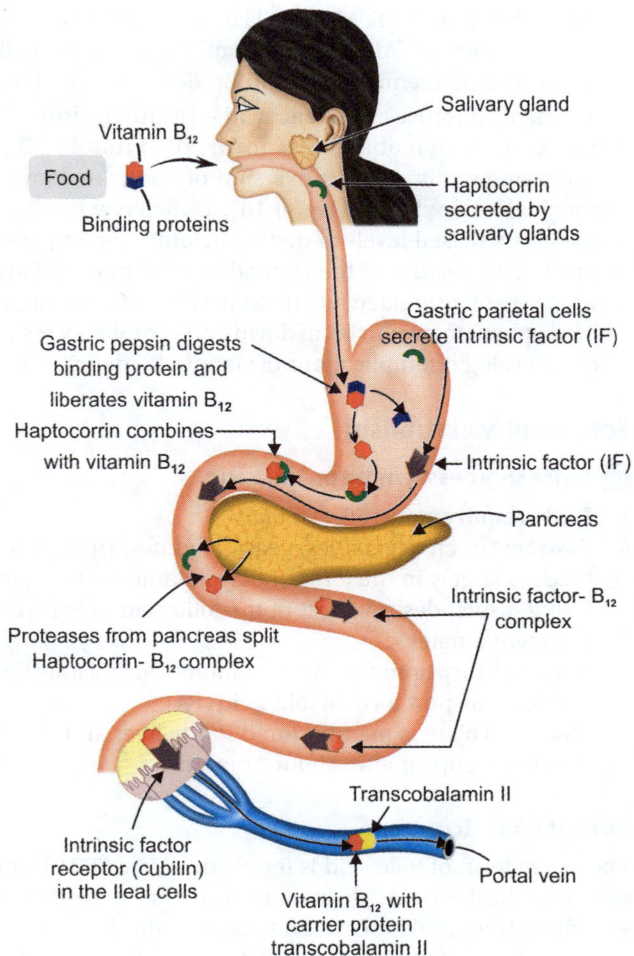

FIG. 8.11: Mechanism of vitamin B12 absorption.

Role of Vitamin B_{12}

Vitamin B_{12} is essential for:

- Normal hemopoiesis
- Maintenance of normal integrity of the nervous system

Vitamin B_{12} is indirectly required for DNA synthesis in various metabolic steps and its deficiency impairs DNA synthesis. There are two biologically active forms of cobalamin in the body; both act as coenzymes, namely: (1) methylcobalamin and (2) adenosylcobalamin.

1. Methylcobalamin is the main form of vitamin B_{12} in plasma and is an essential coenzyme for conversion of homocysteine to methionine and formation of tetrahydrofolate (THF) from methyl THF **(Fig. 8.12)**. During the former reaction, vitamin B_{12} loses its methyl group and this is replaced from methyl THF, the principal form of folic acid in plasma. Tetrahydrofolate is essential for the generation of a precursor of DNA known as deoxythymidine monophosphate (D TMP).

   In vitamin B_{12} deficiency, the main cause of impaired DNA synthesis is that methyl THF is not

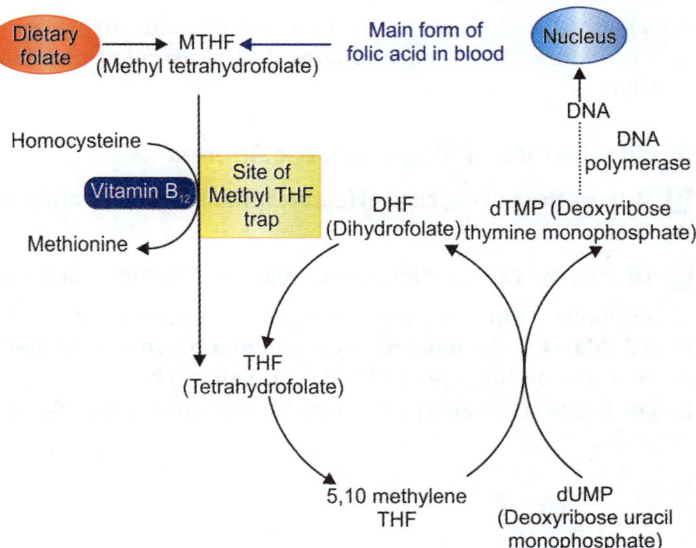

FIG. 8.12: Inter-relation and role of vitamin B12 and folate in DNA synthesis.

converted into THF. Methyl THF accumulates in the cell and is known as "**Methyl THF trap**". Lack of folic acid is the next cause of anemia in vitamin B_{12} deficiency, as the anemia invariably improves with folic acid administration.

2. Deoxyadenosylcobalamin form of vitamin B_{12} is a coenzyme required for conversion of methylmalonyl CoA to succinylmalonyl CoA **(Fig. 8.13)**. Deficiency of vitamin B_{12} causes increased levels of methylmalonic acid in plasma and urine. This results in the formation of abnormal fatty acids which get incorporated into neuronal lipids. Consequently, this predisposes to myelin breakdown and is probably responsible for neurologic complications of vitamin B_{12} deficiency.

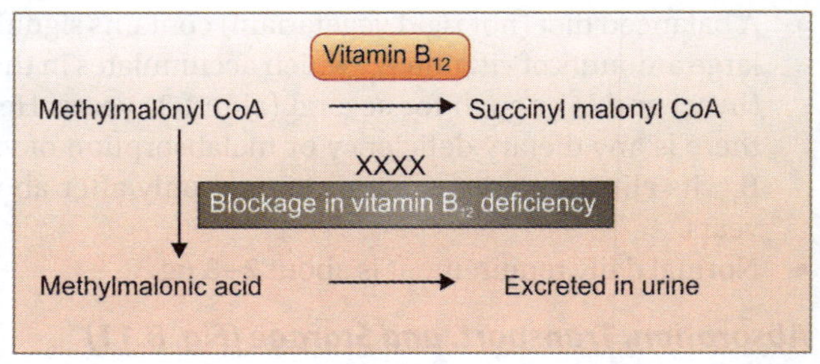

FIG. 8.13: Role of vitamin B_{12} in methylmalonyl CoA metabolism.

Folic Acid Metabolism

Q. Write short essay/note on folic acid.

- **Daily requirement:** 50–200 mg
- **Source:** Green vegetables, yeast, legumes, fruits, and animal proteins are the richest sources. The folic acid in these foods is largely in the form of polyglutamates. Polyglutamates are sensitive to heat (thermolabile), boiling, steaming or frying, which destroy most of the folic acid (destroyed by cooking). Intestinal conjugates split the polyglutamates into monoglutamates.
- **Site of absorption:** Proximal jejunum. During intestinal absorption, they are modified to 5-methyltetrahydrofolate, the normal transport form of folic acid (FA).
- **Storage:** Folate is mainly stored in the liver and is enough for about 3 months and hence the manifestations of folate deficiency appear after about 3 months.

Role of Folic Acid

The active form of folic acid is tetrahydrofolate (THF) which is the biologic "middleman" involved in metabolic processes which synthesize DNA. The various reactions in which folic acid plays a main role are:

- Purine (required for DNA and RNA) synthesis
- Conversion of homocysteine to methionine, a reaction also requiring vitamin B_{12}
- Deoxythymidylate monophosphate synthesis: 5,10-methylene THF polyglutamate is required for conversion of deoxyuridine monophosphate (dUMP) to deoxythymidine monophosphate (dTMP) and DNA, a rate-limiting step in pyrimidine synthesis.

Folic acid is associated with metabolism of histidine: Histidine is metabolized to formiminoglutamic acid (FIGLU) which combines with THF to form glutamic acid **(Fig. 8.14)**. In FA deficiency, this reaction cannot take place and therefore FIGLU accumulates and is excreted as such in urine. This is used as a test to measure folic acid deficiency.

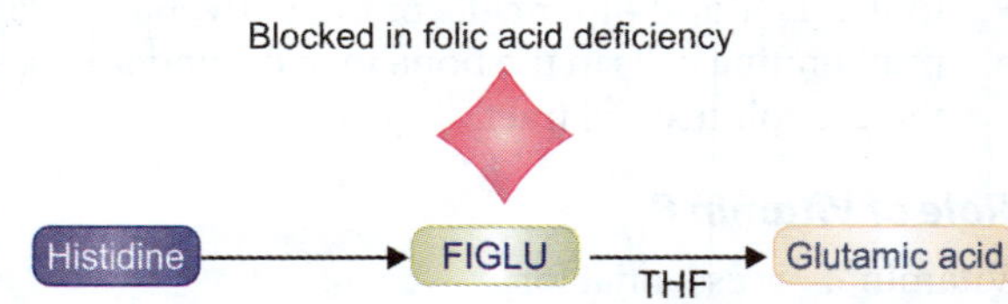

FIG. 8.14: Role of folic acid in metabolism of histidine.

Manifestations of Megaloblastic Anemia

Q. Discuss the causes, clinical features/manifestations, and management of vitamin B_{12} deficiency/megaloblastic anemia.

Q. Discuss the causes, clinical features/manifestations, and management of folate deficiency.

Megaloblastic anemias are a group of disorders characterized by **defective**/impaired **DNA synthesis** and **distinct megaloblasts in the bone marrow** and **macrocytes in the peripheral blood**. Megaloblastic anemias are common among anemias due to impaired red cell production. They are usually caused **due to deficiency of either cobalamin (vitamin B_{12}) or folate (folic acid)** but may occur because of genetic or acquired abnormalities that affect the metabolism of these vitamins.

Etiology of Megaloblastic Anemia (Table 8.8)

TABLE 8.8: Etiology of megaloblastic anemia.

Vitamin B_{12} deficiency	*Folic acid deficiency*
Decreased Intake: Inadequate diet, "pure vegetarians"	**Decreased Intake:** Inadequate diet—alcoholism, malnutrition
Increased Demand: Pregnancy, hyperthyroidism, disseminated cancer	**Increased Loss:** Hemodialysis
Impaired Absorption ➢ Gastric: Deficiency of gastric acid or pepsin or intrinsic factor – Pernicious anemia – Post gastrectomy – Drugs: Prolonged use of H2-receptor blockers and proton-pump inhibitors ➢ Intestinal – Loss of absorptive surface ◆ Malabsorption syndromes ◆ Diffuse intestinal disease—lymphoma, systemic sclerosis ◆ Ileal resection, Crohn disease – Competition for vitamin B_{12}—bacterial overgrowth in blind loops and diverticula of bowel, ***Diphyllobothrium latum***	**Impaired Absorption** ➢ Malabsorption states: Nontropical and Tropical sprue, celiac disease ➢ Diffuse infiltrative diseases of the small intestine (e.g., lymphoma) ➢ Drugs: Anticonvulsant phenytoin, oral contraceptives, metformin, cholestyramine **Increased Demand**: Pregnancy, lactation, infancy, disseminated cancer, markedly increased hematopoiesis (hemolytic anemias), chronic exfoliative skin disease, chronic inflammatory and infective diseases
Abnormal cobalamin transport: Transcobalamin II deficiency	**Impaired Utilization**: Folic acid antagonists (antifolate drugs), such as methotrexate, trimethoprim, pyrimethamine, pentamidine, 5-fluorouracil, hydroxyurea
OTHERS—Antifolate drugs: e.g., methotrexate; Independent of either cobalamin or folate deficiency	

Pathogenesis (Mechanism) of Megaloblastic Anemia

- Megaloblastic anemias are commonly due to deficiency of **vitamin B_{12} (cobalamin) or folic acid**, which are coenzymes required for the synthesis of one of the four bases found in DNA, namely thymidine.
- Deficiency of cobalamin or folate results in failure of DNA synthesis and delayed/arrested nuclear maturation. Synthesis of RNA and protein is normal resulting in normal cytoplasmic maturation. Thus, the **nuclear maturation lags behind the cytoplasmic maturation** producing nucleocytoplasmic asynchrony. This results in abnormal cell proliferation that affects rapidly dividing cells in the bone marrow (erythroid, myeloid, and megakaryocyte series).
- Impaired DNA synthesis causes delay in cell division and increases time between divisions and size of the cells become large and are called as "megaloblasts." The **megaloblasts** have an open, stippled, and lacy chromatin. The megaloblastic changes are most prominent in the early nucleated red cell precursors.
- Erythroid precursor cells show a reduced number of mitoses, and synthesis of hemoglobin is unimpaired. The mature RBCs derived from these megaloblasts are large (**macrocytes**) and **oval** but well hemoglobinized.
- In the bone marrow, a large number of megaloblastic precursors do not mature enough to be released into the blood and are destroyed in the bone marrow (ineffective erythropoiesis). There is also mild hemolysis of red cells in the peripheral blood. This releases large amounts of **lactate dehydrogenase (LDH)** resulting in **raised** levels in the blood.
- In the bone marrow, abnormal proliferation affects myeloid series producing giant metamyelocytes and the megakaryocyte series resulting in dysplastic megakaryocytes.
- All rapidly dividing cells of the body (including skin, GI tract, bone marrow) exhibit megaloblastic changes, and anemia is only a manifestation of a more generalized defect in DNA synthesis.

Pathogenesis of Neurological Changes in Vitamin B_{12} Deficiency

Two mechanisms are responsible for neurologic changes seen of vitamin B_{12} deficiency. Deficiency of vitamin B_{12} causes:

- **Impairment in the conversion of homocysteine to methionine:** Methionine is required for the production of choline and choline-containing phospholipids. These are needed by the neuronal cells.
- **Lack of adenosylcobalamin:** It is a vitamin B_{12}-containing cofactor required for the conversion of methylmalonyl CoA to succinyl CoA. Lack of this cofactor results in increased levels of methylmalonyl CoA and its precursor, propionyl CoA. This causes production of nonphysiologic fatty acids and incorporated into neuronal lipids.

PERNICIOUS ANEMIA

Q. Discuss the etiology of Addisonian pernicious anemia.

Pernicious anemia (PA) is a chronic autoimmune disorder characterized by atrophic gastritis with loss of parietal cells in the gastric mucosa which causes failure of production of intrinsic factor. Absence of intrinsic factor results in failure of absorption of dietary vitamin B_{12} and deficiency which eventually produces megaloblastic macrocytic anemia.

- **Age and gender:** PA is a disease of older age and generally presents in the fifth to eighth decades of life. Females are more involved than males (F:M is 1.5:1).

Etiology

Pernicious anemia is an autoimmune disease causing destruction and permanent atrophy of gastric mucous membrane. The evidences for autoimmune etiology are as follows:

- It is associated with other autoimmune diseases such as Graves' disease, Hashimoto's thyroiditis, vitiligo, and Addison's disease.
- Microscopically, stomach shows **chronic atrophic gastritis** with damage to gastric parietal cells.
- Response to steroids is seen.
- There is presence of autoantibodies in most of the patients. **Two major types** of autoantibodies are found:
    1. **Anti-intrinsic factor (IF) antibody:**
        - Type I (blocking) antibody: This blocks the binding of vitamin B_{12} to IF and is present in 50–75% of the cases and can be detected in both plasma and gastric juice.
        - Type II (binding) antibody: It attaches to the IF–vitamin B_{12} complex and prevents their binding to receptors in the ileal mucosa. They are present in about 40% of patients.
    2. **Parietal cell (type III) antibody:** It is directed against α and β subunits of the gastric proton pump (H^+, K^+-ATPase) in parietal cells but is neither specific for PA nor other autoimmune disorders. They are found in 90% of patients with PA as well as in older patients with chronic nonspecific gastritis.

Role of *Helicobacter pylori*: *H. pylori* gastritis may play a role in PA. There is a **higher incidence of gastric carcinoma** in patients with PA. The incidence is higher in patients with blood group A.

Clinical Features of Macrocytic Anemias (Fig. 8.15)

Q. Discuss clinical manifestations of vitamin B_{12} deficiency/folate deficiency/pernicious anemia.

Onset

The onset is insidious in origin and progresses slowly unless halted by therapy.

Clinical features related to vitamin B_{12} deficiency:

- Classic triad: Weakness, sore throat, and paresthesias
- Tongue: Painful **red "beefy"** tongue due to glossitis and atrophy of papillae **(Fig. 8.15)**. The patient complains of loss of taste and appetite.
- Patients may have a lemon-yellow color due to combination of pallor and mild jaundice caused by excess breakdown of hemoglobin.

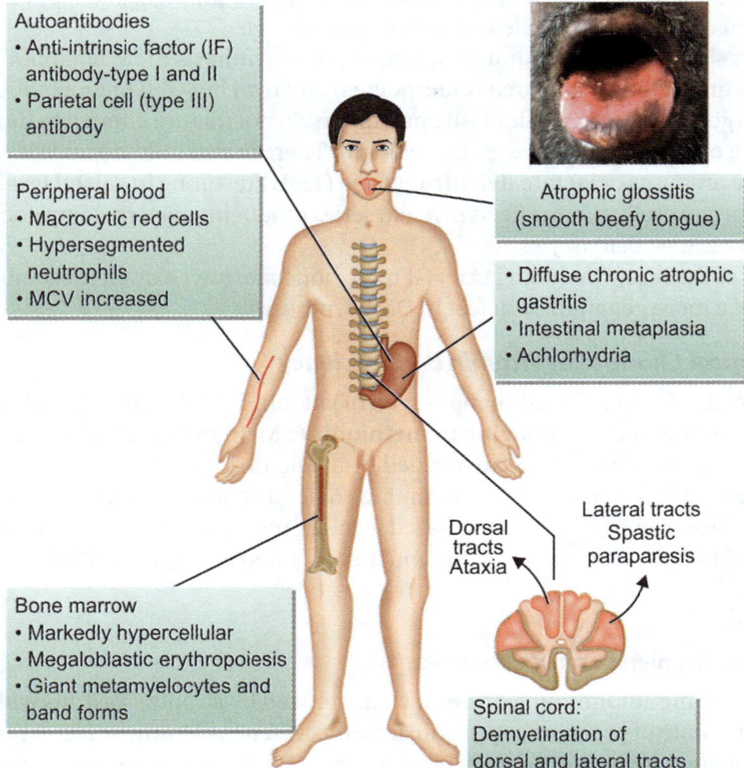

FIG. 8.15: Clinical features and laboratory findings in pernicious anemia.

Pigmentation: Pigmentation of knuckles and creases is common **(Figs. 8.16A and B)**. The generally accepted mechanism of pigmentation is an increase in the melanin synthesis. The other hypotheses proposed are: (1) Deficiency of vitamin B_{12} decreases the level of reduced glutathione, which activates tyrosinase and thus leads to transfer to melanosomes. (2) Defect in the melanin transfer between melanocytes and keratinocytes, resulting in pigmentary incontinence.

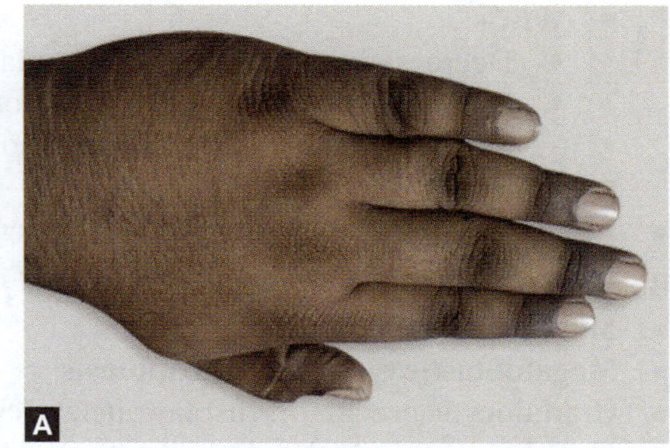

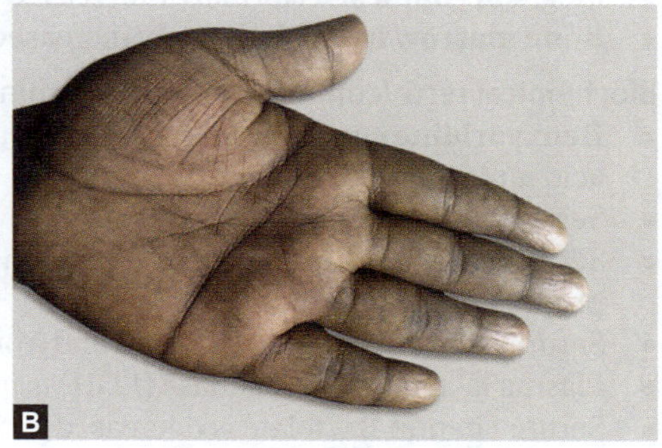

FIGS. 8.16A AND B: (A) Pigmentation of knuckles; (B) Pigmentation of creases.

Neurological Features

Q. Write short essay/note on neurological complications of pernicious anemia/megaloblastic anemia.

- **Peripheral nerves-peripheral neuropathy:** Glove and stocking distribution of numbness or paresthesia. This tingling begins in tips of toes and progresses proximally and is bilateral and symmetric. It is characterized by loss of ankle reflexes.
- **Spinal cord:** Subacute combined degeneration of the cord
  - *Posterior columns:* Impaired/diminished vibration and position sensation
  - *Corticospinal tracts:* Upper motor neuron signs—ataxic, uncoordinated gait. Bilateral extensor plantar with absent ankle jerks
- **Cerebrum:** Depression and loss of memory (dementia), optic atrophy
- A positive Romberg sign and Lhermitte sign may be elicited.
- *Folate deficiency in adults does not give rise to significant neurologic findings.*
- Prematurely gray-haired
- Atherosclerosis: Serum homocysteine level is raised and is a risk factor for **atherosclerosis and thrombosis** (myocardial infarction, stroke).

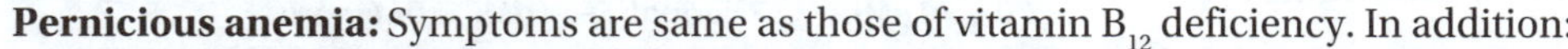

Pernicious anemia: Symptoms are same as those of vitamin B_{12} deficiency. In addition:

- **Hypochlorhydria:** Atrophic gastritis causes decreased secretion of hydrochloric acid and IF. The symptoms include dyspepsia, postprandial fullness, and early satiety.

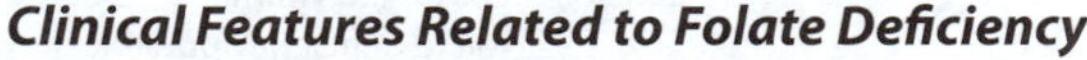

Clinical Features Related to Folate Deficiency

They are similar to those of vitamin B_{12} deficiency except for neurological features.

Diagnosis/Laboratory Findings of Megaloblastic Anemia

Q. Discuss the diagnosis of megaloblastic anemias.

Q. Discuss the diagnosis of anemias due to vitamin B_{12} deficiency.

Blood findings in vitamin B_{12} (including pernicious anemia) and/or folic acid deficiency are similar.

Common Findings

Peripheral blood

Q. Describe the peripheral blood and bone marrow picture in megaloblastic anemia.

- **Hemoglobin and hematocrit (PCV):** Reduced
- **Red cell indices: MCV raised** above 100 fL (normal 82–98 fL)
- RBC, WBC, and platelet count: All are reduced.
- **Peripheral smear (Fig. 8.17): Pancytopenia** (decreased RBCs, WBCs, and platelets)
  - **RBCs:**
    - Macrocytic and oval (egg-shaped macro-ovalocytes) and are diagnostic
    - Marked variation in the size and shape of red cells (anisopoikilocytosis)
    - Evidence of dyserythropoiesis: Basophilic stippling, Cabot ring, and Howell-Jolly bodies

FIG. 8.17: Peripheral blood smear showing macro-ovalocytes (short arrows) and hypersegmented neutrophil (inset).

- **WBCs:**
  - Decreased WBC count (leukopenia)
  - **Hypersegmented neutrophils** (more than five nuclear lobes): First and specific morphological sign of megaloblastic anemia. These neutrophils are also larger than normal.
- **Platelets: Decreased**
- **Reticulocyte count:** Normal or low. Reticulocytosis occurs in response to very small doses of parenteral vitamin B_{12}.

Bone marrow
- **Markedly hypercellular**
- **Megaloblastic type of erythropoiesis**
- Granulocytic precursors display nuclear-cytoplasmic asynchrony in the form of **giant metamyelocytes and band forms**.
- **Megakaryopoiesis:** Normal or increased in number
- **Bone marrow iron:** Moderately increased

Biochemical tests (common for both vitamin B_{12} and folic acid deficiency)
- **Deoxyuridine suppression test:** It is a sensitive measure of deficiency of 5, 10-methylene THF, which occurs in both folic acid and vitamin B_{12} deficiency.
- Serum homocysteine levels are raised.
- Serum bilirubin: Indirect bilirubin is mildly increased due to increased breakdown of red cells in bone marrow and produces mild jaundice.
- Serum iron and ferritin are raised and iron-binding capacity is reduced.
- Plasma lactate dehydrogenase (LDH) is markedly increased.
- Serum vitamin B_{12}/folate is decreased.

Diagnostic/Specific Tests for Vitamin B_{12} Deficiency

- Serum vitamin B_{12} levels: Reduced **and levels are very low** (<200 pg/μL).
- Serum methylmalonic acid (MMA) and homocysteine levels **(Table 8.9)**: Raised.
- Urinary excretion of methylmalonic acid: Raised.
- **Schilling test** (refer below) for vitamin B_{12} absorption, which was discontinued in 2003, once provided invaluable information on the locus and mechanism of cobalamin malabsorption.

TABLE 8.9: Test results on metabolites: Serum methylmalonic acid and total homocysteine in megaloblastic anemia.

Methylmalonic acid (Normal: 70–270 nM)	*Total homocysteine (Normal: 5–14 μM)*	*Diagnosis*
Increased	Increased	Vitamin B_{12} deficiency confirmed; folate deficiency is still possible (i.e., combined vitamin B_{12} plus folate deficiency possible).
Normal	Increased	Folate deficiency is likely; <5% may have vitamin B_{12} deficiency.
Normal	Normal	Vitamin B_{12} and folate deficiencies are excluded.

Diagnostic/Specific Tests for Folic Acid Deficiency

- **RBC folic acid levels: Reduced**
- **FIGLU in urine: Excessively excreted.**

Determining the Cause of the Vitamin (Folate/Vitamin B_{12}) Deficiency

- The cause of folate deficiency is usually determined from the history, physical examination, and clinical features.
- In adults, the cause of vitamin B_{12} deficiency is either due to vitamin B_{12} malabsorption or dietary deficiency of vitamin B_{12}. To determine the basis for malabsorption, one needs additional diagnostic tests (e.g., intestinal biopsy, examination of stool for malabsorption, or *Diphyllobothrium latum* infestation) and requires specific therapy (e.g., gluten-free diet, folate, antibiotics, antihelminthics). A detailed dietary history or past medical history (e.g., gastroduodenal disease, pancreatic insufficiency, impaired bowel motility, or other autoimmune diseases) and physical examination can provide additional clues for other causes.

Schilling Test for Vitamin B_{12} Absorption (Fig. 8.18)

Q. Write short essay on Schilling test/vitamin B_{12} absorption test.

Use: Schilling test helps in distinguishing megaloblastic anemia due to IF deficiency (pernicious anemia) from other causes of vitamin B_{12} deficiency. It is diagnostic of PA, is of historical interest, and is now very infrequently performed.

Method and interpretation

Radioactive vitamin B_{12} (1 μg) is given orally to a fasting patient. This is followed by nonradioactive 1,000 μg of vitamin B_{12} intramuscularly. The injected vitamin B_{12} saturates vitamin B_{12}-binding proteins and flushes out the ingested radioactive vitamin B_{12} which will be excreted in urine. The urine is collected for 24 hours.

- **Stage 1:**
  - Normal persons excrete more than 10% of oral radioactive dose in 24-hour urine.
  - Patients with pernicious anemia excrete less than 5% of the oral dose.

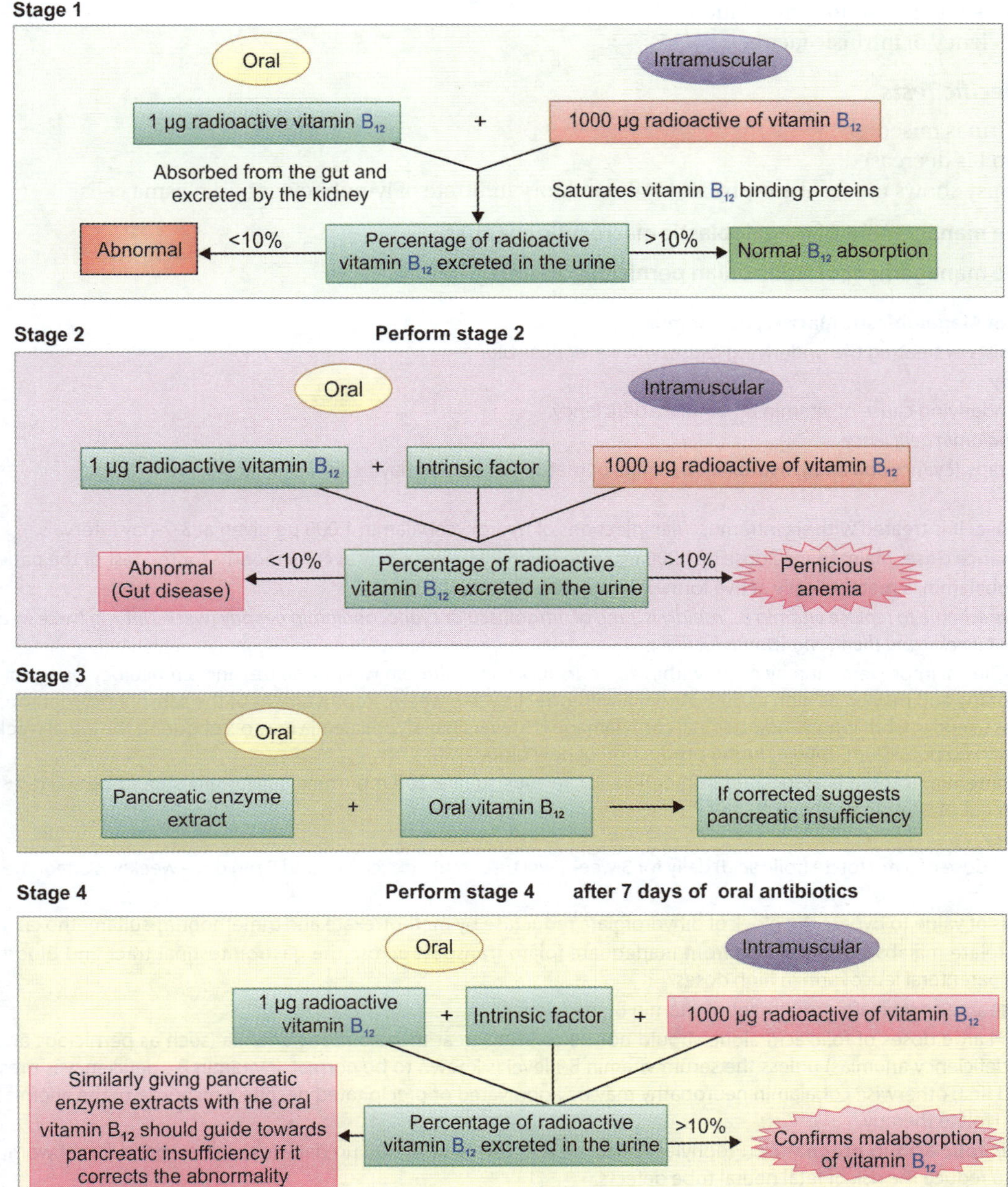

FIG. 8.18: Stages of Schilling test.

- **Stage 2:** If the test is abnormal
  - The test is repeated with addition of oral intrinsic factor to radioactive vitamin B_{12}.
  - If the urinary excretion is now normal, the diagnosis is intrinsic factor deficiency due to either pernicious anemia or gastrectomy.
- **Stage 3:** Giving pancreatic enzyme extracts with the oral vitamin B_{12} should guide toward pancreatic insufficiency if it corrects the abnormality.
- **Stage 4:**
  - If the excretion is still abnormal, the lesion must be in the terminal ileum or there may be bacterial overgrowth. The bacterial overgrowth may be corrected by a 7-day course of oral tetracycline/antibiotics. The test is repeated after a course of oral tetracycline.
  - If the excretion returns to normal, it confirms that malabsorption of vitamin B_{12} is due to bacterial overgrowth in the intestine.

Specific diagnostic tests for pernicious anemia

- Serological tests
  - Anti-intrinsic factor antibodies in serum (in 70% of patients; highly specific for pernicious anemia)
  - Antiparietal cell antibodies (in 85–90%; less specific compared to anti-intrinsic antibodies)

- Achlorhydria with histamine stimulation
- Severe deficiency of intrinsic factor.

Other Nonspecific Tests

- Serum gastrin is raised.
- Pepsinogen I is decreased.
- Gastric biopsy shows mucosal atrophy and inflammatory infiltrate of lymphocytes and plasma cells.

Q. Discuss the management of megaloblastic macrocytic anemias.

Q. Discuss the management of Addisonian pernicious anemia.

Management of Megaloblastic Macrocytic Anemia

Treatment consists of treating the underlying cause, whenever possible.

Specific therapy

Treatment of underlying cause of vitamin B_{12} or folate deficiency.

Vitamin B_{12}/Cobalamin deficiency

Vitamin B_{12} therapy (cyanocobalamin, hydroxocobalamin, or methylcobalamin may be used)

- **Dosage:**
  - **Initial dose:** It is treated with six intramuscular injections of hydroxycobalamin 1,000 µg given at 3-7-day intervals.
  - **Maintenance dose:** Maintenance dose of 1,000 µg to be given intramuscularly every 3 months for the rest of the patient's life. Methylcobalamin, a metabolically active form of vitamin B_{12}, can also be used.
- *An aggressive scheme to replace vitamin B_{12} rapidly is 1 mg of intramuscular cyanocobalamin per day (week 1), 1 mg twice weekly (week 2), 1 mg/week for 4 weeks, and then 1 mg/month for life.*
- **Response:** Clinical improvement may occur within 48 hours (LDH and bilirubin will normalize) and a reticulocytosis peak by the 3–4th day after therapy and may be as high as 50%. Anemia will correct by 4–6 weeks. Improvement of the sensory polyneuropathy may take 6–12 months to correct, but longstanding spinal cord damage is irreversible. Hypokalemia may occur during the initial week of treatment as there is marked potassium uptake during production of new blood cells.
- **Dimorphic anemia:** If there is associated iron deficiency, ferrous sulfate 200 mg thrice daily orally should be started soon after the commencement of vitamin B_{12} therapy.

Folate deficiency

- **Dosage:** Oral dose of 5 mg folate (folic acid) daily for 3 weeks will treat acute deficiency and 5 mg once weekly is adequate maintenance therapy.
- Folinic acid is of value to bypass the block of dihydrofolate reductase by methotrexate and trimethoprim-sulfamethoxazole.
- Congenital folate malabsorption arising from inadequate folate transport across the gastrointestinal tract and blood-brain barrier responds to parenteral leucovorin in high doses.
- **Response** is same as seen after treatment of vitamin B_{12} deficiency.
- **Precaution:** Large doses of folic acid alone should not be given to treat megaloblastic anemia (such as pernicious anemia or other vitamin B_{12} deficiency anemias) unless the serum vitamin B_{12} level is known to be normal. If vitamin B_{12} deficiency is present, it should be corrected first; otherwise cobalamin neuropathy may be aggravated or precipitated despite a response of the anemia of cobalamin deficiency to folate therapy.
- **Prophylactic folic acid in pregnancy:** Prophylactic folic acid in the dose of 400 µg daily is recommended for all women planning a pregnancy to reduce the risk of fetal neural tube defects.

Supportive therapy

- Blood transfusions: Transfusion is usually not necessary and not advisable. It should be given in significantly symptomatic and severely anemic patients with angina or heart failure.
- Other measures: Treatment of infection and physiotherapy in nervous system involvement.

Follow-up

- Clinical and hematological examination should be carried out every 6 months.
- Pernicious anemia: Carcinoma of stomach and gastric carcinoids are more common in patients with pernicious anemia and early detection is important.

Causes of Macrocytosis

Q. Enumerate the causes of macrocytosis/macrocytic anemia.

Macrocytes are large red blood cells with a diameter of more than 9 µ and MCV of more than 95 fL. The macrocytic anemias can be divided into megaloblastic and nonmegaloblastic types, depending on the appearance of developing red cell precursors in the bone marrow.

Megaloblastic Macrocytic Anemia

It is characterized by raised MCV with macrocytosis on the peripheral blood and the presence of abnormal red precursors of the bone marrow known as megaloblasts. Causes of megaloblastic anemia include deficiency of vitamin B_{12}, folate or copper, and drugs that interfere with purine or pyrimidine metabolism. The peripheral blood smear shows macro-ovalocytes and hypersegmented neutrophils.

Nonmegaloblastic Macrocytic Anemia

It is characterized by a raised MCV with macrocytosis on the peripheral blood film with a normoblastic rather than a megaloblastic bone marrow. Common causes are listed in **Box 8.3**. These conditions are associated with normal levels of vitamin B_{12} and folate.

Box 8.3: Causes of nonmegaloblastic macrocytic anemia.

Abnormalities of DNA metabolism

Drugs,
- Zidovudine
- Azathioprine or 6-mercaptopurine
- Capecitabine
- Cladribine
- Cytosine arabinoside
- Hydroxyurea
- Imatinib, sunitinib
- Methotrexate

Shift to immature or stressed red cells
- Reticulocytosis
- Action of erythropoietin—skip macrocytes, stress erythrocytosis
- Aplastic anemia/Fanconi anemia
- Pure red cell aplasia

Primary bone marrow disorders
- Myelodysplastic syndromes
- Congenital dyserythropoietic anemias
- Some sideroblastic anemias
- Large granular lymphocyte (LGL) leukemia

Lipid abnormalities
- Liver disease
- Hypothyroidism

Mechanism unknown
- Alcohol abuse
- Multiple myeloma

HEMOLYTIC ANEMIAS

Q. Define and classify hemolytic anemia. Discuss the clinical features, diagnosis, and management of hemolytic anemias.

Definition

Hemolytic anemias are defined as anemias that result due to increase in the rate of red cell destruction. The life span of red cells (normal life span is 90–120 days) is shortened.

Compensated Hemolytic Disease

Shortening of red cell survival may not always cause anemia as bone marrow can compensate by increased production of red cells by six to eight times.

Classification of Hemolytic Anemias (Table 8.10)

Q. Define and classify hemolytic anemia.

The hemolytic anemias are classified in a variety of ways.

1. **Location of hemolysis:** Depending upon the site of red cell destruction, it can be classified as **intravascular and extravascular** hemolytic disorders.
2. **Source of defect causing hemolysis:** Hemolysis may be due to a defect intrinsic to the red cell itself (**intracorpuscular defect**) or due to an abnormality outside the red cell **(extracorpuscular mechanism).**
3. **Mode of onset: Hereditary and acquired** disorders
4. **Clinical point of view: Acute or chronic**

TABLE 8.10: Classification and causes of hemolytic anemia.

Hereditary	*Acquired*	
Defects in red cell membrane	**Immunohemolytic Anemias**	
Hereditary spherocytosis Hereditary elliptocytosis Stomatocytosis Abetalipoproteinemia (Acanthocytosis)	**Autoimmune Hemolytic Anemias**	
	1. Due to warm antibodies Idiopathic Secondary	**2. Due to cold antibodies** Cold agglutinin disease Paroxysmal cold hemoglobinuria
	3. Hemolytic disease of the newborn	
Red cell enzyme deficiencies	**Fragmentation syndromes**	
Pyruvate kinase deficiency Hexokinase deficiency Glucose-6-phosphate dehydrogenase deficiency (G6PD)	Hemolytic uremic syndrome Thrombotic thrombocytopenic purpura Disseminated intravascular coagulation Prosthetic cardiac valves	
Defects in globin synthesis—Hemoglobinopathies	**Miscellaneous**	
Thalassemia—quantitative Sickle cell syndromes—qualitative Alpha thalassemia Unstable hemoglobin disease	Drugs—oxidant drugs (Primaquine, Dapsone) Chemical—naphthalene, Nitrites and Nitrates, Oxidizing chemicals Thermal injury—burns	
	Paroxysmal nocturnal hemoglobinuria	

Clinical Features of Hemolytic Anemia

Symptoms/History	*Physical findings/Signs*
➢ Mild jaundice ➢ Symptoms due to anemia ➢ Urine color—appears normal (acholuric), turns dark on standing due to oxidation of urobilinogen to urobilin. Black urine (hemoglobinuria) seen in intravascular hemolysis (malaria, mismatched blood transfusion, G6PD deficiency)	➢ Anemia ➢ Mild jaundice ➢ Splenomegaly: Some cases of hemolytic anemia—thalassemia, hereditary spherocytosis ➢ Chronic leg ulcers: Sickle cell anemia

Contd...

Contd...

➤ Infections ➤ Splenic pain: Enlargement or infraction of spleen ➤ Acute crisis: Due to sudden fall in hemoglobin—fever, joint pains, and abdominal pain ➤ Pigment gall stones: Chronic hemolysis ➤ Leg ulcers manifest in adult males: Hereditary spherocytosis and sickle cell anemia ➤ Family history: Congenital hemolytic anemias	➤ Skeletal abnormalities: Expansion of bone marrow in some congenital hemolytic anemias due to increased erythropoiesis, manifests as enlargement of maxillary bones and frontal bossing and malocclusion of the teeth due to overgrowth of upper jaw (thalassemic facies) ➤ Signs of systemic disease: Predisposing to hemolysis ➤ Signs of cholelithiasis: Cholecystitis

Diagnosis of Hemolytic Anemias

Q. Write short essay on laboratory investigations/features of hemolysis/hemolytic anemia.

Recognition of Hemolysis (Table 8.11 and Fig. 8.19)

Features of increased RBC production: As a compensatory mechanism to hemolysis, there is increased production of red cells.

- **Bone marrow** shows **compensatory erythroid hyperplasia.**
- **Peripheral smear** shows **increased reticulocytes** (reticulocytosis), nucleated red cells, and polychromasia. Other findings vary depending on the cause mentioned below.
- **Radiological changes:** Hair-on-end appearance in skull radiograph (thalassemia, sickle cell anemia) is seen.

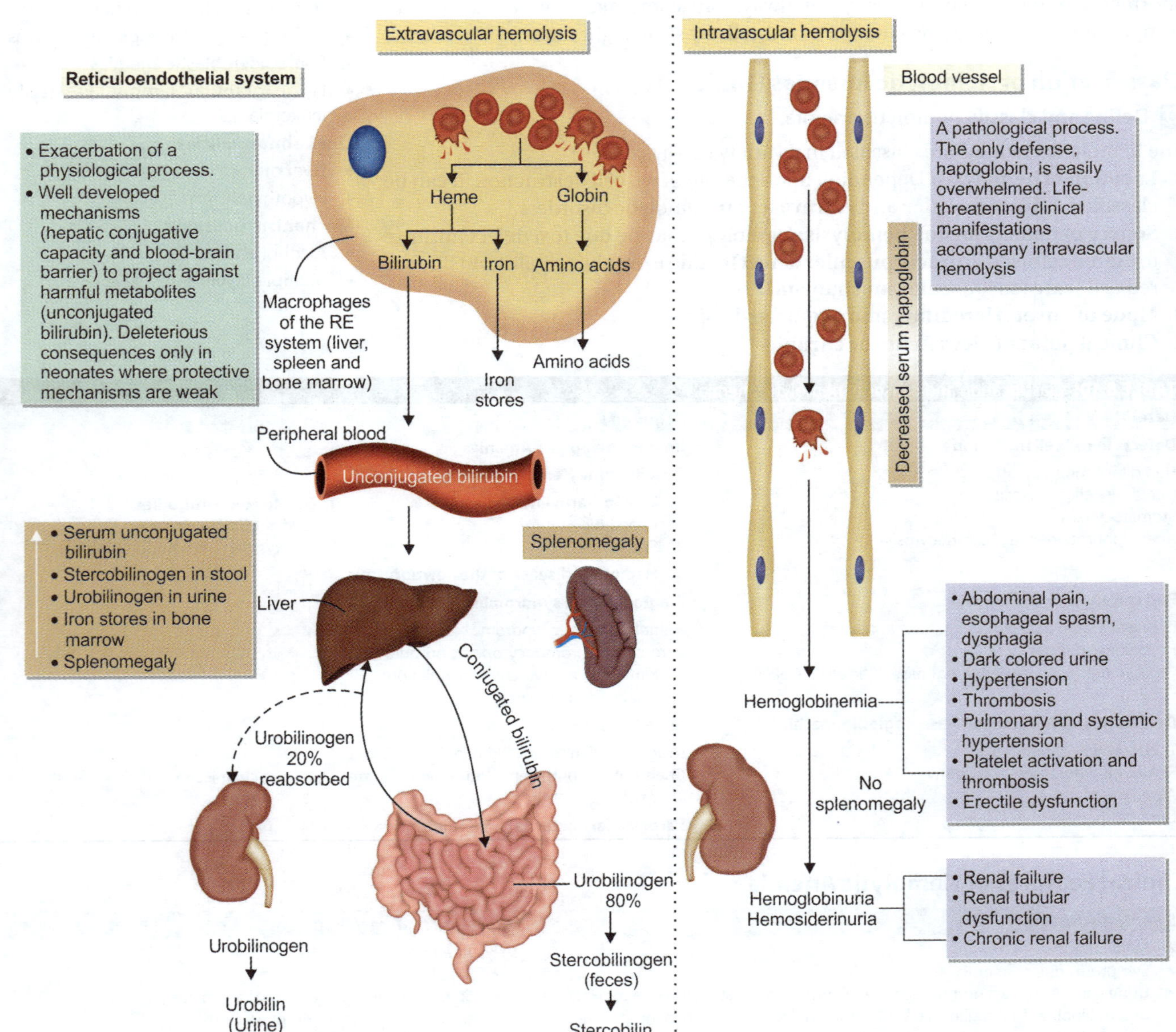

FIG. 8.19: Mechanism and consequences of extravascular and intravascular hemolysis.

Recognition of Cause of Hemolysis

- Common tests:
  - **Peripheral smear examination:** Red cell morphology provides a clue to the underlying hemolytic disorders such as
    (1) spherocyte (hereditary spherocytosis, autoimmune hemolytic anemia), (2) sickle cell (sickle cell anemia), (3) target cell (thalassemia), (4) acanthocyte, (5) schistocyte (intravascular hemolysis-fragmented red cells, helmet cells, triangular cells), and (6) malarial parasite.
  - Coombs test
  - Osmotic fragility, sucrose lysis, and Ham's test
  - Heinz body preparation
  - Hemoglobin electrophoresis
  - High-performance liquid chromatography (HPLC)
  - Measurement of enzyme activity
- Specific tests: Identification of specific cause of hemolysis is dealt under individual diseases.

TABLE 8.11: Summary of laboratory features of hemolytic anemia.

1. Features/consequences of increased RBC destruction/breakdown
- Anemia
- Unconjugated hyperbilirubinemia (jaundice)
- Increased urobilinogen in urine (resulting from bilirubin breakdown in the intestine) leading to high-colored urine
- Shortened red cell life span (demonstrated by ^{51}Cr-labeled red blood cells)
- Other features
  - In extravascular hemolysis: Splenomegaly usual
  - In intravascular hemolysis
    - Decreased plasma haptoglobin and hemopexin
    - Increased plasma lactic dehydrogenase (LDH)
    - Hemoglobinemia, hemoglobinuria, hemosiderinuria, and methemoglobinemia (in some)

2. Consequences of increased RBC production
- **Peripheral smear:** Reticulocytosis
- **Bone marrow:** Erythroid hyperplasia

3. Morphological features of damaged red cells
- **Peripheral smear:** For example, microspherocytes, elliptocytes, red cell fragments

DEFECTS IN HEMOGLOBIN PRODUCTION

Q. Write short note on classification of disorders of hemoglobin (hemoglobinopathies/hereditary disorders of hemoglobin).

Hemoglobin defects may be in the form of production of abnormal (qualitative) or reduced production (quantitative) of normal hemoglobin **(Table 8.12)**. The term hemoglobinopathy, unless specified, usually indicates a qualitative hereditary disorder.

TABLE 8.12: Classification of hemoglobin defects.

Qualitative defect in (structurally abnormal) hemoglobins Hemoglobin S Hemoglobin C Hemoglobin D Punjab	**Combined qualitative and quantitative defects in hemoglobins** Hemoglobin E Sickle-cell β-thalassemia
Quantitative defect in hemoglobins Thalassemias (α, β-thalassemia)	**Acquired hemoglobinopathies** Methemoglobinemia due to toxic exposures Carboxyhemoglobinemia

SICKLE CELL DISEASE

Q. Discuss the etiopathogenesis, clinical features, investigations, and management of sickle cell anemia.

Sickle cell disease (SCD) is an important group of autosomal recessive hereditary disorders of hemoglobin characterized by production of defective hemoglobin synthesis called sickle hemoglobin (HbS). HbS imparts sickle shape to red cells on low oxygen tension or deoxygenation. The term sickle cell disease includes all entities associated with sickling of hemoglobin within the red blood cells. The major entities included are:

- **Sickle cell anemia (SS)** is a homozygous state in which both the β globin chains are abnormal.
- **Sickle cell trait (AS)** is a heterozygous state in which one gene is defective for HbS (abnormal) while the other gene is for HbA (normal).
- **Compound heterozygous** is characterized by both the β-globin chains having different abnormalities (e.g., Hb SC, HbS-β-thalassemia).
  In India, it is seen in certain tribes of South India, Assam, Bihar, and Odisha.

Etiology and Pathogenesis

Sickle cell anemia is caused by production of abnormal hemoglobin called sickle hemoglobin (HbS). In HbS, there is an adenine (A) to thymidine (T) substitution (GAG → GTG) in codon 6 of the β-globin gene. This point mutation results in **replacement of the normal glutamic acid residue by a valine** and alters the solubility or stability of the hemoglobin.

Pathogenesis

The change in the shape is due to dehydration, partly caused by potassium leaving the red cells via calcium-activated potassium channels called the Gárdos channel.

Deoxygenated HbS molecules are insoluble and polymerize to form pseudocrystalline structures known as "tactoids". RBCs become rigid, deformed, and assume a characteristic sickle/crescent shape (sickle-shaped cells). Initially, on reoxygenation this process is reversible. But with repeated episodes of sickling, the RBCs eventually lose their membrane flexibility and become irreversibly sickled cells (ISCs). Factors that favor and hinder sickling are listed in **Table 8.13**.

Consequences of Sickling

Irreversibly sickled cells are dehydrated and dense and will not return to normal when oxygenated. Sickling can produce:

- **Microvascular occlusions:** Impaired passage of ISCs through the microcirculation, produce obstruction of small vessels, and lead to tissue ischemia and infarction
- **Hemolytic anemia:** It is due to shortened survival of the sickle cells which are destroyed by the reticuloendothelial system.

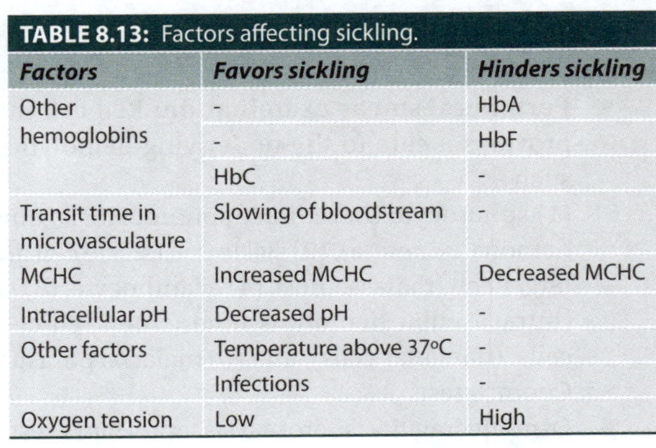

TABLE 8.13: Factors affecting sickling.

Factors	*Favors sickling*	*Hinders sickling*
Other hemoglobins	-	HbA
	-	HbF
	HbC	-
Transit time in microvasculature	Slowing of bloodstream	-
MCHC	Increased MCHC	Decreased MCHC
Intracellular pH	Decreased pH	-
Other factors	Temperature above 37°C	-
	Infections	-
Oxygen tension	Low	High

Clinical Features

Q. Write short essay/note on the complications of sickle cell anemia.

The clinical features change as life advances.

In Children

- An infant till 3 months may be asymptomatic, because of the protective role of HbF. Since HbF disappears after the 3rd month, majority of cases present after 3 months and before the 1st year of life.
- **Prone to infections:** Children are susceptible to acute infections with encapsulated organisms. Common infections are pneumococcal pneumonia, meningitis due to *S. pneumoniae*, and osteomyelitis due to *Salmonella*. Increased susceptibility to infections is because of hypofunction of spleen and defects in the alternative complement pathway which impair opsonization of encapsulated bacteria such as *pneumococci* and *Haemophilus influenzae*. Septicemia and meningitis are the most common causes of death in children. Increased frequency of **osteomyelitis** is because of repeated bone infarcts which act as nidus for infection.
- In children, **bone involvement** may resemble acute osteomyelitis. They manifest as the **hand-foot syndrome and dactylitis** of the bones of the hands or feet or both. It is due to microinfarcts in the carpal and tarsal bones.
- **Sequestration crisis:** It usually occurs in children with chronically enlarged but normal functioning spleen. Sudden trapping of blood in spleen or liver causes rapid enlargement of the organ with resultant drop in hematocrit and hypovolemic shock. This may require blood transfusions.
- **Changes in spleen:** Splenomegaly is observed during early childhood. Repeated episodes of splenic infarct result in atrophy of the spleen **(autosplenectomy)**.
- **Acute chest syndrome** can develop in both children and adults. It is due to infection or infarction in the lung and presents with pain in the chest, fever, respiratory distress, and hypoxemia.
- **Others** include acute coronary syndrome and stroke. Chronic hypoxia in children is responsible for generalized impairment of growth and development.

In Adults (Fig. 8.20)

Anemia: Patients develop severe hemolytic anemia which is exacerbated by secondary folate deficiency. Chronic anemia presents with fatigue, frequent infections, cardiomegaly, and systolic murmurs. Chronic hemolytic anemia causes increased levels of unconjugated (indirect) bilirubin, which predisposes to development of pigmented bilirubin gallstones. Cholelithiasis may lead to cholecystitis.

Q. Write short essay/note on sickle cell crises.

- **Crises:** Irreversibly sickled cells have a shortened survival and plug vessels in the microcirculation. Any new syndrome or episode that develops rapidly in sickle cell anemia is termed crises. The protracted course of sickle cell anemia is frequently exacerbated by a variety of crises. Four types of crises are encountered. These are:

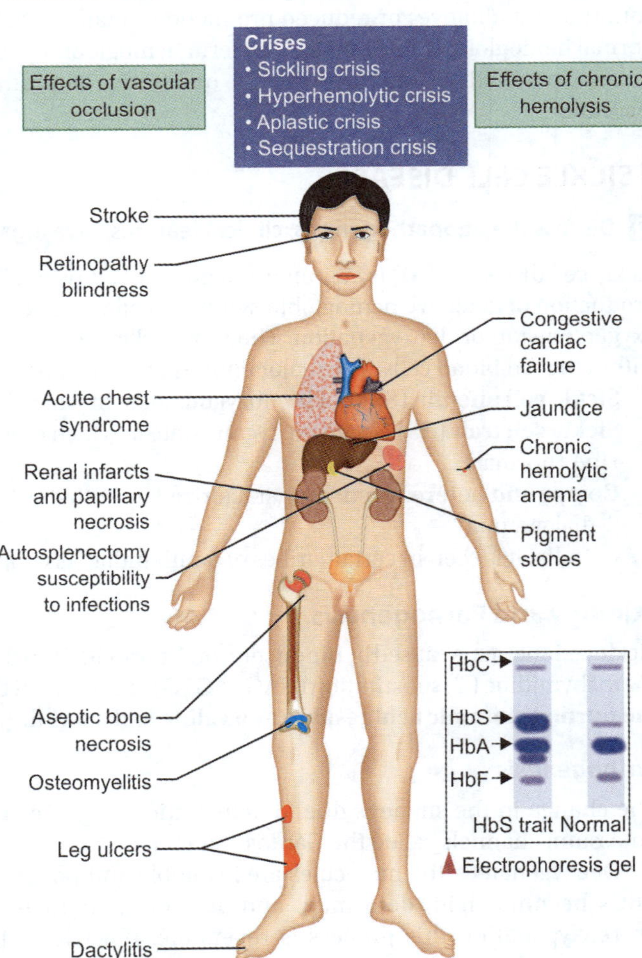

FIG. 8.20: Various effects of vascular occlusion and hemolysis in sickle cell anemia.

- **Infarction (sickling) crisis (vaso-occlusive crisis):** Blockage of microcirculation by sickled red cells causes hypoxic injury and infarction.
  - It is most common and the hallmark of sickle cell disease.
  - It clinically presents with acute, severe pain in the affected region. It commonly involves bones, lungs, liver, and spleen.
  - Bone: Sudden attacks of bone pain are due to ischemia and infarction. Avascular necrosis of the head of femur is also common.
  - Lung: Involvement presents with fever, cough, chest pain, and pulmonary infarcts and is known as *acute chest syndrome (dangerous)*. These are sometimes initiated by a simple lung infection.
  - Spleen: Acute abdominal pain is caused by infarcts of spleen and leads to autosplenectomy.
  - Other sites of infarction: Mesenteric infarction results in acute abdominal pain, cerebral infarctions result in hemiplegia, and infarction of renal papillae results in hematuria. Retinal microinfarcts result in loss of vision.
- **Aplastic crisis:** Temporary suppression of bone marrow erythropoiesis may develop due to an acute infection of erythroid progenitor cells by parvovirus B19.
- **Hemolytic crisis** is characterized by episodes of increased sequestration and destruction of red cells. It presents with marked increase in hemolysis with a sudden lowering of hemoglobin, rapid enlargement of liver and spleen, and reticulocytosis.
- **Sequestration crisis** (described above).
- Other crises encountered rarely are hypoplastic crisis and megaloblastic crisis (due to inadequate folate).

Q. Discuss the long-term complications of sickle cell anemia.

They are described in **Table 8.14**.

TABLE 8.14: Long-term complications of sickle cell anemia.

- **Impaired growth and development** with low weight and delayed sexual maturation
- **Chronic infarcts** of bones
- **Infections** of bones (Salmonella osteomyelitis), lungs, kidneys (pyelonephritis, chronic tubulointerstitial nephritis)
- ***Leg ulcers***
- **Cardiac:** Cardiomegaly, arrhythmias, myocardial infarctions, and iron overload cardiomyopathy
- **Neurological:** Transient ischemic attacks, seizures, cerebral infarction, cerebral hemorrhage, and coma
- **Cholelithiasis**
- **Liver:** Chronic hepatomegaly, liver dysfunction
- ***Priapism***
- **Iron overload** due to repeated transfusions
- **Eye:** Background retinopathy, proliferative retinopathy, vitreous hemorrhages, and retinal detachments
- **Pregnancy:** Spontaneous abortion, intrauterine growth retardation, preeclampsia, and fetal death

Investigations

- **Evidences of hemolysis**
- **Blood count:** Hb is in the range 6–8 g/dL with a high reticulocyte count (10–20%).
- **Peripheral smear:** The characteristic red cell which appears in smear is the **sickle cell (Fig. 8.21).** These appear as long, curved cells with pointed ends. Features of hyposplenism include: Howell-Jolly bodies (small nuclear remnants), **target cells** (due to red cell dehydration), **and ovalocytes.**
- **ESR is low** because sickle cells do not form rouleaux.
- **Sickling test** is induced by adding a reducing (oxygen-consuming) agent like 2% sodium metabisulfite or sodium dithionite to blood sample.
- **Sickle solubility test:** A mixture of HbS in a reducing solution (e.g., sodium dithionite) gives a turbid appearance because of precipitation of HbS, whereas normal Hb gives a clear solution.
- **Hemoglobin electrophoresis:** There is no HbA, 80–95% HbSS, and 2–20% HbF. HbS is slow-moving hemoglobin compared to HbA and HbF. In sickle cell trait (heterozygous state), HbS is 20–40% and the rest is HbA.
- Tests for iron overload: Serum ferritin levels, transferrin saturation, liver iron concentration using liver biopsy specimen, measurement of liver iron using MRI.
- Prenatal diagnosis can be done by analysis of fetal DNA obtained by amniocentesis or chorionic villous biopsy.

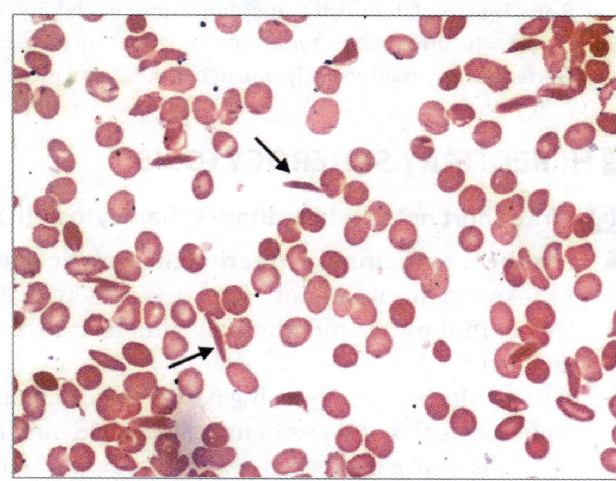

FIG. 8.21: Peripheral blood smear with sickle cells (arrows).

Management

General Measures

Sickle cell disease is a chronic disorder which requires the following general measures:

- **Good nutrition** and folic acid supplementation (5 mg daily) are to be given to all patients with hemolysis.
- **Timely immunizations** against *Streptococcus pneumoniae*, seasonal influenza, *Neisseria meningitidis*, *Haemophilus influenzae type B*, and hepatitis B virus are recommended.
- **Antibiotic prophylaxis** with phenoxymethylpenicillin 500 mg daily starting at the age of 2 months. Older children do not routinely need continued antibiotic prophylaxis.
- Precipitating factors should be avoided or treated quickly. These include avoidance of cold, dehydration, and hypoxia.
- Prevention, prompt identification, and treatment of infections with antibiotics are required.

Anemia

- Transfusions should only be given for clear indications. Transfusion should not be given to patients with chronic stable anemia, those having minor surgery, or those having painful episodes without complications.
- **Indications for blood transfusion:** Transfusion is required to increase the oxygen-carrying capacity, replace the rigid, sickle-shaped RBCs with normal cells, and restore blood flow. Acute transfusions with packed RBCs can be life-saving and chronic transfusions reduce the incidence and severity of most complications.
  - Heart failure, TIAs, strokes, acute chest syndrome, and severe anemia due to aplastic crises and acute splenic sequestration
  - **Repeated transfusions** may be used to reduce the proportion of circulating HbS to less than 20% to prevent sickling, before elective operations and during pregnancy. Chronic RBC transfusion reduces the chance of recurrent ischemic stroke.
  - **Exchange transfusions** may be necessary in patients with severe or recurrent crises or before emergency surgery. Whether exchange transfusion is preferable to simple transfusion in the acute chest syndrome, stroke or other acute complications has not been established by clinical trials.
  - Infarction crises are managed with hydration, oxygen, analgesics, and transfusion with RBC concentrate in selected cases.
- **Iron overload:** With repeated transfusion, iron overload inevitably develops and can result in heart and liver failure and other complications. Iron overload is treated by using iron chelators (deferoxamine or deferasirox).

Hydroxycarbamide (hydroxyurea): It may be used as therapy for patients with severe symptoms. Hydroxyurea (10–30 mg/kg/day) increases HbF and suppresses the neutrophil and reticulocyte counts (which may play a major role in the pathogenesis of sickle cell crisis). Hydroxycarbamide reduces the episodes of pain, the acute chest syndrome, and the need for blood transfusions.

Senicapoc, a Gárdos channel inhibitor, prevented erythrocyte dehydration in clinical trials of patients with sickle cell disease. This drug has antiplasmodium activity.

Acute Painful Crisis

It requires supportive therapy with intravenous fluids, oxygen, antimicrobial agents, and adequate analgesia. Acute severe pain is treated with narcotic and analgesia (morphine) and milder pain can be relieved by codeine, paracetamol, and nonsteroidal anti-inflammatory drugs (NSAIDs). Inhaled nitric oxide inhibits platelet function, reduces vascular adhesion of red cells, and is also a vasodilator. It can provide short-term pain relief and is shown to reduce opiate requirements in acute painful episodes. But it should be restricted to experts to avoid hypoxia and respiratory depression. Nasal oxygen should be employed as appropriate to protect arterial saturation.

Acute chest syndrome is treated with antibiotics, maintenance of arterial oxygenation, pain relief, bronchodilators, and, if required, exchange transfusion.

Chronic leg ulcers: They are treated with elevation of limb, daily dressings with zinc sulfate, and exchange transfusion in extreme cases.

Curative

- **Bone marrow/stem cell transplantation:** In children and adolescents younger than 16 years of age who have severe complications (strokes, recurrent chest syndrome, or refractory pain), bone marrow/stem cell transplantation can provide definitive cure.
- **Gene therapy** is intensively pursued, but no safe measures are currently available.

HEREDITARY SPHEROCYTOSIS

Q. Write short note on hereditary spherocytosis (HS).

- **It is the most common inherited hemolytic anemia in adults**
- **Autosomal dominant** inheritance is present in more than 75% cases
- Defect in the RBC membrane is due to cytoskeleton protein (e.g., **ankyrin, band 3, spectrin, or band protein 4.2**) deficiency.
- This results in red cells losing part of the cell membrane as they pass through the spleen and assume a spheroidal shape (spherocytes) that is less deformable (rigid) and more susceptible to osmotic lysis.
- Red cells have a decreased life span of as low as 10–20 days.

Clinical Features

- Disease may present during anytime from the neonatal period to adulthood.
- **Family history:** Most (75%) HS are inherited as autosomal dominant trait and there is a strong family history of anemia, jaundice, splenomegaly, and cholelithiasis.
- **Anemia** is usually mild to moderate.
- **Jaundice:** There are intermittent attacks of jaundice.
- **Splenomegaly:** Moderate splenic enlargement is characteristic and constant feature.
- **Children:** Growth retardation due to hemolysis and bone changes due to marrow hyperplasia are found in children.
- **Adults:** Anemia, intermittent jaundice, and moderate splenomegaly are found in adults.
- Complications of hereditary spherocytosis are listed in **Box 8.4**.

Box 8.4: Complications of hereditary spherocytosis.

- Cholelithiasis (pigment gallstones)
- Chronic leg ulcers
- Aplastic crises due to parvovirus B19 infection
- Hemolytic crises (rare)

Investigations

- **Anemia:** It is usually mild, but occasionally can be severe.
- **Peripheral blood film** shows **spherocytes (Fig. 8.22)** and reticulocytes. **MCHC is increased**.
- **Demonstration of a hemolytic state:** Raised serum bilirubin and urinary urobilinogen
- Specific diagnostic tests are listed in **Box 8.5**. Increased osmotic fragility may be absent in mild cases and may be positive in autoimmune hemolytic anemia.
- **Negative Coombs test**
- **Strong family history will be present.**

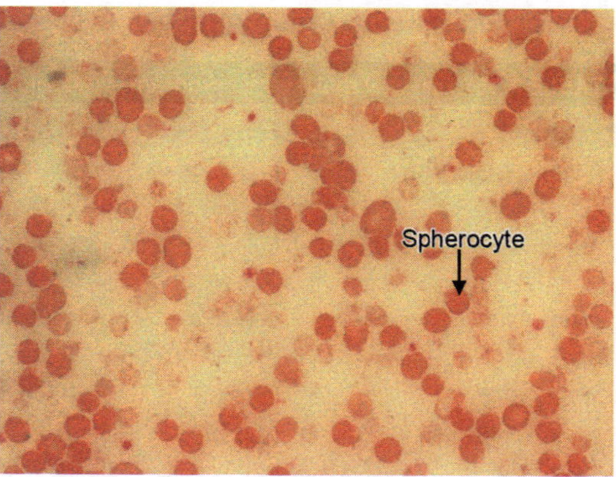

FIG. 8.22: Peripheral blood smear with numerous spherocytes (arrow) in hereditary spherocytosis.

Treatment

- Splenectomy is the treatment of choice and should not be done before the age of 6 years. Splenectomy corrects the anemia and its complications but increases the risk of infections. Hence, it should be preceded by *pneumococcal* and *Haemophilus influenzae* immunization and followed by lifelong penicillin prophylaxis.
- Folic acid supplementation in patients without splenectomy is recommended.
- Regular blood transfusions are required in few patients with severe disease.
- Cholecystectomy is indicated only for symptomatic gallstones.

Box 8.5: Specific diagnostic tests for hereditary spherocytosis.

- Osmotic fragility testing
- Ektacytometry
- Acidified glycerol lysis test
- Cryohemolysis test
- Eosin-5-maleimide binding test

THALASSEMIA SYNDROME

Q. Write short essay/note on definition, common forms, and genetics of thalassemias.

Thalassemia syndrome is a heterogeneous group of inherited disorders which result from reduced or absence of synthesis of one of the globin chains (either α or β globin chain).

Classification

Thalassemic syndromes are mainly classified into two main types depending on the defective globin chain α or β thalassemia **(Box 8.6)**. The mode of inheritance is autosomal recessive. Rarely, HBB gene mutation is inherited as autosomal dominant.

Box 8.6: Classification of thalassemic syndromes.

β-thalassemia syndromes: Based on the genetic defect ($β^+$ or $β^0$):		
β-Thalassemia major (Cooley's Anemia)	**β-Thalassemia intermedia**	**β-Thalassemia minor**
Homozygous disorder. Most severe form Either no production of β-chains ($β^0$) or it is markedly reduced ($β^+$) Anemia—severe, transfusion dependent High level of HbF in the blood	Double heterozygous state Anemia—moderately severe, not transfusion dependent	Also called β-***thalassemia trait*** Heterozygous state Asymptomatic with mild anemia

α-Thalassemia syndromes:			
Each cell has four genes coding for α-globin, two on each chromosome. Each gene contributes to 25% of the total α-globin chains. Severity depends on the number of genes deleted or affected. Deleted genes may vary from 1 to 4.			
1 gene affected	**2 genes affected**	**3 genes affected**	**4 genes affected**
Silent carrier state	α-thalassemia trait	HbH disease	Hb Bart's hydrops fetalis Incompatible with life—stillbirths or die shortly after birth.

α-Thalassemia Syndromes

Each cell has four genes coding for α-globin, two on each chromosome. Each of the four α-globin genes normally contributes 25% of the total α-globin chains. Severity of α-thalassemia depends on the number of α-globin genes deleted or affected. Deleted genes may vary from 1 to 4.

- Silent carrier state develops with deletion of one α-chain gene.
- α-thalassemia trait: It is due to deletion of two α-genes.
- HbH disease: It is due to deletion of three α-genes.
- Hb Bart's hydrops fetalis: It develops if all four genes are absent. It is incompatible with life and the infants are either stillborn or die shortly after birth. They are pale, edematous, and have large liver and spleen.

Classical thalassemia syndromes (genotypes and laboratory findings) are presented in **Table 8.15**.

TABLE 8.15: Classical thalassemia syndromes (genotypes and laboratory findings).

Syndrome	*Genotype*	*Typical findings on CBC*	*Hemoglobin analysis (HPLC or electrophoresis)*
Hydrops fetalis with Hb Barts	(–€–€/ –€–€)	Severe microcytic anemia with hydrops fetalis; usually fatal in utero	Hb Barts (γ globin tetramers); Hb Portland (embryonic hemoglobin); no HbF, HbA, or HbA_2
HbH disease	(α€– / – –) or (α^t –€/ –€–)	Moderate microcytic anemia	HbH (up to 30%); HbA_2 (up to 4%)
Minor	(α€–€/α€–€) or (α α /–€–)	Mild microcytic anemia	Hb Barts (3-8%)
Silent carrier	(α α /α^-)	Normal hemoglobin, normal MCV	Normal
Major (transfusion-dependent)	β^0/β^0 or β^0/β^+	Severe microcytic anemia with target cells (typical Hb 3-4 g/dL)	HbA_2 (5% or more); HbF (up to 95%); no HbA
Intermedia (nontransfusion- dependent)	β^+/β^+	Moderate microcytic anemia	HbA_2 (4% or more); HbF (up to 50%)
Minor (also called trait or carrier)	β/β^0 or β/β^+	Mild microcytic anemia	HbA_2 (4% or more); HbF (up to 5%)

β-*Thalassemia Major*

Q. Discuss the clinical features, salient investigations, diagnosis, and management of β-thalassemia major (Cooley's anemia).

- β-thalassemia major (Mediterranean or Cooley's anemia) is the homozygous form of β-thalassemia characterized by absent or reduced synthesis of β-chain.
- It is most common in Mediterranean countries and parts of Africa and Southeast Asia. In India, it is common among certain communities (e.g., Sindhi, Punjabi, Gujarati, Parsee) in North India and less common in South India.
- **Anemia** is produced due to diminished synthesis of HbA, ineffective erythropoiesis, and extravascular hemolysis.
- **Consequences of ineffective erythropoiesis:**
  - Marked erythroid hyperplasia: Severe hemolytic anemia stimulates erythropoietin (EPO) production by kidney leading to marrow erythroid hyperplasia.
  - Changes in the bone: Thalassemic facies and hair-on-end appearance of skull X-ray
  - Extramedullary hematopoiesis.

Clinical Features

- **Severe anemia:** Infants with thalassemia major are well at birth but develop moderate-to-severe anemia 6-9 months after birth, when hemoglobin synthesis switches from HbF to HbA.
- **Retardation of growth and development:** Untreated/untransfused children **fail to thrive** (growth retardation) and die early within 4–5 years of age from the effects of anemia. They are **susceptible to recurrent bacterial infections.**
- **Changes in bone:** In those who survive longer, bone marrow hyperplasia causes expansion and widening of marrow and gives the **classical X-ray changes**.
  - **Thalassemic (Chipmunk) facies (Fig. 8.23):** Due to enlargement and distortion of craniofacial bones (frontal bossing of the skull, prominent malar eminence, depression of bridge of nose, and hypertrophy of the maxillae, which tends to expose the upper teeth)
  - **Hair-on-end (crew-cut) appearance (Fig. 8.24):** It can be seen in the skull X-ray due to new bone formation.
- **Splenomegaly** may be massive and enlarges up to 1,500 g due to hyperplasia and extramedullary hematopoiesis.
- Liver (hepatomegaly) and lymph nodes also may show extramedullary hematopoiesis.
- **Hemosiderosis:** Although blood transfusions improve the anemia, iron overload will lead to hemosiderosis and secondary hemochromatosis. This may be due to increased gastrointestinal absorption of iron. It damages organs such as heart, liver, and pancreas.
  - Cardiac hemosiderosis results in arrhythmias, heart blocks, and congestive heart failure.
  - Hepatic hemosiderosis results in cirrhosis.
  - Pancreatic hemosiderosis results in diabetes.
  - Pituitary: It leads to hypogonadotropic hypogonadism.
- Treated patients can survive beyond 40 years of age.

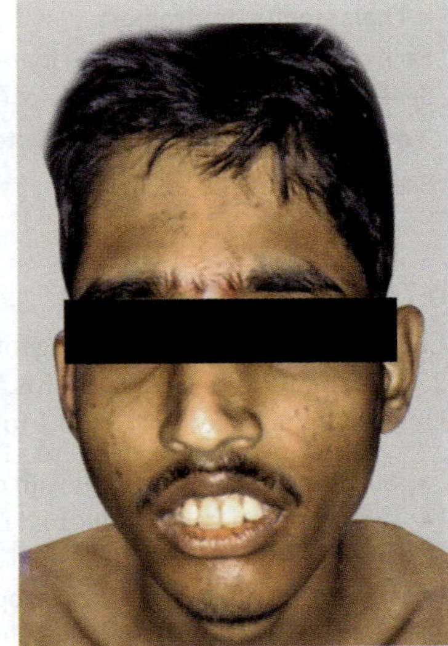

FIG. 8.23: Chipmunk facies in thalassemia.

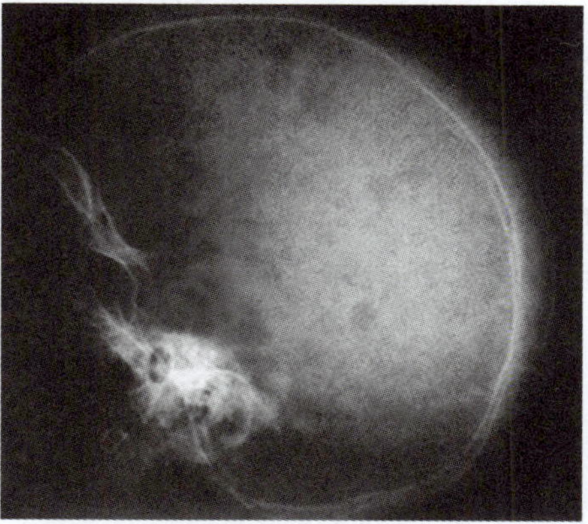

FIG. 8.24: Skull X-ray showing crew-cut appearance due to new bone formation.

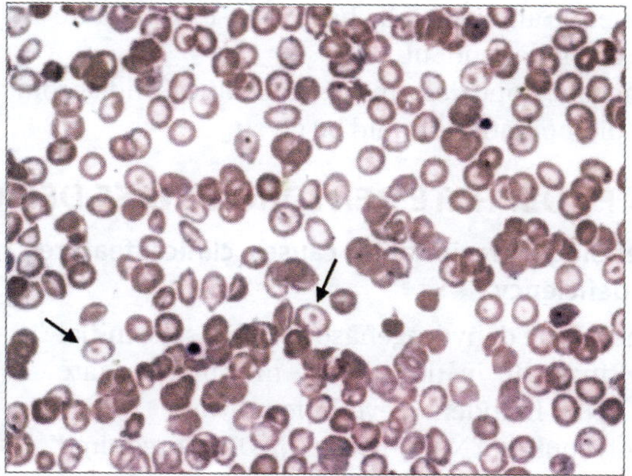

FIG. 8.25: Peripheral blood smear in β-thalassemia showing target cell (arrows).

Investigations

- **Peripheral smear (Fig. 8.25):** Marked **microcytic hypochromic anemia** with moderate to marked anisocytosis and poikilocytosis. Many **target cells** (hemoglobin collects in the center of RBCs) and nucleated red cells are visible.
- **HbF level is increased** (30–92%) on hemoglobin electrophoresis.
- **There is markedly reduced or absent HbA**.
- Osmotic fragility test shows increased resistance to hemolysis.
- Skull radiograph shows a **"hair-on-end"/crew-cut appearance.**
- There is evidence of thalassemia minor in both parents.
- **Red cell distribution width (RDW)** is within normal limits (in contrast to iron deficiency anemia).

Management

- **Aims of treatment:** To suppress ineffective erythropoiesis, prevent deformities of bone, and allow normal activity and development. Blood transfusions may be required every 4–6 weeks. **Hypertransfusion** to maintain Hb level between 10 and 12 g/dL is probably adequate. It decreases the effect of chronic anemia and prevents abnormal growth and development. **Supertransfusion** wherein the Hb level is maintained at 12 g/dL is designed to completely suppress hematopoiesis.
- **Maintenance of Hb level:** Long-term folic acid supplement and regular blood transfusions are recommended to keep the Hb >10 g/dL.
- **Treatment of iron overload:** The iron-chelating agent, **desferrioxamine** (administered parenterally), is indicated if serum ferritin >1,500 μg/L. Ascorbic acid 200 mg daily along with desferrioxamine increases the urinary excretion of iron in response to desferrioxamine. Deferiprone and deferasirox are oral iron chelators.
- **Splenectomy** is indicated in children with massive symptomatic splenomegaly and those with progressively increasing requirement of blood transfusion or hypersplenism.
- **Bone marrow transplantation is done** in young patients.
- **Management of associated complications:** For example, congestive heart failure and endocrinopathies.

β-Thalassemia Minor (Trait)

Q. Write short essay/note on thalassemia minor (trait) and thalassemia intermedia.

- β-thalassemia minor is more common than β-thalassemia major.
- It is a common carrier (heterozygous) state and is usually **asymptomatic.**
- Anemia is mild or absent.
- **Peripheral blood smear** shows severe microcytic and hypochromic red cells with target cells. It may be confused with iron deficiency.
- Serum ferritin and the iron stores are normal.
- **Hb electrophoresis** usually shows a raised HbA_2 (3.5–7.5%) and often a raised HbF.
- Iron should not be given to these patients unless there is associated iron deficiency.
- **Genetic counseling is recommended** to prevent transmission of carrier state from both parents.
- **Prenatal diagnosis** by chorionic villi biopsy at 11 weeks is done.
- It may be associated with other hemoglobin abnormalities. Examples include HbS/β-thalassemia, HbC/β-thalassemia, and HbE/β-thalassemia.

β-Thalassemia Intermedia

- It is a clinical entity in which patients have a clinical spectrum intermediate between thalassemia trait and thalassemia major.

- Patients are anemic and generally have mild-to-moderate anemia (Hb 7–9 g/dL).
- It is not transfusion dependent.
- Mild splenomegaly, bone deformities, gallstones, and chronic leg ulcers may be seen.
- Folic acid supplementation should be given.

GLUCOSE-6-PHOSPHATE DEHYDROGENASE DEFICIENCY

Q. Discuss the etiology, precipitating causes, clinical features, investigations, and management of glucose-6-phosphate dehydrogenase deficiency.

- Glucose-6-phosphate dehydrogenase (G6PD) is the initial and rate-limiting step in the hexose monophosphate (HMP) shunt of the Embden-Meyerhof pathway.
- G6PD is the only source of NADPH, and NADPH is required for the generation of glutathione (GSH), which protects red cells from oxidative stress **(Fig. 8.26)**.
- G6PD-deficient patients may develop acute hemolytic anemia after exposure to any oxidative stress.
- G6PD deficiency is an X-linked disorder and is the most common enzyme deficiency.
- RBCs deficient in G6PD are unable to keep glutathione in a reduced state. These RBCs are susceptible to injury by oxidants of both exogenous and endogenous origins.
- More than 400 G6PD genetic variants are known, but most are harmless. The three common variants are:
  - **G6PD A –:** The minus sign indicates absence of enzyme activity. Hemolysis develops when exposed to oxidant drugs (primaquine) or infections. The hemolysis is mild to moderate and is limited to the older RBCs.
  - **G6PD (B)** or **G6PD Mediterranean/Wild type:** It is prevalent in the Middle East and is the severe form of deficiency. This is the most common variant seen in India. Other variants in India include G6PD Kerala-Kalyan and G6PD Odisha.
  - **G6PD Canton** is seen in Chinese.

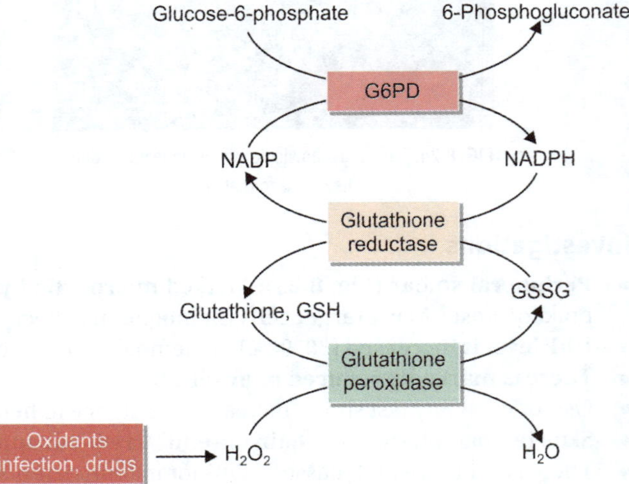

FIG. 8.26: Role of G6PD against injury by oxidants.

Clinical Features

- Most patients with G6PD deficiency remain clinically asymptomatic; however, all of them have an increased risk of developing clinically significant syndromes: (1) acute hemolytic anemia (AHA), (2) neonatal jaundice (NNJ), and rarely, (3) chronic nonspherocytic hemolytic anemia (CNSHA).
- **Acute hemolytic anemia:** Due to intravascular hemolysis, acute hemolytic anemia is the most dramatic clinical presentation of G6PD deficiency. It develops after exposure to an oxidative stress and the triggers include:
  - **Drugs:** Antimalarials (primaquine, quinine, chloroquine), sulfonamides (sulfamethoxazole), antibacterial/antibiotics (cotrimoxazole, nitrofurantoins), antipyretics/analgesics (acetanilide phenazopyridine), dapsone, quinidine, methylene blue, nitrofurantoins, etc.
  - **Fava beans**
  - **Infections:** Viral and bacterial.

  The exposure to triggering agents produces hemolytic attack with rapid development of anemia and hemoglobinuria (cola colored urine). Rarely acute renal failure may develop. The onset can be extremely abrupt, especially following ingestion of the broad beans **(favism)** in children.
- **Neonatal jaundice** is a feature of Mediterranean type. Hemolytic anemia is very rarely severe. Jaundice may be due to decreased hepatic elimination of bilirubin. Severe neonatal jaundice, if not adequately treated with phototherapy, may result in kernicterus or even death.
- **Chronic nonspherocytic hemolytic anemia (CNSHA):** Develops in very small minority of patients. Such a patient is always a male and usually has a history of severe neonatal jaundice and chronic anemia. The degree of chronic anemia is variable and some patients may have required intermittent transfusions. They have reticulocytosis, gallstones, and splenomegaly. Hemolysis is mainly extravascular.

G6PD deficiency (African variety) has a protective effect against *Plasmodium falciparum*.

Laboratory Findings (Investigations)

- **Evidence of intravascular hemolysis:** Raised unconjugated bilirubin, hemoglobinemia, hemoglobinuria, high LDH, and low or absent plasma haptoglobin.

- **Anemia:** It usually ranges from moderate to extremely severe. It is due to both intravascular and extravascular hemolysis.
- **Peripheral blood film:**
    - Normocytic and normochromic with anisocytosis, polychromasia (reticulocytosis), poikilocytes, and spherocytes
    - Bite (blister) cells are red cells in which parts of them appear bitten away.
    - Heinz bodies consist of membrane-bound precipitates of denatured hemoglobin (methemoglobin) and represent oxidative damage. They are seen as dark inclusions within red cells and can be demonstrated by supravital staining with methyl violet.
- **Confirmation of diagnosis:** By estimating G6PD activity of the red cell. This should be estimated several days after the acute hemolytic episode. This is because if done during or immediately after acute hemolysis, it may give a falsely normal value as the young red cells and reticulocytes have near-normal G6PD levels.

Treatment (management) of G6PD deficiency

- **Removal of the triggering agent** and avoiding its further exposure to triggering factors in previously screened patients. Once the cause is recognized, in most cases no specific treatment is required. Management of neonatal jaundice is similar to any other cause of neonatal hyperbilirubinemia.
- Supportive therapy for anemia:
    - Blood transfusion
    - Regular folic acid supplements in CNSHA
- Treatment of infection and genetic counseling

MISCELLANEOUS ANEMIAS

Q. Write short essay/note on the causes and management of normocytic anemia.

Normocytic Normochromic Anemia

Normocytic normochromic anemia is characterized by the normal size of the RBCs and normal MCV **(Table 8.16)**.

TABLE 8.16: Various causes of normocytic normochromic anemia.

Decreased red cell production	*Increased red cell loss or destruction*
➢ Anemia of chronic disease ➢ Chronic renal failure ➢ Chronic liver disease ➢ Endocrine disorders – Hypopituitarism – Hypothyroidism – Hypoadrenalism ➢ Hematological disorders – Marrow hypoplasia or aplasia – Myeloproliferative neoplasms – Myelofibrosis – Sideroblastic anemia	➢ Acute blood loss ➢ Hypersplenism ➢ Hematological disorders – Hemoglobinopathies (sickle cell disease) – Hereditary spherocytosis – Glucose-6-phosphate dehydrogenase (G6PD) deficiency – Microangiopathic anemias [disseminated intravascular coagulation (DIC), thrombotic thrombocytopenic purpura, hemolytic uremic syndromes] – Autoimmune hemolytic anemia – Paroxysmal nocturnal hemoglobinuria
Expansion of plasma volume: Pregnancy.	

Management: Treatment of the underlying disease.

Differential Diagnosis of Hypochromic Microcytic Anemias

Q. Describe the etiology, investigations, and differential diagnosis of hypochromic microcytic anemia.

Table 8.17 shows the differentiating features of hypochromic microcytic anemias.

TABLE 8.17: Various differentiating features of hypochromic microcytic anemias.

	Iron deficiency anemia	*Thalassemia trait*	*Anemia of chronic disease*	*Sideroblastic anemia*
MCV	Reduced	Very low for degree of anemia	Low normal or normal	Inherited—low Acquired—high
Serum iron *(normal 60–170 μg/dL)*	Reduced	Normal to high	Reduced	Raised
Serum total iron binding capacity *(normal 300–350 μg/dL)*	Raised	Normal	Reduced	Normal
Serum ferritin *(normal 15–300 μg/dL)*	Reduced	Normal	Normal or raised	Raised
Serum-soluble transferrin receptors	Increased	Normal or raised	Normal	Normal or raised
Iron in marrow	Absent	Present	Present	Present
Iron in erythroblasts	Absent	Present	Absent or reduced	Ring forms
Hemoglobin A_2 (normal <3%)	Reduced	Increased	Normal	Reduced

Sideroblastic Anemias

Q. Write short essay/note on sideroblastic anemias.

Definition

Sideroblastic anemias are rare inherited or acquired disorders of refractory anemia, characterized by:

- A dimorphic peripheral blood picture. Microcytic hypochromic red cells in hereditary form and macrocytic in the acquired forms of the disease mixed with normochromic cells.
- Presence of ring sideroblasts, excess storage iron in the bone marrow, and increased serum iron concentration. The diagnostic feature is the presence of ring sideroblasts in the bone marrow. The iron-laden mitochondria surround the nucleus of erythroblasts and appear as the pathognomonic "rings" of iron granules with Prussian blue staining (Perls' reaction).
- Tiny iron-containing inclusions, called Pappenheimer bodies, are found in the red blood cells (stain positively by Prussian blue staining).
- Ineffective erythroid hyperplasia due to nonviable sideroblasts.

Classification of Sideroblastic Anemia (Box 8.7)

Microcytosis is often seen in hereditary forms, but normochromic normocytic or even macrocytic RBCs may be seen, especially in the setting of myelodysplasia or in a rare X-linked hereditary form known as Pearson's syndrome.

Box 8.7: Classification of sideroblastic anemia.

Inherited sideroblastic anemia: X-linked disease—transmitted by females	
Acquired sideroblastic anemia	
Primary: Myelodysplasia	
Secondary	Myeloproliferative neoplasms
Drugs, e.g., isoniazid, cycloserine, chloramphenicol, busulfan, D-penicillamine	Myeloid leukemia Primary pyridoxine deficiency
Alcohol abuse	Others (e.g., rheumatoid arthritis, carcinoma)
Lead toxicity	

Treatment

- Withdrawal of causative agent: Some patients respond when the drugs, toxins, or alcohol are withdrawn.
- Occasional cases may respond to pyridoxine or folic acid.
- Supportive treatment with transfusions.
- Erythropoietin can also be given.

Hereditary sideroblastic anemias

Hereditary sideroblastic anemias comprise a clinically, genetically, and hematologically heterogeneous group of rare disorders. It may be inherited as an X-linked or an autosomal (dominant or recessive) disorder. These patients generally have low levels of δ-aminolevulinic acid synthase (ALAS) enzyme in the normoblasts leading to defective synthesis of hemoglobin.

Paroxysmal Nocturnal Hemoglobinuria

Q. Write short essay/note on paroxysmal nocturnal hemoglobinuria (PNH).

Paroxysmal nocturnal hemoglobinuria (PNH) is a rare **acquired nonmalignant, genetic defect due to mutation in the hematopoietic stem cell.** These **clones of red cells are particularly sensitive to destruction by activated complement.** Platelets and granulocytes are also affected and there may be thrombocytopenia and neutropenia.

Etiology and Pathogenesis

The stem cells and their progeny have **deficient synthesis of glycosylphosphatidylinositol (GPI) linked proteins,** namely: (1) decay-accelerating factor or CD55 and (2) membrane inhibitor of reactive lysis or CD59. This is most important and a potent inhibitor of C3 and prevents activation of the alternative complement pathway on their membrane. In PNH, the red cells are abnormally sensitive to complement-mediated intravascular hemolysis. The severity of hemolysis is proportional to the number of these abnormal red cells. The molecular basis of PNH is the mutations in the *pig-A* (phosphatidylinositol glycan protein A) gene responsible for synthesis of the GPI anchor.

Clinical Features

- It is mainly seen in adults, usually in middle age.
- Both sexes are equally affected.
- **Intravascular hemolysis**: Characteristically, only the urine voided at night (nocturnal) and in the morning on waking is dark in color. The hemolysis is due to reduced pH of blood during sleep which enhances the activity of complement. Hemoglobin in acidic urine is converted into acid hematin which colors the urine dark brown. Urinary iron loss may be sufficient to cause iron deficiency. Other features include abdominal pain/dysphagia, erectile dysfunction, pulmonary hypertension, and renal insufficiency.
- Mild jaundice and mild hepatosplenomegaly are often present.

- **Thrombosis:** It is very common involving the hepatic (Budd-Chiari syndrome), portal, or cerebral veins and is often the leading cause of death.
- It may begin or progress to aplastic anemia.

Diagnosis

- **Peripheral smear:** Anemia, reticulocytosis, varying degrees of thrombocytopenia and leukopenia (pancytopenia) are diagnosed.
- Features of **intravascular hemolysis** such as raised bilirubin, hemoglobinemia, hemoglobinuria, and hemosiderinuria are present.
- **Bone marrow** is sometimes hypoplastic (or even aplastic) despite hemolysis.
- Diagnosis is confirmed by Ham's test and sucrose lysis test. These tests cannot reliably detect small populations of affected red cells.
  - **Ham's acidified serum test:** Checks whether red blood cells become more fragile when they are placed in mild acid.
    Ham's test can also be positive in congenital dyserythropoietic anemia.
  - **Sucrose hemolysis test:** A PNH patient's red cell undergoes lysis when incubated in low-tonic-strength solution of sugar sucrose. It can be positive in megaloblastic anemia and autoimmune hemolytic anemia.
- **Flow cytometry:** It detects red cells that are deficient in **GPI-linked proteins (CD55 and CD59).** It is a rapid and sensitive test for diagnosis.
- *Neutrophil alkaline phosphatase* ***(NAP) score:*** *NAP score is reduced (normal 40–100), because NAP is a GPI-linked protein.*
- **Progress:** PNH patients are also at an increased risk for developing aplastic anemia or acute myelogenous leukemia or a myelodysplastic syndrome.

Treatment

- Supportive measures: Blood transfusions (for patients with severe anemia) and control of infections
- Iron therapy is often necessary due to loss in urine.
- **Anticomplement therapy: Eculizumab** is a humanized monoclonal antibody that prevents the cleavage of C5 (thereby the formation of the membrane attack complex) and reduces intravascular hemolysis, hemoglobinuria, and the need for transfusion.
- Long-term anticoagulants may be necessary for patients with recurrent thrombotic episodes.
- Steroids may be useful in some cases.
- Bone marrow (stem cell) transplantation is curative.

Methemoglobinemia

Q. Write short essay/note on methemoglobinemia.

- Normal oxygen transport depends on the maintenance of iron in hemoglobin in ferrous (reduced) form (Fe^{++}).
- **Methemoglobin (Hi)** is a hemoglobin in which the iron is in oxidized ferric form and unable to combine with oxygen. Normal RBCs contain less than 1% methemoglobin. Increased amount of methemoglobin in the RBCs is called methemoglobinemia.
- Clinically, when methemoglobin level is more than 1.5 g/dL, the patient develops cyanosis. At higher levels, it produces headache, weakness, and breathlessness. At higher methemoglobin levels, respiratory depression, altered sensorium, coma, shock, seizures, and death may occur.

Causes of Methemoglobinemia

- Hereditary: Deficiency of methemoglobin reductase, cytochrome B5 reductase deficiency
- Acquired: Exposure to certain drugs and toxins (e.g., nitrites and nitrates, nitrofurantoin, chloroquine, naphthalene, local anesthetics (procaine, lidocaine), primaquine, dapsone, sulfa drugs phenacetin, phenazopyridine, metoclopramide, nitroglycerine], copper sulfate

Treatment

- Methemoglobin reductase deficiency: Oral methylene blue or ascorbic acid
- Severe methemoglobinemia: Intravenous methylene blue. Ensure adequate tissue oxygenation.

Autoimmune Hemolytic Anemia

Autoimmune hemolytic anemias (AIHA) are a group of acquired disorders resulting from increased red cell destruction due to red cell autoantibodies.

Q. Write short essay/note on autoimmune hemolytic anemias.

Classification of Autoimmune Hemolytic Anemia

It may be classified based on:

1. Type of antibody: Interaction of the autoantibody with the red cell antigen is dependent on the temperature, i.e., warm or cold type **(Box 8.8)**.
2. Etiology **(Box 8.9)**.

Warm antibody immunohemolytic anemia

- Warm antibody type is the most common type (50–70%).
- The antibodies are mainly of **IgG** type. The antibodies combine with red cell antigen at 37°C and hence known as **warm antibody**.

Clinical features

- They may occur at all ages and in both sexes, although most frequent in middle-aged females.
- They may present with anemia, jaundice, hepatosplenomegaly, and manifestations and underlying disease.
- Exclude underlying systemic lupus erythematosus, lymphoma, and leukemia.

Investigations

- Evidence of hemolytic anemia
- Spherocytosis (due to red cell damage) and macrocytes in peripheral blood
- Direct antiglobulin (Coombs) test is positive.
- Autoantibodies may have specificity for the Rh blood group system (e.g., for the e antigen).
- In some cases, **autoimmune thrombocytopenia** and/or neutropenia may also be present (Evans' syndrome).

Box 8.8: Classification of autoimmune hemolytic anemia according to type of antibody.

Based on antibody type

Warm Antibody Type (IgG Antibodies Active at 37°C)

- **Primary (Idiopathic)**
- **Secondary**
  - Autoimmune disorders (systemic lupus erythematosus and others)
  - Drugs (e.g., Methyldopa, penicillins, quinidine)
  - Lymphomas—Hodgkin's lymphoma, chronic lymphatic leukemia

Cold Agglutinin Type (IgM Antibodies Active at 4–18°C)

- **Acute**
  - Mycoplasmal infection
  - Infectious mononucleosis
- **Chronic**
  - Idiopathic
  - Lymphomas

Cold Hemolysin Type (Donath-Landsteiner Antibodies)

Rare; seen mainly in children; usually postviral

Box 8.9: Classification of autoimmune hemolytic anemia based on etiology.

Based on Etiology

Idiopathic (50%)

Secondary (50%)

- Drugs, e.g., methyldopa, penicillins, quinidine
- Mycoplasmal infection
- Infectious mononucleosis
- Autoimmune disorders (systemic lupus erythematosus and others)
- Lymphomas

Antiglobulin (Coombs) Test (Fig. 8.27)

Q. Write short essay/note on significance of Coombs test.

There are two types, namely, direct and indirect.

Q. Write short note on Coombs test.

1. **Direct** (Coombs) **antiglobulin test (DAT)** detects the immunoglobulin (IgG) antibody and/or C3 complement (usually C3d) on a patient's RBCs. **A patient's red cells** are washed and suspended in saline. Antiglobulin serum is added. Agglutination of red cells indicates the presence of antibody on the surface of RBCs and interpreted as positive DAT.
2. **Indirect** (Coombs) **antiglobulin test (IAT)** detects the immunoglobulin (IgG) antibody or C3 complement (usually C3d) in the patient's serum. **0 Rh +ve normal red cells and antiglobulin serum are added to the patient's serum.** Agglutination of RBCs indicates the presence of antibodies in the patient's serum and the test is reported as positive for an indirect antiglobulin test.

Treatment

- **Corticosteroids** (e.g., prednisolone in doses of 1 mg/kg daily) are effective in about 80% of patients. Initially for the first 2–4 weeks, prednisolone 60 mg daily is given, followed by gradual tapering of the dose. When a dose of 20–30 mg daily achieves a persistent remission (indicated by the stable Hb level and decreasing reticulocyte count), it is recommended to give prednisone on alternate day. Patients with rapid hemolysis may require intravenous methylprednisolone at a dose of 250–1,000 mg/day for 1–3 days.
- **Avoid blood transfusion** as far as possible, because autoantibodies may cause difficulty in cross-matching the blood.
- Danazol can be used along with prednisone as first-line therapy allowing for a shorter duration of prednisone therapy.
- **Splenectomy** may be necessary.
  - If there is no response to corticosteroids
  - If the remission is not maintained when the dose of prednisolone is reduced
  - If there is requirement of the equivalent of more than 10–15 mg prednisone per day to maintain an acceptable hemoglobin level
- **Intravenous immunoglobulin** may also be used as a temporary measure before performing splenectomy for patients refractory to conventional therapy with corticosteroids.
- **Rituximab** is a monoclonal antibody directed against the CD20 antigen expressed on B lymphocytes.
  - **Use:** Useful in refractory cases and also in secondary type of warm AIHA.
  - **Adverse effects:** Hypotension, fever, chills, rigors, hypertension, bronchospasm, pulmonary infiltrates, acute respiratory distress syndrome, myocardial infarction, cardiogenic shock
  - **Contraindication:** Untreated hepatitis B infection
- **Other immunosuppressive drugs** (e.g., azathioprine, cyclophosphamide, and cyclosporine) may be effective when there is no response to steroids, rituximab, and splenectomy.

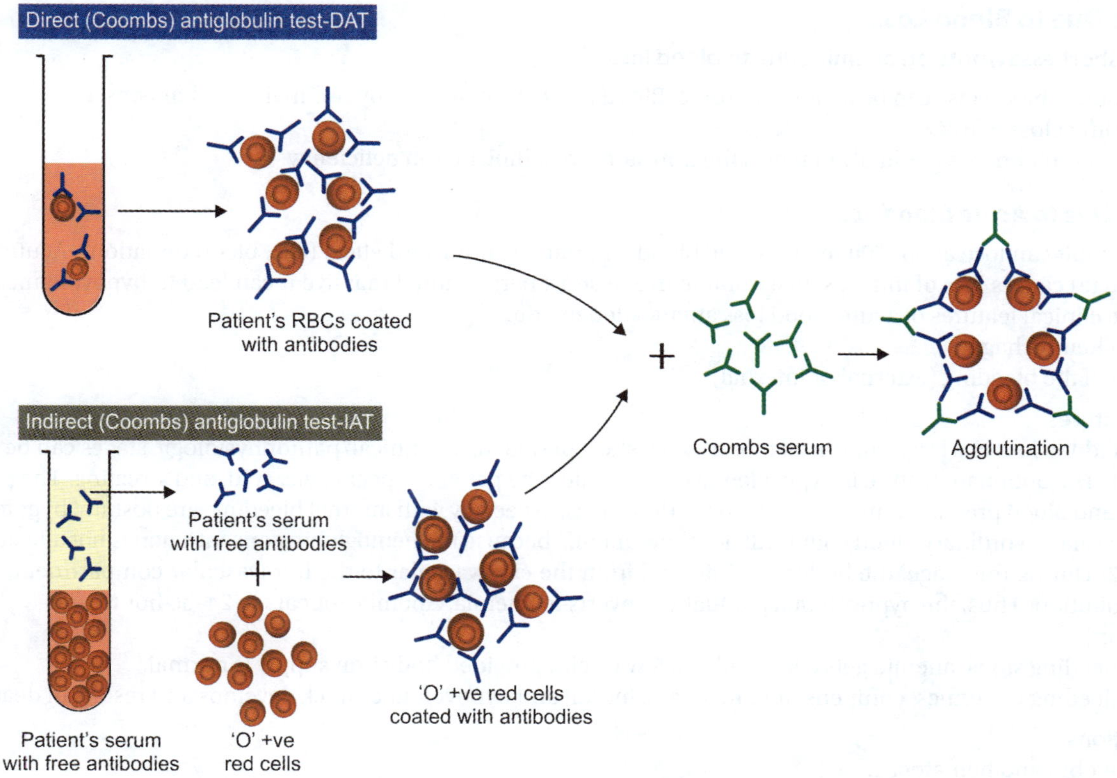

FIG. 8.27: Method of direct and indirect methods of antiglobulin test (Coombs test).

Cold Agglutinin Autoimmune Hemolytic Anemia

Q. Discuss cold hemagglutinin disease (CHAD) in brief.

- It is less common than the warm antibody type and is caused by so-called **cold agglutinins**.
- These antibodies bind to red cell antigens at low temperatures (4–18°C), i.e., avidity of red cell to antibody increases as the temperature falls.
- The antibodies are of IgM type.
- Clinically, it presents acrocyanosis (i.e., blue color of the fingertips, toes, nose, and ear lobes) after exposure to cold. Patients are advised to avoid exposure to cold.

Investigations

- **Red cells** agglutinate in the cold or at room temperature.
- **Direct antiglobulin test** is positive with complement alone.
- **Monoclonal IgM antibodies.**

Treatment
Rituximab (anti-CD20) is successful in some cases. It does not respond to steroids alkylating agents and splenectomy.

Paroxysmal Cold Hemoglobinuria

Q. Write short essay/note on paroxysmal cold hemoglobinuria.

- Paroxysmal cold hemoglobinuria (PCH) is a rare condition which often follows common childhood viral infections (e.g., measles, mumps, and chickenpox).
- The autoantibodies are IgG type and bind to red cells at low temperatures and fix the complement. These are autoantibodies directed against the P antigen system on red cells.
- Since complement cascade functions more efficiently at 37°C, upon warming, complement gets activated resulting in intravascular hemolysis and hemoglobinuria.
- **Donath-Landsteiner test:** Hemolysis is demonstrated in vitro by incubating the patient's red cells and serum at 4°C and then warming it to 37°C.
- Hemolysis is usually transient and found mostly in children. Supportive transfusions of warmed blood may be required.
- DAT is usually negative.

Anemias Due to Blood Loss

Q. Write short essay/note on anemias due to blood loss.

Anemias due to blood loss can be acute or chronic. Blood loss causes anemia by two main mechanisms:
1. By the direct loss of RBCs
2. Continuous blood loss gradually depletes the iron stores resulting in iron deficiency.

Anemias Due to Acute Blood Loss

A healthy adult can lose about 500 mL of whole blood without any untoward effect (e.g., blood donation). Acute blood loss (hemorrhage) causes loss of intravascular volume over a short period and if massive it can lead to hypovolemic shock and death. The clinical features of acute blood loss anemia depend on:
- Rate of hemorrhage
- Nature of the bleeding (external or internal).

Clinical features

After the sudden loss of a large volume of blood over a short period, three clinical/pathophysiologic stages can be identified.
1. Stage 1: The dominant feature is hypovolemia during which the patient appears pale, cold, and sweating. The pulse rate is raised and blood pressure is maintained. The earliest signs, especially with internal bleeding, are postural hypotension and tachycardia. An ordinary blood count will not show anemia because the hemoglobin concentration is not affected.
2. Stage 2: During this stage, the body will shift fluid from the extravascular to the intravascular compartment, producing hemodilution. Thus, the hypovolemia gradually converts to anemia. Anemia appears in 24–36 hours.
3. Stage 3:
   - If bleeding stops, anemia gets corrected in a few weeks, provided body iron supply is normal.
   - If bleeding continues, compensatory mechanisms fail and hypovolemic shock develops and results in death.

Investigations
- Hemoglobin and hematocrit:
  - Normal in early stages (before hemodilution)
  - Reduced in 24–36 hours due to hemodilution
- Peripheral smear shows normocytic normochromic anemia and polychromasia (due to increased reticulocytes). A transient leukoerythroblastic blood picture may be seen in very early stages.

Treatment
Replacement of blood loss by transfusion of whole blood or packed red cells.

Anemia Due to Chronic Blood Loss

In chronic blood loss, compensatory mechanisms replenish the plasma volume and red cell loss. It produces anemia when the rate of blood loss exceeds the regenerative capacity of the bone marrow or when iron reserves are depleted and results in iron deficiency anemia.

Anemia of Chronic Disease

Q. Write short essay/note on anemia of chronic disease.

It is one of the most common types of anemia in developing countries, occurring in patients with chronic infections (also known as anemia of inflammation).

Causes

It occurs in a wide variety of chronic diseases.
- **Chronic infections:** Infective endocarditis, tuberculosis, osteomyelitis
- **Chronic immune disorders:** Crohn's disease, rheumatoid arthritis, systemic lupus erythematosus (SLE)
- **Associated with malignant tumors** (e.g., carcinoma of lung and breast)
  Term anemia of chronic disease is not usually applied to anemias associated with renal, hepatic, or endocrine disorders.

Pathogenesis

- **Impaired iron utilization:** Chronic inflammatory diseases activate macrophages to secrete cytokines such as interleukin-6 (IL-6) and tumor necrosis factor (TNF). There is decreased transfer of iron from the storage pool to bone erythroid precursors.
- **Decreased erythropoietin** (EPO) **production and response:** They result in inadequate proliferation of progenitors.
- **Decreased RBC survival** is due to extracorpuscular defect.

Investigations

- Peripheral smear mainly shows normocytic normochromic red cells.
- **Increased storage iron** in the marrow and revealed by Prussian blue staining

- **Raised serum ferritin** because of the inflammatory process
- **Reduced total iron-binding capacity** (TIBC)
- **Reduced serum iron**
- Reduced transferrin levels
- Normal serum soluble transferrin receptor level.

Management
- Treat the underlying disorder.
- Recombinant erythropoietin therapy may be tried if the anemia is not corrected after treatment of the underlying disorder.

Aplastic Anemia

Q. Define aplastic anemia. Discuss the etiology/causes, clinical features, investigations, and management of aplastic anemia.

Definition

Aplastic anemia is characterized by pancytopenia (anemia, neutropenia, and thrombocytopenia) with hypocellular (aplasia) bone marrow (less than 30% cellularity), and there are no leukemic or other abnormal cells in the peripheral blood or bone marrow.

Causes

See **Table 8.18.**

TABLE 8.18: Common causes of aplastic anemia.

Inherited	
Fanconi anemia Diamond-Black fan anemia Telomerase defects	
Acquired	
Idiopathic Acquired defects in stem cell Immune mediated	
Secondary ➢ ***Chemical Agents*** – **Dose related:** Cytotoxic drugs (alkylating agents, antimetabolites), Benzene, Inorganic arsenicals, Chloramphenicol – **Idiosyncratic:** Chloramphenicol, Phenylbutazone, Penicillamine, Carbamazepine, Gold salts, Organic arsenicals, Methylphenylethylhydantoin	➢ ***Physical Agents:*** Whole-body irradiation ➢ ***Viral Infections*** ➢ Hepatitis (unknown type) – Epstein-Barr virus infections – Cytomegalovirus infections – Herpes zoster (Varicella zoster) – HIV

Clinical Features

It is insidious in onset and the initial presenting feature depends on which cell line is predominantly affected.
- Anemia: Causes progressive weakness, lassitude, fatigability, pallor, and dyspnea
- Neutropenia: Presents as frequent infections (mucocutaneous bacterial) or fatal infections. These include sore throat, oral and pharyngeal ulcers, fever with chills and sweating, chronic skin infections, recurrent respiratory infections, pneumonia, and septicemia.
- Thrombocytopenia: Results in bleeding manifestations in the form of petechiae, bruises, and ecchymoses. These include: bleeding into skin (ecchymoses, petechiae), epistaxis, menorrhagia, bleeding from gums and GI tract, retinal hemorrhage, and cerebral hemorrhage. Bleeding is often the predominant initial presentation with bruising, with minimal trauma or blood blisters in the mouth.

Physical findings: These include ecchymoses, bleeding gums, and epistaxis. Mouth infections are common. Lymphadenopathy and **hepatosplenomegaly** are **rare.** In the presence of splenomegaly, the diagnosis of aplastic anemia should not be made.
- Aplastic anemia may coexist or progress to clonal disorders, such as paroxysmal nocturnal hemoglobinuria (PNH), myelodysplastic syndrome (MDS), or acute myeloid leukemia.

Fanconi's Anemia

- Fanconi's anemia is inherited as an autosomal recessive disorder.
- It is associated with skeletal (short stature), renal (ectopic kidney, horse-shoe kidney), and central nervous system (hydrocephalus) abnormalities. It usually presents between 5 and 10 years of age. Progressive pancytopenia, predisposition to hematologic malignancies (MDS < acute myeloid leukemia), and solid tumors (squamous cell carcinomas of head and neck and anogenital region) are found.

Investigations

Diagnosis is made with: (1) pancytopenia, (2) absence of reticulocytes, and (3) hypocellular or aplastic bone marrow with increased fat spaces.

- **Hemoglobin is decreased.**
- **PCV is decreased.**
- **Reticulocytopenia** (varies from 0.5 to 1%) is a characteristic feature.
- **Peripheral blood** shows pancytopenia.
- **Bone marrow study:** Marked hypocellularity with replacement of more than 70% of the marrow cells by fat. Hematopoiesis: Paucity of all erythroid, myeloid, and megakaryocytic precursors. Initial stages may show focal areas of hematopoiesis. Lymphocytes and plasma cells are prominent. Bone marrow iron stores are usually increased.
- Serum iron and transferrin saturation: Increased
- Ferrokinetic studies: Delayed clearance of radioactive iron from the blood and increased uptake by the liver.

Severe aplastic anemia

The presence of two of the following four features is needed to diagnose severe aplasia: (1) neutrophil count of $<0.5 \times 10^9$/L, (2) platelet count of $<20 \times 10^9$/L, (3) reticulocyte count of $<40 \times 10^9$/L, and (4) marrow cellularity <25%.

Treatment/Management

Removal of the causative factor/agent wherever possible (refer to causes of aplastic anemia in **Table 8.18**).

Providing supportive care while awaiting bone marrow recovery:

- Prevention and treatment of infections
- Treatment of hemorrhage
- Treatment of anemia by red cell transfusion
- **Growth factors:** Granulocyte colony-stimulating factor (G-CSF), Thrombopoietin (TPO) receptor agonists

Severe aplastic anemia

- **Bone marrow (stem cell) transplantation** is the treatment of choice for patients under 40 years of age who have an HLA-identical sibling donor. Patients over the age of 40 years have a high risk of graft-versus-host disease.
- **Immunosuppressive therapy** is used for patients without HLA-matched siblings and those above 40 years of age.
  - Eltrombopag, horse ATG, cyclosporine, and prednisone in combination produce a hematological response rate of 60–80%. These agents destroy activated suppressor cells.
  - Androgens (e.g., oxymetholone) are sometimes useful in patients not responding to immunosuppression and those with moderately severe aplastic anemia.
  - Steroids have little role in severe aplastic anemia but are useful for serum sickness induced by ALG. However, steroids used in children with congenital pure red cell aplasia (Diamond-Blackfan syndrome) and in some adults with pure red cell aplasia are associated with a thymoma.
  - Anti-IL-2 receptor antibody (daclizumab) and arsenic trioxide (ATO) plus cyclosporine have been tried.

Acquired Pure Red Cell Aplasia (PRCA) may develop for unknown reasons, but more commonly it develops in association with specific types of malignancy, infection, or drugs. Most commonly, acquired PRCA develops as a complication of a neoplastic process such as a thymoma B- or T-cell chronic lymphocytic leukemia, non-Hodgkin's lymphoma, or an autoimmune disorder such as rheumatoid arthritis or SLE.

Investigation of a case of anemia is presented in **Flowchart 8.1.**

Pancytopenia

Q. Write short essay/note on the causes of pancytopenia.

Definition: Combination of anemia, leukopenia, and thrombocytopenia.

Causes of Pancytopenia (Table 8.19)

TABLE 8.19: Causes of pancytopenia.

➤ **Decreased bone marrow function** – Aplastic anemia ◆ Idiopathic ◆ Secondary ◆ Inherited ➤ Myelodysplastic syndromes (MDS) ➤ Bone marrow infiltration with: – Leukemia (e.g. Hairy cell leukemia) – Lymphoma – Myeloma	◆ Tumors (carcinoma) ◆ Granulomatous diseases (e.g., disseminated tuberculosis, sarcoidosis) – Nutritional deficiencies: ◆ **Megaloblastic anemia** (vitamin B_{12} and folic acid deficiency) – Paroxysmal nocturnal hemoglobinuria – Myelofibrosis (rare) – Others: Hemophagocytic syndrome, overwhelming sepsis, systemic lupus erythematosus – Drugs ➤ **Increased peripheral destruction** – Hypersplenism

FLOWCHART 8.1: Investigation of a case of anemia.

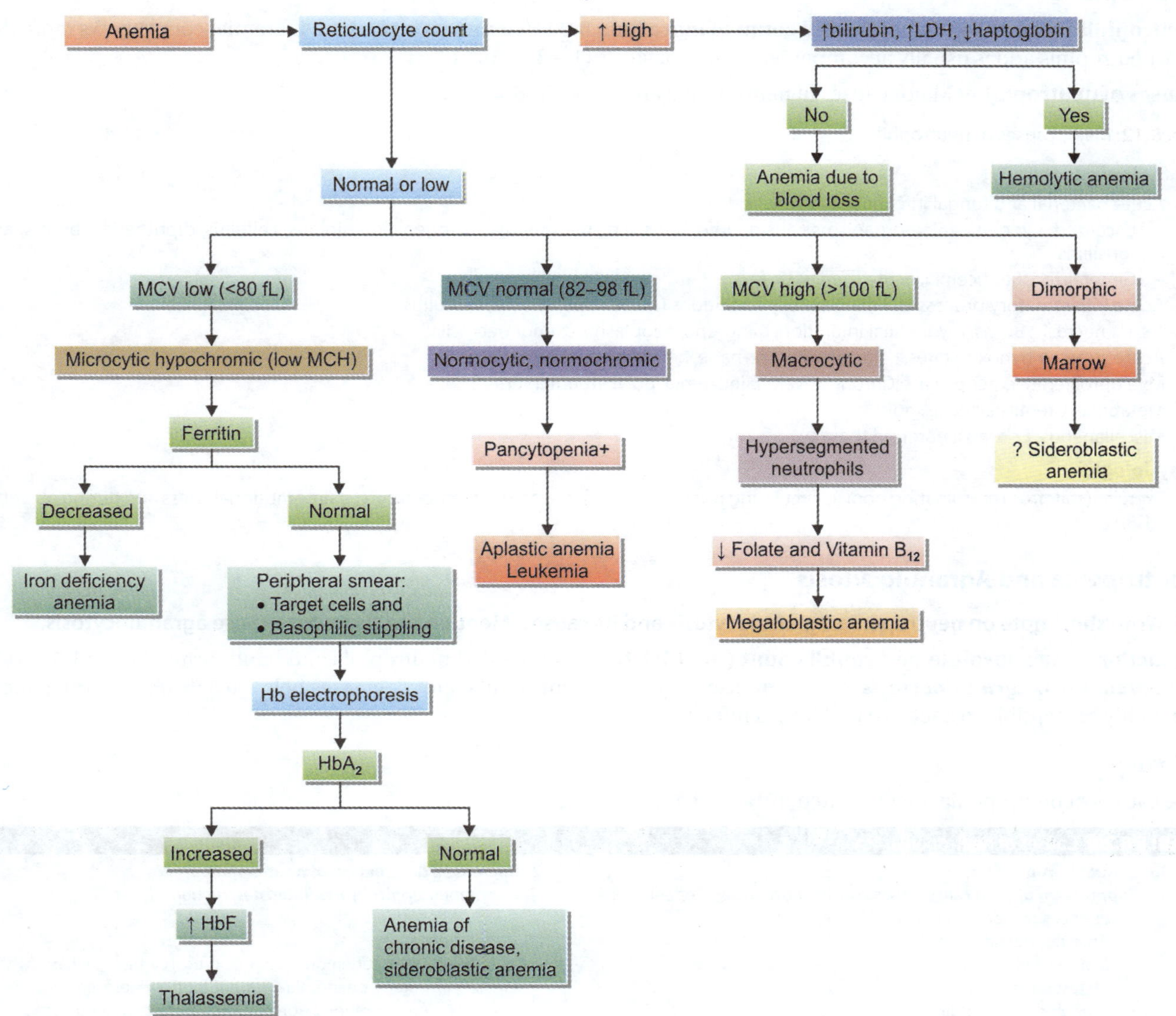

DISORDERS OF WHITE BLOOD CELL

NON-NEOPLASTIC DISORDERS OF WBC LEUKOCYTOSIS

Q. Write short note on leukocytosis.

An increase in the **total** number of **leukocytes** in the blood **more than 11,000/cu mm** (11×10^9/L). It is usually due to increase in the neutrophils but may also be due to increased lymphocytes (or rarely monocytes and eosinophils).

Causes: Common causes of leukocytosis are shown in **Box 8.10**.

Box 8.10: Common causes of leukocytosis.

- Infections
  - Bacterial
  - Viral infections (e.g., infectious mononucleosis)
- Leukemia
  - Acute
  - Chronic: Chronic lymphocytic leukemia and chronic myeloid leukemia
- Leukemoid reactions
- Physiological
  - Pregnancy
  - Exercise

Leukopenia

Total leukocyte count is less than 4,000/cu mm (4×10^9/L).

Causes: Common causes of leukopenia are shown in **Box 8.11**.

Box 8.11: Common causes of leukopenia.

- Typhoid and paratyphoid
- Anemia
  - Aplastic anemia
  - Megaloblastic anemia
- Hypersplenism
- Drugs including cytotoxic drugs
- Radiation
- Rarely leukemia

Neutrophilia

Neutrophilia is an absolute neutrophil count of more than 8,000/cu mm (8 × 10^9/L). Differential count shows more than 70% neutrophils and is usually accompanied by leukocytosis (15–30 × 10^9/L).

Causes of neutrophilia: Major causes of neutrophilia are shown in **Box 8.12**.

Box 8.12: Major causes of neutrophilia.

Pathological:
- Acute bacterial and fungal infections:
  - Localized: Pyogenic microorganisms causing infections, e.g., pneumonias, pyogenic meningitis, cellulitis, diphtheria, abscess, and tonsillitis
  - Generalized: Septicemia, acute rheumatic fever
- Acute inflammatory processes: Inflammatory conditions (acute appendicitis), vasculitis
- Tissue necrosis: Burns, myocardial infarction, gangrene, neoplasms (tumor necrosis)
- Acute stress or hypoxic states: Following hemorrhage, hemolysis and surgery
- Myeloproliferative neoplasms: Chronic myeloid leukemia, polycythemia vera
- Metabolic: Uremia, acidosis, gout
- Miscellaneous: Eclampsia, steroid therapy

Physiological:
- Exercise (shift from marginating pool to circulating pool), newborns, extremes of temperature, pain, emotional stress and during obstetric labor

Neutropenia and Agranulocytosis

Q. Write short note on neutropenia/agranulocytosis and its causes. Mention the drugs that cause agranulocytosis.

Reduction in the absolute neutrophil count (total WBC × % segmented neutrophils and band forms) below 1.5 × **10^9/L (1,500/cu mm).** ***Agranulocytosis*** is the term used when the neutrophil count decreases below 0.5 × 10^9/L. These patients are highly susceptible to bacterial and fungal infections.

Etiology

The causes of neutropenia are presented in **Table 8.20**.

TABLE 8.20: Causes of neutropenia.

1. Inadequate production: ➢ ***Suppression of stem cells:*** In these disorders, granulocytopenia represents a component of pancytopenia – Aplastic anemia – Marrow infiltration – Metastatic tumors – Granulomatous disorders ➢ ***Suppression of committed granulocytic precursors*** – Drugs and chemicals (e.g., sulfonamides, analgesics, arsenicals) – Ionizing radiation ➢ ***Diseases associated with ineffective hematopoiesis*** – Megaloblastic anemias: Vitamin B_{12} or folate deficiency – Myelodysplastic syndromes ➢ ***Congenital:*** Kostmann syndrome (rare) ➢ ***Severe infections*** – Bacterial (e.g., typhoid, paratyphoid, septicemia) – Viral (e.g., influenza, infectious mononucleosis, hepatitis, measles) – Rickettsial (e.g., scrub typhus) – Protozoal (e.g., malaria, kala-azar)	**2. Increased destruction of neutrophils:** ➢ ***Immunologically mediated destruction*** – Idiopathic – Secondary ◆ Drugs (Chemotherapeutic drugs, carbimazole, propylthiouracil, phenothiazines, antibiotics, naproxen) ◆ Autoimmune disorders: For example, systemic lupus erythematosus ➢ **Splenic sequestration** may be associated with pancytopenia. **3. Shift from the circulating pool to marginating pool:** Hemodialysis and cardiopulmonary bypass **4. Idiopathic:** ➢ Hodgkin and non-Hodgkin lymphoma ➢ Chronic lymphocytic leukemia ➢ Viral infections (HIV, hepatitis) ➢ Cyclic neutropenia

Treatment of neutropenia/agranulocytosis (*refer* Oncology Chapter).

Eosinophilia

Q. Define eosinophilia and mention the causes of eosinophilia.

Eosinophilia is an absolute **eosinophil count of more than 450/cu mm** (0.45 × 10^9/L). Causes of eosinophilia are presented in **Table 8.21**.

Lymphocytosis

Q. Write short note on lymphocytosis and its causes.

Lymphocytosis is lymphocyte count more than 4,000/cu mm (4 × 10^9/L) in adults and more than 8,000/cu mm (8 × 10^9/L) in a child. The common causes of lymphocytosis are given in **Table 8.22**.

TABLE 8.21: Causes of eosinophilia.

➢ **Allergic/atopic conditions** – Asthma – Urticaria – Hay fever – Drug reactions – Allergic rhinitis ➢ **Parasitic/helminthic infestations (with tissue invasion)** – Roundworm infestation – Hookworm infestation – Filariasis ➢ **Fungal infections** (e.g., coccidioidomycosis) ➢ **Skin diseases** – Dermatitis (eczema) – Pemphigus – Scabies – Dermatitis herpetiformis	➢ **Hematological diseases** – Chronic myeloid leukemia – Polycythemia – Hodgkin lymphoma – Acute myelomonocytic leukemia – Eosinophilic leukemia ➢ **Miscellaneous** – Tropical eosinophilia – Pulmonary eosinophilia – *Löffler syndrome* – Hypereosinophilic syndrome – Eosinophilic granuloma – Drugs: Sulfonamides, aspirin, penicillins, cephalosporins, allopurinol, carbamazepine

TABLE 8.22: Causes of lymphocytosis.

1. Acute infections – Viral infections – Infectious mononucleosis, mumps, measles, chickenpox, infectious hepatitis – Toxoplasmosis
2. Chronic infections/inflammatory diseases – Tuberculosis – Syphilis – Brucellosis – Inflammatory bowel disease: Crohn's disease and ulcerative colitis
3. Hematologic malignancies – Acute lymphoblastic leukemia – Chronic lymphocytic leukemia – Non-Hodgkin lymphoma with spillover – Adult T-cell leukemia/lymphoma – Hairy cell leukemia

Basophils

Conditions associated with alterations in numbers of blood basophils are presented in **Table 8.23**.

TABLE 8.23: Conditions associated with alterations in numbers of blood basophils.

➢ **Decreased numbers (basopenia)** – Hereditary absence of basophils (very rare) – Elevated levels of glucocorticoids – Hyperthyroidism or treatment with thyroid hormones	– Ovulation – Hypersensitivity reactions – Leukocytosis (in association with diverse disorders)
➢ **Increased numbers (basophilia)** – Allergy or inflammation ◆ Ulcerative colitis ◆ Drug, food, inhalant hypersensitivity ◆ Erythroderma, urticaria ◆ Juvenile rheumatoid arthritis	– Endocrinopathy ◆ Diabetes mellitus ◆ Estrogen administration ◆ Hypothyroidism (myxedema)
➢ Infection – Chickenpox – Influenza – Smallpox – Tuberculosis ➢ Iron deficiency	– Exposure to ionizing radiation – Neoplasia ◆ Basophilic leukemia ◆ Myeloproliferative neoplasms (especially chronic myelogenous leukemia; also polycythemia vera, primary myelofibrosis, essential thrombocythemia) ◆ Carcinoma

ACUTE LEUKEMIAS

Q. Define leukemia.

Definition

Leukemia is defined as a group of malignant stem cell neoplasms characterized by:
- Failure of cell maturation and proliferating of leukocyte precursors (blast/immature cells) which fill the bone marrow
- Abnormal numbers and forms of immature white blood cells which ultimately spill over into the peripheral blood.

Classification of Leukemias

Q. Write short essay/note on classification of leukemias.

1. **General/traditional classification:** According to the light microscopic appearance of the cell and the speed of evolution **(Table 8.24)**
2. **Revised French-American-British (FAB) classification of acute leukemias (Table 8.25)**
   - According to FAB, the marrow should show a blast count of 30% or more.
   - It includes parameters which affect morphology, cytochemistry, immunophenotyping, cytogenetics, and molecular genetics.
3. **WHO classification (2016) of acute myeloid (Table 8.26) and lymphoid leukemia (Table 8.27)**.
   - WHO classification of acute leukemia incorporates parameters, namely morphology, cytochemistry, cytogenetic, molecular genetics (which are related to prognosis), and clinical features.
   - The number of blasts necessary for the diagnosis is more than 20% in bone marrow when compared to 30% in FAB classification.

TABLE 8.24: Traditional classification of leukemia.

Acute	*Chronic*
Acute myeloblastic/myelocytic leukemia (AML)	Chronic myeloid leukemia (CML)
Acute lymphoblastic/lymphocytic leukemia (ALL)	Chronic lymphocytic leukemia (CLL)

TABLE 8.25: Revised FAB classification of acute leukemias.

Type of AML	*Type of ALL*
M0: Minimally differentiated AML M1: AML without differentiation M2: AML with maturation M3: Acute promyelocytic leukemia M4: Acute myelomonocytic leukemia M5: Acute monocytic leukemia M6: Acute erythroleukemia (Di Guglielmo's disease) M7: Acute megakaryocytic leukemia	L1: Small cells with homogeneous nuclear chromatin and scanty cytoplasm L2: Large, heterogeneous cells with variable amount of cytoplasm L3: Large, homogeneous cells with prominent nucleoli, abundant, and deeply basophilic vacuolated cytoplasm

TABLE 8.26: WHO classification (2016) of acute myeloid leukemia and related precursor neoplasms.

Class	*FAB category*	*Prognosis*
➢ **AML with recurrent genetic abnormalities**		
AML with t(8;21)(q22;q22); *RUNX1-RUNX1T1*	M2	Favorable Favorable
AML with inv(16)(p13;1q22) or t(16;16)(p13.1;q22); *CBFB-MYH11*	M4eo M3, M3v M4,	Intermediate
APL with t(15;17)(q22;q12); *PML-RARA* AML with t(9;11)(p22;q23); *MLLT3-MLL* AML with t(6;9)(p23;q34);	M5	Intermediate Poor
DEK-NUP214	–	Poor Variable
AML with inv(3)(q21q26.2) *or t(3;3)(q21.3;q26.2); GATA2, MECOM*	–	Favorable Favorable
AML (megakaryoblastic) with t(1;22) (p13;q13); *RBM15-MKL1*	–	
AML with mutated *NPM1*	Variable	
AML with mutated *CEBPA*		
➢ **AML not otherwise specified**		
AML minimally differentiated	M0 M1 M2 M4	Intermediate
AML without maturation	M5a, M5b M6a, M6b	Intermediate
AML with maturation	M7	Intermediate
Acute myelomonocytic leukemia	–	Intermediate
Acute monoblastic and monocytic leukemia	–	Intermediate
Acute erythroid leukemia		Intermediate
Acute megakaryoblastic leukemia		Intermediate Poor
Acute basophilic leukemia		Poor
Acute panmyelosis with myelofibrosis		
➢ **Myeloid sarcoma**	–	–
➢ **Myeloid proliferation related to Down syndrome**		
Transient abnormal myelopoiesis	–	–
Myeloid leukemia associated with Down syndrome	–	Variable

(AML: acute myeloid leukemia; APL: acute promyelocytic leukemia; MDS: myelodysplastic syndrome)

TABLE 8.27: WHO classification (2016) of acute lymphoblastic leukemia.

B-cell lymphoblastic leukemia/lymphoma, not otherwise specified
B-cell lymphoblastic leukemia/lymphoma, with recurrent genetic abnormalities
➢ B-cell lymphoblastic leukemia/lymphoma with hypodiploidy ➢ B-cell lymphoblastic leukemia/lymphoma with hyperdiploidy ➢ B-cell lymphoblastic leukemia/lymphoma with t(9;22)(q34;q11.2)[*BCR-ABL1*] ➢ B-cell lymphoblastic leukemia/lymphoma with t(v;11q23)[*MLL* rearranged] ➢ B-cell lymphoblastic leukemia/lymphoma with t(12;21)(p13;q22)[*ETV6-RUNX1*] ➢ B-cell lymphoblastic leukemia/lymphoma with t(1;19)(q23;p13.3)[*TCF3-PBX1*] ➢ B-cell lymphoblastic leukemia/lymphoma with t(5;14)(q31;q32)[*IL3-IGH*] ➢ B-cell lymphoblastic leukemia/lymphoma with intrachromosomal amplification of chromosome 21 (iAMP21) ➢ B-cell lymphoblastic leukemia/lymphoma with translocations involving tyrosine kinases or cytokine receptors ("BCR-ABL1–like ALL")
T-cell lymphoblastic leukemia/lymphomas
➢ Early T-cell precursor lymphoblastic leukemia

(ALL: acute lymphoblastic leukemia; WHO: World Health Organization)

Etiology of Leukemias

Q. Discuss the etiology of leukemias.

Risk Factors

In the majority of acute leukemias, the cause is not known. Numerous risk factors may cause mutations in the genes involved in regulating cell proliferation and differentiation.

These genes include oncogenes and tumor suppressor genes. Sophisticated molecular techniques such as fluorescent in situ hybridization (FISH) and gene array technology have led to the understanding of leukemia at the molecular level.

Environmental factors

- **Ionizing radiation:** Ionizing radiation and X-rays are associated with increased risk of leukemias. The evidence for this association is:
  - **Atomic bombing:** Survivors of atomic bomb explosions in Hiroshima and Nagasaki, who had high incidence of AML and CML (chronic myeloid leukemia).
  - **Therapeutic radiation:** Increased risk of AML (secondary leukemia) in patients with malignancies/neoplasms treated by radiation.
  - **X-ray exposure to fetus during pregnancy**.
- **Drugs:** Drugs can cause secondary hematopoietic neoplasms.
  - Secondary AML can develop after exposure to chemotherapy drugs.
  - Alkylating agents such as cyclophosphamide can lead to AML that develops after a median duration of 5-7 years, is usually preceded by myelodysplastic syndrome, and is associated with chromosome 5 or 7 abnormalities.
  - Topoisomerase inhibitors such as anthracyclines lead to AML after a median duration of 1–3 years and are associated with MLL gene abnormalities.
- **Chemicals:**
  - Benzene used in paint industry, plastic glues, etc. It causes chromosomal abnormalities resulting in a higher incidence of acute leukemia, myelodysplastic syndrome, and aplastic anemia.
- **Retroviruses: Human T-cell leukemia virus (**HTLV-1) is associated with adult T-cell leukemia/lymphoma.
- **Immunological:** Immune deficiency states (e.g., hypogammaglobulinemia).

Genetic disorders

A few genetic disorders may be associated with acute leukemias, e.g., Down's syndrome (ALL or AML), Fanconi's anemia (AML), ataxia telangiectasia (ALL, NHL), and Klinefelter syndrome.

Acquired disorders

- Acquired stem cell disorders such as PNH and aplastic anemia may transform into acute leukemia.
- Myelodysplastic syndrome (MDS): AML may develop de novo or secondary to MDS.

Clinical Features

Q. Discuss the clinical features, investigations, diagnosis, and management of acute leukemias.

- Though ALL and AML are distinct (immunophenotypically and genotypically), they usually have similar clinical features. A patient usually presents with nonspecific "flu-like" symptoms.
- Majority of patients with acute leukemia, regardless of subtype, present with symptoms arising from:
  - **Bone marrow failure:** It is due to replacement of normal marrow hematopoietic cells by leukemic blast cells.
    - **Anemia**
      - It causes shortness of breath on effort, excessive tiredness/fatigue, and weakness.
    - **Neutropenia**
      - It results in life-threatening infections by bacteria or opportunistic fungi, *Pseudomonas* and commensals. Fever is due to septicemia.
      - The infection may develop in the oral cavity, skin, lungs, kidneys, urinary bladder, and colon. The common presentations include respiratory infections (pneumonia), cellulitis, or sepsis.
    - **Thrombocytopenia**
      - It presents as bleeding manifestations in the form of petechiae, atraumatic ecchymosis, gum bleeding, epistaxis, urinary tract, and fundal hemorrhages.
      - Intracranial bleeding is a serious and fatal complication, usually associated with headache, fundal hemorrhages, and focal neurological deficits.
    - Marrow expansion and infiltration of the subperiosteum cause:
      - Bone pain (more common in ALL) and sternal tenderness.
  - **Leukostasis:** Stasis of blood flow may develop when the blast count is above 50,000/cu mm.
    - Cerebral leukostasis may cause headache, confusion, and visual disturbances.
    - Pulmonary leukostasis can cause dyspnea at rest, tachypnea, chest pain, pulmonary infarction, and acute respiratory distress syndrome.
  - **Coagulopathy:** Both disseminated intravascular coagulation (DIC) and primary fibrinolysis may lead to hemorrhagic diathesis. DIC is observed in AML-M3 (promyelocytic leukemia).
  - **Extramedullary leukemic infiltration:**
    - Gingival hypertrophy and infiltration of skin (leukemia cutis/chloroma) **(Figs. 8.28A and B)**
- Hepatosplenomegaly
- Generalized lymphadenopathy

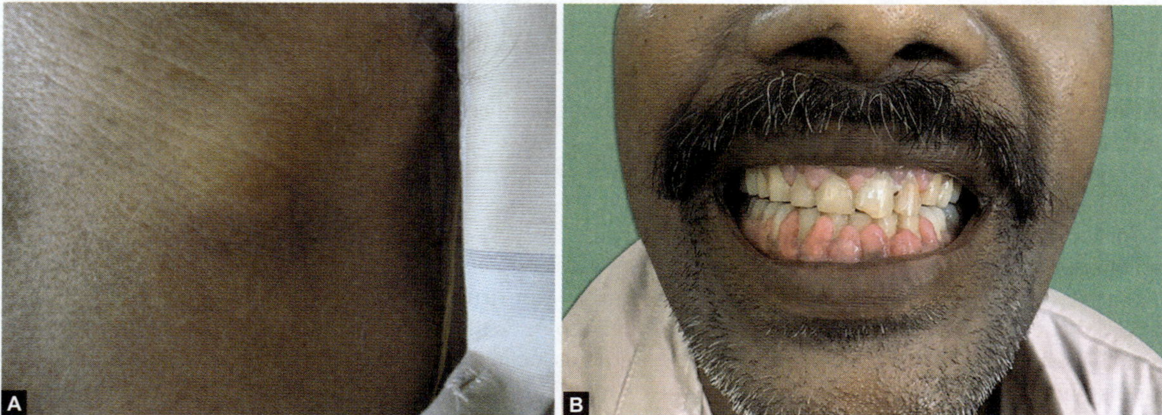

FIGS. 8.28A AND B: Choroma and gingival hyperplasia.

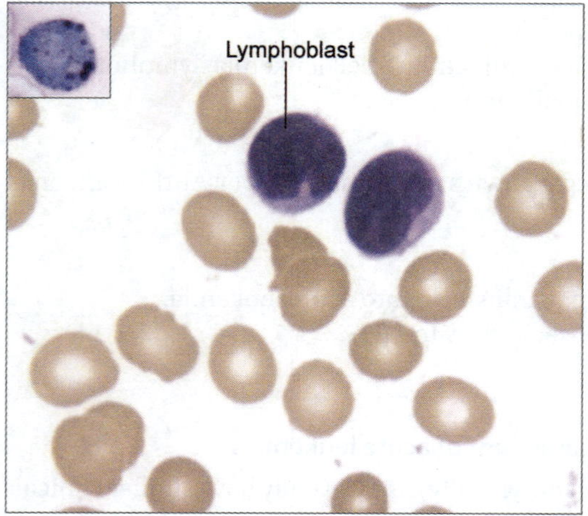

FIG. 8.29: Peripheral blood smear in acute lymphoblastic leukemia showing lymphoblasts. Inset shows lymphoblast with block positivity with PAS stain.

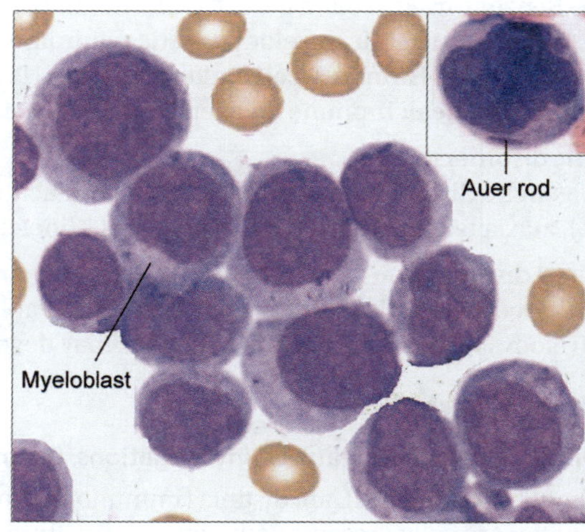

FIG. 8.30: Peripheral smear in AML with myeloblasts. Inset shows myeloblast with Auer rod.

- Leukemic meningitis is rare. It presents as headache and nausea. As the disease progresses, papilledema, cranial nerve palsies, seizures, and altered consciousness develop. CSF characteristically shows leukemic blast cells, elevated proteins, and reduced glucose levels.
- **Chloromas** are localized, solid, soft-tissue tumor masses known as myeloblastomas, granulocytic sarcomas, or chloromas.
  - **Metabolic abnormalities:** Hyperuricemia, elevated serum liver transaminases, and serum LDH are found in patients with acute leukemia.

Investigations

Q. Write short essay on laboratory diagnosis of acute myeloid leukemia. What are Auer rods?

Confirmation of Diagnosis

- **Blood count**
  - Hemoglobin is low.
  - Total leukocyte count: Markedly raised, but usually less than 100×10^9/L (range 1×10^9/L to 500×10^9/L). Leukopenia is common in AML.
  - Platelet count: It is markedly decreased.
- **Peripheral blood smear**
  - It shows numerous **blast cells (Figs. 8.29 and 8.30)**, and types of blasts can be identified morphologically and confirmed with immunophenotyping.
  - **Auer rods** are seen as rod-shaped red inclusion in the cytoplasm of myeloblast.
  - It shows severe normochromic anemia.
- **Bone marrow aspirate:** Hypercellular with reduced erythropoiesis and reduced megakaryocytes. **Blast cells >20%** (often approaching 100%) and type of blast is confirmed by flow cytometry, immunophenotyping (FISH), cytogenetic, and molecular genetics.

Flow cytometry

Q. Write short note on flow cytometry in leukemias.

- Flow cytometric immunophenotyping is useful in diagnosing the lineage in acute leukemia by the expression of lineage-specific CD markers.
- Flow cytometry allows the detection of 1 leukemic cell among 10,000 normal cells **(0.01%)**.
- Common antibodies used in flow cytometric immunophenotyping of acute leukemia are: stem cell/hematopoietic precursors (CD34, HLA-DR, terminal deoxynucleotidyl transferase/TdT), myeloid markers (cMPO, CD13, CD33, CD117, CD15), monocytic markers (CD64, CD14, CD11b,CD11c, lysozyme), erythroid (CD71, CD235a), megakaryocytic (CD41, CD61, CD36), B lymphoid markers (CD19, CD10, CD20, CD22, cCD79a), T lymphoid markers (CD3, CD5, CD7, CD1a,CD2, CD4, CD8), and natural killer (NK) cells (CD56).
  - Therapeutic application—targeted therapy (e.g., Rituximab if anti-CD20 positive, Alemtuzumab if anti-CD52 positive), purging malignant cells from autografts before transplantation

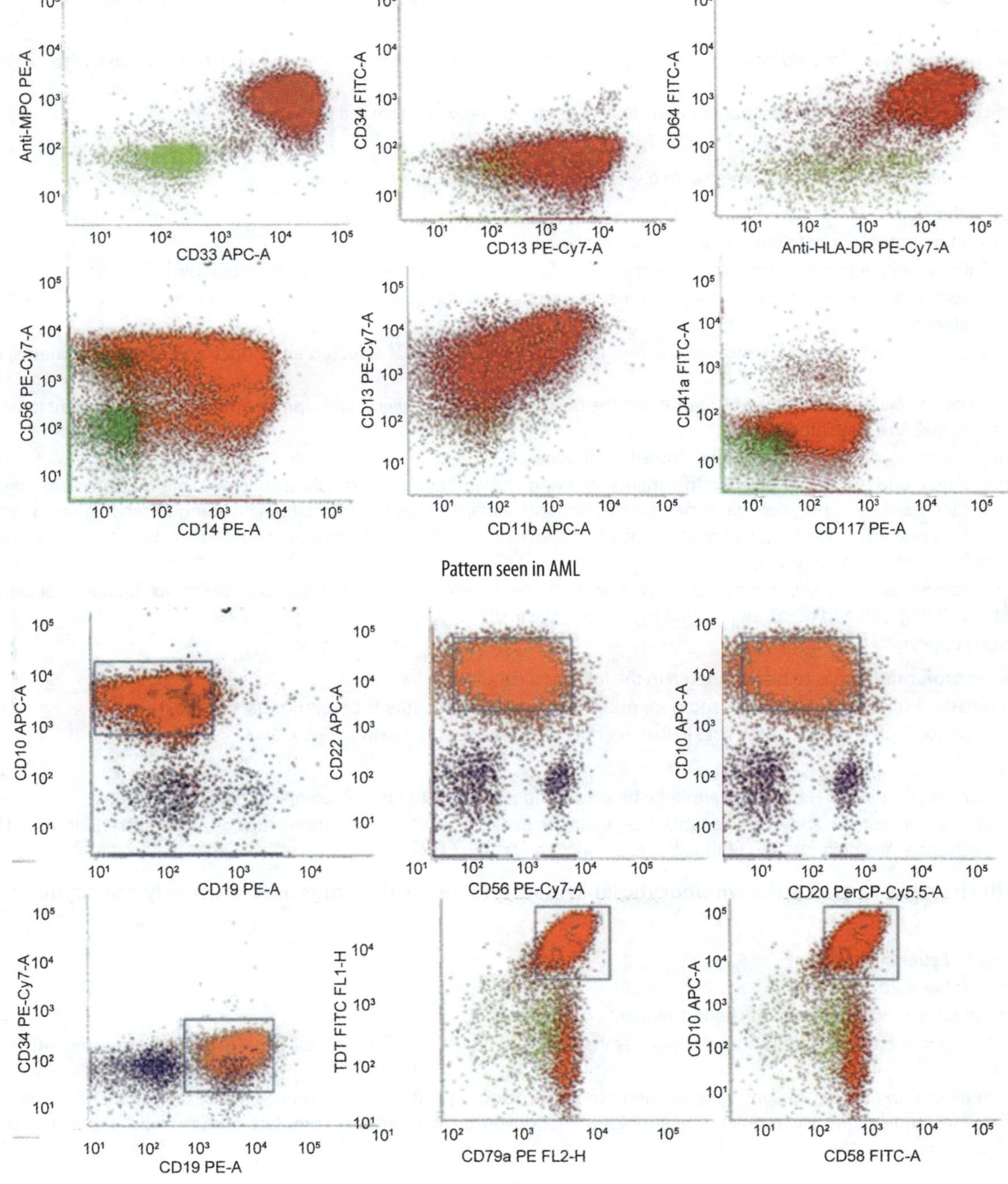

Flow cytometry pattern seen in ALL

- **Chest X-ray:** Mediastinal widening is often seen in T lymphoblastic leukemia.
- **CSF examination:** This is done to rule out occult CNS involvement.

For Planning Therapy

- Biochemical parameters: Serum urate, liver function tests, renal function tests, coagulation studies, serum LDH, etc.
- Cardiac function: ECG and direct tests of left ventricular function (e.g., echocardiogram or MUGA scan)

Q. Discuss the management of acute leukemias.

Management

Principles of Management

At initial presentation, acute leukemia may be:

- Probably curable (childhood acute lymphoblastic leukemia)
- Possibly curable (de novo low-risk AML)
- Probably incurable (AML with adverse cytogenetic features in the elderly, secondary AML, recurrent acute leukemia).

Type of Therapy

- **Palliative therapy:** It is directed toward symptomatic benefit by means of medications and transfusions with or without chemotherapy.
- **Curative intent:** The goal is to cure the patient and involves chemotherapy +/- stem cell transplant.

Active therapy

The first and major decision to be taken is whether to give specific therapy or supportive therapy.

Supportive care/therapy

It forms the basis of treatment for both curative and palliative therapy.

- Treatment of anemia with repeated transfusion of packed red cells to avoid symptoms of anemia (hemoglobin >10 g/dL)
- Prevention or control of bleeding due to thrombocytopenia with platelet transfusions
- Treatment of infection:
  - *Prophylactically:* Education about handwashing and isolation facilities. Use of selected antibiotics and antifungal agents, barrier nursing
  - *Therapeutically:* Management of fever by identifying the microorganism and giving appropriate antimicrobial treatment in bacterial, fungal, protozoal, and viral infections
- Continuous monitoring of liver, kidney, and hemostatic functions
- Maintenance of fluid and electrolyte balance: In patients receiving chemotherapy, rapid lysis of leukemic cells may produce tumor lysis syndrome characterized by hyperuricemia, hyperkalemia, hypocalcemia, and hyperphosphatemia leading to renal injury, arrythmias, and seizures and is potentially life-threatening. It can be prevented by close attention to hydration, urine alkalinization, and prophylactic allopurinol before starting chemotherapy.
- Treatment of hyperleukocytosis: Reduction in leukocyte counts can be achieved by using chemotherapy or hydroxyurea, and leukapheresis (removal of circulating cells and re-infusion of leukocyte-poor plasma).
- Psychological support.

Bone marrow transplantation has to be considered in the following conditions:

1. Acute myeloblastic leukemia (Intermediate and poor risk) in first remission in patients below 60 years of age
2. Acute lymphoblastic leukemia (ALL) (high risk) in first, second, or subsequent remission

Specific therapy

The specific therapy is intended to return the peripheral blood and bone marrow to normal (complete remission—CR).

The survival outcomes of acute leukemia are variable; they could be in excess of 90% in situations such as APML and childhood ALL to as low as 10% in recurrent acute leukemia and high-risk AML.

Q. Discuss the management of acute lymphocytic leukemias. Enumerate the drugs used in acute lymphocytic leukemia.

Acute Lymphocytic Leukemia

Specific therapy **(Table 8.28)** involves:

- **Remission induction** with combination chemotherapy
  - Goal of induction therapy: To induce morphologic remission and to restore normal hematopoiesis in the bone marrow with less than 5% blasts.
  - Remission induction consists of combination chemotherapy including vincristine, prednisolone (dexamethasone), asparaginase (crisantaspase), and usually an anthracycline antibiotic, e.g., doxorubicin. It induces complete morphologic response within 4–6 weeks.

TABLE 8.28: Treatment for ALL (acute lymphoblastic leukemia).

Induction therapy
t(9;22)/BCR-ABL1 negative ALL ➢ Weekly administration of vincristine for 3–4 weeks, daily corticosteroids (prednisone, prednisolone, or dexamethasone), and asparaginase t(9;22)/BCR-ABL1 positive ALL ➢ Tyrosine kinase inhibitors (TKI) such as imatinib or dasatinib Patients with trisomy 21 ➢ High-dose methotrexate
CNS preventive therapy
➢ Triple intrathecal chemotherapy (cytarabine/methotrexate/hydrocortisone) or 1,800 cGy cranial radiation
Postremission therapy
Consolidation ➢ Cytarabine, methotrexate ➢ Anthracyclines (daunorubicin, doxorubicin) ➢ Alkylating agents (cyclophosphamide, ifosfamide) ➢ Epipodophyllotoxins (etoposide, etopophosphamide) **Allogeneic hematopoietic cell transplantation**
Maintenance therapy
➢ Daily oral 6-mercaptopurine, weekly methotrexate with periodic vincristine, prednisone, and intrathecal therapy

Recent Advances

Q. Discuss CAR-T cell therapy.

CAR T-cell therapy is an important new option for pediatric and young adult patients.

- Tisagenlecleucel is an autologous anti-CD19 **chimeric antigen receptor (CAR) T-cell therapy** recently approved by the US Food and Drug Administration for patients with refractory leukemia or those with second or later relapse.
- In this treatment strategy, a patient's own T cells are transduced to express an anti-CD19 CAR that, when reintroduced into the patient, directs specific binding and killing of CD19+ B cells.

CAR T-cell Therapy

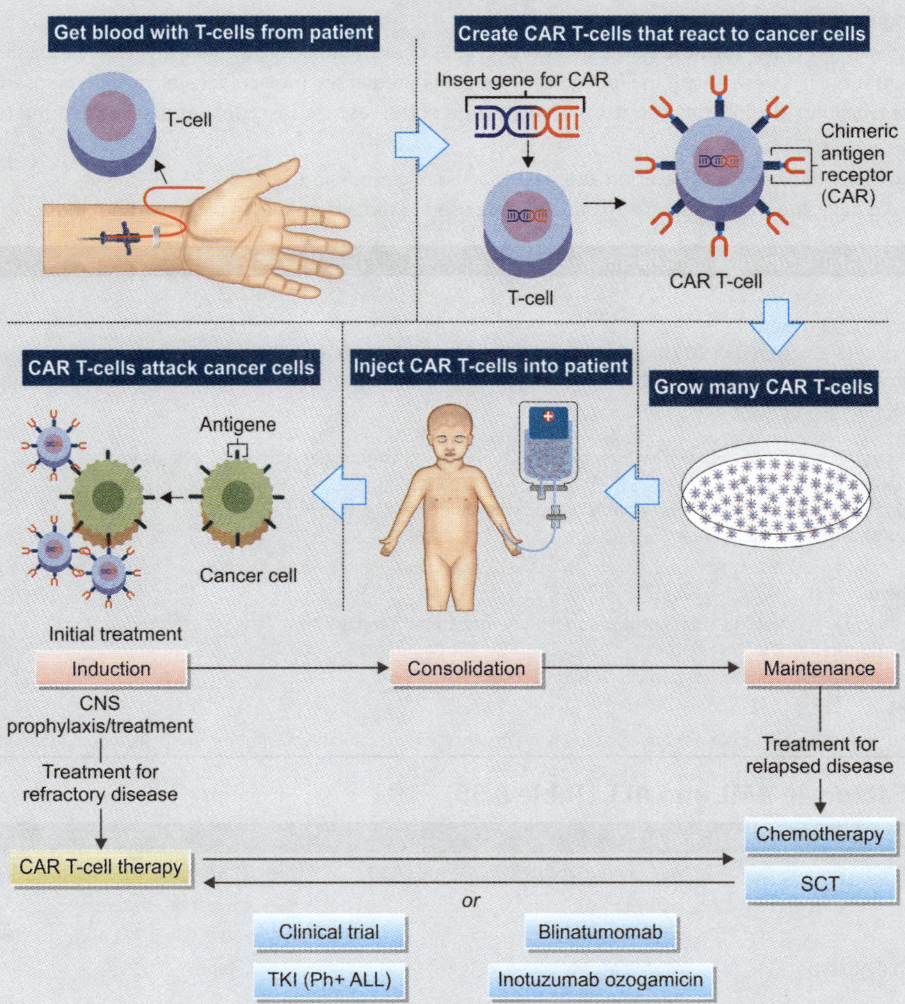

- **CNS preventive therapy** that includes administration of high-dose systemic therapy and CNS-directed treatment
  - **Aim:** To eliminate disease in the CNS and to reduce systemic minimal residual leukemic burden
  - **CNS-directed therapy:** Triple intrathecal chemotherapy (cytarabine/methotrexate/hydrocortisone) or 1,800 cGy cranial radiation
- **Postremission therapy,** similar to induction phase, reduces chances of relapse.
- **Remission maintenance** to prevent relapse and affect cure. It involves administering drugs for 2 years or more and consists of daily 6-mercaptopurine and weekly methotrexate.

Q. Discuss the management of acute myeloid leukemias.

Acute myeloid leukemia (Table 8.29)

Initial therapeutic goal is to quickly induce complete remission (CR) and further therapy to prolong survival and achieve cure. Curative therapy is given to the majority of adults below the age of 60 years (without any significant comorbidity).

Specific therapy (Table 8.29) of the newly diagnosed patient with AML is usually divided into two phases: (1) induction and (2) consolidation phase (postremission) therapy.

- **Induction chemotherapy:**
  - Moderately intensive combination chemotherapy that includes an anthracycline (e.g., daunorubicin or idarubicin) and cytosine arabinoside (cytarabine) ± etoposide.
  - "High risk"patients (include patients <70 years with high-risk karyotype) may only be treated with curative intent if an HLA-identified sibling is available for stem cell transplantation.
- **Consolidation or postremission therapy:** For patients achieving remission with induction therapy in young patients (<60 years) consists of 3 to 4 cycles of high-dose cytosine arabinoside.
  - Low-risk patients in AML; patients with t(8;21) or inv(16) (i.e., low risk karyotype) do not benefit from allogeneic stem cell transplantation during their first complete remission.
  - Patients with high-risk karyotypes should have stem cell transplantation because they respond poorly to conventional chemotherapy.

Acute promyelocytic leukemia (M3)

- It is an uncommon variant of AML associated with severe coagulation complications.
- It has favorable prognosis.
- Induction therapy is with **all-trans-retinoic acid** and anthracyclines or a combination of ATA with arsenic trioxide.
- Allogeneic transplantation: It is necessary if the leukemia is not eliminated at the molecular level, only in relapsed/refractory cases.
- In relapsed cases, arsenic trioxide (induces apoptosis via activation of the caspase cascade) has been also found to be effective.

Alternative chemotherapy

- It is used to curb excessive leukocyte proliferation and not for achieving remission.
- Hydroxyurea up to 4 g daily and L asparaginase 10,000 units are used to reduce leukocyte count without inducing bone marrow failure.

TABLE 8.29: Treatment for AML (acute myeloid leukemia).

Initial treatment for AML
Intensive remission induction (7+3 therapy) ➢ Continuous infusion of cytarabine (100 or 200 mg/m^2 daily for 7 days) together with daunorubicin (by short infusion or bolus for the first 3 days) ➢ Alternative remission induction approaches Gemtuzumab ozogamicin (GO) 6 mg/m^2 on day 1, and 3 mg/m^2 on day 8, and continue treatment with GO for up to eight monthly cycles ➢ Other regimens – FLAG (fludarabine, cytarabine, G-CSF), FLAG-IDA (idarubicin), MITO-FLAG (mitoxantrone), and FLAMSA (amsacrine) – CLAG (cladribine, cytarabine, G-CSF) – Vorinostat (histone deacetylase inhibitor) plus idarubicin and cytarabine – Bortezomib, daunorubicin, and cytarabine – Lenalidomide
Postremission management
➢ Consolidation chemotherapy—cytarabine + daunorubicin or with gemtuzumab ozogamicin ➢ Hematopoietic cell transplantation (HCT) ➢ Maintenance therapy—with gemtuzumab ozogamicin Or Midostaurin
Relapsed or resistant AML
Gemtuzumab ozogamicin, midostaurin, enasidenib, lower intensity treatments (e.g., azacitidine, decitabine), or palliative management

Poor Prognostic Factors in AML and ALL (Table 8.30)

TABLE 8.30: Poor prognostic factors in AML and ALL.

Features	*Acute myeloblastic leukemia (AML)*	*Acute lymphoblastic leukemia (ALL)*
Age	>60 years	<1 year or >9 years
TLC	>1,00,000/mm^3	>30,000 in B-ALL and >100,000 in T-ALL
French-American-British (FAB) type	M_0, M_5, M_6, M_7	L_3 type

Contd...

Contd...

Chromosomal abnormality	High-risk karyotype [t(6;9), inv(3)]	Hypodiploidy (<45 chromosomes), pH positive ALL t (1:19) MLL rearranged
Other features	➤ Secondary cause present ➤ Following myelodysplastic syndrome (MDS) ➤ Relapsed disease ➤ Secondary leukemia ➤ Extramedullary disease	➤ Male gender ➤ Mediastinal mass ➤ CNS involvement ➤ pH-like ALL

Differences Between Acute Lymphoblastic Leukemia and Acute Myeloblastic Leukemia (Table 8.31)

Q. How do you differentiate acute lymphoblastic leukemia from acute myeloblastic leukemia?

TABLE 8.31: Differences between acute lymphoblastic leukemia and acute myeloblastic leukemia.

Clinical features	*Acute lymphoblastic leukemia*	*Acute myelogenous leukemia*
Age	Predominantly children	Predominantly adults
Coagulopathy (DIC)	Absent	Seen in M_3
Gingival hypertrophy and dermal infiltrate (chloromas)	Absent	Seen in M_4 and M_5
Hepatosplenomegaly	In majority (50–75%)	Frequent
Lymphadenopathy	More common	Less common
Leukemic meningitis	More common	Less common
Testicular involvement	In 10–20%	–
Eye involvement	More common	Less common
Investigations		
Type of leukemic blasts	Lymphoblasts (10–15 µm) are smaller than myeloblasts, with a thin rim of agranular cytoplasm and round or convoluted nucleus	Myeloblasts (12–20 µm) are larger than lymphoblasts, with discrete nuclear chromatin and multiple nucleoli
Auer rods (in the cytoplasm)	Absent	Present in 10–20% (diagnostic)
Terminal deoxynucleotidyl transferase (Tdt) in leukemic blasts	In more than 90%	Rare
Cytochemistry		
Myeloperoxidase	–ve	+ve
Sudan Black B	–ve	+ve
Nonspecific esterase	–ve	+ve in M_4 and M_5
Periodic acid Schiff (PAS)	+ve in >50% of cells (Block positivity)	Negative

Subleukemic Leukemia/Aleukemic Leukemia

Q. Write short note on subleukemic leukemia.

- In acute leukemia, the immature neoplastic leukemic "blast" cells proliferate and accumulate but fail to mature. The blasts diffusely replace the normal bone marrow, and a variable number of these accumulate in the peripheral blood.
- Acute leukemia should be diagnosed when the blast cells constitute more than 20% of the nucleated cells in the marrow (normally blast cells < 5%) with an increase in total leukocyte count.
- **Subleukemic/aleukemic leukemia** is characterized by a total leukocyte count which is normal or lower than 4×10^9/L, and peripheral blood shows very few abnormal blasts. It is observed in a small percentage of patients with acute leukemia.
- Diagnosis is confirmed from the bone marrow examination which shows replacement by leukemic cells.

Leukemoid Reaction

Q. Write short note on leukemoid reaction (including its definition).

- Extreme neutrophilia is sometimes associated with the presence of immature white cells and is called leukemoid reaction.
- A **leukemoid reaction** is a benign leukocytic proliferation characterized by a total leukocyte count of more than 50×10^9/L with many immature white cells (such as metamyelocytes, myelocytes, and promyelocytes and even a few myeloblasts) in the peripheral smear.
- Leukemoid reaction is the response of the normal healthy bone marrow to various stresses.
- Causes: Include infections (including tuberculosis), acute hemorrhage, hematological and nonhematological malignancies, and various toxic states.
- Bone marrow is normal with accelerated leukopoiesis.
- LAP source is increased.
- Philadelphia chromosome is negative.

- There is no absolute eosinophilia or basophilia (versus CML).
- Treatment of underlying disorder corrects the blood picture.
- Types of leukemoid reactions are listed in **Box 8.13**.
- It should be differentiated from chronic myelocytic leukemia **(Table 8.32)**.

Box 8.13: Types of leukemoid reactions.

- Myeloid
- Lymphoid

TABLE 8.32: Differences between leukemoid reaction and chronic myeloid leukemia.

Clinical features	*Leukemoid reaction*	*Chronic myeloid leukemia*
Peripheral blood findings	Features of causative disease	Splenomegaly, lymphadenopathy, and bone pain are common
WBC series		
Total WBC count	Moderately increased, rarely exceeds 50 × 10^9/L	Markedly increased and usually exceeds 50 × 10^9/L
Differential leukocyte count	➢ Shift to the left with few immature forms ➢ Toxic granulation seen	➢ Shift to the left with numerous immature forms ➢ Myelocyte and neutrophil peak
Eosinophilia and basophilia	Variable	Present
Leukocyte alkaline phosphatase (LAP)	Increased	Decreased
RBC series		
Anemia	Usually minimal or absent	Severe and progressive
Platelets		
Number	Variable	Normal or increased
Extramedullary myeloid tumors	Absent	Present
Philadelphia chromosome	Absent	Present

Hairy Cell Leukemia

Q. Discuss the clinical features, investigations, and management of hairy cell leukemia.

Clinical Features

- Hairy cell leukemia **(HCL)** is an uncommon chronic malignant disorder of mature B-cells with characteristic fine cytoplasmic projections.
- The term **hairy cell leukemia** is derived from the appearance of fine hairlike cell membrane projections on the leukemic cells, under the phase-contrast microscope.
- Hairy cell leukemia affects middle-aged to elderly men, with a male-to-female ratio of 5:1.
- Clinical features are mainly due to leukemic infiltration of bone marrow, liver, and spleen.
  - **Massive splenomegaly** is the most common finding, hepatomegaly is less common, and lymphadenopathy is distinctly rare.
  - **Pancytopenia** is due to marrow failure and splenic sequestration and is found in more than 50% of cases.
  - **Infections:** About one-third of patients present with infections, especially with atypical mycobacteria, which may be due to monocytopenia. Infections are the most common cause of death.
  - Risk of secondary malignancies such as Hodgkin's lymphoma, non-Hodgkin's lymphoma, and thyroid cancer is there.

Investigations

- Total leukocyte count: It is normal or low. Majority of patients have pancytopenia.
- Peripheral smear: It shows the characteristic hairy cells. These are the medium-sized malignant B lymphocytes with filamentous hairy structures on the surface of the cell. They have a reniform nucleus and abundant pale blue cytoplasm. Cytochemically, these hairy cells stain positively for **tartrate-resistant acid phosphatase (TRAP).**
- Bone marrow: Aspirate yields a dry tap and biopsy shows fibrosis with infiltration by mononuclear cells and hairy cells (fired-egg or honeycomb appearance).
- LAP score is very high. Flow cytometry reveals CD11c, 25, 103, 123 positivity.

Treatment

- Indications for treatment: If the patient develops
  - Cytopenia
  - Symptomatic splenomegaly
  - Constitutional symptoms (e.g., fever, night sweats, and fatigue).
- Treatment of infections with antibiotics.
- Chemotherapy: The purine analogs 2-chloroadenosine acetate (2-CDA) (cladribine) and pentostatin are highly effective with just one cycle of treatment. Rituximab is used in patients who do not respond to the above drugs. Pentostatin, interferon alfa, and splenectomy are other treatment options available.
- Contraindicated drugs: Corticosteroids and myelotoxic drugs

Prognosis: Follows an indolent course and prognosis is excellent.

CHRONIC MYELOID LEUKEMIA

Q. Define chronic myeloid leukemia. Write a short note on Philadelphia chromosome and its significance.

Definition: Chronic myeloid leukemia (CML) is one of the **myeloproliferative neoplasms** (MPN) of **pluripotent hematopoietic stem cell** characterized by **overproduction** of cells of the **myeloid series** (results in marked splenomegaly and leukocytosis) and the presence of the Philadelphia chromosome.

Molecular Pathogenesis

- **Philadelphia (Ph) chromosome**
  - Acquired chromosomal abnormality of **hematopoietic stem cells**
  - **Balanced reciprocal translocation between the long arms of chromosomes 9 and 22 (t 9,22)** increases the length of chromosome 9 and shortening of 22. The **shortened chromosome 22** is known as Philadelphia chromosome **(Ph).**
- ***BCR-ABL1* fusion gene**
  - Translocation results in fusion of the breakpoint cluster region (*BCR*) gene on chromosome 22q with the *ABL1* (named after the Abelson murine leukemia virus) gene located on chromosome 9q.
  - It produces a new hybrid oncogene, namely *BCR-ABL1* fusion gene. The products of this gene are oncoproteins which have uncontrolled kinase activity and trigger the excessive proliferation and reduced apoptosis of CML cells.
  - **Significance:** Apart from CML, Philadelphia (Ph) chromosome can be found in ALL (25–30% in adult and 2–10% in pediatric cases) and occasionally in AML. In patients with Ph positive/negative and *BCR-ABL1* positive, the survival rate and therapeutic response are better than those with both Ph- and *BCR-ABL1*-negative patients.

Natural Course of CML

Q. Discuss the natural course and clinical features of chronic myeloid leukemia.

It has three phases:

1. **Chronic stable phase:** Most of the CML are diagnosed in this phase and lasts for about 3–5 years if untreated.
2. **Accelerated phase:** It is more aggressive and lasts for few months.
3. **Blast crisis phase:** It resembles acute (myeloid or lymphoid) leukemia and has poor prognosis.

Parameter	*Chronic Phase*	*Accelerated Phase*	*Blast Crisis*
White blood cells	≥20	↑	↑
BM Blasts MO	<15%	15–20%	20%
Basophils	<20%	20%	–
Platelets	↑ or normal	↓ or ↑	↓
Marrow cellularity	↑	↑	↑
Cytogenetics	Ph+	Ph+	Ph+
Bcr-abl	+	+	+

Clinical Features in Chronic Stable Phase of CML

Q. Discuss the clinical features in chronic stable phase.

- **Age: It usually occurs between 40 and 60 years** of age.
- **Onset: It is insidious.**

Symptoms

Many patients are asymptomatic during the early stage of CML and may be diagnosed during routine peripheral blood examination.

- **Nonspecific symptoms:** Fatigue, weakness, weight loss, anorexia.
- **Symptoms due to massive splenomegaly: Fullness of abdomen** (abdominal distension, postprandial fullness), reflux esophagitis, dyspnea, and dragging discomfort in the left hypochondrium due to splenomegaly (caused by leukemic infiltration and extramedullary hematopoiesis). Splenomegaly is moderate to severe and is a characteristic feature in majority (80–90%) of patients.
- **Symptoms of hypermetabolic state:** Due to rapid turnover of cells, it may result in symptoms such as fatigue, weakness, fever, sweating, heat intolerance weight loss, and anorexia.
- **Priapism:** It is painful penile erection due to leukostasis (associated with marked leukocytosis or thrombocytosis).
- Bleeding tendencies occur late in the disease.

Signs

- **Pallor** due to anemia.
- **Splenomegaly:** Moderate to massive, nontender splenomegaly. It is due to leukemia infiltration and extramedullary hematopoiesis. Presence of tender spleen and splenic friction rub indicate splenic infarction.

- Mild **hepatomegaly** as a result of leukemic infiltration may develop in 60–70% of cases.
- **Sternal tenderness and bone pain:** They are due to hypercellularity of marrow and irritation of periosteum.

Investigations

Q. Discuss the investigations/laboratory investigations/diagnosis of chronic myeloid leukemia.

- **Hemoglobin** is usually less than 11 g/dL.
- **Total leukocyte count** is markedly raised, almost always more than 20,000/μL, often exceeding 1,00,000/μL. In untreated patients, the leukocyte count progressively increases.

Peripheral Smear (Fig. 8.31)

- **RBC** shows a moderate degree of **normocytic normochromic anemia**.
- **WBC:**
  - **Shift to left (shift to immaturity)** with granulocytes at all stages of development (neutrophils, metamyelocytes, myelocytes, promyelocytes, and occasional myeloblasts). **Predominant cells** are **neutrophils and myelocytes** in an untreated patient. **Blasts** are usually **less than 10%** of the circulating white blood cells.
  - There is increase in basophils (<20%) and eosinophils.
- **Platelets:** Count may be normal, increased, or decreased. Automated analyzers may give falsely elevated platelet counts due to disruption of granulocytes.

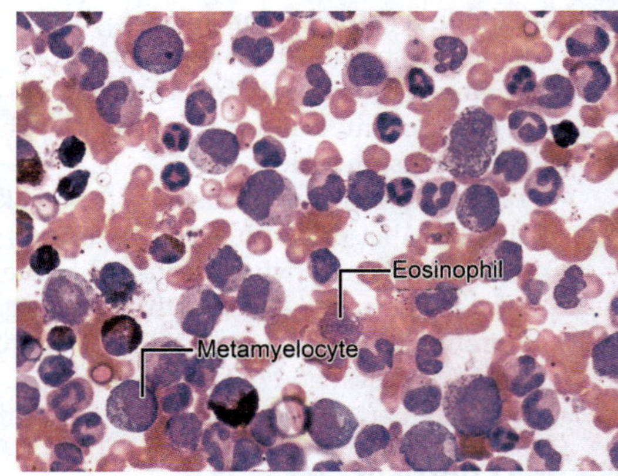

FIG. 8.31: Peripheral blood picture in chronic stable phase of chronic myeloid leukemia.

Bone Marrow Study

- It is markedly hypercellular due to marked hyperplasia of all granulocytic elements.
- About 20–30% of the patients may develop bone marrow fibrosis in late stages.

Philadelphia Chromosome (Ph)

- It is positive in more than 95% of cases, in all three phases. In Ph-negative cases, evidence of translocation can be demonstrated by cytogenetics, reverse transcription-polymerase chain reaction (RT-PCR), and fluorescence *in situ* hybridization (FISH).
- ***BCR-ABL1* fusion gene** can be demonstrated in peripheral blood or bone marrow.

Decreased NAP/LAP Score

It is usually below 20 (normal score ranges from 40 to 100) in majority of patients. This is helpful in differentiating CML from leukemoid reaction.

Biochemical Findings

- Serum LDH and uric acid are increased.
- Serum alkaline phosphatase is increased.
- Serum vitamin B_{12} is markedly elevated due to production of binding protein (transcobalamin) by the granulocyte series.
- Marked thrombocytosis may raise serum potassium spuriously as platelets release potassium during clotting.
- Blood sugar may be falsely decreased due to glucose uptake and metabolism by leukocytes.

Q. Write short essay/note on the treatment and complications of chronic myeloid leukemia. Enumerate the drugs used in chemotherapy.

Q. Write short note on Imatinib.

Treatment of CML

Goal of therapy in CML (Table 8.33)

TABLE 8.33: Response criteria in CML.

Level of response	*Definition*
Complete hematologic response	Normal CBC and differential
Minor cytogenetic response	35–90% Ph metaphases
Partial cytogenetic response	1–34% Ph metaphases
Complete cytogenetic response	0% Ph-positive metaphases
Major molecular response	≥ 3-log reduction of BCR-ABL mRNA
Complete molecular remission	Negativity by qPCR

Chemotherapy (Table 8.34)

Tyrosine kinase inhibitors (TKIs)

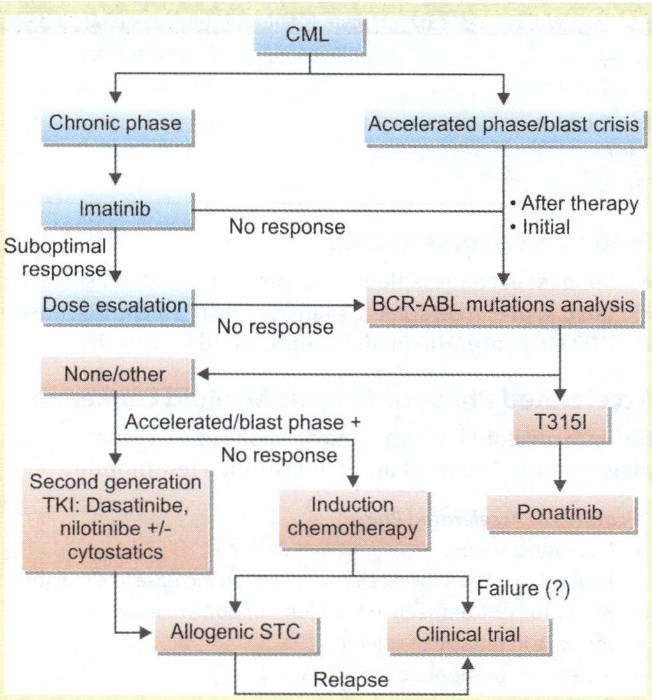

- ***Imatinib mesylate*** is the first-line treatment for the chronic phase of CML.
- If there is failure of response or progress on imatinib, options include:
  - second-generation tyrosine kinase inhibitors (such as dasatinib, bosutinib, or nilotinib),
  - allogeneic bone marrow transplantation, or
  - classical cytotoxic drugs such as hydroxycarbamide (hydroxyurea) or interferon-α or melphalan, and busulfan
  - Omacetaxine/homoharringtonine (plant alkaloid).

Imatinib mesylate

- Imatinib mesylate is a tyrosine kinase inhibitor (TKI) which provides targeted therapy, i.e., high specificity blocks the enzymatic action of the *BCR-ABL* fusion, providing a broader therapeutic window with less toxicity.
- In all newly diagnosed CML, imatinib (400 mg/d) is more effective and has replaced IFN-α and cytarabine. It reduces the uncontrolled proliferation of white cells, producing apoptosis of cancer cells.
- In chronic stable disease, it can produce complete hematological response in >95% of cases and complete cytogenetic response (disappearance of the Ph chromosome and *BCR-ABL* transcripts in the blood) in >76% at 18 months of therapy. Imatinib can be continued indefinitely.
- Overexpression of the *BCR-ABL* chimeric gene or genetic alteration can produce resistance to imatinib mesylate.
  - Side effects of imatinib: Nausea, headaches, fluid retention, muscle cramps, diarrhea, skin rash, and myelosuppression (causing cytopenias).

Ponatinib is the only approved TKI capable of inhibiting BCR-ABL with the gatekeeper *T315I kinase domain mutation*, known to be the cause for 20% of resistant or relapsed CML cases.

Recombinant interferon-α

- **Recombinant interferon-α (rINF-α)** was considered first-line treatment before the invention of imatinib.
- It was given alone or combined with the chemotherapy agent cytosine arabinoside, and induced remission and controlled chronic stable phase of CML in about 70% of cases. But it has no role as a single agent in most patients.
- It should be considered in patients not responding to imatinib.
- It is not effective in accelerated phase or blast crisis phase.
- Dosage: 3–9 mega units/day intramuscularly or subcutaneously.
- Actions of rINF-α:
  - Reduces cellularity of the bone marrow.
  - Reduces the number of Philadelphia-positive tumor cells in 20% of patients.
  - Total eradication of Philadelphia chromosome in ~5% of patients.
  - Reduces platelet count when it is very high.
- Side effects: Flu-like syndrome, weight loss, fatigue, nausea, vomiting, and headache

Hydroxyurea

- It is used to reduce white blood cell counts while awaiting confirmation of a suspected diagnosis of CML in a patient with significant leukocytosis (e.g., >100 x10^9 white cells/L) or in patients with systemic symptoms or with symptomatic splenomegaly.

Splenectomy

- It is indicated to relieve the symptoms due to massive splenomegaly and in repeated splenic infarctions.

Stem cell transplantation (SCT)

- Indication:
  - Patients under the age of 60 years who have a suitable donor
  - Those who do not respond to second-line TKI and those who present with accelerated phase or blast crisis
- Best results are obtained if SCT is done in early chronic stable phase and can cure about 70% of cases.
- It can result in permanent disappearance of the Ph-positive clone.
- Disadvantages: These include risk of complications and death due to graft-versus-host disease (GVHD) and opportunistic infections.

Monitoring

- Bone marrow biopsy: It is done at 6-month intervals to determine the cytogenetic response.
- Quantitative RT-PCR (qPCR): It should be done from peripheral blood at 3–6-month intervals once cytogenetic response has been achieved.

TABLE 8.34: Drugs used and their dosage for induction and maintenance in chronic stable phase of CML.

Drug	Induction dose	Maintenance dose
Imatinib mesylate	300–400 mg/day	300–400 mg/day
Hydroxyurea (hydroxycarbamide)	0.5–2.0 g/day	0.5–2.0 g/day
Melphalan	4–12 mg/day	2–4 mg/day
Busulfan	4 mg/day	2–4 mg/day

Prognostic Scores in CML

- **Sokal score:** Age, spleen size, platelet count, blast cell counts
- **Euro score:** Age, spleen, platelet, blast cell counts, basophil counts, eosinophil counts
- **EUTOS score/Hasford:** Basophils and spleen size.

Accelerated Phase of Chronic Myeloid Leukemia

Chronic myeloid leukemia may transform to a more aggressive blastic phase with or without going through an accelerated phase after 1–5 years of onset. It lasts for a few months.

Features of Accelerated Phase

- Increasing anemia
- Increasing white blood cell count with an increase in circulating immature cells unresponsive to therapy
- Blasts 10–19% are seen in the blood or bone marrow
- Increase in the size of spleen
- Increase in basophil count (<20%)
- Persistent thrombocytopenia or persistent thrombocytosis unresponsive to therapy
- Hydroxyurea is the most effective drug in accelerated phase.

Blast Crisis Phase of Chronic Myeloid Leukemia

- Blast crisis phase of CML represents the transformation of CML into an acute leukemia.
- This final phase lasts for a few weeks to months and has a poor prognosis.
- Blasts constitute 20% or more and may be:
  - Myeloid blast crisis that occurs in 70% when the disease transforms into acute myeloblastic leukemia.
  - Lymphoid blast crisis that occurs in 30% when the disease transforms into acute lymphoblastic leukemia.

Treatment of blast crisis is the same as that for acute myeloblastic or lymphoblastic leukemia. Complications of chronic myelogenous leukemia are enlisted in **Box 8.14**.

Features of Blast Crisis

- Refractory to treatment
- Abrupt increase in the size of spleen
- Bone pain and sternal tenderness
- Anemia and bleeding tendencies
- Generalized lymphadenopathy may appear.
- Peripheral smear and bone marrow showing >30% cells simulating acute leukemia
- Basophils may increase to 20%.
- Thrombocytopenia may result in bleeding episodes.

Box 8.14: Complications of chronic myelogenous leukemia.

- Fatigue due to anemia
- Excess bleeding due to thrombocytopenia
- Bone pain or joint pain due to expansion of bone marrow
- Enlarged spleen
- Vulnerable to infection due to impaired immune system
- Death

CHRONIC LYMPHOCYTIC LEUKEMIA

Q. Discuss the types, clinical features, investigation, clinical staging, and management of chronic lymphocytic leukemia.

Definition

Chronic lymphocytic leukemia (CLL) is a tumor of immature small round lymphocytes characterized by the accumulation of neoplastic mature-looking lymphocytes in the peripheral blood, bone marrow, and lymphoid organs (spleen and lymph nodes).

Types

- B-cell origin: More than 95% of the cases of CLL express the pan B-cell markers CD19 and CD20 and also present is the aberrant expression of T-cell antigen CD5 (found only in a small subset of normal B-cells).
- T-cell origin: It constitutes less than 5%.

Clinical Features

- It is the most common form of chronic leukemia.
- **Age:** Most of the patients at the time of diagnosis are over 50 years of age.
- **Sex:** It is more common in males than in females with a ratio of 2:1.

- **Asymptomatic:** It is found in about 25% of patients and is detected either because of nonspecific symptoms or routine blood examination for some other diseases.
- **Nonspecific symptoms:** This includes fatigue, loss of weight, and anorexia.
- **Painless generalized lymphadenopathy:** Initially, the cervical lymph nodes are enlarged and in later stages there may be generalized lymphadenopathy. Involved nodes are rubbery, discrete, nontender, small, and mobile.
- **Splenomegaly and hepatomegaly:** Mild degree is observed in very few cases.
- **Presenting symptoms** may be:
  - Slowly developing anemia: Due to immune hemolysis and bone marrow infiltration
  - Recurrent infections: Develop due to hypogammaglobulinemia. *Streptococcus pneumonia*, *Staphylococcus*, and *Haemophilus influenzae* cause most of the infections. Herpes zoster is also common.
  - Bleeding manifestations: They are uncommon.

Transformation

CLL may transform to:
- Prolymphocytic transformation with appearance of "prolymphocytes" in the peripheral blood (>10%).
- Transformation to diffuse large B-cell lymphoma (Richter syndrome).
- **Monoclonal B-cell lymphocytosis (MBL):** WHO criteria for monoclonal B-cell lymphocytosis (MBL) are the presence of monoclonal B-cell populations in the peripheral blood (PB) of up to 5×10^9/L either with the phenotype of chronic lymphocytic leukemia (CLL), atypical CLL, or non-CLL (CD52) B cells in the absence of other lymphomatous features. It has been found that MBL precedes almost all cases of CLL/SLL. In 2016, the WHO subdivided MBL into "low count" MBL (characterized by PB CLL count of $<0.5 \times 10^9$/L) and "high count" MBL. The distinction is important because low-count MBL does not require routine follow-up whereas high-count MBL requires routine/yearly follow-up.

Investigations

- **Hemoglobin:** Usually below 13 g/dL and as the disease progresses, it may decrease below 10 g/dL. This is due to marrow failure, but associated autoimmune hemolysis may also be contributory, when present.
- **Blood counts:**
  - Total leukocyte count is increased and varies from 20×10^9/L to 50×10^9/L.
  - Platelet count may be normal or low.
- **Peripheral blood smear (Fig. 8.32):**
  - Mild-to-moderate normocytic normochromic anemia.
  - Lymphocytosis is the characteristic feature and constitutes more than 50% of the white cells, and absolute lymphocyte count should be more than $5,000 \times 10^9$/L.
  - Lymphocytes are of mature type in majority of the cases.
  - **Smudge cells or basket cells** are disintegrated lymphocytes and are due to the rupture of neoplastic lymphocytes while making the peripheral smear due to its fragile nature.
  - Platelets: Normal or reduced in number (autoimmune thrombocytopenia).
- **Bone marrow:** It is involved in all cases of CLL and its infiltration by mature lymphocytes results in hypercellular marrow.
- **Direct Coombs test:** About 15–20% of patients manifest autoimmune hemolytic anemia and have positive direct Coombs test.
- **Lymph node** biopsy shows well-differentiated, small, noncleaved lymphocytes.
- **Immunoglobulins:** They are low or normal.
- Serum folic acid levels are low.

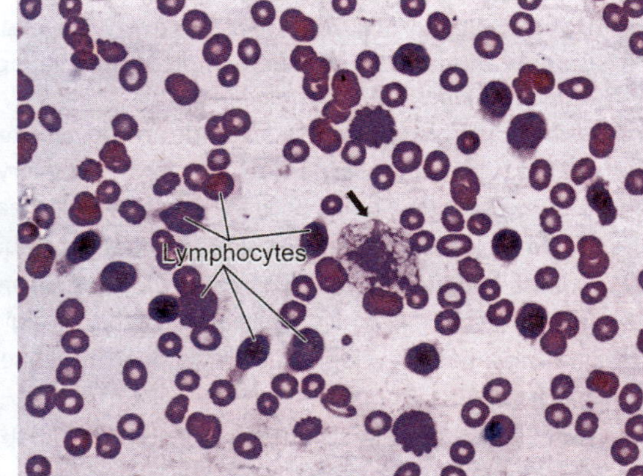

FIG. 8.32: Peripheral blood smear in chronic lymphocytic leukemia showing numerous small lymphocytes and few smudge cells (arrow).

Diagnostic Criteria for Chronic Lymphocytic Leukemia (Table 8.35)

TABLE 8.35: Diagnostic criteria for chronic lymphocytic leukemia.

Lymphocytosis	Immunophenotype
Absolute lymphocyte count should be more than $5,000 \times 10^9$/L	Positive for B-cell surface antigens (CD19, CD20, CD23)
	Aberrant expression of T-cell antigen CD5
Lymphoid cells ≤55% prolymphocytes	Evidence of monoclonality in the form of "light chain restriction"

Clinical Staging

Binet staging and Rai staging of CLL are presented in **Tables 8.36 and 8.37**, respectively.

Lymphoid enlargement includes cervical, axillary, and inguinal lymph nodes.

TABLE 8.36: Binet staging of CLL.

Stage	*Features*	*Survival*
A	No anemia or thrombocytopenia Less than three lymphoid areas enlarged	>10 years
B	No anemia or thrombocytopenia Three or more lymphoid areas enlarged	7 years
C	Anemia (Hb <10 g/dL) and/or thrombocytopenia (<10,000/mm^3) present, regardless of the number of areas of lymphoid enlargement	2 years

TABLE 8.37: Rai staging of CLL.

Stage	*Features*	*Survival*
0	Peripheral blood lymphocytosis alone	>10 years
I	Lymphocytosis with lymphadenopathy	9 years
II	Lymphocytosis with splenomegaly or lymphadenopathy or both	7 years
III	Lymphocytosis with anemia (hemoglobin <11 g/dL) and organomegaly	5 years
IV	Lymphocytosis with anemia, thrombocytopenia, and organomegaly	5 years

Treatment

Absolute indications for treatment: When any of the following features is present:

- Anemia or thrombocytopenia that can be attributed to CLL
- Recurrent fever, extreme fatigue, night sweats, and weight loss
- Bulky or progressive lymphadenopathy; massive or progressive splenomegaly with discomfort
- Autoimmune cytopenias not responsive to corticosteroids
- Symptomatic or functional extranodal involvement (e.g., skin, kidney, lung, spine)
- Progressive disease manifests by doubling of the lymphocyte count in 6 months

Treatment options based on Binet staging (Table 8.38)

Regimen—single-agent fludarabine or combination therapy with fludarabine, cyclophosphamide, and rituximab (FCR)

Chlorambucil: Two regimens

1. Continuous low-dose therapy: 5 mg/day orally
2. Intermittent high-dose therapy (pulse therapy): 0.4 mg/kg for every 2 weeks
   - Complications: Development of myelodysplasia and acute myeloid leukemia

Fludarabine: It is a purine nucleoside analog that is drug of choice in young patients.

- Dose: 25–30 mg/m^2 IV/day for 5 days every 4 weeks
- Complications: Autoimmune hemolytic anemia, opportunistic infections (e.g., *Legionella pneumophila*, *Pneumocystis jiroveci*, *Listeria monocytogenes*, and *Cytomegalovirus*)

Cladribine: It is also a purine nucleoside analog, an alternative to fludarabine. Dose:

- 0.2 mg/kg continuous infusion daily for 7 days every 4 weeks or
- 0.14 mg/kg over 2 hours daily for 5 days every 4 weeks

Pentostatin: It is *a* purine nucleoside analog that can be used instead of fludarabine or cladribine.

Rituximab and alemtuzumab: They are monoclonal antibodies against CD20 and CD52, respectively.

- **Side effects:** Fever, chills, nausea, headache, myalgias

Alkylating agents: Cyclophosphamide, bendamustine.

Newer drugs:

1. Anti CD20 antibodies: Ofatumumab, obinutuzumab
2. BCL2 inhibitor: Venetoclax
3. Bruton tyrosine kinase (BTK) inhibitors: Ibrutinib, acalabrutinib
4. Phosphoinositide 3′-kinase (PI3K) inhibitors: Idelalisib, duvelisib

Chimeric antigen receptor (CAR)—T-cell therapy is an investigational therapy.

TABLE 8.38: Treatment options based on Binet and Rai staging.

Stage	*del (17p) or p 53 mut*	*Fitness*	*IGVH*	*Therapy*
Binet A-B, Rai 0-II, inactive disease	Irrelevant	Irrelevant	Irrelevant	None
Active disease or Binet C or Rai III-IV	Yes	Irrelevant	Irrelevant	Ibrutinib or Venetoclax + Obinutumab or Idelalisib + Rituximab (if contraindications for ibrutinib)
	No	Go go	M	FCR (BR above 65 years) or ibrutinib
			U	Ibrutinib or FCR (BR above 65 years)
		Slow go	M	Venetoclax + Obinutuzumab or Chlorambucil + Obinutuzumab or ibrutinib
			U	Venetoclax + Obinutuzumab or ibrutinib or Chlorambucil + Obinutuzumab

CLL first line treatment (updated June 2019)

MYELOPROLIFERATIVE NEOPLASMS

Q. Define and write short essay/note on myeloproliferative diseases (disorders) or myeloproliferative neoplasms and enumerate myeloproliferative neoplasms.

Definition

Myeloproliferative neoplasms (MPN) (old synonym myeloproliferative disorder/diseases) are clonal hematopoietic stem cell disorders which are characterized by proliferation of one or more of the myeloid lineages (erythroid, granulocytic, megakaryocytic, and mast cells).

It is seen usually in adults with a peak in the 5th to 7th decade. Splenomegaly and hepatomegaly occur commonly due to sequestration of excess hematopoietic cells or proliferation of abnormal hematopoietic cells.

WHO Classification (2016) of Myeloproliferative Neoplasm

WHO classification of MPN has been shown in **Box 8.15**.

Mastocytosis is no longer listed under the broad heading of MPN in WHO (2016) classification.

Box 8.15: WHO classification of myeloproliferative neoplasm.

- Chronic myelogenous leukemia, *BCR-ABL1* positive
- Chronic neutrophilic leukemia
- Polycythemia vera (PV)
- Essential thrombocythemia (ET)
- Primary myelofibrosis (PMF)
- Chronic eosinophilic leukemia not otherwise specified
- Myeloproliferative neoplasm, unclassifiable

POLYCYTHEMIA

Q. Write short essay/note on polycythemia and its classification.

Definition

Polycythemia, or erythrocytosis, refers to an *increase in the number of RBCs above normal* in the circulating blood, usually with a corresponding increase in hemoglobin and PCV level. PCV is a more reliable indicator of polycythemia than is hemoglobin.

Classification and Causes of Polycythemia

Q. Write short note on causes of secondary polycythemia.

Pathophysiological classification of polycythemia has been shown in **Box 8.16**.

Box 8.16: Pathophysiologic classification of polycythemia.

Relative
- Reduced plasma volume with normal red cell mass (hemoconcentration) due to dehydration—low fluid intake, vomiting, diarrhea, sweating, acidosis
- Gaisböck syndrome (spurious polycythemia)

Absolute (increased red cell mass)

Primary (low erythropoietin level)
- Polycythemia vera (erythremia)

Secondary (high erythropoietin level)—erythrocytosis

Compensatory
- Lung disease (e.g., COPD—chronic obstructive pulmonary disease)
- Living in high-altitude
- Cyanotic congenital heart disease (Tetralogy of Fallot, Eisenmenger's complex)
- Chronic carbon monoxide poisoning
- Sleep apnea syndrome
- Smokers

As a consequence of local hypoxia: Renal artery stenosis, end-stage renal disease, hydronephrosis, renal cysts (polycystic kidney disease), postrenal transplant erythrocytosis

Paraneoplastic: Erythropoietin-secreting tumors—renal cell carcinoma, hepatocellular carcinoma, cerebellar hemangioblastoma, uterine leiomyoma, pheochromocytoma

Clinical Features of Polycythemia

- Usually appears insidiously, in late middle age (median age at onset: 60 years).
- Most symptoms are due to the increased red cell mass and hematocrit.
- Plethora and cyanosis due to stagnation and deoxygenation of blood in peripheral vessels are early findings. Headache, dizziness, and visual problems result from vascular disturbances in the brain and retina.
- Increased incidence of thrombotic episodes and bleeding.
- Secondary polycythemia, in addition shows manifestations of the underlying disease.

Polycythemia Vera

Q. Discuss the clinical features, diagnosis, and management of polycythemia vera.

Definition

- Polycythemia vera (PV) is an **acquired myeloproliferative neoplasm** arising from malignant transformation of **hematopoietic stem cell**.
- It is characterized by **trilineage** (erythroid, granulocytic, and megakaryocytic) **hyperplasia** in the bone marrow.
- It leads to **uncontrolled production of red cells, granulocytes and platelets** (panmyelosis) and leads to **erythrocytosis** (polycythemia) and or granulocytosis and thrombocytosis.

Etiology

The etiology of PV is not known. PV is partly due to a failure of apoptosis as a result of deregulation of the *Bcl-x* gene (antiapoptotic gene), in addition a mutation in the tyrosine kinase **JAK 2 V617F** (which causes the substitution of phenylalanine for valine at position 617) has been found; this stimulates low-grade erythropoiesis.

Clinical Features

- Onset is insidious.
- Age and gender: Late middle age (median age at onset is 60 years) and more common in males.
- Features due to increased viscosity and/or decreased cerebral perfusion
  - Plethora (excessive fullness of blood) and deep dusky cyanosis due to stagnation and deoxygenation of blood in peripheral vessels are early findings.
  - Headache, dizziness, vertigo, a sense of fullness in the head, rushing in the ears, visual problems, tinnitus, tiredness, syncope, and even chorea result from vascular disturbances in the brain and retina.
- Severe itching (pruritus) after a hot bath or when the patient is warm is frequent and may be disabling.
- Thrombotic episodes: For example, deep venous thrombosis, myocardial infarction, thrombosis of hepatic veins (producing Budd-Chiari syndrome).
- Bleeding manifestations include epistaxis, bleeding from peptic ulcer, bruising, and intramuscular hemorrhages.
- Peptic ulcer is seen in few patients and is five times more frequent than general population.
- Hyperuricemia: May result in urate stones, gout, and uric acid nephropathy.

Physical findings

- Injection of the conjunctivae, deep red palate, dusky red hands, and retinal venous engorgement.
- Splenomegaly is very common (~70%) and is useful in distinguishing PV from secondary polycythemia.
- Hepatomegaly occurs in ~50%.

Diagnosis

- **Hemoglobin increased ranging from** 14 to 28 g/dL.
- **PCV (hematocrit)** increased to about 60%. However, in many patients, the plasma volume is also increased giving rise to near normal hematocrit. Hence, it is important to determine the red cell mass.
- **Red cell count:** Increased and usually about 6 million/mm^3 (6×10^{12}/L)
- **Increased red cell volume and blood viscosity:** Isotope dilution using the patient's ^{51}Cr-tagged red cells (>36 mL/kg in males and 32 mL/kg in females).
- Total white cell count (~70%) and platelet count (~50%) usually increased.
- Absolute basophil count: Increased to >100/μL in majority of patients.
- **Arterial oxygen saturation** (PO_2) is normal and is useful for differentiating it from secondary polycythemia.
- **Erythropoietin (EPO) levels are decreased** in urine and serum, in contrast to secondary polycythemia.
- **Bone marrow** shows either erythroid hyperplasia or hyperplasia of all elements (trilineage hyperplasia) and depletion of iron stores.
- **Leukocyte alkaline phosphatase (LAP):** Increased in majority of patients.
- **Serum vitamin B_{12} and vitamin B_{12}-binding protein** transcobalamin I (TC I) levels: Increased (not routinely measured)
- **Serum uric acid:** Increased indicating increased cell turnover.
- Abnormal liver function tests.
- Janus kinase 2 (JAK2) mutations (e.g., **JAK2V617F mutation**)
  - In ~95% patients with polycythemia vera, and in ~50% of essential thrombocytosis (ET) and primary myelofibrosis.
  - Janus kinases belong to tyrosine kinase family located on chromosome 9.
  - JAK2 is used by the EPO, thrombopoietin, and granulocyte colony stimulating factor (G-CSF) receptors to transmit signals and are involved in hematopoiesis.
  - JAK2 inhibitors are used for managing these patients.

WHO Diagnostic Criteria for Polycythemia Vera

WHO diagnostic criteria for PV have been shown in **Table 8.39**.

TABLE 8.39: WHO (2016) diagnostic criteria for polycythemia vera (PV).

Major criteria	*Minor criteria*
➢ Hb >18.5 g/dL (men), >16.5 g/dL (women) **OR** Hb or PCV>99th percentile of reference range **OR** Hb >17 g/dL (men) or >15 g/dL (women) if associated with a documented and sustained increase of ≥2 g/dL from baseline that cannot explained otherwise. **OR** Elevated red cell mass >25% above mean normal predicted value	➢ BM showing hypercellularity with trilineage (panmyelosis) myeloproliferation ➢ Subnormal serum EPO level
➢ Presence of JAF2V617F (a mutation in JAK2) or similar mutation	➢ Endogenous erythroid colony (EEC) growth
Diagnostic criteria for PV **Either both major criteria +1 minor criterion or first major criterion + 2 minor criteria**	

(BM: bone marrow; EPO: erythropoietin)

Clinical Course

The clinical course tends to proceed as a series of phases.
- Proliferative phase: Erythroid proliferation with increased red cell mass.
- Spent phase: Excessive proliferation of erythroid cells ceases, resulting in stable or decreased erythrocyte mass
- Progression to myelofibrosis
- Acute myelogenous leukemia in 2–5% of cases.

Complications of PV

Complications of PV have been shown in **Box 8.17**.

Box 8.17: Complications of polycythemia vera (PV).

- Thrombotic and bleeding episodes
- Peptic ulcer
- Hyperuricemia (gout)
- Sudden increase in splenic size
- Acute nonlymphocytic leukemia
- Myelofibrosis and myeloid metaplasia
- Erythromelalgia (thrombocytosis, involving the lower extremities with erythema, warmth, and pain and occasionally digital infarction)

Treatment (Fig. 8.33)

PV generally has a very slow course.

Aim of treatment: To maintain a normal blood count, PCV below 0.45 L/L and the platelet count below 400 x 10^9/L and to prevent the complications (mainly thrombosis and hemorrhage).

- **Venesection:** Repeated venesection (phlebotomy) is the treatment of choice and relieves many of the symptoms of PV.
- **Chemotherapy:** Chemotherapy is indicated if the patient is intolerant to venesection, or thrombocytosis occurs, or symptomatic or progressive splenomegaly develops.
  - Continuous or intermittent treatment with **hydroxycarbamide (hydroxyurea)** is the treatment of choice in patients above 40 years. It controls thrombocytosis and generally safer than alkylating agents (e.g., busulfan) and ^{32}P (Phosphorus) which carry an increased risk of acute leukemia
  - In younger patients, interferon-α is used
- **Radioactive ^{32}P:** One dose may give control for up to1½ years, but carries an increased risk to acute leukemia. In elderly patients (>70 years), ^{32}P or low-dose intermittent busulphan may be more convenient
- **Other measures:**
  - Low-dose aspirin: May be used to reduce thrombotic episodes
  - Anagrelide (inhibits platelet aggregation): May be used if thrombotic features develop despite above treatment.
  - Itching should be treated with antihistamines. If do not relieve, hydroxyurea, interferon-α and psoralens with UV light in 'A' range (PUVA) may be helpful
  - Asymptomatic hyperuricemia does not require treatment

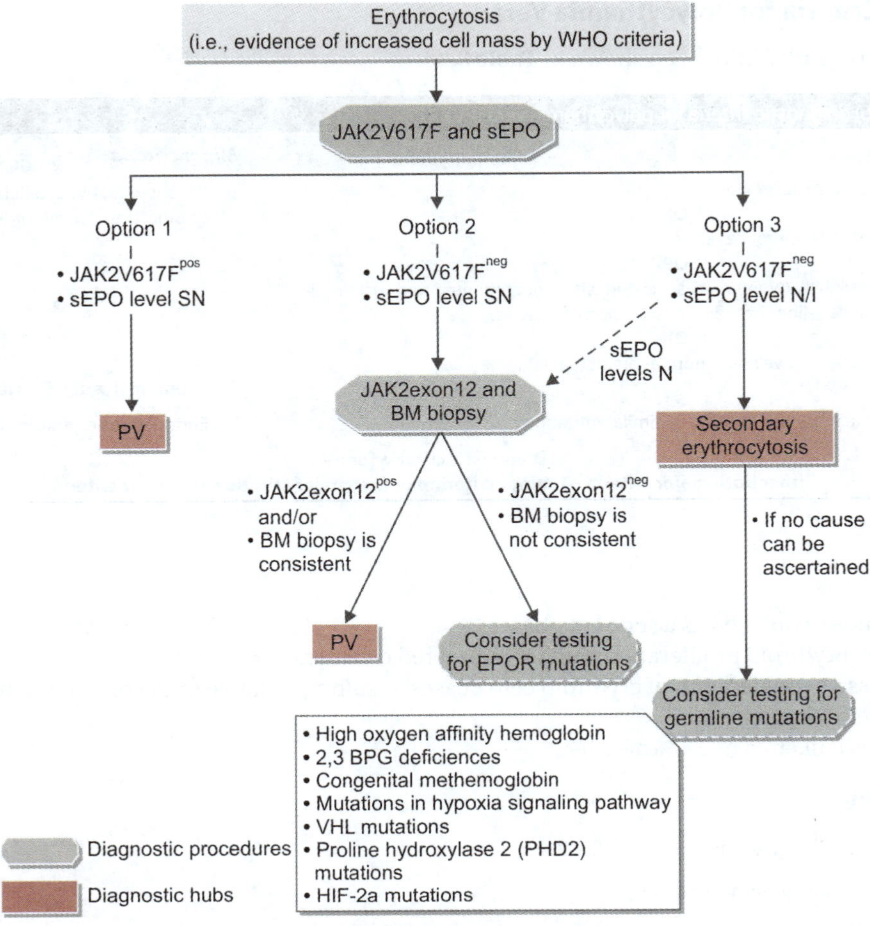

FIG. 8.33: Approach to polycythemia.
(PV: polycythemia vera)

Q. How will you differentiate primary polycythemia (polycythemia vera) from secondary polycythemia with hypoxia [(e.g., chronic obstructive pulmonary disease (COPD)]?

Differences between polycythemia vera and secondary polycythemia have been shown in **Table 8.40**.

TABLE 8.40: Differences between polycythemia vera and secondary polycythemia.

Feature	Polycythemia vera	Secondary polycythemia
➤ Oxygen saturation	Normal	Low
➤ EPO (erythropoietin) levels	Decreased	Increased
➤ Blood counts		
– Total white cell count	Increased	Normal
– Absolute basophil count	Increased	Normal
– Platelet count	Increased	Normal
➤ Leukocyte alkaline phosphatase (LAP)	Raised	Normal
➤ Vitamin B_{12} levels	Increased	Normal
➤ Bone marrow	Trilineage (panhyperplasia)	Erythroid hyperplasia
➤ Splenomegaly	Present	Absent

PRIMARY MYELOFIBROSIS

Q. Discuss the clinical features, investigations, and management of primary myelofibrosis (agnogenic myeloid metaplasia, myelofibrosis with myeloid metaplasia).

Definition

Primary myelofibrosis is a clonal MPN characterized by increased fibrosis within the marrow, which replaces hematopoietic cells leading to cytopenias, splenomegaly, and extensive extramedullary hematopoiesis. The extramedullary hematopoiesis is seen in the spleen, liver and at times in lymph nodes, kidneys, and adrenals.

- It can arise from PV or ET.

Clinical Features

- Usually found above 60 years of age.
- A significant number of cases develop acute myeloid leukemia.

Symptoms

- Symptoms due to progressive anemia: Fatigue, weakness, and anorexia.
- Symptoms due to massive splenomegaly: Abdominal distension, postprandial fullness, reflux esophagitis, dyspnea, and dragging discomfort in the left hypochondrium.
- Symptoms resulting from hypermetabolic state: Fever, fatigue, weight loss, night sweats, and heat intolerance.
- Bleeding tendencies due to thrombocytopenia develops at late stages.
- Death usually occurs due to portal hypertension and infections.
- Median survival is about 5 years.

Signs

- Massive splenomegaly and hepatomegaly.
- Anemia, lymphadenopathy, bleeding manifestations, ascites, cardiac failure, and jaundice.
- Hyperuricemia and secondary gout due to a high rate of cell turnover.
- Extramedullary hematopoiesis: May produce paraspinal masses with spinal cord compression, ascites, and effusions (pleural and pericardial).

Investigations

- Hemoglobin level: Normal in the early stages, but markedly reduced in the late stages.
- Total leukocyte count: Normal/increased (early stages)/decreased (late stages).
- Platelet count: Increased in early stages and decreased in the late stages.
- Peripheral smear:
  - **RBC series**
    - Moderate-to-severe degree of normochromic normocytic anemia accompanied by **leukoerythroblastic blood picture** (precursors of granulocytes and nucleated RBCs being present simultaneously).
    - **Many tear drop-shaped red cells** (dacryocytes) probably due to damage in the fibrotic marrow.
    - Basophilic stippling.
  - **Giant platelets** with vacuoles.
- **Bone marrow:** The peripheral smear findings are not specific and bone marrow biopsy is diagnostic.
  - Cellularity: Early stages (cellular phase), it is often hypercellular and in later stages (hypocellular phase), it becomes hypocellular and diffusely fibrotic.
  - Megakaryocytes are large, dysplastic, and abnormally clustered.
- **LAP score:** Raised
- **Philadelphia chromosome:** Negative.
- JAK2 V617F mutation occurs in ~50% patients. CALR mutation is also present.
- **Serum vitamin B_{12}:** Moderately increased.
- **Radiological examination shows** increased bone density of vertebrate and proximal ends of long bones.

Treatment

No specific therapy exists for primary myelofibrosis

- **Treatment of anemia**
  - Correct other causes of anemia like gastrointestinal blood loss and folic acid deficiency (folic acid 5 mg daily)
  - Packed red cell transfusions
  - Neither recombinant erythropoietin nor androgens (such as danazol) is consistently effective in controlling anemia but can be tried in some patients
  - Glucocorticoids (prednisolone) may control constitutional symptoms and autoimmune complications
  - Combination with low-dose thalidomide (50–100 mg/day) with prednisolone can control anemia and splenomegaly in a significant number of patients

- **Treatment of splenomegaly**
  - **Patients with cellular bone marrow and marked leukocytosis**: Busulphan 2 mg daily
  - Indications for splenectomy in selected cases
    - With hypersplenism
    - If splenomegaly impairs alimentation and should be performed before cachexia sets in
  - Splenic irradiation: To reduce splenic size is reserved for patients, who cannot undergo splenectomy. Patients often develop severe cytopenias
  - Hydroxyurea is useful to control splenomegaly, but can produce myelosuppression that may exacerbate underlying anemia.
- **Treatment of extramedullary hematopoiesis:** By low-dose irradiation
- **Curative treatment: Allogeneic bone marrow transplantation** is the only curative treatment. It should be performed in younger patients as most patients in IMF are above 60 years of age
- **Others**
  - Allopurinol can control hyperuricemia
  - Etanercept (TNF-α antagonist) used in patients with severe constitutional features
  - JAK2 inhibitors ruxolitinib is used in clinical practice

Prognosis

Median survival varies from 27 to 135 months and depends on prognostic factors **(Box 8.18)**.

Box 8.18: Shows poor prognostic factors.

- Age >65 years
- Presence of blasts in peripheral blood
- Hemoglobin level <10 g/dL
- Presence of constitutional symptoms
- Total WBC count >25,000/mm^3

(WBC: white blood cell)

Myelophthisis

Q. Write short note on myelophthisis and its causes.

Fibrosis of the bone marrow can occur as a primary hematologic disease is known as primary myelofibrosis (myeloid metaplasia), and as a secondary reactive process, known as myelophthisis (secondary myelofibrosis).

Causes of myelophthisis (other causes of myelofibrosis) are presented in **Box 8.19**. These causes may also produce splenomegaly.

Box 8.19: Causes of secondary myelofibrosis.

Malignant conditions		***Nonmalignant conditions***
Hematological • Leukemia – Acute leukemia (lymphoid/myeloid) – Chronic myeloid leukemia – Hairy cell leukemia • Multiple myeloma • Polycythemia vera • Hodgkin's lymphoma • Essential thrombocytosis	Nonhematological • Metastasis to marrow – Carcinoma breast, lung or prostate – Neuroblastoma	• Infections • Human immunodeficiency virus (HIV) infection • Tuberculosis • Exposure to thorium dioxide • Systemic lupus erythematosus • Renal osteodystrophy • Hyperparathyroidism • Radiation therapy or treatment with radiomimetic drugs • Gaucher disease

Q. How will you differentiate chronic myeloid leukemia from myelofibrosis?

Differences between chronic myeloid leukemia from myelofibrosis have been shown in **Table 8.41.**

TABLE 8.41: Difference between chronic myeloid leukemia from myelofibrosis.

Features	***Chronic myeloid leukemia***	***Myelofibrosis***
Total leukocyte count	Markedly raised usually more than 20,000/μL	May be raised, but always less than 20,000/μL
Peripheral blood		
Peripheral smear	Shows full range of granulocyte precursors, predominantly mature forms	Shows leukoerythroblastosis with tear drop cells
Nucleated red cells	Few or absent	Numerous
Thrombocytopenia	Occurs late	Common
Marrow fibrosis	Uncommon and minimal	Common and dense
LAP (leukocyte alkaline phosphatase) score	Very low, usually <5	High, usually >100
Philadelphia chromosome	Positive	Negative
Serum vitamin B_{12} levels	Very high	Moderately raised

MYELODYSPLASTIC SYNDROMES

Q. Describe the etiology, classification, clinical features, diagnosis and treatment of myelodysplastic syndrome (MDS).

Definition

Myelodysplastic syndromes are a heterogeneous group of acquired clonal stem cell disorders characterized by:
- Progressive cytopenias (low blood cell counts)
- Dysplasia in one or more major cell lines (erythroid, myeloid and megakaryocytic forms)
- Ineffective hematopoiesis
- Increased risk of development of AML
- A subtype of myeloid neoplasms.

Etiology

- In primary MDS the exact cause is not known, however genetic factors may play a role.
- Causes of secondary/t-MDS: Exposure to radiation, benzene, postchemotherapy (particularly alkylating agents and topoisomerase inhibitors), viruses, cigarette smoking, and PNH.
- Median age is 65 years.

WHO (2016) Classification of MDS

The revised WHO (2016) diagnosis and classification of MDS introduce refinements in morphologic interpretation, cytopenias assessment, and genetic information. Cytopenia is necessary for diagnosis of any MDS and in WHO (2008) classifications, MDS nomenclature included references to "cytopenia" or to specific types of cytopenia (e.g., refractory anemia). Present WHO (2016) classification depends mainly on the degree of dysplasia and blast percentages and specific cytopenias have only minor impact. Hence, the terminology for adult MDS has replaced the terms such as "refractory anemia" and "refractory cytopenia" with "myelodysplastic syndrome" followed by the appropriate modifiers: Single versus multilineage dysplasia, ring sideroblasts, excess blasts, or the del (5q) cytogenetic abnormality **(Table 8.42)**.

Clinical Features

- Usually found in patients above 60 years and slightly more common in males.
- Detected incidentally on routine blood examination in about 50% of patients.

TABLE 8.42: WHO (2016) classification, peripheral smear and bone marrow findings of myelodysplastic syndromes.

Disease	*Dysplastic lineages*	*Cytopenias*[1]	*Ring sideroblasts as % of marrow erythroid elements*	*Bone marrow (BM) and peripheral blood (PB) blasts*
➢ MDS with single lineage dysplasia (MDS-SLD)	1	1 or 2	<15%/<5%[2]	BM <5%, PB <1%, no Auer rods
➢ MDS with multilineage dysplasia (MDS-MLD)	2 or 3	1–3	<15%/<5%[2]	BM <5%, PB <1%, no Auer rods
➢ MDS with ring sideroblasts (MDS-RS)				
– MDS-RS with single lineage dysplasia (MDSRS-SLD)	1	1 or 2	≥15%/≥5%[2]	BM <5%, PB <1%, no Auer rods
– MDS-RS with multilineage dysplasia (MDS-RS-MLD)	2 or 3	1–3	≥15%/≥5%[2]	BM <5%, PB <1%, no Auer rods
➢ MDS with isolated del (5q)	1–3	1–2	None or any	BM <5%, PB <1%, no Auer rods
➢ MDS with excess blasts (MDSEB)				
– MDS-EB-1	0–3	1–3	None or any	BM 5–9% or PB 2–4%, no Auer rods
– MDS-EB-2	0–3	1–3	None or any	BM 10–19% or PB 5–19% or Auer rods
➢ MDS, unclassifiable (MDS-U)				
– With 1% blood blasts	1–3	1–3	None or any	BM <5%, PB = 1%[3], no Auer rods
– With single lineage dysplasia and pancytopenia	1	3	None or any	BM <5%, PB <1%, no Auer rods
– Based on defining cytogenetic abnormality	0	1–3	<15%[4]	BM <5%, PB <1%, no Auer rods
➢ Refractory cytopenia of childhood	1–3	1–3	None	BM <5%, PB <2%

[1]Cytopenias defined as hemoglobin <10 g/dL, platelet count <100 × 109/L, and absolute neutrophil count <1.8 × 109/L; rarely, MDS may present with mild anemia or thrombocytopenia above these levels. PB monocytes must be <1 × 109/L.

[2]If *SF3B1* mutation is present.

[3]1% PB blasts must be recorded on at least two separate occasions.

[4]Cases with ≥15% ring sideroblasts by definition have significant erythroid dysplasia, and are classified as MDS-RS-SL.

- Symptoms are due to cytopenias which may be single-lineage cytopenia, bicytopenia, or pancytopenia. Symptoms include:
  - Weakness (anemia)
  - Infections (leukopenia)
  - Hemorrhage (thrombocytopenia).
- Extramedullary hematopoiesis may cause hepatomegaly and splenomegaly but is uncommon.
- About 10–40% progresses to AML because of which MDS was referred to as preleukemic syndrome.

Diagnosis

- Minimal morphologic criterion for the diagnosis of an MDS: Dysplasia in at least 10% of cells of any one of the myeloid lineages.
- Complete blood count: May give clues to this diagnosis.
- **Peripheral smear:**
  - **RBC:** Mild-to-moderate degree of macrocytic or dimorphic anemia with evidence of dyspoiesis.
  - **WBC** count may be normal or low. Neutropenia with few blasts. Number of blasts determines the type of MDS (**Table 8.42**). The cytoplasm of neutrophils is hypogranular or agranular. The nuclei of neutrophils may show hyposegmentation with only two nuclear lobes (Pseudo-Pelger-Hüet cells), hypersegmentation or ringed neutrophils.
  - **Platelets:** Variable thrombocytopenia, presence of large hypogranular or giant platelets is seen.
  - **NAP score** is moderately or severely decreased.
- **Bone marrow:** The most characteristic features are varying degree of dyspoietic (disordered) differentiation affecting all nonlymphoid lineages (erythroid, granulocytic, monocytic, and megakaryocytic) associated with cytopenias.
- Cytogenic study of the marrow: Most important for establishing the diagnosis. Chromosome abnormalities of chromosome 5 or 7 are frequent.

Treatment

- Therapy is supportive:
  - Packed red cell transfusion for anemia
  - Platelet transfusions for bleeding due to thrombocytopenia
  - Antibiotic therapy for infections
  - Iron chelators to reduce iron overload from multiple transfusions
- EPO and G-CSF may be useful in some patients, to ameliorate symptoms
- Others: Use of thalidomide, lenalidomide (a derivative of thalidomide), 5-azacitidine and decitabine. 5-azacytidine and decitabine (hypomethylating agents) may reduce requirements of blood transfusion and to retard the progression of MDS to AML. Lenalidomide is found useful in the 5q-syndrome
- Allogeneic hematopoietic stem cell transplantation: Curative. However, it may be performed in less than 5–10% of patients because MDS is most common during seventh or eighth decade of life

PLASMA CELL NEOPLASMS

Q. Write short essay/note on plasma cell neoplasms/disorders.

Classification of plasma cell proliferative disorders has been shown in **Table 8.43**.

TABLE 8.43: Classification of plasma cell proliferative disorders.

Monoclonal gammopathies of undetermined significance (MGUS) ➢ Benign (IgG, IgA, IgD, IgM, and rarely, free light chains) ➢ Associated neoplasms or other diseases not known to produce monoclonal proteins ➢ Biclonal gammopathies ➢ Idiopathic Bence Jones proteinuria **Heavy chain diseases (HCDs)** ➢ γ-HCD ➢ α-HCD ➢ μ-HCD	**Malignant monoclonal gammopathies** ➢ Multiple myeloma (IgG, IgA, IgD, IgE, and free light chains) - Overt multiple myeloma - Smoldering multiple myeloma - Plasma cell leukemia - Nonsecretory myeloma - IgD myeloma - Osteosclerotic myeloma (POEMS syndrome) - Solitary plasmacytoma of bone - Extramedullary plasmacytoma ➢ Waldenström's macroglobulinemia ➢ Other lymphoproliferative diseases
Cryoglobulinemia	**Primary amyloidosis (AL)**

MULTIPLE MYELOMA

Q. Discuss the immunopathology, pathology, clinical features, investigations, diagnosis, and treatment of multiple myeloma.

- Multiple myeloma is a malignant plasma cell neoplasm derived from a single clone plasma cells of the bone marrow and produces multiple, lytic bone lesions.
- Plasma cells are derived from B lymphocytes.
- Normal plasma cells secrete equal quantities of heavy and light chains. But the neoplastic plasma cells frequently synthesize excess of light (L) or heavy (H) chains along with complete Igs. Rarely, only light chains or heavy chains are produced.
- The excess of free light chains are small with low molecular weight and therefore excreted in the urine. They are known as Bence-Jones proteins.
- **Classification of myeloma:** It is based on the type of paraprotein secreted namely: (1) IgG (55%), (2) IgA (25%), (3) IgD (uncommon), (4) IgE (uncommon), and (5) light chain disease (20%). In nonsecretory myeloma, there is no M-protein in the blood or urine but bone marrow shows plasmacytosis.
- The cause of multiple myeloma is unclear. Exposure to radiation, benzene, and other organic solvents, herbicides, and insecticides may play a role. Multiple myeloma has been reported in familial clusters of two or more first-degree relatives and in identical twins.

Clinical Features

- Insidious in onset.
- Age and gender: Peak incidence is seen during 6th to 7th decade, and males are more affected than females.
- Symptoms **(Flowchart 8.2 and Table 8.44)**.
  - Some patients may be asymptomatic, and is accidentally detected during the preclinical phase.

FLOWCHART 8.2: Clinical features and laboratory findings in myeloma.

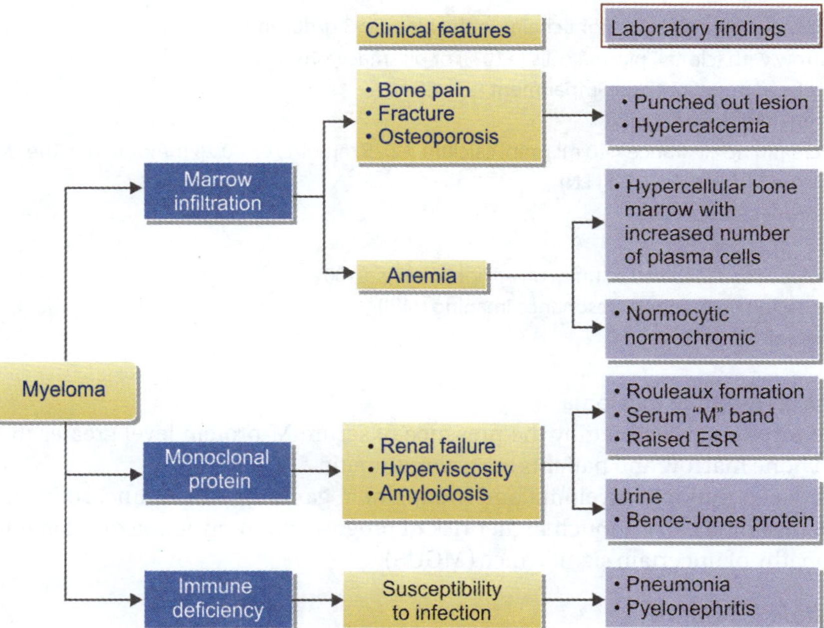

TABLE 8.44: Clinical features in multiple myeloma based on involved organ/system.

Involved organ/system	*Features (Box 8.20)*
Bone	➢ Localized bony swellings over vertebrae, skull, sternum, ribs, and clavicle ➢ Bone pain due to pathological fractures, backache due to involvement of vertebra (60%) ➢ Neurological symptoms of sensory and/or motor loss due to lesion in the vertebra compressing the spinal cord nerve root
Bone marrow	Anemia, leukopenia, and thrombocytopenia
Immune system	Humoral immune deficiency leading to increased susceptibility to infections (recurrent infections), particularly of the respiratory system and urinary tract

Contd...

Contd...

Renal damage is multifactorial due to Bence-Jones proteinuria, hypercalcemia, humoral immune deficiency	Nephrocalcinosis, amyloidosis, renal insufficiency (renal failure in 20–30%), infections, or nephrotic syndrome
Bleeding tendency due to thrombocytopenia	Purpura, epistaxis, gastrointestinal bleeding
Cryoglobulinemia and hyperviscosity (uncommon) syndrome	Hyperviscosity may affect the: ➢ CNS (leading to confusion, headache, vertigo, nystagmus, postural hypotension, and dizziness) ➢ Retina (producing blurred vision, retinal venous congestion, papilledema) ➢ Congestive cardiac failure (CVS)
Neurological manifestations	Amyloid peripheral neuropathy, carpal tunnel syndrome, and compressive myelopathy

(CNS: central nervous system)

Mnemonic to remember common symptoms of multiple myeloma **(Box 8.20)**.

Box 8.20: Mnemonic to remember common symptoms of multiple myeloma.

CRAB: C = Calcium (elevated), **R** = Renal failure, **A** = Anemia, **B** = Bone lesions.

Osteosclerotic Myeloma (POEMS Syndrome)

This syndrome is characterized by polyneuropathy, organomegaly, endocrinopathy, M-protein, and skin changes (POEMS). The major clinical features are a chronic inflammatory-demyelinating polyneuropathy with predominantly motor disability and sclerotic skeletal lesions.

Diagnosis of Multiple Myeloma

Q. Write short essay/note on diagnosis and management of multiple myeloma.

Requires at least two of the following:

- Monoclonal immunoglobulin (M protein) or light chains in the blood (>3 g/dL) and/or urine
- Infiltration of bone marrow with (clonal) plasma cells (≥10%) or plasmacytoma
- Evidence of myeloma-related organ or tissue impairment (≥1)-CRAB
  - Hypercalcemia: Serum (ionized) >5.5 mEg/L
  - Renal insufficiency creatinine clearance <40 mL/min, calcium >2.75 mmol/L, or >0.25 mmol/L than the ULN
  - Anemia (hemoglobin or 2 g/dL below the LLN)
  - Lytic bone lesions and/or osteoporosis
- Other criteria
  - Free light chain ratio between involved to uninvolved light chains >100
  - Presence of >1 bone lesion on magnetic resonance imaging (MRI)
  - Bone marrow plasma cell percentage >60

Smoldering (asymptomatic) multiple myeloma

- Smoldering multiple myeloma is defined by the presence of serum M-protein level greater than 3 g/dL and/or 10% or more plasma cells in bone marrow and patients are asymptomatic.
- This entity lies in between multiple myeloma and monoclonal gammopathy of uncertain significance. Patients with smoldering multiple myeloma carry a much higher risk of progression to myeloma or related malignancy compared to monoclonal gammopathy of uncertain significance (MGUS).

Investigations in Multiple Myeloma

- **Peripheral blood**
  - Usually shows anemia, leukopenia, thrombocytopenia, and raised erythrocyte sedimentation rate (ESR).
  - Peripheral blood smear: May show **rouleaux formation** due to increased immunoglobulins.
- **Bone marrow examination** is important. Normal bone marrow contains 2–10% plasma cells. In myeloma, the bone marrow is **hypercellular** as a result of increased number of plasma cells and **myeloma cells** (neoplastic plasma cells). Increased number of **myeloma cells, more than 30%** of the cellularity is diagnostic.
- **Urine: Bence-Jones proteins** may be present
- **Serum findings:**
  - **Serum β_2 microglobulin:** It is a useful **prognostic marker** and **high values signify poor prognosis.**
  - **Hypercalcemia** is due to extensive osteolytic lesions and osteoporosis and there are also increased levels of serum phosphate.
  - Serum alkaline phosphatase: Usually normal in the absence of complications.
  - Blood urea and serum creatinine raised in 20% of cases and along with electrolytes are used to assess renal function.

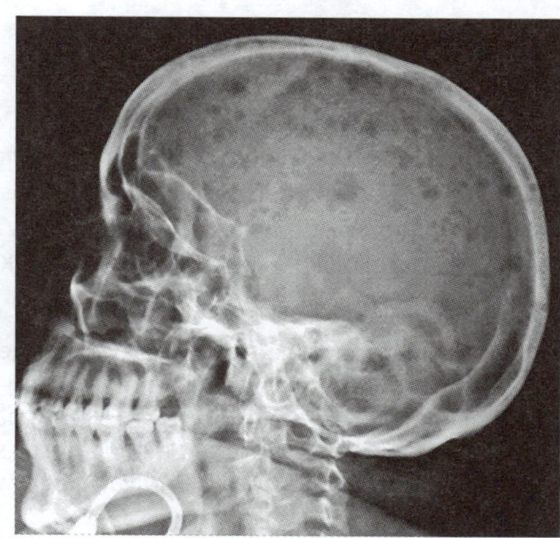

FIG. 8.34: X-ray of skull in myeloma showing punched out lesions.

- Serum proteins: Total serum protein level is increased, albumin is decreased and globulins are markedly increased.
- Serum uric acid: Raised.
- Serum immunoglobulin estimation reveals a reduction of normal immunoglobulins below normal levels.

- **Electrophoretic studies on serum and urine:** Electrophoretic studies reveal raised levels of immunoglobulins in the blood and/or light chains (Bence-Jones proteins) in the urine. The monoclonal immunoglobulin (M-protein) is identified as abnormal protein "spikes" in serum or urine electrophoresis. The type of immunoglobulin can be determined by immunofixation. The most common M-protein is IgG type, followed by IgA.
- **Radiological examination:**
  - Reveals generalized osteoporosis.
  - Radiographs of flat bones: Such as **skull (Fig. 8.34), vertebral bodies, ribs, and pelvis** show the characteristic **punched-out osteolytic lesions.**
  - Collapse of multiple vertebrate is a common finding.
- MRI and positron emission tomography (PET): May detect bone involvement when skeletal survey is normal.

Staging (Tables 8.45 and 8.46)

TABLE 8.45: Modified from Durie-Salmon staging.

Stage	*Criteria*
Stage-I	➢ Low M-component: IgG <5 g/dL, IgA <3 g/dL, urine Bence-Jones protein <4 g/24 hours ➢ Normal hemoglobin, serum calcium, Ig levels (non-M protein)
Stage-II	Overall values between stage I and III
Stage-III	One or more of the following: ➢ Hemoglobin <8.5 g/dL, serum calcium >12 mg/dL ➢ High M-component: IgG >7 g/dL, IgA >5 g/dL, urine light chain >12 g/24 hours ➢ Advanced multiple lytic lesions on X-rays
Subclassification based on renal function ➢ Subclass A = Serum creatinine <2 mg/dL ➢ Subclass B = Serum creatinine >2 mg/dL	

TABLE 8.46: International staging system.

Stage	*Characteristic features*	*Median survival*
I	Serum β2-microglobulin <3.5 mg/dL and serum albumin >3.5 g/dL	62 months
II	Serum β2-microglobulin <3.5 mg/dL and serum albumin <3.5 g/dL and or serum β2-microglobulin <3.5–5.5 mg/dL	44 months
III	β2-microglobulin <5.5 mg/dL	29 months

Treatment

General measures

- High fluid intake of about 3 L/day to treat renal impairment and hypercalcemia
- Prompt treatment of infections with antibiotics
- Treatment of anemia may require blood transfusion and erythropoietin often helps
- Analgesics to be given for relief of bone pain
- Allopurinol 300 mg daily should be given to reduce/prevent hyperuricemia and urate nephropathy
- Hyperviscosity syndrome is managed by plasmapheresis
- Bisphosphonates (e.g., zoledronate, pamidronate, clodronate) which inhibit osteoclast activity. Long-term treatment with this, reduce skeletal events such as pathological fracture, cord compression, and bone pain. An important complication of bisphosphonates is osteonecrosis of jaw
- Orthopedic assistance and physiotherapy can significantly improve the quality of life
- Renal failure: Treated by rehydration and oral prednisolone **(Fig. 8.35)**

Autologous stem cell transplantation

- Young patients (<65 years) without renal failure: Standard treatment is first-line high-dose chemotherapy for myeloablation (melphalan 200 mg/m^2 intravenously) to maximum response and then an autologous stem-cell transplantation

Chemotherapy

Regimen used

- Bortezomib, lenalidomide, dexamethasone (VRd)
- Daratumumab, lenalidomide, dexamethasone (DRd)
- Bortezomib, cyclophosphamide, dexamethasone (VCd)
- Bortezomib, thalidomide, dexamethasone (VTd)
- Carfilzomib, lenalidomide, dexamethasone (KRd)

Older patients

- Thalidomide combined with the alkylating agent (melphalan or cyclophosphamide or chlorambucil) and prednisolone. Thalidomide is teratogenic. Recent studies have suggested that combination with thalidomide, results in improved response rates and overall survival, albeit with increased toxicity **(Box 8.21)**
- Bortezomib is a proteasome inhibitor, which is used for upfront and relapsed is combined with doxorubicin and dexamethasone
- Lenalidomide in combination with steroids has been tried

Younger patients (<65 years)

- Bortezomib, cyclophosphamide and dexamethasone. OR Newer drugs include carfilzomib, Ixazomib, pomalidomide, daratumumab, and elotuzumab
- Orally active cyclophosphamide, thalidomide, and dexamethasone-based induction (CTD) followed by a high-dose melphalan autograft

Radiotherapy

- Effective for local problems like severe bone pain, pathological fractures, and tumorous lesions

As an emergency treatment of spinal cord compression complicating extradural plasmacytomas

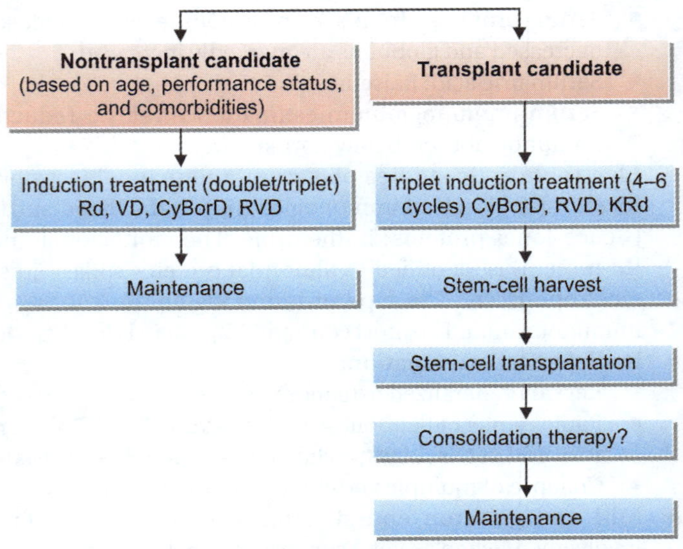

FIG. 8.35: Initial approach to treatment of symptomatic multiple myeloma.

(CyBorD indicates cyclophosphamide, bortezomib, and dexamethasone; KRd, carfilzomib, lenalidomide, and low-dose dexamethasaone; Rd: lenalidomide and low-dose dexamethasone; RVD: lenalidomide, bortezomib, and dexamethasone; VD: bortezomib and dexamethasone.

Box 8.21: Median survival.

- Patients with advanced myeloma: 7–8 months
- With good supportive care and chemotherapy: 3–5 years. Asymptomatic stage I patients are generally not given chemotherapy
- Young patients with intensive therapy may live longer

Renal Involvement in Multiple Myeloma

Q. Write short note on the cause of renal failure of multiple myeloma.

- Renal involvement is observed in 50% of myeloma patients.
- Renal failure develops in ~25% of patients with multiple myeloma.
- Various factors contributing to renal failure in multiple myeloma are:
  - **Tubular damage** from excretion of light chains (Bence-Jones proteinuria).
  - Hypercalcemia resulting in **nephrocalcinosis** and renal damage.
  - **Amyloid deposition** in the glomeruli (renal amyloidosis).
  - Hyperuricemia producing in **urate nephropathy**.
  - **Recurrent urinary tract infections.**
  - **Infiltration** of the kidney **by myeloma cells.**

Poor Prognostic Factors in Multiple Myeloma

Q. Write short note on the indications of poor prognosis in multiple myeloma.

Poor prognostic factors in multiple myeloma have been shown in **Box 8.22**.

Box 8.22: Poor prognostic factors in multiple myeloma.

High levels of β2-microglobulin	Low serum albumin
High serum calcium >12 g/dL at presentation	Low hemoglobin (<8.5 g/dL)
Advanced lytic bone lesions	Thrombocytopenia
Renal failure	Plasma cell leukemia

Radiographic Features in Multiple Myeloma

Q. Write short note on the role of radiographic examination in the diagnosis of multiple myeloma.

Radiographic features in multiple myeloma have been shown in **Table 8.47**.

TABLE 8.47: Radiographic features helpful in the diagnosis of multiple myeloma.

Site of X-ray	*Appearance*
Skull and pelvis	Multiple punched out osteolytic lesions osteoporosis
Chest	Pathological fractures and punched out lesions of ribs, clavicle, and scapulae osteoporosis
Spine	Collapse of multiple vertebrae osteoporosis
Kidney, ureter, and bladder (KUB)	Nephrocalcinosis

Monoclonal Gammopathy of Uncertain Significance

Q. Write short essay/note on monoclonal gammopathy of uncertain significance (MGUS).

Definition: MGUS is defined as presence of serum M-protein concentration lower than 3 g/dL, bone marrow clonal plasma cells <10% plasma cells, and no end organ damage [CRAB (*refer* **Box 8.20**) no hypercalcemia, no renal impairment, no anemia, or no osteolytic lesions] or no evidence of other B-cell neoplasms.

- MGUS is one of the most common plasma cell dyscrasias, occurring in about 3–5% of general population above the age of 50 years.
- **Progression:** MGUS should be considered as preneoplastic condition. It can progress to multiple myeloma, Waldenstrom's macroglobulinemia, primary AL amyloidosis, or a lymphoproliferative disorder at a rate of 1–1.5% per year. Risk of progression to multiple myeloma and related disorders depends upon:
  - Size of M-component (risk of progression with an M-protein value of 1.5 g/dL almost twice that of a patient with an M-protein value of 0.5 g/dL)
  - Type of M-component (IgM and IgA increased risk compared to IgG), and
  - Abnormal free light chain ratio (kappa; lambda ratio-normal being 0.26–1.65).
- Follow-up: Patients should be followed with serum protein electrophoresis at 6 months and, if stable, can be followed every 1–2 years.
- No treatment is indicated.

Differences between multiple myeloma and monoclonal gammopathy of undetermined significance have been shown in Table 8.48.

TABLE 8.48: Differences between multiple myeloma and monoclonal gammopathy of undetermined significance (MGUS).

Characteristic features	*Multiple myeloma*	*MGUS*
M-protein	Found in serum and/or urine except in patients with nonsecretory	Intact immunoglobulin (e.g., IgG, IgM, IgA)
Bone marrow	Clonal plasma cells 10% or more	➢ Clonal plasma cells <10% ➢ No evidence of other B-cell proliferative disorders
Organ/tissue involvement	At least one of the following: ➢ Serum calcium (ionized) >5.5 mEq/L ➢ Renal insufficiency (creatinine >2 mg/dL) ➢ Anemic (hemoglobin <10 g/dL) ➢ Bone involvement—osteolytic bone lesions and/or osteopenia	➢ No hypercalcemia, renal impairment, anemia or bone involvement

Solitary Plasmacytoma

Q. Write short essay/note on solitary plasmacytoma of bone.

- Solitary plasmacytoma (osseous plasmacytoma) is a solitary tumor occurring in the bone consisting of collection of monoclonal plasma cells.
- Comprises 3–5% of plasma cell neoplasms.
- Sites: Common sites are bones with active hematopoiesis and usually occur in the same sites as in multiple myeloma (vertebrae, ribs, skull, pelvis, femur, clavicle, and scapula).
- Clinical features: Localized bone pain or pathological fracture. Vertebral lesions may produce neurologic symptoms secondary to spinal cord or root compression.
- Investigations:
  - M-protein in serum or urine observed 24–72% of patients by immune fixation
  - MRI is useful to rule out occult systemic disease.
- Treatment: Local control is achieved by radiotherapy. Up to two-thirds of patients develop systemic disease.
- Prognosis: Median survival is 7–12 years.

Solitary Extraosseous Plasmacytoma

Q. Write short essay/note on solitary extraosseous plasmacytoma.

- Extraosseous (extramedullary) plasmacytoma are localized plasma cell neoplasms that arise in tissues other than bone.
- Comprises 3–5% of all plasma cell neoplasms.

- Sites:
  - Upper respiratory tract (80%): Oropharynx, nasopharynx, sinuses, and larynx.
  - Other sites: GI tract, lymph nodes, bladder, central nervous system (CNS), breast, thyroid, testis, parotid, and skin.
- Only about 20% of patients have M protein (most commonly IgA).
- Diagnosis: Requires exclusion of occult systemic disease by extensive radiographic imaging.
- Treatment: Eradicated with local radiation therapy.
- Prognosis:
  - About 15% of patients subsequently develop multiple myeloma.
  - About 70% of patients remain disease free at 10 years.

Plasma Cell Leukemia

Q. Write short essay/note on plasma cell leukemia.

- Plasma cell leukemia (PCL) is the term used when the peripheral blood has more than 20% plasma cells with an absolute plasma cell count of 2000/μL or greater.
- Classification: Plasma cell leukemia may be classified as:
  - Primary plasma cell leukemia: It develops without any preceding evidence of multiple myeloma. It is diagnosed in the leukemic phase (60%). It develops in younger individuals and presents with hepatosplenomegaly and lymphadenopathy, a higher platelet count, few bone lesions, mild serum M-protein component, and longer survival rate when compared to those with secondary plasma cell leukemia.
  - Secondary: When leukemic transformation develops in a patient with multiple myeloma (40%).
- It is an aggressive disease associated with a high tumor burden and extramedullary dissemination.

Waldenstorm Macroglobulinemia

Q. Write short essay/note on Waldenstrom macroglobulinemia.

- Waldenstrom macroglobulinemia is a syndrome characterized by IgM monoclonal gammopathy sufficient to cause a hyperviscosity of the blood and bone marrow infiltration.
- Most commonly occurs in association with lymphoplasmacytic lymphoma. The tumor cells undergo terminal differentiation to plasma cells and secrete monoclonal IgM.
- It occurs in older adults (median age 60 years).

Clinical Features

May be asymptomatic.

- Usual presenting complaints are nonspecific and include weakness, fatigue, and weight loss. Symptoms develop due to:
  - **Tumor infiltration:** Most patients present with weakness and fatigue due to anemia caused by marrow infiltration. Other features include fever, night sweats, weight loss, lymphadenopathy, hepatomegaly, and splenomegaly.
  - **Monoclonal protein:** About 10% of patients have autoimmune hemolysis caused by cold agglutinins (monoclonal IgM bind to red cells at temperatures of less than 37°C). IgM may be associated with systemic amyloidosis. IgM-secreted by the tumor, because of its large size, at high concentrations increases the viscosity of the blood, giving rise to hyperviscosity syndrome. Features of hyperviscosity syndrome are:
    - Visual impairment associated with venous congestion (e.g., blurring or loss of vision)
    - Neurologic problems (e.g., dizziness, headache, vertigo, nystagmus, hearing loss, ataxia, paresthesias, diplopia)
    - Bleeding
    - Cryoglobulinemia produces symptoms such as Raynaud phenomenon and cold urticaria
  - Tumor cells can infiltrate organs and result in hepatomegaly, splenomegaly, and lymphadenopathy in about 20% patients.

Diagnosis

- Demonstration of monoclonal IgM: By serum electrophoresis, sample may require warming to 37°C, to avoid interference of cold agglutinins. Immunofixation is required to characterize monoclonal protein.
- Bone marrow aspirate and biopsy: It shows more than 10% lymphoplasmacytic cells (CD20^{+}).

Prognosis: Transformation to large-cell lymphoma occurs but is uncommon. Median survival is 4 years.

Treatment

- It is a chemotherapy- and immunotherapy-sensitive disease controllable with currently available therapies.
- No specific treatment needed for patients who do not have systemic symptoms.
- Single agent therapy with rituximab alone is used in symptomatic patients with modest hematologic compromise, IgM-related neuropathy, or hemolytic anemia unresponsive to corticosteroids.
- Combination chemotherapy and rituximab (anti-CD20): Patients with severe constitutional symptoms, profound hematologic compromise, bulky disease, or hyperviscosity syndrome should be treated with the dexamethasone, rituximab and cyclophosphamide Or bortezomib, dexamethasone, and rituximab or bendamustine rituximab.
- **Plasmapheresis:** Most of IgM secreted by tumor cells is intravascular. Patient with symptoms due to high IgM levels (such as hyperviscosity and hemolysis) should first undergo plasmapheresis which helps in alleviating these symptoms.

HODGKIN LYMPHOMA

Q. Discuss the pathological classification, clinical features, clinical staging, investigations, diagnosis, and treatment/ management of Hodgkin's lymphoma.

- Hodgkin lymphoma (HL) is a malignant lymphoma characterized by a heterogeneous cellularity comprising of **minority** (1–3%) of specific **neoplastic cells** (Hodgkin cells and Reed-Sternberg cells—**Figs. 8.36A and B)** in a "characteristic background" of reactive non-neoplastic cells (majority) of various types.
- **Cell of origin:** The neoplastic Reed-Sternberg cells are derived from germinal center or immediate post-germinal center B-cells indicating that most HLs are unusual tumors of B-cell origin.
- **Age:** Bimodal age incidence
  - One pack in young adults (15–35 years)
  - Other peak in older adults (45–75 years)
- The neoplastic cells in HL are **Reed-Sternberg cells (Figs. 8.36A and B)** and its variants.
- Immunophenotype:
  - Reed-Sternberg cells in classical forms of HL are $CD15^+$ and $CD30^+$.
  - Reed-Sternberg cells in lymphocyte predominance HL are CD15-ve and CD30-ve.

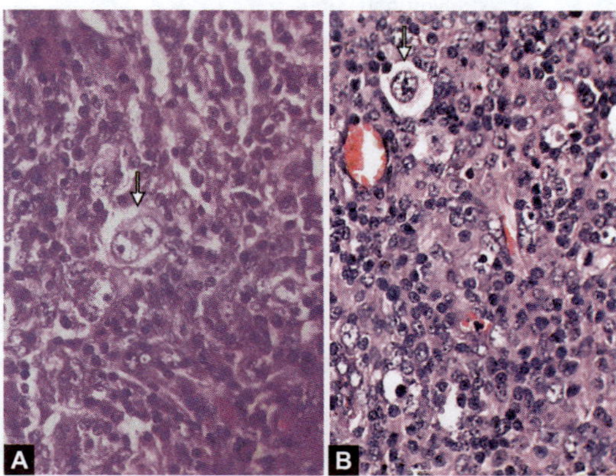

FIGS. 8.36A AND B: Microscopic appearance of Hodgkin lymphoma showing RS cells and Hodgkin cells within the background of mixed population of reactive cells.

Etiology

- **EBV:** Young adults, who have had previous EBV infection (infectious mononucleosis), have an increased risk of developing HL and the EBV genome is frequently identified in the Reed-Sternberg cells.
- **Genetic factors** may play a role because HLA subtypes, particularly HLA-B18, are higher in patients with HL.
- **Immune status:** HL seems to be more frequent in immunocompromised patients or those with autoimmune diseases, such as rheumatoid arthritis.

Classification of Hodgkin Lymphoma

Rye classification (Table 8.49): According to this HL was divided into four types and the prognosis varies depending upon the histological type. The nodular sclerosing type is the most common.

WHO classification of Hodgkin lymphoma has been shown in Box 8.23. It is the presently followed classification.

TABLE 8.49: Rye classification of Hodgkin lymphoma.

Histological type	*Prognosis*
Lymphocyte predominant	Very good
Nodular sclerosing	Good
Mixed cellularity	Fair
Lymphocyte depleted	Poor

Box 8.23: WHO classification of Hodgkin lymphoma.

- Classical Hodgkin lymphoma (>95%)
- Nodular sclerosis (NS) classic Hodgkin lymphoma
- Mixed cellularity (MC) classic Hodgkin lymphoma (most common type in India)
- Lymphocyte-rich (LR) classic Hodgkin lymphoma
- Lymphocyte depletion (LD) classic Hodgkin lymphoma
- Nodular lymphocyte predominance (LP) Hodgkin's lymphoma (<5%)

Clinical Manifestations

- **Most common presentation:** Painless enlargement of one lymph node group (unifocal origin) usually of cervical lymph node, consistency of lymph nodes is described as "Indian rubber" consistency. Then it spreads in a predictable manner to the adjacent lymph node group (contiguous spread).
- **Other presentation**
  - Localized disease of the mediastinum (often young women), with cough due to mediastinal lymphadenopathy or axillary nodes, and rarely in the abdominal, pelvic or inguinal nodes.
  - Generalized disease: With hepatosplenomegaly and constitutional "B" symptoms is uncommon in the beginning, but may become prominent as the disease advances.
  - Rare sites: It includes Waldeyer's ring, mesenteric, epitrochlear, and popliteal nodes.
  - Involvement of extralymphatic organs: Not common and may occur in the later stages.
- Classical **Pel-Ebstein fever:** It occurs in a cyclical pattern, characterized by several days or weeks of fever alternating with afebrile periods. It is rarely seen.
- Alcohol-induced pain at the site of lymphadenopathy.
- Pruritus is troublesome at times.

TABLE 8.50: Clinical staging of Hodgkin lymphomas (Cotswold revision of Ann Arbor staging classification).

Stage	*Definition*
I	Involvement of a single lymph node region or lymphoid structure (e.g., spleen, Waldeyer's ring, thymus) or involvement of a single extralymphatic site.
II	Involvement of two or more lymph node groups on same side of diaphragm (mediastinum is a single site; hilar nodes, when involved on both sides, constitute stage II disease). Localized contiguous involvement of only one extranodal organ or site and lymph node region(s) on the same side of the diaphragm (IIE). Number of anatomic sites should be indicated by suffix (e.g., II_3).
III	Involvement of lymph node regions or structures on both sides of the diaphragm, which may also be accompanied by involvement of the spleen (IIIS) or by localized involvement of only one extra nodal organ site (IIIE) or both (IIISE)
III_1	With or without splenic, hilar, celiac, or portal nodes.
III_2	With paraaortic, iliac, or mesenteric nodes.
IV	Diffuse or disseminated involvement of one or more extranodal organs or tissues, with or without associated lymph node involvement

***E:** Involvement of a single extranodal site, or contiguous or proximal to known nodal site of disease.*
***A:** No "B" symptoms*
***B:** Place the patient in the "B" category when at least one of the following is observed:*
- *Unexplained weight loss >10% of bodyweight during 6 months before staging*
- *Recurrent unexplained fever >38° C during the previous month*

Recurrent heavy night sweats during the previous month
***Lymphatic structures:** Lymph nodes, spleen, thymus, Waldeyer's rings, appendix and Peyer's patches. Liver and bone marrow are excluded.*
Each stage is further divided into A or B based on the absence or presence of systemic symptoms (B symptoms), respectively.

- Nephrotic syndrome: It may develop due to immune complex deposition in the kidneys. It is associated with depressed cell-mediated immunity and increases the risk of infections like herpes zoster, tuberculosis, and infections with Cryptococci/*Cytomegalovirus* and *Candida* species.
- Symptoms due to compression of various organs by lymph node masses or infiltration of various organs may develop with mediastinal involvement. These include dysphagia, dyspnea, Horner's syndrome, hoarseness of voice, superior vena cava syndrome, and inferior vena cava obstruction.

Clinical staging: It is currently according to the Cotswolds modification of the Ann Arbor classification **(Table 8.50)**.
- Lymphatic structures: It includes lymph nodes, spleen, thymus, Waldeyer's rings, appendix and Peyer's patches; liver, and bone marrow are excluded.
- Each stage is further divided into A or B based on the absence or presence of systemic symptoms (B symptoms), respectively.

Investigations

- **Peripheral blood:** Normocytic normochromic anemia is common and in advance stage, microcytic anemia develops due to defective utilization of iron. Total leukocyte count is usually normal, but sometimes may show neutrophil leukocytosis. Eosinophilia is observed in ~20% of patients and thrombocytosis in some patients. Lymphopenia (indicates lymphocyte depletion) is associated with bad prognosis. In the terminal stages, there may be leukopenia and thrombocytopenia.
- **Serum alkaline phosphatase:** If raised usually indicate bone marrow or liver involvement.
- ESR: It may be raised
- **Biopsy:** Fine needle aspiration of involved lymph node may be helpful in the diagnosis.
  - Lymph node biopsy: Surgically or by percutaneous needle biopsy under radiological guidance will establish the diagnosis.
  - Liver biopsy may be useful for diagnosis in patients with hepatomegaly.
- **Staging of HL (Table 8.50):** It is important not only for predicting the prognosis but also for guiding the choice of therapy. This involves careful physical examination and investigations such as: (1) Chest radiographs, (2) liver function tests, (3) renal function tests, (4) abdominal ultrasound, (5) bone marrow trephine and aspirate (indicated in patients with clinically advanced disease, i.e., stage III, IV, those with "B" symptoms and those who are HIV-positive) and (6) CT scans of neck, chest, abdomen, and pelvis.

PET scan: It is utilized for staging as well management of HL.

Management

Aim of treatment: Curative intent with expectation of success. Patients with localized or good-prognosis disease receive a brief course of chemotherapy followed by radiotherapy to sites of node involvement and cured HD in >90% of cases. Presently, patients with all stages of HL are treated initially with chemotherapy. Patients with more extensive disease or those with B symptoms receive a complete course of chemotherapy.

Chemotherapy: Combination chemotherapy has been shown to be highly effective. Popular chemotherapy regimens **(Table 8.51, Fig. 8.37)** used is as follows:

TABLE 8.51: Popular chemotherapy regimens used in the treatment of Hodgkin lymphoma.

Regimen	Drugs used
ABVD	Doxorubicin (adriamycin), biomycin, vinblastine, dacarbazine
MOPP	Mechlorethamine (mustine hydrochloride), vincristine (oncovin), procarbazine, and prednisone
ABVD/MOPP	Alternating cycles of MOPP and ABVD
BEACOPP escalated	Bleomycin, etoposide, adriamycin, cyclophosphamide, vincristine, procarbazine, prednisone in escalated dose

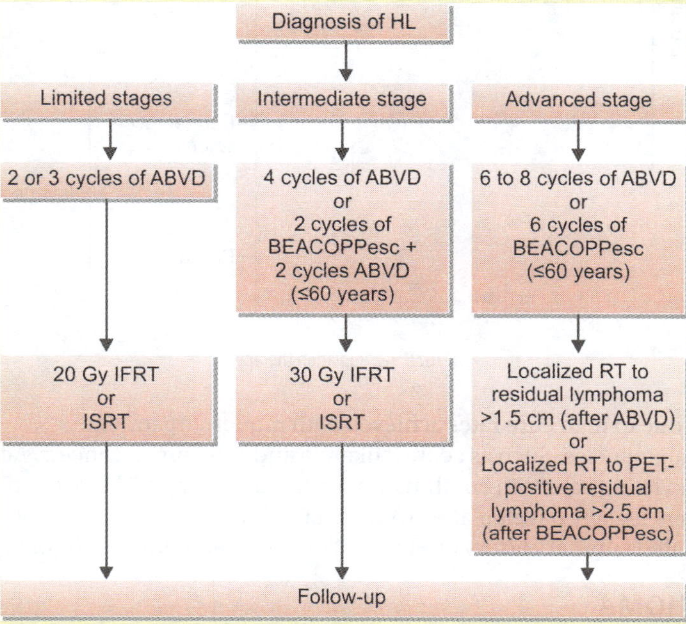

FIG. 8.37: Popular chemotherapy regimens used in the treatment of Hodgkin lymphoma (HL).

Treatment plan for adults with HL (Table 8.52)

Early stage, "low-risk": Moderate chemotherapy, consisting of 2–4 cycles of ABVD followed by involved field irradiation (20–30 Gy). It has a 90% cure rate.

Advanced disease (including locally advanced unfavorable early stage):

- Cyclical chemotherapy with 6–8 cycles of ABVD with involved field irradiation to sites which were initially bulky
- ***Stanford V* for ABVD:** Consists of weekly chemotherapy regimen of doxorubicin, vinblastine, mechlorethamine, etoposide, vincristine, bleomycin, and prednisone) administered for 12 weeks and includes radiation therapy
- Escalated BEACOPP (bleomycin, etoposide, doxorubicin, cyclophosphamide, vincristine, prednisone, and procarbazine)

TABLE 8.52: Treatment plan for adults with Hodgkin lymphoma.

Stage of Hodgkin lymphoma	Prognostic category	Choice of treatment
IA or IIA, no bulky disease*		ABVD × 4 if complete remission after 2 cycles or ABVD × 2 + involved-region radiation therapy (IRRT)
IB, IIB, or any stage III or IV or bulky disease, any stage	≤3 adverse factors**	ABVD until 2 cycles past complete remission (minimum 6, maximum 8)
	≥4 adverse factors**	BEACOPP escalated

*Bulky = largest diameter of any single mass equal to or greater than 10 cm.

**Adverse factors: Male sex, older than 45 years of age, stage IV, hemoglobin less than 10.5 g/dL, WBC count greater than 15,000/mL, lymphocyte count less than 600/mL or less than 8% of the white cell count, or serum albumin less than 4 g/dL.

Autologous bone marrow transplantation is successful in about 40% cases even after the failure of chemotherapy.

Radiation therapy (Fig. 8.38)

- Extended-field radiation (EFRT): Radiation field includes not only the clinically involved nodes, but also the adjacent, clinically uninvolved sites (e.g., mantle field or inverted-Y field).
- Involved-field radiation (IFRT): Radiation field is limited to the clinically involved regions (e.g., mediastinal plus low bilateral supraclavicular field which covers the entire mediastinum)
- Involved-site radiation (ISRT): Radiation field includes only pre- and postchemotherapy tumor volumes plus a margin of healthy tissue to accommodate uncertainties in determining the prechemotherapy tumor volume
- Involved-node radiation (INRT): Radiation field includes pre- and postchemotherapy nodal volumes plus a very limited margin of healthy tissue (0.5–1 cm)

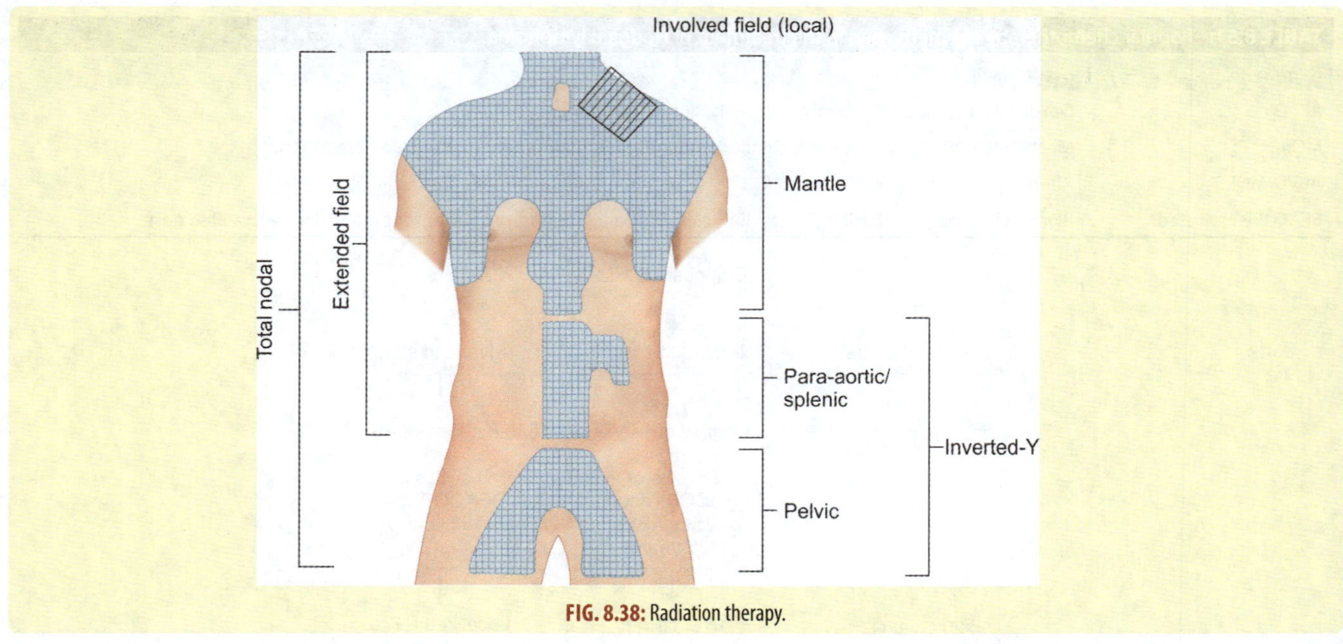

FIG. 8.38: Radiation therapy.

Late complications: Develop due to high cure rates achieved with modern treatment.

- Development of second malignancies: Such as acute leukemia and solid organ cancers. Acute leukemia usually develops within 10 years of use of alkylating agents in combination with radiotherapy. The risk is higher with MOPP as compared to ABVD. Solid organ cancers usually develop after 10 years of radiotherapy.
- Cardiac failure and accelerated coronary artery disease: Following radiotherapy pulmonary fibrosis and hypothyroidism.

NON-HODGKIN LYMPHOMA

Q. Discuss the pathological classification, clinical staging, clinical features, investigations, and management of non-Hodgkin lymphoma (NHL).

- Lymphomas represent solid tumors of the immune system.
- Lymphomas can be divided into two major categories: (1) NHL and (2) HL.
- About 80% of NHL are of B-cell origin and 20% of T-cell origin.

Etiology

Various factors associated with the development of NHL have been shown in **Table 8.53**.

TABLE 8.53: Various factors associated with the development of non-Hodgkin lymphoma.

Genetic factors/inherited immune disorders	Acquired immune disorders
➢ Wiskott-Aldrich syndrome ➢ Ataxia-telangiectasia	➢ Solid organ transplantation ➢ Acquired immunodeficiency syndrome (AIDS) ➢ Rheumatoid arthritis, systemic lupus erythematosis (SLE) ➢ Sjogren syndrome ➢ Hashimoto thyroiditis
Infectious agents	**Occupational and environmental exposure**
➢ **Human T-lymphotropic virus type 1** with adult T-cell leukemia/lymphoma ➢ **Human herpesvirus 8** (Kaposi's sarcoma) associated with primary effusion lymphoma ➢ **Hepatitis C virus:** Lymphoplasmacytic lymphoma and splenic marginal zone lymphoma ➢ ***Helicobacter pylori*:** Associated with gastric lymphoma of extranodal marginal zone/ mucosa ➢ **Epstein-Barr virus:** Associated with Burkitt lymphoma and HL, mucosa-associated lymphoid tissue (MALT)	➢ Ionizing radiation ➢ Herbicides ➢ Organic solvents ➢ Hair dyes ➢ Ultraviolet light ➢ High-fat diets and nitrates in drinking water ➢ Heavy smoking associated with follicular lymphoma

Pathology and Classification

Grading of NHL (Box 8.24)

- Size of the lymphoid cells is a guide to prognosis. NHL with small lymphoid cells (mature lymphocytes) is associated with low-grade and those with large lymphoid cells (immature lymphoid cells) are found in high-grade disease.
- Follicular lymphomas are low grade and have good prognosis, and most diffuse lymphomas are high grade and have poor prognosis.

Box 8.24: Grading of non-Hodgkin lymphoma (NHL).

Indolent or low grade	Highly aggressive/high grade	Aggressive/intermediate grade
• Small lymphocytic • Follicular, predominantly small cleaved cells • Follicular, mixed, small cleaved and large cleaved cells	• Large cell, immunoblastic (B or T cell type) • Lymphoblastic • Small noncleaved cell (Burkitt's and non-Burkitt's)	• Follicular, predominantly large cell, cleaved and/or noncleaved • Diffuse, small cleaved cell • Diffuse, large cell, cleaved or noncleaved

TABLE 8.54: WHO classification of the lymphoid neoplasms (2016).

Precursor B-cell neoplasms (immature B cells)	**Precursor T-cell neoplasms** (immature T cells)
Precursor-B lymphoblastic leukemia/lymphoma	Precursor-T lymphoblastic leukemia/lymphoma
Peripheral B-cell neoplasms (mature B cells)	**Peripheral T-cell and NK-cell neoplasms** (mature T cells and natural killer cells)
Chronic lymphocytic leukemia	T-cell prolymphocytic leukemia
B-cell prolymphocytic leukemia	Large granular lymphocytic leukemia
Lymphoplasmacytic lymphoma	Mycosis fungoides/Sezary syndrome
Mantle cell lymphoma	Peripheral T-cell lymphoma, unspecified
Follicular lymphoma	Anaplastic large cell lymphoma
Marginal zone lymphoma	Angioimmunoblastic T-cell lymphoma
Hairy cell leukemia	Adult T-cell leukemia/lymphoma
Plasmacytoma/plasma cell myeloma	Extra nodal NK/T-cell lymphoma
Diffuse large B-cell lymphoma	
Burkitt lymphoma	

WHO classification of lymphoid neoplasm (Table 8.54)

It requires immunophenotyping, cytogenetics, fluorescent in situ hybridization (FISH), and antigen receptor gene rearrangement studies.

Clinical Features

- **Age:** NHL can occur at any age, but the peak incidence is around 60 years.
- **Most common presentation:**
  - Painless firm, lymph node enlargement or symptoms due to lymph node mass.
  - Extranodal involvement is more common in T-cell lymphoma and involves the bone marrow, gut, thyroid, lung, skin, testis, brain and more rarely, bone.
  - Bone marrow involvement is more common in low-grade (50–60%) than high-grade (10%) NHL and can produce cytopenia.
  - Primary extranodal lymphomas present with soft tissue masses and symptoms relevant to the site. Waldeyer's ring and epitrochlear lymph nodes are frequently involved.
  - Pressure effects: Due to NHL includes gut obstruction, ascites, superior vena cava obstruction, and spinal cord compression.
  - Involvement of liver and spleen results in hepatosplenomegaly.
  - Patients with lymphoblastic lymphoma often present with an anterior mediastinal mass.
  - Burkitt lymphoma typically disseminates to the bone marrow and meninges and involves extranodal sites.
- It may be associated with "B" or systemic symptoms. These include weight loss, sweats, fever, and itching.
- Immunologic abnormalities: For example, autoimmune hemolytic anemia and immune thrombocytopenia.
- Paraneoplastic neurologic complications of NHL include demyelinating polyneuropathy, Guillain-Barré syndrome, autonomic dysfunction and peripheral neuropathy. Paraneoplastic syndromes associated with NHL can affect the skin (e.g., pemphigus), kidney (e.g., glomerulonephritis), and miscellaneous organ systems (e.g., vasculitis, dermatomyositis, and cholestatic jaundice).

Clinical Staging (Ann Arbor Classification)

- Same staging system **(Table 8.50)** is used for both HL and NHL.
- Ann Arbor classification is also used for the clinical staging of NHL but is more useful in HL. However, 'B' symptoms are not included as they are not useful in predicting prognosis.

Investigations

Investigations required for staging the disease are the same as that for HL. Laparotomy is rarely required, only when retroperitoneal nodes are involved.

- **Peripheral blood:** Moderate degrees of anemia may be observed when there is significant bone marrow involvement.
  - Blood counts: Usually normal, but few patients may show lymphocytosis.
  - Splenomegaly with hypersplenism or autoimmune hemolytic anemia may lead to reduced hemoglobin level, reticulocytosis, and positive Coombs test.
- **Bone marrow aspiration and trephine biopsy:** It should be performed early, since marrow involvement is common with NHL.
- **Others investigations:**
  - **Immunophenotyping** of surface antigens to distinguish T- and B-cell tumors. This may be done on blood, marrow or lymph node material. It can be performed by flow cytometry and/or immunohistochemistry utilizing a minimal antibody panel (CD45, CD20, and CD3) to identify B, T or NK subtypes.
  - **Immunoglobulin determination:** Some lymphomas are associated with IgG or IgM paraproteins.
  - **Measurement of uric acid levels:** Few very aggressive high-grade NHLs are associated with very high uric acid levels that can precipitate renal failure when treatment is started.
- Human immunodeficiency virus (HIV) testing.
- Serum levels of LDH, β2-macroglobulin, and serum protein electrophoresis are often needed.
- **Diagnostic spinal tap:** Required when a first prophylactic instillation of cytarabine and or methotrexate is indicated in high-risk patients, especially with involvement of CNS, orbit, bone marrow, testis, spine or base of the skull. It is also indicated in HIV-associated lymphoma and highly aggressive lymphoma.

Management (Box 8.25)

Low-grade NHL:	**High-grade NHL:**
Radiotherapy	
Localized stage I disease	• In few stages I patients without bulky disease • Residual localized bulk disease after chemotherapy • Spinal cord and other compression syndromes
Chemotherapy	
• Oral therapy—chlorambucil (not curative). • Intensive IV chemotherapy in younger patients—better quality of life without any survival benefit	>90% of patients—IV combination chemotherapy—CHOP regimen (cyclophosphamide, doxorubicin, vincristine and prednisolone
Humanized monoclonal antibody therapy	
• Rituximab, ^{131}I-Tositumomab, ^{90}Y-Ibritumomab • Anti-CD20 antibody rituximab(R) alone or with chemotherapy i.e., R-CVP-recommended as first-line therapy.	• Combination with CHOP chemotherapy, rituximab(R) improves overall survival • R-CHOP: First-line therapy for those with stage II or greater diffuse large-cell lymphoma
Autologous bone marrow transplantation:	
	In relapsed chemosensitive disease

Box 8.25: Regimen for non-Hodgkin's lymphoma.

Regimen

CHOP-R	CVP-R	FCR
• Cyclophosphamide • Doxorubicin • Vincristine • Prednisone • Fixed dose rituximab	• Cyclophosphamide • Vincristine • Prednisone • Fixed dose rituximab	• Fludarabine • Cyclophosphamide • Rituximab

Diffuse Large B-Cell Lymphoma (DLBCL)

- Most common lymphoma in the adult population and constitutes about 30–50% of all NHL.
- Present with painless lymphadenopathy at one or several sites. Intra-abdominal disease presents with bowel symptoms due to compression or infiltration of the GIT.
- Treatment: Refer treatment of high-grade NHL mentioned earlier.

Q. How do you differentiate Hodgkin's lymphoma from non-Hodgkin's lymphoma?

Differences between HL and NHL have been shown in **Table 8.55**.

TABLE 8.55: Differences between Hodgkin and non-Hodgkin lymphoma.

Characteristics	*Hodgkin lymphoma*	*Non-Hodgkin lymphoma*
Age	Bimodal peak incidence, 15–35 years and 45–70 years	Peak incidence around 60 years
"B" symptoms	More common	Less common
Alcohol-induced discomfort in lymph nodal region	Common	Not observed
Disease at the time of diagnosis	Usually well localized	Usually widespread
Site of involvement	Unifocal origin and arises in a single node or chain of nodes (cervical, mediastinal, para-aortic)	Mostly involves multiple peripheral nodes (multicentric origin)
Pattern of spread	Orderly spread by contiguity in a predictable fashion	Noncontiguous spread in an unpredictable fashion
Epitrochlear node	Rarely involved	Commonly involved
Mediastinal involvement	Common	Uncommon
Mesenteric nodes and Waldeyer's ring	Rarely involved	Commonly involved
Bone marrow involvement	Late	Early
Extranodal involvement	Uncommon	Common
Characteristic of neoplastic cells	Neoplastic cells—Hodgkin or Reed-Sternberg cells form minor tumor cell mass (1–5%)	Neoplastic cells form the major tumor cell mass
Number of neoplastic cells	Few neoplastic cells (RS cells)	Majority of the cells are neoplastic

Burkitt Lymphoma

Q. Write short note on Burkitt lymphoma/leukemia.

- Burkitt lymphoma is a highly aggressive, often extranodal B-cell lymphoma.
- Most common childhood malignancy worldwide and majority in children, but can occur in all ages.
- Male:female ratio is 3:1.
- Often presents with extranodal involvement or as leukemia.
- Burkitt lymphoma (about 80% of cases) is associated with a specific chromosomal translocation involving *myc* oncogene from chromosome 8 to the immunoglobulin (Ig) heavy chain region on chromosome 14.[t(8;14)].
- Categories of Burkitt lymphoma are explained in **Box 8.26**.

Box 8.26: Three categories of Burkitt lymphoma.

1. Endemic (African)
2. Sporadic (nonendemic) Burkitt lymphoma
3. Immunodeficiency-associated (HIV) lymphomas

Clinical Features

- **Endemic form:** Occurs in Africa. Affects children and adolescents.
  Associated with Epstein-Barr virus infection and corresponds to the distribution of malaria. Involves extranodal sites, particularly the jaw, gastrointestinal tract and gonads. Commonly presenting as a rapidly growing jaw tumor in a young child (4–7 years). Involvement of mandible and maxillary bone leads to deformity, loosening of teeth, and extrusion of the eye with loss of vision.
- **Sporadic from:** It presents as an abdominal mass.
- **Immunodeficiency-associated** (HIV) form: It usually occurs with CD4 counts above 200/mm^3. It again presents with abdominal involvement.
- **Abdominal involvement:** It presents as mass due to bilateral involvement of kidneys adrenals, ovaries, bowel, and lymph nodes.
- **Other sites of involvement:** CNS (common in adults), long bones, salivary glands, thyroid, testes, heart, breast, and bone marrow.

Investigations

- **Histological examination:** Involved tissues show diffuse monotonous infiltrate of medium-sized (intermediate-sized) lymphoid cells, numerous mitoses, and plenty of tumor cells undergoing apoptosis. The nuclear remnants of these apoptotic cells are phagocytosed by benign macrophages creating a characteristic **"starry sky" pattern** (resembling stars in the sky) **(Fig. 8.39)**.
- **Chromosome analysis:** The most common form of translocation results in the movement of the *MYC*-containing segment of chromosome 8 to chromosome 14q32, placing it close to the *IGH* gene. The genetic notation for the translocation is t(8:14) (q24; q32). As a result of translocation, MYC protein is overexpressed and results in cell proliferation and stimulates apoptosis.
- **Antibodies to EB viral capsid antigen:** It may be detected (in endemic type, and in many with sporadic and HIV-associated tumors).

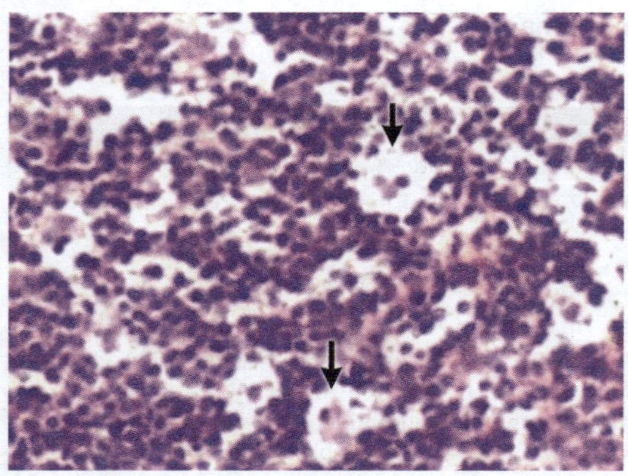

FIG. 8.39: Burkitt lymphoma composed of medium-sized lymphoid cells admixed with benign macrophages (arrows) giving a "starry sky" appearance.

Management
- Treatment must be initiated urgently with curative intent whenever feasible.
- Adequate hydration prior to the initiation of specific therapy to prevent the risk of tumor lysis syndrome.
- Standard treatment comprises of high-intensity, brief-duration cyclical combination chemotherapy. Regimens include:
  - CHOP (cyclophosphamide, hydroxydoxorubicon or doxorubicin, oncovin (vincristine), prednisolone) regimen **OR**
  - Rituximab plus EPOCH (etoposide, prednisolone, oncovin (vincristine), cyclophosphamide and doxorubicin) **OR**
  - CODOX-M/IVAC regimen (cyclophosphamide, vincristine, doxorubicin, methotrexate/ifosfamide, etoposide, or VP-16, cytarabine)
- Prophylactic CNS therapy is essential, intrathecal methotrexate or cytosine arabinoside is given in addition to high-dose systemic administration.
- Cure rates: High as 70–80%.

Adult T-Cell Lymphoma/Leukemia

Q. Write short note/essay on adult T-cell lymphoma/leukemia.

- Adult T-cell leukemia/lymphoma is a neoplasm of CD4+ T-cells and develops in adults infected by *human T-cell leukemia virus type 1 (HTLV-1)*.
- Mode of infection of HTLV-1: Transplacental transmission, blood transfusion, or sexual contact.
- Latency period between infection and development of lymphoma is long (10–30 years).
- Four major presentations:
  1. Acute aggressive form: It is characterized by peripheral blood lymphocytosis, lymphadenopathy, hepatosplenomegaly, skin infiltration, hypercalcemia, lytic bone lesions, and raised LDH levels in blood. Opportunistic infections are common. Peripheral smear usually reveals characteristic, neoplastic cells with multilobulated nuclei, and petal-like nuclear lobules connected by thin chromatin strands, known as "cloverleaf" or "flower" cells are found in the involved tissues and peripheral blood. Bone marrow involvement is usually not prominent.
  2. Lymphomatous form: Constitute ~20% of cases and is associated with generalized lymphadenopathy without leukemia.
  3. Chronic form: Constitute ~15% of cases and may have a low level absolute lymphocytosis in the peripheral blood associated with an exfoliative skin rash.
  4. Smoldering form: Constitute ~5% of cases and have a normal peripheral blood lymphocyte count and a small number of circulating tumor cells and skin rashes.

Prognosis: Most cases progress rapidly and are fatal.

Treatment
- Combination chemotherapy prolongs life but does not produce remissions.
- Combination antiretroviral drugs (zidovudine + interferon-α) may be helpful in some patients.

Mucosa-associated Lymphoid Tissue Lymphoma

Q. Write short note/essay on mucosa-associated lymphoid tissue lymphoma or primary gastric lymphoma.

- It is a small-cell NHL of B-cells that is extranodal in origin.
- **Sites:** MALT lymphoma is often localized to the organ from which it arises in ~40% cases and to the organ and surrounding lymph nodes in ~30% cases. Bone marrow involvement is uncommon and occurs in ~15% cases.
  - Gastric type of MALT lymphoma is associated with *H. pylori* infection. Salivary gland MALT is associated with Sjogren's syndrome.
  - Other sites: It may occur in the stomach, orbit, intestine, lung, skin, soft tissue, bladder, kidney, salivary gland, and CNS.
- Age: Mainly in elderly patients with median age of 60 years.
- Gastric type of MALT lymphoma
  - It may present as a mass or produce local symptoms such as upper abdominal discomfort and dyspepsia.
  - Endoscopy: Often mimic benign conditions like chronic gastritis or a peptic ulcer. Multiple biopsies are required for establishing diagnosis.
  - Endoscopic ultrasound (EUS) useful for staging of gastric MALT lymphoma.
  - Low-grade gastric MALT lymphoma can achieve remission in 80% of cases with eradication of the infection.
- Prognosis: Good in most cases with 5 year survival of 75%.

Treatment
- Localized MALT lymphomas can be treated with surgery or local radiotherapy.
  - Anti *H. Pylori* therapy in gastric MALToma.
- Extensive disease is treated with single chemotherapy agents like chlorambucil, cyclophosphamide, fludarabine, or cladribine. Combination regimens that include rituximab are also highly effective.

Mycosis Fungoides

Q. Write a short note on mycosis fungoides.

- Mycosis fungoides is a rare type of cutaneous T-cell NHL composed of small to medium-sized lymphoid cells with irregular nuclear outlines.
- Insidious in onset and are derived from CD4+T cells of skin-associated lymphoid tissue.
- Age: They usually present between 55 and 60 years.
- The tumor cells show epidermotropism (predilection for the epidermis) and dermis.
- Clinical features: There are three stages:
    1. *Patch stage* (inflammatory *premycotic phase)*, characterized by erythematous macules usually occurring on areas not exposed to sunlight.
    2. *Plaque stage*, with elevated scaly plaques which may be pink or red/brown and are often intensely pruritic.
    3. *Tumor stage*, with dome-shaped firm tumors which may ulcerate.
- **Sézary syndrome:** Patients with mycosis fungoides may develop generalized erythroderma and malignant T-cells with serpentine nuclei are found in the peripheral blood and this condition is known as *Sézary's syndrome.*
- **Immunophenotype:** Tumor cells express pan-T-cell markers CD3, CD5 and CD2.
- **Prognosis:** These are indolent tumors with a median survival rate of 8–9 years.

Treatment
- Localized early-stage mycosis fungoides: Can be cured with radiotherapy, often total-skin electron beam irradiation.
- More advanced stage: Palliative treatment such as topical glucocorticoids, topical nitrogen mustard, phototherapy, psoralen with ultraviolet A (PUVA), and systemic cytotoxic therapy.

Several rare lymphoproliferative disorders other than lymphoma have distinctive clinical courses.

GENERALIZED LYMPHADENOPATHY

Q. Discuss the differential diagnosis (causes) of generalized lymphadenopathy in an adult.

Q. Assessment of the extent of lymph nodal enlargement.

- Generalized lymphadenopathy is defined as significant enlargement of more than 2 or more noncontiguous lymph node groups. Various lymph node areas are depicted in **Figure 8.40**.
- Clinical examination of lymph nodes: (1) Sites of lymph node enlargement, (2) size, (3) consistency, (4) mobile/fixed, (5) presence or absence of tenderness, and (6) draining area.

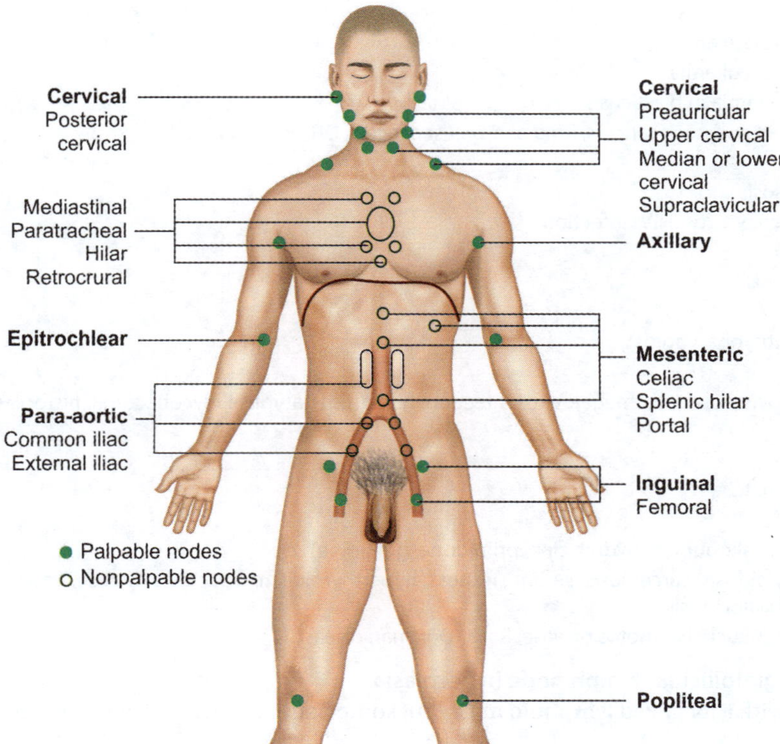

FIG. 8.40: Lymph node areas.

- Systemic abnormalities if any.
- Investigations:
  - Chest X-ray and CT scan of thorax: To detect lymphadenopathy in the mediastinal, hilar, and paratracheal region.
  - Ultrasound scanning and CT scan of abdomen: To detect intra-abdominal lymph nodes.
  - Lymph node groups: Location, lymphatic drainage, and differential diagnosis are mentioned in **Table 8.56.**

TABLE 8.56: Lymph node groups: Location, lymphatic drainage, and differential diagnosis.

Location	*Lymphatic drainage*	*Causes*
Submandibular	Tongue, submaxillary gland, lips and mouth, conjunctivae	Infections of head, neck, sinuses, ears, eyes, scalp, pharynx
Submental	Lower lip, floor of mouth, tip of tongue, skin of cheek	Mononucleosis syndromes, Epstein-Barr virus, cytomegalovirus, toxoplasmosis
Jugular	Tongue, tonsil, pinna, parotid	Pharyngitis organisms, rubella, tuberculosis
Posterior cervical	Scalp and neck, skin of arms and pectorals, thorax, cervical, and axillary nodes	Tuberculosis, lymphoma, head and neck malignancy
Suboccipital	Scalp and head	Local infection
Postauricular	External auditory meatus, pinna, scalp	Local infection
Preauricular	Eyelids and conjunctivae, temporal region, pinna	External auditory canal
Right supraclavicular node	Mediastinum, lungs, esophagus	Lung (right lung and left lower lobe), retroperitoneal or gastrointestinal cancer, tuberculosis
Left supraclavicular node	Thorax, abdomen via thoracic duct	➢ Lymphoma, lung (left upper lobe) ➢ Carcinoma of bronchus, bowel (gastric), bladder, breast and testes, tuberculosis
Axillary	Arm, thoracic wall, breast, parietal pleura	Infections, cat-scratch disease, lymphoma, breast cancer, brucellosis, melanoma, tuberculosis
Epitrochlear	Ulnar aspect of forearm and hand	Infections, NHL, sarcoidosis, tularemia, cat-scratch disease secondary syphilis, disseminated tuberculosis, HIV
Inguinal	Penis, scrotum, vulva, vagina, perineum, gluteal region, lower abdominal wall, lower anal canal	Infections of the leg or foot, STDs (e.g., herpes simplex virus, gonococcal infection, syphilis, chancroid, granuloma inguinale, lymphogranuloma venereum), lymphoma, pelvic malignancy, bubonic plague

Differential Diagnosis (Box 8.27)

Box 8.27: Differential diagnosis of generalized lymphadenopathy.

Cause

- **Malignant neoplasms**
  - Lymphomas (Hodgkin and non-Hodgkin)
  - Leukemias
    - Acute lymphoblastic leukemia
    - Chronic lymphocytic leukemia
    - Chronic myeloid leukemia in blast crisis
  - Metastatic disease (head and neck cancers, lung and breast cancers, GIT malignancies)

  Infections
  - Disseminated tuberculosis
  - Human immunodeficiency virus (HIV) infection
  - Secondary syphilis
  - Infectious mononucleosis
  - Brucellosis
  - Local infections (cellulitis, pharyngitis)
  - Plague
  - Other infections: Toxoplasmosis, cytomegalovirus infection, hepatitis B, atypical mycobacteria, histoplasmosis, coccidioidomycosis, cryptococcosis
- **Autoimmune diseases**
  - Systemic lupus erythematosus
  - Rheumatoid arthritis
- **Drugs induced** (phenytoin, allopurinol, hydralazine, primidone, quinidine)
- **Systemic disorders:** Amyloidosis, sarcoidosis, serum sickness, hyperthyroidism, Gaucher's disease, Kawasaki disease, Kimura disease, hemophagocytic lymphohistiocytosis
- **Rare:** Castleman's disease, Kikuchi Fujimotos disease, Rosai-Dorfman disease

Castleman's disease, or angiofollicular lymph node hyperplasia

- Patients often present with a localized lymphoid mass, but some patients have a systemic illness with fevers, night sweats, weight loss, and fatigue.
- Frequently, the systemic symptoms of Castleman's disease are related to excessive production of IL-6.

- Castleman's disease in HIV-infected patients is frequently associated with HHV-8.
- Patients with disseminated and plasma cell–rich forms of Castleman's disease may occasionally progress to lymphoma.
- Patients with localized Castleman's disease can be treated with surgical removal or radiotherapy. Patients with systemic disease may respond to treatment with high-dose corticosteroids.

Sinus histiocytosis with massive lymphadenopathy, also known as Rosai-Dorfman disease

- Manifests as bulky lymphadenopathy in children and young adults.
- Extranodal sites such as the skin, upper airways, gastrointestinal tract, and CNS can be involved. There is a characteristic pattern of lymphoid proliferation with a thick fibrous capsule, distention of lymphoid sinuses, accumulation of plasma cells, and proliferation of large, often atypical histiocytes.
- The disease is usually self-limited, but it has been associated with autoimmune hemolytic anemia.

Kikuchi's disease (histiocytic necrotizing lymphadenitis)

- Disease of unknown origin that most commonly affects young women.
- Symptoms most commonly consist of painless cervical lymphadenopathy that is often accompanied by fever, flu-like symptoms, and rash.
- Sometimes associated with SLE. Treatment is symptomatic, and symptoms usually resolve within weeks or months.
- Lymph node biopsies reveal foci of necrotic histiocytes.

Kimura disease: Lymphadenopathy; peripheral eosinophilia; and elevated levels of serum immunoglobulin E (IgE).

HEMOSTASIS

Q. Discuss the mechanism of hemostasis.

Q. Write short essay/note on platelets and their functions.

Components of Hemostasis

Three major components namely: (1) Platelet component, (2) vascular component (endothelium), and (3) coagulation component participate in normal hemostatic mechanism. The first two components are involved in primary hemostasis while the last component is involved in secondary hemostasis.

Coagulation System

Coagulation factors are listed in **Table 8.57**. Coagulation can be activated by two pathways namely *extrinsic* and *intrinsic* (**Fig. 8.41**). Both the pathways converge on the activation of factor X to produce factor Xa (activated X).

- **Extrinsic pathway:**
    - It requires an exogenous trigger; hence the name extrinsic. But now it is observed that released tissue factor (a protein-phospholipid complex normally present on vascular cells and activated monocytes) from vascular injury can initiate this pathway. It converts factor VII into activated factor VII (VIIa) in presence of calcium. Activated tissue factor VII complex activates factors IX and X.

TABLE 8.57: Coagulation factors.

Factor	Synonym
I	Fibrinogen
II	Prothrombin
III	Thromboplastin
IV	Calcium
V	Proaccelerin
VI	No specific name or function
VII	Proconvertin
VIII	Antihemophilic factor
IX	Christmas factor
X	Stuart-Prower factor
XI	Plasma thromboplastin antecedent
XII	Hagemen factor
XIII	Fibrin-stabilizing factor

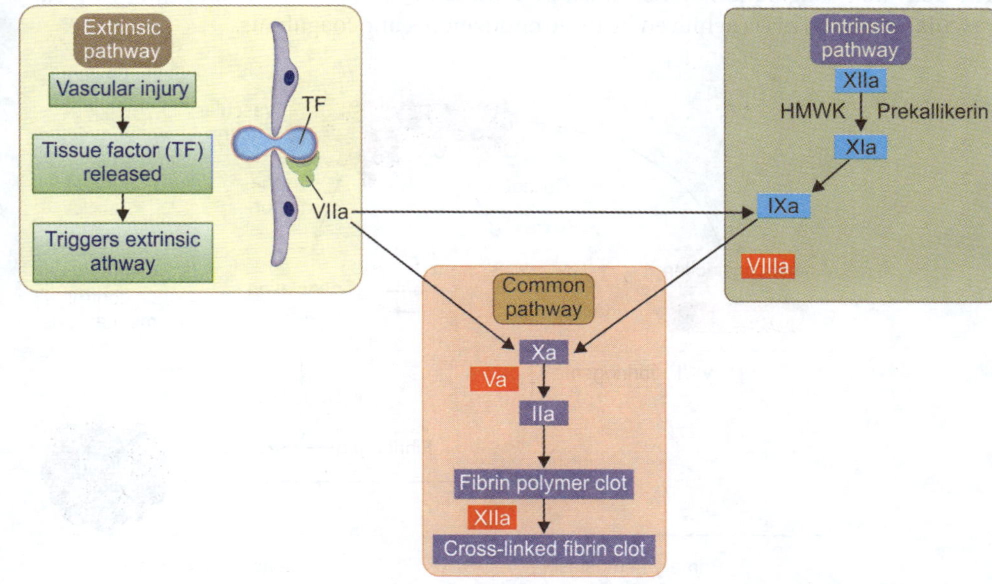

FIG. 8.41: Different pathways of coagulation (extrinsic, intrinsic, and common) pathways.

- The coagulation factors utilized in extrinsic pathway are factors VII, X, II, V, and fibrinogen.
- **Prothrombin time (PT)** is the laboratory test which assesses the function of the coagulation factors involved in the extrinsic pathway.

- **Intrinsic pathway:**
    - This gets activated with exposure of prekallikrein, high-molecular weight kininogen, and factor XII (Hageman factor) to any thrombogenic (negatively charged) surfaces (including glass beads).
    - Prekallikrein is converted to kallikrein and factor XII becomes activated factor XII (XIIa).
    - Factor XIIa converts factor XI into XIa.
    - Factor XIa activates factor IX, and factor IXa with its co-factor FVIIIa activates X to Xa.
    - The coagulation factors utilized in intrinsic pathway are, in order of reaction, factors XII, pre-K, HMWK, XI, IX, VIII, X, V, II, and fibrinogen.
    - The **partial thromboplastin time (PTT)** assesses the function of the coagulation factors utilized in the intrinsic pathway. PTT is initiated by adding negatively charged particles like ground glass.
- **Common pathway:**
    - Above two pathways have in common factors X, V, prothrombin and fibrinogen; and this part of coagulation pathway is known as the common pathway.
    - Common pathway is initiated by factor Xa. Factor Xa converts prothrombin to thrombin (Factor IIa). This is facilitated by Va.
    - Factor IIa converts fibrinogen into fibrin and also activates factor XIII to XIIIa that cross links fibrin to fibrin polymers.

Mechanism of Hemostasis (Fig. 8.42)

- **Primary hemostatic plug:** The platelet component undergoes three different events—platelet adhesion and shape change, platelet secretion (release of granule contents) and platelet aggregation.
- **Secondary hemostatic plug:**
    - Exposure of tissue factor at the site of injury activates the extrinsic coagulation system **(Box 8.28)**.
    - The process generates thrombin, which cleaves circulating fibrinogen into insoluble *fibrin*, creating a fibrin meshwork at the injured site.
    - The platelets contract and form an irreversibly fused mass known as secondary hemostatic plug.
    - The sequence of conversion of the initial temporary primary *hemostatic* (platelet) plug into a permanent secondary hemostatic plug is known as *secondary hemostasis*.

Box 8.28: Functions of platelets.

- Maintain vascular integrity
- Spontaneously arrest bleeding through platelet plug formation
- Participate in the intrinsic coagulation system
- Promote repair and healing through release of growth factors

Coagulation Regulatory Mechanism

Coagulation regulatory mechanism has been shown in **Figure 8.43**.

Q. Briefly outline the natural inhibitors of coagulation.

The activated coagulation system must be limited to the site of vascular injury so as to prevent coagulation in the entire vascular system. This is achieved by three endogenous anticoagulants.

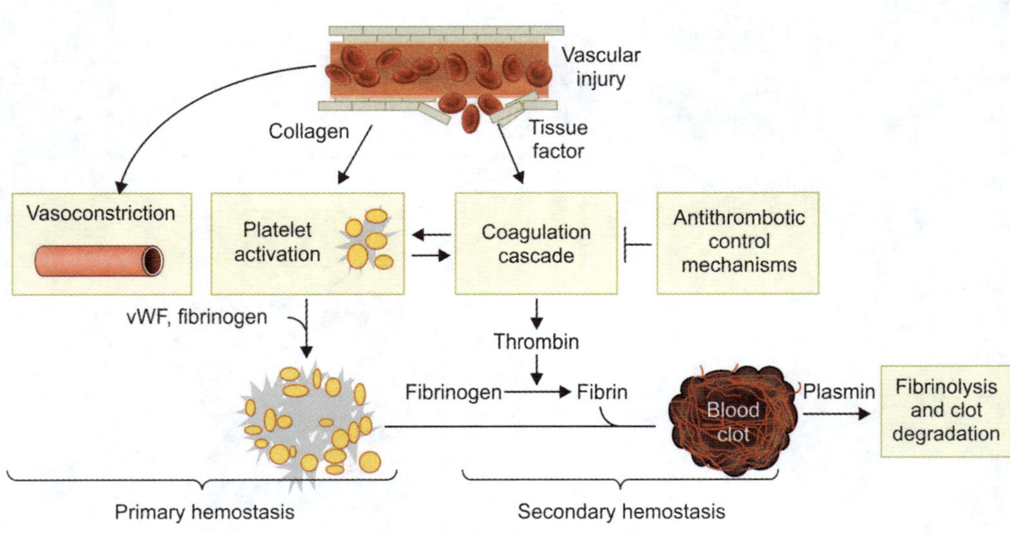

FIG. 8.42: Mechanism of hemostasis.

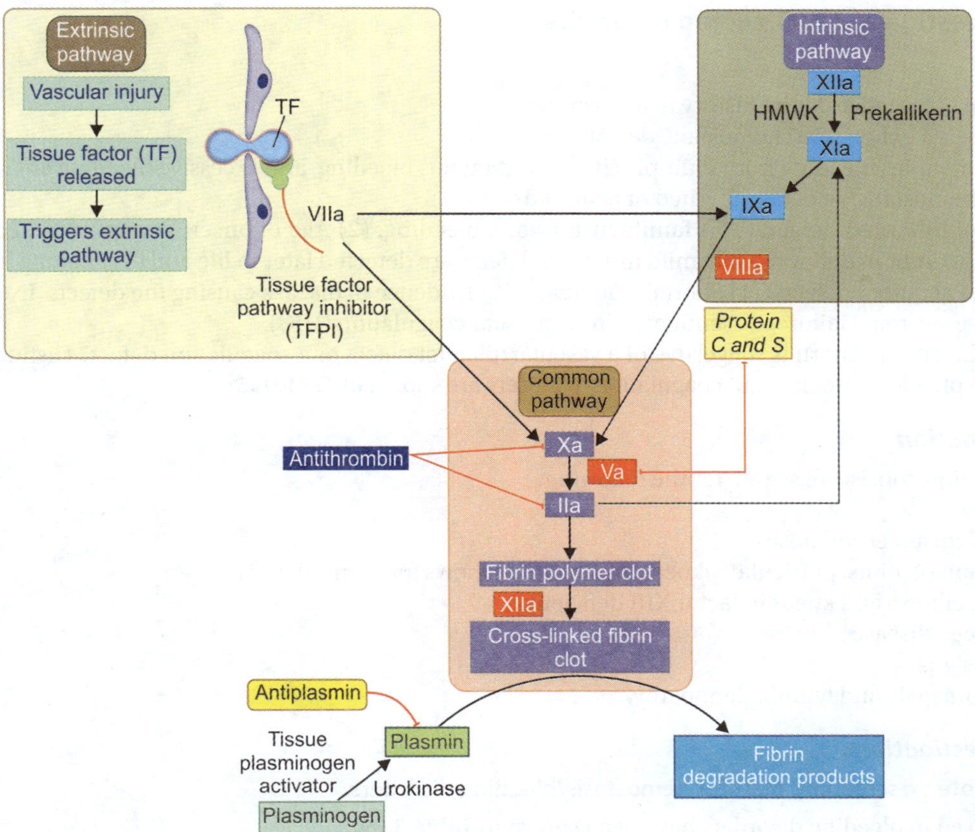

FIG. 8.43: Coagulation regulatory system consisting of antithrombin, protein C and S, and tissue factor pathway inhibitor.

Inhibitors of Coagulation

- **Antithrombin** is a circulating serine protease inhibitor (serpin) which inhibits the activity of thrombin and factors IXa, Xa, XIa and XIIa. One of these is antithrombin III which gets activated by binding to heparin-like molecules on endothelial cells. The heparin used to minimize thrombosis acts by activating antithrombin III.
- **Proteins C and S** are vitamin K-dependent proteins that act in a complex. Thrombin generated by activation of coagulation cascade, binds with thrombomodulin present on the endothelial cell membrane, and activates the coagulation regulatory system called protein C system. Activated protein C (APC) binds with protein S to form APC-protein S complex. This complex inactivates factors Va and VIIIa. Impaired activity of protein C as occurs in factor V Leiden produces thrombophilia.
- **Tissue factor pathway inhibitor (TFPI):** It is a protein which inactivates tissue factor—factor VIIa complexes and inactivates factor VIIa.
  Endothelial cells produce prostacyclin and nitric oxide which inhibit platelet aggregation.

Fibrinolytic System

Q. Describe fibrinolytic system.

- Activation of the coagulation also initiates the fibrinolytic system so that the size of the clot is limited. Fibrinolytic system does this by removal of fibrin from the clot. Otherwise, the clot may progress and involve the entire circulation with its consequences.

BLEEDING DISORDERS (HEMORRHAGIC DIATHESES)

Q. Discuss the evaluation of a patient with bleeding disorder.

Definition

Increased tendency to hemorrhage (usually with insignificant injury) are collectively called as bleeding disorders (hemorrhagic diatheses). Broad classification of bleeding disorders is listed in **Box 8.29**.

Box 8.29: Broad classification of bleeding disorders.

- Coagulation defects
- Platelet disorders
- Vessel wall abnormalities

Evaluation/Investigation of Bleeding Disorders

History

Information to be obtained from the history to determine:
- Whether there is a generalized hemostatic defect?
  - Evidence includes bleeding from multiple sites, spontaneous bleeding, and excessive bleeding after injury.
- Whether the hemostatic defect is inherited or acquired?
  - Features of inherited defect: (1) A family history of a bleeding, (2) Age of onset: Severe inherited defects usually become apparent in infancy, while mild inherited defects are detected later in life and (3) Lifelong history.
  - Features of acquired defects: (1) Short duration and (2) Evidence of disease causing the defects. Examples, evidence of liver disease, renal failure, disseminated intravascular coagulation (DIC).
- Whether the bleeding pattern is suggestive of a vascular/platelet defect or a coagulation defect? Distinguishing features of bleeding in platelet, vascular, and coagulation disorders are shown in **Table 8.58**.

Physical Examination

Physical examination consists of search for the following:
- Type of lesions
  - Purpura, bruises, ecchymoses.
  - Examination of joints, particularly knees, ankles, and elbows for hemarthrosis.
  - Scars over elbows and knees in factor XIII deficiency.
- Signs of liver cell disease
- Neurological signs
- Hepatosplenomegaly and lymphadenopathy.

Laboratory Investigations

Q. Write short note on screening tests for hemostasis/bleeding disorders.

Screening tests used in bleeding disorders have been shown in **Table 8.59.**
- **Bleeding time**
  - Normal range: 4–9 minutes.
  - Prolonged in platelet disorders.
- **Prothrombin time**

TABLE 8.58: Distinguishing patterns of bleeding in platelet, vascular, and coagulation disorders.

Characteristics	*Platelet/vascular disorders*	*Coagulation disorders*
Onset	Spontaneous and develops immediately after trauma/surgery	Delayed bleeding after trauma/surgery
Type of lesion	Petechiae **(Fig. 8.44A)**, purpura **(Fig. 8.44B)**, ecchymosis **(Fig. 8.44C)**	Hematomas
Sites	Skin, mucous membrane	Deep tissues
Mucous membrane	Common from nose, mouth, gastrointestinal and genitourinary tracts	Uncommon except from gastrointestinal or genitourinary tract
Into the joint	Absent	Common in severe factor deficiencies
Into the muscle	Following trauma	Spontaneous
Local pressure	Effective	Ineffective

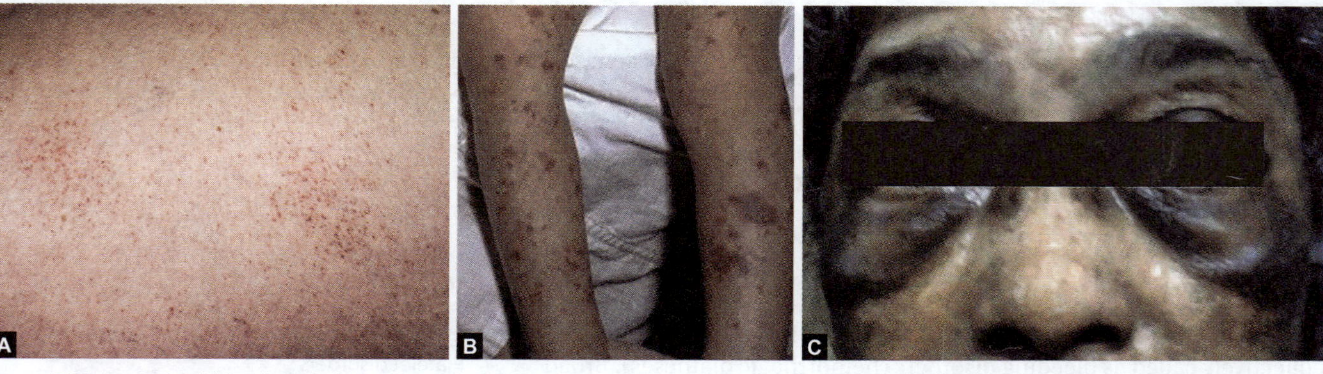

FIGS. 8.44A TO C: (A) Petechiae which appear as small (1–2 mm in diameter), red to purple hemorrhagic spots in the skin, mucous membranes or serosal surfaces; (B) Purpura—slightly larger (>3 mm) than petechiae; (C) Ecchymoses are larger (>1–2 cm) and result from blood escaping.

TABLE 8.59: Screening tests used in bleeding disorders.

Name of the test	*Evaluation*
Blood count and film	Show the number and morphology of platelets and any blood disorder
Platelet count (Normal count: 150 to 450 × 10^9/L)	Platelets
Bleeding time (Normal: <9 minutes)	Platelets
Prothrombin time (Normal: 12–14 seconds)	Platelet function, von Willebrand factor
Activated partial thromboplastin time (Normal 33–45 seconds)	Extrinsic pathway, factors II, V, VII, X
Thrombin time (Normal: 3–5 second > control)	Intrinsic pathway, factors II, V, VIII, IX, X, XI, XII
Clot retraction	Common pathway, factors I, II
Fibrinogen concentration	Platelets
Fibrin degradation products (FDPs)	Fibrinogen

Q. Write short note on prothrombin time.

- It is measured by adding tissue factor (thromboplastin) and calcium to the patient's plasma.
- Normal is 12–16 seconds
- Measures VII, X, V, prothrombin, and fibrinogen (classic "extrinsic" pathway)
- Prolonged
  - With abnormalities of above factors (II, V, VII, and X)
  - In liver disease, DIC, vitamin K deficiency and if the patient is on oral warfarin therapy.

- **Activated partial thromboplastin time (APTT)**
  - Also known as the PTT and is performed by adding a surface activator (such as kaolin, micronized silica or ellagic acid) phospholipid (to mimic platelet membrane) and calcium to the patient's plasma.
  - Normal APTT is 26–37 seconds
  - APTT measures XII, XI, IX, VIII, X, V, prothrombin, and fibrinogen (classic "intrinsic" pathway).
  - **Causes of prolonged APTT**
    - With deficiencies of one or more of above factors (II, V, VIII, IX, X, XI and XII including hemophilia A and B, von Willebrand disease)
    - DIC, heparin therapy, and presence of lupus anticoagulant and acquired factor inhibitors.
- **Correction tests/mixing studies:** It may be used to differentiate various causes of prolonged PT, APTT, and TT
  - Prolonged PT, APTT or TT due to coagulation factor deficiencies can be corrected by addition of normal plasma to the patient's plasma.
  - Failure to correct after addition of normal plasma indicates the presence of an inhibitor of coagulation.
- **Factor assays:** It confirms coagulation defects.

Special tests of coagulation

To confirm the precise hemostatic defect and includes estimation of fibrinogen and FDPs. Various laboratory tests in bleeding disorders are presented in **Table 8.60**.

TABLE 8.60: Laboratory tests in various bleeding disorders.

Disorder	*PT*	*APTT*	*Platelets*	*Bleeding time*
Vit K deficiency	Prolonged	Prolonged	Normal	Normal
vWF dz	Normal PT	Prolonged	Normal	Prolonged/normal
DIC	Prolonged	Prolonged	Reduced	Prolonged
ITP	Normal	Normal	Reduced	Prolonged
Aplasia and leukemia	Normal	Normal	Reduced	Prolonged
Factor VII deficiency	Prolonged	Normal	Normal	Normal
Factor VIII deficiency (Hemophilia A)	Normal	Prolonged	Normal	Normal
Factor IX deficiency (Hemophilia B)	Normal	Prolonged	Normal	Normal
Factor XI, XII deficiency	Normal	Prolonged	Normal	Normal
Factor XIII deficiency (bleeding especially from umbilicus)	Normal	Normal	Normal	Normal

(PT: prothrombin time; APTT: activated partial thromboplastin time; vWF: von Willebrand factor; DIC: disseminated intravascular coagulation; ITP: immune thrombocytopenic purpura)

DISORDERS OF PLATELETS

THROMBOCYTOPENIA

Q. Define thrombocytopenia. Enumerate the common causes, clinical manifestations, investigations, and management of thrombocytopenia.

Definition

Decrease in the platelet count below the lower limit of 150,000/μL is known as thrombocytopenia.
Causes of thrombocytopenia are given in **Table 8.61**.

General Clinical Manifestations

- Bleeding into skin: It presents as purpura, petechiae, ecchymoses.
- Bleeding into mucous membranes: It presents as epistaxis, hemorrhagic bullae in oral mucosa, genitourinary bleeding, and gastrointestinal bleeding.
- Severe thrombocytopenia produces fundal hemorrhage and intracranial bleeding **(Table 8.62)**.
  Approach to the differential diagnosis for petechiae/purpura is presented in **Flowchart 8.3**.

Laboratory Investigations

- **Platelet count**: Reduced and clinical manifestations roughly correlate with the platelet count.

- **Hess test** (capillary fragility test/tourniquet test) may be positive
  - **Principle:** It measures the ability of capillaries to withstand the increased stress.
  - **Procedure:**
    - Sphygmomanometer cuff is tied to the upper arm above the elbow and the cuff is inflated to 80 mm Hg for 5 minutes.
    - Release the pressure after 5 minutes.
    - The number of petechiae present in a circle of 5 cm diameter on the flexor aspect of forearm (below the bend of the elbow) is noted.
  - **Normal:** 0–5 petechiae.
  - **Interpretation:** Positive test is indicated by more than 10 petechiae and is observed in:
    - Vascular purpura
    - Defective platelet function
    - Thrombocytopenia
    - Scurvy.

Bleeding time (BT): Prolonged, and it bears a close relationship to platelet count.

TABLE 8.61: Causes of thrombocytopenia.

Increased platelet destruction	Decreased production of platelets
Immune mediated ➢ **Primary:** Idiopathic thrombocytopenic purpura—acute and chronic ➢ **Secondary:** – Autoimmune: Systemic lupus erythematosus – Alloimmune: Post-transfusion or during pregnancy – Drugs: Quinidine, heparin, sulpha compounds – Infections: HIV, infectious mononucleosis, cytomegalovirus **Nonimmune mediated** ➢ Disseminated intravascular coagulation ➢ Thrombotic thrombocytopenic purpura ➢ Hemolytic uremic syndrome ➢ Mechanical destruction ➢ Microangiopathic hemolytic anemias	**Generalized diseases of bone marrow** ➢ **Aplastic anemia:** Congenital, acquired ➢ **Marrow infiltration:** Leukemia, disseminated cancer **Selective impairment of platelet production** ➢ **Drugs:** Alcohol, thiazides, cytotoxic drugs, alcohol ➢ **Infections:** Measles, HIV **Ineffective megakaryopoiesis** ➢ Megaloblastic anemia ➢ Myelodysplastic syndromes
Sequestration	**Dilutional**
Hypersplenism: Portal hypertension, lymphomas, myeloproliferative disorders	

TABLE 8.62: Clinical features associated with decreased platelet count.

Platelet count/μL	*Clinical features*
30,000–50,000	Post-traumatic bleeding
<30,000	Spontaneous bleeding
<10,000	Intracranial bleeding

FLOWCHART 8.3: Approach to the differential diagnosis for petechiae/purpura.

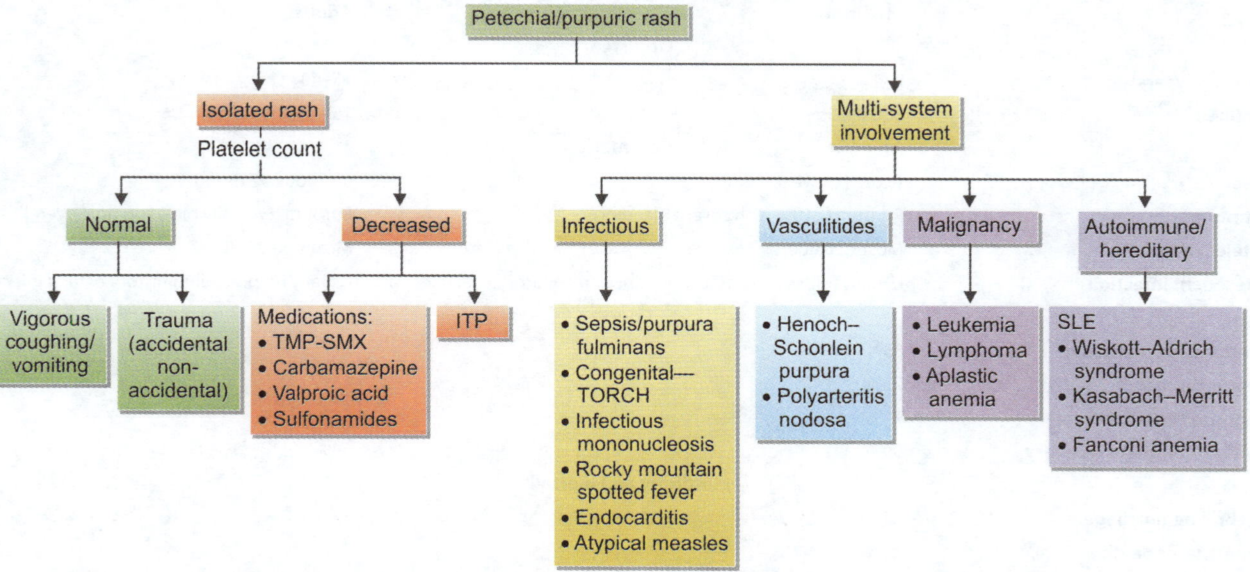

(ITP: immune thrombocytopenic purpura; TMP-SMX: trimethroprim-sulfameathoxazole; SLE: systemic lupus erythematosus)

- **Bone marrow:**
  - Normal or increased number of megakaryocytes indicates increased platelet destruction, hypersplenism, or ineffective platelet production.
  - Decreased number of megakaryocytes indicates reduced production of platelets.

Qualitative Platelets Defects

Qualitative defects of platelet function can be hereditary/ congenital or acquired **(Box 8.30 and Fig. 8.45)**.

Box 8.30: Classification of platelet function disorders.

A. Hereditary
- **Disorders of platelet adhesion**
  - Bernard-Soulier syndrome
- **Disorders of platelet secretion**
  - Storage pool deficiency
- **Disorders of platelet aggregation**
  - Glanzmann thrombasthenia

B. Acquired
- Drugs: Aspirin, nonsteroidal anti-inflammatory drugs (NSAIDs), dipyridamole, sulfinpyrazone
- Renal failure (uremia)
- Hematologic malignancies: Myeloproliferative and myelodysplastic disorders

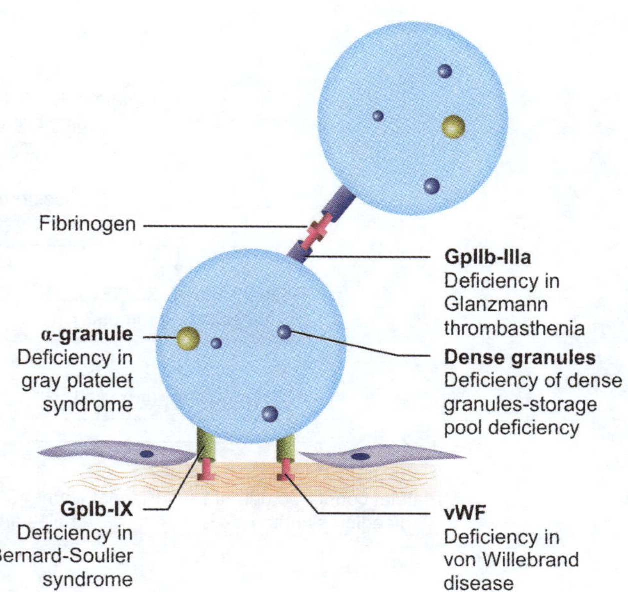

FIG. 8.45: Qualitative/functional disorders of platelets.

IMMUNE THROMBOCYTOPENIC PURPURA

Definition

Immune (idiopathic) thrombocytopenic purpura (ITP) is an autoimmune disorder characterized by increased destruction of platelets by **autoantibodies directed against platelet membrane GPIIb/IIIa and GPIb/IX.**

Pathogenesis

Q. Discuss the pathogenesis, clinical features, investigations/ diagnosis, and management of immune (idiopathic) thrombocytopenic purpura (ITP).

- ITP is *an autoimmune* disorder with formation of antiplatelet antibodies, directed against membrane glycoproteins most often IIb/IIIa or Ib/IX of platelets.
- The antiplatelet antibodies can be demonstrated in approximately 80% of patients and are of the IgG type.

Clinical Features

ITP can be primary or secondary:
- **Primary:** Most cases are primary. There are two major subtypes of primary ITP, acute and chronic **(Table 8.63)**.
  - Acute form is more common in children
  - Chronic form is characterized by the persistence of thrombocytopenia for more than 6 months and is more common in adults.

TABLE 8.63: Differences between clinical features of idiopathic thrombocytopenic purpura in children (acute) and adults (chronic).

	Children	Adults
	Occurrence	
Peak age (years)	2–4	15–40
Sex (F:M)	Equal	1.2–1.7
	Presentation	
Onset	Acute (<1 week)	Insidious >2 months)
Symptoms	Purpura (<10% with severe bleeding)	Purpura (typically bleeding not severe)
Platelet count	Most <20,000/L	Most <20,000/L
Antecedent infection	Usually follows an antecedent upper respiratory viral infection	Usually no preceding history of viral infection
	Course	
Spontaneous remission	83%	2%
Chronic disease	24%	43%
Response to splenectomy	71%	66%
Eventual complete recovery	89%	64%
	Morbidity and mortality	
Cerebral hemorrhage	<1%	3%
Hemorrhagic death	<1%	4%
Mortality of chronic refractory disease	2%	5%

- **Secondary:** Observed in several diseases such as systemic lupus erythematosus, acquired immunodeficiency syndrome (AIDS), hepatitis C, following viral infections and as a complication of drug therapy.
  - Clinical features are not specific but are due to thrombocytopenia in general.
  - Patient has no physical signs other than those due to bleeding and anemia (following menorrhagia and epistaxis), intracranial hemorrhage (ICH), overt gastrointestinal bleeding, and hematuria, are uncommon.
  - Splenomegaly and lymphadenopathy are uncommon in primary ITP and in their presence one should consider the diagnoses other than ITP.
  - May be associated with hemolysis **(Evan's syndrome)**.
  - Majority of patients with acute ITP recover within 6 months.

Investigations and Diagnosis

The diagnosis of ITP is one of exclusion. It requires only isolated thrombocytopenia (i.e., without anemia or leukopenia) without another apparent cause **(Flowchart 8.4)**.

FLOWCHART 8.4: Diagnosis of immune thrombocytopenic purpura (ITP).

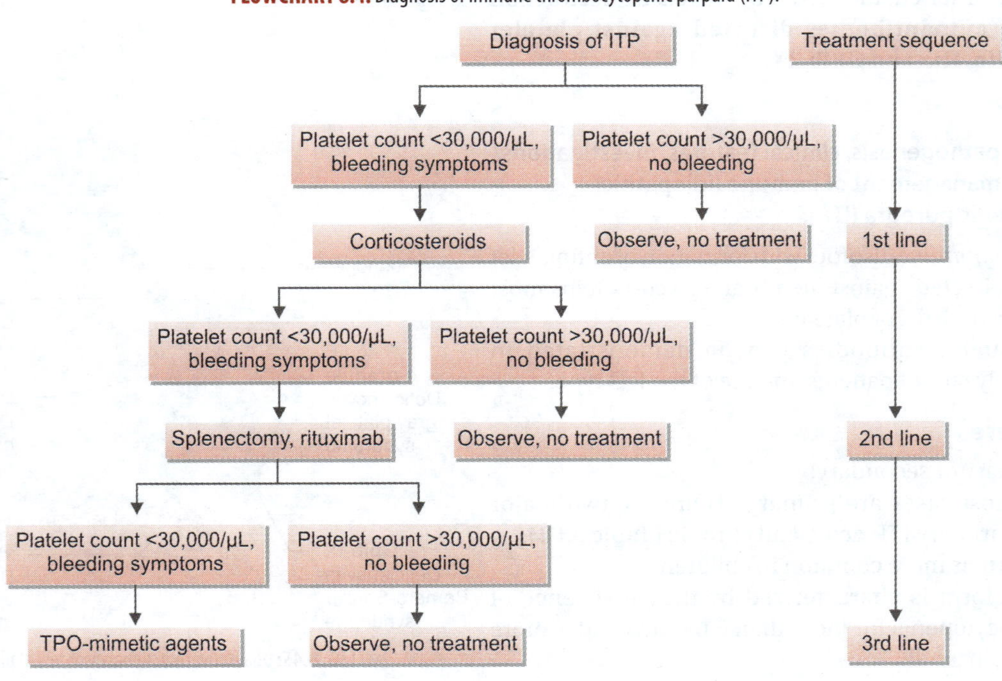

- **Platelet count** is usually **markedly reduced** (thrombocytopenia) and is below 80 × 10^9/L. Platelet count should be repeated using sodium citrate (anticoagulant) to exclude pseudothrombocytopenia caused by platelet aggregation and clumping in the presence of EDTA anticoagulant.
- **Tourniquet test (Hess test):** Positive
- **Bleeding time (BT):** Prolonged
- **Bone marrow examination:** Usually not performed in acute ITP, unless treatment becomes necessary on clinical grounds. It is important in chronic ITP to rule out thrombocytopenia resulting from bone marrow failure. Bone marrow shows moderate increase in number of both immature and mature forms of megakaryocytes. A decrease in the number of megakaryocytes argues against the diagnosis of ITP.
- **Antiplatelet antibodies:** Tests for platelet autoantibodies are not widely available but may be demonstrated in blood. However, a negative test does not exclude ITP.
- In chronic ITP, secondary causes such as HIV, hepatitis C virus infection, etc. should be excluded.

Treatment

- Children with mild acute ITP usually do not require treatment
- Adults with platelet counts >30 × 10^9/L usually do not require treatment. Patients with even lower platelet counts may require treatment, if they have spontaneous bruising or bleeding
- Indications for treatment:
  - Overt hemorrhage (treated with platelet concentrates)
  - Platelet counts below 20,000/mm^3
  - Organ or life-threatening bleeding irrespective of the circulating platelet count
- **Platelet transfusion:** If platelet counts <20,000/mm^3 or bleeding manifestations
- **Single-donor platelets** have a shelf life of 3–5 days, and one unit will raise platelets 30,000 to 50,000/µL
- **First-line therapy:** Consists of treatment with **oral corticosteroids**
  - Indications for corticosteroids:
    - To induce remission
    - To maintain remission in chronic ITP
    - Postoperatively, in patients where splenectomy failed to achieve the result
    - Pregnant women after the 5th month of pregnancy
  - Dosage of corticosteroids:
    - Both adults and children: Initial dose is 1–2 mg/kg of prednisolone/day. Initial dose is continued for at least 2 weeks (or if necessary 3–4 weeks), and then reduced slowly and stopped
    - About 66% respond to prednisolone but relapse is common when the dose is reduced
- **Second-line therapy:**

  Splenectomy: Majority of patients respond well and achieve a normal platelet count
  - **Indications of splenectomy:**
    - Chronic ITP in adults who fail to responded to corticosteroids
    - Patients requiring unacceptably high doses of corticosteroids to maintain a safe platelet count
    - When there is severe bleeding or threatening cerebral hemorrhage (despite adequate corticosteroid therapy)
    - In the first 4–5 months of pregnancy, if steroids do not induce full remission
  - Mechanism of action of splenectomy:
    - Spleen being the major site of platelet destruction, splenectomy prevents its destruction
    - Reduces the concentration of circulating antiplatelet antibodies

  Rituximab
  - 375 mg/m^2 intravenously once a week for four consecutive weeks
  - ADR- immunosuppression, progressive multifocal leukoencephalopathy
- **Third-line therapy:**

  Patients who fail to respond to splenectomy, a wide range of other therapies are available. Major drawbacks of these therapies are modest response rates and slow onset of action. The therapies include:
  - **High-dose corticosteroids**
  - **Intravenous immunoglobulin** (i.e., IgG): It is effective. Responses are only transient (3–4 weeks)
    - Indications:
      - Acute situation prior to surgery and child birth, and in patients with intracranial bleed
      - Patients with ITP where corticosteroid therapy and splenectomy are contraindicated
    - Side effects: Nausea, vomiting, fever, and headache. Uncommonly neutropenia and hemolytic anemia
    - Dose: 1–2 g/kg
  - **RhO(D) immune globulin (anti-D)**
    - Indications: Patients who do not respond to steroids and may be tried before splenectomy
    - Should be given only to Rh-positive patients

- Effective in patients with ITP but the effect is usually temporary, and nearly 50–75% patients relapse
- Dose is 75 µg/kg intravenously
- Side effects: Nausea, vomiting, fever, chills and intravascular hemolysis

– **Immunosuppressive therapy**
  - Indications:
    - Refractory cases which fail to respond to corticosteroids and splenectomy
    - Patients with ITP where corticosteroid therapy and splenectomy are contraindicated
  - Agents used are vinca alkaloids (vincristine, vinblastine), azathioprine, cyclophosphamide, cyclosporine, and combination chemotherapy, mycophenolate mofetil

– **Plasmapheresis:** Employed as an emergency measure to remove antibodies from the plasma

– **Thrombopoietin (TPO) mimetic drugs:**
  - **Romiplostim,** 500 µg subcutaneously once weekly
  - **Eltrombopag** 50 mg, once-daily pill
  - **Avatrombopag** once-daily pill
    - Serious ADRs: Thrombocytosis, thrombosis, bone marrow fibrosis

– **Fostamatinib:** A tyrosine kinase inhibitor that inhibits the spleen tyrosine kinase Syk

– Others:
  - Danazol is an androgen with low virilizing activity has been tried in idiopathic thrombocytopenic purpura
  - Dapsone
  - Platelet transfusions are reserved for intracranial or other extreme hemorrhage, where emergency splenectomy may be justified

- Emergency treatment: Necessary in case of life-threatening bleeding. It consists of intravenous administration of methylprednisolone (30 mg/kg, maximum dose 1 g) over 20 to 30 minutes along with platelet transfusion. This is followed by intravenous immunoglobulin (1 g/kg)

THROMBOCYTOSIS

Q. What are the common causes of thrombocytosis?

Definition

Platelet count more than 450,000/mm^3 is known as thrombocytosis.

Causes

Causes of thrombocytosis have been shown in **Table 8.64**.

TABLE 8.64: Causes of thrombocytosis.

Idiopathic/primary (autonomous production)	*Secondary (reactive thrombocytosis)*
➢ Myeloproliferative neoplasms – Essential thrombocytosis – Polycythemia vera – Chronic myeloid leukemia ➢ Myelodysplastic syndrome	➢ Iron deficiency ➢ Malignancy (paraneoplastic feature) ➢ Following hemorrhage: Acute or chronic blood loss ➢ Following splenectomy ➢ Following major surgery ➢ Inflammatory disorders, e.g., rheumatoid arthritis and inflammatory bowel disease

DISORDERS OF COAGULATION (CLOTTING)

Q. Write short note on congenital bleeding disorders.

Hereditary coagulation disorders are listed in **Box 8.31**.

Box 8.31: Hereditary coagulation disorders.

- von Willebrand disease
- Hemophilia A
- Hemophilia B
- Hemophilia C: Inherited deficiency of factor XI (factor 11); also called Rosenthal syndrome; an autosomal recessive disorder

HEMOPHILIA A (FACTOR VIII DEFICIENCY)

Q. Discuss the etiology, classification, clinical features, diagnosis, and management of hemophilia A.

- Hemophilia A is the most common hereditary X-linked recessive disease with a reduction in the amount or activity of factor VIII (antihemophilic factor). About 30% of hemophiliacs have no family history and may be due to acquired mutations.
- Males are affected and females are carriers.
- Incidence: 1 in 10,000 males.

Mode of Inheritance

- Hemophilia A is an X-linked recessive disorder.
- Usually males are the sufferers and females are the carriers.
- Females can be hemophilic if:
  - She is born to an affected father and a carrier mother (25% risk).
  - Females with inactivation of the X-chromosome such as Turner's syndrome (45, XO)
  - She has inactivation of normal X-chromosome due to unfavorable lyonization (rare).

- Degree of deficiency of factor VIII and severity of bleeding tends to be similar in all the affected members of the same family.
- Normal level of factor VIII in the blood is 0.50–1.50 IU/mL. Hemophilia A may be classified based on the factor VIII activity in blood.

Clinical Features

- Clinical severity depends on the level of factor VIII activity and is presented in the **Table 8.65**.
- Excessive bleeding: Hemophilia A is characterized by excessive bleeding, but is unusual until the child is about 6 months old.
- Post-traumatic bleeding: Bleeding following trauma is characteristically "delayed."
- Severity of bleeding: Range from mild to severe.
- Petechiae observed in platelet and vascular disorders are not seen in hemophilia.

Bleeding into joints (hemarthrosis)

- Frequent and spontaneous hemorrhages occur into the large joints, especially knees, elbows, ankles, wrists and hips, and are known as hemarthrosis.
- Nature of bleeding: Usually spontaneous or follows minor trauma.
- Acute stage: Affected joint is swollen, hot and tender and movements severely restricted. These changes gradually subside over a period of days.
- Consequences: Recurrent bleeding into the joints will lead to crippling deformities and disuse atrophy of muscles around the joint.

Bleeding into muscles

- Common sites: Calf and psoas muscles.
- Consequences:
  - Psoas hematomas may compress the femoral nerve resulting in sensory disturbances over thigh and weakness of quadriceps.
  - Calf hematomas can result in contraction and shortening of the Achilles tendon.

Other manifestations

- Easy bruising
- Massive bleeding following trauma (from wounds) or operative procedures (e.g., bleeding from sockets after dental extraction)
- Cerebral hemorrhage
- Hematuria and ureteric colic due to passage of blood clots.

Laboratory Investigations

- **Bleeding time is normal.**
- **Clotting time is prolonged.**
- **Platelet count is normal.**
- **PT is normal.**
- **APTT is increased** (normal 35–45 seconds) from 50 seconds to a few minutes.
- **Factor VIII assay** is required for the confirmation of diagnosis and to assess the Factor VIII levels and severity of disease.

Antenatal Diagnosis

- **Chorionic villous sampling (CVS):** Done at 8–9 weeks of gestation, sexing the fetus, and using informative factor VIII probes. It is the preferred method.
- **Amniocentesis:** Sexing the fetus at 16 weeks of gestation by amniocentesis and, if fetus is male, a fetal blood sampling is done at about 19–20 weeks of gestation.

TABLE 8.65: Clinical classification of hemophilia A.

Classification	*Factor VIII level*	*Clinical features*
Mild	6–30% of normal (0.06–0.30 U/mL)	➢ Hemorrhage secondary to trauma or surgery ➢ Rare spontaneous hemorrhage
Moderate	1–5% of normal (0.01–0.05 U/mL)	➢ Hemorrhage secondary to trauma or surgery ➢ Occasional spontaneous hemarthrosis
Severe	≤1% of normal (≤ 0.01 U/mL)	➢ Spontaneous hemorrhage from early infancy ➢ Frequent spontaneous hemarthrosis and other hemorrhages, requiring clotting factor replacement

Management

- **Local treatment**
  - **Wounds and bleeding from mucous membrane:** Apply local pressure and pressure bandages or sutures. Immobilize wounds by bandages, splinting, etc.
  - **Hematomas and hemarthrosis:**
    - **During acute stage:** Elevate the affected part and immobilize by splinting and bandages. Pain is relieved by analgesics like acetaminophen or codeine.
    - **During recovery phase:** Physiotherapy.
- **Replacement therapy**
  - Agents used: **Factor VIII concentrate** is available as plasma-derived and recombinant products. Recombinant products are the treatment of choice and are replacing the plasma-derived factor VIII concentrate **(Table 8.66).**
  - Route of administration: Intravenous infusion to correction of deficiency of factor VIII and to achieve normal levels.
  - **Indications of replacement therapy:**
    - Early treatment of spontaneous bleeding.
    - Severe or prolonged wound and tissue bleeding.
    - Control of bleeding during and after surgery and trauma.
    - Prophylaxis: In all patients with severe hemophilia so as to prevent recurrent bleeding into joints and subsequent joint damage (arthropathy).
  - Calculation of dose: Plasma factor VIII, 1 unit/kg will increase activity by 2% (0.02 IU/mL). The desired factor VIII level is about 50% (presuming the initial level to be 0). The dose is calculated as:
    - Dose of factor VIII = Desired factor level (%) × body weight (in kg) × 0.5.
  - **Complications of replacement with factor VIII concentrate therapy:** Former replacement therapy with clotting factor concentrates prepared from pooled human plasma has led to other diseases in patients receiving such treatment.
    - Viral hepatitis (hepatitis B virus, delta virus and hepatitis C virus).
    - Infection with HIV.
    - Development of factor VIII inhibitors.
- **Nontranfusion therapy in hemophilia**
  - **DDAVP (1-Amino-8-D-Arginine Vasopressin)**
    - Desmopressin (DDAVP) is a synthetic vasopressin analog that causes a transient rise in factor VIII activity by 3–5 times. It is given at a dose of 0.3 µg/kg body intravenously over 15 minutes.
    - Indication: Minor bleeding and minor surgery.
  - Antifibrinolytic drugs
    - Indications: To control local hemostasis/bleeding in the gums, nasal bleeding, gastrointestinal tract, during oral surgery (e.g., dental extraction) and menstruation.
    - Drugs used: **Epsilon (ε) aminocaproic acid (EACA) and tranexamic acid.**
    - **Action:** Inhibit the proteolytic activity of plasmin and results in inhibition of fibrinolysis.
    - Dose:
      - Tranexamic acid: 25 mg/kg three to four times a day.
      - EACA: Requires a loading dose of 200 mg/kg (maximum of 10 g) followed by 100 mg/kg per dose (maximum 30 g/d) every 6 hours.
    - Contraindication:
      - Not indicated to control hematuria because of the risk of formation of an occlusive clot in the lumen of genitourinary tract structures.
      - DIC.
      - Thromboembolic disease.

TABLE 8.66: Doses of factor VIII for treatment of hemorrhage.

Site of hemorrhage	*Desired factor VIII level (% of normal)*	*Factor VIII dose (U/kg body weight)*	*Frequency of dose (every no. of hours)*	*Duration (days)*
Hemarthrosis	30–50	~25	12–24	1–2
Superficial intramuscular hematoma	30–50	~25	12–24	1–2
Gastrointestinal tract	~50	~25	12	7–10
Epistaxis	30–50	~25	12	Until resolved
Oral mucosa	30–50	~25	12	Until resolved
Hematuria	30–100	~25–50	12	Until resolved
Central nervous system	50–100	50	12	At least 7–10 days
Retropharyngeal	50–100	50	12	At least 7–10 days
Retroperitoneal	50–100	50	12	At least 7–10 days

Complications

About 15% of the patients receiving factor VIII therapy develop inhibitory antibodies that bind and inhibit factor VIII.

- **Treatment for patients with factor VIII inhibitors:** Immune tolerance induction (ITI) is the most effective strategy of eradication of inhibitors with steroids or other immunosuppressants. Emicizumab, a bifunctional monoclonal antibody that can substitute for factor VIII is used in these cases.
- **Antibodies to AHG may occur de novo in nonhemophiliacs as part of an immunological disorder such as systemic lupus erythematosus.**
- Chronic complications
  - Arthropathy
  - HIV and HCV infection
  - Inhibitor development.

Preventive Therapy for Hemophilia
- Gene therapy
- Concizumab-monoclonal antibody directed against tissue factor pathway inhibitor

Hemophilia B

Q. Write short essay/note on hemophilia B (Christmas disease) and its management.

- Hemophilia B is caused by a deficiency of factor IX.
- Mode of inheritance: X-linked disorder
- Clinical features: Similar to hemophilia A.
  - Patients with severe disease: Present with muscle hematomas and hemarthrosis which progresses to crippling joint deformities.
- Diagnosis: Factor IX assay shows deficiency of factor.

Management

Management is similar to hemophilia A.
- Replacement therapy:
  - Fresh frozen plasma to treat mild-to-moderated bleeding.
  - Recombinant factor IX: To treat moderate-to-severe bleeding.
    - Gene therapy: It may be effective in managing severe disease.
    - Desmopressin is ineffective.

VON WILLEBRAND'S DISEASE

Q. Discuss the etiology, clinical features, investigations, and treatment of von Willebrand's disease.

- von Willebrand's disease (vWD) is characterized by defective platelet function as well as factor VIII deficiency, and both are due to a deficiency or dysfunction of vWF.
- **Major categories:** The vWF gene is located on chromosome 12 and numerous mutations of the gene produce vWD.
  - **Quantitative deficiency in vWF:**
    - Type 1 is an autosomal dominant, relatively mild disorder.
    - Type 3 is an autosomal recessive disorder and is severe.
  - **Qualitative defects (dysfunction) in vWF:** Type 2 von Willebrand disease accounts for 25% of all cases and is usually an autosomal dominant disorder. There are several subtypes.
    - Type 2a is most commonly characterized by defective assembly of multimers.
    - Type 2b is caused by synthesis of an abnormal vWF with increased affinity for platelets which results in thrombocytopenia.

von Willebrand Factor (Fig. 8.46)

- vWF is a protein synthesized by endothelial cells and megakaryocytes.
- **Main functions:**
  - vWF acts as a **carrier protein** which binds to **factor VIII** and forms plasma factor VIII-vWF complex. vWF protects factor VIII and is important for its stability. It has no role in the coagulation cascade, but deficiency of vWF causes a secondary reduction of factor VIII causing coagulation defect.
  - vWF is the most important cofactor for adhesion of platelets to the exposed subendothelial collagen matrix by GpIb/IX. Hence, the deficiency of vWF results in a defect of platelet function.

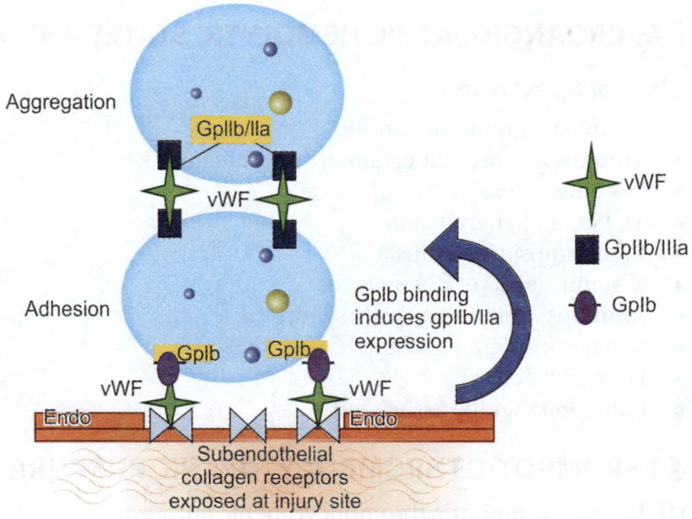

FIG. 8.46: Functions of von Willebrand factor (vWF).

Clinical Features

- Variable and ranges from mild asymptomatic conditions to a severe hemorrhagic disorder.
- The common symptoms are spontaneous bleeding from mucous membranes (e.g., epistaxis), excessive bleeding from wounds or menorrhagia. In severe cases, manifestations may be similar to hemophilia A.

Acquired causes of vWF deficiency are listed on **Box 8.32**.

Laboratory Findings

- **Platelet count** is **normal.**
- **Bleeding time** is **prolonged** despite a normal platelet count because of defect in platelet function.
- **Tourniquet test (Hess test): Positive** due to defect in platelet adhesion.
- **APTT: Prolonged** because vWF stabilizes factor VIII by binding to it. A deficiency of vWF gives rise to a secondary decrease in factor VIII levels.
- **vWF assay:** Plasma level of active vWF is **decreased**.
- **Platelet function test:** Function of vWF is assessed by **ristocetin aggregation test**. Ristocetin induces multivalent vWF multimers to bind platelet glycoprotein Ib-IX and results in bridging of platelets to each other. The resultant clumping (agglutination) of platelets is measured by aggregometer. The degree of ristocetin-dependent platelet agglutination is a measure of vWF activity. Defective ristocetin induced platelet aggregation is diagnostic of vWF.

Box 8.32: Acquired causes of vWF deficiency.

- Hematologic disorders
  - Lymphoproliferative disorders
- Myeloproliferative neoplasms including essential thrombocytosis (ET), systemic lupus erythematosis (SLE) and other autoimmune disorders, and cardiovascular disease
  - Congenital heart disease
  - Aortic stenosis
  - Left ventricular assist device or extracorporeal membrane oxygenation
- Wilms tumor hypothyroidism
- Valproic acid and other medications

Management

Management of bleeding:

- Mild bleeding: Managed with desmopressin.
- Severe bleeding: Controlled by intravenous cryoprecipitate or plasma-derived concentrates containing vWF and factor VIII. Recombinant activated factor VII (rFVIIa,) has also been successfully used in vWD patients with severe hemorrhage refractory to vWF replacement therapy.

Vitamin K deficiency:

- Clinically, it manifests as ecchymoses, bleeding from injection sites, bruises, gum bleeding, hematemesis, melaena, or hematuria.
- Both the PT and activated partial thromboplastin time are prolonged.
- Administration of vitamin K in a dose of 5–10 mg stops bleeding within 1–2 days.
- If blood loss is severe or response to vitamin K is inadequate, transfusion of fresh blood or fresh frozen plasma is indicated.

FIBRINOLYSIS

Causes of excessive fibrinolysis have been shown in **Table 8.67**.

TABLE 8.67: Causes of excessive fibrinolysis.

- Obstetric: Abruptio placentae, amniotic fluid embolism
- Surgical: Gastrectomy, lung resection, nephrectomy, prostatectomy, cardiopulmonary bypass, splenectomy, pancreatectomy
- Medical:
  - Liver diseases (cirrhosis of liver)
  - Leukemias (acute leukemia, chronic granulocytic leukemia type IV)
  - Anaphylactic shock
  - Autoimmune diseases (systemic lupus erythematosus)

MICROANGIOPATHIC HEMOLYTIC STATES AND THROMBOCYTOPENIAS

Clinical Spectrum

- Hemolytic uremic syndrome
- Thrombotic thrombocytopenic purpura (TTP)
- Systemic sclerosis
- Malignant hypertension
- Preeclampsia–eclampsia
- Systemic lupus erythematosus
- Antiphospholipid antibody syndrome
- Renal transplant associated
- Drug induced
- Radiation therapy associated.

THROMBOTIC THROMBOCYTOPENIC PURPURA

Q. Discuss thrombotic thrombocytopenic purpura.

Thrombotic thrombocytopenic purpura (TTP) is a severe microangiopathic hemolytic anemia (MAHA), characterized by systemic platelet aggregation, organ ischemia, profound thrombocytopenia (with increased marrow megakaryocytes), fragmentation of erythrocytes, fever, and renal failure.

Etiology and Pathogenesis

- Normally endothelial cells and megakaryocytes secrete normal vWF multimers into the plasma. These multimers spontaneously develop into unusually large multimers which are most effective in mediating platelet adhesion.
- A plasma protease enzyme called ADAMTS 13 ("vWF metalloprotease") regulates the activity of vWF by cleaving the hemostatically active unusually large multimers into normal multimers. Thus, ADAMTS-13 regulates the size of vWF multimers and prevents platelet adhesion.
- TTP patients have an inherited or acquired deficiency of ADAMTS-13. The deficiency leads to accumulation of unusually large multimers of vWF in plasma.
- These large multimers promote platelet adhesion or promote intravascular platelet aggregation and cause spontaneous activation of the coagulation cascade.
- This results in hyaline thrombi throughout the microcirculation, leading to tissue ischemia, and infarction that are characteristic of TTP.
- Secondary causes of acute TTP: These include pregnancy, oral contraceptives, SLE, infection, and drugs (ticlopidine and clopidogrel). They may or may not have associated antibodies to ADAMTS-13.

Clinical Features

The classic five symptoms of TTP are (1) MAHA with schistocytosis (at least 3 cells per 100), (2) severe thrombocytopenia, (3) transient neurologic symptoms secondary to CNS ischemia, (4) fever and (5) renal abnormalities including hematuria and/or proteinuria.

Laboratory Findings

- **Platelet count markedly reduced** often below 20,000/μL (thrombocytopenia).
- Peripheral blood smear shows fragmented red cells (called **schistocytes**) and numerous reticulocytes.
- PT, PTT, and fibrinogen concentration: Normal, because the coagulation system is not activated.
- Urine shows moderate proteinuria and both gross and microscopic hematuria.
- **Serum LDH: Raised** due to release from ischemic tissues.
- **ADAMTS-13 activity: Reduced** below 5–10% of normal.

Diagnosis

Schistocytes and elevated serum LDH (out of proportion to the degree of hemolysis) suggest the diagnosis of TTP.

Treatment

- **Plasma exchange**
  - Daily plasma exchange (removing 40 mL/kg body weight of plasma and replacing it with equal volume of fresh frozen plasma) is the treatment of choice.
  - Provides ADAMTS-13 and removes associated autoantibody in acute TTP.
  - Continued for at least 2 days after remission, which is defined as stabilization of clinical symptoms and return to normal of platelet count and LDH levels along with rising hemoglobin level.
  - Cryoprecipitate and fresh frozen plasma (FFP) also contain ADAMTS-13 can be used.
- **Corticosteroids:** Pulsed intravenous methylprednisolone is given acutely and is generally added to plasma exchange to suppress formation of antibody.
- **Rituximab:** It is a monoclonal antibody against CD20, suppresses antibody-producing cells. It is used in those patients who are refractory to plasma exchange and corticosteroids.
- **Splenectomy:** Performed in resistant cases which remove antibody-producing cells.
- **Platelet concentrates are contraindicated**.

Prognosis: Untreated cases have a mortality of up to 90% but with modern management it has been reduced to about 10%.

HEMOLYTIC-UREMIC SYNDROME

Q. Discuss the clinical features, investigations, and treatment of hemolytic-uremic syndrome (HUS).

Hemolytic-uremic syndrome is distinguished from TTP by the absence of fever and neurological symptoms, the prominence of acute renal failure (uremia), frequent affection of children, and different pathogenesis.

Etiology and Pathogenesis

- HUS develops following damage to the endothelium by toxins, drugs or radiation. One main cause of HUS in children and the elderly is infectious gastroenteritis caused by ***Escherichia coli* strain 0157:H7**.
- *E. coli* produces a Shiga-like toxin which is absorbed from the inflamed gastrointestinal mucosa.

- The toxin enters circulation and damages endothelial cells of microvasculature, mainly in the renal glomerular capillaries and initiates platelet activation and thrombi formation.
- *Pneumococcus* associated HUS-streptococcal neuramidase exposes a novel antigen [Thomsen-Freidenreich (T) antigen] on RBCs/platelets/glomeruli
- **"Atypical" HUS**
    - Non-STEC, non-pneumococcal
    - Genetic and acquired factors leading to dysregulation of the alternative complement pathway
        - C3/C4
        - Factor H, factor I, factor B
        - MCP (CD46) expression on PBMCs
        - Factor H autoantibodies
        - Mutations
        - Direct exon sequencing of CFH, MCP, CFI, CFB, C3
        - Copy number variation across CFH-CFHR locus
- Red cells get trapped in the formed thrombi, undergo fragmentation resulting in schistocytes.
- Splenic trapping of the fragmented red cells causes extravascular hemolysis.

Differences between thrombotic thrombocytopenic purpura and hemolytic uremic syndrome are presented on **Table 8.68.**

TABLE 8.68: Differences between thrombotic thrombocytopenic purpura and hemolytic uremic syndrome.

Features	*Thrombotic thrombocytopenic purpura (TTP)*	*Hemolytic uremic syndrome (HUS)*
Age	Adults between 20 and 50 years	Children <5 years
Hemolytic anemia	With RBC fragmentation	With RBC fragmentation
Renal dysfunction	Mild to moderate	Acute renal failure
Thrombocytopenia	Present	Present
CNS symptoms	Severe	Mild
Fever	+	—

Clinical Features

- Age: HUS develops most commonly in children between 1 and 5 years of age few days after an episode of bloody diarrhea. HUS can also develop in adults following certain drugs and radiation therapy that damage endothelial cells.
- Classical presentation: **Triad of microangiopathic hemolytic anemia, thrombocytopenia and renal failure** (oliguria). Hematuria and hypertension are also common. Despite thrombocytopenia, bleeding manifestations are rare.
- Complications: Fluid overload may result in pulmonary edema and hypertensive encephalopathy.

Investigations

- Hemoglobin levels: Decreased (anemia).
- Platelet count: Markedly reduced often below 20,000/μL (thrombocytopenia).
- Peripheral blood smear shows fragmented red cells (called schistocytes) and numerous reticulocytes.
- LDH: Elevated.
- Blood urea and creatinine: Elevated.
- Urine: May show proteinuria and red blood cells.
- PT and aPTT: Normal
- Stool: Culture for enterohemorrhagic *E. coli*—positive; shiga toxin—positive.

Treatment

- Supportive care: For the renal and hematological complications.
- Antibiotics: If shigellosis is suspected/detected.
- Experimental: Eculizumab, monoclonal antibody to C5.

Prognosis

With appropriate supportive care, they usually recover completely, but in more severe cases renal damage may result in death.

DISSEMINATED INTRAVASCULAR COAGULATION

Q. Discuss the causes, pathogenesis, clinical features, laboratory features, and management of disseminated intravascular coagulation (DIC: defibrination syndrome: consumption coagulopathy).

Disseminated intravascular coagulation is a widespread acute or chronic thrombohemorrhagic disorder in which a **combination of thrombosis and hemorrhage** develops as a secondary complication of a wide variety of disorders **(Table 8.69).**

TABLE 8.69: Major disorders associated with disseminated intravascular coagulation.

1. Infections	**4. Massive tissue injury**
➢ Gram-negative bacterial sepsis ➢ Meningococcemia and other bacteria ➢ Fungi, viruses, Rocky mountain spotted fever, malaria	➢ Traumatic ➢ Burns ➢ Fat embolism ➢ Surgery
2. Obstetric complications	**5. Vascular disorders**
➢ Retained dead fetus ➢ Septic abortion ➢ Abruptio placentae ➢ Amniotic fluid embolism ➢ Toxemia and preeclampsia	➢ Aortic aneurysm, giant hemangioma
3. Neoplasms	**6. Miscellaneous**
➢ Carcinomas of pancreas, prostate, lung, and stomach ➢ Acute promyelocytic leukemia	➢ Snakebite, liver disease, acute intravascular hemolysis, shock, heat stroke, hypersensitivity, vasculitis

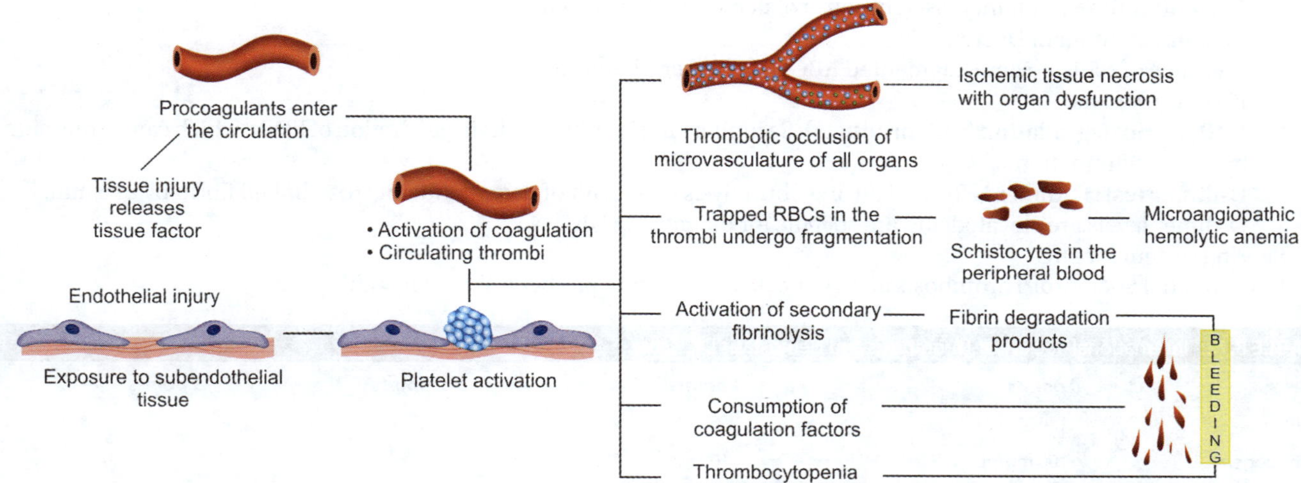

FIG. 8.47: Pathogenesis of thrombosis, ischemic tissue necrosis, and bleeding in disseminated intravascular coagulation.

Pathogenesis (Fig. 8.47)

Clinical Features

- DIC is a serious, often fatal, important clinical condition which needs an immediate diagnosis and management. The symptoms of DIC depend on the nature, intensity and duration of the underlying disorder.
- Signs and symptoms are related to the tissue hypoxia and infarction caused by the microvascular thrombosis; or with bleeding diathesis due to the depletion of factors and the activation of fibrinolytic mechanisms; or both **(Table 8.70)**.
- Bleeding is the most common clinical feature in acute **DIC**. It may manifest as ecchymoses, petechiae, or bleeding from mucous membranes or at the sites of venipuncture.
- Microvascular thrombi cause ischemic necrosis of the organ with resultant dysfunction of the involved organ and occur most often with chronic underlying diseases. Organ dysfunction may manifest as hepatic, renal, cardiac, or respiratory failure or neurological disturbances. It may also result in gangrene of extremities and hemorrhagic necrosis of the skin.

TABLE 8.70: Effects and signs of disseminated intravascular coagulation.

Organ/site	*Due to thrombi in microvasculature*	*Due to hemorrhagic diathesis*
Central nervous system	Multifocal, delirium, coma	Intracerebral bleeding
Renal system	Cortical necrosis—oliguria, azotemia	Hematuria
Skin	Focal ischemic necrosis, gangrene	Petechiae, ecchymoses, bleeding at the sites of venipuncture
Gastrointestinal tract	Acute ulceration	Massive bleeding
Respiratory tract	Acute respiratory distress syndrome	
Mucous membranes		Epistaxis, gingival bleeding
Peripheral circulation	Fragmentation of trapped RBCs—microangiopathic hemolytic anemia	

- Waterhouse-Friderichsen syndrome: Occult thrombosis of adrenal vein thrombosis resulting in adrenal hemorrhage.
- Trousseau sign: Migratory venous thrombosis in cancers.
- Multiorgan dysfunction syndrome (MODS): Frequent consequence of DIC and is usually due to bleeding into organs or thrombotic alteration in various organs (hepatic, cardiac, central nervous, renal, and pulmonary systems).

Laboratory Findings (Investigations) in DIC (Table 8.71)

Q. Write short note on investigations to diagnose DIC.

- ESR: Low
- Peripheral smear: Presence of schistocytes.
- **Screening assays**
  - **Platelet count:** Decreased because of utilization of platelets in microthrombi.
  - **PT:** Increased.
  - **APTT: Increased** because of consumption and inhibition of the function of clotting factors.
  - **Thrombin time (TT):** Increased because of decreased fibrinogen.
  - **Plasma fibrinogen:** Decreased.
  - Presence of schistocytes (fragmented RBCs) in the peripheral smear.
- **Confirmatory tests**
  - **FDP (fibrin degradation/split products):** Secondary fibrinolysis results in generation of FDPs, which can be measured by latex agglutination.
  - **D-dimer test:** D-dimer is formed during fibrinolysis as a result of degradation of cross-linked fibrin by plasmin. D-dimer levels are elevated and are specific for diagnosing DIC.
- Scoring system for DIC
- International Society of Thrombosis and Hemostasis DIC score has been shown in **Table 8.72**.

TABLE 8.71: Routine laboratory value abnormalities in DIC.

Test	*Abnormality*
Platelet count	Decreased
Prothrombin time	Prolonged
aPTT	Prolonged
Fibrin degradation products	Elevated
Protease inhibitors (e.g., protein C, AT, protein S)	Decreased

TABLE 8.72: International Society of Thrombosis and Hemostasis DIC score.

Test	*0 points*	*1 points*	*2 points*	*3 points*
INR	<1.25	1.25–1.5	>1.5	
Fibrinogen	>100 mg/dL	<100 mg/dL		
D-dimer	<400 ng/dL		400–4,000 ng/mL	>4,000 ng/mL
Platelets	>100,000	50,000–100,000	<50,000	

Interpretation of total score:
- ≥5 points: Overt DIC
- <5 points: Patients may still have non-overt DIC, could evolve into overt DIC

Q. Write short note on management of DIC.

Management

- Control or elimination of the underlying cause (e.g., removal of a dead fetus, placenta, etc.).
- Correction of precipitating factors, e.g., acidosis, dehydration, sepsis and hypoxia.
- Management of hemorrhagic symptoms: It is necessary to maintain blood volume and tissue perfusion. Hemorrhagic symptoms are managed by transfusions of platelet concentrates, FFP, cryoprecipitate and red cell concentrates.
  - Dose:
    - Platelet concentrates: 1–2 units/10 kg.
    - Fresh frozen plasma: 15–20 mL/kg.
    - Cryoprecipitate: 1 unit/10 kg.
- Drugs to control coagulation such as heparin or antifibrinolytic drugs have been tried in DIC.
  - Heparin: Low doses of continuous infusion heparin (5–10 U/kg/h) are often used in patients with thrombotic manifestations. It should be given after the correction of bleeding. Major indications for heparin therapy are:
    - Purpura fulminans during the surgical resection of giant hemangiomas and during removal of a dead fetus.
    - Acute promyelocytic leukemia.
  - Antifibrinolytic drugs: For example, EACA, or tranexamic acid prevent fibrin degradation by plasmin may reduce bleeding episodes. However, they increase the risk of thrombosis and concomitant use of heparin is indicated.
  - **Antithrombin III, protein C concentrate, TFPI** have been tried

TRANSFUSION MEDICINE

Q. Discuss blood transfusion, blood component transfusion, and indications for transfusion therapy.

Transfusion medicine comprises of blood and blood component/products transfusion. Blood cannot be synthesized artificially. So the source of blood is from a healthy human donor.

Whole Blood

- One unit of blood collected from a donor contains 450 mL ± 10% of blood and citrate anticoagulant that also contains phosphate and dextrose.
- Whole blood provides both oxygen-carrying capacity and volume expansion. However, it is rarely used because within a few hours or days, some coagulation factors (especially factors V and VIII) and platelets decrease in quantity or lose viability.

Red Cell Concentrates (Packed Red Cells)

- Packed red cells are obtained by centrifugation/sedimentation of the whole blood. All the plasma is removed and is replaced by about 100 mL of an optimal additive solution, such as SAG-M, which contains sodium chloride, adenine, glucose, and mannitol.
- In the packed red cell unit, the hematocrit is between 55% and 65%. Since, the volume is about 330 mL; there is less risk of volume overload.
- One unit of packed red blood cells raises hemoglobin concentration by 1 g/dL.

General indications for RBC transfusion are mentioned in **Box 8.33**.

Box 8.33: General indications for RBC transfusion.

- Replace acute blood loss due to hemorrhage or during surgery to relieve clinical features caused by insufficient oxygen delivery
- Symptomatic anemia in an euvolemic patient
  - β-thalassemia major
  - Sickle cell anemia
  - Aplastic anemia
  - Severe anemia of any cause

Platelet Concentrate

- Platelet concentrate may be obtained from a single donor or pooled plasma. Platelets can also be obtained from a single donor by platelet apheresis SDP-single donor platelets.
- Platelets have ABO antigens on their surface but do not express Rh antigen. Hence, ABO matching required. But it is advisable to transfuse Rh negative persons with platelets only from Rh negative persons. One platelet concentrate (PC) should increase the platelet count by 5,000–10,000/µL. Six units of pooled platelets or one apheresis unit should increase the platelet count by approximately 30,000/µL.
- Indications for platelet concentrate transfusion are mentioned in **Box 8.34.**

Box 8.34: Indications for platelet concentrate transfusion.

Bleeding due to:

- Severe thrombocytopenia (when platelet count is less than 20,000/mm^3).
  - Immune mediated: In patients with autoimmune thrombocytopenia, it should be reserved for patients with life-threatening bleeding.
  - Secondary to bone marrow failure
    - Chemotherapy induced
    - Due to leukemia
    - Dilutional
- Abnormal platelet function
- Disseminated intravascular coagulation (DIC)
- Surgical or invasive procedures in thrombocytopenic patients

- Contraindication to platelet concentrate transfusion
  - Thrombotic thrombocytopenic purpura (TTP)
  - Heparin-induced thrombocytopenia (HIT).
  - Relative contraindication: Idiopathic thrombocytopenic purpura (ITP) or post-transfusion purpura (PTP) because the survival of transfused platelets is very brief.

Granulocyte Concentrates

- Indications: Severe neutropenia with definite evidence of bacterial infection.
- It is not frequently employed, because it is preferable to administer the growth factors for myelopoiesis like G-CSF/GM-CSF. But it is indicated when granulocyte count is less than 500/mm^3 (agranulocytosis), and to combat infections (in neonatal sepsis and chronic granulomatous disease).

Fresh Frozen Plasma

- The volume is about 200 mL and contains all the coagulation factors (including vWF). Present in fresh plasma. The volume transfused depends on the clinical situation and patient size, and should be guided by laboratory assays of coagulation function. The general guide is 10–15 mL/kg per dose.
- ABO matching is essential before infusion of FFP. Rh compatibility is not required

- **Indications:** For replacement of coagulation factors in acquired coagulation factor deficiencies
  - Patients on anticoagulant drug therapy (Coumarin)
  - Antithrombin deficiency
  - Coagulopathy of liver diseases
  - Vitamin K deficiency
  - Microangiopathic hemolytic anemia including TTP, hemolytic uremic syndrome, and HELLP syndrome
  - DIC.

Cryoprecipitate

- Contains concentrated precipitate of factor VIII, XIII, vWF, and fibrinogen.
- Does not require cross-matching before transfusion.
- **Indications:**
  - DIC and other conditions where the fibrinogen level is very low (hypofibrinogenemia).
  - It was used for hemophilia, factor XIII deficiency, and von Willebrand disease. However, it is no longer used for these disorders because of the greater risk of virus transmission compared with virus-inactivated coagulation factor concentrates.
- Various coagulations factors and their amount in one unit of cryoprecipitate are mentioned in **Table 8.73**.

TABLE 8.73: Various coagulations factors and their amount in one unit of cryoprecipitate.

Coagulation factor	*Quantity per unit*
Fibrinogen	150–250 mg
Factor VIII	80–150 units
Von Willebrand factor	100–150 units
Factor XIII	50–75 units

Factor VIII and IX Concentrates

- These are freeze-dried preparations of specific coagulation factors prepared from large pools of plasma from many donors.
- **Indications:** For patients with hemophilia and von Willebrand's disease, where recombinant coagulation factor concentrates are unavailable.

Saline-washed Red Blood Cells

Saline washing of red cells is an effective means of removing leukocytes and plasma (up to 99%). This product is largely restricted to patients with antibodies to IgA or IgE, and those requiring red cells with minimal plasma as in **thalassemia and paroxysmal nocturnal hemoglobinuria.**

Frozen Red Blood Cells

Red blood cells can be freezed and stored up to 3 years by addition of glycerol as an endocellular cryoprotective agent. This procedure is used for storage of rare blood groups. Frozen red cells may be indicated for patients with history of severe allergic reactions to plasma or leukocyte factors, e.g., patients sensitized to IgA.

Irradiated Blood Products

Cellular blood products (red cells, platelets, granulocytes) can be irradiated to a dose of 1,500 rads before transfusion in order to minimize the risk of transfusion-**acquired graft-versus-host disease** in immunocompromised individuals.

Immunoglobulins

Rh Immune Globulin

Indications

- Known or suspected inoculation of Rh– mother with unknown or Rh+ fetal red cells, e.g., abortion, threatened abortion, ectopic pregnancy, amniocentesis, abdominal trauma in 2nd or 3rd trimester, postpartum if new born is Rh+.
- Following transfusion of Rh+ cellular blood products (e.g., platelets) to an Rh– female of child bearing age or younger.
- Acute ITP resistant to steroids.

Safe Transfusion Procedures

Q. Write short note on precautions to be observed in blood transfusion.

Pretransfusion Testing

Before transfusion of any blood or its components, it is necessary to know whether they are compatible with the recipient's blood.

- **Donor blood:** The tests routinely carried out on donor's blood include ABO and Rh grouping, tests for HBsAg, anti-HCV, anti-HIV-1 and HIV-2 and serum alanine aminotransferase (ALT), malaria, and syphilis.
- **Recipient blood:** The recipient's ABO and Rh grouping is also carried out.

Compatibility Testing

These are set of procedures which include: Review of patient's past blood bank history and records (if done earlier), ABO and Rh typing of the recipient and donor, antibody screening test of recipient's and donor's serum followed by cross-matching. It is sometimes referred to as cross-matching. However, cross-match is only a part of compatibility test.

Cross-matching: Cross-matching is very important before any blood transfusion. Cross-matching should be carried out to ensure that there are no antibodies in patient's serum that will react with the donor's cells when transfused. Full cross-matching requires about 45 minutes if no red cell antibodies are present, but may need hours if a patient has multiple antibodies.

- **Importance of cross-matching:**
  - It is the final check of ABO compatibility between donor and recipient.
  - Detects the presence of any clinically significant, unexpected antibodies in the recipient's serum that may react with donor's cells, thereby preventing any transfusion reaction.
- **Types:** Cross-matching procedure may involve **major and minor** cross-matching. Major cross-matching consists of mixing donor's red cells with recipient's (patient's) serum; whereas minor cross-matching consists of mixing patient's red cells with donor's serum.

Bedside Procedures for Safe Transfusion

- An error of patients receiving the wrong blood is important avoidable cause of mortality and morbidity in transfusion medicine.
- Most incompatible transfusions are due to failure to adhere to standard procedures for taking correctly labeled blood samples and ensuring that the correct pack of blood component is transfused into the intended recipient.
- It is always necessary to monitor the recipient during and after transfusion so that any complications can be dealt with accordingly.

COMPLICATIONS OF BLOOD TRANSFUSION

Q. Write short essay/note on the complications of blood transfusion.

Complications of blood transfusion have been shown in **Table 8.74.**

TABLE 8.74: Complications of blood transfusion.

Immunological complications	*Nonimmunological complications*
➤ **Immediate reactions** – Acute hemolytic transfusion reactions – Febrile nonhemolytic reaction – Allergic reaction—urticaria – Anaphylactic reactions – Transfusion-related acute lung injury (TRALI) ➤ **Delayed reactions** ♦ Alloimmunization ♦ Delayed hemolytic transfusion reactions (mostly asymptomatic) ♦ Transfusion associated graft versus host disease ♦ Post-transfusion purpura	➤ **Immediate** – Circulatory overload – Air embolism ➤ **Late** – Iron overload: Transfusion hemosiderosis – Thrombophlebitis – Infections: ♦ Hepatitis (HBV, HCV, and HDV) ♦ HIV (AIDS) ♦ Malaria ♦ Cytomegalovirus ♦ Syphilis

Immunological Complications/Reactions

Acute Hemolytic Transfusion Reaction

- Most serious complication of blood transfusion.
- Cause: Occurs due to transfusion of incompatible donor red cells resulting in destruction of donor cells. Usually due to ABO incompatibility.

Clinical features

- The initial symptoms may **occur within few minutes after starting the transfusion**. Patient typically develops fever with chills, pain in the lumbar region, dyspnea, pruritus, burning sensation at the site of transfusion and centrally along the vein, and chest pain.
- In an unconscious patient, more severe features like hypotension, shock, intravascular hemolysis which results in hemoglobinuria and oliguria with acute renal failure and excessive bleeding due to DIC may develop.

Diagnosis

In majority of cases, this results from clerical errors like wrong labeling of the cross-match sample, improper checking or transfusion to the wrong recipient, confirmed by finding evidence of hemolysis (e.g., hemoglobinuria), and incompatibility between donor and recipient.

Management

- Stop the transfusion immediately if there is any suspicion of serious transfusion reaction.
- Change the blood transfusion set and maintain the venous access using normal saline.
- Perform physical examination such as blood pressure, urine output and evidence of bleeding. Emergency treatment may be needed to maintain the blood pressure and renal function.
- Withdraw new blood samples from the opposite arm of the patient and send it to the blood transfusion laboratory along with the donor units to exclude a hemolytic transfusion reaction.
- Centrifuge one more blood sample from the recipient of transfusion and look for any free hemoglobin in the supernatant.
- Perform coagulation screening tests including partial thromboplastin time, platelet count, fibrinogen levels and fibrin-degradation products to exclude DIC. Laboratory evaluation for hemolysis includes the measurement of serum haptoglobin, lactate dehydrogenase (LDH) and indirect bilirubin levels.
- If hypotension develops, administer intravenous fluids and if required, vasopressors.
- Administer diuretic furosemide to maintain urine output.

Febrile Nonhemolytic Transfusion Reactions (FNHTR)

- Common complication of blood transfusion.
- Cause: Usually develop due to presence of leukocyte antibodies in patients who have previously been transfused or pregnant. Can also occur due to release of cytokines from donor leukocytes in platelet concentrates.
- Time of occurrence: Usually occur toward the end of infusion or within hours of completing the transfusion.
- Typical signs: Flushing and tachycardia, fever (>38°C), chills, and rigors.

Allergic Reactions—Urticaria

- Common but rarely severe.
- Cause: Urticarial reactions are mostly result from plasma-protein incompatibility due to the presence of antibodies in the recipient's blood to infused plasma proteins or infusion of allergens that react with IgE antibodies in the patient.

Treatment: Stop or slow the transfusion and administer 10 mg of chlorphenaramine (chlorpheniramine) intravenously.

Anaphylactic Reactions

- These are severe reactions which develop after transfusion of only a few milliliters of the blood component.
- Severe reactions are seen in patients who have antibodies against IgA and are often deficient in IgA. The antibodies react with IgA present in the donor blood.
- Symptoms and signs: Difficulty in breathing, coughing, nausea and vomiting, hypotension, bronchospasm, loss of consciousness, respiratory arrest, and shock.
- Treatment: Stop transfusion and maintain vascular access. Immediately administer 0.5 mg epinephrine (adrenaline) IM, and 10 mg chlorpheniramine, IV glucocorticoids, and endotracheal intubation may be required in severe cases.

Transfusion Related Acute Lung Injury (TRALI)

- Cause: TRALI usually develops from the transfusion of donor plasma that contains high-titer anti-HLA antibodies that bind recipient leukocytes. This produces aggregation of leukocytes in the pulmonary vasculature and release mediators that increase capillary permeability. Such antibodies are most frequently found in females after pregnancy and are not found in plasma of males unless they have been transfused.
- Patient develops an acute respiratory distress, either during or within 6 hours of transfusing the patient. It is characterized by fever, cough, shortness of breath, and typical bilateral interstitial infiltrates on chest X-ray. The reaction occurs during or soon after transfusion and may be life-threatening.

Treatment: Supportive and patients usually recover without any sequelae.

Delayed Hemolytic Transfusion Reactions (DHTRs)

- These are not completely preventable.
- Cause:
  - May occur in patients previously sensitized to RBC alloantigens (such as Rh, Kidd, Kell, Duffy) by previous transfusions or pregnancies.
  - The antibody level is too low to be detected by pretransfusion compatibility testing.
  - When the patient is transfused with antigen-positive blood, there is early production of alloantibody (usually by IgG antibodies) that binds donor RBCs, resulting in destruction of the transfused donor cells.
- Occurs 3–21 days after transfusion with the incompatible blood.
- Direct Coombs' test (DAT): Positive, if carried out during hemolysis. Later, patient may show only positive indirect Coombs' test.

Treatment: Usually no specific therapy is required.

Transfusion–associated Graft-versus-Host Disease (TA-GVHD)

- Rare but potentially fatal complication.
- Develops 8–10 days, and death occurs at 3–4 weeks after transfusion.
- **Mechanism:** Donor blood products contain mature T lymphocytes that recognize host HLA antigens as foreign and mount an immune response and attack upon recipient's tissues. It is observed more commonly in immunocompromised recipients.
- Clinical features include fever, generalized characteristic skin rash, jaundice (with abnormalities of liver function), diarrhea, and features of pancytopenia (due to marrow failure).

- **Prevention:** TA-GVHD can be prevented by transfusing the irradiated blood/components in patients at risk.
- It is highly resistant to treatment with immunosuppressive therapies, including glucocorticoids, cyclosporine, antithymocyte globulin, etc.

Post-transfusion Purpura

- It is an immune-mediated thrombocytopenia that usually occurs predominantly in parous women.
- Antibodies against human platelet antigens (HPAs) are found in the patient's serum.
- It occurs 7–10 days after platelet transfusion.
- Thrombocytopenia is usually severe and may cause bleeding.
- Platelet transfusions are usually ineffective and can worsen the thrombocytopenia and hence should be avoided.

Treatment: Treatment with high-dose (0.4 g/kg/day for 5 days). Intravenous immunoglobulin may neutralize the effector antibodies, or plasmapheresis can be used to remove the antibodies.

Alloimmunization

- Alloimmunization usually does not cause clinical problems with the first transfusion but these may occur with subsequent transfusions. Delayed consequences of alloimmunization, include HDN (hemolytic disease of the newborn) and rejection of tissue transplants.
- Types:
  - Alloantibodies to RBC antigens
    - Detected during pretransfusion testing and may delay finding antigen-negative cross-match-compatible products for transfusion.
    - Alloimmunization may develop during pregnancy to fetal RBC antigens (i.e., D, c, E, Kell, or Duffy) inherited from the father and not shared by the mother.
  - Alloimmunization to antigens on leukocytes and platelets: It can lead to refractoriness to platelet transfusions.

Nonimmune Complications/Reactions

Q. Write short note on infections transmitted by blood transfusion.

- **Circulatory overload:** Significant in the elderly, pregnant women, those with reduced cardiac function (e.g., cardiac failure) or renal failure resulting in acute pulmonary edema.
- **Air embolism:** It used to develop in olden days when transfusion was given from the glass bottle.
- **Iron overload (transfusion siderosis)**
  - This is seen in patients who receive multiple transfusions over a period of few years (e.g., thalassemia). The excess iron gets deposited in reticuloendothelial cells of spleen, bone marrow, liver, heart and endocrine glands.
  - Iron overload can be prevented or reduced by giving iron chelating agents
- **Thrombophlebitis:** Inflammation of vein may develop in patients with indwelling catheters.
- **Infectious complications:** Transfusion of infected blood may transmit few diseases like AIDS, hepatitis (HBV, HCV and HDV), HTLV-I and II, malaria, and cytomegalovirus infection. This is prevented by screening the donors for these common and ominous infections.

Massive transfusion is defined as transfusion of more than 10 units of red cells or replacement of 1 blood volume in 24 hours. The use of large quantities of stored blood in massive transfusions may lead to a number of complications. Among these are dilutional coagulopathy, circulatory overload, hyperkalemia, hypoglycemia, hypothermia, and rarely, citrate-induced hypocalcemia.

Blood Groups and Diseases

- The first established disease relationship was between carcinoma of the stomach and group A.
- Duodenal ulcer is 1.4 times more common in group O patients.
- It is also reported that group A individuals have greater levels of factor VIII than group O, and hence greater complications of bleeding are seen in group O than A.
- A relationship between the Duffy (Fy) blood group and malaria is well established. It is seen in West Africa where the frequency of Fy a-b- is about 90%; these individuals are resistant to *Plasmodium vivax*. Experimentally, it has been shown that antigens Fya and Fyb act as receptors for the parasite to enter the cell.
- The Kell (K) group is associated with chronic granulomatous diseases and Rh null is implicated in autoimmune hemolytic anemia.

STEM CELLS

Q. Define and classify stem cells. Discuss their clinical applications.

Definition

Stem cells are characterized by their ability of self-renewal and capacity to generate differentiated cell lineages.

Properties

- Self-renewal capacity
- Asymmetric replication: This is characterized by division of stem cell into:
  - One daughter cell which gives rise to differentiated mature cells and regenerating tissues
  - Other remains undifferentiated stem cells which retain the self-renewal capacity.

Types

- **Embryonic stem cells:** During development of embryo, the blastocysts contain undifferentiated pluripotent stem cells which are called as embryonic stem cells or ES cells. These cells can form cells of all three germ cell layers.
  - Normal function: To give rise to all cells of the body.
- **Adult (somatic) stem cells:** Adult stem cells are less undifferentiated than ES cells found in adults. They are found among differentiated cells within a tissue. They are multipotent and have more limited capacity to generate different cell types than ES cells.
  - Normal function: Tissue homeostasis.
  - Use: Adult stem cells include hematopoietic stem cells (HSC) in bone marrow, peripheral blood or cord blood. They are currently the only type of stem cells commonly used to treat human diseases.
  - **Induced pluripotent stem cells (iPS cells):** This is achieved by transferring the nucleus of adult cells to an enucleated oocyte.
    - **Use:** For therapeutic cloning in the treatment of human diseases.

Clinical Application

Some diseases in which marrow transplantation has been utilized are presented in **Box 8.35**.

Box 8.35: Diseases treated with marrow transplantation.

Genetic diseases (allogenic BMT)
- *Red cell disorders*
  - Thalassemia major
  - Sickle cell disease
- *Immunodeficiencies*
  - Severe combined immunodeficiency
  - X-linked agammaglobulinemia
- *Granulocyte disorders*
  - Chediak-Higashi syndrome
  - Chronic granulomatous disease
  - Kostmann syndrome
- *Enzyme deficiencies*
  - Gaucher's disease
  - Mucopolysaccharidoses
  - Leukodystrophies
- *Platelet disorders*
  - Wiskott-Aldrich syndrome
  - Glanzmann's thrombasthenia
- *Other*
  - Osteopetrosis

Marrow failure syndromes allogenic or syngenic BMT
- Severe aplastic anemia
- Fanconi's syndrome
- Paroxysmal nocturnal hemoglobinuria

Malignant diseases

Autologous, syngenic or allogenic BMT
- Acute leukemias
- Chronic leukemias
- Myelodysplastic syndromes
- Hodgkin's disease
- Non-Hodgkin lymphomas
- Other solid tumors

Therapeutic

Other possible uses:
- Ischemic heart disease: Stem cells are injected either into the coronary arteries or directly into the myocardium. They can differentiate into myocardial cells or new blood vessels.
- Spinal cord lesions
- Nonunion of fractured bones
- Parkinson disease
- Huntington disease
- Muscular dystrophy
- Type 1 diabetes mellitus
- Motor neuron disease
- Alzheimer's disease

Other Applications

- Useful in understanding the pathology of disease and origin of cancers.
- Monitor the development of genetic disorders.
- Test the efficacy of drugs.

HEMATOPOIETIC STEM CELL TRANSPLANTATION

Q. Write short essay/note on hematopoietic stem cells (HSC).

Q. Write a short note on peripheral blood stem cell transplantation.

Q. Write short essay/note on bone marrow transplantation and its indications.

- **Bone marrow transplantation** was the original term used to describe the collection and transplantation of hematopoietic stem cells.
- **Hematopoietic stem cell transplantation** is a preferred term, because the peripheral blood and umbilical cord blood are also used as sources of stem cells.
- **Definition:** Hematopoietic stem cell transplantation is defined as the process of collecting and infusing hematopoietic stem cells obtained from bone marrow (bone marrow transplantation) or peripheral blood (peripheral blood stem cell transplantation).
- **Purpose of HSC transplantation:** To repopulate or replace totally or partly recipient's hematopoietic system. HSC are self-renewing cells which can repopulate all the cell lineages in the blood.
- Major sources of hematopoietic stem cells:
  - Bone marrow: Obtained directly from bone marrow by multiple aspirations from the pelvic bones.
  - Peripheral blood (peripheral blood stem cells).
  - Umbilical cord blood.

Indications for Hematopoietic Stem Cell Transplantation

Q. Write short essay/note on indications for bone marrow/stem cell transplantation.

Indications for hematopoietic stem cell transplantation have been shown in **Box 8.36**.

Categories/Types of Hematopoietic Cell Transplantation

- **Autologous ("from self"):** Stem cells obtained from the recipient (same person). The patient's own HSCs are removed and stored in the vapor phase of liquid nitrogen until required. The source of stem cells may be bone marrow or from the blood. It does not require immunosuppression. However, there is no graft-versus-tumor effect and therefore, there is increased risk of disease relapse or progression compared to allogenic HSC transplantation.
- **Allogeneic ("from different genes"):** HSCs are obtained from a donor-either related (usually an HLA-identical sibling) or from a closely HLA-matched volunteer unrelated donor (VUD).
- **Syngeneic ("from same genes"):** HSCs are obtained from an identical twin.
  Main factor for a successful allogenic transplantation is finding of an HLA-matched donor, because it reduces the risk of graft rejection and graft-versus-host disease (GVHD).

Box 8.36: Indication for hematopoietic stem cell transplantation.

Red blood cell disorders
- Severe aplastic anemia
- Thalassemia major
- Fanconi anemia
- Sickle cell disease
- Pure red cell aplasia

WBC disorders
- Leukemia
  - Acute lymphoblastic leukemia—relapse after initial chemotherapy induced remission
  - Chronic myeloid leukemia, acute myeloid leukemia
- Myelodysplastic syndromes, myelofibrosis
- Lymphomas: HL, NHL
- Multiple myeloma

Solid tumors, e.g., germ cell tumors, neuroblastoma

Immunological disorders
- Severe autoimmune disorders: Scleroderma, lupus erythematosus
- Immune deficiency syndromes

Peripheral Blood Stem Cell Transplantation

Definition

It is defined as transplantation of stem cells derived from the peripheral blood of a donor to a recipient (allogenic) or from the patient's own blood (autologous).

Steps

- Hematopoietic stem cells are present in the peripheral blood but in very low concentration (<0.1% of all nucleated cells). To increase their numbers, hematopoietic growth factor (G-CSF or GM-CSF) is administered to the donor (for allogenic stem cell transplant) or to the patient during recovery from intensive chemotherapy (for autologous transplant).

- Stem cells are collected from the blood by apheresis and are infused in the recipient.
- Stem cells engraft in the recipient and is characterized by the recovery of neutrophil count to >500 mm^3 for 3 consecutive days.
- Hematopoietic recovery is more rapid in peripheral hematopoietic stem cell transplantation when compared to bone marrow hematopoietic stem cell transplant.

Umbilical cord blood: It is a good source of HSC with no risk to either infant or mother. Possible contamination of cord blood with CMV and Epstein-Barr virus is also low due to poor transmission from placenta. However, the major disadvantage is that the number of HSCs that can be collected from cord blood is small and an adult might require multiple cord blood donors.

Origin and source of hematopoietic stem cells used for transplantation are presented in **Box 8.37**. Comparison among bone marrow, peripheral blood and cord blood stem cells are presented in **Table 8.75**.

Box 8.37: Origin and source of hematopoietic stem cells used for transplantation.

- ***Origin of hematopoietic stem cells***
  - Autologous
  - Syngeneic
  - Allogeneic
  - Genotypically HLA-identical siblings
  - Phenotypically HLA-identical or HLA-mismatched family members
  - Unrelated volunteer donors
- ***Source of hematopoietic stem cells***
  - Bone marrow
  - Peripheral blood
  - Combination of blood and marrow
  - Umbilical cord blood

TABLE 8.75: Comparison among bone marrow, peripheral blood and cord blood stem cells.

Characteristic	*Bone marrow*	*Peripheral blood*	*Cord blood*
Stem cell content	Adequate	Good	Low
Risk of tumor cell contamination	High	Not applicable	Not applicable
HLA matching	Close matching	Close matching	Less restrictive
Engraftment	Medium	Fastest	Slowest
Risk of acute graft-versus-host disease (GVHD)	High	High	Lowest
Risk of chronic GVHD	Medium	Highest	Lowest

Conditioning Regimens

- Necessary before HSC transplantation.
- Types: **Myeloablative or nonmyeloablative** (or reduced intensity).
  - **Myeloablative regimens:** Eliminates malignant cells in the marrow so that transfused HSC can populate the bone marrow and develop.
  - **Nonmyeloablative regimens:** To induce immunosuppression in recipient so that engraftment of donor cells can take place. It is less toxic.
- Complications of conditioning regimens:
  - Usually develop within 30 days and includes infections, nausea, vomiting, alopecia, mucositis and interstitial pneumonia.
  - Veno-occlusive disease of liver characterized by jaundice, ascites, and tender hepatomegaly.
  - Late complications: Infertility, ovarian failure, and secondary malignancies (AML and solid organ malignancies).

Autologous Stem Cell Transplant

Marrow or peripheral stem cells are obtained from the patient before the high-dose therapy, frozen (cryopreserved) and then reinfused after the high-dose therapy to reconstitute marrow function.

Different steps of autologous stem cell transplantation (Fig. 8.48)

- **Harvesting:** During harvesting, bone marrow and/or peripheral HSCs (identified as CD34+ by immunophenotyping) are collected.
- **Processing of HSCs:** The collected bone marrow or peripheral blood stem cells are suspended in dimethyl sulfoxide (prevents ice crystallization in the cells) and frozen in liquid nitrogen. The HSCs can survive in frozen state for at least 5 years.
- **Conditioning:** Before the autologous transplant, the patient is given a high-dose chemotherapy and/or radiation therapy, sometimes total body irradiation (TBI). This procedure is called conditioning, the purpose of which is to eradicate the recipient's hematopoietic and immune system and also malignant tumor cells if any. Conditioning also makes physical space available for HSCs to engraft. In contrast to allogeneic transplantation, autologous transplantation does not require immunosuppression to prevent GVHD.

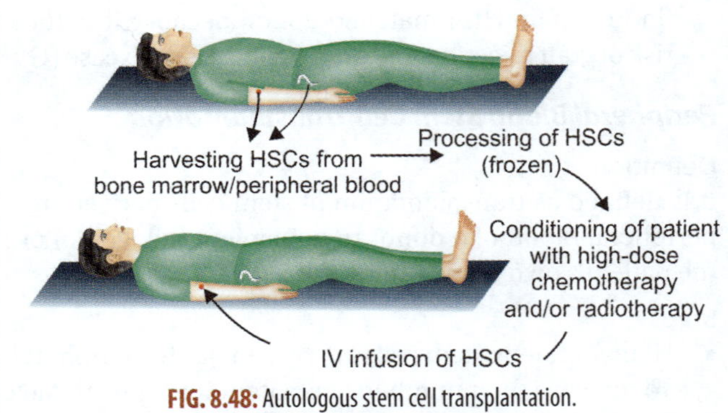

FIG. 8.48: Autologous stem cell transplantation.
(HSC: hematopoietic stem cell)

- **Stem cell transplant:** The collected frozen bone marrow or peripheral HSCs are thawed and infused intravenously like a blood transfusion. These stem cells home from the peripheral circulation to the conditioned empty marrow space. Because of conditioning the patient is pancytopenic and requires critical care. The high-dose chemotherapy also causes breakdown of the normal mucosal barriers in the mouth and gut resulting in increased susceptibility to infections and painful ulcerations.
- **Post-transplant engraftment:** During which the hematopoietic cells produce all the three formed elements of the blood.

Allogenic Bone Marrow Transplantation

The HSCs are obtained from an HLA-matched or HLA-mismatched family member (usually a sibling) or an unrelated donor.

Different steps of allogenic stem cell transplantation (Fig. 8.49)

- **Harvesting:** During harvesting, collected bone marrow and/or peripheral HSCs are mixed with mature WBCs, important being lymphocytes. Mature T lymphocytes are the principal effectors of cell-mediated immunity and both therapeutic benefit and toxicities of allogeneic HSC transplant are due to immunologic reactions between donor T-cells and recipient cells.
- **Conditioning:** This step is similar to autologous HSC transplant. Immunosuppression is to allow engraftment of the transplanted HSCs. The patient's endogenous lymphocytes must be suppressed by immunosuppression so as to prevent GVHD.

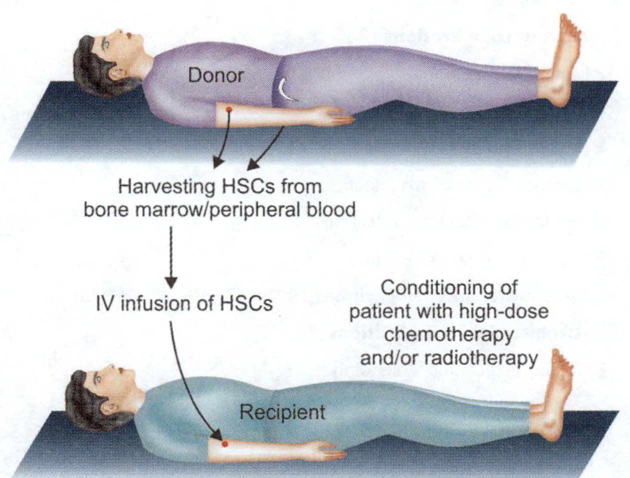

FIG. 8.49: Allogeneic stem cell transplantation.
(HSC: hematopoietic stem cell)

- **Stem cell transplant:** The harvested HSCs are infused into the vein just like a blood transfusion. The stem cells travel and reside in the marrow and produce erythrocytes, granulocytes and platelets. This usually takes 3–4 weeks. Patient requires utmost care during this period similar to autologous transplant.
- **Engraftment:** Donor T lymphocytes help donor HSCs engraft. These T lymphocytes are mostly CD8+ and they destroy any remaining host immune cells which may reject the donor HSCs. Depletion of donor T lymphocytes before allogeneic HSC transplant significantly increases the risk of graft failure. But the greatest disadvantage due to the donor T lymphocytes is development of GVHD.

Complications of Hematopoietic Stem Cell Transplantation (Table 8.76)

Autologous HSC transplants have fewer immunologic complications but have higher rates of relapse of the disease after transplant. Allogeneic HSC transplants have lower rates of relapse but have more immunologic complications, including GVHD, which can be fatal.

- **Infections:** Patients are susceptible to a variety of infections (bacterial, viral, and fungal) due to lack of granulocytes, as well as lack of a functioning immune system. Infections may occur during three different phases after HSC transplantation.
  1. **First phase:** Infections develop due to neutropenia and damage to gastrointestinal mucosal barrier induced by conditioning agents used during transplantation. Source of infection is from oral, skin and gastrointestinal flora.
  2. **Second phase:** It develops during GVHD where T-cell function gets impaired. Patients may develop opportunistic viral and fungal infections.
  3. **Third phase:** It occurs due to chronic GVHD where both B-cell and T-cell functions are impaired. Patients may develop bacterial as well as opportunistic viral and fungal infections.
- **Organ toxicity:** The other complications include damage to GI tract, liver, and lungs.
- **Interstitial pneumonitis:** This is seen in 30–40% of patients and may be fatal in some. Toxicity of radiation and chemotherapy, GVHD and viral, and pneumocystis infections are responsible.
- **Veno-occlusive disease:** VOD results from injury to hepatocytes and endothelium in zone 3 of the liver acinus and obstruction of hepatic sinusoids and venules. The clinical manifestations include jaundice, ascites, and painful hepatomegaly. Tissue plasminogen activator has been used to treat VOD successfully. Severe VOD is often fatal.
- **Graft-versus-host disease:** GVHD is the major complication that follows allogeneic HSC transplant. This is caused by cytotoxic activity of infused donor T lymphocytes reacting against the recipient's tissues/organs (which are considered as foreign to donor T cells).
  - Forms: GVHD can occur in two forms
    1. Acute GVHD: If GVHD occurs before 100 days, it is termed as acute GVHD. It often affects three primary target organs simultaneously, namely skin, gastrointestinal (GI) tract and liver. It causes exfoliative dermatitis, diarrhea, hepatitis and cholestasis. It develops due to production of cytokines by Th1 cells. HLA mismatch is

TABLE 8.76: Complications of hematopoietic cell transplantation.

Vascular access complications	Hepatic complications
Graft failure	➢ Sinusoidal obstructive syndrome
➢ **Blood group incompatibilities and hemolytic complications**	➢ Hepatitis: Infectious versus noninfectious
➢ Acute graft-versus-host disease (GVHD)	**Cardiac toxicity:** Structural (e.g., valvular abnormalities or coronary artery disease) or functional (e.g., cardiomyopathies)
➢ Chronic GVHD	**Lung injury**
Infectious complications	➢ Interstitial pneumonitis: Infectious versus noninfectious
➢ Bacterial infections	➢ Diffuse alveolar hemorrhage
➢ Fungal infections	➢ Engraftment syndrome
➢ Cytomegalovirus infection	➢ Bronchiolitis obliterans
➢ Herpes simplex virus infections	**Kidney and bladder complications:** Hemorrhagic cystitis, nephrotoxicity
➢ Varicella-zoster virus infections	**Endocrine complications**
➢ Epstein-Barr virus infections	➢ **Drug-drug interactions, gonadal dysfunction, thyroid dysfunction**
➢ Adenovirus, respiratory viruses, HHV-6, -7, -8, and other viruses	Growth and development: Growth retardation
Gastrointestinal complications	**Late onset nonmalignant complications**
➢ Mucosal ulceration/bleeding	➢ Osteoporosis/osteopenia, avascular necrosis, dental problems, cataracts, chronic fatigue, psychosocial effects, and rehabilitation
➢ Nutritional support	**Secondary malignancies:** Lymphoma, solid tumors of the tongue, salivary glands, brain, thyroid, bone, malignant melanoma, squamous cell carcinoma, and basal cell carcinoma
	Neurologic complications

one of the important risk factor for its development. Treatment includes methotrexate, cyclosporine, antithymocyte globulin, corticosteroids and monoclonal antibodies against T-cells.

2. Chronic GVHD: Occurs after day 100 following transplantation and can affect the skin, GI tract, liver, eyes, lungs, and joints. GVHD is difficult to treat and in severe cases it is usually fatal. It develops due to cytokine production by Th2 cells. Treatment includes cyclosporine and corticosteroids.

- Three conditions are necessary for the development of GVHD:
  1. An immunocompetent graft (i.e., one containing T-cells)
  2. HLA mismatch (minor or major) between donor and recipient
  3. An immunosuppressed recipient who cannot mount an immune response to the graft.

DRUGS USED IN HEMATOLOGICAL DISEASES

Antiplatelet Drugs (Table 8.77)

Q. Write short essay/note on antiplatelet drugs.

Cyclooxygenase Inhibitors

- **Aspirin** is cheap, effective and most widely used antiplatelet agent.
- **Mechanism of action:** Aspirin inhibits platelet enzyme cyclooxygenase (COX-1 and COX-2) and prevents the synthesis of thromboxane A_2. This results in impairment of platelet secretion and aggregation.
- **Duration of action:** Effects of aspirin on platelet function develop within an hour and lasts for the whole life span of platelets (~7 days).
- **Indications:** Arthritis, secondary prevention of cardiovascular events (acute coronary syndromes, stable angina) in patients with coronary artery, cerebrovascular (transient ischemic attack), or peripheral vascular disease (intermittent claudication).
- **Dose:** Usual dose is 75–325 mg once daily.
- **Side effects:** Dyspepsia to erosive gastritis or peptic ulcers with bleeding and perforation.

TABLE 8.77: Antiplatelet agents by mechanism of action and clinical use.

Cyclooxygenase inhibitors	
Aspirin	Coronary and cerebrovascular disease
Agents that increase cAMP	
Dipyridamole	Coronary, cerebrovascular, peripheral arterial disease
Pentoxifylline	Peripheral arterial disease
Cilostazol	Peripheral arterial disease
ADP receptor blockers	
Ticlopidine	Cerebrovascular disease
Clopidogrel	Coronary, cerebrovascular disease, PCI
Prasugrel	Coronary, cerebrovascular disease, PCI
ADP mimetic	
Cangrelor	Coronary, cerebrovascular disease
Glycoprotein IIb/IIIa inhibitors	
Abciximab	ACS
Eptifibatide	ACS
Tirofiban	ACS

(ADP: adenosine diphosphate; ACS: acute coronary syndrome; cAMP: cyclic adenosine monophosphate; PCI: percutaneous coronary intervention)

Adenosine Diphosphate (ADP) Receptor Antagonists on Platelets (Thienopyridines)

- Thienopyridines are drugs that selectively inhibit ADP-induced platelet aggregation by irreversibly blocking P2Y12.
- Thienopyridines include **ticlopidine, clopidogrel, and prasugrel**.
- Indications: Reduces the risk of cardiovascular death, MI, and stroke in patients with atherosclerotic disease.
- **Dose:**
  - Ticlopidine: 250 mg twice daily
  - Clopidogrel: 75 mg once daily. Loading dose of 300 mg of clopidogrel is given when rapid ADP receptor blockade is needed such as patients undergoing coronary stenting.
  - Prasugrel: A loading dose of 60 mg, prasugrel produces much more rapid, potent, and consistent inhibition of platelet function than clopidogrel loading dose. It is followed by a maintenance dose of 10 mg once daily.
- **Side effects:**
  - Ticlopidine: Gastrointestinal and hematologic (neutropenia, thrombocytopenia, and thrombotic thrombocytopenic purpura). These side effects usually occur within the first few months of starting treatment.
  - Clopidogrel and prasugrel: Gastrointestinal and hematologic side effects are rare.

Adenosine Reuptake Inhibitors

- **Dipyridamole** is a relatively weak antiplatelet agent.
- Mechanism of action:
  - Inhibits phosphodiesterase and blocks the breakdown of cyclic AMP.
- Dose: 25–75 mg three to four times a day. Dipyridamole is more commonly used along with aspirin.
- Indications: Coronary artery disease, ischemic stroke or transient ischemic attack. Rarely used at present because of dose inconvenience and side effects.
- Side effects:
  - Due to **vasodilatory effect**, it can lower the blood pressure and must be used with caution in patients with coronary artery disease.
  - Others: Gastrointestinal complaints, headache, dizziness and hypotension.

Glycoprotein IIb/IIIa Receptor Antagonists (Inhibitors)

- It includes three agents: **Abciximab, eptifibatide, and tirofiban.**
- Uses: Parenteral GPIIb/IIIa receptor antagonists are used in acute coronary syndromes, unstable angina and non-ST-elevatin MI percutaneous coronary interventions.
- **Side effects:** Bleeding tendencies and thrombocytopenia. Eptifibatide may produce hypotension.

Anticoagulants

Q. Classify anticoagulants. Write short essay/note on the commonly used anticoagulants.

Q. Write short note on:
- **Indication for anticoagulants**
- **Contraindication for anticoagulants.**

Classification of Anticoagulants

Classification of anticoagulants has been shown in **Table 8.78.**

TABLE 8.78: Classification of anticoagulants.

Parenteral (rapidly acting)	*Oral (slow acting)*
➢ Heparin (unfractionated and low-molecular weight heparins) ➢ Hirudins ➢ Heparinoids ➢ Indirect factor Xa inhibitors (fondaparinux and idraparinux)	➢ Coumarin derivatives: Warfarin sodium, dicoumarol. These are most commonly used. Bishydroxycoumarin dicoumoral, acenocoumarol (nicoumalone), ethylbiscoumacetate ➢ Indandione derivatives: Phenindione, diphenindione (not used clinically) ➢ Direct thrombin inhibitors: Ximelagatran

Indications for Anticoagulant Therapy

Q. Write short note on indications for long-term anticoagulation.

Indications for anticoagulant therapy have been shown in **Table 8.79.**

Contraindications for anticoagulation therapy are listed in **Box 8.38.**

TABLE 8.79: Indications for anticoagulant therapy.

Purpose	*Clinical situations*
Urgent and for long-term anticoagulation: It is initiated with heparin and taken over by oral anticoagulants	Thrombosis and thromboembolism: ➢ Atrial fibrillation and cardiac disorders with thromboembolism ➢ Deep venous thrombosis ➢ Stroke in evolution and resistant transient ischemic attacks ➢ Pulmonary thromboembolism Others: ➢ Unstable angina and non-ST-elevation myocardial infarction ➢ Prosthetic valves ➢ Peripheral vascular disease
Anticoagulants for brief periods: Heparin alone is used	Cardiac bypass surgery: ➢ Hemodialysis ➢ Disseminated intravascular coagulation (DIC)

Box 8.38: Contraindications for anticoagulant therapy.

- Bleeding disorders, heparin-induced thrombocytopenia
- Severe hypertension, threatened abortion, hemorrhoids, peptic ulcers
- Subacute bacterial endocarditis, tuberculosis
- Ocular and neurosurgery, lumbar puncture
- Chronic alcoholics, cirrhosis, renal failure

Heparin

Unfractionated heparin

Q. Write short note on (unfractionated) heparin.

Mechanism of action: Heparin acts as anticoagulant by activating antithrombin (previously known as antithrombin III) thereby potentiating its action. The activated antithrombin inhibits clotting enzymes, particularly thrombin and factor Xa.

- **Mode of administration:** Heparin is given parenterally. It is usually administered SC or by continuous IV infusion.
- **Dose:** Initial loading dose of 5,000–10,000 units intravenously, followed by maintenance by any one of the following:
  - Continuous intravenous.
  - Intermittent intravenous/subcutaneous.
- **Methods of anticoagulation:**
  - Total anticoagulation: Continuous intravenous maintenance using an infusion pump at a rate of 1,000 units/hour.
  - Low-dose heparinization (e.g., prophylaxis of DVT): 5,000 units 12 hourly or 8 hourly subcutaneously.
  - For prophylaxis: Fixed doses of 5,000 units SC two or three times daily.
- **Duration of therapy:** Variable, but usually ranges from 7 to 10 days.
- **Monitoring:** Heparin therapy is monitored using activated partial thromboplastin time (aPTT), which is maintained at 1.5 to 2 times the control value.
- **Antidote of heparin:** Protamine sulfate
- **Complications of heparin therapy:** Includes bleeding, heparin-induced thrombocytopenia (HIT), osteoporosis, and osteomalacia (in long-standing therapy). HIT is of two types:

Heparin-induced thrombocytopenia

- **HIT type I:** Benign form develops immediately and often resolves after heparin is discontinued and is probably due to direct platelet-aggregation induced by heparin.
- **HIT type II:** The heparin binds to platelet factor 4 (PF4) released from platelets and forms a complex (heparin/PF4 complex) in the circulation. The antibodies formed against these complexes activate platelets, promoting thrombosis even in the presence of marked thrombocytopenia. It develops 5–10 days after starting heparin therapy. Can occur with all types of heparin.

Treatment of HIT Type II

- Immediately stops all heparin administration.
- Start nonheparin anticoagulants, e.g., lepirudin—a recombinant hirudin, argatroban, danaparoid, fondaparinux and bivalirudin.
- Do not administer warfarin as it can produce gangrene of limb or necrosis of skin. Vitamin K is administered if HIT diagnosed after warfarin has already been started.
- Do not administer platelet transfusion even though there is severe thrombocytopenia.

Low-molecular weight heparins (LMWH)

- LMWH are biologically active forms of conventional heparin. The molecular weights ranging from 3,000 to 8,000 Daltons.
- **Mode of action:** They act as anticoagulant primarily by inhibiting activated factor X (Xa) rather than activated factor II (IIa).
- **Advantages:**
  - Can be administered subcutaneously once or twice/day.
  - Pharmacokinetics is predictable and aPTT monitoring is not needed.
  - Less immunogenic and less likely to produce thrombocytopenia.
  - Many patients with DVT (deep vein thrombosis) can be treated on an outpatient basis.
- **Disadvantage:** Higher cost.
- **Commonly available LMWH:** Enoxaparin, dalteparin and tinzaparin.

Warfarin

Q. Write short essay/note on oral anticoagulants.

- Water-soluble vitamin K antagonist.
- **Mode of action:** Vitamin K is necessary for the synthesis of coagulation factors such as prothrombin (factor II) and factors VII, IX and X and also protein C and protein S. Warfarin type anticoagulants prevents the conversion of vitamin K to its active hydroquinone form and interferes with the synthesis of the above vitamin K-dependent coagulation factors.
- **Monitoring:** Warfarin therapy is monitored using the **PT.**
- **Dose:**
  - Starting dose: Warfarin is started at a dose of 5 mg oral on the first day. Subsequent daily doses are adjusted according to PT (INR) which is maintained at 1.5–3 times the control value.
  - Maintenance dose: Varies from 2.5 to 7.5 mg/day.
- **Duration of therapy:** Variable and may range from 3 months to lifelong.
- **Side effects:** These include bleeding and rarely skin necrosis.
- **Antidotes of warfarin:** Injections of vitamin K_1, 5 mg intravenously or fresh frozen plasma or prothrombin complex concentrate.
- **Contraindications:**
  - Severe uncontrolled hypertension
  - Severe renal or liver failure
  - Pre-existing hemostatic disorders
  - Pregnancy: It crosses the placenta and can cause fetal abnormalities. Therefore, should not be used during pregnancy.

Reversing warfarin therapy (Table 8.80)

TABLE 8.80: Reversing warfarin therapy.

Indication	*Action*
INR <6	➢ Lower the dose, consider withholding one or more doses ➢ Recheck in 3–7 days
INR 6–10	➢ Lower the dose and withhold 1–3 doses ➢ Consider administering vitamin K, 1–2 mg orally ➢ Recheck INR in 24–48 hours
INR >10	➢ Withhold doses until INR in desired range and cause of elevation ascertained ➢ Give vitamin K, 2–4 mg orally ➢ Recheck INR in 24 hours
Serious bleeding and major overdose	➢ Consider fresh-frozen plasma or prothrombin complex concentrate and give 5–10 mg vitamin K intravenously

Direct thrombin inhibitors

- **Parenteral: Hirudin**
  - Source: Derived from a medicinal leach.
  - Recombinant form of hirudin, e.g., lepirudin, bivalirudin, and desirudin.
  - Mode of action: Acts directly on thrombin.
  - Monitoring: By measuring aPTT.

Clinical indications and use of direct thrombin inhibitors is presented in **Table 8.81**.

TABLE 8.81: Clinical indications and use of direct thrombin inhibitors.

Agent	*Clinical indication*	*aPTT*
Lepirudin	HIT	ACT
Bivalirudin	Angioplasty, PCI with HIT	aPTT
Argatroban	HIT HIT with PCI	ACT (activated) clotting time

Oral

Q. Discuss novel oral anticoagulants (NOACs).

- **Dabigatran** being used for prophylaxis after hip and knee replacement. The major side effect of dabigatran is hemorrhage.
- ***Idarucizumab:*** *Humanized monoclonal antibody fragment (Fab) indicated in patients treated with dabigatran when reversal of the anticoagulant effects is needed for emergency surgery or urgent procedures, or in the event of life-threatening or uncontrolled bleeding.*
- **Rivaroxaban** and **apixiban** are orally administered drug, factor Xa inhibitor available orally administered direct factor Xa inhibitor that produces its anticoagulant effect through reversible binding with the factor Xa molecule. Rivaroxaban can inhibit both free and thrombus associated factor Xa **(Table 8.82)**.

TABLE 8.82: Potential advantages and disadvantages of NOACs.

Potential advantages	*Potential disadvantages*
➢ Lower rates of intracranial bleed and hemorrhagic strokes than warfarin ➢ No need for routine laboratory monitoring ➢ Fewer drug or food interactions than warfarin	➢ Higher drug cost; may require prior insurance approval ➢ Lack of availability of a reversal agent ➢ Increased risk of gastrointestinal bleeding ➢ Higher rebound rate of VTE events in patients with poor adherence ➢ No clear efficacy data in certain patient populations (e.g., patients with malignancy)

Indirect factor Xa inhibitors

- These include fondaparinux and idraparinux.
- Mode of action: Increases the rate of inactivation of factor Xa by antithrombin, thereby blocking production of thrombin.
- Use: HIT-type II.

Fibrinolytic or Thrombolytic Agents

Q. Write short essay/note on fibrinolytic agents.

Q. Write short essay/note on thrombolytics.

- Goal of therapy: To produce rapid dissolution of thrombus and restore the blood flow.
- Most fibrinolytic or thrombolytic agents are recombinant forms having plasminogen activator activity.
- Mechanism of action: They convert the proenzyme, plasminogen to active enzyme plasmin. Plasmin then degrades the fibrin of thrombi and produces soluble fibrin degradation products.
- Currently approved fibrinolytic agents are:
  - Streptokinase (STK):
    - Source: It is obtained from β-hemolytic streptococci. It is not an enzyme and does not directly convert plasminogen to plasmin. Instead it forms a complex with plasminogen, it converts other/additional molecules of plasminogen into plasmin. Since it is obtained from bacteria, it can produce allergic reactions in about 5% of patients.
    - Uses: In acute ST-elevation myocardial infarction and pulmonary embolism.
  - Urokinase (UK): It is used in patients who received STK in the past 6 months and require a thrombolytic agent for MI or pulmonary embolism. It does not produce allergic reaction.
  - Acylated plasminogen streptokinase activator complex (APSAC)(anistreplase).
  - Recombinant tissue-type plasminogen activator (rtPA): Also known as alteplase or activase is useful in acute thrombotic strokes (within 3 hours of onset) besides acute MI and pulmonary embolism.
  - Prourokinase (pro-UK) like rtPA.
  - Others: Tenecteplase, desmoteplase and reteplase.
- Indications for use of fibrinolytic agents are listed in **Box 8.39**.

Box 8.39: Indication for use of fibrinolytic or thrombolytic agents.

- Acute myocardial infarction
- Massive pulmonary embolism with hypotension
- Acute ischemic stroke (thrombotic or embolic)
- Acute peripheral artery occlusion

Erythropoietin

Q. Write short essay/note on erythropoietin (EPO), recombinant human erythropoietin (rHuEPO) and darbepoietin alpha.

Q. List the ectopic sources of erythropoietin.

- **Site of production:** This hormone is predominantly produced by the juxtatubular interstitial cells of the renal cortex and to a lesser extent in the liver.
- **Stimulus:**
  - **Hypoxia** is the most potent stimulus for EPO production. In the presence of tissue (renal) hypoxia, kidneys respond by increased production of EPO.
  - **Anemia:** Erythropoietin levels are inversely related to hemoglobin concentrations in the blood. Anemia is another important stimulant.
- **Mode of action:**
  - EPO stimulates erythropoiesis by acting on the marrow erythroid progenitors to enhance their survival, proliferation and differentiation.
  - EPO may also protect neuronal cells from noxious stimuli.

  Ectopic sources of EPO are presented in **Table 8.83.**

TABLE 8.83: Ectopic sources of EPO.

Polycystic kidneys	Cerebellar hemangioblastoma	Uterine leiomyoma
Renal cell carcinoma	Hepatocellular carcinoma	Pheochromocytoma

Recombinant Human Erythropoietin (rHuEPO)

- It has same biological effects of endogenous erythropoietin and is available as erythropoietin-α and erythropoietin-β.
- **Indications:** In the treatment of:
  - Anemia associated with chronic renal failure.
  - Anemia of chronic inflammation.
  - Anemia (hemoglobin <10 g/dL) in cancer patients given chemotherapy.
  - Zidovudine-induced anemia in HIV patients.
  - Anemic patients undergoing nonvascular surgery to reduce the need for allogeneic blood transfusions.
- **Side effects:** Hypertension, bleeding, headache, arthralgia, nausea, edema, diarrhea, increased risk of thrombosis, pure red cell aplasia, and progression of cancers.

Darbepoietin Alpha

- Produced by recombinant DNA technology in Chinese hamster ovary cells.
- Half-life about 3 times rHuEPO and hence needs to be given less frequently.

- Side-effects similar to rHuEPO.
- Not approved for the treatment of zidovudine-induced anemia and for blood loss during perioperative period.

Hemopoietic Growth Factors

Q. Write short note on hematopoietic growth factors.

Erythropoietin

Refer above discussion.

Granulocyte Colony Stimulating Factor

- **Indications:**
  - **Primary prophylaxis**
    - To reduce chances of febrile neutropenia following chemotherapy: When the risk of febrile neutropenia is high (>20%) as determined by age, disease characteristics, and myelotoxicity of drugs used.
    - Accelerate hemopoietic recovery after chemotherapy and autologous hemopoietic cell transplantation.
  - **Secondary prophylaxis:** In patients with solid tumors with a previous history of the febrile neutropenia who require high-dose chemotherapy and any dose reduction may compromise treatment outcome.
  - **Patients with neutropenia and fever:** It may be administered to those patients with high risk of infection-related complications, prolonged (>10 days), and severe neutropenia (<100/μL), hypotension, multiorgan dysfunction, or invasive fungal infections. It is not recommended in afebrile patients with neutropenia.
  - **Mobilizing stem cells from bone marrow:** For stem cell transplantation. Both G-CSF and GM-CSF have been used.
- **Disadvantage:** Patients undergoing chemotherapy for breast carcinoma, if treated with G-CSF may develop acute myeloid leukemia or myelodysplastic syndrome. However, the benefit outweighs the possible risks.
- **Dosage:** 15 mg/kg daily by subcutaneous injection. Its pegylated form has a longer duration of action and requires to be given once a day.
- **Adverse effects:** Fever, bone, and joint pains.

Granulocyte-Macrophage Colony-stimulating Factor (GM-CSF)

- **Action:** Increase in neutrophil, eosinophil, macrophage, and sometimes lymphocyte counts.
- **Dosage:** Daily subcutaneous injection of 250 $\mu g/m^2$.
- Both G-CSF and GM-CSF have similar efficacy and indications (refer G-CSF above).

Thrombopoietin

- **Site of production:** Liver and kidney and marrow stromal cells.
- **Action:**
  - Stimulates the survival, proliferation, and differentiation of megakaryocytes and their precursors.
  - Primes mature platelets to aggregate in response to subthreshold levels of thrombin, collagen and ADP.
  - In cancer patients receiving chemotherapy, it has been shown to reduce the duration of postchemotherapy thrombocytopenia.
  - Thrombopoietin is undergoing clinical trials in patients with immune thrombocytopenic purpura.
- **Disadvantage:** Most patients produce antibodies against TPO and therefore, it is not recommended in treatment of any condition.

Vitamin K

Q. Write short note on vitamin K.

- Vitamin K is a fat-soluble vitamin and requires bile for its absorption.
- Vitamin K is required by liver for the production of factors II, VII, IX and X, protein C, and protein S.

Treatment: Shows a dramatic response to parenteral vitamin K therapy. Vitamin K may not be effective in the presence of liver cell disease.
Dose: Daily 10 mg of injections of vitamin K.

Causes of Vitamin K Deficiency

- **Inadequate stores:** As in hemorrhagic disease of the newborn (vitamin K levels are low and are due to lack of gut bacteria and low concentrations of the vitamin in breast milk) and severe malnutrition (especially when combined with antibiotic treatment).
- **Defective absorption:** Diseases that interfere with fat absorption, e.g., obstructive jaundice owing to the lack of intraluminal bile salts, pancreatic disease or small bowel disease.
- **Oral anticoagulant drugs** which are vitamin K antagonists (warfarin therapy).

Clinical manifestation: Deficiency manifests as bleeding/hemorrhagic state.

BONE MARROW EXAMINATION

Q. Write short note on indications for and complications of bone marrow aspiration.

Bone marrow examination is essentially done to confirm or rule out a hematologic disorder. It also helps in evaluation of nonhematological disorders (e.g., metastasis).

Bone marrow may be obtained by:

- **Aspiration:** Bone marrow aspiration is a simple, easy, and safe procedure
- **Trephine biopsy** is indicated in conditions where the aspiration either fails to yield marrow or to confirm some of the diseases (where biopsy findings are diagnostic).

Sites for bone marrow aspiration are listed in **Box 8.40**. Indications for bone marrow aspiration **(Table 8.84)**.

Contraindications for bone marrow aspiration: Hemophilia and congenital hemorrhagic disorders. Complications of bone marrow aspiration and biopsy are listed in **Box 8.41**.

Box 8.40: Sites for bone marrow aspiration.

Usual sites for bone marrow aspiration are:
- Sternum
- Posterior superior iliac spine
- Iliac crest
- Anterior superior iliac spine
- Spinous process of lumbar vertebra

In **infants**, upper end of the tibia is the ideal site for marrow aspirate

Box 8.41: Complications of bone marrow aspiration and biopsy.

- Local infection
- Hemorrhage
- Cardiac tamponade or mediastinitis

TABLE 8.84: Indications for bone marrow aspiration.

- ***Diagnostic***
  - **Primary hematolymphoid disorders**
    - **Red cell disorders:** Nutritional anemia (e.g., megaloblastic anemia), pure red cell aplasia
    - **White cell disorders:** Subleukemic/aleukemic leukemia, diagnosis and classification of acute leukemias
    - **Megakaryocytic disorders:** ITP and other thrombocytopenias
    - **Myeloproliferative neoplasms:** Polycythemia vera, chronic myeloid leukemia, idiopathic thrombocythemia
    - **Myelodysplastic syndromes**
    - **Plasma cell neoplasms:** Multiple myeloma, Waldenström macroglobulinemia
  - **Systemic diseases:** Storage disorders (e.g., Gaucher's, Niemann-Pick's disease)
  - **Staging of lymphoid malignancies and solid tumors:** Lymphoma, metastatic deposits (e.g., carcinoma prostate, breast, lung, kidney)
  - **Detection of infection and/or source of PUO**
    - **Parasitic disorders:** Kala-azar
    - **Fungal disorders:** Histoplasma
    - **Mycobacterial infection**
  - **Iron store**
  - **Miscellaneous disorders:** Pancytopenia or unexplained cytopenias
- ***Post-treatment follow-up:*** To know the response to therapy and follow up in cases of leukemia, aplastic anemia, and agranulocytosis
- ***Therapeutic:*** Bone marrow transplant

SPLEEN

The spleen is a hematopoietic organ capable of supporting elements of the erythroid, myeloid, megakaryocytic, lymphoid, and monocyte-macrophage (i.e., reticuloendothelial).

Splenomegaly

Q. Write short essay/note on splenomegaly.

Definition: The "gold-standard" definition of splenomegaly is splenic weight: The normal adult spleen weighs about 50–250 g. The weight can only be established at splenectomy or postmortem examination. The clinical finding of a palpable spleen was considered as splenic enlargement, but up to 16% of palpable spleens have been found to be of normal size on radiological assessment.

On ultrasound examination, "craniocaudal length" is commonly used to measure splenic size. This correlates with splenic volume. However, the upper limit of normal size varies from 11 to 14 cm.

Mechanisms of Splenomegaly

Many of the mechanisms represent exaggerated forms of normal function of spleen **(Table 8.85 and Box 8.42)**.

Box 8.42: Functions of spleen.

- Clearance of microorganisms and particulate antigens from the blood
- Synthesis of immunoglobulin and properdin factors
- Destruction of senescent or abnormal RBCs
- Embryonic hematopoiesis, which can be reactivated as extramedullary
- hematopoiesis in certain diseases (e.g., primary myelofibrosis)

TABLE 8.85: Mechanisms of splenomegaly.

Mechanism	*Examples*
Immune response work hypertrophy	Subacute bacterial endocarditis, infectious mononucleosis
RBC destruction work hypertrophy	Hereditary spherocytosis, thalassemia major
Congestive	Splenic vein thrombosis, portal hypertension
Myeloproliferative	Chronic myeloid metaplasia
Infiltrative	Sarcoidosis, some neoplasms
Neoplastic	Chronic lymphocytic leukemia, lymphomas
Miscellaneous	Trauma, cysts

Diseases Associated with Splenomegaly

Diseases associated with splenomegaly have been shown in **Table 8.86**.

TABLE 8.86: Diseases associated with splenomegaly.

Infection

- **Acute:** Infectious mononucleosis, viral hepatitis, septicemia, typhoid, cytomegalovirus, toxoplasmosis
- **Subacute/chronic:** Miliary tuberculosis, subacute bacterial endocarditis, brucellosis, syphilis, HIV
- **Tropical/parasitic:** Malaria, leishmaniasis/kala-azar, schistosomiasis

Hematological disorders

- **Myeloproliferative disorders:** Myelofibrosis, chronic myeloid leukemia (CML), polycythemia vera, essential thrombocytosis
- **Lymphoma:** NHL, HL
- **Leukemia:** Acute leukemia, chronic lymphocytic leukemia (CLL), hairy cell leukemia, prolymphocytic leukemia
- **RBC disorders**
  - **Congenital:** Hereditary spherocytosis, thalassemia, HbSC disease
  - **Others:** Autoimmune hemolysis, megaloblastic anemia
- **Congestive:** Cirrhosis, splenic/portal/hepatic vein thrombosis or obstruction, congestive cardiac failure

Inflammatory diseases

- **Collagen diseases:** Systemic lupus erythematosus, rheumatoid arthritis (Felty's)
- **Granulomatous:** Sarcoidosis
- **Neoplastic:** Hemangioma, metastasis (lung/breast carcinoma, melanoma)
- **Infiltrative:** Gaucher's disease, amyloidosis
- **Miscellaneous:** Cysts

Causes of Asymptomatic Splenomegaly

Causes of asymptomatic splenomegaly have been shown in **Table 8.87**.

TABLE 8.87: Causes of asymptomatic splenomegaly.

- Liver disease with portal hypertension
- Splenic vein thrombosis
- Agnogenic myeloid metaplasia
- Gaucher's disease
- Splenic cysts
- Sarcoidosis
- Amyloidosis
- Mild hereditary spherocytosis
- Early stages of polycythemia vera

Causes of Massively Enlarged Spleen (Table 8.88 and Fig. 8.50)

Causes of massively enlarged spleen have been shown in **Table 8.88**.

TABLE 8.88: Causes of massively enlarged spleen.

- Chronic myeloid leukemia
- Myelofibrosis (primary or secondary to polycythemia vera or essential thrombocytosis)
- Hyper-reactive malarial splenomegaly syndrome (tropical splenomegaly syndrome)
- Gaucher's disease
- Lymphoma (mantle cell lymphoma, marginal B cell lymphoma), hairy cell leukemia
- Kala-azar (visceral leishmaniasis)
- Beta thalassemia major
- AIDS with *Mycobacterium avium* complex
- Splenic cysts

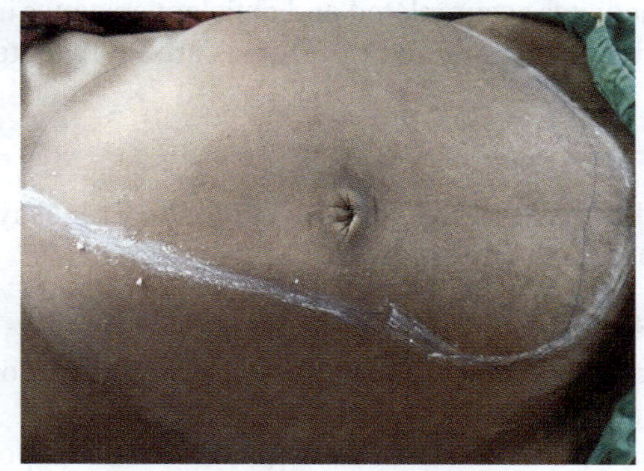

FIG. 8.50: Massively enlarged spleen.

Q. Write short essay/note on causes of massive splenomegaly.

A spleen is considered as massively enlarged when its lower pole is within the pelvis or which has crossed the midline into the right lower or right upper abdominal quadrants.

Indications for Splenectomy

Indications for splenectomy have been shown in **Box 8.43**.

Hypersplenism

Splenomegaly is often accompanied by hypersplenism. This is a complication of splenomegaly and not a diagnosis. The specific cause of the splenomegaly must be determined. Classical features of hypersplenism are listed in **Box 8.44**.

Causes of Splenic Rupture

Causes of splenic rupture have been shown in **Box 8.45**.

Box 8.43: Indications for splenectomy.

- **Hematological:** Isolated thrombocytopenia, immune thrombocytopenic purpura (ITP), hemolytic anemia, autoimmune hemolytic anemia, warm type (AIHA), hereditary spherocytosis, thalassemia major or intermedia, neutropenia, primary myelofibrosis
- Hairy cell leukemia, splenic marginal zone lymphoma, chronic lymphocytic leukemia
- Painfully enlarged spleen
- Traumatic or atraumatic splenic rupture, blunt abdominal trauma with splenic contusion or rupture
- Splenic artery aneurysm
- Hypersplenism
- Primary treatment of an isolated splenic vascular or parenchymal lesion
- Splenic abscess, acute splenic torsion with infarction due (e.g., "wandering spleen syndrome") splenic infarction
- Splenic vein thrombosis with bleeding esophageal varices
- Splenorenal shunting for portal hypertension

Box 8.44: Classical features of hypersplenism.

- Splenomegaly
- Any combination of anemia, leukopenia, and/or thrombocytopenia
- Compensatory bone marrow hyperplasia
- Improvement after splenectomy

Box 8.45: Causes of splenic rupture.

Traumatic splenic rupture: Blunt abdominal trauma

Atraumatic splenic rupture
- Neoplasm, e.g., leukemia, lymphoma
- Infection, e.g., infectious mononucleosis, CMV, HIV, endocarditis, malaria
- Inflammatory disease/noninfectious disorders, e.g., acute and chronic pancreatitis, primary amyloidosis
- Drug and treatment related, e.g., anticoagulation, G-CSF, thrombolytic therapy, dialysis
- Mechanical causes, e.g., pregnancy-related, congestive splenomegaly
- Idiopathic (normal spleen)

DISORDERS OF HEME SYNTHESIS: THE PORPHYRIAS

- The porphyrias are caused by deficiencies of enzymes involved in heme synthesis, which lead to blockade of the porphyrin pathway and subsequent accumulation of porphyrins and their precursors.
- **Cause:** Most of the porphyria is due to partial enzyme deficiencies. These enzyme deficiencies may be inherited as autosomal dominant, autosomal recessive, or X-linked traits, with the exception of porphyria cutanea tarda (PCT), which usually is sporadic.

Classification

Due to deficiency of an enzyme involved in the synthesis of heme, there is build-up of porphyrins and metabolites in various tissues. It is classified depending on site of overproduction and accumulation of porphyrin but overlapping features are common. It may be classified as follows:
- Depending on the major primary site of excess production and accumulation of their respective porphyrin precursors or porphyrins: (1) **Hepatic** (in the liver) or (2) **erythropoietic** (in the red cell).
- Based on the clinical manifestations **as acute or cutaneous.**

Structure of porphyrins: It consists of four pyrrole rings. Two molecules of δALA condense to form a pyrrole ring. Depending on the structure of the side chain, porphyrins can be divided into uroporphyrins, coproporphyrins, or protoporphyrins.

Intermediates accumulated and deficient enzymes in various porphyrias are depicted in **Figure 8.51**.

The three most common porphyrias are PCT, acute intermittent porphyria (AIP), and erythropoietic protoporphyria (EPP).

Clinical Features

Two broad patterns of symptoms occur in the various types of porphyria **(Table 8.89)**: (1) Cutaneous photosensitivity, and (2) acute neurovisceral syndrome.

Cutaneous Photosensitivity

- These are due to excess production and accumulation of porphyrins in the skin and occur predominantly on areas of the skin that are exposed to sunlight.
- Two main patterns of skin damage are seen in the porphyrias:
  1. Due to accumulation of water soluble uro- and coproporphyrins leads to blistering.
  2. Due to accumulation of the lipophilic protoporphyrins leads to burning sensations in the exposed skin.

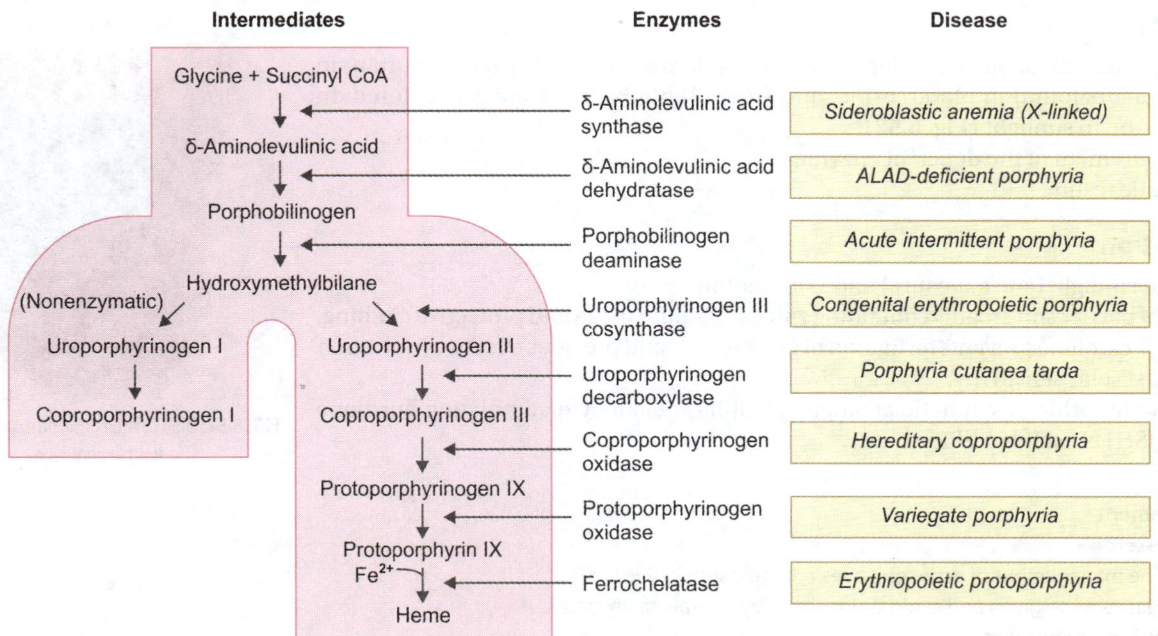

FIG. 8.51: Intermediates accumulated and deficient enzyme in various porphyrias.

TABLE 8.89: Major porphyrias and their laboratory findings.

Porphyria	Deficient enzyme	Principal symptoms	Elevated porphyrins and precursors		
			RBCs	Urine	Stool
Hepatic porphyrias					
5-ALA dehydratase-deficient porphyria (ADP)	ALA-dehydratase	Neurovisceral	Zn-Protoporphyrin	ALA, Coproporphyrin III	
Acute intermittent porphyria (AIP)	HMB (hydroxy methyl bilane)-synthase	Neurovisceral		ALA, PBG, Uroporphyrin	
Porphyria cutanea tarda (PCT)	Urodecarboxylase	Cutaneous photosensitivity		Uroporphyrin, 7-carboxylate porphyrin	Isocoproporphyrin
Hereditary coproporphyria (HCP)	Copro-oxidase	Neurovisceral and cutaneous photosensitivity		ALA, PBG, Coproporphyrin III	Coproporphyrin III
Variegate porphyria (VP)	Proto-oxidase	Neurovisceral and cutaneous photosensitivity			Coproporphyrin III Protoporphyrin
Erythropoietic porphyrias					
Congenital erythropoietic porphyria (CEP)	Urosynthase	Cutaneous photosensitivity	Uroporphyrin I Coproporphyrin I	Uroporphyrin Ib Coproporphyrin Ib	Coproporphyrin I
Erythropoietic protoporphyria (EPP)	Ferrochelatase	Cutaneous photosensitivity			
X-linked protoporphyria (XLP)	ALA-synthase 2	Cutaneous photosensitivity	Protoporphyrin	—	Protoporphyrin

- They produce pain, erythema, bullae, skin erosions, hirsutism and hyperpigmentation. Skin also becomes sensitive to damage from minimal trauma.

Acute Neurovisceral Syndrome

This presents with acute abdominal pain and features of autonomic dysfunction (e.g., tachycardia, hypertension, and constipation). Acute motor polyneuropathy may cause qaudriparesis mimicking GB syndrome. Neuropsychiatric manifestations include insomnia, anxiety, restlessness, agitation, hallucinations, hysteria, disorientation, delirium, apathy, depression, and phobias.

Triggering factors: Porphyria can relapse and remit or follow a prolonged and unremitting course. Sometimes, it may be triggered by alcohol, fasting, or drugs such as anticonvulsants, sulphonamides, estrogen, and progesterone.

Diagnosis

- Diagnosis and classification depends on the pattern of the porphyrins and porphyrin precursors found in blood, urine, and stool **(Table 8.89)**. Urine gets colored on exposure to sunlight **(Fig. 8.52)**.
- Measurement of the deficient enzymes.
- Genetic testing

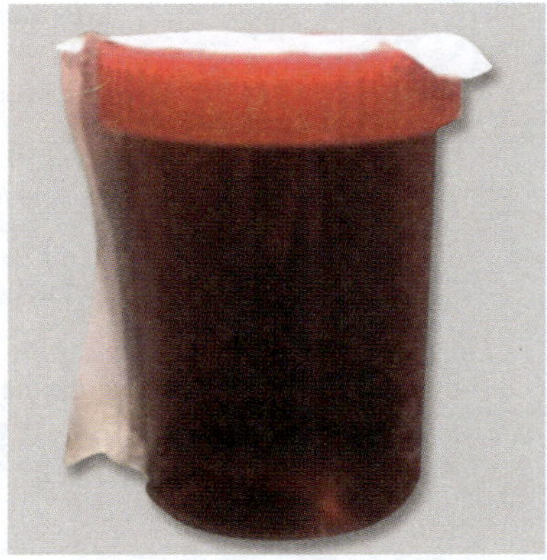

FIG. 8.52: High colored urine on exposure to sunlight in porphyria.

Prevention

- Avoid sunlight (sun exposure) and skin trauma.
- Use of barrier sun creams containing zinc or titanium oxide and protective clothing.
- Oral β-carotene prevents formation of free radicals and provides effective protection against solar sensitivity.
- **Afamelanotide**, a synthetic analogue of alpha-melanocyte-stimulating hormone (α-MSH) is useful in EPP.

Management

Neurovisceral

Acute: The management of acute episodes is largely supportive.

- Analgesics to be given and avoid drugs that may aggravate an attack.
- **Specific management:**
  - **Intravenous glucose** inhibits ALA synthase activity leading to reduced ALA synthesis. In some cases, it can terminate acute attacks.
  - **Intravenous heme** (in various forms such as human hematin or heme arginate) infusion reduces ALA and PBG excretion by having a negative effect on ALA synthase N activity. It relieves pain and accelerates recovery and decreases the duration of an attack and is useful in a severe attack.
  - Maintain calorie and fluid intake.
  - Cyclical acute attacks in females may respond to suppression of the menstrual cycle using gonadotropin-releasing hormone analogs.

Cutaneous Photosensitivity Episodes

Acute attack

- Treated symptomatically.
- Venesection (reduces urinary porphyria) can be used for PCT in both acute and remission phases. A prolonged course of low-dose chloroquine is effective as it helps in excretion by forming a water-soluble complex with uroporphyrins.
- Liver transplantation may be useful for severe cases.

Pseudoporphyria

- In certain settings, patient develops blistering and skin fragility identical to PCT with the histological features but with normal urine and serum porphyrins. Hypertrichosis, dyspigmentation, and cutaneous sclerosis do not occur. This condition is called pseudoporphyria.
- Most commonly due to medications especially NSAIDs, usually naproxen other NSAIDs and tetracycline can cause similar picture.
- Some patients on hemodialysis develop a similar PCT-like picture.

CHAPTER

9

Rheumatology and Connective Tissue Disorders

INTRODUCTION

Q. Develop a systematic clinical approach to joint pain based on pathophysiology.

Q. Prioritize based on clinical features for arriving at an etiological diagnosis in polyarthritis.

Clinical approach to polyarthritis is important and the diagnosis is often challenging due to the extensive differential diagnosis. Thorough history and physical examination is the cornerstone for diagnosis. The clinical factors helpful in narrowing the diagnosis are the ***chronology of symptoms, features of inflammation, joint distribution, extra-articular manifestations, disease course*** and ***patient demographics***.

- **Chronology**
  - Acute polyarthritis may be due to a self-limited disease.
  - It could be due to infectious, crystal induced or reactive causes.
  - Rarely chronic polyarticular arthritides, like rheumatoid arthritis (RA), systemic lupus erythematosus (SLE) can have acute presentation in the early course of illness.
  - Chronic arthritis may be due to immunologic arthritides like RA, noninflammatory and nonarticular causes.
- **Inflammation**
  - Features of inflammation make it inflammatory arthritis and in the absence it is called athralgia.
  - Erythema, warmth, pain and swelling are the cardinal features of inflammation. Fatigue, fever and weight loss can also be present.
  - Morning stiffness lasting for longer than an hour is another clue.
  - Palpate the joint capsule for synovial thickening, soft tissue swelling effusions.
  - Presence of crepitus indicates underlying injury, osteoarthritis (OA) or previous inflammation. Heberden's and Bouchard's nodes indicate osteoarthritis.
  - Subjective sense of swelling without objective sign of synovitis is seen in patients with fibromyalgia.

Q. Determine the potential causes of joint pain based on the presenting features of joint involvement.

- **Joint distribution**
  - Crystal and infectios arthritides are often mono or oligoarticular whereas OA and RA are polyarticular.
  - Joint involvement in RA tends to be symmetrical and polyarticular whereas spondyloarthropathy, gout and reactive arthritis involvement is asymmetric and oligoarticular.
  - Psoriatic arthritis and OA can be either mono or polyarticular and symmetric or asymmetric.
  - Upper extremities are commonly affected in RA and OA, whereas lower extremities are affected commonly in reactive arthritis, spondyloarthropathies and gout.
  - Axial skeleton is involved in ankylosing spondylitis (Sp A) and OA. Osteoarthritis usually spares wrist, elbow and ankle unless there is a past history of trauma.
  - Osteoarthritis involves distal interphalangeal (DIP) and proximal interphalangeal (PIP) joints with sparing of metacarpophalangeal joints. Rheumatoid arthritis spares DIP but affects PIP and metacarpophalangeal (MCP) joints. Psoriasis and crystal arthropathies affect all three joints.
- **Extra-articular manifestations**
  - SLE can present with malar rash and oral ulcers.
  - Psoriatic skin and nail changes accompany psoriatic arthritis.

- Polymyositis is suggested by proximal muscle weakness.
- Reactive arthritis is suggested by a history of recent gastrointestinal or genitourinary infection, conjunctivitis and oral ulcers.
- Spondyloarthropathies can present with enthesitis or dactylitis causing sausage-shaped digits.

- **Disease course**
  - Intermittent arthritis is a feature of crystal arthropathies, Lyme arthritis and palindromic rheumatism that may progress to rheumatoid arthritis later.
  - Migratory arthritis can be a feature of rheumatic fever, bacterial endocarditis, gonococcal infection and viral fever.
- **Patient demographics**
  - Incidence of RA, SLE, fibromyalgia are more among premenopausal women compared to men of same age group.
  - Spondyloarthropathies occur equally in males and females.
  - Gout usually occurs 20 years after puberty in men and 20 years after menopause in women. Rare among premenopausal women unless associated with renal failure.
  - RA, SLE, reactive arthritis and sponyloarthropathies occur more among younger individuals whereas OA, polymyalgia rheumatic and giant cell arthritis occur more among elderly.
  - Family history is important in spondyloarthropathies, rheumatoid arthritis and Heberden's nodes of osteoarthritis.

Table 9.1 discusses the classification of arthritis with examples.

TABLE 9.1: Classification of arthritis with examples.

	Musculoskeletal Complaint				
	Distribution				
	Polyarthritis (≥ 4 joints)		***Monoarthrltis /Oligoarthritis (1-3 joints)***		***Nonarticular***
	Acute	***Chronic***	***Acute***	***Chronic***	
Non-inflammatory	➢ Hemoglobinopathies ➢ Amyloid arthropathies	➢ Osteoarthritis	➢ Meniscal tear ➢ Osteoarthritis flare ➢ Reflex sympathetic dystrophy	➢ Osteoarthritis ➢ Osteonecrosis ➢ Neuropathic arthritis ➢ Hemochromatosis ➢ Pigmented villonodular synovitis	➢ Trauma ➢ Fracture ➢ Fibromyalgia ➢ Reflex sympathetic dystrophy
Inflammatory	➢ Viral arthritis ➢ Serum sickness ➢ Drug induced arthritis ➢ Early onset connective tissue disease (CTD) ➢ Rheumatic fever ➢ Palindromic rheumatism ➢ Remitting seronegative symmetrical synovitis with pitting edema (RS3PE)	➢ Rheumatoid arthritis ➢ Undifferentiated polyarthritis ➢ Inflammatory osteoarthritis ➢ Mixed connective tissue disease ➢ Lupus, scleroderma ➢ Polyarticular juvenile idiopathic arthritis (JIA) ➢ Adult Still's disease	➢ Infectious arthritis ➢ Gout ➢ Pseudogout ➢ Reactive arthritis ➢ Chlamydial arthritis	➢ Psoriatic arthritis ➢ Spondyloarthropathies ➢ Pauciarticular JIA ➢ Indolent infectious arthritis	➢ Bursitis ➢ Tendinitis ➢ Polymyalgia rheumatica

Differences between inflammatory versus noninflammatory arthritis is presented in **Table 9.2**.

TABLE 9.2: Inflammatory versus noninflammatory arthritis.

Features	***Inflammatory (rheumatoid arthritis)***	***Noninflammatory (osteoarthritis)***
➢ Age of onset	➢ Usually 20 to 40 years but may begin at any age	➢ Most commonly over 50 years of age
➢ Speed of onset	➢ Rapid over weeks to months	➢ Slow; over years
➢ Systemic symptoms	➢ Fatigue, low-grade fever, anorexia. Extra-articular manifestations: rheumatoid nodules, Sjögren's syndrome, Felty syndrome	➢ No systemic symptoms
➢ Joint affection	➢ Symmetrical	➢ Asymmetrical
➢ Joint symptoms	➢ Painful, swollen stiff joints and muscle aches	➢ Joints painful without swelling
➢ Joints involved	➢ Primarily affects small joints [metacarpophalangeal (MCP) and proximal interphalangeal (PIP)]	➢ Affects large weight-bearing joints (hip, knee or the spine). Affects proximal interphalangeal (PIP) and distal interphalangeal (DIP) joints
➢ Stiffness	➢ Morning stiffness for >1 hour. Stiffness occurs after periods of rest/inactivity (the so-called 'gel phenomenon')	➢ Morning stiffness for <30 minutes. Stiffness is generally mild and occurs after periods of activity
➢ Relation of movement with pain	➢ Movement or mild to moderate activity decreases pain	➢ Movement increases the pain (worsens with activity) and improves with rest
➢ Examination of joint	➢ Swollen, red, warm, tender and painful	➢ Swollen, cool and hard on palpation. When severely inflamed (as in acute gout or septic arthritis), can have erythema of the overlying skin
➢ Radiological findings	➢ Bony erosion, soft tissue swelling, angular deformities, periarticular osteopenia	➢ Loss of joint space and articular cartilage, routine wear and tear, osteophytes

Contd...

Contd...

➢ Laboratory findings		
Rheumatoid factor (RF), antinuclear antibody	➢ Positive	➢ Negative
Erythrocyte sedimentation rate (ESR) and C-reactive protein (CRP)	➢ Both are often raised	➢ Usually normal but transient elevation of ESR may occur due to synovitis
White blood cell (WBC) count in the synovial fluid	➢ WBC count is >2000/mm³ in septic arthritis and not in rheumatoid arthritis	➢ – <2000/mm³

Q. Describe the appropriate diagnostic work up based on the etiology.

Rheumatological diagnostic tests should be interpreted in the appropriate clinical context **(Table 9.3)**.

- A complete blood count, urine analysis, renal and liver functions test may provide dignostic clues.
- ANA can be positive in 5–10% of general population and may increase with age. Due to the high sensitivity a negative result rules out systemic lupus erythematosus but due to lack of specificity, positive result should be analyzed with caution.
- HLA-B27 positivity with a positive family history is highly suggestive of ankylosing spondylitis. However, relying only on HLA-B27 reports may lead to overdiagnosis as it can be seen in 8% of caucasians.
- Rheumatoid factor lacks sensitivity and specificity; hence both positive and negative results should be interpreted cautiously. Not useful if the patient lacks other criteria for diagnosis.
- Synovial fluid analysis helpful in diagnosing septic and crystal induced arthritis (*Refer* **Table 9.9**).
- Dignostic imaging is helpful in rheumatological disorders.

TABLE 9.3: Diagnostic investigations in rheumatic diseases.

Investigations	***Disease conditions***
Complete blood count	Inflammatory arthritides
Anemia	SLE, RA, IBD, human parvovirus infection B19 infection
Thrombocytopenia	SLE, parvovirus B19 infection
Thrombocytosis	Acute phase reactants, vasculitis, infection
Leukopenia	SLE, RA, Felty's syndrome, Sjögren's syndrome, human parvovirus B19 infection
Leucocytosis	RA, vasculitis, reactive arthritis, infection
Eosinophilia	SLE, RA, IBD, sarcoidosis, dermatomyositis, scleroderma, Churg-Strauss syndrome, PAN, eosinophilic fasciitis, cholesterol emboli
Chest radiograph	
Infiltrates or nodules	RA, sarcoidosis, Wegener's granulomatosis, Churg-Strauss syndrome
Serositis	SLE, RA
Upper lobe fibrosis	Ankylosing spondylitis
Diffuse fibrosis	RA, scleroderma, polymyositis
Rheumatoid factor	Healthy persons; RA, SLE, Sjögren's syndrome, sarcoidosis, reactive arthritis, PMR, polymyositis, psoriatic arthritis, endocarditis, chronic infections, cancer, chronic liver disease, nonrheumatic causes
Joint aspiration	
Culture	Infection
Crystals	Gout, pseudogout
White blood cell count	Inflammation: >2,000 per mm³ Probable infection: >50,000 per mm³
Inflammatory markers Elevated erythrocyte sedimentation rate or C-reactive protein	Infection, most inflammatory arthritides, advanced age, PMR, giant cell arteritis, cancer, anemia, pregnancy
Antinuclear antibody	Healthy persons; SLE, RA, scleroderma, Sjögren's syndrome, vasculitis, polymyositis, medications, many nonrheumatic causes
Hepatic transaminase Elevated aspartate transaminase or alanine transaminase	SLE, PAN, sarcoidosis, hemochromatosis, Sjögren's syndrome, infectious hepatitis, polymyositis
Urinalysis Hematuria	SLE, Wegener's granulomatosis, PAN
Proteinuria	SLE, Wegener's granulomatosis, amyloidosis
Elevated alkaline phosphatase	Bone metastases, Paget's disease, osteomalacia, PMR, ankylosing spondylitis, hyperparathyroidism
Electrocardiogram AV block	Lyme disease, neonatal lupus, ankylosing spondylitis

Contd...

Contd...

Anti-double stranded DNA antibody	SLE, especially lupus nephritis
Anti–SS-A (anti-Ro) and anti–SS-B (anti-La) Antibodies	Sjögren's syndrome, SLE; healthy persons
HLA-B27	Healthy persons; spondyloarthropathies, reactive arthritis
Elevated uric acid	Gout, psoriatic arthritis, Paget's disease; healthy persons
False-positive VDRL	SLE, anticardiolipin antibody syndrome
Cytoplasmic antineutrophil cytoplasmic autoantibody(c-ANCA)	Wegener's granulomatosis
Elevated creatinine	SLE, Wegener's granulomatosis, vasculitis
Elevated creatine kinase	Polymyositis, dermatomyositis, hypothyroidism
Elevated calcium	Hyperparathyroidism, cancer, sarcoidosis

Rheumatoid Factor (RF)

Q. Write short note on rheumatoid factor and mention its significance.

Rheumatoid factor is an autoantibody (IgM, IgG and IgA) directed against the Fc fragment of human immunoglobulin G (IgG).

Significance

- RF has poor specificity and is positive in 70 to 80% of patients with rheumatoid arthritis (RA). It is appropriate and helpful only in patients suspected of having RA. It is not helpful in cases of low clinical suspicion.
- **High RF** titers are observed **with more severe disease** and **extra-articular disease**. The titers generally correlate with severity of disease. However, RF titers are not useful in assessing disease progression.
- It can **also be positive in many other conditions (Table 9.4)**.
- 10–30% of patients with long-standing RA are seronegative.

TABLE 9.4: Conditions associated with a positive rheumatoid factor.

Autoimmune rheumatic diseases (percentage)	*Other conditions*
➢ Rheumatoid arthritis (RA) with nodules and extra-articular manifestations (100)	➢ **Chronic infections:** Infective endocarditis, tuberculosis, leprosy, syphilis
➢ Rheumatoid arthritis (overall 70)	➢ **Viral infections:** Hepatitis, infectious mononucleosis
➢ Sjögren's syndrome (75–95)	
➢ Systemic lupus erythematosus (SLE) (15–35)	➢ **Hyperglobulinemia:** Chronic liver disease, sarcoidosis
➢ Systemic sclerosis (20–30)	
➢ Mixed essential cryoglobulinemia (40-100)	➢ Interstitial lung disease, silicosis, asbestosis
➢ Polymyositis/dermatomyositis (5–10)	➢ Primary biliary cholangitis
➢ Polyarteritis nodosa (PAN)	➢ **Normal population**
➢ ANCA associated vasculitis	- Age >65 years
➢ Juvenile idiopathic arthritis	- Relatives of people with RA
➢ Mixed connective tissue disease (50–60)	➢ B-cell neoplasms

Anticyclic Citrullinated Peptide Antibodies (Anti-CCPs, ACPA)

Q. Enumerate the significance and indications for anticitrullinated peptide antibody (Anti-CCP).

Citrullinated Peptide Antigens

- These include fibrinogen, type II collagen, alpha enolase and vimentin.
- CCPs are derived from proteins in which arginine residues are converted to citrulline residues by an enzyme peptidyl arginine (which is abundant in inflamed synovium and in a variety of mucosal structures) during a variety of biological processes.

Anticyclic Citrullinated Peptide Antibodies (ACPA)

- These antibodies are **useful for diagnosis of RF** and may be involved in tissue injury. Many patients (about 70%) of RF have antibodies against cyclic citrullinated peptides (CCPs).
- These antibodies have **much high specificity** (93–98%) but **less sensitive** (60%) for diagnosis of RA.
- Anti-CCPs may be **detected even in asymptomatic patients** several years before the development of RA and are **associated with severe disease**. Thus, anti-CCP positive patients may require an aggressive treatment.
- Antibodies against CCPs (anti-CCPs) from immune complexes and deposit in various tissues mainly being the joints.
- Positive results can occur in several autoimmune rheumatic diseases (SLE, Sjogren), tuberculosis, hepatis C infection, and chronic lung diseases.
- Antibodies to mutated citrullinated vimentin (**anti-MCV**) is associated with more severe disease than anti-CCP antibodies.
- Serum **14-3-3ε**, which is an intracellular chaperonin protein, has been used diagnostically in RA.

Autoantibodies in Various Connective Tissue Diseases (CTD) (Table 9.5)

Q. Enlist the various antibodies seen in patients with connective tissue diseases and mention its significance.

TABLE 9.5: Autoantibodies in various connective tissue diseases.

Autoantibodies	***Importance***
Rheumatoid factor	*Refer* Table 9.4
Anticyclic citrullinated peptide	*Refer* above
Antinuclear antibodies (ANA)	*Refer* Table 9.6
Anti-double-stranded DNA (anti-dsDNA)	➢ **Highly specific for SLE**, positive in about 60% cases, positivity correlates with lupus nephritis ➢ Low titers are seen in Sjögren's syndrome, RA (rheumatoid arthritis) ➢ Levels often correlate with disease activity ➢ Usually absent in drug-induced SLE
Antihistone	➢ Sensitive for **drug-induced lupus** but not specific ➢ Useful in patients with a positive ANA ➢ Specific for SLE but positive in only 20–30% of cases
Anti-Smith (anti-Sm)	➢ Positive in 20–30% cases of SLE. **Highly specific** for SLE
Anti-U1 ribonucleoproteins (RNP)	➢ High titers in syndromes with features of polymyositits, lupus, scleroderma and mixed CTD (connective tissue disease)
Anti-Ro (anti-SS-A)	➢ Positive in **Sjögren's syndrome** with extraglandular features ➢ Positive in 40% cases of SLE and is associated with photosensitive rash and pulmonary disease. May be positive in ANA-negative lupus. Indicates higher risk of lupus nephritis ➢ May be positive in neonatal lupus or congenital heart block due to maternal antibodies
Anti-La (anti-SS-B)	➢ Present in 10–15% cases of SLE and indicates low-risk of nephritis ➢ Associated with Sjögren's syndrome
Antiphospholipid	➢ Diagnosis of APLAs. Present in nearly 50% cases of SLE ➢ Three types: Lupus anticoagulant (LA), anticardiolipin (aCL) and anti-β_2-glycoprotein-I (anti-β2-GPI) antibody
Anticentromere	➢ Systemic sclerosis (20–35% cases) ➢ CREST syndrome (calcinosis, Raynaud's phenomenon, esophageal dysfunction, sclerodactyly and telangiectasia) ➢ Primary biliary cirrhosis
Antitopoisomerase I (anti-scl-70)	➢ Highly specific for systemic sclerosis, found in 20–40% cases of systemic sclerosis and associated with diffuse cutaneous, pulmonary and cardiac involvements
Anti-jo1	➢ Present in 30% cases with polymyositis or dermatomyositis ➢ Associated with Raynaud's phenomenon
Antineutrophil cytoplasmic antibodies (ANCA)	Refer below

Antinuclear Antibodies

Q. Enumerate the indications, significance and staining patterns of antinuclear antibodies.

Antinuclear antibodies (ANA) are **directed against one or more components of the cell nucleus**. The component of the nucleus includes DNA, RNA, proteins as well as complexes of proteins with nucleic acid.

TABLE 9.6: Conditions associated with a positive ANA test.

Diseases where ANA is useful in diagnosis	***Diseases where ANA is not useful in diagnosis***
➢ Systemic lupus erythematosus (95–100%) ➢ Systemic sclerosis (60–80%) ➢ Sjögren's syndrome (40–80%) ➢ Drug-induced lupus (>95%) ➢ Mixed connective tissue disease (100%) ➢ Polymyositis/dermatomyositis (30–80%) ➢ Autoimmune hepatitis (100%)	➢ Rheumatoid arthritis (30–50%) ➢ Autoimmune thyroid disease (30–50%) ➢ Malignancy varies widely ➢ Infectious diseases varies widely

Note: About 5% of healthy individuals have an ANA titer >1:80.

Significance

- **High titers** of ANA (>1:160) are of **more diagnostic** significance than low titers.
- Circulating **levels of ANA do not correlate with severity or activity** of the disease.
- ANA is **positive in several conditions (Table 9.6)**.
- ANA is used as a **screening test for systemic lupus erythematosus (SLE) and systemic sclerosis (SSc).** ANA has high sensitivity for SLE (100%) but low specificity (10–40%). A negative ANA almost rules out SLE but a positive result does not confirm it. It should not be used to monitor the course of SLE or other diseases.

Tests for detection: ANAs are detected by indirect immunofluorescent staining **(Table 9.7)** of fresh-frozen sections of rat liver or kidney or Hep-2 cell lines (a line of human epithelial cells).

TABLE 9.7: Pattern of antinuclear antibody staining.

Pattern of staining	***Diagrammatic appearance***	***Staining pattern due to***	***Associated conditions***
Homogeneous or diffuse staining of the entire nucleus with or without apparent masking of the nucleoli		Antibodies to nucleosomes (anti-DNP), histones (anti-histone) and occasionally double-stranded DNA (anti-dsDNA)	Rheumatoid arthritis, systemic lupus erythematosus (SLE) and miscellaneous disorders (anti-ssDNA)

Contd...

Contd...

Rim or peripheral staining		Antibodies to double-stranded DNA (anti-DNA) and sometimes to nuclear envelope proteins. Not seen on HEp-2	SLE
Speckled (may be coarse or fine) pattern—the presence of uniform or variable-sized speckles throughout the nucleus. Most common pattern and is least specific		Antibodies to non-DNA nuclear constituents such as Sm antigen (anti-Sm), ribonucleoprotein (anti-RNP), and SS-A (anti-SS-A) and SS-B reactive antigens (anti-SS-B)	SLE, systemic sclerosis (SS), polymyositis (PM)/ dermatomyositis (DM)
Nucleolar pattern—presence of a few discrete spots within the nucleus-stains nucleoli within the nucleus, sharply separated from the unstained nucleoplasm		Antibodies to RNA (anti-nucleolar)	Most often seen in systemic sclerosis
Centromeric pattern—discrete uniform speckles throughout the nucleus. The number of speckles corresponds to a multiple of the normal chromosome number		Antibodies specific for centromeres (anti-centromere)	Systemic sclerosis, Sjögren syndrome, and other diseases

(ds: double stranded; ss: single stranded)

Extractable Nuclear Antibodies

Q. Write short essay/note on extractable nuclear antibodies.

- These are antibodies to extractable nuclear antigens (ENA) and are directed against small ribonuclear proteins (RNA).
- **Types of antibodies and associated conditions are listed in Table 9.8.**
- Their sensitivity and specificity are poor. Though used for diagnostic confirmation, they do not exclude a specific CTD.
- They do not correlate with disease activity and may be found in patients without active disease.

TABLE 9.8: Types of antibodies and associated conditions.

Type of extractable nuclear antibody	*Associated conditions*
➢ Anti-Sm	➢ Only in SLE and represent a serologic marker in disease classification. They are associated with renal involvement
➢ Antiuracil-rich 1 ribonucleoprotein (U1RNP)	➢ SLE and in mixed connective tissue disease
➢ Anti-SS-A/Ro and anti-SS-B/La	➢ SLE and in Sjögren's syndrome
➢ Anti-tRNA synthetases	➢ Polymyositis/dermatomyositis
➢ Antitopoisomerase-1 antibodies (Scl-70)	➢ Diffuse systemic sclerosis
➢ Anticentromere antibodies	➢ Limited systemic sclerosis

Antineutrophil Cytoplasmic Antibodies

Q. Write short essay/note on antineutrophil cytoplasmic antibodies (ANCA), their significance/ANCA associated disorders.

Antineutrophil cytoplasmic antibodies (ANCAs) are heterogeneous group of IgG **autoantibodies directed against certain proteins** (mainly enzymes) **in the cytoplasmic granules of neutrophils and** lysosomes of **monocytes.**

Patterns: On the basis of the target antigens and pattern of immunofluorescence staining, two common patterns of ANCA have been distinguished.

1. **Anti-proteinase-3 (PR3-ANCA):** It is also called cytoplasmic or cANCA. PR3 is a constituent of neutrophil azurophilic granule. It shares homology with many microbial peptides and antibodies against microbial peptides. Antibodies against proteinase-3 (PR3) form PR3-ANCAs. They produce cytoplasmic fluorescence (**cANCA**). They are associated with **Wegener's granulomatosis.**
2. **Anti-myeloperoxidase (MPO-ANCA):** It is also called perinuclear or pANCA. MPO is a lysosomal enzyme normally involved in producing oxygen-free radicals. Antibodies to myeloperoxidase (MPO) forms MPO-ANCAs which produces perinuclear fluorescence (**pANCA**). It can be induced by drugs (e.g. propylthiouracil). They are associated with **microscopic polyangiitis and Churg-Strauss syndrome**.

Significance

- ANCA are **strongly associated with small-vessel vasculitis** and are useful in the diagnosis and monitoring of systemic vasculitis. For their significance in vasculitis, ANCA should be assayed both with indirect immunofluroscence (screening test) and direct ELISA for proteinase-3 or myeloperoxidase.

- **ANCA are not specific for vasculitis.** They may be positive in autoimmune liver disease, malignancy, infection [bacterial and human immunodeficiency virus (HIV)], inflammatory bowel disease, chronic hepatitis, primary sclerosing cholangitis, Felty's syndrome, rheumatoid arthritis, SLE and pulmonary fibrosis.

Synovial Fluid in Disease States (Table 9.9)

Q. Differentiate the synovial fluid features in various arthritis.

Q. Enumerate the indications for arthrocentesis.

- Arthrocentesis helps in the diagnosis of septic/infective arthritis and crystal arthropathies and the indications are as below.
  - Monoarthritis (acute or chronic)
  - Monoarthritis in a patient with chronic polyarthritis
  - Suspicion of joint infection
  - Crystal-induced arthritis
  - Hemarthrosis or trauma with joint effusion.
- Hemorrrhagic effusion may suggest trauma or mechanical derangement, coagulopathy or others.
- Counts less than 2,000 per mm³ may suggest noninflammatory causes like osteoarthritis or trauma.
- WBC count of at least 2,000 per mm³ in synovial fluid suggests inflammation, whereas a count higher than 50,000 per mm³ indicates infection. In later cases, synovial fluid needs to be cultured for ruling out infection.
- Crystal identification by polarized microscopy useful for diagnosis of gout and pseudogout.

TABLE 9.9: Features of synovial fluid in various disease states.

	Normal	*Noninflammatory*	*Inflammatory*	*Pyogenic*
Appearance	Clear	Clear	Cloudy, yellow	Turbid
Viscosity	High	High	Low	Variable, infection usually low
Mucus clot	Good	Good	Poor	Poor
Total WBC/mm³	<200	200–5000	5000–50,000	>50,000
Predominant cell	Monocytes	Monocytes	Polymorphs >60%	Polymorphs >80%. Bacteria present
Protein	<2–3 g/dL	<2–3 g/dL	>3 g/dL	>3 g/dL
Sugar	Equal to blood sugar (BS) taken simultaneously	Equal to blood sugar (BS)	25–50% less than blood sugar	>50% less than blood sugar

Q Describe the role of diagnostic imaging in rheumatological disorders.

Currently available modalities include conventional radiography, computed tomography (CT), magnetic resonance imaging (MRI), arthrography, nuclear medicine scans (bone scintigraphy), and ultrasound.

- **Conventional radiography**
  - Presence of sacroiliitis indicates ankylosing spondylitis.
  - Periarticular osteopenia with erosions, narrowing of the joint space and juxta-articular osteoporosis suggestive of rheumatoid arthritis.
  - "Pencil-in-cup" deformities are suggestive of psoriatic arthritis.
  - Chest radiographs may reveal underlying systemic disease. Radiographs showing infiltrates or nodules are suggestive of rheumatoid arthritis, sarcoidosis, Wegener's granulomatosis or microscopic polyangitis. Serositis on radiograph suggests RA or SLE. Ankylosing spondylitis may present with upper lobe fibrosis whereas RA, scleroderma and polymyositis may present with diffuse fibrosis.
- **Magnetic resonance imaging** is sensitive for diagnosing soft tissue injuries. MRI done in the early course of RA may reveal cartilage destruction that may not be picked up in routine radiographs. MRI can also be used to demonstrate tophi, synovial changes and erosions.
- **Ultrasound** is useful in the detection of soft tissue abnormalities such as tendinitis, tenosynovitis, bursitis, enthesitis and entrapment neuropathies.
- **CT** is useful in the diagnosis of low back pain syndromes. Also HRCT lung can help diagnosis of ILD.
- **Nuclear medicine scans** have great sensitivity for detecting many disease processes because they image and quantify physiologic biochemical processes, as well as provide anatomic information. The combination with single photon emission computer tomography (SPECT) increases anatomical resolution. Whole-body bone scintigraphy might also help differentiate inflammatory spondyloarthropathies from other inflammatory disorders such as SAPHO (synovitis, acne, pustulosis, hyperostosis, osteitis).

RHEUMATOID ARTHRITIS

Q. Discuss the etiology, pathogenesis, clinical manifestations, diagnosis, investigations, complication, and management of rheumatoid arthritis.

Rheumatoid arthritis (RA) is the most common form of chronic inflammatory, potentially crippling arthritis with multisystem involvement affecting approximately 1% of the adult population.

Etiology

The cause is multifactorial and genetic, epigenetic and environmental factors play a part in the pathogenesis of RA.

- **Genetic factors:** Genetic susceptibility is a **major factor** in the pathogenesis of rheumatoid arthritis.
  - **HLA genes:** RA is linked to specific **HLA-DRB1 locus**.
  - **Non-HLA genes:** Polymorphism in *PTPN22* gene, which encodes a tyrosine phosphatase.
  - Abnormal DNA methylation, histone modifications, and microRNA regulation play a key role.
- **Environmental arthritogenic agents:** They are thought to **initiate the disease** process. **Smoking** and several **microbial agents** (e.g. virus, mycobacteria porphyromonas gingivalis, and *Mycoplasma)* have been suggested but not proved.
- **Autoimmunity:** The initial inflammatory synovitis, an autoimmune reaction with T cells is responsible for the chronic destructive nature of rheumatoid arthritis.

Pathogenesis

The rheumatoid synovium (**Pannus**) behaves like a locally-invasive tumor. A cascade network of cytokines like granulocyte macrophage colony-stimulating factor (GM-CSF), interleukin (IL)-2, IL-15, IL-13, IL-17, IL-18, interferon-gamma (IFN-gamma), tumor necrosis factor (TNF) and transforming growth factor-beta (TGF-beta) are involved in the disease progression. B cells, CD4+ T cells, compliment mediated immune activation play a contributory role.

Clinical Features

Q. Enumerate the clinical features of rheumatoid arthritis.

- **Gender:** Female to male ratio is 3:1.
- **Age:** Most common age of onset is between 30 and 50 years, but the disease can occur at any age. In women in late childbearing years and in men during sixth to eighth decade.

Onset

The presenting symptoms result from inflammation of the joints, tendons, and bursae. The onset varies:

- **Slow and insidious in onset:** Presents with malaise, fatigue, anorexia, weakness and generalized musculoskeletal pain.
- **Acute onset:** Sometimes RA may be very acute in onset, with morning stiffness, polyarthritis and pitting edema. This type occurs more commonly in old age.
- **Palindromic onset:** Occasionally, patient present with relapsing and remitting episodes of pain, stiffness and swelling that last for only a few hours or days alternating with symptom-free periods.
- **Systemic onset/extra-articular involvement:** Nonarticular symptoms, which will antedate the onset of arthritis
- Rarely, onset may be monoarticular.

Articular Manifestations

Q. Describe the articular manifestations of rheumatoid arthritis.

- **Joints involved (Fig. 9.1A):** RA can affect any of the synovial (diarthrodial) joints and involvement is usually in a **symmetric distribution**. Most commonly, RA starts in the small joints, namely metacarpophalangeal (MCP), proximal interphalangeal (PIP), and metatarsophalangeal (MTP) joints, followed by the involvement of large joints (wrists, knees, elbows, ankles, hips, and shoulders). Pitting edema over the dorsum gives rise to the **"boxing glove"** appearance. In RA, the hypertrophied synovium (also called pannus) invades and erodes contiguous cartilage, ligaments and bone.
- **Symptoms:** These include pain, swelling, and stiffness. Stiffness dominating in the mornings ('morning stiffness') lasting more than 1 hour is characteristic. Routine activities early in the morning like brushing teeth and combing hair may be very difficult.

Q. Write short note on rheumatoid hand.

Hand and wrist (Figs. 9.1B and C): Hands are a major site of involvement and produces significant disability.

- **The DIP joint is characteristically always spared** unless the patient also has osteoarthritis (both coexist, particularly in elderly patients).
- **Spindling of the fingers:** It is the earliest finding characterized by swelling of the proximal, but not the distal interphalangeal joints.
- **Deformities:** Destruction of the joints and soft tissues may lead to chronic, irreversible deformities.
  - **Ulnar deviation (Figs. 9.1B and C):** It results from subluxation of the metacarpophalangeal (MCP) joints, with subluxation of the proximal phalanx to the volar side of the hand.
  - **'Swan-neck' deformity (Figs. 9.1B and C):** It is due to hyperextension of the proximal interphalangeal joints (PIP) with flexion of the distal interphalangeal joints (DIP). At DIP joint there is elongation or rupture of attachment of the extensor tendon to the base of the distal phalanx; this results in mallet deformity of distal joint and in addition, an extensor tendon imbalance, leading to hyperextension deformity at PIP joint.
  - **'Boutonniere' or 'button-hole' deformity (Fig. 9.1C):** This deformity is due to flexion of the proximal interphalangeal (PIP) joints and extension of the distal interphalangeal (DIP) joints. Disruption of the central slip of the extensor

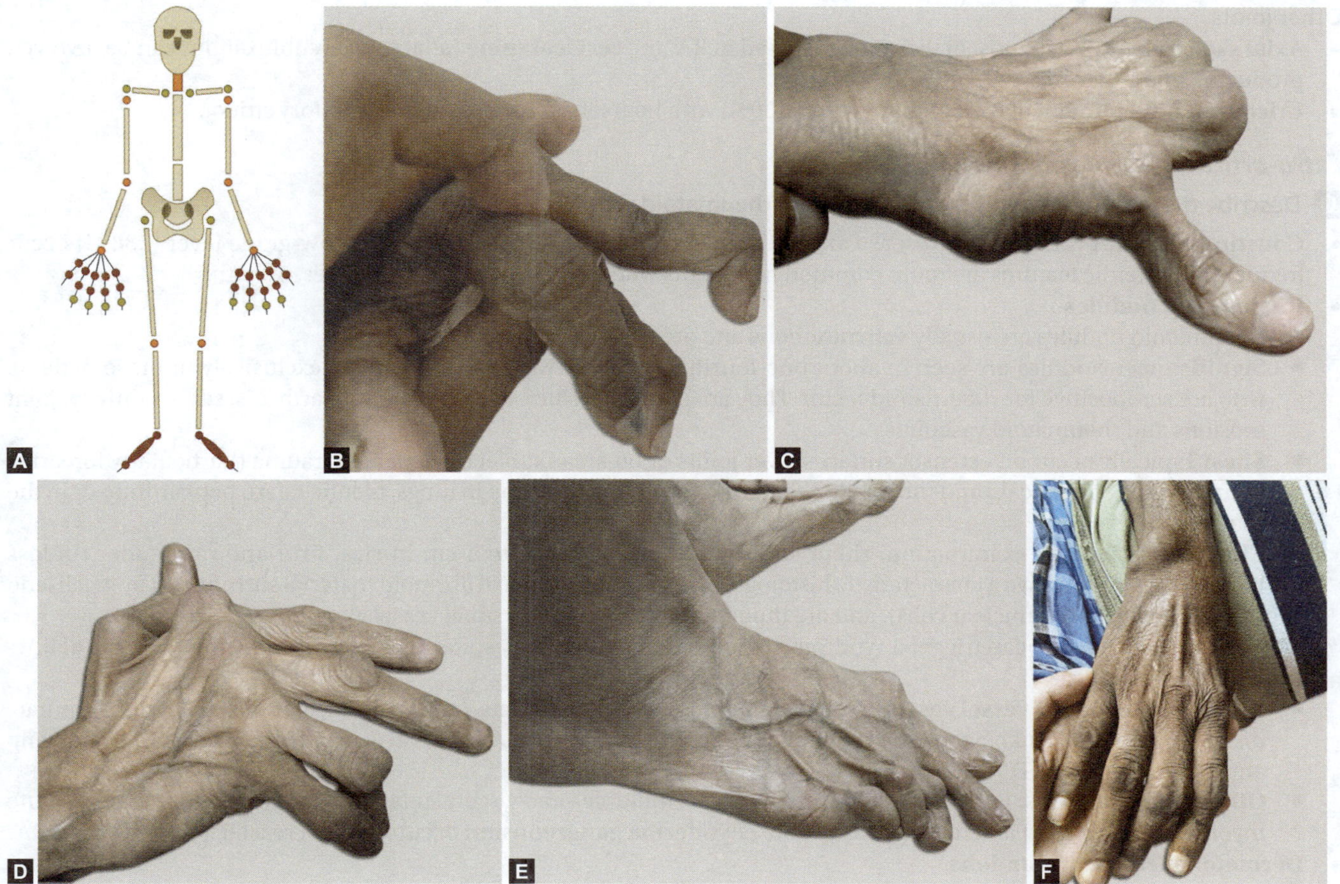

FIGS. 9.1A TO F: Rheumatoid arthritis. (A) Pattern of joint involvement; (B) Swan neck deformity; (C) Boutonniere deformity; (D) Z deformity and ulnar deviation; (E) Hammer toes and hallux valgus; (F) Bow string sign.

tendon and the triangular ligament allows each of the conjoint lateral bands of the digit to slide volarly resulting in a pathologic flexion force and an extension lag; all tendons traversing the PIP joint in this setting elicit flexion of the joint.

- **'Gamekeepers thumb':** It is the result of hyperextension of the first interphalangeal joint and flexion of the first metacarpophalangeal joint. This leads to loss of thumb mobility and occurrence of pinch.
- **Hitchhiker's thumb** (Z-shaped deformity) in which the thumb flexes at the metacarpophalangeal joint and hyperextends at the interphalangeal joint.
- Inflammation of the carpometacarpal joint leads to volar subluxation during contracture of the adductor hallucis.
- **'Z' deformity (Fig. 9.1D):** It is due to radial deviation of the wrist, ulnar deviation of the digits with palmar subluxation of the first MCP joint with hyperextension of the first interphalangeal (IP) joint.
- **Carpal tunnel syndrome:** Due to synovial proliferation in and around the wrists producing compression of the median nerve.
- The **"bow string" sign (Fig. 9.1F)** (prominence of the tendons in the extensor compartment of the hand).

Feet and ankle: In most patients, feet (particularly the MTP joints) are involved early.

- **'Broadening' of the forefoot:** Due to swelling of the metatarsophalangeal joints.
- **Subluxation of the toes at the MTP joints ("cock-up" deformities):** Leads to skin ulceration on the top of the toes and painful ambulation because of loss of the cushioning pads which protect the metatarsals heads.
- **Hallux valgus deformity** and **hammer toes** may be seen **(Fig. 9.1E)**.

Larger joints

- **Involvement of large joints (knees, ankles, elbows, hips and shoulders)** is common but generally occurs somewhat later than small joint involvement.
- Shoulder joint involvement may present as glenohumeral arthritis, rotator cuff fraying and rupture.
- **Synovial cysts:** They present as fluctuant masses around involved joints (large or small). Best examples of synovial cyst is **popliteal ('Baker's) cysts** which develops in the knee joint. The knee synovitis produces excess synovial fluid that communicates posteriorly with the cyst (between the knee joint and the popliteal space) but is prevented from returning to the joint by a one-way valve-like mechanism. Ruptured Baker's cysts can resemble a deep vein thrombosis.

Other joints

- **Axial skeleton:** Although most of the spine is spared in RA, the **cervical spine** (atlantoaxial subluxation) can be involved producing quadriparesis.
- **Cricoarytenoid joint** involvement may present (30%) with hoarseness of voice and inspiratory stridor.

Extra-articular Manifestations (Fig. 9.2)

Q. Describe the various systemic manifestations of rheumatoid arthritis.

- **Constitutional:** RA is a systemic disease and features such as fatigue, weight loss, and low-grade fever (<38°C) occur frequently. Systemic features are more common in patients who have RF or ACPA antibodies, or both.
- **Rheumatoid nodules**
  - Rheumatoid nodules are usually **subcutaneous** and are typically benign.
  - **Significance:** Nodules are seen in about one-fourth of patients with RA and, almost exclusively in those patients who are seropositive for rheumatoid factor. They are clinical predictors of more severe arthritis, sero-positivity, joint erosions and rheumatoid vasculitis.
  - **Sites:** Typically occur on extensor surfaces, over joints or on areas subject to repeated trauma (particularly forearms sacral prominences, scalp and the Achilles tendon). Rarely, they develop in lungs, pleura, heart, pericardium or in the sclera of the eye.
  - **Characteristics:** On examination, rheumatoid nodules are 2 mm to 5 cm in size, firm and nontender (unless traumatized). They have a characteristic histologic picture (central area of fibrinoid material surrounded by a palisade of proliferating mononuclear cells), and are thought to be triggered by small vessel vasculitis.
  - Methotrexate therapy can trigger a syndrome of increased nodulosis despite good control of the joint disease of RA.
- **Rheumatoid vasculitis**
  - **RA-associated small vessel vasculitis:** It can manifest as digital infarcts, cutaneous ulcerations, palpable purpurae, distal gangrene and leukocytoclastic vasculitis. They require prompt more aggressive treatment with disease-modifying antirheumatic drugs (DMARDs).
  - **Other manifestations:** Polyneuropathy, mononeuritis multiplex and visceral infarction (resulting in stroke and acute myocardial infarction) and mesenteric arteritis. **Pyoderma gangrenosum** occurs with increased frequency with RA.
- **Dermatological manifestations**
  - Rhematoid nodules
  - Skin ulcers

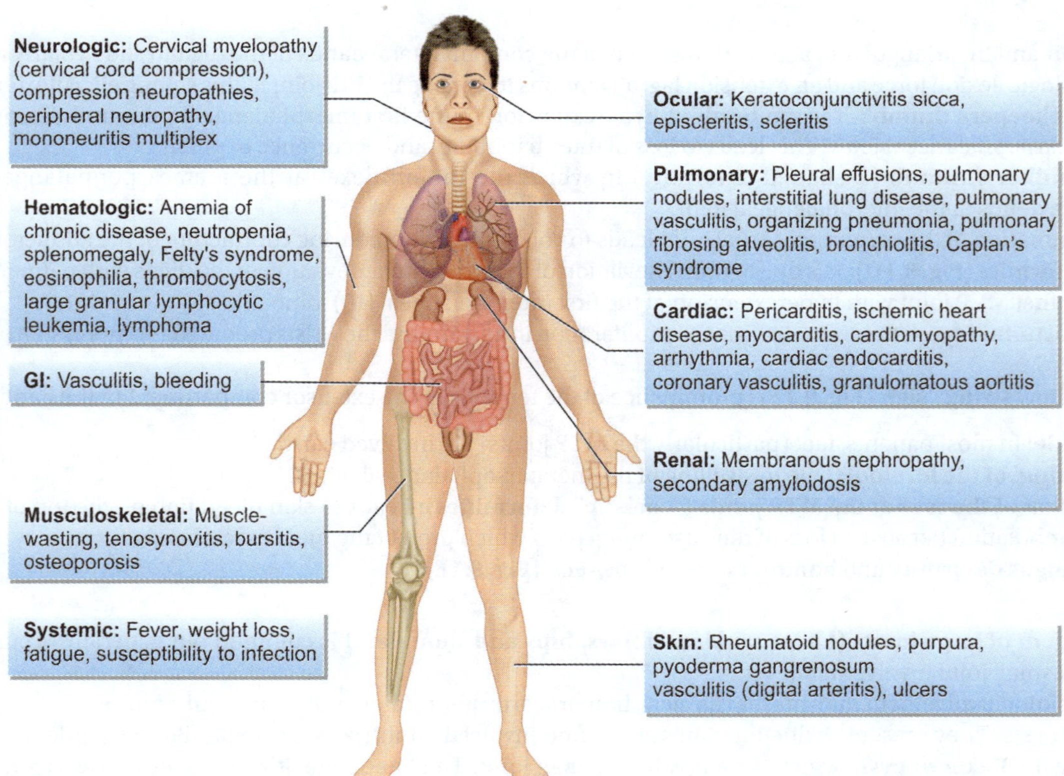

FIG. 9.2: Extra-articular manifestations of RA.

- Neutrophilic dermatosis (Sweet syndrome), pyoderma gangerenosum
- Skin atrophy, petechiae, Raynaud's phenomenon.

Pleuropulmonary Manifestations

Q. Enlist the pleuropulmonary manifestations of rheumatoid arthritis.

- **Pleural lesions: Pleural effusions (exudative)** occur more commonly in men and are usually small and asymptomatic. Pleural fluid is characterized by low glucose and pH.
- Pulmonary lesions:
  - **Rheumatoid nodules** especially in men; usually solid, but may calcify, cavitate or become infected.
  - **Diffuse interstitial fibrosis** causes dyspnea and may progress to cor pulmonale.
  - **Bronchiolitis obliterans** with or without organizing pneumonia.
  - **Granulomatous pneumonitis.**
  - **Pulmonary arteritis** (vasculitis) may result in infarction.
  - **Caplan's syndrome:** It is characterized by the coexistence of seropositive RA and rounded fibrotic, peripherally located nodules of 0.5–5 cm diameter in the lung along with coal worker's pneumoconiosis (CWP)/silicosis.
  - **Treatment induced:** Methotrexate induced lung fibrosis, immunosuppression related infections like TB.
- **Cardiac manifestations**
  - **Pericardial effusions** are common. Rarely, long-standing pericardial disease results in a fibrinous pericarditis and constrictive pericarditis.
  - Coronary artery disease due to **premature atherosclerosis**. Rarely, myocarditis, **valvular involvement** and **conduction defects.**
- **Neurological manifestations**
  - **Peripheral nerve entrapment syndromes:** For example, carpal tunnel syndrome (median nerve at the wrist), and tarsal tunnel syndrome (anterior tibial nerve at the ankle).
  - **Myelopathy:** Due to spinal cord compression produced by acquired atlanto-axial dislocation.
  - **Mononeuritis multiplex:** Due to vasculitis.
- **Ophthalmological manifestations**
  - **Sjögren's syndrome/Sicca complex:** Comprising keratoconjunctivitis sicca, xerostomia and salivary (parotid) gland enlargement.
  - **Scleritis,** episcleritis may progress to perforation of the orbit (scleromalacia perforans).
  - **Brown's syndrome:** Diplopia due to tendinitis of the superior oblique muscles.
- **Osteoporosis:** Osteoporosis secondary to rheumatoid involvements is very common especially with corticosteroid therapy and immobilization.
- **Hematological manifestations**
  - **RBC:** Normocytic normochromic anemia. Causes of anemia in RA include anemia of chronic disease, anemia due to gastrointestinal bleed secondary to NSAIDs/steroids, methotrexate induced folate deficiency, marrow suppression due to disease/drugs and part of hypersplenism if splenomegaly present.
  - **WBC:** Eosinophilia and mild leukocytosis. Neutropenia in cases of Felty's syndrome and large granular lymphocyte syndrome. Patients with RA are at an **increased risk for infections,** and this risk is further increased by some therapies.
  - **Platelets:** Thrombocytosis.
  - **Felty's syndrome:** It is the triad of RA, splenomegaly, and neutropenia.
- **Renal involvement:** In the form of glomerulonephropathy, vasculitis, drug toxicities and secondary amyloidosis.
- **Malignancies:** RA patients have an increased risk of **lymphomas**.

Diagnosis

Q. Enumerate the ACR (American College of Rheumatology)/EULAR criteria for the diagnosis of rheumatoid arthritis.

- Diagnostic criteria of rheumatoid arthritis: In 2010, a collaborative effort between the American College of Rheumatology **(Box 9.1)** and the ACR/European League against Rheumatism presented the criteria for the diagnosis of RA **(Table 9.10)**.
- The Disease Activity Score in 28 joints **(DAS28)** is used to grade severity of RA.
- Simplified Disease Activity Index **(SDAI)** and Clinical Disease Activity Index **(CDAI)** are also used in monitoring.

Box 9.1: American College of Rheumatology (ACR) criteria for rheumatoid arthritis.

- Morning stiffness*
- Arthritis of 3 joint areas*
- Arthritis of the hands*
- Symmetric arthritis*
- Rheumatoid nodules
- Serum rheumatoid factor positive
- Radiographic changes

* These criteria must be present for more than 6 weeks. Presence of 4 criteria favors definite diagnosis of RA.

Investigations

Q. Discuss the diagnostic work up for rheumatoid arthritis.

- **Serology**
  - **Rheumatoid factor**
  - **Anticyclic citrullinated protein antibodies** (ACPA)
- **Markers of acute inflammation**
  - **Anemia of chronic disease** is seen in majority of patients, and the degree of anemia is proportional to the activity of the disease.
  - **Thrombocytosis** is common, and platelet counts return to normal as the inflammation is controlled.
  - **Acute phase reactants, erythrocyte sedimentation rate and C-reactive protein levels** parallel the activity of the disease, and their persistent elevation carries poor prognosis (joint destruction and mortality).
  - **WBC counts** may be raised, normal, or profoundlydepressed (Felty's syndrome).
- **Other autoantibodies:** RA is associated with other autoantibodies, such as antinuclear antibodies (30% of patients) and antineutrophilic cytoplasmic antibodies, particularly of the perinuclear type (30% of patients).
- **Radiographs of the affected joints:** Radiological changes include symmetrical pattern of involvement, juxta-articular osteoporosis, soft tissue swelling, bone erosions and narrowing of the joint space.
- **Ultrasonography and MRI:** More sensitive than plain radiographs and detects soft-tissue synovitis before joint damage. *Doppler ultrasound* is useful for demonstration persistent synovitis when deciding on the need for DMARDs or assessing their efficacy.
- **Synovial fluid analysis:** White blood cell counts typically range from 5000–50,000 per microliter with approximately two-third of the cells being neutrophils with no crystals or organism. None of the synovial fluid findings are pathognomonic.
- **Testing for latent tuberculosis:** Before starting biological agents.

TABLE 9.10: American College of Rheumatology (ACR)/European League against Rheumatism (EULAR) classification criteria for rheumatoid arthritis, 2010.

Features	*Score*
A. Joint involvement	
➢ 1 large joint (shoulder, elbow, hip, knee, ankle)	0
➢ 2–10 large joints	1
➢ 1–3 small joints (MCP, PIP, thumb IP, MTP, wrists) + involvement of large joints	2
➢ 4–10 small joints + involvement of large joints	3
➢ >10 joints (at least 1 small joint)	5
B. Serology (at least one test result is needed for classification)	
➢ Negative RF and negative ACPA	0
➢ Low-positive RF or low-positive ACPA (≤ 3 times ULN)	2
➢ High-positive RF or high-positive ACPA (≥ 3 times ULN)	3
C. Acute-phase reactants (at least one test result is needed for classification)	
➢ Normal CRP and normal ESR	0
➢ Abnormal CRP or abnormal ESR	1
D. Duration of symptoms	
➢ < 6 weeks	0
➢ ≥ 6 weeks	1

(MCP: metacarpophalangeal joint; PIP: proximal interphalangeal joint; IP: interphalangeal joint; MTP: metatarsophalangeal joint; RF: rheumatoid factor; ACPA: anticitrullinated protein antibodies; ULN: upper limit of normal; CRP: C-reactive protein; ESR: erythrocyte sedimentation rate)

- Above criteria yields a score of 0–10. **A score of ≥ 6 required for definitive diagnosis of RA.**
- A score of < 6/10 are not classifiable as RA, but their status to be reassessed over time.

Q. Develop an appropriate treatment plan for patients with rheumatoid arthritis.

Q. Describe the various treatment options for rheumatoid arthritis.

Management

The early recognition of inflammatory arthritis, before irreversible injury has occurred, is the most important element in the effective management

General Measures

The goal of therapy is **disease remission** and **to maintain this remission** by continuing therapy.

- **Rest and splinting** of the involved joints during the acute stage.
- **Physiotherapy:** Helps in mobilization and prevention of contractures.
- **Smoking cessation, control of cardiovascular risks, screening for osteoporosis**

Medical Therapy

Three types of medical therapies are used in the treatment of RA: (1) NSAIDs, (2) glucocorticoids, and (3) DMARDs (both conventional and biologic).

1. **Nonsteroidal anti-inflammatory drugs (NSAIDs):** NSAIDs produce **symptomatic relief** because of its **analgesic and anti- inflammatory properties**. However, they do not alter the underlying disease process. Therefore, they are not used without the concomitant use of DMARDs. Their **chronic use should be minimized** because of its side effects such as gastritis/peptic ulcer disease and impairment of renal function.
2. **Glucocorticoids:** These are the most potent anti-inflammatory treatments available and cause dramatic and rapid improvement. Not only they produce symptomatic improvement, but also significantly decrease the radiographic progression of RA. However, the longterm therapy is associated with mulltisystem toxicities.
   - **Prednisolone** is the most commonly used glucocorticoid and is administered orally.
   - **Bridge therapy:** In 'bridge therapy', glucocorticoids are used first to shut off inflammation rapidly and then to taper them as the DMARD is taking effect.
   - **Pulse therapy:** Remission is induced with IM (intramuscular) depot methylprednisolone 80–120 mg if synovitis persists beyond 6 weeks. Intra-articular long-acting glucocorticoids (e.g. triamcinolone hexacetonide) are used to reduce synovitis.

3. **Disease modifying antirheumatic drugs (DMARDs).**

Q. Describe the basis for biologics and DMARDs in rheumatologic diseases.

Q. Describe the role and current status of various disease modifying antirheumatic drugs (DMARDs).

Patients with RA must be started on DMARD therapy as soon as possible. DMARDs have the ability to inhibit greatly the disease process to modify or change the disabling potential of RA. DMARDs are so named because in most of the cases they are able to slow or prevent structural (radiographic) progression of RA.

Box 9.2: Conventional DMARDs used in RA.

- Methotrexate (MTX)
- Hydroxychloroquine
- Sulfasalazine
- Leflunomide
- Azathioprine
- Gold (auranofin)
- Minocycline
- D-penicillamine

Conventional DMARDs used in RA (Box 9.2)

- Conventional DMARDs exhibit a delayed onset of action and take 2–6 months to exert their full effect.
- Start DMARD therapy early in the disease process. Early in the course of disease, most patients should be started on a combination of DMARDs and analgesics. Before using DMARDs, complete blood count, serum creatinine, aminotransferases, and screening for hepatitis C, hepatitis B, and latent tuberculosis infection. A chest radiograph should be obtained prior to initiating treatment with MTX.

Methotrexate: Currently, methotrexate is the DMARD of choice (considered as 'gold standard' drug) for RA and is the anchor drug for most combination therapies.

- **Mechanism of action** in RA: At the dosages used for RA, methotrexate stimulates extracellular release of adenosine from cells, which has anti-inflammatory and immunomodulatory properties. Enzymes inhibited by methotrexate in RA include **thymidylate synthetase (TS) and 5-aminoimidazole-4-carboxamide ribonucleotide (AICAR) transformylase**. It should not be prescribed in pregnancy.
- **Dose:** Usually given orally in the starting dose of 2.5–7.5 mg/**week** as a single dose. **If there is nopositive response** within 4–8 weeks, and there is no toxicity, the dose should be **increased by 2.5–5 mg/week** each month to 15–25 mg/week before considering, the treatment a failure. Oral absorption of methotrexate is variable. If oral treatment is not effective, it is given by subcutaneous injections. It should be monitored with full blood counts and liver biochemistry.
- **Folic acid**, 1 to 4 mg/day (or 5 mg once a week, on the day following methotrexate dose), reduces most methotrexate associated toxicities (e.g. gastrointestinal intolerance, stomatitis, hepatotoxicity, hyperhomocysteinemia, alopecia) without apparent loss of efficacy.

If methotrexate alone does not sufficiently control RA, it is combined with other DMARDs.

Other DMARDs

- **Hydroxychloroquine** is used usually in combination with other DMARDs, particularly methotrexate. It is given orally at a dose of 200–400 mg daily. It is the least toxic DMARD but also the least effective as monotherapy. Regular monitoring (every 6 months to a year) by ophthalmoscopy to detect any signs of retinopathy, bull's eye maculopathy should be done.
- **Sulfasalazine:** It is effective when given in doses of 1–3 g daily. Monitoring of blood cell counts is recommended, particularly WBC counts, in the first 6 months. Combination of sulfasalazine + hydroxychloroquine + methotrexate is referred to as triple therapy.
- **Leflunomide** is a pyrimidine antagonist, also inhibits enzyme **dihydroorotate dehydrogenase**, interfering with cell signal transduction. It has a very long half-life and is given daily in a dose of 10–20 mg. The most common toxicity is diarrhea, which may respond to dose reduction. Leflunomide is teratogenic and hepatotoxic. It is used as monotherapy or in combination with methotrexate and other DMARDs.
- **Others:** These include minocycline, gold salts, penicillamine and cyclosporine are used sparingly now.

Biologic DMARDs/Biologicals

Q. List the biologicals used in the treatment of rheumatoid arthritis (RA).

- They are usually given along with methotrexate or other conventional DMARDs.
- **Disadvantages: High cost** and **long-term toxicities,** notably **infections** (especially cellulitis, septic joints, tuberculosis, histoplas- mosis, coccidioidomycosis, and *Listeria*) and **demyelinating syndromes**.

TNF-α Blockers

- **Etanercept,** a recombinant TNF receptor fusion protein. Administered subcutaneously in a dose of 25 mg twice weekly.
- **Infliximab** is a mouse/human chimeric monoclonal antibody against TNF-α. It is given intravenously (3–10 mg/kg) every 4–8 weeks.
- **Adalimumab** is a recombinant human IgG1 monoclonal antibody directed against TNF-α. It is administered subcutaneously in a dose of 40 mg every other week.
- Newer TNF inhibitors, certolizumab pegol and golimumab, are also effective.

IL-1 Receptor Blocker

- **Anakinra,** a recombinant human interleukin-1 receptor antagonist. It is given subcutaneously in a dose of 100 mg daily.
- **Tocilizumab and sarilumab** are two newer agents.

Anti-CD20 Antibodies.

- **Rituximab** is a genetically engineered chimeric murine/human monoclonal antibody directed against the CD20 molecule found on the surface of B cells. It is given intravenously as two infusions 2 weeks apart for the treatment of patients with refractory RA.

T-cell Agent

- **Abatacept** is a recombinant fusion protein of the extracellular domain of human CTLA4 and a fragment of the Fc domain of human IgG1. It is administered by intravenous infusion every 4 weeks in a dose of approximately 10 mg/kg.

JAK inhibitors

- **Tofacitinib, baricitinib, peficitinib, and upadacitinib,** can also be used in combination with MTX or as monotherapy.

Immunosuppressants: These are used as third-line drugs for RA that recurs or does not respond to second-line agents. These include cyclophosphamide and azathioprine. However, in RA with acute vasculitis causing serious organ involvement, intravenous administration of cyclophosphamide may be lifesaving.

Surgery

Surgical therapy may improve pain and disability when there is failure of medical therapy. It is useful in maintenance of joint function, and prevention and correction of deformities. Surgical procedures of the joint include (a) synovectomy of the inflammed joint before joint damage; (b) osteotomy to correct the deformity and relieve pain in the upper end of the tibia, and excision of the lower end of the ulna; (c) arthrodesis of the joint to relieve pain in the atlanto-axial joint, wrists, ankle and subtalar joints; (d) excision arthroplasty and (e) joint replacement.

Physiotherapy, Rehabilitation and Assistive Devices

Exercise and physical activity improve muscle strength. Judicious use of wrist splints can decrease pain.

Treatment algorithm for rheumatoid arthritis is presented in **Flowcharts 9.1 and 9.2**.

FLOWCHART 9.1: Treatment algorithm for rheumatoid arthritis (<6 months of symptoms).

Disease activity level: Low | Moderate | High

Start DMARD monotherapy (MTX preferable +/- steroids)

Disease activity level: Low | Moderate | High

Low → Continue current therapy

Moderate, High → Use DMARD combinations TNFi +/- MTX or non-TNFi +/- MTX

Disease activity level: Low | Moderate | High

Low → Continue current therapy

Moderate, High → Treat as established RA

FLOWCHART 9.2: Treatment algorithm for established rheumatoid arthritis (≥6 months of symptoms).

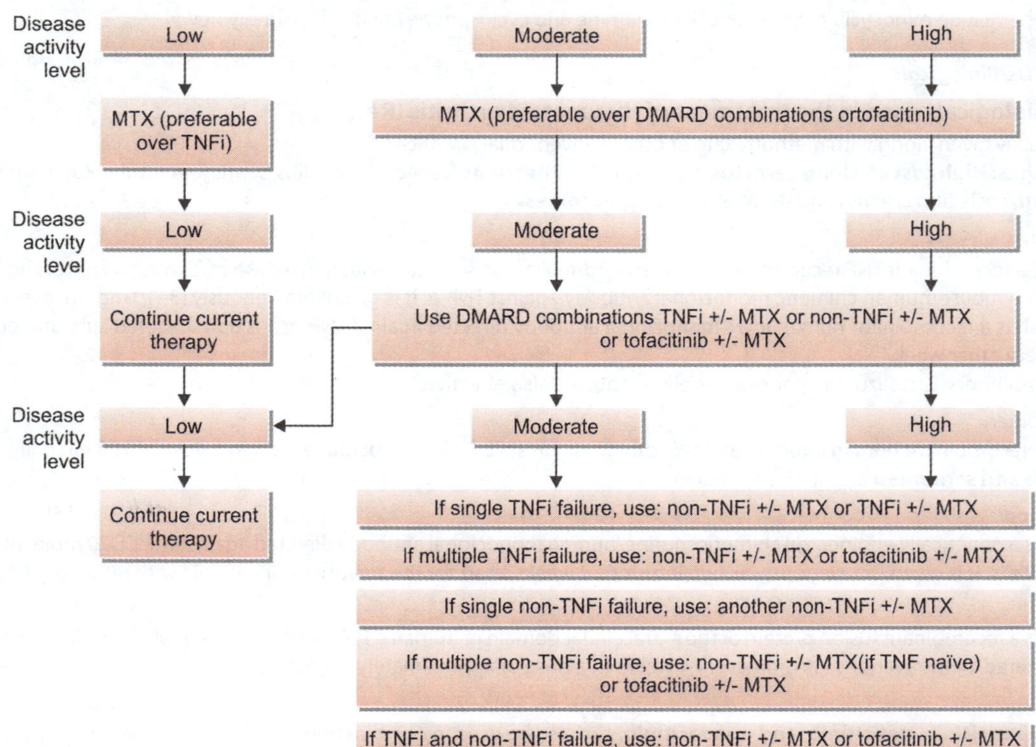

Felty's Syndrome

Q. Write short essay/note on Felty's syndrome and its components.

- Felty's syndrome is the triad of RA, neutropenia and splenomegaly.
- It is seen in patients with long-standing chronic, severe and seropositive RA.
- Autoantibodies to deiminated histones (predominantly histone H3) and neutrophil extracellular chromatin traps (NETs) are postulate as the cause.

Box 9.3: Clinical features of Felty's syndrome.

- Features of RA (rheumatoid arthritis)
- Splenomegaly
- Lymphadenopathy
- Skin pigmentation
- Fever
- Weight loss
  - Rarely recurrent infections and chronic leg ulcers
  - Vasculitis
  - Subcutaneous nodules
  - Portal hypertension
  - Higher risk of Hodgkin's lymphoma

Clinical Features

See **Box 9.3**.

Laboratory Findings

- **Blood:** Neutropenia 3 (absolute neutrophil count below 2000/microL), anemia and thrombocytopenia.
- **Rheumatoid factor (RF):** High titers.
- **Circulating immune complexes (CIC):** Increased levels.

Treatment

- Do not require special specific therapy; instead **treat underlying severe RA**. Immunosuppressive agents particularly methotrexate and azathioprine are beneficial.
- G-CSF and GM-CSF can be tried.
- **Splenectomy is indicated in:** Severe and persistent neutropenia (< 500 cells/mm^3), recurrent or serious bacterial infections, chronic, nonhealing leg ulcers, hypersplenism producing severe anemia or thrombocytopenic hemorrhage.

Prognosis

Poor with an increased mortality due to increased incidence of severe infection.

Nonsteroidal Anti-inflammatory Drugs (NSAIDs)

Nonsteroidal anti-inflammatory drugs are the most widely used drugs, but they have an increased risk of cardiovascular disease. Oral NSAIDs are used for the management of pain due to inflammation.

Mechanism of NSAID action: Arachidonic acid (AA) is derived from membrane phospholipid and its **metabolism occurs along two major enzymatic pathways namely; cyclooxygenase pathway** (produces prostaglandins by the cyclooxygenase) (COX) **and lipoxygenase pathway** (produces leukotrienes by 5-lipoxygenase).

Q. Write briefly on COX enzymes and COX-2 inhibitors.

Traditional NSAIDs versus COX-2 Inhibitors

- **Traditional NSAIDs** (e.g. ibuprofen, diclofenac, and naproxen) exert their anti-inflammatory effect by inhibiting synthesis of prostaglandin from arachidonic acid by blocking both COX enzymes. They do not have a disease-modifying effect in either osteoarthritis or inflammatory rheumatic diseases. Inhibition of COX-1 is required for anti-inflammatory and analgesic effects, but can damage the mucosa of stomach and duodenum and is associated with an increased risk of upper gastrointestinal ulceration, bleeding and perforation. Simultaneous administration of omeprazole (20 mg daily) or misoprostol (200 μg twice or 3 times daily) reduces the risk of NSAID-induced ulceration and bleeding. Other side-effects include fluid retention, renal impairment due to inhibition of renal prostaglandin production, and rashes.
- **COX-2 (cyclooxygenase-2) selective NSAIDs** (e.g. celecoxib, etoricoxib, etodolac, rofecoxib and valdecoxib) selectively inhibit COX-2. They have **analgesic** and **anti-inflammatory properties similar to traditional NSAIDs**. However, they are much less **likely to cause gastrointestinal toxicity** and have **minimal antiplatelet effects**. Similar to traditional NSAIDs, they can produce significant changes in renal function, and hence, should be cautiously used in patients with diabetes, dehydration and congestive heart failure. They **play an important role in the management of inflammation and pain caused by arthritis**. It has been observed that there is a higher risk of myocardial infarction and stroke (thromboembolic complications) in patients using COX-2 inhibitors compared to traditional NSAIDs. Hence, two COX-2 inhibitors namely rofecoxib and valdecoxib have been withdrawn. NSAIDs like diclofenac, nabumetone, meloxicam, and etodolac, are also relatively selective for COX-2 at lower doses.

Differences between Rheumatic Arthritis and Rheumatoid Arthritis (Table 9.11)

Q. Differentiate between rheumatic arthritis from rheumatoid arthritis.

TABLE 9.11: Differences between rheumatic arthritis and rheumatoid arthritis.

	Rheumatic arthritis	*Rheumatoid arthritis*
Onset	Acute	Subacute/chronic
Joints involved	Major joints (e.g. knee), rarely involves small joints of hands/wrists/feet	Small joints, e.g. palm-finger (MCP) joints, joints of the wrist/feet
Joints spared	Spares hip joints	Spares distal interphalangeal (DIP) joint
Spine	Not involved	C1, C2 involved
Presentation	Migratory	Non-migratory, static
Morning stiffness	+/–	+++
Pattern of involvement	Asymmetrical	Symmetrical
Cause	Poststreptococcal	Immune
Deformities	Rare (Jaccouds)	Common
Nodules	Rare, located only subcutaneously, painless	Common, painful, located periarticular, pleura, internal organs
Criteria used for diagnosis	Jones	ACR/EULAR
Antibodies	ASO	RF/ACPA
Treatment	Penicillin/aspirin +/– steroids	DMARDs/biologics
Other systems involved	Cardiac, basal ganglia	All systems involved

(ASO: antistreptolysin O; ACR: American College of Rheumatology; EULAR: European League against Rheumatism; RF: rheumatoid factor; ACPA: anticyclic citrullinated protein antibodies; DMARD: disease modifying antirheumatic drugs)

SYSTEMIC LUPUS ERYTHEMATOSUS

Q. Describe the clinical manifestations, diagnosis and management of systemic lupus erythematosus (SLE).

- Systemic lupus erythematosus (SLE) is a chronic, **multisystemic autoimmune** disease that results from **immune system-mediated tissue damage** and is characterized by the presence of **broad spectrum of autoantibodies**.
- **Arthralgia and rashes** are the **most common clinical features,** whereas **cerebral and renal diseases** constitute **most serious problems**.
- **Age:** It usually occurs in young women between **20 to 30 years**, but may manifest at any age.
- **Sex:** It predominantly affects **women**, with female-to-male ratio of 9:1.

Clinical Features (Table 9.12)

Q. Write short essay/note on clinical features of systemic lupus erythematosus (SLE).

TABLE 9.12: Common clinical manifestations of SLE.

		Clinical manifestations	
System involved	*%*	*Common*	*Uncommon*
Systemic	95	Fatigue, malaise, fever, anorexia, nausea, weight loss	Generalized lymphadenopathy
Musculoskeletal	95	Arthralgias/myalgias, non-erosive polyarthritis, myopathy	Myositis, erosive (Jaccoud's) arthritis
Mucocutaneous	80	Photosensitivity, malar rash ('butterfly' rash), oral ulcers, alopecia, discoid rash, Raynaud phenomenon, livedo reticularis, panniculitis, splinter hemorrhages	Angioedema, bullous lupus, cutaneous vasculitis thromboembolic manifestations
Hematological	85	Anemia, leukopenia (<4000/µL), lymphopenia (<1500/ µL), thrombocytopenia (100,000/µL), lymphadenopathy, splenomegaly, hemolytic anemia	
Neuropsychiatric	60	Delirium, psychosis, seizures, mono/polyneuropathy, mood disorder, headache, Stroke (thromboembolic)	Cranial neuropathy, chorea
Cardiopulmonary	60	Pericarditis/pericardial effusions, coronary artery disease, pleurisy/pleural effusions, lupus pneumonitis, pulmonary hypertension, intestitial lung disease	Myocarditis, Libman-Sacks endocarditis, pulmonary hemorrhage Congenital heart block (neonatal lupus) shrinking lung syndrome
Renal	30–50	Proteinuria 500 mg/24 h, cellular casts, nephrotic syndrome, renal failure	
Gastrointestinal	40	Non-specific symptoms (nausea, mild pain, diarrhea), bleeding or perforation, abnormal live enzymes	Mesenteric vasculitis (with or without ischemia), colitis, splenomegaly
Thrombosis	15	Venous and arterial	
Ocular	15	Sicca syndrome, conjunctivitis, episcleritis, retinal vasculitis	Optic neuritis, uveitis, retinitis
Vasculitis	11–36	Cutaneous , visceral, retinal, pulmonary vasculitis	
Others		Antiphospholipid antibody syndrome, osteoporosis	Inmmunodeficiency

Musculoskeletal Manifestations

- Arthralgia and nonerosive arthritis are most common (>85%). Commonly involves proximal interphalangeal and metacarpophalangeal joints of the hand, along with the knees and wrists.
- In about 10% of patients, **deformities result from damage to periarticular** tissue, a condition termed **Jaccoud's arthropathy**.

Cutaneous Manifestations

- **Classic malar rash** consists of erythematous (flat or raised) facial rash with a **butterfly distribution** across the malar and nasal prominences and sparing of the nasolabial folds **(Fig. 9.3)** and is seen in 30–60% of patients. Butterfly rash is **often triggered by sun exposure**.
- **Discoid lupus** is a benign variant of lupus in which **only the skin is involved**. Discoid rash consists of erythematous, slightly raised patches with adherent keratotic scaling and follicular plugging. Discoid rash without any systemic features occurs in discoid lupus erythematosus (DLE). Only 5% of patients with DLE have SLE; however, as many as 20% SLE patients have DLE. This rash is primarily seen on the face and scalp.
- Generalized **photosensitivity** (skin rash on exposure to sunlight) and alopecia.

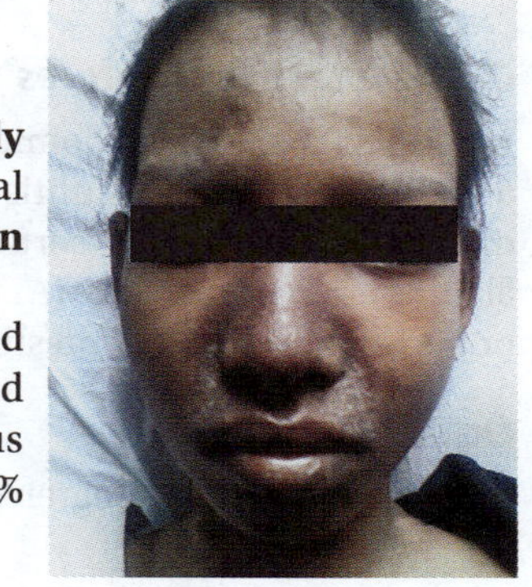

FIG. 9.3: Systemic lupus erythematosus with malar rash and alopecia.

Mucous Membrane Manifestations

Recurrent crops of small, painful ulcerations on the oral or nasal mucosa. Dryness secondary to Sjögren's syndrome.

Hematologic Manifestations

Antibodies that target each of the cellular blood elements are responsible for hematological changes.

- RBC: Normocytic normochromic **anemia**, reflecting chronic illness. **Hemolytic anemia:** Coombs' test positive or microangiopathic hemolysis.
- WBC: **Leukopenia**, particularly lymphopenia.
- Platelets: **Idiopathic/immune thrombocytopenic purpura** induced by antiplatelet antibodies.
- Antibodies to clotting factors can contribute to impaired clot formation and hemorrhage.

Renal Manifestations

Q. Enumerate the renal manifestations of SLE.

- Kidney may be **involved in 30–50%** of SLE patients and is one of the most important organs involved.
- **Often asymptomatic** in most lupus patients, particularly initially. Hence, **urinalysis should be done** in any person suspected of having SLE followed by regular urinalysis and blood pressure monitoring.
- Characterized by proteinuria (>500 mg/24 hours) and/or cellular (red cell) casts.
- Histological classification of lupus nephritis **(Table 9.13)**.

TABLE 9.13: ISN/RPS classification of lupus nephritis.

Class	Histological type
I	Minimal mesangial lupus nephritis (light microscopy: normal glomeruli)
II	Mesangial proliferative LN (few isolated subepithelial/ endothelial deposits visible by IF or electron microscopy)
III	Focal lupus nephritis (<50% glomeruli, subendothelial deposits)
➢ IIIA	Active lesions
➢ IIIA/C	Active and chronic lesions
➢ IIIC	Chronic lesions
IV	Diffuse lupus nephritis >50% glomerul involved, segmental and global lesions
➢ IV-S (A)	Active lesions—diffuse segmental proliferative lupus nephritis
➢ IV-G (A)	Active lesions—diffuse global proliferative lupus nephritis
➢ IV-S (A/C)	Active and chronic lesions—diffuse segmental proliferative and sclerosing lupus nephritis
➢ IV-G (A/C)	Active and chronic lesions—diffuse global proliferative and sclerosing lupus nephritis
➢ IV-S (C)	Chronic in active lesions with scars—diffuse segmental sclerosing lupus nephritis
➢ IV-G (C)	Chronic in active lesions with scars—diffuse segmental global lupus nephritis
V	Membranous lupus nephritis
VI	Advanced sclerosing lupus nephritis

Neuropsychiatric Features

- Nervous system involvement in SLE produces both neurologic and psychiatric manifestations.
- Clinical features include cognitive dysfunction (due to SLE cerebritis), headache and seizures, psychiatric features including depression and psychosis. Peripheral nervous system involvement can cause neuropathy. Cranial nerve and ocular involvement due to vasculopathy.

Cardiac Manifestations

- **Pericarditis most frequent**; serious manifestations are myocarditis and **Libman-Sack (**noninfective endocarditis involving the mitral valve) **endocarditis.**
- **Increased risk for myocardial infarction**, usually due to accelerated atherosclerosis and vasculitis.

Pulmonary Manifestations

- **Pleural lesions:** Pleurisy with or without pleural effusion—most common pulmonary manifestation. Pleural effusion is exudative with low C3 and ANA test positive in the pleural fluid.
- **Lung lesions:** Pneumonitis (exclude infection before ascribing a lung lesion to SLE), shrinking lung syndrome, interstitial inflammation leading to fibrosis and intra-alveolar hemorrhage.

Gastrointestinal Features

Non-specific diffuse abdominal pain (caused by autoimmune peritonitis and/or intestinal vasculitis), nausea sometimes with vomiting and diarrhea. Increases in serum aspartate aminotransferase (AST) and alanine aminotransferase (ALT). Mesenteric vasculitis can cause infarction or perforation of small intestine.

Ocular Manifestations

- Sicca syndrome (Sjogren's syndrome) and nonspecific conjunctivitis are common.
- Serious manifestations are retinal vasculitis (can cause infarcts and cytoid bodies) and optic neuritis. Complications of glucocorticosteroid therapy include cataracts (common) and glaucoma.

Other Manifestations

Kikuchi-Fujimoto disease (splenomegaly, lymphadenopathy), antiphospholipid syndrome, osteoporosis, and complement deficiencies are associated with SLE. Increased risk of hematologic malignancies (particularly non-Hodgkin's lymphoma) and possibly lung and hepatobiliary cancers.

Poor progmnostic factors in SLE include diffuse proliferative glomerulonephritis, male sex, older age at presentation, black race, hypertension and antiphospholipid antibody syndrome.

Clinical features are summarized diagrammatically in **Figure 9.4**. Causes of death in SLE are listed in **Box 9.4**.

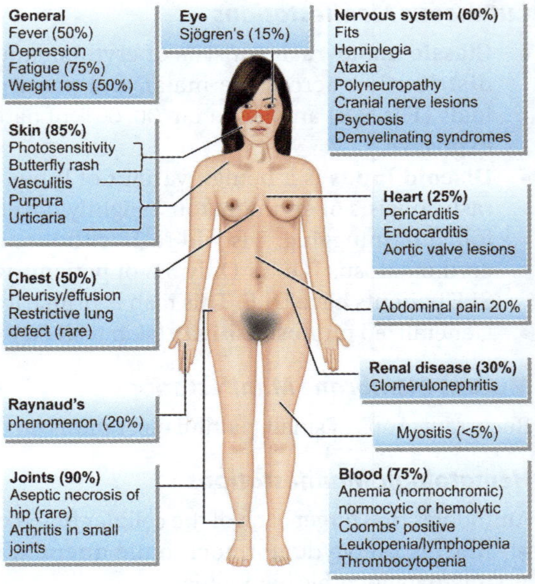

FIG. 9.4: Clinical features of systemic lupus erythematosus (SLE).

Box 9.4: Causes of death in SLE.

- **Infections and renal failure:** Cause of death in the first decade of disease
- **Thromboembolic events:** Cause of death in the second and later decades
- **Cardiovascular:** Due to premature atherosclerosis

Laboratory Findings

Purpose: (1) To establish or rule out the diagnosis, (2) follow the course of disease, and (3) to identify adverse effects of therapies.

Autoantibodies in SLE

Q. Describe the diagnostic work up and the role of autoantibodies in systemic lupus erythematosus (SLE).

- SLE is characterized by the production of **several diverse autoantibodies**. Some antibodies are against different nuclear and cytoplasmic components of the cell that are not organ specific. Other antibodies are directed against specific cell surface antigens of blood cells.
- **Importance of autoantibodies:** (1) **Diagnosis and management** of patients with SLE, and (2) responsible for **pathogenesis of tissue damage.**

Types of Antibodies (Table 9.14)

- **Antinuclear antibody (ANA):** Best screening test and >90% of the patients show a positive test. However, a positive test is not specific for SLE. It can be positive in some normal individual (especially elderly), other autoimmune diseases, acute viral infections, chronic inflammatory processes and with certain drugs.
- **Anti-double-stranded DNA** (anti-dsDNA) antibodies are common in SLE. **Anti-Sm antibodies are highly specific** for SLE. Rising levels of anti-dsDNA and low levels of complement (C3 and C4) usually reflect disease activity.
- **Rheumatoid factor** is positive in 30%.

TABLE 9.14: Autoantibodies in patients with systemic lupus erythematosus (SLE).

➢ Antinuclear antibodies (ANA)	➢ Antihistone
➢ Anti-dsDNA (ds = double stranded)	➢ Antiphospholipid
➢ Anti-Sm (Anti-Smith)	➢ Antierythrocyte
➢ Anti-RNP	➢ Antiplatelet
➢ Anti-Ro (SSA)	➢ Antineuronal
➢ Anti-La (SSB)	➢ Antiribosomal

Other Tests

- **Complete blood count:** Essential and aids in diagnosis and management. **Anemia** (normocytic normochromic and Coombs' positive), **leucopenia, lymphopenia** and **thrombocytopenia** may be present.
- **Activated partial thromboplastin time (aPTT): Prolonged** in the presence of pathogenic **antiphospholipid antibodies**. These antibodies give a false-positive result in the serologic test for syphilis.
- **Erythrocyte sedimentation rate (ESR):** Nonspecific indicator of systemic inflammation. It is often monitored in many patients to know the disease activity.
- **C-reactive protein (CRP):** It is an acute phase reactant which is relatively uninformative and normal in SLE. It does not usually rise with disease activity unless there is infection, arthritis or serositis.
- **Urinalysis:** When there is active nephritis, urinalysis shows proteinuria, hematuria and cellular (red and white blood cell casts in the urinary sediment suggest proliferative glomerulonephritis) or granular casts. Blood urea nitrogen and serum creatinine are elevated in acute kidney injury. If there is proteinuria, urine albumin/creatinine ratio should be measured. Renal biopsy confirms renal involvement.
- **Complement levels:** Low levels of C3 indicate active disease especially nephritis.
- **LE cell:** Phagocytic leukocyte (neutrophil or macrophage) that has engulfed the denatured nucleus of an injured cell is positive. Rarely done nowadays.

Imaging

- Chest X-ray: To exclude other pathology, for pulmonary and cardiac pathology.
- High resolution CT: To demonstrate fibrotic lung.
- Magnetic resonance imaging (MRI) of brain or spinal cord in cases with central nervous system disease involvement.
- Echocardiography to diagnose pericardial and endocardial involvement.

Diagnostic Criteria for Systemic Lupus Erythematosus

Q. List the diagnostic criteria/revised American Rheumatism Association criteria for systemic lupus erythematosus (SLE).

The clinical presentation of SLE is so variable that the American College of Rheumatology has established a complex set of criteria **(Table 9.15)**.

TABLE 9.15: 2019 European League Against Rheumatism (EULAR)/American College of Rheumatology (ACR) classification criteria for systemic lupus erythematosus.

Entry criterion ***Antinuclear antibodies (ANA) at a titer of ≥:80 on HEp-2 cells or an equivalent positive test (ever)***			
If absent, do not classify as SLE; If present, apply additive criteria			
Additive criteria			
Do not count a criterion if there is a more likely explanation than SLE. Occurrence of a criterion on at least one occasion is sufficient. SLE classification requires at least one clinical criterion and ≥10 points.		Criteria need not occur simultaneously. Within each domain, only the highest weighted criterion is counted toward the total score§	
Clinical domains and criteria	**Weight**	**Immunology domains and criteria**	**Weight**
Constitutional Fever	 2	**Antiphospholipid antibodies** Anti-cardiolipin antibodies **OR** Anti-β2GP1 antibodies **OR** Lupus anticoagulant	 2
Hematologic Leukopenia Thrombocytopenia Autoimmune hemolysis	 3 4 4	 **Complement proteins** Low C3 **OR** low C4 Low C3 **AND** low C4	 3 4
Neuropsychiatric Delirium Psychosis Seizure	 2 3 5	**SLE-specific antibodies** Anti-ds DNA antibody* **OR** Anti-Smith antibody	 6
Mucocutaneous Non-scarring alopecia Oral ulcers Subacute cutaneous OR discoid lupus Acute cutaneous lupus	 2 2 4 6		
Serosal Pleural or pericardial effusion Acute pericarditis	 5 6	**NOTE:** §= additional criteria within the same domain will not be counted; * = in an assay with 90% specificity against relevant disease controls. Anti = β2GPI = anti-β2-glycoprotein I; antl-ds-DNA = anti-double stranded DNA.	

Contd...

Contd...

Musculoskeletal Joint involvement	
Renal	
Proteinuria >0.5g/24h	4
Renal biopsy Class II or V lupus nephritis	8
Renal biopsy Class III or IV lupus nephritis	10
Total score	
Classify as Systemic Lupus Erythematosus with a score of 10 or more if entry criterion fulfilled	

Systemic Lupus International Collaborating Clinics (SLICC) Classification 2012 criteria* **(Table 9.16)**.

TABLE 9.16: Systemic Lupus International Collaborating Clinics (SLICC) Classification 2012 criteria.

Lupus nephritis proved by biopsy and ANA or anti-DNA or at least 4 criteria (1 needs to be immunological)	
Clinical	***Immunological***
➢ Acute cutaneous LE	➢ ANA
➢ Chronic cutaneous LE	➢ Anti-dsDNA
➢ Oral ulcer	➢ Anti-Sm
➢ Alopecia	➢ aPL antibodies
➢ Synovitis	➢ Low complement
➢ Serositis	➢ Direct Coombs' test positive
➢ Renal	
➢ Neurologic	
➢ Hemolytic anemia	
➢ Leukopenia/lymphopenia	
➢ Thrombocytopenia	

Differences between rheumatoid arthritis and systemic lupus erythematosus are presented in **Table 9.17**.

TABLE 9.17: Differences between rheumatoid arthritis and systemic lupus erythematosus.

Features	***Rheumatoid arthritis***	***Systemic lupus erythematosus***
Smoking	Predisposing factor	No relation
Female:Male	3:1	9:1
Type of arthritis	Erosive	Non-erosive
Deformities	Common	Rare, Jaccoud's arthropathy (10%)
Systemic involvement	Relatively less	Marked
Nodules	Rheumatoid nodules	Absent
Malar (skin) rash	Nil	Striking feature: malar rash, discoid rash
Photosensitivity	Absent	Photosensitivity present
Oral ulcer and alopecia	Absent	Present
Spine involvement	Involves cervical spine	Rare
Pyoderma gangrenosum	May develop	Rare
Renal involvement	Uncommon	Common and severe
Platelet abnormality	Thrombocythemia	Thrombocytopenia
Serology	RA factor and ACPA	ANA and anti-dsDNA
Criteria for diagnosis	ACR/EULAR	SLICC/ACR
Response to DMARDs	Present	Less response

(ACPA: anticyclic citrullinated peptide antibodies; ANA: antinuclear antibodies; ds: double stranded; ACR: American college of rheumatology; EULAR: European league against rheumatism; SLICC: systemic lupus international collaborating clinics classification)

Management (Flowchart 9.3)

Q. Describe the management principles of systemic lupus erythematosus.

General

- To avoid known triggers of disease exacerbation, such as ultraviolet light, smoking cessation.
- Need for adequate rest.

Conservative therapies for management of non-life-threatening disease

In patients with fatigue, pain, and autoantibodies of SLE, but without major organ involvement are managed by analgesics (**NSAIDs**), antimalarials (**hydroxychloroquine**, chloroquine, and quinacrine) and **low-dose corticosteroids**. Skin lesions and arthritis also respond to hydroxychloroquine. Photosensitive skin lesions need application of sun-screen lotions.

FLOWCHART 9.3: Treatment algorithm for systemic lupus erythematosus.

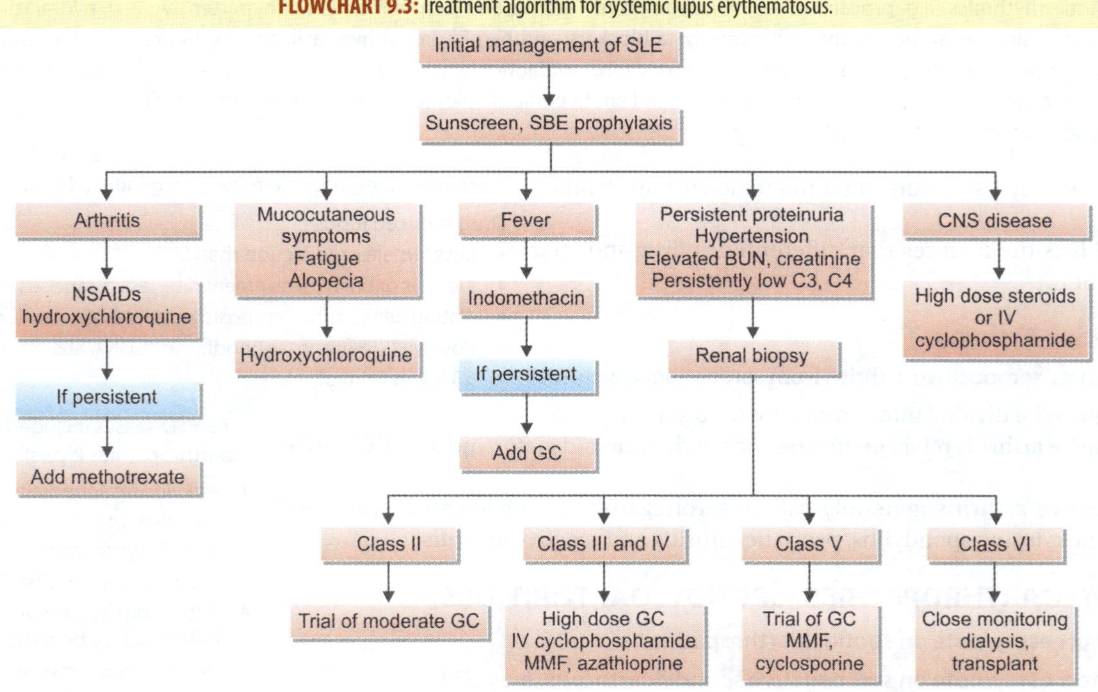

Mild SLE		Moderate to severe SLE	
Constitutional symptoms	HCQ with or without low dose systemic GC or methotrexate; then azathioprine, methotrexate or mycophenolate; then Rituximab or Belimumab	**Alveolitis**	Systemic GC + Mycophenolate or IV Cyclophosphamide; then add rituximab or IV immunoglobulin, maintain with azathioprine or mycophenolate
		Antiphospholipid syndrome	Anticoagulation, with or without HCQ, then add direct thrombin inhibitor
Discoid lupus	Sunscreen, topical corticosteroids, tacrolimus, topical acitretin, with or without HCQ, with ow without systemic glucocorticoids, then add azathioprine or switch with mycophenolate or methotrexate	**Mononeuritis**	Systemic GC with or without IV cyclophosphamide, then add rituximab, IV immunoglobulin or plasmapheresis
		Thrombocytopenia	Systemic GC with or without HCQ, then add azathioprine or mycophenolate, then add rituximab or IV cyclophosphamide or IV immunoglobulin
Polyarthritis	HCQ with or without low dose systemic glucocorticoids, then add methotrexate or rituximab, NSAIDs-adjunctive therapy	**Lupus nephritis**	Systemic GC + mycophenolate, then IV cyclophosphamide, then add rituximab or switch to azathioprine; angiotensin-converting enzyme inhibitor and HCQ as adjunctive therapy
Uncomplicated digital or cutaneous vasculitis	Systemic glucocorticoids, with or without HCQ, with or without methotrexate then add azathioprine or mycophenolate, then switch to IV cyclophosphamide	**Myocarditis**	Systemic GC + IV cyclophosphamide, with or without HCQ, then rituximab, belimumab or IV immunoglobulin
		Pericarditis	NSAIDs, systemic GCs + HCQ, then add mycophenolate, azathioprine or methotrexate; then add belimumab or rituximab
		Pulmonary artery hypertension	Systemic GC + IV cyclophosphamide, or mycophenolate + endothelin receptor antagonist, then add rituximab and PDE-5 inhibitor, then add prostaglandin analogue and maintain with it.

Life-threatening SLE: Proliferative forms of lupus nephritis

- Life-threatening SLE or patients with severe symptoms should receive **corticosteroids**.
- Acutely ill patients and patients with active proliferative glomerulonephritis may be treated with prednisone at 60 mg daily or 1 g of intravenous methylprednisolone administered daily for 3 days.
- **Immunosuppressive agents:** These include azathioprine, methotrexate, cyclophosphamide, my cophenolate mofetil and are also useful in controlling severe disease. They are particularly useful in patients with renal involvement. A combination of intravenous cyclophosphamide and steroids is the most effective regimen. Following intravenouscyclophosphamide, oral mycophenolate mofetil is an alternative to maintain remission.
- Drugs targeting B-cell pathways, such as belimumab and rituximab are used in refractory cases.

Drug-induced Lupus

Q. Write short essay/note on drug-induced lupus.

It is a syndrome consisting of positive ANA associated with symptoms such as fever, malaise, arthritis or intense arthralgias/myalgias, serositis, and/or rash.

Etiology: The syndrome develops during therapy with certain medications and includes:

- **Drugs:** Antiarrhythmics (e.g. procainamide, diltiazem, disopyramide, and propafenone), antihypertensive (e.g. hydralazine), methyl dopa, angiotensin-converting enzyme inhibitors, beta blockers, antithyroid propylthiouracil, antipsychotics (e.g. chlorpromazine and lithium), anticonvulsants (e.g. carbamazepine and phenytoin), antibiotics (e.g. isoniazid, minocycline, and macrodantin), antirheumatic (e.g. sulfasalazine), diuretic (e.g. hydrochlorothiazide) and antihyperlipidemics (e.g. lovastatin and simvastatin).
- **Biologic agents:** Interferons and TNF inhibitors.

Symptoms: Usually resolve after discontinuation of the offending drug.

Box 9.5 lists the features that differentiates drug-induced lupus from SLE.

Box 9.5: Features that differentiate drug-induced lupus from SLE.

Drug-induced lupus
- Less female predilection than SLE
- Kidneys or brain involvement rare, less cutaneous involvement
- Antinuclear antibodies positive; antihistone antibodies
- Positive (95%); autoantibodies to dsDNA absent
- C3 levels normal

Seronegative Arthritis

Q. Differentiate seropositive arthritis from seronegative arthritis.

- Arthritis can be divided into seropositive and seronegative.
- Seropositive arthritis refers to the presence of rheumatoid factor and anti-CCP in the blood.
- Seronegative arthritis generally called 'seronegative spondyloarthropathy' and include ankylosing spondylitis, psoriatic arthritis and reactive arthritis.

Box 9.6: Diseases included under spondyloarthropathies (SpAs).

1. Ankylosing spondylitis (AnS)
2. Reactive arthritis (ReA) (including Reiter's syndrome)
3. Psoriatic arthritis (PsA)
4. Arthropathy associated with inflammatory bowel disease
5. Undifferentiated spondyloarthritis

SPONDYLOARTHROPATHIES (SPONDYLOARTHRITIDES)

Q. Write short essay/note on spondyloarthropathies.

Q. Write short essay/note on seronegative spondyloarthropathies (SSA).

Definition: The spondyloarthropathies (SpAs) are a group of related inflammatory joint diseases **(Box 9.6)** that share clinical features and genetic susceptibility.

Common Features of SpAs

1. **Common clinical features:**
   - Strong predilection for the **spine**, in particular the **sacroiliac joints. Inflammatory back pain** due to sacroiliitis and spondylitis.
   - **Tendency for new bone formation** at sites of chronic inflammation, with **joint ankylosis** as a consequence.
   - If **peripheral arthritis** occurs, it is usually in the **lower extremity and asymmetrical**.
   - **Predilection for sites of tendon insertion into bone (enthesis). Enthesitis** is inflammation at sites where tendons, ligaments or joint capsules attach to bone and is one of the **most specific clinical manifestations** of the SpAs.
   - RF negative; hence, known as **'seronegative'**.
2. **Common genetic predisposing factor:** All subsets have an association with **HLA-B27 allele.**

Ankylosing Spondylitis

Q. Discuss the clinical features, diagnosis and management ankylosing spondylitis, rheumatoid spondylitis or Bekhterev-Strümpell-Marie disease.

Ankylosing spondylitis (AnS) is a chronic inflammatory disorder of unknown causes that primarily affects the axial skeleton (predominantly sacroiliac joints and spine). The peripheral joints and extra-articular structures are also frequently involved.

Age and gender: Usually begins in the second or third decade; male to female ratio is between 2:1 and 3:1.

Clinical Features

Targets in ankylosing spondylitis (Fig. 9.5): Mainly involves spine, sacroiliac joints and large peripheral joints (hip, shoulder) in an asymmetrical pattern.

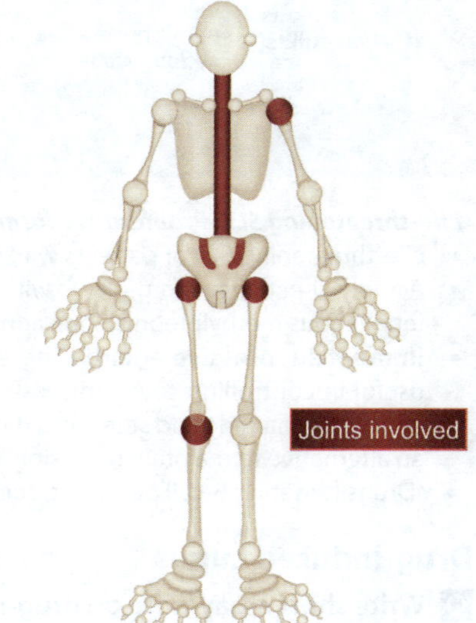

FIG. 9.5: Pattern of joint involvement in ankylosing spondylitis.

Involvement of lumbar spine

- Classical presentation is the **insidious onset of inflammatory low back pain**. The pain is dull and located in the lower lumbar regions or gluteal region and shows nocturnal exacerbation.
- Back pain persists for >3 months. It is accompanied by **early-morning stiffness** that typically **improves with activity**/exercise and **exacerbated by inactivity**.
- "Inflammatory back pain" typically exhibits at least four of the following five features:
  - Age of onset <40 years
  - Insidious onset

    - Improvement with exercise
    - No improvement with rest
    - Pain at night
- **Physical examination:** Physical examination of the spine shows loss of spinal mobility in all directions and pain on sacroiliac stressing.
- **Modified Schober test:** Used to measure lumbar spine flexion. The patient stands upright with heels together. Two marks are made on the spine; one at the lumbosacral junction (identified by a horizontal line between the posterosuperior iliac spines) and another 10 cm above. The patient then bends forward maximally with knees fully extended. The distance between the two marks is measured. This distance increases by >5 cm in the case of normal mobility and by <4 cm in the case of decreased mobility.

Involvement of sacroiliac joint

The tests mentioned below produce stress and pain in the sacroiliac joint.

- **Patrick's test** (figure of 4 test): Pain in the sacroiliac joints may be elicited either by direct pressure or by maneuvers that stress the joint, namely, Patrick's test. One leg is guided into 'figure of 4' position with the ipsilateral ankle resting across the contralateral thigh. The ipsilateral knee is then pressed downwards with one hand while providing counter pressure with the other hand on the contralateral anterior superior iliac spine.
- **FABER (flexion abduction external rotation) maneuver:** Patient lies supine while the examiner flexes and externally rotates the hip.
- **Gaenslen's maneuver:** The examiner extends the hip by letting the leg dangle off the side of the examining table.
- Occiput to wall test **(Flesch test):** Normally zero, in AnS it is increased.

Enthesitis

- Enthesitis is inflammation at the sites of tendon/ligament insertions.
- **Heel pain** due to inflammation at the **Achilles tendon** (Achilles tendinitis) and **plantar fascia** (plantar fasciitis) at calcaneal insertions is common. Like arthritis, enthesitis is also aggravated by rest and improved with activity.
- Other sites of enthesitis include superior and inferior aspects of patella, metatarsal heads and spinal ligament insertions on vertebral bodies.

Other sites

- Involvement of the thoracic spine, costovertebral joints and costosternal joints leads to chest pain, reduced expansion of chest (<5 cm) and thoracic kyphosis.
- Involvement of the cervical spine produces neck pain and a forward stoop of the neck.
- Peripheral arthritis usually occurs late and asymmetric. Involvement of hips and shoulders result in pain and limitation of movement.
- **Dactylitis (sausage digits)** is characterized by diffuse swelling of toes or fingers.

Extra-articular manifestations

See **Table 9.18.**

TABLE 9.18: Extra-articular manifestations of ankylosing spondylitis.

➢ Acute anterior uveitis (iritis) ➢ Inflammatory bowel disease ➢ Aortic insufficiency, cardiac conduction defects and heart failure ➢ Psoriasis ➢ Pulmonary fibrosis and cavitation (apical)	➢ Osteoporosis ➢ Myelopathy secondary to atlantoaxial subluxation and spinal fracture ➢ Cauda equina syndrome ➢ Amyloidosis

Investigations

Describe the diagnostic work up and management of ankylosing spondylitis.

- Erythrocyte sedimentation rate (ESR) and C-reactive protein: Raised.
- Tests for rheumatoid factor (RF): Negative.
- Anti-cyclic citrullinated peptide (CCP) and antinuclear antibodies (ANAs): Negative.
- **HLA-B27: Present in >90% cases.** High sensitivity and specificity.
- MRI and bone scan: They can detect early sacroiliitis.

Radiographic Findings

X-ray

- **Sacroiliac joint:** The medial and lateral cortical margins of both sacroiliac joints lose definition owing to erosions. They show irregularity and loss of cortical margins (blurring of the cortical margins of the subchondral bone), erosions in the joint line, and 'pseudowidening' of the joint space. Subsequently, it shows subchondral sclerosis, joint space narrowing and fusion, bony ankylosis reflecting complete bony replacement of the sacroiliac joints.
- **Lumbar spine:** Radiographs of the spine may show anterior '**squaring**' (loss of the normal anterior concavity of the lumbar vertebra), 'shiny corners' (subchondral sclerosis at the upper edge of the vertebral body), or even 'barreling' of one or more vertebral bodies due to erosion and sclerosis of the anterior corners of vertebrae with subsequent erosion. These are manifestations of enthesitis.

- **Bridging syndesmophytes** are areas of calcification that follow the outermost fibers of the annulus and may also be seen in AS. Progressive ossification may lead to formation of **marginal syndesmophytes** make the diagnosis clear. They are observed as bony bridges connecting successive vertebral bodies anteriorly and laterally. In advanced disease, ossification of the anterior longitudinal ligament and facet joint fusion may also be seen. Eventually, the changes may result in a **'bamboo spine' (Fig. 9.6)**, so called because the multiple bridging syndesmophytes (bridging the intervertebral spaces) can mimic the appearance of bamboo.
- Diffuse osteoporosis of spine and atlantoaxial dislocation can be seen as late feature. Erosive changes may be observed in the symphysis pubis, the ischial tuberosities and peripheral joints.

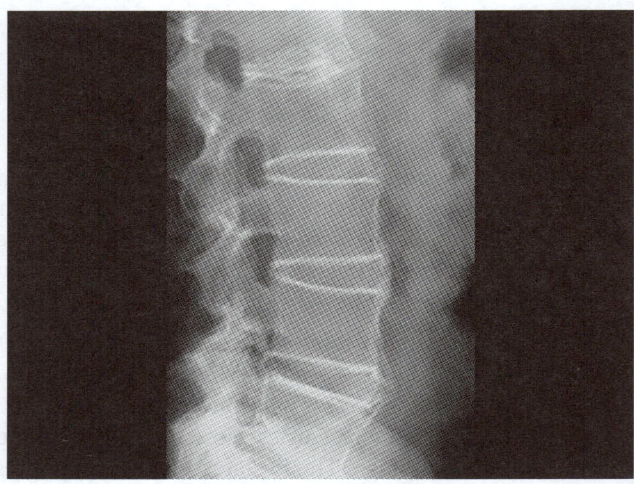

FIG. 9.6: Bamboo spine in ankylosing spondylitis.

Magnetic resonance imaging (MRI)

MRI is **much more sensitive** for detection of early sacroiliitis than X-ray and can also detect inflammatory changes in the lumbar spine.

Diagnostic Criteria (Box 9.7)

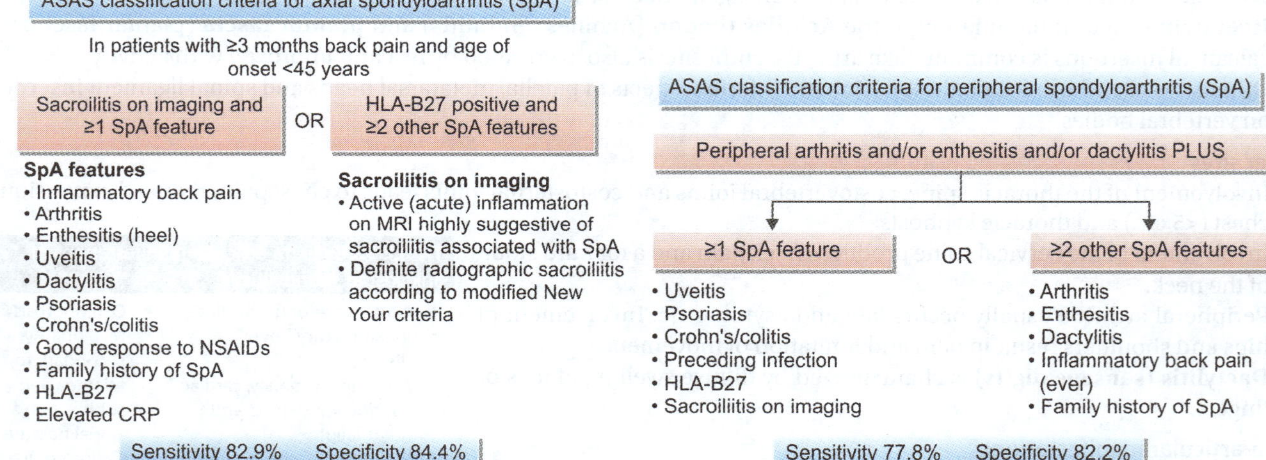

Management

- Early diagnosis is important to maintain posture and range of motion.
- Regular exercise is started with active and passive physiotherapy before syndesmophytes have formed.
- Symptomatic relief of pain and stiffness can be obtained with long-acting or slow-release NSAID or an NSAID suppository improves sleep, peripheral arthritis and enthesitis are managed with NSAIDs or local steroid injections. Indomethacin is the most effective drug and may be given up to a maximum dose of 100 mg/day. Systemic glucocorticoids have limited role.
- **Sulfasalazine and methotrexate** are useful to control effective for peripheral arthritis but not for spinal disease.
  - Peripheral arthritis and enthesitis are managed with NSAIDs or local steroid injections. Rarely systemic corticosteroids may be necessary.

Anti-tumor necrosis factor therapy

Biologic agents, such as monoclonal antibodies to TNF-α **(infliximab, adalimumab, certolizumab, golimumab)** or the soluble TNF receptor **(etanercept)** are options for patients with active ankylosing spondylitis who are not satisfactorily responded to NSAIDs. Duration of treatment is 2–3 years.

Box 9.7: Modified New York Criteria (1984) for ankylosing spondylitis.

Clinical criteria

- Low back pain and stiffness for >3 months that improve with exercise but are not relieved by rest
- Limitation of motion of the lumbar spine in both sagittal and frontal planes
- Limitation of chest expansion

Radiologic criteria

- Sacroiliitis: Grade ≥2 bilateral *or* grade 3 or 4 unilateral

Grading

Definite AS (ankylosing spondylitis) if the radiologic criterion is associated with at least one clinical variable.

Probable ankylosing spondylitis (AS) if:

- The three clinical criteria are present
- The radiologic criterion is present without the clinical criteria

Dosage
- Infliximab: 3–5 mg/kg body weight intravenously every 6–8 weeks.
- Etanercept: 25 mg subcutaneously twice a week initially/50 mg once weekly.
- Adalimumab: 40 mg biweekly by subcutaneous injection.
- Golimumab: 50 or 100 mg every 4 weeks, given by subcutaneous injection.

Secukinumab is an interleukin-17 monoclonal antibody that has been approved for treatment of ankylosing spondylitis.

Others
- Reconstructive surgery
- Pamidronate
- Control of uveitis by local steroids.

Reactive Arthritis

Q. Describe the etiology, clinical features, diagnosis and management of reactive arthritis.

Q. Write a short note on Reiter's syndrome.

- Reactive arthritis (ReA) refers to **acute nonpurulent arthritis** (aseptic arthritis) **complicating an extra-articular infection** elsewhere in the body, most typically enteric (GIT) or urogenital (GU tract) infections.
- **Classical triad of Reiter's syndrome** is (1) **nonspecific urethritis**, (2) **conjunctivitis** and (3) **arthritis.** However, the term is no longer in common use.

Etiology

- **GIT infections:** Common enteric organisms that trigger include *Salmonella typhimurium, Shigella flexneri, Yersinia enterocolitica, Escherichia coli, Clostridum difficile*, and *Chlamydia*.
- **GUT infection:** Common urogential organisms are *Chlamydia trachomatis* or *Ureaplasma urealyticum*.
- More than 75% of ReA patients have the histocompatibility antigen HLA-B27.

Clinical Features

- **Age and gender:** Predominantly a disease of young (18–40 years) men, with a male preponderance of 15:1.
- **Constitutional symptoms** are common and include fatigue, malaise, fever, and weight loss.
- **Arthritis:** Arthritis is typically an acute, asymmetrical, lower limb (e.g. knees, ankles, midtarsal and MTP joints) arthritis and occurs 1 to 3 weeks after the GIT or GUT infection, arthritis usually persists for 3–5 months.
- **Enthesitis** is common.
- **Dactylitis** or **'sausage digit,'** is a diffuse swelling of a solitary finger or toe may also be seen. It is the result of inflammatory changes affecting the joint capsule, entheses, periarticular structures, and periosteal bone.
- Sacroiliitis may be seen in 25% patients.
- **Extra-articular features**
  - **Urogenital lesions:** Urethritis and prostatitis in males, cervicitis or salpingitis in females.
  - **Mucocutaneous lesions:** *Circinate balanitis* (a painless erythematous lesion of the glans penis), *keratoderma blennorrhagica* (hyperkeratotic lesions on the palms of the hands or the soles of the feet) and nail dystrophy.
  - **Ocular disease:** Common and includes conjunctivitis, anterior uveitis and acute iritis.
  - **Others:** Cardiac conduction defects, aortic regurgitation, central or peripheral nervous system lesions, and pleuropulmonary infiltrates.
- Usually a self-limiting course of 3–12 months. About 50% of patients develop recurrent bouts of arthritis and 15–30% develop chronic arthritis or sacroiliitis.

Investigations

- Erythrocyte sedimentation rate (**ESR**) and acute-phase reactants: Usually **raised**.
- **Peripheral blood:** Anemia and polymorphonuclear leukocytosis.
- **Synovial fluid:** Characteristic synovial fluid is **leukocyte-rich** (>2000 white blood cells/mL with a predominance of neutrophils) and may contain multinucleated macrophages (Reiter's cells).
- **HLA-B27: Positive** in more than 75% of cases.
- Serum tests for rheumatoid factor and antinuclear antibodies: Negative.
- **Urethritis:** Confirmed in the 'two-glass test' by demonstration of mucoid threads in the first-void specimen that clears in the second specimen.

Radiological features
- Shows periarticular osteoporosis, joint space narrowing and proliferative erosions in chronic or recurrent disease.
- Periostitis, especially of metatarsals, phalanges and pelvis, and large, fluffy calcaneal spurs at the insertion of the plantar fascia. Sacroiliitis (less common than ankylosing spondylitis) is often asymmetrical and sometimes unilateral.

Syndesmophytes are predominantly coarse and asymmetrical, often extending beyond the contours of the annulus ('non-marginal').

Management
- **Acute attack:**
  - Treated with rest, oral NSAIDs and analgesics. Indomethacin, 75–150 mg/d in divided doses, is the initial treatment of choice.
  - Intra-articular or local steroid injections and rarely systemic steroids in severe cases.
- **Non-specific chlamydial urethritis:** Treated with **doxycycline or ciprofloxacin** or a single dose of azithromycin course.
- No role of antibiotics in reactive spondyloarthropathy secondary to enteric infections.
- **Sulfasalazine, azathioprine and methotrexate** may be useful in patients with disabling relapsing and remitting arthritis.
- **DMARDs:** For patients with persistent marked symptoms, recurrent arthritis or severe keratoderma blennorrhagica.
- Anterior uveitis is a medical emergency and treated by topical, subconjunctival or systemic corticosteroids.
- **TNF-α blocking agents** are the drugs of next choice in severe and persistent disease.

Psoriatic Arthritis

Q. Write short note on psoriatic arthritis.

- Psoriatic arthritis (PsA) is a seronegative inflammatory arthritis that characteristically occurs in patient with psoriasis, a past or family history of psoriasis or with characteristic nail changes.
- Occurs in about 7–20% of patients of psoriasis.

Types: Wright and Moll described five patterns of psoriatic arthritis **(Box 9.8)**

Newer pattern of psoriatic arthritis is described in **HIV patients.**

Box 9.8: Patterns of psoriatic arthritis.

1. Asymmetric inflammatory oligoarthritis
2. Symmetric polyarthritis similar to RA (rheumatoid arthritis)
3. Arthritis of the DIP (distal interphalangeal) joints
4. Spondyloarthropathy (sacroiliitis and spondylitis)
5. Arthritis mutilans

Clinical Features

It presents with pain and swelling affected joints and enthesitis.

- **Asymmetrical inflammatory oligoarthritis:** Most characteristically occur in the hands and feet, when synovitis is associated with tenosynovitis, enthesitis and inflammation of intervening tissue resulting in a **'sausage-shaped digit' or dactylitis**. Usually, less than four joints are involved (oligoarthritis).
- **Symmetrical polyarthritis:** It is more common in women and may strongly resemble RA.
- **Arthritis of the DIP joints:** Uncommon and affects men more than women. It involves finger DIP joints and surrounding periarticular tissues, and is accompanied by nail dystrophy.
- **Psoriatic spondylitis:** Presents similar to AS but with less severe involvement. It is typically unilateral or asymmetric in severity.
- **Arthritis mutilans** is a severe, deforming erosive arthritis accompanied by prominent cartilage and bone destruction results in marked instability of fingers and toes. The encasing skin appears invaginated and 'telescoped' and the finger can be pulled back to its original length.
- ***Enthesitis and tenosynovitis is common.***
- **Skin lesions:** Characteristic skin lesion of psoriasis may be present.
- **Nail changes (Fig. 9.7):** Psoriatic nail dystrophy, onycholysis, pitting, and hyperkeratosis observed in nearly 80% patients with arthritis.
- **Uveitis:** Unilateral or bilateral and is generally chronic.

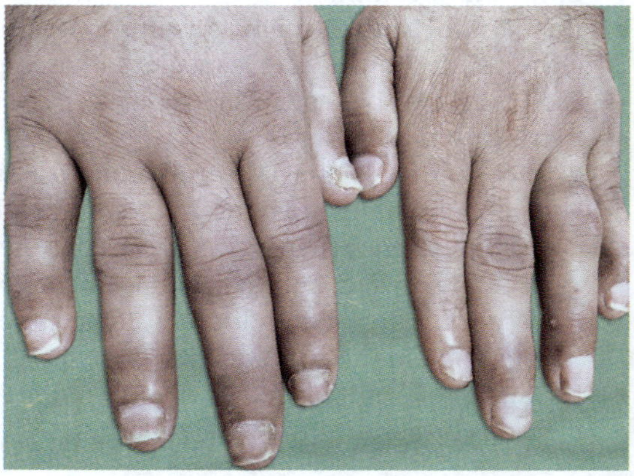

FIG. 9.7: Sausage digits in psoriatic arthritis and psoriatic nails.

Q. Differentiate psoriatic arthritis from rheumatoid arthritis (Table 9.19).

Diagnosis

- Acute phase reactants (ESR and CRP): Raised in active disease.
- Rheumatoid factor and antinuclear antibodies: Negative.
- Radiological findings: May be normal or show erosive change with joint space narrowing similar to those of RA, but osteoporosis is relatively less common. Distal interphalangeal joints may show **'pencil-in-cup' changes (Fig. 9.8)** because of marked resorption of bone. Other findings include enthesitis with periosteal reaction, sacroiliitis and spondylitis.
- MRI and ultrasound with power Doppler are used to detect synovial inflammation and inflammation at the enthuses (enthesitis). *Classification of Psoriatic Arthritis (CASPAR)* criteria is used for diagnosis which include *skin lesions, nail changes, negative RF, dactylitis and juxta-articular bone formation*—3 out of 5 need to be present.

Management

- NSAIDs and analgesics may be sufficient to control symptoms in mild disease.
- Local synovitis may be treated by intra-articular corticosteroid injections.
- DMARDs for persistent synovitis unresponsive to conservative treatment. Sulfasalazine or methotrexate slows the development of joint damage.
- Anti-TNF-α agents (e.g. etanercept, golimumab, infliximab and adalimumab) should be considered for patients with active synovitis who respond inadequately to standard DMARDs.
- Hydroxychloroquine must be avoided as it can cause exfoliative skin reactions.
- **Alefacept** is a fusion protein of soluble lymphocyte function antigen 3 with Fc fragments of IgG1. It is used for moderate-to-severe psoriasis and associated arthritis.

TABLE 9.19: Distinguishing clinical features of psoriatic arthritis from rheumatoid arthritis.

	Psoriatic arthritis	***Rheumatoid arthritis***
Psoriasis	+	-
Symmetric involvement	+	++
Asymmetric involvement	++	+
Enthesopathy	+	-
Dactylitis	+	-
Nail dystrophy, psoriatic skin lesions	+	-
HIV association	+	-
DIP (distal interphalangeal) involvement	+	-
Inflammatory LBA (low backache)	+	-
Sacroiliac joint involvement	+	-

(+: present; –: absent)

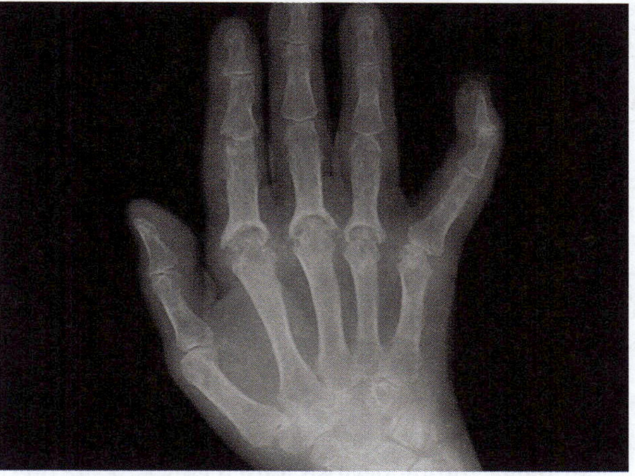

FIG. 9.8: X-ray of hand shows pencil-in-cup appearance in psoriatic arthritis.

Enteropathic Arthritis

Q. Write short note on spondyloarthropathy associated with inflammatory bowel disease.

Also called as enteropathic arthritis associated with inflammatory bowel disease (ulcerative colitis and Crohn's disease).
An acute inflammatory oligoarthritis occurs in 10–20% of patients with inflammatory bowel disease (IBD).
More often in patients with Crohn's disease than in those with ulcerative colitis.

Clinical Features

Peripheral arthritis

- The arthritis is asymmetrical, inflammatory, nonerosive polyarthritis and mainly involves lower-limb joints (knees, ankles, hips).
- The clinical activity of the peripheral arthritis parallels the activity of the gut inflammation. Effective treatment of the GI disease usually controls the joint disease as well.
- It is not associated with HLA-B27 and follows a transient course.

Sacroiliitis

- It is clinically and radiologically similar to classic AS.
- It can manifest before or after the onset of IBD and there is no correlation between activity of the spondylitis and bowel disease.
- HLA-B27 is found in 50% of patients and it follows a chronic course.

Others: Enthesitis, dactylitis and extra-articular manifestations of IBD.

Treatment

- NSAIDs to be used cautiously because they may worsen diarrhea.
- Monoarthritis is treated by intra-articular corticosteroids.
- Sulfasalazine more effective as it may help both bowel and joint disease. Azathioprine and methotrexate may also be used.
- TNF-α blocking drug infliximab used for IBD can help the arthritis.

Differences between inflammatory and mechanical low back pain (LBP) (Table 9.20).

Q. Describe the clinical clues to differentiate inflammatory low back pain of ankylosing spondylitis from mechanical low back pain?

Q. Differentiate between inflammatory versus mechanical back pain.

TABLE 9.20: Differences between inflammatory and mechanical low back pain (LBP).

Features	*Inflammatory LBP*	*Mechanical LBP*
Age at onset	< 40 years	Any age
Type of onset	Insidious	Acute
Symptom duration	>3 months	<4 weeks
Morning stiffness	>60 minutes	<30 minutes
Nocturnal pain	Frequent	Absent
Effect of exercise	Improvement	Exacerbation
Sacroiliac joint tenderness	Frequent	Absent
Back mobility	Loss in all planes	Abnormal flexion
Chest expansion	Often decreased	Normal
Neurologic deficits	Unusual	Possible

ADULT ONSET STILL'S DISEASE (AOSD)

Q. Discuss the clinical features of adult onset still's disease.

AOSD is a rare inflammatory multisystem disease occurring in adults presenting as fever (quotidian/double quotidian), rash, arthritis, sore throat, hepatosplenomegaly and serositis (pleural and pericardial effusion).

The rash is classically evanescent, salmon-colored, macular or maculopapular which is usually nonpruritic and occurs with the fever. Arthritis and arthralgia mostly involve the knee, wrist and the ankle. Myalgia is seen in more than 50 percent of the cases. Macrophage activation syndrome, a rare and fatal complication of Adult Onset Still's disease characterized by leukopenia, hypertriglyceridemia, transaminitis and intavascular coagulation.

Diagnosis

- Adult Onset Still's disease (ASOD) is primarily a diagnosis of exclusion.
- Neutrophilia, thrombocytosis, raised ESR, CRP are present. Increased LDH and liver enzymes are seen
- Marked elevation of ferritin (>3000 mg/ml) found in more than 70 % of patients. Reduced level (<20%) of glycosylated fraction of ferritin is a more useful marker.
- RF and ANA are negative.
- Yamaguchi criteria is the accepted diagnostic criteria.

Treatment

- Often a self limited disease, rarely can have an intermittent flares and chronic articular form.
- NSAID's and glucocorticoids can be given to reduce systemic inflammation.
- DMARD's like methotrexate may be used as steroid sparing agents.
- Anti-TNF alpha antagonist and IL-1 antagonist (Anakinra) and cyclosporine can be used for patients presenting with macrophage activation syndrome.

JUVENILE IDIOPATHIC ARTHRITIS/JUVENILE RHEUMATOID ARTHRITIS

- Formerly called Still's disease
- Onset is before 16 years of age, manifestations persist for at least 6 weeks, and the etiology is unknown.
- JIA can manifest with following clinical types
  - Systemic arthritis associated with fever, rash, lymphadenopathy and organomegaly
  - Polyarthritis, involvement of 4 or more joint areas. RF may be positive or negative
  - Oligoarthritis, involving 4 or less joint areas
  - Enthesitis related arthritis
  - Psoriatic arthritis
  - Undifferentiated arthritis
- Other features include polyserositis and macrophage activation syndrome
- Mild to disease responds to NSAIDs and steroids
- Biologic agents, such as anakinra, canakinumab, or tocilizumab are useful in severe disease and systemic complications.

VASCULITIS

Q. Define and classify vasculitis.

Definition: Vasculitis refers to a heterogeneous group of disorders that is characterized by destructive inflammation of blood vessel walls. The lumen of the inflamed blood vessels is liable to occlude or rupture or develop a thrombus, and this is associated with ischemia of the tissues supplied by the involved vessel.

Classification (Fig. 9.9)

Vasculitis may involve a single organ (e.g. skin), or it may involve several organ systems. One of the basis for classifying the vasculitides is the size of the predominant blood vessels involved (**Box 9.9**).

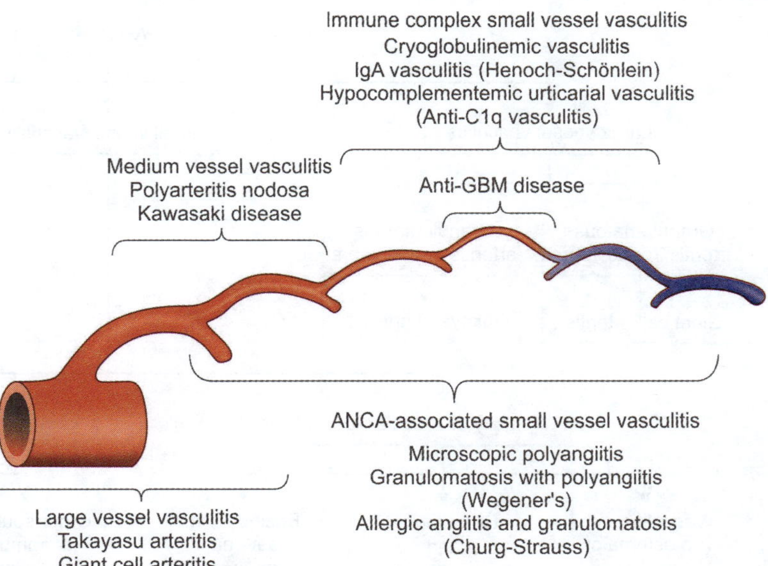

FIG. 9.9: Classification of vasculitis.

Box 9.9: Classification of the primary vasculitides according to size of predominant blood vessels involved (Chapel Hill Consensus Conference).

Predominantly large-vessel (aorta and its major tributaries) vasculitis
- Giant cell arteritis
- Takayasu arteritis
- Cogan syndrome

Predominantly medium-vessel (medium and small-sized arteries and arterioles) vasculitis
- Polyarteritis nodosa
- Primary central nervous system disease
- Buerger disease

Predominantly small-vessel (small arteries, arterioles, venules and capillaries) vasculitis
- ANCA-associated small-vessel vasculitis
  - Granulomatosis with polyangiitis (Wegener granulomatosis)
  - Microscopic polyangiitis
  - Churg-Strauss syndrome (allergic angiitis and granulomatosis)
  - Drug-induced ANCA-associated vasculitis
- Immune complex mediated
  - Cutaneous leukocytoclastic angiitis ('hypersensitivity' vasculitis)
  - Henoch-Schönlein purpura
  - Urticarial vasculitis

Clinical Manifestations

Q. Write short essay/note on clinical features of vasculitis.

Constitutional symptoms: Fever, weight loss, malaise, arthralgias/arthritis (common to vasculitides of all vessel sizes). Typical clinical manifestations of large, medium, and small vessel vasculitis are presented in **Table 9.21** and vasculitis associated with granulomatous inflammation is listed in **Table 9.22**.

TABLE 9.21: Typical clinical manifestations of vasculitis.

Large	*Medium*	*Small*
Limb claudication	Cutaneous	Purpura
Assymetric blood pressure	Nodules	Vesiculobullous lesions
Absence of pulses	Ulcers	Urticaria
Bruits	Livedo reticularis	Glomerulonephritis
Aortic dilation	Digital gangrene	Alveolar hemorrhage
Renovascular hypertension	Mononeuritis multiplex	Cutaneous extravascular necrotizing granulomas
	Microaneurysms	Splinter hemorrhages
	Renovascular hypertension	Uveitis/episcleritis/scleritis

TABLE 9.22: Vasculitis associated with granulomatous inflammation.

Giant cell arteritis	Churg-Strauss syndrome
Takayasu's arteritis	Primary angiitis of the central nervous system
Cogan's syndrome	Buerger's disease
Wegener's granulomatosis (granulomatosis with polyangiitis)	Rheumatoid vasculitis

Giant Cell Arteritis (GCA)

Q. Write short essay/note on temporal arteritis, cranial arteritis or giant cell arteritis.

Giant cell arteritis (temporal arteritis, Horton disease or cranial arteritis) is **inflammatory granulomatous arteritis** of large and medium sized **arteries in the head and neck.** It can involve aorta and its primary and secondary branches.

Age and gender: It is a disease of the elderly and average age at onset is 70. It is extremely rare below 60 years of age. Female to male ratio is about 3:1.

Vessels involved: One or more branches of the carotid artery (e.g. temporal artery, occipital, ophthalmic, posterior ciliary arteries and vertebral arteries). It can involve multiple arteries, aorta and its branches.

Clinical Features

- **Onset** may be gradual or sudden.
- **Systemic manifestations:** Severe malaise, tiredness, **fever, anemia, fatigue** and weight loss.
- **Severe headache:** Most severe and often localized along the course of the superficial temporal artery or occipital region. Arteritis often occurs in the carotid/temporal arteries. On palpation, **the involved artery is tender, thickened** and cord-like or **nodular.** It may be accompanied by tenderness of the scalp or of the temple.
- **Jaw claudication:** When chewing, eating or talking, due to ischemia of the masseter muscles.
- **Visual symptoms:** These include loss of visual acuity, reduced color perception and pupillary defects. It can even present as **sudden blindness** in one eye due to occlusion of the posterior ciliary artery.
- **Neurological manifestations:** It occurs in about 30% of patients and includes transient ischemic attacks, brainstem infarcts and hemiparesis.

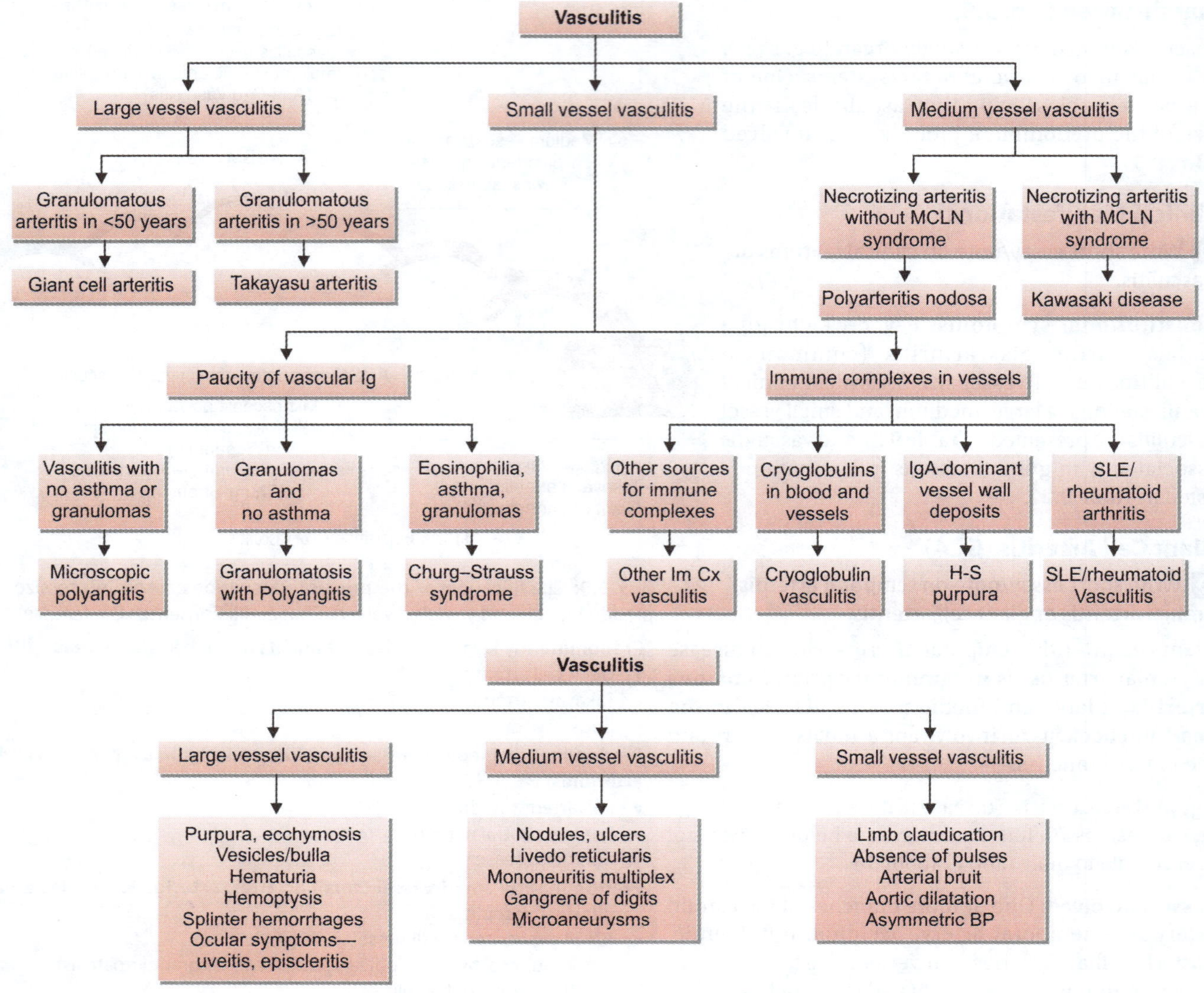

(MCLN: mucocutaneous lymph node; Im Cx: Immune complex; H-S: Henoch-Schönlein)

Investigation

- **Normochromic, normocytic anemia.**
- **ESR** is **raised** (50–120 mm/h) and the **CRP very high.**
- **Temporal artery biopsy** from the affected side is the **definitive diagnostic test**. Characteristic biopsy findings are fragmentation of the internal elastic lamina with necrosis of the media, mixed inflammatory cell infiltrate and granulomatous inflammation of the intima and media with giant cells.
- Color Doppler Ultrasound or arteriography: It may be used for guiding the biopsy. Duplex ultrasonography can detect the characteristic appearance.

Treatment

Corticosteroids are the treatment of choice and should be commenced urgently in suspected giant cell arteritis to prevent the risk of visual loss. It responds dramatically within 24–48 hours of starting corticosteroids. Prednisolone is given at a doseof 40–60 mg/day. NSAIDs should not be used.Tociluzumab and methotrexate have been used as steroid sparing agents.

Polymyalgia Rheumatica (PMR)

Q. Write short note on polymyalgia rheumatica.

PMR is characterized by pain, aching, and stiffness in the muscles of the neck, shoulders, and hip-girdle area that are usually much worse in the morning. PMR is closely associated with GCA (giant cell arteritis).

Criteria for the Diagnosis of PMR (Box 9.10)

Treatment

Corticosteroids: Prednisolone (10–15 mg/day) is rapidly effective. Symptoms are relieved within 48–72 hours and the ESR normalizes after 7–10 days.

Box 9.10: Criteria for the diagnosis of PMR (polymyalgia rheumatica).

- Age >50 years
- Aching and stiffness for at least 1 month, affecting at least two of the three areas (i.e. shoulders, neck, and pelvic girdle)
- Morning stiffness lasting at least 1 hour
- ESR >40 mm/hour
- Exclusion of other diseases except GCA (giant cell arteritis)
- Rapid response to prednisone (20 mg/day)
- All of the above criteria must be met to diagnose PMR

Classic Polyarteritis Nodosa (PAN)

Q. Describe the clinical features, diagnosis and management of classic polyarteritis nodosa (PAN).

Definition: Polyarteritis nodosa is also called classic polyarteritis nodosa is a **systemic, necrotizing vasculitis of small and medium-sized muscular arteries** that **spares the smallest blood vessels** (e.g. arterioles, venules or capillaries). It characteristically involves the **renal and visceral arteries** and is not associated with glomerulonephritis.

Two additional features that distinguish PAN from other forms of systemic vasculitis are:

1. **Confinement of the disease to the arterial rather than the venous circulation.**
2. **Absence of granulomatous inflammation**.

Organ systems involved: Commonly involves **skin, kidneys, heart, liver, and gastrointestinal tract. PAN does not involve pulmonary arteries.**

About 30% of patients with PAN have **chronic hepatitis B** with HBsAg-HbsAb complexes in affected vessels.

Clinical Features

- Age and gender: Peak incidence between **40 to 50 years of age**. Predominantly affects middle aged males (M:F=2:1).
- **Subacute onset** of **constitutional vague symptoms** such as fever, weight loss, weakness, malaise and arthralgias are present in >50% of cases. Others include testicular pain or tenderness, mononeuritis multiplex, and intestinal angina (postprandial pain caused by the involvement of mesenteric vessels). Renal involvement produces renal insufficiency and hypertension. Cutaneous manifestations include erythema nodosum, purpura, livedo reticularis, and ulcers.
- **Absence of pulmonary artery involvement** helps distinguish PAN from most cases of vasculitis. However bronchial arteries may be involved.

Diagnosis

- Anemia, thrombocytosis, and raised acute phase reactants.
- **Hepatitis B surface antigen (HBsAg):** It may be positive.
- p-ANCA: Present in about 20% of cases.
- **Arteriograms:** Demonstrates **aneurysms of small and medium-sized arteries** in the kidney, liver, and visceral vasculature.
- **Biopsy:** Presence of characteristic findings of **vasculitis** of involved organ confirms the diagnosis. Biopsy of symptomatic organs such as nodular skin lesions, painful testes, and nerve/muscle reveals vasculitis. Microscopy shows destruction of the blood vessel wall by inflammatory cells, accompanied by **fibrinoid necrosis**.

Treatment

- **Glucocorticoids and cytotoxic agents:** In idiopathic PAN, remissions or cures is achieved by high doses of glucocorticoids alone. Cyclophosphamide, mycofenolate, rituximab and azathioprine is indicated when PAN is refractory to corticosteroids or when there is serious involvement of major organs.
- PAN with hepatitis B: Antiviral therapy used in combination with glucocorticoids and plasma exchange.

Microscopic Polyangiitis

Q. Write short note on microscopic polyangiitis.

Definition: Microscopic polyangiitis (MPA) is the most common **ANCA-associated necrotizing vasculitis** with **few or no immune complexes** in the involved vessels. It affects **small vessels** (capillaries, venules or arterioles).

Clinical Features

- **Age and gender:** Most common age of onset is 40–60 years. More common in males than females.
- Microscopic polyangiitis is the most common cause of the **pulmonary-renal syndrome,** i.e. alveolar hemorrhage and glomerulonephritis. Alveolar hemorrhage associated with hemoptysis and respiratory compromise.
- The five most common clinical manifestations of MPA are: (1) **glomerulonephritis** (~80% of patients), (2) **weight loss** (>70%), (3) **mononeuritis multiplex** (60%), (4) **fever** (55%), and (5) a variety of **cutaneous findings**-cutaneous vasculitis (>60%).
- **Other features:** Migratory arthralgias or arthritis (either pauciarticular or polyarticular), **palpable purpura,** sometimes with skin ulcerations, nodules, livedo reticularis, and digital gangrene may be seen.

Diagnosis

p-ANCA is positive in most patients, although c-ANCA may also be present in 40% cases.

Treatment

- **Glucocorticoids in combination with either rituximab or cyclophosphamide:** It is the cornerstone of treatment regimens, because most patients with MPA have major organ involvement such as glomerulonephritis, alveolar hemorrhage, or vasculitic neuropathy. Cyclophosphamide may be administered on either a daily or intermittent basis.
- **'Pulse' methylprednisolone** (1 g/d for 3 days) may be considered for patients with severe organ involvement at diagnosis.
- In severe cases (e.g. renal failure or diffuse alveolar hemorrhage), additional use of plasmapheresis is beneficial.
- Other treatment regimens includes mycofenolate, methotrexate, azathioprine and intravenous immunoglobulin.

Churg-Strauss Syndrome

Q. Write short essay/note on Churg-Strauss syndrome/Eosinophilic granulamatosis with polyangitis (EGPA).

- Churg-Strauss syndrome (CSS) or *eosinophilic granulamatosis with polyangitis.*is a rare syndrome that affects small to medium-sized arteries and veins of multiple organ systems.
- **Hallmarks:** It is characterized by **asthma, peripheral and tissue eosinophilia, extravascular granuloma** formation,and **systemic vasculitis**.

Classic Clinical Features

See **Box 9.11**.

Box 9.11: Classic clinical features of Churg-Strauss syndrome.

- Allergic rhinitis and nasal polyposis (75%)
- Asthma (90%)
- Peripheral eosinophilia (10–60% of all circulating leukocytes)
- Fleeting pulmonary infiltrates and occasional alveolar hemorrhage
- Cutaneous nodules, GI bleed, eosinophilic gastroenteritis
- Acute renal insufficiency, acute glomerulonephritis, mononeuritis multiplex, venous thromboembolism, and stroke
- Coronary arteritis pericarditis, rhythm abnormalities myocarditis and heart failure

Investigations

- Striking **eosinophilia** >10% (>1000 cells/µL) in peripheral blood.
- Raised ESR fibrinogen, or α_2-globulins and CRP. Increased IgE levels.
- Urine: RBC casts and proteinuria.
- Positive antinuclear cytoplasmic antibodies against myeloperoxidase (**p-ANCA**) in ~48% of cases.
- Chest X-ray: May show infiltrates and pleural effusion.
- Biopsy: Three histologic criteria for the diagnosis: (1) the presence of necrotizing vasculitis, (2) tissue infiltration by eosinophils, and (3) extravascular granuloma.

Treatment

- High-dose steroids and cyclophosphamide, followed by maintenance therapy with low-dose steroids. Some cases may require addition of cyclophosphamide, mycofenolate and leflunomide
- In severe cases, anti-TNF-α agents like infliximab and etanercept are used
- Anti-interleukin (IL)-5 monoclonal antibodies (mepolizumab, reslizumab) and an anti-IL-5 receptor antibody (benralizumab) are approved for use in severe asthma

Granulomatosis with Polyangiitis (Wegener's Granulomatosis)

Q. Write short essay on clinical features, diagnosis and treatment of granulomatosis with polyangiitis (Wegener's granulomatosis).

Definition: Granulomatosis with polyangiitis is a distinct clinicopathologic entity characterized by **necrotizing vasculitis**, which involves the **upper respiratory tract**, the **lungs**, and the **kidneys.**
It is one of the most common forms of systemic vasculitis. It involves small to medium-sized blood vessels. It affects both the arterial and venous circulations.

Clinical Features

Age and gender: It usually presents during **fourth to fifth decade. Males** are affected more often than females.

- **Nasal involvement:** Found in about 90% of patients. These include nasal crusting, epistaxis (bleeding), paranasal sinus pain, sinusitis, nasal mucosal ulceration and obstruction. Inflammation of nasal cartilage may lead to nasal septal perforation and collapse of the nasal bridge ('saddle nose' deformity). Erosive sinus disease and subglottic stenosis (narrowing of the trachea due to inflammation just below the vocal cords) are highly characteristic of granulomatosis with polyangiitis.
- **Lesions in the mouth:** Two classic mouth lesions are **gum inflammation** ('strawberry gums') and **tongue ulcers**.
- **Deafness** both conductive and sensorineural hearing loss are typical of the disease and **proptosis** due to inflammation of the retro-orbital tissue, diplopia due to entrapment of the extra-ocular muscles, and loss of vision due to optic nerve compression may occur.

- **Lung involvement** may produce cough, hemoptysis (due to alveolar hemorrhage) and dyspnea.
- **Renal involvement** occurs in the form of rapidly progressive glomerulonephritis, resulting in proteinuria, hematuria, red blood cell casts in the urine and renal failure.
- **Other manifestations:** These include palpable purpura, conjunctivitis, episcleritis, scleritis, cranial neuritis and mononeuritis multiplex.

Diagnosis

- **ESR: Markedly elevated.**
- **Non-specific abnormalities:** These include mild anemia, leukocytosis and mild hypergammaglobulinemia (particularly of the IgA class). Complement levels will be normal or elevated.
- **Serum antiproteinase-3 ANCA** (c-ANCA): **Positive** in about 90% of patients.
- **Chest radiograph:** It may show pulmonary infiltrates and **nodules that may cavitate.**
- **Imaging** of the upper airways or chest with MRI: It can be useful in localizing abnormalities.
- **Lung biopsy:** Used for confirmation of the diagnosis. It shows the characteristic necrotizing granulomatous vasculitis.
- **Renal biopsy:** It may show a segmental necrotizing crescentic glomerulonephritis, with no immunoglobulin deposition ('Pauci-immune').

Treatment: Treatment is similar to that for microscopic polyangiitis.

Behçet's Disease/Syndrome

Q. Describe the symptoms, diagnosis and treatment of Behçet's disease.

Behçet's syndrome is characterized by triad of (1) **recurrent episodes of oral/mouth** ulcers, (2) **genital ulcers, and (3) eye inflammation (i.e. iritis).**

Pathologic process is a vasculitis (leukocytoclastic) that may affect small, medium, and large vessels in either the venous or the arterial circulation in any organ.

Clinical Features

Diagnostic criteria: Diagnostic criteria of International Study Group for Behçet's syndrome is presented in **Box 9.12**. However, the spectrum of Behçet's syndrome consists of many manifestations (e.g. neurological involvement seen in 5% of patients, recurrent vascular thrombosis) that are not included in these criteria. Patients can have non erosive arthritis and cutaneous nodules too.

- **Positive pathergy test:** Highly specific to Behçet's disease but may be positive in only 50% of Behçet's patients. It involves pricking the skin with a needle and looking for evidence of pustule development within 48 hours.
- ESR and CRP raised but not autoantibodies.

Box 9.12: Diagnostic criteria for Behçet's syndrome.

One required manifestation

- Recurrent oral ulceration: Aphthous or herpetiform, at least three times in 12 months, usually deep and multiple, and last for 10–30 days. This is the cardinal clinical feature.

plus

At least two of the following:

- Recurrent genital ulceration occurs in 60–80% of cases.
- Characteristic eye lesions: Anterior or posterior uveitis or retinal vasculitis or cells in vitreous on slit-lamp examination.
- Characteristic skin lesions: Erythema nodosum, pseudofolliculitis, papulopustular lesions and acneiform nodules.
- Positive pathergy test.

Treatment

- Oral and genital ulceration: Topical steroid preparations (soluble prednisolone mouthwashes, steroid pastes). Thalidomide (100–300 mg/day for 28 days initially) is very effective for resistant oral and genital ulceration but is teratogenic and neurotoxic.
- Colchicine can be effective for erythema nodosum and joint pain. Apremilast is an alternative to colchicine
- Steroids and immunosuppressants and ciclosporin are indicated for chronic uveitis and rare neurological complications. Anti-TNF agents can be used to control severe uveitis and serious neurological manifestations and gastrointestinal Behçet's disease.

Henoch-Schönlein Purpura/IgA Vasculitis

Q. Write short note on Henoch-Schönlein purpura and anaphylactoid purpura.

- Henoch-Schönlein purpura (also referred to as IgA vasculitis or **anaphylactoid purpura**), is the commonest systemic small-vessel vasculitis in children. It is caused by IgA dominant immune complex deposition following an infectious trigger. It often occurs after upper respiratory tract infections.
- Usually occurs in **children** (>90% of cases) and young adults.

Diagnostic Criteria

Usual presentation: Often present with the **tetrad** of:

1. **Purpura (vasculitic/non-thrombocytopenic/palpable purpura):** Palpable and found over the **buttocks and lower legs (Fig. 9.10).**

2. **Arthralgia or arthritis:** Most patients develop a transient non-migratory polyarthralgias in the absence of frank arthritis and resolves without permanent damage to joints.
3. **Gastrointestinal involvement:** Seen in about 70% of pediatric patients. It is characterized by recurrent colicky abdominal pain associated with nausea, vomiting, diarrhea, or constipation, and the **passage of blood** and mucus per rectum. In some cases, there may beintussusceptions.
4. **Renal involvement:** Seen in 10–50% of patients. It usually produces mild glomerulonephritis causing proteinuria, microscopic hematuria, with red blood cell casts in the urine. It usually resolves spontaneously without treatment.

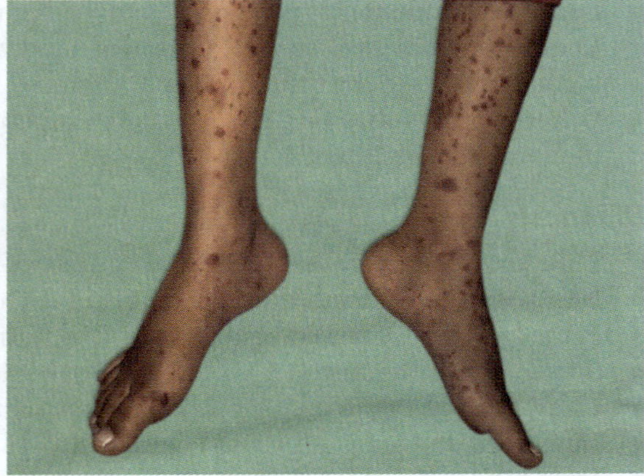
FIG. 9.10: Palpable purpura over lower legs in Henoch-Schönlein purpura.

Other manifestations include scrotal pain keratitis, uveitis, respiratory and neurological involvement.

Prognosis: HSP is self-limited most of the time. The vast majority of cases resolve within 6–8 weeks. Adult cases are sometimes more recalcitrant (not responsive to treatment).

Investigations

- Acute phase reactants are elevated. Serum IgA levels are elevated.
- **Skin biopsy:** Findings are **pathognomonic**. It demonstrates leukocytoclastic vasculitis in capillary venules and direct immunofluorescence of the skin biopsy shows **IgA** immune complexes deposit in the small vessels.

Treatment
- Usually a self-limiting disorder that settles spontaneously without specific treatment.
- Patients respond to bed rest and NSAIDs.
- Corticosteroids and immunosuppressive therapy may be indicated when HSP is severe disease, particularly in the presence of nephritis.

Cogan's Syndrome (CS)

An immune-mediated condition that primarily affects young adults, is associated with ocular inflammation (usually interstitial keratitis) and audiovestibular dysfunction. Maybe associated with large- or medium- to small-sized vessel vasculitis or an aortitis.

Buerger's Disease (Thromboangiitis Obliterans)

- Nonatherosclerotic, segmental, inflammatory disease that affects the small to medium-sized arteries and veins of the extremities.
- Classic patient is a **young male smoker**.
- Identification of the typical pattern of vascular involvement by angiography.
- Major risk factor is tobacco exposure.
- Absence of fibrinoid necrosis (it is a hallmark of most systemic vasculitides).
- Initially, nonspecific pains in the calf, foot, or toes.
- Later, the progression of thrombosis and vasculitis can lead to horrific pain in the digits and limbs and ultimately to gangrene and tissue loss, through either autoamputation or elective amputation.
- The only effective intervention in Buerger disease is **complete smoking cessation**.
- Intermittent pneumatic compressions, calcium channel blockers, phosphodiesterase inhibitors may help in pain relief.

Takayasu Arteritis

Q. Write short essay/note on Takayasu arteritis.

- Takayasu arteritis, named for the Japanese ophthalmologist who first described the ocular manifestations in 1908.
- It is a **large-vessel vasculitis of unknown** cause that chiefly affects **women during their reproductive years.**
- **Sites:** Most common sites are the **aorta** (65%) and the **left subclavian arteries** (93%).
- **Presentation:**
  - Vascular manifestations include: **Bruit, claudication, hypertension, light-headedness** (associated with vertebral or carotid artery disease), **unequal blood pressures in the extremities**, carotidynia, aortic regurgitation, and loss of a pulse. Absence pulses in upper limbs (called **reverse coarctation).**
  - **Bruits:** Most frequent over the carotid arteries, but also often develop in the supraclavicular or infraclavicular space (reflecting subclavian disease), along the flexor surface of the upper arm (from axillary artery disease), or in the abdomen (from renal or mesenteric artery vasculitis). Many patients have multiple bruits.

- A **widened pulse pressure** and diastolic murmur along the right sternal border may signal the aortic regurgitation that develops in 20% of patients. Stroke, angina, and congestive heart failure affect a significant minority of patients.
- **Cardiac complications:** Hypertension, congestive heart failure, angina, and aortic regurgitation.
- About 50% of patients develop **constitutional or musculoskeletal symptoms**. Asthenia, weight loss, fever, myalgia, and arthralgia occur commonly.
- Criteria for the diagnosis of Takayasu arteritis **(Box 9.13)**.

Box 9.13: American College of Rheumatology classification criteria for Takayasu arteritis.

1. Onset at age <40 years
2. Limb claudication
3. Decreased brachial artery pulse
4. Unequal arm blood pressures (>10 mm Hg)
5. Subclavian or aortic bruit
6. Angiographic evidence of narrowing or occlusion of the aorta or its primary branches, or large limb arteritis

Note: The presence of three or more of the six criteria is sensitive (91%) and specific (98%) for the diagnosis of Takayasu arteritis.

Investigations

- Elevated erythrocyte sedimentation rates or C-reactive protein values during phases of active disease.
- Anemia and thrombocytosis
- Vascular abnormalities can be imaged by conventional angiography, MRI, MRA, CT angiography, or ultrasonography. Conventional angiography is the 'gold standard' for precisely delineating the stenosis, occlusions, and aneurysms.

Treatment

- High-dose glucocorticoids in combination with a glucocorticoid-sparing agent (methotrexate, mucophenolate, leflunomide)
- Vascular intervention—for treatment of stenosed arteries leading to organ ischemia or hypertension and for aneurysmal disease.

Q. Differentiate between giant cell arteritis and Takayasu's arteritis.

Differences between giant cell arteritis and Takayasu's arteritis **(Table 9.23)**.

OSTEOARTHRITIS

Q. Discuss the pathogenesis and clinical features and management of osteoarthritis/degenerative joint diseases.

Osteoarthritis (OA) is the most common form of arthritis. OA refers to a **clinical syndrome of joint pain** accompanied by **varying degrees of functional limitation** and reduced quality of life.

OA is a **noninflammatory**, **slowly progressive joint disease**, mainly **involving the cartilage**. It shows **progressive destruction of articular cartilage** of weight-bearing joints of **genetically susceptible older persons**. It leads to narrowing of joint, subchondral bone thickening, and finally **nonfunctioning, painful joints**.

Joints Affected

- **Weight bearing joints** (knee, hips and cervical and lumbar segments of the spine).
- **Non-weight bearing** distal interphalangeal (DIP) joints, thumb bases (first CMC joints and trapezioscaphoid joints), first MTP joints, lower cervical and lumbar facet joints, knees, and hips.

Etiology

Osteoarthritis (OA) is a **multifactorial disease** having both genetic and environmental components **(Table 9.24)**.

TABLE 9.23: Comparison of giant cell arteritis and Takayasu's arteritis.

Feature	*Giant cell arteritis*	*Takayasu's arteritis*
Female-male ratio	2:1	8:1
Age range (years)	50	< 40
Average age of onset (years)	72	25
Visual loss	10–30%	Rare
Involvement of aorta or its major branches	25%	100%
Pathology	Granulomatous arteritis	Granulomatous arteritis
Pulmonary artery involvement	No	Possible
Renal hypertension	Rare	Common
Claudication	Uncommon	Common
Ethnic groups with highest incidence	Scandinavians	Asians
Corticosteroid responsive	Yes	Yes
Bruits present	Minority	Majority
Surgical intervention	Rarely needed	Commonly needed

TABLE 9.24: Risk factors for incidence and progression of osteoarthritis.

Risk factors	
Age	➢ Normal ageing process causes increased progression
Trauma	➢ Collateral ligament, meniscal tears and joint fractures
Occupation	➢ Heavy physical work (e.g. dockers, miners and farmers)
Exercise	➢ High impact sports
Gender	➢ Men under the age of 50 and women over 50
Genetics	➢ Genetic susceptibility to the disease. Genes involved in **prostaglandin** metabolism and **Wnt** (Wingless-related integration site) signaling pathway
Obesity	➢ Strongest modifiable risk factor
Diet	➢ Lower vitamin C and D blood levels
Bone density	➢ Increasing bone density

Types of Osteoarthritis (Box 9.14)

Box 9.14: Types of osteoarthritis.

Idiopathic or primary osteoarthritis: It develops as aging process and may affect few (oligoarticular) or many joints.
- **Localized:** Most commonly affects the hands, feet, knee, hip, and spine.
- **Generalized:** Involves three or more joint sites

Secondary osteoarthritis: It appears in younger individuals with predisposing condition.
- Previous injuries/trauma to a joint
- Congenital or developmental deformity of a joint(s)
- Secondary to systemic disease [e.g. diabetes, marked obesity, acromegaly, hypothyroidism, neuropathic (Charcot) arthropathy]
- Calcium pyrophosphate dihydrate deposition disease (CPPD)
- Bone and joint disorders including rheumatoid arthritis, gouty arthritis, septic arthritis, and Paget disease of bone and osteonecrosis

Identifiable Causes of Osteoarthritis

See **Table 9.25.**

Clinical Manifestations

Age of onset: Usually after age 40.
Joints affected in osteoarthritis **(Table 9.26 and Fig. 9.11)**

Signs, Symptoms and Diagnostic Features of Osteoarthritis (Box 9.15)

TABLE 9.25: Identifiable causes of osteoarthritis.

Congenital disorder (hip) ➢ Legg-Calvé-Perthes disease ➢ Acetabular dysplasia ➢ Slipped capital femoral epiphysis	**Metabolic disorders** ➢ Hemochromatosis ➢ Wilson disease ➢ Ochronosis (alkaptonuria)
Inborn error of connective tissue ➢ Ehlers-Danlos syndrome ➢ Marfan syndrome	**History of a septic joint**
Post-traumatic (knee) ➢ Anterior cruciate ligament tear ➢ Meniscus tear with or without prior meniscectomy surgery	**Postinflammatory** ➢ Underlying rheumatoid arthritis

TABLE 9.26: Joints affected in osteoarthritis.

Commonly affected joints		***Uncommonly affected joints***
Cervical and lumbar spine	Hip	Shoulder
First carpometacarpal joint	Knee	Wrist
Proximal interphalangeal joint	Subtalar joint	Elbow
Distal interphalangeal joint	First metatarso-phalangeal joint	Metacarpophalangeal joint "Missouri metacarpal syndrome"

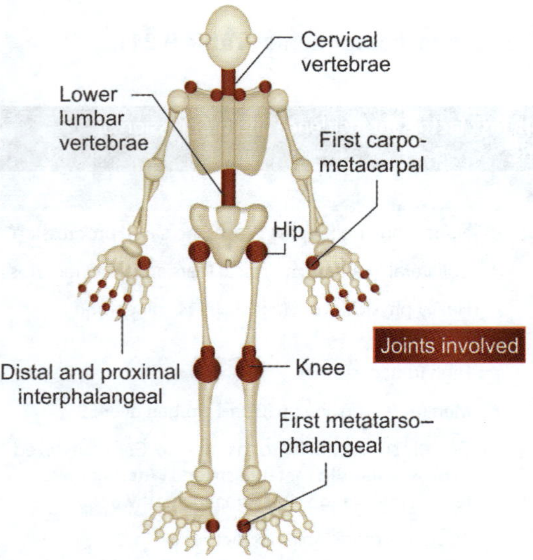

FIG. 9.11: Pattern of joint involvement in osteoarthritis.

Box 9.15: Signs, symptoms and diagnostic features of osteoarthritis.

Symptoms
- Joint pain that increases with activity
- Stiffness: Morning stiffness relatively brief (for <30 minutes) and self-limited
- Gelling

Physical findings
- Crepitus (a grating sensation) on active motion
- Bony enlargement at the joint margin, hard bony enlargements, called **Heberden's nodes** (on DIP) and/or **Bouchard's nodes** (on PIP) **(Fig. 9.12)**
- Decreased range of motion
- Malalignment
- Tenderness to palpation over the joint
- Absence of warmth

Synovial fluid analysis
- Clear fluid
- Noninflammatory synovial fluid (<1000 WBC/mm^3)
- Normal viscosity

Erythrocyte sedimentation rate normal for age

Negative serologic tests for **antinuclear antibody** and **rheumatoid factor**

Radiographic features

Nonuniform joint space narrowing **(Fig. 9.13)**. Subchondral eburnation (bony sclerosis), marginal osteophytes (spur) formation subchondral cysts

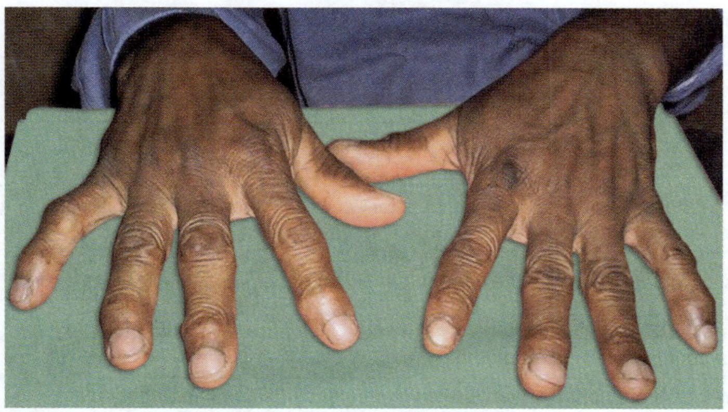

FIG. 9.12: Osteoarthritis showing Heberden's nodes (on DIP) and Bouchard's nodes (on PIP).

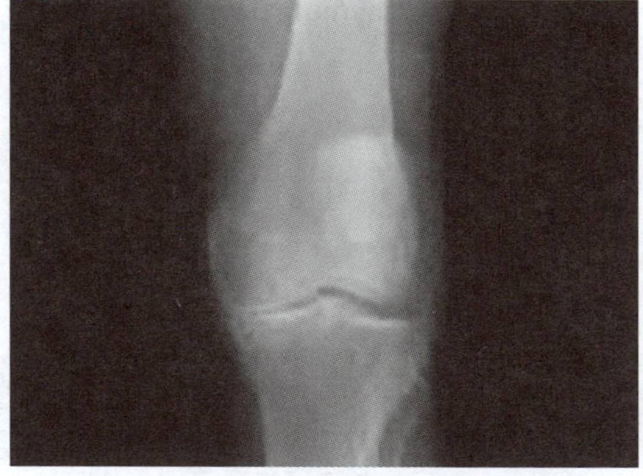

FIG. 9.13: Radiological features of osteoarthritis.

Diagrammatic representation of joint changes in osteoarthritis is shown in **Figure 9.14**.

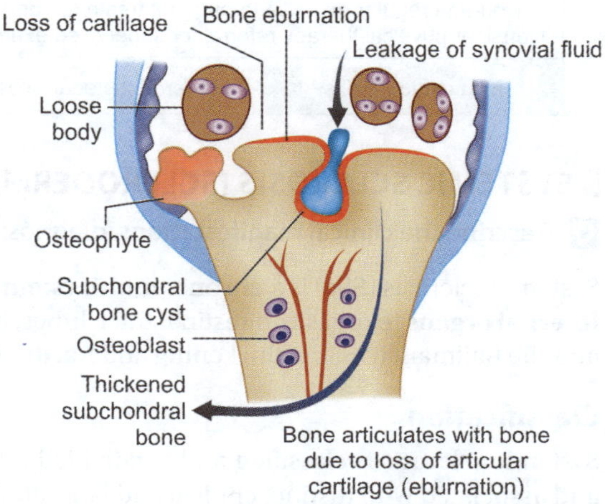

FIG. 9.14: Diagrammatic representation of joint changes in osteoarthritis.

Prevention

Preventing the onset of OA requires lifestyle changes.

- **Primary prevention:** These include:
  - Weight control: Maintaining or reducing weight.
  - Occupational injury prevention: Avoiding repetitive joint use and its injuries.
  - Sports injury prevention: Precautions to prevent injury such as warming up and using proper equipment.
- **Secondary prevention:** Early diagnosis so that appropriate early intervention can be utilized. **However, this is difficult in OA since no effective biomarkers are available to determine the progression of the disease.**
- **Tertiary prevention**: Reduce, delay the onset of complications and disability. The strategies include: self-management (weight control, physical activity, education); home help programs; cognitive behavioral interventions; rehabilitation services and medical surgical treatments.

Therapeutic Options in Osteoarthritis (Table 9.27)

TABLE 9.27: Therapeutic options in osteoarthritis.

Nonpharmacological treatment Education (patient and spouse or family) Social support Physiotherapy (physical therapy) Occupational therapy Weight loss Exercise Orthotic devices Laser Pulsed EMF (electromagnetic field therapy) Ultrasound Transcutaneous electrical nerve stimulation (TENS) Acupuncture Nutrients Herbal remedies Vitamins/minerals	Hormones Psychotropic drugs SYSADOA [symptomatic slow acting drugs for OA : avocado/soybean unsaponifiables (ASU), chondroitin, diacerein and glucosamine] Topical NSAIDs Topical capsaicin **Intra-articular treatment:** Corticosteroids, hyaluronans, tidal irrigation **Surgical** Arthroscopy Osteomy Unicompartmental knee replacement (UKR) Total knee replacement (TKK) Total hip replacement (THR)
Pharmacological treatment Paracetamol/acetaminophen NSAIDs (Non-steroidal anti-inflammatory drugs) COX-2 inhibitors (cyclo-oxygenase-2 selective non-steroidal anti-inflammatory drugs) Opioid analgesics	**Drugs in the pipeline** *Inhibition of breakdown of cartilage by collagenolytic enzymes or matrix metalloproteinases (MMPs)—* ➢ *Doxycycline* ➢ *Therapy that stimulates repair activity by chondrocytes* ➢ *Bisphosphonates* ➢ *Growth factors* ➢ *Cathepsin K inhibition*

Q. Write short essay/note on management of osteoarthritis.

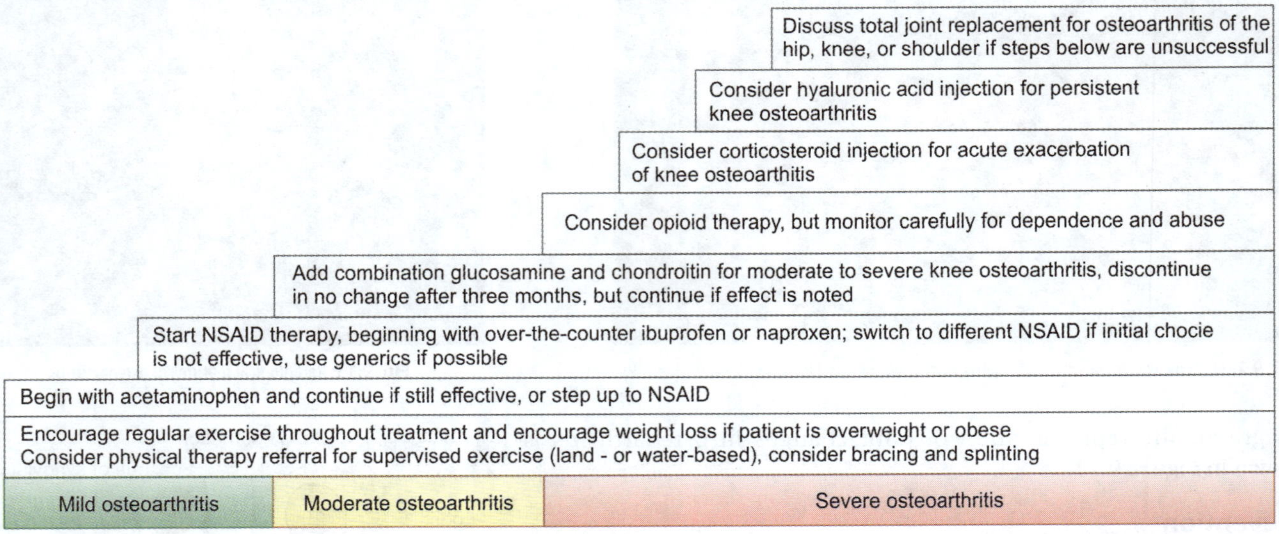

Discuss total joint replacement for osteoarthritis of the hip, knee, or shoulder if steps below are unsuccessful

Consider hyaluronic acid injection for persistent knee osteoarthritis

Consider corticosteroid injection for acute exacerbation of knee osteoarthritis

Consider opioid therapy, but monitor carefully for dependence and abuse

Add combination glucosamine and chondroitin for moderate to severe knee osteoarthritis, discontinue in no change after three months, but continue if effect is noted

Start NSAID therapy, beginning with over-the-counter ibuprofen or naproxen; switch to different NSAID if initial chocie is not effective, use generics if possible

Begin with acetaminophen and continue if still effective, or step up to NSAID

Encourage regular exercise throughout treatment and encourage weight loss if patient is overweight or obese
Consider physical therapy referral for supervised exercise (land - or water-based), consider bracing and splinting

Mild osteoarthritis	Moderate osteoarthritis	Severe osteoarthritis

SYSTEMIC SCLEROSIS (SCLERODERMA)

Q. Describe the clinical manifestations, diagnosis and management of systemic sclerosis.

Systemic sclerosis (SSc) is a **chronic multisystem disease** of connective tissue **affecting the skin, musculoskeletal system, internal organs** (e.g. gastrointestinal tract, lungs, heart and kidneys) and vasculature. Scleroderma literally means 'hard skin' and the hallmark of SSc is thickening and **hardening of the skin** (scleroderma) due to skin fibrosis.

Classification

Systemic sclerosis is classified and subdivided into two principal subsets defined largely by the anatomic skin distribution and associated with distinct clinical and laboratory manifestations.

- **Diffuse cutaneous systemic sclerosis (DCSS:** 30% of cases): It is associated with progressive skin thickening, starting in the fingers and ascending from distal to proximal extremities, the face, and the trunk. These patients have a risk of early pulmonary fibrosis and involvement of kidney and other systems.

Q. Write short note on CREST syndrome and its clinical features.

- **Limited cutaneous systemic sclerosis (LCSS:** 70% of cases). Usually these patients have long-standing Raynaud's phenomenon before other manifestations. Skin involvement progresses slowly and remains limited to the fingers (sclerodactyly), distal extremities, and face, without involvement of trunk. Few of these patients have prominent **C**alcinosis cutis, **R**aynaud's phenomenon, **E**sophageal dysmotility, **S**clerodactyly (scleroderma of the fingers), and **T**elangiectasia, which is termed **CREST syndrome**. CREST syndrome generally show slow progression.
- Other two types are
  1. **Systemic sclerosis sine scleroderma:** A small group of patients have no detectable skin involvement but have clinical features such as Raynauds, digital ulcers, and autoantibodies for SSc.
  2. **Systemic sclerosis with overlap syndrome:** SSc with overlap or features of another systemic rheumatic disease such as systemic lupus erythematosus (SLE), rheumatoid arthritis, polymyositis, or Sjögren's syndrome.

Age and gender: Peak incidence is between 30 and 50 years of age with female to male ratio of 3:1.

Etiology: The cause is poorly understood. There is associations with alleles at the HLA locus have been found. There is immunological dysfunction of T lymphocytes, especially Th1 and Th17 subtypes.

Clinical Features

Q. Write short note on symptoms and signs of systemic sclerosis.

Skin Manifestations

- **Limited disease or CREST syndrome:** Skin involvement restricted to sites distal to the elbow or knee (apart from the face).
- **Diffuse disease:** Skin involvement proximal to the knee and elbow and on the trunk.

Changes in skin (Figs. 9.15A to C)

- Symmetrical and bilateral skin thickening is the hallmark of SSc.
- **Early stage:** Shows non-pitting edema of fingers and flexor tendon sheaths.

- **Later stages:** Skin becomes shiny, firm, thickened, and distal skin creases disappear. After many years, the skin may become thin, atrophic and tightly bound to underlying subcutaneous tissue.
- **Hyperpigmentation:** Skin generally becomes hyperpigmented. In dark-skinned individuals, vitiligo-like areas of hypopigmentation may occur. Because pigment loss spares the perifollicular areas, the skin may develop a **'salt-and-pepper'** appearance most prominently on the upper back and chest.
- **Changes in facial skin:** Produces a beak-like nose, 'mask-like' face, and decreased oral aperture (microstomia).
- **Other manifestations:** These include flexion contractures, ulcers over fingertips and bony prominences (due to breakdown of atrophic skin), telangiectasia, calcinosis cutis and dry coarse skin.

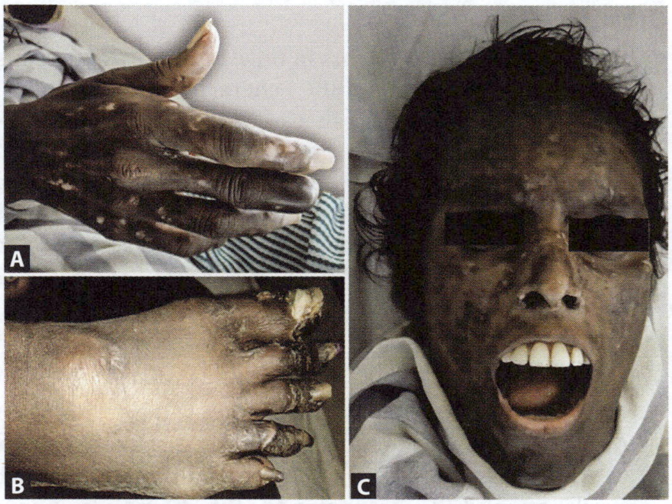

FIGS. 9.15A TO C: Systemic sclerosis. (A and B) Show shiny, thickened skin of hands and feet; (C) Shows mask like face with decreased oral aperture.

Musculoskeletal Manifestations

- Range from mild arthralgias to frank nonerosive arthritis with synovitis resembling rheumatoid arthritis.
- Generalized arthralgia, morning stiffness and flexor tenosynovitis are common.
- Muscle weakness and wasting due to disuse atrophy, myopathy and myositis.
- Restricted hand/limb function associated with contractures of the joints is due to sclerosis of skin rather than joint disease.
- Bone resorption is most common in the terminal phalanges, where it causes loss of the distal tufts (acro-osteolysis) (pseudoclubbing).

Vascular Manifestations

- Involvement of the vasculature is **universal feature** of SSc.
- **Raynaud's phenomenon** is an **episodic reversible vasoconstriction of the vessels of the digits** (fingers and toes) that can result in ischemia of the digits. It occurs in all patients with SSc and can precede other features by many years. This is the first manifestation of the disease in almost every patient.
  - **Triggering factors:** Factors which trigger attack include exposure to cold, a decrease in temperature, emotional stress, and vibration. Typical attacks start with pallor (vasoconstriction), followed by cyanosis (ischemia) of variable duration and erythema (reperfusion) develops spontaneously or with rewarming of the digit.
- A **diffuse vasculopathy of peripheral arteries** (in the extremities) may cause narrowing or occlusion of the vessel lumen leading to tissue ischemia. This may produce skin ulceration over pressure areas, localized areas of infarction and pulp atrophy at the fingertips.
- Vascular disease is fundamental to organ damage and subsequent malfunction of the heart (cardiomyopathy), lung (pulmonary hypertension), kidney [scleroderma renal crisis (SRC)], and other organs in SSc.

Gastrointestinal Manifestations

Gastrointestinal disease in scleroderma usually involves both the upper and lower gastrointestinal tract but clinical expression is highly variable.

- **Esophageal involvement:** It can manifest as reflux with erosive esophagitis, dysphagia and odynophagia, strictures, and dilatation and atony of lower esophagus.
- **Stomach involvement:** It results in dilatation, atony and delayed gastric emptying. Recurrent occult upper gastrointestinal bleeding may occur due to gastric antral vascular ectasia (GAVE) (**'watermelon' stomach**) (**Fig. 9.16**).
- **Small and large bowel involvement:** It results in intermittent abdominal distension, abdominal pain, constipation, intestinal obstruction, malabsorption (due to bacterial overgrowth) and steatorrhea. **Pseudo-obstruction** is a known complication.

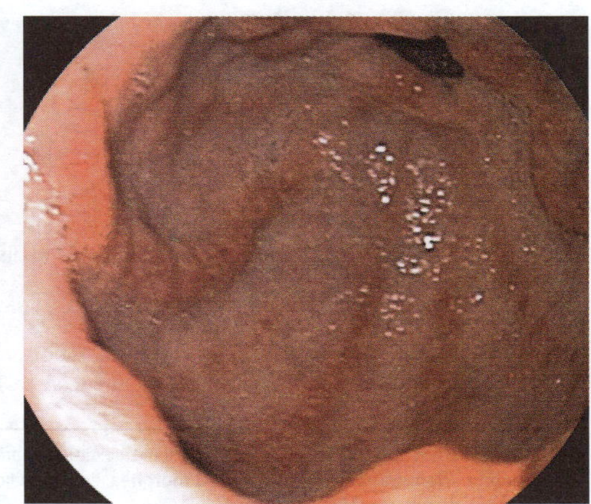

FIG. 9.16: Gastric antral vascular ectasia (watermelon stomach) in scleroderma.

Pulmonary Manifestations

It is a major cause of morbidity and mortality. Main forms of lung disease: inflammatory alveolitis leading to interstitial fibrosis and pulmonary arterial hypertension.

Other Manifestations

- **Renal involvement:** Occurs in only a minority of patients and can be acute or chronic. Acute hypertensive renal crisis (scleroderma renal crisis-SRC) characterized by sudden onset of malignant hypertension and renal failure was used to be the most common cause of death. At present, this is not the case because ACE inhibitors with dialysis and renal transplantation have improved the outlook.
- **Cardiac involvement:** Myocardial fibrosis may cause arrhythmias, conduction defects and cardiomyopathy. Occasionally, pericarditis with or without effusion may develop.

Localized scleroderma: Localized form without systemic involvement **(morphea)**.

Diagnosis (Box 9.16)

Box 9.16: Criteria for diagnosis of scleroderma.

- Thickened (sclerodermatous) skin changes proximal to the metacarpophalangeal joints

OR

- At least two of the following:
  - Sclerodactyly
  - Digital pitting (residual loss of tissue on the finger pads due to ischemia)
  - Bibasilar pulmonary fibrosis

Investigations

- **ESR:** Elevated.
- **IgG levels:** Raised.
- **Anemia:** It may be due to: (1) **chronic disease, (2) iron deficiency** due to gastrointestinal bleed, (3) **folate and B_{12} deficiency** due to blind loop syndrome and (4) m**icroangiopathic hemolytic anemia** due to renal involvement.
- **Urea and creatinine:** Raised in acute kidney injury.
- **Urine** microscopy and if there is proteinuria, measurement of urine albumin/creatinine ratio.
- **Autoantibodies associated with scleroderma (Table 9.28)**
- **Rheumatoid factor:** Positive in 30%.
- **Nail-fold capillary changes:** Visualization of capillaries of the skin at the nail-fold by diascopy gives insight into a patient's microvasculature status. Nail-fold capillary dropout and dilated capillary loops are seen in nearly every patient with scleroderma but are not specific for scleroderma.
- **Imaging**
  - **Chest X-ray:** For changes in cardiac size and evidence of lung disease.
  - **X-ray of hands:** For deposits of calcium around fingers. In severe cases, erosion and absorption of the distal phalanges (acro-osteolysis).
  - **Barium swallow:** To demonstrate impaired esophageal mo- tility. Scintigraphy, manometry, impedance, and upper GI endoscopy are also useful.
  - **High-resolution CT:** To demonstrate interstitial lung disease.
- **Other investigations:** Echocardiography for cardiac involvement and pulmonary hypertension.

TABLE 9.28: Autoantibodies associated with scleroderma.

Autoantibody	*Prevalence*
Antinuclear antibody	>95%
Anti-Scl-70 (anti-topoisomerase I)	20–40%
Anti-centromere	20–40%
Anti-RNA polymerases	4–20%
Anti-B23	10%
Anti-Pm-Scl	2–10%
Anti-U3-RNP (anti-fibrillarin)	8%
Anti-U1-RNP	5%
Anti-Th/To	1–5%

ACR/EULAR critera for classification of systemic sclerosis provided in **Table 9.29**.

TABLE 9.29: 2013 ACR/EULAR criteria for the classification of systemic sclerosis (scleroderma).*

Item	*Sub-item(s)*	*Weight/score*†
Skin thickening of the fingers of both hands extending proximal to the metacarpophalangeal joints (*sufficient criterion*)	–	9
Skin thickening of the fingers (*only count the higher score*)	Puffy fingers Sclerodactyly of the fingers (distal to the metacarpophalangeal joints but proximal to the proximal interphalangeal joints)	2 4
Fingertip lesions (*only count the higher score*)	Digital tip ulcers Fingertip pitting scars	2 3
Telangiectasia	–	2
Abnormal nail-fold capillaries	–	2
Pulmonary arterial hypertension and/or interstitial lung disease (*maximum score is 2*)	Pulmonary arterial hypertension Interstitial lung disease	2 2
Raynaud's phenomenon	–	3
SSc-related autoantibodies (anticentromere, anti–topoisomerase I [anti–Scl-70], anti–RNA polymerase III) (*maximum score is 3*)	Anticentromere 3 Anti–topoisomerase I Anti–RNA polymerase III	3

* The criteria are not applicable to patients with skin thickening sparing the fingers or to patients who have a scleroderma-like disorder that better explains their manifestations (e.g., nephrogenic sclerosing fibrosis, generalized morphea, eosinophilic fasciitis, scleredema diabeticorum, scleromyxedema, erythromelalgia, porphyria, lichen sclerosis, graft-versus-host disease, diabetic cheiroarthropathy).

† The total score is determined by adding the maximum weight (score) in each category.
Patients with a total score of ≥9 are classified as having definite scleroderma.

Treatment

There is no cure and no treatment can halt or reverse the fibrotic changes produced in systemic sclerosis. Treatment should be organ-based to ameliorate the effects of the disease on target organs.

- **General measures:**
  - Education, counseling and family support.
  - Regular exercises and skin lubricants.
  - Monitoring of blood counts, renal functions and analysis of urine on regular basis.
- **Control of Raynaud's syndrome and digital ulcers**
  - Raynaud's phenomenon: **Avoid triggering factors.** Use hand warmers, and oral vasodilators (**calcium-channel blockers**, ACE inhibitors, angiotensin receptor blockers). Parenteral vasodilators (prostacyclin analogues and calcitonin gene-related peptide) may be beneficial in severe digital ischemia.
  - **Digital ulcers:** Endothelin 1 antagonist bosentan promotes healing of digital ulcers. If ulcers become infected, antibiotics may be required.
  - **Surgical management:** Lumbar **sympathectomy**, radical micro-arteriolysis (digital sympathectomy), and thoracic sympathectomy may be beneficial.
- **Hypertension:** Treated aggressively with **ACE inhibitors**, even if renal impairment is present.
- **Esophageal reflux:** Treated with **proton pump inhibitors** and anti-reflux agents, but prokinetic drugs are rarely useful.
- **Intestinal involvement:** Symptomatic malabsorption requires nutritional supplements. Antibiotics may be necessary for small intestinal bacterial overgrowth syndromes, and metoclopramide or domperidone may be useful for symptoms of pseudo-obstruction.
- **Joint involvement:** Treated with analgesics and/or NSAID. If synovitis is present, immunosuppressants such as methotrexate can be used.
- **Pulmonary hypertension:** Treated with oral vasodilators, oxygen and warfarin. Advanced cases require prostacyclin therapy (inhaled, subcutaneous or intravenous) or the oral endothelin-receptor antagonists (bosentan and sitaxsentan). Low-dose oral corticosteroids and cytotoxic drugs (e.g. cyclophosphamide or azathioprine) are indicated when myositis or pulmonary fibrosis is co-exist.
- D-Penicillamine: May reduce skin thickening and also systemic involvement.
- Progressive and diffuse skin involvement without visceral involvement, methotrexate (MTX) or mycophenolate mofetil (MMF).

Prognosis

Prognosis is highly dependent on the extent of major organ disease. Can be predicted to some extent by the degree of skin involvement:

- Limited scleroderma has a normal life expectancy, about 90% 5-year survival rate.
- Diffuse skin disease have only about a 70–80% 5-year survival rate.

SJÖGREN'S SYNDROME

Q. Discuss the clinical manifestations, diagnosis and management of Sjögren's syndrome (SS).

It **mainly affects the exocrine** (salivary and lachrymal) **glands** and is characterized by the immune-mediated destruction of exocrine glands with secondary development of **keratoconjunctivitis sicca** (dry eyes) and **xerostomia** (dryness of the mouth).

Classification

- **Primary:** Sjögren's syndrome (sicca syndrome): It occurs in the absence of any underlying connective tissue disorder.
- **Secondary:** It occurs in association with other autoimmune disorders. These include rheumatoid arthritis, systemic lupus erythematosus, systemic sclerosis (scleroderma), mixed connective tissue disease, primary biliary cirrhosis, vasculitis and chronic active hepatitis.

Age and gender: Usual age of onset is **40 to 50 years**, with **female** to male ratio of 9:1. Mechanisms of tissue destruction: Lymphocytic infiltration and immune-complex deposition.

Clinical Features (Table 9.30)

Q. Write short note on keratoconjunctivitis sicca.

Laboratory Investigations

- **Schirmer tear test:** This is the most commonly used test for the diagnosis of SS. It measures wetting of standardized tear test strip by tear flow over 5 minutes. A standard tear test (absorbent) paper strips is placed between the eyeball and inside of the lower eyelid. Normal result is more than 10 mm of wetting in 5 minutes and if wetting is <10 mm in 5 minutes it indicates defective tear production.
- **Rose Bengal staining**. Staining of the eyes with rose Bengal may show punctate or filamentary keratitis over the area not covered by the open eyelid.

- **Biopsy:** If the diagnosis remains in doubt, it can be confirmed by biopsies of the salivary gland or of the lip (labial minor salivary gland). They show a focal infiltration by lymphocytes and plasma cells. Minor salivary gland biopsy remains a highly specific test for the diagnosis of SS.
- **Tests for salivary gland involvement:** Other diagnostic tests include sialometry (to measure salivary flow), sialography, and scintigraphy. Newer imaging techniques such as ultrasound, MRI or MR sialography of the major salivary glands are also useful.
- **Common laboratory abnormalities**
  - Most patients have an elevated ESR, raised immunoglobulin levels (hypergammaglobulinemia), and circulating immune complexes.
  - Autoantibodies
    - Rheumatoid factor: Usually positive (75–90%).
    - Antinuclear antibodies: Positive in 80% of cases.
    - Anti-mitochondrial antibodies: Positive in 10%.
    - Anti-Ro (SSA) antibodies: Positive in 60–90% (in 10% of cases of RA and secondary Sjögren's syndrome). This antibody can cross the placenta and cause congenital heart block.
    - Anti-La (SSB) antibodies: Present in 40%.
  - Others: Leukopenia, thrombocytosis.

TABLE 9.30: Major clinical manifestations of Sjögren syndrome.

Organ	*Manifestations*
Mouth	Oral dryness (xerostomia), soreness, caries, periodontal disease, oral candidiasis, parotid swelling
Eyes (keratoconjunctivitis sicca)	Ocular dryness (xerophthalmia), corneal ulcers, conjunctivitis and blepharitis (lack of lubricating tears)
Nose and throat	Nasal dryness, chronic cough
Extraglandular manifestations	
Skin	Cutaneous dryness, palpable purpura, urticarial lesions, Raynaud phenomenon
Joints	Arthralgias, non-erosive symmetric arthritis
Lungs	Obstructive chronic lung disease, interstitial pneumopathy
Cardiovascular	Raynaud phenomenon, pericarditis, autonomic disturbances
Liver	Associated hepatitis C virus infection, primary biliary cirrhosis, type 1 autoimmune hepatitis
Kidneys	Renal tubular acidosis type I (distal), glomerulonephritis
Peripheral nerve	Mixed polyneuropathy, pure sensitive neuropathy, mononeuritis multiplex
Central nervous system	White matter lesions, cranial nerve involvement (V, VIII, and VII), myelopathy
Ears	Sensorineural hearing loss
Thyroid	Autoimmune (Hashimoto's) thyroiditis
General symptoms	Low-grade fever, generalized pain, myalgias, fatigue, weakness, fibromyalgia, polyadenopathies, depression, anxiety, increased risk of non-Hodgkin's lymphoma

Treatment

- Management is symptomatic.
- **Ocular symptoms:** Symptomatic treatment is with artificial tears. Lachrymal substitutes (e.g. hypromellose) during the day and more viscous ophthalmologic lubricating ointment at night. Cyclosporine emulsion may be useful in ocular dryness.
- **Oral symptoms:** Best replacement for xerostomia is water, lubricating agents and saliva-replacement solutions. Stimulation of saliva flow by sugar-free chewing gum or lozenges may be helpful. Vaginal dryness is treated with lubricants such as K-Y jelly.
- **Muscarinic agonists** (pilocarpine and cevimeline) have been recently used for the treatment of sicca symptoms in SS. They stimulate the M1 and M3 receptors present on salivary glands and tear glands leading to increased secretory function.
- Hydroxychloroquine is helpful for fatigue and arthralgia.
- Glucocorticoids and immunosuppresive agents are reserved for potentially severe disease. Corticosteroids are used to treat persistent salivary gland swelling or neuropathy. Other agents that can be used are hydroxychloroquine, methotrexate, leflunomide, azathioprine, sulfasalazine, mycophenolic acid, and cyclosporine.
- Biological agents, including infliximab, interferon-α and anti-CD20 antibodies (rituximab) are tried.

Overlap Syndromes and Mixed Connective Tissue Disease (MCTD)

Q. Define mixed connective tissue disease/overlap syndromes.

Overlap syndromes are diseases in which clinical or laboratory signs and symptoms of another defined connective tissue disease occur, such as systemic lupus erythematosus, scleroderma, rheumatoid arthritis, Sjogren's syndrome, Churg-Strauss arteritis, thrombotic thrombocytopenic purpura, antiphospholipid antibody syndrome and autoimmune thyroid disease. **Mixed connective-tissue disease** (MCTD) is a disorder with overlapping clinical features of systemic lupus erythematosus, scleroderma, and myositis, with the presence of a distinctive antibody against **U1-ribonucleoprotein (RNP)**. U1 RNP consists of ribonucleic acid (RNA) plus three proteins (A', C, and a 68-70 kD protein).

CRYSTAL ARTHROPATHIES

Gout

Q. Describe the etiology, clinical manifestations, diagnosis and management of gout.

Q. Discuss the causes, clinical manifestations, investigations and management of hyperuricemia.

Gout is a **heterogeneous group of inflammatory diseases** characterized by **hyperuricemia** (plasma urate level above 6.8 mg/dL) and monosodium **urate crystal deposition in** and around synovial **joints and kidneys**.

Etiology of Gout and Hyperuricemia (Box 9.17)

Q. Write short note on causes of hyperuricemia.

Uric acid is the end product of purine metabolism, which is eliminated only in the urine. Humans do not have uricase, an enzyme which degrades uric acid. Usually, there is a balance between uric acid production and tissue deposition of urates.

Box 9.17: Classification of hyperuricemia.

Urate overproduction
- ***Primary hyperuricemia***
  - Idiopathic
  - Complete or partial deficiency of HGPRT
  - Superactivity of PRPP synthetase
- ***Secondary hyperuricemia***
  - Excessive purine consumption
  - Myeloproliferative or lymphoproliferative disorders
  - Hemolytic diseases
  - Psoriasis
  - Glycogen storage diseases: types 1, 3, 5, and 7

Uric acid under excretion
- ***Primary hyperuricemia***
  - Idiopathic
- ***Secondary hyperuricemia***
  - Decreased renal function
  - Metabolic acidosis (ketoacidosis or lactic acidosis)
  - Dehydration
  - Diuretics
  - Hypertension
  - Hyperparathyroidism
  - Drugs including cyclosporine, pyrazinamide, ethambutol and low-dose salicylates
  - Lead nephropathy

Overproduction and under excretion
- Alcohol use
- Glucose-6-phosphatase deficiency
- Fructose-1-phosphate-aldolase deficiency

(HGPRT: hypoxanthine-guanine phosphoribosyltransferase; PRPP: 5-phosphoribosyl-1-pyrophosphate)

Clinical Features

The natural history of gout has four stages:

1. **Asymptomatic hyperuricemia:** It is a state in which serum urate exceeds the level of solubility but symptoms of crystalline deposition have not occurred. Appears at puberty in males and after menopause in females.
2. **Acute gouty arthritis:**
   - Acute gouty arthritis usually follows decades of asymptom- atic hyperuricemia. Usually the **first attack** occurs in a **mid- dle-aged male.**
   - **Presentation:** It appears as **sudden excruciating** (agonizing) **joint pain, swelling, intense redness** and tenderness of the **first metatarsophalangeal (MTP) joint (termed *podagra*) (Fig. 9.17).** Other joints that can be involved are tarsal joints, ankles, knees and wrists. Gout can also cause bursitis and tenosynovitis. 20% patients can present with a polyarticular pattern is the initial manifestation.
   - **Systemic symptoms:** The acute attack may be accompanied by fever, chills, and malaise, leukocytosis and raised ESR.
   - **Factors which precipitate acute attack** are those that cause fluctuations (rapidly raising or lowering) in serum urate levels. These include overindulgence in certain high-purine foods, alcohol ingestion, starvation, dehydration, certain drugs (e.g. diuretic, salicylates, urate-lowering drugs allopurinol and radiographic contrast agents), trauma and surgery.
   - **Termination of attack:** Even if not treated, acute attacks of gout are usually self-limited, subside spontaneously and first several acute attacks last for 5 to 8 days. Recovery is usually associated with desquamation of the overlying skin. There is no damage to any organ system during the acute attack.
3. **Intercritical gout:** With resolution of the attack, patients enter an interval termed the 'intercritical period'. It is the asymptomatic period between the first acute attack and subsequent attacks. During this period, the previously affected joints are free of symptoms. Despite this, monosodium urate crystal deposition continues.

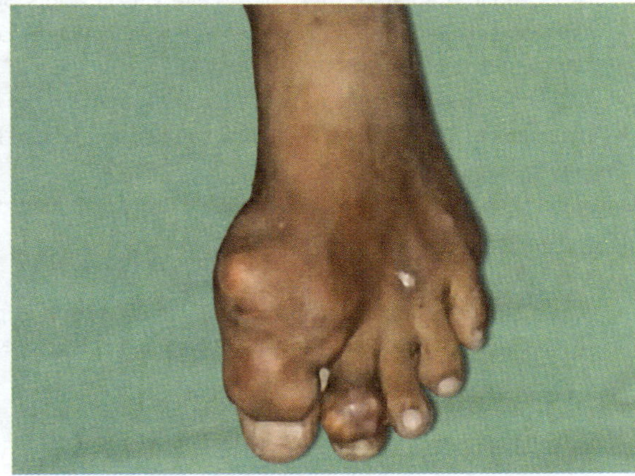

FIG. 9.17: Acute gouty arthritis involving the first metatarsophalangeal (MTP) joint (termed podagra).

Q. Write short essay/note on chronic tophaceous gout.

4. **Chronic tophaceous gout** (tophi and chronic gouty arthritis)
   - Eventually the untreated patient progresses to chronic polyarticular gout (advanced gout). This stage usually develops after several years (10 or more years) of acute gouty arthritis, which may lead to severe crippling disease.
   - The intensity of pain in chronic is not severe compared to that of acute attacks.
   - **Most characteristic lesion** of advanced gout is **subcutaneous tophus**. It results from deposition of crystals in cartilage, synovial membranes, tendons and soft tissues. It can occur anywhere in the body but is most common in the fingers, wrists, ears (helix and antihelix), knees, and olecranon bursa.

Nephropathy

Occurs in 90% of patients with gouty arthritis. Two types of parenchymal renal damage can occur.

1. **Urate nephropathy:** It is characterized by deposition of urate crystals in the interstitial tissue. It may lead to albuminuria, isosthenuria or renal failure.

2. **Obstructive uropathy (nephrolithiasis):** Chronic hyperuricemia may be complicated by formation of uric acid renal stone with blockage of urine flow. The factors favoring stone formation are hyperuricosuria, overproduction of purine, increased ingestion of purine, uricosuric drugs and acidic urine.

Other features: Hypertension is a risk factor for development of gout and gout may be associated with increased incidence of hypertension and cardiovascular disorders.

Investigations

- **Joint fluid microscopy:** Most specific and diagnostic test but is technically difficult. Synovial fluid examined by compensated polarized microscopy shows **urate crystals**. These crystals are bright yellow in color and appear as slender, **needle shaped, negatively birefringent structures.**
  - **Acute gout:** Synovial fluid is turbid due to the greatly elevated cell count (>90% neutrophils).
  - **Chronic gout:** More variable but occasionally it appears white due to the high crystal load. Crystals may be seen between attacks.
- **Serum uric acid:** Raised hyperuricemia (>7.0 mg/dL in males and >6.0 mg/dL in females) does not confirm the diagnosis. However, levels may be normal (in 50% cases) during an acute attack.
- **Serum urea, creatinine:** Monitoring is needed to detect any signs of renal impairment.
- Raised ESR and CRP and neutrophilia are observed during acute gout, and they return to normal as the attack subsides.
- **Plain radiographs:** Usually normal in acute gout. In chronic or tophaceous gout, well-demarcated rounded or oval punched out erosions with hypertrophic calcified 'overhanging edge' **(Martel sign)** are characteristically observed. RA causes marginal erosions within the limits of the joint capsule.
- **Dual-energy computed tomography (DECT):** Identifies urate deposits in articular and periarticular locations and can distinguish urate from calcium deposition.

Q. Write short note on management of acute attack of gout.

Management

Treatment of acute attack

- **NSAIDs:** They rapidly relieve pain and swelling during the acute attack and are the agents of choice. Commonly used drugs include indomethacin (75 mg immediately, then 50 mg 6–8 hours), naproxen (750 mg immediately, then 500 mg every 8–12 hours), *diclofenac* (75–100 mg immediately, then 50 mg every 6–8 hours) and fenoprofen. NSAIDs may cause renal impairment.
- Local icepacks can produce symptomatic relief.
- **Oral colchicine:** It is the second drug of choice which acts by inhibiting microtubule assembly in neutrophils. It is very effective at a dose of 1.2 mg immediately, then 0.6 mg every 6–12 hours. Side effects include diarrhea or colicky abdominal pain.
- **Corticosteroids:** If patient cannot tolerate NSAIDs or colchicine, oral prednisolone (20–30 mg/day) or intramuscular or intra-articular depot methylprednisolone may be tried.
- **ACTH gel:** A single injection of intramuscular ACTH gel (25 to 80 IU) is useful for terminating an acute attack of gout.
- **Interleukin 1 inhibitors:** Anakinra, canakinumab have been tried.

Prophylaxis

Indicated in patients with reccurent flares, tophi with joint damage and patients with renal insufficiency.

Dietary advice

- Avoid alcohol intake, especially beer, which is high in purines and fructose. Carbonated soft drinks are also rich in fructose.
- Avoid meat and shellfish.
- Controlled weight reduction if patient is obese.
- Avoid use of thiazides or loop diuretics.

Drugs for Prophylaxis

Urate-lowering therapy

It is indicated **(Box 9.18)** in patients who develop more than one acute attack within one year and those with complications. Xanthine oxidase inhibitors are used in urate overproducers while uricosuric agents are used in urate underexcretors.

Box 9.18: Indications for urate-lowering drugs.

Hyperuricemia associated with increased uric acid production
- Urinary uric acid excretion of 1000 mg or more in 24 hours
- Very high levels of serum uric acid
- Hyperuricemia associated with HGPRT deficiency or PRPP synthetase overactivity
- Uric acid nephropathy
- Nephrolithiasis
- Prophylaxis before cytolytic therapy
- Evidence of bone or joint damage

(HGPRT: hypoxanthine guanine phosphoribosyl-transferase; PRPP: 5'-phosphoribosyl-1-pyrophosphate)

- **Allopurinol** is the drug of first choice. It is an xanthine oxidase inhibitor that blocks the conversion of xanthine into uric acid. Thus it reduces uric acid production and serum uric acid levels rapidly.
  - **Indication:** Should be used when the attacks are frequent and severe (despite dietary changes), associated with renal impairment or tophi, or when NSAIDs or colchicine are difficult to tolerate.
  - **Dosage:** 300–900 mg daily.
  - **Common side effects:** These include gastrointestinal intolerance and skin rashes. Allopurinol hypersensitivity syndrome is the most severe reaction characterized by fever, skin rash, eosinophilia, hepatitis, progressive renal insufficiency, and death.

- **Febuxostat** is a non-purine selective inhibitor of xanthine oxidase, is a new urate lowering drug that is possibly well-tolerated, safer in renal impairment and superior to allopurinol. Dose is 40–120 mg/day.
- **Uricosuric agents** like **probenecid, benzbromarone, lesinurad,** and **sulfinpyrazone** are indicated in selected cases (when uric acid excretion in the urine is below 600 mg/day). Uricosuric drugs are risky if urinary urate excretion is already >800 mg/24 hours. These are contraindicated in those with urate calculi. Uricosurics are ineffective in renal impairment (creatinine clearance < 50 mL/minute).
- Uricase, analogs as **pegloticase and rasburicase** are used to promote depletion of body urate pools.

Q. Write short note on Lesch–Nyhan syndrome.

- Lesch–Nyhan syndrome is an X-linked recessive disorder characterized by three major clinical elements—overproduction of uric acid, neurological disability and behavioral problems.
- Hyperuricemia may lead to nephrolithiasis, renal failure, gouty arthritis and tophi.
- Neurological disability is characterized by dystonia or other movement disorders like choreoathetosis, ballismus, spasticity and hyperreflexia.
- Behavioral abnormalities include intellectual disability and aggressive and impulsive behaviors.
- Hypoxanthine guanine phosphoribosyltransferase (HPRT) that plays a key role in recycling purine bases is deficient in these individuals due to mutation of HPRT gene on X chromosome.
- Prognosis is bad as the treatment options are limited.
- Allopurinol is useful for treating hyperuricemia.
- Motor disabilities managed by baclofen and benzodiazepines and behavioral abnormalities managed by behavioral therapy and medications.

Calcium Pyrophosphate Dihydrate Deposition Disease/Pseudo-gout

Q. Write short essay/note on pseudo-gout; calcium pyrophosphate dihydrate deposition disease; pyrophosphate arthropathy.

Calcium pyrophosphate dihydrate (CPPD) deposition disease is a condition associated with deposition of calcium pyrophosphate dihydrate (CPPD) crystals within articular and hyaline cartilage.

Common Causes

See **Box 9.19.**

Box 9.19: Common causes of calcium pyrophosphate dihydrate crystal deposition disease.

- Idiopathic (most frequent): Occurs in association with aging
- Complication of primary osteoarthritis
- Long-term consequence of mechanical joint trauma or knee meniscectomy
- Familial
- Associated with systemic metabolic disease, e.g. hyperparathyroidism, dialysis-dependent renal failure, hemochromatosis, hypomagnesemia.

Clinical Features

- May be asymptomatic or may result in a variety of clinical presentations.
- A **common presentation** is **acute inflammatory arthritis** that resembles acute gout. Hence, also known as '**pseudogout**'. However, in contrast to gout it is more common in elderly women and usually affects the knee followed by the wrist, shoulder, ankle and elbow. Examination of joint reveals a warm, tender erythematous joint with signs of a large effusion. Fever is common.
- **Trigger factors:** These include trauma, intercurrent illness and surgery.
- **Chronic arthropathy:** It may also occur in association with CPPD crystal deposition disease.

Investigations

- **Examination of synovial fluid:** CPPD crystals can be demonstrated using compensated polarized microscopy and helps in differentiation from gout. CPPD crystals are generally **rhomboid-shaped and positively birefringent.** They appear blue when parallel to the long axis of the compensator and yellow when perpendicular. The synovial fluid is turbid and may be uniformly blood-stained.
- **X-rays of the affected joint:** It may show calcification in hyaline cartilage and/or fibrocartilage (chondrocalcinosis).

Basic Calcium Phosphate Crystal Deposition

- Basic calcium phosphate (BCP) deposition disease is due to the deposition of **hydroxyapatite or apatite crystals** and other basic calcium phosphate salts (e.g. octacalcium phosphate, tricalcium phosphate) in soft tissues.
- **Main sites of deposits:** BCP crystal deposits are mainly seen in tendons, ligaments and hyaline cartilage. In the shoulder, it may manifest as calcific tendinitis of the rotator cuff.
- **Fluids for crystal detection:** BCP crystals may be detected as **nonbirefringent globular clumps within leukocytes** in synovial and bursal fluids. Under light microscopy BCP crystal clumps stain positive with the calcium-binding dye such as alizarin red S.

Therapeutics for Crystal Deposition Disease

See **Table 9.31**.

TABLE 9.31: Therapeutics for crystal deposition disease.

NSAIDs or COX-2 inhibitors	**Novel therapy** ➢ Phosphocitrate ➢ Caspase-1 or IL-1 antagonism for CPPD crystal-induced inflammation. Hydroxychloroquine for refractory chronic inflammation ➢ TLR2 antagonism for CPPD-associated degenerative arthropathy ➢ Oral calcium supplementation to suppress PTH levels ➢ ANKH anion channel blockade (probenecid) ➢ NPP1 inhibition ➢ TG2 inhibition ➢ Polyphosphates ➢ Promotion of crystal dissolution by alkaline phosphatase or polyamines
Intra-articular corticosteroids	
Systemic corticosteroids	
ACTH	
Prophylactic low-dose colchicine	
Methotrexate for refractory chronic inflammation and recurrent pseudogout	
Oral magnesium (for patients with hypomagnesemia)	

MISCELLANEOUS

Relapsing Polychondritis (RP)

- **Immune-mediated** condition associated with **inflammation in cartilaginous structures and other connective tissues** throughout the body.
- **Sites:** These include **ears**, nose, joints, respiratory tract, and others. Unilateral or bilateral external ear inflammation that characteristically spares the earlobe. episcleritis, scleritis, nasal bridge collapse, larynx and tracheal involvement with respiratory distress is seen.
- The **McAdam's criteria** require at least three criteria out of six of the following: 1) bilateral auricular chondritis, 2) non-erosive seronegative polyarthritis, 3) nasal chondritis, 4) ocular inflammation, 5) respiratory tract chondritis, and 6) cochlear and/or vestibular dysfunction.
- **Associated with diseases:** Thirty percent occur in association with disease such as systemic vasculitis (particularly Wegener granulomatosis), connective tissue disorder (e.g. rheumatoid arthritis or systemic lupus erythematosus), or a myelodysplastic syndrome.
- **Presentation:** Patients can present with respiratory obstruction, aortitis and mitral regurgitation.

Treatment: Steroids and in severe disease immunosuppresive agents (Dapsone, Methrotrexate) are used.

Nonarticular Rheumatism

Q. Differentiate articular from nonarticular disorders.

- Nonarticular rheumatism is not actually a true arthritis. It refers to aches and pains that arise from structures outside of joints.
- **Forms:** Four forms namely **tendinitis, bursitis, FMS (fibromyalgia syndrome), and the myofascial pain syndrome.**
- **Common types of tendinitis and bursitis:**
  1. **Tennis elbow:** Pain over the lateral epicondyle of the elbow due to inflammation of the tendons of the wrist extensor muscles that insert at this location.
  2. **Golfer's elbow:** Pain over the medial epicondyle due to inflammation of the wrist flexor tendons that insert at this location.
  3. **Shoulder impingement syndrome:** It is due to impingement of the tendons of the rotator cuff with shoulder abduction or flexion. It can be associated with supraspinatus tendinitis, subacromial bursitis, or rotator cuff tears.
  4. **Housemaid's knee:** It is prepatellar bursitis produced due to repetitive trauma or overuse such as kneeling. Another common region for bursitis is over the greater trochanter of the lateral hip.

Fibromyalgia Syndrome

Q. Write short note on the criteria for diagnosis of fibromyalgia syndrome (FMS).

Fibromyalgia syndrome is characterized by chronic widespread pain, and is defined as pain for more than three months both above and below the waist.

- **Diagnostic criteria for FMS**
  - At least 3 months of widespread pain that is bilateral, above and below the waist.
  - It includes axial skeletal pain and pain to palpation at a minimum of 11 of 18 predefined tender points **(Fig. 9.18)**.
  - The diagnosis of other diseases does not exclude the diagnosis of FMS.

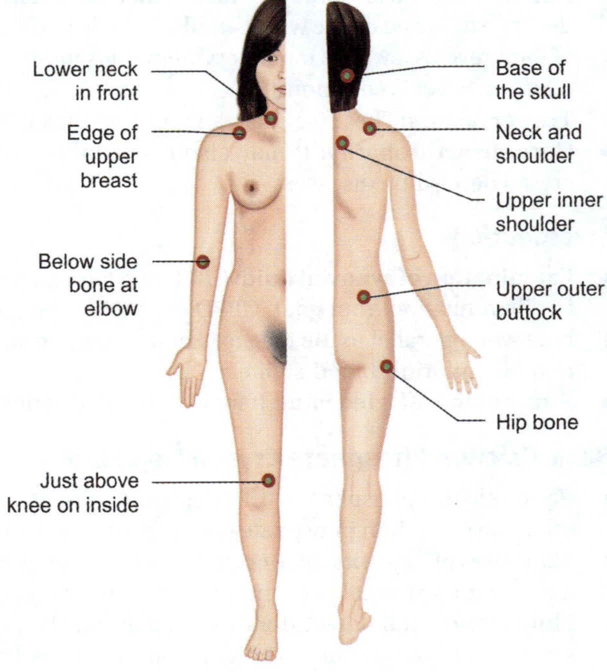

FIG. 9.18: Trigger points in fibromyalgia.

- **Physical examination:** Normal except for tender points in precise locations. Usually these points are tender bilaterally.
  - **Tender points (Fig. 9.18)**: Typically located at the occiput, at the midportion of the trapezius, the origin of the supraspinatus, low anterior cervical region, second costochondral junction, lateral epicondyle, outer upper quadrant of the buttocks, greater trochanter region, and medial knee area.
- **Differential diagnosis:** Medical illnesses that may exhibit symptoms similar to those of FMS include: Celiac sprue, hepatitis C, hyperparathyroidism, hypothyroidism, and polymyalgia rheumatica (PMR).
- Nonpharmacological treatment includes patient education and initiation of exercises
- Amitriptyline, duloxetine, milnacipran, or pregabalin can be used as mono or combination therapy

OSTEOPOROSIS

Q. Describe the risk factors, prevention and treatment of osteoporosis.

Osteoporosis is the most common bone disorder and is a component of the fragility syndrome.

Definition

- It is a bone disease characterized by low bone mass and micro-architectural disruption of bone tissue that leads to increased bone fragility and fracture risk.
- **WHO definition:** Osteoporosis is defined as a bone mineral density (BMD) of 2.5 standard deviations (SDs) below the young healthy adult mean value (T-score ≤–2.5) or lower as measured by DXA (dual-energy X-ray absorptiometry). The term 'established osteoporosis' includes the presence of a fragility fracture. There is inverse relationship between bone mineral density and fracture risk in postmenopausal women and older men. However, this definition should not be applied to young women, men or children.
- **National Institute of Health (NIH) definition:** Osteoporosis is defined as a skeletal disorder characterized by compromised bone strength, which predisposes an individual to an increased risk of fracture.
- **Osteopenia:** It is the term used when the BMD values lies between –1 and –2.5 SDs below the young adult mean.

Epidemiology

Most common bone disorder. More common in women (4:1). More common in Caucasian population than in other races.

Pathogenesis

- In osteoporosis, there is **loss of bone mass,** despite **normal mineralization. In contrast, *osteomalacia*** occurs when **bone is not being properly mineralized,** despite the normal production of bone matrix.
- Osteoporosis develops due to an **imbalance in bone remodeling**. It can be due to increased breakdown of bone (**absorption of bone)** by osteoclasts and/ or decreased bone formation by osteoblasts. The process of **mineralization of new bone matrix** remains normal.
- Osteoporosis affects both **trabecular** (long thick bones, e.g. femur) and **cortical bone** (high surface area, think bones, e.g. spine). When it affects trabecular bones, **reabsorption of bone** is the main mechanism.
- Genetic factors play important role and multiple genes are involved, including collagen type 1A, vitamin D receptor and estrogen receptor genes.
- Nutritional factors, sex hormone status and physical activity also play a role. Cigarette smoking is an independent risk factor.

Classification of Osteoporosis

- **Generalized osteoporosis (Table 9.32):** It involves the entire skeleton. It may be:
  - **Primary** or
  - **Secondary** to variety of conditions
- **Localized:** Limited to certain bone or region (e.g. disuse osteoporosis of a limb).

TABLE 9.32: Causes of generalized osteoporosis

Primary
- Idiopathic
- Postmenopausal
- Senile

Secondary
- Endocrine disorders
  - Addison disease
  - Type 1 diabetes mellitus
  - Hyperparathyroidism
  - Hyperthyroidism
  - Hypothyroidism
  - Pituitary tumors
  - Cushing's syndrome
  - Acromegaly
- Hypogonadal states
  - Turner's syndrome
  - Klinefelter's syndrome
  - Female hypogonadism
  - Premature and primary ovarian failure
  - Anorexia nervosa
  - Hypothalamic amenorrhea
  - Hyperprolactinemia
- Nutritional and gastrointestinal disorders
  - Hepatic insufficiency, severe liver disease, especially biliary cirrhosis
  - Pernicious anemia
  - Subtotal gastrectomy
  - Malabsorption syndromes
  - Malnutrition
  - Parenteral nutrition
  - Vitamin C, D deficiencies
- Rheumatologic disorders
  - Rheumatoid arthritis
  - Ankylosing spondylitis
- Hematologic disorders/malignancy
  - Multiple myeloma
  - Lymphoma and leukemia
  - Malignancy with parathyroid hormone (PTHrP) production
  - Hemolytic anemias (e.g. thalassemia)
  - Systemic mastocytosis
  - Hemophilia
  - Disseminated carcinoma
- Drugs
  - Alcohol
  - Anticoagulants (e.g. heparin)
  - Anticonvulsants
  - Chemotherapy
  - Corticosteroids
  - Proton pump inhibitors
  - Ciclosporin, tacrolimus
- Miscellaneous
  - Homocystinuria
  - Immobilization
  - Osteogenesis imperfecta
  - Pulmonary disease

Clinical Features

- **Risk of fracture:** Osteoporosis can be clinically silent and does not have specific symptoms. However, it increases the risk of bone fractures and fracture is the only cause of symptoms and thereby **increases the morbidity and mortality** in elderly.
- **Fragility fracture:** It is a low-trauma fracture, i.e. mechanical forces (situations) that would not ordinarily result in fracture in healthy people. They typically occur in trabecular bone. The most common sites are:
  - **Spine (vertebrae):** Sudden severe back pain (in the spine) that radiates around to the front suggests **vertebral crush fracture** (compression fracture).
  - **Hip (proximal femur):** Fractures of the **proximal femur** usually occur in elderly persons falling on their side or back. Usually requires prompt surgery.
  - **Wrist (distal radius): Colles' fractures** follow a fall on an outstretched arm.
  - Other sites include arm (humerus), pelvis, ribs, and other bones.

Investigations and Diagnosis

Conventional plain radiograph: It is useful along with CT or MRI, for detecting complications of osteopenia (reduced bone mass; pre-osteoporosis), such as fractures. However, radiography is relatively insensitive for detection of early disease as it requires a substantial amount of bone loss (about 30%) to be apparent on X-ray images. The radiographic features of osteoporosis are cortical thinning and increased radiolucency.

Bone biopsy: Tetracycline labeling of the skeleton on bone biopsy determines the rate of skeletal growth. However, the current use of BMD tests, in combination with hormonal evaluation and biochemical markers of bone remodeling, has replaced the bone biopsy.

Biochemical markers: They provide an index of the overall rate of bone remodeling. Markers for bone formation include serum bone-specific alkaline phosphatase, serum osteocalcin, serum propeptide of type I procollagen. Markers for bone resorption urine and serum cross-linked N-telopeptide, urine and serum cross-linked C-telopeptide and urine total free deoxypyridinoline.

Bone mineral density (BMD): It is a measure of the mineral content of bone. It is mostly calcium, but also comprises potassium, manganese, magnesium, strontium, selenium, and other minerals. The diagnosis of osteoporosis can be made by measuring the bone mineral density (BMD).

- **Dual energy X-ray absorptiometry (DXA):** It is the most commonly used technique to measure BMD. Two low dose X-rays are directed to the area of interest. It measures areal bone density (mineral/surface area rather than a true volumetric density), usually spine (lumbar) and hip (proximal femur). It uses low doses of radiation and is the 'gold standard' for the diagnosis of osteoporosis. Results from DXA are expressed as either the T-score or the Z-score.

- T-score that is 2.5 SD or more below the young adult mean BMD is defined as osteoporosis, provided that other causes of low BMD have been ruled out (such as osteomalacia)
- T-score that is 1 to 2.5 SD below the young adult mean is termed low bone mass (osteopenia)
- Normal bone density is defined as a value within 1 SD of the mean value in the young adult reference population
- Z-score is a comparison of the patient's BMD to an age-matched population.
- A Z-score of -2 or lower is considered below the expected range for age

- **Quantitative ultrasound:** This has many advantages in assessing osteoporosis being quick, easy and cheaper than other methods and does not need ionizing radiation. It is used as a screening procedure prior to DXA assessment and is not used for diagnostic purposes. The calcaneus is the most common skeletal site for quantitative ultrasound assessment.
- **Quantitative CT scanning:** It assesses true volumetric mineral density in mg/cm^3. It gives separate estimates of BMD for trabecular and cortical bone. It is more expensive and requires higher radiation than other techniques.
- **Other investigations:** These may be necessary to exclude other diseases or identify contributory factors associated with osteoporosis. These include complete blood count, thyroid function test, vitamin D levels and myeloma screen. Additionally renal function test, serum calcium, phosphorus, serum PTH, cortisol may be indicated.

Treatment of Osteoporosis

The aim of treatment is to reduce the risk of fracture. Treatment plan for osteoporosis includes: (1) diagnosis of individuals at highest risk, (2) exclusion of secondary causes of osteoporosis and (3) selecting appropriate treatment.

Prevention

Lifestyle changes: Methods to prevent osteoporosis include:

- **Nutrition:** Sufficient daily **calcium** intake (1200–1500 mg/day) and vitamin D.
- **Cessation of smoking.**
- Reduction in alcohol intake.

- **Increase weight bearing exercise:** They increase bone mass density and also helps to prevent falls. At least 30 minutes weight bearing exercise 3x per week is needed to increase bone density. Osteoporosis orthosis helps to prevent spine fractures and support the building up of muscles.
- Fall prevention can help prevent osteoporosis complications.

Pharmacological Management

Q. Write short note on drugs used in osteoporosis.

Drug treatments can reduce the risk of fracture **by up to 50%.**

The two main classes of drugs used namely: 1) antiresorptive agents and 2) anabolic agents.

1. ***Antiresorptive agents:*** They block bone resorption by inhibiting the activity of osteoclasts. These include bisphosphonates, denosumab, raloxifene, and calcitonin.
   - **Bisphosphonates:** These drugs are essentially analogues of pyrophosphate and include alendronic acid, risedronate, clodronate, pamidronate, etidronate. Usually taken **weekly**, and with plenty of water. **Poorly absorbed from the gut.**
     - Should be taken on an empty stomach, as they can bind to calcium in food, after which, the drug cannot be absorbed.
     - Only about 10% of the oral dose is absorbed under normal circumstances.
     - **Adverse drug reactions:** GI upset, esophagitis, bone pain, headache and fever rarely osteonecrosis of jaw. Oral and IV bisphosphonates should not be used in CKD and eGFR <30 to 35 mL/min.
   - **Hormone-replacement therapy (HRT)**
     - No longer used as mainstream treatment. Used if other treatments are not tolerated or effective.
     - It may be useful in women in post-menopausal osteoporosis. Most effective when started early in menopause, and to be continued for >5 years.
     - Disadvantages: (1) Bone loss continues, and is possibly increased upon stopping HRT and (2) increases the risks of cardiovascular disease and stroke.
     - Estrogen analogs: Estrogen replacement therapy is good for prevention of osteoporosis. However, it is not recommended unless there are other indications for its use. In hypogonadal men testosterone has been shown to give improvement in bone quantity and quality.
     - **Raloxifene, Bazedoxifene:** It is a selective estrogen receptor modulators (SERMs) that act on the estrogen receptors throughout the body in a selective manner. Raloxifene has an advantage of reducing the risk of invasive breast cancer. SERMs have been proven effective in clinical trials.
   - **Calcitonin:** It directly inhibits osteoclastic bone resorption activity via the calcitonin receptor on the surface of osteoclasts. It acts by inhibiting actin cytoskeleton which is needed for the osteoclastic activity.
2. ***Bone anabolic agents:*** They stimulate bone formation by acting primarily on osteoblasts. These include parathyroid hormone and teriparatide.
   - **Teriparatide and abaloparatide:** It acts like parathyroid hormone and stimulates osteoblasts and increases their activity. Mostly used for patients with established osteoporosis, those with low BMD or several risk factors for fracture or cannot tolerate the oral bisphosphonates. It is given as a daily injection with the use of a pen-type injection device.
   - **Sodium fluoride:** It produces skeletal changes such as pronounced bone density with increased number and thickness of trabeculae, cortical thickening, and partial obliteration of the medullary space.
3. ***Other agents***
   - **RANKL inhibitors: Denosumab** is a fully human monoclonal antibody that mimics the activity of osteoprotegerin. It binds to RANKL, thereby preventing RANKL from interacting with RANK and reducing its bone resorption.
   - **Romosozumab,** a monoclonal anti-sclerostin antibody has been approved
   - **Strontium ranelate:** It is an alternative oral treatment, belonging to a class of drugs called 'dual action bone agents' (DABAs). It has proven efficacy, especially in the prevention of vertebral fracture. Strontium ranelate is taken as a 2 g oral suspension daily.

Supplements: Dietary supplements are given as adjuncts to pharmacological therapy. These include **(1) calcium and (2) vitamin D.**

ANTIPHOSPHOLIPID ANTIBODY SYNDROME (HUGHES SYNDROME)

Q. Write short note on antiphospholipid antibody (APLA) syndrome and antiphospholipid antibodies.

- Antiphospholipid antibody (APLA) syndrome or antiphospholipid syndrome (APS) is characterized by the **presence of a family of antibodies** in the patient's plasma known as antiphospholipid antibodies (autoantibodies directed against phospholipids) and a syndrome of **hypercoagulability.** This prothrombotic disorder is also associated with thrombocytopenia.
- *The term **antiphospholipid antibody is misleading** because these antibodies react with plasma proteins which themselves bind and form complexes with negatively charged phospholipids. So, in contrast to the terminology antiphospholipid, there is no direct binding of antibodies to phospholipids.*

Types of Antiphospholipid Antibody Syndrome

1. **Primary antiphospholipid syndrome:** They do not have any predisposing cause and their only manifestation is hypercoagulable state.

2. **Secondary antiphospholipid syndrome:** These are found in association with autoimmune diseases, like systemic lupus erythematosus. Because of this association, they were formerly known as lupus anticoagulant syndrome.

Clinical Features

It is the most common acquired hematologic cause of recurrent thromboembolic events. Clinical manifestations chiefly are due to a direct or indirect effect of venous or arterial thrombosis and/or pregnancy morbidity **(Table 9.33)**.

TABLE 9.33: Clinical manifestations of antiphospholipid antibody syndrome.

Organ/System	*Manifestation*
Venous thrombosis and related consequences	Deep vein thrombosis **Cutaneous:** Livedo reticularis **(Fig. 9.19)** **Lung:** Pulmonary embolism, pulmonary hypertension, superficial thrombophlebitis, thrombosis in various other sites
Arterial thrombosis and related consequences	**Neurologic:** Stroke, transient ischemic attack **Cardiac:** Myocardial ischemia (infarction or angina), valvular vegetation (Libman-Sacks endocarditis) **Cutaneous:** Leg ulcers and/or digital gangrene. Arterial thrombosis in the extremities **Ophthalmologic:** Retinal artery thrombosis/amaurosis fugax ischemia of visceral organs or avascular necrosis of bone Multi-infarct dementia
Neurologic manifestations of uncertain etiology	Migraine; epilepsy; chorea; cerebellar ataxia; transverse myelopathy
Renal manifestations	**Renal artery/renal vein/glomerular thrombosis,** renal microangiopathy, renal infarction, acute renal failure, hematuria
Osteoarticular manifestations	Arthralgia; arthritis
Obstetric manifestations	Preeclampsia; eclampsia
Fetal manifestations	Early fetal loss (<10 weeks); late fetal loss (10 weeks); premature birth among the live births
Hematologic manifestations	Thrombocytopenia, autoimmune hemolytic anemia
Others	Osteonecrosis, adrenal infarction
Catastrophic Antiphospholipid Syndrome ➢ History of APS and/or aPL. ➢ Three or more new organ thromboses within a week.	

Diagnosis

Types of antiphospholipid antibodies: Antiphospholipid antibodies are a heterogeneous group of autoantibodies directed against phospholipids-binding proteins. Many plasma proteins (e.g. prothrombin, β_2-glycoprotein) bind to anionic phospholipids resulting in different antiphospholipid antibodies. Antiphospholipid antibodies (APAs) may include (1) **lupus anticoagulant** (LA) **antibody,** (2) **anticardiolipin antibody** (aCL), or (3) **anti-β_2-glycoprotein-I** (anti-β_2-GPI) **antibody.**

1. **Lupus anticoagulant (LA) antibody:**
   - It is named lupus as it was first detected in patients with systemic lupus erythematosus (SLE).
   - It was called anticoagulant because it paradoxically prolongs the clotting times by coagulation assays in vitro (e.g. prolongation of APTT).
   - However, the term lupus anticoagulant is a misnomer, because it is more frequently found in patients without lupus and is not anticoagulant and is associated with a hypercoagulable state rather than bleeding.
   - For LA screening, two or more phospholipid-dependent coagulation tests are necessary. These include (1) activated partial thromboplastin time, (2) dilute Russell viper venom time *(DRVVT)* and (3) kaolin clotting time.
2. **Anticardiolipin antibody (aCL):** They target cardiolipin (a bovine cardiac protein) and are detected by immunoassays.
3. **Anti-β_2-glycoprotein-I (anti-β_2-GPI) antibody:** They are directed against β_2-glycoprotien I and may be causal in APLA syndrome.

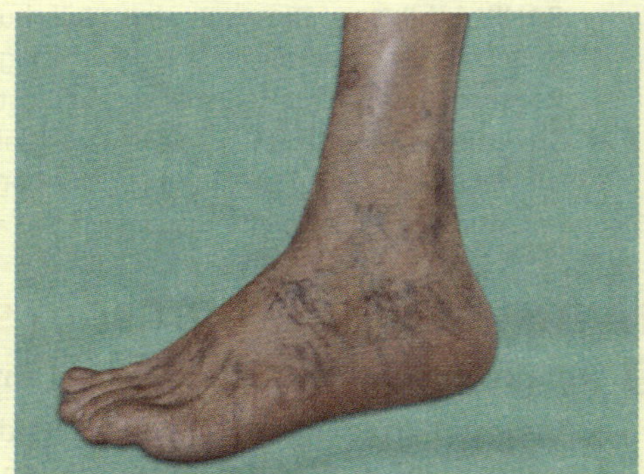

FIG. 9.19: Livedo reticularis-mottled reticulated vascular pattern that appears as a lace-like purplish discoloration of the skin. It is due to swelling of the venules caused by obstruction of capillaries.

Significance

- LA antibodies are more specific, whereas aCL antibodies are more sensitive for antiphospholipid syndrome. IgG aCL antibodies are more specific than IgM type.
- Antiphospholipid antibodies may be detected in 10% of normal population and 30–50% of SLE patients. They can also be found in patients with infections such as human immunodeficiency virus and during therapy with medications (e.g. chlorpromazine).

Criteria for Diagnosis: APLA Syndrome (Box 9.20)

Management

Treatment of Venous Thrombosis

- Patients with APS have a high risk of recurrent thromboembolism. Hence, they should receive antithrombotic therapy.
- **Anticoagulation** with unfractionated heparin or low-molecular-weight heparin (LMWH), and oral warfarin, for acute venous thromboembolism (VTE). This is followed by long-term oral warfarin to a target international normalized ratio (INR) of 2 to 3, alone or in combination with 80 mg of aspirin daily. Duration of treatment is probably lifelong.
- Catastrophic APSis treated with anticoagulation, glucocorticoids, and, in severe cases, plasma exchange and/or intravenous immune globulin (IVIG).

Prevention of Recurrence of Arterial Thrombosis

- Aspirin 325 mg/day or warfarin (INR between 1.4 to 2.8).

Prophylaxis of any Thrombotic Episode

- Aspirin for preventing thrombosis in females with previous pregnancy loss.
- Modification of other risk factors (e.g. hypercholesterolemia, smoking).

Box 9.20: Antiphospholipid antibody syndrome classification criteria (revised **Sapporo classification criteria**).

Vascular thrombosis
- Arterial, venous, or small vessel

Pregnancy morbidity
- One or more fetal deaths
- One or more premature births due to severe preeclampsia or placental insufficiency
- Three or more first trimester losses

PLUS
- Lupus anticoagulant
- Anticardiolipin IgG or IgM (medium to high titer)
- Anti-beta$_2$ glycoprotein-1 IgG or IgM on two occasions 12 weeks (or more) apart
- A definite diagnosis of antiphospholipid syndrome is made if the patient has one clinical and one laboratory criteria.

Management of Pregnancy in patients with Antiphospholipid Syndrome

- **Attempted conception:** Start aspirin 80 mg daily.
- **Confirmed intrauterine pregnancy** by ultrasound, start heparin (5,000–10,000 units every 12 hours) or low-molecular-weight heparin in prophylactic doses (enoxaparin 1 mg/kg, dalteparin 5000 units once a day) and continue till late in the third trimester.
- **Females with a history of pregnancy losses:** The goal is to prevent recurrent pregnancy loss. Two or more early pregnancy losses, or one or more late pregnancy losses without any previous history of thrombosis should receive combination of aspirin and heparin (unfractionated or low molecular weight) during pregnancy.

Treatment

- Intravenous heparin along with high-dose corticosteroids.
- Early addition of plasma exchange and/or intravenous immunoglobulin (400 mg/kg qd) or CD20 monoclonal antibody rituximab, ofatumumab, veltuzumab, and ocrelizumab (375 mg/m^2 per week for 4 weeks) in patients who do not respond promptly to heparin and corticosteroids.

- **Prognosis:** Despite treatment, mortality is about 50%.

INFLAMMATORY MUSCLE DISEASES

Q. Write short note on inflammatory muscle diseases.

Common Inflammatory Muscle Diseases (Table 9.34)

Idiopathic inflammatory myopathies consist of three major types: (1) **polymyositis,** (2) **dermatomyositis** and (3) **inclusion body myositis.**

TABLE 9.34: Common inflammatory muscle diseases.

	Autoimmune (idiopathic)	
Infective forms	***Generalized forms***	***Focal forms***
➢ Viral: Coxsackie B, influenza, Epstein-Barr virus, HIV ➢ Bacterial: *Streptococcus, Staphylococcus,* ➢ clostridia, mycobacteria ➢ Fungal: Candidiasis, coccidioidomycosis, ➢ cryptococcosis ➢ Protozoal: Toxoplasmosis ➢ Helminthic: Trichinosis, cysticercosis	➢ Dermatomyositis ➢ Polymyositis ➢ Inclusion body myositis ➢ Overlap syndromes ➢ Eosinophilic myositis ➢ Granulomatous myositis ➢ Necrotizing myopathy (paraneoplastic)	➢ Monomelic myositis ➢ Eosinophilic myositis ➢ Macrophagic myofasciitis ➢ Orbital myositis

Polymyositis and Dermatomyositis

Q. Write short note on polymyositis and dermatomyositis.

Differentiate polymyositis from dermatomyositis.

Idiopathic Polymyositis

Onset: Gradual. Commonly between 40 and 60 years of age.

Clinical Manifestations

- **Symmetrical proximal muscle weakness:**
  - **Sites affected:** Usually affects the **lower limbs** (hips and thighs) **than the upper limbs** (shoulder girdle muscles). The distal muscles, facial muscles are not usually affected.
- **Others:** Involvement of pharyngeal, laryngeal and respiratory muscles can lead to dysphonia and respiratory failure.
- **Systemic features:** Fever, weight loss and fatigue are common.
- **Investigation:** Muscle biopsy shows fiber necrosis, regeneration and inflammatory cell infiltrate.

Idiopathic Dermatomyositis

Q. Write short note on dermatomyositis.

- Dermatomyositis characterized by **polymyositis** along **with** characteristic **skin changes**. The skin changes may occur before or after the muscle syndrome.
- **Skin changes:** These include
  - **Gottron's papules:** Scaly, erythematous or violaceous, psoriasiform plaques occurring over the extensor surfaces of PIP and DIP joints.
  - **Heliotrope rash:** Violaceous discoloration of the eyelid may be seen along with periorbital edema.
  - **Shawl sign or the V sign:** Occurrence of erythematous macules distributed in a 'shawl' pattern over the upper back, chest and shoulders.
  - **Holster sign:** Poikiloderma on the lateral aspects of the thighs.
  - **Periungual telangiectasias:** Periungual nail-fold capillaries are enlarged and tortuous.
  - **Mechanic's hand:** Fissured, scaly and hyperkeratotic hand (in cases of antisynthetase syndrome).
- **Others:** Ulcerative vasculitis and calcinosis (calcium deposition) of the subcutaneous tissue seen in about 25% of cases. In the long-term, muscle fibrosis and contractures of joints occur.
- **Increased risk of malignancy:** Few patients with dermatomyositis above 60 years of age have an underlying malignancy. The most common being ovarian and gastric carcinoma, and lymphoma.
- **Amyopathic dermatomyositis or dermatomyositis sine myositis:** Presence of pathognomonic skin lesion without muscle involvement.
- **Investigation:** Muscle biopsy shows necrosis of muscle (single fibers or in groups), perifascicular atrophy, and infiltration with lymphocytes.

Table 9.35 lists the differences between dermatomyositis, polymyositis and inclusion-body myositis.

TABLE 9.35: Differences between dermatomyositis, polymyositis and inclusion-body myositis.

Features	*Dermatomyositis*	*Polymyositis*	*Inclusion-body myositis*
Sex	F > M	M = F	M >> F
Age of onset	Any	20 years +	50 years +
Onset	Subacute/acute	Chronic	Chronic
Distribution of weakness	Proximal	Proximal	Proximal + distal + asymmetric (typically quadriceps + finger flexors)
Muscle pain/swelling	In acute cases	No	No
Skin involvement	Often	No	No
Raynaud's , Arthralgia	Frequent	Infrequent	No
Dysphagia	In severe cases	Infrequent	Occasional
Association with cancer	Up to 20%	Probably no	No
Cardiac involvement	Yes	No	No
Interstitial lung disease	Associated with anti-Jo	Associated with anti-Jo	No

Diagnosis

- **ESR** and **CRP:** Usually raised.
- **Serum autoantibody studies: Antinuclear antibodies** frequently positive.
- **Muscles enzymes:** Raised levels of **serum creatine kinase** (CK), **aldolase,** serum glutamic oxaloacetic transaminase (SGOT), lactate dehydrogenase (LDH) and serum glutamic pyruvate transaminase (SGPT).
- **Autoantibodies** directed against cytoplasmic RNA synthetases, other cytoplasmic proteins and RNP found in about 30% of patients. Only antihistidyl-tRNA synthetase (anti-Jo-1 antibody) is a diagnostic marker and is found in 20% of patients with polymyositis/dermatomyositis.
- **Electromyography (EMG):** It can confirm the presence of myopathy and exclude neuropathy.
- **MRI:** It can be used to detect abnormally inflamed muscle.
- **Needle muscle biopsy:** Characteristic changes: fiber necrosis, regeneration and lymphocytic inflammatory cell infiltrate. Open biopsy helps in more thorough assessment.
- **Screening for malignancy:** These include CXR (chest X-ray), mammography, pelvic/abdominal ultrasound, PET scan, urine microscopy and circulating tumor markers.

Management

- **Corticosteroids:** The treatment of choice is prednisolone (dose of 1 mg/kg daily) till patient shows significant improvement. High-dose intravenous methylprednisolone (1 g/day for 3 days) may be necessary in patients with respiratory or pharyngeal weakness.
- **Additional immunosuppressive therapy:** If no improvement with prednisolone, azathioprine (2–3 mg/kg/day) may be added. It also has some steroid-sparing effect. Other steroid-sparing agents include methotrexate, azathioprine, ciclosporin, cyclophosphamide mycophenolate mofetil, tacrolimus and MMF.
- **Intravenous immunoglobulin:** It may be effective in refractory or rapidly progressive cases.

CHAPTER

10

Gastroenterology

SYMPTOMATOLOGY AND EVALUATION OF GASTROINTESTINAL DISEASE

Anorexia (Table 10.1)

Q. List common causes of loss of appetite (anorexia).

TABLE 10.1: Common causes of anorexia.

Infections: Viral fever and tuberculosis	**Renal disease:** Chronic renal failure
Endocrine diseases: Hypothyroidism, hyperparathyroidism, Addison's disease, and panhypopituitarism	**Malignancies:** Any malignant tumors, e.g., carcinoma stomach, pancreas. Leukemias and lymphomas
Liver disease: Hepatitis and cirrhosis	**Psychiatric causes:** Depression, and **anorexia nervosa**

VOMITING

Q. List common causes of persistent vomiting.

- **Vomiting** is the forceful oral expulsion of gastric contents. It is a complex reflex and involves both autonomic and somatic neural pathways.
- **Nausea** is a feeling of wanting to vomit and often precedes actual vomiting.
- **Retching** is a strong involuntary unproductive effort to vomit. It is associated with contraction of abdominal muscles but without expulsion of stomach contents through the mouth.

Mechanism of vomiting: Synchronous contraction of the diaphragm, intercostal muscles, and abdominal muscles raises intra-abdominal pressure. This is combined with relaxation of the lower esophageal sphincter and causes forcible ejection of contents of the stomach.

Common Causes of Nausea and Vomiting (Table 10.2)

TABLE 10.2: Common causes of nausea and vomiting.

Abdominal causes	
Mechanical obstruction Gastric outlet obstruction and small bowel obstruction* **Motility disorders** ➢ Functional dyspepsia gastroesophageal reflux disease (GERD)* ➢ Gastroparesis*	**Other intra-abdominal causes** Acute appendicitis, acute cholecystitis, acute hepatitis, acute mesenteric ischemia, eosinophilic gastroenteritis, and gastric and duodenal ulcer disease*
Drugs	
Aspirin and other nonsteroidal anti-inflammatory drugs **Antidiabetic agents** **Antigout drugs** **Antimicrobials:** Acyclovir, antituberculosis drugs, erythromycin, sulfonamides, and tetracycline **Cancer chemotherapy:** Cisplatin, cytarabine, dacarbazine, etoposide, 5-fluorouracil, and methotrexate	**Cardiovascular drugs:** Antiarrhythmics, antihypertensives, beta-blockers, calcium channel blockers, digoxin, and diuretics **Central nervous system drugs:** Antiparkinsonian drugs (levodopa and other dopamine agonists, anticonvulsants **Others:** Theophylline
Infectious causes	
Acute gastroenteritis: Viral and bacterial	Nongastrointestinal (systemic) infections
Metabolic and endocrine causes	
Acute intermittent porphyria, diabetes mellitus, diabetic ketoacidosis, hyperparathyroidism, and other causes of hypercalcemia*	Addison's disease, hyperthyroidism, hyponatremia, hypoparathyroidism, and pregnancy
Central nervous system causes	
Demyelinating disorders, disorders of the autonomic system, hydrocephalus, meningitis, and migraine headaches*	Intracerebral lesions with edema (projectile vomiting): Abscess, hemorrhage, infarction, and neoplasm*

Contd...

Contd...

Labyrinthine disorders	
Labyrinthitis* Motion sickness	Meniere's disease*
Other causes	
Anxiety and depression* Cyclic vomiting syndrome* Ethanol abuse* Functional disorders and bulimia nervosa*	Cardiac disease: Congestive heart failure Myocardial infarction Myocardial ischemia

*Indicates causes of persistent vomiting

Rumination Syndrome/Mercyism

See **Box 10.1**

Box 10.1: Features of rumination syndrome.

- Rumination is a functional disorder resembles vomiting but does not involve an integrated somatovisceral response coordinated by the emetic center
- It consists of the repetitive effortless regurgitation of small amounts of recently ingested food into the mouth followed by rechewing and reswallowing or expulsion

Complications of Chronic Vomiting

Emetic injuries to the esophagus and stomach:

- Lesions may range from mild erythema to erosions and ulcerations
- Abrupt retching or vomiting episodes may produce longitudinal mucosal and even transmural lacerations at the level of the gastroesophageal junction. When the lacerations are associated with acute bleeding and hematemesis, the clinical condition is described as the **Mallory-Weiss syndrome.**
- **Boerhaave's syndrome** refers to spontaneous rupture of the esophageal wall, with free perforation and secondary mediastinitis.
- **Dental caries** and erosions may result from chronic vomiting.

Spasm of the glottis and aspiration pneumonia:

In patients with diminished consciousness, or in an older person or patient with a depressed cough reflex, may be associated with aspiration of gastric contents into the bronchi, resulting in acute asphyxia and a subsequent risk of **aspiration pneumonia**.

Fluid, electrolyte, and metabolic alterations:

Hypochloremic alkalosis is usually the first metabolic abnormality to develop and is attributable to loss of fluid and hydrogen and chloride ions. Hypokalemia, hypernatremia, and dehydration can occur.

Nutritional Deficiencies

Nutritional deficiencies may result from reduced caloric intake or loss of nutrients in the vomitus.

Q. Discuss treatment of persistent vomiting.

Treatment

1. **Supportive measure: Correction of fluid and electrolyte balance**
2. **Medication:**
   - **Phenothiazines and related drugs:** Prochlorperazine 5–10 mg thrice daily
   - **Dopamine antagonists:** Metoclopramide 10 mg 30 minutes before meals and at bedtime. Side effects include drowsiness and extrapyramidal effects. Domperidone (10 mg thrice daily) has no central nervous system (CNS) side effects
   - **Antihistaminic agents**, e.g., diphenhydramine
   - **Serotonin 5-HT3 receptor antagonists:** Useful in chemotherapy associated emesis. Examples ondansetron and granisetron
   - **Neurokinin-1(NK-1) receptor antagonist**, e.g., aprepitant (oral) and fosaprepitant (parenteral) indicated only in chemotherapy-induced nausea and vomiting
   - **Motilin receptor agonists:** Erythromycin intravenously in boluses of 200–400 mg every 4–5 hours
   - **Muscarinic receptor agonist:** Bethanechol
   - **Synthetic cannabinoids:** Nabilone and dronabinol
   - **Glucocorticoids:** Especially in raised intracranial tension (ICT), and chemotherapy-induced emesis
   - **Gastric electrical stimulation** in refractory cases

Hiccough

Q. List the common causes of hiccough.

The symptom of hiccups (hiccoughs, singultus) is an involuntary, intermittent, and spasmodic contraction of the diaphragm and intercostal muscles and glottic closure. Its causes are listed in **Table 10.3.**

TABLE 10.3: Causes of hiccough.

➢ Hasty ingestion of food and fluids ➢ **Hyponatremia** ➢ **Uremia** ➢ Irritation of the phrenic nerve: Due to compression by tumors, esophagitis, pericarditis, mediastinitis, and surgery of thorax and abdomen ➢ Cerebrovascular accidents (especially **lateral medullary syndrome**), encephalitis, and brain tumors	➢ Diabetic ketoacidosis, renal failure, respiratory failure, and electrolyte imbalance ➢ Local irritation of the diaphragm: Due to gaseous distension of stomach and intestines, subphrenic abscess, peritonitis, and acute myocardial infarction ➢ Psychogenic ➢ Unknown

Symptomatic treatment
- Advised to drink cold water, swallowing a teaspoon of dry sugar
- Apply pressure over the eyeballs
- Perform Valsalva maneuver
- Rebreathing into a paper bag
- Drugs (**Box 10.2**)
- Local infiltration of phrenic nerve with procaine
- Acupuncture

Box 10.2: Drugs used for the treatment of hiccough.
- Chlorpromazine 25–50 mg orally or intramuscularly
- Domperidone 10 mg thrice daily
- Metoclopramide 10 mg thrice daily
- Xylocaine viscus 15 mL thrice a day
- Baclofen 5–10 mg thrice a day
- Nifedipine, haloperidol, phenytoin, olanzapine, nefopam, and gabapentin can be used

Constipation

Q. Define constipation (Rome IV criteria). List the common causes.

Definition: Constipation is defined as persistent, difficult, infrequent passage of hard stools, or seemingly incomplete defecation/evacuation. Many patients may also complain of excessive straining or lower abdominal fullness/discomfort.

Criteria for Functional Constipation (Box 10.3)

Box 10.3: Rome IV criteria for functional constipation.
1. Two or more of the following six must be present*
   a. Straining during at least 25% of defecations
   b. Lumpy or hard stools in at least 25% of defecations
   c. Sensation of incomplete evacuation for at least 25% of defecations
   d. Sensation of anorectal obstruction/blockage for at least 25% of defecations
   e. Manual maneuvers to facilitate at least 25% of defecations (e.g., digital evacuation, support of the pelvic floor)
   f. Fewer than three defecations/week
2. Loose stools are rarely present without the use of laxatives
3. There are insufficient criteria for irritable bowel syndrome (IBS)

*Criteria fulfilled for the previous 3 months with symptom onset at least 6 months prior to diagnosis.

Risk factors: Advanced age, female gender, low level of physical activity, low socioeconomic status, nonwhite ethnicity, and use of certain medications.

Causes of Constipation

See **Table 10.4.**

TABLE 10.4: Causes of constipation.

Primary causes of constipation	*Secondary causes of constipation*
Gastrointestinal disorders: ➢ **Dietary:** Lack of fiber and/or fluid intake ➢ **Motility:** Irritable bowel syndrome, slow-transit constipation ➢ **Structural:** Carcinoma colon, diverticular disease, and Hirschsprung's disease ➢ **Defecation:** Anorectal disease such as Crohn's, fissures, and hemorrhoids	***Medications:*** ➢ Antacids ➢ Anticholinergic agents (e.g., antiparkinsonian drugs, antipsychotics, antispasmodics, and tricyclic antidepressants) ➢ Anticonvulsants (e.g., carbamazepine, phenobarbital, and phenytoin) ➢ Calcium-channel blockers (e.g., verapamil) ➢ Diuretics (e.g., furosemide) ➢ Iron supplements ➢ Nonsteroidal anti-inflammatory drugs (e.g., ibuprofen) ➢ Mu-opioid agonists (e.g., fentanyl, loperamide, and morphine) ***Metabolic and endocrinologic disorders:*** ➢ Diabetes mellitus ➢ Heavy metal poisoning (e.g., arsenic, lead, and mercury) ➢ Hypercalcemia ➢ Hyperthyroidism ➢ Hypokalemia ➢ Hypothyroidism ***Neurologic and myopathic disorders:*** ➢ Amyloidosis ➢ Autonomic neuropathy ➢ Dermatomyositis ➢ Multiple sclerosis ➢ Parkinsonism ➢ Progressive systemic sclerosis ➢ Shy-Drager syndrome ➢ Spinal cord injury

Investigations

It is neither possible nor appropriate to investigate all patients with constipation.

Initial visit:
- Routine biochemistry: Serum calcium, serum glucose, and thyroid function tests
- Complete blood count
- Examination of stool including occult blood
- Digital rectal examination
- Proctoscopy and sigmoidoscopy or colonoscopy: To detect anorectal disease or exclude carcinoma colon (in patients older than 50 years or those with alarm situations such as blood in stool or anemia or weight loss or new onset of symptoms).

If these investigations are normal, a 1 month trial of dietary fiber and/or laxatives is advised.

Next visit: If symptoms persist, barium studies or CT colonography is indicated to look for structural disease. Colonic transit studies, anorectal manometry, and defecography are performed in only in resistant cases without a structural disease.

Q. Discuss management of constipation.

Treatment
- Regular exercise and adequate fluid intake
- Treat the underlying cause or eliminate offending medication
- **Fiber supplementation:** If there is no secondary cause, increasing the fiber content of the diet and fluid intake. A fiber supplement such as wheat bran or psyllium and mucilaginous seeds and seed coats (e.g., ispaghula husk) with water two to four times per day
- **Laxatives (Table 10.5):** They should be restricted to severe cases. Osmotic laxatives act by increasing colonic inflow of fluid and electrolytes by osmotic activity. This softens the stool and stimulates colonic contractility. The stimulatory laxatives act by stimulating colonic contractility and by causing intestinal secretion. Prucalopride is effective in refractory constipation

TABLE 10.5: Various laxatives.

Bulk laxatives	Emollient laxatives (stool softeners)	Stimulant laxatives (stimulate motility and intestinal secretion)	Osmotic laxatives	Others
➢ Soluble (ispaghula, psyllium) ➢ Insoluble (methyl cellulose)	➢ Docusate salts ➢ Mineral oil ➢ Other agents, e.g., polyethylene glycol	➢ Phenolphthalein ➢ Bisacodyl ➢ Anthraquinones—senna and dantron (only for the terminally ill) ➢ Sodium picosulphate ➢ Castor oil	➢ Magnesium sulfate ➢ Lactulose/lactitol ➢ Macrogols	➢ Guanylate cyclase-C receptor agonists (linaclotide and plecanatide) ➢ Lubiprostone (chloride channel activator) ➢ Misoprostol ➢ Colchicine ➢ Prucalopride (5HT4 receptor agonist)

Chronic Blood and Mucus in the Stools

Q. List causes of chronic blood and mucus in the stools. How will you investigate such a case?

Causes

See **Table 10.6**.

TABLE 10.6: Causes of chronic blood and mucus in the stools.

➢ Dysentery – Amebic dysentery – Bacillary dysentery	➢ Inflammatory bowel disease – Ulcerative colitis – Crohn's disease ➢ Intestinal tuberculosis	➢ Carcinoma: Large bowel (rectum, sigmoid and colon) ➢ Diverticulitis ➢ Mesenteric vascular disease ➢ Necrotizing enterocolitis

Investigations

- **Stool examination**
  - Macroscopy: Fresh blood/altered blood/foul smelling/bulky/floats in water/mucus
  - Microscopy (**Table 10.7**)
- **Stool culture and sensitivity**: Grows the organism
- **Proctoscopy:** To detect any ulcers or tumors of rectum and hemorrhoids
- **Sigmoidoscopy:** To detect any ulcers/tumors in the sigmoid colon
- **Colonoscopy:** To visualize colon
- **Barium enema:** To identify any growth or filling defects, strictures, ulcers, and diverticula
- **Biopsy:** Of an ulcer or growth

TABLE 10.7: Microscopic components that can appear in stool.

➢ Ova ➢ Trophozoites ➢ Red blood cells ➢ Bacteria	➢ Cysts ➢ Pus cells ➢ Macrophages

Occult Blood in the Stool

- Stool may appear normal (i.e., no melena) in patients with gastroduodenal bleeding of up to 50–100 mL/day.
- Blood loss in stool of a normal individual varies from 0.5 mL/day to 1.5 mL/day. Occult blood tests begin to become positive usually when blood loss is around 2 mL/day.
- **Test for detection of occult blood** in stool:
  - **Guaiac test:** Gastrointestinal tract bleeding is often intermittent. Hence, this test should be performed for several successive days. This test is negative in a person on iron or bismuth.
  - **Other tests:** Fecal immunochemical tests and heme-porphyrin test.

Conditions with Occult Blood in Stool (Table 10.8)

TABLE 10.8: Conditions with occult blood in stool.

Upper gastrointestinal bleeding	Esophageal varices, esophagitis, peptic ulcer disease, gastritis, and malignancy
Lower gastrointestinal bleeding	Hemorrhoids, malignancy, diverticulitis, inflammatory bowel disease, and celiac sprue
Drugs	Aspirin or steroids (rare)
Others	Hookworm infestation and mesenteric vascular disease

Weight Loss (Table 10.9)

TABLE 10.9: Common causes of weight loss.

Types of weight loss:

➢ **Physiological:** Due to dieting, exercise, starvation, or decreased nutritional intake (e.g., old age)

➢ **Pathological/involuntary**

- Endocrine and metabolic disorders: Diabetes mellitus, hyperthyroidism, pheochromocytoma, Addison's disease, and panhypopituitarism
- Gastrointestinal disorders: Malabsorption, tropical sprue, chronic pancreatitis, inflammatory bowel disease (ulcerative colitis and Crohn's disease), and parasitic infestations
- Chronic infections: Tuberculosis, human immunodeficiency virus (HIV), fungal infections, amebic abscess
- Malignancy: Stomach, colon, pancreas, liver, lung, lymphoma, and leukemia
- Psychiatric illness: Anorexia nervosa, depression, and schizophrenia
- Renal disease: Chronic renal failure and infective endocarditis
- Cardiac disorders: Chronic congestive heart failure
- Respiratory disorders: Emphysema, empyema, chronic obstructive pulmonary disease (COPD)
- Rheumatological: Rheumatoid arthritis
- Idiopathic

Glossitis

Q. List the causes of glossitis.

Definition: Glossitis is defined as inflammation of the tongue.

Causes

B-complex deficiency, megaloblastic anemia (pernicious anemia), oral candidiasis, herpes, cirrhosis, iron deficiency anemia, pellagra, scarlet fever, syphilis, chemical irritants, drug reactions, amyloidosis, sarcoidosis, infections, and vesiculo-erosive diseases.

Clinical Features

- Patients may complain of lingual pain (glossodynia) or burning sensation (glossopyrosis).
- Atrophic glossitis is a sign of protein-calorie malnutrition and muscle atrophy and is commonly found in older adults.
- Median rhomboid glossitis manifests as an asymptomatic, well-defined erythematous patch in the mid-posterior dorsum of the tongue.

Dyspepsia

Q. List the causes and differential diagnosis of dyspepsia.

Dyspepsia is derived from the Greek words *dys and pepse* and literally means "difficult digestion".

- Dyspepsia is a collective description of a variety of gastrointestinal symptoms (**Table 10.10**).
- **Ulcer dyspepsia:** Dyspeptic symptoms associated with peptic ulcer
- **Non-ulcer dyspepsia** (functional dyspepsia): No cause can be found
- **Flatulent dyspepsia:** Usually due to a functional disorder

TABLE 10.10: Symptoms of dyspepsia.

Postprandial fullness	Bloating in the upper abdomen
Early satiation	Nausea
Epigastric pain	Vomiting
Epigastric burning	Belching

Symptoms include early satiety, flatulence, bloating, and belching predominate.

Causes (Table 10.11)

TABLE 10.11: Causes of dyspepsia.

Luminal gastrointestinal tract	*Medications*
➢ Chronic gastric or intestinal ischemia ➢ Food intolerance ➢ Functional dyspepsia ➢ Gastroesophageal reflux disease ➢ Gastric or esophageal neoplasms ➢ Gastric infections (e.g., cytomegalovirus, fungus, tuberculosis, and syphilis) ➢ Gastroparesis (e.g., diabetes mellitus, postvagotomy, scleroderma, chronic intestinal pseudo-obstruction, postviral, and idiopathic) ➢ Irritable bowel syndrome ➢ Peptic ulcer disease ➢ Parasites (e.g., *Giardia lamblia* and *Strongyloides stercoralis*)	Acarbose, aspirin, other nonsteroidal anti-inflammatory drugs (including cyclooxygenase-2 selective agents), colchicine, digitalis preparations, estrogens, ethanol, glucocorticoids, iron, levodopa, niacin, narcotics, nitrates, orlistat, potassium chloride, quinidine, sildenafil, and theophylline ***Pancreaticobiliary disorders*** ➢ Biliary pain: Cholelithiasis, choledocholithiasis, and sphincter of Oddi dysfunction ➢ Chronic pancreatitis ➢ Pancreatic neoplasms ***Systemic conditions*** Adrenal insufficiency, congestive heart failure, diabetes mellitus, hyperparathyroidism, myocardial ischemia, pregnancy, renal insufficiency, and thyroid disease

Nonulcer Dyspepsia (Functional Dyspepsia, Nervous Dyspepsia; Nonorganic Dyspepsia)

Q. Discuss the etiology clinical features, investigations, and management of nonulcer dyspepsia.

Definition: Chronic dyspepsia in the absence of organic disease.
Second most common functional gastrointestinal disorder (after irritable bowel syndrome).

Etiology

- It is dyspepsia in the absence of organic disease and even on detailed investigation, no cause can be found.
- Etiology is poorly understood but probably due to a spectrum of mucosal, motility and psychiatric disorders.
- Symptoms are probably due to disturbances in the motor function of the gastrointestinal tract similar to that occurring in the irritable bowel-syndrome. Both irritable bowel syndrome and nonulcer dyspepsia often exist together in the same patient.
- *Helicobacter pylori* infection should be excluded, because it may be responsible for symptoms in few patients.

Clinical Features

- Usually occurs in young (<40 years of age) females.
- Symptoms and subtypes are described in **Table 10.12**.
- Morning symptoms of pain and nausea on walking are characteristic.
- Features suggestive of irritable bowel syndrome such as pellet-like stools and feeling of incomplete evacuation after defecation may be observed.

TABLE 10.12: Rome IV criteria for functional dyspepsia.

Includes *one* or *more* of the following: 1. Bothersome postprandial fullness 2. Bothersome early satiation	3. Bothersome epigastric pain 4. Bothersome epigastric burning
And	
No evidence of structural disease (including at upper endoscopy) that is likely to explain the symptoms.	
Subgroups according to Rome IV criteria	
➢ **Epigastric pain syndrome (EPS):** Pain centered in the upper abdomen as the predominant symptom ➢ **Postprandial distress syndrome (PDS):** Unpleasant or troublesome nonpainful sensation (discomfort) centered in the upper abdomen is the predominant symptom. This may be accompanied by upper abdominal fullness, early satiety, bloating, and nausea	
Any one of the first two criteria (1 and/or 2, at least 3 days/week) is for PDS while any one of the last two criteria (3 and/or 4, at least 1 day/week) is for EPS	

- History may reveal stress factors such as worries, financial problems, employment, and family affairs.
- On examination, no diagnostic signs, except for inappropriate abdominal tenderness on abdominal palpation.
- All the organic causes of dyspepsia such as peptic ulcer disease (PUD), drug ingestion, depression, pregnancy, alcohol abuse, etc., should be excluded.
- In older patients intra-abdominal malignancy should be excluded which may present with alarming features such as weight loss, anorexia, dysphagia, and hematemesis or melena.

Investigations

The history often suggests the diagnosis.

- *Helicobacter pylori* infection should be serologically excluded in all patients.
- Exclusion of organic causes by following investigations:
  - Blood count, erythrocyte sedimentation rate (ESR) and occult blood in stools
  - Liver function tests (to exclude alcoholism)
  - Pregnancy test
  - Barium meal
  - Ultrasound scan may detect gallstones.
- Indications for endoscopy in patients with chronic dyspepsia/red flags are listed in **Box 10.4**.

Box 10.4: Indications for endoscopy in patients with chronic dyspepsia/red flags.

- Age >60 years
- Dysphagia/previous peptic ulcer disease and odynophagia
- Clinically significant weight loss (>5% usual body weight over 6–12 months)
- Protracted vomiting
- Melena
- Anemia
- Palpable mass
- Jaundice
- Family history of stomach cancer

Management (Fig. 10.1)

- Explanation, reassurance, and lifestyle changes
- Advice to avoid cigarette smoking and alcohol use
- Symptoms if associated with an identifiable cause of stress resolve with appropriate counseling
- Psychological factors influencing on gut function should be explained and may require psychological treatment
- Idiosyncratic and restrictive diets are not beneficial, but reducing intake of fat and coffee may help
- If endoscopy is noncontributory, empirical treatment is advised
  - Prokinetic drugs, such as metoclopramide (10 mg three times daily) or domperidone (10–20 mg three times daily), may be given before meals for nausea, vomiting, or bloating
  - Mosapride or itopride may also be tried
  - H_2-receptor antagonists or proton-pump inhibitors if night pain or heartburn is troublesome
  - *Helicobacter pylori* eradication therapy, if test is positive and may be effective in some patients with functional dyspepsia
  - Selective serotonin reuptake inhibitors may be effective in some patients
  - Low dose tricyclic agents (e.g., amitriptyline) may be of help in up to two-thirds
  - SSRI (selective serotonin re-uptake inhibitor) medication is tried in refractory cases

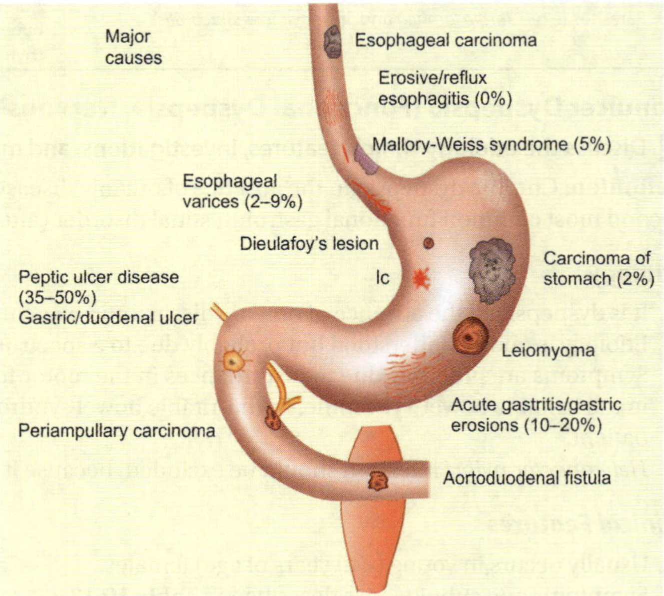

FIG. 10.1: Causes of acute upper gastrointestinal hemorrhage.

Distinguishing Features of Nonulcer Dyspepsia and Ulcer Dyspepsia (Table 10.13)

TABLE 10.13: Distinguishing features of nonulcer dyspepsia and ulcer dyspepsia.

Characteristics	*Nonulcer dyspepsia*	*Ulcer dyspepsia*
Nature of pain	Not episodic	Episodic (periodicity)
Duration of pain	Throughout the day	Occurs only on empty stomach
Relief of pain	Not affected by antacids	Relieved by antacids
Relation of pain with vomiting	Pain is not relieved by vomiting and patient cannot eat afterwards	Pain relieved by vomiting and patient can eat immediately
Relation pain to food	Pain provoked by food	Pain relieved by food
Location of abdominal pain	Diffuse referred to more than one site	Localized referred to epigastrium
Relation of pain to sleep	Pain at night, waking the patient from sleep is rare	Pain at night, waking the patient from sleep is common

GASTROINTESTINAL BLEEDING

Upper Gastrointestinal Bleeding

Q. Enumerate the etiology/causes and investigations of hematemesis upper gastrointestinal bleeding. Discuss how you will manage a case of esophageal varices.

Hematemesis is the bleeding proximal to the duodenojejunal junction (ligament of Treitz).

Etiology (Table 10.14 and Fig. 10.1)

TABLE 10.14: Various causes of upper gastrointestinal (UGI) bleeding.

Esophageal causes
- Esophageal varices (e.g., due to portal hypertension) usually occur from the lower 5 cm of esophagus.
- Erosive esophagitis
- Esophageal carcinoma
- Mallory-Weiss syndrome

Gastroduodenal causes
- Peptic ulcer (gastric and duodenal) disease
- Erosive gastritis (e.g., after ingestion of NSAIDs and alcohol) or duodenitis
- Stress ulcers occurring with shock, sepsis, or severe trauma
- **Curling ulcers** in the proximal duodenum with **severe burns or trauma**
- Carcinoma stomach
- Gastric antral vascular ectasia (GAVE), also described as *watermelon stomach, Dieulafoy's lesion*
- Angiodysplasia or vascular malformations (*Heydes syndrome* in aortic stenosis)
- Rupture of aortic aneurysm or aortic duodenal fistula following aortic graft. Cushing ulcer associated with elevated intracranial pressure

Other cause
- Coagulation defects
- *Cameron's lesions:* Linear erosions or ulcerations in the proximal stomach at the end of a large hiatal hernia, near the diaphragmatic pinch
- Hemobilia
- Hemosuccus pancreaticus

Peptic ulcers are the most common cause of upper gastrointestinal (UGI) bleeding (up to about 50%).

Clinical Features (Table 10.15)

Q. Discuss the appropriate history and clinical features that identify the source of bleeding, quantity, volume loss, etiology, and risk factors of UGI bleed.

Q. List the differential diagnosis for UGI bleed based on presenting symptoms and clinical features.

Presentation: Patient usually presents with either hematemesis (vomiting of blood or coffee-ground material) and/or melena (black, tarry stool).

- **Hematemesis: Color of the vomitus** depends on how long the blood has been in the stomach and the severity of bleeding.
  - **Red** with clots when bleeding is severe and bright red indicates rapid and sizeable bleeding.
  - **Black** ("coffee grounds") when less severe and bleeding is small.

TABLE 10.15: Features suggesting probable source of upper GI bleeding.

History	*Probable source of bleeding*
➤ Features suggestive of peptic ulcer	Peptic ulcer disease
➤ Jaundice, pedal edema, abdominal distension, splenomegaly, ascites, and dilated abdominal veins ➤ Features of liver cell failure, e.g., spider nevi, palmar erythema, jaundice, and gynecomastia	Esophageal varices
➤ Alcohol or drug (NSAIDs) ingestion, trauma, burns, or sepsis	Gastric erosions
➤ Heavy alcohol intake or vomiting	Mallory-Weiss tear
➤ Dysphagia and weight loss prior to bleeding ➤ Tenderness or a mass	Malignant (stomach or esophageal cancer)/intra-abdominal tumor

- **Melena:** It is the passage of **black, tarry,** foul-smelling **stools** containing altered blood. The characteristic color and smell are due to the action of digestive enzymes and bacteria on hemoglobin. It usually occurs when more than 60 mL blood is lost and blood has been present in the UGI tract for at least 14 hours (and as long as 3–5 days). Occasionally, it develops due to hemorrhage from the right side of the colon.
  - Severe/massive acute UGI bleeding can sometimes cause maroon or bright red stool due to passage of frank blood per-rectum **(hematochezia).**
- **Occasionally**, presentation with **symptoms of blood loss only**. These include:
  - **Acute loss with intravascular volume depletion:** Dizziness, extreme pallor, and shock.
  - **Chronic loss:** With symptoms of anemia

Differences between hematemesis and hemoptysis are presented in **Table 10.16**.

TABLE 10.16: Differences between hematemesis and hemoptysis.

Features	*Hemoptysis*	*Hematemesis*
Definition	Coughing out of blood	Vomiting out of blood
Content and color	Mixed with sputum and bright red in color	Mixed with food particles and coffee-ground in color
Contents	Frothy, associated sputum	No froth, associated food particles
Associated symptoms	Cough, dyspnea	Nausea, vomiting, retching, and abdominal discomfort
Melena	Rare	Common
Reaction	Alkaline (blue litmus remains unchanged)	Acidic (blue litmus remains unchanged)

Q. Discuss evaluation and treatment/management of upper gastrointestinal bleeding.

History

Physical Examination: Look for

- Vital signs, orthostatic hypotension
- Abdominal tenderness
- Skin, oral examination
- Stigmata of liver disease
- *Rectal examination:*
  - Objective description of stool/blood
  - Assess for mass, hemorrhoid

Q. Distinguish between upper and lower GI bleed based on clinical features.

Differences between upper and lower GI bleed are presented in **Table 10.17**.

TABLE 10.17: Differences between upper and lower GI bleed.

Features	*Upper GI tract bleed*	*Lower GI tract bleed*
Site of bleeding	Above ligament of Treitz	Below ligament of Treitz
Clinical presentation	Hematemesis or melena	Hematochezia/rarely melena
Nasogastric aspiration shows	Blood	Clear fluid
Bowel sounds	Hyperactive	Normal
BUN (blood urea nitrogen)/creatinine ratio	Increased	Normal

Basic Investigations

- **Complete blood count**
  - Chronic bleeding leads to anemia, but the hemoglobin concentration and the hematocrit level may be normal after sudden, major bleeding until hemodilution occurs.
  - Low platelet count: Suggests chronic liver disease, dilution, or hematologic disorder.
- **Blood urea nitrogen (BUN) and creatinine:** The blood urea nitrogen level increases to greater extent than the creatinine level because of increased intestinal absorption of urea after breakdown of blood proteins. An elevated blood urea with normal creatinine concentration implies severe bleeding.
- **Liver function tests.** They may show evidence of chronic liver disease.
- **Prothrombin time:** It may be prolonged in patients with chronic liver disease or in coagulation disorders or patients on anticoagulated therapy.
- **Cross-matching:** Potential infusion of packed red blood cells.

Q. Write short essay on management and drugs used in upper gastrointestinal bleeding.

Assessment of upper GIT bleed is presented in **Flowchart 10.1.**

FLOWCHART 10.1: Assessment of upper gastrointestinal bleed (UGIB).

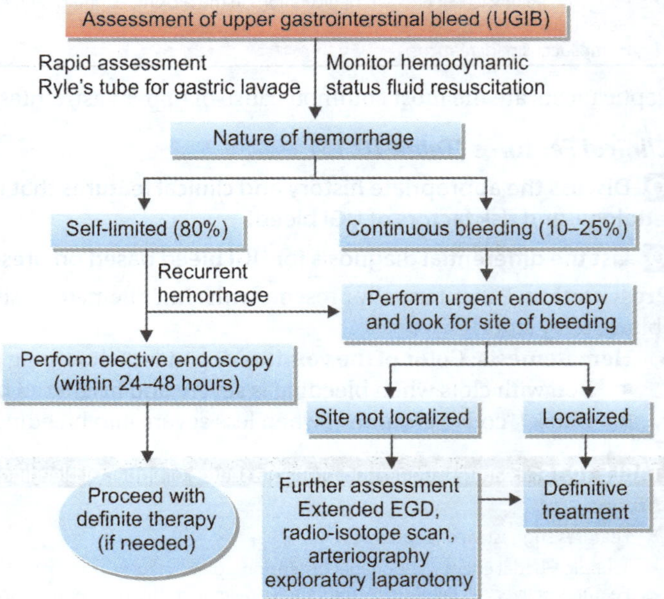

Management

Medical resuscitation and replenishment of intravascular volume: In case of massive bleeding, resuscitation measures should be initiated simultaneously with the initial assessment

- **Intravenous access:** The first step is to gain intravenous access using at least one large-bore (14- or 16-gauge) intravenous catheters for essentially all patients so that normal saline can be infused as fast as necessary to maintain hemodynamic stability
- **Fluid resuscitation:** Adequate resuscitation and hemodynamic stabilization are essential prior to endoscopy (saline). Vasopressors if persistent hypotension
- **Blood product transfusions:** Initiate blood transfusions if the hemoglobin is <7 g/dL to maintain the hemoglobin at a level of ≥9 g/dL. Patients with active bleeding and a low platelet count (<50,000/μL) should be transfused with platelets. Patients with a coagulopathy with a prolonged prothrombin time with INR >1.5 should be transfused with fresh frozen plasma (FFP).

Initial clinical assessment:

- Circulatory status: Severe bleeding causes tachycardia, hypotension, and oliguria. Closely observe with hourly pulse, blood pressure, postural hypotension urine output, and level of consciousness
- Evidence of liver disease: May be present in patients with decompensated cirrhosis
- Comorbidity: Such as cardiorespiratory, cerebrovascular, or renal may be worsened by acute bleeding and also increase the hazards of endoscopy and surgical operations

Gastric lavage: This procedure has been abandoned in present day

- **Procedure:** Gastric lavage is performed by instilling 500 mL of ice-cold or tap water every 30–60 minutes
- **Advantages** of nasogastric or orogastric tube help to localize the site of upper GI bleeding. Determine the type of material whether red blood or coffee-ground. Assess the rate, severity, persistency, and recurrence of the bleeding. Clear the blood from stomach for better endoscopic visualization prior to endoscopy. Remove blood → reduces the risk of encephalopathy in patients with liver disease. Dilute acid-pepsin in stomach → reduces bleeding from erosions. Minimize the risk of aspiration
- **Prognostic score:** Rockall score is based upon age, the presence of shock, comorbidity, diagnosis, and endoscopic stigmata of recent hemorrhage

Endoscopy

Pre-endoscopic pharmacotherapy

For nonvariceal UGIB (upper gastrointestinal bleeding)

- IV proton pump inhibitor: 80 mg bolus, 8 mg/h drip (esomeprazole)
- Rationale: Suppress acid, facilitate clot formation, and stabilization

Goal of endoscopic therapy: To stop acute bleeding and reduce the risk of recurrent bleeding

- Early endoscopy (within 24 hours) is recommended for most patients with acute UGIB
- Achieves prompt diagnosis, provides risk stratification and hemostasis therapy in high-risk patients

Endoscopic hemostasis therapy

It includes (1) epinephrine injection, (2) thermal electrocoagulation, and (3) mechanical (hemoclips). Combination therapy is superior to monotherapy

Nonvariceal UGIB: Postendoscopy management (**Box 10.5**)

Box 10.5: Postendoscopy management of nonvariceal UGIB.

- Patients with ulcers requiring endoscopic therapy should receive PPI x 72 hours
- Determine *H. pylori* status in all ulcer patients
- Discharge patients on PPI (once to twice daily), duration dictated by underlying etiology and need for nonsteroidal anti-inflammatory drugs (NSAIDs)/aspirin
- In patients with cardiovascular disease on low dose aspirin: Restart as soon as bleeding has resolved

Management of upper GI tract bleeding is summarized in **Flowchart 10.2**.

Q. Enumerate the indications for endoscopy, colonoscopy, and other imaging modalities in the investigation of Upper GI bleed.

Endoscopy: It is the diagnostic modality of choice for acute upper GI bleeding. Endoscopy has a high sensitivity and specificity for locating and identifying bleeding lesions in the upper GI tract. Therapeutic endoscopy can in most cases achieve acute hemostasis and prevent recurrent bleeding once a bleeding lesion has been identified. Early endoscopy, within 24 hours is recommended for most patients with acute upper GI bleeding. For patients with suspected variceal bleeding, endoscopy should be performed within 12 hours of presentation.

Colonoscopy: It is indicated in patients with hematochezia and a negative upper endoscopy. It is also frequently performed in patients with melena and a negative upper endoscopy, to rule out right-sided colonic lesions which may also present with melena.

Imaging: Plain radiographs may be useful to demonstrate bowel obstruction/perforation in patients who present with pain abdomen and distention. Barium studies are contraindicated in the acute setting of UGI bleed as it may interfere with the subsequent endoscopy/surgery. USG abdomen is particularly useful in patients with suspected liver disease with clinical signs of portal hypertension.

FLOWCHART 10.2: Management of upper GI tract bleeding.

- Management of upper gastrointestinal bleeding (UGIB)
  - General medical management
  - Types of bleeding
    - Variceal bleeding
      - Medical
      - Pressure techniques
      - Endotherapy
      - Surgical intervention
    - Non-variceal bleeding
      - Endoscopic management
        - Injection adrenaline, fibrin glue, human thrombin, sclerosants alcohol
        - Thermal heater probe, bicap probe, gold probe, argon plasma coagulation, laser therapy
        - Mechanical hemoclips, banding endoloops, staples sutures
      - Other:
        1. Interventional radiological procedures
        2. Transcathetral arterial embolization
        3. Surgical intervention—with or without endoscope

Variceal Bleeding

Occurs in one-third of patients with cirrhosis. In one-third initial bleeding episodes are fatal. Among survivors, one-third will rebleed within 6 weeks. Only one-third will survive 1 year or more. Management of variceal bleed is discussed in Chapter 11.

Lower Gastrointestinal Bleed

Q. List causes of lower gastrointestinal bleeding.

Lower GI bleeding generally signifies bleeding from the colon or anorectum. In patients with severe **hematochezia**, first consider possibility of UGIB. About 10–15% of patients with presumed LGIB are found to have upper GIB.

Etiology (Table 10.18 and Fig. 10.2)

TABLE 10.18: Causes of lower gastrointestinal bleeding.

Diverticulosis (main cause)	Angioectasias
Hemorrhoids anal fissures, ulcer	Colitis (IBD, infectious, and ischemic)
Neoplasms	Postpolypectomy
Dieulafoy's lesion	Radiation colitis, small bowel bleed
	Unknown causes—10%

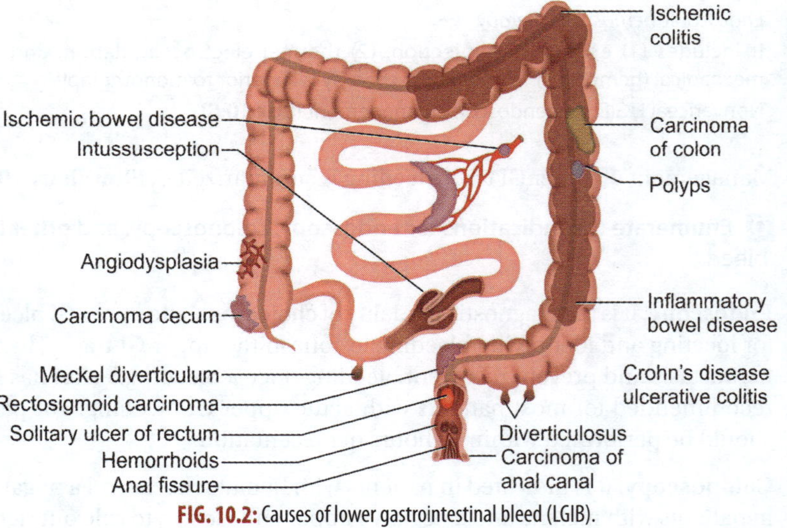

FIG. 10.2: Causes of lower gastrointestinal bleed (LGIB).

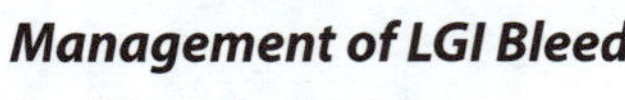

Management of LGI Bleed

See **Flowchart 10.3.**

APPROACH TO DIARRHEA

Q. Enumerate the common cause of diarrhea in the tropics.

Definition: Daily bowel movements of three or more times are considered to be abnormal. The upper limit of stool weight is 200 g daily. Although stool weight usually considered as a "scientific" definition of diarrhea, diarrhea should not be defined solely in terms of fecal weight.

- **Acute diarrhea** is defined as abrupt onset of increased frequency and/or fluidity of bowel movements.
- **Chronic diarrhea** is defined as passage of loose stools with or without increased stool frequency for more than 4 weeks.

FLOWCHART 10.3: Management of lower gastrointestinal bleeding.

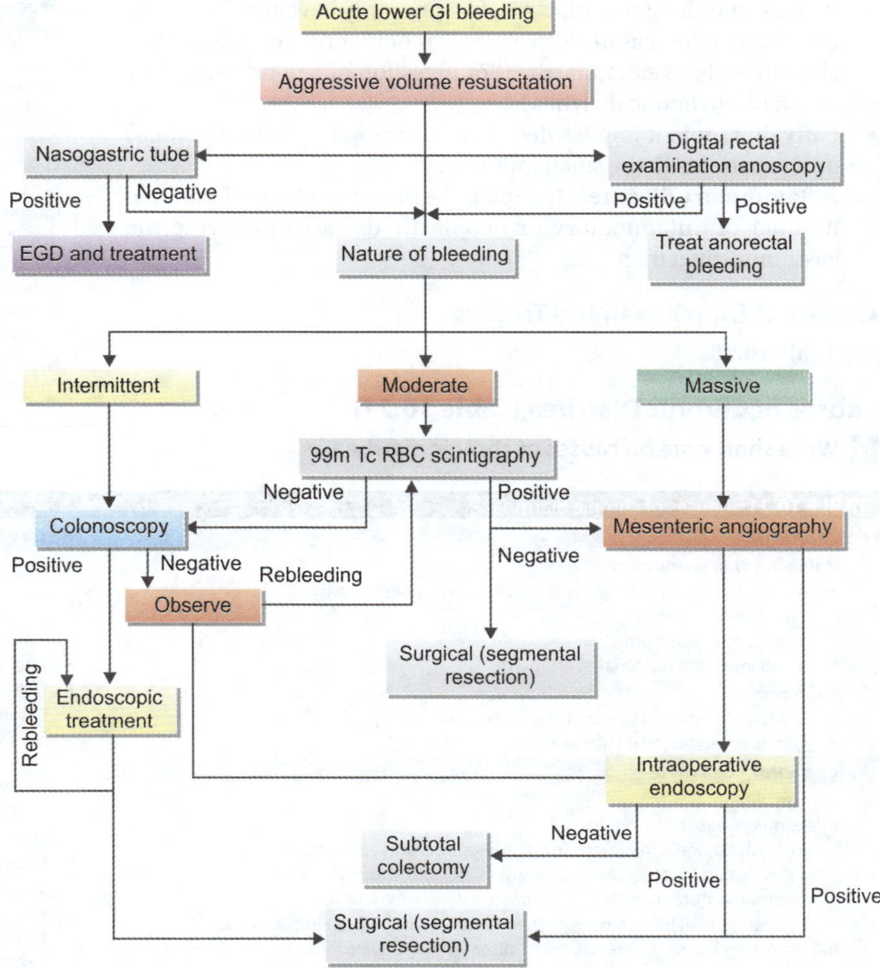

Large-volume versus Small-volume Diarrhea

- Normal rectosigmoid colon functions as a storage reservoir.
- **Left colonic disorders:** Inflammatory or motility disorders involving the left colon compromises this rectosigmoid reservoir capacity and results in **frequent small-volume bowel movements.**
- **Right colonic or small bowel disorders:** In diarrhea due to disorders of the right colon or small bowel and if the rectosigmoid reservoir is intact, individual **bowel movements are less frequent and larger.**

Frequent, small, painful stools may point to a source in the distal colon, whereas painless large-volume stools suggest a right colonic or small bowel source.

Secretory versus Osmotic Diarrhea (Table 10.19)

- **Secretory diarrhea:** It results from malabsorption or secretion of electrolytes (secretory diarrhea).
- **Osmotic diarrhea:** It results from intestinal malabsorption of ingested nonelectrolytes.
- Osmotic diarrhea constitutes small number of cases whereas secretory diarrhea forms the much larger number of cases.
- In secretory diarrhea, sodium, potassium, and accompanying anions account almost entirely for stool osmolality. In contrast, in osmotic diarrhea poorly absorbable solutes within the lumen of the intestine account for much of the osmotic activity of stool water.

TABLE 10.19: Secretory versus osmotic diarrhea.

Type of diarrhea	*Causes*	*Examples*
Secretory diarrhea	Exogenous secretagogues	Enterotoxins (e.g., cholera)
	Endogenous secretagogues	Neuroendocrine tumors (e.g., carcinoid syndrome)
	Absence of ion transporter	Congenital chloridorrhea
	Loss of intestinal surface area	Intestinal resection, diffuse intestinal mucosal disease
	Intestinal ischemia	Diffuse mesenteric atherosclerosis
	Rapid intestinal transit	Intestinal hurry following vagotomy
Osmotic diarrhea	Ingestion of poorly absorbed agent	Magnesium ingestion
	Loss of nutrient transporter	Lactase deficiency

Watery versus Fatty versus Inflammatory Diarrhea

- **Watery diarrhea:** It implies a defect primarily in water absorption as a result of increased electrolyte secretion or reduced electrolyte absorption (secretory diarrhea) or ingestion of a poorly absorbed substance (osmotic diarrhea).
- **Fatty diarrhea:** It implies defective absorption of fat and perhaps other nutrients in the small intestine.
- **Inflammatory diarrhea:** It implies the presence of one of a limited number of inflammatory or neoplastic diseases involving the gastrointestinal tract.

Causes of Diarrhea in the Tropics

See **Table 10.20**.

TABLE 10.20: Causes of diarrhea in tropics.

Gastroenteritis induced by toxin	*Gastroenteritis induced by changes in mucosa*
➢ Performed toxins: *Staphylococcus aureus* and *Bacillus cereus* ➢ Enterotoxins produced in the intestine, *Clostridium perfringens*, *Vibrio cholerae*, enterotoxigenic *Escherichia coli*, enterohemorrhagic *E. coli*, and *Clostridium difficile*	➢ Mucosal changes without invasion: Rotavirus, Norwalk agent ➢ Invasion of mucosa/ inflammatory (invasion or cytotoxin) dysentery – *Salmonella* species, *Shigella* species, enterohemorrhagic *E. coli*, enteroinvasive *E. coli*, *Campylobacter jejuni*, *Yersinia enterocolitica*, and *Entamoeba histolytica* ➢ Other causes: Mushrooms, heavy metals (arsenic), monosodium glutamate

Causes of Chronic Diarrhea (Table 10.21)

Q. Write short note on causes of chronic diarrhea.

TABLE 10.21: Causes of chronic diarrhea.

Fatty diarrhea	*Watery diarrhea*
1. ***Malabsorption syndromes*** – Mucosal diseases (e.g., celiac disease and Whipple's disease) – Mesenteric ischemia – Short bowel syndrome – Small intestinal bacterial overgrowth 2. ***Maldigestion*** – Inadequate luminal bile acid concentration – Pancreatic exocrine insufficiency ***Inflammatory diarrhea*** ➢ Diverticulitis ➢ Infectious diseases – Invasive bacterial infections (e.g., tuberculosis and yersiniosis) – Invasive parasitic infections (e.g., amebiasis and strongyloidiasis) – Pseudomembranous colitis (*Clostridium difficile* infection) – Ulcerating viral infections (e.g., cytomegalovirus, herpes simplex virus) ➢ Inflammatory bowel diseases: Crohn's disease, ulcerative colitis ➢ Ischemic colitis ➢ Neoplasia: Carcinoma of colon, lymphoma ➢ Radiation colitis	➢ Osmotic diarrhea – Carbohydrate malabsorption – Osmotic laxatives ➢ Secretory diarrhea ➢ Bacterial toxins ➢ Congenital syndromes (e.g., congenital chloridorrhea) ➢ Disordered motility, regulation – Diabetic autonomic neuropathy – Irritable bowel syndrome – Postsympathectomy diarrhea – Postvagotomy diarrhea ➢ Diverticulitis ➢ Endocrinopathies: Addison's disease, carcinoid syndrome, gastrinoma, hyperthyroidism, mastocytosis, medullary carcinoma of thyroid, pheochromocytoma, somatostatinoma, and VIPoma ➢ Laxative abuse (stimulant laxatives) ➢ Medications and toxins

Approach to the Patient with Acute Diarrhea

Q. Discuss the evaluation and management of acute diarrhea.

Assessment of the Patient

- Degree of dehydration
- Evidence of specific cause
- Necessity of any diagnostic tests
- Requirement for any treatment

History (Table 10.22) Physical Examination

- Examine for signs of dehydration to assess the severity of the diarrhea. These include examination of pulse, blood pressure (including postural change), skin turgor, dryness of mucous membranes (e.g., mouth), mental status, and breathing.
- Severity of dehydration (**Table 10.23**)
- Electrolyte imbalances: Assess muscle strength and muscle reflexes which may be reduced in hypokalemia.
- Examination of abdomen to exclude any surgical cause (e.g., intestinal obstruction).

TABLE 10.22: Features to be noted during taking history in a patient with acute diarrhea.

1. Duration of diarrhea
2. Travel or use of antibiotics
3. Having food outside in the recent past and time since consumption
4. Any other family member or close associated affected
5. *Associated features:* Pain abdomen, fever, vomiting, and tenesmus
6. *Stool:* Frequency of loose stools, volume, appearance of stools (e.g., rice water), presence of blood or mucus in the stools
7. Urine output
8. Any alteration in the level of consciousness
9. Occupation of the patient

TABLE 10.23: Severity of dehydration.

Features	*Mild*	*Moderate*	*Severe*
Urine output	Decreased	Decreased	Markedly decreased
Physical examination			
Level of consciousness	Normal	Normal	Depressed
Mental status	Normal/irritable	Lethargic	Comatose
Skin	Normal	Cool	Cool and mottled
Skin turgor	Normal	Reduced with skin tenting	Markedly reduced
Mouth/oral mucosa	Dry	Markedly dry	Parched
Eyes	Normal	Sunken (sunken fontanel in infants)	Markedly sunken
Pulse rate	Normal or mild increase	Tachycardia, feeble	Marked tachycardia
Blood pressure	Normal	Postural/orthostatic fall	Hypotension and frank shock
Respiration	Normal	Normal	Acidotic
Investigations			
Urine specific gravity	<1.020	>1.020	>1.035
Blood urea	Normal	Normal to raised	High

Q. Enumerate the indications for stool cultures and blood cultures in acute diarrhea.

Laboratory Investigations

Laboratory investigations usually do not help in the management acute diarrhea.

- **Total white blood cell (WBC) count:** Presence of high leukocyte count with shift to left suggests invasive bacterial infection.
- **Electrolytes and acid-base status:** It should be done in patients with severe dehydration. Severe diarrhea produces metabolic acidosis.
- **Blood cultures:** To be performed when bacteremia or a systemic infection is suspected.
- **Stool examination:** Grossly bloody or mucus in the stool suggests an inflammatory process. In severe cases stool should be examined for the presence of leukocytes, red cells, and cysts or trophozoites/parasites. In cholera *V. cholerae* show the characteristic darting motility. Stool with leukocytes considers inflammatory causes (*Shigella*, *Salmonella*, *Campylobacter*, *E. coli*, *Entamoeba*, and *Clostridium difficile*).
- **Stool culture:** Specific indications **for** stool cultures **include bloody** stools, stools **that** test **positive for occult** blood **or leukocytes, prolonged course of** diarrhea **that has not been treated with** antibiotics, immunocompromised host, or for epidemiologic purposes, such as cases involving food handlers.

Q. Describe and discuss the acute systemic consequences of acute diarrhea including its impact on fluid balance.

Systemic complications of acute diarrheal disease are presented in **Table 10.24**.

TABLE 10.24: Systemic complications of acute diarrheal disease.

Complication	*Associated organism*
Sepsis	*Shigella* species, nontyphoidal *Salmonella enterica*, and *Campylobacter* fetus
Hemolytic-uremic syndrome	*Shigella* species, Shiga toxin-producing *Escherichia coli*
Guillain-Barré syndrome	*Campylobacter jejuni*
Reactive arthritis	*Campylobacter* species, *Salmonella* species, and *Shigella flexneri*

Effect on fluid balance: Usually, more than 90% of the fluid entering the small intestine is absorbed. Only about 1 liter reaches the large intestine. Further absorption occurs in the large intestine and only 100–200 milliliters of water is excreted each day in formed stools. When there is increased secretion and/or decreased absorption in the small intestine, large volumes enter the large intestine. Diarrhea occurs when this volume exceeds the absorptive capacity of the large intestine. Diarrhea stools contain large amounts of water, sodium, chloride, bicarbonate, and potassium. These losses cause dehydration (due to the loss of water and sodium chloride), metabolic acidosis (due to the loss of bicarbonate), and hypokalemia (due to potassium depletion). Among these, dehydration (negative fluid balance) is the most dangerous because it can cause decreased blood volume (hypovolemia), cardiovascular collapse, acute renal failure, mental confusion, and death if not treated promptly.

Small Bowel versus Large Bowel Diarrhea

See **Table 10.25**.

TABLE 10.25: Differences between small bowel and large bowel diarrhea.

Features	*Small bowel diarrhea*	*Large bowel diarrhea*
Characteristic of diarrhea	Large-volume, watery diarrhea	Frequent, small volume, often painful bowel movements
Associated clinical features	Abdominal cramping, bloating and gas formation	Gripping pain in lower abdomen
Fever	Uncommon	Present
Tenesmus	Absent	Present
Blood or mucus stools	Not common	Common
Inflammatory cells and red blood cells in stools	Absent	Present

Management (Flowchart 10.4)

Most of acute diarrhea is self-limited and fluid and electrolyte replacement are of most important in all cases

Rehydration

- Severe diarrhea produces dehydration especially in the very young and very old
- Toxin-induced diarrhea produces stools that are usually isotonic. Concentrations of sodium and chloride are slightly less than that of plasma while bicarbonate concentration is double that of plasma. The stools also contain significant amount of potassium
- In inflammatory diarrhea the electrolyte loss is of less compared to toxigenic diarrhea

Oral rehydration solution (ORS)

Used for mild-to-moderate dehydration

Intravenous fluids

- Used when there is moderate-to-severe dehydration
- Usually Ringer's lactate is administered
- In severe cases, fluids are administrated at a rate of 20 mL/kg/hour for the first 2–3 hours. If the patient improves, reduce the rate to 10 mL/kg/h for the next 2–4 hours
- Concurrently start oral rehydration therapy

FLOWCHART 10.4: Approach to the management of acute diarrhea.

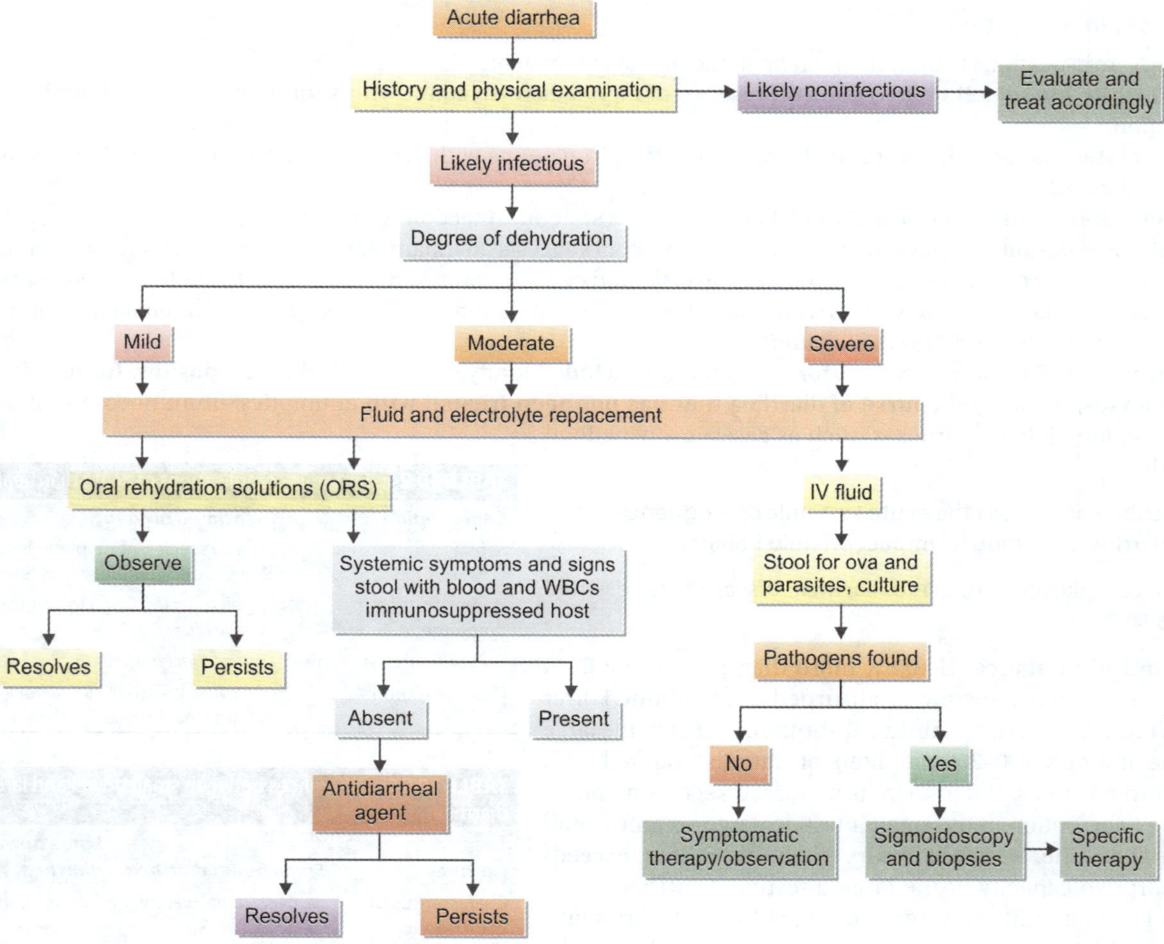

Absorbents

Kaolin absorbs the toxin and may be of use in few patients. However, it does not affect the course of the disease

Antimotility drugs

- Used for symptomatic treatment of toxin-induced diarrhea in adults only. It should not be used in young children and elderly
- It can be given in inflammatory diarrhea along with antibiotics. These include:
  - Opiates (e.g., morphine and codeine): They may cause respiratory depression
  - Diphenoxylate/atropine combination: May cause respiratory depression and anticholinergic side effects
  - Loperamide: Dose is two tablets of 4 mg each initially, then 2 mg after each unformed stool, not to exceed 16 mg/day for ≤2 days
  - Bismuth subsalicylate: It acts as an antisecretory agent. Dose is one tablet every 30 minutes for a total of eight doses or 60 mL every 6 hourly

Antisecretory agents: Racecadotril
- Reduces the hypersecretion of water and electrolytes into the intestinal lumen
- Inhibits enkephalinase (an enzyme that degrades enkephalins)
- Dose: 100 mg thrice daily. To be given to patients with acute, watery diarrhea only
- Contraindication: Renal insufficiency, pregnancy, and breastfeeding

Antispasmodics

Mild antispasmodics such as dicyclomine, hyoscine may be used in patients with significant abdominal cramps

Antibiotics: Indications
- Symptomatic patients with inflammatory diarrhea (high fever, toxicity, and abdominal pain)
- Acute febrile dysentery illness
- Diarrhea caused by *Campylobacter jejuni*. Early use of erythromycin or azithromycin limits the duration of illness
- Commonly used antibiotics: Quinolones (norfloxacin 400 mg and ciprofloxacin 500 mg both given twice daily or levofloxacin 500 mg given once a day) for 3–5 days
- Cholera: Doxycycline in a dose of 300 mg as single dose. Alternatives include trimethoprim-sulfamethoxazole, furazolidone, and norfloxacin

Specific treatment once cause identified

Nonspecific drug therapy for chronic diarrhea is presented in **Table 10.26**.

TABLE 10.26: Nonspecific drug therapy for chronic diarrhea.

Drug class	Agent
Opiates (mu opiate receptor selective)	Codeine, diphenoxylate, loperamide, morphine, and tincture of opium
Enkephalinase inhibitor (delta opiate receptor effects)	Racecadotril
Alpha-2 adrenergic agonist	Clonidine
Somatostatin analog	Octreotide
Bile acid-binding resin	Cholestyramine, colesevelam, and colestipol
Fiber supplements	Calcium polycarbophil, psyllium

Traveler's Diarrhea

Q. Write short note on traveler's diarrhea.

Traveler's diarrhea is the leading cause of illness in travelers. Usually a short-lived and self-limited.

Etiology

- Causative agents: Various pathogens causing travelers' diarrhea are listed in **Table 10.27**. Most important pathogens are *Escherichia coli* and Enteroaggregative *E. coli*: rotavirus and norovirus.
- Source of infection: Main sources of infection are food and water contaminated with fecal matter.

TABLE 10.27: Various causes of traveler's diarrhea.

Bacteria (50–75%)	Viruses (0–20%)	Parasites (0–10%)
Enterotoxigenic *Escherichia coli*	Norovirus (winter vomiting bug)	*Giardia lamblia*
Enteroaggregative *E. coli*	Rotavirus	*Cryptosporidium*
Campylobacter jejuni		*Entamoeba histolytica*
Shigella		
Salmonella (nontyphoid)	No pathogens (10–50%)	

Clinical Features

- Usually involves intercontinental travelers.
- Symptoms: Abrupt in onset, watery diarrhea lasting 2-5 days, abdominal cramps, nausea, vomiting, anorexia, and fever.
- Signs: Diffuse tenderness over abdomen.

Treatment
- Usually self-limited and requires no treatment
- Dehydration is corrected by oral rehydration supplements
- Drugs:
  - Antidiarrheal agents and antibiotics are only rarely required
  - If there is fever or bloody diarrhea advise norfloxacin or ciprofloxacin. Azithromycin is used in patients who are allergic to quinolones
  - Rifaximin (a poorly absorbed rifampicin derivative) is very effective against noninvasive bacterial pathogens

Prevention
- Drugs: Doxycycline 100 mg/day for a few weeks. Norfloxacin/ciprofloxacin/rifaximin once a day
- Probiotics may be useful

DISEASES OF THE ESOPHAGUS

Dysphagia

Q. Discuss causes and investigation (evaluation) and management of dysphagia.

Dysphagia, from the Greek dys (difficulty, disordered) and phagia (to eat), refers to the sensation that food is hindered in its passage from the mouth to the stomach.

Causes of Dysphagia

Oropharyngeal dysphagia

Processes that affect the mouth, hypopharynx, and upper esophagus. The patient often is unable to initiate a swallow and repeatedly has to attempt to swallow. Patients frequently describe coughing or choking when they attempt to swallow. Causes of oropharyngeal dysphagia are listed in **Table 10.28**.

TABLE 10.28: Causes of oropharyngeal dysphagia.

Neuromuscular causes	*Structural causes*
➢ Amyotrophic lateral sclerosis (ALS) ➢ Multiple sclerosis ➢ Muscular dystrophy ➢ Myasthenia gravis ➢ Parkinson's disease ➢ Polymyositis or dermatomyositis ➢ Stroke ➢ Thyroid dysfunction	➢ Carcinoma ➢ Infections of pharynx or neck ➢ Osteophytes and other spinal disorders ➢ Prior surgery or radiation therapy ➢ Proximal esophageal web ➢ Plummer–Vinson syndrome ➢ Thyromegaly ➢ Zenker's diverticulum

TABLE 10.29: Common causes of esophageal dysphagia.

Motility (neuromuscular) disorders	*Structural (mechanical) disorders*
Primary disorders ➢ Achalasia ➢ Diffuse esophageal spasm ➢ Hypertensive LES ➢ Ineffective esophageal motility ➢ Nutcracker (high-pressure) esophagus	**Intrinsic** ➢ Carcinoma and benign tumors ➢ Diverticula ➢ Eosinophilic esophagitis ➢ Esophageal rings and webs (other than Schatzki ring) ➢ Foreign body ➢ Lower esophageal (Schatzki) ring ➢ Medication-induced stricture ➢ Peptic stricture
Secondary disorders ➢ Chagas' disease ➢ Reflux-related dysmotility ➢ Scleroderma and other rheumatologic disorders	**Extrinsic** ➢ Mediastinal mass ➢ Spinal osteophytes ➢ Vascular compression

*Esophageal dysphagia (**Table 10.29**)*

Differential Diagnosis of Dysphagia

Approach to the patient with dysphagia is presented in **Flowchart 10.5.**

Investigations

- Hemoglobin and peripheral smear for anemia
- Chest radiograph detects retrosternal goiter, mediastinal lymph nodes, aortic aneurysms, and primary and secondary malignancy of lungs.
- Esophagoscopy allows removal of foreign body, visualization and biopsy of tumors, ulcers, strictures, etc.
- Computed tomography (CT) scan of thorax
- Biopsy from the growth, ulcer, or inflamed mucosa
- Barium swallow detects tumors as filling defects or strictures (rat tail appearance).
- Esophageal motility studies (esophageal manometry)

FLOWCHART 10.5: Approach to the patient with dysphagia.

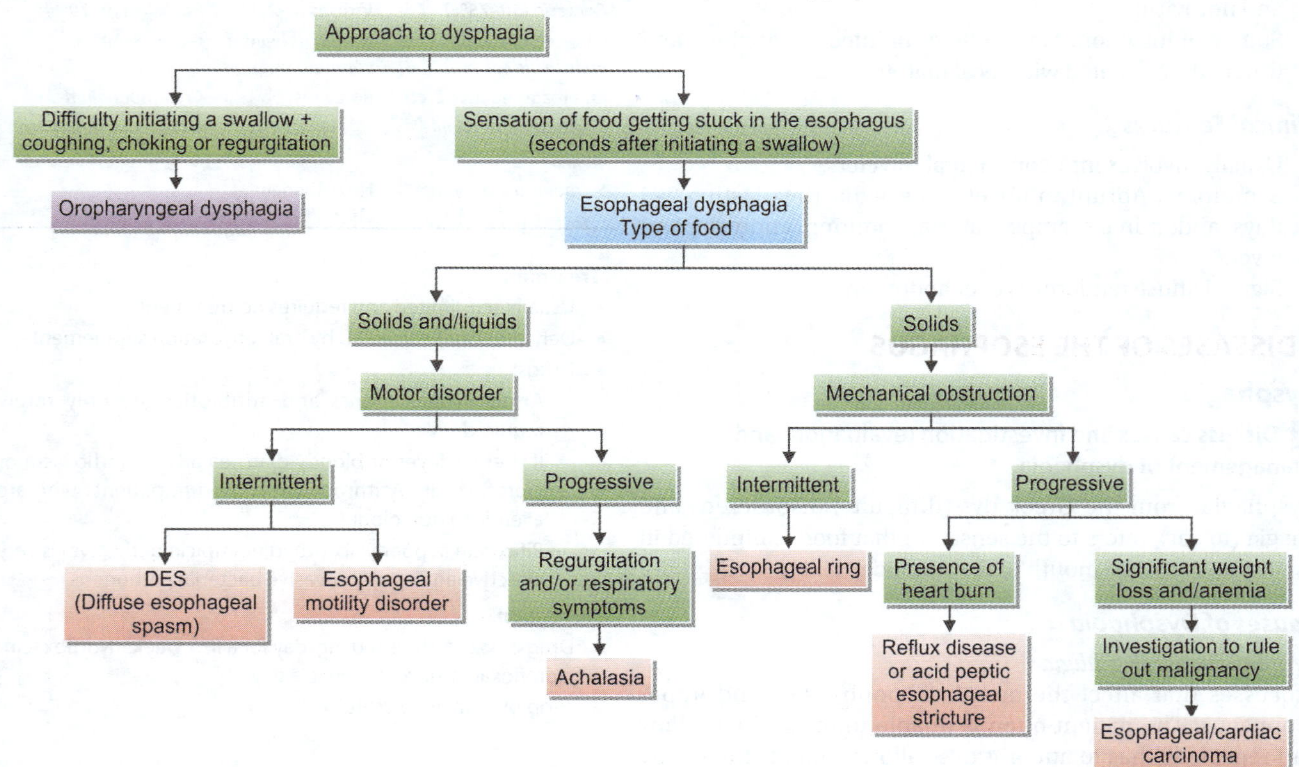

Odynophagia

Q. Write short note on the causes for odynophagia.

Odynophagia, or painful swallowing, is specific feature for esophageal involvement. It usually reflects an inflammatory process in the esophageal mucosa. Its severity varies. It may be a dull retrosternal ache on swallowing to a stabbing pain with radiation to the back so severe that the patient cannot eat or even swallow their own saliva.

Causes of Odynophagia

See **Table 10.30**.

TABLE 10.30: Causes of odynophagia.

Caustic ingestion: Acid, alkali **Pill-induced injury** ➢ Alendronate and other bisphosphonates ➢ Aspirin and other NSAIDs ➢ Iron preparations ➢ Potassium chloride (especially slow-release form) ➢ Tetracycline and its derivatives ➢ Quinidine ➢ Zidovudine	**Infectious esophagitis** ➢ *Viral*: Cytomegalovirus, Epstein-Barr virus, herpes simplex virus, and human immunodeficiency virus ➢ *Bacteria*: Mycobacteria (tuberculosis or *Mycobacterium avium* complex) ➢ *Fungal: Candida albicans*, histoplasmosis ➢ *Protozoan: Cryptosporidium* and *Pneumocystis* **Severe reflux esophagitis** **Esophageal carcinoma**

Plummer-Vinson Syndrome

Discussed in Chapter 8.

Treatment
- Iron deficiency anemia is treated with iron. It may resolve dysphagia
- Endoscopy:
  - Dysphagia may require endoscopic dilatation
  - Follow-up endoscopy at regular intervals to detect development of carcinoma

Gastroesophageal Reflux Disease

Q. Describe the etiopathogenesis, complications, and management of gastroesophageal reflux disease (GERD).

Q. Write short essay on reflux esophagitis and its management.

Definition

- Gastroesophageal reflux disease (GERD) is a consequence of the failure of the normal antireflux barrier to protect against frequent and abnormal amounts of gastroesophageal reflux (GER; i.e., gastric contents moving retrograde effortlessly from the stomach to the esophagus).
- Spectrum of injury to the esophagus includes *esophagitis, stricture, Barrett's esophagus, and adenocarcinoma.*

Pathophysiology

Normal defense mechanisms preventing reflux and reflux esophagitis

Several defense mechanisms prevent the reflux of gastric contents into the esophagus.

- **Antireflux barrier at the gastroesophageal junction (Fig. 10.3):** This consists of (1) lower esophageal sphincter (LES), at the lower end of esophagus, below the diaphragm, (2) striated muscles of the crural diaphragm, (3) phrenoesophageal ligament, (4) oblique entrance of the esophagus into the stomach (angle of His), and (5) attachment of the lower esophageal sphincter (LES) to the crural diaphragm: Intra-abdominal pressure reinforces the LES tone.
- **Esophageal clearance mechanisms:** Reflux of gastric contents into the esophagus occurs in healthy persons and is normally cleared by esophagus in a two-step process:
  1. Volume clearance by peristaltic function: After acid reflux from stomach, the esophageal peristalsis returns the refluxed fluid to the stomach.
  2. Neutralization of acid by bicarbonate in the swallowed saliva: The small amounts of residual acid refluxed into the esophagus are neutralized by weakly alkaline (bicarbonate) contained in swallowed saliva.

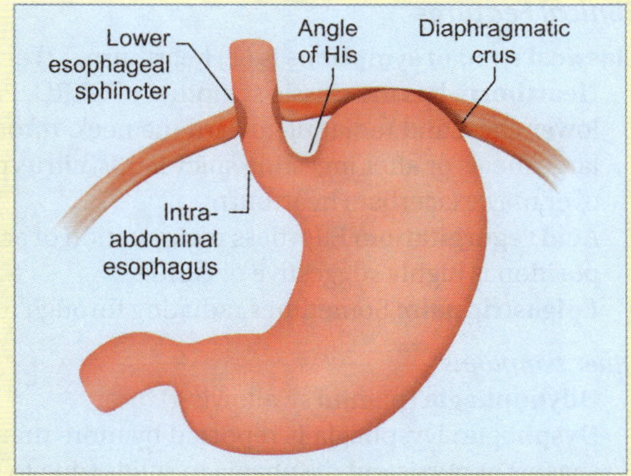

FIG. 10.3: Anatomy of normal antireflux barrier at the lower esophagus.

- **Epithelial defensive factors:** The esophageal mucosa contains mainly three lines of defense.
  1. **Pre-epithelial barrier:** Consisting of (1) small unstirred water layer, (2) bicarbonate from swallowed saliva, and (3) secretions of submucosal glands.
  2. **Epithelial defense:** Consisting of cell membranes and tight intercellular junctions, buffers, and ion transporters.
  3. **Postepithelial defense:** Consists of the blood supply to the esophagus.

Causes of Disruption of Normal Defense Mechanisms (Fig. 10.4)

- **Defective antireflux barriers**
  - **Hiatus hernia (sliding type):** This is characterized by sliding of the esophagogastric junction through the diaphragm. This results in increased exposure of the esophagus to acid and may lead to esophagitis, Barrett's esophagus or peptic strictures.
  - **Abnormalities of lower esophageal sphincter (LES):** Transient relaxation and reduced tone of LES can result in regurgitation, especially when intra-abdominal pressure is increased.
    - Cigarette smoking, chocolate, alcohol, fatty foods, and caffeine cause relaxation and reduction of tone of LES.
    - Cardiomyotomy and vagotomy reduce the efficiency of the LES.
    - Drugs (aminophylline, β-agonists, nitrates, and calcium channel blockers) reduce the tone of LES.
  - Crural diaphragm
  - **Increased the intra-abdominal pressure:** It may occur during pregnancy, obesity, ascites, weight lifting, and straining.

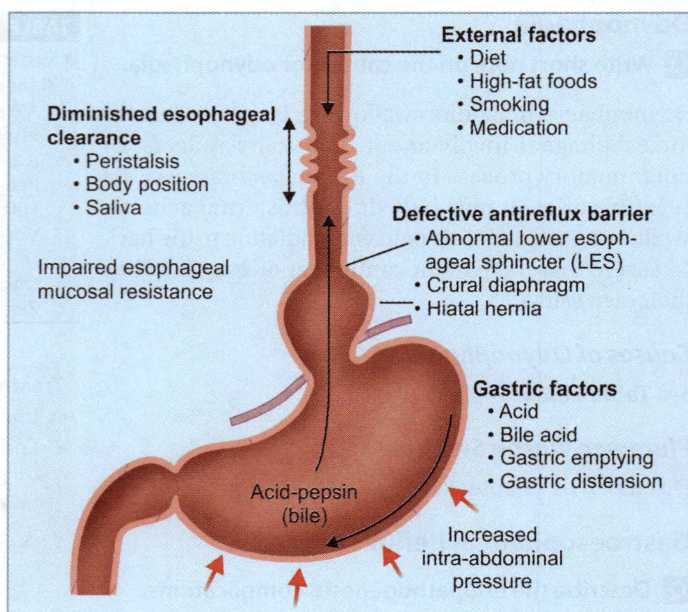

FIG. 10.4: Pathophysiological factors associated with the development of gastroesophageal reflux disease (GERD).

- **Prolonged/delayed esophageal clearance of refluxed acid:** It may be due to (1) impaired peristalsis, (2) reduced salivation, and (3) body position. Poor esophageal clearance leads to increased acid exposure time. Impaired production of saliva may be observed in smokers and Sjogren's syndrome.
- **Defective gastric emptying:** It increases the gastric content available for reflux. It may be due to gastric outlet obstruction, anticholinergic drugs, and fatty food.

Clinical Features

Classical triad of symptoms is (1) heartburn, (2) acid regurgitation, and (3) epigastric pain.

- **Heartburn:** It is the classic symptom of GERD. Patients usually complain of a burning feeling, rising from the stomach or lower chest and radiating toward the neck, throat, and occasionally the back. It occurs postprandially, particularly after large meals or after ingesting spicy foods, citrus products, fats, chocolates, and alcohol. The supine position and bending over may exacerbate heartburn.
- **Acid regurgitation:** Effortless regurgitation of acidic fluid, especially after meals and worsened by stooping or the supine position is highly suggestive of GERD.
- **Epigastric pain:** Sometimes radiating through to the back.

Other symptoms

- **Odynophagia** (painful swallowing)
- **Dysphagia:** Dysphagia is reported by more than 30% of individuals with GERD. Transient to solids (due to esophageal spasm) or persistent dysphagia to solids (due to strictures).
- Less common symptoms associated with GERD include water brash, burping, hiccups, nausea, and vomiting.
- Iron deficiency anemia may occur due to blood loss.

Extraesophageal symptoms

- Atypical chest pain which may be severe and can mimic angina.
- Upper respiratory tract: Hoarseness, sore throat, sinusitis, otitis media, chronic cough, and laryngitis
- Pulmonary: The prevalence of GERD in asthmatics is estimated between 34% and 89%. Other pulmonary diseases associated with GERD include aspiration pneumonia, interstitial pulmonary fibrosis, chronic bronchitis, and bronchiectasis.

*Alarm symptoms or signs (**Table 10.31**)*

Associated conditions: Pregnancy (reducing LES pressure due to the effects of estrogen and progesterone and possibly mechanical factors from the gravid uterus), scleroderma, achalasia cardia, and Zollinger-Ellison syndrome.

TABLE 10.31: Alarm symptoms or signs of GERD.

➢ Dysphagia	➢ Persistent heartburn
➢ Weight loss	➢ Odynophagia
➢ Gastrointestinal bleeding	➢ Anemia
➢ Nausea and vomiting	➢ Family history of cancer early satiety

Complications of GERD

See **Table 10.32.**

TABLE 10.32: Complications of GERD.

➢ Esophagitis	➢ Adenocarcinoma esophagus
➢ Hemorrhage and bleeding (hematemesis, melena)	➢ Aspiration pneumonia
➢ Esophageal ulceration	➢ Iron deficiency anemia
➢ Esophageal strictures	➢ Dental caries
➢ Barrett's esophagus	

Investigations (Table 10.33)

Diagnostic endoscopy should be performed in patients who fail to respond to therapy or have alarm symptoms or signs.

- **Endoscopy:** It is useful for the detection of:
  - **Erosive esophagitis** which would be visualized and confirmed by biopsy.
  - **Complications:** Peptic stricture and Barrett's esophagus (confirmed by biopsy)
- **Barium radiography:** It has no role in the diagnosis of GERD. Barium swallow and meal examination is useful for appreciation of gastroesophageal anatomy and may be important in the diagnosis of hiatus hernia.
- **24-hour pH recording:** It is the "gold standard" for diagnosis of GERD. Prolonged measurement of pH is the most accurate method for the diagnosis of gastroesophageal reflux **particularly** in patients with atypical symptoms and with normal endoscopies.
- **Esophageal manometry:** Useful to exclude achalasia and other motility disorders.
- **Resting ECG and stress ECG:** To rule out ischemic heart disease (IHD).

TABLE 10.33: Diagnostic tests for gastroesophageal reflux disease.

Tests for reflux
- ➢ Intraesophageal pH monitoring (catheter or catheter-free system)
- ➢ Ambulatory impedance and pH monitoring (nonacid reflux)
- ➢ Barium esophagogram

Tests to assess symptoms
- ➢ Empirical trial of acid suppression
- ➢ Intraesophageal pH monitoring with symptom analysis

Tests to assess esophageal damage
- ➢ Endoscopy
- ➢ Wireless capsule endoscopy
- ➢ Esophageal biopsy

Tests to assess esophageal function
- ➢ Esophageal manometry
- ➢ Esophageal impedance

Q. Write short note on management/treatment of gastroesophageal reflux disease (GERD)/reflux esophagitis.

Treatment

General measures

These are lifestyle modifications as listed in **Box 10.6**.

Box 10.6: Lifestyle modifications in the treatment of GERD.

- Avoid foods such as fatty food, alcohol, mint, tomato-based foods, spicy foods, coffee, tea, and acidic foods
- Avoid late night meals before retiring
- Avoid weight lifting, stooping, and bending at waist
- Elevation of the head of the bed in patients with regurgitation or heartburn during night
- Weight reduction
- Stop smoking, alcohol
- Frequents feeds of small volume

Medical treatment

Inhibition of gastric acid secretion is the cornerstone of the treatment of acute GERD.

Antacids (for details refer page 760): Liquid antacids buffer acid and increase LESP. They are used in the dose of 10–15 mL, 1 and 3 hours after meal and at bedtime or as needed. They relieve heart burn in mild cases.

Histamine (H_2)-receptor antagonists (for details refer page 760): They decrease acid secretion. These drugs include cimetidine (800 mg bid, 400 mg qid) or ranitidine (150 mg qid), or famotidine (20–40 mg bid) daily to be given with meals and before bed time, for at least 6 weeks (in mild cases).

Proton-pump inhibitors (PPIs) (for details refer page 760): They decrease acid secretion and gastric volume. They are superior to histamine (H_2)-receptor antagonists. These include omeprazole (20–40 mg/day), lansoprazole (15–30 mg/day), pantoprazole (40 mg/day), esomeprazole (20–40 mg/day), and rabeprazole (10–20 mg/day). Maintenance doses may be necessary for 6–8 months.

- Present evidence does not support the common practice of using metoclopramide or domperidone 10 mg thrice daily either as monotherapy or an adjunct to acid suppression therapy. Its significant adverse effects argue against the use of this drug in GERD.
- *Helicobacter pylori* eradication does not have any therapeutic value.
- Dilatation of esophageal strictures
- Anemia is treated with oral iron or blood transfusion.

Surgical treatment

Indications: (1) failure to respond to medical therapy, (2) patients not willing to take long-term PPIs or intolerant to PPIs, (3) patients with severe symptom, and (4) patients with regurgitation.

Surgical measures

- **Surgical resection of esophageal strictures:** For patients with PPI-refractory GERD, anti-reflux mucosectomy (ARMS) or anti-reflux mucosal ablation (ARMA) can be tried.
- **Antireflux surgery:** Laparoscopic fundoplication for patients with PPI-refractory GERD, anti-reflux mucosectomy (ARMS) or anti-reflux mucosal ablation (ARMA) can be tried. (additional valve mechanism) yields results comparable to continued PPI therapy.

Barrett's Esophagus

Q. Write short answer on Barrett's esophagus.

Barrett's esophagus is a **premalignant condition**, in which the **normal squamous lining of the lower esophagus is replaced by columnar mucosa** (columnar lined esophagus; CLO). The columnar mucosa may show areas of intestinal metaplasia (with goblet cells). It is an adaptive response to chronic gastroesophageal reflux and is often asymptomatic. The risk of esophageal cancer depends on the severity and duration of reflux and it may be detected when the patient presents with esophageal cancer. It is more common in men, obese, and above the age of 50. It is weakly associated with smoking but not with alcohol intake.

Diagnosis: It needs multiple systematic biopsies which may show intestinal metaplasia and/or dysplasia.

Management

Regular endoscopic surveillance to detect dysplasia at an early stage. Currently recommendation are as follows:

- Barrett's esophagus with intestinal metaplasia, but without dysplasia: Should undergo endoscopy at 3–5 yearly intervals, if the length of the Barrettic segment is 3 cm and at 2–3 yearly intervals if the length is >3 cm.
- *Low-grade dysplasia:* It should be endoscoped at 6-monthly intervals. Treatment is indicated only for symptoms of reflux or complications (e.g., stricture).

Endoscopic therapies: Such as radiofrequency ablation or photodynamic therapy, can induce regression. However, they are used only for patients with dysplasia or intramucosal cancer.

High-grade dysplasia or intramucosal carcinoma: Treatment options are either esophagectomy or endoscopic therapy, with a combination of endoscopic resection of any visibly abnormal areas and radiofrequency ablation of the remaining Barrett's mucosa, as an "organ-preserving" alternative to surgery.

Hiatus Hernia

Q. Write short note on hiatus hernia.

It is the herniation of elements of the abdominal cavity (part of stomach) through the diaphragm into the thoracic cavity.

Types (Figs. 10.5A to D)

- **Sliding or type I hiatus hernia:** It is the most common type. In this type, the gastroesophageal junction and the fundus of stomach slide upward above the diaphragmatic hiatus.
- **True paraesophageal (rolling) or type II hiatus hernia:** It is uncommon. In this type, location of gastroesophageal junction is in its normal position, but the fundus and parts of the greater curvature of the stomach herniate into the mediastinum alongside the esophagus.
- **Mixed paraesophageal hernia or type III:** In this type, gastroesophageal junction and a large part of the stomach herniate into the mediastinum.

Predisposing factors: Obesity, pregnancy and ascites. Occurs in 33% of normal adults and 50% of elderly.

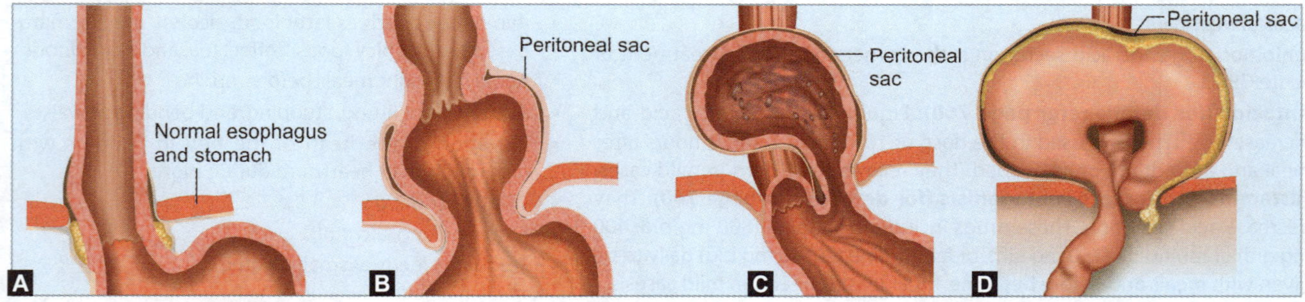

FIGS. 10.5A TO D: Types of hiatus hernia. (A) Normal esophagus and stomach; (B) type I (sliding); (C) type II (paraesophageal/rolling); (D) type III (mixed paraesophageal) hiatus hernia.

Clinical Features

- Majority of hiatus hernia are asymptomatic. Hiatus hernia predisposes to gastroesophageal reflux disease (GERD), and hence, symptoms of GERD may be present.
- Type I: Usually asymptomatic or present with symptoms of heartburn or acid regurgitation.
- Type II and III may present with epigastric pain, chest pain, substernal fullness, shortness of breath, nausea, or vomiting.

Investigations

- **Plain radiograph of the chest:** Hernia may be visible as a gas bubble, often with a fluid level behind the heart.
- **Barium swallow/meal:** It is the best method of diagnosis and demonstrates the presence of gastroesophageal junction in the thorax.
- **Endoscopy**

Management

- Asymptomatic hiatus hernias do not require any treatment. Surgical repair of hernia is required in selected cases with gastroesophageal reflux
- Symptomatic rolling hiatus hernias require surgical repair because it is potentially liable to undergo volvulus as a dangerous complication. **Surgical treatment:** (1) Repair of the diaphragmatic defect and (2) fixing the stomach in the abdominal cavity (fundoplication) combined with an antireflux procedure

Achalasia of the Esophagus

Q. Write short note on achalasia cardia and its diagnosis/investigations.

Achalasia is characterized by **esophageal aperistalsis** and results from progressive degeneration of ganglion cells in the myenteric plexus in the esophageal wall, causing failure of relaxation of the hypertonic lower esophageal sphincter in response to the swallowing wave. Failure of propagated esophageal contraction results in progressive dilatation of the gullet.

Cause: Unknown. Autoimmune, neurodegenerative, and viral etiologies have been suggested. Reduction in nitric oxide synthase containing neurons is detected by immunohistochemical staining in the lower esophageal sphincter. There is degeneration of ganglion cells within the sphincter and the body of the esophagus. Infection with *Trypanosoma cruzi* in Chagas' disease causes a syndrome that is clinically similar to achalasia.

Clinical Features

- **Age and gender:** Occurs equally in males and females and at all ages but is rare in childhood.
- **Dysphagia:** It develops slowly, is initially intermittent and characteristically for both liquids and solids from the onset (worse for solids). Dysphagia is eased by drinking liquids, and by standing and moving around after eating.
- **Episodes of chest pain:** Spontaneous chest pain occurs due to esophageal spasm which may be misdiagnosed as cardiac.
- **Regurgitation of food from the dilated esophagus:** As the disease progresses, dysphagia worsens and caused poor emptying of the esophagus. This may produce nocturnal pulmonary aspiration and aspiration pneumonia.
- Heartburn does not occur because the closed esophageal sphincter which prevents gastroesophageal reflux.
- Achalasia **predisposes to squamous carcinoma of the esophagus.**

Investigations

- **Chest X-ray:** It shows a dilated esophagus. Sometimes fluid level may be observed behind the heart. There is **absence of fundic gas shadow.**
- **Barium swallow:** There is absence of peristalsis and often synchronous contractions in the body of the esophagus. There is tapered narrowing of the lower esophagus producing a **"bird's beak"** appearance due to failure of the sphincter to relax.
- **Manometry** shows high-pressure, nonrelaxing lower esophageal sphincter with poor contractility of the esophageal body.
- **Endoscopy:** It should be performed because carcinoma of the cardia can mimic the presentation and radiological and manometric features of achalasia ("pseudo-achalasia").

Management

Treatment for achalasia is palliative

Endoscopic

- **Endoscopic dilatation of the LES (lower esophageal sphincter)**
- **Endoscopically directed injection of botulinum toxin** into the lower esophageal sphincter (intersphincteric injection)

Surgical

- **Surgical myotomy (Heller's operation)**
- **Peroral endoscopic myotomy (POEM)**

EOSINOPHILIC ESOPHAGITIS

Q. Write short note on eosinophilic esophagitis.

- Eosinophilic esophagitis is characterized by eosinophilic infiltration of esophageal mucosa.
- Atopy (allergic rhinitis, eczema, and asthma) is common, and food allergens may trigger the process.
- Dysphagia is prominent, but symptoms can also mimic GERD.
- Endoscopy reveals—include corrugated mucosa, longitudinal mucosal furrows, fixed esophageal rings or **trachealization (Fig. 10.6)** whitish mucosal plaque or exudate, stricture, and mucosal friability giving the appearance of crepe paper.
- Biopsy ≥15 eosinophils per HPF
- Treatment:
  - First-line therapy consists of PPIs, which also treats concomitant GERD.
  - Topical steroids (swallowed fluticasone, 880–1760 µg/d in two to four divided doses, or swallowed budesonide, 1–2 mg/d in two to four divided doses) are options; prednisone is an alternate option if topical steroids are ineffective.
  - Six food elimination diet (SFED) (eggs, milk, soy, gluten, tree nuts, and seafood).
  - If no response higher doses of topical steroids, systemic steroids, elimination diet trials, or cautious esophageal dilation

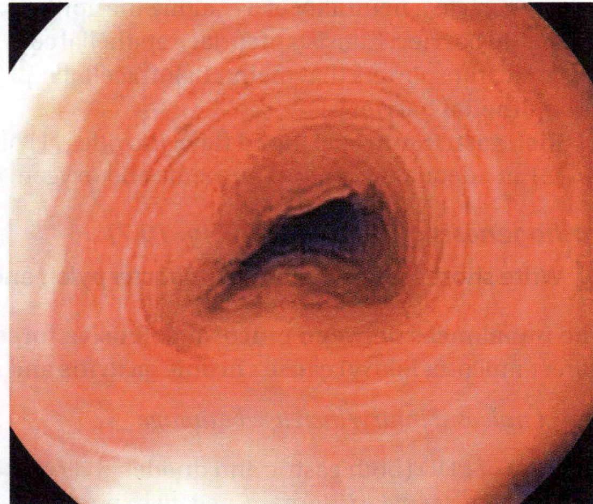

FIG. 10.6: Endoscopy showing trachealization.

DISEASES OF THE STOMACH AND DUODENUM

Peptic Ulcer Disease

Q. Discuss the etiology, pathogenesis, pathology, clinical features, investigations, and management of peptic ulcer disease or acid peptic disease.

Definition

An ulcer in the gastrointestinal (GI) tract may be defined as a break in the lining of the mucosa, with appreciable depth at endoscopy or histologic evidence of involvement of the submucosa.

Sites of Peptic Ulcer

Any portion of the GI tract exposed to acidic gastric juices

- **Duodenum: More common in the first portion of the duodenum** (anterior or posterior wall) **than in the stomach**. Occasionally occurs at both anterior and posterior sites ("kissing" ulcers)
- **Stomach:** Lesser curvature near the junction (transitional zone) of the body and antrum
  - Proximal ulcers: Located in the body of the stomach
  - Distal ulcers: Located in the antrum and angulus of the stomach
- **Gastroesophageal junction of esophagus**
- **Anastomotic site:** Occurs in patients who have undergone a distal gastric resection. Occur at margins of the gastroduodenal anastomosis/gastrojejunostomy (anastomotic ulcer)
- **Multiple ulcers:** In the duodenum, stomach, and/or jejunum in Zollinger-Ellison syndrome
- **At metaplastic or heterotopic gastric mucosa**, e.g., Meckel diverticulum within an ileum having ectopic gastric mucosa

Incidence: ~12% in males and 10% in females.

Etiology

Q. Write short essay/note on risk factors for peptic ulcer disease.

Normal process in the stomach

Two opposing sets of forces keep stomach in a normal state: (1) damaging forces and (2) defensive forces.

1. **Damaging forces:** Capable of inducing mucosal injury are two gastric secretory products: (1) hydrochloric acid, and (2) pepsinogen.
2. **Defensive forces** is a three-level barrier composed of pre-epithelial, epithelial, and subepithelial elements.

Pre-epithelial barrier is a mucus-bicarbonate layer of the stomach.

- **Surface mucus secretion:** Mucin is secreted by surface foveolar cells. Actions of mucus are: (1) Mucus layer promotes formation of an "unstirred" protective layer of fluid on the mucosa. (2) Prevents the direct contact of large food particles with the epithelium. (3) Impedes the diffusion of ions and molecules such as pepsin.
- **Bicarbonate secretion into mucus** by surface epithelial cells → diffuse into the unstirred mucus → buffer the hydrogen ions entering from the luminal aspect → result in a pH gradient, ranging from 1 or 2 at the gastric luminal surface, and reaching to a neutrality of 6–7 along the epithelial cell surface.

Epithelial barrier: Consists of surface epithelial cells act through several factors, such as (1) production of mucus, (2) epithelial cell ionic transporters that maintain intracellular pH, (3) bicarbonate production, and (4) intracellular tight junctions.

Subepithelial barrier

- **Rich gastric mucosal blood flow:** Provides (1) bicarbonate (HCO_3^-), which neutralizes the acid generated by parietal cell, (2) an adequate supply of nutrients and oxygen, and (3) removes toxic metabolic by-products.

Pathogenesis of Peptic Ulcer (Fig. 10.7)

Q. Write short essay/note on *Helicobacter pylori* and its role in pathogenesis (pathophysiology) of gastric ulcer.

The imbalances between mucosal defensive forces (disruption of any of protective mechanisms) **and damaging forces** (direct mucosal injury) **cause chronic gastritis** and also **PUD**.

Direct mucosal injury/increased damage

Majority of PUD (both gastric and duodenal ulcers) can be attributed to NSAIDs and *H. pylori.*

- *Helicobacter pylori* is a gram-negative spiral bacteria with multiple unipolar flagella that allow them to move freely through the gastric mucus layer, where they remain protected from low gastric pH. It is one of the most important, common, primary causes of PUD. It is associated with ~85–90% of duodenal and ~65% of gastric ulcers. *Helicobacter pylori* infection remains one of the most common chronic bacterial infections in humans more than 50% of the world's population is infected with the bacterium. *H. pylori* also plays a role in the development of gastric and duodenal ulcer, gastritis, MALT (mucosal-associated lymphoid tissue) lymphoma, and gastric adenocarcinoma.

- **Mode of spread:** Oral-oral or feco-oral route either by kissing or ingestion of contaminated vomitus.

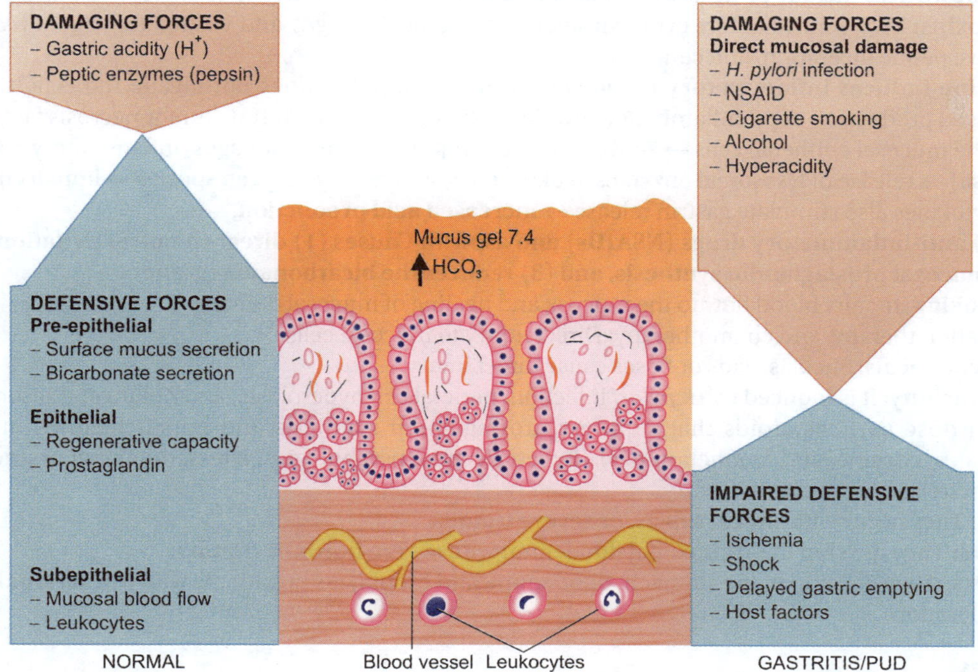

FIG. 10.7: Components involved in mucosal defense and repair in normal (left side) and in acute or chronic gastritis. Gastric mucus barrier consists of viscid mucus (which forms an unstirred layer between the epithelium and the gastric lumen) and bicarbonate.

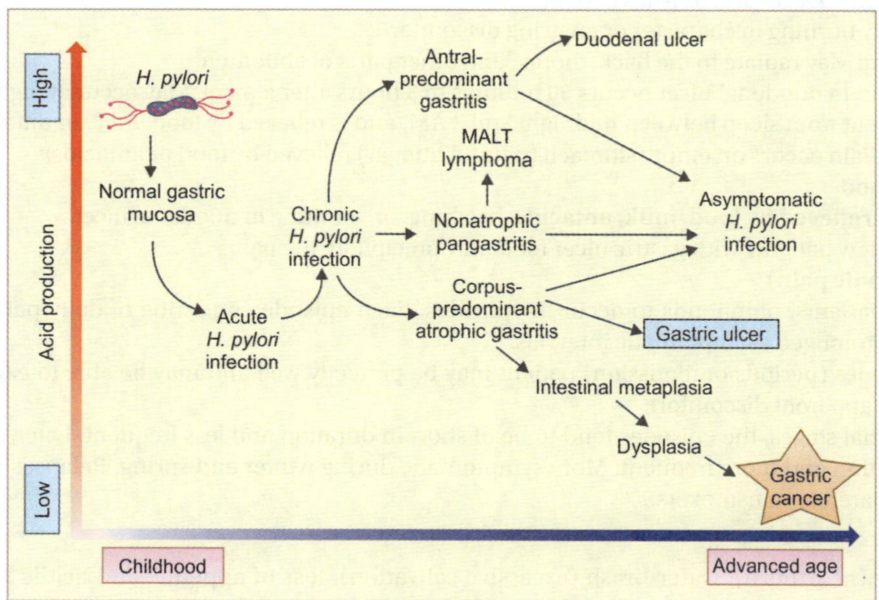

FIG. 10.8: Natural history of *H. pylori* infection.

- **Lesions produced:** *H. pylori* may attach to gastric epithelium causing damage to the mucosa. Causes chronic antral gastritis with high acid production → may progress to pangastritis → resulting multifocal atrophic gastritis → increased risk of gastric adenocarcinoma. Natural history of *H. pylori* infection is shown in **Figure 10.8**.

- **Nongastric diseases and *H. pylori* infection:** Raynaud's, scleroderma, idiopathic urticaria, acne rosacea, migraine, thyroiditis, Guillain-Barré syndrome, coronary artery disease, immune thrombocytopenic purpura.

- **Mechanism of action by *H. pylori*:**
    - **Flagella:** It makes them motile, allows them to burrow and live beneath the mucus layer above the epithelial surface.

- **Urease:** It is produced by *H. pylori* → converts urea into ammonia (strong alkali) → raises the local gastric pH, acts on the antral G cells → release of gastrin → hypergastrinemia → result in hypersecretion of gastric acid.
- **Adhesion molecule:** It helps it to bind to gastric epithelial (surface foveolar) cells.
- **Enzymes:** These include proteases and phospholipases act on the mucous gel → reduce the mucosal defense.
- **Cytotoxins:** Two genes namely cytotoxin-associated gene A *(CagA)* and vacuolating agent (*vacA)* gene cause gastritis, peptic ulceration, and cancer.
- **Cytokine induces inflammatory response:** Normally *H. pylori* does not invade the cells/tissues. It causes increased production of proinflammatory cytokines [interleukin (IL)-1, IL-6, tumor necrosis factor (TNF) and IL-8] by the mucosal epithelial cells → activation of neutrophils and macrophages (inflammatory response to gastric mucosa) → release of lysosomal enzymes, leukotrienes, and reactive oxygen species → impairs mucosal defense. The cytokines also stimulate gastrin release → **increased acid production**.

- **Nonsteroidal anti-inflammatory drugs (NSAIDs) and aspirin: Causes (1) direct chemical irritation of mucosa, (2) suppresses mucosal prostaglandin synthesis, and (3) reduces the bicarbonate secretion.**
- **Cigarette smoking** impairs blood flow to the mucosa and healing of mucosal damage.
- **Alcohol**, radiation therapy, and chemotherapy: Direct injury to mucosal cells.
- **Ingestion of chemicals:** Such as acids or bases cause direct injury.
- **Gastric hyperacidity:** It is induced by *H. pylori* infection, parietal cell hyperplasia, and Zollinger–Ellison syndrome.
- **Others:** High-dose corticosteroids that suppress prostaglandin synthesis and impair healing, other drugs (e.g., bisphosphonates, cocaine, and amphetamines), hypercalcemia, psychological stress, duodenal gastric reflux, Crohn's disease, and systemic mastocytosis.
- **Stress ulcers:** They occur with **shock, sepsis, or severe trauma**.
- **Curling ulcers:** They develop in the proximal duodenum with **severe burns or trauma**.
- **Cushing ulcers:** They develop in the stomach, duodenum, and esophagus in patients with **intracranial disease**. Highly prone for perforation.

Clinical Features

Recurrent episodes of abdominal pain: It is the **most common presentation** and has three notable characteristics:

1. **Localization to the epigastrium:** Pain is referred to epigastrium and the patient will be able to localize the site with one finger (pointing sign). The characteristics of pain are:
   - **Nature:** Usually burning in character or gnawing discomfort.
   - **Radiating pain:** May radiate to the back, thorax, and other parts of abdomen.
   - **Nocturnal:** Pain in duodenal ulcer occurs 90 minutes to 3 hours after a meal. May occur at night (most specific) and wakes the patient from sleep between midnight and 3 AM, and is relieved by food, milk, or antacids.
   - **Hunger pain:** Pain occurs on empty stomach (painful hunger) relieved by food or antacids.
2. **Relationship to food**
   - Pain is usually **relieved by food, milk, antacids**, belching, or vomiting in duodenal ulcer.
   - In contrast, in few patients with gastric ulcer food may precipitate the pain.
3. **Periodicity (episodic pain)**
   - In untreated patients, pain tends to occur in episodes. Each episode consisting of daily pain **lasting 2–8 weeks**, separated by prolonged asymptomatic intervals.
   - Between episodes (periods of remission) patient may be perfectly well and may be able to eat even heavy or spicy meals without apparent discomfort.
   - During the initial stages, the episodes tend to be of short in duration and less frequent. Later, the episodes become longer in duration and more frequent. More symptomatic during winter and spring. Relapses are more common in smokers compared to nonsmokers.

Other symptoms

Retrosternal burning (heartburn), water-brash (excessive salivation), loss of appetite, and acidic regurgitation into the throat and vomiting. Persistent daily vomiting suggests gastric outlet obstruction. Fullness, bloating, anorexia, nausea, and dyspepsia. Tarry stools or coffee-ground vomitus indicate bleeding. Rarely, with anemia due to chronic blood loss, abrupt hematemesis, acute perforation, or gastric outlet obstruction.

Difference between gastric ulcer and duodenal ulcer is shown in **Table 10.34**.

TABLE 10.34: Difference between gastric ulcer and duodenal ulcer.

Features	*Gastric ulcer*	*Duodenal ulcer*
Commonest site	Along the lesser curvature	First part of duodenum
Incidence	Less common	More common
Age	Beyond 6th decade, M > F	Between 25 and 50 years, M > F
Association with *H. pylori* infection	Less common	Strong association
Acid level	Usually normal	High
Clinical features		
Relationship of pain to antacids	Relief of pain not consistent	Prompt relief of pain
Relationship of pain to food	Aggravates the pain	Relieves the pain
Night pain	Not observed	Common
Heartburn	Not common	Common
Hematemesis/melena	Hematemesis more common	Melena more common
Vomiting	Common	No vomiting
Weight loss	Present	Absent
Anorexia and nausea	More common	Less common
Duration of episodes of pain	Relatively longer in duration	Relatively shorter in duration
Course of the illness	Less remission	More remission
Complication	Rarely undergo malignant change	No malignant change

Box 10.7: Complications of peptic ulcer.

- Upper gastrointestinal bleeding (20%)
- Perforation of ulcer (6–7%)
- Gastric outlet obstruction 1–2% (with fluid and electrolyte imbalance), gastrocolic or duodenocolic fistulas
- Rarely malignant transformation
- Rarely pancreatitis due to posterior penetration of ulcer

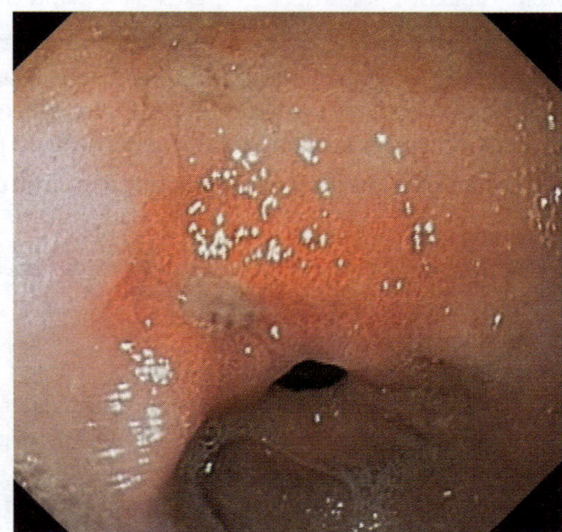

FIG. 10.9: Endoscopic picture of a benign gastric ulcer.

Complications (Box 10.7)

Q. List complications of peptic ulcer disease.

Investigations/Diagnosis

Q. Discuss diagnosis of peptic ulcer disease.

Anatomic diagnosis: Documentation of a peptic ulcer needs either a radiographic (barium study) or an endoscopic examination.

- **Endoscopy (Fig. 10.9):** It is most sensitive and specific for the detection of ulcer disease of the upper GI tract. Typical location of peptic ulcer is duodenal bulb and lesser curvature of stomach. Advantages of endoscopy are: (1) direct visualization of mucosa (to determine if an ulcer is a source of blood loss) and the ulcer (even lesions too small to detect by radiographic examination), (2) useful for photographic documentation of a mucosal defect, and (3) biopsy can be taken to rule out malignancy (about 10% of gastric ulcers are malignant) or *H. pylori.*
- **Endoscopic ultrasound:** It may be useful in detecting an unsuspected submucosal component or enlarged lymph nodes (e.g., in gastric malignancies such as lymphoma and linitis plastica).
- **Etiologic diagnosis:** The cause of the ulcer must be established. The major risk factor for peptic ulcers is either H. *pylori* or NSAID.
- **Tests for *Helicobacter pylori* (Table 10.35)**

Q. Discuss the investigation done in *Helicobacter pylori* infection.

TABLE 10.35: Diagnostic tests for *Helicobacter pylori* (HP).

	Advantages	*Disadvantages*
Nonendoscopic tests		
Serology [qualitative or quantitative immunoglobulin G (IgG)]	Widely available, economical. Good NPV (negative predictive value)	Poor PPV (positive predictive value) if HP prevalence is low. Not useful after treatment
Urea breath test (^{13}C or ^{14}C)	Detects active infection. Accuracy (PPV, NPV) not affected by *H. pylori* prevalence. Useful both before and after treatment	Accuracy affected by PPI and antibiotic use, small radiation dose with ^{14}C test
Stool antigen test	Detects active infection. Accuracy (PPV, NPV) not affected by *H. pylori* prevalence. Useful both before and after treatment (monoclonal test)	Accuracy affected by PPI and antibiotic use

Contd...

Contd...

Endoscopic tests		
Microscopic examination	Excellent sensitivity and specificity, especially with special and immune stains; provides additional information about gastric mucosa	Expensive (endoscopy and histopathology costs), interobserver variability, accuracy affected by PPI and antibiotic use
Rapid urease test	Rapid results, accurate in patients not using PPIs or antibiotics, no added histopathology cost	Requires endoscopy, less accurate after treatment or in patients using PPIs
Culture	Specificity 100%, allows antibiotic sensitivity testing	Difficult and tedious to perform; not widely available; expensive
Polymerase chain reaction (PCR) assay	Excellent sensitivity and specificity, permits detection of antibiotic resistance	Not widely available; technique not standardized; expensive

- **Nonsteroidal anti-inflammatory drugs**: Diagnosis is established based on history of drug use and symptoms of pain.
- **Hypersecretory syndromes:** Zollinger-Ellison syndrome should be considered in patients with multiple ulcers. **Serum gastrin and gastric acid analysis should be** performed in these patients.

Q. Discuss the medical management of peptic ulcer disease and mention the new drugs used in its treatment.

Treatment/Management

Treatment may be divided into short-term management and long-term management (intermittent, maintenance, and surgical treatment).

A. ***Short-term management***

- **General measures (Box 10.8)**
- **Acid neutralizing/inhibitory drugs**

Box 10.8: General measures in peptic ulcer disease.

- **Avoid:** Cigarette **smoking, aspirin, and NSAIDs**
- **Alcohol** to be avoided
- **No special dietary advice** is necessary

a. **Antacids:** Neutralizes the secreted acid and rarely used at present.
  - Mainly used for symptomatic relief of dyspepsia.
  - Preparation: Tablet or liquid preparations
  - Dose: 15–30 mL liquid antacid 1 and 3 hours after food and at bed time for 4–6 weeks.
  - **Commonly used antacids:** Combination of aluminum hydroxide and magnesium hydroxide. Others include calcium carbonate and sodium bicarbonate.
  - **Side effects**
    - Aluminum compounds cause constipation, phosphate depletion and interfere with the absorption of digoxin and tetracycline
    - Magnesium compounds cause diarrhea, hypocalcemia, and hypermagnesemia.
    - Calcium carbonate causes milk-alkali syndrome and sodium bicarbonate produces systemic alkalosis.

b. **Histamine H_2-receptor antagonists:**
  - **Drugs:** These include four agents namely cimetidine (400 mg BD or 800 mg at night), ranitidine (150 mg BD or 300 mg at night), famotidine (20 mg BD or 40 mg at night), and nizatidine (150 mg BD or 300 mg at night). All are equally effective.
  - **Mechanism of action:** Inhibit acid and pepsin secretion by blocking H_2-receptors.

  Duration of treatment:
  - **Duodenal ulcer:** Usually for 4 weeks. Smokers and patients with recent major complications (e.g., hematemesis, perforation), treatment is prolonged to 6–8 weeks.
  - **Gastric ulcer:** For 6 weeks, followed by endoscopy and further treatment if necessary.

c. **Proton pump (H^+, K^+-ATPase) Inhibitors (PPIs)**
  - These agents are substituted benzimidazole derivatives that covalently bind and irreversibly inhibit H^+, K^+-ATPase.
  - They include omeprazole (20 mg/d), esomeprazole (20–40 mg/d), lansoprazole (15–30 mg/d), rabeprazole (20 mg/d), and pantoprazole (40 mg/d). All have similar efficacy in the treatment of various acid-peptic disorders.
  - **Mechanism of action**
    - Proton-pump inhibitors are lipophilic compounds that cross the parietal cell membrane and enter the acidic parietal cell canaliculus.
    - Upon entering the acidic parietal cell, the PPIs are protonated, and trapped within the acid environment of the tubulovesicular and canalicular system. They become activated and bind covalently with the H^+/K^+ ATPase enzyme and potently inhibit all phases of gastric acid secretion by the proton pump.
  - **Side effects:** Headache, diarrhea, abdominal pain, and nausea. The use of PPI may predispose to an increased risk of *Clostridium difficile* infection, community acquired pneumonia, hip fracture, and vitamin B_{12} deficiency.
  - **Advantages:** Superior healing rates, shorter healing time, and faster relief of symptom compared to H_2-blockers.
  - **Indications (Box 10.9)**

Box 10.9: Indications for proton pump inhibitors (PPIs).

- GERD and reflux esophagitis
- Peptic ulcer not responding to other medical measures.
- As an adjunct to anti-*H. pylori* treatment.
- Zollinger-Ellison syndrome

d. **Cytoprotective agents**
  - **Sucralfate:** It is a complex sucrose salt insoluble in water and becomes a viscous paste within the stomach and duodenum. It binds to sites of active ulceration. Sucralfate acts as a protective barrier, over the ulcer and increases the mucosal defense and repair. Standard dose 1 g qid.

- **Bismuth-containing preparations:** Colloidal bismuth subcitrate (CBS) and bismuth subsalicylate are used to induce healing of peptic ulcers. Side effects include black stools, constipation, darkening of the tongue, and neurotoxicity. They are commonly used as one of the agents in an anti-*H. pylori* regimen.
- **Prostaglandin analogs:** They enhance mucosal defense and repair and useful in preventing NSAID-induced mucosal injury. Dose (e.g., Misoprostol) is 200 μg qid.

Q. Discuss management of *Helicobacter pylori* infection/*Helicobacter pylori* eradication regimens.

e. **Treatment for *H. pylori* infection (Tables 10.36 and 10.37; Flowchart 10.6)**
- **Indications:** Consensus of opinion is that all patients with proven acute or chronic duodenal ulcer and those with gastric ulcers who are *H. pylori*-positive should be administered drugs against *H. pylori* (even without documenting the presence of bacteria).
- **Advantages:** It reduces the risk of recurrence of ulcer.
- **Type of therapy:** Triple or quadruple therapy (**Tables 10.36 and 10.37**).

B. ***Long-term management***

1. **Intermittent treatment:** When the symptoms relapses < four times a year, 4 weeks course of one of the ulcer-healing agents are prescribed.
2. **Maintenance treatment**
   - Continuous maintenance treatment is not required after successful eradication of *H. pylori*.
   - If symptoms relapses for more than four times per year or history of complications (e.g., repeated bleeding or perforation) require the lowest effective dose of PPI.
   - Long-term maintenance is with H_2-receptor antagonists (cimetidine 400 mg at night, ranitidine 150 mg at night, famotidine 20 mg at night or nizatidine 150 mg at night).

   New Treatments
   - Cholecystokinin 2 receptor antagonists (CCK2): Itriglumide
   - Potassium competitive acid blockers (P-CABs): Revaprazan
3. **Surgical treatment**
   - Most of peptic ulcers are cured by *H. pylori* eradication therapy and by acid-suppressing drugs. Elective surgery is reserved for the treatment of medically refractory disease (recurrence of ulcer following surgery, gastric outlet obstruction), or urgent/emergency surgery for the treatment of an ulcer-related complication (e.g., perforation and hemorrhage).
   - **Indications for surgery**
     - **Chronic non-healing gastric ulcer:** Persistent ulceration despite adequate medical therapy. The procedure of choice is partial gastrectomy with a Billroth I anastomosis, in which the ulcer and the ulcer-bearing area of the stomach are resected.
     - **Gastric outflow obstruction**
     - **Recurrent ulcer following gastric surgery**
     - **Duodenal ulcer:** Most commonly performed procedures are:
       - ❑ Vagotomy and drainage (by pyloroplasty, gastroduodenostomy, or gastrojejunostomy)
       - ❑ Highly selective vagotomy (which does not require a drainage procedure)
       - ❑ Vagotomy with antrectomy
     - As an emergency for complications namely **perforation and hemorrhage.**

TABLE 10.36: First-line treatment of *Helicobacter pylori* infection.

Treatment regimen	*Duration*	*Eradication rate*
PPI (omeprazole/lansoprazole/pantoprazole/rabeprazole/esomeprazole), clarithromycin 500 mg, amoxicillin 1,000 mg (each twice daily)	10–14 days	70–85%
PPI, clarithromycin 500 mg, metronidazole 500 mg (each twice daily)	10–14 days	70–85%
Sequential therapy PPI, amoxicillin 1000 mg (each twice daily) for 5 days **followed by** PPI, clarithromycin 500 mg, tinidazole 500 mg (each twice daily) for next 5 days.	10 days	90%
Bismuth subsalicylate 525 mg, metronidazole 500 mg, tetracycline 500 mg (each four times daily) **plus** PPI or H_2RA (Ranitidine twice daily)	10–14 days	75–90%

(H_2RA: histamine H_2- receptor antagonists; PPI: proton pump inhibitor)

TABLE 10.37: Rescue treatment for persistent *Helicobacter pylori* infection.

Regimen	*Duration*	*Eradication rate*
Quadruple therapy: Bismuth subsalicylate 525 mg, metronidazole 500 mg, tetracycline 500 mg (each four times daily) **plus** PPI or H_2RA (twice daily)	14 days	70%
PPI, amoxicillin 1,000 mg, levofloxacin 250 mg (each twice daily)	10–14 days	57–91%
PPI amoxicillin 1,000 mg, rifabutin 150 mg (each twice daily)	14 days	60–80%

(H_2RA: histamine H_2- receptor antagonists; PPI: proton pump inhibitors)

FLOWCHART 10.6: Initial approach to antibiotic treatment for *H. pylori* infection.

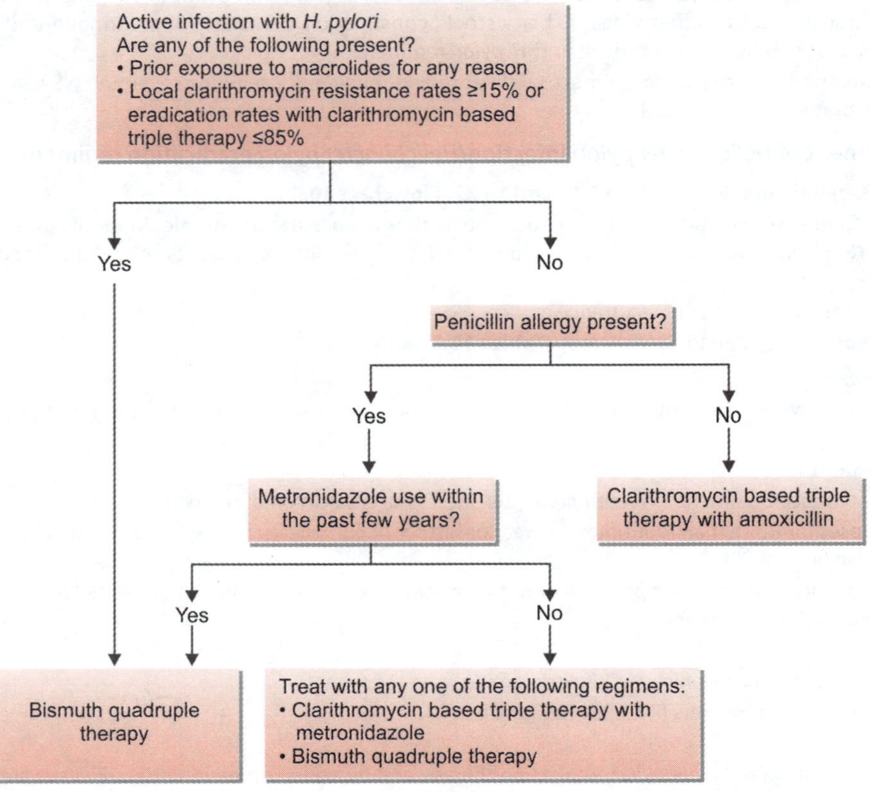

Dumping Syndrome

Q. Write a short note on dumping syndrome.

- It is a series of vasomotor and GI signs and symptoms that occur when food reaches the small bowel too rapidly and usually develops in patients who have undergone vagotomy and drainage (especially Billroth procedures).

Triggering factor: It usually occurs after meals rich in simple carbohydrates (especially sucrose) and high osmolarity. Ingestion of large amounts of liquids may also contribute.

Phases: There are two phases of dumping namely early and late.

1. **Early dumping:**
   - **Time of occurrence:** Occurs 15–30 minutes after meals.
   - **Signs and symptoms:** Consists of crampy abdominal discomfort, nausea, diarrhea, belching (bloating), borborygmi, tachycardia, palpitations, diaphoresis, light-headedness, and, rarely, syncope.
   - **Mechanism:** The signs and symptoms are due rapid emptying of hypertonic gastric contents into the small intestine that draws the fluid into lumen of the gut and leads to distension of small intestine. This leads to reduced volume of plasma and acute intestinal distention. Release of vasoactive GI hormones (vasoactive intestinal polypeptide, neurotensin, and motilin) may also play a role.
2. **Late phase of dumping:**
   - **Time of occurrence:** Occurs 90 minutes to 3 hours after meals.
   - **Signs and symptoms:** Consists of vasomotor symptoms such as light-headedness, diaphoresis/sweating, palpitations, tachycardia, and occasionally syncope.
   - **Mechanism:** Possibly secondary to hypoglycemia from excessive insulin release.

Provocative Test

- After an overnight fast, a solution of 50–75 g glucose given orally.
- Measure blood glucose, hematocrit, pulse rate, and blood pressure at 30 minutes intervals, immediately before and up to 180 minutes after ingestion of glucose.
- Positive test: Characterized by an early (30 minutes) increase in pulse rate (>10/minutes) or hematocrit >3% and late (120–180 minutes) hypoglycemia.

Treatment

- Patient should be asked have small, multiple (six) meals and avoid simple carbohydrates and liquids during meals.
- Antidiarrheals and anticholinergic drugs are complementary to diet.
- Guar and pectin: They increase the viscosity of intraluminal food contents, thereby slowing down gastric emptying.
- Acarbose: It is an α-glucosidase inhibitor that delays digestion of ingested carbohydrates. It appears beneficial in the treatment of the late phases of dumping.
- Octreotide: It is a somatostatin analog given subcutaneously (50 g tid), before the meal may be used in diet-refractory cases. A long-acting octreotide may be given once every 28 days.

DISEASES OF THE INTESTINE

Malabsorption Syndrome

Q. Discuss the classification, etiology, clinical features, investigations (diagnosis), and management of malabsorption syndrome.

Q. List the investigation of a case of steatorrhea.

Definition: Malabsorption is defined as defective/diminished intestinal absorption of one or more dietary nutrients.

TABLE 10.38: Drugs causing malabsorption and systemic diseases associated with malabsorption.

Drug	*Systemic diseases*
Colchicine, neomycin, methotrexate, cholestyramine, and laxatives	Addison's disease, thyrotoxicosis, hypothyroidism, diabetes mellitus, and collagen vascular disease

Classification and Etiology (Fig. 10.10)

Drugs causing malabsorption and systemic diseases associated with malabsorption are presented in **Table 10.38**.

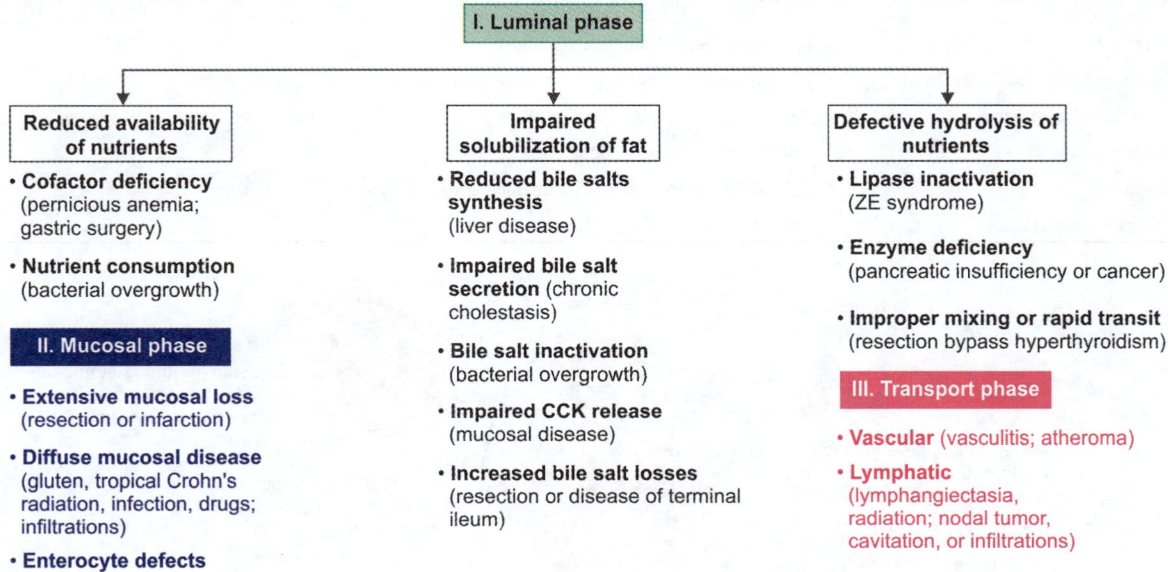

FIG. 10.10: Classification and causes of malabsorption.

Clinical Features

- Onset: Insidious and gradually progresses.
- General features: Diarrhea, abdominal pain, distension, loss of weight, and anemia.
- Symptoms and signs and relevant pathophysiology are presented in **Table 10.39** and **Figure 10.11**.

Q. Discuss the chronic effects of diarrhea including malabsorption.

TABLE 10.39: Signs and symptoms of malabsorption and relevant pathophysiology.

Symptom or sign	*Pathophysiology*
Gastrointestinal	
Diarrhea	➢ Osmotic activity of carbohydrates or short-chain fatty acids ➢ Secretory effect of bile acids and fatty acids ➢ Decreased absorptive surface ➢ Intestinal loss of conjugated bile acids
Abdominal distention, flatulence	Bacterial gas production from carbohydrates in colon, small intestinal bacterial overgrowth
Foul-smelling flatulence or stool	Malabsorption of proteins or intestinal protein loss
Pain	Gaseous distention of intestine
Ascites	Protein loss or malabsorption
Musculoskeletal	
Tetany, muscle weakness, and paresthesias	Malabsorption of vitamin D, calcium, magnesium, and phosphate
Bone pain, osteomalacia, and fractures	Protein, calcium, or vitamin D deficiency; secondary hyperparathyroidism
Cutaneous and Mucosal	
Easy bruisability, ecchymosis, and petechiae	Vitamin K deficiency and vitamin C deficiency
Glossitis, cheilosis, and stomatitis	Vitamin B complex, vitamin B_{12}, folate, or iron deficiency

Contd...

Contd...

Edema	Protein loss or malabsorption
Ichthyosis, acrodermatitis, and scaly dermatitis	Zinc and essential fatty acid deficiency
Follicular hyperkeratosis	Vitamin A deficiency
Hyperpigmented dermatitis	Niacin deficiency (pellagra)
Koilonychia	Iron deficiency
Perifollicular hemorrhage	Malabsorption of vitamin C
Other	
Weight loss and hyperphagia	Nutrient malabsorption
Growth and weight retardation, infantilism	Nutrient malabsorption in childhood and adolescence
Anemia	Iron, folate, or vitamin B_{12} deficiency
Kidney stones	Increased colonic oxalate absorption
Amenorrhea, impotence, and infertility	Multifactorial (including protein malabsorption, secondary hypopituitarism, and anemia)
Night blindness, xerophthalmia	Vitamin A deficiency
Peripheral neuropathy	Vitamin B_{12} or thiamine deficiency
Fatigue, weakness	Calorie depletion, iron and folate deficiency, and anemia
Neurologic symptoms, ataxia	Vitamin B_{12}, vitamin E, or folate deficiency

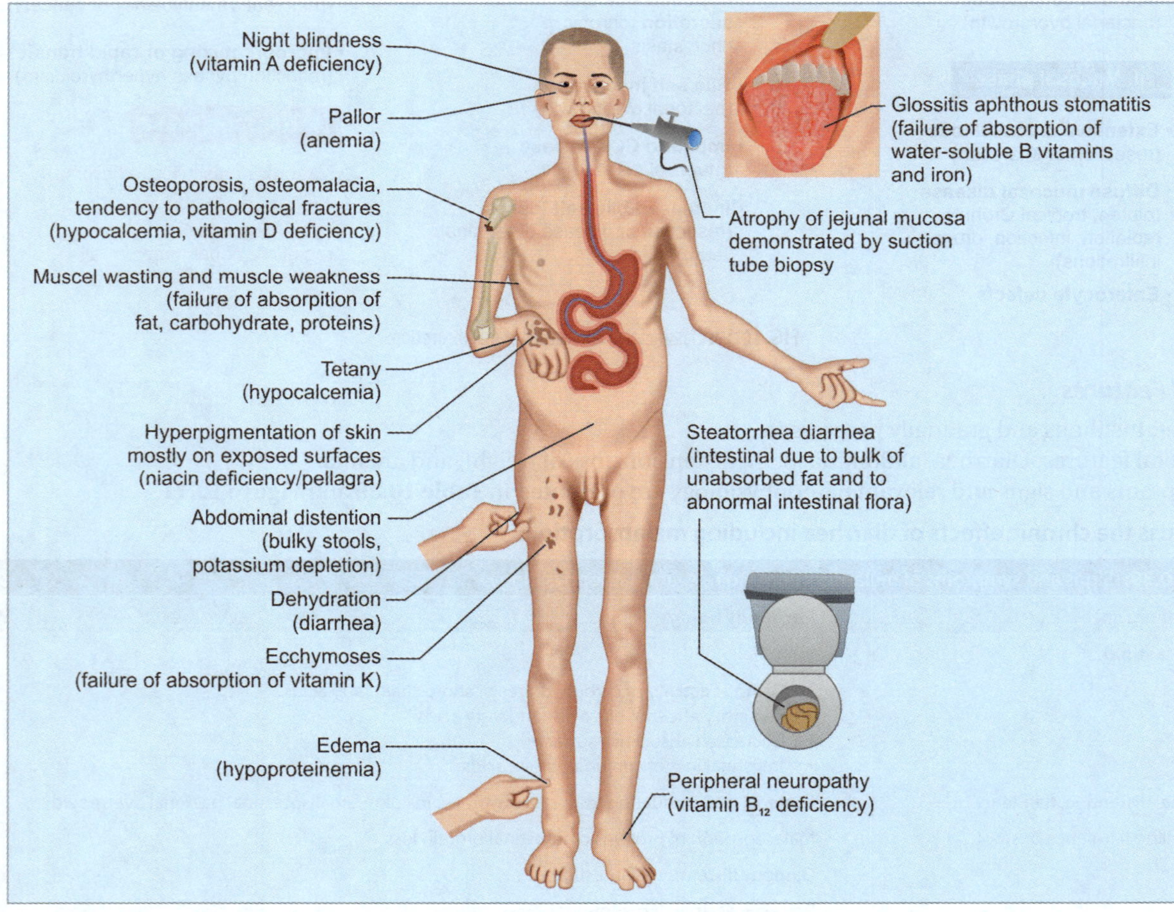

FIG. 10.11: Signs and symptoms of malabsorption.

Clinical features of specific malabsorption disorders are presented in **Table 10.40.**

TABLE 10.40: Clinical features of specific malabsorption disorders.

Disorder	*Cardinal clinical features*
Adrenal insufficiency	Skin darkening, hyponatremia, and hyperkalemia
Amyloidosis	Renal disease, nephrotic syndrome, cardiomyopathy, neuropathy, carpal tunnel syndrome, macroglossia, and hepatosplenomegaly
Carcinoid syndrome	Flushing, cardiac murmur

Contd...

Contd...

Celiac disease	Variable symptoms: Dermatitis herpetiformis, alopecia, aphthous mouth ulcers, arthropathy, neurologic symptoms, and (life-threatening) malnutrition; abnormal liver function test results, and mild iron deficiency
Crohn's disease	Arthritis, aphthous mouth ulcers, episcleritis, uveitis, pyoderma gangrenosum, erythema nodosum, abdominal mass, fistulas, primary sclerosing cholangitis (PSC), and laboratory signs of inflammation
Cystic fibrosis	Chronic sinopulmonary disease, meconium ileus, distal intestinal obstruction syndrome (DIOS), and elevated sweat chloride
Diabetes mellitus	Long history of diabetes and diabetic complications
Glucagonoma	Migratory necrolytic erythema
Hyperthyroidism, hypothyroidism	Symptoms and signs of thyroid disease
Lymphoma	Enlarged mesenteric or retroperitoneal lymph nodes, abdominal mass, abdominal pain, and fever
Pancreatic insufficiency	History of pancreatitis, abdominal pain; or alcoholism; large-volume fatty, and oily stools
Parasitic infection	History of travel to endemic areas
Primary biliary cirrhosis	Jaundice, itching
Scleroderma	Dysphagia, Raynaud's phenomenon, and skin tightening
Tropical sprue	History of travel to endemic area
Tuberculosis	Specific history of exposure, living in or travel to endemic area, immunosuppression, abdominal mass or intestinal obstruction, and ascites
Whipple's disease	Lymphadenopathy, fever, arthritis, cerebral symptoms, and heart murmur
Zollinger-Ellison syndrome	Peptic ulcers and diarrhea

Investigations (Table 10.41 and Flowchart 10.7)

TABLE 10.41: Laboratory tests useful in patients with suspected malabsorption.

Test	*Comment*
Peripheral blood findings	
Hematocrit, hemoglobin	Decreased in iron, vitamin B_{12}, and folate malabsorption or with blood loss
Mean corpuscular hemoglobin or mean corpuscular volume	Decreased in iron malabsorption; increased in folate and vitamin B_{12} malabsorption
White blood cells, differential	Decreased in vitamin B_{12} and folate malabsorption
Biochemical tests (serum)	
Triglycerides	Decreased in severe fat malabsorption
Cholesterol	Decreased in bile acid malabsorption or severe fat malabsorption
Albumin	Decreased in severe malnutrition, protein-losing enteropathy
Alkaline phosphatase	Increased in calcium and vitamin D malabsorption (severe steatorrhea); decreased in zinc deficiency
Calcium, phosphorus, and magnesium	Decreased in extensive small intestinal mucosal disease, after extensive intestinal resection, or in vitamin D deficiency
Zinc	Decreased in extensive small intestinal mucosal disease or intestinal resection
Iron and ferritin	Decreased in celiac disease, in other extensive small intestinal mucosal diseases, and with chronic blood loss
Other serum tests	
Prothrombin time	Prolonged in vitamin K malabsorption
Folic acid	Decreased in extensive small intestinal mucosal diseases, with anticonvulsant use, in pregnancy; may be increased in small intestinal bacterial overgrowth
Vitamin B_{12}	Decreased after gastrectomy, in pernicious anemia, terminal ileal disease, and small intestinal bacterial overgrowth
Endoscopy and biopsy stool tests	
Fat	Qualitative or quantitative increase in fat malabsorption
Elastase, chymotrypsin	Decreased concentration and output in exocrine pancreatic insufficiency
pH	<5.5 in carbohydrate

Tests for fat absorption

Quantitative test

- 72-hour-stool fat collection: Gold standard
- 6 g/day: Pathologic, patients with steatorrhea >20 g/day.

Qualitative tests

- **Sudan III stain** for fat globules in stool: Detect clinically significant steatorrhea in >90% of cases. Acid steatocrit: A gravimetric assay. Sensitivity
  - 100%, specificity—95%, PPV—90%
- NIRA (near infrareflectance analysis): Equally accurate with 72 hours stool fat test. Allows simultaneous measurement of fecal fat, nitrogen, and CHO (carbohydrate)
- Measurement of blood levels of fat-soluble vitamins (A, D, E, and K); prothrombin time.
  - Plasma vitamin A level after 2–3 days of oral retinol: It will be lower than normal.

Tests for carbohydrate absorption

- **Glucose tolerance test:** It reveals absence of rise in blood glucose levels.
- **Blood sugar level:** Low
- **D-xylose absorption test:** D-xylose is a pentose monosaccharide absorbed exclusively at the proximal small intestine. This test is used to assess proximal small intestine mucosal function. The procedure is as follows:
  - After overnight fast, administer 25 g D-xylose perorally.
  - Urine collected for next 5 hours and urinary excretion of D-xylose is estimated.
  - Abnormal test: <4.5 g is abnormal and suggest intestinal malabsorption (duodenal/jejunal mucosal disorders) and excludes pancreatic cause.
- **Lactose tolerance test (LTT):**
  - Orally 50 g of lactose is given.
  - Blood glucose levels measured at 0, 60, and 120 minutes.
  - Normally, blood glucose shows a rise of >20 mg/dL.
  - Blood glucose <20 mg/L + development of symptoms favor diagnosis.
- **Hydrogen breath test:** It is used for the diagnosis of lactase deficiency. 50 g lactose given orally and breath hydrogen measured every hour for 4 hours. Normal value is <10 ppm increase above baseline.

Tests for protein absorption

- **Serum albumin:** Low
- **Nitrogen in the 24-hour stool:** >2.5 g.
- **α_1-Antitrypsin content in stool:** Normally no antitrypsin in stool. A 3 days collection of stools is estimated for α_1-antitrypsin content.

Test for bile acid malabsorption

Selenium-homocholic acid taurine (SeHCAT) test: In this test, Se-labeled bile acid is given orally. After 7 days, total body retention is measured with a gamma camera. Retention value of <10% is abnormal.

Tests for absorption of other substances

- Serum B_{12} level: Reduced
- **Schilling test for absorption of B_{12}:** To determine the cause of cobalamin (B_{12}) malabsorption (discussed in Chapter 8).

FLOWCHART 10.7: Step-wise investigation in a suspected case of malabsorption.

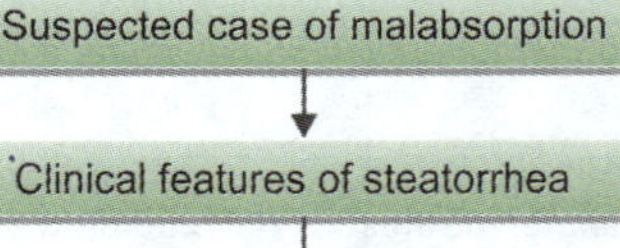

Test for bacterial overgrowth

- Quantitative bacterial count from aspiration from small intestine. Normal count is <10 U/mL (jejunum), >10 U/mL (ileum).
- **Breath tests:** Cholyl-14 C-glycine, e.g., bacterial overgrowth. Lactose H_2 for lactose intolerance, e.g., in bacterial overgrowth.
- **Small intestinal biopsy (duodenal or jejunal):** Lesions seen can be classified into three:
  1. Diffuse and specific, e.g., Whipple's disease
  2. Patchy and specific, e.g., Crohn's disease, lymphoma, and infectious causes
  3. Diffuse and nonspecific, e.g., celiac sprue, tropical sprue, and autoimmune enteropathy

Barium studies: Important information about the gross anatomy and morphology of small intestine.

Treatment of Malabsorption Syndrome

- **General measures**
  - Dehydration and electrolyte deficiency is treated by intravenous infusion
  - Replacement therapy for anemia, bone disease and coagulation defects. Vitamin D, B complex, and calcium supplements
- **Specific therapy depending on the cause**
  - Celiac disease: Gluten-free diet
  - Pancreatic insufficiency: Pancreatic supplements
  - Bile acid deficiency/malabsorption: Low-fat diet and cholestyramine (bile acid binder)

Celiac Disease

Q. Write short essay/note on celiac disease (nontropical sprue/gluten-induced enteropathy).

Definition

Celiac disease is characterized by small intestinal malabsorption of nutrients after the ingestion of wheat gluten or related proteins from rye and barley, villus atrophy of the small intestinal mucosa, prompt clinical and histologic improvement following strict adherence to a gluten-free diet, and clinical and histologic relapse when gluten is reintroduced.

Etiology

Exact etiology is not known, but environmental, immunologic, and genetic factors play important role.

- **Environmental factor:** Gluten is the protein present in the cereals wheat, barley and rye. **Gliadin** is a component of gluten. There is a clear cut association of the celiac disease with gliadin. Gluten restriction results in morphologic changes within hours in patient with celiac disease.
- **Immunologic factor:** It involves both adaptive and innate immune responses. Presence of serum antibodies such as IgA antigliadin, IgA antiendomysial (90–95% sensitivity and specificity), and IgA anti-tTG antibodies in patients with celiac disease. It is not known whether they represent primary or secondary to the tissue damage.
- **Genetic factor(s):** Increased incidence of celiac disease is observed within families but the exact mode of inheritance is unknown. All patients express the HLA-DQ2 or HLA-DQ8 allele.

Pathology

- **Site of lesion:** Biopsy from the **second portion of the duodenum or proximal jejunum** (which are exposed to the highest concentrations of dietary gluten) is diagnostic.
- **Microscopic changes:** Characterized by **increased numbers of intraepithelial CD8+ T lymphocytes** (intraepithelial lymphocytosis), crypt hyperplasia, and **villous atrophy.** Increased numbers of **plasma cells, mast cells, and eosinophils** within the upper part of the **lamina propria**.

Clinical Features

Age and gender: It can manifest at any age. Usually manifests early in childhood at about 2 years of age (after wheat is introduced into the diet), or later in the second to fourth decades of life with a female preponderance.

Symptoms: Many patients are asymptomatic (silent). The symptoms are very variable and often nonspecific.

- Symptoms due to malabsorption of multiple nutrients, with diarrhea, steatorrhea, weight loss, and the consequences of nutrient depletion (i.e., anemia and metabolic bone disease).
- Symptoms due to the depletion of a single nutrient (e.g., iron or folate deficiency or vitamin B_{12} deficiency, osteomalacia, edema from protein loss, and tetany).

Associated diseases

See **Box 10.10**.

Complications

See **Box 10.11**.

Investigations and Diagnosis

- Small-intestinal biopsy: Duodenal/jejunal biopsy is required and is considered as "gold standard" to establish a diagnosis.
- Serologic tests (**Box 10.12**)
- Tests for malabsorption of proteins, carbohydrate, fat, and vitamins
- HLA typing. HLADQ2 is observed in 90–95% of patients and HLADQ8 in about 8%.

Treatment/Management of Celiac Disease

- **Diet: Lifelong gluten-free diet.** Avoid wheat, rye, and barley. Oats not contaminated with flour are tolerated by most patients. Rice, meat, dairy products, vegetables, and fruits are safe. Completely avoid beer and whisky obtained from malt distillation procedures. Lactose-free diet is advisable because of secondary lactase deficiency associated with celiac disease
- **Supplementation of** vitamins and minerals in cases patients with these deficiencies, folic acid supplements for women of childbearing age
- **Pneumococcal vaccinations** (because of splenic atrophy) once in every 5 years
- **Corticosteroids:** They are rarely required. Used in critically ill patients who present with acute celiac crisis characterized by severe diarrhea, dehydration, weight loss, acidosis, hypocalcemia, and hypoproteinemia. May be used in gliadin shock after a gluten challenge

Box 10.10: Diseases associated with celiac disease.

- Insulin-dependent diabetes mellitus (2–8%)
- Thyroid disease (5%)
- Primary biliary cirrhosis (3%)
- Sjögren's syndrome (3%)
- IgA deficiency (2%)
- Pernicious anemia

Box 10.11: Complications of celiac disease.

- Gastrointestinal malignancies: An increased incidence of both gastrointestinal (e.g., *carcinoma of the esophagus)* and nongastrointestinal neoplasms as well as enteropathy associated *T cell lymphoma (EATCL)*
- Development of intestinal ulceration independent of lymphoma (ulcerative jejunitis*)*, refractory sprue, and collagenous sprue
- Nonresponsive celiac disease: Few patients do not improve on a strict diet
- Refractory celiac disease (RCD)
- Pneumococcal infections
- Dermatitis herpetiformis
- Osteomalacia

Box 10.12: Serologic tests in celiac disease.

Serologic tests

- IgA antiendomysial antibody
- IgA antitissue transglutaminase antibody (anti-tTG)
- IgA antigliadin antibody
- IgG antigliadin antibody

Tropical Sprue

Q. Write short essay on tropical sprue (idiopathic tropical malabsorption syndrome).

Definition: Tropical sprue is a condition presenting with chronic diarrhea and malabsorption (of two or more substances) that occurs in residents or travelers to certain, but not all tropical areas (especially India and Southeast Asia) in the absence of other intestinal diseases or parasites.

Etiology

- Etiology and pathogenesis of tropical sprue are unknown.
- **Role of infectious agents:** Because tropical sprue responds to antibiotics, it is possible that it may be caused by one or more infectious agents (e.g., *Klebsiella pneumoniae, Enterobacter cloacae,* or *E. coli*) or a toxin produced by these agents.
- **Role of folic acid deficiency:** Folic acid is absorbed in the duodenum and proximal jejunum, and most patients with tropical sprue show evidence of folate malabsorption and depletion.

Clinical Features

- Clinical features vary in different parts of the world.
- **Intensity:** Vary and consist of diarrhea, anorexia, abdominal distension fatigue, and weight loss.
- **Onset:**
  - **Acute:** Sometimes acute with sudden severe diarrhea and accompanied by fever. It occurs either a few days or many years after being in the tropics.
  - **Chronic phase:** Onset may also be insidious, with chronic diarrhea and evidence of nutritional deficiency. Features of megaloblastic anemia (folic acid malabsorption) and other deficiencies, including ankle edema, glossitis, and stomatitis, are common. Remissions and relapses may occur.

Treatment of Tropical Sprue

- **Broad-spectrum antibiotics:** Tetracycline or oxytetracycline 1 g daily in four divided doses for up to 6 months and produces improvement within 1–2 weeks
- **Folic acid: Dose of 5 mg daily** along with tetracycline is most often curative. It induces a hematologic remission and improvement in appetite, weight gain, and also morphological changes in small intestinal biopsy
- **Correction of deficiencies:** Severely ill patients require resuscitation with fluids and electrolytes for dehydration. Nutritional deficiencies should be corrected such as vitamin B (1,000 μg)
- **Symptomatic treatment for diarrhea**
- **Prognosis:** Excellent. Mortality is usually due to water and electrolyte depletion

Diagnosis and Investigations

- **Abnormal jejunal mucosal biopsy:** It shows partial villous atrophy and mononuclear cell infiltrate in the lamina propria. The lesion is less severe than that of celiac disease.
- **Stool examination**
- **Demonstration of malabsorption**

Lactose Intolerance

Q. Write short note on lactose intolerance.

Etiology

- Lactose is the disaccharide present in milk and it is digested to monosaccharides (glucose and galactose) by the brush border lactase.
- **Classification:** There are two types of lactase deficiency namely primary and secondary.
  - *Primary lactase deficiency:* It is due to genetic deficiency or absence of lactase and both intestinal absorption and brush border enzymes are normal.
  - *Secondary lactase deficiency:* It occurs in association with both structural and functional disorder of brush border enzymes and transport processes, e.g., celiac disease, tropical sprue, and Crohn's disease.
- Lactose intolerance develops due to the deficiency of lactase and lactose present in the milk cannot be hydrolyzed. Hence, lactose gets fermented by bacteria causing gastrointestinal symptoms.

Clinical Features

- Diarrhea, abdominal pain, cramps, and/or flatus develops after ingesting milk or milk products.
- Symptoms improve on withdrawal of milk or milk products.

Investigations

- **Hydrogen breath test:** This is used as a screening test to measure transit time and detect bacterial overgrowth in the small intestine. Appearance of breath hydrogen peak after

Treatment

- Lactose free diet. Avoid milk and dairy products. However, it may lead to nutritional deficiencies, particularly calcium deficiency.
- **Administration of exogenous β-galactosidase**
  - Enzyme replacement therapy with microbial exogenous lactase (obtained from yeasts or fungi)
  - Enzymes supplement to milk and dairy products
  - Use of yogurt and probiotics (source of β-galactosidase)

oral lactulose indicates that the undigested lactose is fermented by the colonic microflora and produces hydrogen which can be detected in expired air.
- Measurement of lactase activity in a jejunal biopsy.

Whipple's Disease

Q. Write short note on Whipple's disease and its important clinical features.

Whipple's disease is a chronic, rare, multisystemic infectious bacterial disease caused by ***Tropheryma whipplei*** (gram-positive).

Clinical Features

- Gender: More common in males than in females.
- Whipple's disease is a chronic multisystem disease associated with diarrhea, steatorrhea, weight loss, arthralgia, and central nervous system (CNS) and cardiac problems.
- Migratory arthralgias of the large joints
- Dementia and other CNS findings (such as supranuclear ophthalmoplegia, nystagmus, and myoclonus)
- Cardiac disease (dyspnea, pericarditis, and culture-negative endocarditis)
- Pleuropulmonary (pleural effusion)

Investigations

Biopsy: Jejunal biopsy and biopsy of other involved tissues show numerous **PAS—positive macrophages with small bacilli**. In the small intestine, these macrophages produce lymphatic blockade in the lamina propria causing malabsorption.

Treatment: Trimethoprim-sulfamethoxazole (double strength tablet): Dose twice a day for 1 year. This should be preceded by a 2-week course of parenteral therapy with ceftriaxone (2 g daily) or by meropenem.

Giardiasis

Q. Write short essay/note on clinical features, diagnosis, and treatment of Giardiasis.

- Giardiasis is an infection caused by flagellate *Giardia lamblia (Giardia intestinalis).*
- Giardiasis is found worldwide and is one of the most common parasitic diseases in both developed and developing countries, causing intestinal disease, and diarrhea.
- It mainly affects children, tourists and immunosuppressed individuals (agammaglobulinemia).
- **Incubation period:** 1–3 weeks
- **Mode of infection:** By ingesting **contaminated water**. In cystic form, it is viable in water for up to 3 months.
- Malabsorption may develop due to loss of brush-border enzyme activities and few patients may show flattering of villi.

Clinical Features

- Range from asymptomatic carrier stage to fulminant diarrhea and malabsorption.
- After ingestion of flagellar trophozoite form, it attaches to the mucosa of duodenum and jejunum and causes inflammation. It produces disease of small intestine.
- **Acute giardiasis:** Starts as **diarrhea, abdominal pain**, nausea, vomiting, anorexia, belching, flatus, weakness, and abdominal pain. Fever and blood in stool are rare. The duration is usually >1 week.
- **Chronic giardiasis:** May present with or without having experienced antecedent acute episode. Diarrhea may not be a prominent symptom and they may have increased flatus, and loose stools. It may produce steatorrhea; malabsorption if illness is prolonged may result in marked weight loss. Symptoms may be continuous or episodic and can persist for years. Chronic giardiasis in children from developing countries may develop retardation of growth.
- **Severe disease:** Giardiasis may be severe in patients with hypogammaglobulinemia, resulting in malabsorption, weight loss, growth retardation, and dehydration.
- Physical examination may reveal abdominal distension and tenderness.
- **Extraintestinal manifestations:** These include urticaria, anterior uveitis, and arthritis.

Investigations/Diagnosis

- **Stool examination: Demonstration of protozoal parasite**
- **Duodenal or jejunal aspiration** by endoscopy or with a luminal capsule gives a higher diagnostic yield.

Treatment/Management

- **Tinidazole** 40 mg/kg (2 g/day) once by mouth and repeated after 1 week
- **Metronidazole** 2 g daily for 3 days or metronidazole 200 mg thrice daily for 5–7 days is usually curative in >90% of cases
- **Nitazoxanide** 500 mg twice a day for 3 days. Other drugs include mepacrine and albendazole
- **Paromomycin** is an oral aminoglycoside and is not well absorbed. It can be given to symptomatic pregnant patients
- **Refractory cases:** Prolonged therapy with metronidazole 800 mg thrice daily for 3 weeks

- **String test:** In this one, end of a piece of string is passed into the duodenum by swallowing and retrieved after an overnight fast. The fluid is expressed from this and examined for the presence of *G. lamblia* trophozoites.
- **Biopsy:** Biopsy and histological examination of jejunal mucosa may show *G. lamblia* on the epithelial surface.
- **Stool antigen detection tests: Detection of parasite antigens in the feces** is sensitive and specific and easier to perform.
- **Other tests:** Chronic cases may show steatorrhea, malabsorption of xylose, and vitamin B_{12} and lactose intolerance.

Carcinoid Tumors (Neuroendocrine Tumors)

Q. Write short note on carcinoid tumors (neuroendocrine tumors) and carcinoid syndrome.

- Neuroendocrine cells are amine- and acid-producing cells located throughout the body.
- Neuroendocrine tumors (NETs) are tumors derived from the diffuse neuroendocrine system of the GI tract.
- Location of carcinoid tumors: Appendix (25%), small intestine (25%), and rectum (15%). Stomach (5%) and lung (15% of all carcinoid tumors).

Classification of Carcinoid Tumors

According to their anatomic area of origin:
- Foregut (lungs, bronchi, and stomach)
- Midgut (small intestine, appendix, and proximal large bowel
- Hindgut (distal large bowel, rectum).

Ultrastructurally, they possess electron-dense neurosecretory **granules which may contain various substances. These include: 5-hydroxytryptamine (serotonin), histamine, tachykinins, motilin, prostaglandins, bradykinins, adrenocorticotropic hormone, and corticotropin-releasing factor.**

Carcinoid Syndrome

It is symptom complex in which systemic symptoms are produced when the vasoactive substances are secreted by carcinoid tumors into the systemic circulation. Carcinoid syndrome occurs in only 8–10% of patients.
- **Midgut carcinoids** (usually ileal carcinoid) with hepatic metastasis can produce carcinoid syndrome. Because, normally liver is able to metabolize these secretory products into inactive forms and with hepatic metastasis the product can reach systemic circulation.
- **Foregut (bronchial and extraintestinal) carcinoids** can present with carcinoid syndrome without hepatic metastases. This is because bioactive products can bypass liver and can be released directly into systemic circulation.
- **Hindgut carcinoids** seldom produce syndrome since they do not secrete these products.
- Intestinal carcinoids have an increased tendency for liver metastasis.

Clinical Features (Table 10.42)

Characterized by cutaneous flushing, involving head and neck (blush area) associated with lacrimation, sweating, bronchospasm, colicky abdominal pain, diarrhea, and right-sided cardiac valvular fibrosis.

TABLE 10.42: Clinical features of carcinoid tumors.

Intestinal obstruction by tumor	Intestinal ischemia due to either mesenteric infiltration or vasospasm
Hepatic metastases may produce pain and jaundice	Features of carcinoid syndrome: Flushing, wheezing, diarrhea, etc.
Cardiac involvement (e.g., tricuspid regurgitation, pulmonary stenosis) leading to heart failure	Facial telangiectasia

Diagnosis

Diagnosed by measuring urinary or plasma serotonin or its metabolites in the urine.
- **Measurement of 5-hydroxyindoleacetic acid (5-HIAA):** Increased (>9 mg) urinary excretion in 24-hour sample collection.
- **Serum chromogranin A levels** are elevated in 56–100% of patients.
- Serotonin level in blood and platelets is high, because it is overproduced in 92% of patients.
- Plasma neuron-specific enolase levels are increased but are less sensitive than chromogranin A.
- **Others:** CT, MRI, and somatostatin receptor scintigraphy, PET (positron emission tomography) with radiolabeled 5-hydroxytryptophan may be helpful.

Treatment
- Avoid conditions and diets that precipitate flushing and diarrhea
- Supplementation of diet with nicotinamide
- Wheezing is treated with oral bronchodilators
- Treatment of heart failure with diuretics
- Control of the diarrhea with antidiarrheal agents (e.g., loperamide and diphenoxylate). If not controlled advise serotonin receptor antagonists (cyproheptadine, methysergide, and ondansetron) to control diarrhea
- Analogs of somatostatin (e.g., octreotide and lanreotide) to control flushing
- Surgical resection of the carcinoid tumor
- Excision of liver metastases or hepatic artery embolization with or without chemotherapy

Ischemic Colitis

Q. Write short note on ischemic colitis.

Etiology

- **Transient nonocclusive hypoperfusion of a segment of the colon**, e.g., systemic hypoperfusion
- **Occlusion of the inferior mesenteric artery or its branches**, e.g., atherosclerotic or thrombotic occlusion
- **Less common causes,** e.g., hypercoagulable states (in young persons), iatrogenic ligation of the inferior mesenteric artery (e.g., with aortic surgery), embolism, vasculitis, and colonic obstruction (e.g., colonic cancer).
- **Drugs and chemicals:** Medications, illicit drugs, and chemicals may also produce chemical picture identical or similar to ischemic colitis (e.g., digitalis, vasopressin, pseudoephedrine, amphetamines, cocaine, estrogens, ergot alosetron, etc.).

Clinical Features

- **Age:** Occur in persons older than 60 years without any apparent cause.
- **Onset:** Many cases are acute and self-limited.
- **Symptoms:** Colicky lower abdominal pain (mostly left lower quadrant), diarrhea, and passage of bright red blood per rectum, nausea, and vomiting. Though the blood loss is not usually enough to require transfusion, some patients may progress to shock because of loss of blood and fluid.
- **Physical examination:** Abdominal tenderness and guarding over the affected portion of the colon (especially left iliac fossa), and abdominal distention fever and tachycardia.

Laboratory Findings/Investigation

- Nonspecific findings such as leukocytosis and hemoconcentration
- Plain radiographs of the abdomen: It may show "**thumbprinting**" at splenic flexure and descending colon or may be normal.
- Computed tomography (CT) scanning of abdomen: Useful to exclude other disorders.
- Double contrast barium enema demonstrates involvement of splenic flexure and descending colon. Mucosal abnormalities are **thumbprinting** and ulceration.
- Colonoscopy has replaced barium studies as it is more sensitive. Sigmoidoscopy shows normal rectal mucosa and bleeding descending from above.
- Arteriography confirms the diagnosis in patients with obstructive lesions.

Treatment

- **For right-sided ischemic colitis:** It requires visceral angiography which is needed for both diagnosis and intra-arterial administration of vasodilators (e.g., papaverine as a 60-mg intravenous bolus followed by an infusion of 30–60 mg/hour). Some patients may need urgent surgery
- **Left-sided acute ischemic colitis:** It accounts for most cases and most cases resolve within hours to a few days with supportive therapy. Therapy includes volume replacement, correction of any low-flow state, broad-spectrum antibiotics (similar to those recommended earlier for patients with small bowel ischemia), avoidance of vasoconstrictive medications, and rarely, blood transfusion. Surgery is required only in patients with signs and symptoms of transmural necrosis, perforation, or massive bleeding
- **Conservative management:** Intravenous fluids, hemodynamic stabilization, discontinuation or avoidance of vasoconstrictive agents, bowel rest, and empiric antibiotics
- **Surgical treatment:** Peritonitis and strictures

Pseudomembranous Colitis

Q. Write short note on pseudomembranous colitis (antibiotic-associated colitis).

Pseudomembranous colitis also referred to as antibiotic-associated colitis or antibiotic-associated diarrhea, generally caused due to toxin produced by *Clostridium difficile*, when the normal bacterial flora is altered or suppressed by antibiotics.

- Antibiotic-associated diarrhea may (**Table 10.43**) also be caused by other organisms such as *Salmonella*, *C. perfringens* type A, or *Staphylococcus aureus* but only *C. difficile* causes pseudomembranous colitis.
- In the colon, the vegetative form of *C. difficile* multiplies and produces **two major toxins** namely toxin A (an enterotoxin) and toxin B (a cytotoxin).

TABLE 10.43: Antimicrobial agents that predispose to *Clostridium difficile*-associated diarrhea and colitis.

Most frequently	Less frequently
➤ Ampicillin and amoxicillin	➤ Macrolides (including erythromycin)
➤ Cephalosporins	➤ Other penicillins
➤ Clindamycin	➤ Sulfonamides
➤ Fluoroquinolones	➤ Trimethoprim/ sulfamethoxazole

Clinical Features

- **Age:** Pseudomembranous colitis usually develops in adults and about 80% of cases occur in people over 65 years of age.
- Patient is on antibiotics or has received antibiotics within last 8 weeks. Clinical symptoms range from asymptomatic to severe and sometimes life-threatening fulminant pseudomembranous colitis.
- **Diarrhea:** It is the most common manifestation.
  - Stool: Soft and unformed to watery or mucoid in consistency and has a characteristic odor. Stools are almost never grossly bloody.
  - Frequency: Patients may have as many as 20 bowel movements/day.
  - Profuse watery diarrhea with abdominal cramps
  - Substantial fluid and protein losses combined with fever, cramps, hypoalbuminemia, leukocytosis, and hypotension.
- **Laboratory findings:** Leukocytosis is common (observed in up to 50% of patients) and is a marker of severe disease. Leukocytosis often >15,000/mm³ white blood cells (WBCs)/L. Extremely high level (>50,000/mm³ indicates fulminant and potentially fatal illness.
- **Complications:** Dehydration, electrolyte disturbances, hypoalbuminemia, toxic megacolon, bowel perforation, hypotension, renal failure, hypotension, lactic acidosis sepsis, and death.

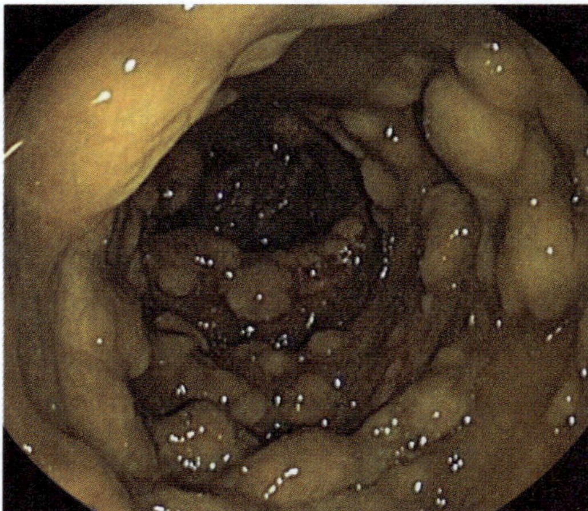

FIG. 10.12: Endoscopic appearance of pseudomembranous colitis.

Investigations and Diagnosis

- Enzyme immunoassay for *C. difficile* glutamate dehydrogenase
- Enzyme immunoassay for *C. difficile* toxins A and B
- Real-time PCR tests detect the critical gene is tcdB.
- Stool culture for *C. difficile*
- **Sigmoidoscopy or colonoscopy:** Endoscopy is a rapid diagnostic tool in seriously ill patients and characteristically shows erythema, white plaques or an adherent pseudomembrane (**Fig. 10.12**). Biopsy can be done.

Treatment/Management

Treatment consists of (1) discontinuation of the implicated antibiotic, (2) supportive care, and (3) avoidance of antiperistaltic agents and opiates

- **Withdraw/discontinue** the precipitating antibiotic/antimicrobial drug and isolate the patient
- **Supportive care:** Oral or intravenous rehydration

  Mild-to-moderate cases: Oral metronidazole 500 mg thrice daily for 10–14 days. Rifaximin can be added
  - **Severe cases:** Oral vancomycin 125 mg 6 hourly for 14 days
  - **Severe complicated or fulminant cases:** Vancomycin (500 mg orally or via nasogastric tube) plus intravenous metronidazole (500 mg q8h) *plus consider* rectal instillation of vancomycin (500 mg in 100 mL of normal saline as a retention enema q6–8h). Intravenous vancomycin not effective. Newer drug fidaxomicin (200 mg twice daily) is as efficacious as vancomycin. If ileus develops vancomycin administered by enema
    - **Oral probiotic therapy:** Use of live nonpathogenic bacteria to re-establish the gut flora often used in resistant or relapsed cases. Probiotics use organisms resistant to gastric acid. However, its clinical benefits are not proved
- **Avoidance of antiperistaltic agents and opiates:** Antiperistaltic drugs such as loperamide or diphenoxylate should not be administered because they can precipitate toxic megacolon
- Colectomy may be necessary in severely ill and refractory cases
- Newer treatment modalities: **Fecal microbiota transplantation** (fecal enemas or infusion of donor feces through a nasoduodenal tube)

Psychosomatic Disorders of the Gastrointestinal Tract

Classification

See **Table 10.44.**

TABLE 10.44: Classification of the functional disorders of gastrointestinal tract.

➢ Bad taste (cacogeusia)—foul smell of breath (halitosis) ➢ Functional heartburn—noncardiac chest pain due to esophageal dysmotility ➢ Functional dyspepsia—functional bloating aerophagia	➢ Globus hystericus ➢ Unspecified excessive belching ➢ Functional or psychogenic vomiting and cyclic vomiting syndrome ➢ Irritable bowel syndrome ➢ Functional diarrhea and functional constipation

Irritable Bowel Syndrome

Q. Write short essay/note on irritable bowel syndrome, its clinical features and management.

Definition

- Irritable bowel syndrome (IBS) is a functional disorder of the gastrointestinal tract characterized by abdominal pain or discomfort and altered bowel habits in the absence of detectable structural, infective or biochemical abnormalities.
- Irritable bowel syndrome is benign, chronic symptom complex of altered bowel habits, and abdominal pain.

Pathophysiology

Exact cause not known and pathogenesis of IBS is poorly understood. However, the following factors have been proposed.

Gastrointestinal motor abnormalities: GI motility is quantitatively different in 25–75% of IBS patients compared with healthy controls.

- Patients with diarrhea as a predominant symptom exhibit rapid jejunal contraction waves, rapid intestinal transit, an increased number of colonic contractions (colonic transit is accelerated), and rectosigmoid motor activity.
- Patients with predominant constipation have decreased orocecal transit and a reduced number of colonic contraction waves.

Visceral hypersensitivity: IBS is associated with increased sensory responses to visceral stimulation induced by intestinal distension. The mechanism for visceral hypersensitivity is not known. This is more common in females and in diarrhea-predominant IBS.

Central neural dysregulation: There is a clinical association of emotional disorders and stress with symptom exacerbation in IBS. MRI has shown that in response to distal colonic stimulation, the mid-cingulate cortex (brain region concerned with attention processes and response selection) shows greater activation in IBS patients. This cerebral dysfunction may lead to the increased perception of visceral pain.

Abnormal psychological features: Abnormal psychiatric features are found in up to 80% of IBS patients. These include anxiety, tension, depression, excessive worry, somatization, and neurosis.

Altered intestinal flora: Bacterial overgrowth (shown by positive lactulose hydrogen breath test) in the small bowel has been observed in IBS patients and may contribute to symptoms.

Abnormal serotonin pathways: Serotonin is a neurotransmitter that plays an important role in the regulation of GI motility and visceral perception.

Post-infectious IBS: IBS may be induced by initial GI infection by *Campylobacter*, *Salmonella*, and *Shigella*.

Immune activation and mucosal inflammation: Certain diet/foods may precipitate an attack.

Clinical Features

- **Age:** IBS affects all ages. Most patients present before age 45 (20–40 years).
- **Gender:** More common in women compared to men (3:1).
- **Abdominal pain** is the most common key symptom (prerequisite clinical feature) for the diagnosis of IBS. Characteristics of pain:
  - **Location:** Pain is most typically referred to the lower abdomen (left or right iliac fossa) or hypogastrium.
  - **Aggravation:** Pain may be aggravated by emotional stress or poor sleep, and intake of food.
  - **Relief:** Abdominal symptoms are relieved by defecation or passage of flatus, but this relief may be temporary.
- **Altered bowel habits:** Most consistent clinical feature in IBS. Bowel pattern subtypes/**variants** are:
  - **Irritable bowel syndrome-constipation predominant (IBS-C):** Patient reports that abnormal bowel movements are usually constipation (>25% Bristol stool types 1 or 2; <25% Bristol stool types 6 or 7).
  - **Irritable bowel syndrome-diarrhea predominant (IBS-D):** Patient reports that abnormal bowel movements are usually diarrhea (>25% Bristol stool types 6 or 7; <25% Bristol stool types 1 or 2).
  - **Mixed IBS (IBS-M):** They have features of alternating diarrhea and constipation (>25% Bristol stool types 1 or 2; >25% Bristol stool types 6 or 7).
  - **Irritable bowel syndrome-unclassified (IBS-U)** includes those patients who meet the diagnostic criteria for IBS but cannot be accurately categorized into one of the other three subtypes.

Most common alteration in the bowel habit is constipation alternating with diarrhea.

- **Diarrhea:** Frequent defecation, often painless, but produce low-volume stools and rare/never at night. Diarrhea usually consists of small volumes of loose stools. Sense of incomplete evacuation, leading to repeated attempts at defecation in a short time span.
- **Constipation:** Pass infrequent pellet-like (ribbon-like or pencil-like) stools usually in association with abdominal pain or proctalgia.
- **Stools:** Usually hard with narrowed caliber. May be accompanied by passage of large amounts of mucus.
- **Gas and flatulence:** Abdominal distention and increased belching or flatulence more common among female patients. Postprandial tenesmus is common and is due to an exaggerated gastrocolic reflex.
- **Other symptoms:** Dyspepsia, heartburn, nausea, and vomiting
- **Extraintestinal symptoms:** Headache, back pain, fatigue myalgia, dyspareunia, and urinary frequency are often observed.
- **Physical examination:** Usually unremarkable, except for abdominal tenderness (most often in the left lower quadrant) or a tender, palpable sigmoid colon. In IBS-C, rectal examination may show paradoxical contraction of the puborectalis muscle or decreased descent of the pelvic floor when simulating a bowel movement.

Investigations

Aim of investigations is to exclude organic gastrointestinal diseases.

- **Full blood count**
- **Stool examination:** For parasites, ova, leukocytes, and occult blood.
- **Sigmoidoscopy:** Usually normal. There may be difficulty in negotiating rectosigmoid curve due to spasm. There may be marked motor activity of bowel and may show abundant mucus.
- **Colonoscopy:** Should be performed to exclude colorectal cancer, in older patients and those with history of rectal bleeding.
- **Barium enema:** Usually normal but may show spasticity of sigmoid, exaggerated haustral markings and a tubular appearance of the descending colon.
- In diarrhea-predominant patients investigations to exclude microscopic colitis, lactose intolerance, bile acid malabsorption, celiac disease, and thyrotoxicosis.

TABLE 10.45: Rome IV diagnostic criteria for irritable bowel syndrome.

Recurrent abdominal pain on average at least 1 day per week in the last 3 months (with symptom onset at least 6 months prior to diagnosis) associated with *two or more* of the following:

1. Related to defecation
2. Associated with a change in frequency of stool
3. Associated with a change in form (appearance) of stool

Symptoms that support the diagnosis of irritable bowel syndrome:

- Abnormal stool frequency: ≤3 bowel movements per week or >3 bowel movements per day
- Abnormal stool form: Lumpy/hard stool or loose/watery stool
- Defecation straining
- Urgency
- Feeling of incomplete bowel movement
- Passing mucus
- Bloating or feeling of abdominal distention

TABLE 10.46: Red flag signs of IBS.

➢ More than minimal rectal bleeding ➢ Weight loss ➢ Unexplained iron deficiency anemia ➢ Nocturnal symptoms	➢ Family history of selected organic diseases including colorectal cancer, inflammatory bowel disease (IBD), or celiac sprue ➢ Fever

Diagnostic Criteria

Rome IV diagnostic criteria for irritable bowel syndrome are presented in **Table 10.45**.

Red flag signs of IBS are presented in **Table 10.46**.

Treatment (Flowchart 10.8)

Patient counseling and dietary alterations

- **Reassurance** and thorough careful explanation of the functional nature and benign prognosis of the disorder
- **Dietary modification:** Avoid obvious foods that precipitate symptoms. The role of probiotics is not well established
  - Many IBS patients have nonspecific intolerance to foods
  - The dietary restriction of fermentable carbohydrates popularly termed the low FODMAP (fermentable oligosaccharides, disaccharides, monosaccharides, and polyols) diet
  - Exclusion of gas-producing foods/foods that increase flatulence (e.g., beans, onions, celery, carrots, raisins, bananas, apricots, prunes, brussels sprouts, wheat germ, pretzels, and bagels), alcohol, and caffeine
  - Irritable bowel syndrome patients should avoid foods that trigger an onset of their symptoms, consume a minimum of high fat foods, and take part in regular physical activity

FLOWCHART 10.8: Management of irritable bowel syndrome.

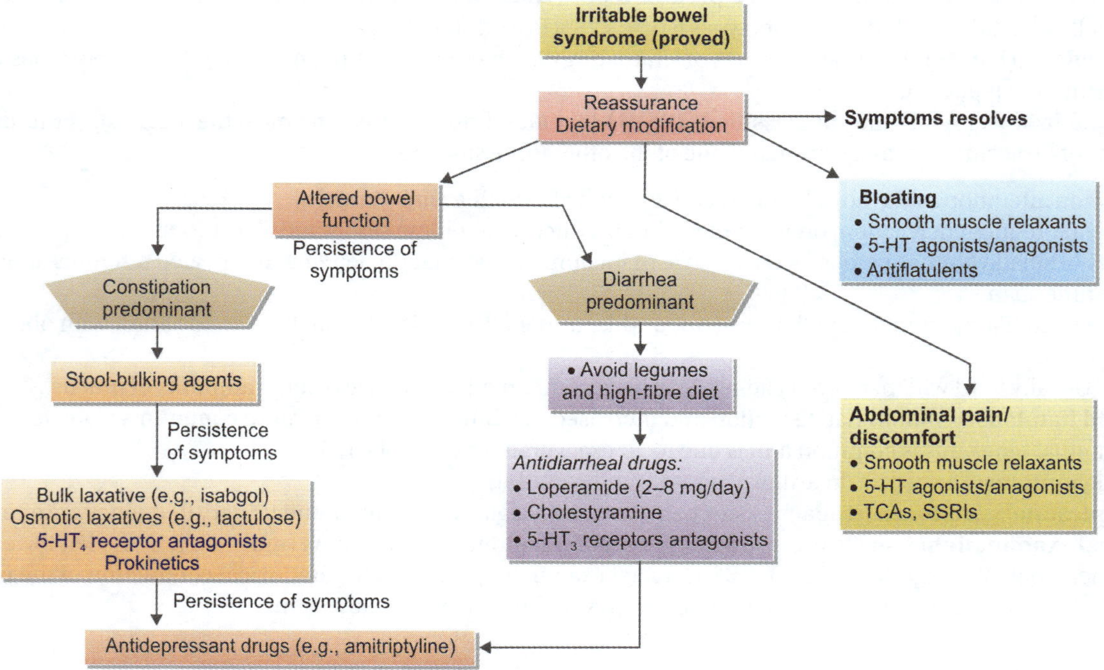

(5-HT: 5-hydoxytryptamine; TCAs: tricyclic antidepressants; SSRIs: selective serotonin reuptake inhibitors)

Constipations-predominant IBS

- **Stool-bulking agents:** High-fiber diets and bulking agents (e.g., bran or hydrophilic colloid) increase the roughage content of the diet (increases the fecal output of bacteria) and delay colonic transit. If symptoms persist add a bulk laxative (methylcellulose, isabgol husk, psyllium fiber supplement, and corn fiber). Osmotic laxatives (e.g., polyethylene glycol, lactulose, and milk of magnesia) or secretory stimulators (e.g., lubiprostone) may be tried, if high-fiber supplementation fails.
- **Prokinetic agents**
  - Tegaserod is a 5-HT_4 receptor agonist and a prokinetic drug, stimulates intestinal peristalsis. However, tegaserod has been withdrawn from the market; because of serious cardiovascular events.
  - Cisapride and mosapride are not useful in most patients.
- **Antispasmodics:** If abdominal pain is not adequately relieved, synthetic anticholinergic agent (dicyclomine 10 mg TID) or an antispasmodic (mebeverine 135 mg TID) may be given.
- **Antidepressant drugs:** Patients with intractable symptoms may be benefited from tricyclic antidepressant drugs such as amitriptyline (10–25 mg orally at bedtime) or desipramine (10–25 mg orally at bedtime).
- **Antiflatulence therapy:** Advised to eat slowly and avoid chew gum or carbonated beverage drinks. Antibiotic rifaximin (400, three times a day) may also help in relieving bloating.
- **Chloride-channel activators:** Lubiprostone activates chloride channels in the intestinal epithelial cells. This in-turn induces passive movement of sodium and water into the lumen of the intestine and improves bowel function.

Diarrhea-predominant IBS

- Advised to avoid legumes and high-fiber diet.
- **Anti-diarrheal drugs**
  - Loperamide (2–4 mg up to four times a day maximum of 12 g/day).
  - Cholestyramine resin is a bile acid-binding agent used as a second-line agent (4 g four to six times a day).
- **Serotonin receptor antagonists:** Serotonin acts on 5-HT_3 receptors and increases the sensitivity of afferent neurons of the gut. Alosetron (others drugs include ondansetron, granisetron, alosetron, and cilansetron) is a 5-HT_3 receptor antagonist reduces abdominal visceral pain, induces rectal relaxation, increases rectal compliance, and delays colonic transit. But it is of little use because of danger of producing ischemic colitis.
- **Antispasmodics:** For the control of pain.
- **Antibiotics:** Nonabsorbable antibiotics such as rifaximin 400 mg BID for 5–6 weeks has been tried.
- **Probiotics use:** The bifidobacteria, *Saccharomyces boulardii,* and other combinations of probiotics demonstrate some efficacy in IBS.
- **Asimadoline:** Kappa-opioid receptor agonist has been in trials for IBS.

Abdominal Tuberculosis

Q. Describe the etiology, pathology, clinical features, complications, differential diagnosis, investigations, and treatment of abdominal tuberculosis.

It includes gastrointestinal tuberculosis, peritoneum, and abdominal lymph nodes, either individually or in combinations.

Gastrointestinal Tuberculosis

Intestinal tuberculosis commonly involves ileocecal region (about 70% of cases) probably because this region has: (1) increased rate of absorption of fluid and electrolyte; (2) increased physiological stasis; (3) prominent lymphoid tissue; and (4) minimal digestive activity.

Other rare regions: These include ascending colon, jejunum, sigmoid colon, rectum, duodenum, stomach, and esophagus.

Etiology

- **Causative agent:** *Mycobacterium tuberculosis* human or bovine strain.
- **Routes of spread of intestinal tuberculosis**
  - **Hematogenous spread:** Primary or secondary tuberculosis of lung may spread through blood into the intestine.
  - **Ingestion:** Mycobacteria in sputum from active pulmonary focus may be ingested and cause intestinal tuberculosis.
  - **Direct spread:** From nearby or adjacent organs.
  - **Through lymphatics:** From infected lymph nodes
- **Routes of spread of peritoneal tuberculosis:** Infection may spread to peritoneum from lymph nodes or intestinal lesions or tuberculous salpingitis (fallopian tube) in females.

Pathology

Intestinal tuberculosis: Three types:

1. **Ulcerative (60%):** More often observed in malnourished adults.
   - **Gross:** Characteristics of tuberculous ulcers are: (1) multiple superficial ulcers mainly found in the ileocecal region; (2) long axis of ulcers is perpendicular to the long axis of the intestine (in typhoid fever, long axis of ulcers lies parallel to the long axis of the intestine).

- **Consequences:** Fibrosis occurring during healing of ulcers produces strictures. Rarely, endarteritis may lead to massive bleeding.

2. **Hypertrophic (10%):** This is a variant of secondary tuberculosis observed in ileocecal region. More often found in relatively well-nourished adults.
   - **Gross:** The lesions are seen mainly in cecum and/or ascending colon. These regions become thick-walled due to scarring, fibrosis, and local hypertrophy) and show mucosal ulceration.
   - Clinically, the lesion present as a palpable and may be mistaken for carcinoma.
3. **Ulcerohypertrophic (30%):**
   - It represents combination of both ulcerative and hypertrophic types.
   - Right iliac fossa mass due to hypertrophic ileocecal region, and involved mesenteric fat and lymph nodes.

Peritoneal Tuberculosis

- **Gross appearance of peritoneum:** Shows multiple yellow-white tubercles. Peritoneum is thick and hyperemic with a loss of its shiny appearance. Omentum is also thickened.
- **Forms:**
  1. *Wet type:* It presents with ascites.
  2. *Encysted (loculated) type:* It presents with a localized abdominal swelling.
  3. *Fibrotic type:* It presents with abdominal masses. They consist of thickening of mesentery and omentum with matted bowel loops. Adhesions may produce intestinal obstruction.

A combination of above types is also can be seen.

Solid Organ Tuberculosis

These include: (1) Spleen, (2) liver, (3) adrenal tuberculosis, and (4) genitourinary tuberculosis.

Tuberculosis of Mesenteric Lymph Nodes

Usually observed in young adults. Involves mesenteric lymph nodes and these nodes may become palpable as rounded mass (tabes mesenterica). May be confused with lymphoma.

Clinical features

- Usually found in young adults.
  - It may present as acute, chronic, or acute on chronic condition.
  - *Common symptoms:* Fever, abdominal pain, anorexia, malaise, weight loss, diarrhea, constipation, alternating constipation and diarrhea, and gastrointestinal bleeding or obstruction.
  - Abdominal pain may be either colicky (due to luminal compromise) or dull and continuous when there is involvement of mesenteric lymph nodes.
- *Physical examination of the abdomen:* It is described as "**doughy**" because matted loops of bowel may be palpable. A well-defined, firm, mobile mass may be found in the right lower quadrant of the abdomen. Mesenteric lymphadenitis produces mass. Abdominal distention due to ascites.

*Complications and differential diagnosis are described in **Box 10.13** and **Table 10.47**.*

Investigations (Flowchart 10.9)

Hematological investigations: ESR is raised, anemia, and hypoalbuminemia.

Box 10.13: Complications of intestinal tuberculosis.

- Intestinal hemorrhage
- Subacute intestinal obstruction
- Fistula formation (between skin and intestine or between loops of intestines)
- Intestinal perforation
- *Malabsorption:* Ileocecal tuberculosis is the common cause of malabsorption in India

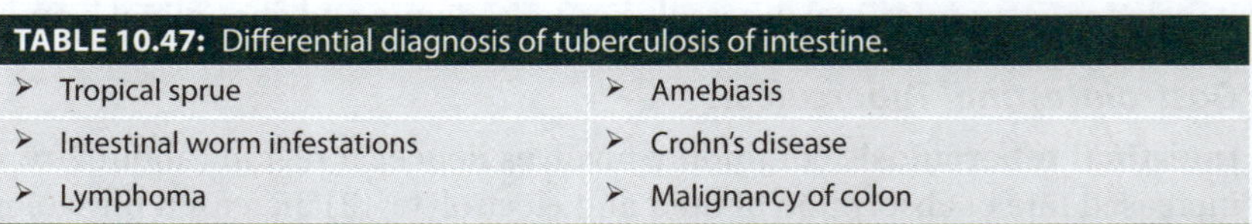

TABLE 10.47: Differential diagnosis of tuberculosis of intestine.

➤ Tropical sprue	➤ Amebiasis
➤ Intestinal worm infestations	➤ Crohn's disease
➤ Lymphoma	➤ Malignancy of colon

FLOWCHART 10.9: Diagnostic algorithm for abdominal tuberculosis.

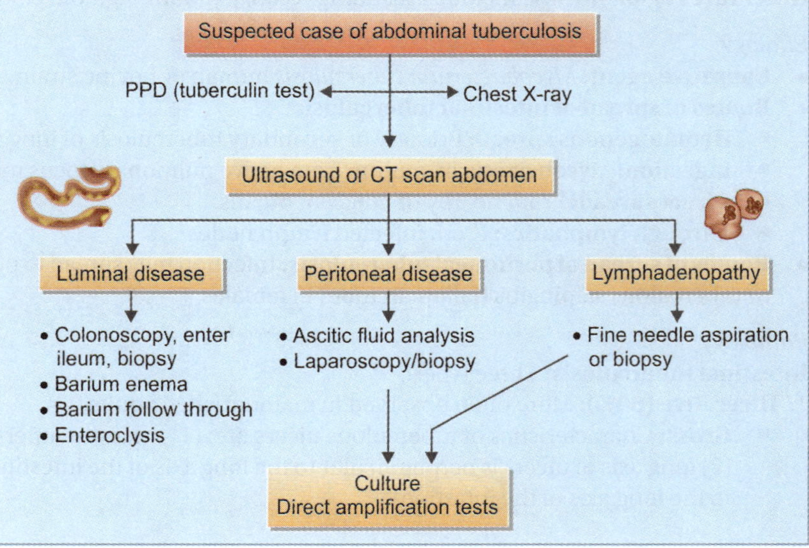

Radiological investigations

- Chest X-ray: May show evidence of active or old tuberculosis.
- Plain X-ray of abdomen: It may reveal calcified lymph nodes.
  - **If there is intestinal obstruction:** Dilated bowel loops with multiple air-fluid levels may be seen.
  - **If intestinal perforation:** Air under diaphragm and dilated loops.
- **Barium meal**
  - May show hypermotility (accelerated intestinal transit)
  - Hypersegmentation of the barium column ("chicken intestine")
  - Precipitation, flocculation, and dilution of the barium
  - Luminal stenosis with smooth but stiff contours ("hour-glass stenosis")

Multiple strictures with segmental dilatation of bowel loops:
Stierlin sign: A defect characterized by failure of the diseased segment to retain barium that is otherwise normally retained by adjacent uninvolved segments. Appears as a narrowing ileum with rapid emptying into a shortened cecum.
String sign: A thin stream of barium seen in the terminal ileum.
Note: Both Stierlin and string sign can also be seen in Crohn's disease, and hence, are not specific for tuberculosis.

- **Barium enema**
  - Wide gaping of ileocecal valve with narrowing of the terminal ileum ("Fleischner" or "inverted umbrella sign"). Fold thickening and contour irregularity or terminal ileum shrunken in size ("conical cecum").
  - Pulled up cecum due to contraction and fibrosis of the mesocolon.
  - Loss of normal ileocecal angle and dilated terminal ileum, appearing suspended from a retracted, fibrosed cecum. Localized stenosis opposite the ileocecal valve with a rounded off smooth cecum and a retracted fibrosed cecum.
- **Abdominal ultrasound**
  - Intra-abdominal fluid (free or loculated; with or without debris and septae).
  - Localized fluid between rapidly oriented bowel loops due to local exudation from the inflamed bowel (interloop ascites; "club sandwich" or "sliced bread" sign).
  - Lymphadenopathy, discrete or matted with heterogeneous echotexture due to caseation.
  - Uniform and concentric bowel wall thickening in the ileocecal region (versus eccentric thickening at the mesenteric border found in Crohn's disease and variegated appearance of malignancy).
- **Contrast-enhanced CT scan**
  - Symmetric circumferential thickening of cecum and terminal ileum. Ulceration or nodularity within the terminal ileum, along with narrowing and proximal dilatation
  - *Regional lymph nodes:* Caseating lymph nodes with hypodense centers and peripheral rim enhancement. Retroperitoneal nodes (periaortic and pericaval) almost never seen in isolation, unlike lymphoma.
  - *Mesenteric thickening:* Omental thickening seen as an omental cake appearance. Thickened peritoneum and enhancing peritoneal nodules.
  - Ascitic fluid of high-attenuation value
- **Ascitic fluid examination lymphocytic ascites with serum-ascites albumin gradient (SAAG) (1.1 g/dL and elevated ascites ADA level)**
- **Biopsy of peritoneum:** Punch or laparoscopic biopsy
- **Colonoscopy:** It may show mucosal nodules and ulcers in colon and is used for taking biopsy from the edge of ulcers.
- **Biopsy from other organs involved:** Liver, lymph node

Treatment

- Antitubercular treatment similar to treatment of pulmonary tuberculosis
- Surgery
- Strictureplasty for strictures that reduce the lumen by 50% or more and that cause proximal dilation
- Resection of segment having multiple strictures

TABLE 10.48: Conditions causing ulcers in intestine.

Predominantly small intestine	*Predominantly large intestine*	*Both small and large intestine*
➤ Enteric/typhoid fever ➤ Tuberculosis ➤ Zollinger-Ellison syndrome ➤ Mesenteric artery occlusion	➤ Amebiasis ➤ Ulcerative colitis ➤ Gram-negative bacillary dysentery ➤ Ischemic colitis	➤ Crohn's disease ➤ Malignant ulcers

Ulcers in Intestine

Q. Write short note on ulcers in intestine.

Conditions causing ulcers in intestine are presented in **Table 10.48**.

INFLAMMATORY BOWEL DISEASE

Q. Describe the etiology, pathology, clinical features, investigations, and management of inflammatory bowel diseases (ulcerative colitis and Crohn's disease).

Inflammatory bowel disease (IBD) is an immune-mediated chronic intestinal condition. It **results from inappropriate mucosal immune activation.**

These include several conditions:

1. Ulcerative colitis (UC) } Most important
2. Crohn disease (CD) }
3. *Others (uncommon) nonspecific inflammatory bowel disease:* Indeterminate colitis (15% patients with IBD) microscopic ulcerative, microscopic lymphocytic, and microscopic collagenous colitis.

Etiology and Pathogenesis of IBD

Genetic Factors

Genetic predisposition/susceptibility contributes to IBD

1. **Familial:**
   - **Crohn's disease:** Genetic factors **play a prominent role**. The concordance rate for monozygotic twins is about 50%.
   - **Ulcerative colitis:** Genetic factors are **less prominent than in Crohn's disease**. The concordance of monozygotic twins is only 16%. Concordance for dizygotic twins for both Crohn's disease and ulcerative colitis is less than 10%.
2. **Susceptibility genes:**
   - **Genes associated with innate immunity and autophagy (e.g., *NOD2/CARD15, ATG16L1, and IRGM*):** Actions of NOD2/CARD15 protein are: (1) **prevents the entry of microbes** into the wall of the intestine; (2) **regulates innate immune responses;** and (3) prevents excessive immune response by luminal microbes.

Environmental Factors

Include both the local microenvironment (intestinal microflora) and the nutritional environment.

1. **Intestinal microflora/microbiota:**
   - **Hygiene hypothesis:** The **gut lumen** contains **abundant commensal bacteria** and its composition within individuals remains stable for several years. This intestinal microflora **can be modified by diet and disease**. **IBD is associated with an alteration in the bacterial flora.**
   - **Improved food storage conditions and decreased food contamination:** It has **reduced frequency of enteric infections**, with "clean" environment in the intestinal lumen → the **immune system may not be exposed to microorganisms** (pathogenic or non-pathogenic) → **inadequate development of regulatory processes** to limit mucosal immune responses.
2. **Smoking:** CD patients are more likely to be smokers, and smoking exacerbates CD. In contrast, an increased risk of UC is observed in non- or ex-smokers.

Host Factors

These include epithelial defects, impaired mucosal barrier, abnormal intestinal defensins, and immune dysregulation.

Psychosocial Factors

It can contribute to worsening of symptoms in IBD. Major life events (e.g., illness or death in the family, divorce, or separation) are associated with an increase in symptoms such as pain, bowel dysfunction, and bleeding.

Ulcerative Colitis

Definition

Ulcerative colitis is a severe-ulcerating inflammatory disease. It is limited to large intestine (the **colon and rectum).** It is characterized clinically by recurrent attacks (exacerbations and remissions) of bloody diarrhea. Pathologically, the inflammatory response is found only in the **mucosa and submucosa** of the intestinal wall and shows chronic destruction of crypts.

Pathology

Site (Fig. 10.13): Ulcerative colitis primarily involves the colonic mucosa. Usually **involves the rectum** (involved in 95% of cases) **and extends proximally** for a variable distance in a continuous fashion to involve part or the entire colon. Skip lesions are not seen in UC.

- **Pancolitis:** If entire colon is involved by the disease, then it is termed **pancolitis.**
- **Left-sided colitis:** When disease involves only the left-side of colon.
- **Extensive colitis:** When disease involves colon up to the hepatic flexure.

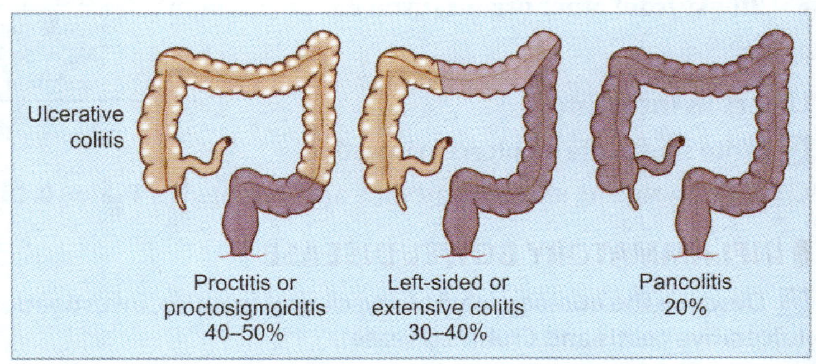

FIG. 10.13: Patterns of distribution in ulcerative colitis.

- **Proctitis/proctosigmoiditis:** When the disease is limited to the rectum alone, then it is known as **ulcerative proctitis.** When the process involves rectum and sigmoid colon, then it is termed **ulcerative proctosigmoiditis.**
- **Backwash ileitis:** The small intestine is normal. However, in severe cases of pancolitis mild mucosal inflammation of the distal ileum may be present and is termed as **backwash ileitis**.

Microscopy

- **Chronic inflammatory infiltrates: Lymphocytes, plasma cells, and macrophages in the lamina propria.** The density of plasma cells is more in the basilar region of the lamina propria (**basal plasmacytosis**) and extends into the muscularis mucosae.
- **Changes in the crypt:** These include **cryptitis, crypt abscesses, destruction of crypts, and distortion of crypt architecture.** Chronic UC may show epithelial dysplasia.
- **Toxic megacolon:** In **severe cases** (fulminant disease-toxic megacolon), inflammation may damage the muscularis propria and disturbs neuromuscular function and leads to **colonic dilation** and **toxic megacolon** that can undergo perforation. The colon is dilated, walls are thin, and with denuded mucosa and colon may rupture.

Clinical Features of UC

Q. Write short essay/note on clinical features of ulcerative colitis.

Major symptoms of UC: The first attack is usually the most severe and the disease is later characterized by relapses and remissions.

- **Diarrhea:** Colonic motility is altered due to inflammation. When the disease is severe, patients develop diarrhea and pass liquid stool containing blood, mucus, pus, and fecal matter. Diarrhea is often nocturnal and/or postprandial.
- **Rectal bleeding:** Patients with proctitis usually pass fresh blood. When the disease extends beyond the rectum, blood is usually mixed with stool or grossly bloody diarrhea may be noted.
- **Tenesmus** or urgency with a feeling of incomplete evacuation.
- **Passage of mucus**
- **Crampy abdominal pain:** Severe pain is not a prominent symptom, but some patients with active disease may present with vague lower abdominal discomfort or mild central abdominal cramping. Severe cramping and abdominal pain can develop when the attack is severe.
- **Others:** These include anorexia, nausea, vomiting, malaise, fever, and weight loss. There may be symptoms and signs of dehydration and anemia. In severe cases, the patient is toxic with fever, tachycardia, and signs of peritoneal inflammation.

Severity of symptoms: It reflects the extent of disease and the intensity of inflammation.

Duration of symptoms: Although UC can present acutely, symptoms are usually present for weeks to months. **Exacerbations and remissions:** They are characteristic features. Relapses are provoked by emotional stress, intercurrent infection, gastroenteritis, antibiotics, or NSAID therapy.

Q. Write short note/essay on extraintestinal manifestations of ulcerative colitis.

Extraintestinal manifestations (*refer* **Table 10.57** and **Fig. 10.15**).

Risk of carcinoma colon: The incidence is high, especially in patients with total colitis, disease of more than 10 years duration and early age of onset.

Signs:

- Tenderness on palpation directly over the colon, especially in the left iliac fossa.
- Signs of proctitis include tender anal canal and blood on rectal examination.
- *Signs of toxic megacolon:* It is a serious complication and its signs include severe pain and bleeding, and signs of peritonitis, if there is associated perforation.

Investigations

Q. Write short essay/note on investigation of ulcerative colitis.

They are required for confirmation of the diagnosis, know the distribution and activity, and identify complications.

Laboratory findings

- **Anemia:** Decrease in hemoglobin may be due to blood loss or malabsorption (nutritional deficiencies) of iron, folic acid, or vitamin B_{12}. It may be associated with raised platelet count.
- **Raised ESR and acute-phase reactants** [C-reactive protein (CRP)], are nonspecific serum inflammatory markers and are observed during exacerbations. They are sometimes used to monitor the activity of disease.
- **Total WBC count:** Moderate leukocytosis is observed in active disease, but a marked leukocytosis suggests an abscess or another suppurative complication.
- **Hypoalbuminemia:** Reduced serum albumin concentration may be due to protein-losing enteropathy, inflammatory disease, or malnutrition (poor nutrition).

- **Stool examination**
  - *Stool microscopy and culture:* To exclude infective pathology and *C. difficile* toxin.
- Blood cultures in patients with septicemia.
- **Serological tests:** These are supportive and not used independently as markers for diagnose IBD.
  - ***Anti-Saccharomyces cerevisiae* antibodies (ASCA):** These are antibodies to yeast. They are observed in 40–70% of patients with Crohn's disease and in less than 15% of patients with ulcerative colitis. Presence of raised ASCA immunoglobulin A (IgA) and IgG titers is highly specific for Crohn's disease.
  - **Perinuclear antineutrophil cytoplasmic antibodies (pANCA):** They are detected in 10–20% of colon-predominant Crohn's disease, and in 55–70% of patients with ulcerative colitis.
  - **Antigoblet cell autoantibodies:** Found in 30–40% cases of ulcerative colitis and Crohn's disease.
- **Other tests:**
  - **Fecal lactoferrin:** It is a very sensitive and specific marker for detecting intestinal inflammation.
  - **Fecal calprotectin:** Its levels correlate with inflammation and helpful in predicting relapses.

Endoscopy

Endoscopy with mucosal biopsy is the gold standard investigation for ulcerative colitis.

Colonoscopy: For mild-to-moderate disease and patient not having an acute flare, colonoscopy is preferable to flexible sigmoidoscopy because it can assess the disease extent and activity. Colonoscopy helps in assessing the extent and activity of ulcerative colitis.

Sigmoidoscopy:

- **During early phase of the mild disease:** (1) Uniform continuous involvement of the mucosa, (2) diffuse mucosal erythema/hyperemia, (3) loss of the normal mucosal vascular pattern, granularity, and edema, and (4) exudate of mucus, pus and blood on the mucosa.
- **As the disease becomes severe:** Mucosa becomes more friable, bleeds easily on touch, and may ulcerate. Pseudo-polyps represent epithelial regeneration and may develop after recurrent attacks in patients with long-standing disease.

Biopsy

Histological changes develop more slowly than clinical features. Biopsies help in diagnosis and to know the disease extent. Rectal biopsy shows mucosal inflammation and histological abnormalities are most severe in the distal colon and rectum.

Chromoendoscopy: Used for diagnosis of dysplasia in patients with long-standing UC.

Radiological features

- **Plain abdominal X-ray:** Useful to exclude toxic dilatation of colon.
- **Barium enema in ulcerative colitis:**
  - Earliest change in UC: Fine mucosal granularity
  - Later, the mucosa shows thickening and superficial ulcers. Deep ulcers appear as 'collar-button' ulcers, which indicate that the ulcer has penetrated the mucosa.
  - Haustral folds may be normal in initial phase of the disease, but later become edematous and thickened.
  - Long-standing disease may show loss of haustration, pseudopolyps, narrowing and shortening of the colon.
- **CT scan:** It is not so helpful when compared to endoscopy and barium enema in UC. CT scanning shows: mild mural thickening (<1.5 cm), inhomogeneous wall density, no thickening of small bowel, increased perirectal and presacral fat and target appearance of the rectum.

Biochemical abnormalities

- Electrolyte abnormalities
- Abnormal liver function tests

Q. Discuss severity staging of ulcerative colitis.

Q. Write short essay/note on management of ulcerative colitis.

Q. Describe and enumerate the indications, pharmacology, and side effects of pharmacotherapy in UC, including immunotherapy.

Treatment (Flowchart 10.10) of Ulcerative Colitis

Whenever possible, IBD should be approached by a multidisciplinary team consisting of physicians, surgeons, radiologists, and dietitians. IBDs are life-long conditions and have psychosocial implications. Truelove and Witts' severity index of ulcerative colitis is presented in **Table 10.49**.

Medical Management of UC

- Aims of medical therapy (**Box 10.14**)

Box 10.14: Aims of medical therapy in ulcerative colitis.

- Treat acute attacks and reduce inflammation
- Prevent relapses and maintain clinical remission
- Detect carcinoma at an early stage
- Select patients for surgery

FLOWCHART 10.10: Algorithm for treatment of ulcerative colitis.

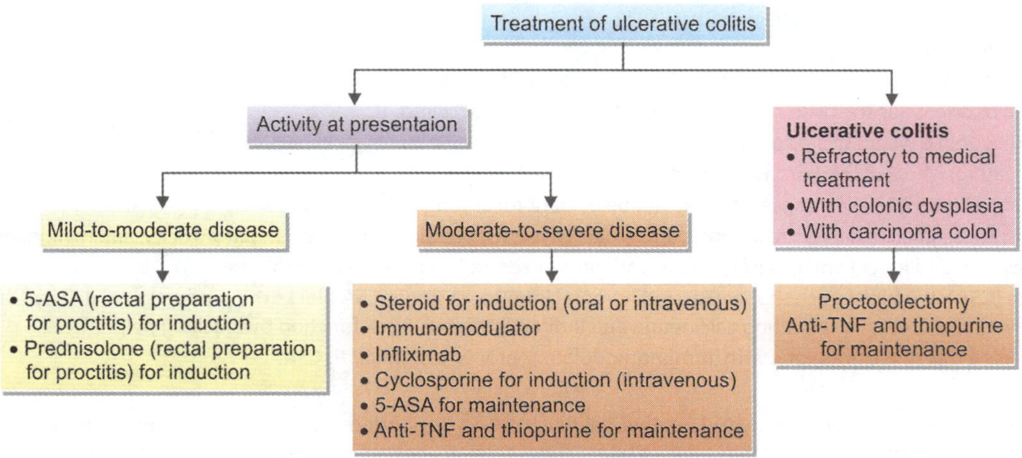

(5-ASA: 5-aminosalicylate agents; TNF: tumor necrosis factor)

- **5-Aminosalicylate (5-ASA) agents (Table 10.50):**
  - Available as oral tablets or topical (enema/suppository) preparation (for rectal and sigmoid disease).
  - These agents include 5-aminosalicylic acid (5-ASA) or mesalazine alone, or combination of 5-ASA with a carrier which releases 5-ASA after splitting by bacteria in colon (sulfasalazine, olsalazine, and balsalazide).
  - Topical mesalazine is the initial preferred agent in mild-to-moderate Ulcerative proctitis/proctosigmoiditis, for induction as well as maintenance of remission. It acts as a topical anti-inflammatory within the lumen of the intestine, controls acute exacerbation, maintains remission, and prevents relapses. Maintenance therapy may decrease the risk of colorectal cancer.
  - Patients who are unwilling or unable to tolerate topical mesalazine can be started an oral 5-ASA medication. Oral 5-ASA should also be added in those patients who do not show remission after 4 weeks of topical therapy.
  - For patients with left-sided or extensive mildly-to-moderately active UC a combination of an oral 5-ASA agent plus rectal mesalazine is used. **Sulfasalazine** and high dose **mesalazine** are the most frequently used oral agents. Sulfasalazine is the combination of a sulfapyridine (acting as a "carrier" that allows 5-ASA to be delivered into the colon) with 5-ASA (active agent). Side effects include: nausea, dyspepsia, hair loss, headache, worsening diarrhea, and hypersensitivity reactions.
  - Sulfa-free aminosalicylate preparations (e.g., olsalazine and balsalazide): They deliver higher amounts of the active ingredient of sulfasalazine (5-ASA, mesalamine) to the site of active disease in the bowel and have limited systemic toxicity.
  - Remission is usually within 2–4 weeks of therapy. If remission is not induced with oral/topical ASA combination within 2–4 weeks, then a topical steroid (Budesonide) is added.

Corticosteroids

- Oral or parenteral corticosteroids are beneficial in inducing remission in moderate-to-severe ulcerative colitis.
- They have no role in maintaining remissions. During clinical remission, steroids should be tapered according to the clinical activity.

Local Treatment

- Topical applications of steroid are also beneficial for distal colitis and as an adjunct in patients with involvement of rectal involvement associated with involvement of proximal colon.
- Hydrocortisone or prednisolone enemas, suppositories or foam may control active disease. Budesonide-MMX uses colonic release technology to extend the application of budesonide throughout the colon.
- **Duration of treatment:** 3–6 weeks.

Systemic Treatment

- **Oral:** Active UC that is unresponsive to 5-ASA therapy is treated with oral prednisone at doses of 40–60 mg/day for 3–6 weeks.
- **Parenteral:**
  - **Intravenous:** Hydrocortisone 300 mg/day or methylprednisolone, 40–60 mg/day are given as a constant infusion in severe cases.
  - **Intramuscular or subcutaneous injection:** Long-acting corticotrophin is used in the treatment of relapses.
- **Tapering of dose:** Steroids once started are gradually tapered and withdrawn, normally at a rate of no more than 5 mg/week.

Antibiotics

No role in the treatment of active or quiescent UC.

Immune Modulators

Indications:

- Patients who remain symptomatic despite 5-ASA therapy.
- Patients who have moderate-to-severe ulcerative colitis.

Drugs

1. **Azathioprine and 6-mercaptopurine (6-MP):**
   - *Usefulness are as follows:*
     - Patients who require two or more corticosteroid courses within a year.
     - Relapse of disease as the dose of prednisolone is reduced below 15 mg.
     - Relapse within 6 weeks of stopping corticosteroid.
   - *Dosage:* Azathioprine 2–3 mg/kg/day and 6-mercaptopurine 1.5 mg/kg/day.
   - *Disadvantage:* Slow clinical response and may not be evident for as long as 12 weeks.
   - *Side effects:* These include allergic reactions, pancreatitis, myelosuppression, infections, hepatotoxicity, and malignancy (lymphoma).
2. **Methotrexate:** It is a folic acid antagonist useful in patients who do not respond to azathioprine.
3. **Cyclosporine (CSA):** It inhibits both the cellular and humoral immune systems. CSA blocks the production of IL-2 by T-helper cells. CSA prevents activation of T cells by inhibiting calcineurin and indirectly inhibits B cell function by blocking helper T cells.
4. **Tacrolimus:** It is a macrolide antibiotic with immunomodulatory properties similar to CSA.

Biologics

Used to treat moderately to severely active ulcerative colitis that has responded inadequately to conventional therapy including corticosteroids and mercaptopurine or azathioprine, or who cannot tolerate, or have contraindications for, such therapies. Common side effects include headaches, nausea, vomiting, diarrhea, skin rash, weight gain from fluid retention, muscle aches, etc. Another important side effect is reactivation of TB. Hence, prior screening for dormant/active TB is mandatory. Screening is using Mantoux test or Quantiferon-TB Gold assay (in WHO—BCG Vaccine countries).

Drugs

1. **Ant-TNF agents: Infliximab** (given IV) is the most commonly used agent. Antitumor necrosis factor (anti-TNF) therapy can prevent or reduce rates of colectomy. Other agents include adalimumab and golimumab (both given subcutaneously).
2. **Vedolizumab**—MAB against aplha4-beta7 integrin. Preferred in elderly (>65 years), and those with history of malignancy or infectious complications.
3. **Ustekinumab**—MAB against interleukin 12/23.

Small Molecule Drugs

Tofacitinib—oral small molecule Janus kinase inhibitor, used for treating adults with moderate to severe UC who have failed or are intolerant to anti-TNF agent-based therapy.

General supportive measures

- *Parenteral nutrition:* It is necessary in seriously ill patients and parenteral broad-spectrum antibiotics may be required in septicemia.
- Correction of dehydration and electrolyte imbalance
- Antispasmodic medications and antidiarrheal (loperamide) for mild diarrhea (to be avoided in severe colitis)

Surgical management (Table 10.51)

- Surgery involves removal of the entire colon (colectomy) and rectum and is a curative procedure. It is indicated UC does not responded adequately to medical therapy. Emergency colectomy may be necessary for toxic megacolon.
- Elective surgical procedure is either panproctocolectomy with ileostomy, or proctocolectomy with ileal-anal pouch anastomosis.

Follow-up

- Extensive colitis of more than 10 years duration: Colonoscopy with multiple biopsies is recommended every 3 years to assess for dysplasia or malignant changes.
- UC for more than 20 years: Colonoscopy is recommended every 2 years. Biopsies from entire colon and samples from suspicious areas. If the biopsy shows high-grade dysplasia, total colectomy is performed.

TABLE 10.49: Truelove and Witts' severity index of ulcerative colitis.

Features	*Mild*	*Moderate*	*Severe*
Bowel movements (number per day)	Fewer than 4	4–6	6 or more plus at least one of the features of systemic upset (marked with * below)
Blood in stools	No more than small amounts of blood	Between mild and severe	Visible blood
Pyrexia (temperature greater than 37.8°C)*	No	No	Yes
Pulse rate greater than 90 bpm*	No	No	Yes
Anemia*	No	No	Yes
Erythrocyte sedimentation rate (mm/hour)*	30 or below	30 or below	Above 30

TABLE 10.50: Various oral 5-ASA (5-aminosalicylate agents) preparations used in ulcerative colitis.

Preparation	*Dosage*
Azo-bond	
Sulfasalazine	3–6 g (acute) 2–4 g (maintenance)
Olsalazine	1–3 g
Balsalazide	6.75–9 g
Delayed-release	
Mesalamine	2.4–4.8 g (acute) 1.6–4.8 g (maintenance)
Controlled-release	
Mesalamine	2–4 g (acute) 1.5–4 g (maintenance)
Delayed and extended-release	
Mesalamine	1.5 g (maintenance)

Crohn's Disease

Q. Discuss the etiology, pathology, clinical features, investigations, and management of Crohn's disease.

Q. Write short note on Crohn's disease.

TABLE 10.51: Indications for surgery in ulcerative colitis.

Intractable/ extensive colitis	Toxic megacolon	Colonic perforation
Severe colonic hemorrhage	Colon cancer prophylaxis	Colon dysplasia/ cancer
Frequent relapses	Chronic damage to bowel-strictures	

Etiology and Pathogenesis

Refer etiology and pathogenesis of IBD.

Pathology

Gross

- **Site (Fig. 10.14):** It can involve any area of the gastrointestinal (GI) tract from mouth to anus. Unlike UC, rectum is spared in CD. Most commonly involved sites are:
    - Terminal ileum and right side of colon (40–55%)
    - *Small intestine/bowel disease alone (30–40%):* Terminal ileum alone or ileum and jejunum.
    - Colon alone (15–25%)

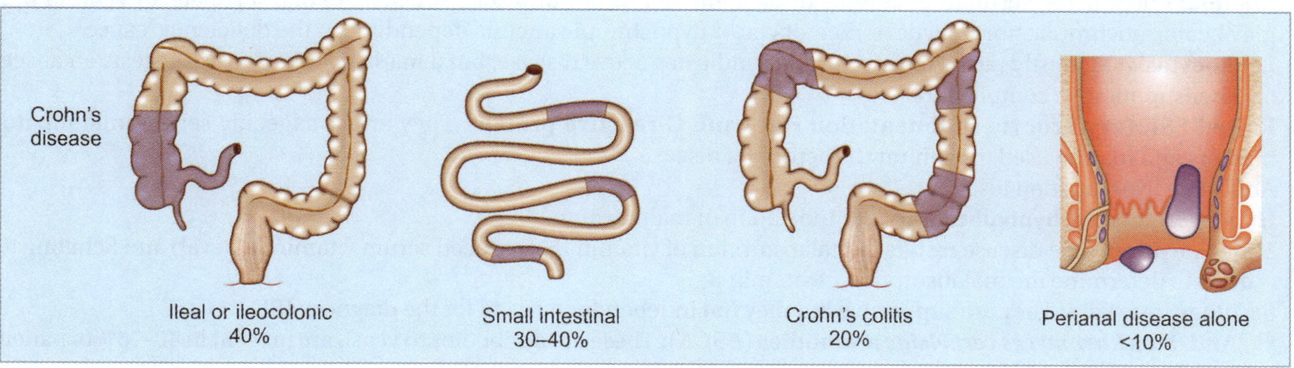

FIG. 10.14: Patterns of distribution in Crohn's disease.

- **Number of lesions:** Usually, the lesions are **multiple.**
- **Skip lesions:** The intestinal involvement is **discontinuous in which inflamed segments of intestine are** sharply demarcated/**separated by apparently normal** intervening bowel/**intestine** in between.
- **Intestinal wall:** The involved intestinal wall shows **fibrotic thickening and is rubbery** and appears like a hosepipe and produces a characteristic radiological sign known as the "**string sign**".
- **Transmural inflammation:** Inflammation involves all layers of the bowel wall.
- **Mucosal lesions***:* The earliest lesion is the **aphthous ulcer** which becomes deeper, transmural, and discrete. Multiple lesions may coalesce longitudinally to form linear or **serpentine** (snake-like) ulcers and produce characteristic **"cobblestone"** appearance. Later the ulcer becomes deeper and form linear clefts or **fissures.** Similar to UC, pseudopolyps may also form in CD.
- **External surface:** The fat may encircle around the antimesenteric serosal surface producing a pattern known as **creeping fat.**
- **Adhesion and fistulae:** Involved loops of bowel are often adherent to each other. **Fissures** frequently develop between mucosal folds. They may extend deeply to become **fistula tracts or sites of perforation**. These fistulas may also penetrate from the bowel into other organs, including the bladder, uterus, vagina, and skin.

Microscopic features

- **Chronic inflammation** by **lymphocytes, plasma cells, and macrophages**
- **Mucosal ulcerations:** Which are small, superficial (aphthous ulcers).
- **Crypt abscesses:** Clusters of neutrophils within a crypt and are often associated with crypt destruction.
- **Noncaseating granulomas**

Clinical Features of Crohn's Disease

Symptoms due to involvement of small intestine or ileum and right colon (ileocolitis). CD present with one of two patterns of disease: (1) penetrating fistulous pattern or (2) fibrostenotic obstructing pattern. The clinical manifestations depend on the site of disease.

- Crohn's disease is a chronic disease with exacerbations and remissions.
- Major symptoms include abdominal pain (typically in the right lower quadrant), diarrhea, and weight loss (due to malabsorption and patients avoid food because eating provokes pain).

- Ileal Crohn's disease may cause subacute or acute intestinal obstruction and patients present with recurrent episodes of colicky abdominal pain, abdominal distention, nausea, vomiting, and excessive borborygmi.
- Sparing of rectum and the presence of perianal disease are observed in about 30% of patients in the form of fistulas, abscesses, fissures, and skin tags. It presents with pain, discharge, and fever (if there is an abscess).

Physical examination

- Signs depend on the location and severity of the disease process.
- Abdominal tenderness in the right lower quadrant (classical), accompanied by fullness, guarding, or a mass depending on the severity of inflammation.
- Palpable mass per abdomen and rectally reflects adherent loops of intestine and abscess.
- Features of malabsorption such as weight loss and anemia (iron, folic acid, and vitamin B_{12} malabsorption)
- Sodium, potassium, water, magnesium and zinc deficiency may develop due to chronic diarrhea.
- Stool usually does not show frank blood, mucus or pus unless colon is involved.
- Oral ulcers

Investigations

- **Anemia:** Anemia may result from chronic disease, blood loss or nutritional deficiencies of iron, folate, or vitamin B_{12}. It may be normochromic normocytic or macrocytic or hypochromic anemia depending on the deficiency/cause.
- **Leukocytosis:** Modestly raised leukocyte count indicates active disease, but a marked leukocytosis suggests an abscess or other suppurative complication.
- **Raised ESR (erythrocyte sedimentation rate) and C-reactive protein:** They are nonspecific serum inflammatory markers and may be used to monitor the activity of disease.
- Abnormal liver function tests
- **Hypoproteinemia/hypoalbuminemia:** Indication of malnutrition.
- **Malabsorption:** Ileal disease results in malabsorption of vitamin B_{12} (reduced serum vitamin B_{12} level) and Schilling test is done to determine the malabsorption of vitamin B_{12}.
- **Serologic markers:** They are supportive but may not independently used for the diagnose IBD.
  - **Anti-*Saccharomyces cerevisiae* antibodies (ASCA):** These are antibodies to yeast, are present in 40–70% of patients with Crohn's disease (positive in only 10–15% cases of ulcerative colitis).
  - **Perinuclear antineutrophil cytoplasmic antibodies (pANCA):** They are present in 20% of patients with CD (colon predominant disease), and in 55% of patients with ulcerative colitis.
  - Antigoblet cell autoantibodies in 30–40% cases of Crohn's disease.
  - Antiglycan antibodies in about 40–50% cases (e.g., antilaminaribioside, antimannobioside antibodies).
- **Stool examination:** Stool microscopy and culture to exclude infectious causes of diarrhea.
- **Sigmoidoscopy and colonoscopy in Crohn's disease:**
  - Segmental inflammation with normal mucosa between (skip lesions).
  - Discrete, aphthous, or deep ulcers and occasionally connected to one another, forming longitudinal stellate, serpiginous, and linear ulcers.
  - Perianal disease (fissures, fistulas and skin tags) or sparing of the rectum.
  - Strictures are common.
  - Biopsy of involved region (e.g., colonic mucosa, ileal mucosa, anal skin tags, and perianal inflammatory lesions) shows typical noncaseating granulomatous inflammation (tuberculosis must be excluded) and infiltration by lymphocytes and plasma cell.
  - Wireless capsule endoscopy (WCE) allows direct visualization and identification of inflammation in the entire small bowel mucosa. However, it should be avoided in the presence of small bowel strictures.

Radiological Findings in Crohn's disease

Barium meal follow thorough and barium enema

- *Early radiographic findings in the small bowel:*
  - Thickened folds and aphthous ulcerations
  - Cobblestone appearance of mucosa resulting from longitudinal and transverse ulcerations.
- *More advanced disease:*
  - Transmural inflammation leads to decreased luminal diameter and limited distensibility.
  - Rigidity of involved segments and multiple strictures.
  - As ulcers progress deeper, they can lead to fistula formation. Radiographic "string sign" is due to long areas of transmural inflammation and fibrosis, producing narrowing of lumen of involved small intestine.
  - *Segmental nature of CD:* It results in wide gaps of normal or dilated bowel between involved segments (skip lesions).
  - Inflammatory masses and abscesses may be found.
  - Fistulous tracts

High-resolution ultrasound and spiral CT scanning

- It helps in defining thickness of the bowel wall and intra-abdominal abscesses.

Radionuclide scan

- Using gallium-labeled polymorphs or indium-labeled leukocytes identify intestinal and colonic disease and localize extraintestinal abscesses.

Q. Discuss Crohn's disease severity index.

Crohn's Disease Activity Index

Clinical readout	*Weighting*
Number of liquid or soft stools each day for 7 days	× 2
Abdominal pain/graded from 0–3 on severity each day for 7 days	× 5
General well-being subjectively assessed from 0 (well) to 4 (terrible) each day for 7 days	× 7
Presence of complications* *One point each is added for each set of complications: ➤ The presence of joint pains of frank arthritis ➤ Inflammation of the iris or uveitis ➤ Presence of erythema nodosum, pyoderma gangrenosum, or aphthous ulcers ➤ Anal fissures, fistulae or abscesses ➤ Fever (>100°F) during the previous week	× 20
Taking Lomitil or opiates for diarrhea	× 30
Abdominal mass (0 as none, 2 as questionable, 5 as definite)	× 10
Absolute deviation of hematocrit from 47% in men and 42% in women	× 6
% deviation from standard weight	× 1

Remission of Crohn's disease is defined as a CDAI of less than 150.
Severe disease was defined as a value of greater than 450.
Response defined as a fall of the CDAI of greater than 70 points.
Source: Best WR et al., Gastroenterology. 1976;70(3):439-44.

Treatment (Flowchart 10.11)

Medical Management of Crohn's Disease

General Considerations

- Stop cigarette smoking
- Diarrhea can be controlled with loperamide, codeine phosphate, or cophenotrope.
- Long-standing diarrhea may be due to bile acid malabsorption and is treated with bile salt sequestrants (e.g., cholestyramine).
- *Anemia:* Due to vitamin B_{12}, folic acid, or iron deficiency, should be treated accordingly.

Induction and Maintenance of Remission

- **Glucocorticosteroids:** Used to induce remission in moderate and severe Crohn's disease. Oral prednisolone 30–60 mg/day, which is gradually tapered and withdrawn. Mild-to-moderate ileocecal, CD should be treated by controlled-release steroids such as budesonide (9 mg by mouth once a day).

FLOWCHART 10.11: Treatment approach to Crohn's disease.

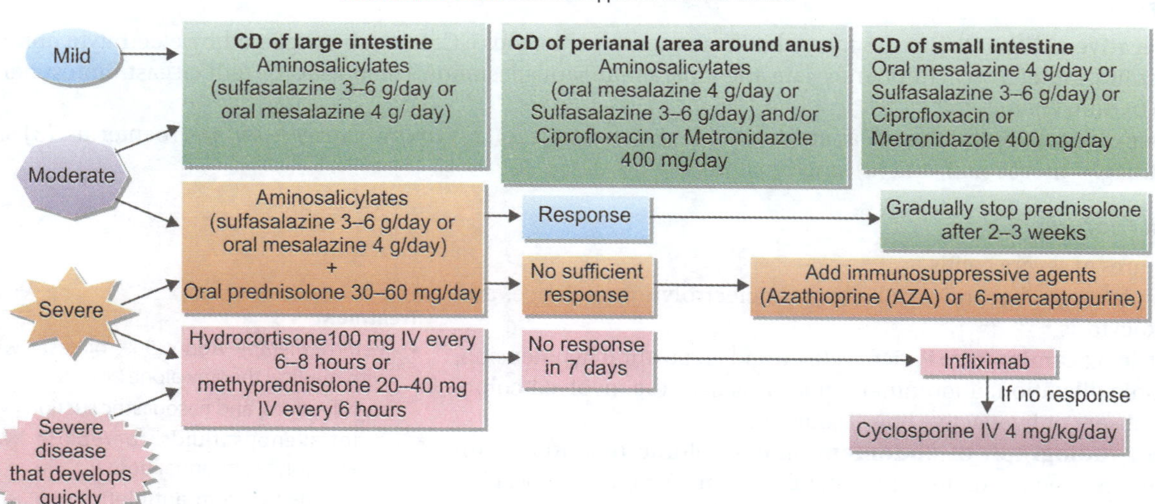

- **Aminosalicylates:** 5-ASA (e.g., mesalazine 4 g/day or sulfasalazine 3–6 g/day) as maintenance in mild-to-moderate ileocolonic disease. However, they are not effective for maintaining remission.
- **Antibiotics:** Ciprofloxacin and metronidazole 400 mg are used in abscess and perineal Crohn's disease.
- **Nutritional therapy:** Dietary antigens may stimulate the immune response in the intestinal mucosa. Bowel rest and total parenteral nutrition (TPN) are effective in inducing remission but are not effective as maintenance therapy. Enteral diets with a low fat and a low linoleic acid content (not palatable) may induce remission are similar to steroids.
- **Immunosuppressive agents:** Azathioprine (AZA) and its metabolite 6-mercaptopurine (6MP) and newer drugs (e.g., mycophenolate mofetil) suppress the proliferation of T- and B-lymphocytes. They are effective in inducing and maintaining remission and have steroid-sparing properties.
- **Biologic therapy:** Anti-TNF therapy is reserved for moderate-to-severe Crohn's disease that failed to respond to other therapies (infliximab, adalimumab, and peg certolizumab) and in CD with refractory perianal and enterocutaneous fistulas. Vedolizumab an integrin antibody is preferred in elderly and in those with malignancies or infectious complications. Another MAB ustekinumab (anti IL 12/23) is used when standard Anti-TNF therapy fails.

Maintenance of Remission

- Aminosalicylates
- Azathioprine, 6MP, and mycophenolate mofetil

Surgical Management (Table 10.52)

- **Small intestine:** Strictures can be widened (stricturoplasty)/ minimal resection and anastomosis.
- **Colorectal:**
  - Subtotal colectomy and ileorectal anastomosis, if rectum is spared.
  - Pancolectomy with ileostomy, if whole colon and rectum are involved

Assessment of severity of Crohn's disease is presented in **Table 10.53.**

TABLE 10.52: Indications for surgery in CD.

Small intestine	*Colon and rectum*
➤ Stricture and obstruction not responding to medical therapy ➤ Severe hemorrhage ➤ Refractory fistula ➤ Abscess	➤ Intractable/fulminant disease ➤ Perianal disease not responding to medical therapy ➤ Refractory fistula ➤ Colonic obstruction/perforation ➤ Colon dysplasia/cancer

TABLE 10.53: Severity of Crohn's disease.

Mild–moderate	*Moderate–severe*	*Severe/fulminant*
CDAI 150–220	*CDAI 220–450*	*CDAI >450*
Ambulatory Able to tolerate oral alimentation without manifestations of dehydration Systemic toxicity (high fevers, rigors, and prostration) abdominal tenderness painful mass Intestinal obstruction, or >10% weight loss	Failed to respond to treatment for mild–moderate disease or Has more prominent symptoms of fever, significant weight loss, abdominal pain or tenderness, intermittent nausea or vomiting (without obstructive findings), or significant anemia	Persistent symptoms despite treatment with corticosteroids/ biologics as outpatients or Has high fevers, persistent vomiting, intestinal obstruction, significant peritoneal signs, cachexia, or abscess

(CDAI: Crohn's disease activity index)

Toxic Megacolon

Q. Give a brief account of toxic dilatation of colon (toxic megacolon).

Definition: Toxic megacolon is defined as a transverse or right colon with a diameter of greater than 6 cm, with loss of haustration.

Causes

- **Ulcerative colitis:** One of the most significant complications of UC. It can be triggered by electrolyte abnormalities, narcotics, antidiarrheal (diphenoxylate and loperamide) antispasmodics medications (reduce gastrointestinal motility), and barium enema.
- **Other rare causes:** (1) Diarrheas are due to *Clostridium difficile*, (2) *Campylobacter jejuni* gastroenteritis, (3) Shigellosis, (4) Chagas' megacolon, and (5) amebic colitis.

Clinical Features

- Features of severe colitis
- High fever, tachycardia, dehydration, electrolyte imbalance, and leukocytosis
- **Physical examination:** Patient is toxic and ill, postural hypotension, colonic dilatation, abdominal tenderness over the involved colon, and absent or hypoactive bowel sounds.
- **Plain radiograph of abdomen:** Shows colonic dilatation with transverse colonic diameter greater than 6 cm. Air may be observed in the wall of the colon.

Complications

Perforation is the most dangerous of the local complications.

Treatment

- *Medical therapy:* About 50% of cases will resolve with medical therapy alone
  - Nil mouth, and nasogastric suction
  - Intravenous fluids to replace water and electrolyte abnormalities
  - Broad-spectrum antibiotics (e.g., ampicillin-sulbactam) plus metronidazole
- Urgent colectomy may be necessary when there is no improvement with medical therapy

Complications of Inflammatory Bowel Disease

Q. Write short note on the complications of inflammatory bowel disease.

It may be local and systemic (extraintestinal).

Local Complications (Tables 10.54 and 10.55)

Conditions that mimic inflammatory bowel disease (ulcerative or Crohn's colitis) are presented in **Table 10.56.**

Extraintestinal Manifestations (Table 57 and Fig. 10.15)

Q. Write short note/essay on extraintestinal manifestations of inflammatory bowel disease.

TABLE 10.54: Local complications of Crohn's disease.

- **Fistula formation:** It may develop between loops of intestine and surrounding structures such as urinary bladder, vagina, and abdominal or perianal skin. Perforations and peritoneal abscesses are common
- **Stricture formation:** May produce intestinal obstruction
- **Iron-deficiency anemia** with colonic disease
- **Malabsorption:** Extensive involvement of the small intestine may result in loss of **protein and hypoalbuminemia, generalized nutrient malabsorption, or malabsorption of vitamin B_{12}, and bile salts**
- **Fibrosing strictures** in the terminal ileum are common
- **Acute complications:** Perforation abscesses and hemorrhage
- **Development of carcinoma** is rare. Risk of carcinoma colon is increased in patients with long-standing colonic disease
- Gallstones and **urinary oxalate stones**
- **Systemic secondary amyloidosis** rare

TABLE 10.55: Local complications of UC.

- **Toxic megacolon:** In fulminant cases, the inflammation and inflammatory mediators can damage the muscularis propria and disturb neuromuscular function. This may lead to colonic dilation and toxic megacolon, which may lead to perforation
- **Colorectal cancer:** Long-standing ulcerative colitis may develop colorectal cancer than the general population
- Hemorrhage leading to blood loss
- Electrolyte disturbances due to diarrhea

TABLE 10.56: Conditions that mimic inflammatory bowel disease (ulcerative or Crohn's colitis).

Infective
- **Bacterial:** Salmonella, *Shigella*, pseudomembranous colitis, *Campylobacter jejuni*, gonococcal proctitis, *Chlamydia proctitis E. coli* O157
- **Viral:** Herpes simplex proctitis, cytomegalovirus
- **Protozoal:** Amoebiasis

Noninfective

Ischemic colitis, collagenous colitis, radiation proctitis, Behçet's disease, diverticulitis, carcinoma colon, and NSAIDs

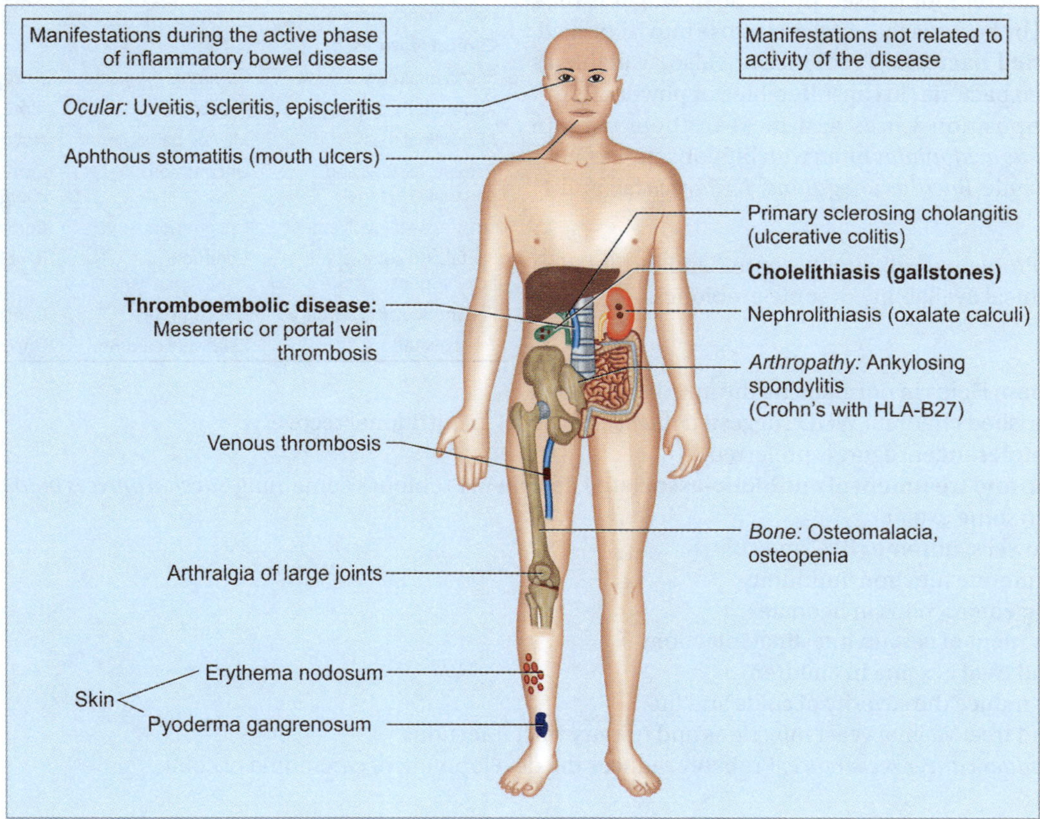

FIG. 10.15: Systemic complications of inflammatory bowel disease.

Q. Describe and enumerate the indications for surgery in IBD.

Indications for surgery in IBD have been described in **Tables 10.51 and 10.52**.

Differences between Ulcerative Colitis and Crohn's Disease of the Colon (Table 10.58)

Q. Write short note on the differences between ulcerative colitis and Crohn's disease of the colon.

TABLE 10.57: Extraintestinal manifestations of IBD.

Complication	*Crohn's disease*	*Ulcerative colitis*
Ocular: Uveitis, scleritis, and episcleritis	+	+
Arthropathy: Pauciarticular, polyarticular, and ankylosing spondylitis	+	+
Skin: Erythema nodosum, pyoderma gangrenosum	+	+
Primary sclerosing cholangitis	+	+
Thromboembolic disease	+	+
Renal: Nephrolithiasis	+	+
Bone: Osteomalacia, osteoporosis	+	–
Oral ulcers	+	–
Vitamin B_{12} deficiency	+	–

TABLE 10.58: Differences between ulcerative colitis and Crohn's disease of the colon.

Characteristics	*Ulcerative colitis*	*Crohn's disease*
Pathological features		
Involvement of bowel	Continuous involvement	Segmental involvement (skip lesions)
Inflammation	Restricted to mucosa and submucosa	Transmural
Noncaseating granulomas	Absent	Common
Crypt abscess	Common	Uncommon
Goblet cell depletion	Seen	Absent
Strictures, fissures and fistulae	Uncommon	Common
Mesenteric and lymph nodal involvement	Absent	Common
Clinical features		
Rectal bleeding	Common	Uncommon
Abdominal pain	Less common	More common
Abdominal masses	May be palpable	Not usually palpable
Fistulae, fissures and perianal skin tags	Uncommon	Common and characteristic
Small bowel involvement	Uncommon	Common
Rectal and colonic involvement	Common	Rare
Recurrence after surgery	Not common	Common
Toxic dilatation	Relatively common	Uncommon

PROBIOTICS AND PREBIOTICS

Q. Discuss briefly about probiotics and prebiotics.

Probiotics

Definition: Probiotics are defined as live microorganisms which are beneficial to its host. Throughout their journey in the digestive tract, they need to be intact, so they can reach the intestines where they act to give their beneficial effects to the body.

Nature

- **Bacteria:** Probiotics are usually bacterial components of the normal intestinal flora of human beings (e.g., *lactobacilli* and *Bifidobacterium infantis*). They produce lactate and short-chain fatty acids (e.g., acetate and butyrate) as end products of metabolism.
- **Yeast:** *Saccharomyces boulardii* is yeast.

Preparation

- **Yogurt:** It is commonly used probiotic in which is milk fermented by bacteria that convert lactose into lactic acid.
- **Freeze-dried bacteria:** Probiotics are also available as freeze-dried bacteria (in capsule, tablet, or powder form). Their composition varies and most of them contain *Lactobacillus acidophilus* often with bifidobacteria. Other strains include *Bacillus coagulans, L. Paracasei,* and *L. johnsonii.*

Limitations: Problems with quality control and formulation restrict the clinical availability of some probiotics.

Uses

- **Malnutrition:** Helps in normalizing the nutritional status of malnourished children. WHO suggested the use of yogurt in nutritional recovery.
- **Lactose intolerance:** Yogurt is preferred.
- **Prevention and treatment of antibiotic-associated diarrhea:** Probiotics containing *Saccharomyces boulardii* yeast may be useful to some extent.
- Irritable bowel syndrome (IBS) and colitis
- Improve immune function/immunity
- Necrotizing enterocolitis in neonates
- Speed treatment of certain intestinal infections
- Prevent and treat eczema in children
- Prevent or reduce the severity of colds and flu
- Prevent and treat vaginal yeast infections and urinary tract infections
- *Reduce bladder cancer recurrence:* Probably reduces the development of carcinoma of colon.

Prebiotics

Definition

Prebiotics are referred to as a dietary fiber or carbohydrates that act as the food of probiotics. This is why it triggers bacterial growth and activity in the intestinal microflora. Therefore, it promotes good health of the host.

- Chemical substances (usually oligosaccharides) which beneficially nourish and act as a fertilizer to promote growth of the host's intrinsic probiotic bacteria. They encourage their growth.
- Prebiotics are special form of dietary fiber.
- Prebiotics are not digested (nondigestible) by the small intestine and nonmetabolized by nonprobiotic gut flora such as *Bacteroides* species and *Escherichia coli* present in the host.
- Synthetic prebiotics are oligosaccharides containing fructose or galactose, known as fructose oligosaccharides (FOS) and galactose oligosaccharides (GOS), respectively. Lactulose is also a prebiotic.
- These oligosaccharides are enriched with the combination of inulin.
- They may be added to foods, or combined with a probiotic.

Box 10.15: Potential uses of prebiotics.

- Relief of constipation
- Reduce intestinal pH
- Restore intestinal bacterial balance
- Increase in the absorption of calcium and magnesium
- Effect on blood cholesterol level
- Reduction of fasting glucose level in type 2 diabetes patients
- Reduce risk on colorectal cancer
- Effects on the immune system
- Better intestinal flora in infants
  - Lactulose: Useful in hepatic encephalopathy
  - Prevention of osteoporosis: Prebiotics may increase calcium absorption
  - Chronic constipation

Potential Uses of Prebiotics

See **Box 10.15**.

Synbiotics

- Synbiotics refer to the combination of the prebiotics and probiotics within a single product.
- Prebiotics are targeted to act on the large intestines while the probiotics are most effective in doing its role in the small intestine.
- The two agents have been said to act synergistically. So, the term synbiotics is used.

MISCELLANEOUS TOPICS

Gardner's Syndrome

- Condition in which familial adenomatous polyposis (FAP) is associated with predominant extraintestinal manifestations.
- Autosomal dominant disorder
- *Adenomatous polyps:* Numerous in colon and few in the stomach and duodenum
- *Extraintestinal lesions:* These include:
  - **Osteomas of mandible, skull, and long bones**
  - **Epidermal cysts, desmoid tumors, thyroid tumors, etc.**

Treatment: Prophylactic total colectomy.

Peutz-Jeghers Syndrome

- It is a rare autosomal dominant syndrome.
- Median age of presentation is 11 years
- It is characterized by:
  - **Multiple GI hamartomatous polyps:** Involves the entire GIT but are most common in the small intestine. Usually, present in the dozens.
  - **Mucocutaneous hyperpigmentation:** The melanotic pigmentation is seen in the mouth, buccal mucosa, and genitalia region.
- Peutz-Jeghers syndrome is associated with an **increased risk** of **several malignancies.** These include cancers of the colon, pancreas, breast, lung, ovaries, uterus, and testicles.
- **Genetics:** Inactivation (loss-of-function mutations) of the *STK11/LKB1* gene (tumor suppressor gene) detected in about 70% of affected families. The **hamartomas are not preneoplastic precursor lesions**.
- **Clinical presentation:** Abdominal pain, rectal bleeding, anemia, intestinal obstruction, and intussusception.
- **Diagnosis and treatment:** Intraoperative enteroscopy (IOE) and remove all small intestinal polyps by double balloon enteroscopy (DBE).

Indications, Contraindications and Complications of Upper Gastrointestinal Endoscopy (Table 10.59)

Q. List indications, contraindications, and complications of upper gastrointestinal endoscopy.

TABLE 10.59: Indications, contraindications, and complications of upper gastrointestinal endoscopy.

Diagnostic indications	Therapeutic indications
➤ *Upper gastrointestinal bleeding:* Past or present; acute or chronic patients with splenomegaly or suspected chronic liver disease: For presence and grading of esophagogastric varices ➤ Upper abdominal distress that persists despite an appropriate trial of therapy ➤ Dysphagia or odynophagia ➤ Esophageal reflux symptoms that are persistent or recurrent despite appropriate therapy ➤ Persistent nausea and vomiting of unknown cause surveillance for malignancy, abnormal CT scan or barium meal gastric or esophageal ulcers ➤ Familial adenomatous polyposis adenomatous gastric polyps Barrett's esophagus ➤ Occult gastrointestinal bleeding ➤ After caustic ingestion to assess for acute injury dyspepsia over 55 years of age or with alarm symptoms atypical chest pain ➤ Weight loss ➤ Duodenal biopsies in the investigation of malabsorption and to confirm a diagnosis of celiac disease prior to commencement of gluten-free diet	➤ Treatment of bleeding lesions ➤ Sclerotherapy or banding of varices ➤ Removal of foreign bodies ➤ Removal of selected polypoid lesions or superficial neoplasms ➤ Placement of feeding or drainage tubes ➤ Dilation of stenotic lesions ➤ Palliative treatment of stenosing neoplasms ➤ Drainage of pancreatic pseudocysts **Contraindications** ➤ **Absolute contraindications** - Severe shock - Possible visceral perforation ➤ **Relative contraindications** (can be performed by experienced hands) - Recent myocardial infarction, unstable angina, and cardiac arrhythmia - Severe respiratory disease - Atlantoaxial subluxation **Complications** ➤ Cardiorespiratory depression due to sedation ➤ Aspiration pneumonia ➤ Perforation

Indications for Colonoscopy (Table 10.60)

Q. List indications for colonoscopy.

TABLE 10.60: Indications for colonoscopy.

Diagnostic	*Therapeutic*
➤ Unexplained rectal bleeding ➤ Unexplained lower gastrointestinal symptoms and signs, such as recent onset constipation or feeling of incomplete evacuation, especially in the elderly ➤ Polyp and cancer screening or follow-up ➤ Inflammatory bowel disease ➤ Stricture or colonic narrowing (with and without inflammatory bowel disease) ➤ Diverticular disease ➤ Infectious colitis ➤ Radiation colitis ➤ Ischemic colitis ➤ Endometriosis ➤ *Pneumatosis cystoides intestinalis*	➤ Polypectomy ➤ Foreign body removal ➤ Dilation of strictures in colon or terminal ileum ➤ *Therapeutic:* Hemostasis ➤ Tumor resection (palliative) ➤ Colonic decompression (volvulus and pseudo-obstruction)

Protein-losing Enteropathy

Q. Write short note on protein-losing enteropathy.

It is characterized by excessive loss of protein into the gut lumen, sufficient to cause hypoproteinemia.

Causes (Table 10.61): Most common in diseases with mucosal ulceration.

Clinical features: Peripheral edema and hypoproteinemia.

Investigations: Liver function tests are normal liver function and no proteinuria. Diagnosis can be confirmed by measuring fecal clearance of a1-antitrypsin or ^{51}Cr-labeled albumin after intravenous injection. Other investigations depend on the underlying cause.

TABLE 10.61: Causes of protein-losing enteropathy.

With erosions or ulceration of mucosa: Crohn's disease, ulcerative colitis, cancer of esophagus, stomach or colon, radiation damage, and lymphoma
Without erosions or ulceration of mucosa: Menetrier's disease, Celiac disease, bacterial overgrowth, eosinophilic gastroenteritis, systemic lupus erythematosus, and tropical sprue
With obstruction of lymphatics: Intestinal lymphangiectasia, lymphoma, Whipple's disease, and constrictive pericarditis

Treatment of the underlying disorder, with nutritional support and measures to control peripheral edema.

Generalized Abdominal Distension (Box 10.16)

Q. List causes of abdominal distension.

Box 10.16: Causes of abdominal distension (7Fs).

Fat, fluid (ascites), flatus (obstruction/ileus), fetus (pregnancy), feces (constipation), full bladder, fatal neoplasm (organomegaly)

Differences between Diarrhea and Dysentery (Table 10.62)

Q. Distinguish between diarrhea and dysentery based on clinical features.

TABLE 10.62: Differences between diarrhea and dysentery.

Diarrhea	*Dysentery*
➢ Voluminous fluid feces	➢ Scanty sticky feces
➢ No blood in feces	➢ Blood in feces
➢ No mucus in feces	➢ Mucus in feces
➢ Less pus cells	➢ Abundant pus cells
➢ Less straining during defecation	➢ Severe straining during defecation (tenesmus)

Causes of Oral Ulceration

Q. List causes of oral ulceration and aphthous ulcer.

Aphthous Ulceration

Aphthous ulcers are superficial and painful ulcers which can develop in any part of the mouth. Recurrent ulcers are common in women prior to menstruation. The cause is unknown. Other causes of oral ulceration are presented in **Table 10.63**.

TABLE 10.63: Causes of oral ulcers.

➢ **Aphthous:** Idiopathic Infection, premenstrual	➢ **Gastrointestinal diseases:** Crohn's disease, Celiac disease
➢ **Infection:** Fungal (candidiasis), viral (herpes simplex, HIV), bacterial (e.g., syphilis, tuberculosis)	➢ **Dermatological conditions:** Lichen planus, dermatitis herpetiformis
➢ **Drugs:** Nicorandil, NSAIDs (nonsteroidal anti-inflammatory drugs), methotrexate, cytotoxic drugs, Stevens–Johnson syndrome	➢ **Systemic diseases:** Systemic lupus erythematosus, Behçet's syndrome, vitamin deficiencies
➢ **Neoplasia:** Carcinoma, leukemia, Kaposi's sarcoma	➢ Traumatic ulcers

CHAPTER 11

Hepatobiliary System

FUNCTIONS OF LIVER

Q. Enumerate important functions of liver.

Important functions of liver are listed in **Box 11.1**.

Box 11.1: Important functions of liver.

- Protein metabolism and urea formation
- Carbohydrate metabolism: Includes gluconeogenesis, glycogenolysis, and glycogenesis
- Lipid metabolism
- Bilirubin formation from hemoglobin degradation
- Metabolism of vitamins and minerals
- Hormone metabolism
- Drug and alcohol metabolism
- Cholesterol metabolism
- Bile acid formation and bile secretion
- Synthesis of plasma proteins including coagulation factors
- Immunological function: Removal of gut endotoxins and foreign antigens
- Maintains core body temperature
- Maintains pH balance and correction of lactic acidosis

LIVER FUNCTION TESTS

Q. Discuss the liver function tests. Discuss approach to jaundice.

Liver Biochemistry

No single test alone can be used to assess liver function.

Serum Bilirubin

- Normal values of total serum bilirubin are between 0.3 and 1.3 mg/dL, with 95% of a normal population falling between 0.2 and 0.9 mg/dL (almost all unconjugated). Bilirubin is a degradation product of hemoglobin and hem-containing proteins. Bilirubin metabolism is summarized in **Figure 11.1**.
- Total serum bilirubin = Conjugated (direct) + unconjugated (indirect) bilirubin.

Type	*Bilirubin level*	*Causes*	*Bilirubinuria, liver function test (LFT)*
Unconjugated Hyperbilirubinemia	Usually <6 mg/dL	➢ Hemolytic anemia ➢ Ineffective erythropoiesis ➢ Gilbert's syndrome	Absent LFT otherwise normal
Conjugated hyperbilirubinemia	Higher levels	➢ Parenchymal liver diseases ➢ Biliary tract obstructions	Present LFT deranged

- The presence of conjunctival icterus suggests a total serum bilirubin level of at least 3.0 mg/dL level below which is called **anicteric jaundice**, but does not allow differentiation between conjugated and unconjugated hyperbilirubinemia.
- Tea or cola-colored urine may indicate the presence of bilirubinuria and thus conjugated hyperbilirubinemia.
- **Fluctuating hyperbilirubinemia** is observed in gallstones, carcinoma of ampulla of Vater, chronic hepatitis, hemolytic anemias, and Gilbert's syndrome.

Serum Enzymes

Enzymes that reflect damage to hepatocytes—aminotransferases (transaminases)

- These enzymes are present in hepatocytes and leak into the blood with liver cell damage. These include two enzymes, namely: (1) aspartate aminotransferase (AST/SGOT), and (2) alanine aminotransferase (ALT/SGPT).
- Present in hepatocytes and leak into the blood with liver cell damage
- **Normal value:** 10–40 U/L.
- Poor correlation between the degree of liver cell damage and level of aminotransferases
- **Aspartate aminotransferase:** Mitochondrial and cytoplasmic isoenzymes. High concentration also in heart, muscle, kidney, and brain. Raised in hepatic necrosis, myocardial infarction, muscle injury, and congestive cardiac failure.
- **Alanine aminotransferase:** Cytosolic enzyme. More specific for liver injury.

AST: ALT ratio:
- AST: ALT >1: Chronic viral hepatitis and nonalcoholic fatty liver disease (NAFLD).
- AST: ALT ratio >2:1 is suggestive, while a ratio >3:1 is highly suggestive of alcoholic liver disease. A low level of ALT in the serum in alcoholic patients is due to an alcohol-induced deficiency of pyridoxal phosphate.

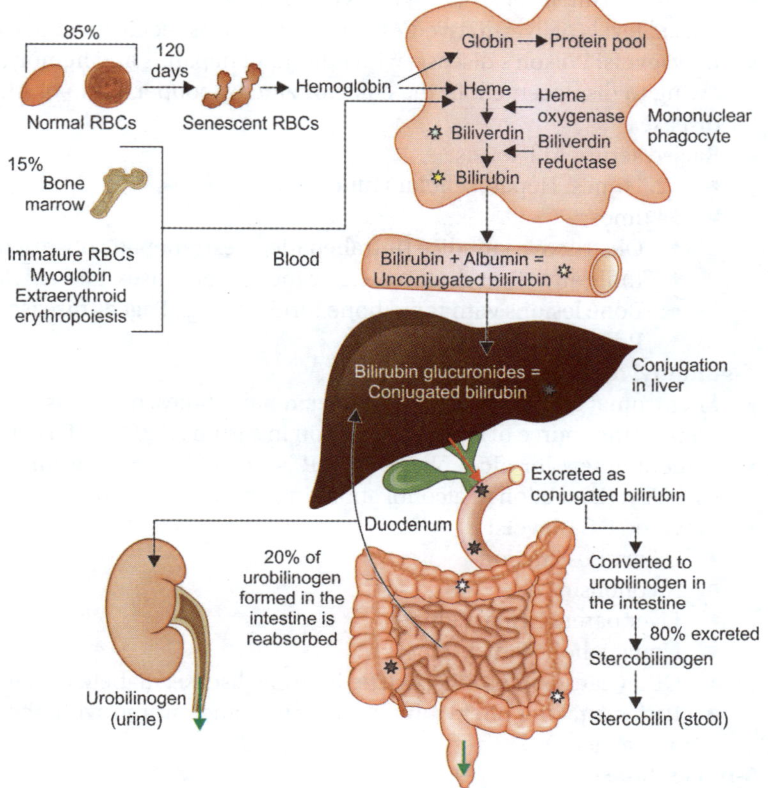

FIG. 11.1: Bilirubin metabolism.

Causes of Elevated Serum Aminotransferases (Tables 11.1A and B)

TABLE 11.1A: Chronic mild elevations (<150 U/L).

ALT > AST		AST > ALT	
Hepatic	**Nonhepatic**	**Hepatic**	**Nonhepatic**
➤ α1-antitrypsin deficiency ➤ Autoimmune hepatitis ➤ Chronic viral hepatitis (B, C, D) ➤ Hemochromatosis ➤ Medications and toxins ➤ Steatosis and steatohepatitis	➤ Celiac disease ➤ Hyperthyroidism	➤ Alcohol-related liver injury ➤ Cirrhosis ➤ Wilson's disease	➤ Hypothyroidism ➤ Macro-AST ➤ Myopathy ➤ Strenuous exercise

(ALT: alanine aminotransferase; AST: aspartate aminotransferase)

TABLE 11.1B: Acute severe elevations (>1,000 U/L).

ALT>AST		AST>ALT	
Hepatic	**Nonhepatic**	**Hepatic**	**Nonhepatic**
➤ Acute bile duct obstruction ➤ Acute Budd–Chiari syndrome ➤ Acute viral hepatitis ➤ Autoimmune hepatitis ➤ Hepatic artery ligation ➤ Ischemic hepatitis ➤ Medications/toxins ➤ Wilson's Disease	None	Medications or toxins in a patient with underlying alcoholic liver injury	Acute rhabdomyolysis

(ALT: alanine aminotransferase; AST: aspartate aminotransferase)

Enzymes that reflect cholestasis

These include three enzymes: (1) alkaline phosphatase (ALP), (2) 5′-nucleotidase, and (3) ϒ-glutamyl transpeptidase (GGT).

Q. Write short answer on causes/diseases with elevated/very high serum alkaline phosphatase.

Alkaline phosphatase:
- Many distinct isoenzymes—liver, bone, kidney, placenta, small intestine, origin can be determined by electrophoretic separation.

- Normal serum level: 3–13 KA units (80–240 IU/L).
- Raised levels of liver-derived ALP are not totally specific for cholestasis.
- **Low levels:** Wilson's disease, with fulminant hepatitis and hemolysis, possibly because of reduced activity of the enzyme owing to displacement of the cofactor zinc by copper. Ratio of ALP to total bilirubin of <2 is quite specific for Wilson's disease.
- Raised serum ALP levels:
  - <2.5 times: Hepatocellular jaundice
  - >4 times:
    - Obstructive jaundice (intrahepatic or extrahepatic obstruction)
    - Infiltrative liver diseases, e.g., cancer, metastases, and amyloidosis
    - Bone lesions with rapid bone turnover, e.g., Paget's disease
    - Primary biliary cirrhosis

ϒ-glutamyl transpeptidase (GGT)

- Microsomal enzyme is present in liver, renal tubules, pancreas, and intestine.
- Identify the source of isolated elevation in serum ALP (GGTP is normal in bone disease)
- Screening test for alcoholism: If ALP is normal, raised serum γ-GT is a good guide to alcohol intake of more than 60 g/day. (Detection of alcohol abuse in patients who deny it).
- **Elevated GGT levels:**
  - Biliary obstruction
  - Alcoholism
  - Liver parenchymal damage
  - Nonalcoholic fatty liver
  - Other causes: Chronic obstructive lung disease, diabetes mellitus, hyperthyroidism, obesity, and renal failure.
  - Patients taking phenytoin, barbiturates, and antiretroviral therapy—nonnucleoside reverse transcriptase inhibitors and abacavir

5-nucleotidase:

- Microsomal enzyme has similar significance as that of GGT.
- 5′NT levels are not increased in bone disease but are increased in hepatobiliary disease.

Lactate dehydrogenase (LDH): Not useful in diagnosis of liver diseases

- Moderate elevations: Ischemic hepatitis and hepatic metastasis.
- ALT/LDH ratio >1.5 suggests ischemic hepatitis while ratio <1.5 is seen with paracetamol toxicity.

Biosynthetic Function of the Liver

Tests that measure synthetic function of the liver.

Plasma Proteins

Serum albumin:

- It is **synthesized exclusively in liver** and used as a marker of synthetic function.
- **Normal serum albumin level:** 4–5.5 g/100 mL and albumin has a half-life of around 20 days.

Significance:

- **Low levels:** Serum albumin is an **excellent marker of hepatic synthetic function**. Hypoalbuminemia is observed in chronic liver diseases such as cirrhosis and chronic hepatitis and usually reflects severe liver damage and decreased albumin synthesis. A **falling serum albumin level in liver disease is a bad prognostic sign.**
- **Apart** from chronic liver disease, it may be observed in chronic inflammation, sepsis, expanded plasma volume, and renal or gastrointestinal (GI) loss.

***Serum globulins*:**

- **They** constitute a group of proteins made up of ϒ-globulins (immunoglobulins) synthesized by B lymphocytes and α- and β-globulins synthesized primarily by hepatocytes.
- **Normal serum globulin level:** 1.5–3.5 g/100 mL.
- **Significance:** ϒ-globulins are **increased in chronic liver disease** (e.g., chronic hepatitis and cirrhosis). Increase in the concentration of specific isotypes of ϒ-globulins (immunoglobulins) is helpful in the recognition of certain chronic liver diseases (**Table 11.2**).
- **Cirrhosis:** Plasma proteins show decrease in albumin and increase in ϒ-globulin.

TABLE 11.2: Specific types of elevated immunoglobulin and its associated conditions.

Specific type of immunoglobulin	Condition in which it is raised
IgG	Chronic hepatitis, autoimmune hepatitis (AIH), and cryptogenic cirrhosis
IgA	Alcoholic liver disease
IgM	Primary biliary cholangitis

Coagulation factors:
- **Liver produces all the coagulation factors, except factor VIII.**
- Vitamin K is required for the activation of coagulation **factors II, VII, IX, and X.**
- The coagulation factors have short half-life time. Thus, measurement of the clotting factors is the **single best measure of hepatic synthetic function** and useful in both the diagnosis and assessing the prognosis of acute parenchymal liver disease.
- **Prothrombin time:**
  - Prothrombin time depends on factors I, II, V, VII, and X.
  - Normal value is 11–12.5 seconds.
  - Prothrombin time collectively measures factors II, V, VII, and X.
  - Causes of prolonged prothrombin time are listed in **Box 11.2**.
- *Unlike the serum albumin, the prothrombin time allows an assessment of current hepatic synthetic function; factor VII has the shortest serum half-life (6 hours) of all the clotting factors.*

Box 11.2: Causes of prolonged prothrombin time.
- Severe liver damage: Acute hepatitis (e.g., viral hepatitis), cirrhosis
- Deficiency of vitamin K
  - Obstructive jaundice that reduces vitamin K absorption
  - Fat malabsorption
  - Poor intake
  - Antibiotic therapy which produces destruction of vitamin
  - Producing commensals
- Disseminated intravascular coagulation
- Drugs and toxins: Warfarin, rivaroxaban, apixaban, edoxaban, dabigatran, viper envenomation, anticoagulant rodenticide poisoning

Ceruloplasmin:
- It is an **acute-phase reactant** synthesized by the liver.
- In blood, it binds to copper and acts as a major carrier for copper.
- **Normal plasma level:** 20–60 mg/dL
- **Causes of elevated levels:** Infections, liver diseases, obstructive jaundice, rheumatoid arthritis, and pregnancy.
- **Causes of decreased levels:** Wilson's disease (due to decreased rate of synthesis), neonates, Menkes disease, kwashiorkor, marasmus, protein-losing enteropathy, and copper deficiency.

Cholesterol:
- It is synthesized in the liver. Advanced liver disease may be associated with very low cholesterol. However, primary biliary cholangitis (PBC) may be associated with markedly raised cholesterol. Similarly, a low urea level also indicates severe liver dysfunction.

  Liver functions tests and their significance are summarized in **Table 11.3**.

TABLE 11.3: Summary of main liver function tests and its significance.

Test	*Function determined/assessed*
Serum bilirubin	Transport
Serum enzymes ➢ Serum aminotransferases (ALT and AST) ➢ Serum alkaline phosphatase (ALP) ➢ ϒ-glutamyl transpeptidase (GGT)	 ➢ Hepatocellular damage ➢ Biliary tract obstruction ➢ Enzyme induction
Plasma proteins	Synthesis
Prothrombin time	Synthesis

Serum autoantibodies:
- ***Antimitochondrial antibody (AMA):*** *Antinuclear, smooth muscle (actin), liver/kidney microsomal antibodies, antinuclear cytoplasmic antibodies (ANCA).*

Urine Tests

Bilirubin in urine:
- Normally, bilirubin cannot be detected in urine.
- In unconjugated hyperbilirubinemia, urine does not contain bilirubin **(acholuric jaundice)**. Thus, **absence of bilirubin in urine in a jaundiced patient suggests unconjugated hyperbilirubinemia.**
- In conjugated hyperbilirubinemia, urine contains bilirubin. Thus, **bilirubinuria in a jaundiced patient points to conjugated hyperbilirubinemia** (hepatobiliary disease).
- Urinary bilirubin is detected by Fouchet's test.

Urine urobilinogen:
- Urobilinogen is **normally present in urine in trace amounts** (1–2 mg/dL) and is insufficient to cause a significant positive reaction.
- **Causes of increased urobilinogen in urine (Box 11.3)**
- **Causes of absent urobilinogen:** In **obstructive jaundice** (bilirubinuria present), bilirubin does not reach the intestine and so is not converted into urobilinogen.
- Urinary urobilinogen is detected by Ehrlich's aldehyde test.

Box 11.3: Causes of increased urobilinogen in urine.

Hemolytic anemias (without bilirubin in urine)
- Thalassemia
- Sickle-cell anemia
- Hereditary spherocytosis

Liver diseases (bilirubinuria present)
- Preicteric phase of infective hepatitis
- Drugs or toxic hepatitis
- Cirrhosis

α-Fetoprotein (AFP)

- α-fetoprotein is normally produced by fetal liver cells and its levels falls to low levels after birth.
- **Causes of elevated levels** of α-fetoprotein are:
  - **Hepatocellular carcinoma** (HCC)
  - **Carcinomas of stomach, pancreas, gallbladder, bile ducts, and lungs**
  - **Teratomas**

DIAGNOSTIC PROCEDURES

Endoscopic Retrograde Cholangiopancreatography

Q. Write short note on endoscopic retrograde cholangiopancreatography.

Endoscopic retrograde cholangiopancreatography (ERCP) is a technique used to **outline the biliary and pancreatic ducts**.

Procedure

An endoscope is passed into the second part of the duodenum and cannulation of the ampulla. Contrast is injected into the biliary tree and the patient is screened radiologically. **Figure 11.2** shows ERCP with stone in the common bile duct (CBD).

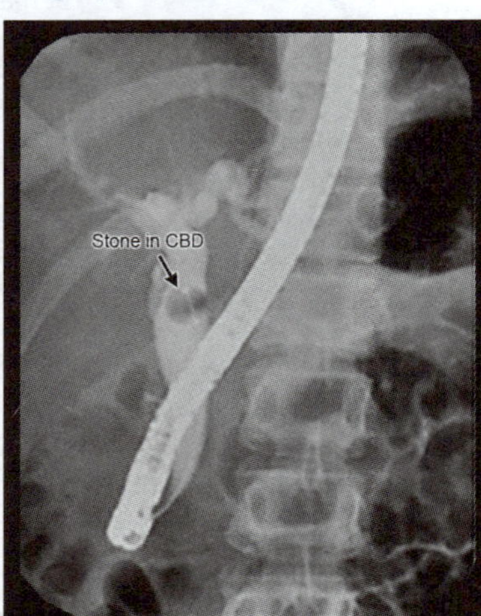

FIG. 11.2: ERCP shows stone in the common bile duct (CBD).

Uses of ERCP

See **Table 11.4**.

TABLE 11.4: Uses of ERCP.

Diagnostic procedure	*Therapeutic procedure*
Evaluation of acute/ chronic pancreatitis	Removal of CBD stones
Evaluation of patient with obstructive jaundice	Sphincterotomy
Cholangitis	Dilatation of benign strictures
Biopsy for periampullary carcinoma	Placement of nasobiliary catheters and biliary stents
	Brachytherapy for cholangiocarcinoma

Complications

The complication rate in diagnostic ERCP is 2–3%. Complications include pancreatitis, cholangitis, bleeding, and duodenal perforation.

Magnetic Resonance Cholangiopancreatography

Q. Write short note on magnetic resonance cholangiopancreatography.

Magnetic resonance cholangiopancreatography (MRCP) is a noninvasive technique largely replacing diagnostic (but not therapeutic) ERCP.

Technique

A heavily T2-weighted sequence enhances visualization of the water-filled biliary (intrahepatic ducts) and pancreatic ducts (extrahepatic ducts). It produces high-quality images of ductal anatomy.

Advantages of MRCP over ERCP (Box 11.4) Indications

- Diagnosis of bile duct obstruction and pancreatic duct abnormalities, e.g., choledocholithiasis, malignant obstruction of bile and pancreatic ducts, congenital anomalies, and chronic pancreatitis.
- Unsuccessful ERCP or a contraindication to ERCP (as in patients with cardiorespiratory compromise, renal failure).

Box 11.4: Advantages of MRCP over ERCP.

- No need for contrast media or ionizing radiation
- Images can be acquired faster
- Less operator dependent
- No risk of pancreatitis

Endoscopic Ultrasound

Q. Write a short note on endoscopic ultrasound.

Procedure

In endoscopic ultrasound (EUS), a small high-frequency ultrasound probe is placed on the tip of an endoscope and placed by direct vision into the duodenum.

Advantages

Gradually replacing diagnostic ERCP:

- Close proximity of the ultrasound probe to the pancreas and biliary tree allows high-resolution ultrasound imaging.
- Accurate staging of small, potentially operable, pancreatic tumors (e.g., neuroendocrine tumors) can be done.
- It is less invasive method for bile duct imaging.

Uses

Diagnostic

- Imaging pancreatic and biliary diseases, e.g., choledocholithiasis, pancreatic and biliary cancers, and cystic lesions of the pancreas
- Ampullary carcinoma: To know the local extension of tumor and regional lymph node metastasis that cannot be evaluated by ERCP
- Performing fine-needle aspiration under EUS guidance from suspicious lesions for confirmation of malignancy

Therapeutic

- Increasingly used for guided interventions:
  - To reduce pain in patients with unresectable pancreatic carcinoma, for injecting bupivacaine and alcohol into the celiac ganglia.
  - Endoscopic management of pancreatic pseudocysts.

Disadvantages

- Cost is high.
- High degree of training is required.

LIVER BIOPSY

Q. Write short note on the indications, significance, and complications of liver biopsy.

Percutaneous liver biopsy is an invasive procedure that can be performed with or without radiographic guidance.

Indications, contraindications, and complications of liver biopsy (Table 11.5).

TABLE 11.5: Indications, contraindications, and complications of liver biopsy.

Indications	*Contraindications*	*Complications*
➢ Cirrhosis of liver ➢ Unexplained hepatomegaly, splenomegaly, Jaundice ➢ Hepatitis: Chronic or acute ➢ Tumors: Primary or secondary ➢ Granulomatous diseases: Tuberculosis, leprosy, sarcoidosis ➢ Storage and metabolic disorders: amyloidosis, storage disorders, hemochromatosis, Wilson's disease ➢ After liver transplantation: Assess for rejection, disease recurrence ➢ Brucellosis ➢ Pyrexia of unknown origin (with hepatomegaly) ➢ Malignancy ➢ Miliary tuberculosis ➢ Lymphoma staging	➢ Hepatocellular failure ➢ Congenital coagulation disorders ➢ Hepatobiliary infections ➢ Massive ascites ➢ Obstructive jaundice ➢ Severe jaundice ➢ Prolonged prothrombin time: More than 3 seconds over control ➢ Relative contradictions: ➢ Hydatid cyst liver ➢ Hemangioma liver	➢ Pleurisy, perihepatitis ➢ Hemorrhage ➢ Intrahepatic hematoma ➢ Biliary peritonitis ➢ Hemobilia ➢ Arteriovenous fistula ➢ Infection ➢ Organ perforation ➢ Carcinoid crisis

JAUNDICE

Q. List the causes of jaundice. How will you arrive at the etiology of jaundice? Give the points of differentiation in clinical features and investigations.

Definition

Jaundice (icterus) is defined as **yellowish pigmentation** of **skin, mucus membranes, and sclera** due to **increased levels of bilirubin** in the blood. The scleral involvement is because of its rich elastic tissue that has special affinity for bilirubin.

- **Normal serum bilirubin level:** In normal adults, it ranges from 0.3 to 1.2 mg/dL.
- **Jaundice** is clinically detected when the **serum bilirubin level is above 2.0–2.5 mg/dL.** With severe disease, the levels may be as high as 30–40 mg/dL.
- **Latent jaundice** is the term used when serum bilirubin is more than 1.2 mg/dL but less than 2.5mg/dL.
- *Carotenemia is characterized by yellowish pigmentation of skin by carotene but not of sclera. Quinacrine consumption also causes yellowish discoloration of skin and mucus membranes.*

Classification of Jaundice

Q. Write short note on causes of indirect/unconjugated hyperbilirubinemia.

Jaundice can be classified in two ways:

1. **Based on the underlying cause (Table 11.6):**
   - Predominantly unconjugated hyperbilirubinemia
   - Predominantly conjugated hyperbilirubinemia.

TABLE 11.6: Classification of jaundice.

Predominantly unconjugated hyperbilirubinemia	*Predominantly conjugated hyperbilirubinemia*
1. **Increased production of bilirubin**	1. **Decreased hepatocellular excretion**
Hemolytic anemias	Liver damage or toxicity (e.g., hepatitis)
Resorption internal hemorrhage (e.g., GI bleeding, hematomas)	Deficiency of membrane transporters- Dubin–Johnson syndrome, Rotor syndrome
Ineffective erythropoiesis	
2. **Reduced hepatic uptake**	2. **Impaired intra/extrahepatic bile flow**
Drug that interference with membrane carrier systems	Inflammatory destruction of bile ducts (e.g., primary biliary cirrhosis)
Diffuse liver disease (hepatitis, cirrhosis)	Gall stones
Some cases of Gilbert syndrome	Carcinoma: Head of pancreas, periampullary carcinoma, cholangiocarcinoma
3. **Impaired bilirubin conjugation**	
Physiologic jaundice of the newborn	
Crigler–Najjar syndrome types I and II	
Gilbert syndrome	
Diffuse liver disease (hepatitis, cirrhosis)	

2. **Based on pathological mechanism (Table 11.7):**
   - Hemolytic (prehepatic) jaundice
   - Hepatocellular jaundice (hepatic)
   - Obstructive jaundice (posthepatic).

TABLE 11.7: Classification of jaundice based on the pathological mechanism.

Hemolytic jaundice	
Intracorpuscular defects	**Extracorpuscular defects**
➢ Hereditary: Spherocytosis, sickle cell disease, thalassemia, G6PD deficiency ➢ Acquired: Vitamin B_{12} and folate deficiency	➢ Autoimmune, alloimmune hemolytic anemias ➢ Fragmentation syndromes: Prosthetic valves ➢ Drugs, e.g., sulfasalazine, dapsone ➢ Infections of RBCs: Malaria
Hepatocellular jaundice	
➢ Viral, alcoholic hepatitis ➢ Chronic hepatitis ➢ Cirrhosis—any type ➢ Infiltrations	➢ Ischemic liver ➢ Drug-induced hepatitis: Chlorpromazine, imipramine, INH, rifampicin, erythromycin, amitriptyline, halothane, methyldopa
Cholestatic (obstructive) jaundice	
Intrahepatic (small duct obstruction)	**Extrahepatic (large duct obstruction)**
➢ Primary biliary cirrhosis ➢ Primary sclerosing cholangitis ➢ Alcohol, drugs ➢ Viral hepatitis ➢ Cirrhosis ➢ Chronic hepatitis ➢ Secondaries in liver ➢ Severe bacterial infections ➢ Inherited cholestatic liver disease ➢ Pregnancy	➢ Gallstones in the common bile duct (CBD) ➢ Parasitic: Helminths in the CBD ➢ Carcinoma – Head of pancreas – Ampulla of Vater – Bile duct (Cholangiocarcinoma) – Liver metastases ➢ Stricture of bile ducts ➢ Sclerosing cholangitis ➢ Chronic pancreatitis

Hemolytic Jaundice

Q. Write short note on prehepatic jaundice.

- **Increased destruction of red blood cells or their precursors** causes increased production of bilirubin.
- **Unconjugated bilirubin** accumulates in the plasma and results in jaundice.
- **Jaundice is usually mild (Fig. 11.3)** because normal liver can easily handle the increased bilirubin production.

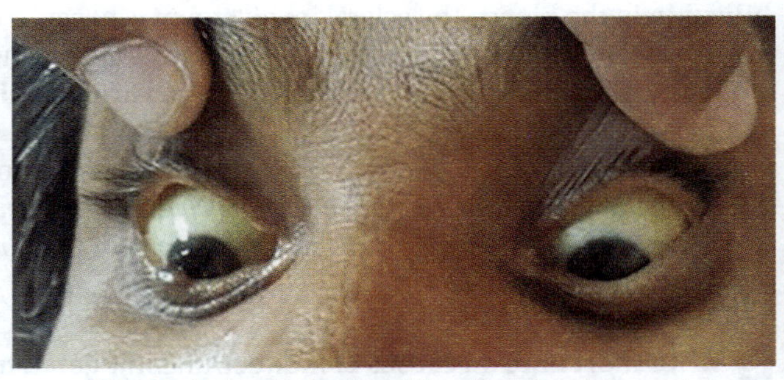

FIG. 11.3: Conjunctiva showing mild jaundice in hemolytic anemia.

Q. How do you clinically differentiate hemolytic jaundice, hepatocellular jaundice, and obstructive (cholestatic) jaundice?

Clinical features

- **Pallor** due to anemia
- **Mild jaundice** without any signs of liver disease

- **Hepatosplenomegaly** due to increased activity of reticuloendothelial system.
- Gallstones and leg ulcers may be seen depending on the cause of anemia.
- **Dark stools** due to increased stercobilinogen in stool
- **Urine turns dark yellow** on standing. This is due to increased urobilinogen being converted to urobilin in urine.

Investigations
- Peripheral smear—shows features of hemolysis
- **Predominantly unconjugated hyperbilirubinemia.** Serum bilirubin is raised (<6 mg%).
- **No bilirubin in urine**, because the unconjugated bilirubin is not water soluble and cannot pass into the urine; hence the term "**acholuric jaundice**"
- **Urinary urobilinogen is increased** (more than 4 mg/24 hours).
- Other LFTs (e.g., serum ALP, transferases, and albumin) are normal; however, LDH is increased.

Hepatocellular Jaundice

- Hepatocellular jaundice occurs as a **consequence of parenchymal liver disease** which leads to an inability of the liver to transport bilirubin across the hepatocyte into the bile.
- Defect in bilirubin transport across the hepatocyte may occur at any point between the uptake of unconjugated bilirubin into the hepatocyte and transport of conjugated bilirubin into biliary canaliculi.
- In hepatocellular jaundice **(Fig. 11.4)**, **both unconjugated and conjugated bilirubin level rise** in the blood.

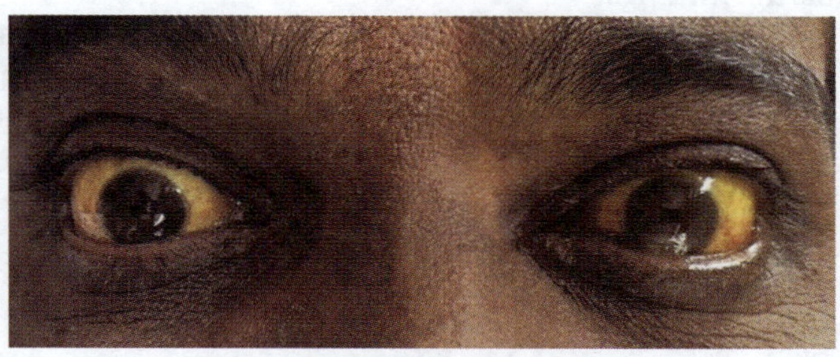

FIG. 11.4: Deep jaundice in viral hepatitis.

Investigations
- **Raised transaminases** (AST and ALT): Acute jaundice with AST > 1000 U/L is highly suggestive of an **infectious cause** (e.g. hepatitis A, B), **drugs** (e.g., paracetamol) or **hepatic ischemia.**
- Imaging
- Liver biopsy

Cholestatic (Obstructive/Surgical) Jaundice

Q. Write short note on causes and features of obstructive jaundice.

- **Cholestasis means failure of bile flow.** Its cause may be anywhere between hepatocyte and duodenum (**Fig. 11.5**).
- Cholestatic jaundice is usually a "**surgical jaundice**" meaning a cause that requires surgical intervention.
- Cholestasis can be intrahepatic or extrahepatic.
- **Consequences of cholestasis:**
  - **Retention of bile acids and bilirubin** in the liver and blood
  - **Deficiency of bile acids in the intestine**

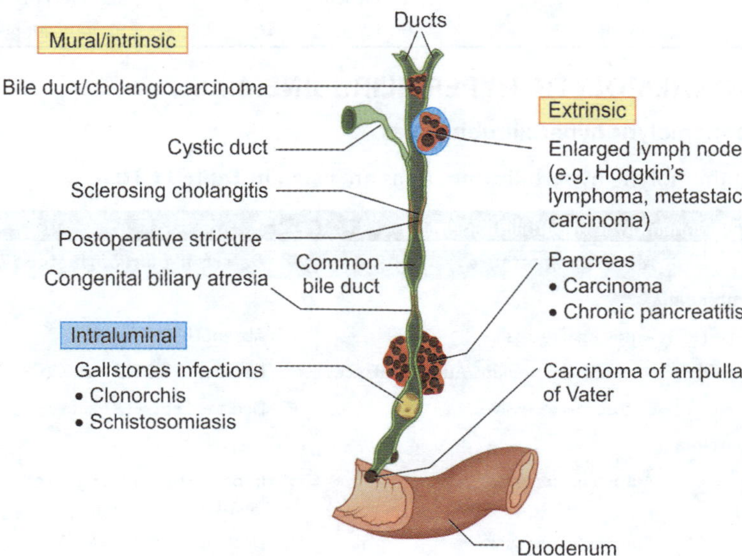

FIG. 11.5: Causes of obstructive jaundice.

Clinical features (Table 11.8)

TABLE 11.8: Symptoms and signs of cholestatic jaundice.

Symptoms	*Signs*
➤ Jaundice (gradually progressive/fluctuating) ➤ Pruritus ➤ Pale, clay-colored stools ➤ Dark urine (increased conjugated bilirubin)	➤ Deep jaundice with a greenish hue ➤ Scratch marks ➤ Xanthelasmas on eyelids and xanthomas over tendons
Depending on the cause ➤ Fever with chills and rigors (cholangitis) ➤ Weight loss (malabsorption) ➤ Bleeding tendency (vitamin K deficiency) ➤ Bone pains (calcium and vitamin D deficiency) ➤ Abdominal pain (gall stones)	**Depending on the cause** ➤ Palpable gallbladder in carcinoma head of pancreas ➤ Large hard irregular liver (malignancy) ➤ Late features: Secondary biliary cirrhosis and signs of liver cell failure

Investigations

***Serum findings*:**
- **Serum bilirubin is markedly raised** and is predominantly conjugated hyperbilirubinemia
- **Serum ALP is markedly raised** (3–4 times that of normal).
- Minimal biochemical changes of liver parenchymal damage.
- Antimitochondrial antibody (in primary biliary cholangitis).

***Urine findings*:**
- Bilirubin present
- Urobilinogen absent

Clinical features useful in differentiating different types of jaundice are listed in **Table 11.9**.

TABLE 11.9: Clinical features useful in differentiating different types of jaundice.

Feature	*Hemolytic (prehepatic)*	*Hepatocellular (intrahepatic)*	*Obstructive (posthepatic)*
Jaundice Color Depth	Lemon yellow—mild	Orange yellow—variable	Greenish yellow—deep
Pruritus	-	Variable	+
Bleeding tendency	-	+	+ (late)
Anemia	+	-	-
Splenomegaly	+	Variable	Absent (may develop later when cirrhosis develops)
Palpable gallbladder	-	-	May be present
Features of hepatocellular failure	-	+ (early)	+ (late)
Conjugated bilirubin	Absent	Raised	Raised
AST or ALT	Normal	Increased	Normal
ALP	Normal	Normal	Raised
Urine bilirubin	Absent	Present	Present
Urine urobilinogen	Present	Present	Absent

CONGENITAL NONHEMOLYTIC HYPERBILIRUBINEMIAS

Q. List congenital nonhemolytic hyperbilirubinemias.

Various congenital nonhemolytic hyperbilirubinemias are listed in **Table 11.10**.

TABLE 11.10: Congenital nonhemolytic hyperbilirubinemias.

Hereditary disorder	*Mode of inheritance*	*Defects in bilirubin metabolism*	*Characteristics*
Unconjugated hyperbilirubinemia			
Crigler–Najjar syndrome type I	Autosomal recessive	Absent UGT1A1 activity	Fatal
Crigler–Najjar syndrome type II	Autosomal dominant/Autosomal recessive	Decreased UGT1A1 activity	Usually mild
Gilbert syndrome	Autosomal recessive	Decreased UGT1A1 activity	Harmless
Conjugated hyperbilirubinemia			
Dubin–Johnson syndrome	Autosomal recessive	Impaired biliary excretion of bilirubin glucuronides	Liver with pigmented granules in cytoplasm. Harmless
Rotor syndrome	Autosomal recessive	Decreased hepatic uptake Decreased biliary excretion	Harmless

(UGT: uridine diphosphate-glucuronyl transferase)

Individuals with Crigler-Najjar or Gilbert syndrome cannot ConjuGate bilirubin.
Individuals with Rotor syndrome or Dubin-Johnson syndrome cannot get RiD of DiRect bilirubin.

Gilbert Syndrome

- Relatively **common,** autosomal **recessive, harmless,** inherited disorder
- **Etiology: Mutations in *UGT1* gene**—inadequate synthesis of UGT1A1 enzyme (about 30% of normal)
- **Clinical features:**
  - More common in males
  - Usually asymptomatic, jaundice is incidentally detected.
  - **Mild, chronic unconjugated fluctuating hyperbilirubinemia.**
  - No other functional derangements
  - Severity of jaundice increases with infections, fatigue, exertion, and fasting
  - Physical examination is otherwise normal.
- **Investigations:**
  - Unconjugated hyperbilirubinemia (less than 6 mg %)—raised bilirubin levels during fasting is the most common diagnostic tool.
  - Urine: Increased urobilinogen and absent bilirubinuria
  - Peripheral smear, reticulocyte count, and serum haptoglobin: Normal

Treatment: Usually no treatment is required. Glucuronosyltransferase activity may be increased by administering phenobarbital 60 mg BD.

Crigler–Najjar Syndrome Type I

- Rare, **autosomal recessive** disorder, invariably fatal
- Etiology: Due to **complete absence of hepatic UGT1A1**.
- Chronic, severe, **unconjugated hyperbilirubinemia** with severe jaundice, icterus and **death** secondary to kernicterus **within 18 months** of birth.
- **Bile** does contain conjugated bilirubin; hence it is **colorless**.
- **Liver** is **morphologically normal** by light and electron microscopy.

Treatment: Daily phototherapy and **liver transplantation.** Phenobarbital has **no effect**.

Crigler–Najjar Syndrome Type II

- Less severe, nonfatal disorder, also known as **Arias syndrome**
- Autosomal recessive inheritance in most cases
- Partial deficiency of UGT1A1 enzyme (10% of normal).
- Jaundice is milder than type I and does not develop kernicterus

Treatment: Treatment includes ultraviolet light therapy and liver transplantation. Phenobarbital treatment can improve bilirubin glucuronidation by inducing hypertrophy of hepatocellular endoplasmic reticulum.

Dubin–Johnson Syndrome

- Benign autosomal recessive disorder
- **Etiology: Complete absence** of the **multidrug resistance protein 2 (MRP2)** which is required for secretion of conjugated bilirubin from hepatocytes into canaliculi. This leads to defect in hepatocellular excretion of bilirubin glucuronides across biliary canalicular membrane.
- **Clinical features:** Chronic, recurrent conjugated hyperbilirubinemia, generally after puberty.
- **Investigations:**
  - Conjugated hyperbilirubinemia (usually 2–5 mg/dL)
  - Bromosulfthalein (BSP) clearance—impaired with reflux into blood at 90 minutes
  - Bilirubinuria
  - Gallbladder is usually not visualized on oral cholecystography.
  - Liver biopsy: **Dark pigment** in centrilobular hepatocytes, **coarse melanin-like pigmented granules** within the enlarged lysosomes, present in the cytoplasm. Pigment composed of polymers of epinephrine metabolites.

No treatment is required in most cases. Most of the patients have a normal life expectancy.

Rotor Syndrome

- Rare, autosomal recessive, asymptomatic conjugated hyperbilirubinemia.
- Defective organic anion transport proteins; (OATP) 1B1 and 1B3 in hepatocytes → impaired transport and reduced storage capacity of conjugated bilirubin
- Clinical presentation—mild jaundice.

- ***Investigations:***
  - Conjugated hyperbilirubinemia
  - Bilirubinuria
  - BSP clearance test—impaired without reflux back into blood
  - Gallbladder is visualized on oral cholecystography.
- Liver is morphologically normal. No pigmentation

Charcot's Triad

Q. Write short note on Charcot's triad.

It consists of following in the presence of stones in bile ducts:
- Pain in the right hypochondrium
- Intermittent or persistent jaundice
- Fever with chills and rigors due to acute cholangitis

Reynolds' pentad adds mental status changes and sepsis to the triad.

Courvoisier's Law

Q. Describe Courvoisier's law.

In obstruction of CBD due to a stone, the gallbladder as a rule is impalpable (no distension). This is because the gallbladder is usually already shriveled, fibrotic, and nondistensible and hence will not be palpable.

In obstruction from other causes (e.g., carcinoma head of pancreas) distension of the gallbladder is common and hence gallbladder may be palpable.

Exceptions of Courvoisier's law
- Double impaction: Stones, simultaneously occluding the cystic duct and the distal.
- Pancreatic calculus obstructing the ampulla of Vater
- Oriental cholangiohepatitis
- Periampullary carcinoma in patients with cholecystectomy
- Mirizzi syndrome

VIRAL HEPATITIS

Q. Describe the etiology, epidemiology, pathogenesis, clinical features, and treatment of viral hepatitis.

Q. Write short note on the diagnosis, prevention, and management of acute viral hepatitis.

Etiology

Q. List the viruses causing acute hepatitis.

Various causes of acute hepatitis and types and causes of viral hepatitis are listed in **Box 11.5** and **Table 11.11**, respectively.

TABLE 11.11: Types of viral hepatitis.

Hepatitis caused by common (hepatotropic) viruses		***Other viruses***
Type of hepatitis	**Causative agent**	Cytomegalovirus Epstein–Barr virus Herpes simplex virus Yellow fever virus Hepatitis G virus Dengue Virus
Hepatitis A	Hepatitis A virus (HAV)	
Hepatitis B	Hepatitis B virus (HBV)	
Hepatitis C	Hepatitis C virus (HCV)	
Delta hepatitis	Hepatitis D virus (HDV)	
Hepatitis E	Hepatitis E virus (HEV)	

Box 11.5: Causes of acute hepatitis.

- Viral hepatitis **(Table 11.11)**
- Other infections: Leptospirosis, malaria, dengue, brucellosis
- Alcohol
- Drugs: Paracetamol, isoniazid (INH), rifampicin, halothane
- Ischemic and vascular:
  - Cardiogenic shock
  - Hypotension
  - Cocaine, methamphetamine, and ephedrine
  - Acute Budd–Chiari syndrome
- Toxins: Amanita, carbon tetrachloride, and yellow phosphorous
- Pregnancy-related:
  - Preeclampsia
  - Acute fatty liver of pregnancy
  - HELLP syndrome
- Immunological: Autoimmune hepatitis, primary sclerosing cholangitis
- Metabolic or hereditary:
  - Nonalcoholic fatty liver disease
  - Hemochromatosis
  - Wilson's disease

HEPATITIS A

Q. Discuss the clinical features, investigations, and management of hepatitis A infection.

Etiology

- Caused by hepatitis A virus (HAV) which is a nonenveloped, 27-nm, **RNA virus** belonging to the Picornavirus group.
- Hepatitis A is the **most common type of viral hepatitis,** often occurs in epidemics.

- It most commonly affects children and young adults.
- **Overcrowding and poor sanitation** facilitate the spread.

Source of Infection

The only source of infection is **acutely infected person.**

- Virus replicates in the liver, is excreted in bile and then excreted in stool/feces of infected persons for about 2 weeks before the onset of symptoms and then for a further 2 weeks or so.

Mode of Spread

Fecal-oral route (either via person-to-person contact or consumption of contaminated food or water). In outbreaks, it spreads through water, milk, and shell fish.

Incubation Period

15–45 days (average 28 days).
There is no carrier state.
Clinical features are discussed together.

Extrahepatic Manifestations

Extrahepatic manifestations are less frequent in acute HAV infection than in acute hepatitis B virus (HBV) infection. Most common manifestations are quickly fading rash (14%) and arthralgias (11%) while uncommon are myocarditis, thrombocytopenia, aplastic anemia, red cell aplasia, leukocytoclastic vasculitis, glomerulonephritis, and arthritis, in which immune-complex disease is believed to play a pathogenic role.

Prevention and Prophylaxis

- Maintain good hygiene and improve social conditions. HAV is resistant to chlorination but is killed by boiling water for 10 minutes.
- **Active immunization:** A formaldehyde-inactivated HAV vaccine (contains the single HAV antigen) for active immunization and can be used in individuals above the age of 2 years. It probably provides lifelong immunity.
- **Passive immunization:** Normal human immunoglobulin [0.02 mL/kg intramuscularly (IM)] made from pooled human plasma is used if exposure to HAV is <2 weeks and can protect from HAV infection for 3 months. HAV vaccine should also be administered.

Hepatitis B

Q. What are the common causes of viral hepatitis? Discuss the clinical features, complications and management of hepatitis B infection.

Etiology

Hepatitis B is caused by HBV which is a **hepatotropic DNA virus** belonging to the family Hepadnaviridae.

Structure and Genome of HBV

Complete infective virion (HBV virion) is called as Dane particle. It is spherical 42-nm particle and **double-layered** comprising an inner core or nucleocapsid (27 nm) surrounded by an outer envelope of surface protein (HBsAg).

Viral genome: It consists of partially double-stranded circular DNA and has four genes.

1. **HBsAg (hepatitis B surface antigen) (*S* gene): HBsAg** is a product of *S gene* which is secreted into the blood in large amounts. HBsAg is immunogenic.
2. **HBcAg (hepatitis B core antigen) (*C* gene):** The *C* gene produces two antigenically different products:
   i. **Hepatitis B core antigen (HBcAg):** It remains intracellular within the hepatocytes and does not circulate in the serum. Hence, it is not detectable in the serum of patients.
   ii. **(HBeAg) (hepatitis B e antigen):** It is secreted into serum and is a **surrogate (substitute) marker for high levels of viral replication.** It is essential for the establishment of persistent infection.
3. **HBV polymerase (*P* gene): A polymerase (Pol)** is a product of *P gene* and DNA polymerase enzyme is needed for virus replication.
4. **HBxAg (*X* gene): HBx protein** is necessary for virus infectivity and has been **implicated in the pathogenesis of liver cancer** in HBV infection.

Source of infection: Human suffering from hepatitis (acute/chronic) or carriers is the only source of infection. HBV is100 times as infectious as human immunodeficiency virus (HIV) and 10 times as infectious as hepatitis C virus (HCV).

Mode of Transmission

Q. Write short note on mode of transmission of hepatitis B (serum hepatitis).

1. **Vertical/congenital transmission:** Transmission from mother [who is carrier for HBV (90% HBeAg+ve, 30% HBeAg–ve)] to child may occur in utero, during parturition, or soon after birth. It not transmitted by breastfeeding.
2. **Horizontal transmission:** It is the **dominant mode** of transmission.
   - **Parenteral:** It is the major route of transmission but occasionally nonparenteral.
     - By **percutaneous and mucus membrane** exposure to infectious body fluids, through minor cuts/abrasions in the skin or mucus membranes. In children, it can be transmitted through minor abrasions or close contact with other children. HBV can survive for long periods on household articles, e.g., toys, toothbrushes, and may transmit the infection.
     - **Intravenous route:** HBV can transmitted through transfusion of unscreened infected blood or blood products. This mode of spread is rare now, because of routine screening of all blood donors for HBV and HCV. Intravenous drug abuse with sharing of needles and syringes, tattooing, and acupuncture are other ways of developing infection.
   - **Close personal contact:** Nonparenteral route of transmission includes spread through body fluids (virus can be found in these fluids) such as saliva, urine, semen, and vaginal secretions. However, this requires close personal contact, unprotected **heterosexual or homosexual intercourse**.

Incubation period: 30–180 days (mean, 8–12 weeks)

Chronic carrier state can develop with HBV infection (1–20%).

Prevention and Prophylaxis

Q. Write short on prevention and prophylaxis of HBV.

- **Avoiding risk factors:**
  - Not to sharing of needles
  - Having safe sex
  - Transfuse safe blood and blood products
  - Enforced strict standard safety precautions in laboratories and hospitals to avoid accidental needle punctures and contact with infected body fluids
- **Active immunization:** By using recombinant vaccines (containing HBsAg). It is advised in following individuals:
  - **Children:** In India, nonpercutaneous routes of transmission are quite prevalent and active immunization using vaccine is recommended in all children.
  - **High-risk groups:** For example, healthcare personnel, hemodialysis patients, injection drug users, hemophiliacs and sexual contacts of HBsAg carriers.
- **Dosage regimen:** Three injections are given into the deltoid muscle at 0, 1, and 6 months. Dose is 10 µg for children under 10 years and 20 µg in children above 10 years. More frequent and larger doses are required in individuals over 50 years of age or clinically ill and/or immunocompromised (including HIV infection or AIDS). Side-effects are very few.
- **Combined prophylaxis:** This consists of vaccination and immunoglobulin. It should be given to individuals with:
  - Accidental needle-stick injury, gross personal contamination with infected blood and exposure to infected blood in the presence of cuts and grazes
  - All newborn babies of HBsAg-positive mothers
  - Regular sexual partners of HBsAg-positive patients, who have been found to be HBV negative
  - Dosage: For adults, a dose 0.05–0.07 mL/kg bodyweight hepatitis B immunoglobulin (HBIG) (200 IU to newborns) and the vaccine (IM) given at another site.

Treatment: Pegylated interferon alpha, lamivudine, adefovir, entecavir, telbivudine, or tenofovir may be used as initial therapy but lamivudine and telbivudine are not preferred because of high rates of resistance.

Hepatitis C

Etiology

- Previously called bloodborne non-A, non-B hepatitis.
- It is a small**, enveloped**, **single-stranded RNA virus** belonging to the family Flaviviridae.
- A characteristic feature is emergence of an endogenous, newly mutated strain. Because of **genomic instability and antigenic variability, producing an effective HCV vaccine is difficult**.
- HCV has six genotypes and in India, most prevalent is **HCV3**.
- **Mode of spread:** HCV is not transmitted by breastfeeding.
  - It is mainly transmitted by the **parenteral route (transfusion** of blood and blood products, and in drug addicts) as a bloodborne infection
  - Sexual contact (low chances of transmission)
  - Perinatal/vertical transmission

- **Incubation period: 15–160 days** (mean, 7 weeks)
- Nearly 80% infected individuals develop chronic hepatitis.

Hepatitis D

Q. Write short note/essay on etiology and epidemiology of delta hepatitis.

Etiology

- Caused by hepatitis D virus (HDV or delta virus), which is a **defective/incomplete RNA virus** and belongs to the Deltaviridae family. The RNA genome is covered by an outer coat/shell of HBsAg.
- It has no independent existence and requires HBV for its replication and expression.
- Because HDV is dependent on HBV, the duration of HDV infection is determined by the duration of HBV infection. It causes **delta hepatitis (Hepatitis D)** with two clinical patterns.
  - **Acute coinfection:** It develops when individual is exposed simultaneously to serum, containing both HDV and HBV. The HBV infection first becomes established and the HBsAg is necessary for development of complete HDV virions.
  - **Superinfection:** It occurs when an individual is already infected with HBV (chronic carrier of HBV) is exposed to a new dose HDV.
- **Mode of spread:** Parenteral route and sexual contact.
- Fulminant hepatitis can follow both patterns of infection but is more common after coinfection.

Hepatitis E

Q. Write short note/essay on transmission, clinical features, and management of hepatitis E infection.

It was previously called epidemic or enterically transmitted non-A, non-B hepatitis.

Etiology

- Hepatitis E virus (HEV) is an unenveloped, single-stranded RNA virus in the *Hepevirus* genus.
- Viral particles are 32–34 nm in diameter.
- Hepatitis E occurs primarily in young to middle-aged adults.
- **Source of infection:** HEV is a **zoonotic disease with animal reservoirs**, such as monkeys, cats, pigs, rodents, and dogs. Virions are shed in stool during the acute illness.
- **Mode of transmission:** An **enterically transmitted, waterborne** infection. It is common after contamination of water supplies such as after monsoon flooding.
- **Incubation period:** 14–60 days (mean, 5–6 weeks).

Outcome of Infection

- HEV infection is responsible for more than 30–60% of cases of sporadic acute hepatitis (clinically very similar to hepatitis A) in India. It **produces self-limiting acute hepatitis**.
- It **does not cause chronic liver disease**.
- **High mortality** rate (about 20%) among **pregnant women.**

Prevention and Control

- Good sanitation and hygiene similar to hepatitis A
- Vaccine has been developed and used successfully in China.

Clinical Features of Viral Hepatitis

Q. Write short note/essay on clinical features of acute hepatitis/hepatitis A/hepatitis B.

Phase 1: Incubation period
Varies according to the virus
Phase 2: Symptomatic preicteric phase
Lasts for 1–2 weeks before onset of jaundice Prodromal symptoms–systemic and variable Constitutional symptoms—anorexia, nausea, vomiting, poor appetite, fatigue, malaise, headache, etc. Low-grade fever—more in hepatitis A and E than in hepatitis B or C Hepatitis B may be present with serum sickness-like immunological syndrome consisting of rashes and small joints polyarthritis Upper vague abdominal pain due to stretching of liver capsule Dark urine and clay-colored stools

Contd...

Contd...

Phase 3: Symptomatic icteric phase
With the onset of clinical jaundice, the constitutional prodromal symptoms usually diminish. Liver becomes enlarged and tender. Pruritus may develop due to bile salt retention. Splenomegaly and cervical lymphadenopathy may be observed in about 10–20% of patients Dark urine and pale stool
Phase 4: Recovery (convalescence) phase
Symptoms disappear, appetite improves, jaundice decreases, stools and urine normal, and liver size decreases. Duration is variable, 2–12 weeks. It is more prolonged in acute hepatitis B and C. Complete clinical and biochemical recovery within 1–2 months in A and E and 3–4 months in B and C.

Fulminant Hepatitis

It can develop in hepatitis B, D, and E. It is uncommon with hepatitis C and rare in hepatitis A. With hepatitis E, fulminant hepatitis occurs in nearly 20% cases in pregnant females.

Summary of various hepatotropic viruses are presented in **Table 11.12**.

TABLE 11.12: Summary of various hepatotropic viruses.

Features	*HAV*	*HBV*	*HCV*	*HDV*	*HEV*
Incubation period in days (range)	30 (15–45)	90 (30–180)	50 (15–160)	90 (30–180)	40 (14–60)
Onset	Acute	Insidious or acute	Insidious	Insidious or acute	Acute
Age group affected	Children, young adults	Young adults, babies, toddlers	Adults, but any age	Any age (similar to HBV)	Young adults
Mode of transmission	Fecal-oral	Parenteral, sexual contact, perinatal	Parenteral, sexual contact, perinatal	Parenteral	Fecal-oral
Clinical					
Severity	Mild	Occasionally severe	Moderate	Occasionally severe	Mild
Chronicity	Never	10%	80%	5% with coinfection; ≤70% for superinfection	Never
Carrier state	None	1–30%	1.5–3.2%	Variable	None
Progression to cancer	None	+ (Neonatal infection)	+	±	None
Prognosis	Good	Worse	Moderate	Good in acute and poor in chronic	Good
Prophylaxis	Immunoglobulin Inactivated vaccine	Hepatitis B immunoglobulin, recombinant vaccine	None	HBV vaccine (none for HBV carriers)	Vaccine

Investigations

- **Urine**
  - **Bilirubinuria** (in early stages) and **increased urinary urobilinogen** slight microscopic hematuria and mild proteinuria
- **Hematological tests**
  - **Leukopenia with a relative lymphocytosis**
  - Prothrombin time (PT) is prolonged in severe cases which signifies extensive hepatocellular damage. This is one of the best indices of prognosis.
  - **Erythrocyte sedimentation rate (ESR) is raised**
- **Biochemical investigations**
  - **Aminotransferases (AST, ALT): Raised** and maximum levels are observed during the prodromal phase (400–4,000 IU/L). They progressively decline during icteric and recovery phases.
  - **Bilirubin:** Both conjugated and unconjugated bilirubin levels are equally **raised**.
  - **ALP:** It may be **raised** but usually less than two times the normal.
  - Serum protein: Normal
  - Blood glucose: It may below.
- **Serological tests:** During prodromal phase, low titers of antismooth muscle antibody, rheumatoid factor, antinuclear antibody, and heterophil antibody may be observed.

Serological Markers for Viral Hepatitis

Hepatitis A	
IgM anti-HAV	It appears at the onset of symptoms and is **reliable marker of acute infection.**
IgG anti-HAV	It persists for years and **provides lifelong immunity** against reinfection.

Contd...

Contd...

Hepatitis B	
HBsAg	It is the **first** marker to appear in serum before symptoms, and is undetectable in 3–6 months. **Significance**: Presence in acute and chronic hepatitis B indicates **infectious state**. Loss of HBsAg with development of anti-HBs denotes recovery.
Anti-HBs	Antibody to HBsAg, appears after disappearance of HBsAg. It is present on vaccination. **Significance**: **Protective antibody** may persist for life, providing protection.
IgM anti-HBc	It appears in serum 1–2 weeks after appearance of HBsAg. **Significance: Earliest antibody marker** indicates recent infection (first 6 months). High titers in acute hepatitis B and low titers in chronic hepatitis B.
IgG anti-HBc	**Significance: It indicates remote infection** (beyond 6 months) and previous infection with HBV even when all the other viral markers are not detectable.
HBeAg	It is detected transiently, early in the course. **Significance: Persistence** of 6 weeks after the onset **indicates infectivity, severe disease** progressing to **chronic hepatitis**. Absence is a favorable serologic finding.
Anti-HBe	**Significance:** It is found in **recovery phase** and **seroconversion.**
HBV DNA, DNA polymerase	It is found in serum and liver soon after HBsAg appears. **Significance:** It is not helpful in diagnosis of hepatitis B but valuable in **assessing the prognosis**. It indicates **active viral replication.**
Hepatitis C	
Anti-HCV	It appears after infection, disappears after recovery, and persists in chronic hepatitis C.
HCV RNA	It appears after exposure.
Hepatitis D (Delta Hepatitis)	
HDV RNA	It is detectable in the blood and liver before and in the early days of acute disease.
Anti-HDV	IgM anti-HDV is the most reliable indicator of recent HDV exposure.
Hepatitis E	
HEV RNA, HEV virions	Before the onset of clinical illness, it can be detected in stool and serum.
IgM anti-HEV	After the onset of clinical illness, serum aminotransferases rises and elevated titers also occur simultaneously.
IgG anti-HEV	After recovery, the IgM is replaced with a persistent IgG anti-HEV titer.

*Hepatitis B (**Figs. 11.6 and 11.7**)*

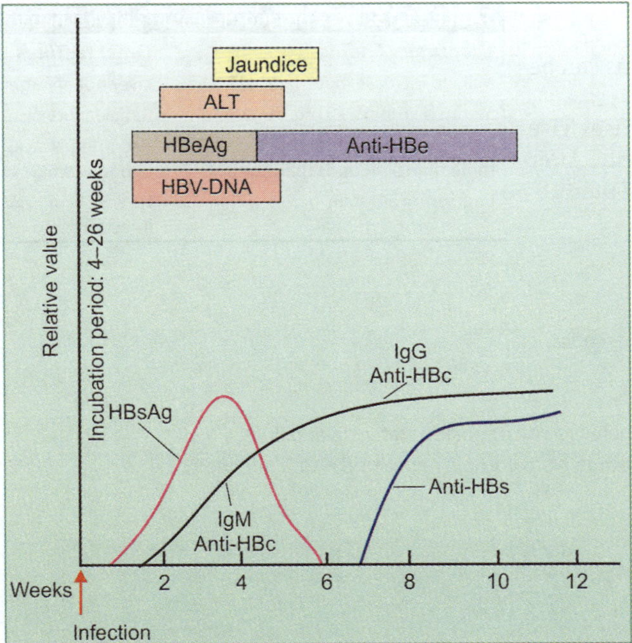

FIG. 11.6: Sequence of serologic markers in acute hepatitis with resolution caused by hepatitis B virus (HBV).
(ALT: alanine aminotransferases; Anti-HBc: antibodies against Hepatitis B core antigen; Anti-HBe: antibodies against Hepatitis B e antigen; Anti-HBs: antibodies against Hepatitis B surface antigen; DNA: deoxyribonucleic acid; HBeAg: Hepatitis B e antigen; HBsAg: Hepatitis B surface antigen; Ig: immunoglobulin)

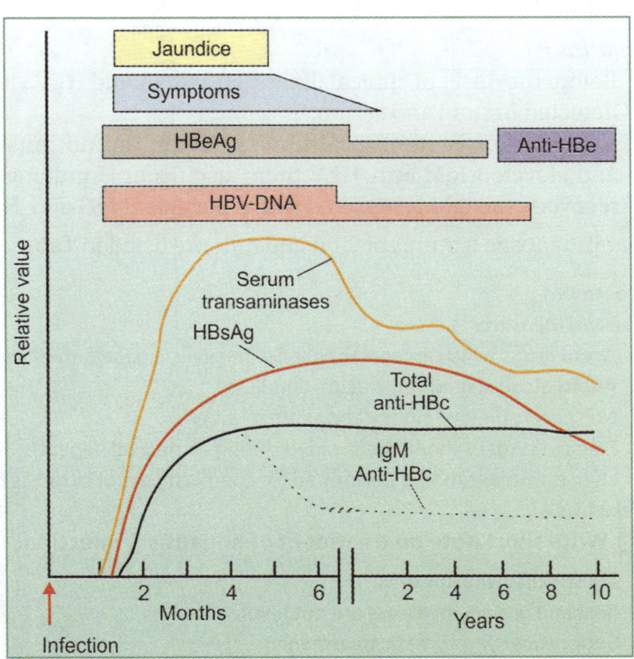

FIG. 11.7: Sequence of serologic markers in chronic hepatitis caused by hepatitis B virus (HBV).
(Anti-HBc: antibodies against Hepatitis B core antigen; Anti-HBe: antibodies against Hepatitis B e antigen; DNA: deoxyribonucleic acid; HBeAg: Hepatitis B e antigen; HBsAg: Hepatitis B surface antigen; IgM: immunoglobulin M)

Q. Write short note on HBsAg/Australia antigen/hepatitis B surface antigen.

Interpretations of serological findings and its significance in HBV are summarized in **Table 11.13**.

HBV viral DNA (HBV DNA): Most accurate marker of virus replication.

TABLE 11.13: Interpretation of serological findings and its significance in HBV.

Antigens		*Antibodies*			*Interpretation*
HBsAg	HBeAg	Anti-HBc	Anti-HBs	Anti-HBe	
–	–	–	–	–	Susceptible
–	–	–	+	–	Immunity to HBV caused by previous exposure or vaccination
+	+	IgM +ve and IgG –ve	–	–	**Acute hepatitis B**, highly infectious High titer in acute hepatitis B and low titer in chronic hepatitis B
–	–	IgM –ve and IgG +ve	+	+	**Resolved acute hepatitis B, seroconversion, low infectivity**
+	+	IgM –ve and IgG +ve	–	–	**Chronic infection** or carrier state, **high infectivity**
+	–	IgG +ve	–	+/–	**Chronic infection** or carrier state, **low infectivity**
–	–	–	+	–	**HBV vaccination**
–	–	+	–	–	**Interpretation unclear***
HBV DNA: (i) indicative of active viral replication, (ii) detected in both serum and liver, and (iii) indicates response to treatment					

*May be most commonly resolved infection, resolving acute infection, false +ve anti-HBc (thus susceptible) or chronic infection (low level).

Q. Write short note on complications of acute viral hepatitis.

Complications of Acute Viral Hepatitis (Table 11.14)

Hepatitis C

- **Anti-HCV:** It appears after the infection, disappears after the recovery, and persists in chronic hepatitis C.
- **HCV-RNA:** It appears after the exposure.
- **Anti-HCV** (antibodies against HCV) does not confer immunity.

Hepatitis D

- **HDV RNA:** Detectable in the blood and liver before and in the early days of acute disease.
- **Anti-HDV:** IgM anti-HDV is the most reliable indicator of recent HDV exposure.

Hepatitis E

- Before the onset of clinical illness, HEV RNA and HEV virions can be detected in stool and serum.
- After the onset of clinical illness, serum aminotransferases rise and elevated **IgM anti-HEV** titers also occur simultaneously. After recovery, the IgM is replaced with a persistent IgG anti-HEV titer.

Poor prognostic features of viral hepatitis are listed in **Table 11.15**.

TABLE 11.14: Complications of acute viral hepatitis.

Hepatic complications	*Extrahepatic complications*
Fulminant hepatic failure	Aplastic anemia
Cholestatic viral hepatitis	Renal failure
Relapsing hepatitis	Polyarteritis nodosa
Posthepatitis syndrome	Henoch–Schönlein purpura
Chronic hepatitis	Myocarditis
Cirrhosis	Transverse myelitis
Hepatocellular carcinoma	Peripheral neuropathy

TABLE 11.15: Poor prognostic features of viral hepatitis.

Laboratory findings	*Other features*
Marked increase in AST and ALT levels	Liver not enlarged
Serum bilirubin >20 mg/dL	Renal failure
Prolongation prothrombin time by more than 5 seconds than control	Recurring attacks of hypoglycemia
Low serum albumin	HBV, HCV, or HDV infections

Treatment

General Measures

- Avoid drugs which are metabolized in the liver, e.g., sedatives and narcotics.
- **Avoid alcohol** during the acute illness.
- No specific dietary modifications are required.
- Elective surgery should be avoided during acute viral hepatitis, as there is a risk of postoperative liver failure.
- Liver transplantation is performed for complications of cirrhosis resulting from chronic hepatitis B and C infection.

Hepatitis A

Q. Write short note on treatment of hepatitis A infection.

- **No specific treatment**
- Rest and dietary measures are not helpful.
- Supportive symptomatic treatment
- Corticosteroids do not have benefit.

Hepatitis B

Q. Write short note on treatment of hepatitis B infection.

Therapeutic goal

- It prevents the progression to end-stage liver disease, hepatocellular carcinoma (HCC), and death with improvement in quality of life.
- Clearance of HBV DNA
- Absence of HBeAg and HBsAg and appearance of antibody
- Normalization of liver enzymes and histology

Acute Hepatitis B
- In previously healthy adults, recovery occurs in ~99%; therefore, antiviral therapy is not required.
- Mainly symptomatic.
- Monitor HBV markers.
- Entecavir (ETV) or tenofovir (TDF) to be given when HBeAg persists beyond 12 weeks, and in patients who are very ill.

Postexposure Prophylaxis to Prevent Hepatitis B Virus Infection (Described in detail in Chapter 5).

Hepatitis C
- Goals of treatment of HCV: (1) Eradication of virus, (2) reduce progression of disease, (3) histological improvement, and (4) decrease frequency of HCC.
- Interferon-∝ is used in acute hepatitis C to prevent chronic disease.
- HCV: Progression of fibrosis determines the prognosis and liver biopsy is the gold standard to assess fibrosis.

Hepatitis D
Active liver disease (raised ALT levels and/or inflammation on biopsy) is treated with peginterferon ∝-2a and adefovir for 12 months.

Transfusion-associated Hepatitis (TAH):
- It includes HCV and/or HBV (discussed above).

CHRONIC HEPATITIS

Q. Discuss the classification, etiology, pathology, clinical features, complications, prevention, and management of chronic hepatitis/chronic hepatitis B infection.

Q. Write short essay on chronic active hepatitis.

Definition

Chronic hepatitis is defined as **symptomatic, biochemical, or serologic evidence of hepatic disease** for **more than 6 months**. Microscopically, there should be inflammation and necrosis in the liver.

Classification

Older classification: Previously chronic hepatitis was classified into:
- Milder forms: (i) Chronic persistent hepatitis (CPH), and (ii) chronic lobular hepatitis (CLH)
- Severe forms: Chronic active hepatitis (CAH)

However, this classification is not very helpful in determining the prognosis.

Present classification: In order to assess response to therapy and prognosis, present classification is based on combination of three factors **(Box 11.6)**.

Box 11.6: Basis of present classification of chronic hepatitis.
- Etiology: Cause of hepatitis
- Grade: Histologic activity
- Stage: Degree of progression

Classification Based on the Causes of Chronic Hepatitis
See **Table 11.16**.

TABLE 11.16: Classification based on the causes of chronic hepatitis.

Chronic viral hepatitis	Chronic hepatitis B ± hepatitis D, Chronic hepatitis C
Drug-associated chronic hepatitis	Methyldopa, isoniazid, ketoconazole, and nitrofurantoin
Autoimmune hepatitis	
Hereditary	Wilson's disease
Unknown cause	Cryptogenic chronic hepatitis
Others	Ulcerative colitis, rarely alcohol

***Classification*: Based on the grade of chronic hepatitis**
- Histological assessment of inflammation and necrosis observed on liver biopsy. Indicates severity of liver disease.
- Scoring system: Histologic activity index (HAI) and METAVIR score can be graded as mild, moderate, and severe.
  - **Interface hepatitis** (piecemeal/periportal necrosis)**: Spillover of inflammatory cells** (lymphocytes and plasma cells) from **portal tract into the adjacent** periportal hepatocytes at the limiting plate, with degenerating and apoptosis of periportal hepatocytes.
  - **Bridging necrosis:** Confluent necrosis of hepatocytes is observed in severe acute hepatitis. Forms bridges between **portal tract to portal tract, central vein to central vein, or portal-to-central** regions of adjacent lobules.
  - Degree of hepatocyte degeneration and focal intralobular necrosis
  - Degree of portal inflammation
  - **Fibrosis: Hallmark of chronic liver damage.**
- **Classification based on stage of chronic hepatitis:** It indicates level of progression and based on the degree of hepatic fibrosis **(Table 11.17)**.

TABLE 11.17: Modified histological activity index—Staging.

Degree of fibrosis	Stage
No fibrosis	0
Mild fibrosis of some portal areas	1
Moderate fibrosis of most portal areas	2
Severe fibrosis of most portal areas with occasional portal–portal (P–P) bridging	3
Fibrous expansion of portal areas with marked bridging of P-P and portal–central (P–C)	4
Marked bridging (P–P and/or P–C) with occasional nodules (incomplete cirrhosis)	5
Cirrhosis	6

Autoimmune Hepatitis

Q. Write short note on clinical features and treatment of autoimmune hepatitis.

Autoimmune hepatitis (AIH) is a **chronic and progressive (unresolving) hepatitis** of unknown cause. No features are absolutely diagnostic and are associated with **circulating autoantibodies and hypergammaglobulinemia.**

Clinical Features

- **It may be asymptomatic or** present with **fatigue** (most common), **anorexia, jaundice, myalgia, and diarrhea.**
- **Acute hepatitis:** In about 30% of cases, it may present as acute hepatitis similar to viral hepatitis, which does not resolve with time.
- **Fulminant hepatic failure (FHF)** or **asymptomatic elevation of serum ALT.**
- **Cirrhosis:** In about 25% patients.
- **Jaundice** may be mild to moderate and is found in 69% of patients.

Investigations

Biochemical findings

- **Serum aminotransferases:** High and more than 10 times during relapses
- **Serum bilirubin:** Mildly raised usually less than 6 mg/dL
- **Serum ALP:** Mildly raised
- **Serum γ-globulins:** High; hypergammaglobulinemia is polyclonal; the IgG fraction predominates.
- **Serum albumin:** Low
- Serum al-antitrypsin, serum ceruloplasmin, iron and ferritin levels: Normal.

Autoantibodies

Classification of autoimmune hepatitis based on immunological markers and autoantibodies is presented in **Box 11.7.**

Other tests

- HBsAg and other viral markers: Negative
- Prothrombin time: Prolonged

Liver biopsy

Chronic hepatitis, variable amounts of interface hepatitis, Cirrhosis, bridging necrosis

Box 11.7: Classification of autoimmune hepatitis based on immunological markers.

Based on the differences in immunological markers AIH is divided into:

- **Type 1 AIH** is characterized by **anti-smooth muscle antibodies** (SMAs) and **antinuclear antibodies** (ANA), or both. Most commonly seen in females and associated with extrahepatic immunologic diseases such as autoimmune thyroiditis, Graves' disease, ulcerative colitis, rheumatoid arthritis, and Coombs-positive hemolytic anemia.
- **Type 2 AIH** is characterized by **antibodies to liver/kidney microsome type 1 (anti-LKM1).** Most affected persons are children.
- **Type 3 AIH: Presence of antibodies to** soluble liver antigen/liver pancreas (anti-SLP/LP)

Treatment

- Prednisolone: 30 mg given orally daily for 2 weeks. Gradually tapering dose as LFT improves. Maintenance dose of 10–15 mg daily for at least 2 years after LFT has become normal.
- Azathioprine: Dose of 1–2 mg/kg daily, added as a steroid-sparing agent and some patients for sole long-term maintenance therapy or if dose of prednisolone is more than 10 mg/day.
- Other immunosuppressive agents: Mycophenolate, ciclosporin and tacrolimus for resistant cases.
- Duration of treatment: Lifelong in most cases
- Liver transplantation: If treatment fails

Course and Prognosis

- Exacerbations and remissions are common. Progression of steroid and azathioprine therapy produces remission in over 80% of patients.
- It may progress to hepatic failure and death.
- Some may develop cirrhosis and its complications.
- Hepatocellular carcinoma is uncommon.

Chronic Hepatitis B

Q. Write short note on complications of HBV infection.

- Chronic HBV infection occurs following an acute HBV infection (may be subclinical) and occurs **in about 1–10%** of patients.
- HBV infection is considered as chronic when the HBsAg (hepatitis B surface antigen) persists for more than 6 months.
- **It may progress to cirrhosis and HCC.**

- **Risk of chronic hepatitis:** Depends on:
  - **Age at which the contact of acute infection:** Chronic hepatitis occurs **more commonly with neonatal** (90%) **or childhood** (20–50% below the age of 5 years) **infection** rather than in adult life (<10%).
  - **Immune status:** In immunocompetent adults, the incidence of acute hepatitis is high while chronic infection is rare (1–2% of cases).

Other conditions where incidence of chronic hepatitis B infection is high are given in **Table 11.18**.

TABLE 11.18: Conditions associated with chronic hepatitis B state.

Down syndrome	Polyarteritis nodosa
Lepromatous leprosy	Patients on chronic hemodialysis
Leukemias	Needle using drug addicts
Hodgkin lymphoma	HIV infection

Phases of Chronic HBV Infection

1. **Immune-tolerant phase:** Characteristic features are:
   - **Asymptomatic** and frequent **in children**. Infection during birth or in early childhood develop prolonged immune-tolerant phase, and disease progresses even after the disappearance of HBeAg in some of these patients.
   - **Active viral replication** in liver but **little or no evidence of disease activity**.
   - **HBsAg and HBeAg positive** and **very high levels of serum HBV DNA.**
   - Normal LFTs
   - Liver biopsy shows no inflammation or fibrosis.
   - It may **lasts for decades**. Therefore, lifelong monitoring is necessary.
2. **Immune-active phase (chronic hepatitis):** Most patients with immune-tolerant phase progress to the immune-active phase.
   - **Vigorous immune response.**

   Criteria for chronic HBV active hepatitis are:
   - Liver biopsy shows **chronic hepatitis** with moderate or severe necroinflammation and fibrosis.
   - **Evidence of active HBV replication: High levels of HBV DNA and HBeAg**
   - Persistent or intermittent **elevation of serum aminotransferases** (ALT/AST)
3. **Inactive chronic Hepatitis B—carrier phase with low replication:** Incidence varies. Most patients with chronic HBV infection will eventually enter inactive carrier phase.
   - **Criteria for carrier phase:**
   - **Serological findings:**
     - **HBsAg positive** in the serum > 6 months.
     - **HBeAg negative** and **HBe antibody positive** (seroconversion from HBeAg to HBeAb).
     - **Undetectable or low levels** (below 400 IU/L) **of HBV DNA** in the serum.
     - **Normal aminotransferase** (ALT) levels.
   - **Liver biopsy** does not show any significant hepatitis.
   - **Low-risk for hepatocellular carcinoma**
   - Liver abnormalities generally do not progress to more severe disease.
   - Disease may be reactivated by severe immunosuppression (e.g., during chemotherapy for cancer or with bone marrow transplantation).

   Individuals **infected during adults or adolescents** usually **become inactive carriers** after they clear HBeAg.
4. **Chronic HBeAg-negative immune reactivation:**
   - Patients harbor HBV variants with mutations that prevent production or have low HBeAg.
   - HBV DNA levels are high, liver enzymes are raised, and active histological activity is present.
   - Late phase in the natural history of chronic HBV and often seen in older patients with advanced disease

   HBV genotype C infection (prevalent in India) has an increased chance of developing cirrhosis and HCC.

Clinical Features

- Asymptomatic or may develop severe end-stage liver disease.
- **Symptoms: Fatigue, malaise, and anorexia**, persistent or intermittent jaundice.
- **During end-stage liver disease:** Symptoms due to complications of cirrhosis occur.
- **Extrahepatic manifestations:** Arthralgias, arthritis, vasculitis, glomerulonephritis, and polyarthritis nodosa.
- Mild hepatomegaly
- Long-standing cases **may develop HCC.**

Phases of Chronic Hepatitis B Infection

Phase	*ALT*	*HBV DNA*	*HBeAg*	*Liver histology*
Immune tolerant	Normal	Elevated typically >1 million IU/mL	Positive	Minimal inflammation and fibrosis
HBeAg-postive immune active	Elevated	Elevated ≥20,000 IU/mL	Positive	Moderate-to-severe inflammation or fibrosis
Inactive chronic Hepatitis B	Normal	Low or undetectable <2,000 IU/mL	Negative	Minimal necroinflammation but variable fibrosis
HBeAg-negative immune reactivation	Elevated	Elevated ≥2,000 IU/ml	Negative	Moderate-to-severe inflammation or fibrosis

Investigations

Biochemical investigations:

- **Serum aminotransferase: Mildly elevated** but may be as high as 1,000 units. ALT (SGPT) tends to be more raised than compared to AST (SGOT). Once cirrhosis develops, AST levels exceeds ALT.
- **Serum bilirubin:** It may be normal or raised up to 10 mg/dL.
- **Serum proteins: Hypoalbuminemia** in severe cases and hyperglobulinemia

Prothrombin time: Prolonged

Serological markers **(Box 11.8)**

Box 11.8: Serological markers of chronic hepatitis B.

- Positive HBsAg
- Positive IgG anti-HBc, negative IgM anti-HBc
- Positive HBe antigen or rarely, positive anti-HBe
- Positive HBV DNA

Treatment for Chronic Hepatitis B (Flowchart 11.1)

Criteria: Three criteria are used namely: (1) serum levels of HBV DNA, (2) serum levels of ALT, and (3) histological grade and stage.

- Serum HBV DNA above 2000 IU/mL (about >10,000 copies/mL)
- Serum ALT level greater than two times the normal
- Moderate-to-severe active necroinflammation and/or fibrosis in the liver biopsy

In **presence of cirrhosis** (compensated or decompensated), **oral antiviral agents** are recommended but liver transplantation may be necessary.

Patients without cirrhosis: Pegylated interferon, tenofovir, and entecavir are the preferred agents in **patients with clinically compensated cirrhosis**, entecavir or tenofovir (tenofovir alafenamide or tenofovir disoproxil fumarate) is preferred.

For patients with decompensated cirrhosis, interferon is **contraindicated**, and either entecavir or tenofovir should be used.

Immunotolerant patients, usually young with normal ALT and high HBV DNA levels, without evidence of liver disease do not need therapy, but be regularly followed-up.

Aim of treatment (Box 11.9)

Antiviral agents: Most commonly used drugs **(Box 11.10)** are:

- **Pegylated α-2a interferon**
  - Response (defined as loss of HBeAg and HBV DNA) occurs in 25–40% of cases.
  - **Dose:** 180 µg once a week subcutaneously and produces response after 48 weeks of treatment.
  - **Side effects:** Acute flu-like symptoms, malaise, headache, depression, reversible hair loss, bone marrow depression, thrombocytopenia, and infection
  - Patients with HIV respond poorly and it should not be given to patient with cirrhosis.
- ***Entecavir:***
  - A cyclopentyl guanosine analog that is a very effective and quickly reduces HBV DNA by 48 weeks.
  - 0.5–1 mg daily
- ***Tenofovir:***
  - It is a cytosine nucleoside analog which is also very effective and has a similar potency to entecavir. It is used for HIV patients with HBV infection.
  - Tenofovir alafenamide (25 mg daily) OR tenofovir disoproxil fumarate (300 mg daily)
- ***Lamivudine:***
  - It is well tolerated. However, rate of development of viral resistance (80%) is high and itself may cause hepatitis. Hence, lamivudine monotherapy is no longer recommended.
  - Dosage is 100 mg/day given orally once a day until HBeAg becomes negative.
  - Used if coinfection with HIV
- ***Adefovir dipivoxil:***
  - A nucleotide reverse transcriptase inhibitor.
  - 10 mg daily is used in treatment of patients with lamivudine-resistant HBV
- ***Telbivudine:***
  - An L-nucleoside that may cause myopathy and neuropathy.
  - The recommended dose is 600 mg once daily.

Box 11.9: Aim of treatment of chronic hepatitis B.

- Seroconversion of HBeAg when present to anti-HBe. When HBeAg disappears, remission is usually attained for several years.
- Reduction of HBV DNA to 400 IU/L or less.
- Achieve normal levels of serum ALT.
- Histological improvement in inflammation and fibrosis in the liver biopsy
- Patients usually remain HBsAg positive, but loss of serum HBsAg indicates a good response.

Box 11.10: Drugs used for chronic hepatitis B.

- Peginterferon in combination with other agents:
  - Lamivudine plus peginterferon
  - Entecavir plus peginterferon
  - Tenofovir plus peginterferon
  - Adefovir plus peginterferon
  - Telbivudine plus peginterferon
- Lamivudine plus adefovir dipivoxil
- Tenofovir disoproxil plus entecavir
- Tenofovir disoproxil plus emtricitabine

Prognosis

- Development of chronic hepatitis depends on the age at which infection is acquired.
- Development of cirrhosis is associated with a poor prognosis.
- Hepatocellular carcinoma is one of the most common carcinomas in HBV-endemic areas.

FLOWCHART 11.1: Treatment algorithm for HBeAg-negative and HBeAg-positive chronic hepatitis B.

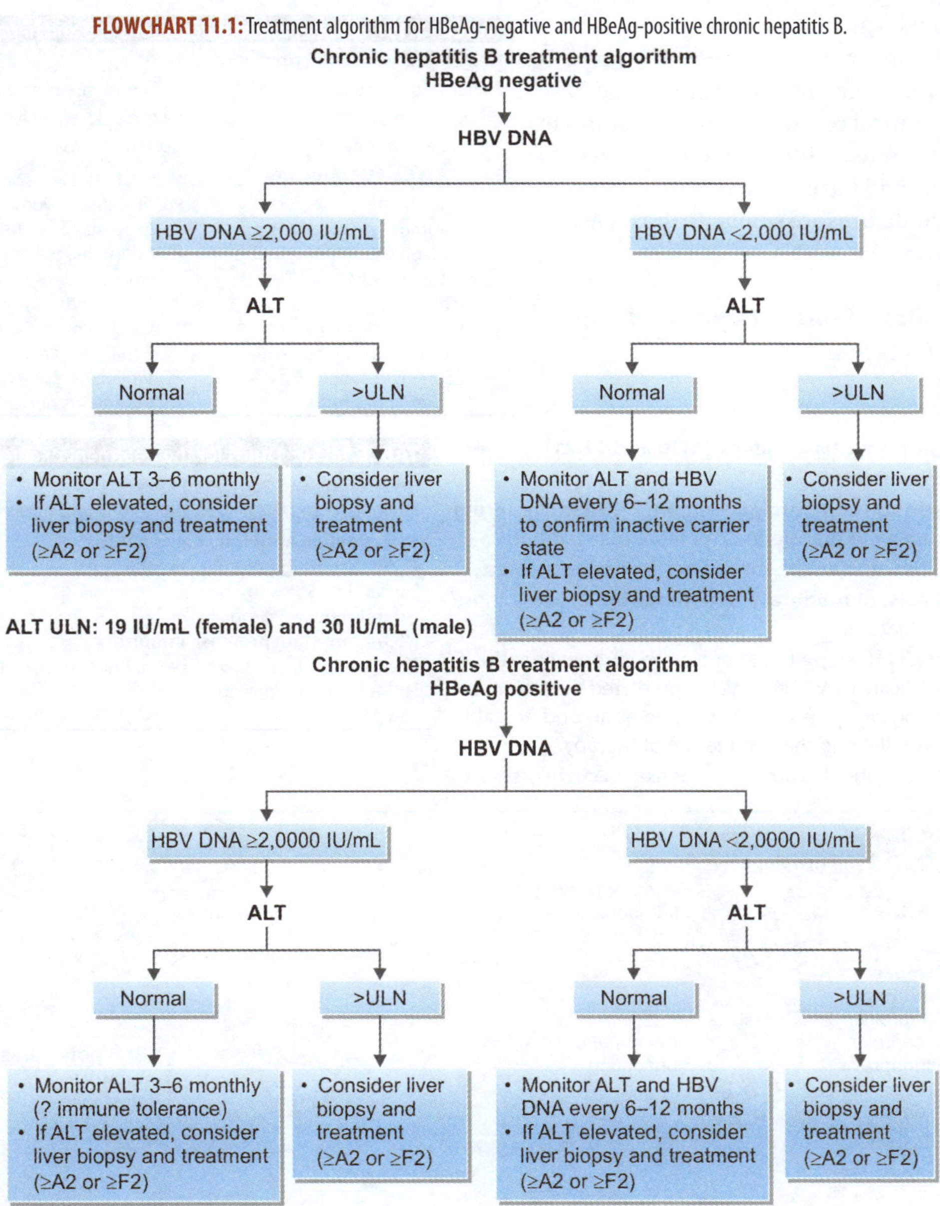

(HBeAg: hepatitis B e antigen; HBV DNA: hepatitis B DNA; ALT: alanine transaminase; ULN: upper limit normal)

Chronic Hepatitis C

Q. Write short note on complications of HCV.

- **Chronic hepatitis occurs in the majority** (70–85%) **of individuals infected by HCV** and is the hallmark of HCV infection.
- **Cirrhosis** develops **over 5–20 years in 20–30%** of patients, while HCC also develops in several patients, especially with cirrhosis.
- **Factors that accelerate progression** to advanced liver disease includes: **Alcohol consumption**, **coinfection with HIV or HBV**, and **older age** at the time of acquiring the infection.

Clinical Features

- **Usually asymptomatic**. Detected following a routine biochemical test when mild elevations in the aminotransferases (usually ALT) are detected.
- Clinical features **when present** are **similar to chronic hepatitis B**. Most common being fatigue and jaundice being rare.
- Extrahepatic features (**Table 11.19**).

Investigations

- **HCV antibody** in the serum is detected in more than 95% cases.

- **HCV RNA** detectable in all patients
- **Liver biopsy** is performed if active treatment is being considered. The histological changes are highly variable. It most commonly shows features of chronic hepatitis, often with **lymphoid follicles in the portal tracts**, and **fatty change.**
- Other laboratory features are similar to those seen in chronic hepatitis B.

Extrahepatic Manifestations of Hepatitis B and Hepatitis C Virus Infection

See **Table 11.19**.

TABLE 11.19: Extrahepatic manifestations of B and hepatitis C virus infection.

Hepatitis B virus infection	
Polyarteritis nodosa	Glomerulonephritis
Cryoglobulinemia	Serum sickness-like symptoms
Papular acrodermatitis (in children)	Aplastic anemia
Hepatitis C virus infection	
Proven associations	*Possible associations*
➢ Autoimmune thyroiditis	➢ Chronic polyarthritis
➢ B-cell nonHodgkin's lymphoma	➢ Idiopathic pulmonary fibrosis
➢ Diabetes mellitus	➢ Noncryoglobulinemic nephropathies
➢ Lichen planus	➢ Sicca syndrome
➢ Mixed cryoglobulinemia	➢ Carcinoma of thyroid
➢ Monoclonal gammopathies	➢ Renal cell carcinoma
➢ Porphyria cutanea tarda	➢ Vitiligo
➢ Glomerulonephritis	➢ Cutaneous necrotizing vasculitis

Treatment of Chronic Hepatitis C (Tables 11.20 and 11.21)

- **Indications for treatment:**
  - **Chronic hepatitis** on liver histology with **HCV RNA in the serum** and raised serum aminotransferases for more than 6 months.
  - Chronic hepatitis with persistently normal aminotransferases.
  - **Cirrhosis, fibrosis,** or **moderate inflammation** on liver biopsy (biopsy not mandatory).
- **The goal of antiviral therapy** in patients with chronic hepatitis C virus (HCV) is to eradicate HCV RNA, which is predicted by attainment of a sustained virologic response (SVR), defined as an undetectable RNA level 12 weeks following the completion of therapy.
- **Liver transplant:** For patients with decompensated **cirrhosis**.

TABLE 11.20: Drugs for the treatment of chronic hepatitis C.

Interferons and Pegylated Interferons
IFN alfa-2b and IFN alfa-2a Interferons **and Ribavirin**
Direct-acting antiviral agents (DAAs)
NS5B targeting polymerase inhibitors
Nucleotide: Sofosbuvir
Nonnucleotide: Dasabuvir
NS3/4 targeting protease inhibitors
Boceprevir, Telaprevir, Simeprevir, Prataprevir, Grazoprevir, Voxilaprevir
NS5A targeting agents
Ledipasvir, Daclatasvir, Ombitasvir, Elbasvir, Velpatasvir, Pibrentasvir

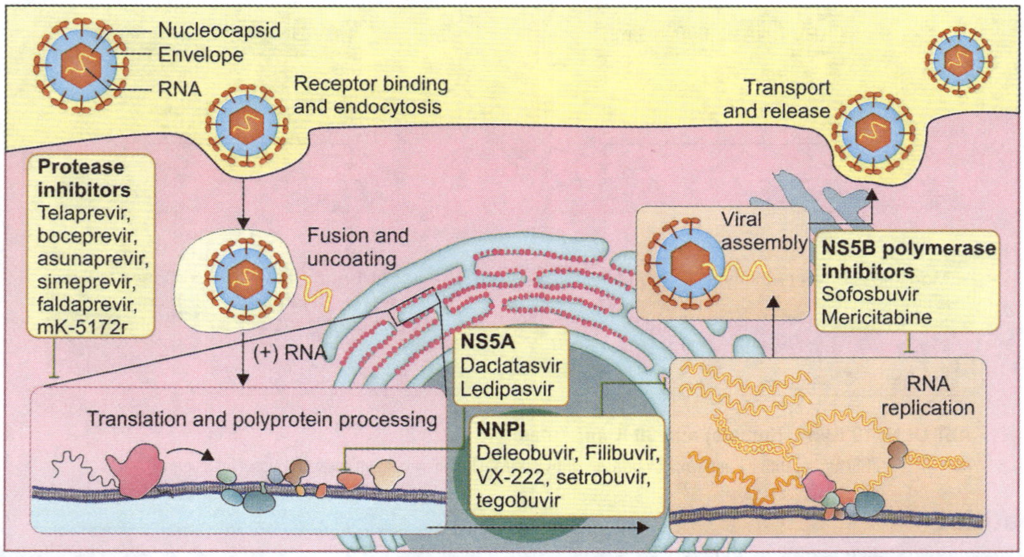

TABLE 11.21: Antivirals for HCV infection in treatment-naive patients.

	Preferred	***Alternative***
Genotype 1 without cirrhosis	Daclatasvir/sofosburvir or ledipasvir/sofosbuvir	Simeprevir/sofosbuvir or ombitasvir/paritaprevir/ritonavir/dasabuvir ± ribavirin
Genotype 1 with cirrhosis	Daclatasvir/sofosburvir ± ribavirin or ledipasvir/sofosbuvir ± ribavirin	Simeprevir/sofosbuvir ± ribavirin or ombitasvir/paritaprevir/ritonavir/dasabuvir ± ribavirin
Genotype 2 with and without cirrhosis	Sofosbuvir/ribavirin	Daclatasvir/sofosbuvir
Genotype 3 without cirrhosis	Daclatasvir/sofosburvir or sofosbuvir/ribavirin	
Genotype 3 with cirrhosis	Daclatasvir/sofosburvir ribavirin	Sofosbuvir/pegylated interferon/ribavirin
Genotype 4 without cirrhosis	Daclatasvir/sofosburvir or ledipasvir/sofosbuvir	Simeprevir/sofosbuvir or ombitasvir/paritaprevir/ritonavir/ribavirin
Genotype 4 with cirrhosis	Daclatasvir/sofosburvir ± ribavirin or ledipasvir/sofosbuvir ± ribavirin	Simeprevir/sofosbuvir ± ribavirin or ombitasvir/paritaprevir/ritonavir/ribavirin
Genotype 5 or 6 with and without cirrhosis	Ledipasvir/sofosbuvir	Simeprevir/pegylated interferon/ribavirin

(HCV: hepatitis C virus; IFN: interferon; P: pegylated interferon-alfa 2a or 2b; R: ribavirin; r: ritonavir)

ACUTE LIVER FAILURE

Q. Define fulminant hepatic failure. Discuss the causes, pathology, clinical features, investigations, complications, and management of fulminant hepatic failure.

Q. Enumerate the precipitating causes of hepatic coma in a case of chronic liver disease. Discuss the diagnosis and treatment of hepatic coma.

Definition

Acute liver failure is defined as the rapid progressive deterioration in the liver function, specifically coagulopathy [elevated prothrombin time/international normalized ratio (INR)] and mental status changes (encephalopathy) in a patient without known prior liver disease.

Classification of Acute Liver Failure

Acute liver failure is subclassified into hyperacute, acute, and subacute, depending on the interval between onset of jaundice and encephalopathy.

1. **Hyperacute hepatic failure:** If encephalopathy develops within 7 days, it is called **hyperacute hepatic failure** and has better prognosis than acute hepatic failure.
2. **Acute/FHF:** In this, encephalopathy develops within 3 weeks (7–21 days) from onset of symptoms in a patient with a previously normal liver.
3. **Subacute hepatic failure:** If hepatic failure develops at a slower pace (>21 days and <26 weeks), it is called **subacute or subfulminant hepatic failure.**

Note: Chronic liver failure is an illness with a duration of >26 weeks.

Fulminant Hepatic Failure

It is defined as severe hepatic failure (insufficiency) in which encephalopathy develops within **8 weeks** from onset of symptoms in a patient with a previously normal liver.

Etiology: FHF is a rare but often life-threatening condition and the various causes of FHF are listed in **Table 11.22**.

TABLE 11.22: Important causes of fulminant hepatic failure.

A. **Viruses:** HAV and HAB. Occasionally, HCV and others
B. **Noninfectious causes**
1. Drugs: Important examples include: ◆ Analgesics (e.g., paracetamol) ◆ Monoamine oxidase inhibitors ◆ Antituberculosis (e.g., isoniazid) ◆ Antiepileptic (e.g., valproate) ◆ Halogenated anesthetics ◆ 'Social' drugs (e.g., "Ecstasy")
2. Toxins: *Amanita phalloides*, rodenticides, heavy metals (copper)
3. Miscellaneous: ◆ Wilson's disease ◆ HELLP syndrome ◆ Eclampsia, preeclampsia ◆ Acute fatty liver of pregnancy ◆ Reye's syndrome ◆ Autoimmune hepatitis ◆ Budd Chiari syndrome ◆ Shock, ischemic hepatitis
4. Unknown (15–30% cases)

Clinical Features

1. **General features:**
   - Jaundice, weakness, nausea, and vomiting
   - Pain in the right hypochondrium
   - Small liver and liver dullness are absent on percussion.
   - Ascites and edema develop later.
2. **Features of hepatic encephalopathy:**
   - **Mental state:** It varies from mild drowsiness, confusion, and disorientation (grades I and II) to unresponsive coma (grade IV) with convulsions.
   - **Fetor hepaticus and flapping tremor** (asterixis) is common.
   - Ascites and splenomegaly are rare.
   - Fever, vomiting, hypotension and hypoglycemia may be observed.
   - Spasticity and extension of the arms and legs and plantar responses remain flexor until late.
3. **Features of cerebral edema:** Cerebral edema develops in ~80% of patients.
   - Bradycardia, intracranial hypertension, and irregular respiration (Cushing's triad).
   - Pupils: Unequal or abnormally reacting or fixed pupils
   - Hyperventilation and hyperreflexia.
   - Consequences: Intracranial hypertension and brain herniation are the most common causes of death.

Investigations

Investigations to determine the cause of acute liver failure:

- **Serum findings:**
  - **Hyperbilirubinemia:** Serum bilirubin is raised.
  - **Serum aminotransferases are raised** but are not useful indicators of the course of the disease as they tend to fall with progressive liver damage.

- **Coagulation factors are decreased** including prothrombin and factor V. Prothrombin time is prolonged.
- Serum proteins: **Hypoalbuminemia**
- **Plasma and urine amino acids are increased.**
- **Blood ammonia levels: Raised.**

- **Urine** shows protein, bilirubin, and urobilinogen.
- **Peripheral blood:** Leukocytosis and thrombocytopenia.
- **EEG:** It may be help in grading the encephalopathy.
- **Ultrasound:** To detect the liver size and for any evidence of underlying liver pathology
- **CSF:** Intracranial pressure is raised, but CSF is normal.

TABLE 11.23: Complications of fulminant hepatic failure.

Encephalopathy	Bacterial and fungal infections
Cerebral edema	Gastrointestinal bleeding, hypotension
Respiratory failure	Hypoglycemia, hypokalemia
Renal failure	Hypothermia
Pancreatitis	Acid–base imbalance
Hypocalcemia, hypomagnesemia	

Complications of FHF are listed in **Table 11.23.**

Pathogenesis and management of major complications of acute liver failure are given in **Table 11.24.**

TABLE 11.24: Pathogenesis and management of major complications of acute liver failure.

Complication	***Pathogenesis***	***Management***
Hypoglycemia	Diminished hepatic glucose synthesis	Blood glucose monitoring Intravenous (IV) glucose supplementation (10–20% dextrose)
Encephalopathy	Cerebral edema	ICP monitoring (if stage 3 or 4 encephalopathy) CT scan (if advanced encephalopathy) Elevate head of the bed > 30° Consider osmotherapy (mannitol) or barbiturates. Treat other contributing factors. Reduce fever (cooling blankets, antibiotics) Avoid benzodiazepines and sedative medications. Moderate hypothermia
Infections	Reduced immune function Invasive procedures	Aseptic medical, nursing care Daily cultures: Blood, urine, and sputum High index of suspicion: Bacterial/fungal infection Antibiotics: Gram-negative, anaerobes, skin flora Consider antifungal therapy if patient worsens, despite antibacterial coverage
GI hemorrhage	Stress ulceration	Nasogastric tube placement IV H_2-receptor antagonist or proton pump inhibitor
Coagulopathy	Reduced clotting factor synthesis Thrombocytopenia Fibrinolysis	Parenteral vitamin K Platelet or plasma infusions for bleeding and before procedures Cryoprecipitate for bleeding with hypofibrinogenemia Recombinant factor VIIa
Hypotension	Hypovolemia Decreased vascular resistance	Hemodynamic monitoring of central venous pressures Volume repletion with blood or colloid α-adrenergic agents
Respiratory failure	ARDS	Hemodynamic monitoring of central venous pressures Mechanical ventilation
Pancreatitis	? Hypoxia	Supportive care, supplemental oxygen if needed Abdominal CT to exclude necrotizing pancreatitis
Renal failure	Hypovolemia Hepatorenal syndrome Acute tubular necrosis	Hemodynamic monitoring of central venous pressures Volume repletion with blood or colloid Avoidance of nephrotoxic agents (e.g., aminoglycosides, NSAIDs, contrast dye) Oral *N*-acetylcysteine prior to IV contrast agent Hemofiltration, dialysis

(ARDS: acute respiratory distress syndrome; CT: computed tomography; ICP: intracranial pressure; GI: gastrointestinal; NSAIDs: nonsteroidal anti-inflammatory drugs)

Prognosis: The mortality is ~80% without liver transplantation, and ~35% with transplantation.

Reye's Syndrome

- Reye/Reye's syndrome is a rapidly progressive encephalopathy with hepatic dysfunction, which begins several days after apparent recovery from a viral illness, especially varicella or influenza A or B. History of aspirin intake may be present.
- **Liver shows severe fatty change.**
- **Raised ammonia levels and liver enzymes**
- Usually no jaundice

FATTY LIVER

Q. List causes of fatty liver.

Fatty liver (steatosis) is **abnormal accumulations of triglycerides within** cytosol of the **parenchymal cells**.

Causes of fatty liver (Table 11.25)

TABLE 11.25: Various causes of fatty liver.
Alcohol
Nonalcoholic fatty liver disease/Nonalcoholic steatohepatitis
Drugs: Glucocorticoids, amiodarone, tetracycline, aspirin, methotrexate, didanosine, zidovudine, tamoxifen, amiodarone
Nutritional: Protein–calorie malnutrition, total parenteral nutrition, and rapid weight loss/obesity
Metabolic: Diabetes, lipodystrophy, and acute fatty liver of pregnancy
Miscellaneous: Inflammatory bowel disease, HIV infection, chronic hepatitis C, toxic mushrooms (*Amanita phalloides*), Reye's syndrome, obstructive sleep apnea, and Indian childhood cirrhosis

Nonalcoholic Fatty Liver Disease, Nonalcoholic Steatosis and Nonalcoholic Steatohepatitis)

Q. Write short note on nonalcoholic fatty liver disease and nonalcoholic steatohepatitis.

Nonalcoholic fatty liver disease is a disease of affluent societies. Its prevalence increases in proportion to the rise in obesity. Its progression accounts for the majority of cryptogenic cirrhosis.

It is increasingly recognized condition and is the most common cause of chronic liver disease after hepatitis B, hepatitis C, and alcohol.

Classification

- **Simple fatty liver disease** with favorable prognosis
- **Nonalcoholic steatohepatitis** (NASH) associated with fibrosis and progression to cirrhosis and sometimes to HCC.

Risk Factors for NAFLD

Increased prevalence in those with the metabolic syndrome.

- **Obesity, hypertension, type 2 diabetes mellitus, hyperlipidemia, and insulin resistance.**
- **Rare causes:** Tamoxifen, amiodarone and exposure to certain petrochemicals.
- **Pathogenesis:** NASH is induced by two consecutive steps: Excess fat accumulation and subsequent necroinflammation in the liver **(Fig. 11.8)**.

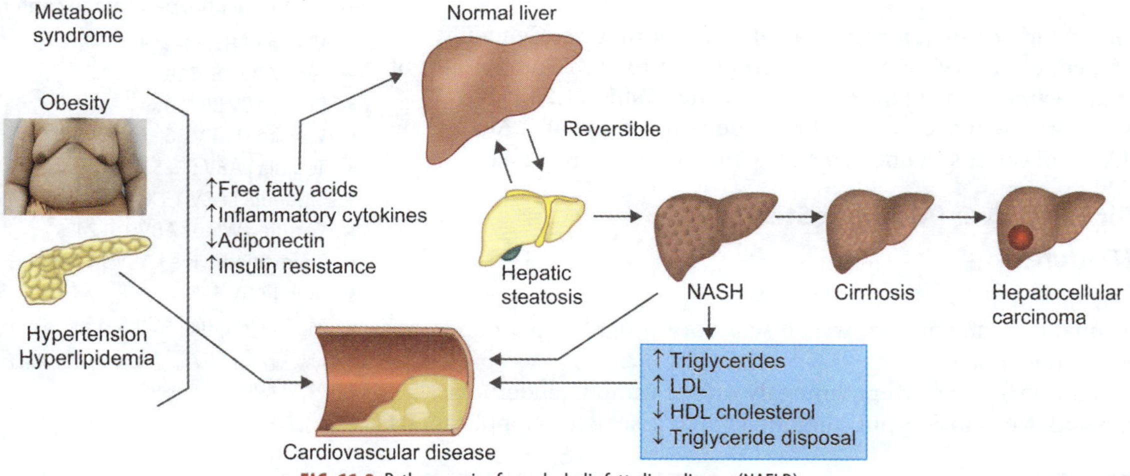

FIG. 11.8: Pathogenesis of nonalcoholic fatty liver disease (NAFLD).
(NASH: nonalcoholic steatohepatitis; LDL: low-density lipoprotein; HDL: high-density lipoprotein)

Clinical Features

- Most are **asymptomatic** at the time of diagnosis and many patients are **obese.**
- Some have fatigue, malaise, and a sensation of fullness in the upper abdomen.
- **Hepatomegaly** is the only sign in most patients.

Diagnosis of NAFLD

Patient with mild-to-moderately elevated serum transaminases, no history of alcohol abuse and a negative chronic liver disease screen.

Investigations

- **Mild elevation of serum aminotransferases** is frequently the sole abnormality with AST: ALT < 1. This ratio increases as fibrosis advances. It may be only isolated elevation of the GGT. ALP is elevated in about 30% of patients.

- **The alcoholic liver disease to NAFLD index (ANI):**
  - ANI = -58.5 + 0.637 (MCV) + 3.91 (AST/ALT) - 0.406 (BMI) + 6.35 for men
  - An ANI greater than zero favors a diagnosis of alcoholic liver disease, whereas an ANI less than zero favors a diagnosis of NAFLD.
- Ferritin levels are increased in 20–50% of patients.
- Autoantibodies are found in about 25% patients with more advanced fibrosis.
- Ultrasound and CT features: Similar to those in alcoholic fatty liver
- **Liver biopsy:**
  - **Best diagnostic tool for confirmation and staging the disease**.
  - Microscopic changes are **similar to those of alcohol-induced** hepatic injury and range from simple fatty change to fat and inflammation (steatohepatitis) and fibrosis. NASH is characterized by fat, Mallory bodies, neutrophil infiltration, and pericellular fibrosis.

Management/Treatment:
- Weight loss, control of diabetes, and hyperlipidemia in the early stages
- Some drugs such as metformin, thiazolidinediones (e.g., pioglitazone), liraglutide, ursodeoxycholic acid (UDCA), vitamin E, orlistat, obeticholic acid, aramchol, betaine, losartan pentoxipylline and atorvastatin have shown some promise.
- Liver transplantation is done for end-stage cirrhosis. Unfortunately, it may recur in the graft.
- Regular follow-up, particularly for steatohepatitis

ALCOHOLIC LIVER DISEASE

List the types of alcoholic liver diseases. Discuss the clinical features and management of alcoholic hepatitis.

Chronic and excessive consumption of alcohol can produce a wide spectrum of liver disease which can be divided mainly into four major lesions:
1. Fatty liver
2. Alcoholic hepatitis
3. Alcoholic cirrhosis (refer later)
4. HCC

Threshold for alcohol and risk of alcoholic liver disease: Generally, the effects of alcohol are worse in women compared to men and amount of alcohol with degree of risk in male are presented in **Table 11.26**.

For women, the above figures should be reduced by 50%. Alcohol by volume (ABV) of various alcoholic beverages is shown in **Box 11.11**.

TABLE 11.26: Amount of alcohol consumption and its associated risk of alcoholic liver disease in male.

Amount of ingestion per day	*Degree of risk*
160 g ethanol (20 single drinks)	High
80 g ethanol (10 single drinks)	Medium
40 g ethanol (5 single drinks)	Low

Box 11.11: Alcohol percentage content.

- Vodka | ABV:40–95%
- Gin | ABV:36–50%
- Rum | ABV:36–50%
- Whiskey | ABV:36–50%
- Tequila | ABV:50–51%
- Liqueurs | ABV:15%
- Fortified Wine | ABV:16–24%
- Unfortified Wine | ABV:14–16%
- Beer | ABV:4–8%
- Malt beverage | ABV:5–15%

Note: ABV: alcohol by volume. ABV: milliliters (mL) of pure ethanol present in 100 mL of solution at 20°C.

Alcoholic Fatty Liver (Alcoholic Steatosis)

Clinical Features

- It is asymptomatic.
- Occasionally, it may present with discomfort in right upper quadrant, nausea, and jaundice.
- Most common feature is **hepatomegaly** with or without tenderness.
- Progression to cirrhosis is not common with its associated complications.

Investigations

- **Biochemical findings:**
  - Moderately **raised ALT and AST with AST: ALT >1.**
  - γ-GT level is a sensitive test to determine whether the individual is taking alcohol.
- Ultrasound: Diffuse increase in echogenicity
- CT scan: Fatty infiltration produces a low-density liver.
- **Liver biopsy: It shows accumulation of fat in perivenular hepatocytes and later in entire hepatic lobule.**

Treatment: Complete cessation of alcohol consumption and nutritional support results in normalization of biochemical findings and histological changes.

Alcoholic Hepatitis

Clinical Features

- It may be **asymptomatic or present with fever, rapid onset of jaundice**, **abdominal discomfort,** and proximal muscle wasting.

- Portal hypertension, spider nevi, ascites, and bleeding due to esophageal varices can occur without cirrhosis.
- Hepatomegaly (tender) and splenomegaly.

Investigations

- Biochemical findings:
  - **Serum aminotransferase (AST and ALT) raised** to 2–7 times of normal (usually < 400 IU)
  - **AST: ALT ratio is >1 (generally >2)**
  - Raised bilirubin
  - Mildly elevated serum ALP
  - Decreased albumin
- Hematological findings: Prolonged prothrombin time and leukocytosis.
- **Liver biopsy: Ballooning degeneration** of hepatocytes with **leukocyte infiltration. Mallory bodies are** often seen. They are potentially reversible but many progress to cirrhosis.

Prognosis

- **Variable** and despite abstinence, the liver disease progresses in many patients. Conversely, a few patients continue to drink heavily without developing cirrhosis.
- Mortality is high in patients with severe alcoholic hepatitis.
- Poor prognostic factors (**Box 11.12**)

Box 11.12: Poor prognostic factors of alcoholic hepatitis.

- Prothrombin time >5 seconds of control
- Anemia
- Albumin <2.5 g/dL
- Serum bilirubin >8 mg/dL
- Progressive encephalopathy
- Renal failure
- Presence of ascites
- Maddrey's discriminant function >32.

Maddrey's discriminant function (DF) = (4.6 x [prothrombin time (sec) – control prothrombin time (sec)]) + (serum bilirubin)

The **ABIC** (age, bilirubin, INR, and creatinine) is a modification of the MELD score. An ABIC score >9 is associated with approximately 80% mortality at 90 days.

Treatment

- It is advised to stop alcohol consumption for life, because this is a precirrhotic condition.
- Severe hepatitis needs bed rest.
- Nutrition: Feeding via a fine-bore nasogastric tube or sometimes intravenously (>3,000 kcal/day; multivitamins mainly vitamins B and C).
- Treatment for encephalopathy and ascites
- Corticosteroids (prednisolone) may be tried in severe cases (discriminant function > 32) in the absence of any infection.
- Antibiotics (pentoxifylline) in severe cases (discriminant function >32) and antifungal prophylaxis.

CIRRHOSIS

Q. LIst the causes of cirrhosis. Discuss the pathology, pathogenesis, classification, clinical features, investigations, complications and treatment/management of cirrhosis.

Q. Describe Laennec's cirrhosis and alcoholic cirrhosis.

Definition

Cirrhosis is an **end-stage** of any chronic liver disease. It is a **diffuse process** (entire liver is involved) characterized by **fibrosis** and conversion of normal architecture to structurally **abnormal regenerating nodules** of liver cells. The three main morphologic characteristics of cirrhosis are: (1) **fibrosis,** (2) **regenerating nodules,** and (3) **loss of architecture** of the **entire liver**.

Classification

Morphological classification (**Box 11.13 and Fig. 11.9**)

Box 11.13: Morphological classification of cirrhosis.

Micronodular cirrhosis (Laennec's cirrhosis)	Macronodular cirrhosis
• Regular, small nodules < 3 mm • Uniform thin regular fibrous connective tissue septa • Involvement of every lobule of whole liver • Most common cause: Alcoholic cirrhosis	• Irregular, coarse nodules of variable size, >3 mm • Fibrous connective tissue septa, broad, vary in thickness. Liver surface is grossly distorted • Most common cause: Chronic viral hepatitis • Increased risk of developing carcinoma of liver
Mixed cirrhosis	
Both micronodular and macronodular cirrhosis	

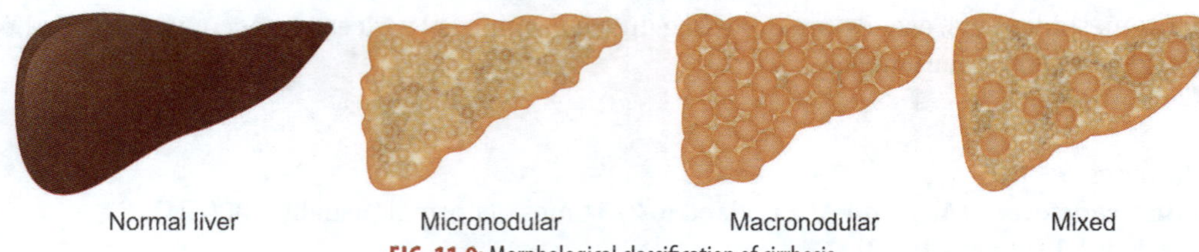

FIG. 11.9: Morphological classification of cirrhosis.

Etiological Classification

Main causes of cirrhosis are listed in **Box 11.14**.

Pathology and Pathogenesis of Cirrhosis

- Chronic injury to the liver results in inflammation and **widespread necrosis of liver cells** and, eventually, **fibrosis**. Fibrosis is due to **activation of the stellate cells (in the space of Disse) by many cytokines** and their receptors, reactive oxygen intermediates, and other paracrine and autocrine signals. TGF-β is the most potent fibrogenic mediator.
- Cirrhotic changes affect the **whole liver**, but not necessarily every lobule.
- **Extensive fibrosis** that distorts and results in loss of liver architecture.
- **Regenerating nodules** are produced due to hyperplasia of the remaining surviving liver cells.
- **Destruction and distortion of hepatic vasculature** by fibrosis lead to obstruction of blood flow. Vascular reorganization leads to portal hypertension and its sequelae (gastroesophageal varices and splenomegaly).
- **Ascites and hepatic encephalopathy** develop due to hepatocellular insufficiency and portal hypertension.
- Hepatocellular damage produces jaundice, edema, coagulopathy, and a various metabolic abnormalities.

Box 11.14: Main causes of cirrhosis.

- Alcohol (one of the most common causes)
- Chronic viral hepatitis (most common cause)
  - Hepatitis B
  - Hepatitis C
  - Delta hepatitis (Hepatitis D) + Hepatitis B
- Nonalcoholic steatohepatitis (NASH) or nonalcoholic fatty liver disease (NAFLD) (earlier was considered as cryptogenic cirrhosis)
- Biliary cirrhosis
  - Primary biliary cholangitis
  - Secondary biliary cirrhosis
  - Primary sclerosing cholangitis
  - Autoimmune cholangiopathy, IgG4 cholangiopathy
- Autoimmune hepatitis
- Budd–Chiari syndrome
- Intrahepatic or extrahepatic biliary obstruction: Recurrent biliary obstruction (e.g., gallstones)
- Inherited metabolic liver disease
  - Hemochromatosis
  - Wilson's disease
  - α1 antitrypsin deficiency
  - Cystic fibrosis
  - Glycogen storage disease
- Drug-induced cirrhosis: For example, methotrexate, methyldopa, isoniazid, phenylbutazone, sulfonamides
- Others: Indian childhood cirrhosis, cardiac cirrhosis, chronic venous outflow obstruction, celiac disease Hereditary hemo-telangiectasia, infection [e.g., brucellosis, syphilis, echinococcosis, porphyria, idiopathic adulthood ductopenia (Caroli disease)]

Alcoholic Cirrhosis

- Safe limits of alcohol are 200 g (20–40 g/day) in males and 140 g (16–30 g/day) in females of alcohol per week. Intake of 180 g of alcohol/day for 25 years increases the risk of cirrhosis by 25 times.
- Development of cirrhosis is six-fold when alcohol consumption is double the safety limit.
- Hepatitis C infection is an important contributory factor for progression to cirrhosis.
- Pathogenesis of alcoholic cirrhosis (**Fig. 11.10**).

Clinical Features

Q. Write the clinical features and treatment of alcoholic cirrhosis.

Symptoms

- **Highly variable** and in some patients it may be completely asymptomatic and is incidentally diagnosed at ultrasound or at surgery.
- **Nonspecific symptoms:** Weakness, fatigue, muscle cramps, weight loss, anorexia, nausea, vomiting, and upper abdominal discomfort.
- **Symptoms of hepatic insufficiency**
- **Symptoms of portal hypertension and its sequelae**
- **Symptoms due to endocrine changes:**
  - Loss of libido, hair loss
  - Females: Irregular menses, amenorrhea, and atrophy of breast
  - Males: Gynecomastia, testicular atrophy, and impotence.
- **Hemorrhagic tendencies:** Due to decreased production of coagulation factors by the liver and thrombocytopenia resulting from hypersplenism. These include easy bruising, purpura, epistaxis, menorrhagia, and GI bleeding.

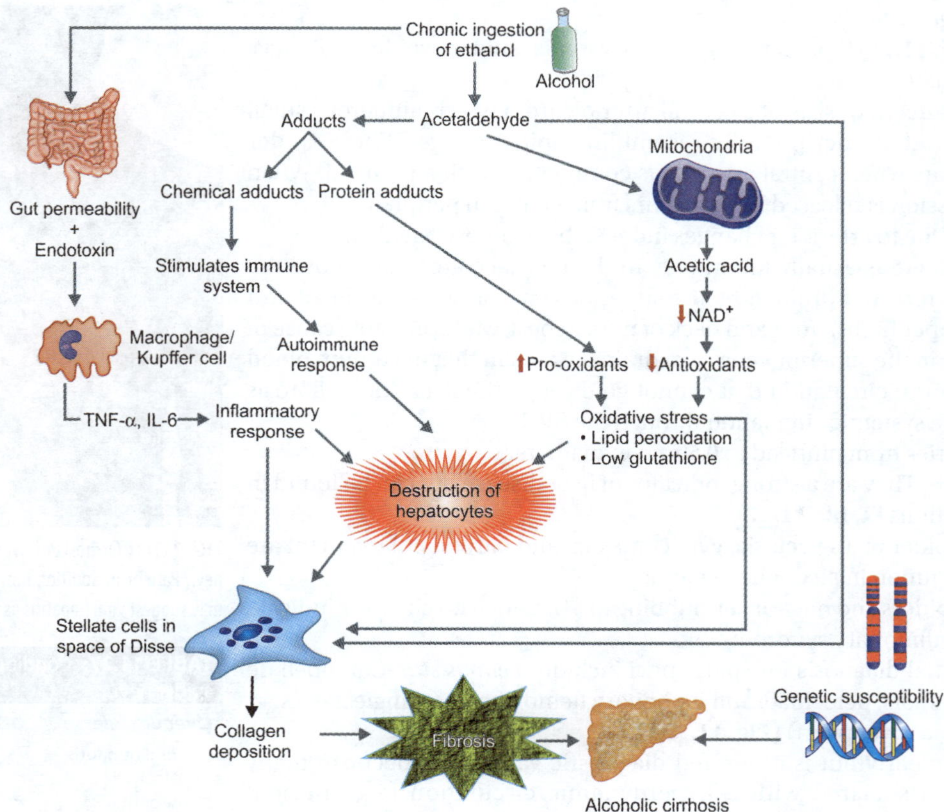

FIG. 11.10: Pathogenesis of alcoholic liver disease.

Signs

Summary of signs of cirrhosis of liver is given in **Box 11.15**.

Box 11.15: Summary of signs of cirrhosis of liver.

Signs	*Symptoms*
Jaundice Hepatomegaly/shrunken liver Ascites **Circulatory changes:** Spider nevi, Palmar erythema **Endocrine changes:** Loss of libido, diminished body hair and hair loss, gynecomastia, testicular atrophy, impotence in males, irregular menses, amenorrhea breast atrophy in females. **Hemorrhagic tendency:** Bruises, purpura, and epistaxis **Portal hypertension:** Splenomegaly, portosystemic collateral vessels, variceal bleeding Flapping tremors Pigmentation, clubbing, cyanosis, white nails, Muehrcke's nails Dupuytren's contracture, parotid enlargement	Asymptomatic, diagnosed at ultrasound. **Nonspecific:** Weakness, fatigue, muscle cramps, weight loss, anorexia, nausea, vomiting, upper abdominal discomfort **Hepatic insufficiency** **Portal hypertension, sequelae** **Endocrine changes:** Males: gynecomastia, loss of libido, hair loss; Females: Irregular menses, amenorrhea, breast atrophy **Hemorrhagic tendency:** Easy bruising, purpura, epistaxis, menorrhagia and gastrointestinal bleeding.

Jaundice

- Jaundice is **not a common** feature of cirrhosis; it is more common with acute diseases.
- Mechanisms of jaundice in cirrhosis:
  - Failure to excrete bilirubin (mainly)
  - Intrahepatic cholestasis (superadded hepatitis/tumor)
  - Hemolysis due to hypersplenism (not a major contributor)

Hepatomegaly

- **Early stages: Liver is enlarged**, firm to hard, irregular, and nontender. Hepatomegaly is **not common** in cirrhosis but common when the cirrhosis is due to alcoholic liver disease, NASH, and hemochromatosis. Hepatomegaly may indicate transformation into HCC.
- **Late stages: Liver decreases in size** and nonpalpable due to progressive destruction of liver cells and accompanying fibrosis.

Ascites

Ascites due to liver failure and portal hypertension signify advanced disease.

Circulatory changes

1. Spider nevi **(Fig. 11.11)** (Spider telangiectasia, vascular spiders, spider angiomas, arterial spiders).
   - ♦ **Appearance:** Consists of a central arteriole from which numerous small vessels radiate peripherally-resembling spider's legs. Whole spider disappears when central arteriole is compressed with a pinhead. When compression is released filling occurs from center to periphery.
   - ♦ **Cause:** Due to arteriolar changes induced by hyperestrogenism.
   - ♦ **Sites affected:** Usually found only in the necklace area, i.e., above the nipples, territory drained by the superior vena cava such as head and neck, upper limbs, front and back of upper chest. Most probable cause of location in the superior vena cava drainage area in that maximum blood in the portal circulation that cannot go through the liver due to fibrosis reach the systemic circulation through the SVC.
   - ♦ **Size:** Varies from pinhead to 0.5 mm in diameter.
   - ▪ **Significance:** They are a strong indicator of liver disease but can be found in other conditions (**Table 11.27**).
     - ♦ Florid spider telangiectasia, gynecomastia, and parotid enlargement are most common in alcoholic hepatitis.
     - ♦ Florid spiders and new-onset clubbing in a patient with cirrhosis indicate hepatopulmonary syndrome.
     - ♦ Differential diagnosis for spider nevi includes *venous star,* Campbell de Morgan spots, petechiae, and hereditary hemorrhagic telangiectasias.
2. Palmar erythema (liver palm) **(Fig. 11.12A)**
   - ▪ Can be seen early but is of limited diagnostic value, as it occur in many conditions associated with a hyperdynamic circulation (e.g., normal pregnancy).
   - ▪ **Cause:** Develops due to increased peripheral blood flow. In cirrhosis, circulatory changes results in increased peripheral blood flow and decreased visceral blood flow (especially to the kidneys).
   - ▪ **Sites involved:** Prominent in the thenar and hypothenar eminences of palm. May be seen on the sole.

FIG. 11.11: Cirrhosis of liver with ascites and spider nevi. Patient in addition has tattoo and keloid, which may suggest viral hepatitis as the cause of cirrhosis.

TABLE 11.27: Conditions associated with spider nevi.

Liver disorders	*Others*
➢ Viral hepatitis ➢ Alcoholic hepatitis ➢ Hepatocellular carcinoma ➢ Treatment with Sorafenib	➢ 2% of healthy individuals ➢ Third trimester of pregnancy ➢ Rheumatoid arthritis ➢ Thyrotoxicosis

Endocrine changes

- **Diminished body hair and loss of hair (Fig. 11.12B)**
  - ▪ Seen mainly in males with loss of male hair distribution
  - ▪ Alopecia affects usually the face, axilla, and chest and is due to hyperestrogenism
  - ▪ *Causes of hyperestrogenism:* Due to increased peripheral formation of estrogen resulting from diminished hepatic clearance of the precursor, androstenedione.
  - ▪ *Effects of hyperestrogenism:* Alopecia, gynecomastia, and testicular atrophy.
- **Hyperglycemia: 80%** of cirrhotics have impaired glucose tolerance, 20% develop diabetes.

In Males

Q. Write short note on gynecomastia and enumerate its causes.

- **Gynecomastia (Fig. 11.12C)**
  - ▪ Found in males (atrophy of breasts in females).
  - ▪ Cause: Due to increased estradiol/free testosterone ratio

  Causes of gynecomastia are listed in **Table 11.28**.

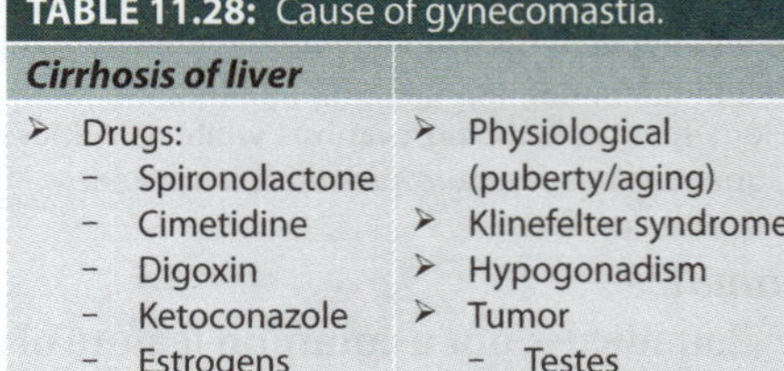

TABLE 11.28: Cause of gynecomastia.

Cirrhosis of liver	
➢ Drugs: – Spironolactone – Cimetidine – Digoxin – Ketoconazole – Estrogens – Isoniazid	➢ Physiological (puberty/aging) ➢ Klinefelter syndrome ➢ Hypogonadism ➢ Tumor – Testes – Lung

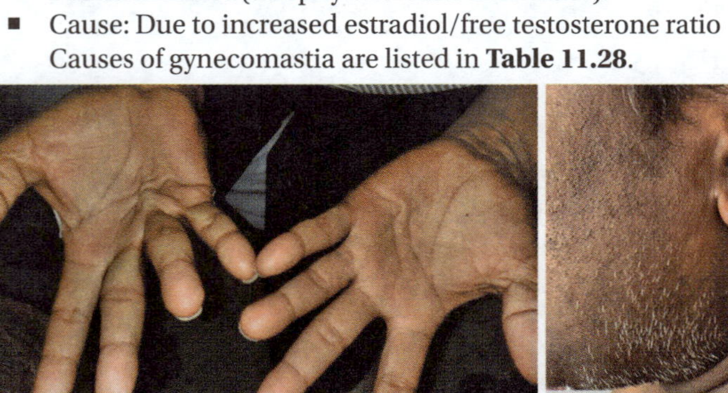

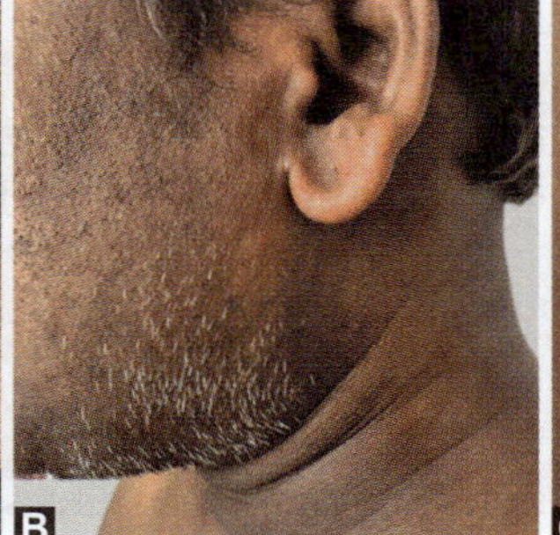

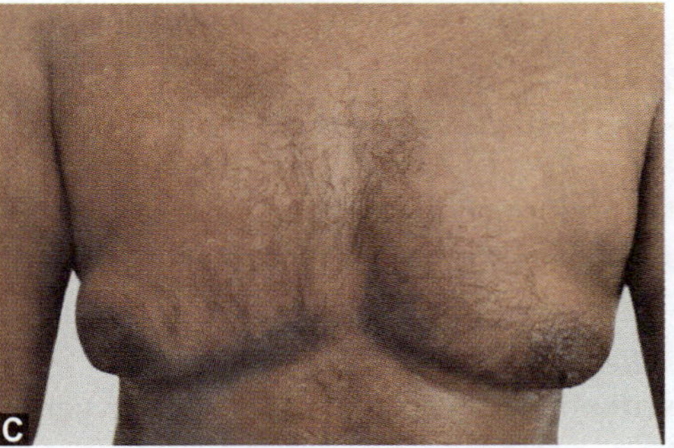

FIGS. 11.12A TO C: Features of cirrhosis. (A) Palmar erythema with Dupuytren's contracture; (B) Diminished facial hair with parotid enlargement; (C) Gynecomastia.

- Appear as palpable nodule (4 cm, subareolar). Microscopy: Proliferation of glandular tissue of breast. *Pseudogynecomastia is accumulation of subareolar fat tissue without palpable nodule.*
- **Testicular atrophy:** Due to hyperestrogenic state, it is characterized by a small size compared with Prader orchidometer **(Fig. 11.13C)**—soft testes with loss of testicular sensation (sickening sensation in epigastrium on squeezing the testes). The dimensions of the average adult testicle is 4.5 × 3.5 × 2.5 cm and the volume is 15–25 mL.

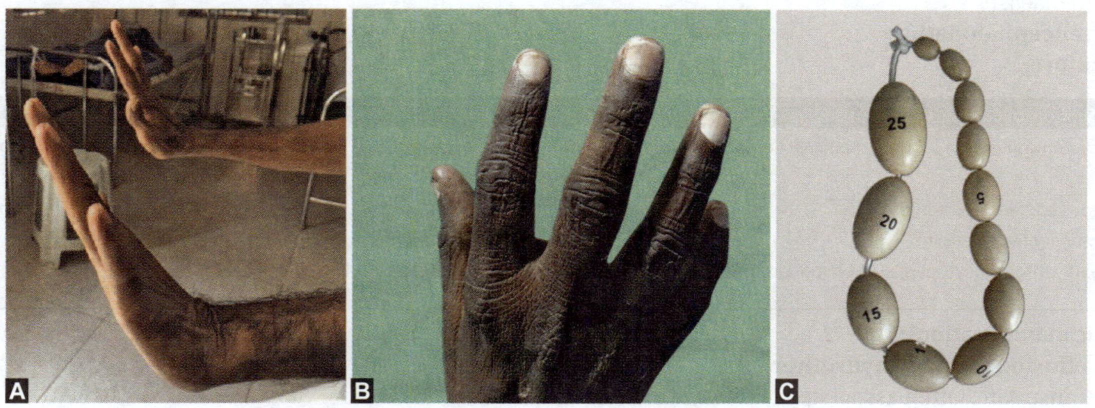

FIGS. 11.13A TO C: (A) Flapping tremor; (B) White nails; (C) Prader orchidometer.

In Females

- Irregular menses, amenorrhea, and atrophy of breast.

Flapping tremors (Fig. 11.13A): Observed in hepatic precoma (refer to hepatic encephalopathy on pages 832–7).

Other features

- **Generalized skin hyperpigmentation:** Due to increased melanin deposition
- **Dupuytren's contracture (Fig. 11.12A)—sign of alcoholism**
  - **Cause:** Fibrosis of palmar aponeurosis is probably caused by local microvessel ischemia. Platelet and fibroblast-derived growth factors promote fibrosis.
  - **Sites involved:** Flexion contracture of the fingers (especially ring and little fingers)
  - **Other causes** of Dupuytren's contracture: Diabetes mellitus, rheumatoid arthritis, and manual labor (workers exposed to repetitive handling tasks or vibration).
- **Clubbing and central cyanosis:** Due to development of pulmonary arteriovenous shunts that lead to hypoxemia
- **Nail changes**
  - White (Terry's) chalky (**Fig. 11.13B**) and brittle nails
  - Muehrcke's nails: Characterized by transverse white lines that disappear on applying pressure and these lines do not move with growth of nail.
  - Clubbing is present in PBC or hepatoma
- **Parotid and lacrimal gland enlargement:** Observed commonly in alcoholic cirrhosis due to associated autonomic dysfunction.
- **Anemia:** Due to various causes **(Box 11.16)**

Box 11.16: Causes of anemia in cirrhosis.

- Acute and chronic blood loss from varices
- Nutritional deficiency of vitamin B_{12} and folate
- Hypersplenism
- Bone marrow suppression by alcohol
- Hemolysis.
- Zeive's syndrome: Alcohol-induced hemolytic anemia with hypercholesterolemia

Signs Pointing the Etiology of Cirrhosis

Signs	*Etiology of Cirrhosis*
Parotid enlargement, Dupuytren's contracture	**Alcohol**
Tattoo marks, jaundice	**Hepatitis B/C**
Metabolic syndrome	**NASH**
Xanthoma, xanthelasma, obstructive jaundice	**Primary biliary cirrhosis**
Association with inflammatory bowel disease	**Primary sclerosing cholangitis**
Skin hyperpigmentation, organomegaly, diabetes	**Hemochromatosis**
Emphysema and cirrhosis	**Alpha1 antitrypsin deficiency**
Longstanding right-sided heart failure, constrictive pericarditis, mitral stenosis, tricuspid regurgitation, cor pulmonale, cardiomyopathy	**Cardiac cirrhosis**
Tender liver with absent abdominojugular reflux	**Budd–Chiari**
Arthritis, skin changes, nephritis	**Autoimmune**
Deforming arthritis on treatment	**Methotrexate induced**
Kayser–Fleischer (KF) ring on cornea, young onset, family history +	**Wilson's disease**

Symptoms and Signs due to Complications

Q. Write short essay on complications/life-threatening complications of cirrhosis of liver.

Three major complications of cirrhosis **(Table 11.29)** are:

1. **Portal hypertension:** Splenomegaly and collateral vessel formation are features of portal hypertension develops in advanced disease.
2. **Hepatic encephalopathy**
3. **Renal failure.**

TABLE 11.29: Complications of cirrhosis.

➢ Portal hypertension and its sequelae (variceal hemorrhage)	➢ Hepatic encephalopathy	➢ Hepatocellular carcinoma
➢ Ascites	➢ Portal gastropathy	➢ Portal vein thrombosis
➢ Spontaneous bacterial peritonitis	➢ Hepatorenal syndrome	➢ Cirrhotic cardiomyopathy
➢ Portopulmonary hypertension	➢ Hepatopulmonary syndrome	➢ Hepatic hydrothorax
➢ Coagulopathy,thrombocytopenia, and hyponatremia	➢ Endocrine dysfunction—adrenal insufficiency, gonadal dysfunction, thyroid dysfunction	➢ Cirrhotic osteodystrophy

Extrahepatic manifestations:

1. **Pleural effusion (hepatic hydrothorax):**
   - It is transudate. Often associated with ascites. Most often seen on right side.
   - **Mechanisms:**
     - Hypoalbuminemia causes decreased colloid osmotic pressure.
     - Leakage of ascitic fluid may occur through diaphragmatic defects.
     - Transdiaphragmatic migration of fluid via lymphatic channels

Treatment: It includes control of ascites, transjugular intrahepatic portosystemic shunt, video-assisted thoracoscopy with pleurodesis, video-assisted thoracoscopy with repair of defects in the diaphragm and liver transplantation.

2. **Hepatopulmonary syndrome**
   - **Definition:** Hypoxemia occurring in patients with advanced liver disease
   - **Cause:** Hypoxemia is due to intrapulmonary vascular vasodilation without any evidence of primary pulmonary disease.
   - Patients show features of cirrhosis with **spider nevi, clubbing, and cyanosis**.
   - **Symptoms:** Most patients have no respiratory symptoms but with more severe disease complain of insidious onset of breathlessness on standing **(orthodeoxia-platypnea)**.
   - **Investigations:**
     - Chest X-ray: May show a bibasilar interstitial pattern that reflects the predominantly basal vascular dilatations.
     - Transthoracic ECHO: Shows intrapulmonary shunting.
     - Arterial blood gases: Confirm the arterial oxygen desaturation. Diagnosis by contrast-enhanced (microbubble) echocardiography, perfusion lung scan, and pulmonary angiography.

Treatment: Oxygen inhalation and coil embolization (in localized shunts). Liver transplantation.

3. **Portopulmonary hypertension:** It is characterized by a raised mean pulmonary artery pressure, increased pulmonary vascular resistance and normal wedge pressure developing in portal hypertension. Dyspnea on exertion is the most common symptom, and can lead to right heart failure.
4. **Cirrhotic cardiomyopathy:** Characterized by systolic and diastolic dysfunction, electrophysiological changes, and gross and microscopic structural changes.
5. **Hepatic osteodystrophy:** Osteoporosis and osteomalacia

Table 11.30 shows noninvasive direct and indirect markers of hepatic fibrosis.

TABLE 11.30: Noninvasive direct and indirect markers of hepatic fibrosis.

Direct markers	
Procollagen type I carboxy terminal peptide (PICP), procollagen type III amino-terminal peptide (PIIINP)	Metalloproteinases (MMPs), tissue inhibitors of matrix metalloproteinases (TIMPs), hyaluronic acid
Indirect serum markers of liver fibrosis	
Indices	**Individual components**
AST/ALT ratio	Aspartate aminotransferase, alanine aminotransferase
PGA	Prothrombin index, GGT, apolipoprotein A1
APRI	AST/platelet count
FibroSpect II	HA, TIMP-1, α2-macroglobulin
FibroTest/FibroSure	γ2 macroglobulin, γ2 globulin, γ globulin, apolipoprotein A1, GGT, total bilirubin
FibroIndex	Platelet count, AST, GGT
FibroMeter	Platelet count, γ2 macroglobulin, AST, age, prothrombin index, HA, blood urea nitrogen
Hepascore	Age, gender, bilirubin, GGT, HA, γ2-macroglobulin
FIB-4	Platelet count, ALT, AST, platelet count, age

(ALT: alanine aminotransferase; APRI: AST/platelet ratio index; AST: aspartate aminotransferase; GGT: gamma-glutamyl transpeptidase; HA: hyaluronic acid; TIMP-1: TIMP metallopeptidase inhibitor 1)

Prognostic Classifications

Q. Write short note on Child–Pugh score or Child–Turcotte–Pugh score.

The Child-Pugh (CP) scoring classification was originally used to risk-stratify patients undergoing shunt surgery. Modifications of Child's-Pugh grading (A, B, and C)/Child-Turcotte-Pugh score is shown in **Table 11.31** and is useful to grade the **severity of liver disease and prognosticate** patients with established cirrhosis. Other scoring system used is **The Model for End-stage Liver Disease (MELD)** which bilirubin, creatinine, and INR for prothrombin time to predict 3-month survival.

$MELD = 3.8 \times log_e(serum\ bilirubin\ [mg/dL]) + 11.2 \times log_e(INR) + 9.6 \times log_e(serum\ creatinine\ [mg/dL]) + 6.4$

Characteristics of end-stage of cirrhosis **(Box 11.17)**.

TABLE 11.31: Modified Child's–Pugh classification or Child–Turcotte–Pugh (CTP) score.

Parameter	Score		
	1	2	3
Encephalopathy	None	Mild	Marked
Ascites	None	Mild or controlled with diuretics	Moderate/ severe
Prolongation of prothrombin time (seconds over normal)	<4	4–6	>6
Serum albumin (mg/dL)	>3.5	2.8–3.5	<2.8
Serum bilirubin (mg/dL)	<2	2–3	>3

CTP class A: Points 5–6; CP class B: 7–9; CP class C: > 9 (range 5–15) 1-year survival rates for patients with Child–Pugh class A, B, and C cirrhosis are approximately 100, 80, and 45%, respectively.

Box 11.17: Characteristics of end-stage of cirrhosis.

- Jaundice
- Progressive, refractory ascites
- Worsening of signs of portal hypertension
- Progressive renal dysfunction hepatic encephalopathy

Poor Prognostic Factors in Cirrhosis (Table 11.32)

TABLE 11.32: Poor prognostic factors in cirrhosis.

Laboratory findings	Clinical findings
➤ Low serum albumin of<2.5 g/dL ➤ Low serum sodium of <120 mmol/L ➤ Rising serum creatinine ➤ Prolongation of prothrombin time more than 1.5 times of control (>6 seconds above normal)	➤ Persistent jaundice (serum bilirubin >20 mg/dL) ➤ Ascites responding poorly to therapy ➤ Encephalopathy not associated with an extensive collateral circulation ➤ Hemorrhage from varices with poor liver function ➤ Neuropsychiatric complications ➤ Persistent hypotension ➤ Small liver ➤ Etiology (e.g., hepatitis C, alcoholic cirrhosis, if the patient continues drinking)

Investigations

Investigations are helpful for assessing the severity and type of liver disease.

Liver Function Tests

- **Hyperbilirubinemia:** Due to rise in both conjugated and unconjugated bilirubin. Not very common with cirrhosis. It could suggest superadded hepatitis, hepatocellular carcinoma, congestive or obstructive etiology.
- **Serum proteins:** Show **reversal of A:G ratio.**
  - **Serum albumin is decreased** (hypoalbuminemia) and is due to reduced synthesis by liver.
  - **Serum globulin is increased** (hyperglobulinemia) due to stimulation of reticuloendothelial system.
- **Serum transaminases**
  - **AST (SGOT) is raised.**
  - **ALT (SGPT) is raised** and usually less than 300 units/dL.
  - **AST:ALT ratio**
    - **More than 2 in alcoholic cirrhosis.**
    - **Less than 2 in cirrhosis complicating viral hepatitis.**
- **ALP:** It may be slightly elevated.
- **Prothrombin time: Prolonged** due to reduced synthesis of clotting (especially vitamin K-dependent) factors.

Hematological Tests

Peripheral blood picture

- **Anemia and acanthocytosis** (spur-like projections on RBC).
- **Leukopenia and thrombocytopenia** (due to hypersplenism and bone marrow suppression by alcohol).

Serological markers: For hepatitis B and C.

Other Biochemical Markers

- Serum electrolytes:
  - Low sodium (hyponatremia) indicates severe liver disease and is due to either defect in free water clearance or to excess diuretic therapy.
  - Hypokalemia, hypomagnesemia, and hypophosphatemia

- **Blood ammonia** estimation: It is a reliable investigation when hepatic encephalopathy is suspected. Raised blood ammonia is due to:
  - Decreased clearance by liver
  - Shunting of portal venous blood to systemic circulation
- Respiratory alkalosis: It may develop due to central hyperventilation.
- Glucose intolerance.

Box 11.18: Ultrasound examination in cirrhosis.

- Changes in size and shape of the liver
- Fatty change and fibrosis produce a diffuse increased echogenicity
- Nodularity of the liver surface
- Distortion of the arterial vascular architecture
- Patency and size of the portal and hepatic veins and their diameters
- Detect hepatocellular carcinoma
- Enlargement of spleen
- Ascites

Imaging

- **Ultrasound examination** can demonstrate features listed in **Box 11.18**.
- **CT scan:** To detect hepatosplenomegaly and dilated collaterals. Arterial phase-contrast-enhanced scans to detect HCC. Other noninvasive markers to detect hepatic fibrosis are Hepascore, FIB-4 index, Fibroindex, AST to platelet ratio, etc. (*refer* **Table 11.32**).
- ***Endoscopy*** for detecting and treating varices and portal hypertensive gastropathy. Barium swallow may also be useful for demonstration of varices.
- **Hepatic elastography**

Q. Write short note on hepatic elastography.

- Hepatic fibrosis represents an early stage of chronic liver disease and cirrhosis.
- Conventional liver tests and imaging studies are not sensitive for detecting hepatic fibrosis.
- Hepatic elastography is a noninvasive method **for measurement of hepatic fibrosis**.
- Methods used are ultrasound and MRI [acoustic radiation force impulse imaging (ARFI), real-time shear wave elastography (SWE)].
- Methods for performing SWE, including transient elastography, point-SWE, and two-dimensional (2D)-SWE.
- Ultrasound-based elastography is primarily used to assess hepatic fibrosis, it can also be used to predict complications in patients with cirrhosis-like development of large varices and HCC.

Liver Biopsy (Box 11.19)

Box 11.19: Usefulness of liver biopsy in cirrhosis.

- **To confirm the diagnosis** of cirrhosis
- **Assesses the severity and type** of liver disease
- Special stains: They may be necessary for iron and copper
- Immunocytochemical stains: They can identify viruses.

Special investigations depending on the etiology:

- Chemical measurement of iron (serum transferrin saturation level and serum ferritin) and copper (ceruloplasmin) are required to confirm diagnosis of iron overload or Wilson's disease.
- Others: Serum α-fetoprotein, α_1-antitrypsin, antinuclear antibodies and anti-smooth muscle antibodies, etc. depending on the etiology.

Ascitic Fluid Examination (Discussed Later)

Investigations for the etiology of cirrhosis: Even in a patient of cirrhosis with chronic consumption of alcohol, rule out other causes (viral serology, etc.) as only 15–18% of alcoholics develop cirrhosis.

Management (Treatment)

- There is **no treatment available to arrest or reverse the cirrhotic changes** in liver. **Liver transplantation** is the specific treatment.
- Progression may be halted by correcting the underlying cause, removal of causative agents such as drugs and alcohol.
- **Diet:**
  - High-protein diet: Minimum 1 g/kg/day; 2,000–3,000 kcal/day
  - Diets with branched-chain amino acids in patients predisposed to hepatic encephalopathy.
  - Multivitamin supplements.
  - Reduce salt intake.
- Avoidance of aspirin, NSAIDs, and other hepatotoxic drugs.
- **Management of the complications:** Specific treatment of complications, e.g., variceal bleeding, hepatic encephalopathy, and ascites (discussed separately).
- **Follow-up:** With 6-monthly ultrasound and serum α-fetoprotein measurements for early detection of development of a HCC.

PORTAL HYPERTENSION

Portal vein is formed by the union of the superior mesenteric and splenic veins. Normally, the pressure within portal vein is 5–8 mm Hg (or 10–15 cm saline).

Definition

- Portal hypertension is defined as **prolonged elevation of portal venous pressure** (>30 cm saline).
- It is better defined as elevation of **hepatic venous pressure gradient** (HVPG-difference in pressure between portal vein and hepatic vein) more than 7 mm Hg. HVPG more than 10 mm Hg defines significant portal hypertension.

Classification of Portal Hypertension (Fig. 11.14)

Q. Define and classify portal hypertension.

Portal hypertension can be classified according to the site of obstruction into **prehepatic, intrahepatic, and posthepatic**.

- **Prehepatic causes:** Obstruction/ blockage of the portal vein before it ramifies within the liver, e.g., portal vein thrombosis, splenic vein thrombosis, and massive splenomegaly (Banti's syndrome).
- **Intrahepatic causes:** Due to distortion of the liver architecture and may be further divided into:
  - **Presinusoidal** (e.g., in schistosomiasis)
  - **Sinusoidal** (e.g., in cirrhosis)
  - **Postsinusoidal** (e.g., hepatic sinusoidal obstruction—veno-occlusive syndrome).
- **Posthepatic causes:** Due to venous blockage outside the liver and are rare, e.g., severe right-sided heart failure, Budd-Chiari syndrome, constrictive pericarditis, and hepatic vein outflow obstruction.

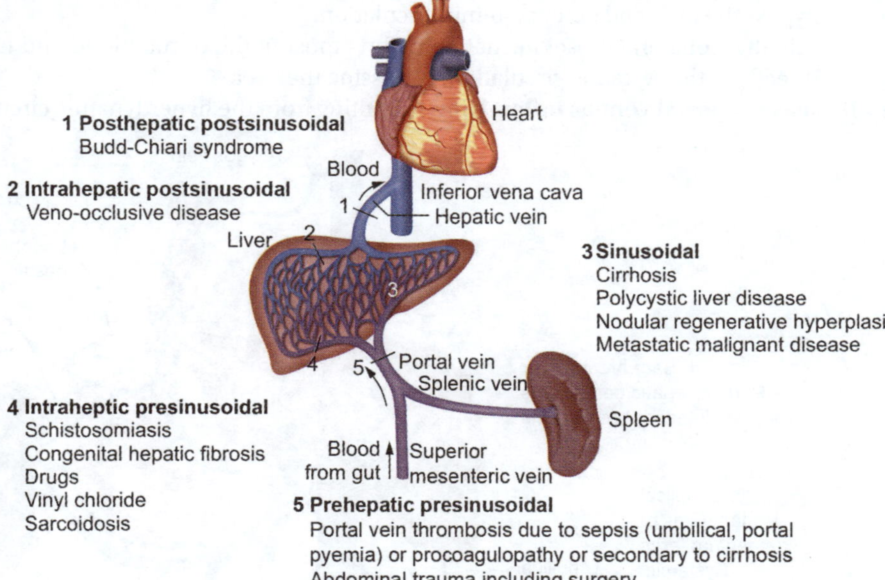

FIG. 11.14: Classification of portal hypertension according to site of vascular obstruction.

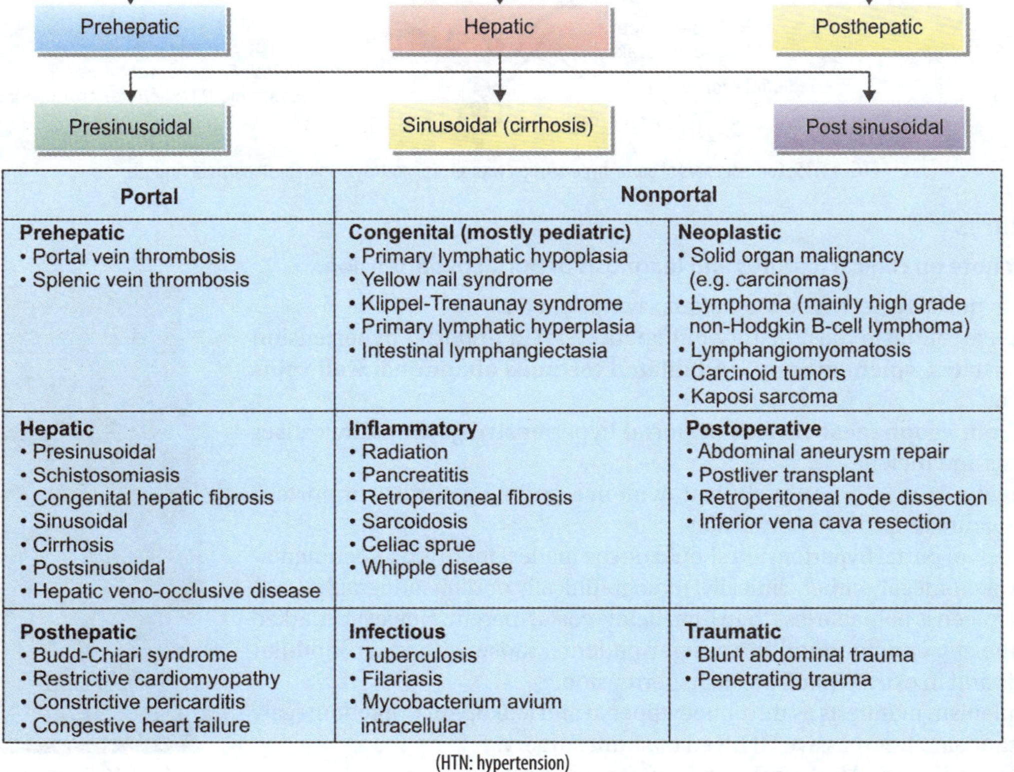

Portal	Nonportal	
Prehepatic • Portal vein thrombosis • Splenic vein thrombosis	**Congenital (mostly pediatric)** • Primary lymphatic hypoplasia • Yellow nail syndrome • Klippel-Trenaunay syndrome • Primary lymphatic hyperplasia • Intestinal lymphangiectasia	**Neoplastic** • Solid organ malignancy (e.g. carcinomas) • Lymphoma (mainly high grade non-Hodgkin B-cell lymphoma) • Lymphangiomyomatosis • Carcinoid tumors • Kaposi sarcoma
Hepatic • Presinusoidal • Schistosomiasis • Congenital hepatic fibrosis • Sinusoidal • Cirrhosis • Postsinusoidal • Hepatic veno-occlusive disease	**Inflammatory** • Radiation • Pancreatitis • Retroperitoneal fibrosis • Sarcoidosis • Celiac sprue • Whipple disease	**Postoperative** • Abdominal aneurysm repair • Postliver transplant • Retroperitoneal node dissection • Inferior vena cava resection
Posthepatic • Budd-Chiari syndrome • Restrictive cardiomyopathy • Constrictive pericarditis • Congestive heart failure	**Infectious** • Tuberculosis • Filariasis • Mycobacterium avium intracellular	**Traumatic** • Blunt abdominal trauma • Penetrating trauma

(HTN: hypertension)

Pathogenesis of Portal Hypertension (Fig. 11.15)

Q. Discuss the etiology, pathogenesis, clinical features, investigations, complications and management of portal hypertension.

Portal hypertension in cirrhosis results from:

- **Increased intrahepatic resistance** to blood flow through the liver and leads to:
    - As portal pressure rises above 10–12 mm Hg, the portal venous system dilates, reduces the portal blood to the liver and collaterals occur within the systemic venous system. Development of collateral vessels allowing portal blood to bypass the liver and enter systemic circulation.
    - Initially, collateral vessel formation diverts most of the portal blood and later almost all of the entire portal blood directly to the systemic circulation, bypassing the liver.
- **Increase in portal venous inflow (flow)** resulting from the hyperdynamic circulation.

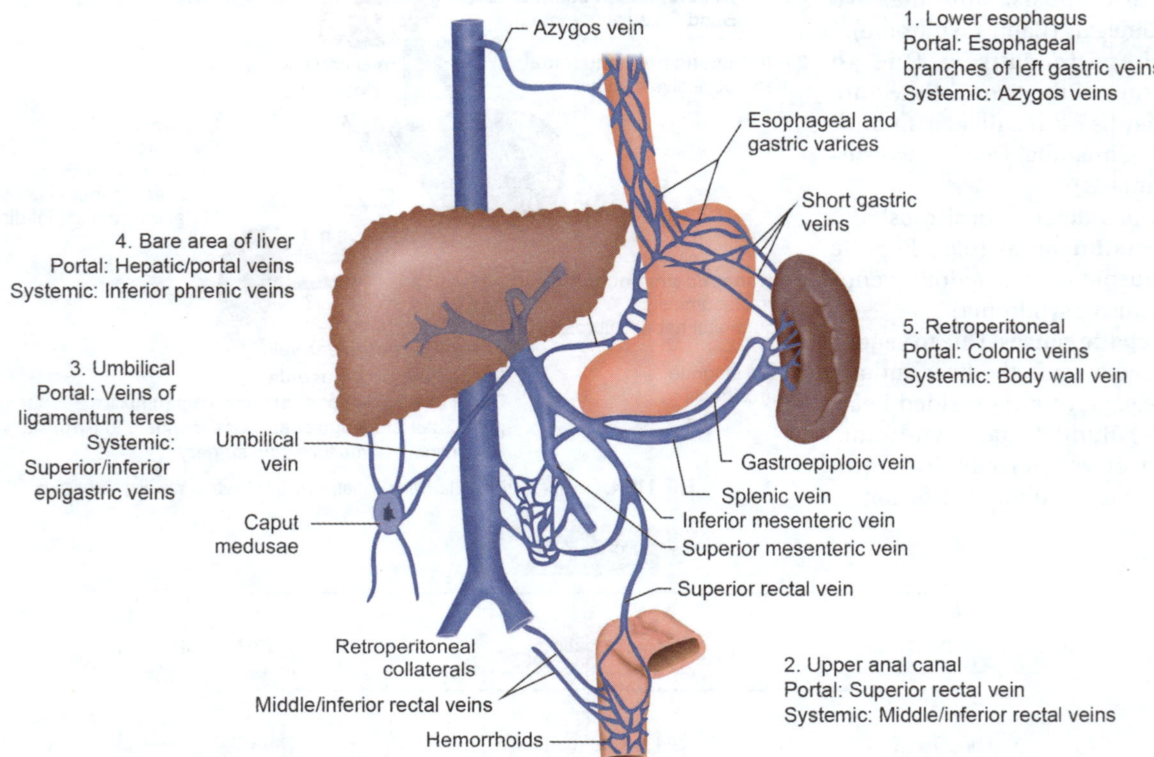

FIG. 11.15: Consequences of portal hypertension with sites of portosystemic anastomosis in cirrhosis.

Clinical Features

Q. Write short note on clinical features and diagnosis of portal hypertension.

- Patients with portal hypertension are often asymptomatic.
- History, e.g., alcoholism, past history of hepatitis. Triad of portal hypertension consists of **ascites, splenomegaly, and dilated tortuous abdominal wall veins (Fig. 11.16).**
- **Bleeding from esophageal varices** or portal hypertensive gastropathy causes hematemesis and melena.
- **Splenomegaly:** It may be only clinical evidence and single most important diagnostic feature of portal hypertension.
    - A diagnosis of portal hypertension should not be made if there is no documentation of splenomegaly either clinically, radiographically or ultrasonography.
    - Usually spleen is palpable less than 5 cm below costal margin. However, marked splenomegaly can be found in younger patients, those with macronodular cirrhosis and in extrahepatic portal hypertension.
    - Hypersplenism manifests as thrombocytopenia and leukopenia. Splenomegaly may disappear after massive GI bleed or shunt surgery.
- **Features due to liver cell failure/hepatic encephalopathy.**
- **Fetor hepaticus:** It is a musty odor of breath due to shunting of blood from portal system to systemic circulation that allows mercaptans to pass directly to the lungs, bypassing the liver.
- **Caput medusae**, suggestive of an intrahepatic cause of portal hypertension, are present around the umbilicus; the flow of blood is away from the umbilicus.
    - In Budd–Chiari syndrome, by contrast, veins are dilated in the flanks and back, and blood flows in a cephalic direction.

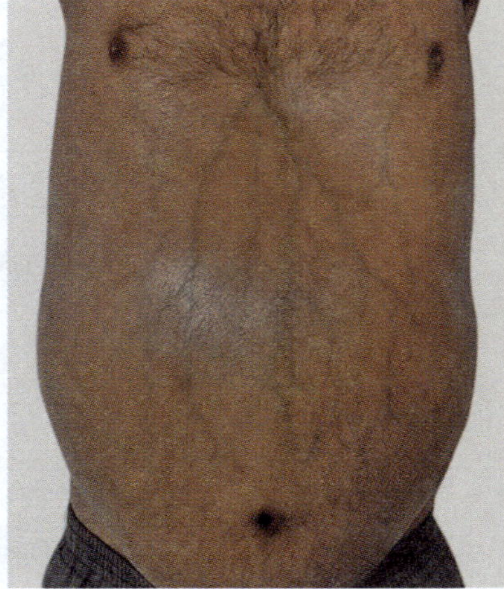

FIG. 11.16: Dilated veins over the anterior abdominal wall and ascites in cirrhosis.

- A bruit may be heard in the left or the right upper quadrant in a patient with a splanchnic arteriovenous fistula.
- **Cruveilhier–Baumgarten syndrome:** A venous hum may be heard in the epigastrium of a patient with portal hypertension and represents collateral flow in the patent umbilical vein in the falciform ligament. A patent umbilical vein excludes an extrahepatic cause of portal hypertension because the umbilical vein arises from the intrahepatic portion of the left portal vein.
- **Rectal varices** may be confused with internal hemorrhoids because of their location. However, hemorrhoids result from a displacement of the anal cushions and hyperperfusion of the arteriovenous plexus vascular cushions without direct communication with any of the major branches of the portal venous system.
- **Liver:** It may be enlarged or shrunken.
  - **Small, contracted, fibrotic** liver is found when the portal venous pressure is very high.
  - Soft liver usually suggestive of extrahepatic portal vein obstruction.
  - Firm liver suggestive of cirrhosis and hence intrahepatic portal hypertension
- **Ascites:** It develops partly due to portal hypertension but mainly due to liver cell failure.

Investigations

The diagnosis of portal hypertension can be made on clinical grounds.

- **Barium swallow:** It shows varices as filling defects in the lower-third of esophagus (**"bag of worms appearance**").
- **Upper GI scopy**
  - Most reliable method of investigation.
  - Esophageal varices appear as blue rounded projections (red spots and red stripes) under submucosa.
  - **"Cherry red spots" indicate impending rupture of varices.**
- **Ultrasonography** (*refer* to **Box 11.22**).
- **Portal venography** (splenoportal venogram) rarely done nowadays.
- **Measurement of portal venous pressure:** By either wedged hepatic venous pressure (WHVP) or transhepatic venous pressure. It is useful for (1) confirmation of portal hypertension, and (2) differentiating sinusoidal from presinusoidal portal hypertension.
- **Proctoscopy and barium enema:** Useful for demonstrating varices in the rectum and colon
- **Liver function tests:** To confirm the liver diseases.

Complications of Portal Hypertension (Box 11.20)

Q. Name the drugs that are used in the reduction of portal venous pressure.

Treatment of Portal Hypertension

- Treatment of underlying disease
- Drugs used in the treatment of portal hypertension **(Box 11.21)**
- Nonselective β-blockers (propranolol, nadolol) produce vasodilatation of both splanchnic arterial bed and portal venous system. Also reduce recurrence of variceal bleed. The usual starting dose of long-acting propranolol is 40 mg once daily and that of nadolol is 20 mg once a daily. **Carvedilol** in addition to reducing portal venous inflow through nonselective beta blockade, the anti-alpha 1 adrenergic activity leads to reduced hepatic vascular tone and hepatic resistance.
- Nitrates (nitroglycerine and isosorbide dinitrate) along with β-blockers reduce the risk of variceal bleed and are used for primary prophylaxis of variceal bleed.

Box 11.20: Complications of portal hypertension.

- Variceal bleeding: Mainly esophageal and gastric
- Hepatic encephalopathy
- Ascites, spontaneous bacterial peritonitis (SBP)
- Hepatorenal, hepatopulmonary syndrome
- Congestive gastropathy
- Hypersplenism
- Iron-deficiency anemia

Box 11.21: Drugs used in the treatment of portal hypertension.

Drugs that decrease portal blood flow:

- Nonselective β-adrenergic blocking agents (propranolol, nadolol, carvedilol)
- Somatostatin and its analogs
- Vasopressin
- Drugs that decrease intrahepatic resistance
- α1-adrenergic blocking agents (e.g., prazosin)
- Angiotensin receptor blocking agents
- Nitrates

Esophageal Varices

Q. Discuss the diagnosis and management of esophageal variceal bleeding.

- About 90% of patients with cirrhosis will develop gastroesophageal varices, but only one-third of these will bleed from them.
- The most common site of bleeding is esophageal varices within 3–5 cm of the esophagogastric junction.
- Factors that predispose to rupture of varices are listed in **Box 11.22.**

Clinical Features

Painless, mild-to-massive hematemesis, with or without associated melena

Signs

- **Depending on the amount of blood loss**, it may vary from mild postural tachycardia to shock.
- **Features of liver cell failure, ascites, and portal hypertension.**

Box 11.22: Factors predisposing varices rupture.

- Large varices
- "Red sign" on varices (diagnosed at endoscopy) suggests imminent rupture.
- Associated with severe liver disease
- High portal venous pressure
- Salicylates and other nonsteroidal anti-inflammatory drugs

Diagnosis

- **Fiberoptic endoscopy:** Performed within 8 hours of bleeding reveals the bleeding site and the presence of varices **(Fig. 11.17)**. This helps in excluding the other causes of bleeding. The descriptors are presented in **Box 11.23**.
- **Ultrasonography:** Useful to confirm the patency of portal vein.

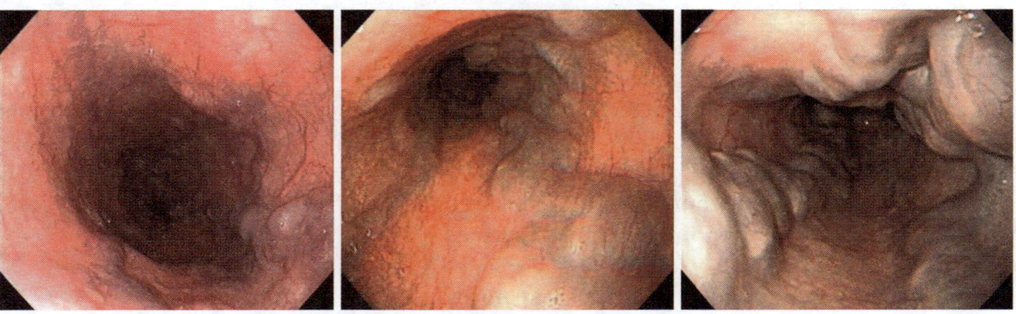

FIG. 11.17: Endoscopy view of esophageal varices (Grade I, II, and III).

Box 11.23: Descriptors of esophageal varices.

- Red color signs (ominous signs) include:
  - Red "wale" markings, which are longitudinal whip-like marks on the varix
  - Cherry-red spots, which usually are 2–3 mm or less in diameter
  - Hematocystic spots are blood-filled blisters 4 mm in diameter
- Color of the varix can be white or blue
- Form (size) of the varix at endoscopy:
  - Grade I: Esophageal varices may be small and straight
  - Grade II: Tortuous and occupying less than one-third of the esophageal lumen
  - Grade III: Large and occupying more than one-third of the esophageal lumen

Q. Describe the management of acute variceal bleeding. Describe the medical management of bleeding of esophageal varices.

Management

Management goal **(Box 11.24)**.

Box 11.24: Management goal in esophageal varices.

- Management of the active bleeding episode
- Prevention of rebleeding
- Prophylactic measures to prevent the first hemorrhage

Management of acute variceal bleeding (Flowchart 11.2)

General measures—resuscitation

- **Immediate hospitalization and nursing:** Patients require intensive-care nursing. Nil by mouth until bleeding stops.
- Assess the general condition of the patient pulse and blood pressure and maintain fluid (intake and output) and electrolyte balance.
- Obtain blood for grouping and crossmatching, hemoglobin, prothrombin time, blood urea, electrolytes, creatinine, LFTs, and blood cultures.
- Grade cirrhosis according to Child-Pugh score (*refer* **Table 11.31**).
- Immediately restore blood volume with blood transfusion and avoid saline infusions as far as possible. Prompt correction of hypovolemia is needed.
- Correction of coagulation factor deficiency by fresh blood or fresh frozen plasma.
- Platelet transfusions to raise platelet count above 50,000/mm^3.
- Vitamin K is administered intramuscularly or intravenously.
- To prevent stress ulcers, give H_2 receptor antagonists (e.g., cimetidine, ranitidine or famotidine) or proton-pump inhibitors (e.g., pantoprazole or omeprazole).
- **Prophylactic antibiotics:** Reduce infection and mortality and prevent spontaneous bacterial peritonitis (SBP). Usually oral and intravenous quinolones are used (e.g., ciprofloxacin 500 mg twice daily).

- **Measures to prevent hepatic encephalopathy:** Portosystemic encephalopathy (PSE) may be precipitated when the amount of bleeding is large because blood contains protein.
- Treatment of ascites by ascitic tap (paracentesis) or by administration of spironolactone or amiloride.
- Monitor for alcohol withdrawal (in case of alcoholic cirrhosis) and give thiamine.

Urgent endoscopy

- Urgent endoscopy is done to confirm the diagnosis of gastroesophageal varices. Varices may or may not be present and it helps to exclude bleeding from other sites (e.g., gastric ulceration).
- **Portal hypertensive (or congestive) gastropathy** is defined as chronic gastric congestion, punctate erythema, and gastric erosions. It can also cause bleeding.
- To reduce esophageal ulceration following endoscopic therapy, sucralfate is given in the dose of 1 g four times daily.

Local measures

Injection sclerotherapy or variceal banding

Acute variceal bleeding may be treated by endoscopic procedure with (1) sclerotherapy and (2) endoscopic variceal banding [endoscopic variceal band ligation (EVBL)]. They arrest bleeding in 80% of cases and reduce early rebleeding.

- **Sclerotherapy:** Injection of sclerosing agent into the varices may arrest bleeding by producing thrombosis of vessel. Commonly used sclerosants are listed in **Box 11.25** and complications of sclerotherapy are mentioned in **Table 11.33**.
- **Banding (Fig. 11.18):** Varices are banded by mounting a band on the tip of the endoscope, sucking the varix just into the end of the scope and dislodging the band over the varix.
- **Cyanoacrylate injection** is used in patients with large gastric varices.

Vasoconstrictor therapy

- **Uses:** This therapy is mainly used for (1) emergency control of bleeding while waiting for endoscopy, and (2) in combination with endoscopic techniques.

Aim: To reduce the portal inflow of blood and portal pressure constricting the splanchnic arterioles.

Drugs used

- **Terlipressin**
  - Action: Terlipressin produces vasoconstriction by releasing vasopressin from it.
  - Dose: 2 mg IV 6-hourly till bleeding stops, and then reduced to 1 mg 4-hourly after 48 hours if a prolonged dosage regimen is used.
  - Contraindication: Patients with ischemic heart disease.
  - Side effects: Abdominal colic, evacuation of bowels, and facial pallor due to the generalized vasoconstriction.
- **Somatostatin and octreotide**
  - Somatostatin and its synthetic analog octreotide stops bleeding from varices in more than 80% patients.
  - Its effects are equivalent to vasopressin and endoscopic therapy.
  - Side-effects: Very few.
  - Dose:
    - Somatostatin: Infusion of 250–500 µg/h followed by 250 µg/h for 2–5 days.
    - Octreotide: 50 µg as bolus followed by 50 µg/h for 2–5 days.
  - Indication: When there are contraindications to terlipressin.
- Vasopressin [0.1–0.5 units/min for 4–12 hours (up to 48 hours)]: It was used in the past but is not commonly used now.

FLOWCHART 11.2: Algorithm for the treatment of bleeding from acute esophageal varices.

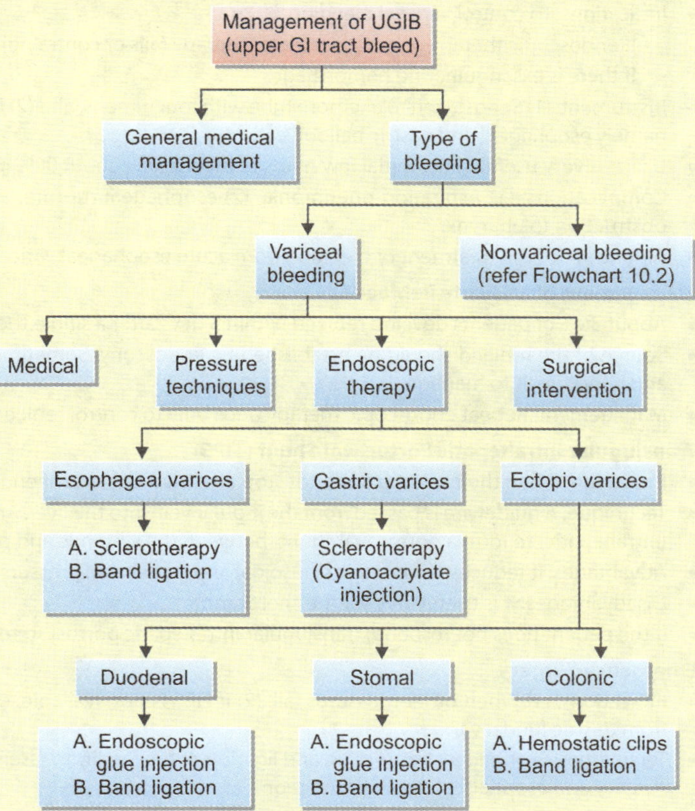

Box 11.25: Commonly used sclerosants in esophageal varices.

- Ethanolamine oleate
- Sodium morrhuate
- Absolute alcohol
- Sodium tetradecylsulfonate

TABLE 11.33: Complications of sclerotherapy.

Esophageal complications	Pulmonary complications
➢ Reappearance of varices ➢ Esophageal ulceration and perforation ➢ Esophageal reflux ➢ Stricture formation	➢ Chest pain, pleural effusion, mediastinitis, and aspiration pneumonia ➢ Acute respiratory failure
Abdominal pain, fever, and dysphagia	Spinal cord paralysis due to anterior spinal artery occlusion
	Mortality: 1%

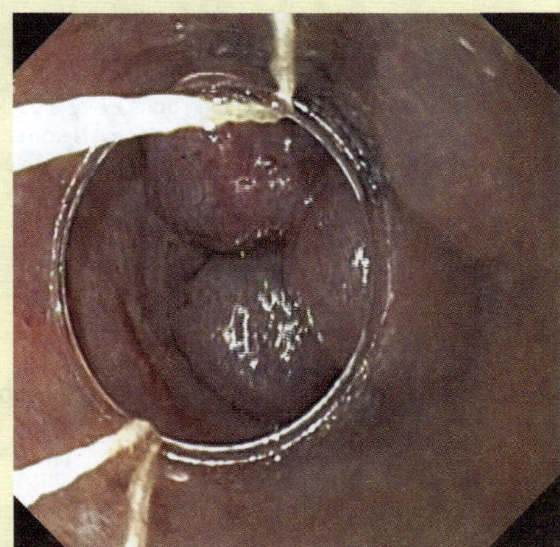

FIG. 11.18: Banding of esophageal varices.

Balloon Tamponade

- Indications: To control variceal bleeding
  - If endoscopic therapy or vasoconstrictor therapy fails or contraindicated
  - If there is exsanguinating hemorrhage
- Instrument: (1) Sengstaken–Blakemore tube with four lumens, and (2) Minnesota tube with four lumens. These tubes have two balloons, namely esophageal and gastric balloons.
- Use: It is very useful in the initial few hours of bleeding in about 90% of cases.
- Complications: (1) Aspiration pneumonia, (2) esophageal rupture, and (3) necrosis and ulcerations of esophageal mucosa, and (4) obstruction to pharynx.
- Algorithm for the treatment of bleeding from acute esophageal varices **(Flowchart 11.2)**

Management of an Acute Rebleed

- About 30% of patients develop rebleed within 5 days after a single therapeutic endoscopy.
- Source of the rebleed should be established by endoscopy. Sometimes it is due to an ulcer developed due to previous sclerotherapy and it is difficult to manage.
- Management: Repeat endoscopic therapy once only to control rebleeding and further sclerotherapy or banding should not be done.

Transjugular Intrahepatic Portocaval Shunt (TIPS)

- Indication: When the bleeding does not stop after two sessions of endoscopic therapy within 5 days.
- Technique: A guidewire is passed from the jugular vein into the liver. An expandable metal shunt is forced over it into the liver substance (intrahepatic) to form a portocaval shunt (between the systemic and portal venous systems).
- Advantages: It reduces the hepatic sinusoidal and portal vein pressure without the risks of general anesthesia and major surgery.
- Disadvantages: It is useful only for the short term.
- If the patient does not respond, transjugular intrahepatic portosystemic shunt (TIPSS) is useful in most patients.

Emergency Surgery

- Indications: (1) When other measures fail, (2) if TIPS is not available, (3) continued or recurrent hemorrhage, and (4) if the bleeding is from gastric fundal varices.
- Techniques: Esophageal transection and ligation of the feeding vessels to the bleeding varices. Infrequently acute portosystemic shunt surgery and esophageal staple transaction.

PREVENTION OF VARICEAL BLEEDING—PROPHYLAXIS

Primary Prophylactic Measures	
Useful in patients with cirrhosis and varices, who have not bled.	
Nonselective β-blockers: Propranolol, nadolol ➢ Reduce chance of upper GI bleeding, cost-effective. Reduce recurrence. ➢ Efficacy is similar to prophylactic banding. ➢ Act by vasodilatation of splanchnic arterial bed and portal venous system.	**Nitrates:** Nitroglycerine, isosorbide dinitrate Given with-blockers—reduced risk of variceal bleed Variceal banding is done if there are contraindications or intolerance to nonselective beta-blockers
Recurrent Variceal Bleeding (Secondary Prophylaxis)	
Bleeding recurs in about 60–80% of patients within 2 years after initial bleed.	
Long-term measures	**Surgical portosystemic shunting**
Nonselective beta-blockers: Treatment of choice. Propranolol: 80–160 mg/day oral, decreases portal pressure, decreases frequency of rebleed (as effective as sclerotherapy or ligation), prevents bleeding from portal hypertensive gastropathy. **Endoscopic treatment:** Injection sclerotherapy or variceal banding. Repeated courses of banding done every 2 weeks until the varices are obliterated. It is superior to sclerotherapy. **Transjugular portosystemic stent shunts:** Reduce rebleeding rates compared to endoscopic techniques but associated with increased rate of encephalopathy. Used if endoscopic or medical therapy fails.	Performed in patients with good liver function (Child–Pugh A, B), when medical therapy, EVBL and sclerotherapy are unsuccessful with very low risk of rebleeding. **Types of portal systemic shunts:** ➢ *Nonselective shunt with end-to-side portocaval anastomosis* decompresses entire portal venous system, produces significant postoperative hepatic encephalopathy. ➢ *Selective distal splenorenal (Warren) shunt*- decompress only varices while maintaining blood flow to liver via superior mesenteric vein, produces less encephalopathy. **Complications of portosystemic shunts** 5% mortality, shunt closure, hepatic encephalopathy due to reduction in portal pressure and hepatic blood flow, postoperative jaundice because of deterioration of liver function. **Esophageal transection:** Devascularization procedure that does not produce encephalopathy. **Liver transplantation:** Treatment of choice when liver function is poor.

HEPATIC ENCEPHALOPATHY

Q. Define hepatic (portosystemic) encephalopathy.

Definition

Hepatic encephalopathy or portosystemic encephalopathy is defined as a **neuropsychiatric syndrome** (alteration in mental status and cognitive function) occurring **secondary to chronic liver disease**. Encephalopathy may be **acute** and potentially reversible, **or chronic** and progressive.

Etiology

Q. Discuss the etiology, pathogenesis, clinical features, precipitating factors, investigations, and treatment/management of hepatic encephalopathy.

Q. Write short essay on alcoholic cirrhosis with acute hepatic encephalopathy.

- More common in patients with chronic liver disease such as **cirrhosis.** In patients with portal hypertension, it develops due to spontaneous "shunting" or in patients following a **portosystemic shunt procedure**, e.g., TIPS (transjugular intrahepatic portocaval shunt). *Adult-onset citrullinemia type II closely mimics hepatic encephalopathy.*
- Acute encephalopathy can occur in **acute fulminant hepatic failure**.

Pathogenesis

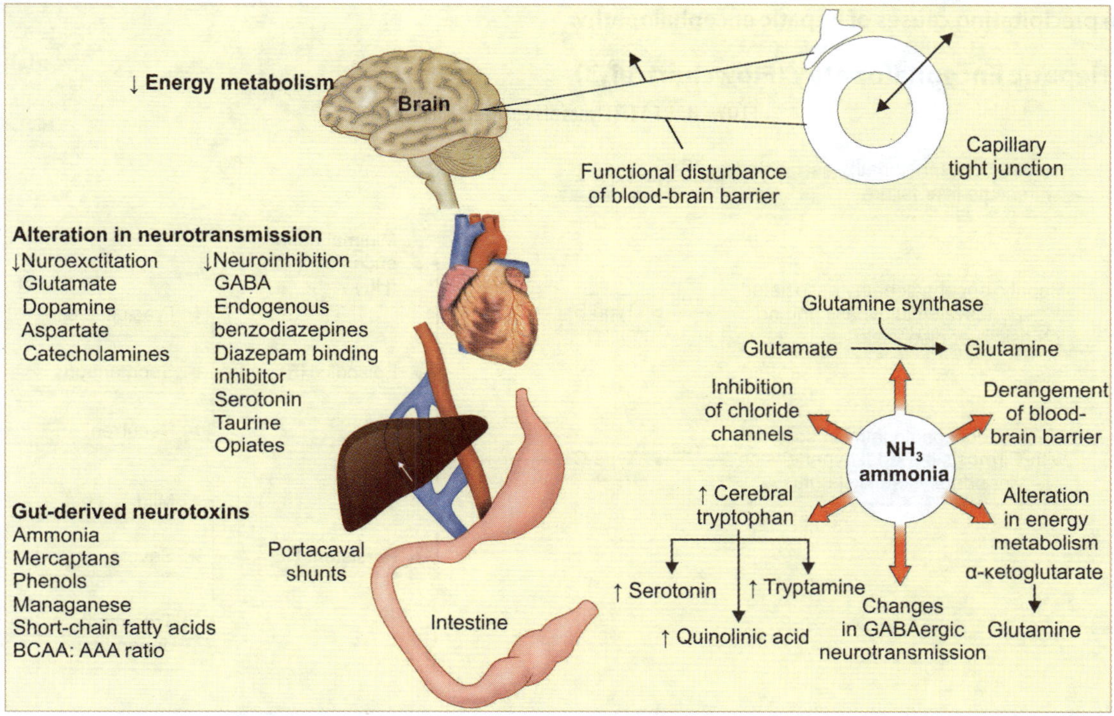

(BCAA:AAA: branched-chain amino acid:aromatic amino acid; GABA: gamma aminobutyric acid)

- **Mechanism is unknown** but many factors play a role. Six pathogenic mechanisms have been proposed.
  1. Gut-derived neurotoxins that are normally metabolized by the liver
  2. Brain water homeostasis
  3. Oxidative/nitrosative stress
  4. Astrocyte dysregulation
  5. Neurotransmitter dysfunction (decreased glutamine, increased GABA, serotonin)
  6. Infection and inflammation
- Hepatic encephalopathy develops **due to disturbance of brain function resulting from various toxic substances reaching the brain**. Normally, these toxic substances are derived from the intestine (gut-derived neurotoxins) and carried by portal circulation to the liver, where they are detoxified. Hence, they neither enter the systemic circulation nor reach the brain.
- In hepatic encephalopathy, these toxic substances are not removed by the liver and reach the brain. **Three factors are responsible** for this are:
  1. **Vascular shunting/bypassing the liver:** The portal blood bypasses the liver via the collaterals into systemic circulation and the "toxic" metabolites pass directly to thebrain.
  2. **Decreased liver mass:** It results in severe hepatocellular dysfunction leading to defective detoxification of the toxic substances.
  3. **Increased permeability of the blood-brain barrier:** Allows the toxins to enter the brain.
- **Toxic substances:** Involved in hepatic encephalopathy is listed in **Table 11.34 Ammonia plays a major role** and is produced by the breakdown of protein by intestinal bacteria.

TABLE 11.34: Toxic substances involved in hepatic encephalopathy.

➤ Ammonia plays major role	➤ Aromatic amino acids (tyrosine and phenylalanine)
➤ Free fatty acids	➤ Reduced branched-chain amino acids (valine, leucine and isoleucine)
➤ Mercaptans derived from methionine	➤ Phenol, Indole (oxindole)
➤ γ-aminobutyric acid (GABA)	➤ False neurotransmitters (octopamine)

*Precipitating Factors for Portosystemic/Hepatic Encephalopathy (**Table 11.35**)*

TABLE 11.35: Precipitating factors for hepatic/portosystemic encephalopathy.	
➢ Increased protein load	➢ Acute infections including spontaneous bacterial peritonitis
– Dietary protein	➢ Drugs, e.g., sedatives, antidepressants, narcotics, alcohol
– Gastrointestinal bleeding	➢ Viral/alcoholic hepatitis
➢ Fluid and electrolyte disturbance such as hypokalemia, hyponatremia, metabolic alkalosis due to:	➢ Surgical procedure: Portosystemic shunt operations
– Large-volume paracentesis	➢ Development of hepatocellular carcinoma, hepatic or portal vein thrombosis
– Overzealous use of diuretics	➢ Uremia
– Vomiting and diarrhea	➢ Constipation

Q. List the precipitating causes of hepatic encephalopathy.

Types of Hepatic Encephalopathy (Flowchart 11.3)

FLOWCHART 11.3: Types of hepatic encephalopathy.

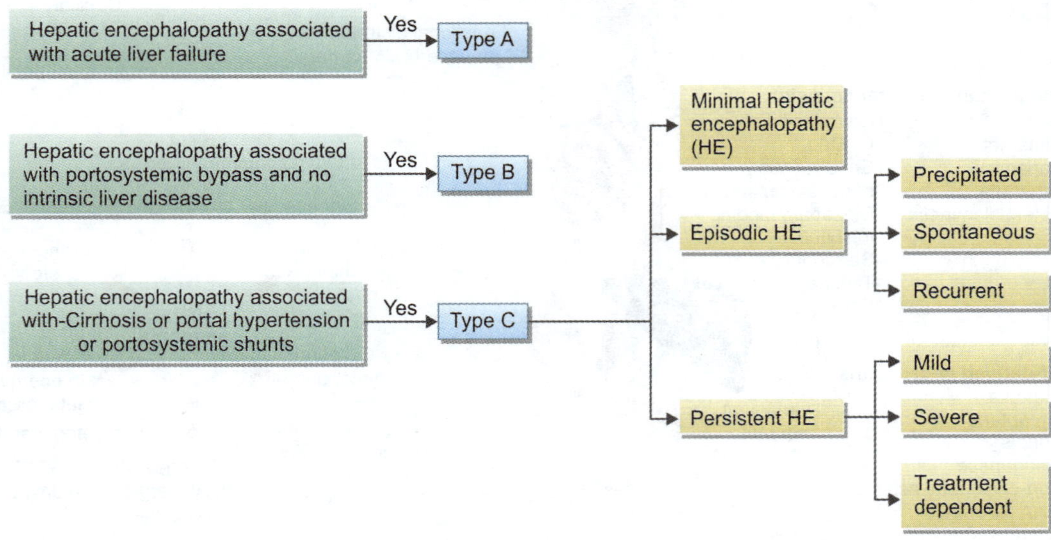

Clinical Features

- **Acute hepatic (portosystemic) encephalopathy** often has a precipitating factor (**Table 11.35**) and the patient becomes drowsy and comatose within weeks to months. Brain edema may occur with severe encephalopathy and may lead to cerebral herniation.
- **Chronic hepatic (portosystemic) encephalopathy**
- **Disturbances in consciousness and behavior** may fluctuate. Hypersomnia is the earliest feature and may progress to **reversion of sleep rhythm (daytime somnolence).** Patient may become quite violent and difficult to manage or may be very sleepy and difficult to rouse. Patients are **irritable, confused, disoriented** with slow slurred speech, later may become drowsy and eventually progress to coma.

Clinical grade of hepatic encephalopathy are presented in **Table 11.36**.

TABLE 11.36: West Haven criteria clinical grade of hepatic encephalopathy.			
Clinical grade	***Clinical signs***		
Grade	**Consciousness**	**Intellect and Behavior**	**Neurological Findings**
0	Normal	Normal	Normal examination or impaired psychomotor testing
1	Mild lack of awareness	Shortened attention span; impaired addition or subtraction	Mild asterixis or tremor
2	Lethargic	Disoriented, inappropriate behavior	Obvious asterixis, slurred speech
3	Somnolent but arousable	Gross disorientation, Bizarre behavior	Muscular rigidity and clonus, Hyper-reflexia
4	Coma	Coma	Decerebrate posturing

- **Change in personality mood and intellect**
- General features: Nausea, vomiting, and weakness

Signs

- **Fetor hepaticus** (a sweet smell to the breath).
- **Asterixis** (flapping tremors) (*refer* **Fig. 11.13A**) is a motor disturbance marked by intermittent lapses of an assumed posture, as a result of intermittency of sustained contraction of groups of muscles. Usually manifests as a bilateral flapping tremor at the wrist, metacarpophalangeal, and hip joints. It may also be seen in tongue, foot, and any skeletal muscle.
  - **Mechanism:** Probably due to interruption of the posture pathway in the rostral reticular formation and abnormal joint proprioception.
  - The lapse of posture has been termed **"negative myoclonus"** because during tonic muscle contraction (i.e., posture), a short electromyography (EMG) silent period precedes the tremor.
  - **Causes:** Hepatic encephalopathy, renal failure, metabolic encephalopathy, CO_2 toxicity, Wilson's disease, electrolyte abnormalities (hypoglycemia, hypokalemia, and hypomagnesemia), drug intoxications [e.g., barbiturate intoxication, alcoholism, phenytoin intoxication ("phenytoin flap") and primidone intoxication] and psychotropic drugs (clozapine, sodium valproate, and risperidone). Lesions in the genu and anterior portion of the internal capsule or ventrolateral thalamus may cause unilateral asterixis.
- Fluctuating neurological signs
- Constructional apraxia with the patient being unable to write or draw
- Hypertonia—later hypotonia
- Hyperreflexia and extensor plantar, later loss of reflexes

International Society for Hepatic Encephalopathy and Nitrogen Metabolism (ISHEN) criteria and Full Outline of Unresponsiveness (FOUR):which assesses four components: eye response, motor response, brain-stem reflex, and respirations are better scoring systems .

Diagnosis: It is based on clinical features. Diagnosis of minimal hepatic encephalopathy is currently based on neuropsychometric tests, including the number connection test, digit symbol test, and the block design test.

Reitan Number Connection Test (Fig. 11.19)

There are 25 numbered circles which can normally be joined together within 30 seconds.

Critical Flicker Frequency

- Critical Flicker frequency (CFF) is a test of retinal gliopathy (that occurs in patients with HE) that can be performed using a portable machine.
- During this test, the patient is asked to indicate the maximum frequency at which they can still perceive the light as flickering while changing the frequency over time.
- A CFF threshold of 38–39 Hz has been shown to differentiate between manifest HE (i.e., early stages of OHE) and no HE

Investigations

- **Blood ammonia levels: Raised** (upper limit of normal is 0.8–1 μg/mL) and can be used for the differential diagnosis of coma and to follow a patient with PSE.
- Serum levels of **3-nitrotyrosine** may be elevated in patients with minimal hepatic encephalopathy
- **Electroencephalography (EEG):** Bilaterally synchronous decrease in wave frequency and an increase in wave amplitude, associated with the disappearance of a readily discernible normal alpha-rhythm (8–13 cps).
- **Cerebrospinal fluid: Glutamine increased,** proteins normal, and cell count normal
- Visual evoked potential abnormalities may be present during subclinical encephalopathy.
- Routine LFTs only confirm the presence of liver disease and not the presence of encephalopathy.
- Imaging is performed to rule out other causes.

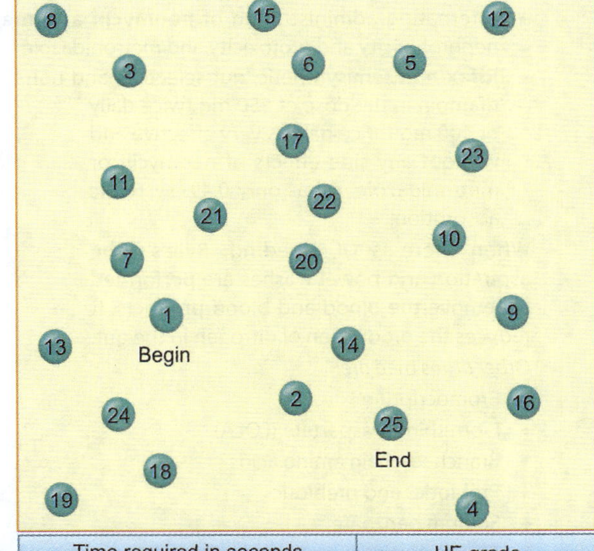

Time required in seconds	HE grade
≤30	None-minimal
31–50	Minimal-I
51–80	I-II
81–120	II-III
Forced termination	III

FIG. 11.19: Number connection test.

Q. Write short note on treatment of hepatic encephalopathy.

Treatment of hepatic encephalopathy

Treatment is multifactorial. Restriction of protein intake is reserved for resistant cases.

General measures:

- Management or removal of the precipitating factors is the most important aspect in the treatment.
- Maintain nutrition with adequate calories 35–40 kcal/kg/day.
- Maintain hydration and correct the electrolyte imbalance.
- **Protein restriction** in the diet. Administer 1.0–1.2 g/kg of proteins daily, preferably vegetable protein.
- Zinc supplementation may be helpful and is relatively harmless.
- Stop or reduce diuretic therapy.
- Treat any infection with **suitable antibiotics** (e.g., ampicillin, rifaximin, metronidazole, or neomycin).
- Stop alcohol. **Avoid sedatives.** For restlessness and excitement, small dose of diazepam or midazolam may be given intravenously.

Evacuation of the bowels and sterilizing the bowel:

- Give purgation and enemas to empty the bowels of nitrogenous substances.
- **Lactulose therapy:** To reduce plasma ammonia level
  - Actions: Lactulose (beta-galactosidofructose) is a nonabsorbable disaccharide, which acts as an osmotic purgative. In the colon, lactulose and lactitol are catabolized by the bacterial flora to lactic acid and acetic acid. It lowers the colonic pH and favors the formation of the nonabsorbable NH^{+} from NH, trapping NH^{+} in the colon and thus reducing plasma ammonia concentrations. Other mechanisms of action include (1) increased incorporation of ammonia by bacteria for synthesis of nitrogenous compounds, (2) modification of colonic flora, resulting in displacement of urease-producing bacteria with nonurease-producing bacteria and cathartic effects that improves GI transit, allowing less time for ammonia absorption, (3) increased fecal nitrogen excretion due to the increase in stool volume, and (4) reduced formation of toxic short-chain fatty acids (e.g., propionate, butyrate, valerate).
  - Dose: 15–30 mL three times orally per day. Dose is increased gradually till there are two to three loose stools per day.
  - **Lactitol** (β-galactoside sorbitol 30 g daily): It has a similar action, more palatable and better than lactulose.
    - Poorly absorbed antibiotics: They are often used as adjunctive to sterilize the gut in patients who have difficulty with lactulose. They reduce the intestinal ammonia production by bacteria.
    - Alternating administration of **neomycin and metronidazole** to reduce the individual side effects of each neomycin for nephrotoxicity and ototoxicity and metronidazole for peripheral neuropathy.
    - **Rifaximin** semisynthetic, gut-selective, and nonabsorbable oral antibiotic, derived from rifamycin and a structural analog of rifampin in the dose of 550 mg twice daily or 400 mg thrice daily is very effective and without any side effects of neomycin or metronidazole. It has only 0.4% systemic absorption.
  - When there is GI bleeding, Ryle's tube aspiration and bowel washes are performed to remove the blood and blood products. It reduces the production of nitrogen in the gut.
  - *Other drugs tried are:*
    - Bromocriptine
    - L-ornithine L-aspartate (LOLA)
    - Branched-chain amino acids
    - Probiotics and prebiotics
    - Sodium benzoate
    - Zinc, polyethylene glycol, acarbose
    - Flumazenil
    - Melatonin
- Novel treatment strategies include use of L carnitine, rivastigmine, endocannabinoids, and mGluR1 antagonists.
  - In acute liver failure, mannitol and judicious use of intravenous fluids to reduce the spontaneous cerebral edema (controversial).
  - Liver transplantation.
  - **MARS**—Molecular Adsorption Reversibility System—purifies the blood by removal of albumin bound as well as water-soluble substrates.

Management of hepatic encephalopathy is summarized in **Flowchart 11.4**.

FLOWCHART 11.4: Management of hepatic encephalopathy.

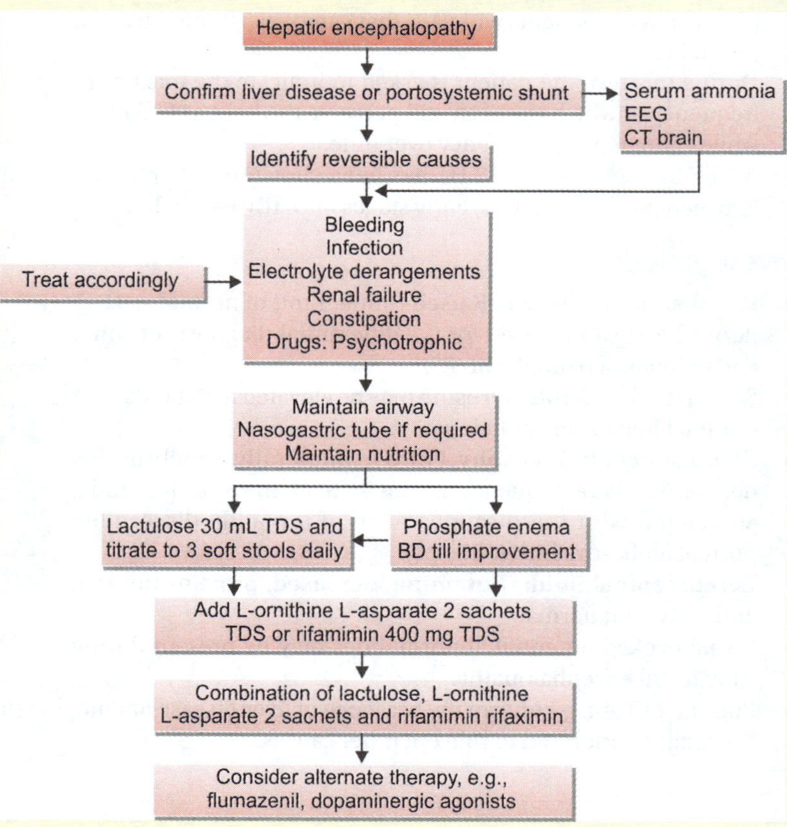

Hepatorenal Syndrome

Q. Write a short note on hepatorenal syndrome.

- Hepatorenal syndrome (HRS) is a form of **functional azotemia without renal pathology in patients with advanced cirrhosis or acute liver failure**.
- The urine output is low, tubular function is normal, and kidneys are histologically normal.
- This occurs in 10% of patients with advanced cirrhosis with jaundice and ascites.

Pathogenesis

- **Initially, severe peripheral vasodilatation** (probably due to nitric oxide), leads to severe **reduction in the effective blood volume and hypotension**.
- This **activates** the homeostatic mechanisms and **rennin-angiotensin-aldosterone system leading to vasoconstriction of the renal vessels**.
- Increased preglomerular vascular resistance directs the flow of blood away from the renal cortex. This leads to a **reduced glomerular filtration rate**.
- **Eicosanoids** are another mediator involved in pathogenesis of HRS.

Box 11.26: Precipitating factors for hepatorenal syndrome (HRS).

- Gastrointestinal bleeding
- Aggressive paracentesis
- Diuretic therapy
- Sepsis including spontaneous bacterial peritonitis
- Diarrhea

Precipitating Factors for HRS

See **Box 11.26**.

Clinical Types

Type 1 hepatorenal syndrome (HRS)	*Type 2 hepatorenal syndrome*
➢ Progressive oliguria, rapid rise of serum creatinine to > 2.5 mg/dL ➢ Very poor prognosis ➢ Precipitated by spontaneous bacterial peritonitis ➢ Without treatment, median survival is <1 month, die within 10 weeks after onset of renal failure	➢ Reduction in glomerular filtration, moderate, stable increase of serum creatinine (>1.5 mg/dL) ➢ Better prognosis than Type 1 HRS ➢ Usually occurs in patients with refractory ascites (resistant to diuretics) ➢ Median survival is 3–6 months

Clinical Features

- Develops in advanced cirrhosis, almost always with ascites
- Anorexia, weakness, fatigue, oliguria, nausea, vomiting, and thirst
- Terminally coma deepens and hypotension develops.

Investigations

- **Urea and creatinine levels: High**.
- Serum sodium: Less than 130 mEq/L.
- Urine sodium excretion: Less than 10 mEq/day
- Urinalysis: Normal
- Urine: Plasma osmolality ratio is more than 1.5.

Diagnosis

Usually made in the presence of a large amount of ascites in patients who have a stepwise progressive increase in creatinine.

Diagnostic criteria HRS (**Table 11.37**)

TABLE 11.37: All of the following must be present for the diagnosis of hepatorenal syndrome (HRS).

➢ Cirrhosis with ascites
➢ Serum creatinine > 1.5 mg/dL
➢ No improvement of serum creatinine (decrease to a level of 1.5 mg/dL or less) after at least 2 days of diuretic withdrawal and volume expansion with albumin
➢ Absence of shock
➢ No current or recent treatment with nephrotoxic drugs
➢ Absence of parenchymal kidney disease as indicated by proteinuria > 500 mg/day, microhematuria (>50 red blood cells per high power field), and/or abnormal renal ultrasonography

Treatment

- **Prevention:**
  - Avoid over vigorous diuretic therapy
  - Slow treatment of ascites
  - Early recognition of electrolyte imbalance, hemorrhage, or infection
- **Stop diuretic therapy.**
- **Correct hypovolemia** by intravenous plasma protein solution or salt-poor albumin
- Screen and **treat infection** including SBP
- An **albumin infusion** (1 g/kg bodyweight/day up to a maximum of 100 g/day) in combination with **terlipressin** (vasopressin analogs) is effective short-term medical therapy
- Currently, **midodrine** (α-agonist) along with octreotide and intravenous albumin is also used.
- Renal replacement therapy
- TIPSS if vasoconstrictors fail

Liver transplantation is the treatment of choice

ASCITES

Q. Discuss the pathogenesis and management of ascites and refractory ascites in cirrhosis.

Q. Discuss the definition, mechanism, causes, clinical features and differential diagnosis of ascites.

Ascites is defined as the **accumulation of excess fluid within the peritoneal cavity**.

The **most common** (85% of cases) **cause** of ascites is **portal hypertension** caused by **cirrhosis**; however, malignant or infectious causes can also produce ascites.

Pathogenesis/Mechanisms

Pathogenesis of Ascites in Cirrhosis (Fig. 11.20)

It is complex, involving the following mechanisms:

- **Portal hypertension:** Increase in portal vein hydrostatic pressure and results in extravasation of fluid from plasma into the peritoneal cavity.
- **Hypoalbuminemia:** Due to decreased synthetic function in a cirrhotic liver, plasma oncotic pressure is reduced. This results in an extravasation of fluid (ascites and edema).
- **Splanchnic vasodilation and hyperdynamic circulation**. It reduces systemic arterial blood pressure, activates **renin-angiotensin-aldosterone system** with the development of **secondary hyperaldosteronism.** Failure of liver to metabolize aldosterone intensifies secondary hyperaldosteronism. It leads to **sodium retention** and **fluid accumulation** and expansion of the extracellular fluid volume.

  The combination of portal hypertension, splanchnic arterial vasodilation, and sodium and water retention increases the hydrostatic pressure as well as permeability of interstitial capillaries. It causes extravasation of fluid into the peritoneal cavity.
- **Percolation of hepatic lymph into the peritoneal cavity:** In cirrhosis, hepatic lymphatic flow exceeds thoracic duct capacity. The excess lymph oozes freely from the surface of cirrhotic liver into the peritoneal cavity and causes ascites.

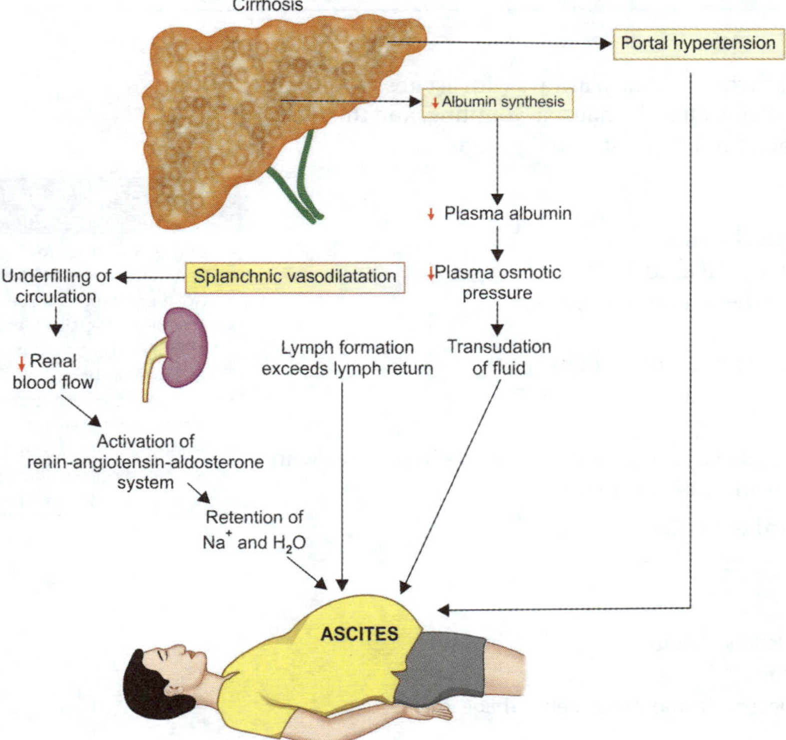

FIG. 11.20: Pathogenesis of ascites in cirrhosis.

Theories of ascites: According to the **underfill theory**, transudation from the liver leads to reduction of the blood volume, thereby stimulating sodium (Na) retention by the kidney.

- According to the **overflow theory**, increased portal pressure stimulates renal Na retention through incompletely defined mechanisms.
- The **vasodilation theory** suggests that portal hypertension leads to vasodilation and relative arterial hypotension.

Pathogenesis in the Absence of Cirrhosis

In Cirrhosis	*Absence of Cirrhosis*
Portal hypertension	**Inflammation of peritoneum**:
Increase in portal vein hydrostatic pressure, cause extravasation of fluid from plasma into the peritoneal cavity.	Peritonitis from bacteria or mycobacteria causes increased vascular permeability and exudation of fluid into peritoneal cavity.
Hypoalbuminemia	**Venous obstruction**
Decreased synthetic function in cirrhosis reduces plasma oncotic pressure, results in extravasation of fluid (ascites and edema).	Inferior vena caval (IVC) obstruction increases the hydrostatic pressure, leads to transudation of fluid into peritoneal cavity.
Splanchnic vasodilation	**Lymphatic obstruction**
Reduction of arterial blood pressure activates **renin–angiotensin–aldosterone system** causing secondary hyperaldosteronism. Liver fails to metabolize aldosterone increased hyperaldosteronism. It causes **sodium and fluid retention.**	Obstruction of lymphatic flow due to involvement of mesenteric lymph nodes, thoracic duct, and abdominal lymphatic ducts can cause leakage of chyle into peritoneal cavity and can lead to chylous ascites.
Percolation of lymph	**Rupture of a viscus**
In cirrhosis, hepatic lymphatic flow exceeds thoracic duct capacity. Excess lymph oozes freely from the surface of cirrhotic liver into the peritoneal cavity causing ascites.	Outpouring of blood, cystic fluid, contaminated material, favoring ascites. Pancreatic ascites results from leakage of pancreatic enzymes into the peritoneum (pancreatitis).
Combination of portal hypertension, splanchnic arterial vasodilation, and sodium and water retention increases the hydrostatic pressure as well as permeability of interstitial capillaries. It causes extravasation of fluid into the peritoneal cavity.	**Malignancy**: Primary peritoneal malignancies (mesothelioma, sarcoma), abdominal malignancies (gastric, colonic adenocarcinoma) or metastatic disease from breast, lung, or melanoma.

Clinical Features

Symptoms

- Distension of abdominal (increase in abdominal girth) and bloated feeling often accompanied by peripheral edema.
- Ascitic fluid may cause elevation of diaphragm and compromise respiratory function and produce dyspnea and orthopnea.
- Indigestion and heart burns due to gastroesophageal reflux may develop because of increased intra-abdominal pressure.
- Malnourishment and patients have muscle wasting and excessive fatigue and weakness.

Signs (Fig. 11.21 and Box 11.27)

- Distension of abdomen and fullness of flanks (bloated feeling)
- Umbilicus appear flat or everted.
- Skin over the abdominal wall appear stretched and shiny.
- In the erect posture, hypogastrium appears prominent.
- Abdominal wall may show two types of distended veins:
  - **Caput medusae** in which veins radiate out from the umbilicus with blood flow away from the umbilicus. They represent collaterals developed due to portal hypertension.

Box 11.27: Five signs of ascites.

1. Horseshoe dullness
2. Shifting dullness
3. Puddle sign
4. Fullness of flank
5. Fluid thrill/fluid wave

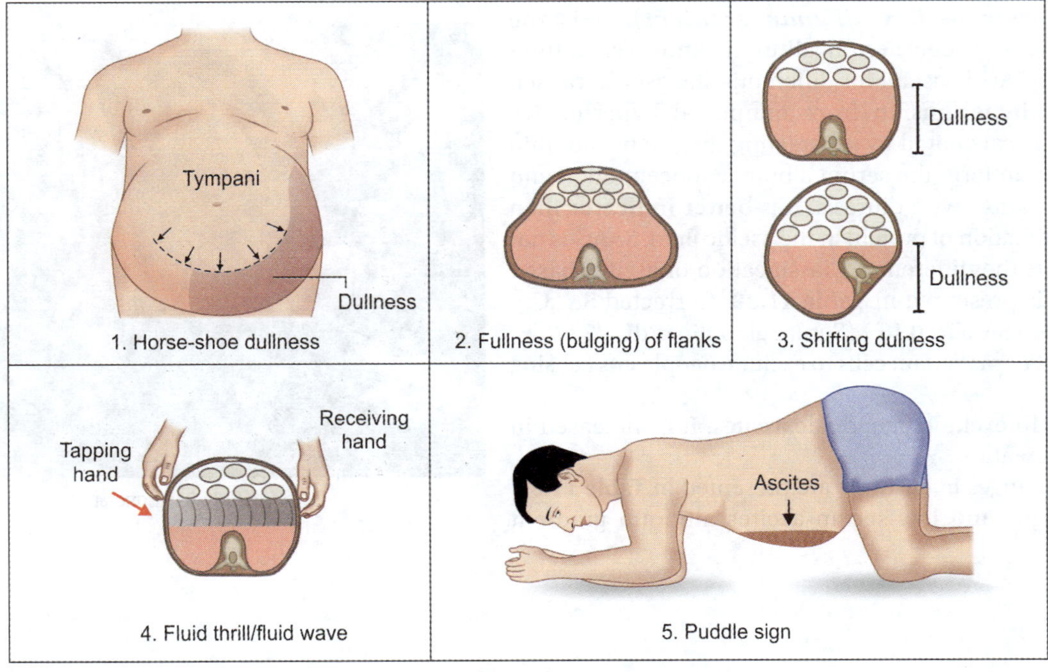

FIG. 11.21: Signs of ascites.

- **Prominent veins in the flanks** with blood flow from below upward. They represent the IVC collaterals developed due to compression of IVC by severe ascites.
- **Abdominal dullness:** It indicates the presence of fluid in the abdominal cavity.
  - Dullness in the paraumbilical zone is detected with smaller amounts of fluid. This is elicited by asking the patient to assume knee elbow position and paraumbilical region percussed. Normally, the percussion note is tympanitic. With mild ascites the dullness is found only in the flanks.

Q. What is Puddle sign?

- **Puddle sign/Lawson's sign:** It can detect even ascites as low as 120 mL. Patient is asked to lie in prone position for 5 minutes, followed by knee elbow position. Place the diaphragm of the stethoscope on the most dependent part of the abdomen. Repeatedly flick one flank lightly. Diaphragm is gradually moved to the opposite flank. A marked change in the intensity and character of percussion note indicates the presence of fluid.
- With moderate ascites, both the flanks and hypogastric areas are dull **(horse shoe-shaped dullness)**. The epigastrium and
- Umbilical regions show resonant note due to floating intestines.
- With massive ascites, the whole of the abdomen is dull, except for a small region over the umbilicus.
- For elicitation, **shifting dullness** at least of 500–1000 mL of fluid is required.
- **Fluid thrill** can be elicited in tense ascites (fluid more than 2,000 mL).

Secondary effects

- **Edema of scrotum**.
- **Pedal edema:** Due to hypoproteinemia and a functional block of IVC caused by tense ascites.
- **Pleural effusion:** Mainly on the right side. Pleural effusion is due to defects in the diaphragm that allows the ascitic fluid to pass into the pleural cavity.
- **Cardiac apex: Shifted upward** because of raised diaphragm
- **Distension of neck veins:** Secondary to a raised right atrial pressure, which follows tense ascites and raised diaphragm.
- **Meralgia paresthetica:** It can develop due to compression of lateral cutaneous nerve of thigh.
- Divarication of recti and hernia

Investigations

Ultrasonography: It is very sensitive and can detect even small amounts of ascitic fluid and also useful in identifying the cause.

- **Paracentesis and evaluation of ascitic fluid** (*refer* **Table 11.40**).
- **Laparoscopy and biopsy of peritoneum**

Aspirate about 10–20 mL of ascitic fluid and ascitic tap (**Fig. 11.22**) the following tests are performed:

- ***Cell count*:** A neutrophil count above 250 cells/mm^3 usually indicates SBP.
- ***Gram stain and culture*:** For bacteria and acid-fast bacilli.
- ***Protein*:** Total ascitic fluid protein less than 1.5 g/dL indicates an increased risk of SBP.
- ***SAAG (Serum ascites albumin gradient)*:** It is the differences between serum albumin and ascitic fluid albumin. SAAG is useful for differentiating ascites caused by portal hypertension from nonportal hypertensive ascites. It is calculated by subtracting the ascitic albumin concentration form the serum albumin concentration and does not change with diuresis. It is **better indicator** than simple estimation of protein in the ascitic fluid. SAAG is not a ratio, it is the difference. Classification of ascites based on SAAG is presented in **Table 11.38**. Corrected SAAG = Uncorrected SAAG × 0.16 × (Serum globulin g/dL + 2.5).
- ***Cytology*:** For malignant cells to exclude neoplasms causing ascites
- ***Amylase*:** To exclude pancreatic ascites. It is increased in acute pancreatitis.

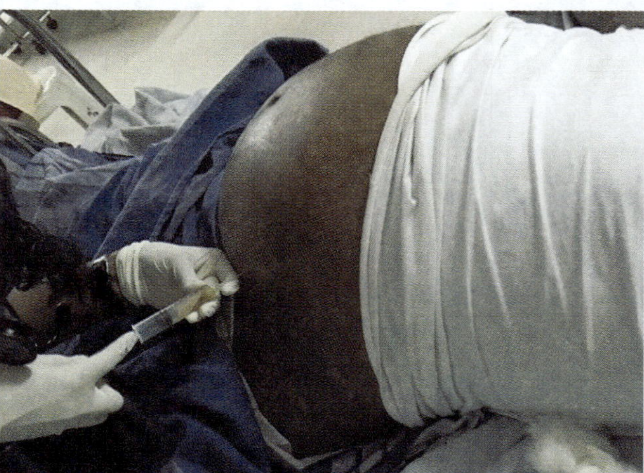

FIG. 11.22: Ascitic tap.

Ascitic fluid changes in cirrhosis are presented in **Table 11.39**. Causes of high- and low-serum-ascites albumin gradient (**Table 11.38**).

TABLE 11.38: Causes of high and low serum-ascites albumin gradient.

Causes of high serum-ascites albumin gradient (> 1.1 g/dL)	*Causes of low serum-ascites albumin gradient (< 1.1 g/dL)*
➢ Portal hypertension, e.g., cirrhosis of liver ➢ Hepatic outflow obstruction ➢ Alcoholic hepatitis ➢ Cardiac failure ➢ Myxedema ➢ Fatty liver of pregnancy ➢ Budd–Chiari syndrome ➢ Hepatic veno-occlusive disease ➢ Right-sided heart failure ➢ Constrictive pericarditis ➢ Massive liver metastasis	➢ Peritoneal tuberculosis ➢ Carcinoma involving peritoneal cavity ➢ Pancreatitis ➢ Nephrotic syndrome ➢ Biliary ascites ➢ Serositis (connective tissue disorders) ➢ Bowel infarction

TABLE 11.39: Ascitic fluid changes in cirrhosis.

Features	*Findings*
Appearance	Clear, straw-colored or light green
Specific gravity	<1.018
Protein	<2.5 g/dL
Total cell count	Normal (<250/L)
Differential cell count	Mesothelial cells and lymphocytes
Gram's stain	Negative
Culture	Negative
Malignant cells	Absent
Serum ascites albumin gradient (SAAG)	1.1 g/dL

Differential Diagnosis of Ascites (Table 11.40)

Nature of Ascitic Fluid

The ascitic fluid may be transudate or exudate. Differences between transudates and exudates are listed in **Table 11.41**.

TABLE 11.40: Examination of ascitic fluid and its interpretation.

Feature	*Interpretation*
Gross appearance	
➢ Clear, straw-colored or light green	➢ Cirrhosis, infective (e.g., tuberculosis, following intra-abdominal perforation), malignancy, chronic pancreatitis, heart disorders (congestive cardiac failure, constrictive pericarditis, hepatic vein obstruction (e.g., Budd–Chiari syndrome), Meigs's syndrome (ovarian tumor), hypoproteinemia (e.g., nephrotic syndrome)
➢ Hemorrhagic	➢ Malignant tumors, tuberculosis, acute pancreatitis, ruptured ectopic pregnancy, trauma to abdomen
➢ Cloudy, turbid	➢ Bacterial peritonitis
➢ Milky white (chylous)	➢ Lymphatic obstruction (e.g., by carcinoma), cirrhosis
➢ Specific gravity	➢ <1.018 in transudates
	➢ >1.018 in exudates
➢ Protein	➢ <2.5 g/dL in transudates
	➢ >2.5 g/dL in exudates
➢ Serum-ascites albumin gradient (SAAG)	*Refer* **Table 11.38**
➢ Glucose	➢ Low in malignancy, tuberculosis, peritonitis
➢ Amylase activity	➢ >1,000 units/L in pancreatitis
Microscopy	
➢ Polymorphs	➢ <250/mm³ in cirrhosis
	➢ >250/mm³ in bacterial peritonitis
➢ Lymphocytes	➢ Tuberculosis, malignancy
➢ Cytological examination	➢ Malignancy
➢ Special stains	
– Gram's stain	➢ Bacterial peritonitis
– Ziehl–Neelsen staining	➢ Tuberculosis
Culture	
➢ Pyogenic bacteria	➢ Bacterial peritonitis
➢ Mycobacteria	➢ Tuberculosis

TABLE 11.41: Differences between transudative and exudative ascites.

Characteristics	*Transudate*	*Exudate*
Cause	Noninflammatory process	Inflammatory process
Mechanism	Ultrafiltrate of plasma, due to increased hydrostatic pressure with normal vascular permeability	Increased vascular permeability
Appearance	Clear, serous	Cloudy/turbid purulent/hemorrhagic/chylous
Color	Straw yellow	Yellow to red
Specific gravity	<1.018	>1.018
Protein	Low, <2 g/dL, mainly albumin	High, >2 g/dL
Clot	Absent	Clots spontaneously because of high fibrinogen
Cell count	Low (<250/μL)	High (>250/μL)
Type of cells	Few lymphocytes and mesothelial cells	Neutrophils in acute and lymphocytes in chronic inflammation
Bacteria	Absent	Usually present
Lactate dehydrogenase (LDH)	Low	High
Examples	Cirrhosis, nephrotic syndrome, heart failure	Peritonitis, malignancy

Causes: Various causes of ascites are listed in **Table 11.42**.

TABLE 11.42: Causes of ascites.

Cause	*Frequency (%)*
Parenchymal liver disease	78
Cirrhosis	77
Fulminant liver failure	1
Malignancy	12
Cardiovascular disease ➢ Congestive heart failure ➢ Constrictive or restrictive cardiomyopathy ➢ Thrombosis of inferior vena cava ➢ Budd-Chiari syndrome ➢ Veno-occlusive disease	5
Infection Tuberculosis Fitz-Hugh-Curtis syndrome (chlamydiae, gonococci) Coccidioidomycosis Whipple's disease (Tropheryma whipplei)	2
Renal	1.5
Nephrotic syndrome Uremia Hemodialysis	
Pancreatic	1
Bacterial peritonitis	0.5
Marked hypothyroidism Collagen vascular disease Familial mediterranean fever Amyloidosis Hereditary angioneurotic edema Menetrier's disease and protein-losing enteropathy Starch peritonitis Trauma	

Management

- **General measures:**
  - Hospitalization is necessary, if there is massive ascites.
  - Check serum electrolytes, renal function tests at the start of treatment and twice a week.
  - Weigh the patient daily. Measure abdominal girth and strict intake and output monitoring daily.
- **Bed rest** alone induces diuresis in a small proportion of people because renal blood flow increases in the horizontal position, but in practice is not helpful. Ascites treatment algorithm is shown in **Flowchart 11.5**.
- **Dietary restriction of sodium** by reducing sodium intake to 40 mmol in 24 hours and maintain an adequate protein and calorie intake with a palatable diet.

First-line treatment of patients with cirrhosis and ascites consists of sodium restriction (88 mmol/day [2000 mg/day]) and diuretics (oral spironolactone with or without oral furosemide).

Fluid restriction is not necessary unless serum sodium is less than 125 mmol/L

- **Drugs:** Many contain significant amounts of sodium (up to 50 mmol daily). Examples include antacids, antibiotics (particularly the penicillins and cephalosporins) and effervescent tablets. Sodium-retaining drugs (nonsteroidal, corticosteroids) should be avoided.
- **Fluid restriction to 1,000–1,500 mL/day** is necessary if the serum sodium is under 128 mmol/L.
- **Diuretics**
  - **Aim of diuretic therapy: To produce a net loss of fluid** of about 700 mL/day (0.7 kg weight loss in patients with ascites alone or

FLOWCHART 11.5: Ascites treatment algorithm.

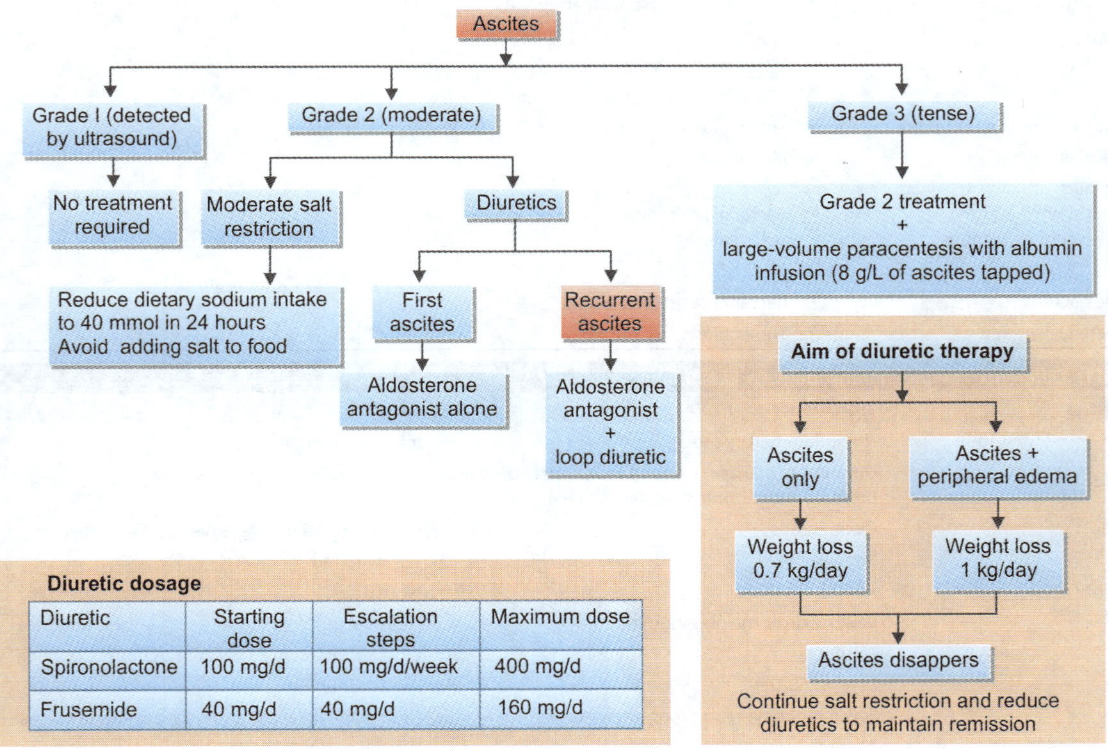

Diuretic	Starting dose	Escalation steps	Maximum dose
Spironolactone	100 mg/d	100 mg/d/week	400 mg/d
Frusemide	40 mg/d	40 mg/d	160 mg/d

- 1.0 kg if both ascites and peripheral edema is present). The maximum rate at which ascites can be mobilized is 500–700 mL/day. This is to prevent diuretic-induced renal failure and/or hypernatremia.
- Diuretics are administered in a step-wise manner.
- **Aldosterone antagonists:** As there is **secondary hyperaldosteronism**, the diuretic of first choice is the one of the aldosterone antagonists (potassium-sparing diuretics), e.g., **spironolactone, triamterene, amiloride.** Spironolactone is started at a low dose of 25 mg QID (100 mg daily), and gradually stepped up every week to a maximum of 400 mg/day (providing there is no hyperkalemia). Chronic administration of spironolactone produces gynecomastia. **Eplerenone** 25 mg once daily does not produce gynecomastia.
- **Loop diuretics:** When a large dose of spironolactone has failed, add a loop diuretic, such as **furosemide 20–40 mg or bumetanide 0.5 mg or 1 mg daily**. Usually spironolactone is combined with furosemide. Disadvantages of loop diuretics include development of hyponatremia, hypokalemia, and volume depletion.
- **Stop all diuretics, if severe hyponatremia** (sodium <120 mEq/L), progressive renal failure or worsening of hepatic encephalopathy occurs. Vaptans may improve serum sodium in patients with cirrhosis and ascites.

Treatment of Refractory Ascites

Q. Write short essay/note on indication, procedure, and complications of abdominal paracentesis.

Refractory ascites is defined as fluid overload that (1) is unresponsive to sodium-restricted diet and high-dose diuretic treatment (400 mg per day of spironolactone and 160 mg per day furosemide), or (2) recurs rapidly after therapeutic paracentesis.

They are managed on the following lines:

1. **Intravenous salt-poor albumin, 25 g in 3 hours.**
2. **Oral midodrine 7.5 mg three times daily.**
3. **Large-volume paracentesis**
   - **Indications (Box 11.28)**
   - **Procedure:**
     - Remove 3–5 L of fluid over 1–2 hours.
     - Salt-free albumin (8 g/L of ascetic fluid removed) if volume is more than 4–5 L is removed. If albumin is not available, dextran-70 may be used. Strict monitoring is necessary.
   - **Complication:** Hypovolemic and renal dysfunction (postparacentesis circulatory dysfunction) more likely with removal of > 5 L and worse liver function.
4. **Shunts:**
   - **TIPSS:** It is used for resistant ascites, if there is no spontaneous portosystemic encephalopathy and no disturbance of renal function.
   - **Le Veen shunt:** It is a peritoneovenous shunt that allows the peritoneal fluid to drain directly into the internal jugular vein.
5. Slow low-dose continuous albumin, Furosemide with or without Terlipressin **SIFA(T)**infusion.
6. Liver transplantation.

Box 11.28: Indications for large-volume paracentesis.

- Refractory ascites
- Used to relieve symptomatic tense ascites, e.g., cardiorespiratory distress due to gross ascites.
- Impending rupture of a hernia.

Bacterial Peritonitis

Types: (1) Acute bacterial peritonitis or (2) chronic bacterial peritonitis.

1. **Acute Bacterial Peritonitis**

   Causes: Appendicitis, perforated peptic ulcer or typhoid ulcer, cholecystitis, diverticulitis, gangrene of the small intestine and ulcerative colitis.

   Symptoms

   Fever, nausea, thirst, vomiting, severe abdominal pain. No flatus.

   Signs

   - Hippocratic facies
   - Tachycardia, hypotension, and shock
   - Board-like rigidity, tenderness, and rebound tenderness
   - Absent peristaltic sounds.

   Investigations **(Box 11.29)**

2. **Chronic Bacterial Peritonitis**
   - Associated with subacute intestinal obstruction
   - Ascitic fluid: Exudate, protein is high, and contains a large number of chronic inflammatory cells.
   - Classification of ascitic fluid infections is listed in **Table 11.43.**

Box 11.29: Investigations in acute bacterial peritonitis.

- **Plain radiograph of abdomen**
  - Dilated loops of intestine
  - Gas under the diaphragm if there is intestinal perforation
- **Ascitic** fluid **(Flowchart 11.6)**
  - Exudate, turbid, or purulent
  - Shows intestinal contents in the fluid
  - Cell counts: Markedly increased, polymorphs > 250/mm^3
  - Gram stain: Positive for bacteria
  - Culture: It shows growth of organism.

Treatment: It is a surgical emergency.

- Correction of fluid and electrolyte balance
- Broad spectrum antibiotic therapy
- Treat the shock
- Surgical treatment depending on the causes

Treatment of the underlying cause.

Spontaneous Bacterial Peritonitis

Q. Write short note on diagnosis and management of spontaneous bacterial peritonitis.

Patients with cirrhosis and ascites are highly susceptible to infection of ascitic fluid.

FLOWCHART 11.6: Approach to the patient with ascites following diagnostic paracentesis.

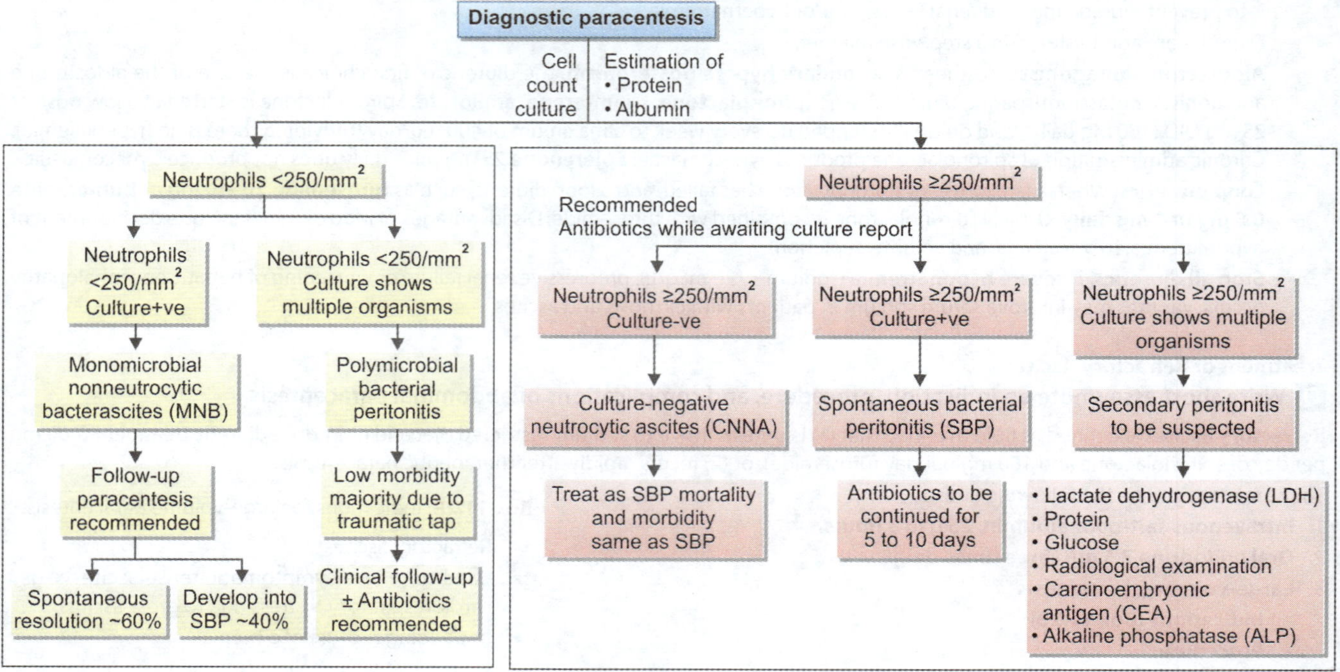

Definition

Spontaneous bacterial peritonitis is a **common and severe complication of ascites** characterized by **spontaneous infection of ascitic without an evident intra-abdominal surgically treatable source**.

TABLE 11.43: Classification of ascitic fluid infection.

➤ Culture-negative neutrocytic ascites
➤ Monomicrobial nonneutrocytic bacterascites
➤ Polymicrobial bacterascites (needle perforation of the bowel)
➤ Secondary bacterial peritonitis
➤ Spontaneous bacterial peritonitis

Pathogenesis

- **Causative agents***:* Most common organisms are *Escherichia coli, Klebsiella,* or enterococci, or other gut bacteria. Others include streptococci and enterococci.
- **Route of infection:** The infecting organisms in the gut flora traverse the intestine into mesenteric lymph nodes, leading to bacteremia and seeding of the ascitic fluid by hematogenous spread.

Clinical Features

- SBP should be **suspected in any patient with ascites who clinically deteriorates.**
- It may present as **sudden deterioration or hepatic encephalopathy in a cirrhotic patient with ascites.**
- Features include **fever, abdominal pain or discomfort and rebound abdominal tenderness** or they may present without any of these features.
- In terms of important predictors for identifying cirrhotic patients at greatest risk for SBP, both a high serum bilirubin (above 2.5 mg/dL) and a low ascitic fluid protein concentration (less than 1.0 g/dL) have been shown to be independent factors for both initial episodes of SBP as well as for recurrence.

Investigations

- **Peripheral blood: Leukocytosis.**
- **Ascitic fluid:**
  - **Cloudy fluid**
  - **Leukocyte count: More than 500/mm³**. A raised neutrophil count of > 250/mm³ in ascites is alone sufficient for diagnosis and to start treatment immediately.
  - pH: Less than 7.3.
  - **Culture: Positive**. Monomicrobial *E. coli* is the most common organism.
- Investigations to rule out abdominal sources of peritonitis by imaging

Diagnosis

With **clinical suspicion, a diagnostic aspiration** (paracentesis) should always be performed in patients with GI bleeding, shock, fever, worsening liver and/or renal function, and hepatic encephalopathy for making the diagnosis.

Treatment

- **Third-generation cephalosporin:** Such as **cefotaxime or ceftazidime** being the most commonly used antibiotic. This is modified on the basis of culture results. Dose of cefotaxime: 2 g IV 8 hourly for 5 days.
- **Alternative therapy** in patients without shock or hepatic encephalopathy
  - **Amoxicillin/clavulanate** (1.2 g IV 8 hourly followed by 625 mg orally)
  - **Ciprofloxacin** (200 mg IV12 hourly followed by 500 mg BID orally)
  - **Ofloxacin** (400 mg twice daily).

Note: Quinolones should not be given if patient is on norfloxacin for prophylaxis.

- Antibiotic therapy and albumin (1.5 g/kg bodyweight within 6 hours of detection and 1 g/kg on day 3) reduces risk of type1 HRS.

Prophylaxis for SBP

Recurrence is common (70% within a year) and prophylaxis is indicated (**Box 11.30**).

- **Drugs:**
  - In **patients with upper GI hemorrhage: cefotaxime or norfloxacin**
  - (400 mg BID for 7 days).
  - In **patients with low ascitic protein content** or previous episode of SBP: Long-term quinolones such as **norfloxacin** (400 mg/day lifelong).
  - Alternative but less effective drugs: Include cotrimoxazole (800 mg sulfamethoxazole + 160 mg trimethoprim once a day) or ciprofloxacin (750 mg once a week).

Box 11.30: Indications for prophylaxis for spontaneous bacterial peritonitis.

- **Patients with acute gastrointestinal bleeding** (antibiotic prophylaxis also reduces the rate of rebleeding)
- Patients with a **previous episode(s) of SBP** and recovered
- Patients with **low total ascites protein content** < 1.5 g/dL or severe liver disease and no prior history of SBP

Tuberculous Peritonitis

- **Pathogenesis:** Tuberculosis spreads to involve peritoneum by or more of the following sources:
  - Through hematogenous seeding of peritoneum
  - Through lymphatics or mesenteric nodes
  - From genitourinary source

Clinical Features

- **Night sweats, weight loss, loss of appetite, malaise, and evening rise of temperature**
- Gradual abdominal distension and **"doughy feel" of the abdomen**.
- Multiple palpable masses in the abdomen produced due to matted omentum and loops of intestine.

Investigations

See **Table 11.44**.

TABLE 11.44: Investigations in tuberculous peritonitis.

Ascitic fluid	
➢ Usually straw colored ➢ **Protein: >2.5g/dL** ➢ **Lymphocytes >70%** ➢ **Ziehl–Neelsen staining:** It may show acid-fast bacilli.	➢ Culture of ascitic fluid for tubercle bacilli ➢ Adenosine deaminase (ADA) levels: Raised ➢ **Peritoneal biopsy under laparoscopy**: Shows **granuloma** and helps in confirmation of diagnosis

Treatment: Antituberculous chemotherapy.

Malignant Ascites

Causes

- Primary tumors of stomach, colon, ovary or other **intra-abdominal tumors may produce exudation fluid into the peritoneal cavity.**
- **Peritoneal metastasis:** From any primary.
- **Periumbilical subcutaneous metastatic tumor** deposits (known "Sister-Joseph's" nodules'), e.g., carcinoma of stomach.

Investigations

- **Ascitic fluid (Box 11.31)**
- **Biopsy of the peritoneum** by laparoscope: **It shows the tumor** and useful for confirmation of diagnosis.

Box 11.31: Ascitic fluid findings in malignant ascites.

- Appearance: **Exudate and hemorrhagic**
- **Protein: High**
- **Specific gravity: High**
- Microscopy: Sediment shows **malignant cells.**

Treatment: Palliative

- Repeated paracentesis.
- Intraperitoneal instillation of chemotherapeutic drugs: It may reduce rate of reaccumulation of ascites. The drugs include methotrexate, nitrogen mustard, or immunotherapy (interferon alfa).

Meigs's Syndrome

Q. Write short note on Meigs's syndrome.

Features of Meigs's syndrome are presented in **Box 11.32**.

Box 11.32: Features of Meigs's syndrome.

- Pleural effusion is most commonly **right sided**, may be exudate or transudate.
- **Ascites**
- **Pelvic tumor** (commonly fibroma of the ovary) in females. Both ascites and pleural effusion resolve following excision of the pelvic tumor.

Chylous Ascites

- Characterized by the **presence of chyle** (intestinal lymph) in the peritoneal cavity. Ascitic fluid is milky or creamy due to the presence of chylomicrons.
- **Causes:**
  - Injury/trauma to the main lymph ducts in the abdomen.
  - Malignancy (e.g., lymphoma) or tuberculosis causing obstruction of the intestinal lymphatics
  - Filariasis
  - Intestinal obstruction associated with rupture of a major lymphatic channel
  - Congenital lymph angiectasia
- **Clinical features:**
  - Acute abdominal pain with signs of peritoneal irritation
  - Distended, nontender, fluid filling the abdomen (chylous ascites).
- **Ascitic fluid:**
  - **Milky or creamy**
  - **High fat (triglycerides > 1,000 mg/dL) content.**
  - **Sudan III staining demonstrates fat globules.**

Ascites Praecox

Q. What is ascites praecox?

- In ascites praecox, ascites occurs early and is disproportionately prominent as well as appears before the edema. It occurs in constrictive pericarditis, acute Budd–Chiari syndrome, tuberculous peritonitis, and malignant peritonitis.
- In constrictive pericarditis, ascites appears first, followed by edema. This sequence is one of the cardinal features, distinguishing ascites from congestive heart failure in which edema appears first and ascites much later. Edema is minimal in constrictive pericarditis and occurs in the later part of the disease.

DRUG AND TOXIN-INDUCED HEPATITIS

Q. Write a short note on drug-induced liver injury.

Types of drug-induced liver injury (DILI)

Variable	*Direct hepatotoxicity*	*Idiosyncratic hepatotoxicity*	*Indirect hepatotoxicity*
Frequency	Common	Rare	Intermediate
Dose-related	Yes	No	No
Predictable	Yes	No	Partially
Latency	Typically rapid (days)	Variable (days to years)	Delayed (months)
Common phenotypes	Acute hepatic necrosis, serum enzyme elevations	Acute hepatocellular hepatitis	Acute hepatitis, immune mediated hepatitis, fatty liver
Most common agents	High doses of acetaminophe, niacin, aspirin	Amoxicillin-clavunate, cephalosporins, macrolide antibiotics	Anti-neoplastic agents, Glucocorticoids
Cause	Intrinsic hepatotoxicity when agent given in high doses	Idiosyncratic metabolic or immunologic reaction	Indirect action of agent on liver or immune system

DILI can also be classified as:

- Immune mediated (allergic)
- Non-immune mediated (non-allergic)

	Immune mediated	*Non-immune mediated*
Latency period	1–6 weeks	1 month to 1 year
Fever, rash, eosinophilia	Yes	Uncommon
Reproduction of liver injury upon drug rechallenge	Yes	Uncommon
Dose Related	No	May be

Investigations

Case definitions for DILI:

- ≥5 × ULN elevation of ALT
- ≥2 × ULN elevation in ALP (particularly with accompanying elevation in concentrations of GGT in the absence of bone pathology driving the rise in ALP).
- ≥3 × ULN elevation in ALT and simultaneous elevation of TB exceeding 2 × ULN.

$$R = \frac{\text{ALT} \div \text{ULN of ALT}}{\text{Alkaline phosphatase} \div \text{ULN of alkaline phosphatase}}$$

- $R \geq 5$ = Hepatocellular injury
- $R \leq 2$ = cholestasis
- $R > 2$ and <5 = Mixed pattern of injury

RUCAM (Roussel Uclaf causality assessment method) is an objective means of assessing causality that it is based on a numerical scoring system.

Hy's law

- ≥3 × ULN elevation of ALT or AST with >2 × ULN elevation of total bilirubin, without initial findings of cholestasis, indicated by elevated ALP.
- It is an indicator of severity.
- It is associated with a 10% higher risk of mortality.

Clinicopathologic Classification of Drug-induced Liver Disease (Table 11.45)

TABLE 11.45: Clinicopathologic classification of drug-induced liver injury (DILI).

Category	*Implicated drugs: Examples*
Hepatic adaptation	Phenytoin, warfarin, rifampin, flavaspidic acid
Dose-dependent hepatotoxicity (necrosis)	Acetaminophen (paracetamol), nicotinic acid, amodiaquine, hycanthone, carbon tetrachloride, mushroom (Amanita phalloides), yellow phosphorus
Other cytopathic toxicity, acute steatosis	Valproic acid, didanosine, HAART agents, fialuridine, L-asparaginase, some herbal medicines
Acute hepatitis	Isoniazid, dantrolene, nitrofurantoin, halothane, sulfonamides, phenytoin, disulfiram, acebutolol, etretinate, ketoconazole, terbinafine, troglitazone, rifampicin, methyldopa, ibuprofen, ketoconazole, fluconazole, zidovudine, chlorothiazide, oxyphenisatin
Chronic hepatitis	Nitrofurantoin, etretinate, diclofenac, minocycline, nefazodone, phenytoin, isoniazid
Granulomatous hepatitis	Allopurinol, carbamazepine, hydralazine, quinidine, quinine, phenylbutazone, sulfonamides, allopurinol
Cholestasis without hepatitis	Oral contraceptives, androgens
Cholestatic hepatitis	Chlorpromazine, tricyclic antidepressants, erythromycin estolate, amoxicillin–clavulanic acid, methimazole, chlorpromazine, chlorpropamide, methyl testosterone, anabolic steroids, cyclosporine, nimesulide
Cholestasis with bile duct injury	Chlorpromazine, flucloxacillin, dextropropoxyphene
Chronic cholestasis	Chlorpromazine, haloperidol, erythromycin, cimetidine/ranitidine, nitrofurantoin, imipramine, azathioprine
Hepatic fibrosis	Methotrexate
Vanishing bile duct syndrome	Chlorpromazine, flucloxacillin, trimethoprim–sulfamethoxazole
Sclerosing cholangitis	Intra-arterial floxuridine, intralesional scolicidals
Steatosis (fatty change)	Zidovudine, amiodarone, indinavir, ritonavir, methotrexate, tetracyclines, valproic acid
Steatohepatitis	Perhexiline, amiodarone,
Vascular disorders	Contraceptive drugs, anabolic steroids, azathioprine
Tumors	Contraceptive pill, danazol

Treatment:

- Discontinue the implicated agent.
- Spontaneous recovery after discontinuation is an important criteria in causality assessment.
- Specific therapy:
  - Cholestyramine is used to decrease the course of hepatotoxicity due to specific drugs such as leflunomide and terbinafine. Dose: 4 g every 6 hourly for 2 weeks.
  - Carnitine is used in valproate toxicity. Dose: 100 mg/kg IV over 30 minutes (maimum dose—6 g), followed by 15 mg/kg every 4 hourly until clinical improvement.
  - N-acetyl cysteine is used in paracetamol poisoning.
- Cholestatic DILI can be treated with UDCA at a dose of 13–15 mg/kg
- Corticosteroids have not proven to be beneficial in idiosyncratic DILI unless accompanied by hypersensitivity features such as eosinophilia, rash, and fever.
- Any sign of acute liver failure requires prompt referral to a liver transplant center.

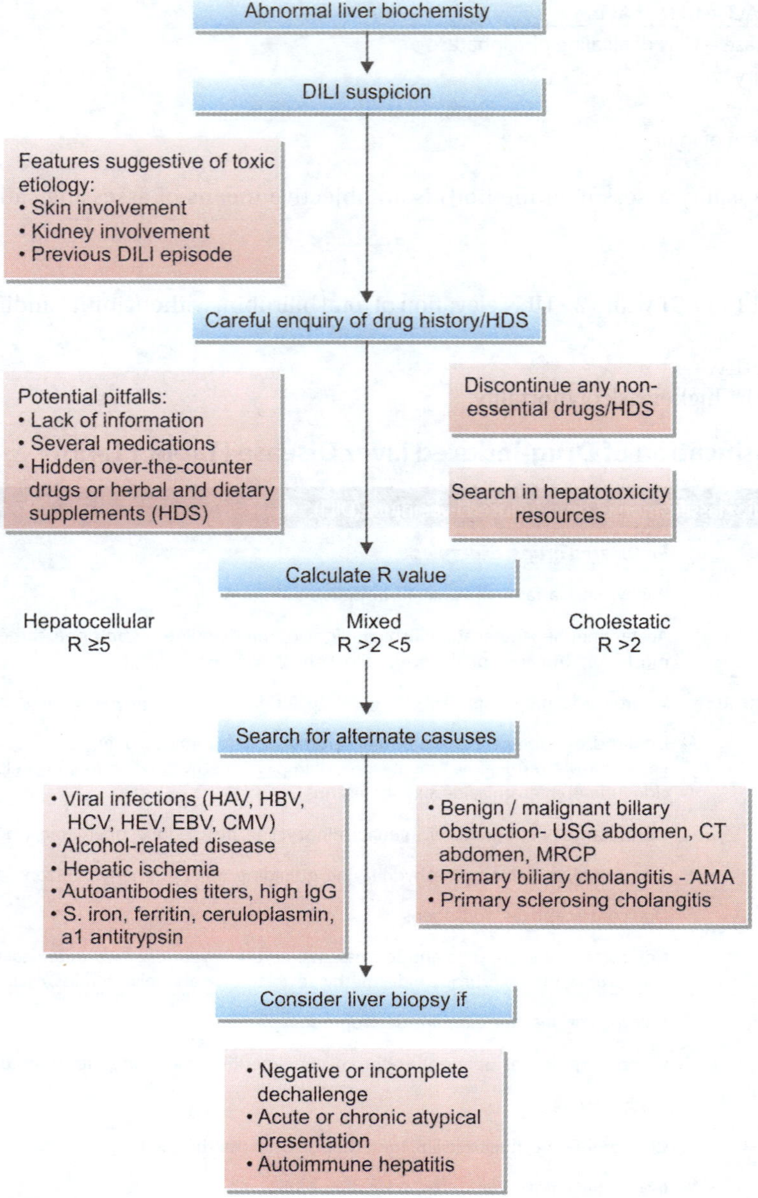

HEPATIC VENOUS OUTFLOW TRACT OBSTRUCTION

Q. Discuss the etiology, pathology, clinical features, investigations, and management of hepatic venous outflow tract obstruction.

Q. Describe veno-occlusive disease or sinusoidal obstruction syndrome.

- Obstruction to the hepatic venous outflow can occur at different levels. These include:
  - Small central hepatic veins: Veno-occlusive disease
  - Large hepatic veins: Budd–Chiari syndrome
  - Inferior vena cava
  - Heart
- *Clinical features:* It depends on the cause and on the speed with which obstruction develops. Common features are congestive hepatomegaly and ascites.

Budd–Chiari Syndrome

Q. Explain briefly about Budd–Chiari syndrome.

- *Definition:* Budd–Chiari syndrome is characterized by obstruction of hepatic venous outflow owing to occlusion of the hepatic vein.

- *Level of obstruction:* It may be at any level from the small hepatic veins to the junction of the IVC with the right atrium.
- Classic Budd–Chiari syndrome results from thrombosis of one or more hepatic veins at their openings into the IVC.

Etiology (Box 11.33)

Box 11.33: Various causes of Budd–Chiari syndrome.

Hepatic vein obstruction

Venous thrombosis

- Hypercoagulability states
  - Hematological disorders
  - Polycythemia vera
  - Paroxysmal nocturnal hemoglobinuria
  - Antithrombin III, protein C, or protein S deficiencies
  - Antiphospholipid syndrome
  - Sickle cell disease
  - Leukemia
  - Pregnancy
  - Use of oral contraceptive pills

Compression (may also produce thrombosis)

- Hepatic infections
- Hydatid cyst
- Liver abscess
- Obstruction due to tumors
- Renal cell carcinoma
- Adrenal tumors
- Hepatocellular carcinoma
- Posterior abdominal wall sarcomas

Radiation injury

Congenital venous webs

Trauma to the liver

Idiopathic (40–50% of cases)

Clinical Features

Budd–Chiari syndrome: It comprises a triad of (1) abdominal pain, (2) ascites, and (3) hepatomegaly with hepatic histology showing centrilobular sinusoidal distension and pooling.

- Acute form (acute Budd–Chiari)
  - Follows sudden venous occlusion (e.g., by renal cell carcinoma, HCC, and polycythemia)
  - Acute upper abdominal pain, nausea, vomiting, tender hepatomegaly, marked ascites, and mild jaundice
  - With total venous occlusion: Delirium, coma, and hepatocellular failure
- Fulminant form (fulminant Budd–Chiari syndrome)
  - Presents with fulminant hepatic failure usually in the setting of an additional predisposing factor (e.g., factor V Leiden mutation)
  - Occurs particularly in pregnant women
- Chronic form (chronic Budd–Chiari)
  - More gradual occlusion and more usual presentation
  - Pain in abdomen, tender hepatomegaly, and gross ascites
  - Enlarged caudate lobe of the liver becomes palpable
  - Jaundice is mild or absent
  - Splenomegaly with portal hypertension
  - Negative hepatojugular reflux, i.e., pressure over the liver fails to fill the jugular veins.
  - Bilateral pedal edema and distended veins over abdomen, flanks, and back **(Fig. 11.23)**, with IVC obstruction
  - Features of cirrhosis and portal hypertension in patients who survive the acute event
  - HCC may develop.

Investigations

- Liver function tests vary considerably.
  - Features of acute hepatitis: Mild hyperbilirubinemia, raised ALP, low serum albumin, and raised transaminases
- *Ascitic fluid examination:* Typically shows a high protein content (>2.5 g/dL, i.e. exudate) in the early stages; however, this often falls later in the disease.
- *Ultrasound*: It may show enlargement of the caudate lobe, intrahepatic collaterals, echogenic areas, and ascites. It also may show compression of the IVC, if present.
- *Pulsed Doppler sonography or a color Doppler:* It may show obliteration of the hepatic veins and reversed flow or associated thrombosis in the portal vein with high accuracy. This may be sufficient to establish the diagnosis. Doppler ultrasonography, with sensitivity and specificity rates >80%, is the diagnostic procedure of first choice.
- *Noninvasive CT or MRI:* It may also demonstrate occlusion of the hepatic veins and IVC with diffuse abnormal parenchyma on contrast-enhancement. It may also demonstrate enlargement of the caudate lobe which has independent blood supply and venous drainage.

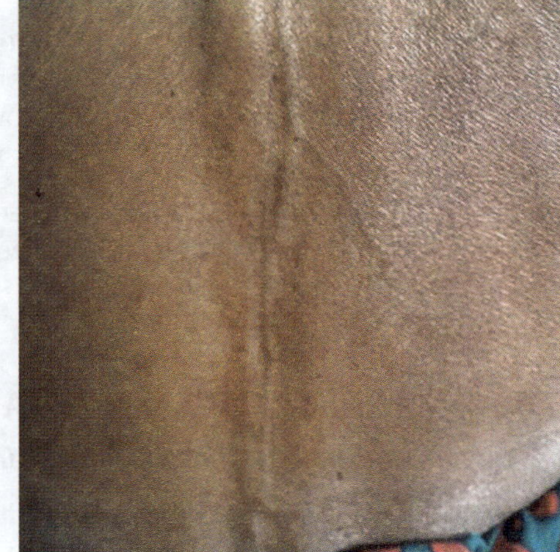

FIG. 11.23: Budd–Chiari dilated veins in back and lumbar region.

- Hepatic venography is only necessary if CT and MRI are unable to demonstrate the hepatic venous anatomy clearly. It helps to determine extent of block and caval pressures.
- *Liver biopsy:* It shows centrilobular congestion hemorrhage, fibrosis, and cirrhosis depending on the duration of the disease.
- *Other investigations:* To identify a cause (e.g., blood tests and coagulation studies).

Management

- Predisposing causes should be removed or treated as far as possible.
- *In the acute situation with recent thrombosis:* Treated with thrombolytic therapy consisting of intrahepatic venous streptokinase (in very early cases of thrombosis), followed by heparin and oral anticoagulation (warfarin).
- *Short hepatic venous strictures:* Treated with angioplasty
- *Extensive hepatic vein occlusion:* Insertion of a covered TIPSS followed by anticoagulation may be useful in opening of the hepatic veins. Direct intrahepatic portocaval shunt (DIPS) is a modification of the TIPS procedure, using intravascular ultrasound-guidance, combined with fluoroscopy.
- *Ascites:* Initially treated medically with low-salt diet, diuretics as well as treating the underlying cause (e.g., polycythemia). If not relieved may be treated with surgical shunts such as Le Veen shunt and portosystemic shunts.
- Percutaneous balloon angioplasty is performed for membranous obstruction of the IVC and hepatic vein.
- Congenital web can be treated radiologically or resected surgically.
- Liver transplantation is indicated for chronic Budd–Chiari syndrome and for progressive liver failure, followed by lifelong anticoagulation.
- Without transplantation or shunting, particularly acute and fulminant types, are associated with poor prognosis.

Veno-occlusive Disease

Veno-occlusive disease (VOD), also known as sinusoidal obstruction syndrome, is a rare condition characterized by widespread occlusion of the small central hepatic veins.

Etiology

- Develops as a complication of:
  - Total body irradiation/myeloablative regimens are used before hematopoietic stem cell transplantation. It carries a high mortality.
  - A variety of antineoplastic drugs have been implicated as causes of sinusoidal obstruction syndrome including gemtuzumab ozogamicin, actinomycin D, dacarbazine, cytosine arabinoside, mithramycin, and 6-thioguanine.
  - Chronic immunosuppression with azathioprine or 6-thioguanine
  - Ingestion of herbal teas made with pyrrolizidine alkaloids in Senecio and Heliotropium plants
  - Ingestion of alkaloids in inadequately winnowed wheat or in "bush tea"
  - Hepatic irradiation

Clinical Features

Clinical features are similar to those of the Budd–Chiari syndrome. Classically, sinusoidal obstruction syndrome manifests with mild hyperbilirubinemia (bilirubin levels >2 mg/dL), painful hepatomegaly, weight gain of >2%, and development of ascites.

Investigations

- Large hepatic veins appear patent radiologically. This is in contrast to Budd–Chiari syndrome.
- Transjugular liver biopsy (with portal pressure measurements) confirms diagnosis.
- Liver biopsy: Evidence of venous outflow obstruction

Treatment

- Supportive and includes control of fluid overload, ascites, and hepatocellular failure.
- Defibrotide is a novel oligodeoxyribonucleotide with anti-ischemic, antithrombotic, and thrombolytic activity but minimal systemic anticoagulant effect. Several studies have shown efficacy of defibrotide in the prevention and treatment of sinusoidal obstruction syndrome with no major toxicity.

HEPATOCELLULAR CARCINOMA

Q. ***Discuss the etiology, clinical features, investigations, and management of hepatocellular carcinoma.***

Hepatocellular carcinoma is the most common primary malignancy of liver from hepatocytes or their precursors. Predominantly in males with M: F ratio of 2.4: 1. The number of men and number of women with HCC in the absence of cirrhosis are almost equal.

Etiology (Table 11.46)

Clinical Features

- Usually develops in patients with underlying cirrhosis
- **Nonspecific symptoms** Include ill-defined upper abdominal pain in the right hypochondrium, malaise, weakness, anorexia, fatigue, weight loss and ascites. Rapid development of these symptoms in a patient with cirrhosis is suggestive of HCC. Fever occurs due to tumor necrosis.

- On examination:
  - **Liver is enlarged, irregular, and nodular with pain or tenderness.**
  - **Friction rub or a hepatic bruit over the liver due to vascularity of tumor**
- Blood-tinged ascites, bone pain, and dyspnea due to metastasis.

TABLE 11.46: Risk factors for hepatocellular carcinoma.

Major risk factors	***Minor risk factors***	
➢ Chronic hepatitis: HBV/HCV	➢ Hereditary hemochromatosis	➢ Oral contraceptives
➢ Alcoholic cirrhosis	➢ Wilson's disease	➢ Cigarette smoking
➢ Aflatoxin B_1(a fungal toxin contaminating food)	➢ Primary biliary cholangitis	➢ Betel quid chewing
➢ Nonalcoholic steatohepatitis (NASH)	➢ Tyrosinemia	➢ Thorotrast and arsenic exposure
	➢ α_1-antitrypsin deficiency	➢ Obesity
	➢ Glycogen storage disease	➢ Ataxia telangiectasia
	➢ Hormones: Anabolic steroids, estrogens and androgens	➢ Hypercitrullinemia
		➢ Acute intermittent porphyria
		➢ Gallstones and cholecystectomy **>one in second column and other in third column**

(HBV: hepatitis B virus; HCV: hepatitis C virus)

Paraneoplastic Syndromes Associated with Hepatocellular Carcinoma (Table 11.47)

All patterns of HCCs have a strong tendency for invasion of vessels. The portal vein and its branches are infiltrated by tumor. Occasionally, long, snake-like tumor masses may **invade the portal vein** and occlude portal circulation. Rarely tumor may invade IVC and extend into the right side of the heart through the hepatic veins. It may metastasize to the lungs.

TABLE 11.47: Paraneoplastic syndromes associated with hepatocellular carcinoma.

Carcinoid syndrome	Porphyria
Hypercalcemia	Sexual changes—isosexual precocity, gynecomastia, feminization
Hypertrophic osteoarthropathy	Systemic arterial hypertension
Hypoglycemia	Thyrotoxicosis
Neuropathy	Thrombophlebitis migrans
Osteoporosis	Watery diarrhea syndrome
Polycythemia (erythrocytosis)	Dermatomyositis, pemphigus foliaceus, pityriasis rotunda

Investigations

- **Serum marker**
  - **Alpha-fetoprotein:** About 50% HCC is associated with high serum (>500 µg/L) or rising levels of alpha-fetoprotein. However, α-fetoprotein levels are often raised in other neoplastic and nonneoplastic liver diseases and in some extrahepatic disorders. AFP concentrations are normal in up to 40% of small HCCs.
  - **α-l-fucosidase:** It is raised in HCC and also in cirrhosis.
  - **Serum des-γ-carboxy prothrombin:** It is raised in a majority of HCC.
  - **Plasma microRNA** expression is also marker of HCC.
  - **Serum ALP: Very high.**
- Ultrasound scans show filling defects.
- CT scan **(triple-phase)** or MRI abdomen has 75–85% sensitivity in picking HCC. Hyperenhancement on late arterial phase images and washout at the portal venous and/or delayed phases of multiphasic contrast material-enhanced imaging are seen.
- **Hepatic artery angiography shows "tumor blushes."**
- Liver scintigraphic scans.
- **Liver aspiration or biopsy** particularly under ultrasonic guidance confirms the diagnosis.

Management/Treatment

Treatment is different for patients with cirrhosis and those without. Therapy depends on tumor size, multicentricity, extent of liver disease (Child–Pugh score) and performance status.

The Barcelona-Clínic Liver Cancer (BCLC) staging system

- Stage 0 with very early HCC are optimal candidates for resection. Stage A - early HCC are candidates for radical therapies (resection, liver transplantation or percutaneous treatments).
- Stage B- intermediate HCC—chemoembolization. Stage C -advanced HCC -new agents in the setting of clinical trials ,
- Stage D-end-stage disease—symptomatic treatment
- Surgical resection: It is indicated when lesions 1–3 in number and <5 cm in size; without metastasis; with child score A. Local or segmental resections are preferred to major resections. After successful resection, tumor recurs in the cirrhotic liver in about 70% of patients after 5 years.

- Nonsurgical therapy: Majority of patients diagnosed in the advanced stage of HCC and cannot be treated by surgical resection. These patients can be treated by following nonsurgical therapy.
  - Local ablation strategies:
    - Radiofrequency ablation (RFA): Percutaneous RFA uses heat to kill tumor cells. A single electrode inserted into the tumor under CT or ultrasound guidance.
    - Transarterial embolization (TAE): Hepatic artery embolization with Gelfoam and doxorubicin
    - Transarterial chemo-embolization (TACE): With drugs such as doxorubicin but is contraindicated in decompensated cirrhosis and when HCC is multifocal can be combined with RFA.
  - Local injection therapy: Numerous agents can be used for local injection into tumors and includes percutaneous ethanol injection (PEI) or percutaneous acetic acid injection (PAI). PEI causes not only direct destruction of tumor cells, but also destroy normal cells in the vicinity. It usually requires multiple injections (average three) and the maximum size of tumor treated is 3 cm.
  - Conventional chemotherapy and radiotherapy are unsuccessful.
  - Chemotherapy using sorafenib: This drug is a multikinase inhibitor with activity against RAF, VEGF, and PDGF signaling.
  - Nivolumab against programmed cell death 1 receptor (PD-1) has been used as immunotherapy.
- Liver transplantation: Indicated in presence of localized tumor and underlying advanced liver disease. Unfortunately, the underlying liver disease (e.g., hepatitis B and C) may recur in the transplanted liver.

Prognosis

Depends on size of tumor, the extent of spread (e.g., presence of vascular invasion), and liver function in those with cirrhosis.

LIVER TRANSPLANTATION

Q. Discuss briefly about liver transplantation.

- Transplantation of liver is useful in treating patient with end-stage liver disease or acute/fulminant liver failure and 5-year survival rate in good centers is about 75%.
- **"Split" livers:** In which one liver is used for two recipients. It is helpful in tackling organ shortage and in shortening the time on the waiting list.
- **Orthotopic liver transplantation:** It is the most common form of liver transplantation. Orthotopic means that the graft is placed in its correct anatomical location. In this technique, donor organ after removal of the native organ is transplanted in the same anatomic location.
- **Auxiliary partial orthotopic liver transplantation** (APOLT) is also called partial or split liver transplantation.
  - In this technique, a segment of donor liver is transplanted in a recipient who has undergone hemihepatectomy to make room for the graft.
  - **Advantage:**
    - If the donor's liver fails, the recipient's own organ can function as a backup until a new liver is found.
- **Living donor liver transplantation:** In this technique, a portion of healthy person's liver is removed and used for transplantation.
  - **Living-related donors: In this,** the donor of the liver segment is a first-degree living relative.
- **Bioartificial liver:** Cultured hepatocytes are used in patients with acute liver failure till donor liver becomes available.

Indications (Table 11.48)

TABLE 11.48: Indications for liver transplantation.

Cirrhosis due to	*In children*
➢ **Acute/fulminant liver failure** (e.g., seronegative hepatitis, drug-induced liver injury). ➢ Chronic viral hepatitis C and B ➢ Alcoholic liver disease (after successful demonstration of abstention) ➢ Other causes of cirrhosis (e.g., nonalcoholic steatohepatitis, autoimmune diseases, primary biliary cholangitis)	➢ **Biliary atresia** ➢ **Inborn errors of metabolism:** Wilson's disease, glycogen storage diseases, Crigler–Najjar syndrome type I, familial hypercholesterolemia, α1-antitrypsin deficiency familial amyloid polyneuropathy, primary hyperoxaluria
➢ **Hepatocellular carcinoma** with no single lesion >5 cm or no more than three lesions with the largest being 3 cm or smaller. ➢ **Failure of previous liver transplant**	

Contraindications

- **Absolute contraindications**
  - Poor expected outcome of transplantation (e.g., multisystem organ failure, malignancy or infection of extrahepatic or extrabiliary tract, HCC with metastatic spread advanced cardiac or pulmonary disease, and HIV infection).
- **Relative contraindications**
  - Comorbidities that reduce survival (e.g., renal insufficiency, primary hepatobiliary malignancy >5 cm, hemochromatosis, SBP, patient older than 65 years).

Complications of Liver Transplantation (Table 11.49) and Immunosuppression (Box 11.34)

TABLE 11.49: Complications of liver transplantation.

Hepatic complications	Nonhepatic complications	
➢ Preservation-reperfusion injury with graft failure due to ischemia ➢ Acute graft rejection ➢ Surgical complications—relating to the anastomosis of bile duct and blood vessels such as failure or obstruction of biliary anastomosis.	➢ Chronic graft rejection ➢ Recurrent disease ➢ Infection and drug-induced liver injury ➢ Jaundice (due to blood transfusion, use of drugs and anesthetic agents, etc.).	➢ Infections/sepsis ➢ Fluid overload ➢ Renal dysfunction ➢ Intraperitoneal bleed

Box 11.34: Complications of immunosuppression.

- Infections
- Metabolic syndrome
  - Hypertension
  - Diabetes mellitus
  - Obesity
  - Dyslipidemia
  - Cardiovascular risk
  - Acute and chronic renal disease
  - Metabolic bone disease
  - De novo malignancy

PYOGENIC ABSCESS

Q. Discuss the etiology, clinical features, investigations, and management of pyogenic liver abscess (bacterial liver abscess).

Etiology

- Bacterial infections in the liver may be manifested as pyogenic abscess. The most common organism includes *E.coli. Streptococcus milleri, Klebsiella pneumoniae,* and *Bacteroides*. Other organisms include *Enterococcus faecalis, Proteus vulgaris,* and *Staphylococcus aureus*. Often the infection is mixed. Tuberculosis and melioidosis can present with liver abscess.
- **Route of infection:** The organisms may reach the liver through one of the following routes:
  1. **Portal vein:** Major source is intra-abdominal infections (e.g., appendicitis, diverticulitis, colitis and perforated bowel).
  2. **Arterial blood supply:** During systemic bacteremia, organism may reach liver via hepatic artery.
  3. **Ascending infection** in the biliary tract (ascending cholangitis).
  4. **Direct invasion** of the liver from a nearby source (e.g., subphrenic abscess, perinephric abscess), or a penetrating injury.

Box 11.35: Indications for ultrasound-guided aspiration of liver abscess.

- Large abscess (>6 cm).
- Abscess in the left lobe.
- Lack of response within 48-72 hours of medical therapy
- Ultrasonography suggestive of large abscess impending rupture

Clinical Features

- **Fever, chills, rigors, and right upper quadrant pain** radiating to right shoulder
- Weight loss, anorexia, nausea, and vomiting; Can manifest as PUO
- Pleuritic chest pain
- **Tender hepatomegaly**
- Mild jaundice may develop when there is extrahepatic biliary obstruction.
- Respiratory findings at the base of right lung (pleural effusion and crepitations) or a pleural rub in the right lower chest.

Investigations

- **Serum bilirubin:** Raised in 25% of cases
- **Serum ALP:** Markedly elevated
- **Blood cultures:** Positive in only 30% of cases.
- **Normochromic normocytic anemia**, usually accompanied by a polymorphonuclear leukocytosis
- **ESR and CRP** are often raised.
- Chest radiograph: Elevation of the right dome of diaphragm, and in severe cases right basilar atelectasis and pneumonia or effusion
- Ultrasonography confirms the diagnosis.
- CT scan of abdomen: helpful when ultrasound is normal.
- Needle aspiration of pus for culture and sensitivity

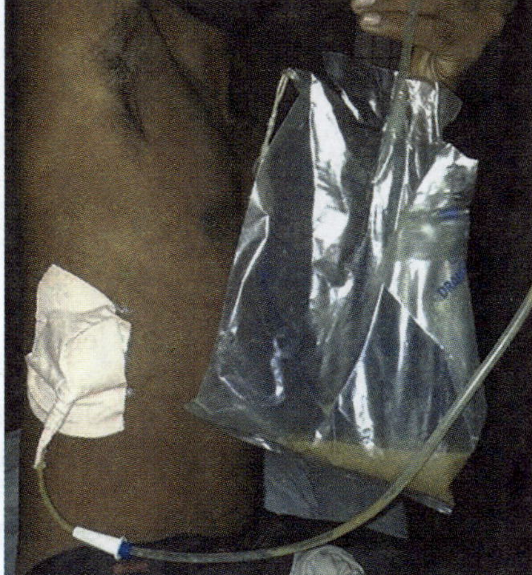

FIG. 11.24: Drainage of abscess with pig tail.

Management

- **Antibiotics:** Initiate treatment with antibiotics (combination of ampicillin, gentamicin, and metronidazole) to cover gram-positive, gram-negative, and anaerobic organisms till the causative organism is identified. Later, change the antibiotic according to the culture and sensitivity reports. Duration of treatment is 4–8 weeks.
- **Ultrasound-guided aspiration of the abscess:** Indications are listed in **Box 11.35**.
- **Surgical drainage** via a large-bore needle for those who fail to respond **(Fig.11.24)**.
- **Treat the underlying cause.**

AMEBIC LIVER ABSCESS

Q. Write short essay/note on diagnosis and management of amebic liver abscess/hepatic amebiasis.

Liver involvement by *Entamoeba histolytica* produces amebic liver abscess. The term amebic hepatitis is not used at present.

Pathogenesis

- ***Entamoeba histolytica*** trophozoites from the base of an amebic ulcer in **colon** may reach liver **through the portal circulation.** The capillary system of the liver acts as an efficient filter and holds these trophozoites. **Trophozoites** multiply, **kill hepatocytes,** cause coagulation necrosis of the liver cells and produce single or multiple abscesses.
- Amebic abscess ranges from 8–12 cm in diameter and appears well circumscribed.
  In most of the cases, the abscess is single and confined to the **posterosuperior aspect of the right lobe of the liver**. This is because right-lobe portal laminar blood flow is supplied predominantly by the superior mesenteric vein, whereas the left-lobe portal blood flow is supplied by the splenic vein. Abscess cavity is filled with a thick, dark brown, odorless, semisolid necrotic material, which resembles **anchovy paste (sauce) in color and consistency.**

Clinical Features

- Symptoms are similar to pyogenic abscesses (such as fever, anorexia, weight loss and malaise). Concurrent diarrhea is present in less than one third of patients.
- **Insidious**/gradual **onset** with low-grade fever, sweats, malaise, weight loss, chills, and rigors. Few may have an acute-onset of fever. In later phase, there may be swinging temperature and sweating usually without marked systemic symptoms or associated cardiovascular signs.
- **Pain:** Patient may have pain in the right hypochondrium due to stretching of the liver capsule. Diaphragmatic irritation by abscess may cause referred pain in the right shoulder.
- Past history of dysentery may be present. Jaundice is rare.
- **Physical examination:** The patient looks ill, shows an enlarged, tender liver, intercostals point tenderness in the posterolateral of a lower right intercostals space (intercostal tenderness) and bulging of the intercostals spaces, upward extension of the liver dullness on percussion. There may be signs of an effusion or consolidation in the base of the right side of the chest.

Complications

1. **Due to rupture of abscess:**
   - Spontaneous external rupture may produce "granuloma cutis."
   - Rupture into bronchus may result in expectorates large amounts of the typical "anchovy-sauce" pus
   - Rupture into pleural space may produce massive pleural effusion
   - Rupture into peritoneal cavity may produce peritonitis
   - Rupture below the diaphragm to produce subdiaphargmatic abscess
   - Rupture into stomach
   - Abscess in the left lobe of liver may rupture into pericardium resulting in pericarditis and rarely cardiac tamponade.
2. **Due to direct extension** into lung, it may produce amebic lung abscess.
3. **Due to hematogenous spread:** Metastatic brain abscess, splenic abscess

Diagnosis

- **Blood:** Polymorphonuclear leukocytosis is a characteristic finding.
- **Liver function tests:** May be abnormal.
  - Most consistent abnormality is raised ALP.
  - Level of AST reflects the severity of the disease. Jaundice is uncommon, and its presence is indicative of a grave prognosis.
- **Chest radiography:** Demonstrate abscess (a raised right hemidiaphragm on chest X-ray). Other findings include right-sided pleural effusion and right basal pneumonitis.
- **Ultrasound:** Ultrasonic scanning of liver is very useful for establishing the diagnosis and localization of the abscess. The defect produced by abscess in the liver usually persists for several months after the complete recovery of the patient.
- **Isotope liver scans and computed tomography:** Can also assist to detect abscess
- **Serologic tests:** For ameba, include indirect hemagglutination test, amebic complement fixation test, ELISA or counter immunoelectrophoresis which can detect antibodies in the blood and are more useful in amebic liver abscess.
- **Amebic fluorescent antibody test:** It is positive in about 90% of patients with liver abscess and in 60–70% with active colitis. **Nested-multiplex PCR** has a sensitivity of 75–100%.

- **Aspiration of amebic liver abscess:** Needle aspiration yields the characteristic "anchovy-sauce" or "chocolate-brown" pus (**Fig. 11.25**). The pus is usually thick in consistency, yellow or green in color, and characteristically odorless. It consists of liquefied necrotic liver tissue and does not contain polymorphonuclear leukocytes. As the parasites are localized in the abscess wall, pus may not show free amebae. Ameba may be demonstrated in the terminal portion of the aspirate, or by a needle biopsy of the abscess wall.

Treatment
- **Metronidazole** 800 mg three times daily for 7–10 days or **tinidazole** 2 g orally daily as a single dose for 5 days is usually adequate in liver abscess. Severe cases may need intravenous administration of metronidazole (500 mg 8 hourly).
- **Chloroquine:** It may be given at a dose of 300 mg twice daily for 2 days, followed by 150 mg twice daily for another 19 days. It is usually administered to those patients who do not respond adequately to metronidazole.
- **Emetine and dehydroemetine** are lethal to the trophozoites of *E. histolytica*. However, because of their toxicity, they are rarely used. Dehydroemetine is less toxic than emetine. Toxicity includes cardiac arrhythmias, muscle weakness, vomiting precordial pain, and diarrhea.
- **Therapeutic aspiration of the abscess:** If a liver abscess is large or likely to burst, or if the response to chemotherapy is not prompt, aspiration is required and repeated if required. Rupture of an abscess into the pleural cavity, pericardial sac or peritoneal cavity needs immediate aspiration or surgical drainage.
- **Percutaneous drainage:** It is achieved by placing a large-bore catheter into the abscesses for draining the abscess. It is usually performed when therapeutic aspiration fails and its indications are:
  - Large abscess and associated risk of spontaneous rupture (especially left-lobe abscesses)
  - If abscess is ruptured already (drainage of both abscess and extraneous collection)
  - Absence of response to medical therapy with signs of persistent sepsis or enlarging abscesses or persistent symptoms
  - Evidence of liver failure
- **After treatment** of the invasive disease, luminal amebicide such as diloxanide furoate 500 mg orally TID for 10 days; or aminosidine (paromomycin) 25–35 mg/kg/day orally in three divided doses for 7–10 days should be given to clear luminal cysts or parasite. Alternative agents include iodoquinol 650 mg orally TID for 20 days, and nitazoxanide.

Clinical comparison between pyogenic and amebic liver abscess (**Table 11.50**)

TABLE 11.50: Pyogenic and amebic liver abscess: clinical comparisons.

Parameter	*Pyogenic liver abscess*	*Amebic liver abscess*
Number	Often multiple	Usually single
Location	Either lobe of liver	Usually right hepatic lobe, near the diaphragm
Presentation	Subacute	Acute
Jaundice	Mild	Moderate
Diagnosis	US or CT-guided aspiration	US or CT and serology

(CT: computed tomography; US: ultrasound)

FIG. 11.25: Anchovy-sauce appearance of amebic abscess.

METABOLIC LIVER DISEASE

Iron Overload

Q. What are various disorders associated with iron overload?

Q. Discuss the etiology, pathology, clinical features, investigations, and management of hereditary (primary) hemochromatosis ("bronze diabetes").

Classification of Iron Overload (Box 11.36)

In secondary iron overload, iron accumulates in Kupffer cells rather than hepatocytes compared to that of hereditary hemochromatosis.

Box 11.36: Classification of iron overload.

Hereditary
- Mutations of genes encoding HFE, transferrin receptor 2 (TfR2), or hepcidin
- Mutations of genes encoding hemojuvelin (HJV)

Hemosiderosis (secondary hemochromatosis)
- Parenteral iron overload
  - Exogenous: Multiple blood transfusions, repeated iron injections, long-term hemodialysis
  - Endogenous: Sickle cell disease
- Ineffective erythropoiesis with increased erythroid activity: β-thalassemia, sideroblastic anemia, porphyria cutanea tarda
- Increased oral intake of iron
- Chronic liver disease: Chronic alcoholic liver disease

Hereditary Hemochromatosis

- Hereditary hemochromatosis (HH) is an inherited **autosomal recessive** disorder characterized by **abnormal (excessive) accumulation of iron** in various parenchymal organs leading to eventual fibrosis and functional organ failure.
- In symptomatic patients of hemochromatosis, the total body iron is increased to 20–40 g, compared with 3–4 g in normal individuals.

- Associated with **high incidence of HCC**
- Most of the hereditary hemochromatosis is inherited as autosomal recessive genetic disorder and associated with HLA-B3, B7 and B14 histocompatibility antigens.

Pathology

The **excess iron is deposited** commonly in the **liver, joint, heart, pancreas, endocrine glands** (e.g., pituitary gland) **and skin.**

Clinical Features

- **Age and gender:** Overt clinical manifestations occur **more frequently in males** over the age of 40 years. About 90% of the patients are males. Females are protected because of loss of iron during menstruation and pregnancy.
- **Symptoms:**
  - It may develop due to toxic damage of cells by accumulated iron and consequent fibrosis.
  - Symptoms may be **vague**-muscle aches, weakness, abdominal and/or joint pain.
  - **Classic triad:** Consists of **bronze skin pigmentation** (**Fig. 11.26**) (due to melanin deposition in exposed parts, axillae, groins and genitalia), **hepatomegaly and diabetes** mellitus (**"bronzed diabetes"**) is observed in patients with gross iron overload.
  - **Late features:** Hypopituitarism, loss of libido, testicular atrophy, cardiac complaints (cardiomyopathy, heart failure and cardiac arrhythmias), hypothyroidism, cirrhosis with hepatosplenomegaly, spiders, loss of body hair, jaundice, and ascites.
  - Cirrhosis

Complications

- **Chondrocalcinosis:** Develops due to asymmetrical deposition of calcium pyrophosphate in both large and small joints and leads to an arthropathy. It has characteristic radiologic findings: Squared-off bone ends and hook-like osteophytes in the second and third metacarpophalangeal (MCP) joints.
- **Hepatocellular carcinoma** in 30% of patients with cirrhosis
- **Multi-organ failure**
- Susceptibility to specific infections (bacteria whose virulence is increased in the presence of excess iron). These include

Listeria monocytogenes, Yersinia enterocolitica, and Vibrio vulnificus.

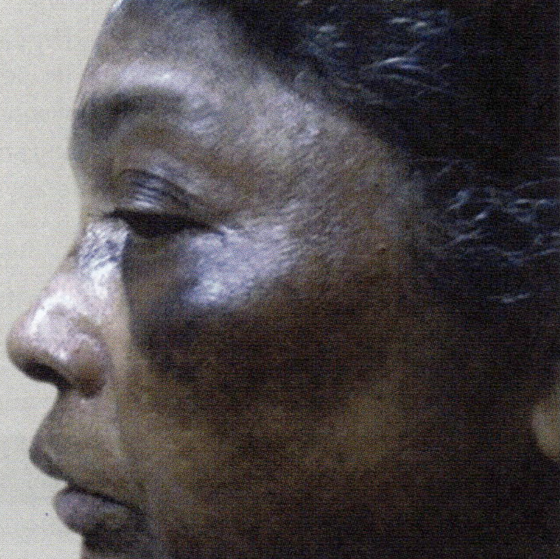

FIG. 11.26: Skin pigmentation in hemochromatosis.

Investigations

- **Serum iron profile:**
  - **Serum iron** is **elevated** (>30 μmol/L).
  - **Total iron binding capacity (TIBC): Reduced**
  - **Fasting transferrin saturation** (serum iron divided by the total iron binding capacity) **is high (>45%)** which is **highly sensitive for diagnosis.**
  - **Serum ferritin is elevated** (usually >500 μg/L or 240 nmol/L). It is less sensitive than transferrin saturation in screening for hemochromatosis because it is also increased in alcoholic liver disease, hepatitis C infection, NASH. It is also an acute-phase reactant and increased in other inflammatory and neoplastic conditions.
- **Biochemical tests** for liver function are **often normal**, even with established cirrhosis.
- **Genetic testing:** It is performed if iron studies are abnormal.
- **CT scan:** Shows **increased density of liver** due to deposits of iron.
- **Magnetic resonance imaging (MRI):** It is **sensitive** to detect liver iron content.
- **Liver biopsy:** Not necessary for diagnosis. It shows **iron deposition** and hepatic **fibrosis** leading on to cirrhosis.
- **Screening**: All first-degree family members of hereditary hemochromatosis must be screened to detect early and asymptomatic disease.

Treatment and Management

- Treatment **should be started before permanent organ damage** occurs due to iron toxicity. The excess iron should be removed as rapidly as possible and prolongs life and may reverse tissue damage.
- **Phlebotomy/Venesection:** Venesection of 500 mL blood (removes 250 mg of iron) is performed twice-weekly until the serum iron is normal. This may take 2 years or more.
- **Chelation therapy:** Rarely in patients who cannot tolerate venesection because of severe cardiac disease or anemia, chelation therapy with **desferrioxamine** can be used. Dose is 40–80 mg/kg/day subcutaneously. It removes about 10–20 mg of iron/day. Deferiprone and deferasirox are other chelators.

- **Erythrocytapheresis** is an apheresis technique whereby red cells are removed in an isovolemic manner and the patient's plasma is returned to the patient, larger amounts of iron can be removed per session than by phlebotomy.
- Treatment of diabetes
- Treatment of cirrhosis: There is a risk of malignancy if cirrhosis is present
- Treatment of congestive heart failure and cardiac arrhythmias
- **Dietary limitations:** (i) Dietary iron intake to be restricted, (ii) agents for reducing iron absorption (tannates in tea, phytates, oxalates, calcium, and phosphates) to be used, (iii) avoidance of excessive ethanol, (iv) avoidance of ascorbic acid (vitamin C) supplements, and (v) avoidance of uncooked seafood.

Wilson's Disease

Q. Discuss the etiology, pathology, clinical features, investigations, and management of Wilson's disease (hepatolenticular degeneration).

Q. Explain in brief about Kayser-Fleischer ring.

- **Wilson's disease (progressive hepatolenticular degeneration)** is a **very rare inborn error of copper metabolism** characterized by **increased total body copper.**
- Excess **copper deposition** in various organs: **(1) liver, (2) basal ganglia of the brain, (3) cornea, (4) kidneys, and (5) skeleton**.
- **Potentially treatable** condition.

Etiology

- **Autosomal recessive** disorder
- Consanguinity is risk factor.
- **Molecular defect within a copper-transporting ATPase** encoded by a gene (***ATP7B***) located on chromosome 13. More than 300 mutations have been identified and is rare in India and Asia.
- **Defect:** Excessive accumulation of copper in the body due to:
  - Failure of incorporation of copper into proceruloplasmin and leads to **low serum ceruloplasmin.**
  - Failure of biliary copper excretion, causing its accumulation in the body.

Pathology

Liver: Microscopic features are **not diagnostic** and vary from that of **chronic hepatitis to macronodular cirrhosis**. Stains for copper show a periportal distribution of copper.

Clinical Features

- **Age of presentation** is usually between **5 and 30 years**.
  - Children usually present with hepatic problems.
  - Young adults usually present with more neurological problems.
- **Features of liver involvement:** Varies from (1) acute hepatitis going on to, (2) fulminant hepatic failure, to (3) chronic hepatitis, or (4) cirrhosis
- **Features of brain involvement: Dysarthria,** involuntary movements, tremors (especially asymmetric, resting and intention tremors, wing beating), **ataxia,** and eventually dementia.
- **Psychiatric manifestations:** Phobia, depression, compulsive behavior

- **Kayser–Fleischer rings**
  - It is a **characteristic sign** due to deposition of **copper in the Descemet's membrane** of cornea.
  - Appears as **greenish-brown or golden-brown ring at the corneoscleral junction** (around the periphery of the cornea), appearing first at the upper periphery gradually disappear with effective medical treatment or liver transplantation.
  - Best identified by slit-lamp examination
  - It may be absent in young children and disappears with treatment.
  - May be associated with "sunflower cataracts."
  - **Kayser–Fleischer rings (Fig. 11.27) are not specific for Wilson's disease**; they are found occasionally in patients with other types of chronic liver disease, usually with a prominent cholestatic component, such as PBC, primary sclerosing cholangitis, or familial cholestatic syndromes, and rarely in patients with nonhepatic diseases.

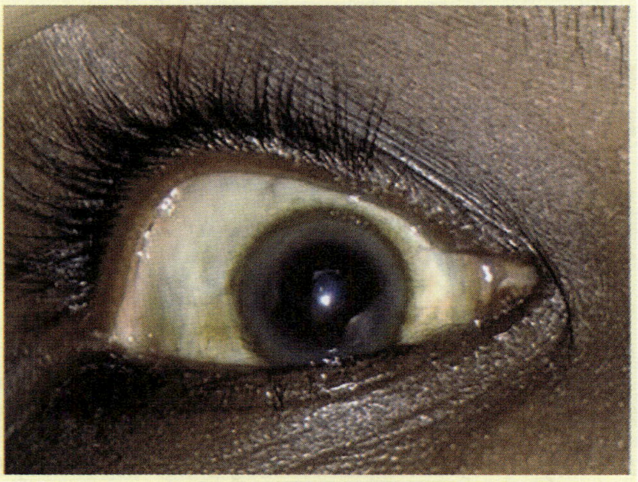

FIG. 11.27: Kayser–Fleischer ring.

Other manifestations: Kidney (renal tubular damage), skeleton (osteoporosis, arthropathy).

Investigations

- **Slit-lamp examination** of the eyes for Kayser–Fleischer ring
- **Serum copper: Reduced** but can be normal.
- **Serum ceruloplasmin levels: Low** and less than 20 mg/dL.
- **Urinary copper: Usually increased** 100–1,000 μg in 24 h (1.6–16 μmol); normal levels <40 μg (0.6 μmol). The **penicillamine challenge:** 500 mg dose of penicillamine at the beginning of the 24-hour urine collection and then again at 12 hours. Urinary copper excretion greater than 1,600 mg per 24 hours (>25 μmol) is diagnostic.
- **Liver biopsy:** Gold standard. Diagnosis depends on the amount of copper in the liver (>250 μg/g dry weight).
- **Hemolysis and anemia** may be found.

Treatment and Management

- Treatment should be started early and will show improvement both clinically and biochemically.
- **Chelating drugs**
  - **Penicillamine with pyridoxine:** It should be given lifetime in the dose of 1–1.5 g daily and effectively chelates copper.
- For asymptomatic cases and maintenance therapy (after maximal improvement with penicillamine)
  - **Trientine dihydrochloride:** In the dose of 1.2–1.8 g/day
  - **Zinc acetate:** Indicated in chronic hepatitis and cirrhosis. Dose 150 mg/day. It blocks absorption of copper from intestine. However, it **should not be administered with penicillamine or trientine** since both these drugs chelate zinc.
  - **Other drugs:** (1) intramuscular **dimercaprol,** (2) **ammonium tetrathiomolybdate,** (3) **potassium sulfide, and** (4) **carbacrylamine resins.**
  - **Liver transplantation:** In fulminant hepatic failure and decompensated/advanced cirrhosis
  - All siblings and children of the patient should be screened for Wilson's disease and treated even if they are asymptomatic, and if there is evidence of copper accumulation.

α1-Antitrypsin Deficiency

Q. Write a short note on α_1-antitrypsin.

Clinical Features

- In neonates, it produces cholestatic jaundice
- **In adults:**
  - **Liver: Chronic hepatitis, cirrhosis, HCC, and cholangiocarcinoma**
  - **Lung: Emphysema, chronic bronchitis**
  - **Others:** Panniculitis, vasculitis, pancreatitis, and glomerulonephritis

Investigations

- **Serum α_1-antritrypsin is low** (normal above 150 mg/dL).
- **Serum protein electrophoresis** shows **absence of $\propto_1$-globulin peak**.
- **Liver biopsy:** α_1-AT accumulates in periportal hepatocytes and can be seen as **periodic acid-Schiff (PAS)-positive, diastase-resistant globular inclusions** in these **hepatocytes**. The injury to these hepatocytes results in progressive fibrosis and cirrhosis.

Treatment

- **No treatment** apart from dealing with the complications of liver disease.
- Stop cigarette smoking and alcohol intake.
- Liver or lung transplantation.

BILIARY CIRRHOSIS

Q. What is biliary cirrhosis? Discuss the etiology, pathology, clinical features, investigations, and management of primary biliary cholangitis.

- It is a type of **cirrhosis** of the liver **secondary to prolonged obstruction of biliary system** (anywhere between the small interlobular bile ducts and the papilla of Vater).
- Obstruction results in progressive destruction of bile ducts.

Classification

Biliary cirrhosis may be subdivided into PBC and secondary biliary cirrhosis.

1. **Primary biliary cholangitis:** It is a probably an **autoimmune disorder** of the intrahepatic biliary tree.
2. **Secondary biliary cirrhosis:** It is due to **prolonged obstruction of the extrahepatic biliary tree.**

Primary Biliary Cirrhosis Presently called as Primary Biliary Cholangitis

Gender: It usually affects **middle-aged women**, with a female to male ratio of more than 6:1.
Age: Peak incidence between **40 and 50 years** of age (perimenopausal).

Etiology and Pathogenesis

- PBC is thought to be an **autoimmune disorder**, but its exact pathogenesis is not known.
- **Genetic and environmental** factors play role in the pathogenesis of the PBC. Probably an environmental factor acts on a genetically predisposed individual via molecular mimicry initiate autoimmunity.

Clinical Features

- It is **insidious in** onset and asymptomatic patients are discovered during routine examination or investigations.
- Commonly present with **pruritus** (often the earliest symptom), **fatigue, and skin pigmentation** (due to melanin deposition) abdominal discomfort.
- **Features of liver involvement:**
  - **Intense pruritus** (probably due to bile salts) occurs months to years before jaundice and is more at night. Scratch marks.
  - **Progressive jaundice (bottle green color)**
  - **Clubbing** of fingers
  - Hepatosplenomegaly
  - Hepatic decompensation, portal hypertension, ascites and variceal bleeding develop.
- **Hypercholesterolemia:**
  - **Xanthelasmas** (cholesterol-rich macrophages) around the eyes **(Fig.11.28)**
  - **Xanthomas** over joints, tendons, hand creases, elbows, and knees
  - Pain, tingling, and numbness over feet and hands due to peripheral neuropathy produced by lipid infiltration of peripheral nerves.

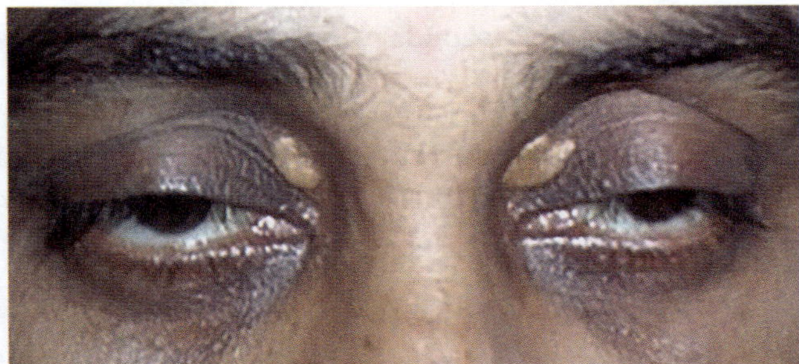

FIG. 11.28: Xanthelasmas around the eyes.

- **Malabsorption**
  - Steatorrhea and diarrhea due to malabsorption of fat
  - Easy bruising and ecchymosis due to vitamin K deficiency
  - Osteomalacia and/or osteoporosis due to malabsorption of vitamin D
  - Night blindness due to vitamin A deficiency
  - Dermatitis due to vitamin E deficiency
- **Extrahepatic manifestations:** These include autoimmune disorders such as Sjögren syndrome, keratoconjunctivitis sicca (dry eyes and mouth), systemic sclerosis, autoimmune thyroiditis, rheumatoid arthritis, Raynaud phenomenon, membranous glomerulonephritis, and celiac disease.

Investigations

- **Antimitochondrial antibodies** are characteristic and are essential for the diagnosis of PBC. They are found in 90–95% of patients. M2 antibody is specific. Other nonspecific antibodies (e.g., **antinuclear factor** and smooth muscle) may also be present.
- **Marked rise of serum 5′-nucleotidase** activity
- **High serum ALP** (markers of cholestasis)**:** Two-to five-fold rise
- **Hyperlipidemia and serum cholesterol** is **raised.**
- **Serum bilirubin:** Hyperbilirubinemia of the conjugated type occurs in late stages.
- **Serum transaminase:** Mild elevation of transaminases.
- **Serum IgM** may be **very high**.
- **Ultrasound:** It shows diffuse alteration in liver architecture.
- **MRCP (or ERCP):** It shows normal biliary tree.
- **Liver biopsy:** Portal tract infiltration by lymphocytes and plasma cells and about 40% have granulomas. Later portal tract fibrosis and, eventually progress to cirrhosis.

Note: Hepatic granulomas are not specific and are also found in sarcoidosis, tuberculosis, schistosomiasis, drug reactions, brucellosis, parasitic infestation (e.g., strongyloidiasis) and other conditions.

Management/Treatment

- **Ursodeoxycholic acid (10–15 mg/kg):** It improves bilirubin and aminotransferase levels. It should be started early in the asymptomatic phase.
- **Steroids:** They improve biochemical and histological disease but may lead to increased osteoporosis.
- **Other therapies** include azathioprine, colchicines, and methotrexate and cyclosporine may be beneficial in few patients.
- **Steatorrhea:** It is treated by limiting intake of fat and substituting long-chain triglycerides with medium-chain triglycerides in the diet.

- **Malabsorption of fat-soluble vitamins** (A, D, and K) is managed **by supplementation.**
- Calcium supplementation
- **Pruritus** is difficult to control but following can be helpful.
  - **Cholestyramine** one 4 g sachet three times daily, but is unpalatable
  - Antihistamines
  - Rifampicin, naloxone hydrochloride, ondansetron, and opiate antagonists (naloxone and naltrexone)
- Liver transplantation

Complications: These include (i) cirrhosis, (ii) osteoporosis and osteomalacia, (iii) polyneuropathy, and (iv) increased risk of HCCs.

Secondary Biliary Cirrhosis

Q. Write short note on secondary biliary cirrhosis.

Definition

Cirrhosis developing **secondary to prolonged** (for months) **obstruction** of the extrahepatic (large biliary duct) biliary tree

Causes of Obstruction

(1) Gallstones, (2) bile duct strictures, and (3) sclerosing cholangitis
Patients with malignant tumors of bile duct or pancreas rarely survive long enough to develop secondary biliary cirrhosis.

Cardiac Cirrhosis

Q. Write short note on cardiac cirrhosis.

- **Cause:** Liver damage primarily due to congestion may develop in all types of **right heart failure.** Examples: valvular heart disease, constrictive pericarditis, or cor pulmonale of long duration (more than 10 years).
- **Mechanism:** Right heart failure causes retrograde transmission of raised venous pressure via the IVC and hepatic vein into the liver. This leads to passive congestion of liver. When passive venous congestion becomes chronic/prolonged, the liver becomes enlarged, tender and shows a "nutmeg appearance" (alternating red-congested and pale-fibrotic areas). Very rarely, prolonged, severe right-sided heart failure and hepatic congestion cause cardiac cirrhosis.
- **Clinical features**
  - Usually dominated by the heart disease
  - Symptoms and signs of severe right heart failure.
- **Diagnosis**
  - Firm enlarged liver with signs of chronic liver disease in a patient with valvular heart disease, constrictive pericarditis, or chronic cor pulmonale
  - Nonpulsatile liver despite the presence of tricuspid regurgitation
  - Liver biopsy confirms the diagnosis (not required in most cases).

Treatment of the underlying cardiovascular disorder.

Noncirrhotic Portal Fibrosis

Q. Write a short note on noncirrhotic portal fibrosis.

- Noncirrhotic portal fibrosis (NCPF) is an idiopathic disease characterized by periportal fibrosis and involvement of small and medium branches of portal vein.
- It leads to development of portal hypertension and splenomegaly without features of liver cell failure.
- Worldwide it accounts for 3–5% of all patients with portal hypertension, but in India it accounts for 15–20% of cases of portal hypertension.

Etiology

Bacterial infections, exposure to toxins (arsenic, vinyl chloride monomer, copper sulfate, methotrexate, hypervitaminosis A, 6-mercaptopurine), immunological abnormalities and hypercoagulable states may play a role.

Clinical Features

- Characterized by upper GI bleed, **massive splenomegaly** with anemia
- Preserved liver function
- **Ascites, jaundice, and hepatic encephalopathy are uncommon.**

Investigations

- *Liver function tests:* Usually normal
- *Peripheral blood:* Pancytopenia may develop due to hypersplenism.
- *Doppler ultrasound:* It shows patent splenoportal axis and hepatic veins.
- *Splenoportovenography (SPV):* It reveals massive dilatation of the portal and splenic veins, and the presence of collaterals.
- *Liver biopsy:* Lobular architecture maintained, portal fibrosis of variable degree, sclerosis and obliteration of small-sized portal vein radicals.

Treatment: Endoscopic sclerotherapy or banding to prevent variceal bleed and shunt surgery.

Differences between extrahepatic portal venous obstruction (EHPVO), NCPF, and cirrhosis are presented in **Table 11.51**.

TABLE 11.51: Differences between EHPVO, NCPF, and cirrhosis.

Features	*EHPVO*	*NCPF*	*Cirrhosis*
Median age	10 years	28 years	40 years
Ascites	Absent	Absent	+++
Encephalopathy	Nil	Nil	Present
Deranged LFT	Nil	Nil	Present
Splenomegaly	Moderate- massive	Moderate	Mild- moderate
Abdominal vein	Nil	Nil	Anterior abdominal veins +
Liver–Gross	Normal	Normal	Shrunken, nodular
Liver biopsy	Normal	Portal fibrosis	Hepatic necrosis, fibrosis, regenerative nodules
Ultrasonography	Portal/splenic vein block and cavernoma	Dilated and patent portal vein	Coarse echotexture of liver. Dilated portal vein, ascites
Site of block	Extrahepatic presinusoidal	Intrahepatic presinusoidal	Intrahepatic sinusoidal and postsinusoidal

(EHPVO: extrahepatic portal venous obstruction; LFT: liver function test; NCPF: noncirrhotic portal fibrosis)

Common Causes of Painful Hepatomegaly (Table 11.52)

TABLE 11.52: Common causes of painful hepatomegaly.

➢ Hepatitis	➢ Amoebic liver abscess	➢ Malignancies
– Viral hepatitis	➢ Pyogenic liver abscess	– Hepatocellular carcinoma
– Drug-induced hepatitis	➢ Actinomycosis	– Secondaries
– Alcoholic hepatitis	➢ Congestive cardiac failure	
– Chronic hepatitis	➢ Acute Budd-Chiari syndrome	

Q. What are the common causes of hepatomegaly with tenderness (tender hepatomegaly)?

Causes of Pulsatile Liver (Box 11.37)

Q. Write short note on causes of pulsatile liver.

Box 11.37: Causes of pulsatile liver.

- Tricuspid regurgitation (systolic)
- Tricuspid stenosis (diastolic)
- Aortic regurgitation

Causes of Splenomegaly (Table11.53)

Q. Enumerate the common causes of splenomegaly.

TABLE 11.53: Classification of splenomegaly and their causes.

Mild splenomegaly (up to 5 cm)	
Acute infections	Septic shock, infective endocarditis, enteric fever, infectious hepatitis, infectious monoculeosis, brucellosis, cytomegalovirus, toxoplasmosis
Chronic infections	Tuberculosis, syphilis, brucellosis, chronic bacteremia, HIV
Parasitic infestations	Malaria, kala-azar, and schistosomiasis
Inflammation	Rheumatoid arthritis, sarcoidosis, SLE
Others	Congestive cardiac failure, thalassemia minor
Moderate splenomegaly (up to umbilicus) (5–8 cm)	
Neoplastic	Lymphomas, acute leukemias, chronic lymphocytic leukemia, chronic myeloid leukemia
Nonneoplastic	Cirrhosis of liver (with portal hypertension), chronic hemolytic anemia, malaria, kala-azar, sarcoidosis, infectious mononucleosis, splenic abscess, amyloidosis, hemochromatosis, polycythemia vera
Massive splenomegaly (below umbilicus) (more than 8 cm) (Fig. 11.29)	
Common causes	Chronic myeloid leukemia, myelofibrosis, kala-azar, hairy cell leukemia, tropical splenomegaly, portal hypertension (extrahepatic portal vein thrombosis), hyperreactive malarial splenomegaly
Uncommon causes	Lymphomas, Gaucher's disease, Niemann–Pick disease, thalassemia major, splenic cysts and tumors of spleen, myeloid metaplasia, hairy cell leukemia, sarcoidosis, *MAC* infection in HIV patients

(MAC: *Mycobacterium avium* complex; SLE: systemic lupus erythematosus)

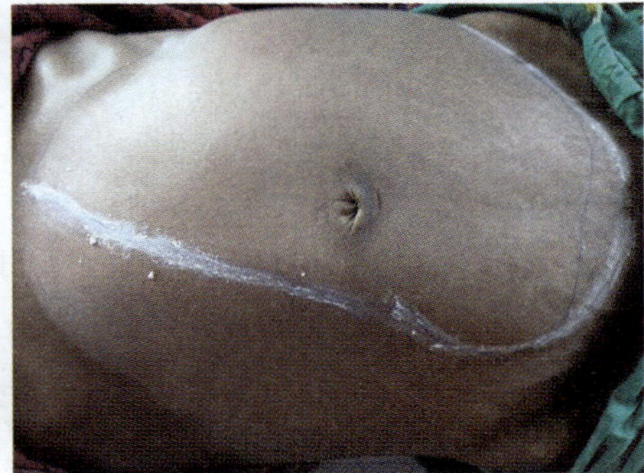

FIG. 11.29: Massive splenomegaly in chronic myeloid leukemia (CML).

Causes of Hepatosplenomegaly (Table 11.54 and Figs. 11.30 and 11.31)

TABLE 11.54: Causes of hepatosplenomegaly.

Infections: Malaria, kala-azar, infective hepatitis, disseminated tuberculosis (TB), bacterial endocarditis, infectious mononucleosis	**Hematological disorders:** Chronic hemolytic anemia, chronic myeloid leukemia, myelofibrosis, Hodgkin and non-Hodgkin lymphoma
Congestive states: Congestive cardiac failure, constrictive pericarditis, cirrhosis of liver with portal hypertension, Budd–Chiari syndrome	**Storage disorders:** Gaucher's disease, glycogen storage disorders, and amyloidosis

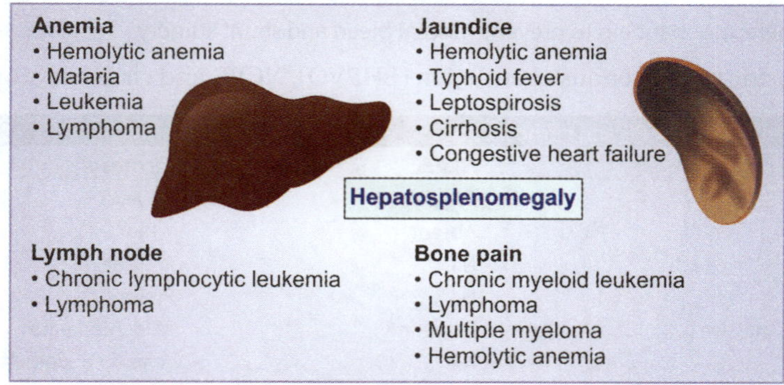

FIG. 11.30: Causes of hepatosplenomegaly according to the associated sign.

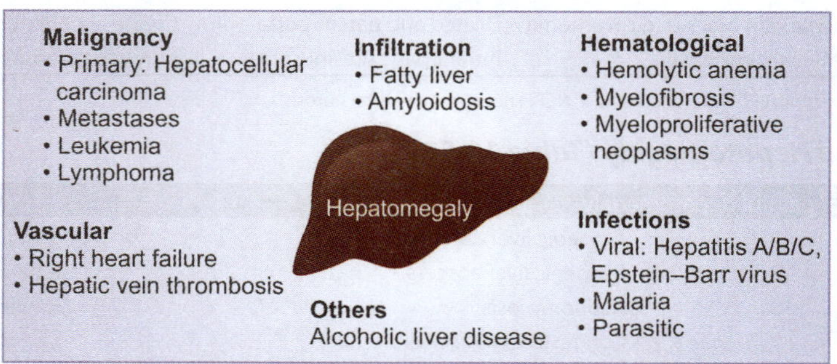

FIG. 11.31: Hepatomegaly according to underlying pathology.

Causes of Hepatosplenomegaly with Lymphadenopathy (Box 11.38)

Box 11.38: Causes of hepatosplenomegaly with lymphadenopathy.

- Lymphomas
- Infectious mononucleosis
- HIV
- Sarcoidosis
- Lymphocytic leukemia
- Disseminated tuberculosis
- Disseminated histoplasmosis

HEPATIC DISORDERS OF PREGNANCY

Q. List the differential diagnosis for liver diseases during pregnancy.

Disease	*Hyperemesis gravidarum*	*Liver failure due to preeclampsia*	*Intrahepatic cholestasis*	*AFLP*	*HELLP*
Trimester	1st	>20 weeks	2nd to 3rd	2nd to 3rd	3rd to postpartum
Frequency	0.3–2%	<10%	0.1–5%	0.01%	0.2–0.6%
Clinical features	Nausea, vomiting, dehydration, weight loss, features of ketosis	Hypertension, proteinuria, headache, blurring of vision, edema of extremities	Jaundice rarely, pruritus	Abdominal pain, proteinuria, encephalopathy	Abdominal pain, vomiting, proteinuria, headache, edema of extremities
Ascites	Nil	Nil	Nil	May be present	Nil
Platelet count	No change	Decreased	No change	Decreased	Decreased
Hemolysis	No change	Increased	No change	No change	May be increased

Contd...

Contd...

Bilirubin and bile acids	Bilirubin remains low. No change in bile acids	Bilirubin remains low. No change in bile acids	Bile acids may be increased 50–100 times.	Mildly increased bilirubin; no change in bile acids	Bilirubin remains low. No change in bile acids
AST/ALT	1–2 times normal	1–100 times normal	1–5 times normal	5–10 times normal	1–100 times normal
LDH	No change	Mildly increased	No change	Mildly increased	Usually above 600 IU/L
ALP	No change	Mildly increased	Increased	Increased	Increased
Uric acid	No change	Increased	No change	Highly increased	Increased
Treatment	Supportive therapy, antiemetics, vitamin replacement, admission if dehydration is severe	Good control of blood pressures, careful monitoring for progression into eclampsia	Ursodeoxycholic acid may be administered. Delivery preferably at 36–37 weeks	Delivery to be done early preferably at 34–36 weeks.	Delivery to be done early. May need to go as early as 24–34 weeks as long as antenatal corticosteroids are given
Complications	Resolves spontaneously by 18 weeks	Maternal and perinatal mortality	Late IUDs	Liver rupture, necrosis, maternal and perinatal mortality	Maternal and perinatal mortality

(AFLP: acute fatty liver of pregnancy; ALT: alanine aminotransferase; ALP: alkaline phosphatase; AST: aspartate aminotransferase; HELLP: hemolysis, elevated liver enzyme levels, and low platelet levels; LDH: lactate dehydrogenase)

CHAPTER 12

Pancreas

PANCREATITIS

Acute Pancreatitis

Q. Discuss the etiology, clinical features, investigations, diagnosis, complications and management of acute pancreatitis.

Definition

Acute pancreatitis is best defined clinically by a patient presenting with two of the three criteria listed in **Box 12.1**.

Box 12.1: Criteria for diagnosis of acute pancreatitis.

- Symptoms: Epigastric pain, consistent with the disease.
- Laboratory findings: Serum amylase or lipase three times greater than the upper limit of normal.
- Radiologic imaging: Findings consistent with the diagnosis, by either computed tomography (CT) or magnetic resonance imaging (MRI).

Classification of Acute Pancreatitis

Atlanta classification of acute pancreatitis

- **Interstitial edematous acute pancreatitis:** Characterized by acute inflammation of the pancreatic parenchyma and peripancreatic tissues, but without tissue necrosis.
- **Necrotizing acute pancreatitis:** Characterized by inflammation associated with pancreatic parenchymal necrosis and/or peripancreatic necrosis.

Classification of acute pancreatitis according to the severity

- **Mild acute pancreatitis:** Not associated with organ failure and local or systemic complications.
- **Moderately severe acute pancreatitis:** No organ failure or transient organ failure (<48 hours) and/or local complications.
- **Severe acute pancreatitis:** Persistent organ failure (>48 hours) that may involve one or multiple organs.

Box 12.2: Mnemonic for causes of pancreatitis.

I GET SMASHED
Idiopathic
Gallstones
Ethanol
Trauma
Steroid
Mumps
Autoimmune
Scorpion bite
Hyperlipidemia
ERCP
Drugs

Etiology (Table 12.1) (Box 12.2)

Q. Describe etiology of acute pancreatitis.

TABLE 12.1: Causes of acute pancreatitis.

Obstructive Causes	Toxins
➤ Gallstones (40-70%) ➤ *Obstruction of the pancreatic duct system:* Ampullary or pancreatic tumors ➤ *Parasites:* Ascaris lumbricoides and clonorchis sinensis organisms ➤ *Developmental anomalies:* Pancreas divisum, choledochocele, annular pancreas	➤ Ethyl alcohol (25–35%) ➤ Methyl alcohol ➤ Scorpion venom ➤ Snake venom ➤ Organophosphates ➤ Insecticides ➤ Smoking

Contd...

Contd...

Drugs ➢ *Definite association:* Azathioprine, 6-mercaptopurine, valproic acid, estrogens, corticosteroids, didanosine ➢ *Probable association:* Thiazides, ethacrynic acid, phenformin, procainamide, chlorthalidone, L-asparaginase	**Metabolic Causes** ➢ Hyperlipoproteinemia ➢ Hypertriglyceridemia (1–14%) ➢ Hyperparathyroidism ➢ Hypercalcemia ➢ Renal failure ➢ Postrenal transplantation
Trauma ➢ *Accidental*: Blunt trauma to the abdomen ➢ *Iatrogenic injury:* Postoperative, postendoscopic retrograde cholangiopancreatography, endoscopic sphincterotomy, sphincter of Oddi manometry	**Infectious** ➢ *Viral:* Mumps, rubella, viral hepatitis, coxsackie virus B, echovirus, cytomegalovirus, human immunodeficiency virus ➢ *Bacterial:* Mycoplasma, *Campylobacter jejuni*, tuberculosis, *Legionella* species, Leptospirosis ➢ *Fungi: Aspergillus* ➢ *Parasites: Clonorchis sinensis, Toxoplasma, Cryptosporidium, Ascaris, Echinococcus granulosus, Fasciola hepatica*
Vascular ➢ *Ischemia:* Hypoperfusion (e.g. postcardiac surgery) or atherosclerotic emboli ➢ *Vasculitis*: Systemic lupus erythematosus, polyarteritis nodosa, malignant hypertension	**Idiopathic**
Miscellaneous ➢ Penetrating peptic ulcer ➢ Pregnancy associated Reye syndrome ➢ Autoimmune	**Genetic** ➢ Mutations in the pancreatic trypsin inhibitor (*SPINK1*) gene in the cystic fibrosis transmembrane regulator (CFTR) ➢ Gain-of-function mutations in the *PRSS1* gene

Pathogenesis (Fig. 12.1)

Autodigestion of the pancreatic substance is a currently accepted pathogenic theory of acute pancreatitis. According to this theory, acute pancreatitis develops as a consequence of premature and exaggerated activation of proteolytic enzymes within the pancreas itself (e.g. trypsinogen, chymotrypsinogen, proelastase, and lipolytic enzymes such as phospholipase A_2).

Activation of pancreatic enzymes

Activation of trypsin: One of the proenzyme is trypsinogen, which is **prematurely activated to trypsin.** It is an important triggering event. Actions of trypsin are:

- ***Activates other proenzymes:*** Trypsin converts many proenzymes into active forms (such as proelastase and prophospholipase). Activated enzymes elastase (from proelastase) and phospholipase (prophospholipase) can damage the elastic fibers of blood vessels and degrade fat cells.

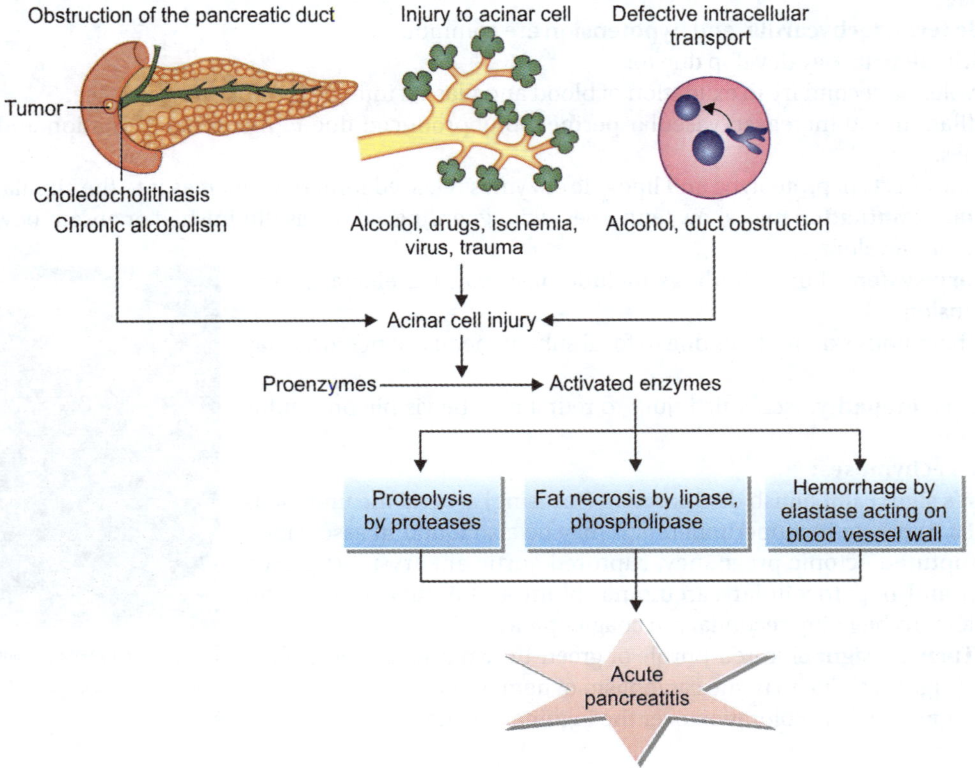

FIG. 12.1: Pathogenesis of acute pancreatitis.

- ***Activation of kinin, clotting and complement system:*** Trypsin acts on kinin system and converts prekallikrein to its activated form kallikrein. This in turn can activate Hageman factor (factor XII), the clotting and complement systems.

The severity of acute pancreatitis depends on the balance of two opposite sets of forces, namely the activity of released proteolytic enzymes and antiproteolytic factors. The latter consists of an intracellular pancreatic trypsin inhibitor protein and circulating β2-macroglobulin, α1-antitrypsin and C1-esterase inhibitors.

Clinical Features

Q. Write short note on signs and symptoms of acute pancreatitis.

Symptoms

- **Abdominal pain:** It is the cardinal and major symptom of acute pancreatitis. Its characteristics are:
  - **Location:** Upper abdominal pain usually located in the **epigastric and periumbilical region** more on the left or right side, depending on the portion of the pancreas is involved.
  - **Onset: Sudden** onset and gradually increases in severity.
  - **Nature: Constant, steady, intense** (over 15–60 minutes)/dull and boring.
    - Pain is relieved by sitting or leaning forward (Mohammedan prayer sign) due to shifting forward of abdominal contents and taking pressure off from inflamed pancreas.
    - When the retroperitoneum is involved, pain often **radiates to the upper back** as well as to the chest, flanks, and lower abdomen.
    - 5–10% of patients with acute severe pancreatitis may have *painless disease* and have *unexplained hypotension*
- **Other symptoms:** These include anorexia, nausea, and vomiting.

Acute pancreatitis may present as acute abdomen as a medical emergency.

Signs

- **Early stages**
  - Distressed and anxious patient.
  - **Marked epigastric tenderness** and **abdominal distension** (due to gastric and intestinal hypomotility). In the **early stages**, rebound **tenderness and guarding are absent** because the inflammation is mainly in the retroperitoneal region.
  - Tachypnea due to ARDS, atelectasis and pleural effusion.
  - In patients with gallstones **jaundice** may develop due to compression of the intrapancreatic portion of the common bile duct caused by edema of the head of the pancreas.
- **Severe disease**
  - **Low grade fever, tachycardia,** and **hypotension** are common.
  - **Shock with oliguria** may develop due to:
    - Hypovolemia secondary to exudation of blood and plasma into the retroperitoneal space.
    - Vasodilation and increased vascular permeability produced due to increased formation and release of kinin peptides.
    - Systemic effects of proteolytic and lipolytic enzymes released from the pancreas into the circulation.
  - **Abdominal examination** may show tenderness with guarding as well as diminished or absent bowel sounds (when paralytic ileus develops).
  - **Respiratory system:** Lungs findings include basal rales, atelectasis, and pleural effusion.
  - **Skin:** Erythematous skin nodules due to focal subcutaneous fat necrosis may be seen.
  - **Purtscher retinopathy:** Ischemic injury to retina may be visible on fundus examination.
  - **Cutaneous echymoses:**
    - **Cullen's sign:** Faint bluish discoloration (bruising) around the umbilicus **(Fig. 12.2)** due to hemoperitoneum. It may be also found in association with ruptured ectopic pregnancy, ruptured aortic aneurysm, ruptured spleen and hepatocellular carcinoma, blunt abdominal trauma and spontaneous bleeding secondary to coagulopathy.
    - **Grey Turner's sign:** Blue-red-purple or green-brown discoloration of the flanks **(Fig. 12.2)** due to tissue catabolism of hemoglobin.
    - **Fox's sign:** Bluish discoloration over the inguinal ligament.

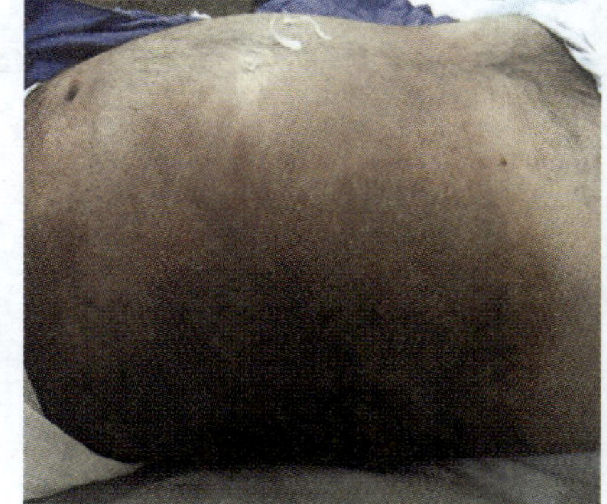

FIG. 12.2: Ecchymotic discoloration in the periumbilical region (Cullen's sign) or along the flank (Grey Turner's sign).

Laboratory Investigations

Q. Write short note on diagnosis and treatment of acute pancreatitis.

Q. Write short note on investigation (including biochemical evaluation) in acute pancreatitis.

Blood

The diagnosis of acute pancreatitis is usually established by the finding of **raised level of serum amylase and lipase** and ultrasound or CT evidence of pancreatic swelling.

1. ***Serum amylase:***
   - Levels markedly (three times the upper limit of normal) raised within 6–12 hours and then decline to normal within 3–5 days.
   - Persistently elevated serum amylase levels indicate development of complications such as pancreatic abscess or pseudocyst formation.
   - Amylase levels may be spuriously normal in 20% patients with alcoholic pancreatitis and 50% patients with hypertriglyceridemia.
   - Peritoneal amylase is massively raised in pancreatic ascites.
   - *Serum amylase concentrations are also elevated in other conditions like perforated bowel, salivary gland obstruction/ infection, ruptured ectopic pregnancy, renal failure, mesenteric infarction macroamylasemia, etc.*
2. ***Urinary amylase:*** Levels may be diagnostic because they remain elevated over a longer period of time.
3. ***Serum lipase:***
   - Preferable to amylase for diagnosis as it remains elevated for a longer period of time (8–14 days) than levels of serum amylase. It has **greater diagnostic accuracy** and is a more useful indicator of acute pancreatitis.
   - Rises within 4–8 hours of the onset of symptoms, peaks at 24 hours.
   - Marked elevation of lipase in pleural or peritoneal fluid (> 5000 IU/dL) suggests acute pancreatitis.
4. ***C-reactive protein level:*** It is useful in assessing severity and prognosis of acute pancreatitis.
5. ***Other blood investigations:***
   - **Low Hb:** Indicates prolonged hemetemesis/melena, internal hemorrhage.
   - **Leukocytosis:** Moderate to severe acute pancreatitis usually show leukocytosis.
   - **Low platelets:** DIC
   - **Hyperglycemia and glycosuria:** It occurs in 10% of cases. Possibly due to hyperglucagonemia, associated with relative hypoinsulinemia.
   - **Hypocalcemia:** It is due to precipitation of calcium soaps in necrotic fat. Persistent hypocalcemia is a poor prognostic sign.
   - **Other baseline investigations:** These include urea and electrolytes, liver biochemistry, (raised bilirubin, AST/ALT/ LDH, ALP, GGTP-gallstone pancreatitis) LDH, triglycerides, and arterial blood gases.

Radiology

The enlarged inflamed pancreas may be directly visualized by radiography.

- ***Plain X-ray (X-ray abdomen and chest):*** Useful for excluding other causes of acute abdominal pain (e.g. gastroduodenal perforation or obstruction). A supine abdominal X-ray may reveal gallstones or pancreatic calcification. Nonspecific signs like 'colon cut-off sign', 'sentinel loop sign' can be seen.
- ***Abdominal ultrasound scan:*** Used as a screening test to evaluate gallbladder and biliary tree (to identify gallstones, biliary obstruction or pseudocyst formation). It may show pancreatic swelling, necrosis and peripancreatic fluid collections. However, the pancreas may not be visualized because of gas-filled loops of bowel.
- ***CT scan of abdomen:*** May show swollen pancreas (phlegmon), pseudocyst **(Fig. 12.3)** or pancreatic abscess. Helpful in **assessing the severity,** the risk of morbidity and mortality and the complications of acute pancreatitis.
  - ***Contrast-enhanced CT scanning:*** Should be performed after 72 hours of onset of symptoms to know the extent of pancreatic necrosis. Necrotizing pancreatitis shows decreased pancreatic enhancement on CT, following intravenous injection of contrast material.
    It can detect complications such as fluid collections, abscess formation, pseudocyst and involvement of the colon, blood vessels and other adjacent structures by the inflammatory process. The presence of gas within necrotic material suggests infection and possible abscess formation.

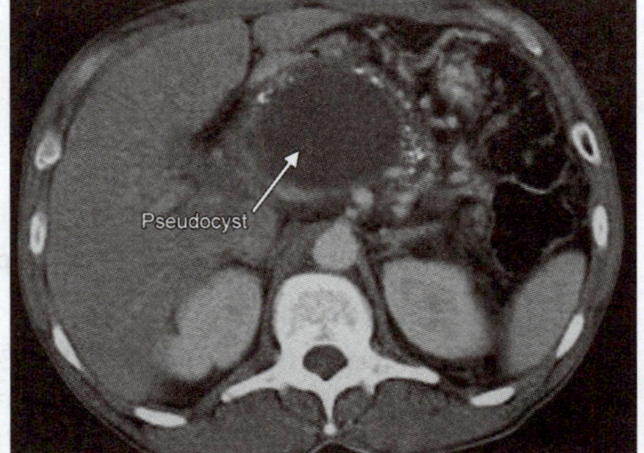

FIG. 12.3: CT image showing pseudocyst.

- ***MRI abdomen and magnetic resonance cholangiopancreatography (MRCP):*** Its uses are:
  - For assessing the degree of pancreatic damage/necrosis.
  - To identify gallstones within the biliary tree.
  - To differentiate between fluid and solid inflammatory masses.
- ***Endoscopic retrograde cholangiopancreatography (ERCP):*** Used for removing bile duct stones in few selected cases of gallstone-related pancreatitis and for sphincterotomy/stent placement.

Determining the Severity of Acute Pancreatitis

- **Course of acute pancreatitis:** Majority of cases of acute pancreatitis are mild and run a short, self-limiting course. About 25% develop a more complicated course and in about 10% this may be life-threatening.
- The **best scoring system** available is: **Ranson scoring system (Table 12.2)**.
- The **modified Glasgow (Box 12.3) or the Imrie criteria** consists of 8 parameters and requires a 48-hour period of observation and scores 3 or more it indicates severe pancreatitis.
- **Acute physiology and chronic health evaluation (APACHE) II score:** It is based on common physiological and laboratory values, adjusted for age and the presence or absence of a number of other chronic health problems (>8 predicts severe disease).
- **Bedside index for severity in acute pancreatitis (BISAP),** also uses the first letter of each parameter for 1 point. *The BISAP score provides a single point for 5 parameters: blood urea nitrogen (BUN) greater than 25 mg/dL, impaired mental status, systemic inflammatory response syndrome, age greater than 60, and/or the presence of a pleural effusion, for a possible total of 5 points.* A BISAP score greater than 3 is associated with a seven- to twelve-fold increase in developing organ failure.
- **Computed tomography (CT) grading system of Balthazar and CT severity index (CTSI)** is presented in **Table 12.3** (added score >5 indicates severe pancreatitis).

Apart from the above scoring systems, individual laboratory tests have been suggested to establish severity.

- These include methemalbumin, alpha-2 macroglobulin, alpha-1 antitrypsin, C3 and C4 levels, phospholipase A2, C-reactive protein, trypsinogen-activated peptide (TAP) and granulocytic elastase.

Differential Diagnosis of Acute Pancreatitis

See **Table 12.4.**

Complications of Acute Pancreatitis

Q. Write short note on complications of acute pancreatitis.

Local (Pancreatic) Complications

- **Acute peripancreatic fluid collections (APFC)** do not have a well-defined wall, usually remain asymptomatic.
- **Pancreatic pseudocyst:** It represents a localized peripancreatic collection of pancreatic juice and debris usually developing in the lesser sac following inflammatory rupture of the pancreatic duct. It may be palpable in the upper abdomen four to six weeks after onset of symptoms.

TABLE 12.2: Ranson criteria for assessing severity of acute pancreatitis.

Factors	Alcoholic pancreatitis	Gallstone pancreatitis
1. On admission		
Age	>55 years	>70 years
WBC count	>16,000/cumm	>18,000/cumm
Blood glucose	>200 mg/dL	>220 mg/dL
Serum lactate dehydrogenase (LDH)	>350 IU/L	>400 IU/L
Serum aspartate aminotransferase (AST)	>250 IU/L	>250 IU/L
2. Within 48 hours		
Hematocrit decreases	>10%	—
Increase of blood urea nitrogen (BUN)	>5 mg/dL	>2 mg/dL
Serum calcium	<8 mg/dL	<8 mg/dL
PaO_2	60 mmHg	—
Base deficit	>4 mEq/L	>5 mEq/L
Fluid deficit	>6 L	>4 L
Number of criteria and approximate mortality (%): 0 to 2 = 0%; 3 to 4 = 15%; 5 to 6 = 50%; >6 = 100%.		

Box 12.3: Modified Glasgow criteria.

P - PaO_2 <8 kPa
A - Age >55-year-old
N - Neutrophilia: WBC >15 × 10^9/L
C - Calcium <2 mmol/L
R - Renal function, urea >16 mmol/L
E - Enzymes: LDH >600 IU/L; AST >200 IU/L
A - Albumin <32 g/L (serum)
S - Sugar: Blood glucose >10 mmol/L

TABLE 12.3: Computed tomography (CT) grading system of Balthazar and CT severity index (CTSI).

Balthazar grades			
Grade A		Normal pancreas consistent with mild pancreatitis	
Grade B		Focal or diffuse enlargement of the gland, including contour irregularities and inhomogeneous attenuation but without peripancreatic inflammation	
Grade C		Grade B plus peripancreatic inflammation	
Grade D		Grade C plus associated single fluid collection	
Grade E		Grade C plus two or more peripancreatic fluid collections or gas in the pancreas or retroperitoneum	
CTSI = Balthazar grade score plus necrosis score*			
Balthazar grade score:		Necrosis score:	
A	= 0	Absence of necrosis	0
B	= 1	Necrosis of up to 33% of pancreas	2
C	= 2	Necrosis of 33% to 50%	4
D	= 3	Necrosis of >50%	6
E	= 4		

*Score = morbidity [%]/mortality [%]: 0 to 3 = 8%/3%; 4 to 6 = 35%/6%; 7 to 10 = 92%/17%.

TABLE 12.4: Differential diagnosis of acute pancreatitis.

➤ Perforation: Peptic ulcer/intestinal	➤ Acute myocardial infarction
➤ Acute cholecystitis	➤ Pneumonia
➤ Acute appendicitis	➤ Abdominal aortic dissection
➤ Bowel ischemia	➤ Diabetic ketoacidosis
	➤ Renal colic
	➤ Acute hepatitis

Small pseudocysts are common and resolve as the pancreatitis recovers, but those larger than 6 cm can persist causing abdominal pain and may compress or erode surrounding structures.

- **Pancreatic necrosis *(sterile or infected)*:** Necrosis may result in an acute necrotic collection (ANC) that contains a variable amount of fluid and necrosis or walled-off necrosis (WON), which consists of a mature, encapsulated collection.
- **Pancreatic abscess:** Localized collection of pus close to the pancreas and containing little or no pancreatic necrotic tissue.
- **Pancreatic ascites:** May develop due to leakage of fluid from a disrupted pancreatic duct into the peritoneal cavity. Systemic complications are listed in **Table 12.5.**

TABLE 12.5: Complications of acute pancreatitis.

Local	*Systemic*
➢ **Acute peripancreatic fluid collections (APFC)** do not have a well-defined wall ➢ **Pseudocyst:** Encapsulated collection of fluid with a well-defined inflammatory wall usually outside the pancreas with minimal or no necrosis ➢ **Necrosis:** Acute necrotic collection **(ANC)** that contains a variable amount of fluid and necrosis but lacks a definable wall walled-off necrosis **(WON),** which consists of a mature, encapsulated collection of pancreatic and/or peripancreatic necrosis that has developed a well-defined inflammatory wall. ➢ **Abscess** ➢ **Pancreatic ascites** – Disruption of main pancreatic duct – Leaking pseudocyst ➢ Involvement of contiguous organs by necrotizing pancreatitis ➢ Massive intraperitoneal hemorrhage ➢ Thrombosis of blood vessels (splenic vein, portal vein) ➢ Pseudoaneurysm ➢ Bowel infarction ➢ Obstructive jaundice ➢ Abdominal compartment syndrome	➢ Systemic inflammatory response syndrome **(SIRS)** due to increased vascular permeability caused by release of cytokine, platelet aggregating factor and kinin ➢ **Respiratory complications:** Pleural effusion, hypoxia—adult respiratory distress syndrome (ARDS) due to microthrombi in pulmonary vessels, pneumonia ➢ **Cardiovascular:** Hypotension and shock, hypovolemia ➢ **Gastrointestinal complications: Upper gastrointestinal bleeding** due to gastric or duodenal erosions and paralytic ileus ➢ **Hepatobiliary complications:** Jaundice, common bile duct obstruction (obstructive jaundice), splenic or portal vein thrombosis, variceal hemorrhage ➢ **Renal:** Oliguria, azotemia renal artery and/or renal vein thrombosis, acute tubular necrosis ➢ **Metabolic:** Hyperglycemia (due to disruption of islets of Langerhans with altered insulin/glucagon release), hypocalcemia: due to sequestration of calcium in fat necrosis ➢ **Hematological complication:** Disseminated intravascular coagulation (DIC), increased factor VII or fibrinogen ➢ Fat necrosis (subcutaneous nodules), polyarthritis ➢ Retinopathy (Purtscher's retinopathy): Sudden blindness ➢ **Central nervous system:** Psychosis, encephalopathy and coma

Q. Write short note on treatment of acute pancreatitis.

Management/Treatment

Steps involved

General supportive care

In about 85–90% of patients, acute pancreatitis is self-limited and subsides spontaneously. The initial management of acute pancreatitis is similar, irrespective of the cause.

- **Intravenous (IV) fluids:** 5 to 10 mL/kg per hour of isotonic crystalloid solution to maintain normal intravascular volume. There may be large amount of fluid loss during early phase of acute pancreatitis.
- **Feeding:**
  - *Nil orally* initially **only in** severe pancreatitis.
  - In the absence of ileus, nausea or vomiting, oral feeding can be initiated early (within 24 hours) as tolerated.
  - Total **parenteral nutrition** may be associated with a high-risk of infection.
  - Nasogastric/nasojejunal administration of feed is possible in most of the patients followed by gradual oral intake.
- **Analgesia for pain:** Tramadol or other opiates (hydroxymorphine, fentanyl, meperidine) are the drugs for pain control. Morphine and diamorphine are avoided, because they may exacerbate pancreatic ductular hypertension by causing contraction of sphincter of Oddi.
- **Nasogastric suction/aspiration:** Indications include (1) continuation of pain, (2) presence of protracted vomiting or (3) obstruction observed on plain X-ray abdomen. It prevents abdominal distension and vomiting and the risk of aspiration pneumonia.
- **Prophylactic antibiotics: Prophylactic antibiotics are not recommended in patients with acute pancreatitis.** Carbapenems (imipenem or meropenem) or ceftazidime/cefuroxime used only for infected pancreatic necrosis.
- **Other drugs:** Proton-pump inhibitors, glucagon, octreotide, pentoxifylline and aprotinin (protease inhibitor).
- **Anticoagulation** with a low molecular weight heparin for prevention of deep vein thrombosis (DVT).
- Management of acute pancreatitis **(Flowchart 12.1).**
- **Indications for surgery (Box 12.4).**
- **Endoscopic retrograde cholangiopancreatography (ERCP)** is indicated within first 36–48 hours in severe pancreatitis associated with gallstone obstruction (particularly when complicated by cholangitis or jaundice).
- Small percentage patients develop multiorgan failure (reflecting the extent of pancreatic necrosis) and all **severe cases** should be managed in a **high-dependency or intensive care unit.**
- Detection and treatment of complications
- Treatment of the underlying cause (e.g. gallstones, hypercalcemia, hypertriglyceridemia).

Box 12.4: Indications for surgery in acute pancreatitis.

- Infected pancreatic necrosis (pancreatic abscess).
- **Complications:** Most patients with complications such as acute peripancreatic fluid collections and/or pseudocysts do not require surgical interventions unless they become infected or cause compression of other organs.
- **Cholecystectomy**: It should be carried out in gallstone related pancreatitis as soon as feasible (within 2 weeks after the resolution of acute episode). This will prevent potentially fatal/recurrent episode of pancreatitis.

FLOWCHART 12.1: Management of acute pancreatitis.

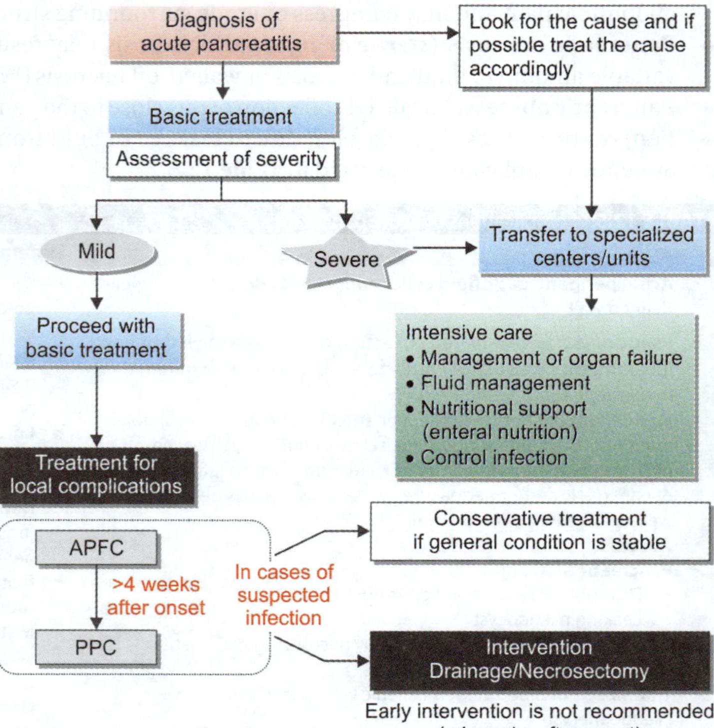

(APFC: acute peripancreatic fluid collections; PPC: pancreatic pseudocyst)

Chronic Pancreatitis

Q. Write short essay/note on chronic pancreatitis.

- Chronic pancreatitis is defined as **chronic inflammation of the pancreas** presenting as recurrent pain, characterized by the presence of **inflammation, fibrosis, and loss of acinar and islet cells.** The pancreas shows **irreversible damage to the exocrine pancreas in the form of fibrosis causing exocrine deficiency** (malabsorption). In the **late stages**, there may be destruction of endocrine parenchyma producing endocrine deficiency (**diabetes mellitus**).

Etiology (Table 12.6)

Q. Write short essay/note on causes and complications of chronic pancreatitis.

Pathogenesis

Repeated attacks of acute pancreatitis may lead to chronic pancreatitis. Four models have been suggested which are responsible for the development of chronic pancreatitis.

1. **Obstruction theory:** Some etiological agents cause increase protein concentrations, precipitation of these proteins; form ductal plugs in pancreatic juice. The ductal plugs may calcify to form calculi which further obstruct the pancreatic ducts.
2. **Necrosis-fibrosis theory:** The inflammation and scarring resulting from bouts of acute pancreatitis cause obstruction and stasis within the duct. It may subsequently form stones in the duct.
3. **Toxic-metabolic theory:** Toxins such as alcohol and its metabolites can cause direct toxic damage to acinar cells, and eventually fibrosis.
4. **Oxidative stress theory:** The pancreas is exposed to 'oxidative stress' either through the systemic circulation or through reflux of bile into the pancreatic duct. It also results in recurrent inflammation, tissue damage and fibrosis, and the activation of lysosomes and proenzymes.

TABLE 12.6: Causes of chronic pancreatitis: ***TIGAR-O*** classification system.

Causes
Toxic-metabolic
➤ **Alcohol abuse (~70%)**
➤ Tobacco smoking
➤ Hypercalcemia (e.g. hyperparathyroidism)
➤ Chronic renal failure
Idiopathic (~20%)
➤ Tropical/Fibrocalculous pancreatitis
Genetic
➤ Hereditary pancreatitis (cationic trypsinogen mutation)
➤ Cystic fibrosis due to cystic fibrosis transmembrane conductance regulator (CFTR) gene mutations
➤ SPINK1 mutations, mutations in the cationic trypsinogen gene (PRSS1)
Autoimmune
➤ Isolated autoimmune chronic pancreatitis (Type 1—IgG4 related, Type 2—idiopathic duct centric)
➤ Part of multi-organ disorders (Sjögren's syndrome, primary biliary cirrhosis)
Recurrent and severe acute pancreatitis
Obstructive
➤ Duct obstruction (e.g. tumor)
➤ Pancreas divisum
➤ Stenosis of sphincter of Oddi

Clinical Features

Q. Discuss the clinical features of chronic calcific pancreatitis.

- Predominantly affects middle-aged alcoholic men. In southern India, severe chronic calcific pancreatitis may develop in nonalcoholics, probably as a result of *malnutrition and cassava consumption*.
- **Abdominal pain:** Due to increased pressure within the pancreatic ducts and direct involvement of pancreatic and peripancreatic nerves by the inflammatory process. Pain is variable in location, severity, and frequency.
  - May be **continuous or intermittent**.
  - May be **referred to back**.

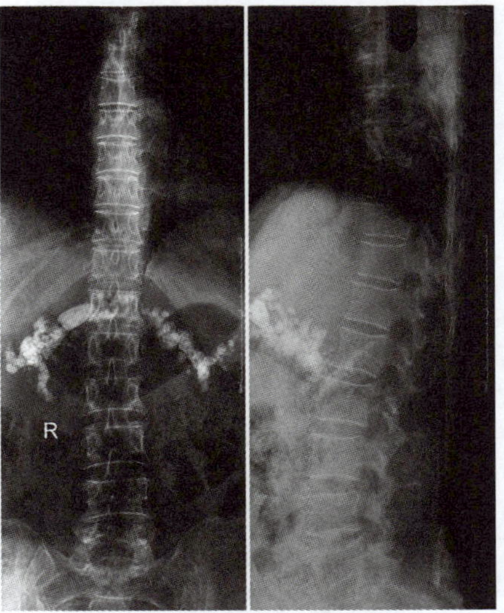

FIG. 12.4: Erect abdominal X-ray AP and lateral views showing calcific pancreatitis.

- Pain is often increased by eating of heavy meals. This may lead to a fear of eating with consequent weight loss.
- No uniform relationship between pain and alcohol. Pain may be either exacerbated by alcohol excess or may be relieved by drinking alcohol.
- It is partially relieved on stooping and bending forwards (Mohammedan prayer sign).

- Features of **maldigestion/malabsorption:** Manifested as chronic diarrhea, **steatorrhea,** weight loss, fatigue.
- **Diabetes mellitus [pancreatogenic (type 3c) diabetes]** develops in about 30% of patients.
- In late stages, mechanical obstruction of the common bile duct due to fibrosed head of pancreas can produce jaundice.

Physical Examination

Thin, malnourished patient with **tenderness in the epigastric region**.

Investigations

- **Serum amylase and lipase:** May be elevated but in advanced disease they are usually normal.
- **Plain X-ray of abdomen (Fig. 12.4):** May show diffuse **calcifications** in pancreatic area (in ~30%) and usually indicate significant damage to the pancreas.
- **Transabdominal ultrasound scan:** Used for initial assessment.
- **Contrast-enhanced spiral CT scan:** Useful for a more detailed assessment. It may show pancreatic calcification, dilated pancreatic duct, pancreatic atrophy and dilatation/stricture of bile duct.
- **Endoscopic retrograde cholangiopancreatography (ERCP)** is the gold standard for accurate diagnosis and demonstrates pancreatic ducts.
- **MRI with MRCP:** Provides a direct view of the pancreatic duct and detects more subtle abnormalities of the pancreatic duct. **MRI and** MRCP are now the diagnostic procedures of choice.
- **Endoscopic ultrasonography (EUS):** It is useful for specifically assessing complications of chronic pancreatitis including pseudocyst formation and possible development of malignancy.
- **Pancreatic exocrine function tests:**
  - Secretin/cholecystokinin (CCK) stimulation test: Collection of pure pancreatic juice after secretin/CCK injection (gold standard but invasive and seldom used).
  - Fecal chymotrypsin or elastase level: Abnormal in the majority of moderate to severe chronic pancreatitis.
  - 24-hour fecal fat, the Lundh test meal, oral glucose tolerance test and pancreolauryl or PABA test.
- **Gene mutation analysis:** In cases where the etiology is not known. Common mutations include PRSS1, SPINK-1 and CFTR encoding genes.

Complications of Chronic Pancreatitis

Pseudocyst formation, bile duct or duodenal obstruction, pancreatic ascites or pleural effusion, splenic vein thrombosis, pseudoaneurysms, osteopenia, osteoporosis and, pancreatic cancer are the complications of chronic pancreatitis.

Treatment

- **Long-term abstinence of alcohol** in patients with alcohol-related chronic pancreatitis may benefit. Smoking cessation prevents progression.
- **Treatment of abdominal pain:** About 60% of patients will become pain-free after about 6–10 years.
  - **Opioids (tramadol) or non-steroidal anti-inflammatory drug (NSAIDs):** Tricyclic antidepressants (e.g. amitriptyline) and membrane stabilizing agents (e.g. pregabalin) may also be used for chronic pain.
  - **Intractable pain** may be treated by **celiac axis nerve block.**
  - **Surgery** includes **pancreatectomy and pancretojejunostomy** performed for unremitting pain.
  - **Endoscopic therapy** is useful in painful chronic pancreatitis to drain pancreatic duct in patients with obstructed ducts and treatment of complications (e.g. pseudocysts and bile duct obstruction with jaundice).
- **Steatorrhea:**
  - The steatorrhea seen in pancreatic insufficiency may be high, with up to 30 mmol of fat lost/24 h. This is treated with **pancreatic enzymes supplements** particularly lipase, 80,000–1,00,000 units before each meal.
  - An **acid suppressor (H_2-receptor antagonist or proton pump inhibitor)** to prevent inactivation of pancreatic enzymes by gastric acid.
  - Diet rich in **medium-chain triglycerides** which do not require lipase for digestion may be given.
  - Vitamin D supplementation (calcifediol)
- **Treatment of diabetes:** With insulin.

FIBROCALCIFIC/TROPICAL PANCREATITIS

Q. Describe the features of tropical pancreatitis.

- **Juvenile form of chronic calcific pancreatitis** and is **not related to alcohol** intake.
- Almost **exclusively** observed **in tropical countries**. In India, it is more common in southern states namely Kerala and Tamil Nadu.

Box 12.5: Risk factors for tropical pancreatitis.

- Malnutrition
- Infections, e.g. coxsackie and viral hepatitis
- Oxidant stress
- Diet rich in cassava, tapioca (contains cyanogenic glycosides)
- Familial.

Etiology

Exact etiology is **not known** and possible risk factors are listed in **Box 12.5**.

Clinical Features

- **Age and gender:** Young males.
- Course: **Accelerated course.**
- **Symptoms: Recurrent abdominal pain**, typically in **epigastric area with radiation to back**. Pain precipitated by heavy meals. Pancreatic exocrine deficiency presents with steatorrhea and malabsorption and endocrine deficiency presents with **diabetes mellitus**. Even without insulin **ketosis is uncommon** and frequent episodes of hypoglycemia with insulin are observed.
- **Signs:** Malnutrition, enlarged parotid glands, abdominal distention and a peculiar cyanotic hue of the lips.

Investigations

- **Plain X-ray and ultrasound of abdomen:** Shows multiple, large intraductal calculi.
- **Blood:** Sugar, serum amylase, lipids, calcium need to be checked.

Treatment

- Similar to chronic pancreatitis described earlier.
- Insulin for diabetes and requires a careful watch for hypoglycemia.

Differences between Alcoholic Pancreatitis and Tropical Pancreatitis (Table 12.7)

Q. How will you differentiate tropical pancreatitis from alcoholic pancreatitis?

TABLE 12.7: Differences between alcoholic pancreatitis and tropical pancreatitis.

Characteristics	*Alcoholic pancreatitis*	*Tropical pancreatitis*
Age	35–45 years	20–40 years
Gender	Commonly males	Males > females
Steatorrhea	More common	Less common
Diabetes mellitus	Less common	More common
Intraductal calculi	Less common	Frequent
Development of pancreatic malignancy	Less common	More common

Autoimmune Pancreatitis (AIP)/Autoimmune Chronic Pancreatitis (ACP)

- Autoimmune pancreatitis is a distinct **chronic inflammatory and sclerosing disease of the pancreas.**
- **Subtypes:**
  - **Type 1—IgG4-related disorder:** It is **one of the IgG4-related disorders** characterized by a **raised serum IgG4 level**. Other IgG4-related disorders are autoimmune cholangitis, Riedel's thyroiditis, aortitis and tubulointerstitial nephritis. Microscopically, IgG4-related disorders show **dense lymphoplasmacytic infiltrate with many IgG4-positive plasma cells**, a mild to moderate infiltration by eosinophils and an obliterative phlebitis in some organs, e.g. pancreas.
  - **Type 2—idiopathic duct-centric pancreatitis or AIP** with a granulocytic epithelial lesion.
- **Age and gender:** It is more **common in men** (2:1) and usually manifests in **middle age** (>85% above the age of 50 years).
- **Clinical presentation:** It presents with **abdominal pain, weight loss** or **painless obstructive jaundice** (due to obstruction of the intrapancreatic bile duct), without acute attacks of pancreatitis. Other symptoms include vomiting, and glucose intolerance.
- **Association with other autoimmune disease:** AIP may also develop in association with other autoimmune disorders. These disorders include Sjögren's syndrome, primary sclerosing cholangitis (PSC), inflammatory bowel disease, retroperitoneal fibrosis (most commonly presenting as hydronephrosis due to entrapment of the ureter).
- **Laboratory findings:** Elevated serum immunoglobulins (IgG or IgG4), and the presence of other autoantibodies including those directed towards nuclear and smooth muscle antigens.
- **Imaging:** It shows diffuse enlargement of pancreas, narrowing of the pancreatic duct and stricturing of the lower bile duct.

The Mayo clinic **HISORt** criteria for the diagnosis of autoimmune pancreatitis **(Table 12.8)**.

Treatment: Glucocorticoid therapy usually produces rather dramatic improvement with rapid resolution of both symptoms and radiographic abnormalities. This is the hallmark of autoimmune pancreatitis. Some patients require azathioprine.

TABLE 12.8: HISORt criteria of autoimmune pancreatitis.

Category	*Criteria*
Histology	One of the following:
	Periductal lymphoplasmacytic infiltrate with obliterative phlebitis and storiform fibrosis (LPSP)
	Lymphoplasmacytic infiltrate with storiform fibrosis showing abundant IgG4 positive cells (>10 cells/HPF)
Imaging (CT)/(MRI)	Typical; diffusely enlarged gland with diffuse rim enhancement, diffusely irregular attenuated pancreatic duct
	Other; focal pancreatic mass or enlargement; focal pancreatic duct stricture; pancreatic duct stricture, pancreatic atrophy; pancreatic calcification or pancreatitis
Serology	Elevated serum IgG4 level
Other organ involvement	Hilar/intrahepatic biliary strictures, persistent distal biliary strictures, parotid or lacrimal gland involvement, mediastinal lymphadenopathy or retroperitoneal fibrosis
Response to steroid **t**herapy	Resolution/marked improvement of manifestations with steroid therapy

PANCREATIC CANCER

- Pancreatic cancer is the fifth most common cause of cancer death in the Western World.
- **Age and gender:** Its incidence increases with age and the majority occur in the **elderly over the age of 60. Males** are affected twice as often as females.

Etiology

- ***Risk factors:***
  - The most important environmental factor is cigarette smoking
  - The second most modifiable risk factor is obesity
  - Excess intake of alcohol, high fat and protein diet, excessive intake of coffee and tea consumption and chronic calcific pancreatitis
  - DM is associate with a 40% ↑ risk of pancreatic cancer.
- **Genetic predisposition:** About 5 to 10% of patients with pancreatic cancer have a family history of the disease. FAMMM (familial atypical multiple mole melanoma syndrome), HNPCC (hereditary nonpolyposis colorectal cancer syndrome), hereditary pancreatitis, MEN, Lynch syndrome and Peutz-Jeghers syndrome have an increased risk of pancreatic cancer.
- Mutational activation of oncogenes, predominantly KRAS, inactivation of tumor suppressor genes such as TP53 (70%), p16/CDKN2A (98%), and SMAD4 (55%) are commonly associated.

Pathology

- Ductal adenocarcinoma accounts for 85–90% of pancreatic tumors. Cystic neoplasms represent 10%–15% of cystic lesions of the pancreas. 5% are endocrine tumors. Only 2% of tumors of the exocrine pancreas are benign.
- **Location:** About 60–70% of these tumors are localized in the head of the gland, 5–10% in the body, and 10–15% in the tail.
- **Spread:** Local spread, lymphatic spread as well as hematogenous spread occurs rapidly.

Clinical Features (Fig. 12.5)

Symptoms

- **Central abdominal pain:** Pain is common symptom and is usually incessant and gnawing, **epigastric, radiate** from the upper abdomen **to the back**, increasing on lying down and relieved by sitting up or bending forwards. Pain is primarily due to invasion of the celiac or superior mesenteric arterial plexus.
- **Others:** Loss of weight and cachexia.
- Symptoms **depend upon the site of the tumor**.
  - **Carcinoma of the head of pancreas:** They present early because of the obstruction to the common bile duct by the tumor produces **obstructive jaundice** present in >50% of patient (due to obstruction of bile flow), often with severe **pruritus** (secondary to cholestasis). Other symptoms include clay-colored stools with or without melena or silver stools. Obstruction of the pancreatic duct may cause episodes of pancreatitis.
  - Less common symptoms include those of diabetes and pancreatitis.
  - **Carcinoma of the body and tail of the pancreas: May be silent** till quite large and widely disseminated.

Physical Signs

- **General: Pallor, jaundice** and weight loss may be present. Scratch marks and **erythema ab igne** is seen.
- **Abdominal mass: A mass may be felt** in the epigastrium; the liver may be enlarged (hepatomegaly) due to biliary obstruction or secondary involvement (hepatic metastasis).

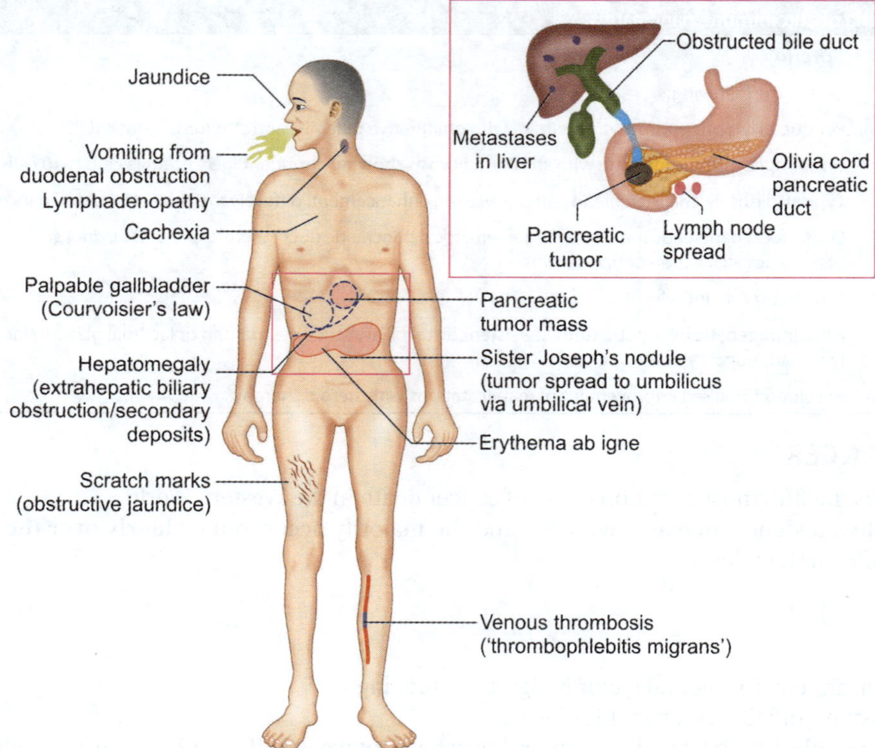

FIG. 12.5: Features of carcinoma of the pancreas.

- **Courvoisier's law:** A distended nontender gallbladder may be palpable in a jaundiced patient due to distal biliary obstruction by a pancreatic cancer.
- **Due to spread of tumor:**
  - With peritoneal involvement and **ascites**, shifting dullness and fluid thrill can be elicited. On per rectal examination, nodules (**Blumer's shelf**) or peritoneal fluid may be felt.
  - Involvement of the left supraclavicular node (**Virchow's node**) and umbilicus (**Sister Mary Joseph's node**) indicates advanced carcinoma.
- **Other presenting physical signs:** Migratory thrombophlebitis—recurrent venous thrombosis (**Trousseau sign**), diabetes, polyarthritis, paraneoplastic syndromes (Cushing syndrome), skin nodules (secondary to localized fat necrosis and associated inflammation) and hypercalcemia may be seen in some cases.

Investigations

- **Blood:** It may show anemia. Liver function tests may show features of obstructive jaundice with elevated alkaline phosphatase. Urobilinogen is absent in urine whereas bile salts and bile pigments are evident. Occult blood may be present in stool.
- **Radiology: Barium meal** shows widening of the 'C' loop (**pad sign**) and reverse '3' sign in periampullary carcinoma. Hypotonic duodenography reveals a 'rose thorn' appearance. Endoscopic retrograde cholangiography increases the diagnostic yield; USG and CT scan are helpful in localizing the tumor.
- Ultrasound, contrast CT and ERCP yield in localization of tumor, assessing the spread as well as operability, guided biopsy/cytology helps to confirm diagnosis.
- **ERCP:** A "double-duct sign," representing strictures in biliary and pancreatic ducts, is classically found in many patients. Tissue sampling can also be obtained during ERCP.
- Endoscopic ultrasonography is the most accurate test for the detection of pancreatic cancer.
- **Tumor markers:** Carcinoembryonic antigen (CEA) and **CA-19-9** [high sensitivity (80%) but a high false-positive rate].

Prognosis

Overall survival is about 3–5%, with median survival of 6–10 months for locally advanced cancer and 3–5 months for those with metastases.

Treatment

- **Surgical resection:** It is the only method of effecting cure. Resectable tumors in the head and periampullary region are removed by Whipple's pancreaticoduodenectomy or its modifications.
- **Chemotherapy:** For inoperable cases chemotherapy with gemcitabine, capecitabine, paclitaxel, cisplatin, docetaxel, oxaliplatin, irinotecan, 5-fluorouracil, mitomycin, streptozotocin and high-dose methotrexate, alone or in combination, may be beneficial. Tyrosine kinase inhibitors of EGFR (e.g. erlotinib) and monoclonal antibodies cetuximab is under trials.
  - FOLFIRINOX is a chemotherapy regimen for treatment of advanced pancreatic cancer (FOL – folinic acid (leucovorin), F – fluorouracil (5-FU), IRIN – irinotecan, OX – oxaliplatin)
- Radiotherapy may be supportive.
- **Palliative treatment:**
  - **Pain:** Palliation for pain may be achieved with either analgesic nerve blocks (coeliac axis block/neurolysis, percutaneous cordotomy) or with duct drainage (pancreaticogastric anastomosis).
  - Jaundice can be relieved by choledochojejunostomy or percutaneous/endoscopic stenting—endoprostheses (elderly and with very advanced disease).

ENDOCRINE TUMORS OF PANCREAS/PANCREATIC NEUROENDOCRINE TUMORS (PNETs)

- Endocrine tumors of pancreas (ETP) are classified as functioning or nonfunctioning according to the type and level of their hormonal secretion.
- Among functioning ETP, insulinomas (50%) and gastrinomas (30%) are the most frequent; tumors secreting vasoactive intestinal peptide (VIPomas), glucagon (glucagonomas), and somatostatin (somatostatinomas) are much rarer (5–10%). These secreting growth-hormone-releasing factor (GHRH), adrenocorticotropic hormone (ACTH) or corticotropin-releasing factor (CRF), and parathyroid hormone related peptide (PTHrp) are anecdotal.
- Conversely, at least 15% of ETP are nonfunctioning or secrete nonclinically active peptides such as human pancreatic polypeptide (PPomas).

Insulinoma (Beta Cell Tumor)

- **Most common** of endocrine tumors; **10% are malignant** and produce pronounced hypoglycemia.

Clinical Features

- Higher incidence in **women**.
- **Whipple's triad (Box 12.6).**

Box 12.6: Whipple's triad.

- **Attack of hypoglycemia** (mental confusion, weakness, fatigue and convulsions) **while fasting.** Neuroglycopenic symptoms (anxiety, nervousness, dizziness and confusion) may develop during fasting. In some psychoses, seizures related to hypoglycemia and weight gain is seen.
- **Blood sugar <50 mg/dL during an attack.**
- **Relief of symptoms by administration of glucose.**

Diagnosis

Fasting blood levels of insulin and glucose:

- **Inappropriately elevated serum level of insulin** (>54 u/mL) for the level of glucose **establishes the diagnosis.**
- Blood **insulin-to-glucose ratio of >0.4 is diagnostic.**
- Blood fasting **C-peptide level** of >1.7 mg/mL is a good indicator.
- **Proinsulin level** is elevated and is used as a tumor marker.
- Suppression and stimulation (tolbutamide, calcium, glucagon) tests may be performed.

Radiology

- **Selective angiography** is best investigation, with few false positive results.
- **USG** is positive in 20–40% of cases.
- **CT with intravenous contrast** shows a dense blush.
- **MRI:** Bright spots are seen on T2 weighted images. In the presence of somatostatin receptors, octreotide scan may be useful. Portal venous sampling has 75% accuracy.
- **Calcium angiography:** It can determine the location of insulinoma whereas endoscopic USG has 80% positivity.

Treatment of Insulinoma

- **Aim:** To localize and remove the tumor safely.
- **Hypoglycemia** can be **managed medically** (by using diazoxide, octreotide, lanreotide).
- **Surgery:**
  - If tumor is **small** and in the **head**: Removed by **enucleation.**
  - If in the **body or tail**: Remove it either by **enucleation** or by **distal** (subtotal) **pancreatectomy.**
  - If the tumor is **malignant and is operable: Resection.**
- **For metastasis** (liver, adjacent lymph nodes):
  - Hepatic artery embolization, RFA and cryoablation or radioembolization.
  - Streptozotocin, chlorozocin, 5-FU, either alone or in combination.

Gastrinoma (Delta Cell Tumor)

(Synonym: **Zollinger-Ellison syndrome)**

- Second most common islet cell tumor (0.1–0.4/million population/year), but with MEN I it is the most common functional pancreatic neoplasm; 20% of ZES have MEN I.

Q. Write short essay/note on etiology, clinical features and treatment of Zollinger-Ellison syndrome.

Pathology

- **Sites:** Most common site of gastrinoma is duodenum (50-88% in sporadic ZES, 70-100% in MEN1 ZES), pancreas (only 25%, and rarely in gastric antrum).
- **Effects:** It produces excessive gastrin.
- **Characteristics:**
  - Often **solitary and malignant**.
  - When occurs as part of **MEN I, they are multiple and less malignant**.
  - Duodenal gastrinomas are less malignant than pancreatic tumors. They are slow growing even in the presence of metastasis.

Gastrinoma Triangle of Passaro (Fig. 12.6)

1. Junction between the cystic duct and common bile duct
2. Junction between the 2nd and 3rd parts of the duodenum
3. Junction between neck and body of pancreas

60–90% of gastrinomas arise within this triangle

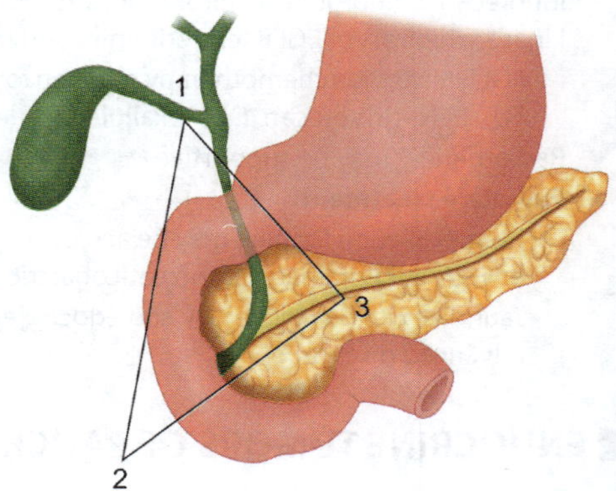

FIG. 12.6: Gastrinoma triangle.

Clinical Features

- More frequent in **middle-aged men**. With MEN I, the symptoms occur earlier (3rd decade).
- **Zollinger-Ellison syndrome** is characterized by **hyperacidity and non-healing ulcers** (gastric, duodenal, jejunal, or in atypical locations). Epigastric pain with duodenal ulcer is seen in 90% of cases; 1/3rd have diarrhea, and weight loss is common (40% of cases). Esophagitis, dysphagia (30%), stricture and perforation may occur.

Diagnosis

- **ZES:** About 30–40% do not have evidence of peptic ulcer disease and 40% have duodenal instead of pancreatic tumor.
- **Gastric acid hypersecretion** (basal acid output >15 mEq/L) and **elevated fasting gastrin** (> 100 pg/mL) are suggestive. Provocative tests using secretin, calcium or gastrin may be used. Gastric pH <2 and fasting serum gastrin level > 1000 pg/mL is diagnostic.
- **Immunohistochemistry:** Demonstration of gastrin in neoplastic cells by immunoperoxidase is confirmatory.
- **Tumor localization:** Using ultrasound, CT scan and endoscopic USG.
  - **Selective angiography** is best for primary and metastatic gastrinomas (40–60% accuracy) and with secretin stimulation, the accuracy increases to 70%.
  - Portal venous sampling for gastrin.

Treatment

Medical

- **Control acid secretion** using H_2 blockers. Dose: 2 grams ranitidine, 0.3 g famotidine or 80 mg omeprazole/pantoprazole per day. Parenteral ranitidine may be used.

Surgery

- Accurately **identification of duodenal or pancreatic tumor** by inspection, palpation and if needed by intraoperative USG or transillumination duodenotomy.
- Surgical management
  - Excision, gastrectomy, enucleation based on tumor size, number and location.
- **Patients with MEN I having gastrinoma:**
  - **Surgery is not indicated.**
  - Four-gland parathyroidectomy with autografts is the initial procedure of choice to control hyperparathyroidism. Gastric acid hypersecretion is controlled as in sporadic gastrinoma (mentioned above).
  - If liver metastasis is present and resectable: Resection.
  - Chemotherapy: Doxorubicin, 5-FU, streptozotocin shows 40% response. Interferon and octreotide may also be used.

Glucagonoma (Alpha Cell Tumor)

Rare α-cell tumor.

Clinical Features

- Functional tumors: They produce the **glucagonoma syndrome** comprising abnormal glucose tolerance test, normocytic normochromic anemia, necrolytic migratory erythema (pathognomonic), red tongue, angular stomatitis, weight loss, tendency to develop infection, and depression.
- **Elevated fasting plasma glucagon >500 pg/mL is diagnostic.**

Treatment: Preoperative control of diabetes, treatment of venous thrombosis and correction of nutritional status with total parenteral nutrition. Surgical resection is done after localizing the tumor.

Somatostatinoma (Delta Cell Tumor)

Rare malignant D cell tumors of the pancreas and 30% occur in the duodenum and small bowel. They affect both the sexes equally, with approximate age of 50 years. They cause diabetes mellitus, gallstones and diarrhea/steatorrhea.

Diagnosis: High fasting serum somatostatin levels.

Treatment: Octreotide therapy may be tried and the tumor surgically resected after localization. Cholecystectomy may be required for cholelithiasis.

VIPoma (WDHA Syndrome; Verner-Morrison Syndrome; Pancreatic Cholera)

- Endocrine pancreatic tumor producing vasoactive intestinal polypeptide (VIP).
- **Symptoms:** Severe secretory diarrhea secondary to the stimulation of adenyl cyclase within the enterocyte (Verner-Morrison syndrome). Large-volume diarrhea (>3 L/day), hypokalemia, and hypo- or achlorhydria form part of the syndrome; hence the term **W**atery **D**iarrhea, **H**ypokalemia, **A**chlorhydria (WDHA) syndrome.

Diagnosis: Presence of severe secretory diarrhea, detection of elevated fasting levels of plasma VIP (>250 pg/mL) and localization of pancreatic islet cell tumor.

Treatment

- Correction of dehydration, hypokalemia and other metabolic abnormalities.
- Octreotide may be tried for symptomatic relief.
- Surgical removal of the tumor.
- For unresectable and metastatic tumors chemotherapy with 5-FU and streptozotocin. Interferon has also been used. Palliative debulking for incurable and metastatic tumors.

CHAPTER

13 Kidney

FUNCTIONAL ANATOMY OF KIDNEY

Q. Describe the nephron with the help of a diagram. What are the functions of the kidney?

Unit of Kidney

The **nephron is the structural and functional unit** of the kidney. It consists of the glomerulus and its tubule, and the common collecting system. Each kidney consists of about 1 million nephrons. Different components of a nephron are shown in **Figure 13.1**.

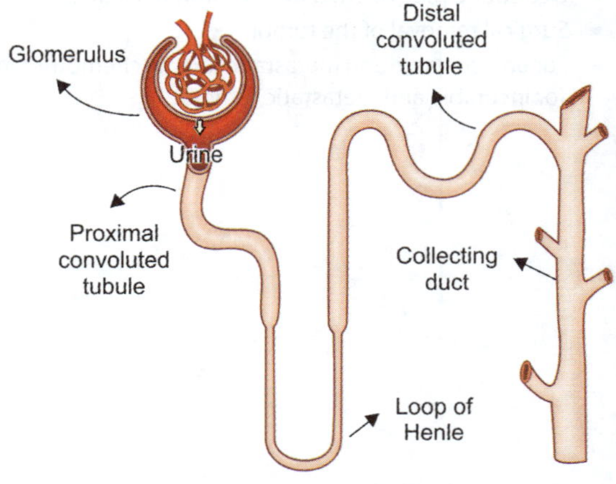

FIG. 13.1: Different components of the nephron.

Functions of Kidney

- **Excretion** of many metabolic breakdown products (including ammonia, urea and creatinine from protein, and uric acid from nucleic acids), drugs and toxins
- Regulation of **water and electrolyte balance**
- Maintenance of **acid-base balance**
- **Reabsorption** of essential substances
- Secretion of hormones such as **erythropoietin and renin**
- Metabolism of **vitamin D**
- **Regulation of blood pressure**

Juxtaglomerular Apparatus

Q. Write a short note on the juxtaglomerular apparatus.

Components of juxtaglomerular apparatus (Fig. 13.2): It consists of (1) macula densa, (2) the extraglomerular mesangium, (3) the terminal portion of the afferent glomerular arteriole (contains renin-producing granular cells), and (4) the proximal portion of the efferent arteriole.

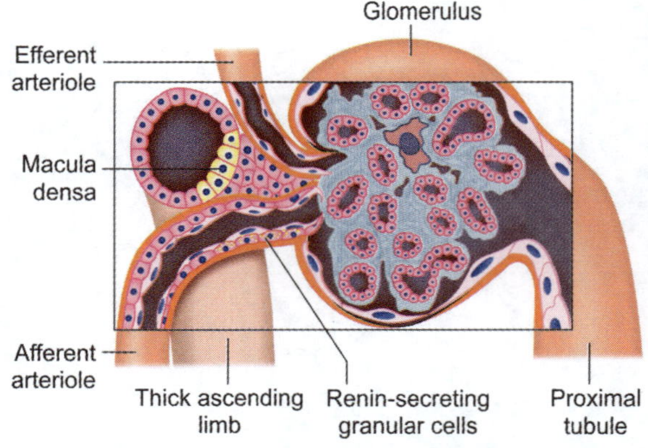

FIG. 13.2: Diagrammatic representation of glomerulus and juxtaglomerular apparatus.

1. **Macula densa:** The afferent arterioles and the thick ascending limb of loop of Henle are in contact for a short distance. The macula densa is a plaque of tall and columnar cells within this thick ascending limb of the loop of Henle and contains large, tightly packed cell nuclei (hence termed macula densa). This anatomical arrangement allows changes in the renal tubule to influence the behavior of the adjacent glomerulus (tubuloglomerular feedback).
2. **Extraglomerular mesangium.**
3. **Terminal portion of the afferent glomerular arteriole:** Shows thickening due to specialized myoepithelioid cells (juxtaglomerular cells) that contain large secretory granules of renin.
4. **Proximal portion of the efferent arteriole.**

RENIN

Renin is **secreted and stored in the juxtaglomerular cells.**

Factors controlling release of renin

- Pressure changes in the afferent arteriole
- Sympathetic tone
- Sodium, chloride, and osmotic concentration of the fluid in the distal convoluted tubule at the macula densa
- Local prostaglandin and nitric oxide release.

Mechanism of action of renin

- **Renin** acts on angiotensinogen in the blood and **converts angiotensinogen to angiotensin I.**
- **Angiotensin I** (decapeptide) is **converted to angiotensin II** (octapeptide) **by angiotensin-converting enzyme (ACE)**, which is present in the lung, luminal border of endothelial cells, glomeruli and other organs.
- **Angiotensin II** has **two major systemic effects: Systemic vasoconstriction** and **sodium and water retention** by release of aldosterone from the adrenal cortex.
- Aldosterone produces constriction of the efferent arteriole of the glomerulus and thereby increases glomerular filtration pressure.

Consequences of renin action

- By above mentioned mechanisms, the kidneys **"defend" circulating blood volume, blood pressure, and glomerular filtration during circulatory shock.**
- However, the same mechanisms can lead to systemic hypertension in renal ischemia.

Renin-angiotensin-aldosterone system (RAAS) is presented in **Figure 13.3**.

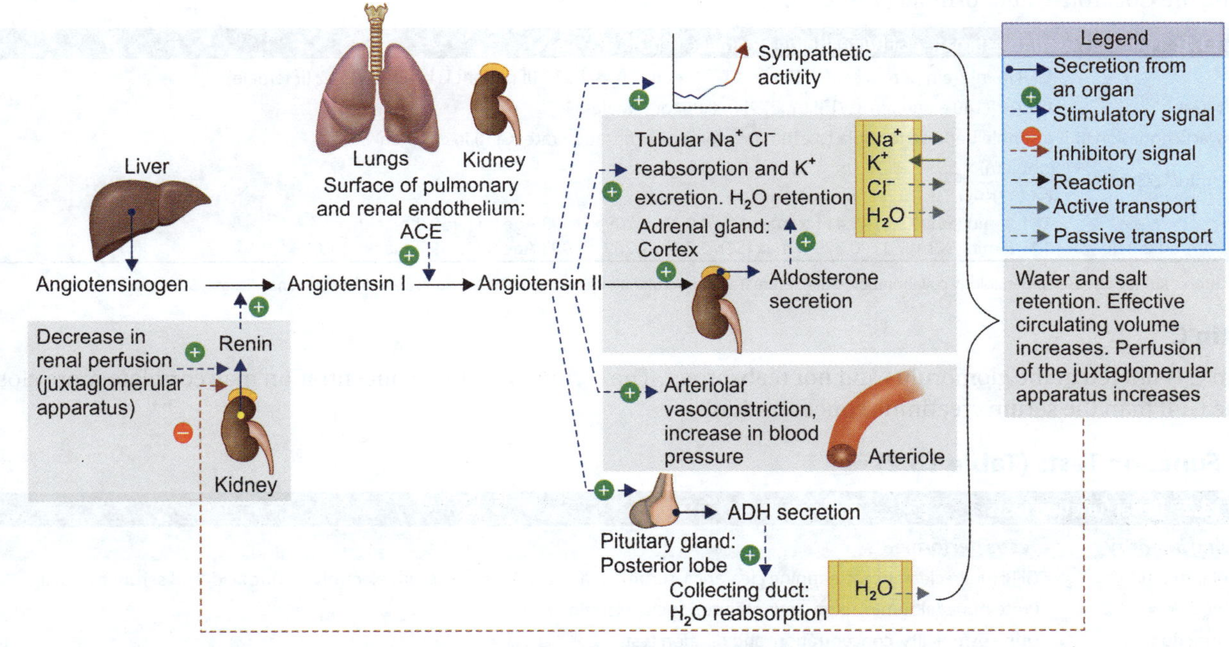

FIG. 13.3: Renin-angiotensin-aldosterone system. (ADH: antidiuretic hormone)

APPROACH TO RENAL DISEASES

Azotemia

Definition: It is a **biochemical abnormality** characterized by an **elevation of the blood urea nitrogen (BUN) and creatinine** levels. It is mainly due to a decreased glomerular filtration rate (GFR).

Causes: Azotemia can be divided into prerenal, renal, and postrenal (discussed later under AKI section).

Glomerular Filtration Rate (GFR)

- Measurement of the GFR is required to know the exact level of renal function. It is necessary to calculate GFR when the serum (plasma) urea or creatinine is within the normal range.
- Glomerular filtration rate for an average adult is about 125 mL/minute. Formula for calculation of GFR is presented in **Table 13.1**.
- The most common methods utilized to estimate the GFR are—measurement of the creatinine clearance and estimation equations based upon serum creatinine such as the Cockcroft-Gault equation, the Modification of Diet in Renal Disease (MDRD) study equations.

Measurement

Renal clearance (C) = $\frac{UV}{P}$

C = renal clearance, U = urinary concentration of any substance, P = plasma concentration of the same substance, V = minute volume of urine.

Inulin Clearance

- It is the **gold standard but is not practical**.
- Inulin is a polysaccharide that **passes freely through the glomerular capillary wall**. It is **neither absorbed nor excreted by the tubules** and hence, the quantity of inulin excreted in urine (UV) is identical to the amount filtered by the glomeruli. Therefore, the **renal clearance of inulin can be used to measure GFR.**

Creatinine Clearance

Q. Write short note on creatinine clearance and mention the formula for its calculation.

- The measurement of creatinine clearance, which approximates to that of inulin is the **most commonly used for measurement of GFR.** Other substances that are used are iohexol, iothalamate, ^{51}*Cr-EDTA*
- **Principle:** Creatinine clearance is based on the fact that **daily production of creatinine** (mainly from muscle cells) is **remarkably constant** and little affected by protein intake. Thus, serum creatinine and urinary output vary very little throughout the day and renal creatinine clearance given an estimate of the glomerular function of the kidney.
- **Cockroft–Gault equation:** If serum creatinine level is stable, creatinine clearance (hence GFR) can also be calculated by using the Cockroft–Gault formula (**Table 13.1**).

TABLE 13.1: Formulas used to estimate eGFR/creatinine clearance (CrCl).

MDRD		GFR in mL/min per 1.73 m^2 = 175 × SCr$^{-1.154}$ × age$^{-0.203}$ × 1.212 (if patient is black) × 0.742 (if female)
Cockroft–Gault		CrCl = [(140 – age) × TBW]/(SCr × 72) (× 0.85 for females)
The Schwartz equation: It is a simple bedside formula to estimate glomerular filtration rate (GFR) in children GFR (mL/min/1.73 m^2) = $\frac{\text{Height (cm)} \times 55}{\text{SCr (mg/dL)}}$		
CKD-EPI	Male	141 × min (SCr/0.9,1) –0.411 × max (SCr/0.9,1) –1.209×0.993 Age × (1.159 if black)
	Female	141 × min (SCr/0.7,1) –0.329 × max (SCr/0.7,1) –1.209×0.993 Age × (1.159 if black) × 1.018

(CKD-EPI: chronic kidney disease epidemiology collaboration; eGFR: estimated glomerular filtration rate; MDRD: modification of diet in renal disease; SCr: serum creatinine)

Cystatin C

Cystatin C is filtered at the glomerulus and not reabsorbed. The serum cystatin C concentration may correlate more closely with the GFR than the serum creatinine concentration.

Renal Function Tests (Table 13.2)

TABLE 13.2: Renal function tests.

Functional integrity	***Test/s performed***
Glomerular function	GFR: Inulin clearance, creatinine clearance, serum urea and creatinine, serum electrolytes,uric acid, and serum osmolality
Renal blood flow	Proteinuria (albumin), para-aminohippuric acid excretion test
Tubular function	Urine osmolality, concentration, and dilution test
	Urine electrolytes, e.g., Na, K, Ca, phosphate, uric acid
	Urine HCO_3, ammonia, pH after acid loading
Structural integrity	
➢ Plain X-ray KUB (kidney, ureter, bladder) ➢ Antegrade and retrograde pyelography ➢ Ultrasound ➢ Renal arteriography	➢ IVP (intravenous pyelogram) ➢ CT scan, CT urogram, MRI ➢ Kidney biopsy

Examination of the Urine

Q. Write short essay on routine examination of urine.

Physical Examination

Appearance: Color and clarity

Q. Write short note on causes of red colored urine.

- **Normal** urine is **straw to amber colored** due to the presence of urochrome pigment, excretion of which is generally proportional to the metabolic rate.

- Urine color interpretation (**Table 13.3**).
- Approach to red urine (**Flowchart 13.1**)
- Clarity
- Cloudy or turbid urine is most commonly associated with urinary tract infections (UTIs). Turbid white urine is sometimes called as albinuria (**Box 13.1**).

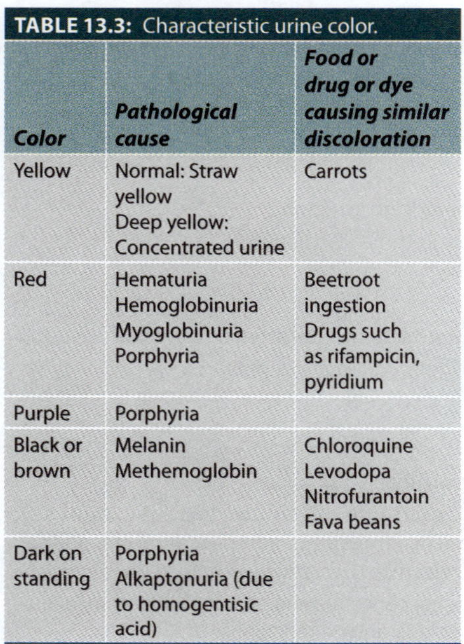

TABLE 13.3: Characteristic urine color.

Color	*Pathological cause*	*Food or drug or dye causing similar discoloration*
Yellow	Normal: Straw yellow Deep yellow: Concentrated urine	Carrots
Red	Hematuria Hemoglobinuria Myoglobinuria Porphyria	Beetroot ingestion Drugs such as rifampicin, pyridium
Purple	Porphyria	
Black or brown	Melanin Methemoglobin	Chloroquine Levodopa Nitrofurantoin Fava beans
Dark on standing	Porphyria Alkaptonuria (due to homogentisic acid)	

FLOWCHART 13.1: Approach to red color or dark urine.

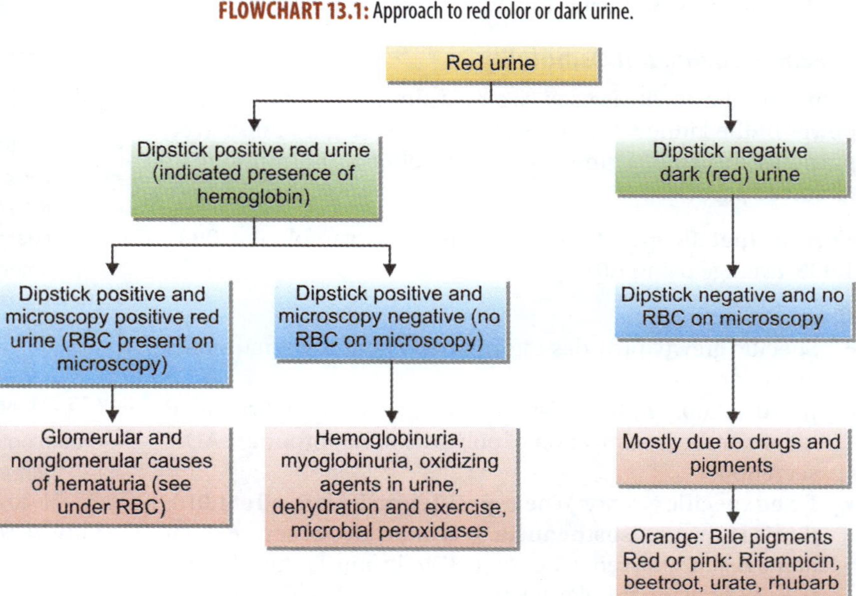

Box 13.1: Causes of turbid urine or albinuria.

- Chyluria
- Filariasis, schistosomiasis,postsurgery, malignancy
- Hyperuricosuria
- Phosphaturia
- Hyperoxaluria
- Proteinuria
- Pyuria
- Lipiduria
- Caseous material from renal tuberculosis
- Congenital malformations of the lymphatic vessels

TABLE 13.4: Characteristic urine odor and condition.

Characteristic urine Odor	*Condition*
Musty odor	Phenylketonuria
Sweet or fruity odor	Diabetes, ketosis, maple syrup urine disease
Sweaty foot or acrid odor	Isovaleric acidemia, glutaric acidemia
Rancid/fishy odor	Hypermethionemia
Swimming pool odor	Hawkinsinuria
Cat urine odor	3-hydroxyl 3-methyl glutaric aciduria
Maple syrup	Maple syrup urine disease
Boiled cabbage	Hypermethionemia
Tomcat urine	Multiple carboxylase deficiency
Hops-like urine	Oasthouse urine disease
Rotting fish	Trimethylaminuria

Odor

The characteristic urine odor and condition has shown in **Table 13.4**.

Urine Volume

A healthy adult excretes about 600–2,000 mL of urine in 24 hours. Volume is measured by collecting 24-hour urine samples in a measuring cylinder.

Q. Define oliguria, anuria, and polyuria. List the causes.

- **Oliguria:** Decreased production of **urine usually <400 mL** of urine **per day or less than 17 mL/hour.** On an average diet, about 300–500 mL urine/day is required to excrete the solute load at maximum concentration.
    - **Causes of oliguria (Table 13.5)**
- **Anuria:** Anuria is defined as urine output that is less than 100 mL/24 h or 0 mL/12 h. Anuria more commonly suggests reduced production of urine or obstruction to urine flow from both kidneys (until proved otherwise). Bladder outflow obstruction must always be considered first.
    - **Causes of anuria (Box 13.2)**

- **Polyuria:** Polyuria is defined as **persistent large increase in urine volume of >3 L/day and 2 L/m^2 in children.** This term should exclude normal individuals who take large amount of fluid and therefore, form large volumes of urine. Polyuria may be either due to increased urinary solute excretion (osmotic/solute diuresis) or pure water diuresis.
  - **Causes of polyuria** (**Box 13.3**)

Specific Gravity and Osmolality

Urine specific gravity is used as a measure of the concentrating power of the kidney. It is a measure of the weight of dissolved particles in urine. Urine osmolality reflects the number of dissolved particles.

Normal specific gravity of a 24-hour urine sample is **1.003–1.035**, average being 1.016.

Uses:
- Specific gravity provides information about the renal status and hydration.
- It is used only in the differential diagnosis of oliguric renal failure or the investigation of polyuria or inappropriate ADH secretion.
- **Fixed specific gravity:** When **specific gravity is fixed** at 1.010, this is known as **isosthenuria**. It is indicative of severe renal damage [chronic renal failure (CRF)/chronic kidney disease (CKD)] or acute tubular necrosis (ATN) with disturbance of both the concentrating and diluting abilities of the kidney.

Urinary pH

Normal urine is usually acidic with pH varying from 4.6 to 8. Measurement of urinary pH is not necessary except in the investigation and treatment of renal tubular acidosis (RTA).

TABLE 13.5: Causes of oliguria.

Nonrenal conditions	*Renal diseases*
➤ Excess loss of fluid ➤ Hypovolemia ➤ Shock ➤ Congestive heart failure ➤ Cirrhosis ➤ Pancreatitis, sepsis ➤ Peritonitis	➤ Acute glomerulonephritis ➤ Acute tubular necrosis (ATN) ➤ Acute interstitial nephritis ➤ Obstructive nephropathy

Box 13.2: Causes of anuria.

- Obstruction:
  - Bilateral ureteric obstruction
  - Prostatic or urethral obstruction
  - Renal stones
  - Tumors
- **Renal ischemia:** Bilateral renal arterial or venous occlusion
- *All causes of oliguria can lead to anuria.*

Box 13.3: Causes of polyuria.

- Pathological polyuria:
  - Increased excretion of solute (osmotic diuresis): Glucosuria—hyperglycemia, administration of mannitol, and hypercalcemia. Urea diuresis and sodium diuresis.
  - Defective renal concentrating ability: Diabetes insipidus, papillary necrosis, and diuretic phase of ATN
  - Failure of production of ADH: Idiopathic (50%), mass lesion, trauma, and infection
  - Drugs/toxins: Diuretics, lithium, and alcohol
- Primary (or psychogenic) polydipsia: Excess fluid intake

(ADH: antidiuretic hormone; ATN: acute tubular necrosis)

Chemical Examination

Urine should be examined for the presence of protein, blood and sugar in all patients suspected of having renal disease.

Proteinuria

Q. Write short note on proteinuria and microalbuminuria and their causes.

- Healthy adults may daily excrete <150 mg of total proteins and <30 mg of albumin.
- Proteinuria is defined as the **urinary excretion of >150 mg of protein/day.** It is one of the most common signs of renal disease. Pyrexia, exercise, and adoption of the upright posture (*postural proteinuria*) may also increase urinary protein output.

The types of proteinuria and causes are described in **Table 13.6**.
- Algorithm approach to proteinuria is presented in **Flowchart 13.2**.
- **Amount of pathological proteinuria:** It may be "mild" (<1.0 g/day), "moderate" (1.0–3.5 g/day) or "massive"/"heavy" (>3.5 g/day).

Microalbuminuria

- Normal urine contains <30 mg of albumin/day (<20 µg of albumin per minute).
- **Definition:** Microalbuminuria is the **presence of albumin (small amounts) in urine about >30 to <300 mg/day.** It is defined as the persistent elevation of the urinary albumin excretion of 30–200 mg/L (or 20–200 µg/min) in an early morning urine sample. It indicates early and possibly reversible glomerular damage.

TABLE 13.6: Types of proteinuria and causes.

Types of proteinuria	*Causes*
Transient proteinuria	Fever, heavy exercise, noradrenaline/albumin infusion
Orthostatic proteinuria	Usually in 2–5% of adolescents, rare above age of 30 years
Overflow proteinuria	Myeloma, hemoglobinuria, myoglobinuria
Glomerular proteinuria	Primary glomerular diseases, secondary glomerular diseases, diabetic nephropathy, hypertensive nephrosclerosis
Tubulointerstitial proteinuria	Heavy metal intoxications, autoimmune or allergic interstitial inflammation, drug-induced interstitial injury
Postrenal proteinuria	Urinary tract infections, nephrolithiasis, tumor

FLOWCHART 13.2: Algorithm approach to proteinuria.

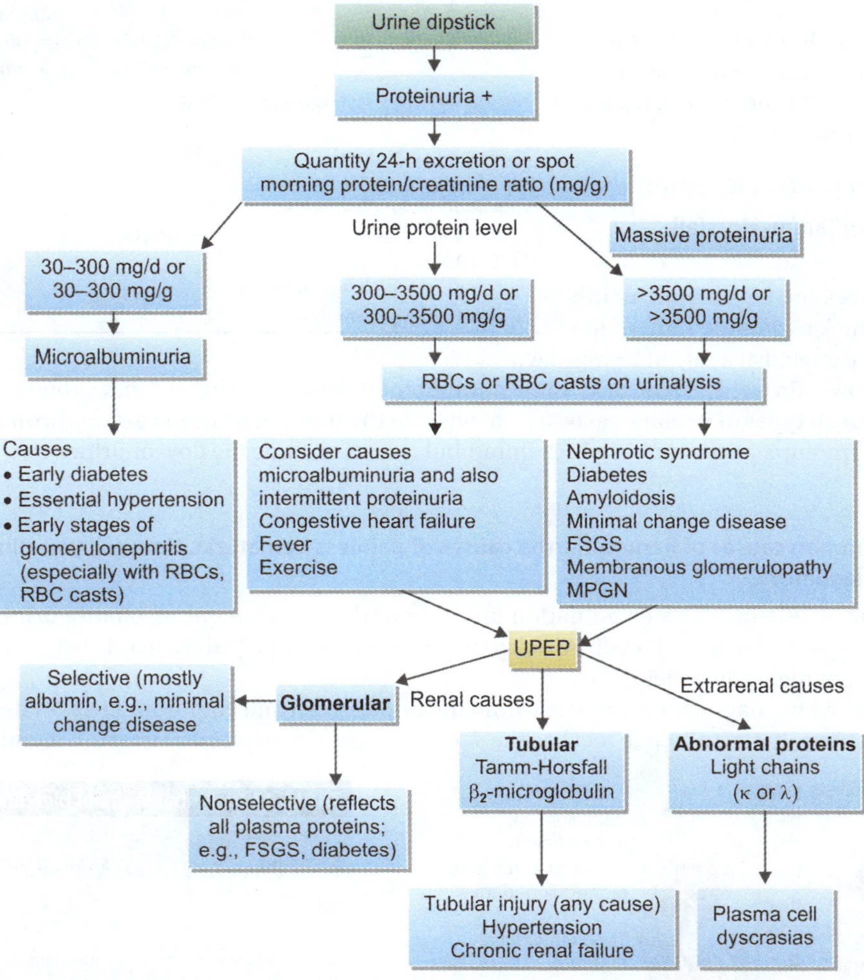

(FSGS: focal segmental glomerulosclerosis; MPGN: membranoproliferative glomerulonephritis; UPEP: urine protein electrophoresis)

- It is so named because conventional dipsticks cannot detect albumin levels of 30–300 mg/day (if urine volume is normal). An increase in albumin excretion between these two levels so-called microalbuminuria.
- **Significance:** The presence of albumin in the urine is a sign of glomerular abnormality.
  - **Diabetes mellitus:**
    - Microalbuminuria is an **early indicator of diabetic glomerular disease**. It is widely used as a predictor of the development of nephropathy in diabetics (raised fractional excretion of magnesium is a more sensitive marker than microalbuminuria in detecting early diabetic nephropathy).
    - In diabetic patients presence of microalbuminuria is associated with **increased cardiovascular mortality**.
  - Essential hypertension: **In hypertensive patients, microalbuminuria predicts cardiovascular morbidity and mortality.**
  - **Normotensive individuals:**
    - **Risk marker for the presence of cardiovascular disease predicts progression of nephropathy** when it increases to frank albuminuria (>300 mg/day).
    - **Atherosclerosis:** Persistent microalbuminuria is also associated with an increased risk of atherosclerosis and cardiovascular mortality.

Treatment

- Microalbuminuria can be reduced, and its progress to overt proteinuria can be prevented or retarded by **aggressive reduction of blood pressure (especially with ACE inhibitors or angiotensin receptor blockers), and control of diabetes mellitus.**
- **Blood pressure should be maintained at or below 130/80 mm Hg in patients with diabetes or kidney disease.**

Albumin-Creatinine Ratio

Measurement of 24-hour urinary excretion rates provides the most precise measure of microalbuminuria. However, it is often difficult to obtain 24-hour urine, it is more convenient to measure urinary albumin: creatinine ratio in a random urine sample and generally **albumin-creatinine ratio (ACR)** of 2.5–20 corresponds to albuminuria of 30–300 mg daily respectively (**Table 13.7**). The adequacy of the collection can be estimated by quantifying the 24-hour urine creatinine and comparing this value to the expected urine creatinine.

TABLE 13.7: Classification of proteinuria.

	Dipstick (not accurate)	Albumin-creatinine ratio (in mg/g)	Protein-creatinine ratio (in mg/g)
Normal to mildly increased *KDIGO A1*	Negative to trace	<30	<150
Moderately increased *KDIGO A2* (Previously microalbuminuria)	Trace to +	30–300	150–500
Severely increased *KDIGO A3* (Previously macroalbuminuria)	+ or greater	>300	>500
Nephrotic-range proteinuria	+++ or ++++	>2,200	>3,500

Tamm–Horsfall Mucoprotein (Uromodulin)

Q. Write short note on Tamm–Horsfall mucoprotein.

- It is a **protein present in normal urine** produced in the thick ascending limb of the loop of Henle. It is excreted at a rate of 25 mg/day.
- Function is not known. Probably it may have some immunomodulatory activity and may protect against UTI.

It is a **constituent of all types of urinary casts.** It is involved **in the pathogenesis of cast nephropathy** (observed in renal failure associated with multiple myeloma) in which intratubular casts occlude the flow or urine.

Hematuria

Q. Enumerate the common causes of hematuria/the causes of painless hematuria. How will you clinically localize and evaluate the site of bleeding?

- Hematuria may be visible on gross examination and reported by the patient as bloody urine (**macroscopic**/overt hematuria), or invisible and detected on dipstick/chemical testing of urine [**microscopic** hematuria—three or more red blood cells (RBCs) per high-power field].
- **Site of bleeding:** Bleeding may occur at any site within the urinary tract and common causes of hematuria are illustrated in **Figure 13.4**. Features that may help to localize the site of bleeding in the urinary tract are mentioned in **Table 13.8**.

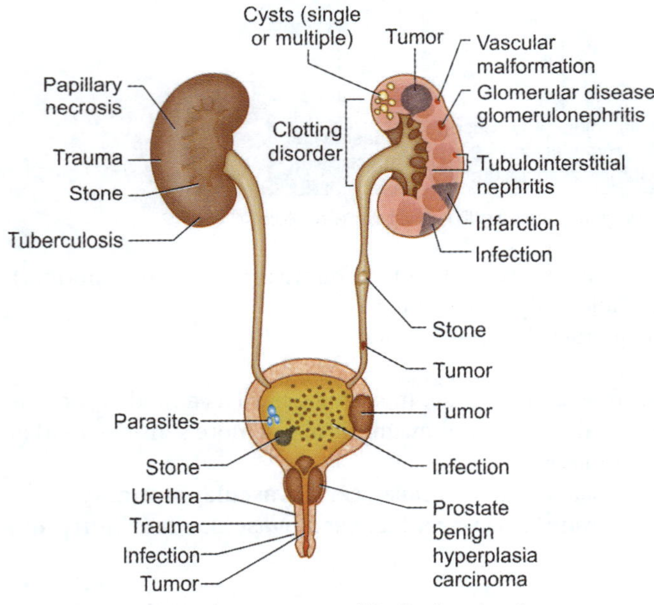

FIG. 13.4: Sites and common causes of bleeding from the urinary tract.

TABLE 13.8: Probable site of bleeding and its features.

Probable site of bleeding	*Suggestive features*
Urethra	Blood is seen at the start of voiding and then the urine becomes clear
Urinary bladder or above	Blood diffusely present throughout the urine
Glomerular origin	➢ Cola colored urine ➢ Red-cell casts (glomerulonephritis) ➢ Dysmorphic erythrocytes (irregular outer cell membrane) ➢ Acanthocytes (erythrocytes with one or more membrane protrusions of variable size and shape)
Renal pelvis and lower urinary tract	Pink or red colored urine
Prostate or bladder base	Blood only at the end of micturition
Lower urinary tract origin	Isomorphic erythrocytes in urine Microscopic clots of clumped erythrocytes in urine

Causes of Painless Hematuria (Table 13.9)

TABLE 13.9: Causes of painless hematuria.

Site of hematuria	*Causes*
Kidney	➢ Glomerulonephritis, IgA nephropathy ➢ Pyelonephritis: Severe acute pyelonephritis, papillary necrosis (more common in diabetes mellitus and sickle cell trait or disease) ➢ Tumors: Renal cell carcinoma ➢ Others: Infective endocarditis, renal tuberculosis, benign familial hematuria, microscopic polyangiitis, Wegener's granulomatosis
Ureter	Neoplasms
Bladder	Neoplasms, trauma, schistosomiasis
Prostate	Prostatitis, neoplasms
Urethra	Trauma

Glycosuria

- Blood glucose level varies between 70 and 120 mg/dL. This may increase to 120–160 mg/dL after a meal. Normally, all the glucose in the blood is filtered through the glomerulus and reabsorbed at the proximal tubules.
- If the renal threshold (the lowest blood glucose level that will result in glycosuria) is exceeded (usually >180–200 mg/dL), the excess glucose will not be reabsorbed into the blood and will be eliminated in the urine as in cases of diabetes mellitus. The presence of detectable amounts of **glucose in urine** is termed **glycosuria**.

Bacteriuria

Dipstick tests used for detection of bacteriuria detect nitrite produced from the reduction of urinary nitrate by bacteria. It is also for the detection of leukocyte esterase, an enzyme specific for neutrophils. *Enterobacteriaceae* species elaborate the enzyme nitrate reductase, which confers the ability to convert urinary nitrate to nitrite. So, nitrite-positive urine may indicate bacteriuria.

Microscopy

Microscopic examination of urine should be done in all patients suspected of having renal disease, on a "clean" midstream sample.

Cells

They are expressed as number of cells per low power or high power field.

- **Red blood cells:** Presence of RBCs (more than 3/hpf) in the urine indicates bleeding at any point in the urinary system from the glomerulus to the urethra. In glomerular diseases, the urine show red cells with cellular protrusions or fragmentation and are named as **dysmorphic** (distorted morphology) RBCs.
- **White blood cells:** Increased number of WBCs (mainly neutrophils more than 5/hpf) in urine is known as **pyuria**. It is indicative of an inflammatory reaction within urinary tract such as UTI, stones, tubulointerstitial nephritis (TIN), papillary necrosis, tuberculosis, and interstitial cystitis. The causative organism of infection may be identified by bacteriological examination. When accompanied by **leukocyte casts** or mixed leukocyte-epithelial cell casts, increased urinary leukocytes are considered to be of **renal origin.**

Patient's Evaluation of Hematuria

Investigations

- **Urine examination:**
  - **Proteinuria**
  - **Culture of urine for acid-fast bacilli**
  - **Microscopy:**
    - **Morphology of RBC** (assessed by phase contrast microscopy of fresh urine)
    - **Urine cytology:** For malignant cells especially in patients with risk factors such as smoking, analgesic abuse, industrial toxin exposure (e.g., aniline, benzidine, aromatic amines), age >50 years, pelvic irradiation, urinary schistosomiasis
- **Renal function tests**
- **Blood:**
  - Platelet count
  - Coagulation studies
  - Autoantibodies (antinuclear antibody, antineutrophil cytoplasmic antibody)
- **Radiological investigations:**
  - **Ultrasound for kidneys, ureters, bladder and prostate, CT, MRI**
  - Intravenous pyelography
- **Cystourethroscopy**

Casts

Casts are one of the organized elements which are **formed only in the kidney** and are **indicative of a renal disease.** They are cylindrical bodies, molded in the shape of the distal tubular lumen formed by solidification of **Tamm–Horsfall protein**, a glycoprotein secreted in the distal convoluted tubules and collecting tubules. These proteins form a fibrillar meshwork (basic matrix) and can trap any elements including cells, cell fragments or granular material.

Types of urinary casts and their significance

See **Figure 13.5.**

Crystals (Figs. 13.6A to C)

They may be found in patients with renal calculi. Calcium oxalate and urate crystals can be found in normal urine that has been left to stand.

ACUTE KIDNEY INJURY (ACUTE RENAL FAILURE)

Q. Discuss the classification, causes, pathogenesis, clinical features, diagnosis, investigations, and management of acute kidney injury/acute renal failure.

Renal failure is the failure of renal excretory function due to reduced GFR. Acute kidney injury (AKI) was previously known as acute renal failure (ARF). The other term used for this is **azotemia**.

Definition

Acute kidney injury is a clinical syndrome, defined as an **abrupt, deterioration of kidney function**, which is usually, but not invariably, reversible over a period of days or rarely over a few weeks. The deterioration in renal function is sufficiently severe to result in retention of nitrogenous wastes in the body (uremia) and other waste products normally cleared by the kidneys.

- It is **usually** but not invariably accompanied by **oliguria**.
- Conventionally the term ARF is often used in reference to the subset of patients with a need for acute dialysis support.

Cast and its appearance	Significance
Hyaline cast	• Nonspecific. Present in normal urine • Acute glomerulonephritis (AGN) • Chronic glomerulonephritis (CGN) • Fever • Congestive heart failure
Waxy cast	• End stage kidney • Chronic/advanced renal failure • Amyloidosis
Cellular casts	
1. Red blood cell (RBC) cast	• Always indicates renal disease • AGN • Lupus nephritis • Goodpasture syndrome • Subacute bacterial endocarditis • Renal infarction
2. Leukocyte (WBC) cast	• Acute pyelonephritis • AGN (proliferative glomerulonephritis) • Interstitial nephritis
3. Epithelial cast	• Acute tubular necrosis/injury • Viral disease (e.g. cytomegalovirus disease) • Drug • Interstitial nephritis • Transplant rejection
Granular cast (finely or coarsely granular) Coarsely granular Finely granular	• Tubular damage • CGN • Nephritis with tubular injury • Renal failure
Fatty cast	• Nephrotic syndrome • Fabry's disease • Other nephritidis
Telescoped (mixed) sediment	• Proliferative GN (systemic lupus erythematosus, polyarteritis nodosa) • Hypersensitivity reaction • Subacute bacterial endocarditis
Bacterial cast	• Diagnostic of acute bacterial pyelonephritis • Intrinsic renal infections
Broad cast (renal failure casts)	• Progressive renal failure with compensatory hypertrophy of nephron (poor prognosis)

FIG. 13.5: Urinary casts and their significance.

Crystal in normal acidic urine	Condition
Amorphous urates	• Normal acidic urine • Concentrated urine as in fever and dehydration
Crystalline urates (sodium, potassium and ammonium)	• Normal acidic urine
Crystalline uric acid	• Normal acidic urine • Post-chemotherapy for lymphoma and leukemia
Calcium oxalate	• Normal acidic urine • Large numbers in severe chronic renal disease or ethylene glycol or methoxyflurane toxicity/poisoning • Nephrolithiasis

FIG. 13.6A: Normal crystals found in acidic urine.

Crystal in normal alkaline urine	
Amorphous phosphates	Calcium carbonate
Ammonium biurate crystals	Crystalline phosphates-triple phosphates

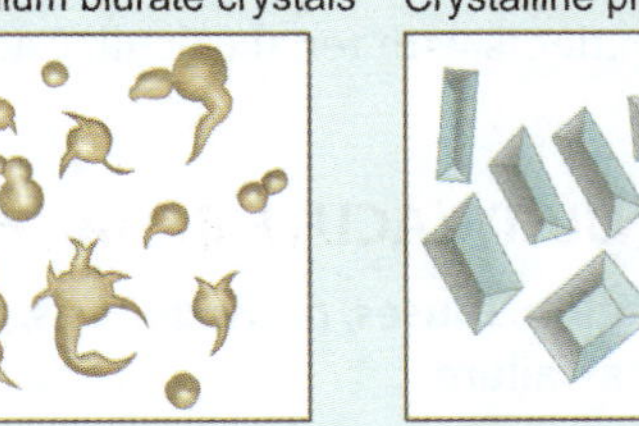

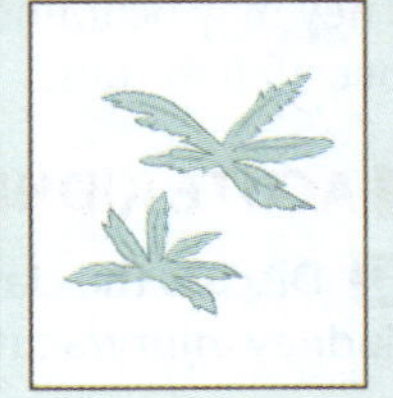

Crystalline phosphates-triple phosphates: It may be found in normal alkaline urine
- Struvite stones (magnesium, ammonium, phosphate) due to urease positive bacteria
- Urinary tract infection

FIG. 13.6B: Normal crystals found in alkaline urine.

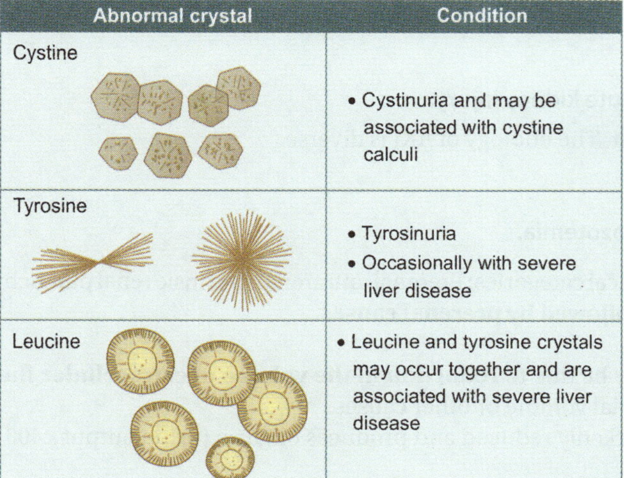

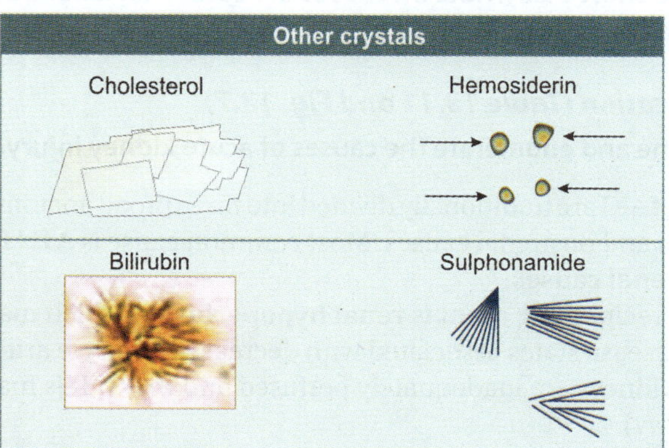

FIG. 13.6C: Abnormal crystals found in urine.

Classification of Acute Kidney Injury

Acute kidney injury is a medical emergency. It may produce sudden, life-threatening biochemical disturbances. ***AKI includes an increase in serum creatinine by ≥0.3 mg/dL (27 µmol/L) within 48 hours or an increase to ≥1.5 times the presumed baseline value that is known or presumed to have occurred within the prior 7 days, or a decrease in urine volume to <3 mL/kg over 6 hours*** [Kidney Disease: Improving Global Outcomes (KDIGO)-AKI].

RIFLE Criteria (Table 13.10)

- The distinction between acute and CKD or acute on chronic kidney disease, cannot easily be done in case of uremia. Acute Dialysis Quality Initiative group proposed the **RIFLE** (**R**isk, **I**njury, **F**ailure, **L**oss, **E**nd-stage renal disease) **criteria** to classify AKI.
- These criteria indicate an increasing degree of renal damage are of predictive value for mortality.

TABLE 13.10: RIFLE criteria for classification of acute kidney injury.

Grade	GFR criteria	Urine output criteria
Risk (Stage 1)	Increased serum creatinine × 1.5 times within 48 hours	Urine output <0.5 mL/kg/hour × 6 hours
Injury (Stage 2)	Increased serum creatinine × 2–3 times	Urine output <0.5 mL/kg/hour × 12 hours
Failure (Stage 3)	Increased serum creatinine × 3 times or serum creatinine (acute rise of = 0.5 mg/dL)	Urine output <0.3 mL/kg/hour × 24 hours OR Anuria for 12 hours OR Initiation of renal replacement therapy
Loss	Persistent AKI = Complete loss of renal function >4 weeks	
End-stage kidney disease	Persistent renal failure >3 months	

(GFR: glomerular filtration rate)

Acute Kidney Injury Network Classification

Acute kidney injury network **(AKIN)** has proposed a modification of the RIFLE criteria. It includes less severe AKI, a time constraint of 48 hours, and gives a correction for volume status before classification. According to this, AKI is classified into **three stages.**

- **Stage 1** is same as risk category of RIFLE with **addition of increase in serum creatinine by 0.3 mg/dL** within 48 hours.
- **Stages 2 and 3 are same as** injury and failure categories of **RIFLE.**

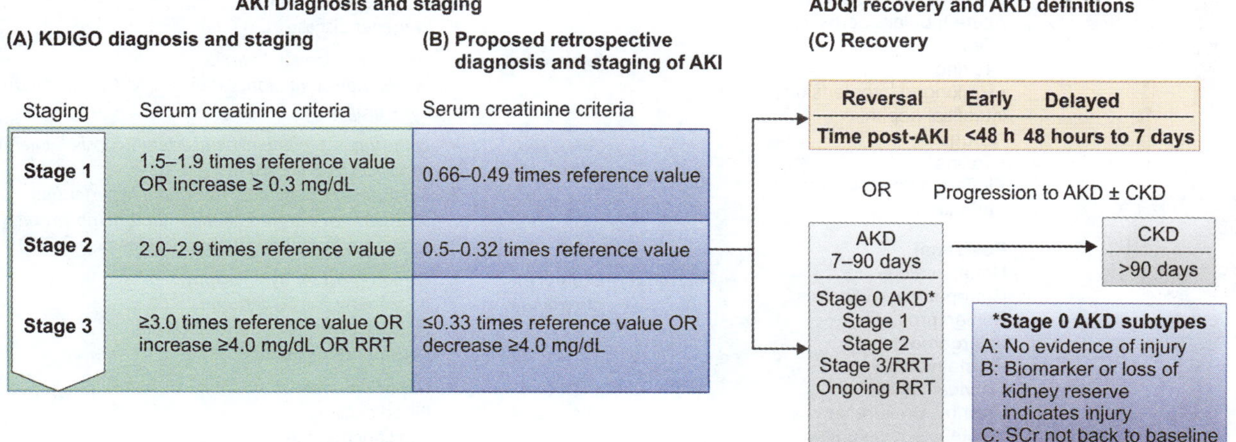

(ADQI: acute disease quality initiative; AKD: acute kidney disease; AKI: acute kidney injury; CKD: chronic kidney disease; KDIGO: Kidney Disease: Improving Global Outcomes)

Etiopathogenesis

Causes

Q. Write short essay/note on causes of acute renal failure/acute kidney injury.

At rest normal kidney receives about 25% of the cardiac output. The etiology of AKI is diverse.

Classification (Table 13.11 and Fig. 13.7)

Q. Define and enumerate the causes of acute kidney injury/azotemia.

Causes of AKI are traditionally divided into three broad anatomical categories: Prerenal, intrarenal (intrinsic renal parenchymal disease), and postrenal causes. Most common cause is **ATN followed by prerenal causes.**

- **Prerenal causes:**
  - Precipitating event is **renal hypoperfusion** which may be due to **reduction in the volume of extracellular fluid** or disease states associated with decreased effective arterial volume or other causes.
  - Kidneys are inadequately perfused and the GFR is markedly reduced and produces oliguria (urine output <400 mL/day).
- **Renal causes:**
  - **Intrinsic diseases of kidney** causing AKI are classified according to the primary histologic site of injury: **tubules, interstitium, vasculature or glomerulus.**
  - **Renal tubular epithelial (RTE) cell injury**, commonly known as **acute tubular necrosis** (ATN) and occurs more commonly due to ischemia of any cause, but can also be damaged by specific renal toxins. ATN results in ischemia and necrosis of the tubular epithelial cells. However, when the causative factors are removed the tubular cells can regenerate.
- **Postrenal causes:** These include obstruction of the urinary tract at any point in its course from the tubule to the urethra.

TABLE 13.11: Classification of causes of acute kidney injury.

Category	*Abnormality*	*Possible causes*
Prerenal	Hypovolemia	➤ Hemorrhage Volume depletion Renal fluid loss (over-diuresis) Third space (burns, peritonitis, muscle trauma)
	Impaired cardiac function	➤ Congestive heart failure Acute myocardial infarction Massive pulmonary embolism
	Systemic vasodilatation	➤ Antihypertensive medications Gram-negative bacteremia Cirrhosis Anaphylaxis
	Increased vascular resistance	➤ Anesthesia ➤ Surgery ➤ Hepatorenal syndrome ➤ NSAID medications ➤ Drugs that cause renal vasoconstriction (i.e., cyclosporine)
Intrinsic	Tubular	➤ Renal ischemia (*shock, complications of surgery, hemorrhage, trauma, bacteremia, pancreatitis, pregnancy*) ➤ Nephrotoxic drugs (*antibiotics, antineoplastic drugs, contrast media, organic solvents, anesthetic drugs, heavy metals*) ➤ Endogenous toxins (*myoglobin, hemoglobin, uric acid*)
	Glomerular	➤ Acute postinfectious glomerulonephritis ➤ Lupus nephritis ➤ IgA glomerulonephritis ➤ Infective endocarditis ➤ Goodpasture syndrome ➤ Wegener disease
	Interstitium	➤ Infections (*bacterial, viral*) ➤ Medications (*antibiotics, diuretics, NSAIDs, and many more drugs*)
	Vascular	➤ Large vessels (*bilateral renal artery stenosis, bilateral renal vein thrombosis*) ➤ Small vessels (*vasculitis, malignant hypertension, atherosclerotic or thrombotic emboli, hemolytic uremic syndrome, thrombotic thrombocytopenic purpura*)
Postrenal	Extrarenal obstruction	➤ Benign prostate hypertrophy ➤ Improperly placed catheter ➤ Bladder, prostate or cervical cancer ➤ Retroperitoneal fibrosis
	Intrarenal obstruction	➤ Nephrolithiasis ➤ Blood clots ➤ Papillary necrosis

(IgA: Immunoglobulin A; NSAIDs: nonsteroidal anti-inflammatory drugs)

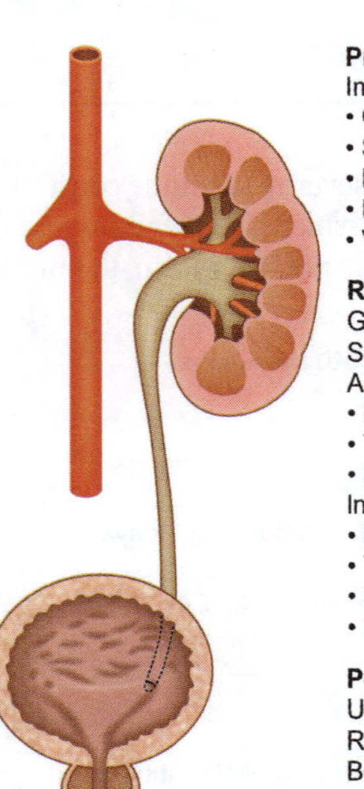

FIG. 13.7: Causes of acute kidney injury.

Clinical Features (Table 13.12)

General Symptoms

- Irrespective of the cause ARF present with symptoms related to uremia. These include **anorexia, nausea, vomiting, intellectual clouding, drowsiness, fits, coma, pruritus, hemorrhagic episodes** (e.g., epistaxis and gastrointestinal hemorrhage), and **dyspnea** due to fluid overload.
- **Physical findings** include asterixis, myoclonus, pericardial rub, and evidence of fluid overload in the form of edema, elevated jugular venous pressure (JVP), and crepitation.

TABLE 13.12: Clinical features of acute kidney injury.

Type of acute kidney injury	*History findings*	*Physical examination findings*
Prerenal	➢ Volume loss (e.g., history of vomiting, diarrhea, diuretic overuse, hemorrhage, burns) ➢ Reduced fluid intake ➢ Cardiac disease ➢ Liver disease	➢ Orthostatic hypotension and tachycardia Poor skin turgor ➢ Dilated neck veins, S3 heart sound, pulmonary rales, peripheral edema ➢ Ascites, caput medusae, spider angiomas
Intrinsic renal		
Acute tubular necrosis	History of receiving nephrotoxic medications (including over-the-counter, illicit, and herbal), hypotension, trauma or myalgias suggesting rhabdomyolysis, recent exposure to radiographic contrast agents	Muscle tenderness, compartment syndrome, assessment of volume status
Glomerular	Lupus, systemic sclerosis, rash, arthritis, uveitis, weight loss, fatigue, hepatitis C virus infection, human immunodeficiency virus infection, hematuria, foamy urine, cough, sinusitis, hemoptysis	Periorbital, sacral, and lower-extremity edema, rash, oral/nasal ulcers, hypertension
Interstitial	Medication use (e.g., antibiotics, proton pump inhibitors), rash, arthralgias, fever, infectious illness	Fever, drug-related rash (skin) eosinophilia
Vascular	Nephrotic syndrome, trauma, flank pain, anticoagulation (atheroembolic disease), vessel catheterization or vascular surgery	Skin changes, livedo reticularis, fundoscopic examination (showing malignant hypertension), abdominal bruits
Postrenal	Urinary urgency or hesitancy, gross hematuria, polyuria, stones, medications, cancer	Bladder distention, pelvic mass, prostate enlargement

Q. How will you differentiate renal from prerenal failure?

Q. Describe clinical and laboratory differences between prerenal and renal azotemia.

AKI Due to a Prerenal Disorder

- Most common form of AKI
- Rise in serum creatinine/BUN due to inadequate renal plasma flow and intraglomerular hydrostatic pressure to support normal glomerular filtration.
- Usually no or reversible parenchymal injury, but may be associated with ATN.
- Renin-angiotensin-aldosterone system responds to decreased effective circulating volume, but renal autoregulation fails once systolic blood pressure falls below 80 mm Hg.
- Nonsteroidal anti-inflammatory drugs—prevent renal afferent vasodilatation.
- Angiotensin-converting enzyme inhibitors/angiotensin receptor blockers (ACEIs/ARBs)—prevent renal efferent vasoconstriction.

ARF Due to Renal Causes

Most common causes—sepsis, ischemia, and nephrotoxins. Prerenal AKI can lead to ATN in some cases.

Acute tubular necrosis is the most important cause of ARF due to intrinsic renal diseases. The clinical course in ATN/ARF is divided into three phases:

1. **Oliguric (initiation) phase:**
   - Clinical features depend on the initiating event that caused the ischemic form of AKI. Patients develop symptoms due to fluid overload and azotemia. Fluid overload results in raised JVP, pedal edema, ascites, and pulmonary edema.
   - Mild reduction of urine output and increase in BUN. Hyperkalemia occurs commonly during this phase. This phase usually **lasts for about 10–14 days**. About 40% of the patients may have normal urine output and is called nonoliguric renal failure. The electrolyte disturbances are less in these patients.
2. **Maintenance phase*:*** During this phase, there is sustained decrease in urine output in the range of 40–400 mL/day **(oliguria), salt and water overload, rising BUN level, hyperkalemia, metabolic acidosis, and other features of uremia**. This phase lasts for days to weeks.

3. **Diuretic (recovery) phase:** During this phase there is a **steady increase in urine output** and in a few days the patient develops **polyuria with a urine output that may reach up to 3 L/day**. During this phase the tubular concentrating capacity is defective, and there is uncontrolled loss of large amounts of water, sodium, and potassium (leading to **hypokalemia**) in the urine. Once the renal tubular function returns to normal, BUN, creatinine levels, and urine volume also return to normal.

- ARF due to glomerulonephritis (GN) presents with hypertension, proteinuria, and hematuria.
- Drug-induced acute tubule-interstitial nephritis patients may present with fever, skin rash, and arthralgia.

Ischemia—associated AKI

- Kidneys receive 20% of cardiac output, account for 10% of oxygen consumption although they constitute only 0.5% of human body mass.
- Renal outer medulla—one of the most hypoxic regions in the body - due to:
- Architecture of blood vessels that supply tubules
- Enhanced leukocyte-endothelial interactions in small vessels causing inflammation
- This causes:
  - Reduced blood flow to metabolically active s3 segment of proximal tubule
  - Mitochondrial dysfunction and release of reactive oxygen species (ROS) leading to tubular injury

Exogenous toxins—contrast agents

- Iodinated contrast agents (CT):
  - Risk of contrast nephropathy increased in presence of CKD, diabetic nephropathy, multiple myeloma, congestive cardiac failure (CCF).
  - Diagnosis: Rise in serum creatinine within 24–48 hours following exposure, peak at 3–5 days, resolving within 1 week.
  - Severe dialysis requiring AKI only occurs in the setting of other coexisting conditions mentioned above.
- Others: High-dose gadolinium (MRI), oral sodium phosphate solutions (bowel purgatives), drugs

Endogenous toxins

- **Rhabdomyolysis**—traumatic crush injuries, muscle ischemia during vascular/orthopedic surgery, compression during come/immobilization, prolonged seizure activity, excessive exercise, heat stroke, malignant hyperthermia, infections, metabolic disorders such as hypophosphatemia and severe hypothyroidism, myopathies—release of **myoglobin**.
- Massive hemolysis—release of **hemoglobin**.
- **Tumor lysis syndrome**—after initiation of cytotoxic therapy (lymphoma, ALL, myeloma)

AKI Due to Postrenal Causes

- Partial or total obstruction to unidirectional flow of urine—leading to increased hydrostatic pressure and interference with glomerular filtration
- Obstruction can be anywhere from renal pelvis to tip of urethra.
- B/L renal obstruction or U/L obstruction of a single functioning kidney, setting of CKD, reflex vasospasm of contralateral kidney.
- Causes:
  - Bladder neck obstruction—prostate disease, neurogenic bladder, and therapy with anticholinergic drugs.
  - Obstructed Foley's catheter
  - Ureteric obstruction—intraluminal obstruction—calculi, blood clots, sloughed renal papillae; infiltration of ureteric wall—neoplasia; external compression—retroperitoneal fibrosis, neoplasia, abscess, and surgical damage.
- If untreated, obstructive nephropathy leads to irreversible tubulointerstitial fibrosis (i.e., intrinsic disease).

Investigations

Serum Creatinine and Urea

- The rate of rise in serum creatinine and urea is determined by the rate of protein catabolism (tissue breakdown).
- **Raised serum creatinine and urea** levels are the most consistent findings. In ARF due to prerenal causes, there is a disproportionate elevation of serum urea in relation to serum creatinine.

Q. List the causes of raised serum creatinine (Box 13.4).

Drawbacks: Rise in creatinine is an unreliable indicator of early renal injury because:

- Normal **serum creatinine level is an influenced by several nonrenal factors** (age, gender, muscle mass, medications, hydration and nutrition status, and tubular secretion).
- **More than 50% loss of renal function must be lost before serum creatinine rises.**

Box 13.4: Causes of raised serum creatinine.

- Azotemia: Prerenal, renal, and postrenal
- Large amount of consumption of meat
- Hypothyroidism, acromegaly, and gigantism
- Rhabdomyolysis
- Drugs: Statins, fibrates

- **Serum creatinine does not reflect true GFR**. This is because several hours to days must elapse before a new equilibrium between presumably steady state production and decreased excretion of creatinine is established.

Newer Novel Biomarkers for AKI

These markers can diagnose early AKI and include (1) neutrophil gelatinase-associated lipocalin (NGAL), (2) kidney injury molecule-1 (KIM-1), (3) interleukin-18 (IL-18), and (4) cystatin C.

Other Investigations

- **Other biochemical findings:** Include **hyperkalemia, hypocalcemia, hyperphosphatemia, and hyperuricemia.**
- **Urine analysis (Tables 13.13 and 13.14)**
  - RBCs/RBC casts: Glomerulonephritis, vasculitis, malignant hypertension, and thrombotic microangiopathy
  - WBCs/WBC casts: Interstitial nephritis, GN, pyelonephritis, allograft rejection, and malignant infiltration of kidney
  - Renal tubular epithelial cells/RTE casts/pigmented casts: ATN, TIN, acute cellular allograft rejection, myoglobinuria, hemoglobinuria
  - Granular casts: ATN, GN, TIN, and vasculitis
  - Eosinophiluria: Allergic interstitial nephritis, atheroembolic disease, pyelonephritis, cystitis, GN
  - Crystalluria: Acute uric acid nephropathy, calcium oxalate (ethylene glycol intoxication), drugs/toxins (acyclovir, indinavir, sulfadiazine, and amoxicillin)

TABLE 13.13: Urine finding in different types of acute kidney injury.

Type of acute kidney injury	*Urine findings*
Prerenal	Normal or hyaline casts
Intrarenal	
Tubular cell injury	Muddy-brown, granular, epithelial casts
Interstitial nephritis	Pyuria, hematuria, mild proteinuria, granular, and epithelial casts, eosinophils
Glomerulonephritis	Hematuria, marked proteinuria, red blood cell casts, granular casts
Vascular disorders	Normal or hematuria, mild proteinuria
Postrenal	Normal or hematuria, granular casts, pyuria

TABLE 13.14: Urinary abnormalities in ARF.

	Prerenal	*Renal*	*Postrenal*
Specific gravity	>1.020	1.010	—
Urine osmolality (mOsm/kg)	>500	250–300	400
Urine/plasma osmolality	>1.1	1–1.1	1–1.1
Urinary sodium (mEq/L)	<20	>40	<30
FENa	<1%	>1%	Variable
Urine/plasma creatinine	>40	<20	<20
Renal failure index	<1	>2	>2
Urinary sediment	Scanty	Active	Scanty
Urinary proteins	Minimal	Moderate to severe	Minimal

(FENa: Fractional excretion of sodium)

- Proteinuria:
  - Mild—<1 g/day—ischemia or nephrotoxin associated AKI
  - Moderate—multiple myeloma, atheroemboli
  - Severe (nephrotic range) >3.5 g/day—GN, vasculitis, toxins that affect both glomerulus and tubulointerstitium such as NSAIDs, minimal change disease
- **Electrocardiogram:** May show features of hyperkalemia.
- **Chest radiograph:** May show pulmonary edema and pleural effusion.
- **Others:**
  - **In rapidly progressive glomerulonephritis (RPGN):** Systemic causes (e.g., Wegener's granulomatosis) must be excluded by appropriate investigations (e.g., cAN-CA). A **kidney biopsy may be necessary**.
  - **In postrenal ARF:** Renal imaging by plain abdominal X-ray and ultrasonography may be useful.
  - Kidney injury molecule 1 (KIM 1): Ischemia or nephrotoxin associated AKI
  - Neutrophil gelatinase-associated lipocalin (NGAL): Cardiopulmonary bypass-associated AKI
  - Insulin-like growth factor-binding protein 7 (IGFBP7): Marker of development of severe AKI
  - Tissue inhibitor of metalloproteinase-2 (TIMP-2): Marker of development of severe AKI
  - **Fractional excretion of sodium (Table 13.15)**: The ratio of sodium clearance to creatinine clearance, increases the reliability of this index. However, it may remain low in some renal diseases. Fraction of filtered sodium load that is reabsorbed by the tubules—measure of kidney's ability to reabsorb sodium as well as endogenously and exogenously administered factors that affect tubular reabsorption.

Helps in differentiating between prerenal azotemia and ATN, but has limited role.

TABLE 13.15: Values of FENa (fractional excretion of sodium) and BUN-to-serum creatinine ratio in various causes of acute kidney injury.

Etiology of acute kidney injury	*FENa*	*BUN-to-serum creatinine ratio*
Prerenal	<1%	>20
Intrarenal		<10–15
➢ Tubular necrosis	≥1%	
➢ Interstitial nephritis	≥1%	
➢ Glomerulonephritis (early)	<1%	
➢ Vascular disorders (early)	<1%	
Postrenal	≥1%	>20

(BUN: blood urea nitrogen)

Complications of Acute Kidney Injury (Box 13.5)

Q. Mention the complications of acute kidney injury (acute renal failure).

Box 13.5: Complications of acute kidney injury.

- **Metabolic:** Hyperkalemia, hypocalcemia, hyperphosphatemia, hypermagnesemia,hyperuricemia, metabolic acidosis (increased anion gap)
- **Cardiovascular:** Cardiac arrhythmias, pulmonary edema, pericarditis/pericardial effusion
- **Gastrointestinal:** Gastrointestinal hemorrhage
- **Neurologic:** Encephalopathy, neuropathy, seizures
- **Hematologic:** Anemia, bleeding—platelet dysfunction
- **Miscellaneous:** Infections (pneumonia, urinary tract infection, septicemia)

Management (Flowchart 13.3)

General measures and management of complications:

- **Fluid balance:** Advisable to **restrict fluid intake.**
  - Amount of fluid to be given **depends upon** the **degree of edema, and fluid loss** through urine, gastrointestinal tract and skin.
  - Usually intake restricted to about **400 mL/day** in addition to the abovementioned fluid losses.
- **Sodium balance: Sodium is restricted** to avoid volume expansion and overhydration
  - **Hyponatremia** is common and is usually **due to excessive fluid administration.**
  - Hypernatremia may occur occasionally, due to excessive administration of sodium bicarbonate for correction of acidosis.
- **Potassium balance: Hyperkalemia is the leading cause of death** in ARF. Treatment is discussed in Chapter 14.
- **Acid-base balance:** In most patients **acidosis** is of moderate degree and does not require treatment. However, in **advanced cases intravenous sodium bicarbonate** may be necessary. Acidosis if accompanied by severe hyperkalemia and fluid overload is best treated with dialysis.
- **Calcium-phosphorus balance:** Both **hypocalcemia and hypercalcemia** are observed **in the maintenance phase** of ARF and are not serious clinical problems. **Phosphate retention** occurs in patients can be **controlled with aluminum hydroxide, lanthanum carbonate, sevelamer, calcium acetate or calcium carbonate** [bind phosphate within the gastrointestinal tract (GIT) and eliminated in stool].
- **Diet:**
  - **Restrict dietary proteins** to about 40 g/day. Suppress endogenous protein catabolism to a minimum level by giving as much energy as possible in the form of carbohydrates and fats. Patients treated by blood purification techniques are given 70 g or more protein/day.
  - **Hypercatabolic patients** may **need higher nitrogen intake** to prevent negative nitrogen balance.
  - **Restrict the salt intake.**
  - **Vitamin supplements** are usually necessary.
- **Systemic complications of ARF: Infections** and **gastrointestinal bleeding** are two important complications.
  - **Infectious complications** [very high (80%)] includes pulmonary, urinary, and wound infections (in post-traumatic and postoperative patients). Infections should be treated promptly by **appropriate antibiotics.**
  - **Gastrointestinal bleeding** (in 40% of patients) may prove fatal and treated by proton pump inhibitors and gastroprotective agents. Qualitative platelet dysfunction, which results in a hemorrhagic diathesis.
- **Use of drugs: Great care is necessary** in the use of drugs and nephrotoxic drugs should be avoided.

Treatment of the underlying cause of the AKI:

- **Identify the cause** (by simple initial investigations such as ultrasound or may require additional investigations, including renal biopsy) and **correct it, if possible.**

Specific therapy:

- **No specific treatment** for ATN, other than restoring renal perfusion.
- **Intrinsic kidney disease may require specific therapy** (e.g., immunosuppressive drugs such as corticosteroids and cyclophosphamide in some causes of **rapidly progressive glomerulonephritis**).
- **"Postrenal" obstruction** requires **urgent relief of obstruction.** Once the blood chemistry returns to normal, the underlying cause should be treated whenever possible.
- **Drug-induced** acute tubule-interstitial nephritis usually recovers after stopping the offending drug, but sometimes, short course of steroids may be helpful.
- **If conservative measures fail, dialysis and hemofiltration** may be necessary. These techniques purify blood and/or remove excess fluid. Main indications of dialysis and hemofiltration in ARF are listed in **Table 13.16. Table 13.17** lists the preventive strategies for conditions with high risk of acute kidney injury.

Q. Write short note on indications for dialysis in acute renal failure.

TABLE 13.16: Indications of dialysis or hemofiltration in acute renal failure (ARF).

1. Fluid overload refractory to diuretics and refractory pulmonary edema	6. ESRD (end-stage renal disease)
2. Severe metabolic acidosis (pH < 7.1)	7. Severe biochemical derangement in the absence of symptoms (especially in an oliguric and hypercatabolic patients)
3. Resistant hyperkalemia	8. Removal of drugs causing the acute renal failure (e.g., gentamicin, lithium, severe aspirin overdose)
4. Complications of uremia (e.g., pericarditis, encephalopathy, neuropathy)	9. Severe hyperphosphatemia (defined as >12 mg/dL)
5. Increased plasma urea (>180 mg/dL) and creatinine (>6.8 mg/dL)	10. Tumor lysis syndrome
	11. Anuria for >12 hours

Contd...

Contd...

Indications for urgent renal replacement therapy:
- Pulmonary edema
- Hyperkalemia:
  - >6.5 mEq/L
  - Signs and symptoms of hyperkalemia such as cardiac conduction defects, muscle weakness
  - >5.5 mEq/L with ongoing muscle breakdown (rhabdomyolysis) or ongoing potassium absorption [gastrointestinal (GI) bleed]
  - Signs of uremia (pericarditis, seizures, severe declining mental status)
  - Severe metabolic acidosis (pH < 7.1), unless it is easily reversible such as diabetic ketoacidosis
  - Acute poisonings

FLOWCHART 13.3: Approach to acute kidney injury.

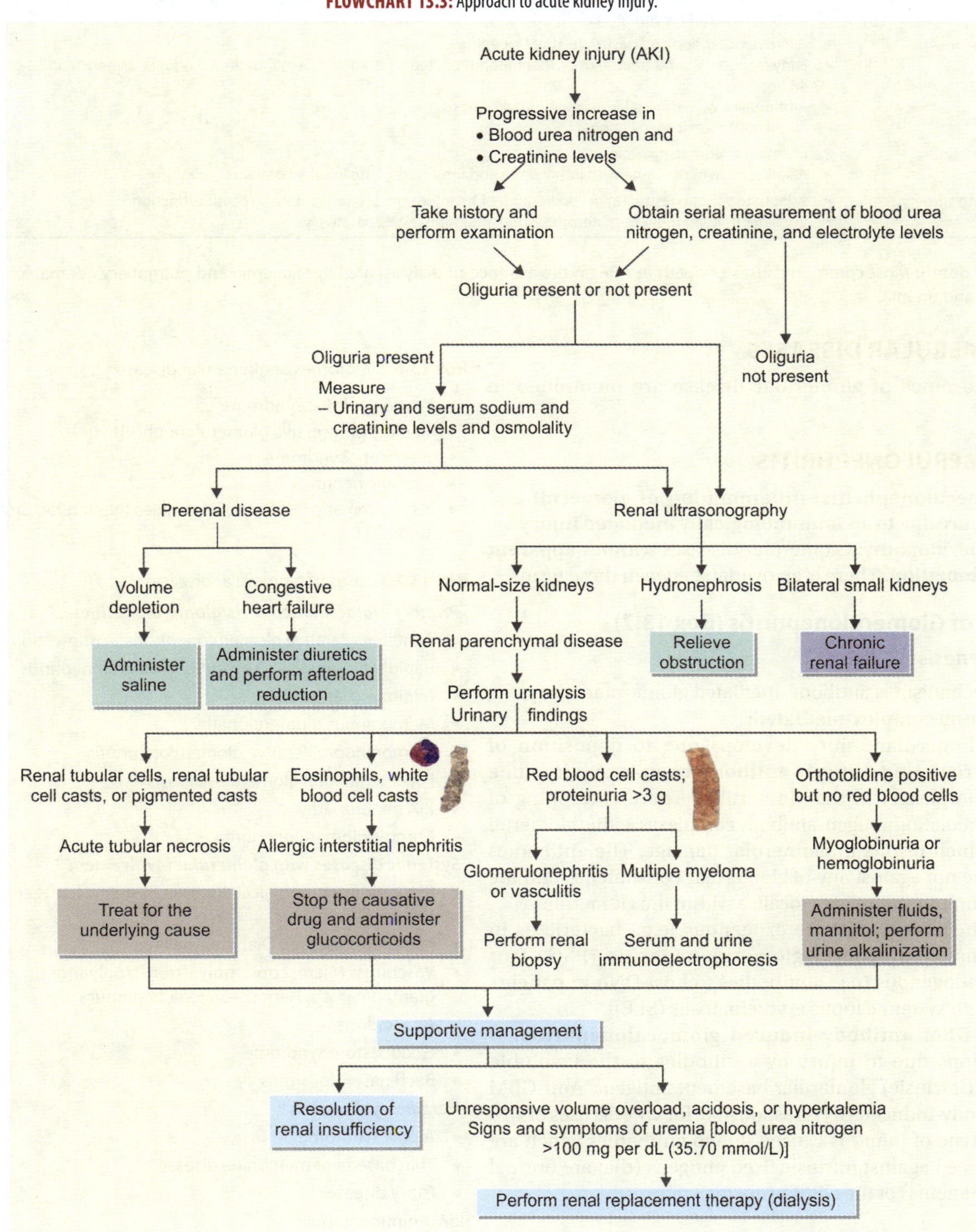

TABLE 13.17: Preventive strategies for conditions with high risk of acute kidney injury.

Risk factors	*Preventive strategies*
Cancer chemotherapy (risk of tumor lysis syndrome)	➢ Hydration and allopurinol administration a few days before chemotherapy initiation
Exposure to nephrotoxic medications	➢ Avoid nephrotoxic medications if possible. Use appropriate dosing, intervals, and duration of therapy
Exposure to radiographic contrast agents	➢ Avoid use of intravenous contrast media when risks outweigh benefits ➢ If use of contrast media is essential, use iso-osmolar or low-osmolar contrast agent with lowest volume possible ➢ Use of N-acetylcysteine may be considered
Hemodynamic instability	➢ Optimal fluid resuscitation, a mean arterial pressure goal of > 65 mm Hg is widely used; isotonic solutions (e.g., normal saline) ➢ Vasopressors are recommended for persistent hypotension (mean arterial pressure <65 mm Hg) despite fluid resuscitation ➢ Dopamine is not recommended
Hepatic failure	➢ Avoid hypotension and gastrointestinal bleeding ➢ Early recognition and treatment of spontaneous bacterial peritonitis; use albumin, 1.5 g/kg at diagnosis and 1 g/kg at 48 hours ➢ Albumin infusion during large volume paracentesis ➢ Avoid nephrotoxic medications
Rhabdomyolysis	➢ Maintain adequate hydration ➢ Alkalinization of the urine with intravenous sodium bicarbonate in select patients
Undergoing surgery	➢ Adequate volume resuscitation/prevention of hypotension, sepsis, optimizing cardiac function ➢ Consider holding renin-angiotensin system antagonists preoperatively

Cause of death: Most common causes of death in ARF (in the absence of dialysis) are hyperkalemia and pulmonary edema, followed by infection and uremia.

GLOMERULAR DISEASES

The syndromes of glomerular disease are mentioned in **Box 13.6**.

GLOMERULONEPHRITIS

- **Glomerulonephritis: Inflammation of glomeruli** and **most are** due to an **immunologically mediated injury**.
- **Glomerulopathy:** Glomerular diseases **without apparent inflammation.** There is an overlap between these terms.

Causes of Glomerulonephritis (Box 13.7)

Pathogenesis

Main mechanism is antibody-mediated glomerular injury.

1. **Immune complex-mediated:**
   - Glomerular injury develops due to deposition of **circulating antigen-antibody complexes** (immune complexes) in the glomerulus. There is trapping of circulating antigen-antibody complexes within glomeruli which results in glomerular damage. The antibodies are not against any of glomerular constituents, and the immune complexes localize within the glomeruli.
   - The antigen may be exogenous [e.g., bacteria as in poststreptococcal glomerulonephritis (PSGN) or endogenous (e.g., antibodies to host DNA in patients with systemic lupus erythematosus (SLE)].
2. **Anti-GBM antibody-induced glomerulonephritis:** It develops due to injury by antibodies to the insoluble fixed (intrinsic) glomerular basement antigens. Anti-GBM antibody-induced GN is responsible for <5% of cases of GN. This type of injury is caused due to antibodies which are produced against intrinsic fixed antigens (that are normal components) of the GBM proper.

Box 13.6: Syndromes of glomerular disease.

- Acute nephritic syndrome
- Rapidly progressive glomerulonephritis
- Nephrotic syndrome
- Chronic nephritis
- Asymptomatic urinary abnormalities (hematuria, proteinuria or both)

Box 13.7: Causes of glomerular diseases.

Primary glomerulonephritis/glomerulopathies

- Acute proliferative glomerulonephritis: Postinfectious, others
- Rapidly progressive (crescentic) glomerulonephritis
- Minimal-change disease
- Membranous glomerulopathy
- Membranoproliferative glomerulonephritis
- Focal segmental glomerulosclerosis
- IgA nephropathy
- Chronic glomerulonephritis

Systemic diseases with glomerular involvement

- Systemic immunological diseases: Systemic lupus erythematosus
- Metabolic diseases: Diabetes mellitus
- Vasculitis: Microscopic polyarteritis/polyangiitis, Wegener granulomatosis, Henoch–Schönlein purpura
- Amyloidosis
- Goodpasture syndrome
- Bacterial endocarditis

Hereditary disorders

- Alport syndrome
- Thin basement membrane disease
- Fabry disease

(IgA: Immunoglobulin A)

Terms used in glomerular diseases
- **Focal:** Some glomeruli, but not all show the lesion.
- **Diffuse (global):** Most of the glomeruli (>75%) show the lesion.
- **Segmental:** Only a part of the glomerulus is affected (most focal lesions are also segmental, e.g., focal segmental glomerulosclerosis).
- **Proliferative:** Increase in cell numbers due to hyperplasia of one or more of the resident glomerular cells with or without inflammation.
- **Membranous:** Capillary wall thickening due to deposition of immune deposits or alterations in basement membrane.
- **Crescent formation:** Proliferation of parietal epithelial cell with mononuclear cell infiltration in Bowman's space.

Characteristics of acute nephritic syndrome are presented in **Box 13.8**.

Spectrum of glomerular diseases are presented in **Flowchart 13.4** and various causes of proliferative and nonproliferative GN are shown in **Figure 13.8**.

Box 13.8: Characteristics of acute nephritic syndrome.
- **Hematuria** (gross or microscopic)
- **Red cell casts in the urine**
- **Azotemia** (temporary)
- **Temporary oliguria** (due to decreased glomerular filtration rate)
- **Hypertension**
- Proteinuria*
- **Edema*** (periorbital, leg or sacral)

*Not as severe as in nephrotic syndrome.

Acute Proliferative Glomerulonephritis

These are immune complexes mediated diseases. The inciting antigen may be:
- **Exogenous,** e.g., postinfectious GN which commonly follows streptococcal infection, but may also associated with other infections
- **Endogenous,** e.g., nephritis of SLE
- It is characterized histologically by cellular proliferation (mesangial and endothelial) associated with infiltration by leukocytes (neutrophils, macrophages).

FLOWCHART 13.4: Spectrum of glomerular diseases.

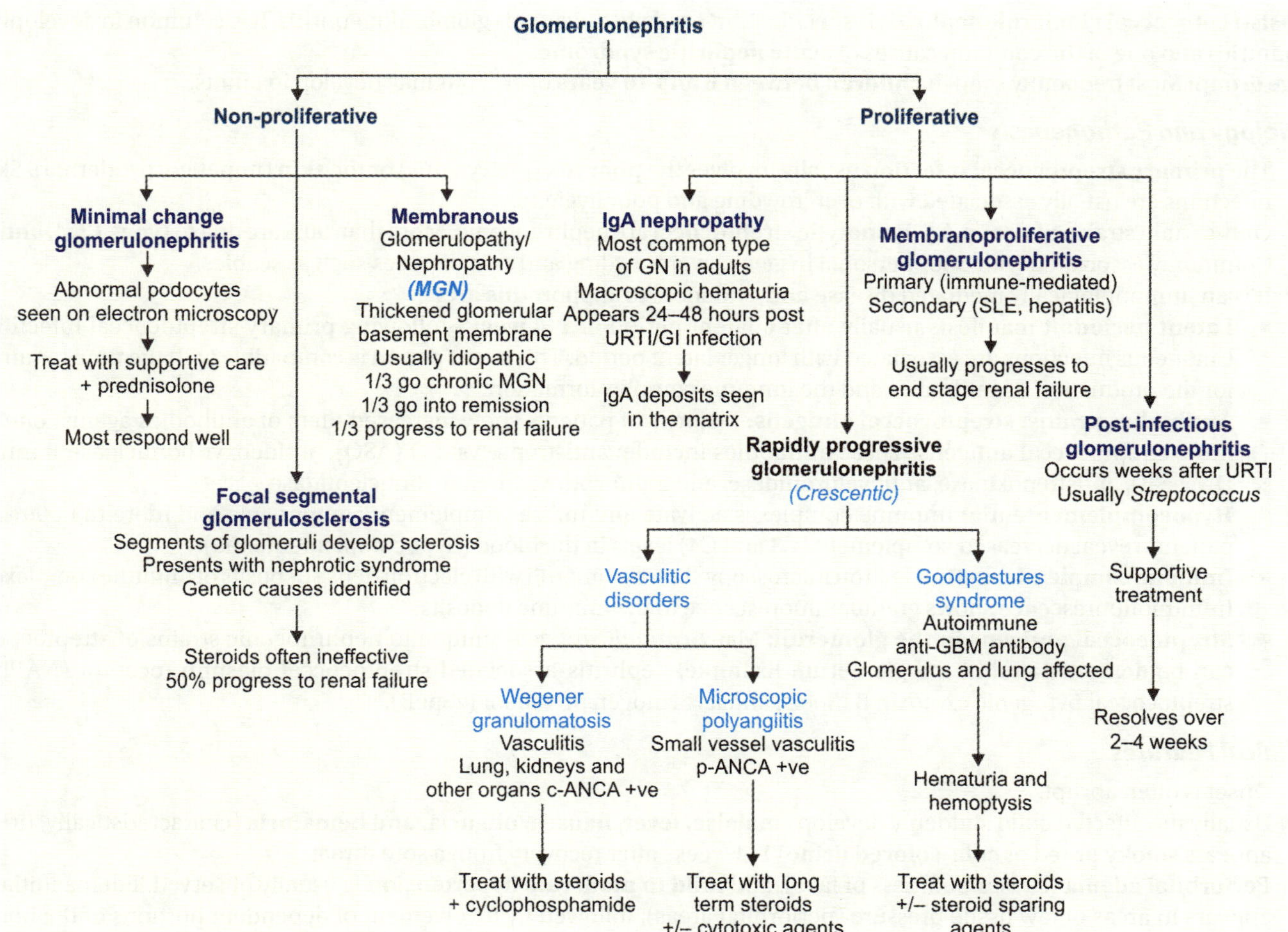

(ANCA: antineutrophil cytoplasmic antibody; GI: gastrointestinal; GN: glomerulonephritis; IgA: immunoglobulin A; SLE: systemic lupus erythematosus; URTI: upper respiratory tract infection)

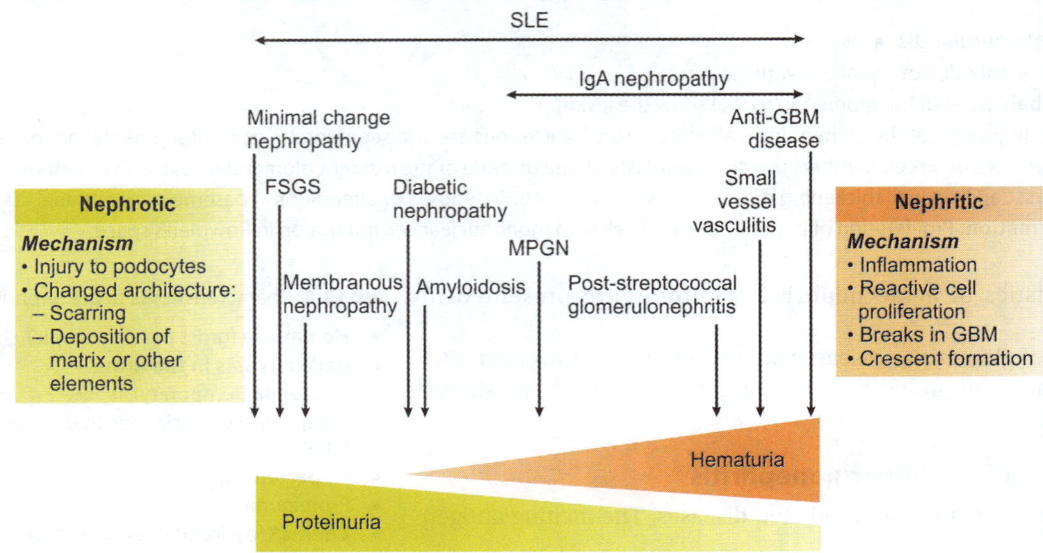

FIG. 13.8: Various causes of proliferative and nonproliferative glomerulonephritis.

(FSGS: focal segmental glomerulosclerosis; IgA: Immunoglobulin A; MPGN: membranoproliferative glomerulonephritis; SLE: systemic lupus erythematosus; GBM: glomerular basement membrane)

Poststreptococcal (Postinfectious) Glomerulonephritis

Q. Write short essay/note on acute glomerulonephritis or acute nephritic syndrome and its causes and clinical features.

Q. Discuss the etiology, pathogenesis, clinical features, diagnosis, complications, and management of acute poststreptococcal glomerulonephritis [acute glomerulonephritis (AGN)].

Poststreptococcal glomerulonephritis is specific subtype of postinfectious glomerulonephritis. It is common in developing countries and one of the common causes of **acute nephritic syndrome.**

Age group: Most frequently seen in **children between 6 and 10 years** of age, but may develop in adults.

Etiology and Pathogenesis

- The **primary streptococcal infection** usually involves the **pharynx** (pharyngitis) or the **skin** (impetigo/pyoderma). Skin infections are usually associated with overcrowding and poor hygiene.
- Only certain strains of **Group A β-hemolytic streptococci** are nephritogenic. More than 90% are due to **types 12, 4, and 1**.
- Commonly associated with poor personal hygiene, overcrowding and skin diseases such as scabies.
- It is an immunologically mediated disease **and** evidences to support **this are:**
  - **Latent period:** It manifests usually after a latent period of **1–4 weeks** following primary streptococcal infection. Cutaneous infections are associated with longer latent period. This latent period is compatible with the time required for the production of antibodies and the immune complex formation.
  - **Antibodies against streptococcal antigens:** Majority of patients show increased titers of antibodies against one or more streptococcal antigens. These antibodies include: antistreptolysin O (ASO), antideoxyribonuclease B (anti-DNase B), antistrepokinase, antihyaluronidase, and antinicotinyl adenine dinucleotidase.
  - **Hypocomplementemia:** Immune complexes activate and utilize complement components and more than 90% of patients reveal decreased complement (C3 and C4) levels in the blood (hypocomplementemia).
  - **Immune complex deposits:** Electron microscopy shows glomeruli with electron dense deposits of immune complexes. Immunofluorescence shows granular fluorescence to the immune deposits.
  - **Streptococcal antigens in the glomeruli:** Many *cationic antigens* unique to nephritogenic strains of streptococci can be demonstrated in the glomeruli. Example, nephritis-associated streptococcal plasmin receptor (NAPlr), streptococcal pyrogenic exotoxin B (SpeB) and its zymogen precursor (zSpeB).

Clinical Features

- Onset is often abrupt.
- Usually the affected child suddenly develops **malaise, fever, nausea, oliguria, and hematuria** (characteristically, urine appears **smoky or** red or **cola-colored urine**) 1–4 weeks after recovery from a sore throat.
- **Periorbital edema** (causes puffiness of face), and **mild to moderate hypertension** is usually observed. Edema initially appears in areas of low tissue pressure (periorbital areas), followed by involvement of dependent portions of the body, and may be associated with ascites and/or pleural effusion.
- In adults clinical features are atypical. They may present with the sudden appearance of **hypertension or edema, and elevation of BUN.**

Investigations (Table 13.18)

TABLE 13.18: Various laboratory findings in acute poststreptococcal glomerulonephritis (PSGN).

Blood findings	*Urinary findings*
➢ Raised **antistreptococcal antibody,** titers, e.g., antistreptolysin O (ASO) titer. ➢ Significant **reduction in serum concentration of complement** (C3) components. ➢ Urea and creatinine: May be elevated and indicates renal impairment.	➢ **Oliguria** ➢ **Mild (variable degree) proteinuria** (usually less than 1 g/day) ➢ **Hematuria (smoky or cola-colored urine)** ➢ Urine microscopy: – Red cells (particularly dysmorphic, i.e., distorted and fragmented red cells) – Red cell casts
Renal biopsy: Diffuse acute inflammation in the glomerulus with neutrophils and deposition of immunoglobulin G (IgG) and complement. Electron microscopy shows electron-dense deposits in the subepithelial aspects of the capillary walls.	

(PSGN: poststreptococcal glomerulonephritis)

Q. Write short essay/note on diagnostic criteria and management of nephritic syndrome.

Q. Write short essay/note on urinary findings in acute glomerulonephritis.

Management/Treatment
- **Supportive treatment during acute PSGN:** These include **rest, salt restriction, diuretics and antihypertensives.**
- **Dialysis is necessary when there is severe oliguria, fluid overload, and hyperkalemia.**
- Steroids and cytotoxic drugs are of no value. However, if recovery is slow or if RPGN develops, corticosteroids (methylprednisolone) may be of some help.

Complications

Q. Write short note on the complications of acute poststreptococcal glomerulonephritis/nephritic syndrome.

(1) Rapidly progressive glomerulonephritis, (2) pulmonary edema, (3) hypertensive encephalopathy, and (4) renal failure.

Prognosis

Majority of patients with the epidemic form of PSGN have an **excellent prognosis.**
- **Children: Prognosis is good** and more than 95% totally recover. Minority may develop a RPGN.
- **Adults: Less benign**. They may recover promptly or develop RPGN or progress to chronic glomerulonephritis (hypertension and/or renal impairment).

Prevention: Pharyngitis caused by streptococci should be treated promptly by antibiotics which protects against development of GN.

Rapidly Progressive Glomerulonephritis/Crescentic Glomerulonephritis

Q. Write short essay/note on the causes, clinical features, investigations, and treatment of rapidly progressive glomerulonephritis.

Q. Write short essay/note on crescentic glomerulonephritis.

Definition: Rapidly progressive glomerulonephritis is a **syndrome**, characterized by **rapid and progressive loss of renal function** (usually a 50% reduction in the GFR within 3 months) associated with **severe oliguria and signs of nephritic syndrome**. If not treated death occurs due to renal failure within weeks to months. Histologically, it is characterized by **extensive crescents** (usually >50%).

Crescent

Crescents are formed by the **proliferation of the parietal epithelial cells** lining Bowman capsule along with the **infiltration of monocytes and macrophages**.

Classification

Rapidly progressive glomerulonephritis classified into three types based on immunological findings (**Table 13.19**). Each type may be idiopathic or associated with a known disorder.

Clinical Features (Table 13.20)

Investigations
- **Blood**
  - Leukocytosis and anemia
  - **Blood urea and serum creatinine** levels: Usually **raised.**

TABLE 13.19: Classification of rapidly progressive glomerulonephritis (GN).

Type of RPGN
Type I (anti-GBM antibody) (linear deposits of IgG and C3 on IF) ➢ Goodpasture syndrome
Type II (immune complex) (granular deposits of immune complex) ➢ Idiopathic immune complex-mediated RPGN ➢ IgA nephropathy ➢ Membranous glomerulopathy ➢ Mesangiocapillary GN ➢ Associated with secondary GN ➢ Post-infectious glomerulonephritis (poststreptococcal GN) ➢ Lupus nephritis ➢ Henoch–Schönlein purpura ➢ Mixed cryoglobulinemia
Type III (pauci-immune) (no deposits on IF) ➢ Idiopathic ➢ Wegener granulomatosis ➢ ANCA-associated ➢ Microscopic polyangiitis ➢ Renal-limited necrotizing crescentic glomerulonephritis ➢ Churg–Strauss syndrome

(ANCA: antineutrophil cytoplasmic antibodies; GBM: glomerular basement membrane; IF: immunofluorescent; IgA: immunoglobulin A; IgG: immunoglobulin G; RPGN: rapidly progressive glomerulonephritis)

TABLE 13.20: Usual clinical features of RPGN.

➢ **Hematuria with RBC casts** in the urine ➢ **Moderate proteinuria**	➢ **Variable hypertension** and edema ➢ **Oliguria and uremia**
In **Goodpasture syndrome** patient may present with recurrent hemoptysis or life-threatening pulmonary hemorrhage	

(RPGN: rapidly progressive glomerulonephritis)

TABLE 13.21: Complement levels in nephritic syndrome.

Low complement	*Normal complement*
➢ Postinfectious glomerulonephritis ➢ Mesangiocapillary glomerulonephritis ➢ Systemic lupus erythematosus ➢ Infective endocarditis ➢ Essential mixed cryoglobulinemia	➢ IgA nephropathy ➢ Idiopathic crescentic glomerulonephritis ➢ Anti-GBM disease ➢ Vasculitides: Henoch–Schönlein purpura, Wegener's granulomatosis, microscopic polyangiitis

(IgA: immunoglobulin A)

- **Urinalysis**
  - **Moderate proteinuria** (1–4 g/day)
  - Microscopic hematuria
  - **RBC and WBC casts.**
- **Others**
  - **Complement levels** (C3 and C4): **May be decreased** in immune-complex mediated RPGN.
  - **Circulating anti-GBM antibodies:** In Goodpasture syndrome.
  - Antineutrophil cytoplasmic antibody: In pauci-immune RPGN.
  - Serum cryoglobulin levels: May be raised in cryoglobulinemia.
- Abdominal ultrasound: Normal sized kidneys**.**
- **Chest X-ray:** Patients with Goodpasture syndrome and vasculitides may show **diffuse opacities** if associated with pulmonary hemorrhage.
- **Renal biopsy:** Shows **crescents**.

Complement Levels in Nephritic Syndrome (Table 13.21)

Algorithm of approach to the patient presenting with acute glomerulonephritis/nephritic syndrome is presented in **Flowchart 13.5.**

Treatment

It depends on the factors involved in the pathogenesis.

- **Supportive therapy:**
  - **Control of infection**
  - **Control of volume status** (dialysis may be needed)
- **Specific therapy:**
  - **Plasma exchange** to remove circulating antibodies and in patients presenting with life-threatening pulmonary hemorrhage.
  - **Steroids methylprednisolone—500–1,000 mg/day for 3 days to suppress inflammation** from antibody already deposited in the tissue.
  - **Immunosuppressive therapy** (e.g., cyclophosphamide, azathioprine, mycophenolate) such as cyclophosphamide to suppress further antibody synthesis.
  - **Infliximab and rituximab.**

NEPHROTIC SYNDROME

Q. Discuss the etiology, pathogenesis, clinical features, diagnosis, and management of nephrotic syndrome.

Q. Define nephrotic syndrome. Discuss the differential diagnosis in a 30-year-old male presenting with anasarca.

Features of nephrotic syndrome are mentioned in **Box 13.9.**

Box 13.9: Characteristics of nephrotic syndrome.

- Massive/heavy proteinuria (>3.5 g of protein/24 hours)
- Hypoalbuminemia
- Generalized edema
- Hyperlipidemia and lipiduria

Pathophysiology (Fig. 13.9)

- **Massive proteinuria** is characterized by **daily loss of 3.5 g or more** of **protein** (less in children) in the **urine**.
  - Normally, the glomerular capillary wall acts as a size and charge dependent barrier for the plasma filtrate.
  - Proteinuria in nephrotic syndrome is due to **increased permeability of glomerular capillary wall to plasma proteins.** This increased permeability is due to glomerular inflammation, change in the surface electrical charge, and an alteration in the pore size.

FLOWCHART 13.5: Algorithm of approach to the patient presenting with acute glomerulonephritis/nephritic syndrome.

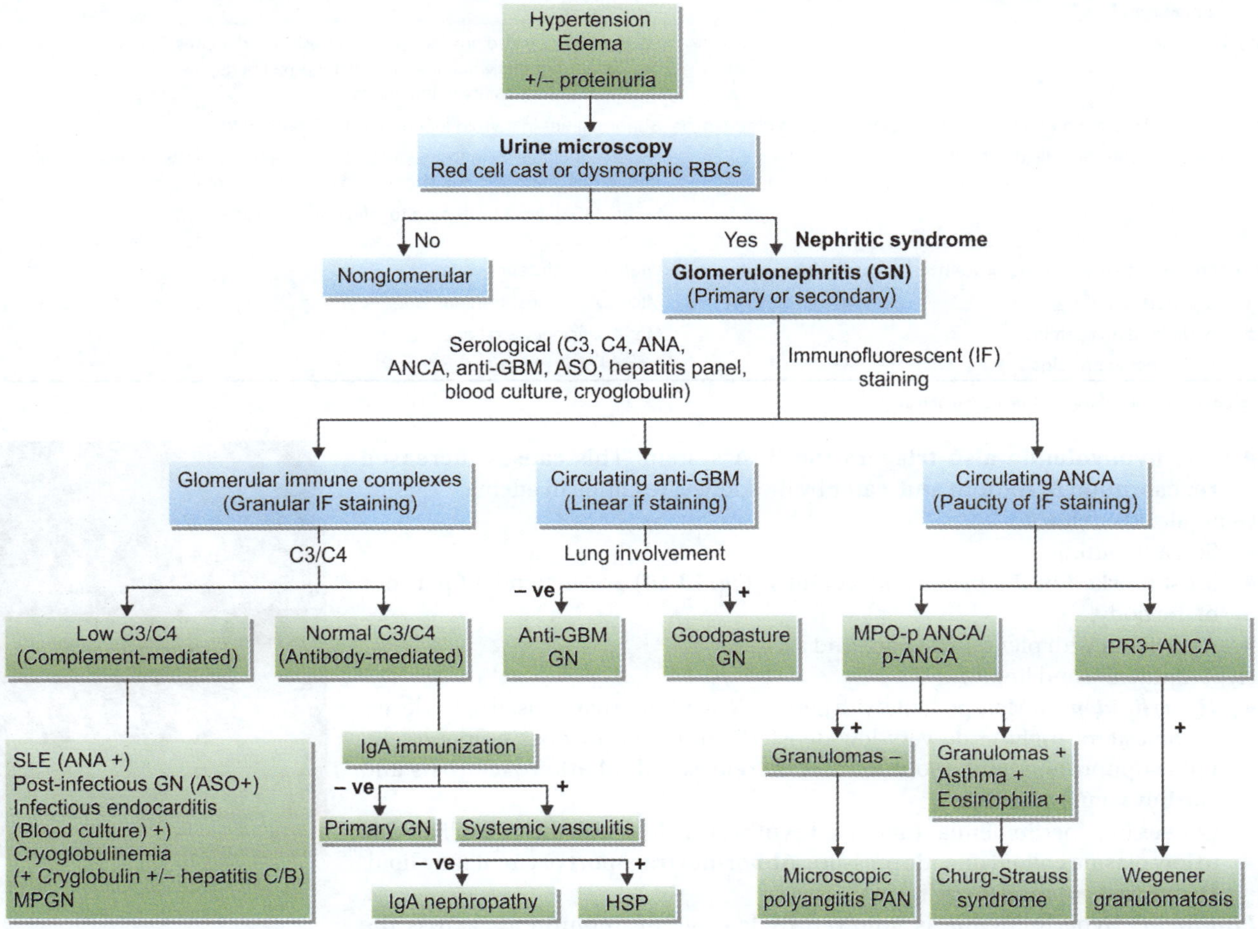

Hypertension
Edema
+/– proteinuria
↓
Urine microscopy
Red cell cast or dysmorphic RBCs
- No → Nonglomerular
- Yes → **Nephritic syndrome** → **Glomerulonephritis (GN)** (Primary or secondary)

Serological (C3, C4, ANA, ANCA, anti-GBM, ASO, hepatitis panel, blood culture, cryoglobulin)
Immunofluorescent (IF) staining

- Glomerular immune complexes (Granular IF staining) → C3/C4
  - Low C3/C4 (Complement-mediated) → SLE (ANA +); Post-infectious GN (ASO+); Infectious endocarditis (Blood culture) +); Cryoglobulinemia (+ Cryglobulin +/– hepatitis C/B); MPGN
  - Normal C3/C4 (Antibody-mediated) → IgA immunization
    - – ve → Primary GN
    - \+ → Systemic vasculitis
      - – ve → IgA nephropathy
      - \+ → HSP
- Circulating anti-GBM (Linear if staining) → Lung involvement
  - – ve → Anti-GBM GN
  - \+ → Goodpasture GN
- Circulating ANCA (Paucity of IF staining)
  - MPO-p ANCA/ p-ANCA
    - \+ Granulomas – → Microscopic polyangiitis PAN
    - Granulomas + Asthma + Eosinophilia + → Churg-Strauss syndrome
  - PR3–ANCA → + → Wegener granulomatosis

[ANA: antinuclear antibody; ANCA: antineutrophil cytoplasmic antibody; ASO: antistreptolysin O; GBM: glomerular basement membrane; HSP: Henoch–Schönlein purpura; MPGN: membranoproliferative glomerulonephritis; MPO-ANCA: anti-myeloperoxidase (previously called p-ANCA); PR3-ANCA: anti-proteinase-3; PAN: polyarteritis nodosa]

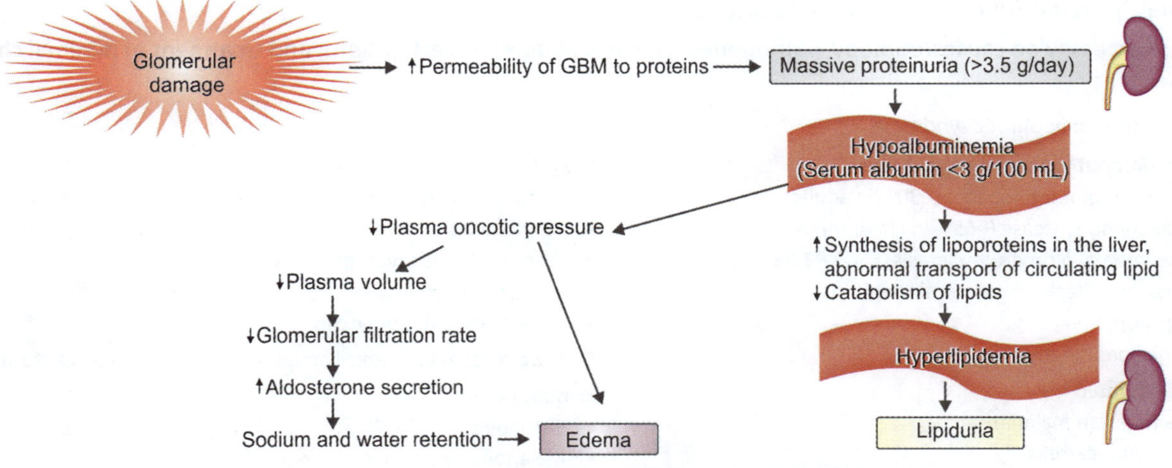

FIG. 13.9: Various characteristic features of nephrotic syndrome and its mechanism. (GBM: glomerular basement membrane).

- The **major proportion of protein** lost in the urine is **albumin,** and rarely globulins. Consequences of protein loss are listed in **Table 13.22.**

• Hypoalbuminemia
  - Massive proteinuria decreases the serum albumin levels (hypoalbuminemia).
  - **Hypoalbuminemia decreases the colloid osmotic pressure** of the blood resulting in a disturbance in the Starling forces acting across peripheral capillaries.

TABLE 13.22: Consequences of protein loss/complications of nephrotic syndrome.

Nature of protein loss	***Consequences***
Hypoalbuminemia	Edema and may also produce pleural effusion and ascites. Subungual edema may manifest as parallel white lines in the fingernail beds Increased susceptibility to infections
Urinary losses of plasma proteins such as thyroxine-binding globulin	Abnormalities in thyroid function tests, hypothyroidism
Deficiency of antithrombin III (due to urine loss)	Hypercoagulable state (consequences include DVT, pulmonary embolism, myocardial infarction, and stroke) and renal vein thrombosis
Loss of globulins in urine	Severe IgG deficiency leading to infections such as spontaneous bacterial peritonitis
Loss of cholecalciferol-binding protein	Vitamin D deficiency state
Loss of transferrin	Microcytic hypochromic anemia
Loss of metal-binding proteins	Metal deficiency, e.g., zinc, copper
Loss of drug-binding proteins	Altered drug pharmacokinetics

(DVT: deep venous thrombosis; IgG: immunoglobulin G)

- The **hypovolemia also triggers the RAA** system. This causes **increased reabsorption of sodium and water** by the kidney, resulting in edema.
- Generalized edema
  - Soft and pitting
  - **Most marked in the periorbital regions** (**Fig. 13.10**) and dependent portions of the body.
  - Associated with pleural effusions and ascites.
- Hyperlipidemia and lipiduria
  - ***Hyperlipidemia:*** Most patients with nephrotic syndrome have raised blood levels of cholesterol, triglyceride, very-low-density lipoprotein, low-density lipoprotein, Lp(a) lipoprotein, and apoprotein. It **increases risk of atherosclerosis** and **cardiovascular disease.**
  - **Causes** of hyperlipidemia: **Increased synthesis** of lipoproteins in the liver due to low plasma colloid oncotic pressure. **Abnormal transport** of circulating lipid. **Decreased catabolism** of lipids

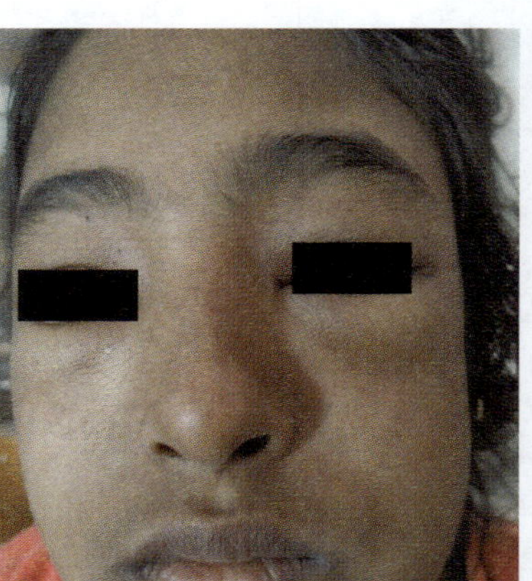

FIG. 13.10: Facial and periorbital puffiness in nephrotic syndrome.

- ***Lipiduria:*** Hyperlipidemia is followed by leakage of lipoproteins across the glomerular capillary wall → leaked lipoprotein is reabsorbed by tubular epithelial cells → then shed along with the degenerated cells → **appears in urine either as free fat or as oval fat bodies.**

Causes of Nephrotic Syndrome (Box 13.10 and Fig. 13.11)

Q. Write short essay on causes/etiology, pathogenesis, clinical features, investigations, and treatment of minimal change disease.

Box 13.10: Causes of nephrotic syndrome.

A. Primary (idiopathic) glomerular disease
- Membranous glomerulopathy (~30% in adults)
- Minimal-change disease (~65% in children)
- Focal segmental glomerulosclerosis (FSGS ~35% in adults)
- Membranoproliferative glomerulonephritis
- IgA nephropathy
- Mesangial proliferative

B. Infection-related
- Malaria (quartan malaria)
- Infective endocarditis
- Hepatitis B and C
- HIV
- Syphilis

C. Systemic diseases
- Diabetes mellitus
- Amyloidosis
- Systemic lupus erythematosus
- Polyarteritis nodosa
- Wegener's granulomatosis

D. Drug and toxins: Penicillamine, gold, street heroin, captopril

E. Malignancy
- Carcinoma
- Melanoma
- Hodgkin's disease, chronic lymphatic leukemia

F. Others: Bee-sting allergy, hereditary nephritis

(FSGS: focal and segmental glomerulosclerosis; IgA: immunoglobulin A)

- Minimal change disease (MCD)
  - Minimal change disease is named so because the **glomerular changes** are **absent or minimal and glomeruli appear normal under light microscopy.** But under electron microscopy, it shows **diffuse effacement (loss) of foot processes** of visceral epithelial cells (podocytes).

- **Minimal change disease is the** major cause of nephrotic syndrome in children (80%), but it is less common in adults (20%).
- **Age:** Peak incidence between 2 and 6 years of age.

- Focal and segmental glomerulosclerosis (FSGS)
  - FSGS is characterized by the **sclerosis** that **involves only part of the capillary tuft** (i.e., segmental) **of some glomeruli** (i.e., focal).
  - Accounts for about **one-third of cases of nephrotic syndrome in adults.**
  - Usually manifest as nephrotic syndrome or heavy proteinuria, hypertension, renal insufficiency, and occasionally hematuria.
  - **Causes (Box 13.11)**
- **Membranous nephropathy**
  - Characterized by **uniform diffuse thickening of the glomerular capillary wall.** This is due to the accumulation of **electron-dense deposits along the subepithelial side** of the glomerular basement membrane.
  - **Common cause (~30%) of the nephrotic syndrome in adults.**
  - **Gender and age:** Male predominance and high incidence between 30 to 50 years of age.
  - **Causes (Box 13.12)**
  - About 75% of patients present with nephrotic-range proteinuria and 50% present with microscopic hematuria.

FIG. 13.11: Etiology of nephrotic syndrome by age.

Box 13.11: Causes of focal and segmental glomerulosclerosis.

Primary (idiopathic)

Secondary

- Viruses: HIV infection
- Drugs: Heroin addiction
- Sickle-cell disease
- Massive obesity
- Congenital (e.g., unilateral agenesis) and acquired (e.g., reflux nephropathy) reductions in renal mass

Hereditary forms: Inherited mutations in genes that encode podocyte proteins, e.g., podocin, α-actinin 4

Box 13.12: Causes of membranous nephropathy.

Primary/idiopathic: No identifiable cause in about 85% of patients

Secondary (20–30% cases): In association with:

- **Therapeutic drugs:** Penicillamine, captopril, nonsteroidalanti-inflammatory drugs (NSAIDs), gold
- **Malignant neoplasms**, e.g., carcinomas of the lung and colon, lymphomas and melanoma
- **Autoimmune disease**, e.g., systemic lupus erythematosus (SLE), thyroiditis
- **Infections:** Chronic hepatitis B, hepatitis C, quartan malaria, syphilis, schistosomiasis

Investigations in Nephrotic Syndrome

Q. Write a short note on urinary findings in nephrotic syndrome.

- **Urine examination**
  - **Proteinuria:** Twenty-four hour urinary protein estimation.
  - **Microscopy:** Red cells and red cell casts and waxy casts may be present. However, in minimal change disease, RBCs and red cell casts are not seen. Shows lipiduria
- **Serum albumin: Reduced**
- **Serum cholesterol: Raised**
- **Renal biopsy: May be necessary** for histological diagnosis.
- **Other investigations:** Depending on the suspected secondary causes appropriate investigations are to be performed.

Management

A. General measures

Measures to reduce proteinuria: These measures are necessary if immunosuppressive drugs and other specific measures against the underlying cause do not benefit.

- **Angiotensin-converting enzyme inhibitors and/or angiotensin II receptor antagonists:** They **reduce proteinuria** in all types of GN and also slow **the rate of progression of renal failure** by lowering glomerular capillary filtration pressure. Blood pressure and renal function should be monitored regularly during their administration.

Measures to control complications

- **Treatment of edema:**
  - Initially, it is treated by **dietary salt (sodium) restriction, rest and a thiazide diuretic** (e.g., chlorthalidone, bendroflumethiazide). The weight loss should not be more than 1 kg/day. Aggressive diuretic therapy may precipitate ARF due to reduction in intravascular volume.
  - **If not responsive, furosemide 40–120 mg daily** with the **addition of amiloride** (5 mg daily), and serum potassium concentration should be monitored.
  - **Gut mucosal edema** in nephrotic syndrome may **cause malabsorption of diuretics** (as well as other drugs). Thus, if there is **resistance to oral diuretic treatment, parenteral administration is required.**
  - In diuretic-resistant patients and those with oliguria and uremia in the absence of severe glomerular damage (e.g., in minimal-change nephropathy) edema may be treated by **infusion of salt-poor albumin as a temporary measure combined with diuretic therapy**. However, most of infused albumin will be excreted by the kidneys within 1–2 days.

- **Dietary proteins:** It is advisable to **take normal protein** and should be about 0.8–1.0 g/kg. A high-protein diet (approximately 80–90 g protein daily) increases proteinuria and may be harmful in the long-term. However, malnutrition should be prevented.
- **Hypercoagulable state:** Develops due to loss of coagulation factors (e.g., antithrombin) in the urine and an increase in production of fibrinogen by liver. It **predisposes to venous thrombosis and thromboembolism.** Therefore, **avoid prolonged bed rest**. Long-term **prophylactic anticoagulant therapy** is desirable and it is indicated in patients who have already developed deep venous thrombosis or arterial thrombosis.
- **Lipid abnormalities:** They **increase in the risk of myocardial infarction or peripheral vascular disease.** Hypercholesterolemia is treated with an **HMG-CoA reductase inhibitor and dietary restrictions of lipids.**
- **Vitamin D supplementation:** To be given if there is biochemical evidence of vitamin D deficiency.
- **Sepsis:** It is a **major cause of death** in nephrotic syndrome. The increased susceptibility to infection is partly due to loss of immunoglobulin in the urine. They are particularly **susceptible to pneumococcal infections** and pneumococcal vaccine should be given to these patients. Early detection and aggressive treatment of infections should be done. Vaccinations prophylactically is advisable.

B. Treatment of underlying cause

Minimal change disease

- **In children:**
  - **Initial treatment** by **high-dose corticosteroid** therapy with prednisolone 60 mg/m² daily (up to a maximum of 80 mg/day) for a maximum of 4–6 weeks.
  - Followed by alternate day prednisolone at a dose of 40 mg/m² (1 mg/kg in adults) for further 4–6 weeks.
  - **More than 95% of children respond** to the above therapy. Children who respond within the first 4 weeks of corticosteroid therapy are termed "steroid responsive." Those who relapse on withdrawal of corticosteroid therapy are termed "steroid dependent."
  - **Relapse:**
    - One-third of patients relapse on steroid withdrawal, and remission is once more induced with **steroid therapy**.
    - In patients who have frequent relapses or develop unacceptable corticosteroid side effects, long-term remission can be achieved by a course of **cyclophosphamide** 1.5–2.0 mg/kg daily is given for 8–12 weeks **with concomitant prednisolone** 7.5–15 mg/day. Steroid unresponsive patients may also benefit by cyclophosphamide. Not more than two courses of cyclophosphamide should be given because of the risk of side-effects (e.g., azoospermia).
    - An alternative to cyclophosphamide is **ciclosporin** 3–5 mg/kg/day (ciclosporin is potentially nephrotoxic).
- **Adults: Response rates are significantly lower** and response may occur late (12 weeks with daily steroid therapy and 12 weeks of maintenance with alternate-day therapy).
- **Prognosis: Excellent,** although it may show remission and relapses.

Focal and segmental glomerulosclerosis

- **Steroids:** It is **beneficial in only 20–30% patients** and usually prednisolone is given in the dose of 0.5–2 mg/kg/day.
- **Cyclosporine** may be effective in reducing or stopping urinary protein excretion.
- **Cyclophosphamide, chlorambucil or azathioprine** may be used **as second-line therapy in adults.**
- About **50% progress to end-stage renal failure**.

Membranous glomerulonephritis

- **Oral high-dose corticosteroids are not useful for** producing either a sustained remission of nephrotic syndrome or preserving renal function.
- **Alkylating agents: Cyclophosphamide and chlorambucil** are effective. However, because of long-term toxicity, these drugs should be reserved for patients who have severe or prolonged nephrosis (i.e., proteinuria >6 g/day for >6 months), renal insufficiency, and hypertension. **Cyclophosphamide, cyclosporine and chlorambucil** in combination with steroids may be helpful.
- **Anti-B lymphocyte therapy is more effective** against T lymphocytes than broad-spectrum immunosuppressive agents. Anti-CD20 antibodies (rituximab, which ablates B lymphocytes) improve renal function, reduce proteinuria and increase the serum albumin.
- **Prognosis:** Spontaneous remission may occur in 40%, 3–40% may develop repeated remissions and relapses and 10–20% patients may develop progressive renal failure.

Immunoglobulin A Nephropathy (Berger's Disease)

Q. Write short essay/note on IgA nephropathy.

- Characterized by **focal and segmental proliferative GN** with **predominant IgA deposition in the glomerular mesangium**.
- **Clinical features:**
  - Occurs in **children and young males**.
  - **Presents with** asymptomatic/painless microscopic hematuria or recurrent macroscopic hematuria **generally within** 1–2 days after an upper respiratory or gastrointestinal viral infection.
  - Proteinuria occurs and in 5% it can be in the nephrotic range.
  - Occasionally, it may present as ARF or nephritic syndrome.

- **Diagnosis by renal biopsy:** Immunofluorescence microscopy shows prominent **IgA deposits** in the mesangial regions.
- **Prognosis:**
  - **Usually good**, especially in patients with normal blood pressure, normal renal function, and absence of proteinuria at presentation.
  - Complete remission uncommon.
  - **Risk of development of end-stage renal failure** in about 25% of patients with proteinuria of more than 1 g/day, elevated serum creatinine, hypertension, ACE gene polymorphism and presence of tubulointerstitial fibrosis on renal biopsy.

Management
- **Steroids:** Used for patients with proteinuria of 1–3 g/day, mild glomerular changes only, and preserved renal function. They reduce proteinuria and stabilize renal function.
- **Use of immunosuppressive therapy is controversial.**
- **Combination therapy:** In patients with progressive disease (creatinine clearance <70 mL/min), **prednisolone with cyclophosphamide** can be used for 3 months followed by maintenance with prednisolone and azathioprine.
- **Tonsillectomy: May reduce proteinuria and hematuria** in patients with recurrent tonsillitis.
- **Combination of ACE inhibitor and angiotensin II receptor antagonist:** Can be given to all patients, with or without hypertension and proteinuria. This combination therapy reduces proteinuria and preserves renal function.

Hereditary Nephritis or Alport's Syndrome

- Most common familial nephropathies, characterized by familial occurrence of **progressive hematuria, nephritis, and sensorineural loss of hearing.**
- Common in females. Male patients develop severe renal disease with progressive renal failure occurring before the fourth decade. Most females have a normal life-span.
- **Pathology:** Electron microscopy—shows irregular thickening of GBM, splitting and splintering of the lamina densa and small, round, electron-dense granulations are present within the lucent zones. GBM lesions are the hallmark but not specific of Alport's syndrome.
- **Clinical presentation**
  - Major presentation: Macroscopic or microscopic hematuria and may be observed at birth.
  - Other presenting features: Proteinuria, edema, hypertension, renal failure, and deafness.
    - Microscopic or recurrent episodes of macroscopic hematuria following upper respiratory infection (or physical exertion) may resemble postinfective glomerulonephritis.
    - Incidental leukocyturia and pyuria may lead to erroneous diagnosis of UTI.
    - Nephrotic syndrome can occur with increasing proteinuria. Hypertension develops with progressive renal insufficiency.
    - Deafness is more frequent in males and progression of hearing loss usually indicates poor prognosis.
    - Ocular changes include anterior lenticonus (most common) and associated posterior or anterior cataract.

Treatment: No specific measure to prevent progression of renal disease. Treatment includes renal replacement therapy, by long-term hemodialysis or renal transplant. Hearing defect can be temporarily compensated by the use of hearing aid.

TUBULOINTERSTITIAL DISEASES

- **Tubulointerstitial nephropathy** is an **inflammatory condition affecting primarily the renal tubules (Fig. 13.12) and interstitium**.
- **Structural changes in the glomeruli develop later** and results in progressive decline in GFR, glomerular proteinuria and volume-dependent hypertension.
- It accounts for **20–40% of cases of CRF** and **10–25% of cases of ARF.**

Acute Tubulointerstitial Nephropathy

- Tubulointerstitial nephritis is a frequent cause of AKI that can lead to CKD.
  - Affects renal tubules and interstitial components of the renal parenchyma
  - *Characterized*: Tubular dysfunction with electrolytes abnormalities (moderate proteinuria, varying degrees of renal impairment)

Two most common causes of acute TIN are **drugs or toxins and infections**.

Etiology (Box 13.13)

Drug-induced acute TIN

- After exposure to a causative drug, **renal dysfunction may occur within a few hours** but can occur after weeks or months.
- Preceded or accompanied by the triad of **fever** (70–100%), **skin rash** (30–50%) and **eosinophilia (transient).** Skin rash and eosinophilia are not found in TIN caused by NSAIDs.
- **Microscopic hematuria, pyuria, and proteinuria** are present in almost all cases. **Eosinophiluria (>50% of WBC) is a sensitive marker of drug-induced TIN.**
- Patients may need steroids (methylprednisolone 500–1000 mg/day for 3 days).

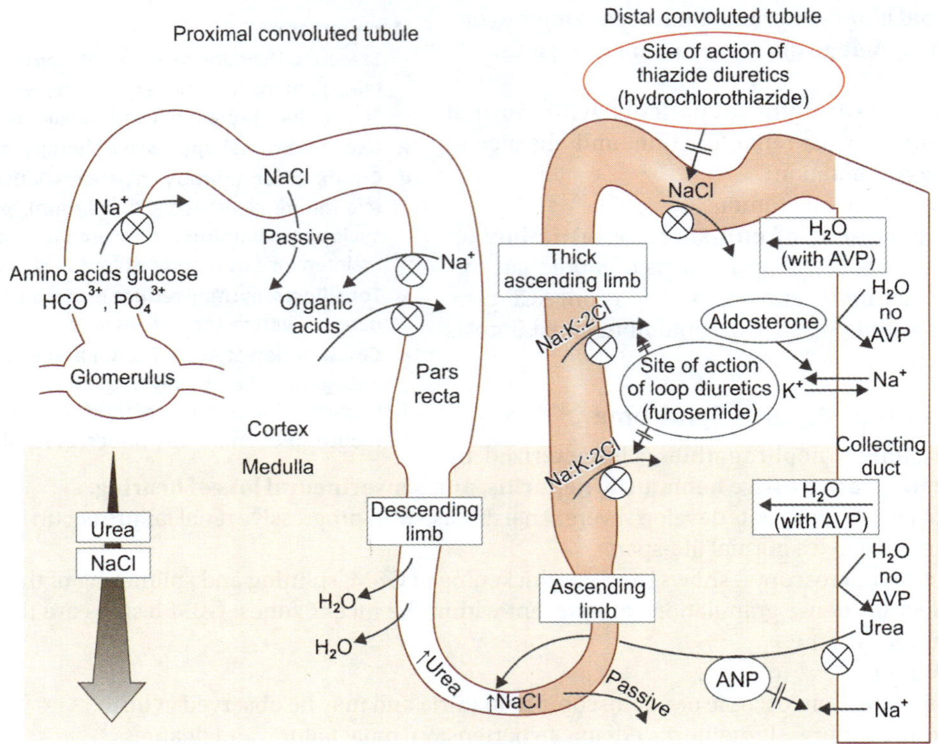

FIG. 13.12: Structure of renal tubules.
(ANP: atrial natriuretic peptide; AVP: arginine vasopressin)

Box 13.13: Etiology of acute tubulointerstitial nephropathy.

Drugs
- Antimicrobials
- Analgesics/NSAIDs
- Diuretics
- Anticonvulsants
- Metabolic salts
- Indigenous medication

Infections
- Viral: Cytomegalovirus, hepatitis, HIV, Epstein–Barr virus, hantavirus, polyomavirus
- Bacterial: Salmonella, Streptococcus, Yersinia, Brucella, leptospirosis
- Fungal: Histoplasmosis
- Parasitic: Leishmania, Toxoplasma

Immunological
- Transplant rejection
- Systemic lupus erythematosus (SLE), Sjögren's syndrome, sarcoidosis

Metabolic
- Hypercalcemia, cystinosis, potassium depletion, hyperoxaluria

Hemopoietic
- Myeloproliferative diseases, plasma cell dyscrasias

Miscellaneous
- Irradiation, heat stroke

Idiopathic

Analgesic Nephropathy

- **Prolonged analgesic abuse** leads to a nephropathic process characterized by **capillary sclerosis, chronic tubulointerstitial diseases and papillary necrosis**.
- Imaging reveals shrunken kidneys with calcification of renal papillae.
- Risk of developing renal disease is **dependent upon** the **frequency and duration of analgesic consumption,** the cumulative amount of individual analgesic exceeding 3 kg (phenacetin, acetaminophen, or aspirin).

Tubulointerstitial Nephritis and Uveitis Syndrome

- Combination of TIN and uveitis
- Abnormal renal function, abnormal urinalysis
- Anterior uveitis—photophobia, eye pain and redness, eyelid edema, rapidly progressive loss of vision, as well as symptoms of systemic illness, including weight loss, fever, and fatigue
- Seen in adolescent girls
- Has good prognosis

Treatment of Interstitial Nephritis

- Stop the offending agent
- Prednisone at a dose of 1 mg/kg/day (to a maximum of 40–60 mg) for a minimum of 1–2 weeks, beginning a gradual taper after the serum creatinine has returned to or near baseline.
- Cyclophosphamide (2 mg/kg/d)
- Mycophenolate
- Plasmapheresis.

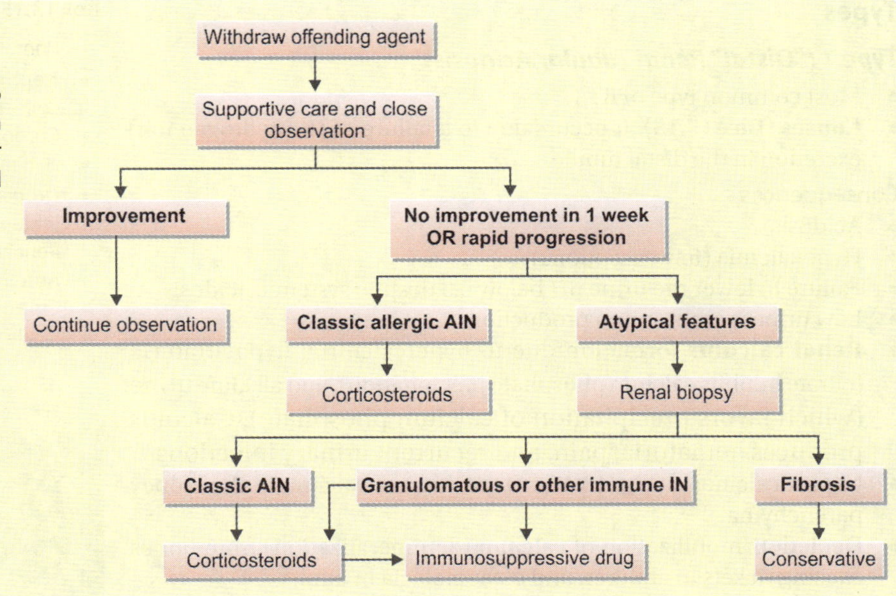

RENAL TUBULAR ACIDOSIS

Q. Write short essay/note on renal tubular acidosis.

- Renal tubular acidosis refers to hyperchloremic (normal anion gap) metabolic acidosis in the presence of normal or almost normal renal function.
- Renal tubular acidosis arises as a result of defects in the tubular transport of HCO_3^- and/or H^+.
- Most forms of RTA are usually asymptomatic; rarely, life-threatening electrolyte imbalances may occur.

Mechanism

Renal tubular acidosis can be due to a defect in one of three processes:

1. **Impaired acid secretion in the late distal tubule** or cortical collecting duct intercalated cells (classical distal RTA).
2. **Impaired bicarbonate reabsorption in the proximal tubule** (proximal RTA).
3. **Impaired sodium reabsorption in the late distal tubule** or cortical collecting duct. It is associated with reduced secretion of both potassium and H^+ ions (hyperkalemia distal RTA).

Box 13.14 lists types of renal tubular acidosis (RTA).

Box 13.14: Types of renal tubular acidosis (RTA).

- Type 1 RTA or distal tubular RTA
- Type 2 RTA or proximal RTA
- Type 3 RTA or mixed RTA
- Type 4 RTA or hypoaldosteronism hyperkalemia RTA

Overview of various forms of renal tubular acidosis

Type of renal tubular acidosis	*Type 1 RTA (distal RTA)*	*Type 2 RTA (proximal RTA)*	*Type 4 RTA (hyperkalemic RTA)*
Incidence	➢ Rare	➢ Very rare	➢ **Common**
Pathophysiology	➢ Inability of intercalated cells of the distal tubule to secrete H^+	➢ Inability of the proximal convoluted tubule cells to reabsorb HCO_3^-	➢ **Aldosterone** deficiency and/or resistance
Serum potassium levels	➢ **Hypokalemia**	➢ Hypokalemia	➢ **Hyperkalemia**
Urine pH	➢ >5.5	➢ <5.5	➢ <5.5
Urine anion gap	➢ Positive	➢ Negative	➢ Positive
Calcium excretion	➢ ↑	➢ Normal	➢ Normal or ↓
Bone involvement	➢ Bone demineralization without overt **rickets** or **osteomalacia**	➢ **Vitamin D**-resistant **rickets/osteomalacia**	➢ Bone demineralization without overt **rickets** or **osteomalacia**
Nephrolithiasis	➢ **Usually present**	➢ Absent	➢ Absent
Treatment	➢ Alkali therapy with **sodium bicarbonate** or sodium citrate (Shohl's solution)	➢ Alkali therapy with orally administered **potassium citrate**	➢ **Furosemide** ➢ Mineralocorticoid replacement (fludrocortisone) ➢ Low-potassium diet

Types

Type 1 ("Distal" Renal Tubular Acidosis)

- Most common type of RTA.
- **Causes (Box 13.15)**: It occurs due to a failure of H^+ (hydrogen ion) excretion in the distal tubule.

Consequences

- Acidosis
- Hypokalemia (few exceptions)
- Failure to lower the urine pH below 5.3 despite systemic acidosis
- Low urinary ammonium production
- **Renal calculus** formation due to hypercalciuria, hypocitraturia (citrate inhibits calcium phosphate precipitation), and alkaline urine (which favors precipitation of calcium phosphate). Calculus produces hematuria, pain, and recurrent urinary infections.
- Nephrocalcinosis (**Fig. 13.13**): Deposition of calcium in the kidney parenchyma.
- Depletion/mobilization of calcium (demineralization) from bones causing rickets in children and osteomalacia in adults.

Diagnosis

- Urinary pH > 5.3 in presence of systemic acidosis
- Plasma bicarbonate (HCO^-) <20 mEq/L
- **Acid load test:**
  - Give ammonium chloride by mouth (100 mg/kg) and check pH of urine hourly and plasma HCO_3^- at 3 hours.
  - Plasma HCO_3^- should drop below 21 mmol/L.
  - Diagnosis is confirmed if urine pH remains >5.3 despite a plasma HCO_3 of 21 mmol/L.

Box 13.15: Causes of type 1 renal tubular acidosis (RTA).

- Primary/hereditary
- Nephrocalcinosis (producing damage of cortical collecting duct)
- Chronic urinary tract obstruction
- Hypergammaglobulinemic states
- Drugs and toxins, e.g., ifosfamide, amphotericin B, lithium, and toluene
- Renal transplant rejection
- Autoimmune disease, e.g., Sjögren's syndrome
- Cirrhosis of liver
- Sickle cell anemia

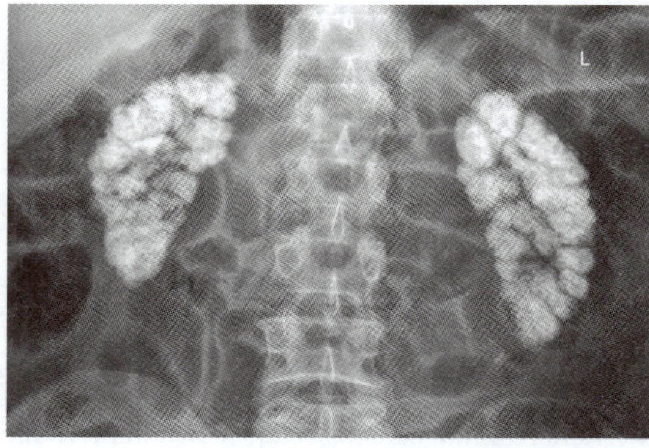

FIG. 13.13: Nephrocalcinosis in type 1 renal tubular acidosis (RTA).

Treatment

- **Correction of the acidosis:** Oral sodium bicarbonate or sodium citrate reverses bone demineralization.
- **Potassium supplements:** Potassium citrate in case of hypokalemia, stone formation, and nephrocalcinosis.
- **Thiazide diuretics:** They cause volume contraction and increased proximal sodium bicarbonate reabsorption.

Type 2 ("Proximal") Renal Tubular Acidosis

- Very rare and is due to **failure of filtered sodium bicarbonate reabsorption** in **the proximal tubule.** It leads to appearance of bicarbonate in urine and subsequent acidosis.
- **Causes of type 2 RTA (Box 13.16)**: Inherited forms of isolated type 2 RTA may show both autosomal dominant and recessive patterns of inheritance.

Consequences: Type 2 RTA usually occurs as part of a generalized tubular defect, together with urinary wasting of amino acids, phosphate, and glucose (Fanconi's syndrome), as well as bicarbonate and potassium.

- Acidosis less severe than type 1 RTA
- Hypokalemia
- Inability to lower the urine pH below 5.5 despite systemic acidosis
- Appearance of bicarbonate in the urine despite a subnormal plasma bicarbonate
- Bone demineralization due to phosphate wasting.

Box 13.16: Causes of type 2 renal tubular acidosis (RTA).

- Inherited
- Paraproteinemia
- Amyloidosis
- Hyperparathyroidism
- Heavy metal toxicity
- Drugs and toxins such as antiretroviral drugs, ifosfamide, lead, and cadmium
- Wilson's disease

Treatment

- **Large/**massive **doses of sodium bicarbonate:** May be required to overcome the renal "leak" of bicarbonate.
- **Potassium supplementation:** Often necessary because loss of bicarbonate in urine potentiates hypokalemia.

Type 3 Renal Tubular Acidosis

- It represents a combination of type 1 and type 2.
- **Inherited type 3 RTA:** It is caused by mutations resulting in carbonic anhydrase type II deficiency. It is characterized by osteopetrosis, cerebral calcification, and mental retardation.

Type 4 Renal Tubular Acidosis

It is also known as "hyporeninemic hypoaldosteronism." Its features are listed in **Box 13.17**.

- Causes of type 4 RTA is presented in **Table 13.23**.

Box 13.17: Features of type 4 renal tubular acidosis.

- Hyperkalemia
- Reduced plasma bicarbonate and hyperchloremia
- Normal ACTH stimulation test
- Low basal 24 hours urinary aldosterone
- Reduced response of plasma renin and plasma aldosterone to stimulation
- Correction of hyperkalemia by fludrocortisone

Treatment of type 4 RTA

- Treatment of aldosterone deficiency: With a mineralocorticoid (e.g., fludrocortisones) and glucocorticoid for cortisol deficiency (if present).
- Hyporeninemic hypoaldosteronism by fludrocortisones and accompanying hypertension and edema are treated by thiazide or loop diuretic. Diuretics are also necessary for the control of hyperkalemia.

TABLE 13.23: Causes of type 4 RTA.

Primary aldosterone deficiency	*Hyporeninemic hypoaldosteronism*	*Aldosterone resistance*
➢ Primary adrenal insufficiency ➢ Congenital adrenal hyperplasia ➢ Deficiency of aldosterone synthase ➢ Potassium sparing diuretics	➢ Renal dysfunction (e.g., diabetic nephropathy) ➢ Angiotensin-converting enzyme (ACE) inhibitors ➢ HIV ➢ Nonsteroidal anti-inflammatory drugs ➢ Cyclosporine	➢ Drugs (e.g., amiloride, spironolactone, trimethoprim, pentamidine) ➢ Pseudohypoaldosteronism

Algorithm approach to RTA is presented in **Figure 13.14**.

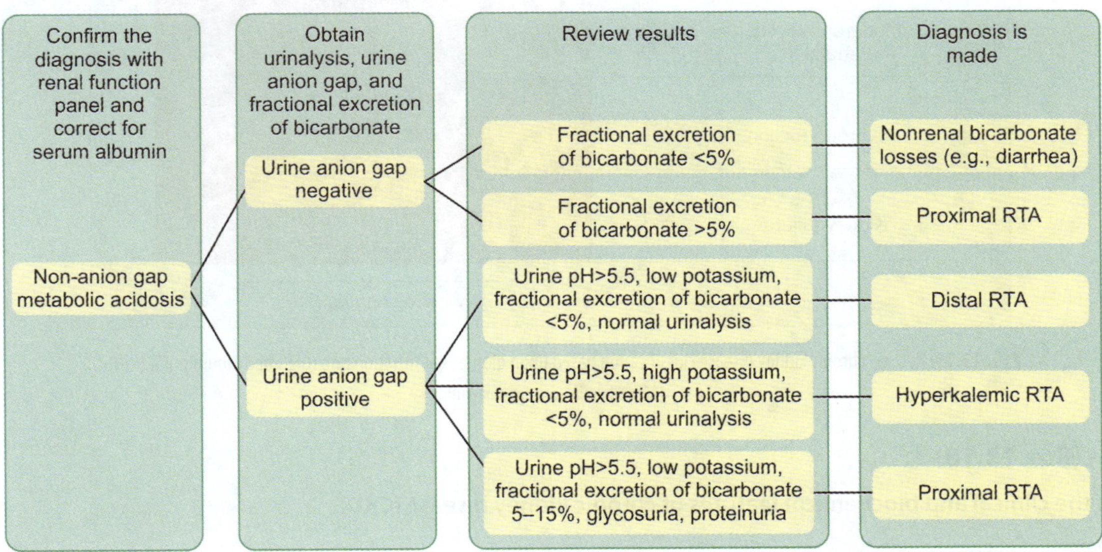

FIG. 13.14: Algorithm approach to renal tubular acidosis (RTA).

CHRONIC KIDNEY DISEASE (TABLE 13.24)

Q. Write a short note on chronic kidney diseases.

Chronic kidney disease previously termed CRF or insufficiency.

Chronic kidney disease refers to a spectrum of **long-standing** (more than 3 months), usually **progressive** processes associated with **irreversible worsening of renal function** and decline in GFR. **CKD spectrum ranges from abnormalities detectable only by laboratory testing to uremia.**

Revised CKD classification based upon GFR and albuminuria KDIGO 2013 is presented in **Figure 13.15**.

TABLE 13.24: Classification of CKD (The National Kidney Foundation-Kidney Disease Outcomes Quality Initiative NKF-KDOQI) working group.

Stage	*Description*	*GFR (mL/minute/1.73 m²)*
1	Chronic kidney damage with normal or increased GFR	>90
2	Mild GFR loss	60–89
3	Moderate GFR loss *stage 3A (GFR: 45–59 mL/min) and stage 3B (GFR: 30–44 mL/min)*	30–59
4	Severe GFR loss	15–29
5	Kidney failure requiring dialysis *(5D)* or transplantation *(5T)*	<15

GFR and ACR categories and risk of adverse outcomes			ACR categories (mg/mmoL), description and range		
			<3 Normal to mildly increased	3–30 Moderately increased	>30 Severely increased
			A1	A2	A3
GFR categories (mL/min/1.73 m^2) description, and range	≥90 Normal and high	G1	No CKD in the absence of markers of kidney damage		
	60–89 Mild reduction related to normal range for a young adult	G2			
	45–59 Mold-moderate reduction	G3a			
	30–44 Moderate-severe reduction	G3b			
	15–29 Severe reduction	G4			
	<15 Kidney failure	G5			

Increasing risk (down the GFR categories) · Increasing risk (across the ACR categories)

FIG. 13.15: Revised chronic kidney disease classification based upon glomerular filtration rate (GFR) and albuminuria (KDIGO). (ACR: albumin-to-creatinine ratio)

Definition (Box 13.18)

Q. Discuss the clinical and biochemical features of chronic kidney disease (CKD).

Box 13.18: Definition of chronic kidney disease (CKD).

- Glomerular filtration rate (GFR) of <60 mL/minute/1.73 m^2 for 3 months or more, with or without kidney damage or a urinary albumin to creatinine ratio >65 mg/mmol or protein creatinine ratio of 100 mg/mmol.
  OR
- Kidney damage for 3 or more months with or without decreased GFR, as evidenced by any of the following:
  - **Microalbuminuria:** Albumin excretion rate 30–300 mg/day in urine or urinary albumin >30 mg/day excretion of creatinine.
  - **Macroalbuminuria:** Albumin excretion rate in urine 300 mg/day.
  - **Pathologic abnormalities** such as abnormal findings on renal biopsy.
  - **Radiologic abnormalities** such as scarring or polycystic kidneys on renal ultrasound scan.

Causes of Chronic Kidney Disease

See **Table 13.25.**

Clinical Approach to Chronic Kidney Disease

History

- Duration of symptoms
- Drug intake: These include nonsteroidal anti-inflammatory agents, analgesic, and other medications (e.g., herbal medicines).
- Previous medical and surgical history, e.g., chemotherapy, SLE, malaria.
- Previous urinalysis or urea and creatinine values if performed.
- Family history of renal disease.

TABLE 13.25: Important causes of chronic kidney disease.

I. **Glomerulopathies*** *Proliferative glomerulonephritis (GN), crescentic GN, membranoproliferative GN, mesangiocapillary GN*	IV. **Obstructive*** *Calculus tumors, retroperitoneal fibrosis, prostatic enlargement*
II. **Systemic and metabolic diseases** *Diabetes** *Systemic lupus erythematosus (SLE), polyarteritis nodosa (PAN), amyloidosis* *Gout*	V. **Vascular** *Essential hypertension (accelerated)*, renovascular vasculitis (SLE, PAN, scleroderma)*
III. **Interstitial** *Chronic interstitial nephritis*, chronic pyelonephritis*, analgesic* *Tuberculosis, nephrocalcinosis*	VI. **Congenital** *Polycystic kidney*, medullary cystic disease, Alport's syndrome*

*Common causes of chronic renal failure

Symptoms

- Unfortunately, **early stages** of CKD **may be asymptomatic**, despite the progressive loss of kidney function and accumulation of numerous metabolites.
- Usually there is a rough correlation between serum urea and creatinine levels and symptoms. Symptoms are common when the serum urea level exceeds 40 mmol/L.

Clinical Features (Table 13.26 and Fig. 13.16)

Q. Write short essay/note on the clinical features of CKD.

TABLE 13.26: Clinical features of chronic kidney disease (CKD).

System	*Clinical features*	*Cause*
Renal	Nocturia and polyuria	Impaired concentrating ability of kidney
Muscle	Generalized myopathy	Combination of poor nutrition, hyperparathyroidism and vitamin D deficiency
Gastrointestinal	Malaise, loss of appetite (anorexia), nausea, vomiting, diarrhea	Nitrogenous waste products
Metabolic	Paresthesia and tetany	Hypocalcemia
Endocrine	Loss of libido in both sexes Women: Amenorrhea, menorrhagia Males: Erectile dysfunction, oligospermia	Hypothalamic-pituitary axis dysfunction
Skeletal	Bone pain	Metabolic bone disease
Respiratory	Pleural effusion, interstitial lung disease, calcification	Salt and water retention
Hematologic	Symptoms due to anemia: Fatigue, lassitude	Anemia is normochromic and normocytic type. Various causes mentioned in **Table 13.32**
Skin	Pruritus/itching, rash, metastatic calcification	Retention of nitrogenous waste products of protein catabolism, hyperparathyroidism, calcium-phosphate deposition
Immune system	Infections	Leukocyte functional defects, reduced cellular immunity
Cardiovascular	Atherosclerosis, heart failure, hypertension	Hypertension, homocysteinemia, calcification of heart valves
Neurologic	Peripheral neuropathy, mental slowing, clouding of consciousness and seizures myoclonic twitching, coma, restless leg syndrome or sensory deficits	Uremic toxins
Serosal inflammation	Pericardial or pleural pain and fluid, peritoneal fluid	Water retention

Complications of Chronic Renal Failure

Q. Write short essay/note on the complications of chronic renal failure.

Anemia: Various causes of anemia in CRF are listed in **Box 13.19**.

Q. Write short essay/note on renal osteodystrophy.

Metabolic Bone Disease: Renal Osteodystrophy

The term "renal osteodystrophy" (bone mineral disorder), constitutes various forms of bone disease that may develop alone or in combination in CRF. It includes (1) hyperparathyroid bone disease (osteitis fibrosa cystica), (2) osteomalacia, (3) osteoporosis, (4) osteosclerosis, and (5) adynamic bone disease.

Box 13.19: Causes of anemia in chronic renal failure (CRF).

- Deficiency of erythropoietin (most important)
- Toxic effects of uremia on bone marrow precursor cells
- Bone marrow fibrosis secondary to hyperparathyroidism
- Deficiency of hematinic: Iron, vitamin B_{12}, folate because of reduced dietary intake due to anorexia. Intestinal absorption of iron is also impaired.
- Increased red cell destruction: Abnormal red cell membranes
- Increased blood loss
  - Occult gastrointestinal bleeding
  - Blood sampling
  - Blood loss during hemodialysis
  - Capillary fragility
  - Due to platelet dysfunction and capillary fragility

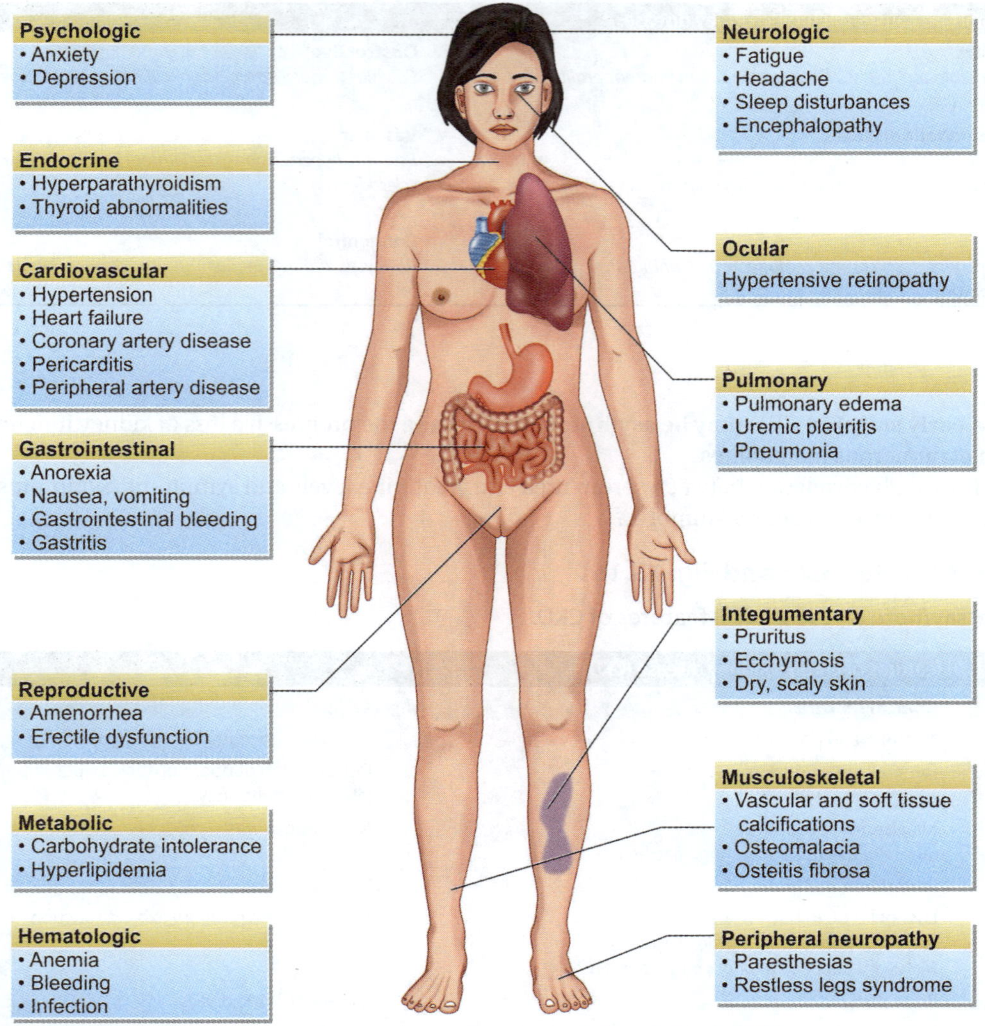

FIG. 13.16: Various clinical manifestations of chronic kidney disease (CKD).

Pathogenesis of bone disease (Fig. 13.17)

- Phosphate retention owing to reduced excretion by the kidneys release of **fibroblast growth factor 23 (FGF 23)** and other phosphaturic agents by osteoblasts as a compensatory mechanism. Actions of FGF 23 are:
  - Causes phosphaturia to normalize the plasma phosphate level.
  - It downregulates 1α-hydroxylase to reduce intestinal absorption of phosphate.
- Decreased production of the lα-hydroxylase enzyme by the kidney results in reduced conversion of 25-$(OH)_2D_3$ (25-hydroxyvitamin D) to the more metabolically active 1,25-$(OH)_2D_3$(1,25-dihydroxycholecalciferol). Its consequences are:
  - Decreased activation of vitamin D receptors (VDRs) in the parathyroid glands leads to increased release of parathyroid hormone (PTH) causing secondary hyperparathyroidism.
  - Decreased intestinal absorption of calcium causes hypocalcemia which leads in turn to increased PTH production by the parathyroid glands.
  - Phosphate retention also indirectly lowers ionized calcium and these together results in an increase in PTH synthesis and release. The raised serum phosphate combine with calcium in the extracellular space, causing ectopic calcification in blood vessels and other tissues.
  - Parathyroid hormone causes reabsorption of calcium from bone and increased reabsorption of calcium from proximal renal tubules.

  This prevents hypocalcemia induced by 1,25-$(OH)_2D_3$ deficiency and phosphate retention.
  - **Secondary hyperparathyroidism** causes increased osteoclastic activity, cyst formation and bone marrow fibrosis (osteitis fibrosa cystica).
  - Long-standing secondary hyperparathyroidism finally causes hyperplasia of the glands with autonomous or **"tertiary" hyperparathyroidism**.

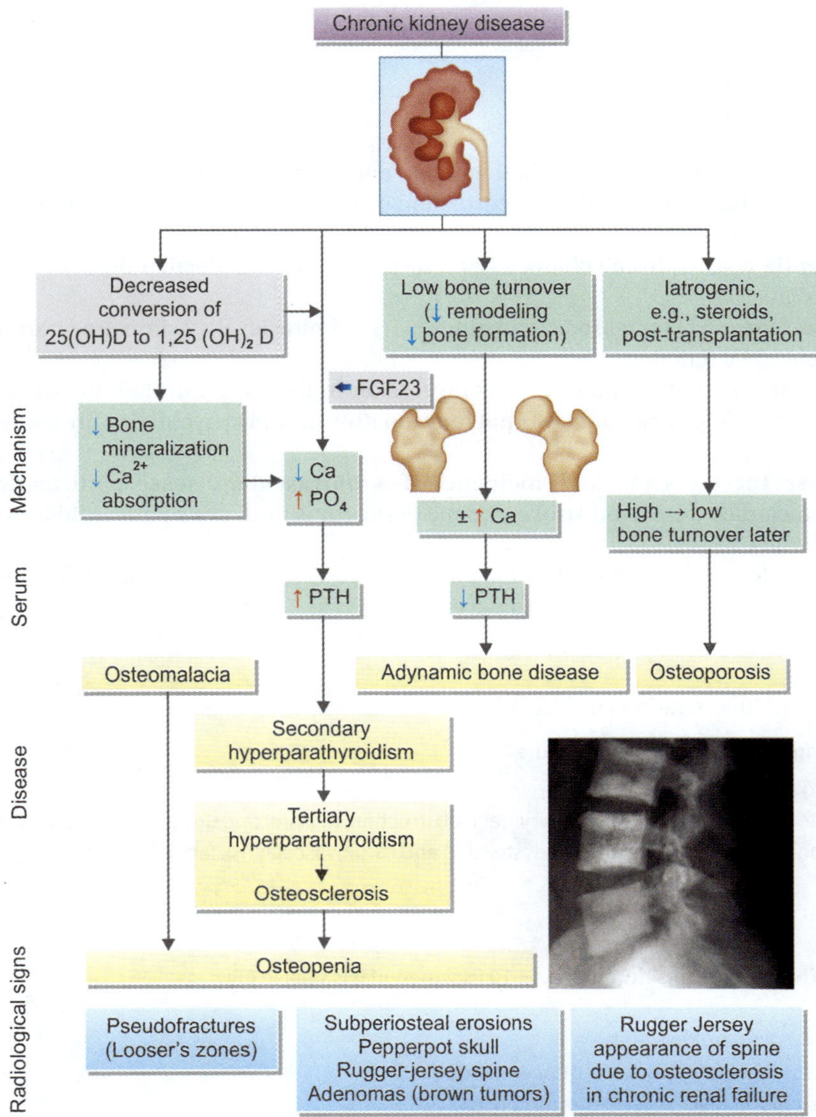

FIG. 13.17: Lateral spine X-ray showing rugger-jersey appearance of spine.

[25-(OH)D_3: 25-hydroxyvitamin D; 1,25-$(OH)_2D_3$: 1,25-dihydroxycholecalciferol; FGF23: fibroblast growth factor 23; Ca: calcium; PO_4: phosphate; PTH: parathormone]

- **Osteomalacia:** It is due to impaired mineralization of osteoid caused by deficiency 1,25-$(OH)_2D_3$ and hypocalcemia.
- **Osteosclerosis:** Literally means "hardening of bone" characterized by increased bone density and is due to the direct result of long-standing PTH excess. Alternating bands of sclerotic and porotic bone in the spine give rise to a characteristic **"rugger-jersey"** appearance on X-ray (**Fig. 13.17**).
- **Osteoporosis** is probably related to malnutrition and is commonly found in CRF, often after transplantation and the use of corticosteroids.
- **Adynamic bone disease** is the condition of in which both bone formation and resorption are depressed.

- **Gastrointestinal complications:** (1) Reduced gastric emptying and increased risk of reflux esophagitis, (2) increased risk of peptic ulceration and acute pancreatitis, and (3) constipation (especially in patients on continuous ambulatory peritoneal dialysis (CAPD), and (4) gastrointestinal bleed.
- **Metabolic abnormalities:**
  - **Gout:** Urate retention is a common in CRF.
  - **Insulin requirement and resistance:** Insulin is catabolized by and to some extent excreted via the kidneys. Thus, insulin requirements in diabetic patients reduce as renal failure progresses. By contrast, end-organ resistance to insulin is observed in advanced renal impairment.
- **Lipid metabolism abnormalities:** Include (1) impaired clearance of triglyceride-rich particles and (2) hypercholesterolemia.
- **Endocrine abnormalities:** Include (1) Hyperprolactinemia, (2) increased luteinizing hormone (LH) levels in both sex, (3) decreased serum testosterone levels, (4) absence of normal cyclical changes in female sex hormones, resulting in

oligomenorrhea or amenorrhea, (5) abnormalities of growth hormone secretion and action, and (6) abnormal thyroid hormone levels.

- **Muscle dysfunction proximal myopathy.**
- **Nervous system**
  - *Central nervous system:*
    - Unusual combination of depressed cerebral function and decreased seizure threshold.
    - **Dialysis disequilibrium** develops if rapid correction of severe uremia is done by hemodialysis owing to osmotic cerebral swelling.
    - **Dialysis dementia** is a syndrome characterized by progressive intellectual deterioration, speech disturbance, myoclonus, and fits.
  - *Autonomic nervous system:* (1) Increased circulating catecholamine level, (2) impaired baroreceptor sensitivity, and (3) impaired efferent vagal function.
  - *Peripheral nervous system:* (1) Median nerve compression in the carpal tunnel due to β_2-microglobulin-related amyloidosis, (2) restless legs syndrome, (3) polyneuropathy, and (4) psychiatric problems (anxiety, depression, phobias, and psychoses).
- **Cardiovascular disease: Increased (16-fold) incidence of cardiovascular disease,** particularly myocardial infarction, cardiac failure, sudden cardiac death and stroke, uremic pericarditis or dialysis pericarditis. Hypertension develops in about 80% of patients with CRF.
- **Malignancy: Raised** incidence of malignancy. Malignant change can occur in polycystic kidney disease. Lymphomas, primary liver cancer, and thyroid cancers can also develop.

Investigations

Box 13.20 lists the purpose of investigations in CKD.

Box 13.20: Purpose of investigations in chronic renal failure.

- To identify the underlying cause wherever possible.
- To identify reversible factors (e.g., hypertension, urinary tract, obstruction, nephrotoxic drugs, and salt and water depletion).
- To screen for complications (e.g., anemia, renal osteodystrophy) and cardiovascular risk factors.

Urinalysis

- **Physical examination:** Fixed specific gravity around 1.010 (isosthenuria) is seen in CRF.
- **Chemical examination**
  - Hematuria may indicate glomerulonephritis.
  - Proteinuria, if heavy, is strongly suggestive of glomerular disease.
  - Glycosuria with normal blood glucose level is common in CRF.
- **Urine microscopy**
  - **White cells** in the urine usually indicate **bacterial urinary infection**, sterile pyuria suggests papillary necrosis or renal tuberculosis.
  - **Eosinophils** indicate **allergic tubulointerstitial nephritis** or cholesterol embolization.
  - **Red cells** source may be from anywhere in the urinary tract between the glomerulus and the urethral meatus.
  - **Red-cell casts** are suggestive of **glomerulonephritis.**
  - **Granular casts** indicate **active renal disease.**
  - **Broad casts** are seen in CRF.
- **Urine culture** should be performed. Early-morning urine samples should be cultured for tuberculosis.

Urine Biochemistry

- **24-hour creatinine clearance** is useful to know the severity of renal failure.
- **Urine osmolality** is a measure of concentrating ability.
- **Urine electrophoresis** and immunofixation for the detection of light chains in myeloma.

Serum Biochemistry

- **Serum urea and creatinine:** The most consistent abnormalities in CRF are **elevated** levels of urea and creatinine. The level of serum creatinine correlates with the degree of renal damage.
- **Electrophoresis and immunofixation for myeloma.**
- Extreme elevations of creatine kinase and a disproportionate elevation in serum creatinine and potassium compared to urea suggestive of rhabdomyolysis.
- Other biochemical abnormalities include hypocalcemia, hyperphosphatemia, hyperuricemia and hyperkalemia.

Hematology

- **Anemia**
- **Eosinophilia** suggestive of allergic TIN, vasculitis, or cholesterol embolism.
- **Peripheral smear** with **fragmented red cells (Burr cells) and/or thrombocytopenia** suggestive of **intravascular hemolysis** due to accelerated hypertension, hemolytic uremic syndrome or thrombotic thrombocytopenic purpura.
- **Markedly raised erythrocyte sedimentation rate (ESR)** is suggestive of **myeloma**.

Immunology

- **Low complement components** may be seen in **active glomerular disease** (e.g., SLE, PSGN).
- **Autoantibody screening** helpful autoimmune diseases (e.g., SLE).
- **Antibodies to streptococcal antigens** (ASOT, anti-DNase B) if PSGN is suspected.
- **Antibodies to hepatitis B and C**
- **Antibodies to HIV** when HIV-associated renal disease is suspected.
- **Malaria** can cause glomerular disease in the tropics.

Radiological Investigation

- **Ultrasound:** Ultrasonography to assess the renal size and to exclude hydronephrosis. Renal ultrasound usually shows shrunken kidneys in CRF. *In diabetic glomerulosclerosis, amyloidosis, polycystic kidney diseases, HIV nephropathy, bilateral hydronephrosis, and myeloma, the kidneys may be of normal size.*
- **Plain abdominal radiography and CT** (without contrast) to exclude low-density renal stones or nephrocalcinosis. CT may also useful for the diagnosis of retroperitoneal fibrosis and useful in some patients with suspected obstructive nephropathy.
- **MRI:** Magnetic resonance angiography is useful in renovascular disease.

Renal Biopsy

Aim: To establish the nature and extent of renal disease, which helps in treatment and predicting prognosis. It should be performed in patient with unexplained renal failure and normal-sized kidneys (exception diabetic glomerulosclerosis), unless there are strong contraindications.

Management of Chronic Renal Failure

Management of CRF can be divided into three parts:

1. Establishing the diagnosis and etiology of CKD and to detect any reversible factors
2. Measures to prevent/slow down the further damage to the kidney (progression of CKD)
3. Supportive measures (e.g., dialysis or transplantation) when necessary

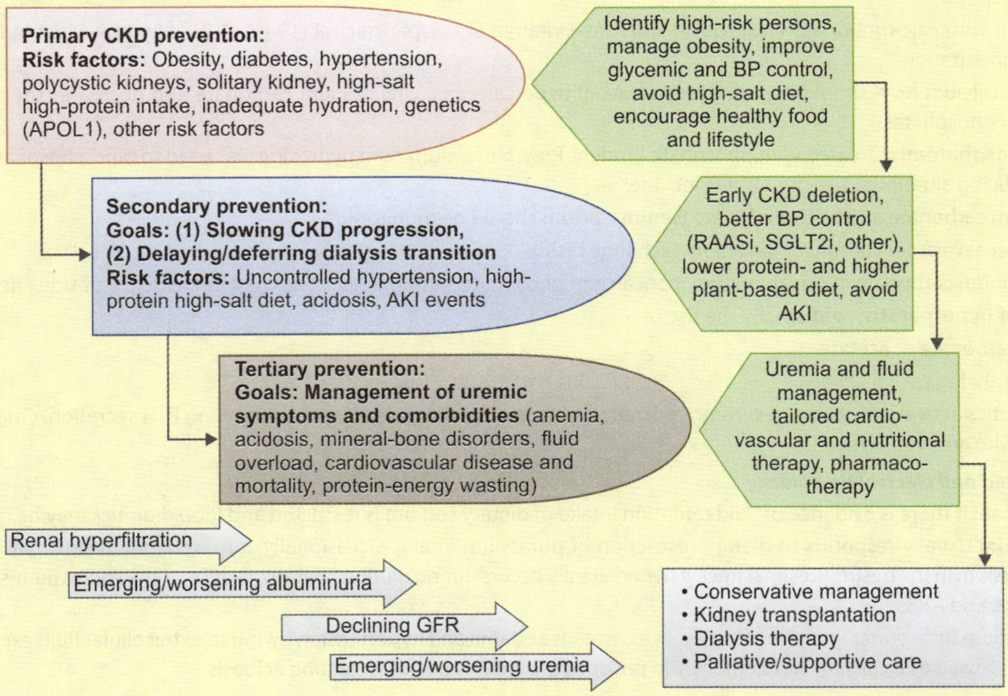

Primary CKD prevention:
Risk factors: Obesity, diabetes, hypertension, polycystic kidneys, solitary kidney, high-salt high-protein intake, inadequate hydration, genetics (APOL1), other risk factors

Identify high-risk persons, manage obesity, improve glycemic and BP control, avoid high-salt diet, encourage healthy food and lifestyle

Secondary prevention:
Goals: (1) Slowing CKD progression, (2) Delaying/deferring dialysis transition
Risk factors: Uncontrolled hypertension, high-protein high-salt diet, acidosis, AKI events

Early CKD deletion, better BP control (RAASi, SGLT2i, other), lower protein- and higher plant-based diet, avoid AKI

Tertiary prevention:
Goals: Management of uremic symptoms and comorbidities (anemia, acidosis, mineral-bone disorders, fluid overload, cardiovascular disease and mortality, protein-energy wasting)

Uremia and fluid management, tailored cardio-vascular and nutritional therapy, pharmaco-therapy

Renal hyperfiltration → Emerging/worsening albuminuria → Declining GFR → Emerging/worsening uremia

- Conservative management
- Kidney transplantation
- Dialysis therapy
- Palliative/supportive care

Treatments aimed at specific causes of CKD: Optimization glucose control in diabetes mellitus, immunomodulatory agents for glomerulonephritis, and emerging specific therapies to retard cytogenesis in polycystic kidney disease. Any reversible factors should be detected and treated (**Table 13.27**).

TABLE 13.27: Reversible factors in chronic kidney disease.

1. Hypovolemia: Vomiting, diarrhea, excessive diuresis, congestive heart failure
2. Urinary tract obstruction: Nephrolithiasis, papillary necrosis, bladder outlet obstruction
3. Infection
4. Uncontrolled or accelerated hypertension
5. Nephrotoxic drugs: Aminoglycosides, cephalosporins, tetracycline, amphotericin, radio-contrast agents, NSAIDs, diuretics
6. Electrolyte and metabolic disorders: Hyperphosphatasemia, hyperuricemia, acidosis
7. Vasculitis: Systemic lupus erythematosus, Wegener's granulomatosis, microscopic polyarteritis
8. Pregnancy: Eclampsia

Measures to Reduce the Symptoms and Progression of CRF

- Following measures may stabilize or slow the decline of renal function.
- **Control of hypertension and proteinuria:** Goals of treatment include: (1) blood pressure should be reduced <130/80 mm Hg and proteinuria < 0.3 g/24 hours. If creatinine is below 3 mg/dL, ACE inhibitors and ARBs (inhibit the angiotensin-induced vasoconstriction of the efferent arterioles of the glomerular microcirculation) are the drugs of choice.
- **Diet**
  - **Protein restriction** to 0.60 and 0.75 g/kg/day, i.e., about 40 g/day (with higher amount of essential amino acids). It reduces symptoms associated with uremia and may also slow the rate of renal decline at earlier stages of renal disease.
  - **Avoid foods with high potassium.**
  - **Salt restriction** is necessary in most of the patients. However, patients with salt-losing nephropathy (tubulointerstitial disease) require a high-salt intake.
- **Slowing progression of diabetic renal disease** by control of blood glucose and maintaining HbA1c in the range of 7.0–7.5.
- **Use of lipid-lowering agents:** Hypercholesterolemia is common in patients with significant proteinuria, and in patients with CKD. Lipid lowering reduces vascular events in nondialysis CKD.
- Cessation of smoking.
- Exercise and weight reduction.
- Avoid nephrotoxic medications.

Corrections of complications

Calcium and phosphate control and suppression of PTH

- **Treatment of hypocalcemia and hyperphosphatemia:** Both should be treated aggressively.
  - **Hypocalcemia:**
    - Treated with calcitriol or alphacalcidol (1-α-hydroxyvitamin D_3) or paricalcitol (19-nor-1,25-dihydroxyvitamin D3) and calcium supplementation.
    - Serum calcium level should be monitored to avoid hypercalcemia. Oral calcium carbonate also decreases the bioavailability of dietary phosphates.
  - **Hyperphosphatemia:** Treated with phosphate binders. Previously, aluminum hydroxide was used to bind phosphate in the gut and was producing aluminum toxicity. Others include:
    - Calcium carbonate and calcium acetate (serum calcium should be monitored).
    - Polymer sevelamer carbonate (an anion-exchange resin).
    - Lanthanum carbonate (a nonaluminum, noncalcium phosphate-binding agent) has higher incidence of side effects.
- **Treatment of hyperparathyroidism:** By the use of
  - Calcium carbonate or acetate.
  - Vitamin D analogs.
  - Calcimimetics activate the calcium-sensing receptor in the parathyroid gland, thereby inhibiting PTH secretion. Cinacalcet is used in patients who are on dialysis.

Maintenance fluid and electrolyte balance

- **Fluid retention:** If there is evidence of fluid retention intake of dietary sodium is restricted and loop diuretics may be necessary.
- **Hyperkalemia:** Usually responds to dietary restriction of potassium intake. Occasionally, ion-exchange resins may be necessary to remove potassium in the gastrointestinal tract. If hyperkalemia occurs during diuretic therapy, reduce or stop potassium-sparing diuretics, ACE inhibitors, and ARBs.
- **Acidosis:** Sodium bicarbonate may be effective, but can cause edema and hypertension owing to extracellular fluid expansion. Calcium carbonate, also used as a calcium supplement and phosphate binder is useful in treating acidosis.

Q. Write short essay/note on the management of anemia in chronic renal failure.

Treatment of anemia in chronic renal failure

- The anemia of erythropoietin (EPO) deficiency is treated with recombinant (synthetic) human EPO (erythropoietin-alpha or -beta, or the longer-acting darbepoetin-alpha). Administration of erythropoietin-alpha through subcutaneous route is contraindicated in CRF and the intravenous route is used, initially 50 U/kg of epoetin-alpha over 1–5 minutes three times/week. EPO is less effective in the presence of iron deficiency, active inflammation or malignancy, and in patients with aluminum overload (found in dialysis).

	Initiation dose in CKD—nondialysis dependent	Initiation dose in dialysis dependent CKD
➤ Erythropoietin	➤ 20–50 U/kg 3 times/week (If given IV, IV dose is 20–30% higher than SC dose)	
➤ Darbepoetin alpha	0.45 mcg/kg every 4 weeks (SC or IV)	0.45 mcg/kg once weekly (SC or IV) Or 0.75 mcg/kg every 2 weeks (SC or IV)
➤ Epoetin beta	➤ 0.6 mcg every 2 weeks (SC or IV)	

- Blood pressure, hemoglobin concentration and reticulocyte count are measured every 2 weeks and the dose adjusted to maintain a target hemoglobin level of 10–12 g/dL.
- Hemoglobin >13 g/dL has been associated with increased incidence of cardiovascular mortality.
- Some newer agents tried in management of anemia in CKD:
  - **Prolyl hydroxylase inhibitors:** Roxadustat, vadadustat
  - **Erythropoietin mimicking peptide:** Peginesatide
- **Specific treatment:** Renal replacement therapy

Table 13.28 lists the differences between AKI and CKD.

TABLE 13.28: Differences between acute kidney injury (AKI) and chronic kidney disease (CKD).

	AKI	*CKD*
Previous history of kidney disease	Absent	Present
Previous elevated creatinine >3 months	Absent	Present
Anemia	Absent	Present
Hypertension	+/–	++
Kidney size (ultrasound)	Not contracted	Contracted
Complications: Hyperphosphatemia, hypocalcemia, neuropathy, osteodystrophy, band keratopathy	Absent	Present

CYSTIC DISEASES OF KIDNEY

Polycystic Kidney Diseases

Types: Two types

1. **Autosomal-recessive (childhood) polycystic kidney disease (ARPKD):**
   - Mutation in PKHD1 gene on chromosome 6, the gene that encodes for fibrocystin and biliary epithelial epithelial tissue
   - A specialized layer of tissue formed by closely aggregated cells that line the outer surface of organs, blood vessels, the skin, and the inner surface of body cavities. Divided into squamous, cuboidal, and columnar types
   - docIcon General histology → Epithelium → cells.
   - All patients also have cysts in the liver and patients who survive infancy may develop **congenital hepatic fibrosis** and intrahepatic bile duct dilatation (Caroli disease).
2. **Autosomal-dominant (adult) polycystic kidney disease (ADPKD):**
   - ADPKD is the MC inherited renal disease
   - ADPKD is caused by mutations in
     - PKD1 on chromosome 16 codes for polycysti n-1 (PC1)
     - PKD2 on chromosome 4 codes for polycysti n-2 (PC2)
     - 10% patients may have no family history; due to spontaneous mutation
     - PKD2: Slower disease progression

- It characterized by **multiple thin-walled, spherical cysts in cortex and medulla of both kidneys.** These cysts expand and cause destruction of kidney parenchyma and leads to renal failure.
- Associated extrarenal anomalies:
  - **Cysts in other organs** such as liver (**polycystic liver disease** in more than 75% of cases) spleen, pancreas, thyroid, ovary, endometrium, seminal vesicles, and epididymis.
  - Intracranial **Berry aneurysms** in the circle of Willis (in 10–30%) which may rupture and cause subarachnoid hemorrhages.
  - **Mitral valve prolapse** and other cardiac valvular anomalies. Colonic diverticula, abdominal or inguinal hernias are associated.
- **Clinical presentation**

Q. Discuss the clinical features and complications of adult polycystic kidney disease.

- May be at **any age** from the second decade and majority of patients remain **asymptomatic until the fourth decade** of life.
- **Presenting manifestations**
  - Acute loin/**flank pain** (heaviness or dragging sensation), and/or hematuria (owing to hemorrhage into a cyst), UTI (pyelonephritis and renal cyst infection) or urinary tract stone formation and renal colic (due to passage of blood clots in the urine).
  - Vague abdominal/loin or discomfort due to increased size of the kidneys
  - **Subarachnoid hemorrhage** due to rupture of berry aneurysm
  - Renal hemorrhage and hematuria
  - **Hypertension** and its complications
  - Complications of associated liver cysts
  - When sufficient quantity of nephrons are destroyed, patient develops **CKD** and symptoms of uremia and/or anemia
  - **Polycythemia** (due to increased erythropoietin production) is a rare complication and presentation of ADPKD.
  - Rarely renal carcinoma
- **Physical examination:** Bilateral large **abdominal masses** of irregular kidneys.
- **Investigation:**
  - **Abdominal ultrasound** is used for establishing the definitive diagnosis.
  - **MRI** is more sensitive than ultrasound and can detect small cysts (**Fig. 13.18**).
  - **IVU:** Rarely performed nowadays and may demonstrate the characteristic "drooping water-lily sign."
- **Screening:** The children of patients with established ADPKD should undergo screening.

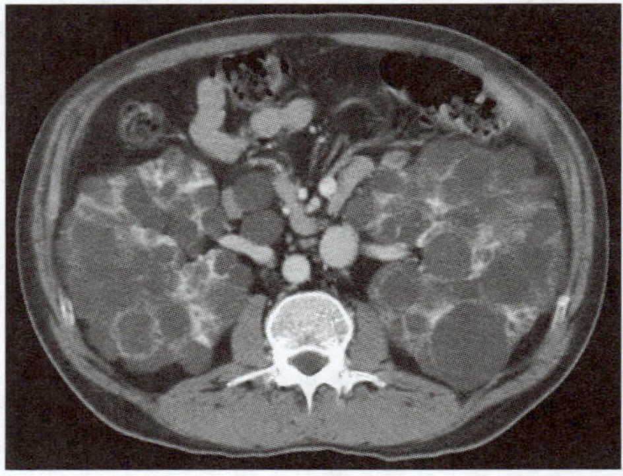

FIG. 13.18: MRI showing polycystic kidney.

Treatment
- Control of hypertension
- Control of pain
- Treatment of infection
- Management of CKD—dialysis or transplantation (if required) and
- Specific treatment—vaptans, mammalian target of rapamycin (mTOR) inhibitors (sirolimus, everolimus), and somatostatin analogs have been tried in treatment of ADPKD.

Medullary Sponge Kidney

- Medullary sponge kidney (MSK) is characterized by nonprogressive dilatation of collecting ducts and tubules.
- Usually inherited as autosomal dominant
- May be associated with other developmental and genetic disorders
- Often asymptomatic, and may manifest with hematuria, nephrolithiasis, and infection.

Medullary Cystic Disease or Juvenile Nephronophthisis

- Two distinct genetic and age-related forms with similar renal morphology. Autosomal recessive manifests during childhood and is frequently associated with extrarenal abnormalities such as ophthalmologic, mental retardation, cerebellar ataxia, skeletal anomalies, and hepatic fibrosis.
- The disease progresses to end-stage renal disease (ESRD) before the age of 25 years.

OBSTRUCTIVE UROPATHY

- **Obstructive uropathy** is a term used for obstruction in the urinary passage involving the urethra, bladder, ureters or pelvicalyceal system. It leads to impedance to urine flow and consequent damage to renal function.
- **Nature of obstruction:** It is acute or chronic.
  - **Acute obstruction:** The changes in kidney function are completely reversible after the relief of obstruction.
  - **Chronic obstruction:** It leads to irreversible structural and functional changes.

Site and Cause of Urinary Tract Obstruction (Table 13.29)

TABLE 13.29: Site and cause of urinary tract obstruction.

Site	*Cause*
Infundibular/pelvis	Congenital, calculi, infection, trauma, tumor
Ureteropelvic junction	Congenital stenosis*, calculi, trauma
Ureter	Obstructive megaureter*, ectopic ureter, ureterocele, calculi*, retroperitoneal tumor (lymphoma), inflammatory bowel disease, retroperitoneal fibrosis, chronic granulomatous disease (tuberculosis)
Bladder	Neurogenic dysfunction*, tumor (rhabdomyosarcoma), diverticula, ectopic ureter
Urethra	Posterior urethral valves*, diverticula, strictures, atresia, ectopic ureter, foreign body, phimosis*, priapism prostatic enlargement*, extrinsic compression due to tumor, lymph nodes

*Relatively common.

NEPHROLITHIASIS

- Nephrolithiasis (also known as kidney stones or renal calculi) is a common disorder characterized by the formation of aggregates of microscopic crystals into solid objects (stones).
- **Constituent:** Usually contain calcium or phosphate along with small amounts of proteins and glycoproteins.
- **Size:** They vary greatly in size from millimeters to centimeters.
- **Age and gender:** It usually appears during middle age and is more common in men than women (M:F = 2:1).
- **Risk of recurrence:** Calculi recur in about 50% of cases within 3–5 years.

Etiology (Box 13.21)

Q. Write short note on predisposing factors for renal stones.

- Normal urine contains inhibitors of crystal formation (citrate, inorganic magnesium, pyrophosphate, glycosaminoglycans and nephrocalcin) that prevent the formation of calculi.
- When the chemical concentration of urine is altered, the calculus forming substances may exceed their maximum solubility in water and may favor crystal formation.

Types

Calcium Stones (Oxalate Calculus/Calcium Oxalate)

- Most (80%) renal stones are **composed of calcium complexed with oxalate** (calcium oxalate) or **phosphate** (calcium phosphate) or a mixture of these (calcium oxalate + calcium phosphate). These stones are **radiopaque**.
- Causes (**Box 13.22**).

Uric Acid Stones

- Commonly found in patients **with hyperuricemia** (e.g., gout) and **diseases involving rapid cell turnover** (e.g., leukemias). However, more than 50% of patients have neither hyperuricemia nor increased urinary excretion of uric acid.
- **Uric acid is insoluble in acidic urine** and **urine pH below 5.5 may predispose to uric acid stones.**
- Uric acid stones are **radiolucent** stones.
- Causes (**Box 13.22**).

Struvite Stones or (Triple stones/Magnesium, Ammonium, Phosphate Stones)

- They are composed of calcium phosphate often with magnesium and ammonium phosphate and are **known as struvite stones or triple phosphate stones**.
- Causes (**Box 13.22**): These stones are unique in that they **develop after infections of the urinary tract by urea-splitting bacteria** (e.g., ***Proteus***), which convert urea to ammonia → produces alkaline pH + slowing of urine flow (people with abnormal urinary drainage, such as those with ureteral reflux, neurogenic bladder, other forms of bladder dysfunction, or ureteral diversions) → precipitation of magnesium, ammonium, phosphate (struvite), and calcium phosphate (apatite).

Cystine Stones

- Cystine stones are uncommon and associated with **cystinuria**, which is due to genetic defects in the renal reabsorption of cystine or other amino acids.
- Stones form at **low urinary pH** (acidic urine)
- Cystine stones also are radiopaque
- Recur frequently in most affected individuals
- Diagnosis is suggested by a positive urine nitroprusside test and confirmed by analysis of the calculus.
- **Urine sediment:** It may show the characteristic **hexagonal cystine crystals** and crystal formation is favored in acidic urine (low pH).

Box 13.21: Predisposing factors for renal stones.

Environmental and dietary factors
- Conditions that favor low volume of urine: High atmospheric temperatures, low intake of fluid
- Diet: High protein, high sodium, low calcium
- High excretion of sodium, oxalate, and urate excretion
- Low excretion of citrate

Acquired causes
- Hypercalcemia
- Ileal disease or resection (increases oxalate absorption and urinary excretion)
- Renal tubular acidosis (RTA) type I (distal)
- Infection: Urinary infection by urea-splitting organisms such as *Proteus, Pseudomonas, Klebsiella, Staphylococcus,* and *Mycoplasma*

Congenital and inherited disorders
- Medullary sponge kidney
- Familial hypercalciuria
- Cystinuria
- Renal tubular acidosis (RTA) type I (distal)
- Primary hyperoxaluria

Box 13.22: Types and causes of renal stones.

Type

1. Calcium oxalate and/or calcium phosphate (~80%)
   - Idiopathic hypercalciuria: Most common
   - Hypercalciuria and hypercalcemia
   - Hyperoxaluria: Enteric (oxalate-containing foods, salt, protein-meat) vitamin C abuse, primary
   - Hyperuricosuria
   - Idiopathic
2. Uric acid (~7%)
   - Associated with hyperuricemia
   - Associated with hyperuricosuria
   - Idiopathic
3. Struvite (magnesium, ammonium, phosphate) ~10%
   - Urinary tract infection
4. Cystine (~2%)
5. Others/unknown (~1%)

Clinical Manifestations

- **Most common** presenting symptoms: (1) **Severe colicky flank and/or abdominal pain** radiating to the anterior abdominal wall and (2) **hematuria** (microscopic or gross). This symptom complex termed renal or ureteric colic. These symptoms are due to partial or full obstruction produced by stones while passing through the ureter.
- **Asymptomatic:** Stone is **incidentally discovered** in an abdominal computed tomography or ultrasound examination for other purposes.
- **Symptoms depending on the site of stone:**
  - **Stones in the renal pelvis usually are painless** unless infection or obstruction is present.
  - **Ureteral stones may cause nausea, vomiting, and severe abdominal** and/or flank pain radiating into the groin, urethra, or genitalia.
  - **Stones at the ureterovesical** junction may produce **dysuria, frequency,** and **urgency**, even in the absence of infection.
  - Once in the bladder, stones are normally passed out without difficulty, but they can remain there and grow to very large sizes in patients with bladder dysfunction.
- Fever and pyuria suggest associated UTI and must be confirmed by urine culture.
- Chronic and complete obstruction can result in hydronephrosis and loss of function in the affected kidney.

Diagnosis/Investigations (Box 13.23)

- **CT-KUB** (CT of kidney, ureter, and bladder) is the **gold standard** for diagnosis. It defines the size and location of any stones (including nonradiopaque stones, such as those containing uric acid and cysteine) in the urinary tract.
- **Abdominal ultrasound or intravenous pyelograms** (IVPs) are generally inferior in sensitivity and specificity compared to the computed tomography scan.
- A **plain X-ray of the abdomen** (**Fig. 13.19**) has limited diagnostic utility, but may be useful to track progression of previously diagnosed radiopaque stones.
- **Urine analysis:** To confirm the presence of **blood** and check for **evidence of infection**. **Urinary sediment** should be examined under the microscope for crystals. Any stones passed in urine should be saved for analysis. Metabolic evaluation of stones should always be performed before starting on a therapeutic regimen. **Urine culture** should be done when clinically indicated.
- **Laboratory tests:** These include serum studies for renal function, electrolytes, calcium, magnesium, phosphate, and uric acid. If there is hypercalcemia, a PTH level should be obtained.

Box 13.23: Important investigations in patients with renal calculi.

1. Routine urine examination (albumin, RBC, WBC, casts and crystals, and pH)
2. Renal functions (blood urea, serum creatinine)
3. Imaging (ultrasonography and IV urography)
4. To find out underlying cause
   - Chemical analysis of calculus passed in urine
   - Plasma calcium, phosphate, and parathormone
   - 24-hour urine for estimation of calcium, oxalate, urate, cysteine

Treatment

Acute Management

- **Acute colic** should be treated with an effective/powerful **analgesic.** Diclofenac orally or IV infusion or as a suppository is very effective. However, opiates may be needed.
- **Increase the water intake** to maintain a daily urine output of 2 L or more. If this is not possible, **intravenous fluids** should be given to **increase urinary output**.
- Stone removal **strategies** are **based on the size of the stone.**
  - Most small calculi (**<5 mm in diameter**) usually **pass spontaneously**.
  - **Alpha blockers** (e.g., tamsulosin) facilitate spontaneous expulsion of distal **ureteral stones of <6 mm size.**
  - **Stones >1 cm diameter** usually need **urological or radiological intervention**. Extracorporeal shock wave lithotripsy (ESWL) causes fragmentation of most of the stones into pieces <5 mm, which then pass spontaneously. Ureteroscopy with a YAG laser (for larger stones) and percutaneous nephrolithotomy also can be used. Open surgery is rarely necessary.
- **Surgical removal** is attempted only if the stone passage becomes complicated. Complicating features include failure to pass stone in 3–7 days, acute renal failure, gross hematuria with clots, or infection. Open surgical procedures are very rarely performed. Endoscopic or surgical removal is recommended for: (a) persistent pain not relieved by analgesia, (b) stone obstructing a single kidney, or bilateral ureteral obstruction and/or pyonephrosis.

Chronic Management

- **Fluid: Increase the urine volumes** (dilution) so that it reduces supersaturation and prevents new stone formation. Increase the fluid intake until daily urine output exceeds 2–3 L.

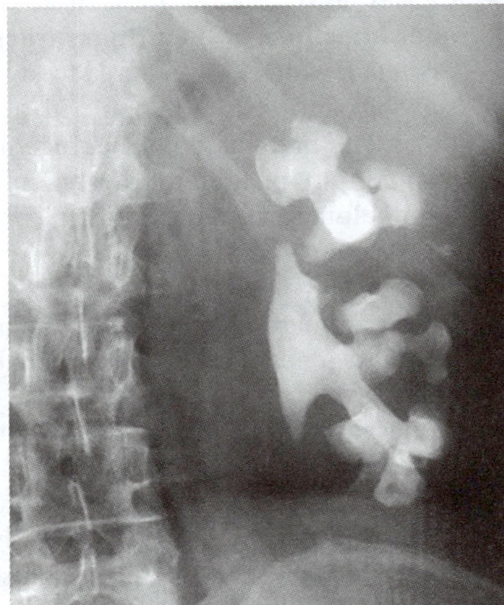

FIG. 13.19: X-ray shows staghorn calculi.

- **Avoid:** Vitamin D supplements (increase calcium absorption and excretion) and vitamin C supplementation (increases oxalate excretion).
- **Calcium-containing stones**
  - **Modification of diet** to reduce risks of stone formation in recurrent stone formers (>5 years between episodes).
  - **Thiazide diuretics** (e.g., 12.5–25 mg of hydrochlorothiazide) reduce urinary calcium excretion and are useful in hypercalciuric calcium stone formers.
  - **Potassium citrate** (60 mEq/day) in divided doses is used in hypocitraturia and also helps to prevent recurrence in patients with normal urinary citrate levels.
  - **Oxalate:** Avoid foods rich in oxalate (spinach, rhubarb).
- **Uric acid stones**
  - In patients with hyperuricosuria (>1,000 mg of uric acid per 24 hours) and normal serum calcium, **allopurinol** in the dose of 100–200 mg/day reduce uric acid synthesis.
  - **Alkalinization of the urine** to a pH of 7 or above to increase uric acid solubility and to dissolve uric acid crystals. This is achieved by supplementation with potassium citrate, potassium bicarbonate, or sodium bicarbonate in divided doses, or acetazolamide to alkalinize the nocturnal urine.
- **Cystine stones:** Decrease the urinary concentration of cystine below the solubility limit of 200–300 mg/L. Apart from the methods already described, alkalinization of the urine to a pH above 7.5 is critical. This usually can be achieved with Shohl's solution (contains sodium citrate).

URINARY TRACT INFECTIONS

Q. Discuss the etiopathogenesis, clinical features, investigations, and management of urinary tract infection.

Definition

A UTI is associated with multiplication of organisms in the urinary tract and is defined as the presence of more than **10^5 organism/mL** in the midstream sample of urine (MSU).

Clinical Presentation

See **Table 13.30.**

TABLE 13.30: Clinical spectrum of urinary tract infection (UTI).

Asymptomatic bacteriuria (ABU)	*Symptomatic (disease)*
Presence of bacteriuria (>10^5/mL or two occasions in females and on one occasion in males) indicating UTI but without symptoms. ➢ Common in pregnancy ➢ Occurs in the absence of symptoms ➢ Does not usually require treatment	➢ Includes – Acute urethritis – Acute cystitis – Acute prostatitis – Acute pyelonephritis – Renal abscess – Septicemia with septic shock ➢ Requires antimicrobial therapy

Anatomic Classification of Urinary Tract Infections

- **Lower urinary tract infections:** Include cystitis (bladder), prostatitis, and urethritis.
- **Upper urinary tract infections:** Include infection of kidneys and their collecting systems (pyelonephritis) and perinephric abscess.

Etiology

Q. What are the predisposing causes of urinary tract infection?

Q. Write short essay on:
- **Etiology and factors responsible for urinary tract infections.**
- **Risk factors for urinary tract infections.**

Causative organisms: Majority (~85%) of UTI are the caused by **gram-negative bacilli** which are normal inhabitants of the intestinal tract (enteric origin).
- **Most common pathogens:** ***Escherichia coli*** (80% cases), *Proteus, Klebsiella, Enterobacter,* and *Pseudomonas.*
- **Less common:** *Streptococcus faecalis*, staphylococci, and fungi.
- **In immunocompromised patients: Viruses** (polyoma virus, cytomegalovirus, and adenovirus).

Pathogenesis (Fig. 13.20)

Q. Differences between male and female urinary tract infection.

Route of infection: Bacteria can reach urinary tract via the bloodstream, the lymphatics or by direct extension (e.g., from a vesicocolic fistula), but in majority of cases via the ascending transurethral (via the urethra) route.

A. **Ascending infection:** It is the **most common route** of infection of the renal parenchyma, i.e., pyelonephritis. It is a form of endogenous infection, where the source of infecting organisms is the **patient's own fecal flora**. The infection ascends from the lower urinary tract into the renal parenchyma. Different steps in the pathogenesis of pyelonephritis are:
   - **Colonization of the distal urethra and introitus** (in the female): By enteric or coliform bacteria from the perineum due to poor hygiene and hormonal effects.

- **Entry from the urethra to the bladder**: Organisms may enter the bladder during **urethral catheterization or other instrumentation.** Urinary infections are more common in females, because of:
  - Shorter urethra (4 cm)
  - Absence of prostatic fluid which has antibacterial properties
  - Hormonal changes in women which affect the adherence of bacteria to the mucosa.
  - Trauma to the urethra during sexual intercourse facilitates entry of introital bacteria into the bladder.
  - Gram-negative enteric organisms residing around the anal region also colonize the periurethral region.
- **Urinary tract obstruction and stasis of urine**

Q. Write short note on causes of urinary tract infection in male.

- **Obstruction/bladder dysfunction:** Causes incomplete emptying and increased residual volume of urine. Examples: benign prostatic hypertrophy, tumors, strictures, or calculi.
- **Neurogenic bladder dysfunction:** Diabetes, spinal cord injury, tabes dorsalis, and multiple sclerosis predisposes to UTI.
- **Stasis:** Organisms introduced into the bladder can multiply when there is stasis.

B. **Hematogenous route:** It is less common route of infection. Because of rich blood supply, bacteria can seed the kidneys during the course of septicemia or infective endocarditis through the bloodstream. It occurs with nonenteric organisms (e.g., staphylococci), fungi, and viruses. Hematogenous infections occur in: (i) the presence of ureteral obstruction, (ii) debilitated patients, and (iii) patients receiving immunosuppressive therapy.

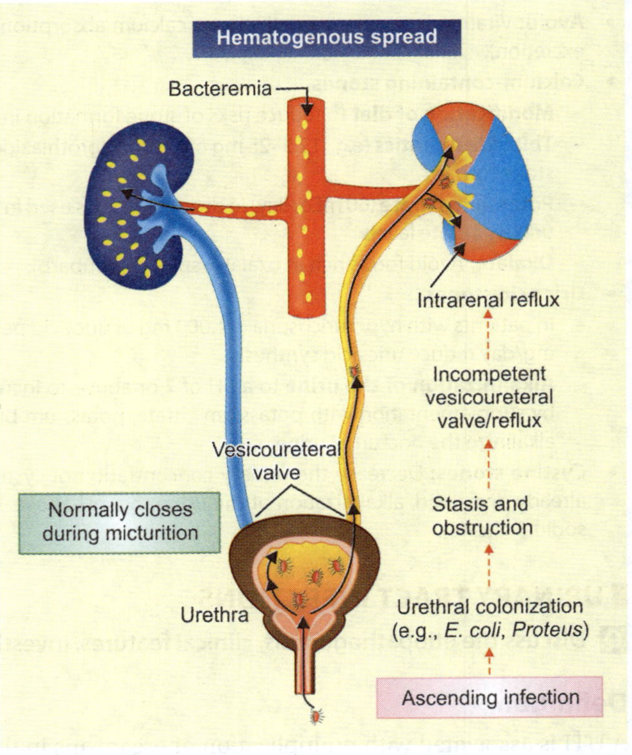

FIG. 13.20: Pathogenesis of acute pyelonephritis. More common mode is ascending infection. Hematogenous infection results from bacteremic spread.

Clinical Features (Table 13.31)

Q. List the differences between complicated and uncomplicated UTI.

TABLE 13.31: Clinical features of UTI.

➢ Fever with chills and rigors	➢ Suprapubic pain and tenderness resulting from cystitis
➢ Micturition abnormalities – Increased frequency of micturition – Dysuria (painful voiding) or scalding micturition – Urgency – Strangury: Intense desire to pass more urine after the bladder has been emptied. It is due to detrusor spasm and occurs in cystitis.	➢ Urine: – Hematuria – Cloudy urine with an unpleasant odor

Uncomplicated versus Complicated UTI (Table 13.32)

TABLE 13.32: Differences between uncomplicated versus complicated urinary tract infection (UTI).

Features	*Uncomplicated urinary tract infection*	*Complicated urinary tract infection*
Characteristics	UTI occurring in patients with functionally normal urinary tracts	UTI occurring in patients with abnormal urinary tracts (e.g., with stones, or associated diseases such as diabetes mellitus) or infection that extends beyond the bladder
Lesions	Includes cystitis or urethritis due to bacterial colonization of the bladder or urethra	Infection of renal parenchyma and renal pelvis (pyelonephritis) or prostate (prostatitis)
Sex affected	Much more in females than in males	Infection in men often considered complicated
Predisposing factors	May not be obvious	Usually occurs in presence of obstructive lesions or following instrumentation on urinary tract
Clinical features	Burning on urination and frequent urination without fever or flank pain	Accompanied by fever or flank pain ➢ Costovertebral angle tenderness ➢ Pelvic or perineal pain in men (prostatitis)
Prognosis	Responds well to treatment and persistent or recurrent infection seldom results in serious kidney damage	May be difficult to treat and relapses after treatment are common
Sequelae	Rare	Common such as sepsis, metastatic abscesses, and renal failure

Acute urethral syndrome: About one-third of females with dysuria and pregnancy have either insignificant bacteria in midstream culture or completely sterile cultures and is known as acute urethral syndrome. It is often due to infection with usual organisms (culture shows only 10^2–10^4 bacteria) or due to unusual organism (*Neisseria gonorrhoeae, Chlamydia trachomatis*).

Causes of Dysuria (Box 13.24)

Factors Determining Symptomatic Infection

- *Virulence:* Ability of the organism to adhere to epithelial cells determines the degree of virulence.
- *Innate host defense:* The following hosts defense mechanisms are required for the prevention of UTI:
  - *Neutrophils:* Activation of neutrophils is necessary for bacterial killing and their impaired function predisposes an individual to severe UTI.
  - *Complement:* Complement activation with IgA production by uroepithelium (acquired immunity) plays a major role in defense against UTI.
  - *Commensal organisms* (e.g., lactobacilli)*: Form* part of the normal host defense and their eradication by spermicidal jelly or disruption by certain antibiotics results in overgrowth of *E. coli.*
  - *Urine flow* and normal micturition: Wash out bacteria and stasis of urine predisposes to UTI.
  - *Uroepithelium*—mannosylated proteins: Such as Tamm-Horsfall proteins (THPs), have antibacterial properties and are present in the mucus and glycocalyx covering uroepithelium. Normally, they interfere with bacterial binding to uroepithelium. Thus, disruption of this uroepithelium by trauma (e.g., sexual intercourse or catheterization) predisposes to UTI.
- Pregnancy is associated with an increased incidence of UTI. Factors that favor UTI include: (1) decreased ureteral tone (progestational activity), (2) decreased ureteral peristalsis, and (3) transient incompetence of the vesicoureteral valves.

Factors that indicate a complicated UTI

- **A**natomical abnormality of the urinary tract
- **B**acterial persistence in spite of adequate therapy
- **C**hildhood UTI
- **D**iabetes
- **E**lderly
- **F**unctional abnormality of the urinary tract [vesicoureteric reflux (VUR); neurogenic dysfunction]
- **G**estational (pregnancy); **G**ender-male
- **H**ospital acquired (catheter induced, instrumentation, stents)
- **I**mmunosuppression

Box 13.24: Causes of dysuria.

- Urinary tract infections (e.g., urethritis, cystitis, vaginitis, pyelonephritis)
- Sexually transmitted infections
- Genital herpes
- Chlamydia
- Gonorrhea
- Inflammation and irritation of bladder and urethra, e.g., stones

Honeymoon Cystitis (or "Honeymoon Disease")

Q. Write short note on honeymoon cystitis.

Honeymoon cystitis is caused as a result of frequent or prolonged sexual activity, as would typically be expected in the honeymoon period of a marriage. It can occur when a woman has sex for the first time, or when a woman has sex after a long period of time without any sexual activity.

Symptoms: Same as with cystitis due to other cause.

During sex, *E. coli* on the skin around your anus can be transferred to urethra of women (for example, via partner's fingers or penis).

Investigations

Urine Examination

- **Dipstick tests:** Most gram-negative organisms reduce nitrates to nitrites and dipstick tests (nitrite test) are used to detect nitrite in urine. Dipsticks that detect significant

Symptoms and Signs of UTI

Constitutional:

- Malaise
- Listlessness
- Fever
- Chills
- Nausea and vomiting

Upper tract—symptoms	Upper tract—signs
• Flank pain	• Flank/CVA tenderness
• Back ache	• Flank mass
• Heaviness in the flank	• Scoliosis
	• Psoas spasm
Lower tract—symptoms	**Lower tract—signs**
• Frequency	• Suprapubic tenderness
• Scalding urination	• Bladder distension (bladder outlet obstruction)
• Urgency	• Urethral discharge
• Strangury	• Urethral tenderness
• Hematuria	
• Turbid urine (pyuria)	
• Foul smelling urine	
• Pneumaturia/fecaluria	
Genital-female—symptoms	**Genital-female—signs**
• Leukorrhea	• Vaginal discharge
• Dyspareunia	• Pelvic organ prolapse
• Pruritus vulvae	• Atrophic vaginitis
Genital-male—symptoms	**Genital-male—signs**
• Pain in the urethra	• Phimosis, balanoposthitis
• Deep perineal pain	• Urethral tenderness
• Orchalgia	• Periurethral abscess
	• Perineal tenderness (cowperitis)
	• Signs of epididymo-orchitis
	• Prostatic enlargement on DRE

(CVA: costovertebral angle; DRE: digital rectal examination)

pyuria depend on the release of esterases from leukocyte (leukocyte esterase test). Positive dipstick tests for both nitrite and leukocyte esterase are highly predictive of acute infection.
- **Microscopic examination:** For leukocytes, leukocyte casts and red cells.
- **Culture and sensitivity** of a freshly voided clean-catch midstream specimen of urine.

Box 13.25 lists causes of sterile pyuria.

Box 13.25: Causes of sterile pyuria.
- Partially treated UTI
- Tuberculosis of urinary tract
- Calculi in urinary tract
- Infection with other organisms (e.g., *Chlamydia, Corynebacterium*, etc.)
- Tumors of bladder
- Chemical cystitis/drugs
- Prostatitis
- Interstitial nephritis
- Appendicitis

Special Investigations

- Prostatitis
  - Per rectal examination of the prostate
  - Prostatic massage followed by urine culture
- Cystitis: Cystoscopy.
- **Renal ultrasonography CT-KUB, MR urogram:** To identify obstruction, cysts, and calculi.
- **Intravenous urography (IVU),** including a postvoid film of bladder: To identify physiological and/anatomical abnormalities of urinary tract.
- Dimercaptosuccinic acid (DMSA) renal scan: For pyelonephritis.
- Micturating cystourethrogram (**MCU**) to identify vesicoureteric reflux and disturbed bladder emptying.
- In females with recurrent UTI, **pelvic examination** to exclude cystocele, rectocele, and uterine prolapse.

Treatment
- **Antibiotic therapy:** The choice of antibiotic depends on the result of urine culture and sensitivity of urine.
  - The commonly employed antibiotics include cotrimoxazole (trimethoprim and sulfamethoxazole 1 double strength tablet two times daily), ampicillin (250 mg three times daily), amoxicillin (250 mg 8-hourly three times daily), oral cephalosporin, nitrofurantoin (50 mg three times daily), and quinolones. Treatment is over 3–5 days in uncomplicated infections (nitrofurantoin for 7 days) and for 7–10 days in complicated infections.
- **Hospitalized patients:**
  - No risk factors for infection with a multidrug-resistant organism → ceftriaxone (1 g IV once daily) or piperacillin-tazobactam (3.375 g IV every 6 hours)
  - At least one risk factor for infection with a multidrug-resistant organism → antipseudomonal carbapenem (imipenem 500 mg IV every 6 hours, meropenem 1 g IV every 8 hours, or doripenem 500 mg IV every 8 hours).
  - *Enterococcus* species or MRSA are suspected → add vancomycin, daptomycin, or linezolid.
  - "Single-shot" treatment with 3 g of amoxicillin or 1.92 g of cotrimoxazole can be used in patients with bladder symptoms of less than 36 hours duration and without any previous history of UTI.
  - If patients has a calculi, catheter or other obstructions, no antibiotic is necessary unless symptomatic.
- **Fluid intake:** A high (2 L daily) fluid intake during treatment and for some subsequent weeks to initiate water diuresis, so as to maintain a high rate of urine flow.
- **Other measures:**
  - Regular complete emptying of urinary bladder at 2- to 3-hour intervals.
  - Alkalinization of urine
  - Urinary analgesics (e.g., phenazopyridine) and antispasmodics (e.g., hyoscyamine) to be given for detrusor spasm.
  - If patients presents for the first time with high fever, loin pain and tenderness, urgent renal ultrasound examination is performed to exclude an obstructed pyonephrosis. If this is present percutaneous nephrostomy is performed to drain it.
  - Cranberry juice inhibits adherence of uropathogens to uroepithelial cells, hence advisable to prevent recurrent UTI.
  - In females: The incidence of UTIs can be reduced by (1) adequate perineal hygiene, (2) emptying the bladder before bedtime and before and after intercourse, and (3) application of 0.5% cetrimide cream to periurethral area before intercourse. Atrophic vaginitis should be identified and treated in postmenopausal women.
  - Avoidance of constipation (may impair bladder emptying).

Asymptomatic bacteriuria: It requires treatment (1) if a patient is pregnant, (2) in case of renal transplantation, or (3) before planning for a urologic surgery. Treatment of asymptomatic bacteriuria in pregnant women decreases the occurrence of pyelonephritis.

ACUTE PYELONEPHRITIS

Q. Discuss the etiology, clinical features, investigations, diagnosis, and management of acute pyelonephritis.

Q. Write short essay/note on common causes, diagnostic features, and management of upper urinary tract infections.

Definition: Acute pyelonephritis is an acute suppurative inflammation of upper urinary tract affecting the tubules, interstitium, and renal pelvis. There is often coincident cystitis.

Clinical Features

Classic triad: (1) loin pain, (2) fever, and (3) tenderness over the kidneys. Presence of this triad and significant bacteriuria usually indicates acute pyelonephritis.

- Sudden onset of pain in one or both loins (costovertebral/renal angle), radiating to the iliac fossa and suprapubic area.
- Fever with chills and rigors, and malaise
- **Tenderness and guarding in the renal angle**
- Dysuria, frequency, and urgency. Frequent passage of small amount of urine accompanied by scalding, cloudy urine.
- Acute pyelonephritis caused by the presence of obstruction (e.g., stone, tumor, bladder neck obstruction, enlarged prostate), can be very severe and may progress to renal abscess.
- Rarely, acute pyelonephritis may be associated with necrotizing papillitis/papillary necrosis. Causes include diabetes mellitus, chronic urinary obstruction, analgesic nephropathy, and sickle-cell disease.

Investigations

Q. Write short note on urinary abnormalities in acute pyelonephritis.

- **Peripheral blood:** Characteristically shows leukocytosis.
- **Urine examination**
  - **Microscopy** shows numerous pus cells and organisms, WBC casts, some red cells, and epithelial cells.
  - **Culture** of midstream urine (MSU) shows growth the causative organism.
- **Other investigations:** When the diagnosis is uncertain, other investigation are required to exclude anatomical abnormalities of the urinary tract. When acute pyelonephritis is severe, the possibility of any obstruction or abscess formation must be excluded. It is also necessary, if there is inadequate response or rapid recurrence of pyelonephritis following appropriate therapy.
  - **Ultrasonography:** Most frequently done, but is relatively insensitive.
  - **Computerized tomography (CT)** is performed if ultrasound is normal. It can detect calculi, obstruction, hemorrhage, gas, enlargement of kidney, and inflammatory masses (damaging renal function).
  - **Intravenous urography** is usually not done at present.
  - **Radionuclide scan:** The radionuclide agent is injected into bladder through suprapubic route may be useful to detect reflux.
  - **Dimercaptosuccinic acid renal scan:** If performed within 2 days DMSA can help diagnosing acute pyelonephritis. It is advisable to scan after 4–6 months of an acute episode to detect renal parenchymal damage.

Management

Intravenous antibiotics: Intravenous ampicillin, amoxicillin plus aminoglycosides (e.g., tobramycin), cephalosporin (e.g., cefuroxime), quinolone (e.g., ciprofloxacin), or a combination beta-lactam/beta-lactamase inhibitor (piperacillin-tazobactam) or carbapenem (meropenem) (discussed above).

Persistent or Recurrent UTI

Q. Write short essay/note on persistent or recurrent urinary tract infection and its management.

- In some patients with UTI, the causative organism persists on repeat culture of urine in spite of treatment, or reinfection develops with any organism after an interval. Such cases, there is more probably an underlying cause is present and hence a more detailed investigation is necessary.
- Recurrent infections are common in females.
- Recurrent UTI, especially in the presence of an underlying cause may produce permanent renal damage. If an underlying cause cannot be treated, suppressive antibiotic therapy can prevent recurrence and reduce the risk of septicemia and renal damage.
- Culture and sensitivity of urine should be at regular intervals.

Treatment: Two or three antibiotics in sequence, rotating every 6 months often reduces the emergence of resistant organisms. Other methods discussed above.

Emphysematous Pyelonephritis

Q. Write short note on emphysematous pyelonephritis.

- It is a type of severe acute pyelonephritis most often caused by *E. coli* and *Klebsiella pneumoniae.*
- The major risk factors for emphysematous UTIs are diabetes and urinary tract obstruction.
- The infections primarily occur in women at a mean age of about 60 years.
- Abdominal pain is the major clinical manifestation with renal angle tenderness. Pneumaturia may be seen after bladder catheterization.
- The diagnosis of emphysematous UTIs is made by abdominal imaging; computed tomography is more sensitive than plain films and can detect obstructing lesions.
- Treatment: Parenteral antibiotics, percutaneous drainage/nephrectomy.

CHRONIC PYELONEPHRITIS

Q. Write short essay on the clinical features, investigations, and management of chronic pyelonephritis (reflux nephropathy).

Chronic pyelonephritis is a chronic inflammation of tubulointerstitial tissue leading to scarring of calyces, pelvis, and renal parenchyma.

Types

- **Reflux nephropathy (chronic reflux-associated pyelonephritis/atrophic pyelonephritis):** It results recurrent UTIs from a combination of factors such as:
  - **Congenital vesicoureteral reflux and intrarenal reflux:** Chronic pyelonephritis is so often associated with vesicoureteric reflux and some feel that it is better named "reflux nephropathy." Reflux may be unilateral or bilateral and accordingly causes scarring of one or both the kidney.
  - **Superimposition of a urinary** infection acquired in infancy or early childhood.
- **Chronic obstructive pyelonephritis:** Develops due to **recurrent infections** superimposed on obstructive lesions, which lead to renal inflammation parenchymal atrophy, and scarring.

Chronic pyelonephritis is an important cause of renal damage and ESRD. Morphological changes are depicted in **Figure 13.21**.

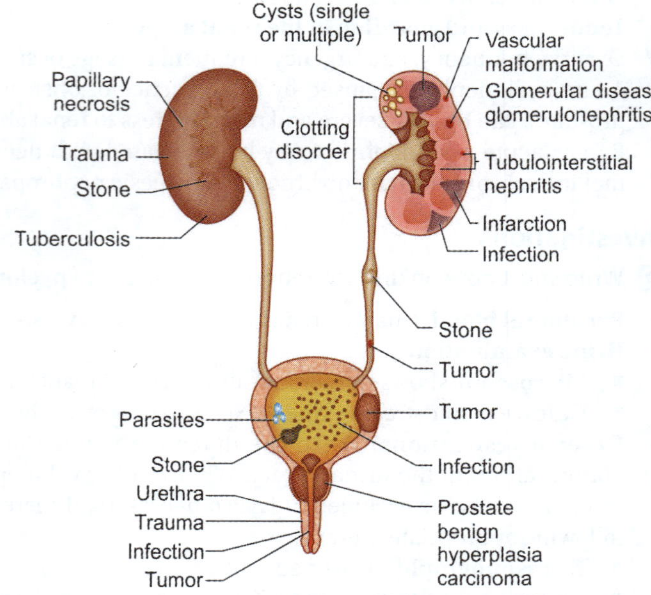

FIG. 13.21: Morphological changes in reflux nephropathy compared with normal.

Clinical Features

- Reflux pyelonephritis may be of silent onset. Clinical features includes back pain, lassitude, or symptoms of uremia or hypertension. Other symptoms include frequency of micturition, dysuria, pyuria, and bacteriuria.
- **Xanthogranulomatous pyelonephritis (XGP):** Predominantly affects elderly women. The condition is commonly associated with renal calculi or obstructive uropathy and is usually unilateral. The kidney is enlarged, and nonfunctioning and may even mimic a tumor.

Investigations

- **Culture of the urine:** *E. coli* is the most common organism causing infection. Other organisms include *Proteus, Pseudomonas aeruginosa,* and staphylococci.
- **Ultrasound of kidneys**
- **CT scan of the kidneys:** Diagnostically, it reveals irregular renal outlines, clubbed calyces, and a variable decrease in the size of kidney. The condition may be unilateral or bilateral and may affect entire or part of the kidney.
- DMSA scan is more accurate than IVU.
- **Intravenous urogram:** Shows localized contraction of the renal substance associated with clubbing of the adjacent calyces.
- **Micturating cystourethrogram (MCU):** Reveals vesicoureteric reflux, but has been replaced by radionuclide cystography scan.
- **Cystoscopy and urography:** May detect any abnormality causing obstruction to the flow of urine.

Management

- Eradicating predisposing factors:
  - Examples include treatment of calculi and malformations.
  - Surgery is performed if the vesicoureteric reflux persists and is indicated only when the disease is confined to one kidney. Most cases of childhood reflux likely to disappear spontaneously. Patients with end-stage renal failure require renal replacement.
- Treatment of infection: Meticulous early detection and control of infection can prevent further scarring and allow normal growth of the kidneys. Unfortunately, once the parenchyma is scarred it becomes susceptible to blood–borne reinfection sometimes with a different and resistant organism. Thus, antibiotics may be of temporary benefit and progressive renal damage is common.
  - Use of appropriate antibiotics for 7 days.
  - If the infection cannot be eradicated suppressive therapy may be given several months with trimethoprim (100 mg at bed time) or nitrofurantoin (50 mg at bed time).

- Other measures:
  - Complete emptying of the bladder should be advised.
  - Double micturition is advised if reflux. This consists of emptying of the bladder and then again second time attempt to empty the bladder, after about 10–15 minutes.
- Control of hypertension because severe hypertension is a relatively common cause of end-stage renal failure in childhood or adult life.

TUBERCULOSIS OF THE URINARY TRACT

Q. Describe renal tuberculosis.

Q. Briefly outline the clinical features, investigations, and treatment of tuberculosis of the urinary tract.

Tuberculosis of the urinary tract results from hematogenous spread from a distant primary focus of infection that is often impossible to identify.

Types of lesions in renal tuberculosis (**Figs. 13.22A to H** and **Table 13.33**).

TABLE 13.33: Types of lesions in renal tuberculosis.

Types	
Tuberculous papillary ulcer	Tuberculous perinephric abscess
Cavernous form	Pseudocalculi
Hydronephrosis	Caseous (putty) kidney
Pyonephrosis	Miliary

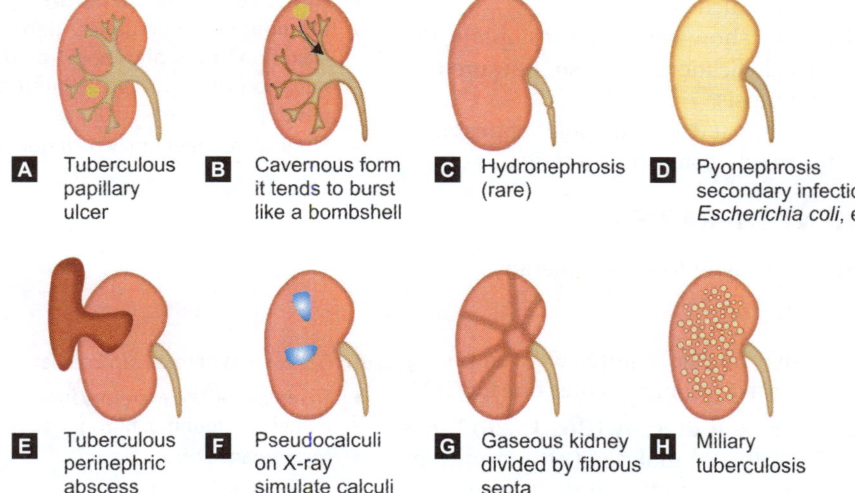

FIGS. 13.22A TO H: Various types of lesions in tuberculosis of kidney.

Etiology and Pathology

- Tuberculosis usually involves one kidney. Rarely, tuberculosis may be bilateral as part of the generalized process of miliary tuberculosis.
- Tuberculous granulomas in the region of renal pyramid may coalesce to form an ulcer and discharge mycobacteria and pus cells into the urine.
- Untreated lesions of renal tuberculosis may enlarge and form tuberculous abscess in the parenchyma.
- Fibrosis at the necks of the calyces and the renal pelvis may cause tuberculous pyonephrosis.
- Extension of tuberculous pyonephrosis or renal abscess may result in perinephric abscess and the kidney may be progressively replaced by caseous material (putty kidney). This may become calcified (cement kidney).
- Renal tuberculosis is often followed by infection of the ureters and bladder leading to ureteral stricture and contraction of bladder.
- Rarely, cold abscesses may form in the loin. In male, tuberculous epididymo-orchitis may develop even without any lesion in bladder.

Clinical Features

- Usually occurs between 20 and 40 years of age
- Affects males more commonly than females (2:1)
- Affects right kidney more commonly than the left

Symptoms

These include a dull ache in the renal angle, increased frequency of micturition, dysuria, and constitutional symptoms such as fever (evening rise of temperature) malaise and weight loss. Tuberculous cystitis present with hematuria and painful micturition.

- **Physical examination:** Shows an enlarged palpable kidney and tenderness in the renal angle.

Investigation

- **Urine examination:**
  - **Microscopic examination: Sterile pyuria** is characterized by urine containing pus cells, but fails to grow any organism on routine culture. This is the **characteristic feature.**
  - **Urine examination for tubercle bacilli:** Five early morning consecutive samples of urine should be examined (because there is usually intermittent excretion of tubercle bacilli). Alternatively, a 24-hour urine collection can be examined for acid-fast bacillus (AFB).
  - **Culture of the urine:** Diagnosis of active tuberculous infection depends on culture of mycobacteria from early-morning urine samples.
- **Radiography**
  - **Plain KUB radiograph:** It may show calcification (pseudocalculi) in the renal parenchyma and ureter.
  - **Chest X-ray:** Should be done in all cases to exclude active or previous evidence of pulmonary tuberculosis.
- **IVU:** May reveal irregular contour of the kidney, hydrocalyx, cold abscess, displacement of adjacent calyces, and small contracted bladder (systolic or thimble bladder).
- **Ultrasonography:** May show dilated calyces, hydronephrosis, small abscesses, and areas of calcification.
- **Excretion urography:** May show cavitating lesions in the renal papillary areas with calcification. May also show ureteral obstruction with hydronephrosis.
- **Cystoscopy:** May show a characteristic "golf hole" appearance of the ureteric orifice due to sclerosing periureteritis.

Treatment

- **Antituberculous chemotherapy:** Similar to that for pulmonary tuberculosis. Renal ultrasonography or excretion urography should be done 2–3 months after initiation of treatment as ureteric strictures may first develop in the healing phase.
- Surgical treatment may be required in selected cases.

RENAL REPLACEMENT THERAPIES

Q. Write short essay/note on renal replacement therapy.

Requirement

Renal replacement therapy (RRT) may be required on a temporary measure in patients with AKI or on a permanent measure for CKD.

Main options of renal replacement therapy (Box 13.26, Table 13.34 and Fig. 13.23): (1) Peritoneal dialysis, (2) intermittent hemodialysis (HD) combined with ultrafiltration, if necessary, (3) intermittent hemofiltration, (4) continuous arteriovenous or venovenous hemoiltration, and (5) hemodiafiltration, and (6) renal transplantation.

Box 13.26: Aim of renal replacement techniques.

- To replace all the excretory functions of the normal kidney namely excretion of nitrogenous wastes
- Maintenance of:
  - Plasma biochemistry
  - Normal electrolyte concentrations
  - Normal extracellular volume (fluid balance)

Note: They do not replace the endocrine and metabolic functions of the kidney

Hemodialysis

Q. Write short note on hemodialysis.

Q. Describe the types and indications for dialysis. Enumerate complications of hemodialysis.

Hemodialysis (**Fig. 13.24**) is the most common form of RRT used in ESRD and also in AKI.

Basic Principles

- In hemodialysis, blood from the patient is pumped through an array of semipermeable membranes (the dialyzer, often called an "artificial kidney").
- This brings the blood into close contact with dialysate (dialysis fluid) flowing countercurrent to the blood on the other side of membrane.
- This allows accumulated uremic toxins (e.g., urea and creatinine) and electrolytes (e.g., potassium) to diffuse across a semipermeable membrane (**Fig. 13.25**) from the blood (where they are in high concentrations), to the dialysis fluid on the other side (where they are in low concentrations). This in turn results in changes in the plasma biochemistry toward that of the dialysate due to the diffusion of molecules down their concentration gradients.

TABLE 13.34: Options of renal replacement therapy.

Options	
Dialysis	Clearance of small molecules and toxins using diffusion occurring across a membrane.
➤ Hemodialysis	Dialysis with clearance occurring across a synthetic membrane.
➤ Peritoneal dialysis	Dialysis with clearance occurring across a native peritoneal membrane.
Ultrafiltration	Fluid removal across a semipermeable membrane during dialysis by convection (solutes are moved under pressure across a membrane)
Hemofiltration	Continuous dialysis therapy which involves removal of plasma water and its dissolved constituents (e.g., K^+, Na^+, urea, phosphate) by convection flow across a high-flux semipermeable membrane, and concurrent reinfusion of an electrolytic solution of the desired biochemical composition
Hemodiafiltration	Combination of hemodialysis and hemofiltration
Continuous renal replacement therapies	Include hemofiltration and hemodiafiltration

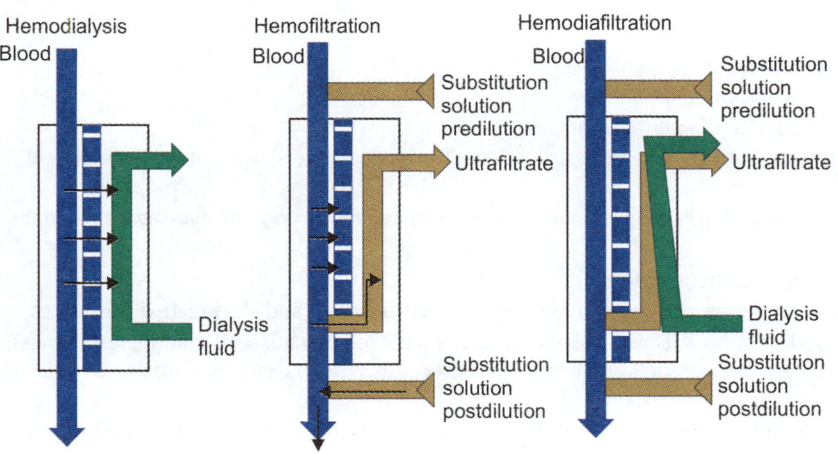

FIG. 13.23: Options of renal replacement therapy.

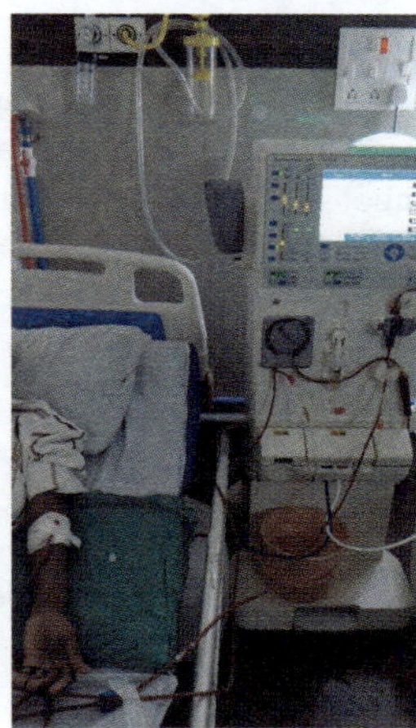

FIG. 13.24: Hemodialysis unit.

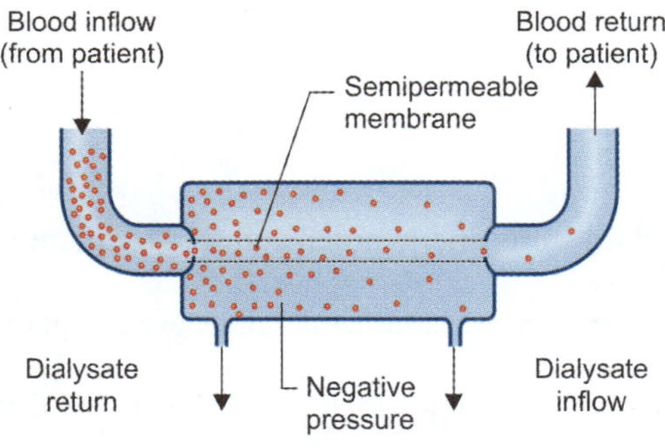

FIG. 13.25: Hemodialysis showing changes across a semipermeable dialysis membrane.

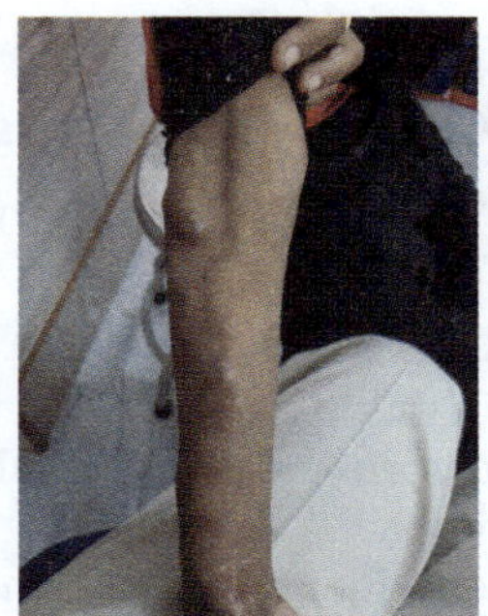

FIG. 13.26: Arteriovenous fistula (AV) created for dialysis.

Access for Hemodialysis

Usually for adequate dialysis, required blood flow is 200–300 mL/minute and the dialysate flow is 500 mL/minute. Hemodialysis involves gaining access to the circulation through:

- **Arteriovenous fistula (Fig. 13.26):** For long-term dialysis access to the bloodstream is achieved by surgical construction of an arteriovenous fistula, usually in the forearm using the radial or brachial artery and the cephalic vein.
- **Arteriovenous shunt:** In patients with poor-quality veins or arterial disease (e.g., diabetes mellitus) access is obtained by interposing a piece of synthetic material [polytetrafluoroethylene (PTFE) grafts] between native artery and native vein.
- **Central venous catheter:** If immediate dialysis is required, a large bore double lumen cannula may be inserted into a central vein (subclavian, jugular or femoral).

Each session of hemodialysis usually lasts for 4–5 hours. Two or three sittings/week may be required. Indications of RRT discussed under AKI.

Types of hemodialysis are depicted in **Figure 13.27**.

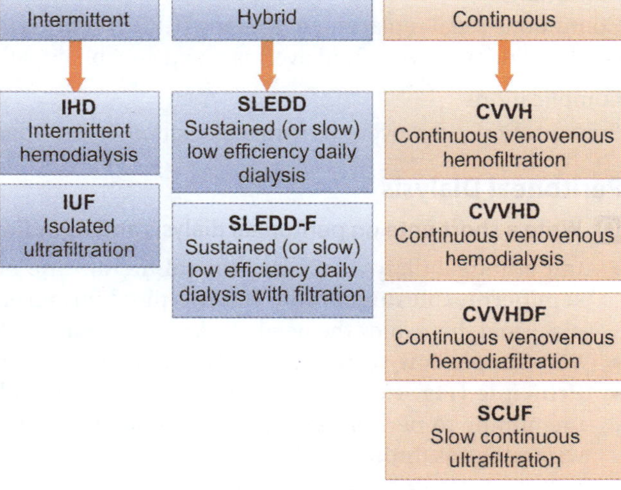

FIG. 13.27: Types of hemodialysis.

Complications

Q. Write short essay/note on complications of hemodialysis.

- **Hypotension during dialysis:** It is the major complication and its contributing factors include: (1) excessive removal of extracellular fluid and hypervolemia, (2) shift of fluid into intracellular compartment (due to rapid reduction in urea in the extracellular compartment) and inadequate "refilling" of the blood compartment from the interstitial compartment, (3) abnormalities of venous tone, (4) autonomic neuropathy, (5) acetate toxicity that causes vasodilatation, and (6) left ventricular failure.

- **Other complications:**
  - Cardiac arrhythmias due to potassium and acid-base shifts
  - Hemorrhage due to anticoagulants and venous needle discontinuation
  - Air embolism due to disconnected or defect lines and equipment malfunction
  - Anaphylactic reactions to the dialyzer may rarely occur to ethylene oxide (used to sterilize most dialyzers) or in patients receiving ACE inhibitors (with polyacrylonitrile dialyzers).
  - Hard-water syndrome due to failure to soften water resulting in a high calcium concentration prior to mixing with dialysate concentrate.
  - Hemolytic reactions
  - Infections usually occur with vascular access devices (catheter or fistula).
  - Pulmonary edema due to fluid overload. Other features include hypothermia, platelet consumption, and electrolyte disturbances.
- **Dialysis disequilibrium syndrome:** May develop following a dialysis session. It is characterized by nausea, vomiting, restlessness, headache, hypertension, myoclonic jerks, and in severe case, seizures and coma. This is because of rapid changes in plasma osmolality leading to cerebral edema.
- **Dialysis dementia:** May develop in patients on long-term hemodialysis. It is characterized by speech dyspraxia, myoclonic jerks, dementia, seizures and later, death. It is mainly due to aluminum toxicity and some may be due to viral infection.

The rate of death from cardiac disease is higher in patients on hemodialysis when compared to patients on peritoneal dialysis or after renal transplantation.

Acute Dialysis in Critically Ill Patients

Continuous Renal Replacement Therapy

Advantages

- It is used in critically ill patients who cannot tolerate large fluid shifts and hypotension that frequently occurs during standard hemodialysis.
- It allows slow and isotonic fluid removal. Thus produces excellent hemodynamic tolerance, even in patients with shock or severe fluid overload.
- Since dialysis is continuous, volume removal and correction of metabolic abnormalities can be modified at any time. This allows rapid adjustment in critically ill patients.

Continuous renal replacement therapy modalities

The most common is continuous venovenous hemodiafiltration. This combines convective and diffusive clearance through a dialyzer with reinfusion of electrolyte-rich solutions.

Indications

Continuous renal replacement therapy (CRRT) is of choice in patients with ARF combined with hemodynamic instability, cerebral edema, severe fluid overload, and encephalopathy.

Complications

Embolization, arteriovenous fistula formation, hemorrhage, and infection from catheter access.

Peritoneal Dialysis

Q. Write a short note on peritoneal dialysis and its indications (Box 13.27).

- In peritoneal dialysis, the **peritoneal membrane of the patient acts as a semipermeable membrane**. Through this diffusion of water and solutes takes place and this avoids the need of extracorporeal circulation of blood.
- **Very simple, low-technology** treatment when compared to hemodialysis.
- **Principle (Fig. 13.28A):** Solutes diffuse from blood across the peritoneal membrane to peritoneal dialysis fluid down a concentration gradient and water diffuses through osmosis.

Box 13.27: Indications for peritoneal dialysis.

- Preferred mode of dialysis for infants and young children
- Patients with severe hemodynamic instability on hemodialysis
- Patients with difficult vascular access

Procedure

- A plastic or silicone tube/catheter is placed into the peritoneal cavity through the anterior abdominal wall (**Fig. 13.28B**).
- Dialysate is instilled into the peritoneal cavity, usually under gravity.
- Urea, creatinine, phosphate, and other uremic toxins pass across the peritoneal membrane into the dialysate because of their concentration gradients.
- Water (with solutes) is attracted into the peritoneal cavity by osmosis.
- The fluid is removed by gravity after 30–60 minutes, and the fluid is changed regularly to repeat the process several times. This is called as intermittent peritoneal dialysis and is mainly used in ARF.

When chronic peritoneal dialysis required, a soft catheter is inserted, with its tip in the pelvis with an exit site in the lateral abdominal wall.

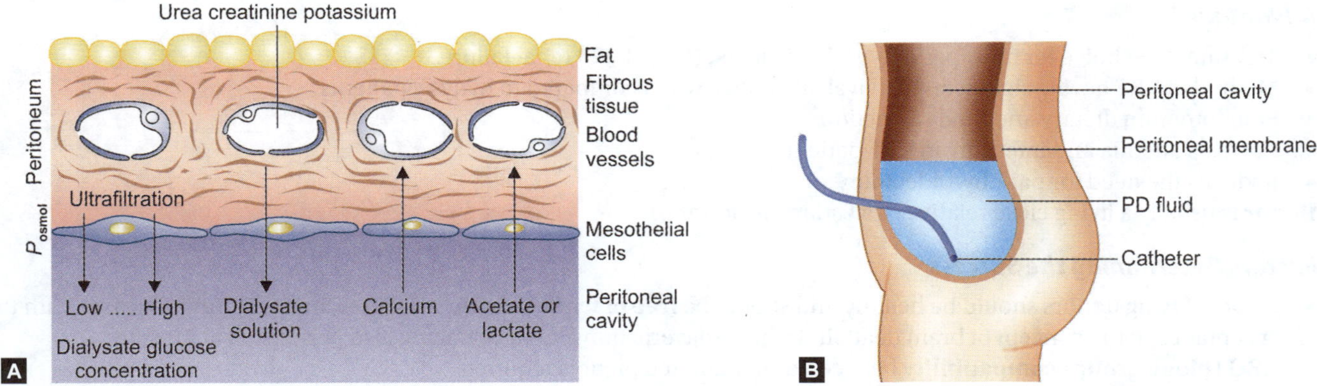

FIGS. 13.28A AND B: (A) Principle of peritoneal dialysis; (B) Peritoneal dialysis.

Complications

- **Technical complications:** Catheter-related exit site infection, tunnel infection, peritonitis, pericatheter leakage, poor drainage, catheter migration rarely bowel perforation.
- **Raised intra-abdominal pressure:** Hernias, fluid leaks, rectal prolapse, vaginal prolapse, low back pain, scrotal edema, and decrease in appetite, **sclerosing encapsulating peritonitis**.

Forms of Peritoneal Dialysis

- **Continuous ambulatory peritoneal dialysis**
  - In this type of peritoneal dialysis, dialysate is present within the peritoneal cavity continuously, except when dialysate is being exchanged.
  - Dialysate exchanges are performed 3–5 times a day.
  - About 1.5–3 L bags of dialysate are infused into the peritoneal catheter using a sterile no-touch technique.
  - Each exchange takes 20–40 minutes.
  - This technique is useful for maintenance of peritoneal dialysis in patients with end-stage renal failure (CRF).
- **Nightly intermittent peritoneal dialysis (NIPD):**
  - In this type of peritoneal dialysis, an automated device is used to perform exchanges each night (while the patient is asleep).
  - Apart from that night, sometimes dialysate is left in the peritoneal cavity during the day, to increase the time during which biochemical exchange is occurring.
- **Tidal dialysis:** In this type of peritoneal dialysis, a residual volume of dialysate is left within the peritoneal cavity with continuous cycling of smaller volumes in and out.

Differences between hemodialysis and peritoneal dialysis are presented in **Table 13.35**.

TABLE 13.35: Differences between hemodialysis and peritoneal dialysis.

Features	*Hemodialysis*	*Peritoneal dialysis*
Efficiency	Efficient	Less efficient
Duration and time interval	4 hours three times per week is usually adequate	Four exchanges per day are usually required. Each taking 30–60 minutes (continuous ambulatory peritoneal dialysis) or 8–10 hours each night (automated peritoneal dialysis)
Interval between dialysis	2–3 day between treatments	A few hour between treatments
Conduction of dialysis	Needs visits to hospital (although home treatment is possible for some patients)	Performed at home
Requirement	Requires adequate venous circulation for vascular access	Requires an intact peritoneal cavity without major scarring from previous surgery
Diet and fluid restriction	Required between treatments	Diet and fluid less restricted
Speed of removal of fluid and associated symptoms	Fluid removal compressed into treatment periods. May cause symptoms and hemodynamic instability	Slow continuous fluid removal. Usually asymptomatic
Infections	Infections related to vascular access may occur	Peritonitis and catheter-related infections may occur
Dependency of patient	Patients are usually dependent on others	Patients can take fully responsibility for their treatment

Renal Transplantation

Q. Write a short essay/note on renal transplantation.

Successful renal transplantation offers the best chance of long-term survival with almost complete rehabilitation in ESRD.

Advantages

- Treatment of choice for most patients with advanced (end-stage) renal failure.
- Method of RRT having significant survival advantage when compared to dialysis patients.
- Freedom from dietary and fluid restriction
- Corrects anemia and infertility in CRF patients
- Reduces the need for parathyroidectomy

Donor is usually a living close relative or a cadaveric donor.

Factors Determining the Success

- **Donor:** Living donors should be healthy and should be **free of hypertension, diabetes, or malignant disease**. With the acceptance of the concept of brain death in India, cadaveric transplants are being also performed at present.
- **ABO (blood group) compatibility** between donor and recipient is required.
- **Matching donor and recipient for HLA type:**
- **Among the 6 HLA types in each person (A/B/C/DP/DQ/DR), three HLA types are matched (HLA DR, HLA-B, HLA-A)**
  - It is preferable to have a donor with a HLA-identical that of the recipient. Matching for HLA-DR antigens (class II) appears to be most important for graft survival. Matching at the HLA-B locus (class I) has only a minor effect on graft outcomes.
  - Complete compatibility at HLA-A, HLA-B, and HLA-DR offers the best chance of long survival of the graft, followed by a single HLA mismatch (i.e., antigen possessed by the donor and not possessed by the recipient).
  - Class I antigens (HLA-A, B, and C) are detected by a lymphocyte assay and class II (HLA-DR) by mixed lymphocyte culture.
- **Cross-matching:** Presensitization (i.e., presence of antibodies against donor ABO blood group and HLA class I antigens) is detected by a cross-matching. Transplantation is contraindicated if it is positive.

Contraindications (Table 13.36)

TABLE 13.36: Absolute and relative contraindications for renal transplantation.

Absolute contraindications	*Relative contraindications*
Renal ➢ Reversible renal involvement ➢ Active glomerulonephritis ➢ Active vasculitis or recent anti-GBM disease ➢ Previous sensitization to donor tissue **Non-renal** ➢ Disseminated or active untreated cancer ➢ Severe occlusive aortoiliac vascular disease ➢ Severe psychiatric disease ➢ Persistent substance abuse ➢ Severe mental retardation ➢ Severe heart disease/refractory congestive heart failure ➢ Active infection	➢ Age: Very young children (<1 year) or older people (>75 years) ➢ Iliofemoral occlusive disease ➢ Diabetes mellitus ➢ Severe diseases of lower urinary tract: Bladder dysfunction or urethral abnormalities ➢ Chronic liver disease ➢ Treated malignancy ➢ Significant comorbidity

Technique

- Before transplantation, the recipient receives a hemodialysis to ensure a relatively normal metabolic state.
- In transplantation, donor human kidney (either from a cadaveric donor or from a living close relative) is placed in an extraperitoneal pouch in the **iliac fossa** of the recipient (**Fig. 13.29**).
- The renal artery and vein of donor kidney are anastomosed to the recipient's iliac vessels. The donor ureter is placed into the recipient's bladder. The recipient's original kidneys are left undisturbed.
- Eighty percent of grafts now survive for 5–10 years in the best centers, and 50% for 10–30 years.

Immunosuppressive therapy

- Unless the donor is genetically identical (i.e., an identical twin), immunosuppressive treatment is required to prevent rejection.
- Immunosuppressive therapy varies from center to center and combination of drugs is often used.
- Commonly used drugs include corticosteroids, antiproliferative agents (e.g., azathioprine, mycophenolate mofetil), calcineurin inhibitor (e.g., ciclosporin, tacrolimus, sirolimus), and antibodies [polyclonal antithymocytic globulin (ATG), antilymphocytic globulin (ALG), and monoclonal (OKT3) antibodies]. Newer drugs include basiliximab and daclizumab (antibodies against interleukin-2 receptor).
- Immunosuppressive agents can be classified as:
  - Induction immunosuppression:
    - Depleting agents:
      - Anti Cd-52 : Alemtuzumab
      - OKT3: Anti-CD3 monoclonal antibodies
      - Rabbit ATG

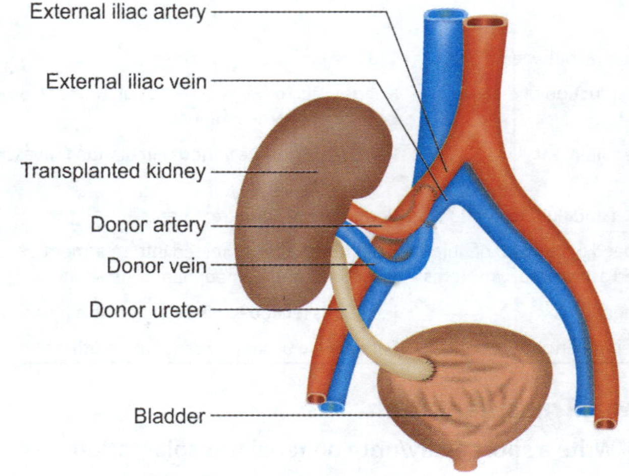

FIG. 13.29: Renal transplantation.

- Nondepleting agents:
  - Anti-CD-25: Basiliximab, daclizumab
- Maintenance immunosuppression:
  - Calcineurin inhibitors: Cyclosporine, tacrolimus
  - Mycophenolate mofetil
  - Steroids
  - mTOR inhibitors: Sirolimus

Complications (Fig. 13.30)

- **Acute tubular necrosis:** It is the most common cause of cadaveric graft dysfunction (up to 40–50%).
- **Technical failures:** These include (1) occlusion or stenosis of the arterial anastomosis, (2) occlusion of the venous anastomosis, and (3) urinary leaks owing to damage to the lower ureter, or defects in the anastomosis between ureter and recipient bladder.
- **Transplantation rejection:** In spite of prophylactic use of immune suppressants before or at the time of transplantation, most recipients undergo one or more type of rejection.
- Types of graft rejection:

- **Hyperacute rejection**
  - A special type of compliment-mediated rejection occurs if the host has **preformed anti-donor** antibodies (for example, anti-ABO blood type antibodies) in the circulation before transplantation. These antibodies bind to endothelium of graft organ, activates complement followed by vascular thrombosis.
  - Occurs within minutes. The transplanted kidney must be removed immediately to prevent a severe systemic inflammatory response and generalized clotting.

Category of infections: Nosocomial and procedure-related **Timeframe:** <1 month	**Category of infections:** Latent, prior, and opportunistic **Timeframe:** 1–6 months	**Category of infections:** Community-acquired **Timeframe:** >6 months
• Donor-related infections – HSV, LCM, rabies, West Nile viurs • Recipient-acquired infections – *Aspergillus* species – *Pseudomonas* species • Wound infections, line/catheter infections, aspiration, C. *difficile* colitis, drug-resistant organisms (MRSA, VRE)	• With PCP and antiviral prophylaxis: – BK polyomavirus, HCV, adenovirus, influenza – *Cryptococcus neoformans* – *Myocobacterium tuberculosis* • Without PCP and antiviral prophylaxis: – *Pnemocystis jirovecii* pneumonia (PCP) – Herpes family (CMV, HSV, VZV, EBV) – Hepatitis B virus – *Listeria, Nocardia, Toxoplasma* species	• Urinary tract infections • Pneumonia • Late viral infections • *Nocardia, Aspergillus, Mucor species* • *Actinomyces* species (rare)

Timeline of post-transplant infectious complications

Early → Intermediate → Late

Timeline of post-transplant noninfectious complications

Antibody-mediated rejection **Timeframe:** Minutes to hours	Borderline T-cell mediated rejection **Timeframe:** >5 days to 6 months	T-cell mediated rejection **Timeframe:** >5 days to years	Interstitial fibrosis and tubular atrophy **Timeframe:** >12 months to years

Perioperative renal artery thrombosis Timeframe: Minutes to hours	Ureteral stricture or obstruction Timeframe: Weeks to 6 months	De novo primary renal neoplasm Timeframe: >1 year

Perioperative acute tubular necrosis Timeframe: <2 days	Perioperative ureteral obstruction Timeframe: <2 days	Renal calculi Timeframe: >3 months	Donor-related malignancy Timeframe: >1 year

Hematoma Timeframe: Immediate to 5 days	Urinoma Timeframe: 10 days	Abscess Timeframe: Weeks to months	Lymphocele Timeframe: 2 weeks to 6 months	PTLD/lymphoma Timeframe: >1 year

Renal allograft compartment syndrome Timeframe: Immediate to 2 hours	Drug-related nephrotoxicity Timeframe: >2 months	Renal artery stenosis Timeframe: >3 months	Abdominopelvic complications Timeframe: Days to years

Renal vein thrombosis Timeframe: Immediate to 5 days	Post-biopsy pseudoaneurysm Timeframe: Anytime post-transplantation	Post-traumatic injury Timeframe: Anytime post-transplantation

FIG. 13.30: Summary of post-transplant infectious and noninfectious complications

- **Acute rejection**
  - **Time of occurrence:** Within days to weeks after transplantation in the nonimmunosuppressed host.
  - **Type:** Either cellular or humoral immune mechanisms may predominate.
    - **Acute cellular rejection:** Occurs within few months after transplantation and develops renal failure.
    - **Acute humoral rejection (rejection vasculitis):** Main target of the antibodies is the graft vasculature → manifest as vasculitis. Caused by anti-donor antibodies
    - **Features:** Acute rejection is characterized by deterioration of renal function, hypertension, weight gain, tenderness and swelling of the graft, fever and appearance of protein, lymphocytes, and renal tubular cells in the urine sediment.
    - If the diagnosis is not clear, percutaneous needle biopsy is performed for histopathological examination.

Treatment
- Use additional immunosuppressant including intravenous pulses of methylprednisolone and antilymphocyte antibody.
- Antibody-mediated rejection is less likely to respond to corticosteroids and may be treated with plasma exchange (to remove the antibody) and intravenous immunoglobulin.

- **Chronic rejection:** Few patients may develop irreversible chronic graft rejection.

- **Other complications**
  - **Infection** is the most important cause of morbidity and mortality. Risk of infections can be divided into three distinct time periods.

1. **First month post-transplant:** These include (a) infections present in the recipient before transplant and aggravated by immunosuppressive therapy (e.g., tuberculosis, systemic fungal infections, hepatitis B or C, HIV or smouldering bacterial infections); (b) infections transmitted through contaminated allograft; and (c) routine postsurgical bacterial infections of the wound, IV lines, and urine catheters.
2. **1–6 months post-transplant:** These include: (a) viral infections (e.g., cytomegalovirus, Epstein–Barr virus, hepatitis viruses, and HIV) and (b) superinfection with opportunistic bacteria or fungi (e.g., *Pneumocystis carinii, Listeria monocytogenes,* and *Aspergillus*).
3. **More than 6 months post-transplant:** These include (a) chronic progressive disease due to viral infections acquired earlier [e.g., progressive cytomegalovirus (CMV) chorioretinitis, progressive liver disease due to hepatitis B or C virus, and EBV-associated lymphoproliferative disorders]; (b) opportunistic infections with pathogens such as *Pneumocystis carinii, Cryptococcus, Listeria monocytogenes,* and *Nocardia asteroides* in patients with chronic graft dysfunction who have received multiple courses of antirejection therapy; and (c) infections similar to those in the community.

  - **Post-transplantation lymphoproliferative disorders:** Epstein–Barr virus-associated malignancies are common in those who received biological agents and in children.
  - **Malignancy:** Immunosuppressive therapy is associated with increases the risk of skin tumors (e.g., basal and squamous cell carcinoma). Incidence is 5–6% in Western countries and lower (2%) in India.
  - **Cardiovascular disease** is responsible for deaths in 20–30% of patients, especially the elderly and diabetics.
  - **Post-transplant hypertension** develops in up to 80% of patients early in the postoperative course and in 50% of stable recipients on maintenance immunosuppression.
  - **Post-transplant osteoporosis** is common due to treatment with steroids.
  - **Recurrent and de novo renal disease** is common (e.g., primary FSGS, type II membranoproliferative glomerulonephritis, diabetic nephropathy and IgA nephropathy, hyperoxaluria).
  - **Vascular:** Renal artery thrombosis and renal artery stenosis.
  - **Urologic:** Ischemic necrosis of the lower end of the ureter may produce urinary leak, calyceal-cutaneous fistula. Vesicoureteric reflux into the graft may lead to increased frequency of UTIs.

RENAL BIOPSY

Q. Write short note on renal biopsy and its indications.

It is used to establish the nature and extent of renal disease. Biopsy is performed transcutaneously with ultrasound guidance. Biopsy material is examined under light microscopy, electron microscopy and by immunofluorescence. Indications for renal biopsy are presented in **Table 13.37** and contraindications and complications of renal biopsy are presented in **Table 13.38**.

TABLE 13.37: Indications for renal biopsy.

Condition	Indication
Nephrotic syndrome	Routinely indicated in adult NS In children: In SRNS—before CyA starting/if CyA given >6 months to detect calcineurin toxicity
Nephritic syndrome	1. Normal C3 at presentation 2. After 6–8 weeks if: - Persistent low C3 - Gross hematuria - Nephrotic proteinuria 3. RPGN-like presentation

Contd...

Contd...

Other glomerular diseases ➢ **Alport** ➢ **IgAN** ➢ **HUS** ➢ **HSP**	to establish diagnosis
CKD	Normal kidney size (e.g., IgA nephropathy in ESRD can still be positive)
Renal transplant	To look for allograft dysfunction Done after ruling out: ➢ Urinary obstruction ➢ Urinary sepsis ➢ RAS ➢ Toxic CNI levels
AKI	To look for unknown etiology of AKI once prerenal and postrenal causes and acute tubular necrosis ruled out
Systemic disease with renal dysfunction	➢ Small vessel vasculitis ➢ Anti-GBM ➢ Lupus ➢ Diabetes: Only if atypical features present

(AKI: acute kidney injury; CKD: chronic kidney disease; CNI: calcineurin inhibitor; ESRD: end-stage renal disease; GBM: glomerular basement membrane; HSP: Henoch-Schönlein purpura; HUS: hemolytic uremic syndrome; IgA: immunoglobulin A; IgAN: IgA nephropathy; RAS: renin-angiotensin system; RPGN: rapidly progressive glomerulonephritis; SRNS: steroid-resistant nephrotic syndrome; CyA: cyclosporin A)

TABLE 13.38: Contraindications and complications of renal biopsy.

Contraindications	***Complications***
➢ Coagulation disorders ➢ Thrombocytopenia ➢ Uncontrolled hypertension ➢ Solitary kidney ➢ Renal neoplasms (to avoid spread along needle track) ➢ Large and multiple renal cysts ➢ Acute urinary tract infections ➢ Urinary tract obstructions ➢ Kidney less than 60% predicted size	➢ Pain ➢ Infection ➢ Bleeding into the urine ➢ Bleeding around kidney ➢ Arteriovenous fistula ➢ Accidental biopsy of other organ or perforation of organs such as liver, spleen ➢ Rarely death

CHAPTER

14

Fluid and Electrolyte Disturbances

DISORDERS OF SODIUM AND WATER BALANCE

Q. Write short note on the normal distribution of water in the body of an average adult male.

Composition of Body Fluids

- Water is the most abundant constituent of the body, accounting for about 50% of body weight in women and 60% of the body weight in men.
- Total body water is distributed in two major compartments:
  1. Intracellular fluid compartment (IFC) = 2/3rd of body water
  2. Extracellular fluid compartment (ECF) = 1/3rd of body water
     ECF consists of:
     - **Intravascular (plasma water)** compartment: 3/4th of ECF or 15% of total body weight.
     - **Extravascular (interstitial)** compartment: 1/4th of ECF or 5% of total body weight.

  For example, the distribution of body fluid in a man of 70 kg is as mentioned in **Table 14.1.**

Normal Water Balance

- In a normal person, daily fluid requirement = sum of urine output + net insensible fluid losses
  - Insensible fluid loss = 500 mL through skin + 400 mL through lung + 100 mL through stool = 1,000 mL
  - Insensible fluid input = 300 mL water through oxidation
  - Net normal daily insensible fluid loss = 1,000 mL - 300 mL = 700 mL
- *Hence, daily fluid requirement = urine output + 700 mL*
- Abnormal fluid loss:
  - 500 mL through moderate sweating
  - 1-1.5 L through severe sweating/high fever
  - 0.5-3 L through exposed wound surface (burns) and body cavity (laparotomy)
  - These parameters help to determine the daily fluid requirement in patients, especially those on intravenous fluids.

TABLE 14.1: Distribution of body fluid in a 70 kg man.

	Total	*ICF*	*ECF*	*Interstitial*	*Plasma*
% of body weight	60%	40%	20%	15%	5%
Volume for 70 kg weight	42.0 L	28.0 L	14.0 L	10.5 L	3.5 L

TABLE 14.2: Normal range of various electrolytes, pH, and osmolality of blood.

Component	*Normal range*	*Component*	*Normal range*
Sodium (Serum)	136–145 mmol/L	Calcium (Plasma)	9–10.5 mg/dL
Potassium (Serum)	3.5–5.0 mmol/L	pH of blood	7.35–7.45
Chloride (Serum)	98–106 mmol/L	Bicarbonate (Blood)	21–28 mmol/L
Magnesium (Serum)	2–3 mg/dL	Osmolality (Serum)	285–295 mOsm/kg water
Phosphorus (Serum)	3–4.5 mg/dL		

Electrolytes (Table 14.2)

- Electrolytes are ions that are either positively charged (cations) or negatively charged (anions).
- Sodium (Na^+) is the main cation, while chloride (Cl^-) and bicarbonate (HCO_3^-) are the major anions in the extracellular (ECF) compartment.
- Potassium (K^+) and magnesium (Mg^{2+}) are the major cations, while phosphate, sulfate, and protein are the major anions in the intracellular (ICF) compartment.
- The normal range of different electrolytes in the blood is as shown in **Table 14.2.**

OSMOLALITY, OSMOLARITY, AND TONICITY

- **Osmolality**: Osmolality of a solution is determined by the amount of solute dissolved in a solvent (i.e., water) measured in weight (kg). When osmolality is high, solution is more concentrated, and when the osmolality is low, solution is diluted.
- **Osmolarity:** Osmolarity is the concentration of osmotically active particles, expressed as milliosmoles per liter (mOsm/L).
- Plasma osmolarity = 2 × Na^+ (mEq/L) + glucose (mg/dL)/18 + BUN (mg/dL)/2.8
- In practice, *osmola'r'ity* is the same as *osmola'l'ity* (mOsm/kg H_2O) because 1 L of water is equivalent to 1 kg of water.
- **Tonicity vs osmolality:**
  - Osmolality refers to all particles in solution
  - Tonicity describes whether the particles are effective or ineffective osmoles.

VOLUME REGULATION AND OSMOREGULATION

Q. What are the factors that determine the control of ECF volume?

Q. Write a note on sodium balance.

Total body sodium is the main determinant of ECF volume: Regulation of the sodium balance, i.e., the difference between sodium intake and output, is crucial to maintaining normal ECF and plasma volume, with the kidney matching the urinary output of sodium with that of sodium intake.

A positive Na^+ balance would lead to ECF volume expansion, while conversely, a negative Na^+ balance would lead to ECF volume contraction.

Sodium intake: Daily sodium consumption varies widely between low-Na^+ diets containing 20 mmol/day (approximately 1.2 g salt/day) and high-Na^+ diets containing 200 mmol/day (approximately 12 g salt/day).

Sodium excretion: Figure 14.1 shows the renal handling of sodium by the nephron.

Na^+ is freely filtered across glomerular capillaries and is subsequently reabsorbed throughout the nephron.

1. *Proximal convoluted tubule (PCT)*: Approximately 2/3rd (67%) of Na^+ is reabsorbed.
2. *The loop of Henle*: About 25–30% is reabsorbed via apical Na^+ K^+ $2Cl^-$ transporter.
3. *Distal convoluted tubule (DCT)*: About 5% by thiazide sensitive Na^+ Cl^- cotransporter.
4. *Collecting ducts*: About 3% of Na^+ reabsorption takes place in the cortical and medullary collecting ducts.

The excretion of Na^+ is less than 1% of the filtered load, with more than 99% of the filtered load being reabsorbed.

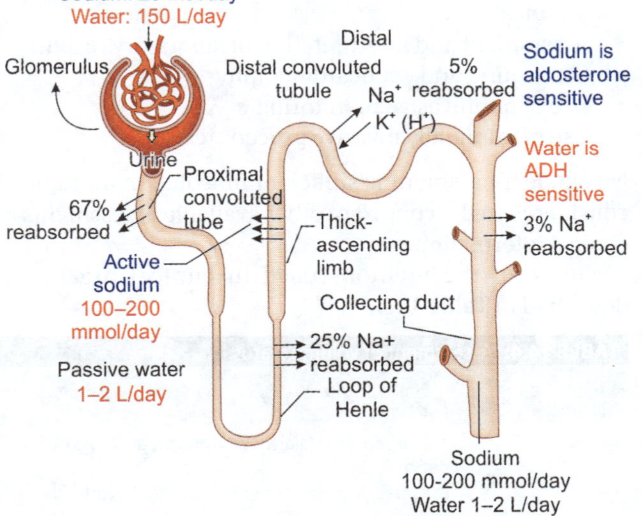

FIG. 14.1: Regulation of sodium excretion by kidney.

Renal excretion of sodium is regulated by four major steps:

1. *Renin-angiotensin-aldosterone system*:
   - The renin-angiotensin-aldosterone system is activated in response to decreased renal perfusion pressure.
   - Angiotensin II stimulates Na^+ reabsorption in the proximal tubule (Na^+–H^+ exchange).
   - Aldosterone stimulates Na^+ reabsorption in the late distal tubule and the collecting duct.
2. *Sympathetic nervous system (SNS) activity*: Baroreceptors sense a decrease in arterial pressure and stimulate the SNS and cause vasoconstriction of afferent arterioles and increased proximal tubular sodium reabsorption.
3. *Atrial natriuretic peptide (ANP)*:
   - ANP, secreted by the atria in response to an increase in ECF volume, causes vasodilation of afferent arterioles, vasoconstriction of efferent arterioles, increased GFR, and decreased Na^+ reabsorption in the late distal tubule and collecting ducts.
   - Other peptides in the ANP family, including urodilatin (secreted by the kidney) and brain natriuretic peptide (BNP) (secreted by cardiac ventricular cells and the brain), have similar effects to increase GFR and decrease renal sodium reabsorption.
4. *Starling forces in peritubular capillaries*:
   - Increase in ECF volume reduces the peritubular capillary oncotic pressure and inhibit proximal tubule Na^+ reabsorption.
   - Decrease in ECF volume increases the peritubular capillary oncotic pressure and stimulate proximal tubule Na^+ reabsorption.

Body fluid osmolarity is maintained at a value of about 285–290 mOsm/L by processes called osmoregulation.

Even minor changes in body fluid osmolarity produce a series of hormonal responses that influence the reabsorption of water by the kidneys, attempting to restore osmolarity back to normal value.

These renal mechanisms for the reabsorption of water are responsible for maintaining constant body fluid osmolarity.

Vasopressin, also known as **arginine vasopressin (AVP)** or **antidiuretic hormone (ADH)**, by its effect on the renal collecting system, is the major determinant which regulates the excretion of free water.

Increased serum osmolality stimulates osmoreceptors in the anterior hypothalamus, which in turn stimulates thirst and the secretion of ADH from the posterior pituitary gland. ADH circulates via the blood to the kidneys, where it leads to the increase in the water permeability of the principal cells of the late distal tubule and the collecting duct, resulting in increased water reabsorption. Because more water is reabsorbed by these segments, the osmolarity of urine increases and the amount of urine decreases. This, along with increased water intake, restores serum osmolarity to normal levels.

Conversely, reduced serum osmolarity, via inhibition of the osmoreceptors in the anterior hypothalamus, suppresses thirst as well as the secretion of ADH, which results in excretion of large amount dilute urine, restoring serum osmolarity to normal levels.

Table 14.3 summarizes the factors which determine volume and osmoregulation.

ASSESSING VOLUME STATUS

Q. How do you asses volume status?

Hemodynamic assessment methods include:

- Interpretation of history and physical examination findings
- Assessment and interpretation of laboratory results
- Ultrasound and echocardiography
- Use of noninvasive monitoring
- Use of minimally invasive procedures

No single assessment is sufficient in isolation and must be considered in the context of other available assessments and clinical information.

Some of the methods used in clinical practice are described in **Table 14.4**.

TABLE 14.3: Determinants of volume regulation and osmoregulation.

Factor	*Volume regulation*	*Osmoregulation*
Factor sensed	Effective arterial blood volume	Plasma osmolality
Sensed by	Baroreceptors	Hypothalamic osmoreceptors
Effectors	Aldosterone, angiotensin II, sympathetic nervous system	ADH, thirst
What is affected	Urine sodium excretion	Urine osmolality, thirst

(ADH: anti-diuretic hormone)

TABLE 14.4: Assessment of volume status.

Method	*Features*	*Invasive/ Noninvasive*	*Static or dynamic*	*Assesses fluid responsiveness*	*Comment*
History	Thirst/vomiting/diarrhea/hemorrhage: Indicate fluid deficit Dyspnea and pedal edema favor fluid overload	Noninvasive	Static	No	–
Charting	Fluid balance charts (input/output charting) 24-hour weighing—best measure of change in water balance	Noninvasive	Dynamic	Yes	Fluid balance charts do not measure insensible loss and may have irregularities in measurement and recording Weighing may be difficult in critically ill
Physical examination	Tachycardia, postural hypotension, low JVP, cold extremities, poor capillary return, dry mouth, sunken facies, altered mentation, and reduced urine output suggest hypovolemia Pulmonary edema, peripheral edema, raised JVP, and S3 gallop suggests volume overload	Noninvasive	Static and dynamic	Yes	Serial examinations may detect changes in organ perfusion
Passive leg raising (PLR)	The head and the upper torso are lowered to a supine position, while simultaneously raising the legs to a 45° angle for 4 minutes. This increases the venous return to the heart and is similar to the administration of 250 mL of fluid bolus. Hemodynamics are assessed before and after the PLR; if cardiac output improves, the patient is "fluid responsive" and administration of IV fluids should improve hemodynamics	Noninvasive	Dynamic	Yes	Unreliable with intra-abdominal hypertension, DVT in the leg, lower limb amputation
Biochemistry	Higher BUN: Creatinine ratio (>20:1), reduced urine sodium levels (<25 mEq/L), increased lactates suggest hypovolemia	Invasive	Static	No	Affected by drugs and other clinical conditions

Contd...

Contd...

Bedside ultrasound and echocardiography	Heart: Measurement of cardiac chamber function, pericardial tamponade Inferior vena cava: Collapse >50% indicates fluid tolerance Lung ultrasonography: More B lines correspond with increasing fluid overload. Also helps to identify pneumothorax, which causes obstructive shock	Noninvasive	Static and dynamic	Yes	Helps to identify various causes of shock such as cardiogenic, hypovolemic or obstructive
Central venous pressure	Central venous catheters through IJV or subclavian vein can be used to measure CVP Normal: 4–8 mm Hg Low CVP—hypovolemia High CVP—volume overload, cardiac causes such as CHF, cardiac tamponade, tricuspid regurgitation, pulmonary causes such as pulmonary embolism, tension pneumothorax, intermittent positive pressure ventilation	Invasive	Static	No	Poor correlation with fluid responsiveness
Pulmonary capillary wedge pressure (Swan-Ganz catheter)	A Swan-Ganz catheter is inserted through the IJV or the subclavian vein, and into the right atrium and ventricle to end in the pulmonary artery Commonly used in the management of postoperative cardiac patients and those with severe pulmonary hypertension	Invasive	Static	No	Poor correlation with fluid responsiveness
Stroke volume or pulse pressure variation	Pulse pressure analysis using data obtained form an arterial line helps to determine fluid responsiveness Steep variation—fluid responsiveness	Invasive	Dynamic	Yes	Requires sedated, mechanically ventilated patient
Transesophageal Doppler	A transducer is inserted into the esophagus to obtain accurate measures of stroke volume and cardiac output	Invasive	Dynamic	Yes	Not useful for continuous measurements
Thoracic electrical bioimpedance	Bioimpedance measures the resistance of electrical current through different body tissue and fluids, and can quantify the amount of tissue and fluid in the body	Noninvasive	Static	No	Not able to assess intravascular volume

DISTURBANCES OF BODY FLUIDS

The disturbances of body fluids can be grouped according to whether they involve volume contraction or volume expansion and whether they involve an increase or a decrease in body fluid osmolarity are described in **Table 14.5** and **Figure 14.2.**

TABLE 14.5: Disturbances in body fluids.

Type	*Example*	*ECF volume*	*ICF volume*	*Osmolarity*	*Hematocrit*	*Plasma (Protein)*
Isosmotic volume contraction	Diarrhea; burn	↓	No change	No change	↑	↑
Hyperosmotic volume contraction	Sweating, fever, diabetes insipidus	↓	↓	↑	No change	↑
Hyposmotic volume contraction	Adrenal insufficiency	↓	↑	↓	↑	↑
Isosmotic volume expansion	Infusion of isotonic NaCl	↑	No change	No change	↓	↓
Hyperosmotic volume expansion	High-NaCl intake	↑	↓	↑	↓	↓
Hyposmotic volume expansion	SIADH	↑	↑	↓	No change	↓

VOLUME DEPLETION (HYPOVOLEMIA)

Q. What is hypovolemia?

Hypovolemia, synonymous with ECF volume contraction, refers to a loss of salt and water.

Q. Describe the causes, clinical features, laboratory features, and treatment of volume depletion.

Causes of Hypovolemia

See **Table 14.6.**

TABLE 14.6: Causes of volume depletion (hypovolemia).

Extrarenal losses	*Renal losses*
➢ *Gastrointestinal losses*: – Diarrhea – Vomiting – Gastrointestinal bleeding – External drain (tube drainage or ostomies) ➢ *Sequestration into third space*: – Pancreatitis – Crush injuries – Intestinal obstruction – Skeletal fractures ➢ *Loss from skin*: – Excessive sweating – Burns	➢ *Excessive use of diuretics*: – Osmotic diuresis – Glycosuria in uncontrolled diabetes – Excessive use of mannitol ➢ *Diabetes insipidus*: Impaired ADH secretion/response to ADH ➢ *Renal disease:* – Tubular disorders – Recovery phase of oliguric kidney injury – Release of urinary tract obstruction – Chronic interstitial renal diseases ➢ *Deficiency of mineralocorticoids*: – Addison's disease

Clinical Features

Mild to Moderate Volume Loss

- Thirst
- Postural dizziness, weakness
- Dry mucous membranes and axillae
- Cold, clammy extremities
- Collapsed peripheral veins
- Delayed capillary refill time
- Tachycardia (pulse rate >100 beats/min)
- Postural increase in pulse of 30 beats/min or more

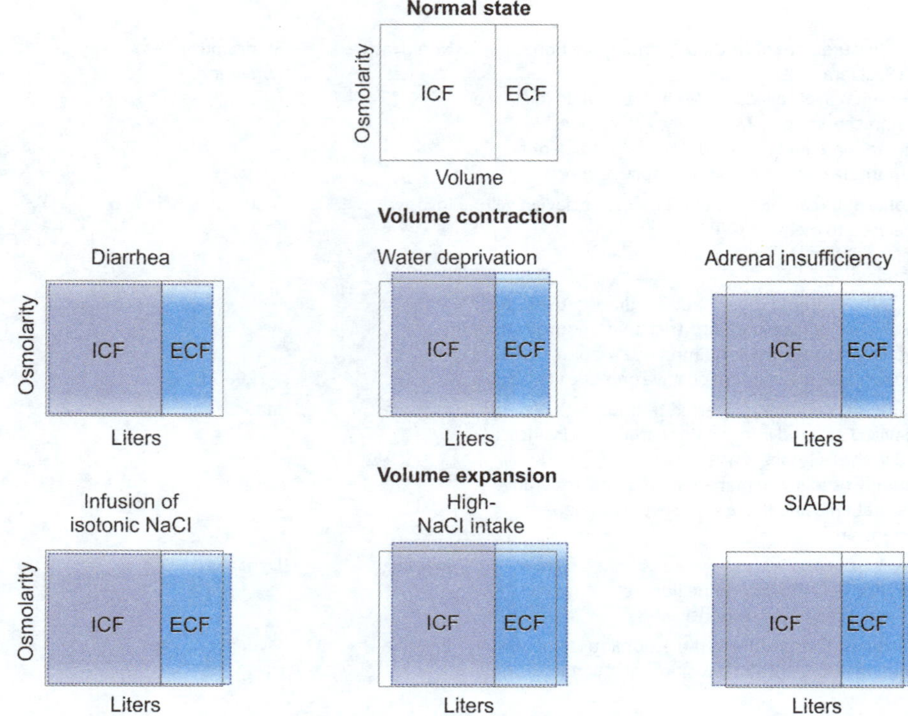

FIG. 14.2: Shifts of water between body fluid compartments.

- Postural hypotension (systolic blood pressure decrease >20 mm Hg on standing)
- Low jugular venous pulse
- Decreased urine output

Severe Volume Loss and Hypovolemic Shock

- Altered mental status (or loss of consciousness)
- Peripheral cyanosis
- Reduced skin turgor (in young patients)
- Marked tachycardia, low pulse volume
- Supine hypotension (systolic blood pressure <100 mm Hg)

Laboratory Features

- **Hematocrit:** Increased due to hemoconcentration. May be reduced if hypovolemia is secondary to hemorrhage.
- **Blood urea nitrogen (BUN) and creatinine:** BUN/creatinine ratio >20:1 is usually seen. This is due to a differential increase in urea reabsorption in the collecting duct. Confounding factors include upper gastrointestinal tract hemorrhage and administration of corticosteroids, which increase urea production, as well as malnutrition and liver disease, which diminish urea production.
- **Serum sodium:** Normal, reduced, or elevated depending on the proportion of loss between water and sodium.
- **Urine osmolality and specific gravity:** These are often elevated in hypovolemic states. However, these may be altered by an underlying renal disease that leads to renal sodium wasting, concomitant intake of diuretics or a solute diuresis.
- **Urinary sodium:** Hypovolemia normally promotes renal sodium reabsorption. Hence, urine sodium is low, typically less than 25 mmol/L in most cases of hypovolemia and states of low effective arterial volume. However, urine sodium concentration may be misleading in cases of:
  - Metabolic alkalosis (e.g. nasogastric suction or vomiting), as bicarbonaturia obligates excretion of a cation. Hence, the urine sodium concentration might not be low. In this circumstance, the urine chloride concentration should be measured, which will typically be <15 mEq/L.
  - Presence of acute tubular necrosis—kidney tubular function is impaired, thus the urine sodium concentration may not be low.
  - Use of diuretics
- **Urine chloride levels (Low):** It follows a similar pattern of urine sodium concentration because sodium and chloride are generally reabsorbed together. Urine chloride is a better measure than urine sodium in cases of volume depletion with metabolic alkalosis, as described above.

- **Fractional excretion of sodium**:
  - $[U_{Na} \times P_{creat} / U_{creat} \times P_{Na}] \times 100$.
  - In an oliguric patient with AKI, FE Na less than 1% is consistent with volume depletion; FE Na greater than 1% is more consistent with acute tubular necrosis.

Treatment
- The goal of treatment is to replace the fluid deficit and ongoing losses with a fluid that resembles the lost fluid.
- The cause of hypovolemia should be treated, where possible.
- Mild-to-moderate volume depletion (often due to gastroenteritis) should be corrected by increasing oral intake of sodium and water by an oral rehydration solution.
- In severe volume depletion, intravenous crystalloids such as normal saline or Ringer's lactate are usually the preferred initial choice for volume resuscitation.
- Transfusion of blood products is crucial for hemorrhage.

Q. What is dehydration? Describe the clinical features of dehydration.
- Dehydration refers to a loss of water.
- This should be differentiated from hypovolemia, which implies a loss of salt and water.
- Dehydration may cause manifestations of hypernatremia.
- **Table 14.7** describes the signs of dehydration depending on the degree of dehydration.

TABLE 14.7: Signs of dehydration depending on the degree of dehydration.

	Degree of dehydration		
Features	***Mild***	***Moderate***	***Severe***
Peripheral pulses	Normal	Slightly decreased	Difficult to palpate
Heart rate	Normal	Slightly increased	Significant increased with tachycardia
Capillary refill	Normal	About 2 seconds	>3 seconds
Mucus membranes and skin	Normal	Dry	Extremely dry
Eyes	Normal	Normal	Shrunken
Production of tears	Normal	Decreased	Absent
Amount of urine excreted	Normal	Decreased	Little or none
Fontanelle (in infants)	Flat	Soft	Shrunken

VOLUME EXPANSION (HYPERVOLEMIA)

- Hypervolemia is an expansion of the ECF compartment, due to an excess of total body sodium and water.
- Hypervolemia is typically due to renal retention of sodium and water.
- This renal retention may be primary or secondary.
- Secondary causes are secondary to reduced effective arterial blood volume depletion (arterial underfilling).
- Major causes of hypervolemia are listed in **Table 14.8.**

TABLE 14.8: Major causes of extracellular fluid volume expansion.

Primary renal sodium retention	***Secondary renal sodium retention***
➢ Acute kidney injury ➢ Advanced chronic kidney disease ➢ Glomerular diseases	➢ Cardiac failure ➢ Cirrhosis ➢ Nephrotic syndrome ➢ Idiopathic edema ➢ Drug-induced edema ➢ Pregnancy

EDEMA

Q. Define edema. What is anasarca?

Q. What are the common causes of generalized edema?

Q. List medications that can cause edema.

Q. Discuss the mechanism of edema formation. How will you differentiate between cardiac, renal and hepatic edema?

Definition

Edema: Edema is an accumulation of fluid in the interstitial space that occurs when local or systemic conditions cause capillary filtration to exceed the limits of lymphatic drainage.

Anasarca: It refers to generalized and massive edema, often accompanied by large effusions into the peritoneal, pleural, and pericardial spaces.

Table 14.9 shows the medications that cause edema.

Differences between the principal causes of edema are described in **Table 14.10.**

TABLE 14.9: Medications that cause edema.

Types of medication	***Class of medication***
Antihypertensive medications	➢ Calcium-channel blockers (nifedipine, felodipine, amlodipine, and verapamil) ➢ Direct vasodilators (hydralazine, minoxidil, diazoxide) ➢ Antiadrenergics (clonidine, reserpine, and methyldopa)
Chemotherapy	Cisplatin and docetaxel
Diabetic medications	Thiazolidinediones (rosiglitazone), insulin
Hormones	Estrogen, progesterone, testosterone, glucocorticoids, and fludrocortisone
Pain relief medications	NSAIDs
Psychiatric medications	Monoamine oxidase inhibitors Antipsychotics (olanzapine)
Immunological/ Immunosuppressant	Cyclophosphamide, cyclosporine, interleukin 2, OKT3 monoclonal antibody
Anticonvulsant	Pregabalin and gabapentin

Causes of Pitting Dependent Edema (Table 14.11)

Pathogenesis of systemic edema from congestive heart failure, renal failure, or reduced plasma osmotic pressure is shown in **Figure 14.3.**

Pitting edema may be divided into two categories:
1. **Rapid pitting** recovery within <40 seconds and is seen with hypoproteinemia.
2. **Slow pitting edema** (>40 seconds) is usually seen in patients with normal albumin levels **(Fig. 14.4).**

TABLE 14.10: Differentiating the principal causes of generalized edema.

Organ system	*History*	*Physical examination*	*Laboratory findings*
Cardiac	➢ Exertional dyspnea ➢ Paroxysmal nocturnal dyspnea ➢ Orthopnea ➢ Bendopnea ➢ Initial site of edema: pedal edema/sacral edema	Pulsus alternans, elevated jugular venous pressure, displaced or dyskinetic apical pulse, S3 gallop	Elevated BNP/NT-pro BNP
Hepatic	➢ Ascites ➢ Dyspnea, when associated with significant degree of ascites ➢ Jaundice	➢ Ascites ➢ Signs of chronic liver disease (jaundice, palmar erythema, spider angiomata, male gynecomastia or female breast atrophy, testicular atrophy; signs of hepatic encephalopathy) may be present ➢ Jugular venous pressure normal or low	➢ Reduced serum albumin, other hepatic proteins (transferrin, fibrinogen) ➢ Elevated PT/INR ➢ Liver enzymes may be elevated, depending on the cause and acuity of liver injury ➢ Thrombocytopenia may be present
Renal (CKD)	➢ Symptoms of uremia, such as decreased appetite, nausea and vomiting, altered (metallic or fishy) taste, altered sleep pattern, difficulty concentrating ➢ Decreased urine output ➢ Dyspnea	➢ Pallor ➢ Hypertension ➢ Uremic fetor ➢ Pericardial friction rub	➢ Elevation of serum creatinine and cystatin C ➢ Proteinuria ➢ Hematuria ➢ Hyperkalemia ➢ Metabolic acidosis ➢ Hypocalcemia ➢ Hyperphosphatemia ➢ Anemia
Renal (nephrotic syndrome)	➢ Periorbital edema ➢ Frothy urine	➢ Periorbital edema ➢ Hypertension	➢ Proteinuria (≥3.5 g/d) ➢ Hypoalbuminemia ➢ Hypercholesterolemia ➢ Microscopic hematuria

TABLE 14.11: Causes of pitting dependent edema.

Mechanism	*Causes*
Increased hydrostatic/ systemic venous pressure	**Systemic venous hypertension:** ➢ Congestive heart failure ➢ Pericardial diseases, constrictive pericarditis, and tricuspid valve disease
	Regional venous hypertension: ➢ Inferior vena cava syndrome ➢ Obstruction (e.g., venous thrombosis*) or compression of veins (e.g., external mass) ➢ Lower extremity venous insufficiency
Decreased plasma oncotic pressure (hypoproteinemia)	**Impaired protein synthesis:** ➢ *Decreased protein intake*: Starvation, kwashiorkor, and malnutrition ➢ *Decreased absorption of proteins*: Malabsorption ➢ Impaired hepatic synthesis due to liver disease **Increased loss of protein:** ➢ *Skin loss*: Burns, weeping skin diseases ➢ *Urinary loss*: Nephrotic syndrome ➢ *Fecal loss*: Bowel disease, malabsorption, protein-losing gastroenteropathy
Inflammation	Acute* and chronic inflammation*
Increased capillary permeability	Vasculitis*, idiopathic cyclic edema of women (varies with menstrual cycle), and postanoxic encephalopathy
Sodium retention	Excessive salt intake with renal insufficiency Increased tubular reabsorption of sodium, e.g., increased renin-angiotensin-aldosterone secretion

*Causes painful edema

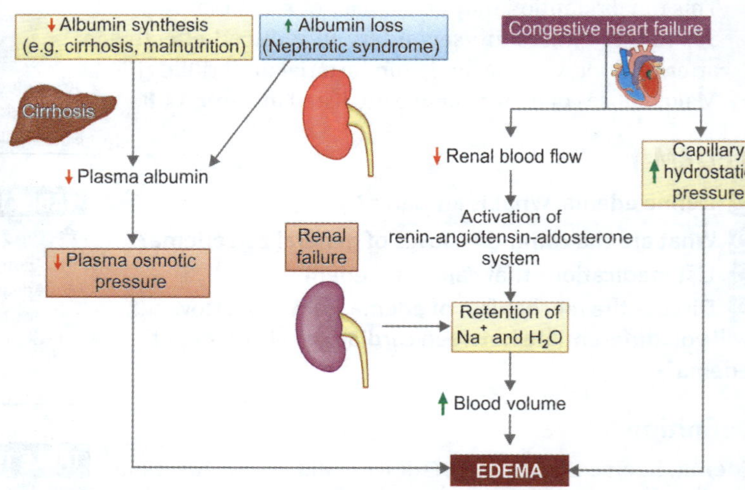

FIG. 14.3: Pathogenesis of systemic edema from congestive heart failure, renal failure or reduced plasma osmotic pressure.

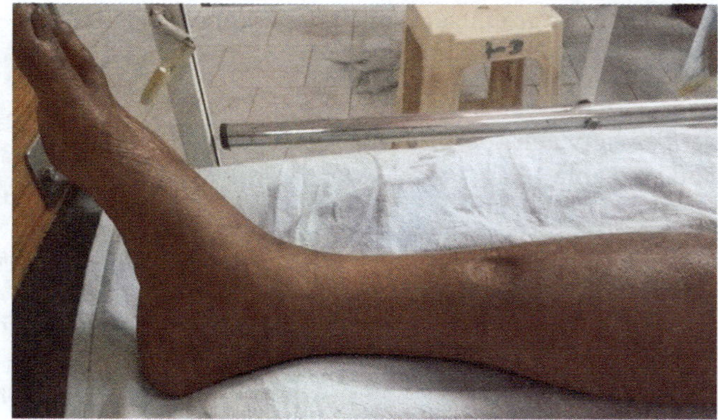

FIG. 14.4: Pitting edema in congestive heart failure.

Treatment of Extracellular Volume Expansion

Q. Discuss the principles of management of extracellular volume expansion/generalized edema.

General Management

- Recognize and treat the underlying cause
- Medications that promote sodium retention (e.g., NSAIDs) should be discontinued.
- Achieving negative sodium balance, by dietary sodium restriction and administration of diuretics.
  - Moderate dietary sodium restriction (2 g Na^{+}/day) should be encouraged.
  - Restriction of total fluid intake in patients with hypervolemic hyponatremia.
  - Diuretic therapy: Cornerstone of management of extracellular volume overload (described later).

Additional specific therapy based on the etiology:

- *Liver cirrhosis:* Large volume paracentesis with albumin infusion, TIPS (Transjugular intrahepatic portosystemic shunt)
- *Heart failure:* Use of ACE inhibitors and angiotensin receptor blockers (ARBs) to inhibit RAAS, ultrafiltration, and left ventricular assist devices
- *Chronic kidney disease:* ACE inhibitors and ARBs, renal replacement therapy (dialysis and kidney transplant)
- *Nephrotic syndrome:* Use of glucocorticoids, ACE inhibitors, and ARBs
- *Edema of nutritional origin:* Thiamine for beriberi, high protein diet.

DIURETIC THERAPY

Q. Describe various diuretics in use.

Q. Add a note on diuretic therapy in edematous patients.

- Diuretics are the cornerstone in the management of extracellular volume overload. They are also used in the management of hypertension.
- They act by inhibiting sodium reabsorption at various locations along the nephron.
- **Table 14.12** provides a summary of the various subclasses of diuretics.
- Caution should be exercised during therapy with diuretics as ECF volume expansion may have occurred in order to compensate for arterial underfilling, as in cirrhosis and heart failure.
- In these cases, overly rapid diuresis may lead to a significant reduction in the vascular space, which leads to decreased venous return to the heart, decreased cardiac filling pressures, decreased stroke volume, decreased cardiac output, and ultimately hypotension. Impaired renal perfusion may lead to prerenal AKI.
- This situation is more commonly seen in those patients with ascites, but without pedal edema.
- Rapid removal of excess fluid is generally necessary only in life-threatening situations, such as pulmonary edema and hypervolemia-induced hypertension.
- Most patients generally tolerate gradual correction of volume overload.

TABLE 14.12: Summary of diuretics.

Subclass, drug	*Site of action*	*Mechanism of action*	*Clinical uses*	*Toxicities*	*Comments*
Loop diuretics					
Furosemide, bumetanide, torsemide (sulfonamide loop diuretics) Ethacrynic acid: Not a sulfonamide but has typical loop activity and some uricosuric action	Ascending limb of Henle's loop	Inhibition of the Na/K/2Cl channel, leading to marked increase in NaCl excretion, K^{+} wasting, metabolic alkalosis, increased urine Ca^{2+} and Mg^{2+}	Pulmonary edema, peripheral edema, heart failure, hypertension, acute hypercalcemia, type IV RTA	Ototoxicity, hypovolemia, K wasting, hyperuricemia, hypomagnesemia	Potent diuretics used in diseases associated with significant edema
Thiazides					
Hydrochlorothiazide, metolazone Chlorothiazide: *Only parenteral thiazide available (IV)* Chlorthalidone	Distal convoluted tubule (DCT)	Inhibition of Na/Cl transporter in the distal convoluted tubule leads to increase in NaCl excretion, some K wasting, metabolic alkalosis, decreased urine Ca^{2+}	Hypertension, mild heart failure, nephrolithiasis, nephrogenic diabetes insipidus, osteoporosis	Hyponatremia, hypokalemia, metabolic alkalosis, hyperuricemia, hyperglycemia	Widely used in the treatment of hypertension and less severe edema. Metolazone is commonly used along with loop diuretic for "sequential blockade"
Potassium-sparing diuretics					
Spironolactone Eplerenone	Collecting tubules	Aldosterone antagonists: Reduce Na retention and K wasting in kidney	Cirrhosis of liver (up to 400 mg/day of spironolactone), heart failure with reduced ejection fraction (25–50 mg/day of spironolactone), hypertension associated	Hyperkalemia, gynecomastia (spironolactone, not eplerenone)	Weak diuretics Interaction with other K-retaining drugs such as ACE-I, ARBs, beta-blockers and NSAIDs

Contd...

Contd...

			with hyperaldosteronism and resistant hypertension (25–50 mg/day of spironolactone)		
Amiloride Triamterene	Collecting tubules	Blocks epithelial sodium channels (ENaC): Reduces Na retention and K wasting	Along with other diuretics to prevent hypokalemia from other diuretics. Prevention of amphotericin-induced hypokalemia and hypomagnesemia Reduces lithium-induced polyuria Liddle's syndrome	Hyperkalemia, metabolic acidosis	
Osmotic diuretics					
Mannitol	Multiple segments	Freely filtered at the glomerulus but not reabsorbed by any part of the tubular system. Retains fluid osmotically within the tubular lumen and limit the extent of sodium reabsorption in multiple segments. Marked increase in urine flow, reduced brain volume, decreased intraocular pressure, initial hyponatremia, then hypernatremia	Renal failure due to increased solute load (rhabdomyolysis, chemotherapy), raised intracranial pressure, raised intraocular pressure	Nausea, vomiting, headache	Not used for generalized edema
Carbonic anhydrase inhibitors					
Acetazolamide	Proximal convoluted tubule (PCT)	Indirectly inhibits Na^+-H^+ exchange by reducing the elimination of secreted H^+ in the PCT	Glaucoma, mountain sickness, edema with alkalosis	Hyperchloremic metabolic acidosis, hypokalemia, renal stones, may worsen hepatic encephalopathy in cirrhotics	Weak diuretic
Other drugs with diuretic action					
➢ SGLT2 inhibitors—refer to Chapter 3 (Diabetes Mellitus)					
➢ Desmopressin, Vasopressin (ADH) antagonists—see section on vasopressin antagonists below					

LYMPHEDEMA: NONPITTING EDEMA

Characteristics: Edema due to impaired ability of the lymphatic vasculature to collect and transport interstitial fluid, which in the latter stages is characterized by nonpitting edema which does not resolve on limb elevation and is often associated with trophic skin changes such as fibrosis, induration, acanthosis, and warty overgrowths **(Fig. 14.5)**.

Lymphedema may be primary or secondary. It may involve the upper limb or the lower limb.

Classification of primary lymphedema: Based on age at lymphedema onset:
- Lymphedema congenital—at or shortly after birth (<1 year old)
- Lymphedema praecox—from ages 1–35 years
- Lymphedema tarda—>35 years old

Causes of lymphedema:
- Primary causes:
  - Milroy disease
  - Lymphedema-distichiasis syndrome
  - Hypertrichosis-lymphedema-telangiectasia syndrome
  - Yellow nail syndrome: Lymphedema, yellow nail beds, pleural effusion, and bronchiectasis
- Secondary causes:
  - Infections:
    - Filariasis—most common secondary cause worldwide
    - Recurrent bacterial infections
    - Tuberculosis
  - Malignancy and malignancy-related treatments—most common secondary cause in developed countries
    - Associated malignancies:
      - Breast cancer—most common
      - Lower extremity melanoma
      - Gynecologic cancer

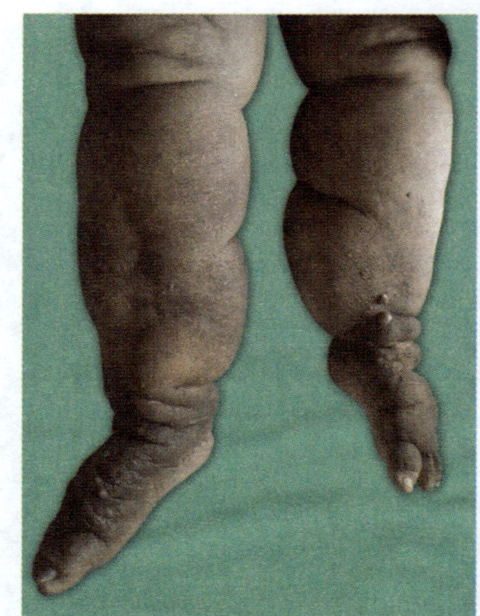

FIG. 14.5: Massive nonpitting edema with elephantiasis caused by filariasis of the leg.

- Genitourinary cancer
- Head and neck cancer
- Mechanism:
  - Neoplastic disruption of lymphatics
  - Radiotherapy-induced damage to lymphatics
  - Surgical removal of lymph nodes
- Inflammatory disorders:
  - Rheumatoid arthritis
  - Psoriatic arthritis
  - Sarcoidosis
- Circumferential wounds to extremities
- Burns

Clinical features and staging of lymphedema:

- Typically unilateral or asymmetric
- Features of underlying etiology
- The International Society of Lymphology (ISL) provides a staging system for staging lymphedema:
  - Stage 0 or Ia: Usually asymptomatic
  - Stage I: Edema present; edema reduced by limb elevation
  - Stage II:
    - Early stage II: Pitting edema present
    - Late stage II: Nonpitting edema
    - Limb elevation does not reduce edema
  - Stage III: Elephantiasis present with fibrotic changes. Nonpitting edema.
- **Kaposi-Stemmers sign:** The thickened skin folds at the base of the second finger/toe, making it difficult for the examiner to lift the dorsum of the fingers/toes of the affected limb. This can be seen at any stage of the lymphedema.
- Peau d'orange appearance
- Look for scrotal swelling in patients with suspected filariasis.

Complications of Lymphedema

- *Infection*: Recurrent cellulitis, lymphangitis
- Lymphangiosarcoma **(Stewart-Treves syndrome)**

Evaluation

- Blood smear to evaluate for presence of microfilaria
- Radionuclide lymphoscintigraphy (isotope lymphography) is the preferred test if diagnosis is unclear.
- Duplex Doppler ultrasound for examining the deep venous system may supplement the evaluation of extremity edema.
- MRI and CT: Both provide objective evidence of structural changes such as cutaneous thickening, presence of edema within the epifascial plain, and can also detect characteristic "honeycomb" pattern of subcutaneous tissue.

Treatment

See **Table 14.13.**

TABLE 14.13: Treatment of lymphedema.

Complex decongestive physiotherapy (CDPT):	*Surgery*:
➢ Manual lymphatic drainage: Mild manual tissue compression ➢ Compression with multilayered bandage wrapping ➢ Skin care ➢ Exercise Weight reduction Limb elevation Diuretics have not been shown to be useful *Control of infection*: ➢ Treatment of cellulitis ➢ An extended period of oral antibiotics may be considered in patients with three or more episodes of cellulitis in a year	➢ Reconstructive surgery: – For early lymphedema – Microsurgical lymphatic-venous anastomosis – Autologous vessel transplantations ➢ Debulking surgery (excisional procedures): – Suction-assisted lipectomy – Staged cutaneous/subcutaneous excision

Localized Edema

See **Box 14.1.**

Box 14.1: Various type of localized edema.

- *Facial edema*: Trichinosis, hypothyroidism, allergies, nephrotic syndrome, and angioedema
- *Pretibial myxedema*: Graves' thyrotoxicosis
- *Neurogenic edema*: Secondary to autonomic dysfunction
- *Lipedema*: Adiposity of the legs
- *Pseudothrombophlebitis*: It is unilateral edema with raised venous pressure caused by a popliteal cyst

DISORDERS OF SODIUM BALANCE

Hyponatremia

Q. Write short essay/note on definition, causes, clinical features, approach, and treatment of hyponatremia.

Q. List causes of drug-induced hyponatremia.

Box 14.2 shows the drugs causing hyponatremia.

Box 14.2: Drugs causing hyponatremia.

- Vasopressin analogs: Desmopressin, oxytocin
- Medications that stimulate release of vasopressin or potentiate the effects of vasopressin: SSRIs, antidepressants, morphine, and other opioids
- Medications that impair urinary dilution: Thiazide diuretics
- Medications that cause hyponatremia by unknown mechanism: Carbamazepine, antipsychotics, NSAIDs, cyclophosphamide, vincristine, nicotine, and chlorpropamide
- Illicit drugs: Ecstasy (MDMA)—associated with acute, life-threatening hyponatremia

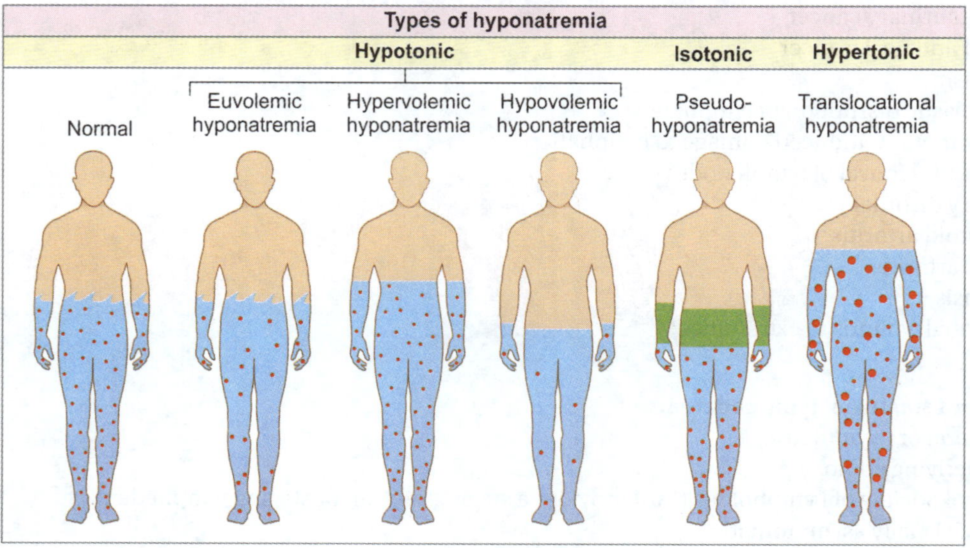

FIG. 14.6: Types of hyponatremia.

Definition: Hyponatremia is defined as a condition in which serum sodium is <135 mEq/L.

- It is a **disorder of water regulation**, i.e., it usually results from increased water retention.
- It is the most common disorder of electrolytes in clinical practice, being reported in 10–30% of acutely or chronically hospitalized patients.

Classification of hyponatremia:

- Based on **duration and rate of development** of hyponatremia:
  - Acute hyponatremia < 48 hours
  - Chronic hyponatremia ≥ 48 hours—more common
- Based on **serum sodium concentration** of hyponatremia:
  - Mild: Serum sodium 130–135 mEq/L
  - Moderate: Serum sodium 125–129 mEq/L
  - Severe: Serum sodium <125 mEq/L
- Based on serum osmolality and volume status, hyponatremia is subdivided into 3 main types **(Fig. 14.6):**

Box 14.3: Alternate classification of hypotonic hyponatremia based on the ability to excrete dilute urine.

- Unimpaired urine dilution (ADH levels are not elevated)
  - Primary polydipsia
  - Low dietary solute intake (beer potomania, tea and toast diet)
- Impaired urine dilution but normal suppression of ADH
  - Advanced renal failure
  - Diuretic-induced hyponatremia
- Impaired urine dilution due to unsuppressed ADH secretion
  - Reduced effective arterial blood volume
    - Hypovolemic hyponatremia
    - Heart failure and cirrhosis (hypervolemic hyponatremia)
    - Addison's disease
  - SIADH
- Disorders with impaired urine dilution due to abnormal V2 receptor (nephrogenic SIADH)
- Abnormally low osmostat which leads to low threshold for release of ADH
- Exercise-induced hyponatremia
- Cerebral salt wasting

Hypotonic Hyponatremia (Box 14.3):

- Serum osmolality < 280 mOsm/kg H_2O
- Most common type of hyponatremia
- Due to:
  - Inadequate solute intake
  - Excess electrolyte-free water intake
  - Retention of electrolyte-free water due to:
    - Presence of AVP
    - Kidney disease
    - Use of diuretics: Diuretics cause volume depletion and release of AVP; and may also lead to diminished sodium transport in renal diluting sites.
- Consequences of hypotonic hyponatremia: Cell edema, predominantly cerebral edema
- Subtypes:
  - Hypovolemic hyponatremia
  - Hypervolemic hyponatremia
  - Euvolemic hyponatremia

Hypovolemic hyponatremia:

- Hypovolemic hyponatremia results from loss of fluids rich in sodium and/or potassium.
- This stimulates thirst and AVP secretion, leading to water retention.

- Causes:
  - GI losses:
    - Diarrhea
    - Vomiting
  - Renal losses:
    - Diuretics (predominantly thiazide diuretics)
    - Cerebral salt wasting
    - Adrenal insufficiency
    - Salt-losing nephropathies
  - Dermal losses:
    - Burns
    - Sweating
  - Third spacing:
    - Pancreatitis
    - Sepsis
    - Bowel obstruction

Hypervolemic hyponatremia:
- Caused by renal sodium and water retention
- Causes:
  - Cirrhosis of liver
  - Heart failure
  - Chronic kidney disease
  - Nephrotic syndrome

Euvolemic hyponatremia:
- Most common dysnatremia in hospitalized patients
- Causes:
  - SIADH
  - Nephrogenic syndrome of inappropriate antidiuresis
    - Due to mutation causing activation of V2 vasopressin receptor (V2R)
  - Low solute intake: "tea and toast" diet, beer potomania
  - Hypothyroidism
  - Glucocorticoid deficiency
  - Exercise associated hyponatremia
    - Due to excessive water intake combined with impaired water excretion due to persistent ADH secretion
  - Water intoxication

Isotonic Hyponatremia

- Serum osmolality 280–295 mOsm/kg H_2O
- Pseudohyponatremia due to hyperlipidemia or hypoproteinemia (e.g. multiple myeloma)

Hypertonic Hyponatremia

Serum osmolality > 295 mOsm/kg H_2O
- Due to presence of additional osmoles (glucose/mannitol)
- Hyperglycemia
- Note: Sodium correction in hyperglycemia: For every 100 mg/dL increase in blood sugar, sodium concentration will fall by approximately 2 mEq/L
- Hypertonic fluid infusion
- Radiocontrast.

Effect of Hypotonic Hyponatremia on Brain (Fig. 14.7)

Hyponatremia induces generalized cellular swelling due to entry of water from ECF to ICF. The symptoms of hyponatremia are primarily neurological and are due to the development of cerebral edema within a rigid skull.
- **Swelling and reduced osmolality:** Within minutes of hyponatremia, the reduced osmolality causes a shift of fluid from the ECF to the ICF, leading to brain swelling. This usually occurs when the hyponatremia develops rapidly.
- **Rapid adaptation:** The brain tries to rapidly adapt to this hypotonic environment by the loss of electrolytes such as sodium, potassium, and chloride. These are osmotically active and help in partially restoring the brain volume.
- **Slow adaptation:** Further loss of osmotically active organic compounds such as glutamate, myoinositol, and taurine from the brain cells also help in restoring brain volume.

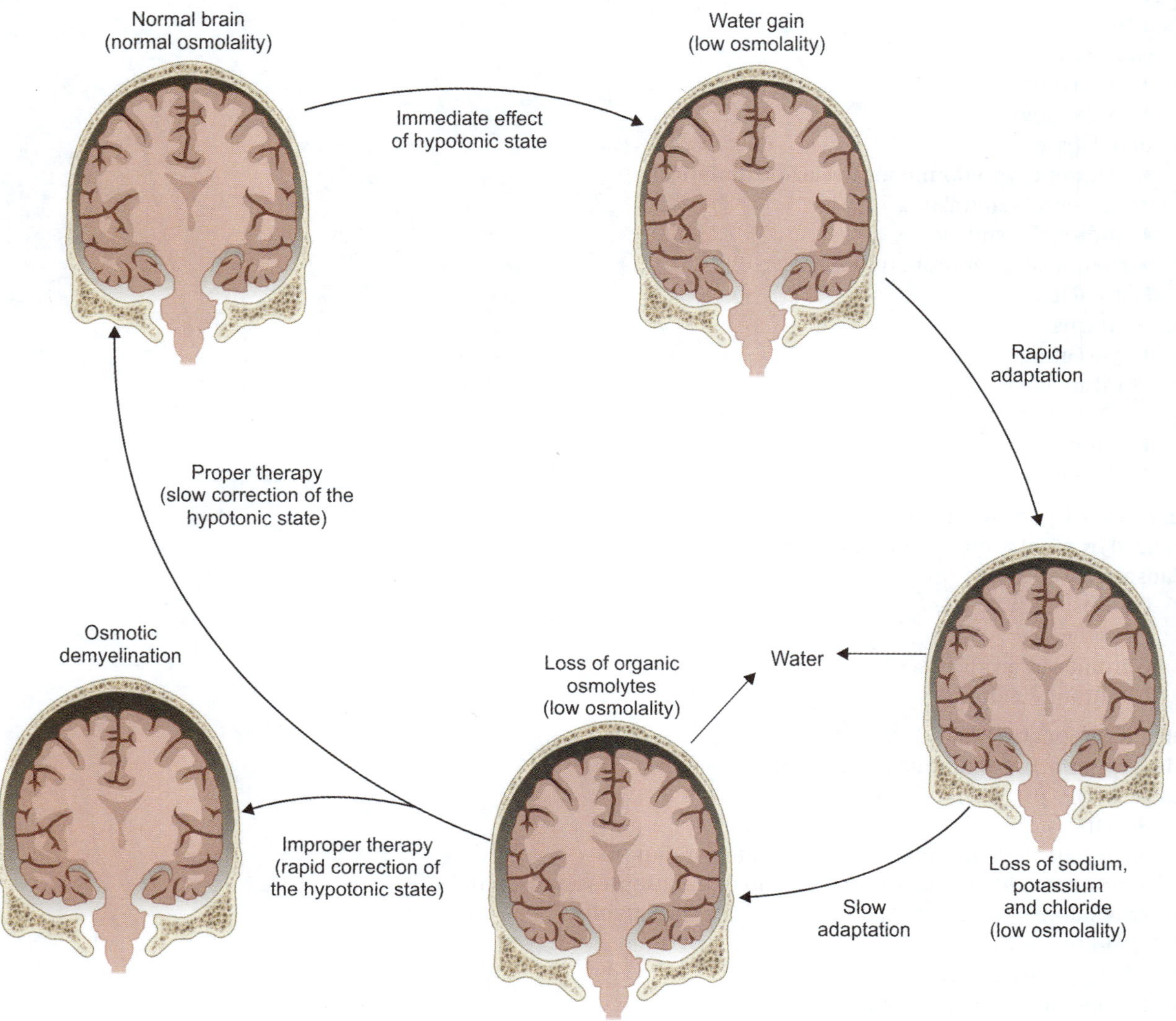

FIG. 14.7: Effects of hyponatremia on the brain.

- The adaptation process takes about 48 hours, which is the basis for the classification of acute and chronic hyponatremia based on the threshold of 48 hours.
- **Slow versus rapid correction of hypotonicity:**
  - Before adaptation (<48 hours), decreased extracellular osmolality triggers water to enter brain cells, increasing the risk of cerebral edema.
  - After adaptation (>48 hours), rapid increase in serum sodium concentration can cause brain cells to release water, increasing the risk of osmotic demyelination. Hence sodium should be corrected at a slow rate in chronic hyponatremia.

Clinical Features

- Hyponatremia is essentially a laboratory diagnosis.
- History and physical examination should determine the volume status of the patient and try to identify the cause of the hyponatremia.
- Symptoms due to hyponatremia depend on the acuity of presentation and the serum sodium levels, as described in **Table 14.14**.

TABLE 14.14: Classification by severity of symptoms of hyponatremia.

Severity	*Serum sodium level*	*Neurologic symptoms*	*Typical duration of hyponatremia*
Mild	<135 mmol/L	Headache, irritability, difficulty concentrating, altered mood, and depression	Chronic
Moderate	Generally <130 mmol/L	Nausea, confusion, disorientation, altered mental status, unstable gait, and falls	Acute or chronic
Severe	Generally <125 mmol/L	Vomiting, seizures, obtundation, respiratory distress, and coma	Acute

Investigations

- **Step 1: Serum sodium:**
  - Hyponatremia is diagnosed when serum sodium is <135 mEq/L
  - Based on severity, hyponatremia is classified as:
    - Mild: Serum sodium 130–135 mEq/L

- Moderate: Serum sodium 125–129 mEq/L
- Severe: Serum sodium < 125 mEq/L

- **Step 2: Serum osmolality:**
  - Serum osmolality < 275 mOsm/kg H_2O indicates hypotonic hyponatremia.
  - Serum osmolality between 280 and 295 mOsm/kg H_2O indicates isotonic hyponatremia (pseudohyponatremia).
  - Serum osmolality > 295 mOsm/kg H_2O indicates hypertonic hyponatremia.
- **Step 3: Urine osmolality:**
  - It should be measured in patients with hypotonic hyponatremia to confirm if urine is appropriately dilute.
  - If urine osmolality is less than 100 mOsm/kg H_2O
    - It indicates that there is no diluting defect.
    - This may be seen in primary polydipsia or due to low solute intake (e.g., beer potomania)
    - Low urine osmolality may also be seen in patients with hypovolemic hyponatremia who have been volume resuscitated, if osmolality is measured after administration of isotonic saline.
  - If urine osmolality is more than 200 mOsm/kg H_2O, assess volume status and urine sodium.
- **Step 4: Urine sodium:**
  - *See* **Table 14.15**
- **Other investigations:**
  - Thyroid function test: To rule out hypothyroidism
  - Serum cortisol ± ACTH: To exclude adrenal insufficiency
  - Serum creatinine: To look for renal insufficiency
  - Serum uric acid: May help assess volume status
  - Other tests to diagnose the underlying cause, as guided by history and physical examination:
    - Serum lipids and serum protein electrophoresis in cases of pseudohyponatremia to look for hypercholesterolemia and multiple myeloma, respectively.
    - Echocardiogram, BNP: For heart failure
    - Ultrasound abdomen: Cirrhosis
    - Urine for proteinuria
    - CT brain/chest/abdomen: To help detect paraneoplastic SIADH.

TABLE 14.15: Differentiating hypotonic hyponatremia based on volume status and urine sodium.

Volume status	*Urine sodium (mEq/L)*	*Etiology*
Hypovolemic	≤20	Nonrenal sodium loss
	>20	Renal sodium loss
Hypervolemic	≤20	Cirrhosis, heart failure, and nephrotic syndrome
	>20	Renal failure
Euvolemic	>20	Most patients with euvolemic hyponatremia

Approach to the diagnosis of the cause of hyponatremia **(Figure 14.8).**

Management

The management of hypotonic hyponatremia depends on the severity, duration of symptoms, and the underlying cause.

Goals of treatment

- To correct serum sodium levels to avoid complications of severe hyponatremia
- To avoid overly rapid correction of hyponatremia, which may lead to osmotic demyelination
- Correct underlying causes

1. **Severe symptomatic hyponatremia:**
   - Goal: Rapid increase of serum sodium by 4–6 mEq/L is recommended irrespective of whether hyponatremia is acute or chronic.
   - This is done by IV infusion of hypertonic saline.
     - Protocol 1: 100 mL bolus of 3% saline is infused over 10 minutes; repeated up to 3 times, as necessary.
     - Protocol 2: 150 mL bolus of 3% saline over 20 minutes. Check serum sodium concentration after 20 minutes. Consider repeating twice or until a target of 5 mEq/L increase in serum sodium concentration.
   - Follow-up management:
     - If symptoms improve:
       - Stop infusion of hypertonic saline
       - Start treatment based on etiology, if identified
     - If symptoms do not improve:
       - Continue IV infusion of 3% hypertonic saline aiming for an increase in sodium concentration by 1 mmol/L/hr
     - Note: Stop hypertonic saline when either:
       - Symptoms improve or
       - Serum sodium concentration increases by 10 mEq/L in total or
       - Serum sodium concentration reaches 130 mEq/L
2. **Mild or asymptomatic hyponatremia:**
   - Treatment depends on whether hyponatremia is acute or chronic and based on the underlying etiology

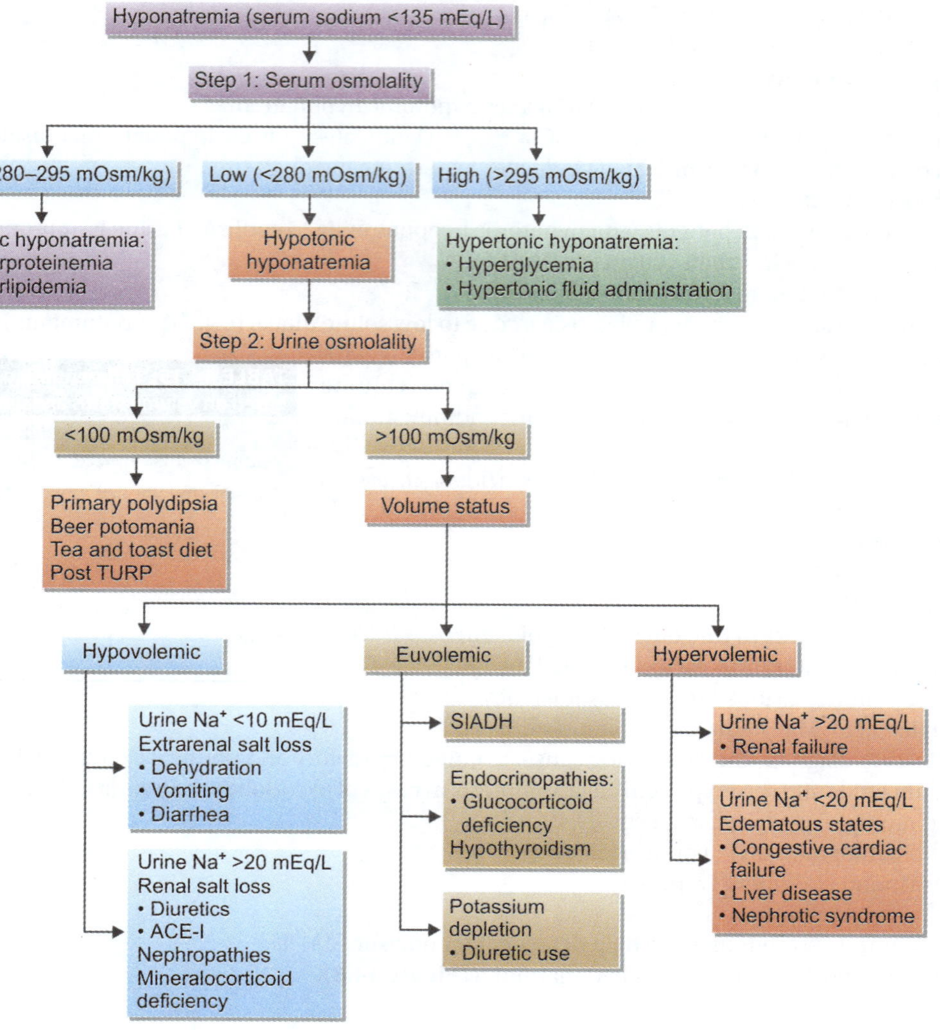

FIG. 14.8: Algorithm for diagnosing the cause of hyponatremia.

- Rate of correction:
  - Acute hyponatremia:
    - Rate of correction does not need to be restricted in well-documented cases of acute hyponatremia
  - Chronic hyponatremia/duration of hyponatremia unknown:
    - Increase serum sodium with a goal of ≤6–8 mEq/L/day and not more than 18 mEq/L in 48 hours
    - Monitor serum sodium every 2–4 hourly

3. **Estimating the effect of 1 L of any IV saline infusion on serum sodium levels:**
   - Change in serum sodium = [(infusion sodium concentration + infusion potassium concentration) – serum sodium concentration/Total body water + 1]
   - The sodium content of various intravenous fluids is mentioned in **Table 14.16.**
   - This formula may be used to determine the amount of saline and the rate of fluid infusion required to correct hyponatremia.
   - However, this formula is only a rough guide and is limited by the fact that it does not account for ongoing electrolyte or water losses.
   - Use of this formula does not serve as a replacement for regular serum sodium monitoring. Sodium levels should be monitored every 2–4th hourly.

TABLE 14.16: Sodium content of various intravenous fluids per liter.

Intravenous fluid	*Sodium content*
7.5% $NaHCO_3$	900 mEq/L
3% NaCl	512 mEq/L
0.9% NaCl normal saline	154 mEq/L
Ringer lactate	130 mEq/L
0.45% NaCl Half NS	77 mEq/L
Isolyte G	63 mEq/L
Isolyte M	40 mEq/L
5% Dextrose	Nil

4. **Additional treatment based on the underlying etiology (in mild or asymptomatic disease)**
   a. Hypovolemic hyponatremia:
   - In patients with asymptomatic hypovolemic hyponatremia, isotonic saline can be used to restore the intravascular volume.
   - Amount of 0.9% saline to be replaced may be calculated by the above formula and overcorrection of chronic hyponatremia should be avoided.
   - Fludrocortisone can be used in cerebral salt-wasting syndrome.

b. Hypervolemic hyponatremia:
- Fluid restriction:
  - The amount of fluid intake should be [urine output – 500 mL]
  - Amount of fluid to be restricted can also be determined by calculating the urine: plasma electrolyte ratio (urinary [Na] + [K]/ Plasma [Na]
    a. If the ratio is more than 1, then the fluid can be aggressively restricted up to less than 500 mL/day.
    b. For approx 1 then the fluid can be restrict up to 500–700 mL
    c. For ratio less than 1, fluids can be restricted up to 1 L.
  - Loop diuretics
  - Vasopressin antagonists may be useful when the above measures fail (see section on Vaptans below)

c. Euvolemic hyponatremia:
- Treat the underlying cause where possible
- Fluid restriction
- Loop diuretics
- Oral salt tablets in patients with SIADH
- Oral urea tablets in patients with SIADH

- Demeclocycline in patients with chronic asymptomatic hyponatremia due to SIADH if unresponsive to fluid restriction
- Vasopressin antagonists

5. **Correction of inadvertent rapid overcorrection of sodium:**
- Discontinue hypertonic saline/other measures of active sodium correction
- Infusion of electrolyte free water (e.g.,5% Dextrose)
- IV desmopressin

Q. Write short note on VAPTANS.

Vasopressin Receptor Antagonists (VAPTANS)

- Nonselective (mixed V1A/V2):
  - *Conivaptan*: Intravenous
- Selective:
  - *V1A selective (V1RA)*: Relcovaptan
  - *V1B selective (V3RA)*: Nelivaptan
  - *V2 selective (V2RA)*: Tolvaptan, lixivaptan, mozavaptan, satavaptan. V2 selective (V2RA) can cause an electrolyte-free aquaresis, reduce urine osmolality and raise serum Na. Their mechanism of action is presented in **Figure 14.9**.
- Tolvaptan and conivaptan are FDA-approved drugs.
- **Tolvaptan**, an oral V2 selective agent, is the most commonly used agent.
  - Indication:
    - Use in euvolemic or hypervolemic hyponatremia (heart failure).
  - Dose:
    - Initially 15 mg/day
    - Maximum 60 mg/day
  - Treatment should be limited to 30 days
  - Monitor serum sodium and volume status
  - Contraindicated in:
    - Hypovolemic hyponatremia
    - Acute hyponatremia and severe symptomatic hyponatremia (urgent need to raise serum sodium levels)
    - Pregnancy
    - Severe liver dysfunction and cirrhosis

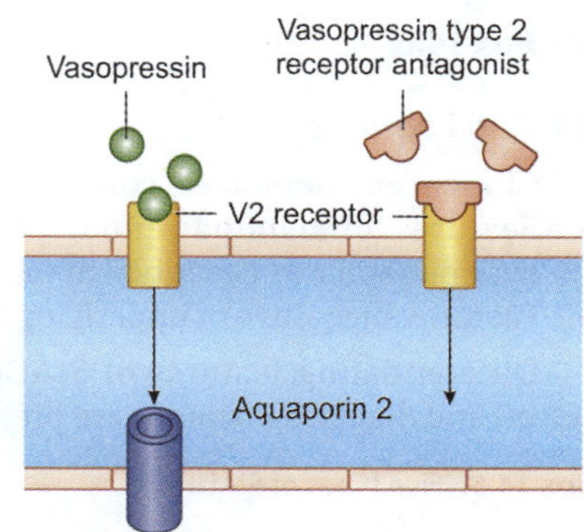

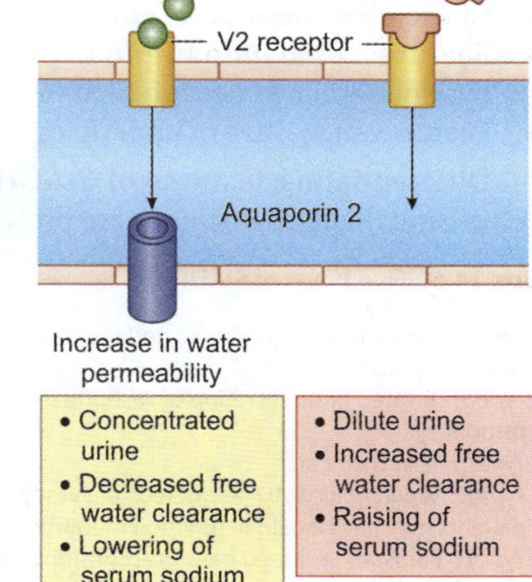

FIG. 14.9: Mechanism of action of vaptans.

- Vaptans are not suitable for hyponatremia due to cerebral salt wasting and psychogenic polydipsia where the ADH level is appropriate.
- Caution: It should **NOT** be used along with hypertonic saline.
- Adverse effects
  - Thirst 8–16%; dry mouth 4–13%, polyuria
  - Hypernatremia develops in 5%.
  - Rapid correction of serum sodium levels may predispose to osmotic demyelination syndrome.
  - Hyperglycemia
  - GI hemorrhage in cirrhosis

Other Uses of Vaptans

- **Polycystic kidney disease:** Polycystin defects may promote cyst development because they increase intracellular cAMP (a second messenger for AVP acting at the V2R), therefore, V2R antagonists may reduce cyst volume.
- **Congenital nephrogenic diabetes insipidus:** Type 2 V2R mutations cause misfolding and interfere with trafficking of the receptor from the endoplasmic reticulum to the cell membrane—VRA can bind to misfolded intracellular V2R and improve transport to the cell membrane.

Syndrome of Inappropriate Antidiuretic Hormone Secretion (SIADH/SIAD)

Q. Write short note on syndrome of inappropriate antidiuretic hormone secretion.

The syndrome of inappropriate antidiuretic hormone is a disorder of water and sodium balance characterized by hypotonic euvolemic hyponatremia due to impaired free water excretion, which is caused by nonphysiologic secretion of ADH which persists in the absence of an osmotic or hemodynamic stimulus.

Criteria for the diagnosis of SIADH are enlisted in **Box 14.4**.

SIADH is the most common cause of hyponatremia.

Plasma levels of arginine vasopressin (AVP) in various types of SIADH are shown in **Figure 14.10** and **Box 14.5.**

Box 14.4: Bartter's criteria for diagnosis of syndrome of inappropriate antidiuretic hormone secretion.

- Hyponatremia
- Serum osmolality < 270 mOsm/kg (hypotonic)
- Euvolemia
- Urinary osmolality > 100 mOsm/kg of H_2O
- Urinary sodium > 30 mEq/L without restricted dietary intake of salt
- Normal renal, cardiac, hepatic, adrenal, pituitary, and thyroid function
- Exclusion of diuretic use

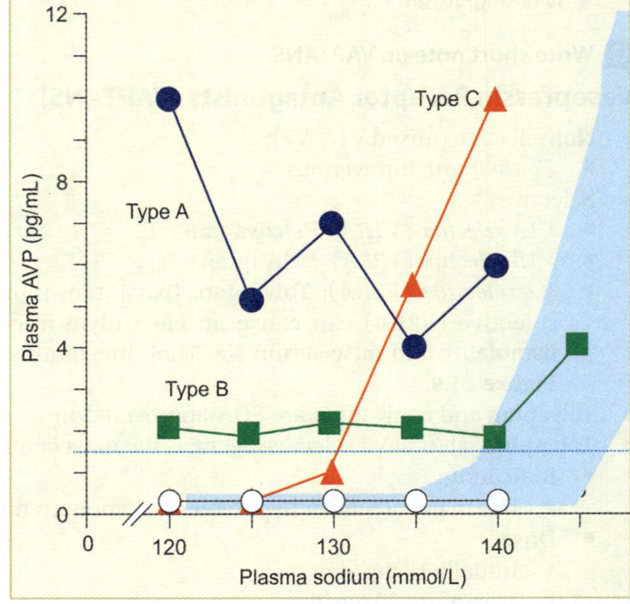

FIG. 14.10: Types of SIADH (syndrome of inappropriate antidiuretic hormone). (AVP: arginine vasopressin)

Etiology of SIADH

See **Box 14.6.**

Clinical Features

- **Clinical euvolemia:** No edema observed
- Features of hyponatremia, based on the severity of hyponatremia, as described in the earlier section
- Features suggestive of underlying etiology.

Differentiating features of SIADH, cerebral salt wasting (CSW) and diabetes insipidus are presented in **Table 14.17.**

Box 14.5: Five types of SIADH.

Type A: Characterized by unregulated secretion of vasopressin—most common pattern
Type B: Elevated basal secretion of vasopressin despite normal regulation by osmolality
Type C: "Reset osmostat"
Type D: *Nephrogenic SIAD*—undetectable vasopressin (AVP) levels (these patients may have a gain of function mutation of the V_2-receptor)
Type E: "Barostat"—altered baroreceptor signaling despite normovolemia. Thus there is a large increase in vasopressin secretion with minor reduction in blood pressure or volume.

Box 14.6: Various causes of SIADH.

- *Malignancies*: Bronchogenic carcinoma (small cell carcinoma), carcinoma of duodenum, stomach, pancreas, prostate, bladder, lymphoma, and mesothelioma
- *Respiratory*: Pneumonia, lung abscess, tuberculosis, aspergillosis, positive pressure ventilation (PPV), pneumothorax, and asthma
- *Neurological*: Encephalitis, meningitis, brain abscess, head trauma, GB syndrome, subarachnoid hemorrhage, subdural hemorrhage, cerebrovascular accident, cerebral and cerebellar atrophy, multiple sclerosis (MS), and hydrocephalus
- Others:
  - AIDS
  - *Drugs*: Chlorpropamide, SSRI, MAOI, tricyclic antidepressants, carbamazepine, oxytocin, vasopressin, desmopressin, cyclophosphamide, and vincristine
  - *Acute intermittent porphyria*
  - *Idiopathic*

TABLE 14.17: Differentiating features of syndrome of inappropriate antidiuretic hormone secretion (SIADH), cerebral salt wasting (CSW), and diabetes insipidus.

	SIADH (euvolemic)	*CSW (hypovolemic)*	*Diabetic insipidus*
Mechanism	Inappropriate ADH secretion leading to free water retention	Inappropriate natriuretic peptide levels which leads to salt and water loss	Deficiency/resistance to ADH
Urine output	Normal–low	Normal–high	Polyuria
CVP	Normal	Low	Can be normal or low
Blood pressure	Normal	Orthostatic hypotension may be present	Orthostatic hypotension may be present
Serum Na	Low	Low	High
Serum osmolality	Low < 285 mOsm/kg	Low < 285 mOsm/kg	Normal or high
Urine Na	High > 30 mmol/L	Higher > 30 mmol/L	Low
Serum urea	Normal–low	Normal–high	Normal–high
Management	Fluid restriction	Fluid administration	Correction of water deficit, desmopressin

Treatment
- Treat the underlying cause
- In severe hyponatremia, infusion of hypertonic saline as described above
- Restrict the fluid intake to 500–1,000 mL/day, as described above
- Oral salt tablets can be advocated
- Oral urea
- Combination of loop diuretics and oral salt tablets
- Vasopressin-2 receptor antagonists (aquaretics: tolvaptan, conivaptan)
- Demeclocycline:
  - It inhibits AVP in the collecting duct.
  - Indicated for chronic asymptomatic hyponatremia due to SIADH if unresponsive to fluid restriction
  - Adverse effects: Nephrotoxicity

Cerebral Salt Wasting

- ***Causes*:**
  - ***Typically described in subarachnoid hemorrhage.***
  - Also seen in other CNS disorders such as closed head injury, CNS surgery, CNS tumors, CNS infections, and meningitis.
- ***Mechanism***: Postulated that brain natriuretic peptide increases urine volume and Na^+ excretion.
- ***Signs/Symptoms*:**
  - ***Typical onset is within the first 10 days following a neurosurgical procedure or event.***
  - Polyuria, weight loss, dehydration/hypovolemia, hypotension, and low CVP.

Laboratory Values

- Hyponatremia due to excessive renal Na loss
- High urine Na >30 mmol/L
- Urine osmolality inappropriately elevated >100 mOsm/kg
- Low serum uric acid concentration

Treatment
- 3% saline to raise the serum sodium levels, as described in the section on hyponatremia
- Volume replacement with 0.9% normal saline
- Salt supplementation
- Fludrocortisone

Hypernatremia

Q. Write short note on hypernatremia.

Definition: It is defined as serum Na^+ concentration >145 mmol/L.

Hypernatremia is usually the result of loss of water in excess of sodium.

Hypernatremia is generally mild unless thirst mechanism is abnormal or access to water is limited, e.g., infants, physically challenged, impaired mental status, postoperative patient, and intubated patients in ICU.

Table 14.18 describes the causes of hypernatremia based on the volume status.

Drugs causing hypernatremia
- Drugs associated with nephrogenic DI:
  - Lithium
  - Cisplatin
  - Aminoglycosides
  - Amphotericin B
  - Demeclocycline
  - Vitamins A and D
- Drugs associated with central diabetes insipidus:
  - Phenytoin
  - Ethanol
- Drugs that lead to renal water loss:
  - Loop diuretics
  - Mannitol
- Other drugs:
  - Lactulose and sorbitol—lead to hypotonic GI losses
  - Hypertonic saline
  - Sodium bicarbonate

TABLE 14.18: Causes of hypernatremia based on volume status.

Volume status	Total body water	Total body Na^+	Causes
Hypovolemic	↓↓	↓	**Extrarenal losses:** Diarrhea, fistulas, burns **Renal losses:** Osmotic or loop diuretics, intrinsic renal disease, postobstruction
Euvolemic	↓	Slight ↓/No change	**Renal losses:** Diabetes insipidus, hypodipsia **Extrarenal losses:** Respiratory/skin insensible losses
Hypervolemic	↑	↑↑	Accidental salt ingestion Administration of hypertonic saline Malfunctioning of hemodialysis equipment Primary hyperaldosteronism Cushing's syndrome

Classification of Hypernatremia based on Duration of Symptoms

- Acute hypernatremia <48 hours
- Chronic hypernatremia >48 hours

Clinical Features

- Features of underlying etiology
- Features due to hypernatremia:
  - Marked thirst
  - Increased urine frequency/volume
  - Lethargy
  - Weakness
  - Irritability
  - Seizures
    - Coma
    - Neurological symptoms are more common with acute hypernatremia, but patients with chronic hypernatremia may progress to altered mental status and coma
- Volume status should be determined to classify hypernatremia.

Investigations

- Serum sodium levels
  - Hypernatremia if serum sodium > 145 mEq/L
- 24-hour urine volume measurement:
  - The appropriate response to hypernatremia is a small amount of concentrated urine.
    - Urine volume <800 mL
    - Urine osmolality >800 mOsm/L
    - May be seen in GI or insensible losses, primary hypodipsia
  - Urine volume >1,000 mL suggests a defect in renal water conservation.
- Urine osmolality and serum osmolality
  - Possible etiologies based on urine osmolality are described in **Table 14.19**.
- Other testing based on etiology:
  - Further testing for DI: Discussed in Chapter 2.
    - Water deprivation test
    - Desmopressin challenge test
    - Serum AVP levels
    - Imaging of the brain with MRI/CT in central DI
      - Renal USG and RFTs: For renal disease
      - Gastric sodium or stool sodium: In salt poisoning
      - CPK: For hypernatremia associated with rhabdomyolysis

TABLE 14.19: Urine osmolality and the possible etiologies of hypernatremia.

Urine osmolality		Etiology
Low	Urine osmolality ≤ serum osmolality	Diabetes insipidus
High	Urine osmolality ≥ serum osmolality	Pure volume depletion not due to diabetes insipidus E.g.: GI or insensible losses Primary hypodipsia
Equal	Urine osmolality = serum osmolality	Partial DI Osmotic diuresis Renal concentrating defect due to renal failure

Management of Hypernatremia

Management depends upon:
- Onset of hypernatremia: Acute vs chronic
- Volume status

Management of chronic hypernatremia

1. Fluid replacement:
   - If hypovolemic, treat with 0.9% saline until vital signs are normal.
   - Once patient is euvolemic, calculate the free water deficit as follows:
   - *Calculation of free water deficit for chronic hypernatremia*

   $$\text{Free water deficit} = \frac{\text{Plasma Na}^{+}\text{ concentration} - 140}{140} \times \text{Total body water}$$

   - Also correct ongoing water losses
   - Choice of fluids for correction of free water deficit includes:
     - Water by NG tube or orally
     - IV 5% dextrose
     - Hypotonic saline: IV quarter or half normal saline
   - Goal of treatment: To lower sodium by 8–10 mmol/day
   - Rapid correction of hypernatremia is dangerous because sudden decrease in osmolality can cause rapid shift of water into the cells resulting in swelling of brain cells.
   - Typical requirements of fluids depending on the degree of fluid depletion are mentioned in **Table 14.20.**
2. Treatment based on volume status and etiology:
   - Hypovolemic hypernatremia:
     - Correct hypovolemia with isotonic saline
     - Treat underlying cause of hypovolemia (e.g., diarrhea)
     - 5% dextrose or hypotonic saline to correct water deficit
   - Euvolemic hypernatremia:
     - Replace water losses
     - For central DI:
       - Desmopressin
     - For nephrogenic DI:
       - Stop causative agent
       - Amiloride for lithium-associated nephrogenic DI
       - Low sodium diet, combined with thiazide diuretics may be useful. This enhances the proximal reabsorption of salt and water, thus decreasing urinary free water loss
     - Hypervolemic hypernatremia:
       - Discontinue salt intake
       - Diuretics—to lower serum sodium and treat volume expansion
       - 5% dextrose to correct water deficit

TABLE 14.20: Requirement of fluids depending on degree of depletion.

Degree of depletion	*Type of fluid and route of administration*	*Quantity and time for replacement*
Mild (1–2 L deficit)	Water by mouth or 5% glucose IV	2 L, over 6–12 hours
Moderate (2–4 L deficit)	5% glucose IV	2–4 L, over 24 hours
Severe (4–10 L deficit)	0.9% NaCl IV 5% dextrose IV 5% dextrose IV	1 L, over 1 hour 3 L, over 2 hours 3 L, over 24–48 hours

Management of acute hypernatremia

Correction of serum sodium by 1 mEq/L/hr in the first 6–8 hours is recommended.

Indicators of adequate correction: Relief of thirst, urine output of more than 1,500 mL/24 hours and normal plasma sodium levels.

Diabetes Insipidus

Discussed in Chapter 2.

Osmotic Demyelination Syndrome or Central Pontine Myelinolysis

Q. Write short note on osmotic demyelination.

- It was first described by Adams et al. in 1959.
- *Risk factors*: Alcoholism, chronically ill patients, elderly/malnourished, cirrhosis predisposes to demyelination (due to depletion of intracellular organic solutes).
- Hypokalemia is a strong predictor.
- Demyelination can be diffuse and not involve the pons. Extrapontine areas include cerebellar and neocortical white/gray junctional areas, thalamus, subthalamus, amygdala, globus pallidus, putamen, caudate, and lateral geniculate bodies.
- Rate of correction over 24 hours more important than rate of correction in any one particular hour.
- More common, if sodium increases by more than 20 mEq/L in 24 hours
- Very uncommon, if sodium increases by 12 mEq/L or less in 24 hours
- Symptoms generally occur 2–6 days after elevation of sodium and usually either irreversible or only partially reversible.

Clinical Features

- Dysarthria, dysphagia, parkinsonism, catatonia, locked-in syndrome, lethargy and coma, seizures, nystagmus, ataxia, emotional lability, akinetic mutism, gait disturbance, myoclonus, behavioral disturbances, paraparesis or quadriparesis.
- MRI with diffusion-weighted imaging will be helpful in early detection.

Treatment
- There is no effective therapy.
- Changes are permanent.
- Mortality is very high.
- Case reports of improvement with aggressive plasmapheresis immediately after diagnosis.
- Case reports of treatment with thyrotropin-releasing hormone. Infusion of myoinositol (a major osmolyte lost in the adaptation to hyponatremia) protects against mortality and myelinolysis from rapid correction of hyponatremia.

DISORDERS OF POTASSIUM BALANCE

Potassium

Q. Write short note on the normal physiology of potassium in the body.

- Potassium is the major intracellular cation.
- *Distribution of potassium*:
  - Total body potassium in a person weighing 70 kg is about 4,000 mEq.
  - 99% of the potassium is located inside the cells, predominantly within muscle cells.
    - 28 L of ICF contains ~4,000 mEq = 150 mEq/L
  - <1% of the total body potassium is extracellular.
    - 14 L of ECF contains ~70 mEq = 4 mEq/L
- Potassium levels are maintained within a narrow range of 3.5–5.5 mEq/L in the ECF.
- The electrochemical gradient of potassium across the cell membrane is maintained by the Na^+/K^+ ATPase system in the cell membrane which actively transports potassium into and sodium out of the cell.
- This gradient is required for the proper functioning of excitable tissues such as nerves and muscles.
- Overall potassium balance:
  - Normal intake: 100 mEq/day
  - Normal excretion:
    - Urine: 90 mEq/day
    - Fecal excretion: 10 mEq/day
- Internal potassium balance: Sudden changes in plasma K^+ is prevented by:
  - Shift of K^+ into the cell via the Na^+/K^+ ATPase under the influence of insulin and beta-adrenergic stimulation
  - Renal K^+ excretion
- Renal excretion:
  - Excretion through kidney is the major route of elimination of dietary and other sources of excess K^+.
  - Potassium reabsorption:
    - About 65% of filtered potassium is absorbed in proximal convoluted tubule. It is absorbed passively with sodium and water, through the paracellular pathway.
    - 25% of the filtered potassium is reabsorbed at the thick ascending limb by the $Na^+/K^+/2Cl^-$ transporter.
  - Only 10% of the filtered potassium reaches the distal nephron.
  - Potassium secretion (and hence excretion):
    - In the distal nephron and the collecting duct
    - Increased distal fluid and sodium delivery increases K^+ secretion
    - Hyperkalemia and metabolic alkalosis also directly increase K^+ secretion
    - However, the most important factor that influences potassium secretion is aldosterone.
  - A negative feedback mechanism exists between plasma potassium concentration and aldosterone.
  - Hyperkalemia leads to increased release of aldosterone (via Renin-angiotensin-aldosterone mechanism or via direct release of aldosterone from adrenal cortex), which then leads to increased K^+ secretion, H^+ secretion, and sodium reabsorption by the kidneys.

Hypokalemia

Q. Write short note on:
- **Normal serum potassium level and causes of hypokalemia.**
- **Hypokalemia**

- Normal serum potassium level is maintained within a narrow range of 3.5–5.5 mEq/L.
- An abnormally low level (<3.5 mmol/L) of serum potassium (K^+) is called hypokalemia.

Causes (Table 14.21)

TABLE 14.21: Various causes of hypokalemia.

1. **Decreased intake**
   a. Starvation, anorexia nervosa
   b. Potassium-free IV fluid
   c. Clay ingestion (bentonite): It binds dietary K^+ and decreases K^+ absorption
2. **Redistribution into cell**
   a. *Metabolic or respiratory alkalosis*: Due to K^+ redistribution into the cell as well as increased K^+ loss (renal)
   b. Hormonal
      i. Insulin
      ii. *β_2 adrenergic agonist*: It causes K^+ influx into the cell as well as stimulates insulin release
      iii. α-adrenergic antagonist
   c. *Anabolic states*:
      i. Vitamin B_{12} or folic acid (red blood cell production)
      ii. Granulocyte macrophage colony-stimulating factor
      iii. Total parenteral nutrition
   d. *Others*:
      i. Pseudohypokalemia
      ii. Barium toxicity
      iii. Hypothermia
      iv. Hypokalemic periodic paralysis
      v. Chloroquine intoxication
3. **Increased loss**
   a. **Gastrointestinal:**
      - Vomiting
      - Nasogastric aspiration
      - Diarrhea
      - Villous adenoma
      - VIPoma
      - Ileal loop/conduit with ureteric implants
      - Sodium phosphate solution used for bowel cleansing
      - Laxative abuse
   b. **Integumentary loss**
   c. **Dialysis and plasmapheresis**
   d. **Renal:**
      Diuresis:
      i. Diuretics—acetazolamide, loop, and thiazide
      ii. Osmotic diuresis
      iii. Recovery from ATN/renal obstruction
      True mineralocorticoid excess:
      i. Primary hyperaldosteronism (Conn's)
      ii. Secondary hyperaldosteronism
      iii. Cushing syndrome, steroid therapy
      iv. Congenital adrenal hyperplasia
      v. Hereditary glucocorticoid responsive aldosteronism
      vi. Renal artery stenosis
      Genetic conditions that cause renal loss of potassium:
      i. Liddle syndrome
      ii. Apparent mineralocorticoid excess
      iii. Bartter syndrome
      iv. Gitelman syndrome
      v. Fanconi syndrome
      Renal tubular acidosis:
      i. Distal (type 1) RTA
      ii. Proximal (type 2) RTA
      Other drugs:
      - Fludrocortisone
      - Antibiotics: Penicillin, ampicillin
      - Sodium bicarbonate
      - Drugs associated with hypomagnesemia
        - Amphotericin B
        - Aminoglycosides
        - Cisplatin
      Others:
      - Hypomagnesemia
      - Licorice ingestion—mineralocorticoid-like effects

Clinical Features of Hypokalemia

- Severity of clinical manifestations depends on degree and duration of hypokalemia.
- Patients with mild hypokalemia (K^+ 3–3.5 mEq/L) are usually asymptomatic.
- Nervous system manifestations:
  - Leg cramps
  - Generalized weakness
  - Fasciculations and tetany
  - Ascending paralysis including respiratory muscle paralysis
- Cardiac manifestations:
  - Arrhythmias
  - ECG changes
- GI manifestations:
  - Paralytic ileus
- Renal manifestations:
  - Metabolic acidosis
  - Rhabdomyolysis in severe hypokalemia
  - Hypokalemic nephropathy—renal tubular damage
  - Cyst formation
  - Nephrogenic diabetes insipidus
  - Polyuria
- Features of the underlying cause of hypokalemia

Investigations

- Initial tests:
  - Measurement of serum electrolytes, including bicarbonate, calcium, and magnesium.
  - Blood glucose testing
  - Urea and creatinine

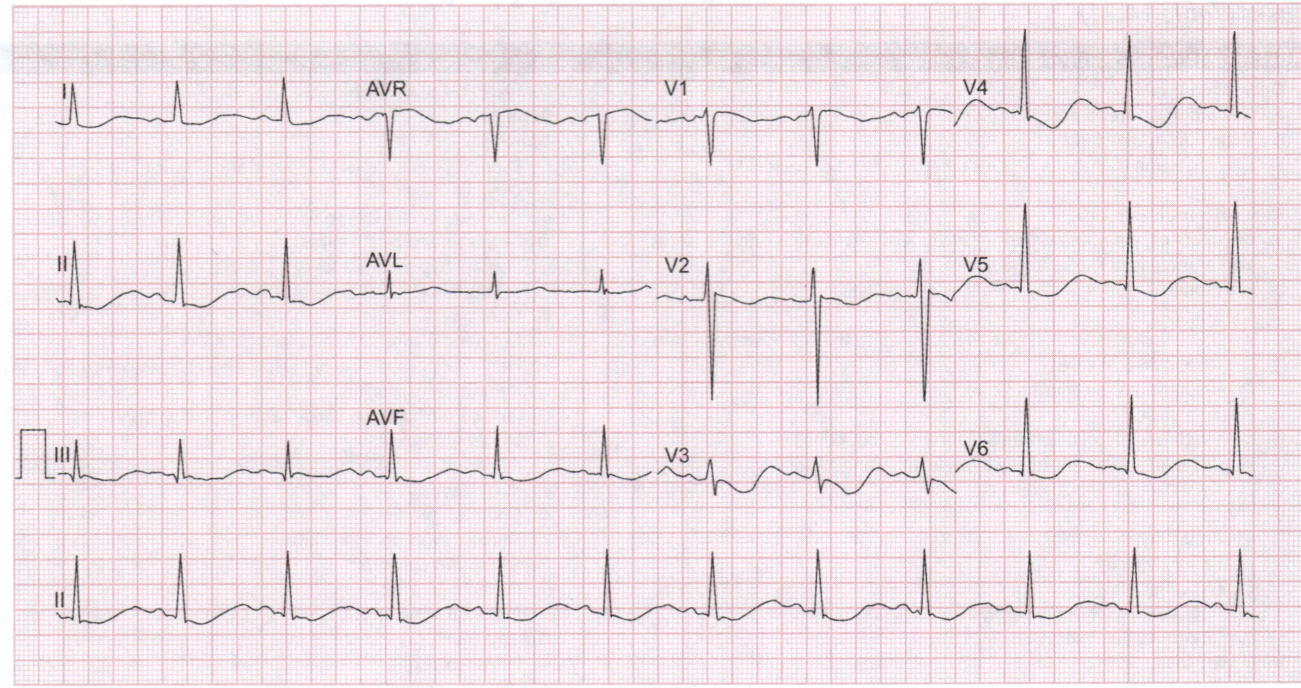

FIG. 14.11: ECG showing QT prolongation and U waves.

- ECG:
  - **ECG changes (Fig. 14.11 and Table 14.22):** The electrocardiographic changes of hypokalemia are due to delayed ventricular repolarization and do not correlate well with plasma-potassium concentration.
- Urine potassium
- Urine potassium to creatinine ratio

TABLE 14.22: Electrocardiographic changes in hypokalemia.

Early changes	*Changes due to severe potassium depletion*
➢ Flattening or inversion of the T wave ➢ Prominent U wave ➢ ST segment depression ➢ Prolonged QU interval	➢ Prolonged PR interval ➢ Decreased voltage and widening of the QRS complex ➢ An increased risk of ventricular, arrhythmias especially in patients with myocardial ischemia or left ventricular hypertrophy

Q. Discuss approach to management of hypokalemia. Add a note on TTKG.

Approach to Diagnosis of a Patient with Hypokalemia

- **Exclude pseudohypokalemia and potassium redistribution** from the ECF to the ICF, e.g., with marked leukocytosis (e.g., AML), recent IV insulin, prolonged storage of samples.
- Thorough history and physical examination to determine the etiology, e.g., diuretic and laxative abuse, vomiting, and severity of symptoms.
- In patients with hypokalemic paralysis, life-threatening ventricular arrhythmias or patients with severe hypokalemia who require emergency surgery, emergency treatment should be initiated.
- In the absence of such life-threatening features:
  - Assess intake of potassium. If low, consider oral replacement of potassium
  - If potassium intake is normal, measure urinary K^+ and creatinine.
    - If 24-hour urinary K^+ is less than 15 mEq/day or spot urine K^+/creatinine ratio is less than 15 mEq/g, it suggests extrarenal potassium loss, such as GI potassium loss.
    - If 24-hour urinary K^+ is more than 15 mEq/day or spot urine K^+/creatinine ratio is more than 15 mEq/g, it suggests abnormal renal potassium loss.
  - If renal loss is present, the next step is to assess the **transtubular potassium gradient (TTKG)**.
    - TTKG is a measurement of net K^+ secretion by the collecting duct after correcting for changes in urine osmolality.
    - TTKG = Urinary K^+ × Plasma osmolality/Serum K^+ × Urinary osmolality
    - In hypokalemia, TTKG should be <3
    - TTKG > 4 suggests increased distal K^+ secretion.
  - The next step would be to assess the **blood pressure and the volume status**.
    - If hypertension is found, then measure plasma renin, aldosterone, and cortisol levels **(Table 14.23)**
    - If no hypertension is found, look for acid-base status.

- If **metabolic acidosis** is present, causes include:
  - Renal tubular acidosis
  - Diabetic ketoacidosis or
  - Acetazolamide use
- If **metabolic alkalosis** is present:
  - Measure **urine chloride** levels.
    - If urine chloride is <10 mmol/L, consider chloride secreting diarrhea or vomiting
    - If urine chloride is >20 mmol/L, measure urine calcium to creatinine ratio
      - Urine calcium to creatinine ratio <0.15: Gitelman syndrome or thiazide diuretic use
      - Urine calcium to creatinine ratio > 0.20: Bartter's syndrome or loop diuretic use

TABLE 14.23: Differentiating hypokalemia with increased distal K^+ secretion and hypertension.

Plasma aldosterone	*Plasma renin*	*Cortisol levels*	*Etiology*
High	High	Normal	Renal artery stenosis Reninoma Malignant hypertension
High	Low	Normal	Primary hyperaldosteronism
Low	Low–normal	Normal	Liddle syndrome Licorice ingestion
Low	Low–normal	High	Cushing syndrome

Additional testing

- Serum digoxin levels if patient is receiving treatment with digoxin
- Thyroid function tests, especially in patients with paralysis, to rule out thyrotoxic periodic paralysis
- Serum magnesium levels, as hypomagnesemia is often associated with hypokalemia, and such patients are often refractory to K^+ replacement alone.
- Other testing as per etiology (e.g., CT of adrenal glands if mineralocorticoid/glucocorticoid/catecholamine excess is suspected).

Treatment

- **Therapeutic goals:**
  - To correct the potassium deficit
  - To minimize the ongoing losses
  - To treat the underlying cause to prevent further episodes
  - To prevent overly rapid correction, which can cause acute hyperkalemia, which in turn can cause ventricular fibrillation and sudden death
- It should be noted that a decrement of 1 mmol/L in the plasma-potassium concentration (from 4.0 to 3.0 mmol/L) may represent a total body potassium deficit of 200–400 mmol.

Oral Therapy

- Oral or enteral therapy is preferred in nonemergent patients who can take orally and has normal GI tract function.
- Potassium chloride (15 mL = 20 mEq) is the preferred agent. Especially useful in Cl-responsive metabolic alkalosis.
- Potassium phosphate is useful when coexistent phosphorus deficiency.
- Potassium bicarbonate, acetate, gluconate, or citrate is useful in metabolic acidosis.
- Usual dose: 40–100 mEq/day in 2–4 divided doses

IV Therapy

- Indicated for patients with severe hypokalemia (<2.5 mEq/L), symptomatic hypokalemia, those with nonfunctioning GI tract or those who are unable to take orally.
  - Note: 1 mL of 15% potassium chloride = 2 mEq/L, 10 mL = 20 mEq/L.
- The maximum concentration of administered potassium should be no more than:
  - 40 mEq/L via a peripheral vein or
  - 100 mEq/L via central vein
- The rate of infusion should not exceed 10–20 mEq/hr unless paralysis or malignant ventricular arrhythmia is present.
  - Maximum rate of infusion should not exceed 40 mEq/hr in these cases.
  - Maximum dose per day: 240–400 mEq/day

Choice of fluid during IV therapy

- KCL should always be administered in saline solutions, rather than dextrose-containing solutions.
- This is because dextrose-containing solutions can stimulate cellular potassium uptake, resulting in worsening of the hypokalemia.

Choice of central line placement for IV therapy

In cases of infusion of potassium chloride through central lines, femoral lines are preferred to internal jugular or subclavian central lines, as the infusion through the latter can lead to rapid changes in the local concentration of potassium and affect cardiac conduction.

Monitoring during IV therapy

- Continuous ECG monitoring should be done, especially if the rate of infusion is more than 10 mEq/hr.
- Serum potassium levels should be monitored 1–4 hours after a dose of 60–80 mEq/L is given, before giving further potassium doses.

Additional therapy

- **Replace magnesium, if magnesium deficiency is present.**
- High potassium diet
- Treat the underlying cause

Hyperkalemia

Q. Write short essay/note on:

- **Causes and treatment of hyperkalemia.**
- **ECG changes in hyperkalemia.**
- **Clinical features, diagnosis, and treatment/management of hyperkalemia.**
- **Drugs used to treat hyperkalemia.**

Definition: Hyperkalemia is defined as plasma **potassium greater than 5.5 mEq/L.**

Based on severity, it may be classified as:

- Mild hyperkalemia: Serum potassium: 5.5–5.9 mEq/L
- Moderate hyperkalemia: Serum potassium: 5.9–6.4 mEq/L
- Severe hyperkalemia: Serum potassium: ≥6.5 mEq/L

Causes of Hyperkalemia

See **Table 14.24**.

TABLE 14.24: Causes of hyperkalemia.

A. *Increased potassium intake*
   - Diet
   - Potassium-containing salt substitutes
   - Potassium supplementation
   - Chewing and ingestion of burnt match heads (cautopyreiophagia)

B. *Decreased renal excretion*
   i. Reduced GFR:
      - Acute kidney injury (AKI)
      - Chronic kidney disease (CKD)
   ii. Tubulointerstitial disease:
      - Interstitial nephritis
      - Sickle cell disease
      - Obstructive uropathy
   iii. Mineralocorticoid deficiency:
      - Primary adrenal insufficiency
      - Type IV RTA
   iv. Drugs:
      - Reduced renin release:
         - Beta-blockers
         - NSAIDs
      - Reduced mineralocorticoid receptor activation:
         - ACE-I
         - ARBs
         - Aldosterone receptor antagonists
         - Heparin
         - Ketoconazole
      - Inhibition of Na^+/K^+ ATPase, necessary for collecting duct K^+ secretion:
         - Calcineurin inhibitors
         - Digitalis
      - Blocking ENaC Na channel, decreasing gradient for K^+ secretion:
         - Amiloride
         - Triamterene
         - Trimethoprim
         - Pentamidine
   v. Other:
      - Gordon syndrome (pseudohypoaldosteronism type 2)

C *Transcellular shift of potassium*:
   - Metabolic acidosis
   - Severe hyperglycemia
   - Insulin deficiency
   - Beta-blockers
   - Hemolysis
   - Rhabdomyolysis
   - Tumor lysis syndrome
   - Hyperkalemic periodic paralysis

D. Pseudohyperkalemia:
   - Hemolysis due to mechanical trauma during venipuncture
   - Repeated fist clenching during blood withdrawal
   - Acute respiratory alkalosis (crying/hyperventilation during blood withdrawal)
   - In vitro hemolysis
   - Leukocytosis

Clinical Features

- **Often asymptomatic** until plasma K^+ concentration is greater than 6.5–7.0 mEq/L, when it may lead to fatal cardiac arrhythmia, hence it is called as **silent killer**. Hence, suspect hyperkalemia as potential cause in all patients presenting with cardiac arrest.
- Signs and symptoms of underlying disease: For example:
  - CKD
  - History of drugs causing hyperkalemia
- Signs and symptoms due to hyperkalemia:
  - Cardiac:
    - Arrhythmias **(Figs. 14.12 and 14.13)**
  - Musculoskeletal:
    - Weakness
    - Paresthesia
    - Ascending paralysis
  - Gastrointestinal:
    - Nausea
    - Vomiting
    - Diarrhea

Investigations

- Initial tests:
  i. Measurement of urea, creatinine, electrolytes, including bicarbonate
  ii. Blood glucose levels
  iii. Blood gas analysis to look for metabolic acidosis
  iv. ECG: ECG changes are shown in **Figures 14.12 and 14.13**. The earliest electrocardiographic changes are increased T-wave, amplitude or peaked T-wave.
  v. Urine electrolytes
- Additional tests:
  i. CPK levels in suspected rhabdomyolysis
  ii. LDH levels in suspected hemolysis

iii. Uric acid and phosphorous levels in suspected tumor lysis syndrome
iv. Plasma cortisol, renin and aldosterone levels to assess mineralocorticoid deficiency
v. Serum digoxin levels in patients receiving digoxin

Approach

- Rule out pseudohyperkalemia, transcellular shifts and excess intake of potassium
- Thorough history and physical examination to determine the etiology (e.g., renal disease, drugs) and severity of symptoms
- In asymptomatic patients with serum potassium >6.5 mEq/L or those with hyperkalemia and additional ECG changes/muscle weakness/paralysis or significant tissue injury, emergency treatment should be initiated **(Table 14.31)**.
- **Urine K⁺** less than 40 mEq/day suggests reduced renal excretion.
- Urine Na⁺ less than 25 mEq/day suggests that distal sodium delivery is a limiting factor in potassium excretion. Volume correction with normal saline or treatment with furosemide may be effective in reducing potassium levels.
- Measurement of **transtubular potassium gradient (TTKG)** helps to determine whether hyperkalemia is caused by aldosterone deficiency/resistance or whether hyperkalemia is secondary to nonrenal cause.

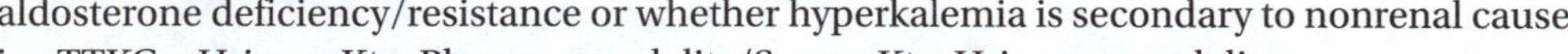

i. TTKG = Urinary K^+ × Plasma osmolality/Serum K^+ × Urinary osmolality

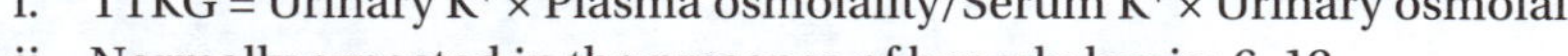

ii. Normally expected in the presence of hyperkalemia: 6–12
iii. If <5: Suggests reduced distal potassium secretion
iv. If >8–10: Suggests reduced tubular flow

- In cases of hypokalemia due to reduced distal potassium secretion, 0.05 g of 9α-fludrocortisone is given:
  - If TTKG < 8, it suggests tubular resistance. Likely causes include:
    - Tubulointerstitial diseases
    - Urinary tract obstruction
    - Pseudohypoaldosteronism type 1 or 2
    - Drugs: Amiloride, triamterene, spironolactone, calcineurin inhibitors, and trimethoprim
  - If TTKG > 8–10, hypoaldosteronism is likely

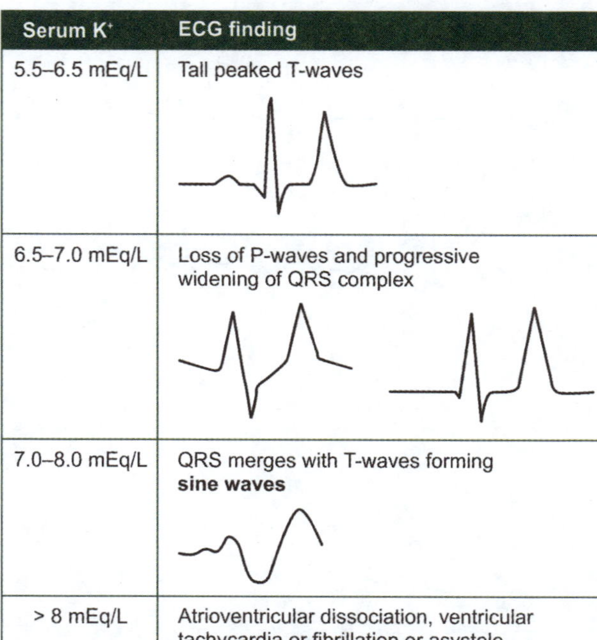

Serum K^+	ECG finding
5.5–6.5 mEq/L	Tall peaked T-waves
6.5–7.0 mEq/L	Loss of P-waves and progressive widening of QRS complex
7.0–8.0 mEq/L	QRS merges with T-waves forming **sine waves**
> 8 mEq/L	Atrioventricular dissociation, ventricular tachycardia or fibrillation or asystole

FIG. 14.12: ECG changes in hyperkalemia in relation to serum potassium.

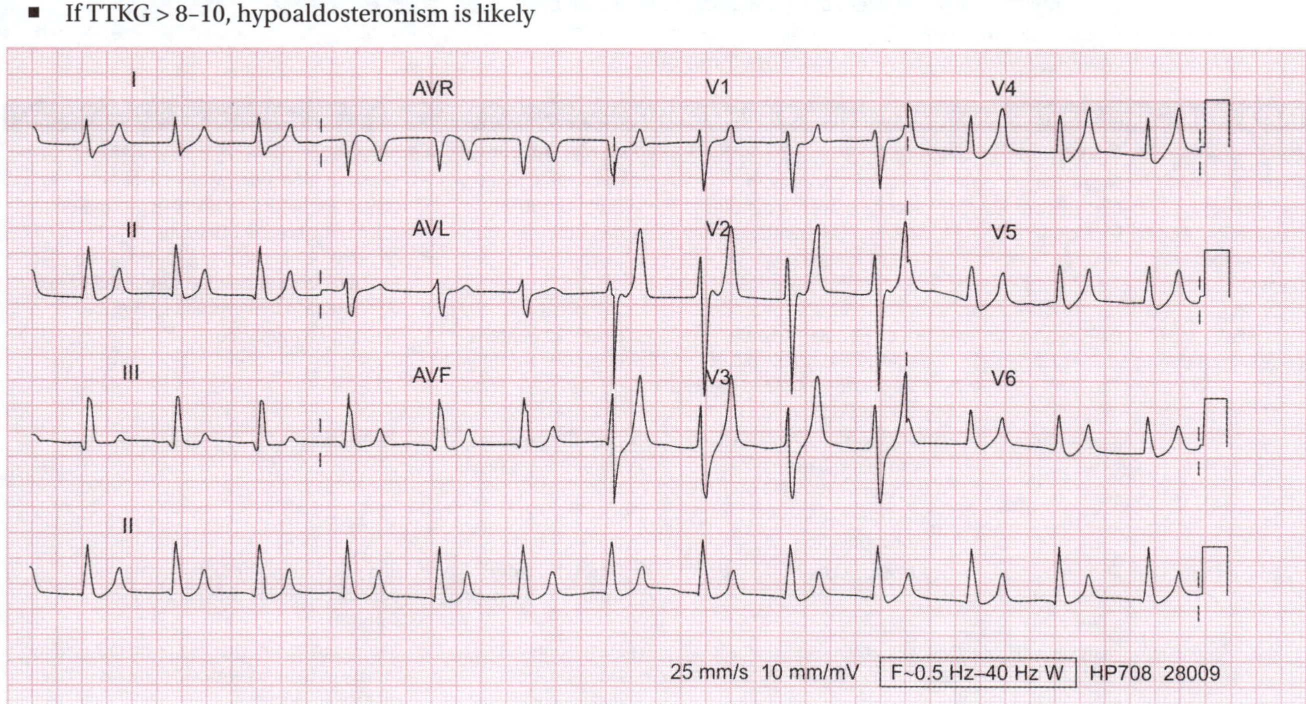

FIG. 14.13A: ECG changes in hyperkalemia (increased T-wave, amplitude or peaked T-wave).

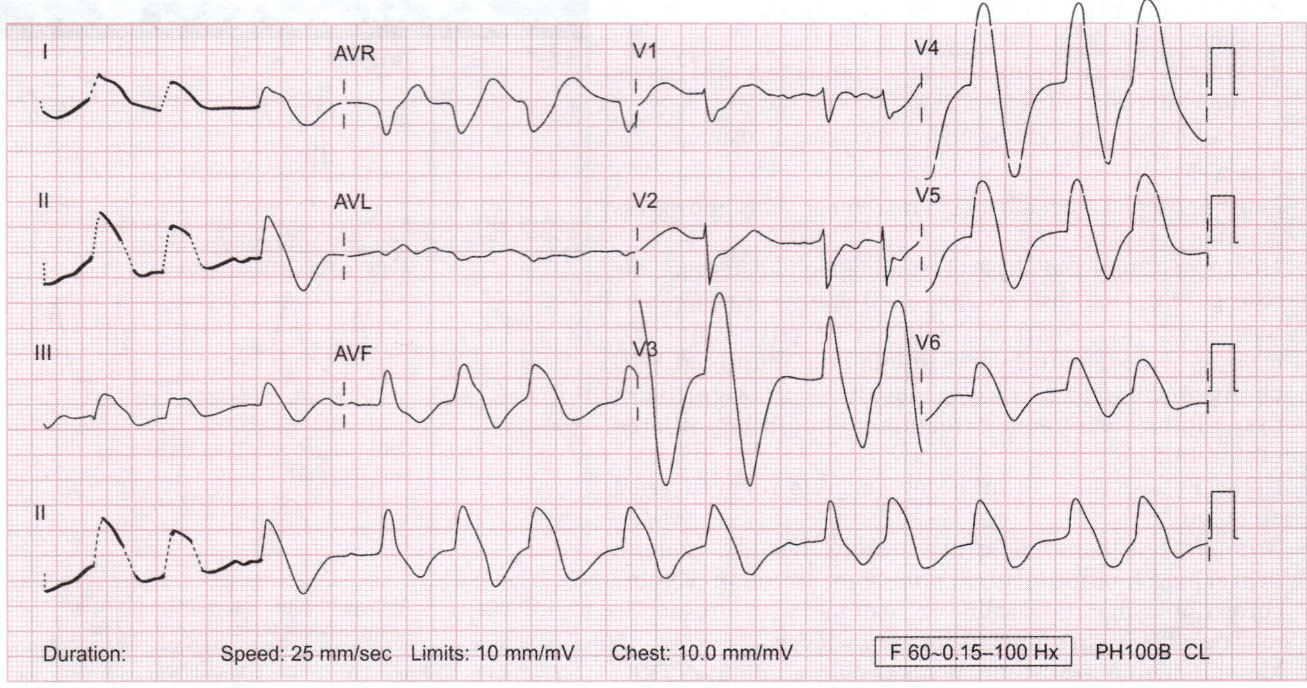

FIG. 14.13B: ECG of severe hyperkalemia showing sine wave pattern.

- In cases of hypoaldosteronism, renin levels should be measured:
  i. Renin high: Primary adrenal insufficiency, isolated aldosterone deficiency, ACE-I, and ARB
  ii. Renin low: Pseudohypoaldosteronism type 2, acute glomerulonephritis, diabetes mellitus, and beta-blockers, and NSAIDs.

Treatment

The urgency and aggressiveness of treatment of hyperkalemia depends on its degree and clinical status.

Emergency treatment (Table 14.25)

- Indications for emergency treatment:
  - Asymptomatic potentially fatal hyperkalemia (serum potassium >6.5 mEq/L)
  - Profound weakness including paralysis
  - Absence of P wave, QRS widening or ventricular arrhythmia on ECG

TABLE 14.25: Drugs used in the emergency treatment of hyperkalemia.

Mechanism	*Intervention*	*Dose*	*Onset and duration*	*Caution*
Myocardial membrane stabilization, if ECG changes are present	IV calcium gluconate or IV calcium chloride	➢ 10 mL of 10% calcium gluconate over 10 minutes ➢ Equivalent elemental calcium dose of 13.6 mEq	➢ Onset: 1–3 minutes ➢ Duration: 30–60 minutes	➢ Should not be administered in $NaHCO_3^-$ containing solutions because precipitation of calcium carbonate can occur ➢ Hypercalcemia can precipitate digoxin toxicity. Hence should be administered over 30 minutes in patients on digoxin
Intracellular potassium shifting	Dextrose/Insulin	➢ Insulin (regular) 10 units intravenous with 50 mL of 50% dextrose, if blood glucose < 250 mg/dL	➢ Onset: 30 minutes ➢ Duration: 4–6 hours	➢ Watch for hypoglycemia
	Beta agonists	➢ Nebulized salbutamol 10 mg ➢ Note that the dose of salbutamol is 2–8 times that usually given for bronchodilation	➢ Onset: 30 minutes ➢ Duration: 2–4 hours	➢ Tachycardia
Potassium removal	Sodium polystyrene sulfonate	➢ 30–60 g PO or PR	➢ Onset: 1–2 hours ➢ Duration: 4–6 hours	➢ Risk of colon perforation when given as enema, especially with concurrent use of sorbitol
	Hemodialysis	Best way of removal	➢ Onset: Immediate ➢ Duration: Until dialysis completed	➢ Serum potassium should not be reduced too rapidly in patients with arrhythmias or heart disease

Other drugs which can be considered in acute hyperkalemia:

- **Sodium bicarbonate:**
  - Useful in patients who have metabolic acidosis (pH <7.2)
  - Mechanism: Shifts potassium into the cell
  - Adverse effects:
    - Can worsen intravascular volume overload, especially in patients with oliguric AKI
    - Acute hypernatremia
- IV normal saline:
  - Mechanism: Increases distal sodium delivery, thus helping in renal excretion
- Diuretics:
  - Useful for chronic or mild hyperkalemia
  - Used in volume expanded patients or along with IV normal saline
  - Mechanism: Increased renal excretion
  - Not very effective in patients with severe renal impairment, who constitute the majority of the population with severe hyperkalemia. Hence, it is not used routinely in the emergency management of hyperkalemia.

Chronic treatment

- Treat the underlying cause
- Stop the offending drug
- Reduction of dietary potassium intake
- Use of medications such as:
  - Diuretics
  - Sodium bicarbonate in patients with acidosis
  - Potassium-binding resins
- Sodium polystyrene sulfonate, Patiromer, Sodium zirconium cyclosilicate
  - Fludrocortisone has been used in patients with chronic hypotension secondary to adrenal insufficiency in patients with normal renal function.

ACID-BASE BALANCE

Q. Write short essay/note on:
- **Physiology of acid-base balance.**
- **Different terminologies used in assessment of acid-base status of a patient.**

Definitions

- **Acid:** Any compound which forms H^+ ions in solution (proton donors), e.g., carbonic acid releases H^+ ions.
- **Base:** Any compound which combines with H^+ ions in solution (proton acceptors), e.g., bicarbonate (HCO^-) accepts H^+ ions.

Regulation of Acid-Base Balance

- Maintenance of blood pH is an important homeostatic mechanism of the body. The pH of the blood is maintained between 7.35 and 7.45.
- Normal pH and its variation is indicated in **Box 14.7**.

Maintenance of Acid-Base Balance/pH

Many physiological mechanisms maintain pH of the ECF within narrow limits **(Box 14.8)**.

Box 14.7: Normal pH and its variation.

- *Normal pH*: 7.35–7.45
- *Acidosis*: Physiological state resulting from abnormally low plasma pH
- *Alkalosis*: Physiological state resulting from abnormally high plasma pH
- *Acidemia*: Plasma pH < 7.35
- *Alkalemia*: Plasma pH > 7.45

Box 14.8: Response of the body to acid-base challenge.

1. *Buffering*: Two most common chemical buffer groups
   i. Bicarbonate
   ii. Nonbicarbonate (hemoglobin, protein, and phosphate):
      - Blood buffer systems act instantaneously
      - Regulate pH by binding or releasing H^+
2. Respiratory acid-base control mechanisms
3. Renal acid-base control mechanisms

APPROACH TO ACID-BASE DISORDER

Step 1: Determine if the patient has academia (plasma pH < 7.35) or alkalemia (plasma pH > 7.45)

Step 2: Determine the primary abnormality and the compensatory response, as described in **Table 14.26**

Step 3: Determine whether the compensation is appropriate, as describe in **Box 14.9**. If the compensation is **not** appropriate, it suggests the presence of a combined acid-base disorder.

- For example:
  - In a patient with metabolic acidosis, the body tries to compensate by lowering the pCO_2.

- ♦ If the pCO_2 is lower than expected: Compensation is excessive. The patient has an additional respiratory alkalosis.
- ♦ If the pCO_2 is higher than expected: Compensation is inadequate. The patient has an additional respiratory acidosis.

Step 4: For patients with metabolic acidosis:
- Determine anion gap.
- Assess the delta ratio.

Classification of Acid-Base Disorders

See **Table 14.26.**

ANION GAP

Q. What is anion gap? Enumerate conditions associated with increased anion gap.

- Anion gap (AG) denotes the concentration of the unmeasured anions in the plasma, namely—phosphates, sulfates, organic acids, and protein anions.
- Anion gap = $\{[Na^+] + [K^+]\} - \{[HCO_3^-] + [Cl^-]\}$
  - Normal cations in plasma: Na^+, K^+, Ca^{2+}, Mg^{2+}
  - Normal anions in plasma are Cl^-, HCO^-, negative charges present on albumin, phosphate, sulfate, lactate, and other organic acids.
  - The sums of the positive and negative charges are equal.
- Normal anionic gap is 8–12 mEq/L.
- **Albumin is the principal unmeasured anion.**
- Hence, if there are gross changes in serum albumin levels, the following correction should be applied.
  - $AG_{corrected} = AG + \{(4 - albumin) \times 2.5\}$
- Elevated anion gap:
  - An elevated anion gap suggests the presence of metabolic acidosis with a circulating anion
  - Usually found in some forms of metabolic acidosis **(Table 14.27)**.
- Normal anion gap:
  - Normal anion gap metabolic acidosis can result from renal or nonrenal causes **(Table 14.28)**.
- **Urinary anion gap (UAG):**
  - UAG *(in mEq/L or mmol/L)* = $(U_{Na}^{+} + U_{K}^{+}) - U_{Cl}^{-}$
  - In cases of normal anion gap metabolic acidosis (NAGMA), urine anion gap is useful to distinguish between renal and extrarenal causes.
  - UAG is normally a positive value: +30 to +50 mmol/L.

TABLE 14.26: Classification of acid-base disorders.

Disorder	*pH*	*[H⁺]*	*Primary abnormality*	*Compensatory response*
Metabolic acidosis	↓	↑	↓ $[HCO_3] < 22$ mmol/L	↓ pCO_2
Metabolic alkalosis	↑	↓	↑ $[HCO_3] > 26$ mmol/L	↑ pCO_2
Respiratory acidosis	↓	↑	↑ $pCO_2 > 42$ mm Hg	↑ $[HCO_3]$
Respiratory alkalosis	↑	↓	↓ $pCO_2 < 38$ mm Hg	↓ $[HCO_3]$

Box 14.9: Determining if the compensation is appropriate.

Expected compensation

Metabolic acidosis:
- ➢ *Winter's formula*: $pCO_2 = 1.5\,[HCO_3] + 8 \pm 2$
- ➢ *Alternate methods*:
  - For decrease of 1 mmol/L of HCO_3^-: 1.2 mm Hg decrease in pCO_2 **or**
  - $pCO_2 = HCO_3^- + 15$ **or**
  - pCO_2 = Last 2 digits of pH
- ➢ Note: If pCO_2 > expected pCO_2 à additional respiratory acidosis
- ➢ If pCO_2 < expected pCO_2 à Additional respiratory alkalosis is also present

Metabolic alkalosis:
- ➢ For every 10 mmol/L increase in HCO_3 • pCO_2 increases by 7
- ➢ Note: If pCO_2 > expected pCO_2 • additional respiratory acidosis
- ➢ If pCO_2 < expected pCO_2 • additional respiratory alkalosis is also present

Respiratory acidosis:
- ➢ ***Acute:*** For every 10 increase in pCO_2 • HCO_3 increases by **1**
- ➢ ***Chronic:*** For every 10 increase in pCO_2 • HCO_3 increases by **3.5**
- ➢ Note: If HCO_3^- > expected HCO_3^- • additional metabolic alkalosis is also present
- ➢ If HCO_3^- < expected HCO_3^- • additional metabolic acidosis is also present

Respiratory alkalosis:
- ➢ ***Acute:*** For every 10 decrease in pCO_2 • HCO_3 decreases by **2**
- ➢ ***Chronic:*** For every 10 decrease in pCO_2 • HCO_3 decreases by **5**
- ➢ Note: If HCO_3^- > expected HCO_3^- • additional metabolic alkalosis is also present
- ➢ If HCO_3^- < expected HCO_3^- • Additional metabolic acidosis is also present

TABLE 14.27: Causes of high anion gap metabolic acidosis (HAGMA).

Lactic acidosis	**Toxins**	Mnemonic: **GOLDMARK**
Ketoacidosis:	Ethylene glycol	**G**—Glycols
Diabetic	Methanol	**O**—Oxoproline
Alcoholic	Salicylates (Aspirin)	**L**—L-Lactate
Starvation	Propylene glycol	**D**—D-Lactate
Renal failure (acute and chronic):		**M**—Methanol
		A—Aspirin
		R—Renal failure
		K—Ketoacidosis

TABLE 14.28: Causes of normal anion gap metabolic acidosis(NAGMA).

Loss of bicarbonate	*Reduced renal acid excretion (retention of HCl)*	*Others*
➢ GI causes: Diarrhea, biliary or pancreatic fistulas ➢ Renal causes: – Proximal renal tubular acidosis (type 2) – Toluene intoxication (>12 hours) – Carbonic anhydrase inhibitors – Spironolactone ➢ Ureter: GI connections (intestinal mucosa exchanges urinary chloride for bicarbonate resulting in urinary bicarbonate loss)	➢ Renal failure ➢ Renal tubular acidosis type 1 (distal) and type 4	➢ Fluid resuscitation with saline (mild dilution of HCO_3^- by addition of Cl^- containing fluid) ➢ Adrenal insufficiency ➢ Drugs: – Prostaglandin inhibitors – Amiloride – Trimethoprim – Pentamidine

- Positive UAG:
  - Renal tubular acidosis (types 1, 2, and 4)
  - Renal failure
- Negative UAG: Increased renal excretion of an unmeasured cation such as NH_4^+
  - Diarrhea
  - Biliary or pancreatic fistulas
  - GI-ureteral connections

"Delta Ratio"/"GAP-GAP"

- Ratio of delta anion gap (difference in anionic gap from the normal anion gap) to delta bicarbonate (the difference in bicarbonate from the normal bicarbonate levels).
- Delta ratio = Δ AG/Δ HCO_3^-
- It can be used to identify concurrent metabolic disorders.
- Interpretation of delta ratio:
  - 0.8–1.2 = Anion gap metabolic acidosis alone
  - 0.3–0.7 = Anion gap metabolic acidosis + Nonanion gap metabolic acidosis
  - >1.2 = Anion gap metabolic acidosis + Metabolic alkalosis

Metabolic Acidosis

Q. Write short note on:
- **Causes of metabolic acidosis (*see* Tables 14.27 and 14.28).**
- **Clinical features and management of metabolic acidosis.**

- Metabolic acidosis is a primary acid-base disorder characterized by fall in both pH of blood (↓ pH) and bicarbonate level in the plasma (↓ HCO_3^-).
- Metabolic acidosis can develop when there is an imbalance between net acid production and net acid excretion **(Fig. 14.14).**
- Metabolic acidosis occurs when an acid other than carbonic acid (due to CO_2 retention) accumulates in the body, leading to fall in the plasma bicarbonate.
- Thus, it is due to gain of strong acid or loss of base (HCO_3^-).

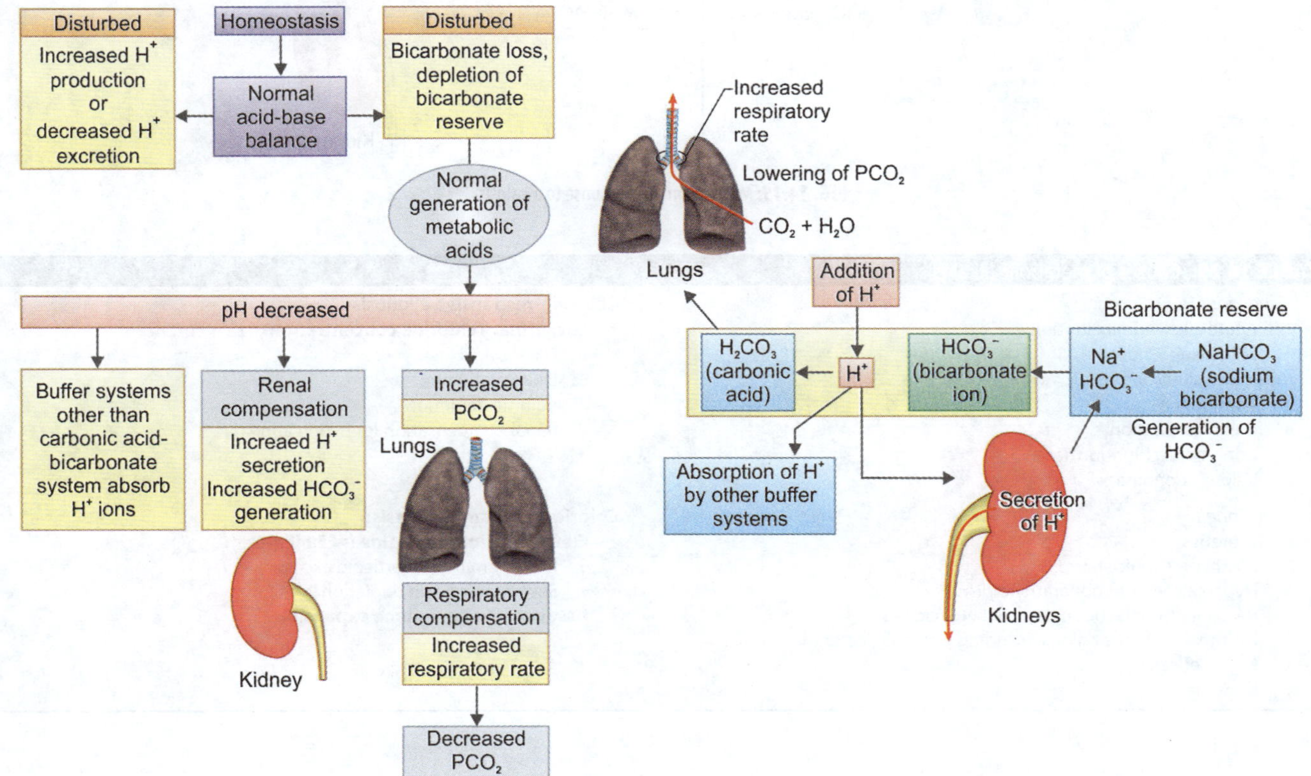

FIG. 14.14: Mechanism and response to acidosis.

Clinical Features (Box 14.10)

Symptoms are specific and a result of the underlying pathology.

Treatment
- Correct the underlying disorder
- Sodium bicarbonate may be administered in severe acidosis.
- Tromethamine (tris-hydroxymethyl aminomethane; THAM) is an alternative to $NaHCO_3$.
- Dialysis may be necessary in renal failure with metabolic acidosis.

Box 14.10: Clinical features of metabolic acidosis.

Respiratory effects: Hyperventilation. In severe cases, there is deep sighing respiration (Kussmaul's breathing or "air hunger").

CVS: ↓ myocardial contractility, sympathetic over activity, resistant to catecholamines

CNS: Lethargy, disorientation, stupor, muscle twitching, coma, and cranial nerve palsies

Others: Hyperkalemia

Metabolic Alkalosis

Q. Write short note on metabolic alkalosis.

Metabolic alkalosis is characterized by rise in both plasma bicarbonate level and plasma pH. The primary event is elevation of pH due to raised plasma bicarbonate concentration (HCO_3^-) or decreased acid **(Fig. 14.15).**

Types: Metabolic alkalosis may be hypovolemic or normovolemic. Causes of metabolic alkalosis are listed in **Table 14.29**.

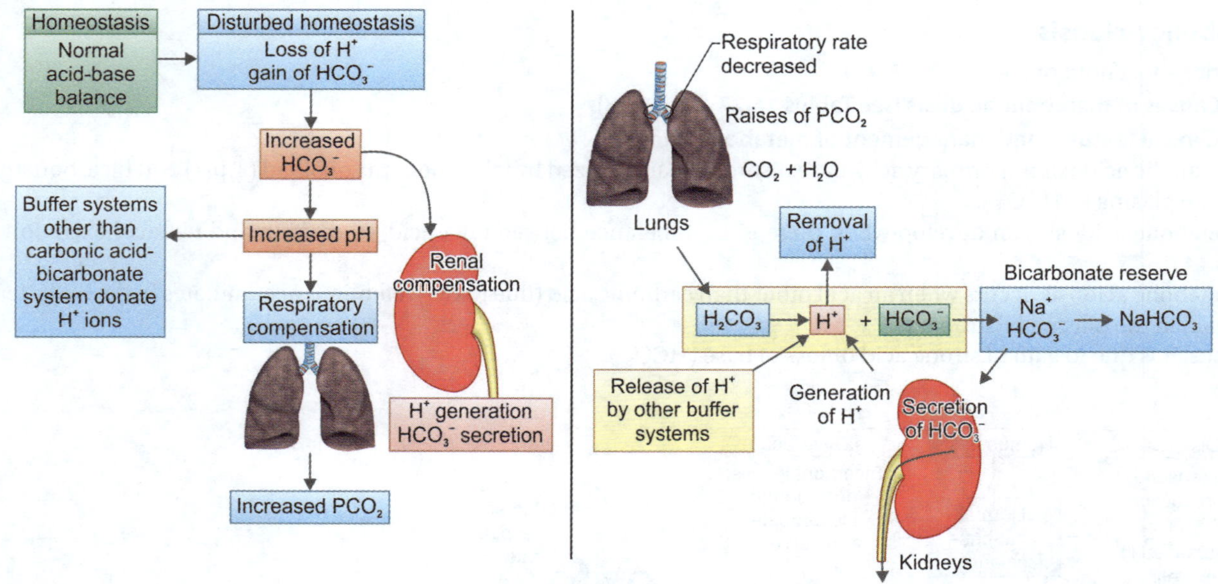

FIG. 14.15: Mechanism and response to alkalosis.

TABLE 14.29: Causes of metabolic alkalosis.

➢ *Exogenous HCO_3^- loads*: - Acute alkali administration - Milk-alkali syndrome ➢ *Gastrointestinal origin*: - Vomiting - Gastric aspiration - Congenital chloridorrhea - Villous adenoma	**Chloride-responsive alkalosis:** ➢ **Low urinary chloride concentration** (<15 mEq/L) - Gastric acid loss - Diuretic therapy - Volume depletion - Renal compensation for hypercapnea
➢ *Renal origin*: - Diuretics - Posthypercapnic state - Hypercalcemia/hypoparathyroidism - Recovery from lactic acidosis or ketoacidosis - Non-reabsorbable anions including penicillin, carbenicillin - Mg^{2+} deficiency - K^+ depletion	**Chloride-resistant alkalosis:** ➢ **Elevated urinary chloride** (>25 mEq/L): - Primary mineralocorticoid excess - Severe potassium depletion ➢ **Associated with volume expansion**

Clinical Features (Table 14.30)

TABLE 14.30: Clinical features of metabolic alkalosis.

➢ Decreased myocardial contractility ➢ Arrhythmias ➢ Decreased cerebral blood flow ➢ Confusion	➢ Mental obtundation ➢ Neuromuscular excitability ➢ Hypoventilation ➢ Pulmonary microatelectasis

Management
- Correct the underlying cause to stop loss of acid
- *Metabolic alkalosis with hypovolemia*: Corrected by intravenous infusions of 0.9% saline with potassium supplements. This reverses the secondary hyperaldosteronism and the kidneys excrete the excess alkali in the urine.
- *Metabolic alkalosis with normal or increased volume*: Treatment of the underlying endocrine cause.
- *Acetazolamide may be considered for patients with posthypercapnic metabolic alkalosis*
- *Dialysis may be required if severe alkalosis or renal failure is present.*

Respiratory Acidosis

Q. Write short note on respiratory acidosis.

Respiratory acidosis is a primary acid-base disorder characterized by ↑ PCO_2 • ↓ pH.
- Acute (<24 hours)
- Chronic (>24 hours)

Causes of Respiratory Acidosis (Table 14.31)

TABLE 14.31: Causes of respiratory acidosis.

CNS depression: ➢ Drugs: Opiates, sedatives, and anesthetics ➢ Obesity hypoventilation syndrome ➢ Stroke **Neuromuscular disorders** ➢ Neurologic: Multiple sclerosis, polio, GBS, tetanus, botulism, and high cord lesions ➢ End plate: Myasthenia gravis, OP poisoning, and aminoglycoside toxicity ➢ Muscle: Hypokalemia, hypophosphatemia, muscular dystrophy **Airway obstruction** ➢ COPD, acute aspiration, and laryngospasm	**Chest wall restriction:** ➢ *Pleural*: Effusions, empyema, pneumothorax, and fibrothorax ➢ *Chest wall*: Kyphoscoliosis, scleroderma, ankylosing spondylitis, and obesity **Severe pulmonary restrictive disorders:** ➢ Pulmonary fibrosis ➢ *Parenchymal infiltration*: Pneumonia and pulmonary edema **Abnormal blood CO_2 transport** ➢ *Decreased perfusion*: Heart failure, cardiac arrest, and pulmonary embolism ➢ Severe anemia ➢ Acetazolamide carbonic anhydrase inhibition ➢ Red cell anion exchange: Loop diuretics, salicylates, NSAID

Clinical Features (Box 14.11)

Box 14.11: Clinical features of respiratory acidosis.

- **RS (respiratory system):**
  - Stimulation of ventilation (tachypnea)
  - Dyspnea
- **CNS (central nervous system):**
  - ↑cerebral blood flow • ↑ ICT, papilledema
  - CO_2 Narcosis (disorientation, confusion, headache, lethargy)
  - Coma (arterial hypoxemia, ↑ ICT, anesthetic effect of ↑ PCO_2 >100 mm Hg)
- **CVS:** Tachycardia, bounding pulse
- **Others:** Peripheral vasodilatation (warm, flushed, sweaty)

Treatment
- The underlying causes should be corrected.
- Consider ventilatory support:
  - Noninvasive positive pressure ventilation
  - Intubation and mechanical ventilation
  - Rapid infusion of alkali is justified only in prolonged cardiopulmonary arrest.
  - Avoid overfeeding as changes in metabolism may worsen acidosis by increasing the rate of elimination of carbon dioxide.

Respiratory Alkalosis

Q. Write short note on respiratory alkalosis and its causes.

- Most common acid-base abnormality in critically ill is characterized by ↓PCO_2 → ↑pH.
- Primary process: **Hyperventilation:**
  - **Acute:** $PaCO_2$ ↓, pH-alkalemic
  - **Chronic:** $PaCO_2$ ↓, pH normal/near normal

Causes of Respiratory Alkalosis (Table 14.33)

TABLE 14.32: Causes of respiratory alkalosis.

A. *Central nervous system stimulation*: 1. Pain 2. Anxiety, psychosis 3. Fever 4. Cerebrovascular accident 5. Meningitis, encephalitis 6. Tumor 7. Trauma B. *Hypoxemia or tissue hypoxia*: 1. High altitude 2. Septicemia	3. Hypotension 4. Severe anemia C. *Drugs or hormones*: 1. Pregnancy, progesterone 2. Salicylates 3. Cardiac failure D. *Stimulation of chest receptors*: 1. Hemothorax 2. Flail chest 3. Cardiac failure 4. Pulmonary embolism	E. *Miscellaneous*: 1. Hepatic failure 2. Mechanical ventilation 3. Heat exposure 4. Recovery from metabolic acidosis

Clinical Features of Respiratory Alkalosis (Table 14.33)

TABLE 14.33: Clinical features of respiratory alkalosis.

➤ **CNS:** – ↑ Neuromuscular irritability (tingling, circumoral numbness) – **Tetany** – ↑ ICT(intracranial tension) – Light headedness, confusion	➤ **CVS:** – CO and SBP ↑ (↑ SVR, HR) – Arrhythmias – ↓ myocardial contractility ➤ **Others** – Hypokalemia, hypophosphatemia – ↓ Free serum calcium—tetany – Hyponatremia, hypochloremia

Treatment
- Elimination of the underlying disorder
- In acute hyperventilation syndrome, sedation and **rebreathing into a bag** may terminate the attack.

GENETIC SYNDROMES WITH ACID-BASE AND POTASSIUM ABNORMALITIES (TABLE 14.34 AND FIG. 14.16)

TABLE 14.34: Genetic syndromes with acid-base and potassium abnormalities.

Syndrome	*Genetics*	*Blood pressure*	*Acid-base disorder and Potassium*	*Renin and aldosterone*	*Other features*	*Treatment*
Liddle syndrome	ENaC gene Chr 16p12 Autosomal dominant	Hypertension	Metabolic alkalosis Hypokalemia	Both suppressed	Salt-sensitive	ENaC inhibitors
Glucocorticoid-remediable aldosteronism (GRA)	CYP11B1 / CYP11B2 Chr 8q24 Autosomal dominant	Hypertension	Metabolic alkalosis Hypokalemia	Renin suppressed Aldosterone normal or elevated	Unusual urine steroid metabolites	Corticosteroid therapy
Apparent mineralocorticoid excess (AME)	11β-HSD 2 Chr 16q22 Autosomal recessive	Hypertension	Metabolic alkalosis Hypokalemia	Both suppressed	Nephrocalcinosis can be seen Elevated urine cortisol:cortisone ratio	Spironolactone and ENaC inhibitors
Mineralocorticoid receptor activating mutation (Geller syndrome)	NR3C2 Chr 4q31 Autosomal dominant	Hypertension	Metabolic alkalosis Hypokalemia	Both suppressed	Exacerbated in pregnancy Spironolactone acts as agonist	ENaC inhibitors
Aldosterone producing adenomas (APA)	KCNJ5 CACNA1D ATP1A1 ATP2B3 De novo or autosomal dominant	Hypertension	Metabolic alkalosis Hypokalemia	Renin suppressed Aldosterone elevated	Imaging shows adrenal adenoma	Spironolactone or Eplerenone Adenomectomy
Congenital adrenal hyperplasia (CAH)	17-β hydroxylase 11-β hydroxylase 10q24 8q24 Autosomal recessive	Hypertension	Metabolic alkalosis Hypokalemia	Both suppressed	ACTH elevated Mineralocorticoids elevated Glucocorticoid deficiency and abnormal sex hormones	Corticosteroid therapy
Pheochromocytoma	Ret NF1 VHL SDHB SDHC Autosomal dominant or de novo	Labile hypertension Orthostatic hypotension	Metabolic alkalosis Hypokalemia	Both elevated	Elevated metanephrines	Alpha blocker Surgery

Contd...

Contd...

Pseudohypo-aldosteronism type 2 (Gordon syndrome)	WNK 1 WNK 4 Kelch-like and Cullin 3 Autosomal dominant/ autosomal recessive or de novo	Hypertension	Metabolic acidosis Hyperkalemia	Renin suppressed Aldosterone normal	Hypercalciuria	Thiazide diuretics
Pseudohypo-aldosteronism type 1	NR3C2 SCNN1A SCNN1B SCNN1G Autosomal dominant/ autosomal recessive	Normal–low	Metabolic acidosis Hyperkalemia	Renin elevated	Failure to thrive Resistance to steroid treatment	Saline infusion Bicarbonate supplementation Dialysis
Bartter syndrome (*similar to loop diuretic*)	Multiple genes such as SLC12A1 KCNJ1 CLCNKB BSND Types 1, 2, 3, 4, 4b: Autosomal recessive Type 5: Autosomal dominant	Normal–low	Metabolic alkalosis Hypokalemia	Renin and aldosterone elevated	Nephrocalcinosis (types 1 and 2) Neonatal manifestation (types 1, 2, 4, and 4b) Deafness (types 4 and 4b) Hypercalciuria	Increase salt intake Potassium supplementation NSAIDs K^+ sparing diuretics
Gitelman syndrome (*similar to thiazide diuretic*)	SLC12A3 Chr 16q13 Autosomal recessive	Normal–low	Metabolic alkalosis Hypokalemia	Both elevated	Hypomagnesemia Hypocalciuria Increased bone density Chondrocalcinosis	Increase salt intake Potassium supplementation Magnesium supplementation NSAIDs K^+ sparing diuretics
EAST (Epilepsy, Ataxia, Sensorineural deafness, Tubulopathy) syndrome	KCNJ10 1q23 Autosomal recessive	Normal–low	Metabolic alkalosis Hypokalemia	Both elevated	Hypomagnesemia Hypocalciuria Seizures Hearing loss	Increase salt intake Potassium supplementation Magnesium supplementation K^+ sparing diuretics

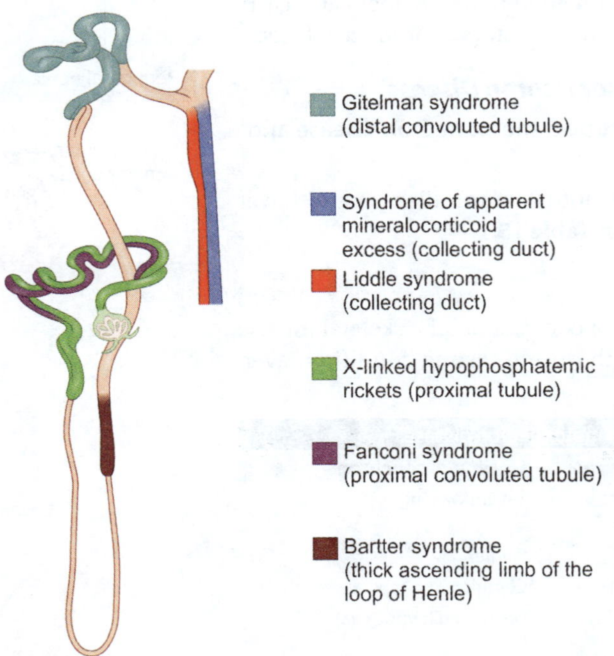

FIG 14.16: Sites of the nephron affected with genetic syndromes with acid-base potassium abnormalities.

CHAPTER

15 Neurology

INTRODUCTION AND SYMPTOMATOLOGY

Weakness and Paralysis

Categories (Flowchart 15.1 and Fig. 15.1)

- **Upper motor neurons:** They consist of corticospinal interneurons which arise from the motor cortex and descend to the spinal cord where they activate the lower motor neurons (anterior horn cells) through synapses.
- **Lower motor neurons:** The term "motor neuron" is usually used only to the efferent neurons that actually innervate muscles (the lower motor neurons). A motor neuron consists of nerve cell (neuron) which is located in the anterior horn cell of the spinal cord and its fibers (axon) project outside the spinal cord to directly or indirectly control effector organs, mainly muscles and glands. Motor neuron axons are efferent nerve fibers and carry signals from the spinal cord to the effectors to produce effects.

FLOWCHART 15.1: Classification of motor neuron.

Upper motor neuron:
Motor cortex → (Corticospinal tract) → Anterior horn cell
Cortex → (Corticonuclear tract) → Clinical nerve nucleus

Lower motor neuron:
Anterior horn cell → Peripheral nerve
Clinical nerve nucleus → Cranial nerves

Signs of Upper and Lower Motor Neuron Disease

Q. List the differences between upper motor neuron disease and lower motor neuron disease.

The differences between upper motor neuron disease and lower motor neuron disease are listed in **Table 15.1**.

Tone

- Muscle tone is a partial state of contraction of a skeletal muscle to maintain its optimal length during resting condition, even

TABLE 15.1: Signs of upper and lower motor neuron disease.

Sign	*Upper motor neuron*	*Lower motor neuron*
Atrophy	None (rarely disuse atrophy)	Severe wasting
Muscles affected	Group of muscles	Single
Fasciculations	None	Common
Tone	Hypertonia—rigidity/ spasticity	Decreased (hypotonia)
Distribution of weakness	Distal predominant/ regional	Predominantly proximal (except neuropathy)/segmental
Tendon reflexes	Exaggerated/hyperactive	Hypoactive/lost
Babinski's sign	Present	Absent
Flexor spasms, clonus	Present	Absent

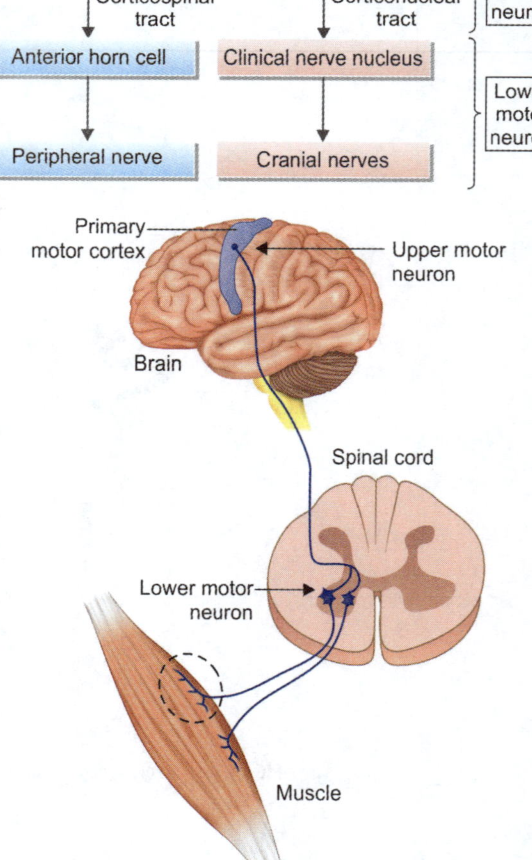

FIG. 15.1: Upper and lower motor neurons—a two-neuron circuit.

when a force is applied to elongate the muscle. It is accomplished by the asynchronous discharge of nervous impulse in the motor neurons in the anterior gray horn of the spinal cord.
- Clinically, it may be defined as the resistance that is encountered when the joint of relaxed muscle is moved passively.
- Increased tone: Associated with disease of upper motor neurons due to loss of inhibition of γ-motor neurons above the site of lesion.
- **Hypotonia:** Causes of hypotonia is listed in **Box 15.1**.

Q. List the causes of hypotonia.

Q. Enumerate the differences between spasticity and rigidity.

The differences between spasticity and rigidity are listed in **Table 15.2**.

Other causes of hypertonia: Tetanus, seizure (tonic phase), tetany, **catatonia, paratonia *(gegenhalten, mitgehen).***

Box 15.1: Causes of hypotonia.
- **Lesions of the motor side of the reflex arc:** Poliomyelitis, polyneuritis, peripheral nerve injuries
- **Lesions of the sensory side of the reflex arc:** Tabes dorsalis, herpes zoster, carcinomatous neuropathy
- **Combined motor and sensory lesion:** Syringomyelia, cord or root compression, gross cord destruction
- Lesions of the muscle (myopathies), neuromuscular junction (NMJ) (myasthenia)
- State of neuronal shock in upper motor neuron lesion
- Cerebellar lesions
- Chorea
- Periodic paralysis
- Rapid eye movement (REM) sleep
- Benzodiazepine overdose, neuromuscular blockers

TABLE 15.2: Differences between spasticity and rigidity.

	Spasticity	*Rigidity*
Lesion	Pyramidal tract lesion	Extrapyramidal tract lesion
Tone	Tone is more in the antigravity group of muscles than in the gravity assisted group of muscles	Tone is equally raised in the gravity assisted and antigravity group of muscles
Character	Clasp knife type of spasticity	Lead pipe or cogwheel type of rigidity
Relation to velocity	Velocity dependent, better appreciated when passive movement of the joint is carried out rapidly	Rigidity is not velocity dependent
Abdominal reflexes	Lost	Preserved
Plantar reflex	Plantar is extensor	Plantar is flexor
Deep tendon reflexes	Brisk or exaggerated	Normal or decreased
Clonus	May be associated sustained clonus	Clonus is absent
Features in limbs	The limb does tend to return toward a particular fixed posture or extreme joint angle	The limb does not tend to return toward a particular fixed posture or extreme joint angle
Reason	Increased gamma-motor activity	Increased alpha- and gamma-motor activity

Fasciculation and Fibrillation

Q. What is fasciculation and fibrillation?

When a motor unit (group of muscle fibers) becomes diseased, especially in anterior horn cell diseases, it may discharge spontaneously, producing **fasciculations** that may be seen or felt clinically or recorded by electromyography (EMG). Fasciculations are visible, fine and fast, sometimes vermicular contractions of fine muscle fibers that occur spontaneously and intermittently.

When motor neurons or their axons degenerate, the denervated muscle fibers also may discharge spontaneously. These single muscle fiber discharges, or **fibrillation** potentials, cannot be seen or felt but can be recorded with EMG.

Causes of fasciculation: Amyotrophic lateral sclerosis, progressive spinal muscular atrophy, post-polio syndrome, hyperthyroidism, organophosphorus poisoning, drugs (e.g., atropine, lithium), mercury, benign fasciculation.

Myotonia

Q. What is myotonia?

- Myotonia is characterized by continued, involuntary muscle contraction even after cessation of voluntary effort (i.e., muscle contraction continues beyond the period of time required for a particular movement to be made and there is failure of normal muscle relaxation).
- It is best seen in the face and hand muscle. When the patient is asked to smile and then relax his facial muscle, a delay in relaxation of the muscle is noted and the smile remains fixed for a longer duration (transverse smile). Similarly, when the patient is asked to grip the examiner's fingers and then let go immediately, a delay in the relaxation of the grip is noted.
- **Myokymia** is a vermicular or continuous rippling movement of a group of muscle fibers that can be seen in neuropathies [Guillain–Barré syndrome (GBS)], plexopathies, and Isaac's syndrome.

Causes of myotonia

See **Box 15.2.**

Box 15.2: Causes of myotonia.
- Myotonic dystrophy type 1
- Myotonic dystrophy type 2/proximal myotonic myopathy
- Myotonia congenita
- Paramyotonia congenita
- Hyperkalemic periodic paralysis

Ataxia

Q. Write a short note on causes of ataxia.

Ataxia is a disorder characterized unsteadiness and impaired coordination of regulating body posture and the rate, range, force, and direction of movement. Types of ataxia are listed in **Box 15.3**.

Reflexes

Plantar Response/Reflex

Q. Write a short note on plantar reflex and extensor plantar reflex/Babinski's sign.

Plantar response/reflex is nociceptive, superficial reflex. Its segmental innervation is S1 segment of the spinal cord. It was first described by Babinski.

Box 15.3: Types of ataxia.

- **Cerebellar:** vasculitis, multiple sclerosis, infection bleeding, infarction, tumors, direct injury, toxins (e.g., alcohol), genetic disorders
- **Sensory:** Posterior column diseases, large fiber neuropathy
- Optic
- Vestibular
- Frontal lobe ataxia (Bruns ataxia)
- Mixed
- Psychogenic
- Pseudoataxia

Technique

- Position the patient in supine with hip and knee extended.
- Fix the ankle joint by holding it and stroke (gentle but firm pressure) the outer aspect of sole with a blunt point (tip of a key). The stroke is directed forward and then curves inward along the metatarsophalangeal joints from the little to the big toe and stopped short of the base of great toe (root value S1).

Interpretation

Normal response is great toe will flex at the metatarsophalangeal joint accompanied by flexion of other toes. Normal response should not be termed "negative Babinski's sign".

Abnormal responses

- **Absent:** No response is seen. Plantar response/reflex may be absent when there is loss of sensation of the sole (L5–S1), thick sole, paralysis of the extensor hallucis, and lesions of reflex arc.
- **Extensor:** Extension (dorsiflexion) of the great toe with or without fanning of others toes (abduction) is known as **Babinski's sign (mediated by L5)**. Fanning of toes without great toe extension has no significance. When fully developed it is accompanied by dorsiflexion of ankle, flexion of hip and knee joint, and slight abduction of thigh with contraction of the tensor fascia lata. Its causes are:
  - Physiological: It may be normally extensor in infants below 6 months, during deep sleep, under general anesthesia.
  - Pathological: Lesion of corticospinal (pyramidal) tract above S1 segment, deep coma, transiently after seizure, alcohol intoxication, hypoglycemia and metabolic encephalopathy.

Alternative ways to elicit Babinski's sign

Chaddock's (lateral malleolus), Gordon's (calf), Oppenheim's (anterior tibia), Schaeffer's (Achilles tendon), Gonda's (press down 4th toe), Stransky's (adduct little toe), Bing's (pinprick on dorsolateral foot).

Deep Tendon Reflex

See **Table 15.3**.

TABLE 15.3: Commonly elicited superficial reflexes and deep tendon reflexes.

Superficial reflexes	*Deep tendon reflexes*
➤ Corneal (cranial nerve V and VII) ➤ Abdominal – Epigastric (T6–T9) – Mid abdominal (T9–T11) – Hypogastric (T11–L1) ➤ Cremasteric (L1, L2) ➤ Anal reflex (S2, S3) ➤ Plantar reflex – Reflexogenic zone—S1 – Afferent nerve—tibial nerve	➤ Jaw jerk (afferent and efferent both 5th nerve, center mid pons) ➤ Biceps (C5, C6) ➤ Brachioradialis/supinator/radial periosteal (C5, C6) ➤ Triceps (C6–C8) ➤ Knee jerk/quadriceps/patellar reflex (L2–L4) ➤ Ankle jerk (L5, S1, S2) **Latent reflexes** (suggest pyramidal lesion if present unilaterally) ➤ Tromner's/finger flexor reflex/ Hoffman's sign ➤ Wartenberg's sign

Vertigo

Q. Write a short note on causes of vertigo.

- **Definition:** Vertigo is defined as an abnormal perception (hallucination/illusion) of movement (a sensation of rotation or tipping) of either the environment or self (body or part of it). The individual feels that the surroundings are spinning or moving. BPPV is the most common cause.
- The perceived movement may be falling down, or rotating or there is a sensation of spinning of the outside world. It is often accompanied by nausea or vomiting.
- **Mechanism:** It develops because of conflicting visual, proprioceptive and vestibular information about a person's position in space. Lesions causing vertigo are listed in **Table 15.4**.

TABLE 15.4: Lesions causing vertigo—the most common cause is benign paroxysmal positional vertigo (BPPV).

Site of lesion	*Example*
Labyrinth	Ménière's disease
VIIIth cranial nerve	Acoustic neuroma
Vestibular neurons	Vertebral artery ischemia, vestibulitis, drugs
Cerebellum/brainstem	Tumor, infarct, multiple sclerosis, drugs, toxins
Temporal lobe	Epilepsy, tumor
Others	Migraine, epilepsy, neurodegenerative diseases

Gait

Observation to be noted while the patient walks: (1) Posture of the body while walking, (2) the regularity of the movement, (3) the position and movement of the arms, (4) the relative ease and smoothness of the movement of the legs, (5) the distance between the feet both in forward and lateral directions, (6) the ability to maintain a straight course, (7) the ease of turning, (8) stopping, and (9) position of feet and posture just before initiation of gait.

Gait Cycle

See **Figure 15.2.**

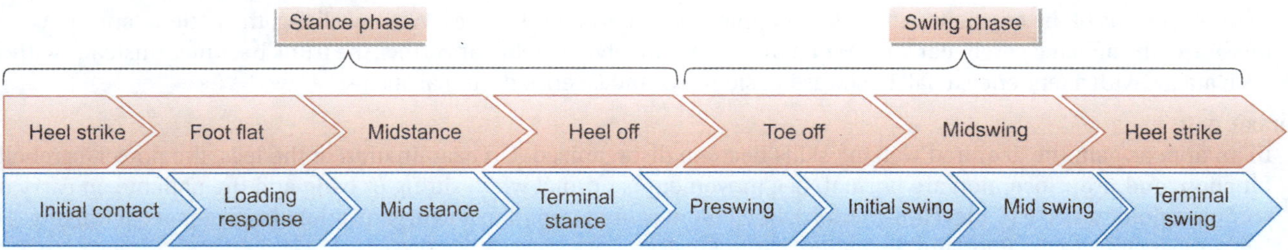

FIG. 15.2: Phases of the gait cycle.

Abnormalities of Gait (Fig. 15.3)

Q. Write a short note on gait abnormalities with examples.

Neurogenic gait disorders should be differentiated from those due to skeletal abnormalities (characterized by pain producing an antalgic gait, or limp). Gait abnormalities incompatible with any anatomical or physiological deficit may be due to functional disorders.

Pyramidal (circumduction/hemiplegic) gait

- Lesions of the upper motor neuron produce characteristic extension of the affected leg. There is tendency for the toes to strike the ground on walking and outward throwing/swing of lower limbs. This movement occurring at the hip joint is called circumduction. There is leaning toward the opposite normal side. The arm of the affected side is adducted at the shoulder and flexed at the elbow, wrist, and fingers.
- In hemiplegia/hemiparesis, there is a clear asymmetry between affected and normal sides on walking, but in paraparesis both lower legs swing slowly from the hips in extension and are stiffly dragged over the ground (walking in mud).

Foot drop (high stepping/slapping gait)

In normal walking, the heel is the first part of the foot to hit the ground. A lower motor neuron lesion affecting the leg will cause weakness of ankle dorsiflexion, resulting in a less controlled descent of the foot, which makes slapping noise as it hits the ground. In severe cases, the foot will have to be lifted higher at the knee to allow room for the inadequately dorsiflexed foot to swing through, resulting in a high-stepping gait. Cause: for example, common peroneal nerve palsy.

Myopathic gait/waddling gait (primary muscle disease)

- During walking, alternating transfer of the body's weight through each leg, needs adequate hip abduction.
  - Causes: Weakness of proximal lower limb muscles (e.g., polymyositis, muscular dystrophy) causes difficulty rising from sitting. The hips are not properly fixed by these muscles and trunk movements are exaggerated, and walking becomes a *waddle or rolling*. The pelvis is poorly supported by each leg. This may be seen with bilateral congenital dislocation of hip (Trendelenburg gait). The patient walks on a broad base with exaggerated lumbar lordosis.

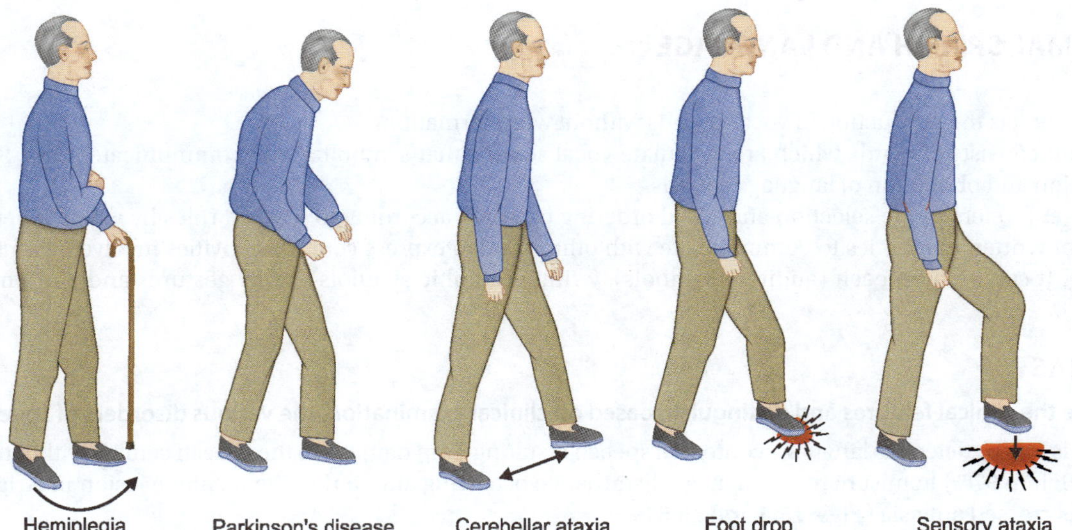

FIG. 15.3: Abnormal gait.

Ataxic gait (cerebellar ataxia: broad-based gait)

- In this type of gait, the patient, unstable, tremulous and reels in any direction (including backward) and walks on a broad base. Ataxia describes this incoordination. The patient finds difficulty in executing tandem walking.
- Causes: Lesions of the cerebellum, vestibular apparatus or peripheral nerves. When walking, the patient tends to veer to the side of the affected cerebellar lobe. When the disease involves cerebellar vermis, the trunk becomes unsteady without limb ataxia, with a tendency to fall backward or sideways and is termed truncal ataxia.

Apraxic gait

- In an apraxic gait, the acquired walking skills become disorganized. On examination of the legs, the power, cerebellar function, and proprioception are normal. Leg movement is normal when sitting or lying and the patient can carry out complex motor tasks (e.g., bicycling motion). But patient cannot initiation and organization the motor act of walking. The feet appear stuck to the floor and the patient cannot walk.
- Causes: Diffuse bilateral hemisphere disease or diffuse frontal lobe disease (e.g., tumor, hydrocephalus, and infarction).

Marche à petits pas

- It is characterized by small, slow steps and marked instability. In contrast to the festination found in Parkinson's disease, it lacks increasing pace and freezing.
- Cause: Small vessel cerebrovascular disease, and accompanying bilateral upper motor neuron signs.

Extrapyramidal gait (shuffling gait)/Festinant gait

- It is characterized by stooped posture and gait difficulties with problems initiating walking and controlling the pace of the gait. Patients make a series of small, flat footed shuffles and become stuck while trying to start walking or when walking through doorways (freezing). The center of gravity will be moved forward to aid propulsion and difficulty stopping. It is characterized by muscular rigidity throughout extensors and flexors. Power is preserved, pace is shortened and slows to a shuffle, and its base remains narrow. There is a stoop and diminished arm swinging and gait becomes festinant (hurried) with short rapid steps. Patient will be having difficulty in turning quickly and initiating movement. Retropulsion, i.e., small backward steps are taken involuntarily when a patient halts.
- Cause: Parkinsonism.

Scissoring gait

It may be seen classically with cerebral palsy due to bilateral spasticity.

Sensory ataxia gait (stamping gait)

- It is characterized by broad based, high stepping, stamping gait and ataxia due to loss of proprioception (position sense). This type of ataxia becomes more prominent by removal of sensory input (e.g., walks with eyes closed) and becomes worse in the dark. Romberg's test is positive.
- Causes: Peripheral sensory (large fiber) lesions (e.g., polyneuropathy), posterior column lesion (vitamin B12 deficiency or tabes dorsalis).

Choreiform gait (hyperkinetic gait)

- The patient will display irregular, jerky, involuntary movements in all extremities. Walking may accentuate their baseline movement disorder.
- Causes: Sydenham's chorea, Huntington's disease, and other forms of chorea, athetosis or dystonia.

ABNORMAL SPEECH AND LANGUAGE

***Definitions*:**

- **Phonation:** It is the production of vocal sounds without word formation.
- **Speech:** It consists of words which are articulate vocal sounds that symbolize and communicate ideas. Speech is the articulation and phonation of language sounds.
- **Language:** It refers to the selection and serial ordering of words according to learned rules by which a person can use spoken or written modalities to communicate with others and to express cerebral activities involved with thinking and learning. It can be by speech (auditory symbols), writing (graphic symbols), or by gestures and pantomime (motor symbols).

APHASIAS

Q. Describe the clinical features and distinguish, based on clinical examination, the various disorders of speech.

- Aphasia is loss or defective language content of speech resulting from damage to the speech centers within the dominant (usually left in 97%) hemisphere. A language disturbance occurring after a right hemisphere lesion in a right hander is known as crossed aphasia **(Figs. 15.4 and 15.5)**.
- It includes defect in or loss of the power of expression by speech, writing or gestures or a defect in or loss of the ability to comprehend spoken or written language or to interpret gestures.
- Aphasia may be categorized according to whether the speech output is fluent or nonfluent.

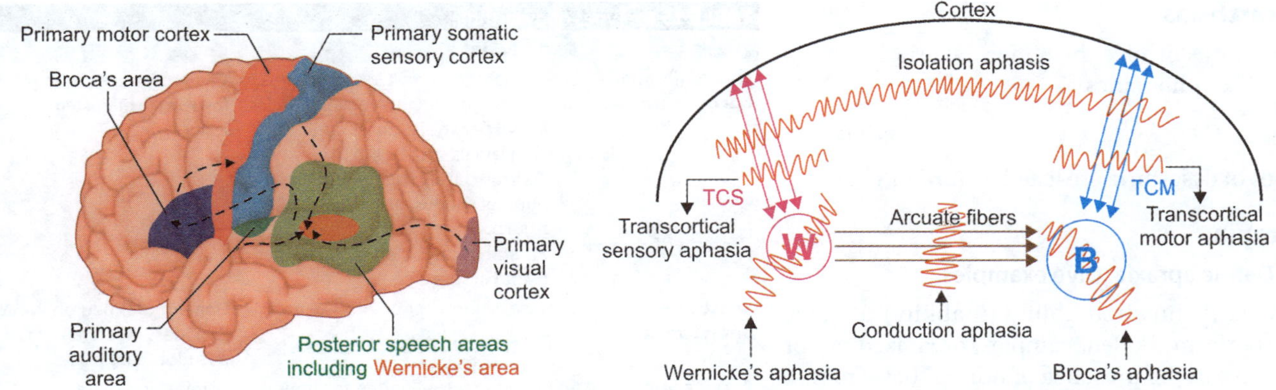

FIG. 15.4: Language and the brain.

FIG. 15.5: Schematic representation of aphasias and associated lesions.

TABLE 15.5: Types of aphasia.

Type of aphasia	*Site of lesion*	*Comprehension*	*Fluency*	*Repetition*	*Reading*	*Writing*	*Naming*
Wernicke's/sensory/receptive/posterior	Infarction of inferior division of middle cerebral artery	Absent	Preserved	Absent	—	—	—
Broca's/motor/expressive/anterior	Infarction of superior frontal branch of middle cerebral artery	Preserved	Absent	Absent	—	—	—
Global	Dominant frontal, parietal and superior temporal lobe	Absent	Absent	Absent	—	—	—
Conduction/arcuate	Arcuate fascicle	Preserved	Preserved	Absent	—	—	—
Transcortical sensory	Posterior watershed zone	Absent	Preserved	Preserved	—	—	—
Transcortical motor	Anterior watershed zone	Preserved	Absent	Preserved	—	—	—
Alexia without agraphia	Occipitotemporal region	Preserved	Preserved	Preserved	Lost	Preserved	—
Alexia with agraphia	Left angular gyrus	Preserved	Preserved	Preserved	Lost	Lost	—
Nominal/anomic/amnesic	Temporoparietal	Preserved	Preserved	Preserved	Preserved	Preserved	Absent

- **Fluent aphasias** (receptive aphasias) are impairments mostly due to the input or reception of language, with difficulties either in auditory verbal comprehension or in the repetition of words, phrases or sentences spoken by others. For example, Wernicke's aphasia.
- **Nonfluent aphasias** (expressive aphasias) are difficulties in articulating, with relatively good auditory, verbal comprehension. For example, Broca's aphasia.

Categories/Varieties of Aphasia (Table 15.5)

- **Alexia:** It is the impairment of visual word recognition, in the context of intact auditory word recognition and writing ability.
- **Agraphia:** It is the inability to write, as a language disorder resulting from brain damage.
- **Anomia:** In this, word approximates the correct answer but it phonetically inaccurate (plentil for pencil)—phonemic paraphasia. When the patient cannot say the appropriate name when an object is shown but can point the object when the name is provided is known as one way or retrieval based naming deficit.

The classification of aphasia has been shown in **Flowchart 15.2**.

FLOWCHART 15.2: Classification of aphasia.

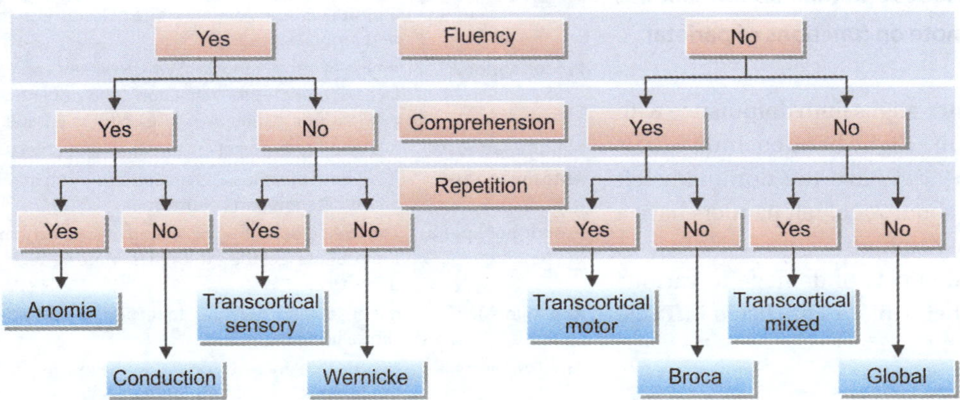

Dysarthrias

Dysarthrias involve the abnormal articulation of sounds or phonemes.

Types

Types of dysarthria are listed in **Table 15.6**.

TABLE 15.6: Types of dysarthria.

Type	*Description*	*Cause*
Flaccid (lingual, buccal, guttural)	Lower motor neuron (LMN) weakness of facial, lingual or pharyngeal muscles ➢ **Facial paralysis** causes difficulty with labials such as b p m w ➢ **Tongue paralysis** affects a large number sounds, particularly l, d, n, s, t, x ➢ **Palatal paralysis** produces a nasal twang in speech	Cerebrovascular accidents (especially brainstem lesions)
Spastic (hot potato voice)	Strained, slurred hot potato-like voice	Upper motor neuron (UMN) weakness (bilateral), e.g., pseudobulbar palsy
Ataxic speech	***Scanning speech***—undue separation of syllables (monosyllable speech)	Cerebellar diseases
	Staccato speech—explosive type of speech with emphasis on syllables	
Hypokinetic	Slow monotonous low voice with inapproprite silence	Extrapyramidal (parkinsonism)
Hyperkinetic dysarthria	Distorted speech with continuous change in articulation	Chorea, athetosis, dyskinesias
Myasthenic dysarthria	Voice is normal in the beginning but becomes weak as sentences progress	Myasthenia gravis

Apraxia

Q. Define apraxia. Give examples.

Apraxia is impaired ability (inability) to carry out (perform) skilled, complex, organized motor activities in the presence of normal basic motor, sensory, and cerebellar function. Examples of complex motor activities: dressing, using cutlery and geographical orientation.

Types

Types of apraxia are listed in **Table 15.7.**

- **Gerstmann's syndrome:** The combination of acalculia (impairment of simple arithmetic), dysgraphia (impaired writing), finger anomia (an inability to name individual fingers such as the index or thumb), and right-left confusion (an inability to tell whether a hand, foot, or arm of the patient or examiner is one the right or left side of the body) is known as Gerstmann's syndrome.
- **Site of lesion:** Inferior parietal lobule (especially the angular gyrus) in the left (dominant) hemisphere.

TABLE 15.7: Types of apraxia.

Type	*Description*
Ideomotor apraxia	Most common. It is the inability to perform a specific motor command/act (e.g., cough, lighting a cigarette with a matchstick) in the absence of motor weakness, incoordination, sensory loss or aphasia. Site of lesion is bilateral parietal lobe. Buccofacial apraxia involves apraxic deficits in movements of the face and mouth. Limb apraxia encompasses apraxic deficits in movements of the arms and legs
Dressing apraxia	Site of lesion is nondominant parietal lobe. It is inability to wear his/her dress
Constructional apraxia	It is inability to copy simple diagrams or build simple blocks. Site of lesion is nondominant parietal lobe
Ideational apraxia	It is a deficit in the execution of a goal-directed sequence of movements even with real object (e.g., asked to pick up a pen and write, the sequence of uncapping the pen, placing the cap at the opposite end). This is commonly associated with confusion and dementia rather than focal lesions associated with aphasic conditions
Gait apraxia (Bruns ataxia)	Seen in normal pressure hydrocephalus (NPH)
Gaze apraxia	Part of Balint's syndrome
Other apraxias	Speech apraxia, conceptual apraxia, and conduction apraxia

Agnosia

Q. Write a short note on agnosia.

Agnosia is failure to recognize objects (e.g., places, clothing, persons, sounds, shapes or smells), despite the presence of intact sensory system.
Site of lesion: Contralateral parietal lobe.

Types

Types of agnosia are listed in **Table 15.8.**

TABLE 15.8: Types of agnosia.

Type	*Description*
Visual agnosia	Failure to recognize what is seen with eyes despite the presence of intact visual pathways. The individual can describe the shape, color, and size without naming it. Site of lesion is in the posterior occipital or temporal lobes
Prosopagnosia	A type of visual agnosia in which patient cannot identify familiar faces, sometimes the reflection of his or her own face in the mirror even including their own. Site of lesion is parieto-occipital lobe
Simultanagnosia	It is inability to perceive more than one object at a time
Autotopagnosia	It is a form of agnosia, characterized by an inability to localize and orient different parts of the body
Pseudopolymelia	The feeling of false—the feeling of false extremities. More frequent the patients feel the extremities. More frequent the patients feel the third-hand
Anosognosia	It is an inability or refusal to recognize a defect or disorder that is clinically evident
Auditory agnosia	Heartfelt deafness: It consists in the loss of ability to know objects on sounds characteristic for them (clock—on ticking)

Functions of Cerebral Hemispheres

Q. Write a short note on normal functions of different cortical lobes and their abnormalities.

Q. Write a short note on functions of parietal lobe.

Cerebral dominance aligns limb dominance with language function. Right-handed individuals almost always (>95%) have the dominant left hemisphere, and about 7% of left handers have a dominant right hemisphere.

Functions and effects of damage to various lobes of cerebral hemispheres are listed in **Table 15.9** and **Figure 15.6**.

TABLE 15.9: Functions and effects of damage to various lobes of cerebral hemispheres.

Lobe	*Function*	*Cognitive/behavioral effects of damage*
Frontal Please **SMILE** (Mnemonic)	**P**ersonality	Disinhibition
	Social behavior	Lack of initiation
	Micturition	Antisocial behavior
	Intelligence	Impaired memory
	Language	Expressive dysphasia
	Emotional response	Incontinence
Parietal: Dominant side	Language	Dysphasia, dyslexia
	Calculation	Acalculia
	Others	Apraxia, agnosia
Parietal: Nondominant side	Spatial orientation	Spatial disorientation, neglect of contralateral side
	Constructional skills	Constructional apraxia, dressing apraxia
Temporal: Dominant side	Auditory perception	Receptive aphasia
	Language	Dyslexia
	Verbal memory	Impaired verbal memory
	Smell	
	Balance	
Temporal: Nondominant side	Auditory perception	Impaired nonverbal memory
	Melody/pitch perception	Impaired musical skills (tonal perception)
	Nonverbal memory	
	Smell	
	Balance	
Occipital	Visual processing	Visual inattention, visual loss, visual agnosia (Anton–Babinski syndrome)

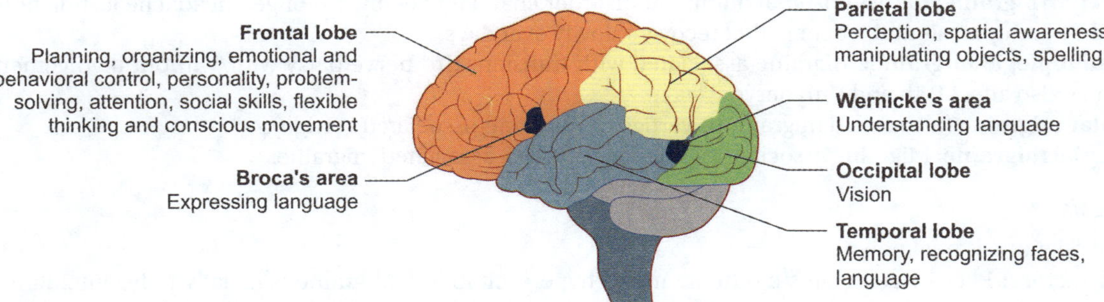

FIG. 15.6: Functions of various lobes of cerebral hemispheres.

HEADACHE

Headache is among the most common reasons, patients seek medical attention.

Classification of Headache (Table 15.10 and Fig. 15.7)

- Primary headaches: Benign, recurrent, no organic disease as their cause. It affects the quality of life of the patient.
- Secondary headaches: Underlying organic disease.

Q. Define and classify headache and describe the presenting features, precipitating factors, aggravating and relieving factors of various kinds of headache.

MIGRAINE

Q. Write a short essay/note on classification, pathogenesis, clinical features, and management of migraine.

Migraine is a neurovascular disease caused by neurogenic inflammation and characterized by severe, recurring headaches.

- It is the second most common cause of headache. It is usually characterized by an

TABLE 15.10: Classification of headache.

Primary headache		*Secondary headache*
Type	***Percent (%)***	➤ Head or neck trauma
Tension-type	69	➤ Cranial or cervical vascular disorder—arterial dissection, cerebral venous thrombosis
Migraine	16	➤ Noninfectious inflammatory disease
Idiopathic stabbing	2	– Intracranial neoplasm
Exertional	1	– High and low cerebrospinal fluid pressure headache
Cluster	0.1	➤ Substance use or its withdrawal
Other primary headache ➤ Paroxysmal hemicrania ➤ SUNCT = Short-lasting unilateral neuralgiform headache attacks with conjunctival injection and tearing ➤ SUNA = Short-lasting unilateral neuralgiform headache attacks with cranial autonomic symptoms		➤ Disorder of homeostasis—hypoxia, hypercarbia, hypoglycemia ➤ Psychiatric disorder—somatization ➤ Cranial neuralgia ➤ Infection—meningitis ➤ Disorder of cranium, neck, face, eyes, ears, nose, sinus, teeth, mouth, or other facial structure

episodic severe pain on one side of the head (headache) and usually associated with certain features such as sensitivity to light, sound or movement; nausea and vomiting often accompany the headache.

- Gender—Female: Male ratio is 5:1.

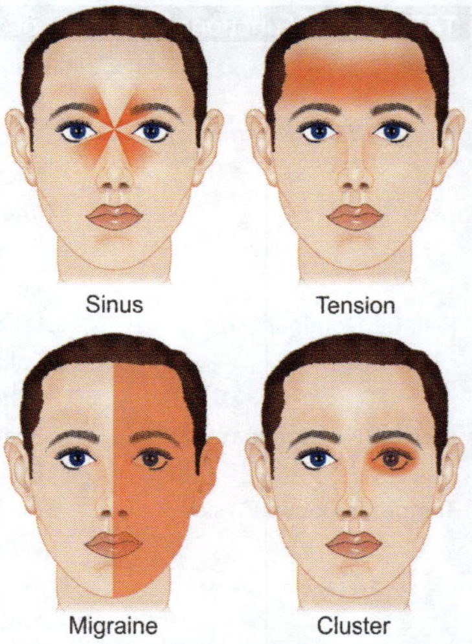

Sinus Tension Migraine Cluster

FIG. 15.7: Headache types.

Classification

Q. Classify migraine and describe the distinguishing features between classical and nonclassical forms of migraine.

- **Migraine without aura or common migraine:** It does not give any warning signs before the onset of headache. It occurs in about 70–80% of migraine patients.
- **Migraine with aura or classical migraine:** It gives some warning signs called "aura" before the actual headache begins. About 20–30% migraine patients experience aura. The most common aura is visual and may include both positive and negative (visual field defects) features.
- **Retinal migraine:** It involves attacks of monocular scotoma or even blindness of one eye for less than an hour and associated with headache.
- **Childhood periodic syndromes:** It involves cyclical vomiting (occasional intense periods of vomiting), abdominal migraine (abdominal pain, usually accompanied by nausea), and benign paroxysmal vertigo of childhood (occasional attacks of vertigo). They may be precursors or associated with migraine.
- **Complicated migraine:** It describes migraine headaches and/or auras that are unusually long or unusually frequent, or associated with a seizure or brain lesion.
- **Basilar migraine:** Occipital headache, preceded by vertigo, diplopia and dysarthria, ±visual and sensory symptoms (brainstem symptoms).
- **Hemiplegic migraine:** Rare autosomal dominant disorder characterized by prolonged headache lasting hours or days, followed by hemiparesis and/or coma that recovers slowly over days.
- **Ophthalmoplegic migraine:** Migraine associated with transient IIrd nerve palsy with/without involvement of pupil; sometimes also affect IVth and VIth nerve.
- **Vestibular migraine** (also called migrainous vertigo or migraine-associated vertigo).
- **Catamenial migraine:** Migraine associated with menstruation-associated migraine.

Pathogenesis

- Cause of migraine is not known.
- **Genetic factors:** Play a role in causing the neuronal hyperexcitability. Migraine is usually polygenic. Rarely, familial migraine is associated with mutations in the $\alpha 1$ subunit of the P/Q-type voltage-gated calcium channel or neuronal sodium channel (SCN1A), and **a dominant** loss of function mutation in a potassium channel gene (TRESK). Migraine is frequently associated with positive family history, and similar phenomena occur in disorders such as CADASIL.
- Genes for **familial hemiplegic migraine**
  - FHM1—CACNA1A: Neuronal P/Q calcium channel—increases neurotransmitter release
  - FHM2—ATP1A2: Astrocyte sodium pump—dysfunction increases extracellular K+
  - FHM3—SCN1A: Neuronal sodium channel—increased action potential firing
- **Hormonal influences:** Female preponderance and the frequency of migraine attacks at certain points in the menstrual cycle due to hormonal fluctuations. Estrogen-containing oral contraception can exacerbate migraine in few patients.
- **Right-to-left cardiac shunt:** Migraine with aura has been associated with patent foramen ovale (PFO), atrial septal defect (ASD), and pulmonary arteriovenous malformations (AVMs) in hereditary hemorrhagic telangiectasia (Osler–Weber–Rendu syndrome).

Several theories have been proposed for the pathogenesis of migraine **(Flowchart 15.3)**.

- *Vascular theory:* Constriction of intracerebral blood vessel produces aura. Vasodilatation of intracranial/extracranial blood vessel produces headache phase.
- *Serotonin theory:* Decreased serotonin levels linked with migraine and specific serotonin receptors found in blood vessels of brain.
- *Neurogenic theory:* The aura (see clinical features below) is thought to be due to spreading cortical depression wave of neuronal depolarization followed by depressed activity spreading slowly anteriorly across the cerebral cortex from the occipital region. This spreading process occurs at a rate of about 3 mm/minute. Dysfunction of activation of cells in the trigeminal nucleus releases vasoactive neuropeptides [e.g., calcitonin gene-related peptide (CGRP), substance P, and other vasoactive peptides including 5-HT] by activated trigeminovascular neurons. They produce painful meningeal inflammation and vasodilation.
- Dopamine plays a role and most migraine symptoms can be induced by dopaminergic stimulation. There is dopamine receptor hypersensitivity in patients with migraine.

FLOWCHART 15.3: Pathogenesis of migraine.

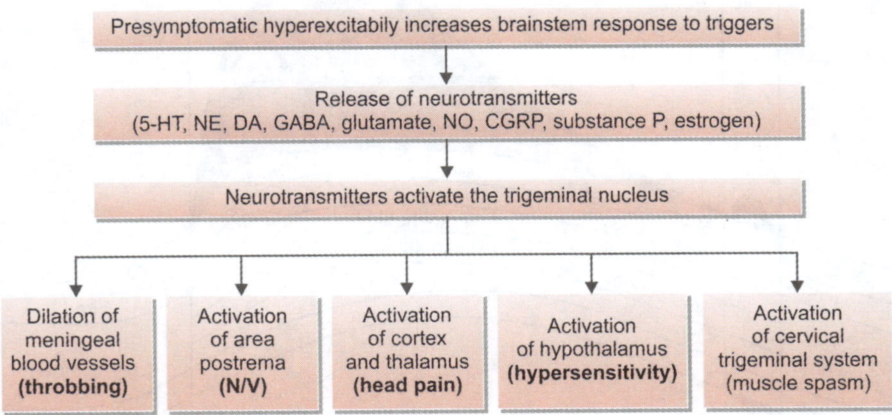

Cortical Spreading Depression

- Wave of activation followed by reduced activity that spreads across the surface of the brain.
- Initial dilation conducted with intrinsic velocity ahead of cortical spreading depression (CSD), subsequent constriction, and eventual dilation.

Astrocyte Calcium Waves

- Slowly propagated waves evoked by wide variety of stimuli
- Associated with active release of: ATP, glutamate, K+, lactate, prostanoids, and interleukins (ILs)

Precipitating factors: Anything can initiate or precipitate or amplify an attack. Common triggers are: excess stress, glare, exposure to bright light, loud noises/sounds, smoke or strong scents, menstruation, lack or excess of sleep, cheese, caffeine, alcohol, chocolate, citrus fruit, food additives such as monosodium glutamate, vasodilators, hunger, physical exertion, stormy weather or barometric pressure changes, contraceptive pills, etc.

Clinical Features

Headache is usually hemicranial, throbbing, and associated with nausea and vomiting.

- **Migraine without aura** (previously called "common" migraine).
  - About 70–80% of patients with migraine have characteristic headache but without aura.
  - Typically attacks are episodic and start at puberty and prevalence increases in 4th decade. It may show variable degree of spontaneous remissions.
  - The scalp may be tender to touch during episodes (allodynia is production of pain from normally nonpainful stimuli) and the patients prefer to be still in a dark and quiet environment.
  - Other symptoms associated with migraine headache are listed in **Table 15.11**.

TABLE 15.11: Symptoms associated with migraine headache.

Nausea	*Vomiting*
Photophobia, prostration	Visual disturbances
Lightheadedness	Paresthesias
Scalp tenderness/cutaneous allodynia	Vertigo

- **Migraine with aura** (previously known as "classical" migraine)
  - Migraine aura: About 20–30% of patients with migraine experience malaise, irritability, behavioral change or focal neurological symptoms for some hours or days immediately preceding the headache phase.

  Type of aura: (1) visual aura, (2) sensory aura, or (3) language aura.
  - **Visual aura:** It is the most common type characterized by positive visual symptoms such as shimmering, teichopsia (silvery zigzag lines also called **fortification spectra**) flashing lights or fragmentation of the image (like looking through a pane of broken glass) or scintillating spots across the visual fields for up to 40 minutes. Sometimes there may be temporary patchy visual field loss which may move across the visual field (scotomas) and even evolve into hemianopia or tunnel vision.
  - **Sensory aura:** It consists of positive sensory symptoms such as tingling followed by numbness, spreading over 20–30 minutes, from one part of the body to another.
  - **Language aura:** Dominant hemisphere involvement may cause transient speech disturbance.
  - Motor aura-transient weakness.
- **Duration of aura:** Usually it evolves over 5–20 minutes with symptoms changing as the wave of spreading neuronal depression moves across the surface of the cortex. It rarely lasts for >60 minutes and is followed immediately by the headache phase **(Fig. 15.8)**.

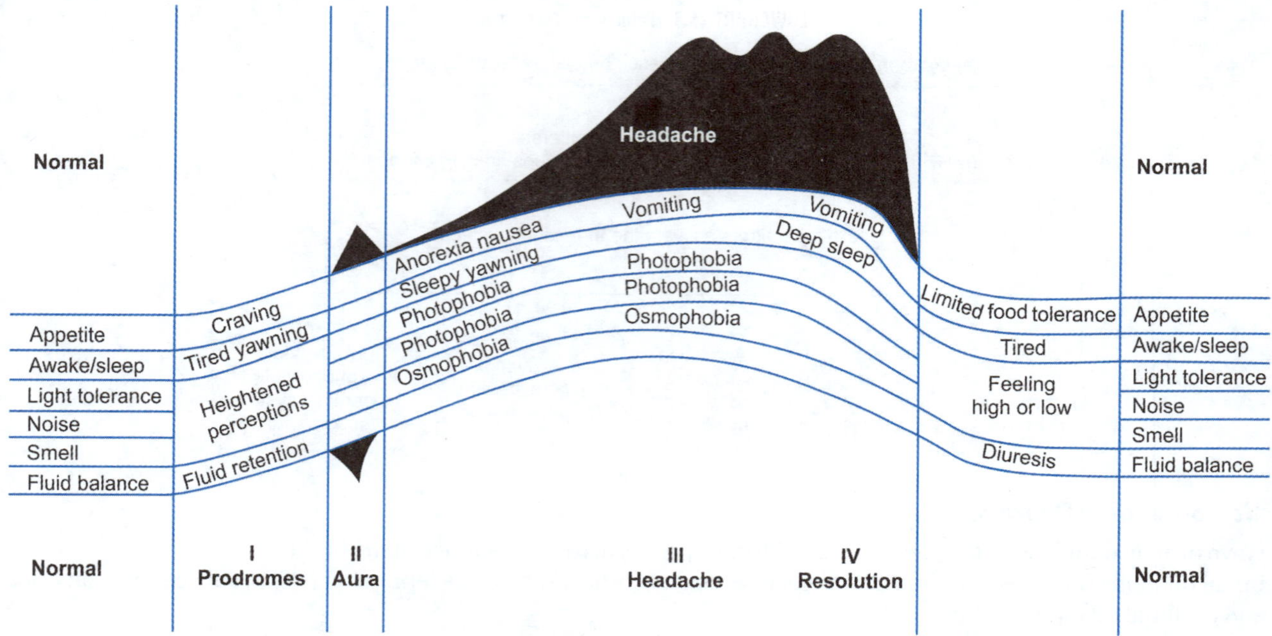

FIG. 15.8: Migraine phases.

Diagnostic Criteria

See **Table 15.12.**

Strongest predictors of migraine

- Are you nauseated or sick to your stomach when you have a headache?
- Has a headache limited your activities for a day or more in the last 3 months?
- Does light bother you when you have a headache?
- Patients who answer positively to two out of three have a 93% chance of having migraines.

TABLE 15.12: Simplified diagnostic criteria for migraine.

Repeated attacks of headache lasting 4–72 hours (untreated) with	
At least two of the following features:	Plus at least one of the following features:
➢ Unilateral pain	➢ Nausea/vomiting
➢ Throbbing pain	➢ Photophobia and phonophobia
➢ Motion sensitivity (headache aggravated with head movement or physical activity)	➢ Normal physical examination, no other reasonable cause for the headache
➢ Moderate or severe intensity	

Complications of Migraine

- **Status migrainosus** is a debilitating migraine attack lasting for >72 hours.
- Persistent aura without infarction is defined by aura symptoms persisting for 1 week or more with no evidence of infarction on neuroimaging.
- Migrainosus infarction: Migraine attack, occurring in a patient with migraine with aura, in which one or more aura symptoms persist for >1 hour and neuroimaging shows an infarction in a relevant brain area.
- Migraine aura-triggered seizure is a seizure triggered by an attack of migraine with aura.

Red Flags of Headache

They have been shown in **Box 15.4**.

Box 15.4: RED flags of headache.

- "Worst" headache ever
- First severe headache
- Subacute worsening over days or weeks
- Altered level of sensorium/consciousness
- Abnormal neurologic examination
- Fever or unexplained systemic signs
- Significant weight loss
- Vomiting that precedes headache
- Pain induced by bending, lifting, cough, worsens with Valsalva maneuvers
- Pain which disturbs sleep or presents immediately upon awakening
- Known systemic illness, history of trauma, cancer or HIV
- New-onset headache in a patient >50 years of age
- Focal neurologic deficits, jaw claudication
- Morning headache associated with nausea and vomiting
- Pain associated with local tenderness (e.g., region of temporal artery)

Mnemonic SNNOOP10

- **S**ystemic symptoms including fever
- **N**eoplasm history
- **N**eurologic deficit (including decreased consciousness)
- **O**nset is sudden or abrupt
- **O**lder age (onset after age 50 years)
- **P10:**
  - Pattern change or recent onset of new headache
  - Positional headache
  - Precipitated by sneezing, coughing, or exercise
  - Papilledema
  - Progressive headache and atypical presentations
  - Pregnancy or puerperium
  - Painful eye with autonomic features
  - Post-traumatic onset of headache
  - Pathology of the immune system such as HIV
  - Painkiller (analgesic) overuse (e.g., medication overuse headache) or new drug at onset of headache

Q. Write a short essay/note on management of migraine in young adults. Mention three drugs used and write short note on prophylactic therapy.

FLOWCHART 15.4: Treatment of migraine.

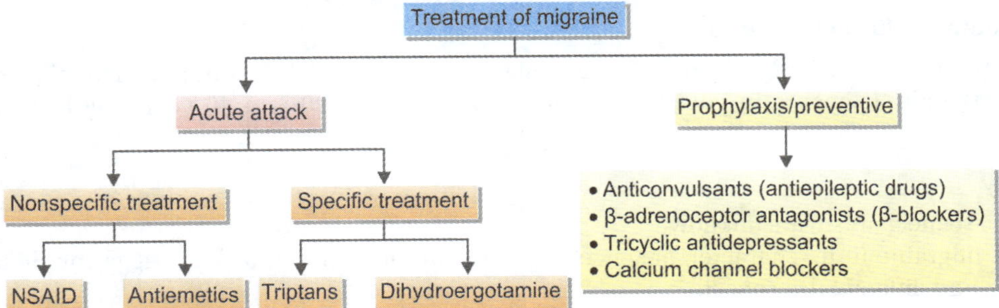

Management (Flowchart 15.4)

Nonpharmacological treatment (General measures)

- Explanation that migraine has no grave prognosis.
- Identification of triggers and avoidance of identified triggers or exacerbating factors to prevent attacks. Women with aura should avoid estrogen treatment (oral contraception or hormone replacement). Lifestyle modification wherever possible.
- Other measures: Meditation, relax techniques, psychotherapy.

Pharmacological treatment

- Abortive treatment: Treatment of acute attack.
- Preventive treatment: Drug prophylaxis.

Treatment of an acute attack

- Analgesic: Simple analgesia such as aspirin, paracetamol or nonsteroidal anti-inflammatory agents.
- Nausea may be treated by an antiemetic (metoclopramide or domperidone).
- Severe attacks: If there is previously no relief with a nonsteroidal anti-inflammatory drug (NSAID), use "triptans".
  - **Triptans** (e.g., *sumatriptan*: 50–100 mg tablet/5–20 mg nasal spray/6 mg S/C; *rizatriptan*: 5–10 mg tablet; *frovatriptan*: 2.5 mg oral; naratriptan: 2.5 mg oral; *almotriptan*: 12.5 mg oral; *eletriptan*: 40–80 mg oral; *zolmitriptan*: 2.5 mg oral/5 mg intranasal spray):
  - **Mode of action:** Potent 5-HT1B/1D agonists, inhibit release of CGRP and substance P, inhibit activation of the trigeminal nerve, and inhibit vasodilation in the meninges.
  - **Administration: Triptans are** available as oral preparations, nasal spray, and subcutaneous injections.
  - **Contraindications:** Ischemic heart disease or stroke, high risk for coronary artery disease, pregnancy, hemiplegic or basilar migraine and use with ergots.
- Calcitonin gene-related peptide antagonists (e.g., **erenumab, fremanezumab, galcanezumab**) are very effective for acute treatment of migraine.
- **Lasmiditan**, a selective serotonin 1F receptor agonist has been tried.
- Single-pulse **transcranial magnetic stimulation** (TMS) has shown good benefits.

Drug prophylaxis

- Indications for drug prophylaxis in migraine are listed in **Box 15.5**. Various drugs can be used and the most frequently used are:
  - Anticonvulsants [antiepileptic drugs (AEDs)]: **Valproate** (800 mg) or **topiramate** (100–200 mg daily) is the most effective option.
  - β-adrenoceptor antagonists (β-blockers), e.g., **propranolol** slow-release 80–160 mg daily.
  - Tricyclic antidepressants, e.g., **amitriptyline** 10 mg increasing weekly in 10 mg steps to 50–60 mg or Dosulepin (10–200 mg at night).
  - Methysergide 1–2 mg TID in resistant cases (prolonged use may produce retroperitoneal and mediastinal fibrosis).
  - Botulinum toxin has been tried as a treatment for chronic migraine.
  - Vasoactive drugs and calcium channel blockers: These include **flunarizine** (5–10 mg OD at bedtime), verapamil (80–160 mg 3 times a day), and methysergide and are used in refractory cases. Pizotifen is rarely used.
  - **Memantine**—N-methyl-D-aspartate (NMDA) receptor antagonist, blocks glutamate
  - Nonprescription medications:
    - Riboflavin (B_2): 400 mg daily
    - Magnesium oxide: 400 mg daily
    - Coenzyme Q10: 150 mg daily
    - Feverfew: 10–30 mg daily
    - Butterbur (Petadolex): 50–75 mg BID
    - Melatonin

Box 15.5: Indications for drug prophylaxis in migraine.

- Patients who have very frequent headaches (>2–3 weeks)
- Attack duration > 48 hours
- Migraine-related disability >3 days/month
- Headache extremely severe
- Migraine accompanied by severe aura
- Contraindication to acute treatment
- Unacceptable adverse effects with acute migraine treatment
- Patients preference

Cluster Headache

Q. Write a short note on cluster headache.

Cluster headache (migrainous neuralgia) is distinct from migraine and is much less common than migraine.
Age and gender: Usually it occurs in young adult in the 3rd decade (20 and 40 years) with male predominance (M:F = 5:1).

Pathophysiology

- Cause and precise mechanism are unknown.
- It differs from migraine in its character, absence of genetic predisposition, lack of triggering dietary factors, male predominance, and different drug effect.
- Abnormal hypothalamic activity is observed on functional imaging studies during an attack. Patients are often smokers and consume more than average alcohol.

Clinical Features

- Cluster headache is **periodic with recurrent bouts** of identical headaches beginning at the **same hour for weeks at a time** (the eponymous "cluster"). Patients may develop either one or several attacks within a 24-hour period.
- Cluster headache causes **severe (excruciating) and worst, stabbing/boring, unilateral periorbital/retro-orbital pain with parasympathetic autonomic features** in the same eye (e.g., unilateral lacrimation, nasal congestion, and conjunctival redness/injection or even a transient Horner's syndrome). The pain is so severe that they may commit suicide.
- **Circadian periodicity:** Usually cluster period lasts for few weeks and followed by remission for months to years. They typically recur a year or more later often at the same time of year.

Diagnostic Criteria for Cluster Headache

Diagnostic criteria for cluster headache have been shown in **Box 15.6**.

Management of Cluster Headache

- **Acute attacks:** Analgesics are not useful and acute attacks are usually halted by:
  - **Subcutaneous injection of sumatriptan** (6 mg) is the drug of choice for acute treatment. It works quickly and usually shortens an attack to 10–15 minutes. There is no evidence of tachyphylaxis. Oral sumatriptan is not effective. Sumatriptan (20 mg) and zolmitriptan (5 mg) nasal sprays are also effective or
  - **Inhalation of 100% oxygen** at 10–12 L/minute for 15–20 minutes. Many respond very well.
  - The brevity of the attack probably prevents other migraine therapies from being effective. **Octreotide** is effective in the treatment of acute cluster headaches.
- **Most prophylactic migraine drugs are often ineffective.** Attacks can be prevented in some patients by sodium valproate, lithium, verapamil, methysergide and/or a short course of **oral corticosteroids.**

Box 15.6: Diagnostic criteria for cluster headache.

At least five attacks fulfilling following:
- Severe or very severe unilateral orbital, supraorbital and/or temporal pain lasting 15–180 minutes if untreated
- Headache is accompanied by at least one of the following:
  - Autonomic features: Unilateral
    - Conjunctival redness/injection and/or lacrimation or
    - Nasal congestion and/or rhinorrhea or
    - Edema of eyelid
    - Sweating on the forehead and face or
    - Miosis and/or ptosis or
  - Restlessness or agitation
- Frequency of attacks: From one every other day to eight/day

Tension-type Headache

Q. Write a short note on tension headache.

It is the most common type of headache.
Pathophysiology is incompletely understood, and few consider this as a milder version of migraine.

Clinical Features

Characteristic features of headache **(Fig. 15.9)** are:
- Pain is "dull" "tight" or like a "pressure", and it may be accompanied by a sensation of a band round the head or pressure at the vertex.
- It is of constant character and generalized, but often radiates forward from the occipital region. It may be episodic or persistent.
- Severity may vary, and is not associated vomiting or photophobia. The pain often progresses throughout the day.
- Tenderness may be present over the skull vault or in the occiput.

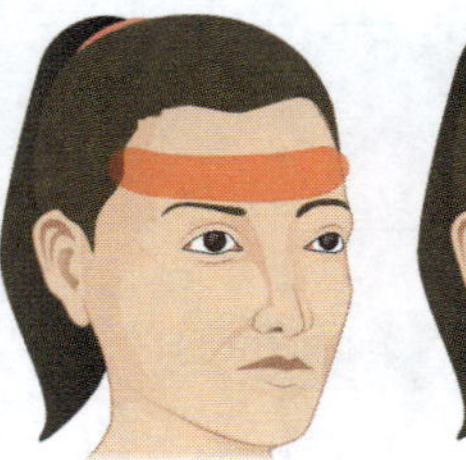

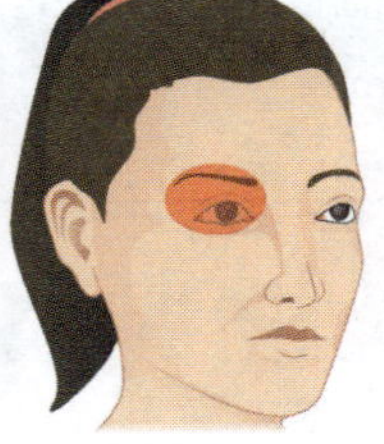

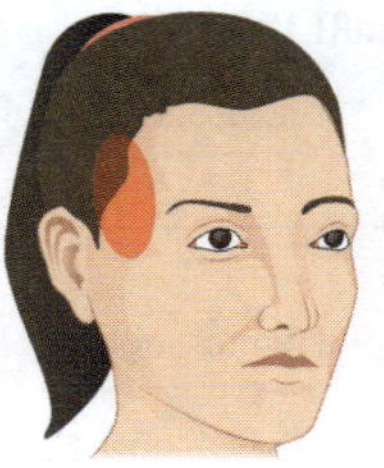

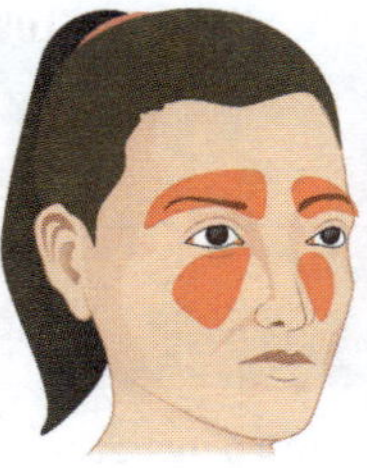

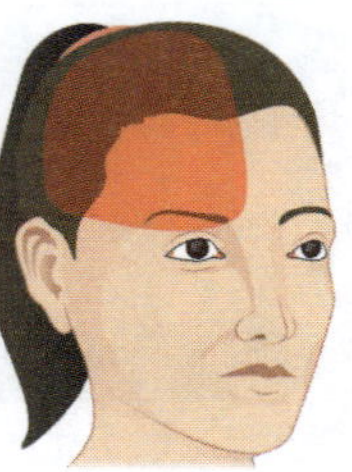

FIG. 15.9: Common primary headaches—characteristic features.

Management
- Carefully assess, followed by discussion of likely precipitants and reassurance that the prognosis is good.
- Physiotherapy (with muscle relaxation and stress management) may be helpful.
- Low-dose amitriptyline may be beneficial. Investigation is rarely required.

The differences between most common primary headaches are presented in **Table 15.13**.

TABLE 15.13: Comparison of most common primary headaches.

Characteristic	*Migraine*	*Tension*	*Cluster*
Age of onset	25–55 years	30–50 years	20–40 years
Location	60–70% unilateral	Bilateral	Unilateral, orbital, supraorbital, temporal
Duration of episode	4–72 hours	30 minutes to 7 days	15–180 minutes
Severity	Moderate to severe	Mild to moderate	Extremely severe
Type	Pulsating, throbbing	Pressing, tightening but not pulsating	Boring, searing
Pattern	1–2 attacks per month	<180 attacks per year (or <15 attacks per month)	1–8 attacks per day separated by pain-free periods
Associated symptoms	Nausea, vomiting, photophobia, phonophobia (two of these)	Either photophobia or phonophobia, but not both, no nausea or vomiting	Conjunctival injection, lacrimation forehead/ facial swelling, nasal congestion, rhinorrhea, ptosis, miosis, eyelid edema

STROKE AND CEREBROVASCULAR DISEASE

Q. Classify cerebrovascular accidents and describe the etiology, predisposing genetic and risk factors, pathogenesis of hemorrhagic and nonhemorrhagic stroke.

Q. Describe clinical features, diagnosis of the cerebral stroke in young, and its management.

Q. Describe the etiology, clinical features, and treatment of cerebral thrombosis.

Q. Write a short essay/note on cerebrovascular accidents/stroke.

Stroke

- **A stroke (cerebrovascular accident is a vague** term which should be avoided) is defined as a syndrome of rapid **(abrupt) onset of a neurologic deficit** that is attributable to a focal vascular cause.
- **World Health Organization (WHO) definition:** Stroke is a defined as a clinical syndrome consisting of **"rapidly developing clinical signs of focal (or global) disturbance of cerebral function, with symptoms lasting for 24 hours or longer or leading to death, with no apparent cause other than of vascular origin".**
- **Progressing stroke (or stroke in evolution):** It is a stroke in which the focal neurological deficit worsens after the patient first presents. It may be due to increasing volume of infarction, secondary hemorrhage in the infarcted area or increasing cerebral edema.
- **Complete stroke:** Rapid onset with persistent focal neurological deficit which does not progress beyond 96 hours.
- **Evolving stroke:** Gradual stepwise development of neurological deficits.

Focal cerebral deficits that develop slowly (over weeks to months) are unlikely to be due to stroke and are more suggestive of tumor or inflammatory or degenerative disease.

Terminologies

Several terms are used to classify strokes, mainly based on the duration and evolution of symptoms.

- **Transient ischemic attack (TIA):** Described later
- **Reversible ischemic neurological deficit (RIND):** In some cases, deficits last for longer than 24 hours but resolve completely or almost completely within a few days.
- **Stuttering hemiplegia:** Internal carotid lesions are characterized by repeated episodes of TIA followed by fully evolved stroke.

FLOWCHART 15.5: Classification of stroke.

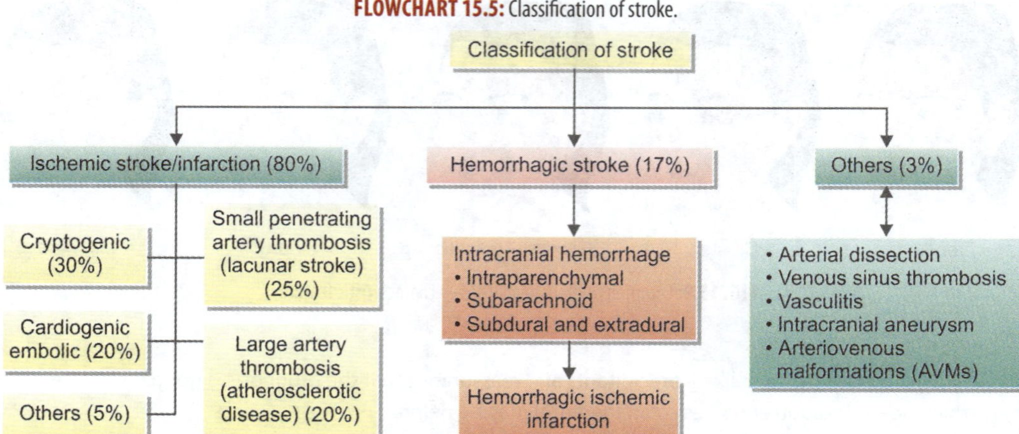

Types of Stroke (Flowchart 15.5)

About 80% of patients develop **cerebral infarction** due to inadequate blood flow to part of the brain, and most of the remainder develops an **intracerebral hemorrhage.**

- **Ischemic stroke: Cerebral infarction is most commonly caused by thromboembolic disease** secondary to atherosclerosis in the major extracranial arteries (carotid artery and aortic arch). About 20% of infarctions are caused by emboli from the heart, and about 20% are caused by thrombosis in situ caused by intrinsic disease of small perforating vessels (lenticulostriate arteries), producing lacunar infarctions.
- **Hemorrhagic stroke: Intracranial hemorrhage** (ICH) is caused by bleeding directly into or around the brain. Neurological symptoms are produced by compression, toxic effects or raised intracranial pressure (ICP).
- **Hemorrhagic conversion of ischemic stroke**
  - This may occur after thrombolytic drugs (alteplase) are administered to patients with an ischemic stroke or where a patient has a large cerebral clot, which tends to be more common with cardioembolic strokes.
  - The major adverse effect of thrombolysis is symptomatic intracerebral hemorrhage, observed in around 6–7% of cases.
  - The risk of symptomatic ICH increases with age, high blood pressure, very severe neurological deficits, severe hyperglycemia, and with early ischemic changes on computed tomography (CT) scans.
- **Cerebrovascular anomalies** such as intracranial aneurysm and AVMs.

Box 15.7: Risk factors for stroke.

Risk factors in patients of all age groups	
High-risk	
• Hypertension (including isolated systolic) • Smoking • Diabetes mellitus • Atrial fibrillation • Drugs: Cocaine, amphetamine • Dilated cardiomyopathy • Endocarditis	• High cholesterol • Obesity • Vasculitis: Systemic vasculitis [e.g., polyarteritis nodosa (PAN)], granulomatosis with polyangiitis (Wegener's, etc.), primary CNS vasculitis, meningitis (syphilis, tuberculosis, fungal, bacterial, zoster)
Low-risk	
• Migraine • Oral contraceptives or alcohol • Patent foramen ovale	• Recent myocardial infarction • Prosthetic valve • Sleep apnea
Additional risk factors that are more common in young patients	
Hypercoagulable disorders	
• Protein C and S deficiencies • Antithrombin III deficiency • Antiphospholipid syndrome • Factor V Leiden mutation • Prothrombin G20210A heterozygous mutation	• Sickle cell anemia • Hyperhomocysteinemia • Thrombotic thrombocytopenic purpura • Arterial dissection • Infections (e.g., syphilis, HIV) • Systemic malignancy

Risk (Predisposing) Factors for Stroke (Box 15.7)

Q. Write a short essay/note on risk factors for stroke.

Pathophysiology (Flowchart 15.6)

- Complete stop of cerebral blood flow (CBF) causes death of brain tissue within 4–10 minutes. The CBF to the ischemic core is <10 mL/100 g/minute.
- Ischemic penumbra **(Fig. 15.10)** is the region surrounding the central core. The tissue of the penumbra is functionally impaired and is at risk of infarction. CBF is 10–18 mL/100 g/minute. It has the potential to be salvaged by revascularization. The

FLOWCHART 15.6: Pathophysiology of ischemic stroke.

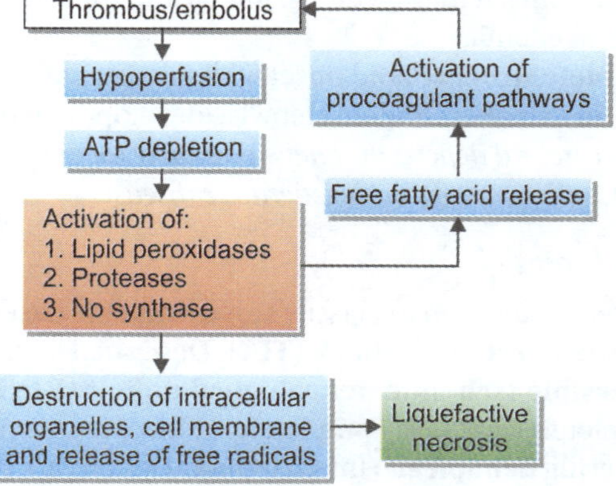

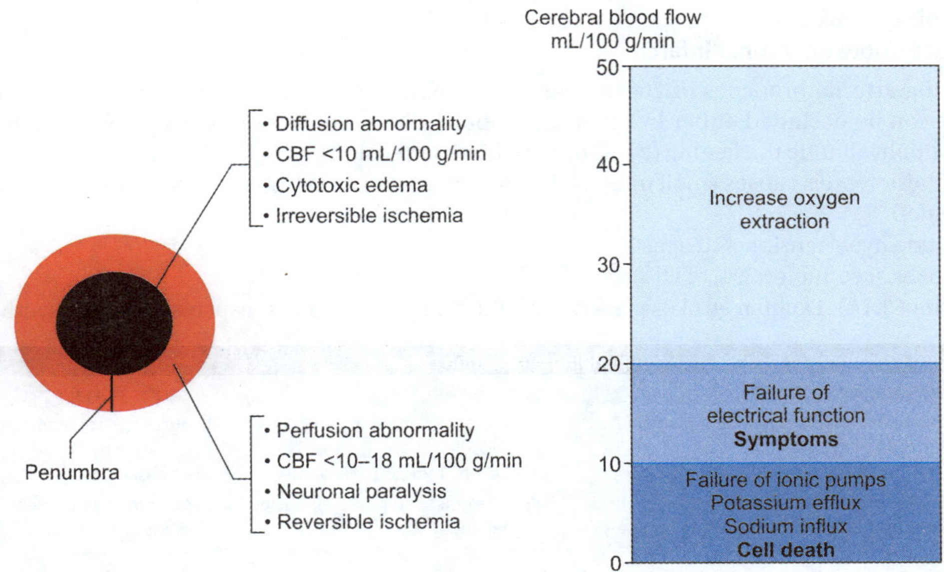

FIG. 15.10: Ischemic penumbra and ischemic core (black center). (CBF: cerebral blood flow)

damage of the penumbra is coupled by inflammation and excitotoxicity mediated by glutamine and sodium. Also, hyperglycemia and fever worsen the penumbra, so need to be controlled.

Etiology of Ischemic Stroke

See **Box 15.8.**

Embolic occlusion

Q. Write a short essay/note on embolic stroke, its causes, and management.

Artery-to-artery embolic stroke

- **Any vessel** may be the source of emboli, including the aortic arch, common and internal carotid, vertebral and basilar arteries.
- **Atherosclerosis within the carotid artery:** Carotid bifurcation atherosclerosis is the most common source of artery-to-artery embolus.
- **In young (age <60 years) patients:** Intracranial atherosclerosis, dissection of the internal carotid or vertebral arteries or even vessels beyond the circle of Willis is a common source of embolic stroke.

Box 15.8: Etiology of ischemic stroke.

Thrombotic occlusion
- Small vessel (lacunar) stroke
- Large vessel thrombosis

Embolic occlusion
- **Artery-to-artery:** Carotid bifurcation, aortic arch, arterial dissection
- **Cardioembolic:** Atrial fibrillation, mural thrombus, myocardial infarction, dilated cardiomyopathy, valvular lesions, mitral stenosis, mechanical valve, bacterial endocarditis
- **Paradoxical embolus:** Atrial septal defect, patent foramen ovale

Venous sinus thrombosis

Subarachnoid hemorrhage due to vasospasm

Cardioembolic stroke

- Heart is a common source of emboli. Emboli from the heart **most often lodge in the middle cerebral artery** (MCA), the **posterior cerebral artery** (PCA), or one of their branches. Infrequently, the anterior cerebral artery (ACA) territory is involved.
- **Nonrheumatic atrial fibrillation** (and other arrhythmias) causing thrombosis in a dilated left atrium is the **most common cause of cerebral embolism.** Other causes include cardiac valvular disease such as congenital valve disorders, infective vegetations; rheumatic and degenerative calcific changes may cause embolization.
- Simultaneous infarcts in different vascular territories are suggestive that heart or aorta is the source of emboli.

Paradoxical embolus

Atrial septal defect or PFO may occasionally allow passage of fragments of thromboemboli [e.g., from a lower limb deep vein thrombosis (DVT)] from the right atrium to the left. This is believed to be the most common cause of cryptogenic strokes.

Other embolism like fat embolism, air embolism, amniotic fluid embolism, tumor embolism is rarely associated with neurological deficits.

Thrombosis occlusion

Large vessel thrombosis

Thrombosis developing at the site of ruptured mural atheromatous plaque may produce occlusion of involved vessel or may be a source of artery-to-artery embolism.

Small Vessel (Lacunar) Stroke

Q. Write a short essay/note on lacunar infarct.

- Small penetrating arterial branches of 200–800 µm in diameter, supply the deep brain parenchyma. Each of these small branches can be occluded either by atherothrombotic disease at its origin or by the development of occlusive vasculopathy—lipohyalinotic thickening (consequence of hypertension).
- Thrombosis of these vessels causes small infarcts that are referred to as lacunes. These infarcts range in size from **0.2 to 15 mm** in diameter.
- Risk factors include hypertension and age.
- Small vessel strokes account for 20% of all strokes.
- Symptoms **(Table 15.14)**: Lacunar strokes present with fluctuating symptoms "capsular warning syndrome".

TABLE 15.14: Signs and symptoms of lacunar stroke depending on location of lesion.

Syndrome	*Signs/Symptoms*	*Localization*	*Vascular supply*
Pure motor	Contralateral hemiparesis or hemiplegia. Affects face, arm, and leg equally	➢ Posterior limb of internal capsule ➢ Corona radiata-basis pontis	Lenticulostriate branches of the middle cerebral artery (MCA) or perforating arteries from basilar artery
Pure sensory	Contralateral hemisensory loss. Persistent or transient numbness and/or tingling on one side of the body	VPL (ventral posterolateral) nucleus of thalamus	Lenticulostriate branches of MCA. Small thalamoperforators of PCA (posterior cerebral artery)
Mixed sensorimotor	Contralateral weakness and numbness. Hemiparesis or hemiplegia with ipsilateral sensory impairment	Thalamus and adjacent posterior limb of internal capsule	Lenticulostriate branches of MCA
Dysarthria-clumsy hand	Slurred speech and weakness of contralateral hand (fine motor)	Basis pontis	Basilar artery perforators
Ataxic hemiparesis	Combination of cerebellar and motor symptoms. Contralateral hemiparesis and ataxia out of proportion to weakness	➢ Internal capsule—posterior limb ➢ Basis pontis ➢ Corona radiata	➢ Lenticulostriate branches of MCA ➢ Perforating arteries of basilar artery
Hemiballismus/hemichorea	Contralesional limb flailing/dyskinesia	Subthalamic nucleus	Perforating arteries of anterior choroidal or PCOM (posterior communicating artery)

Clinicoanatomic Correlation (Table 15.15)

TABLE 15.15: Features of cerebral ischemia depending on the neuroanatomic basis.

Vascular territory	*Signs and symptoms*
Internal carotid artery	➢ Combined ACA (anterior cerebral artery) + MCA (middle cerebral artery) ➢ Ipsilateral monocular visual loss (amaurosis) secondary to central retinal artery occlusion (CRAO)
Left ACA	➢ Right leg numbness and weakness ➢ Transcortical motor aphasia ➢ Ideomotor apraxia
Right ACA	➢ Left leg numbness and weakness ➢ Motor neglect ➢ Possibly ideomotor apraxia
Left MCA	➢ Right face/arm > leg numbness and weakness ➢ Aphasia ➢ Left gaze preference
Right MCA	➢ Left face/arm > leg numbness and weakness ➢ Left hemispatial neglect ➢ Right gaze preference ➢ Agraphesthesia/astereoagnosia

Stroke Localization—Clinical Features (Tables 15.16 to 15.18 and Fig. 15.11)

TABLE 15.16: Commmon localization of hemiplegia.

Site of lesion	*Predominant clinical features*
Cortex	➢ Monoplegia common (brachial—MCA territory; Crural—ACA territory) ➢ Hemiplegia (may be present but never dense) ➢ Contralateral VIIth cranial nerve palsy [upper motor neuron (UMN) variant] ➢ Seizures ➢ Aphasias (in dominant hemisphere) ➢ Apraxias (in nondominant hemisphere)
Subcortical (usually secondary to hypoperfusion)	➢ Monoplegias common ➢ Transcortical aphasias common
Internal capsule lesion	➢ Contralateral hemiplegia (dense) ➢ Contralateral hemisensory loss ➢ Contralateral VIIth cranial nerve palsy (UMN variant)

Contd...

Contd...

	➢ Homonymous hemianopia ➢ Brocas's like aphasia (only site to have subcortical aphasia) *Note:* Most common etiology being ischemic and hence is territory specific. Since different parts of internal capsule has blood supply from different blood vessels, all the above-mentioned features may not be present at same time. However, if present, it suggests hemorrhage or tumor compressing internal capsule.
Brainstem lesion	Discussed separate **Table 15.17**
High cervical cord lesion (Brown–Sequard Syndrome)	➢ Ipsilateral hemiplegia ➢ Ipsilateral loss of posterior column sensation ➢ Contralateral loss of pain and temperature sensation ➢ Usually no cranial nerve involvement

TABLE 15.17: Posterior circulation strokes—brainstem syndromes.

Site of lesion/syndrome	*Blood supply and tracts involved*	*Ipsilateral (I/L) features*	*Contralateral (C/L) features*
Midbrain			
Benedikt's syndrome (Claude's + Weber's)	Interpeduncular branches of basilar artery, PCA—posterior cerebral artery (midbrain tegmentum—CN III fibers; red nucleus; CST; SCP)	Ipsilateral CN III palsy	Ataxia + Hyperkinesia and tremor (rubral tremor) + Hemiparesis
Claude's syndrome	PCA (midbrain tegmentum—CN III fibers; red nucleus; SCP)	Ipsilateral CN III palsy; contralateral	Ataxia + Tremor (rubral tremor)
Weber's syndrome	Paramedian branches of the basilar artery, PCA	Ipsilateral CN III palsy	Hemiparesis
Nothnagel's syndrome	Basilar penetrating artery, mesencephalic artery (midbrain tectum—ipsilateral or bilateral CN III)	Oculomotor palsies; ataxia	
Parinaud's syndrome	Midbrain dorsum (quadrigeminal plate region; pretectum; periaqueductal gray matter)	Impaired upgaze; convergence retraction nystagmus; dilated pupils with light-near dissociation	
Top of basilar artery syndrome	Midbrain Thalamus Portion of temporal and occipital lobe involved	Behavioral abonormalities Ocular finding Visual defects Pupillary abnormalities Motor deficits	
Artery of Percheron stroke	Single thalamic perforating aretery from the proximal PCA	Altered sensorium Vertical gaze palsy Memory impairement	
Pons			
Raymond–Céstan syndrome	Long circumferential branch of basilar artery (CN VI; CST)	VIth nerve palsy	Hemiparesis
Millard–Gubler syndrome	Basilar artery (CN VII; CST)	VIIth nerve palsy (± Lateral rectus palsy)	Hemiparesis
Foville's syndrome	Basilar artery (CN VII; lateral gaze center, CST)	VIIth nerve palsy + Horizontal gaze palsy	Hemiparesis
Pierre Marie–Foix syndrome	AICA	VIth + VIIth nerve palsy Horner's syndrome	Hemiparesis
Medulla			
Wallenberg's syndrome (lateral medullary syndrome)	Vertebral artery > posterior inferior cerebellar artery (PICA) (lateral medullary tegmentum—spinal tract of CN V and its nucleus; nucleus ambiguus; emerging fibers of CNs IX and X; LST; descending sympathetic fibers; vestibular nuclei; inferior cerebellar peduncle; afferent spinocerebellar tracts; lateral cuneate nucleus)	Loss of pain and temperature of face I/L decreased corneal reflex; I/L weakness of soft palate; I/L loss of gag reflex; I/L paralysis of vocal cord; I/L central Horner's syndrome; nystagmus; cerebellar ataxia of I/L limbs; lateropulsion; Hiccups	Loss of pain and temperature of body
Dejerine's syndrome (medial medullary syndrome)	Vertebral > anterior spinal artery	I/L tongue weakness	Hemiparesis
Avellis' syndrome	Medullary tegmentum	I/L palatal and vocal cord weakness	Loss of pain and temperature
Jackson's syndrome	Medullary tegmentum	Ipsilateral flaccid paralysis of soft palate, pharynx, and larynx; flaccid weakness and atrophy of SCM and trapezius (partial), and of the tongue	

Contd...

Contd...

Schmidt's syndrome	Lower medullary tegmentum	Ipsilateral paralysis of soft palate, pharynx, and larynx; flaccid weakness and atrophy of SCM and trapezius (partial)	
Céstan–Chenais syndrome	Due to vertebral artery occlusion below origin of the PICA (nucleus ambiguus; ICP; sympathetics; corticospinal tract, medial leminiscus	Ipsilateral weakness of soft palate, pharynx, and larynx; cerebellar ataxia; Horner's syndrome	Contralateral hemiparesis with loss of posterior column function
Internuclear ophthalmoplegia (INO)	Medial longitudinal fasciculus (MLF) lesion in the midbrain	I/L adduction palsy	Contralateral gaze-evoked nystagmus
Wall-eyed bilateral internuclear ophthalmoplegia (WEBINO)	Bilateral MLF lesion in the brain	Bilateral adduction deficit and primary gaze position exotropia	
Gerstmann's syndrome	Parietal lobe	Inability to write (dysgraphia or agraphia), the loss of the ability to do mathematics (acalculia), the inability to identify one's own or another's fingers (finger agnosia), and inability to make the distinction between the right and left side of the body	
Anton's syndrome	Bilateral occipital cortex involvement due to bilateral PCA infarct	Anton's syndrome describes the condition in which patients deny their blindness despite objective evidence of visual loss, and moreover confabulate to support their stance	Anosognosia (or lack of awareness of defect) and confabulation
Balint's syndrome	Parieto-occipital lobes on both sides of the brain	Inability to perceive the visual field as a whole (simultanagnosia), difficulty in fixating the eyes (oculomotor apraxia), and inability to move the hand to a specific object by using vision (optic ataxia)	

TABLE 15.18: Clinical features of stroke depending on localization (anterior circulation).

Syndrome	*Clinical features*	*Localization*
Middle cerebral artery (M1) syndrome	Produces pure motor or sensory motor stroke contralateral to the side of lesion. If ischemia of putamen, pallidus—predominantly parkinsonian features	Internal capsule, caudate nucleus, putamen, and outer pallidus
Middle cerebral artery (M2) syndrome	Brachial syndrome: Weakness of hand and arm; Frontal opercular syndrome: Broca's aphasia with facial weakness with or without arm weakness	Superior division of MCA-M2 involved
	If dominant hemisphere: Wernicke's aphasia without weakness with contralateral homonymous superior quadrantanopia If nondominant hemisphere: Hemispatial neglect, spatial agnosia without weakness	Inferior division of MCA-M2 involved
Complete MCA syndrome	Contralateral hemiplegia, contralateral hemianesthesia, contralateral homonymous hemianopia, gaze preference to the ipsilateral side. If dominant hemisphere involved—global aphasia. If nondominant hemisphere involved—hemispatial neglect, anosognosia and constructional apraxia	
Unpaired ACA syndrome	Profound abulia and bilateral pyramidal signs with paraparesis or quadriparesis and urinary incontinence	Frontal lobe, entire medial part of cerebral hemispheres
Anterior choroidal artery occlusion syndrome	Contralateral (C/L) hemiplegia, C/L hemianesthesia, C/L homonymous hemianopia	Posterior limb of internal capsule, retrolentiform and sublentiform parts

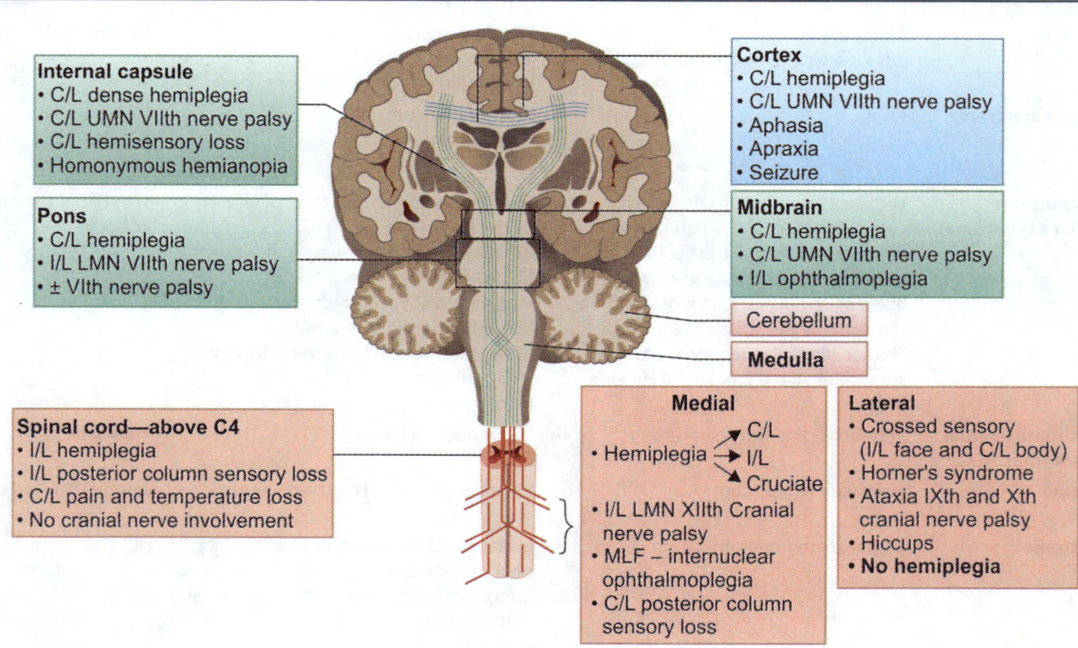

FIG. 15.11: Localization of lesion in hemiplegia.

Lateral medullary syndrome

Q. Write a short note on lateral medullary syndrome.

It is also known as Wallenberg's syndrome and is due to occlusion of the **posterior inferior cerebellar artery or vertebral artery.** Localization/structures involved and associated symptoms are presented in **Table 15.19**.

TABLE 15.19: Localization/structures involved and associated symptoms of lateral medullary syndrome (LMS).

Localization/structures involved	*Symptoms*
➤ Vestibular nuclei and connections ➤ Inferior cerebellar peduncle (Restiform body)	➤ Dizziness and imbalance ➤ Hypotonia ipsilateral side ➤ Diplopia/Oscillopsia ➤ Nystagmus, limb ataxia
➤ Spinal nucleus of CN V ➤ Spinothalamic tract	➤ Loss of pain and temperature sensation in ipsilateral face ➤ Loss of pain and temperature contralateral trunk (crossed sensory loss)
➤ Nucleus ambiguous (CN IX and X)	➤ Ipsilateral paralysis of palate, pharynx, and larynx ➤ Absent gag reflex
➤ Descending sympathetic fibers ➤ Dorsomotor nucleus of vagus	➤ Ipsilateral Horner's syndrome ➤ Autonomic signs—labile BP/tachycardia/sweating/arrhythmias
➤ Ventrolateral medullary tegmentum and the medullary reticular zone (respiratory centers)	➤ Failure of automatic respirations ➤ Hiccoughs
➤ **Corticospinal tracts, medial lemniscus not involved**	➤ **No pyramidal tract signs. Posterior column sensations preserved**

Oxfordshire Community Stroke Project (OCSP)—Bamford classification:

- **TACS (Total anterior circulation syndrome)**
  Hemianopia, hemiparesis, and higher cortical dysfunction
- **PACS (Partial anterior circulation syndrome)**
  Any two of TACS criteria or isolated higher cortical dysfunction
- **LACS (Lacunar syndrome)**
  Pure motor, pure sensory, sensorimotor strokes, dysarthria-clumsy hand syndrome or ataxic hemiparesis
- **POCS (Posterior circulation syndrome)**
  Isolated hemianopia or brainstem or cerebellar signs

TOAST (the Trial of ORG 10172 in Acute Stroke Treatment) classification of subtypes of acute ischemic stroke is presented in **Box 15.9**.

Box 15.9: TOAST classification of subtypes of acute ischemic stroke.

- Large artery atherosclerosis
- Cardioembolism
- Small vessel occlusion
- Stroke of other determined etiology
- Stroke of undetermined etiology

Hypoperfusion and its consequences

- A **generalized reduction in CBF due to systemic hypotension** (e.g., cardiac arrhythmia, cardiac arrest, myocardial infarction, or hemorrhagic shock) usually **produces syncope**.
- If low CBF persists for a longer duration, then **infarction in the border zones** (watershed areas) between the major and PCA distributions may develop (particularly if there is severe stenosis of proximal carotid vessels).
- In **more severe instances, global hypoxia-ischemia causes** widespread brain injury, the constellation of cognitive sequelae that ensues is called **hypoxic-ischemic encephalopathy**.
- **Focal ischemia or infarction**, conversely, is usually by thrombosis of the cerebral vessels themselves or by emboli from a proximal arterial source of the heart.

Carotid and vertebral artery dissection

- About 20% of cases of young (below the age 40 years) stroke are due to dissection of carotid or vertebral artery.
- It may develop sometimes as a **sequel of trivial neck trauma or hyperextension** (e.g., after whiplash, hair washing in a salon, or exercise). Predisposing factors include subtle collagen disorders (e.g., partial forms of Marfan's syndrome).
- **Most dissections occur in large extracranial neck vessels** and are characterized by **penetration of blood into the subintimal region of vessel wall** and form false lumen. However, it is the thrombosis within the true lumen due to tissue thromboplastin release which results in embolization from the site of dissection. This type of stroke sometimes develops days after the initial event.
- Symptoms: Pain in the neck or face is the clue for diagnosis.

Venous stroke

- Only 1% of strokes are due to venous thrombosis (within intracranial venous sinuses).
- **Predisposing factors:** It may occur in **pregnancy, hypercoagulable states** and thrombotic disorders or with dehydration or malignancy.
- **Consequences:** Cortical infarction, seizures, and raised ICP.

Investigations/Diagnosis

Neuroimaging (Figs. 15.12A to C)

- CT scans: To identify or exclude hemorrhage as the cause of stroke.
  - They **identify extraparenchymal hemorrhage,** neoplasms, abscesses, and other conditions mimicking as stroke.
  - Brain CT scans in the first several hours after an infarction generally does not show any abnormality, and the infarct may not be detected reliably for 24–48 hours.

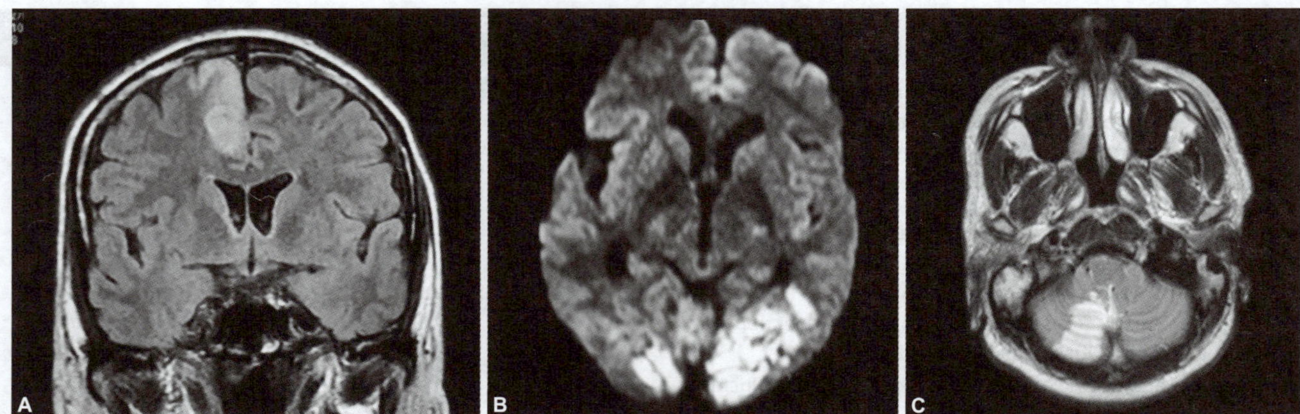

FIGS. 15.12A TO C: Neuroimaging in stroke: (A) Acute right anterior cerebral artery (ACA) infarct; (B) Acute bilateral posterior cerebral artery (PCA) infarct—Anton's syndrome; (C) Right lateral medullary syndrome.

  - CT may fail to show small ischemic strokes in the posterior fossa because of bone artifact; small infarcts on the cortical surface may also be missed.
- Magnetic resonance imaging (MRI): Reliably documents the extent and location of infarction in all areas of the brain, including the posterior fossa and cortical surface. MRI is less sensitive than CT in detecting acute bleeding.
- **Diffusion-weighted imaging and FLAIR** (fluid-attenuated inversion recovery) imaging are more sensitive for early brain infarction than standard MR sequences or CT. It can identify ischemic penumbra and patients showing large regions of mismatch may be better candidates for acute revascularization.

Vascular imaging

- Many ischemic strokes are due to atherosclerotic thromboembolic disease of the major extracranial vessels. Detection of extracranial vascular disease can establish the diagnosis of ischemic stroke and, it may also help for specific treatments (e.g., carotid endarterectomy to reduce the risk of further stroke).
- Extracranial arterial disease can be noninvasively detected by duplex ultrasound, magnetic resonance angiography (MRA) or CT angiography, or occasionally intra-arterial contrast radiography.

Cardiac investigations

- Cardioembolism is responsible for 20% of ischemic strokes. The source of emboli includes atrial fibrillation, prosthetic heart valves, other valvular abnormalities, and recent myocardial infarction.
- Clinical examination and ECG help in identifying the source of cardiac emboli. However, it may be necessary to perform a transthoracic or transesophageal echocardiogram to confirm the cardiac source or for detecting an unsuspected source (e.g., endocarditis, atrial myxoma, intracardiac thrombus or PFO). Such findings will help in providing specific cardiac treatment.

Blood investigations

- Complete blood count, erythrocyte sedimentation rate (ESR), glucose, renal function test (RFT), liver function test (LFT), serum electrolytes, prothrombin time-international normalized ratio (PT-INR), activated partial thromboplastin time (aPTT)
- **Workup for hypercoaguable states.**

- CBC with differential and platelets
- PT/aPTT
- Fibrinogen
- Factor VIII
- Factor VII
- C-reactive protein
- Antithrombin III
- Protein C
- Protein S (total and free)
- Lipoprotein (a)
- Activated protein C resistance (APCR)
- Leiden factor V mutation if APCR negative
- Prothrombin G20210A mutation
- Antiphospholipid antibodies (Abs)
  - Lupus anticoagulant
  - Anticardiolipin Abs
  - Anti-β-2-glycoprotein I Abs
  - Antiphosphatidylserine Abs
- Methyltetrahydrofolate reductase
  - MTHFR C677T and A1298C mutations
- Sickle cell screen

Paramedical personnel and general public are taught how to make the diagnosis of stroke on a simple history and examination—**FAST (Box 15.10)**.

Complications of Acute Stroke (Box 15.11).

Q. Write a short essay/note on complications of stroke.

Differential Diagnosis of Stroke

See **Box 15.12.**

Box 15.11: Complications of acute stroke.

- Cerebral edema
- Cardiac arrhythmias, myocardial infarction, and neurogenic cardiac injury
- Chest infection
- Seizures
- Deep venous thrombosis/pulmonary embolism
- Pressure sores
- Urinary infection
- GI bleed: Stress ulcers, drug induced
- Constipation
- Painful shoulder/contractures
- Depression and anxiety
- Increased ICT and coning

Box 15.10: Diagnosis of stroke on a simple history and examination—FAST.

- **F**ace: Sudden weakness of the face
- **A**rm: Sudden weakness of one or both arms
- **S**peech: Difficulty in speaking, slurred speech
- **T**ime: Sooner the starting of treatment, better the outcome

Box 15.12: Differential diagnosis of stroke.

Structural stroke mimickers

- Tumors: Primary and metastatic cerebral tumors
- Subdural hematoma
- Cerebral abscess
- Demyelinating disorders: Multiple sclerosis
- Peripheral nerve lesions (vascular or compressive)

Functional stroke mimickers

- Seizure and postictal state
- Focal seizures
- Syncope
- Hypoglycemia
- Migrainous aura
- Conversion disorders and other psychiatric disorders
- Ménière's disease/other vestibular disorders
- Encephalitis
- Wernicke's encephalopathy
- Transient global amnesia
- Metabolic encephalopathy

Treatment of Ischemic Stroke—"Time is Brain" (Fig. 15.13)

Treatments designed to reverse or lessen the amount of tissue infarction and improve clinical outcome fall into six categories: (1) IV thrombolysis, (2) endovascular techniques, (3) antithrombotic treatment, (4) medical support, (5) neuroprotection, and (6) stroke centers and rehabilitation.

1. **Intravenous thrombolysis**
   - Intravenous (IV) administration for recombinant recombinant tissue plasminogen activator (r-tPA) within 3 hours of the onset of symptoms reduces disability and mortality from ischemic stroke.
     - Indications and contraindications for r-tPA **(Box 15.13)**.
   - Administration
     - Administer at the rate of 0.9 mg/kg intravenously (maximum 90 mg) as 10% of total dose as an IV bolus and remainder of dose as a continuous IV infusion over 60 minutes.

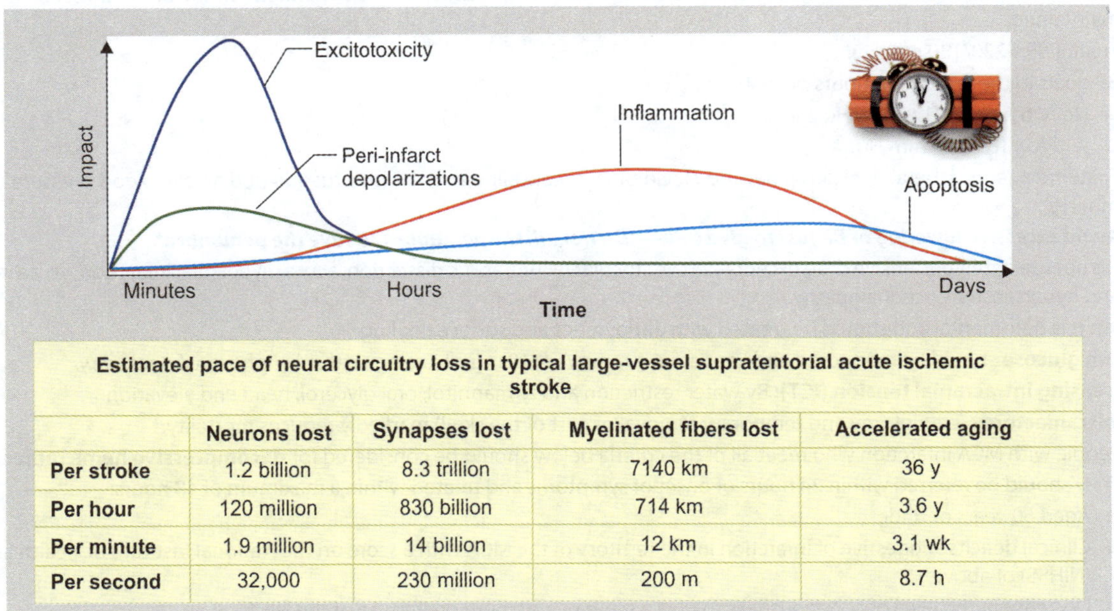

Estimated pace of neural circuitry loss in typical large-vessel supratentorial acute ischemic stroke

	Neurons lost	Synapses lost	Myelinated fibers lost	Accelerated aging
Per stroke	1.2 billion	8.3 trillion	7140 km	36 y
Per hour	120 million	830 billion	714 km	3.6 y
Per minute	1.9 million	14 billion	12 km	3.1 wk
Per second	32,000	230 million	200 m	8.7 h

FIG. 15.13: Treatment of ischemic stroke—"Time is brain".

- No other antithrombotic treatment for 24 hours.
- Avoid urethral catheterization for 2 hours.

– For decline in neurologic status or uncontrolled blood pressure, stop infusion, give cryoprecipitate, and reimage brain emergently.

2. **Endovascular mechanical thrombectomy:** It is an alternative or adjunctive treatment of acute stroke in patients who are ineligible for, or have contraindications to, thrombolytics or in those who have failed to have vascular recanalization with IV thrombolytics.
3. **Antiplatelet therapy**
   – Platelet inhibition: Aspirin 150 mg + clopidogrel 75 mg daily. *Note:* Glycoprotein IIb/IIIa receptor inhibitor abciximab causes excess ICH and should be avoided in acute stroke.
   – Randomized studies of unfractionated heparin, low-molecular-weight heparins, or heparinoids have shown no proven benefits in the reduction of stroke-related mortality, stroke-related morbidity, early stroke recurrence, or stroke prognosis except in the case of cerebral venous thrombosis (CVT).
4. **Anticoagulation for acute ischemic stroke: Routine use of anticoagulation for acute ischemic stroke is not recommended.** Only indications for anticoagulants are:
   – Conditions with potential high risk of early cardiogenic re-embolization (e.g., atrial fibrillation)
   – Symptomatic arteriosclerotic stenosis with crescendo TIAs
   – Known hypercoagulable states
   – Cerebral venous sinus thrombosis.

Box 15.13: Indications and contraindications for recombinant tissue plasminogen activator (r-tPA).

Indications for r-Tpa	
• Clinical diagnosis of stroke • Onset of symptom to time of drug administration ≤3 hours (time window: 3–4.5 hours) • Age ≥18 years	• CT scan showing no hemorrhage or infarct size >1/3rd of the middle cerebral artery (MCA) territory • Consent by patient or surrogate
Contraindications for r-tPA	
• Sustained BP >185/110 mm of Hg despite treatment • Platelets <100,000/μL • Hematocrit <25% • Glucose <50 or >400 mg% • Use of heparin/warfarin within 48 hours and prolonged activated partial thromboplastin time (aPTT) or international normalized ratio (INR) • Prior intracranial hemorrhage	• Prior stroke or head injury within 3 months • Major surgery in preceding 14 days • Minor stroke symptoms • GI bleed in preceding 21 days • Recent myocardial infarction (within 3 months) • Coma or stupor • Pregnancy • Age >80 years

5. **Medical support**
   – **Prevention of the common complications** of bedridden patients:
     - Infections (pneumonia, urinary, and skin): Prophylactic antibiotic.
     - Deep venous thrombosis with pulmonary embolism: Subcutaneous heparin and pneumatic compression stockings to prevent DVT.
     - Others: Catheterization, Ryle's tube (RT) feeding, maintenance of hygiene, etc.
   – **Maintenance of blood pressure:** Collateral blood flow within the ischemic brain is dependent on the blood pressure; hence, it is to be maintained.
     - Treat if BP >220/120 mm Hg.
     - BP goals in the first 24–48 hours post-stroke:
       - No IV tPA: <220/120 mm Hg
       - IV tPA: <185/110 mm Hg.
     - First-line agents: labetalol, nicardipine, and clevidipine; second-line agent: nitroprusside [if diastolic blood pressure (DBP) >120 mm Hg].

       Avoid excessive lowering of BP just to give t-PA—"Do not kill the penumbra to save the penumbra".
     - Do not use antihypertensive drug except—left ventricular failure, aortic dissection, acute myocardial infarction, acute renal failure, and hypertensive encephalopathy.
   – **Fever:** It is detrimental and should be treated with antipyretics and surface cooling.
   – **Serum glucose** should be monitored and kept at <6.1 mmol/L (110 mg/dL) using an insulin infusion if necessary.
   – **Decreasing intracranial tension (ICT):** By water restriction and IV mannitol, oral glycerol, head end elevation.

     Hemicraniectomy (craniotomy and temporary removal of part of the skull) markedly reduces mortality.
     - People with MCA infarction who meet all of the criteria below should be considered for **decompressive hemicraniectomy.**
     - They should be referred within 24 hours of onset of symptoms and treated within a maximum of 48 hours:
       - Aged 60 years or under
       - Clinical deficits suggestive of infarction in the territory of the MCA with a score on the National Institute of Health Stroke Scale (NIHSS) of above 15
       - Decrease in the level of consciousness to give a score of 1 or more on item 1a of the NIHSS
       - Signs on MRI of an infarct of at least 50% of the MCA territory, with or without additional

 - ❑ Infarction in the territory of the anterior or PCA on the same side, or
 - ❑ Infarct volume >145 cm^3 as shown on diffusion-weighted MRI.
- Control of intracranial pressure: In cerebellar strokes, even small amounts of cerebellar edema can acutely increase ICP or directly compress the brainstem. Prophylactic suboccipital decompression of large cerebellar infarcts before brainstem compression is very useful.

 Endovascular treatment approaches:
 - EKOS (ultrasound-enhanced thrombolysis)
 - Neuroflo (perfusion augmentation)
 - Mechanical endovascular thrombectomy
6. **Statins:** Atorvastatin, rosuvastatin—10–20 mg
7. **Neuroprotection:** Drugs that block the excitatory amino acid pathways (nimodipine, magnesium, lubeluzole, basic fibroblast growth factor, and citicoline) protect neurons and glia in animals, but they have not yet been proven to be beneficial in humans.
8. **Rehabilitation:**
 - Proper rehabilitation of the stroke patient includes early physical, occupational, and speech therapy. It is directed toward educating the patient and family about the patients' neurologic deficit, preventing the complications of immobility (e.g., pneumonia, DVT and pulmonary embolism, pressure sores of the skin, and muscle contractures), and providing encouragement and instructions in overcoming the deficit.
 - Goal of rehabilitation: It is to return the patient to home and to maximize recovery. The use of restraint therapy (immobilizing the unaffected side) has been shown to improve hemiparesis following stroke, even years following the stroke.

Secondary Prevention of Stroke and Transient Ischemic Attack

ABCD² score can help in identifying the stroke risk. A score of <4 is associated with a minimal risk whereas >6 is high risk for a stroke **(Table 15.20)**.

Treatment of Atherosclerosis

- **Risk factors:** Treatment of hypertension, diabetes, dyslipidemia, and cessation of smoking. Patients with higher risk scores need to be on anticoagulation while those with lower scores antiplatelet agents would suffice.
- **Atorvastatin:** In the dose of 80 mg/day useful both in secondary and primary prevention even with normal lipid levels.
- **Antiplatelet agents:** Aspirin, clopidogrel or dipyridamole are used.
- **Anticoagulation therapy for embolic stroke:** Anticoagulation (INR range, 2–3) in patients with chronic nonvalvular (nonrheumatic) atrial fibrillation prevents cerebral embolism and is safe. Warfarin, apixaban, dabigatran, rivaroxaban, edoxaban are equally effective.
- **Calculation of CHADS² score:** *One point for age > 75 years, one point for hypertension, one point for congestive heart failure (CHF), one point for diabetes, and two points for stroke or TIA; sum of points is the total CHADS² score.*

TABLE 15.20: Features and ABCD² score useful in assessing the stroke risk.

Clinical feature	*Score*
A: Age > 60 years	1
B: BP systolic >140 mm Hg or diastolic BP > 90 mm Hg	1
C: Clinical symptoms	
➢ Unilateral weakness	2
➢ Speech disturbance without weakness	1
D: Duration of symptoms	
> 60 minutes	2
10–59 minutes	1
D: Diabetes (oral medications or insulin)	1
ABCD² total score	Sum each category

Treatment of Carotid Atherosclerosis

- **High-grade stenosis of carotid artery:** Patient with recent symptomatic (within 2 weeks of symptoms) hemisphere ischemia, high-grade stenosis (>70%) in the appropriate internal carotid artery, and an institutional perioperative morbidity and mortality rate of 6% generally should undergo carotid endarterectomy.
- **Low-grade stenosis of carotid artery:** For asymptomatic stenosis and symptomatic low-grade stenosis (50–70%), medical therapy for reduction of atherosclerosis risk factors, including cholesterol-lowering agents and antiplatelet medications, is generally recommended.
- **Endovascular therapy:** Balloon angioplasty coupled with stenting to open stenotic carotid arteries and maintain their patency.

Treatment of Intracranial Atherosclerosis

- Symptomatic lesions with intracranial angioplasty and stenting.
- Dural sinus thrombosis: By short-term anticoagulants, regardless of the presence of ICH, for venous infarction following sinus thrombosis.

Young Stroke (Box 15.14)

Q. Write a short essay/note on etiology of stroke in a young.

The term "young stroke" is used to denote stroke in individuals <45 years of age.

Box 15.14: Causes for young stroke.

- **Cardiac**
  - Congenital heart disease, patent foramen ovale
  - Atrial myxoma
  - Atrial fibrillation and other arrhythmia
  - Cardiomyopathy, myocarditis, myocardial infarction
  - Cardiac surgery, cardiac catheterization
  - Endocarditis, rheumatic heart disease
  - Prosthetic valve
- **Hematologic**
  - Sickle cell disease, iron deficiency anemias, polycythemia vera
- **Hypercoagulable states**
  - Inherited prothrombotic states, protein C and S deficiency, antithrombin III deficiency, factor V Leiden gene mutation, prothrombin gene mutation
  - Antiphospholipid syndrome
  - Hyperhomocysteinemia
  - Myeloproliferative disorders (e.g., leukemia, lymphoma)
  - Pregnancy
  - Exposure to hormonal treatments such as anabolic steroids and erythropoietin
  - Nephrotic syndrome
- **Vascular**
  - **Noninflammatory**
    - Arterial dissection
    - Secondary to connective tissue disease (Ehlers–Danlos, Marfan)
    - Moyamoya disease
    - Hypertension
    - Radiation vasculopathy
    - Vasculitis and postinfectious vasculopathy
    - Migraine
    - Cerebral autosomal dominant arteriopathy with subcortical infarcts and leukoencephalopathy (CADASIL) Fibromuscular dysplasia, Susac's syndrome, Sneddon's syndrome, Fabry's disease
  - **Inflammatory**
    - Takayasu arteritis
    - Giant cell arteritis
    - Kawasaki disease
    - Polyarteritis nodosa
    - Human immunodeficiency virus (HIV)
    - Bacterial meningitis

Intracranial Hemorrhage

Q. Describe the risk factors, etiopathogenesis, clinical features, investigations, diagnosis, and management of cerebral/intracerebral hemorrhage.

Q. Describe the etiology, clinical features, investigations, and management of hemorrhagic stroke.

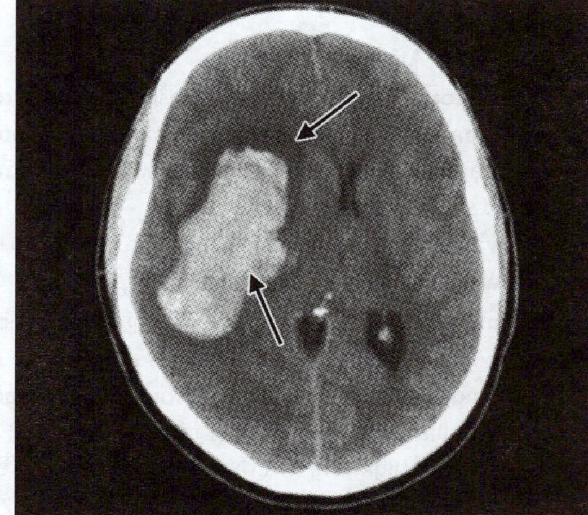

FIG. 15.14: CT showing hemorrhage in internal capsule.

- This includes: (1) intracerebral **(Fig. 15.14)** and cerebellar hemorrhage, (2) subarachnoid hemorrhage (SAH), and (3) subdural and extradural hemorrhage/hematoma.
- It causes about 10% of acute stroke events. It is usually due to rupture of a blood vessel within the brain parenchyma but may also occur in association with an SAH if the artery ruptures into the brain substance as well as into the subarachnoid space.
- **Hypertensive intraparenchymal hemorrhage** (hypertensive hemorrhage or hypertensive intracerebral hemorrhage) usually results from spontaneous rupture of a small penetrating artery deep in the brain. The most common sites are the **basal ganglia (especially the putamen), thalamus, cerebellum, and pons. Cortical bleeds are rare.**
- **Pontine hemorrhages:** 3Ps namely pinpoint pupil, hyperpyrexia, paralysis (quadriplegia). There is prominent decerebrate rigidity and "pinpoint" (1 mm) pupils that react to light. There is impairment of reflex horizontal eye movements evoked by head turning (doll's head or oculocephalic maneuver) or by irrigation of the ears with ice water.
- **Primary versus secondary hemorrhage** (hemorrhage that frequently occurs also into an area of brain infarction)—may be difficult to distinguish from primary intracerebral hemorrhage both clinically and radiologically.

Consequences of Hemorrhage

- **Immediate cessation of function:** The sudden entry of blood into the brain parenchyma causes immediate cessation of function in that area as neurons are structurally disrupted with splitting of white matter fiber tracts.
- **Mass effect:** The hemorrhage may expand over the first minutes or hours, or it may produce a rim of cerebral edema. Progression of neurological deficit occurs due to the mass effect. If large, they can cause shift of the intracranial contents, producing transtentorial coning and sometimes rapid death.
- **Resorption of hematoma:** If the patient survives, the hematoma is gradually absorbed, and produces a hemosiderin-lined slit in the brain parenchyma.

Causes of Intracranial Hemorrhage

See **Table 15.21.**

TABLE 15.21: Causes of intracranial hemorrhage and its location.

Cause	*Location*	*Comments*
Head trauma	Intraparenchymal: Frontal lobes, anterior temporal lobes, subarachnoid	Coup and countercoup injury during brain deceleration
Hypertensive hemorrhage	Putamen (most common), globus pallidus, thalamus, cerebellar hemisphere, pons	Chronic hypertension produces hemorrhage from small (100 µm) vessels in these regions
Metastatic brain tumor	Lobar	Primary tumors in lung, choriocarcinoma, melanoma
Coagulopathy	Any	Uncommon cause: Often associated with prior stroke or underlying vascular anomaly
Drug	Lobar, subarachnoid	Cocaine, amphetamine, phenylpropanolamine
Arteriovenous malformation	Lobar, intraventricular, subarachnoid	Risk is 2–4% per year for bleeding
Aneurysm	Subarachnoid, intraparenchymal, rarely subdural	Mycotic and nonmycotic forms of aneurysms
Cerebral amyloid angiopathy	Lobar	Most common cause for recurrent lobar hemorrhage in elderly

Clinical Features

- **Clinical presentation depends upon** which **arterial territory is involved** and the **size of the lesion**.
- **Rapid-onset:** Occurs over minutes.
- **Most common presentation:** Weakness of the face or arm, or disturbance of speech.
- **Focal deficit of brain function:** Affects an identifiable area of the brain and is "negative" in character (i.e., abrupt loss of function without positive features such as abnormal movement). Features which suggest the location of lesion are:
  - **Lesion in the cerebral hemisphere:** Usually characterized by unilateral motor deficit, a higher cerebral function deficit such as aphasia or neglect, or a visual field defect.
  - **Lesion in the brainstem or cerebellum:** Ataxia, diplopia, vertigo and/or bilateral weakness.
  - **Intracerebral hemorrhage:** Combination of severe headache and vomiting at the onset of the focal deficit.

Management/Treatment

Any identified coagulopathy should be reversed as soon as possible.

- For patients taking VKAs (vitamin K antagonists), rapid reversal of coagulopathy can be achieved by infusing prothrombin complex concentrates which can be administered quickly, followed by fresh frozen plasma and vitamin K.
- When ICH is associated with thrombocytopenia (platelet count < 50,000/µL), transfusion of fresh platelets is indicated.

Control of BP

- BP >185/110 increases the size of hematoma by more bleeding. Hence, maintain a mean arterial pressure (MAP) < 130 mm Hg, unless an increase in ICP is suspected.
- In patients who have ICP monitors in place, keep the cerebral perfusion pressure (MAP-ICP) > 60 mm Hg (i.e., one should lower MAP to this target if blood pressure is elevated).
- Blood pressure should be lowered with nonvasodilating IV drugs such as nicardipine, labetalol, or esmolol.

Hyperosmolar therapy

- Mannitol: Bolus of 0.25 g/kg to 1 g/kg body weight.
- Hypertonic saline, concentrations ranging from 3 to 23.4%.

Hyperventilation decreases $PaCO_2$, which can induce constriction of cerebral arteries by alkalinizing the cerebrospinal fluid (CSF).

Barbiturate coma

Pentobarbital is given in a loading dose of 10 mg/kg body weight followed by 5 mg/kg body weight each hour for three doses.

Hypothermia

Steroids are used for primary and metastatic brain tumors, to decrease vasogenic cerebral edema.

Treatment of raised intracranial tension

- If the hematoma causes marked midline shift of structures with consequent obtundation, coma or hydrocephalus, osmotic agents coupled with induced hyperventilation can be instituted to lower ICP.
- Once ICP is recorded, further hyperventilation and osmotic therapy can be tailored to the individual patient to keep cerebral perfusion pressure (MAP-ICP) above 60 mm Hg.
- If ICP is still found to be high, CSF can be drained from the ventricular space and osmotic therapy continued.
- Persistent or progressive elevation in ICP may prompt surgical evacuation of the clot.
- Glucocorticoids are not helpful for the edema from intracerebral hematoma.
- Most cerebellar hematomas >3 cm in diameter will require surgical evacuation.

Transient Ischemic Attack

Q. Write a short essay/note on TIA including its definition.

Transient ischemic attack is characterized by a brief episode of neurological dysfunction (sudden loss of function) in which symptoms and signs resolve completely after a brief period within 24 hours (usually within 30 minutes).

- Transient ischemic attack is defined as a transient episode of neurologic dysfunction caused by focal brain, spinal cord, or retinal ischemia, without acute infarction. However, TIAs may herald a stroke.
- It may be better to describe as symptoms <1 hour with no evidence of infarction.
- It may have infarct even with symptoms lasting a few hours (~50% of TIA patients have MRI evidence of ischemia).
- **Newer, neuroimaging informed, operational definitions of TIA—"a brief episode of neurological dysfunction caused by focal brain or retinal ischemia, with clinical symptoms typically lasting less than *one hour, and without evidence of acute infarction"***

Clinical Features

Hemiparesis and aphasia are most common. Other features include amaurosis fugax (sudden transient loss of vision in one eye), hemisensory loss, hemianopic visual loss, diplopia, vertigo, vomiting, choking, dysarthria, ataxia, etc.

Types

Types of TIA have been shown in **Box 15.15**.

Box 15.15: Types of transient ischemic attack (TIA).

- Embolic TIA—recurrent, short-lasting episodes of stereotyped symptoms (shotgun TIA)
- Large artery TIA—longer-lasting less frequent episodes with varied symptoms
- Lacunar TIA

*Recurrent same side, same territory TIA is suggestive of vessel disease

*TIA in both anterior and posterior circulation is suggestive of cardioembolism

Diagnosis

Diagnosis of TIA often depends on its description. There may be clinical evidence of a source of embolus (e.g., carotid arterial bruit/stenosis, atrial fibrillation or other dysrhythmia, valvular heart disease/endocarditis, recent myocardial infarction.

- An underlying **risk factor**/condition may be present. These include atheroma, hypertension, postural hypotension, bradycardia or low cardiac output, diabetes mellitus, etc.

Treatment (Flowchart 15.7)

Medical therapy and surgical treatment if appropriate. If patients have $ABCD^2$ (refer **Table 15.20**) score >4, or have had two recent TIAs (especially within the same vascular territory), they should be investigated and advised for secondary prevention of stroke.

FLOWCHART 15.7: Management of transient ischemic attack (TIA).

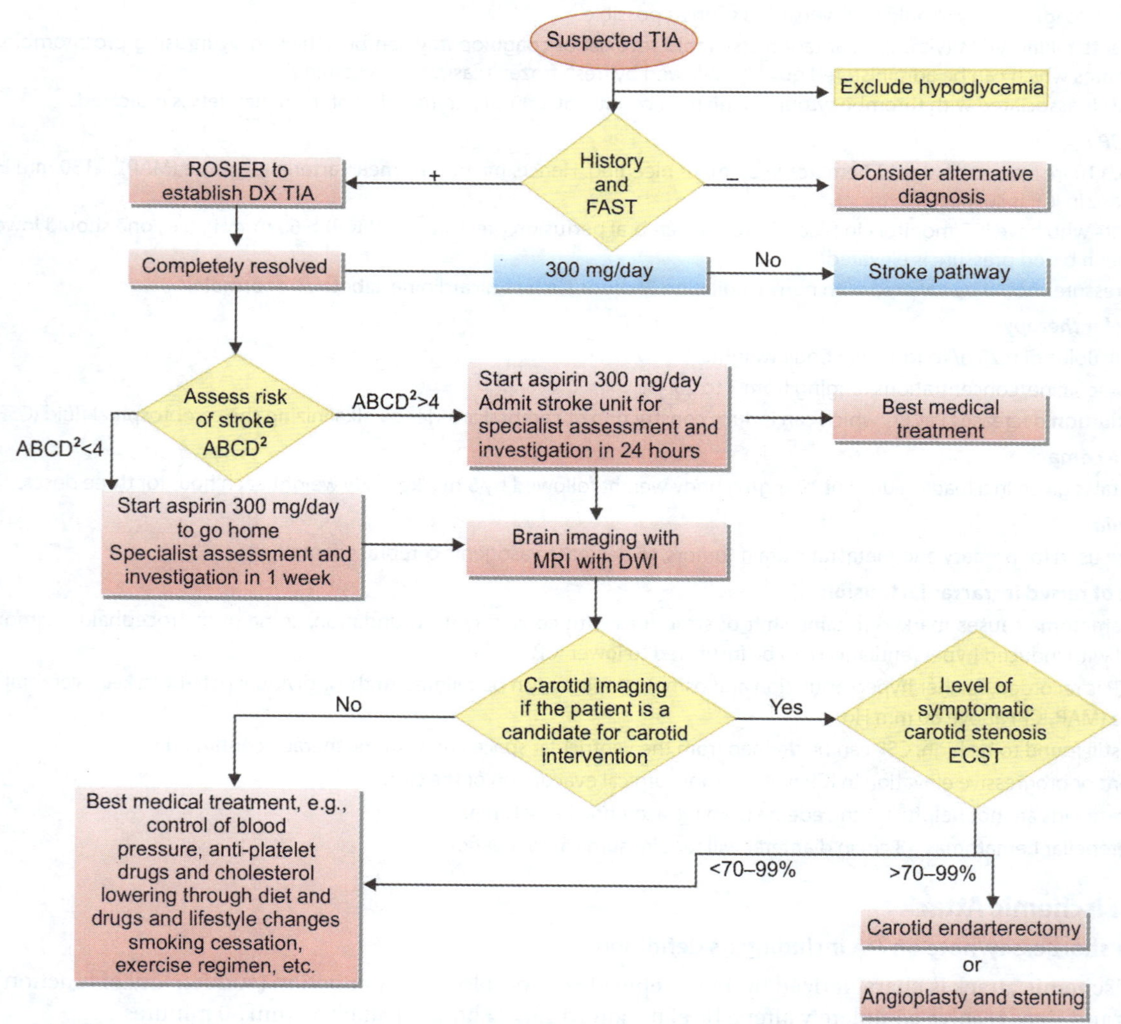

(ROSIER: Recognition Of Stroke In the Emergency Room; FAST: Face Arm Speech Test; DWI: diffusion-weighted imaging; ECST:European Carotid Surgery Trial)

Subarachnoid Hemorrhage

Q. Discuss the clinical manifestations and treatment of primary SAH.

Q. Write a short essay/note on SAH.

Subarachnoid hemorrhage is a pathologic condition in which the **blood enters the subarachnoid space.** SAH is less common than ischemic stroke or intracerebral hemorrhage. It accounts for about 5% of strokes.

Etiology (Table 15.22)

- **Most common cause** of SAH **is trauma.**
- **Most common cause of spontaneous SAH** is an **aneurysmal** (saccular or "berry" aneurysms) **bleed** (65–80%).
- SAH causes intense reductions in CBF, reduced cerebral autoregulation, and acute cerebral ischemia.
- The overall case fatality varied from 32 to 67%.

Risk factors for SAH have been shown in **Box 15.16**.

TABLE 15.22: Causes of subarachnoid hemorrhage.

Category	*Causes*
Trauma	Closed, penetrating, electric, etc.
Vascular	Aneurysms (berry aneurysm), atherosclerosis, arteriovenous malformations (AVMs), vasculitides
Idiopathic	Benign perimesencephalic subarachnoid hemorrhage
Blood dyscrasias	Leukemia, hemophilia, thrombocytopenia
Infections	Dengue, leptospirosis, bacterial meningitis
Toxins	Amphetamines, cocaine, nicotine, anticoagulants
Neoplasms	Gliomas, meningiomas, hemangioblastoma, etc.

Box 15.16: Risk factors for subarachnoid hemorrhage.

- Hypertension
- Cigarette smoking
- Oral contraceptives
- Diurnal variations in blood pressure
- Pregnancy and parturition
- Slight increased risk during lumbar puncture and/or cerebral angiography in patient with cerebral aneurysm
- Slight increased risk with advancing age
- Alcohol consumption (debatable)
- Following cocaine abuse
- Increased incidence of polycystic kidneys, fibromuscular dysplasia of extracranial arteries, Ehlers–Danlos syndrome, moyamoya, AV malformations and coarctation of aorta

Circle of Willis

- Circle of Willis is a circulatory anastomosis that supplies blood to the brain and surrounding structures. This anastomotic pathway is important for the preservation of brain function when major blood flow is disrupted in one of the major feeding vessels.
- Constituents arteries of circle of Willis **(Fig. 15.15 and Box 15.17)**:

The MCAs, supplying the brain, do not form the part of the circle of Willis.

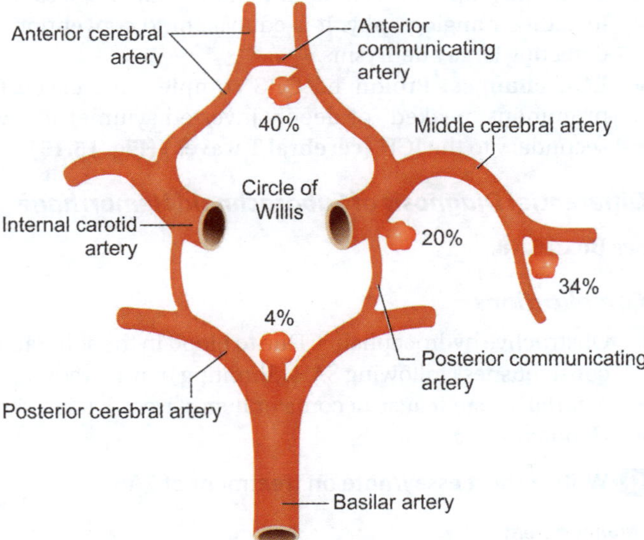

FIG. 15.15: Blood supply to the brain and circle of Willis with common sites of saccular (berry) aneurysms.

Box 15.17: Constituents arteries of circle of Willis.

- Two internal carotid arteries (left and right)
- Anterior cerebral artery (left and right)
- Anterior communicating artery
- Posterior cerebral artery (left and right)
- Posterior communicating artery (left and right)
- Basilar artery formed by joining of two vertebral arteries

Saccular ("berry") aneurysm

- Saccular aneurysms develop within the circle of Willis and adjacent arteries. Three most common locations are—(1) the terminal internal carotid artery, (2) MCA bifurcation, and (3) top of the basilar artery.
- It can undergo spontaneous rupture and cause SAH. If the patient survives, but the aneurysm is not obliterated, the rate of rebleeding is about 20% in the first 2 weeks, 30% in the first month, and about 3% per year afterward.
- The annual risk of rupture for aneurysms <10 mm in size is 0.1%, and for aneurysms >10 mm in size is 0.5–1%.

Clinical Features of Subarachnoid Hemorrhage

- **Headache:** Most common symptom (97%). Usually severe (the worst headache of my life) and sudden **(thunderclap)** in onset. Few patients may have milder warning headaches (sentinel headaches) in 2–8 weeks preceding the major hemorrhage. Headache may pulsate toward the occiput and sometimes may be felt as neck pain. Occipital and posterior cervical pain may signal a posterior inferior cerebellar artery or anterior inferior cerebellar artery aneurysm. If there is expanding MCA aneurysm, pain may be observed in or behind the eye and in the low temple. Headache commonly occurs on physical exertion, straining, and sexual excitement.
- **Vomiting** may be present.
- **Other symptoms:** Decreased consciousness and alertness, seizure (10%) and stiff neck, etc.
- **Rerupture/rebleed:** The rerupture of an untreated aneurysm in the first month following SAH is ~30%, with the peak in the first 7 days.

Physical examination:

- Patient is usually distressed and irritable, with photophobia.
- Neck stiffness (and a positive Kernig's sign) due to subarachnoid blood may be present but this may take few hours to develop. Focal hemisphere signs, e.g., intracerebral hematoma may cause hemiparesis or aphasia.
- Rarely, IIIrd nerve palsy may be developing due to local pressure from an aneurysm of the posterior communicating artery.
- Fundoscopy: It may show **subhyaloid hemorrhage** which is canoe-shaped, (***SAH plus subhyaloid hemorrhage = Terson's syndrome***) produced due to tracking of blood along the subarachnoid space around the optic nerve.

Investigations

Computed tomography scan: It shows blood in the subarachnoid space (if performed in the first few days), intracerebral hematoma, hydrocephalus, associated brain ischemia, and occasionally aneurysmal location.

Q. Write a short essay/note on CSF findings in SAH.

- **Lumbar puncture:** It should be performed when clinical suspicion of SAH is high, CT scan does not reveal subarachnoid blood, and there is no mass effect. In the initial few hours, CSF will be uniformly blood stained. **Xanthochromia** appears within 6 hours of SAH and persists for nearly 2 weeks. Naked inspection of supernatant CSF is usually sufficiently reliable for diagnosis of SAH. Spectrophotometry to estimate bilirubin in the CSF released from lysed cells confirm the diagnosis.
- **Angiography:** It is required to locate the site of bled aneurysm and details that are needed to ligate the aneurysm by the neurosurgeon. It should be done in all patients fit for surgery (i.e., age < 65 years and who are not in coma).
- **Magnetic resonance angiography:** It will accurately identify aneurysms > 5 mm in size.
- **CT angiography:** It is a rapid readily available, less invasive alternative to catheter angiography. It is equivalent to conventional angiography for detecting large aneurysms.
- **ECG changes:** Prolonged QRS complex, increased QT interval, and prominent "peaked" or deeply inverted symmetric T waves are usually secondary to the ICH **(cerebral T waves) (Fig. 15.16).**

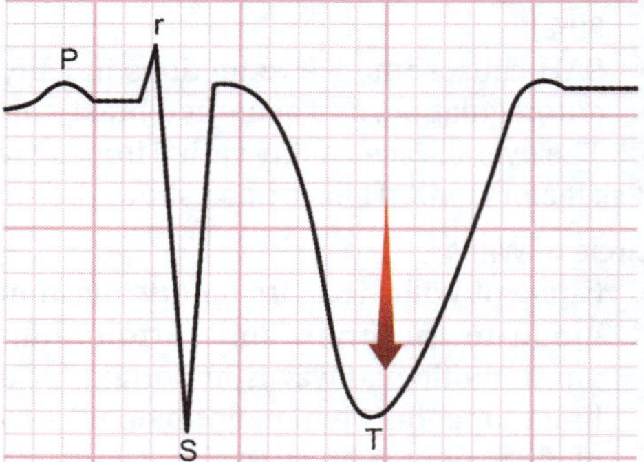

FIG. 15.16: Electrocardiographic (ECG) changes.

Box 15.18: Differential diagnosis of subarachnoid hemorrhage.

- Migraine
- Acute bacterial meningitis
- Cervical arterial dissection

Differential Diagnosis of Subarachnoid Hemorrhage

See **Box 15.18**.

Complications

- Obstructive hydrocephalus: Due to blood in the subarachnoid space. It may be asymptomatic but may cause deteriorating consciousness following SAH. Shunting may be required.
- Arterial spasm (cause of coma or hemiparesis): It is a serious complication and is a poor prognostic feature.
- Hyponatremia.

Q. Write a short essay/note on treatment of SAH.

Management

- Immediate treatment is absolute **bed rest** (for 4 weeks) and **supportive measures.** These include protecting the airway, managing blood pressure and raised ICP, pain management, and sedation. It should be discussed urgently with a neurosurgical team. Patient is advised to gradually resumption of physical activities after recovery.
- **Control of hypertension:** In conscious patients without raised ICP, active treatment of hypertension is necessary. A target MAP of 130 mm Hg is recommended. Drugs include labetalol, esmolol or nicardipine. Sodium nitroprusside should be avoided because may cause increase of ICP.
- **Avoid strictly:** *Hypovolemia, hypotension, hyperthermia, hyperglycemia, and hyponatremia.*
- **Calcium channel blocker:** Nimodipine (30–60 mg IV for 5–14 days, followed by 360 mg orally for a further 7 days) provides a modest but significant improvement in outcome by reducing cerebral arterial vasospasm. It is given for 3 weeks to prevent delayed ischemia in the acute phase and decreases mortality.
- **Prophylactic anticonvulsants**

- **Interventional management:** Early aneurysm repair prevents rerupture/rebleeding and improve blood flow. An aneurysm can be "clipped" by a neurosurgeon or "coiled" by an endovascular surgeon.
  - **Insertion of platinum coils into an aneurysm:** If angiography shows an aneurysm (most common cause of SAH), endovascular treatment by inserting a platinum coils via a catheter in the aneurysm sac to promote thrombosis and ablation of the aneurysm, is the first-line treatment. Surgical clipping of the aneurysm neck also helps in reducing the risk of recurrence (both early and late). Endovascular coiling has fewer perioperative complications and better outcomes than surgery. For unruptured aneurysms > 8 mm in diameter the risk of treatment is less than the risk of hemorrhage if not treated.
- **Treatment of complications:** Managing delayed cerebral ischemia due to vasospasm (may be treated with vasodilators), treating obstructive hydrocephalus (may require drainage via a shunt), treating hyponatremia (managed by fluid restriction), and systemic complications associated with immobility, such as chest infection venous thrombosis and preventing pulmonary embolus.

Q. Identify the nature of the cerebrovascular accident based on the temporal evolution and resolution of the illness.

The differences between hemorrhagic, thrombotic, and embolic strokes are listed in **Table 15.23**.

TABLE 15.23: Differences between hemorrhagic, thrombotic, and embolic strokes.

Feature	*Hemorrhagic stroke (intracerebral or subarachnoid hemorrhage)*	*Ischemic stroke*	
		Thrombotic	*Embolic*
Time of onset of stroke	During activity	Suddenly and often during sleep or in the early morning (4 AM)	Any time
Rapidity of onset and progression	Over minutes and hours	On waking up or over hours	Rapid within seconds deficit maximum at onset
Transient ischemic attacks (TIAs)	Absent	Precedes stroke	Precedes stroke
Vomiting	Recurrent	Absent or occasional	Absent or occasional
Headache	Severe and prominent	Mild or absent	Mild or absent
Early resolution (within minutes or days)	Unusual	Variable	Possible
Meningeal irritation	May be present	Absent	Absent
Carotid bruit and absence of pulse	Not observed	Highly supports the diagnosis	Possible
Valvular heart disease and atrial fibrillation	Not found	Unusual	Highly supports the diagnosis
CT scan findings	Hemorrhage	Early stage: Normal. Later: Pale infarct	Early stage: Normal: Later Pale infarct

Note: It may not be possible always to differentiate stroke of different type with absolute certainly.

Cerebral Venous Thrombosis

Q. Write a short note of cerebral venous thrombosis.

It is the thrombosis of the draining venous sinuses of the cerebral cortex and the least common of all other types of cerebrovascular accidents (1–2% of strokes in young adults).

Thrombosis most commonly involves superior sagittal sinus and it may extend into transverse and sigmoid sinuses.

Thrombosis of deep venous system (e.g., internal cerebral veins, vein of Galen or straight sinus) is less common.

Age and gender: It frequently affects young adults and children. More common in women than men with an F:M ratio of 3:1. It may be due to the presence of gender-specific risk factors such as pregnancy, puerperium, oral contraceptive pills, and hormone replacement therapy (HRT). One of the leading causes of maternal mortality and morbidity with cases of puerperal CVT occurring 10–12 times more frequently in India than the west.

TABLE 15.24: Causes of cerebral venous thrombosis (CVT).

Local causes	*Systemic causes*
➢ Trauma to the dural sinuses ➢ Infection of structures adjacent to the dural sinuses: Otitis media, mastoiditis, sinusitis, tonsillitis ➢ Invasion or compression of venous sinuses by neoplasms	➢ **Hypercoagulable states,** e.g., inherited prothrombotic states, protein C/S deficiency, antithrombin III deficiency, factor V Leiden gene mutation, prothrombin gene mutation, presence of lupus anticoagulant, oral contraceptive use, pregnancy, malignancy ➢ Dehydration

Causes of Cerebral Venous Thrombosis (Table 15.24)

See **Table 15.24.**

Pathophysiology

Two basic mechanisms are responsible for the development of the clinical features in CVT.

1. Thrombosis of cerebral veins or sinuses leading to cerebral parenchymal lesions or dysfunctions.
2. Occlusion of dural venous sinus causes reduced absorption of CSF and raised ICP.

Obstruction of venous structures → increased venous pressure → decreased capillary perfusion → increased cerebral blood volume → disruption of blood brain barrier → plasma leakage into interstitial space → cerebral edema, parenchymal changes, and venous hemorrhage.

Clinical Features

The clinical presentation of CVT is highly variable and it may present as acute/subacute/chronic.

Symptoms and signs: Depends on the sinuses involved, the place of occlusion, and involvement of cortical veins and presence of collaterals, parenchymal changes and the patient's age. Symptoms are grouped under three major clinical syndromes:

1. **Isolated intracranial hypertension syndrome** (headache with or without vomiting, papilledema, and visual problems)
2. **Focal syndrome** (focal deficits or seizures or both)
3. **Encephalopathy** (multifocal signs, mental status changes, stupor or coma).

Diagnosis

- **CT or MR venography:** Direct signs of CVT in CT include:
  - **Dense triangle sign**—seen as hyperdensity with triangular shape at the posterior end of superior sagittal sinus caused by venous thrombus.
  - **Empty delta sign**—seen in head CT with contrast as a triangular pattern of contrast enhancement surrounding a central region lacking contrast enhancement.
  - **Cord sign**—as linear or curvilinear hyperdensity over the cerebral cortex caused by thrombosed cerebral veins.
- **CT or MRI** to detect secondary parenchymal lesions.
- **CSF examination:** To rule out meningitis or SAH.
- Workup for prothrombotic state.

Treatment

Treatment should be started as soon as the diagnosis is confirmed and consists of:

- Treatment of the underlying cause when known.
- Control of seizures and intracranial hypertension.
- **Antithrombotic therapy.**

The main treatment option to achieve these goals is anticoagulation using heparin or LMWH (IV/SC). It is recommended that anticoagulant therapy with warfarin should be given for a minimum of 3 months after acute CVT aiming at an INR target of 2.5 (2–3).

TABLE 15.25: Example of demyelinating diseases.

Central nervous system	*Peripheral nervous system*
➢ **Autoimmune,** e.g., multiple sclerosis (MS), neuromyelitis optica ➢ **Nutritional,** e.g., Wernicke's encephalopathy, subacute combined degeneration ➢ **Infectious,** e.g., acute disseminated encephalomyelitis (ADEM), HIV encephalitis, Creutzfeldt–Jakob encephalitis ➢ **Toxic,** e.g., radiation, chemotherapeutic agents, methanol ➢ **Hypoxic/ischemic,** e.g., vasculitis	➢ Deficiencies of vitamin B1: Dry beriberi ➢ Guillain–Barré syndrome ➢ Vitamin B12 deficiency ➢ Organophosphate poisoning ➢ Chronic inflammatory demyelinating polyneuropathy ➢ Charcot–Marie–Tooth disease ➢ Copper deficiency

DEMYELINATING DISEASES

Q. What are the common demyelinating diseases?

Table 15.25 shows example of demyelinating diseases.

Multiple Sclerosis

Q. Write a short essay on multiple sclerosis (MS) and its clinical features.

- Chronic autoimmune T-cell-mediated inflammatory disorder with selective destruction of myelin of the central nervous system (CNS). It has a **relapsing-remitting** or progressive course. The neurological deficits are disseminated in time and space.
- It is termed multiple sclerosis because of the multiple scarred areas (well-demarcated gray areas termed **plaques)** of demyelination throughout the brain and spinal cord observed on macroscopic examination. The plaques are crucial for diagnosis. The peripheral nervous system (PNS) is generally spared.

Epidemiology

- **Gender:** Female preponderance and female to male ratio is 2:1.
- **Age:** Usually present between 20 and 40 years of age and is rare after 60 years of age.

Pathophysiology

Both genetic and environmental factors play a causative role.

- **Genetic factors:** Risk of familial recurrence in MS is 15%, with highest risk in first-degree relatives. Multiple genes interact and it has a complex polygenic inheritance pattern. HLA-DR2 association. Other autoimmune disorders occur in patients with MS and their relatives, indicating a genetic predisposition to autoimmunity.
- **Environmental factors:** Epidemiologic evidence supports the role of an environment exposure in MS but these factors are still largely unknown. For example, sunlight exposure, vitamin D, and exposure to Epstein–Barr virus (EBV). Viral infections can precipitate MS relapses in genetically susceptible individuals.

Etiology and Pathogenesis

- Etiology is not known.
- It is probably a T-cell-mediated autoimmune disease causing an inflammatory process within the white matter of the brain and spinal cord. MS risk correlates with high socioeconomic status, which may reflect improved sanitation and delayed initial exposures to infectious agents.

Clinical Manifestations

- No single group of signs or symptoms is diagnostic of MS **(Table 15.26)**.
- **Onset:** May be abrupt/insidious, vary from trivial to severe form.
- Presentation varies and depends on the anatomical site of lesions and severity. It has been called as the modern "great imitator". MS commonly involves ***pyramidal tract, optic nerve, posterior cord, cerebellum, and medial longitudinal fasciculus (MLF).***
- **Common symptoms in MS (Box 15.19):** Disability and neurological impairments gradually accumulate over the years.

Clinical course: Main clinical patterns are:

- **Relapsing-remitting MS** (RRMS) (85–90%): Discrete attack and complete recovery.
- **Secondary progressive MS** (SPMS): Begin as RRMS, clinical steady deterioration at some stage.
- **Primary progressive MS** (PPMS) (10–15%): Steady function decline from onset.
- **Progressive relapsing MS** (PRMS)
- **Malignant MS/Aggressive MS** refers to disease with a rapid progressive course, leading to significant disability in multiple neurologic systems in a relatively short time after disease onset.
- **Tumefactive MS** is an acute tumor-like MS variant in which some patients with demyelinating disease present with large (>2 cm) acute lesions, often associated with edema or ring enhancement.

Box 15.19: Common presentations of multiple sclerosis.

- Optic neuropathy (neuritis)
- Relapsing/remitting sensory symptoms, e.g. **Lhermitte's sign** (barber chair phenomenon, is an electrical sensation that runs down the back and into the limb on neck flexion)
- Subacute painless spinal cord lesion
- Acute brainstem syndrome: Sudden diplopia, and vertigo with nystagmus
- Subacute loss of function of upper limb (dorsal column deficit): Clumsy/useless hand or limb
- Fatigue, cognitive impairment
- Sixth cranial nerve palsy, wall-eyed bilateral internuclear ophthalmoplegia **(WEBINO)**
- Unsteadiness or ataxia. **Charcot's triad** of dysarthria, ataxia, and tremor
- Urinary symptoms—bladder hyperreflexia
- Neuropathic pain, fatigue, spasticity, depression, sexual dysfunction
- **Uhthoff's phenomenon:** Worsening of neurologic symptoms (especially vision) when the body gets overheated

Diagnosis

The diagnosis of MS is usually easily made in a young adult with relapsing and remitting symptoms referable to different areas of CNS white matter. No single diagnostic test for definitive diagnosis of MS.

Magnetic resonance imaging (Figs. 15.17A and B)

- Characteristic abnormalities are found in >95% of patients.
- Lesion appears as focal area of hyperintensity on T2-weighted.
- Typical lesions are oval up to 2 cm in diameter, and frequently orientated perpendicular to the lateral ventricular surface, corresponding to the pathologic pattern of perivenous demyelination (Dawson's fingers).
- Lesions are multifocal (periventricular, juxtacortical, infratentorial, or spinal cord).

Evoked potential (EP) or evoked responses

Assesses function in afferent (visual, auditory and somatosensory) or efferent (motor) CNS pathways, abnormalities on one or more EP modalities occur in 80–90% of MS patients. However, they are less important than MRI.

Cerebrospinal fluid examination

- CSF cell count may be raised (5–60 mononuclear cells/mm)—mononuclear cell pleocytosis.
- Increased immunoglobulin G (IgG), total CSF protein, CSF IgG index.
- Protein electrophoresis: Oligoclonal IgG bands detected by agarose gel, but these are not specific.

McDonald criteria for MS are presented in **Table 15.26**.

TABLE 15.26: McDonald criteria for multiple sclerosis (MS).

Attack	*Lesion*	*Additional criteria for diagnosis MS*
2 or more	2 or more	Nonclinical evidence alone will suffice
2 or more	1 lesion	**Dissemination in space of MR (or await further clinical attack implicating a different CNS site)**
1 attack	2 lesions	**Dissemination in time on MR** (or await further clinical attack implicating a different CNS site)
1 attack	1 lesion	**Dissemination in space and time** (or await further clinical attack implicating a different CNS site)
0 attack **Progression from onset**		One year of disease progression (retrospective or prospective) and at least two out of three criteria ➢ Dissemination in space in the brain ➢ Dissemination in space in the spinal cord based on 2 or more T2 lesions ➢ Positive CSF

Treatment of Multiple Sclerosis

- **Treatment of acute attack**
  - **Intravenous methylprednisolone** 500–1,000 mg/day for 3–5 days, followed by a course of oral prednisone beginning at a dose 60–80 mg/day and gradually tapered over 2 weeks. High-dose cyclophosphamide has been used for induction therapy to stabilize aggressive MS.
  - **Plasma exchange:** 5–7 changes are done with 40–60 mL/kg per exchange alternate days for 14 days for cases that are unresponsive to glucocorticoids.

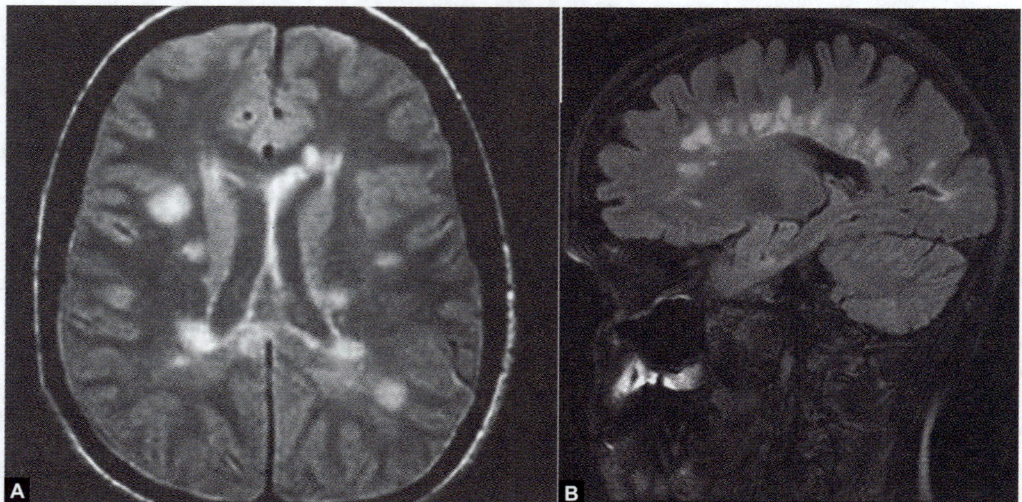

FIGS. 15.17A AND B: Magnetic resonance imaging of multiple sclerosis.

- **Disease-modifying drugs:** For prophylaxis of RRMS and SPMS after acute stage has passed. No effective treatment for PPMS. These include interferon (IFN)-β (1a-1b), glatiramer acetate, natalizumab, mitoxantrone hydrochloride, rituximab, siponimod, fingolimod, and cladribine.
- **Ocrelizumab,** a recombinant human anti-CD20 monoclonal antibody designed to optimize B-cell depletion, is the first drug to significantly reduce the risk of disability progression among patients with PPMS.
- **Symptomatic therapy**
  - **Weakness (heat-induced):** K+ channel blockers—4-aminopyridine, 3,4-diaminopyridine
  - **Spasticity/spasm:** Physiotherapy, avoid trigger factors. Drugs like baclofen, diazepam, tizanidine, and dantrolene can be used.
  - **Pain:**
    - Anticonvulsant: Carbamazepine, phenytoin, gabapentin, pregabalin
    - Antidepressant: Amitriptyline/nortriptyline, desipramine, venlafaxine
    - Antiarrhythmic: Mexiletine
  - Bladder care.

The differences between MS and neuromyelitis optica (NMO) are listed in **Table 15.27**. *It is important to differentiate as IFN is contraindicated in NMO.*

SEIZURES AND EPILEPSY

Q. Classify seizure/epilepsy. Discuss the evaluation of adult seizures and management of seizures.

Q. Describe the types, etiology, clinical features, investigations (evaluation), and management of epilepsy. Enumerate antiepileptic agents.

Q. Classify epilepsy. Describe the clinical features and treatment of grand mal (generalized tonic-clonic) epilepsy.

Q. Write a short essay/note on:
- **Enumerate the causes and investigation of a seizure. Mention drugs used to treat grand mal epilepsy.**
- **Temporal lobe epilepsy.**
- **Management of complex partial seizures.**
- **Complications of status epilepticus (SE).**
- **Causes of convulsion.**
- **Primary epileptic disorders.**
- **Complications of seizures.**
- **Define complex partial seizure.**

TABLE 15.27: Differences between multiple sclerosis and neuromyelitis optica (NMO).

Features	*Devic's disease (NMO)*	*Multiple sclerosis*
Age	Adults	Young adults
F:M	>3:1	<3:1
Distribution of signs and symptoms	Restricted to optic nerves and spinal cord	Any white matter
Attack severity	Usually severe	Usually mild
Brain MRI	Usually normal (rarely lesion around area postrema +)	Multiple periventricular white matter lesions
Cord MRI	Longitudinally extensive transverse myelitis (LETM) central necrotic lesions, 3 or more spinal cord segments involved	Multiple small peripheral lesions
CSF cells	Pleocytosis during attack	Rarely >25 cells
Oligoclonal bands	Usually absent	Usually present
Antibodies	Anti-NMO antibody (46%), anti-AQP4 (aquaporin 4) (85%) present	No antibodies
Coexisting autoimmunity	Frequent (30–40%) (Sjogren's syndrome)	Less common
Recurrence rate	Higher (90%)	Lower
Recurrence interval	Shorter	Longer

- **Seizure:** It is a **paroxysmal event due to abnormal, excessive, hypersynchronous discharges from** an aggregate of CNS **neurons.**
- **Epilepsy** is a chronic neurological disorder defined as the occurrence of 2 or more unprovoked or reflex seizures at least 24 hours apart, the occurrence of a single unprovoked or reflex seizure in an individual with an underlying condition that increases the risk of subsequent seizures (e.g., a brain tumor), or the presence of an epilepsy syndrome.
- An individual with a single seizure or recurrent seizures due to correctable or avoidable circumstances does not necessarily have epilepsy.

Classification of Seizures (Tables 15.28 and 15.29)

Q. Classify seizure/epilepsy.

- Seizures are classified as **"simple"** if there is **no impairment of consciousness** or as **"complex"** if an **alteration in consciousness** occurs. **Seizures may be either focal or generalized.**
  - **Focal seizures:** They originate within networks limited to one cerebral hemisphere across both cerebral hemispheres. They are usually **associated with structural abnormalities** of the brain.
  - **Generalized seizures:** In contrast to focal, they may result from **cellular, biochemical, or structural abnormalities** that have a more widespread distribution. However, there are clear exceptions in both cases.
- Most seizures last seconds to minutes.
- **Status epilepticus** (*discussed later*).

TABLE 15.28: New classification of seizures.

Focal seizures: It can be further described as having motor, sensory, autonomic, cognitive, or other features	
Generalized seizures	
➢ Absence (typical/atypical)	➢ Atonic
➢ Tonic-clonic (in any combination)	➢ Myoclonic
	➢ May be focal, generalized, or unclear
➢ Clonic	
➢ Tonic	
Unknown: Epileptic spasms	

TABLE 15.29: International League Against Epilepsy (ILAE) 2017 classification of seizure types.

Generalized onset seizures	
➢ Tonic-clonic	➢ Typical
➢ Clonic	➢ Atypical
➢ Tonic	➢ Myoclonic
➢ Myoclonic	➢ Eyelid myoclonia
➢ Myoclonic-tonic-clonic	
➢ Myoclonic-atonic	
➢ Atonic	
➢ Epileptic spasms	
Focal onset seizures	
Motor onset	**Nonmotor onset**
➢ Aware	➢ Aware
➢ Impaired awareness	➢ Impaired awareness
➢ Unknown awareness	➢ Unknown awareness
➢ Automatisms	➢ Autonomic
➢ Atonic	➢ Behavior arrest
➢ Clonic	➢ Cognitive
➢ Epileptic spasms	➢ Emotional
➢ Hyperkinetic	➢ Sensory
➢ Myoclonic	
➢ Tonic	
➢ Focal to bilateral tonic-clonic	➢ Focal to bilateral tonic-clonic
Unknown onset seizures	
Motor	**Nonmotor**
➢ Tonic-clonic	Behavior arrest
➢ Epileptic spasms	
Unclassified seizures	

Focal Seizures

Focal Seizures without Dyscognitive Features

- In this type, **consciousness is fully preserved during the seizure** and the clinical manifestation is relatively simple.
- Focal seizures can cause motor, sensory, autonomic, or psychic symptoms without an obvious alteration in consciousness.
- A focal motor seizure arising from the right primary motor cortex near the area controlling hand movement will note the onset of involuntary movements of the contralateral, left hand.
- Three additional features of this seizures are:

Q. Write a short note on Jacksonian epilepsy.

Jacksonian march: Representing the **spread of seizure activity over a progressively larger region of motor cortex.** In Jacksonian seizures, march of symptoms occurs where if it is motor, clonic jerking starts at a point. For example, it may start at face, and spreads to upper limb, then to lower limb and then on to opposite side to become a generalized fit. This denotes the path of spread of the epileptic activity and is called Jacksonian spread/march.

Q. Write a short note on Todd's paralysis.

- **Todd's paralysis** or the **localized paresis:** It is a condition characterized by brief, temporary paralysis that follows a seizure. It may occur **for minutes to hours in the involved region following** the seizure.
- **Epilepsia partialis continua:** Analogous to partial SE. It is often quite refractory to medical therapy.

Other manifestations:
Changes in somatic sensation (e.g., paresthesia), vision (flashing lights or formed hallucinations), equilibrium (sensation of ailing or vertigo), and autonomic function (flushing, sweating, piloerection).

Focal Seizures with Dyscognitive Features

- Focal seizure activity may be accompanied by a transient impairment of the patient's ability to maintain normal contact with the environment.
- Patient is **unable to respond to visual or verbal commands** during the seizure and has impaired recollection or awareness of the ictal phase.
- The seizures **frequently begin with an aura** (i.e., focal seizures without dyscognitive features) that is stereotypic for the patient.
- The start of the ictal phase is often a **sudden behavioral arrest or motionless stare,** and this marks the onset of the event for which the patient will be amnesic.

- The behavioral arrest is usually accompanied by oromandibular or hand automatisms, which are involuntary, automatic behaviors that have a wide range of manifestations.
- **Automatisms** may consist of very basic behaviors such as chewing, lip smacking, swallowing or picking movements of the hands or more elaborate behaviors such as a display of emotion or running.

Complex Partial Seizures (Temporal Lobe Seizures)

Focal seizures arising from the temporal or frontal cortex may also cause alterations in hearing, olfaction or higher cortical function (psychic symptoms-like to sensation of unusual intense odors (e.g., burning rubber or kerosene) or sounds (crude or highly complex sounds) or illusions that objects are growing (metamorphopsia) smaller (micropsia) or larger (macropsia). When such symptoms precede focal seizures with dyscognitive features or secondarily generalized seizure, these seizures serve as a warning, or aura.

Generalized Seizures

- Generalized seizures **arise from both cerebral hemispheres simultaneously.**
- It may be practically defined as **bilateral clinical and electrographic events without any detectable focal onset.**
- Though they arise at some point of the brain they rapidly engage neuronal networks in both cerebral hemispheres.

Absence Seizures (Petit Mal Seizures)

- Sudden, brief lapses of **consciousness without loss of postural control.**
- **It lasts for only a few seconds and consciousness returns rapidly** and there is no postictal confusion.
- Usually accompanied by subtle, bilateral motor signs such as rapid blinking of the eyelids, chewing movements, or small amplitude, clonic movements of the hands. Absence seizures can be typical or atypical.
- Onset usually in childhood (ages 4–8 years) or early adolescence and are the main seizure type in 15–20% of children with epilepsy.
- May occur hundreds of times in a day without the knowledge of parents or the child.
- First clue may be often unexplained "daydreaming" and a decline in school performance recognized by a teacher.
- **Electroencephalography (EEG):** Generalized, symmetric, 3-Hz spike-and-wave discharge that begins and ends suddenly, superimposed on a normal EEG background which can be provoked by hyperventilation.

Generalized Tonic-Clonic Seizures (Grand Mal Seizures)

Q. Write a short essay/note on clinical features and treatment of grand mal (generalized tonic-clonic) epilepsy.

- Main type of seizure in 10% of all individuals with epilepsy.
- Usually **begins abruptly without warning.** Some may develop vague premonitory symptoms which are distinct from the stereotypic auras associated with focal seizures that generalize.
- **Initially,** there is **tonic contraction of muscles throughout the body** leading to **loud moan or ictal cry, cyanosis,** biting of the tongue, etc.
- Marked enhancement of sympathetic tone leads to increases in heart rate, blood pressure, and pupillary size.
- **After 10–20 seconds, clonic phase starts** with **superimposed relaxation** which progressively increases until the end of ictal period.
- **Postictal phase** is characterized by **unresponsiveness, muscular flaccidity, and excessive salivation, bladder or bowel incontinence.**
- Patients **gradually regain consciousness** over **minutes to hours** with accompanying postictal confusion, headache, and muscle ache.
- **EEG:** Generalized high-amplitude, polyspike discharges in tonic phases which in the clonic phase typically interrupted by slow waves to create a spike-and-wave pattern.
- **Other variants** include pure tonic and pure clonic type.

Atonic Seizures

- They are characterized by **sudden loss of postural muscle tone** lasting **1–2 seconds.**
- **Consciousness is briefly impaired,** but there is usually **no postictal confusion.**
- They may cause only a quick head drop or nodding movement, while a longer seizure will cause the patient to collapse.
- They **are rarely seen in isolation** and are usually seen in association with known epileptic syndromes.
- **EEG:** Brief, generalized spike-and-wave discharges followed immediately by diffuse slow waves that correlate with the loss of muscle tone.

Myoclonic Seizures

- **Sudden, brief jerky muscle contraction** that may involve **one part of the body or the entire body.**
- Normal, common physiologic forms of myoclonus are the sudden jerking movement observed while falling asleep and hiccups.

- Most pathologic myoclonus commonly seen in association with metabolic disorders, degenerative CNS diseases, or anoxic brain injury.
- Myoclonic seizures are the predominant feature of juvenile myoclonic epilepsy (JME).
- **EEG:** May show bilaterally synchronous spike-and-wave discharges synchronized with the myoclonus.

Epilepsy Syndromes

Epilepsy syndromes are disorders in which **epilepsy is a predominant feature,** and there is sufficient evidence to suggest a common underlying mechanism.

Juvenile Myoclonic Epilepsy

- Juvenile myoclonic epilepsy is a **generalized seizure** disorder of **unknown cause** that appears in **early adolescence** and is usually characterized by **bilateral myoclonic jerks** that may be single or repetitive.
- The myoclonic seizures are **most frequent in the morning** after awakening and can be provoked by sleep deprivation.
- Unless severe **consciousness is preserved.**
- Many patients also experience generalized tonic-clonic seizures (GTCSs), and up to one-third have absence seizures.
- The condition is otherwise benign, and although complete remission is uncommon, the seizures respond well to appropriate anticonvulsant medication.
- Lifelong treatment is necessary and **sodium valproate** is the drug of choice.

Lennox–Gastaut Syndrome

Lennox–Gastaut syndrome is seen in children between the ages of 1–8 and is characterized by the following triad.

1. **Multiple seizure types** (usually including generalized tonic-clonic, atonic, and atypical absence seizures).
2. **EEG:** Shows **slow (<3 Hz) spike and wave discharges** and a variety of other abnormalities.
3. **Impaired cognitive function** in most but not all patients.

Lennox–Gastaut syndrome is an epileptic encephalopathy **associated with CNS disease or dysfunction** from a variety of causes, including developmental abnormalities, perinatal hypoxia/ischemia, trauma, infection, and other acquired lesions.

- The multifactorial nature of this syndrome suggests that it is a nonspecific response of the brain to diffuse neural injury.
- A similar syndrome in infancy that often evolves into Lennox–Gastaut syndrome is **West syndrome,** characterized by infantile spasms, Salaam attacks, other findings of cerebral dysfunction, and abnormal EEG pattern (hypsarrhythmia).

Mesial Temporal Lobe Epilepsy Syndrome

- Mesial temporal lobe epilepsy (MTLE) is the **most common syndrome** associated with complex partial seizures and is an example of symptomatic, partial epilepsy.
- Characteristic **hippocampal sclerosis** on MRI is an essential element in the pathophysiology of MTLE for many patients.
- Recognition of this syndrome is especially important because it tends to be **refractory to treatment with anticonvulsants but responds extremely well to surgical intervention.**

Febrile Seizures

- Usually occur between **3 months and 5 years of age** and have a peak incidence between 18 and 24 months.
- It **is GTCS** in child **during a febrile illness** in the setting of a common childhood infections.
- The seizure is likely to occur during the rising phase of the temperature curve (i.e., during the first day).
- A **simple febrile seizure** is a **single, isolated** event, brief and symmetric in appearance. **Complex febrile seizures** are characterized **by repeated seizure activity,** duration >15 minutes, or by focal features.
- Simple febrile seizures are not associated with an increase in the risk of developing epilepsy; while complex febrile seizures have a risk of 2–5%. Other risk factors include the presence of pre-existing neurologic deficits and a family history of nonfebrile seizures.

Causes of Seizures According to Age

See **Box 15.20**.

Box 15.20: Causes of seizures according to age.

Neonates (<1 month)
- Perinatal hypoxia and ischemia
- Intracranial hemorrhage and trauma
- CNS infections
- Metabolic

Infants and children (>1 month and <12 years)
- Febrile seizures
- Genetic disorders (metabolic, degenerative, primary epilepsy syndromes)
- CNS infections

Adolescents (12–18 years)
- Trauma
- Genetic disorders
- Infection

Young adults (18–35 years)
- Trauma
- Alcohol withdrawal

Older adults (>35 years)
- Cerebrovascular disease
- Trauma (including subdural hematoma)
- Brain tumor
- Alcohol withdrawal
- Degenerative diseases

Evaluation of the Patient with a Seizure

- When a patient is seen shortly after a seizure, the first priorities are **attention to vital signs, respiratory and cardiovascular support,** and **treatment of seizures if they resume.**
- When the patient is not acutely ill, the evaluation will initially focus on whether or not there is a history of earlier seizures.

First Seizure

If this is the patient's first seizure, then the emphasis will be to **establish whether** the reported **episode was a seizure** rather than another paroxysmal event.

In case of GTCS, features supporting organicity are postictal confusion, tongue bite, history of fall or having sustained injury, etc.

- **Determine the cause of the seizure** by identifying risk factors and precipitating events. Precipitating factors such as sleep deprivation, systemic diseases, electrolyte or metabolic derangements (like hypoglycemia, hyper and hypocalcemia, hyponatremia hypomagnesemia) acute infection, drugs that lower the seizure (like penicillins, quinolones, antipsychotics, lithium, amphetamine, barbiturates, cocaine) threshold or alcohol or illicit drug use should be identified.
- **General physical examination:** Look for signs of system illnesses or infection. Careful examination of the skin may reveal signs of neurocutaneous disorders such as tuberous sclerosis or neurofibromatosis, or chronic liver or renal disease. Organomegaly may indicate a metabolic storage disease, and limb asymmetry may provide a clue to brain injury early in development.
- Finally **decide whether anticonvulsant therapy is required** in addition to treatment for any underlying illness. It is usually not required in case of metabolic or electrolyte derangements and seizures due to alcohol withdrawal.
- If no metabolic or infectious causes found, then look for
  - Focal features of seizure
  - Any focal neurological deficits
  - Any other neurological dysfunction/mental retardation
- Unusual features such as, prolonged duration of seizures (>6 hours), more than six seizures, SE, or a prolonged postictal state.
  - If present, usually antiepileptic therapy is required. Then MRI and EEG are done to find any mass lesion/stroke/degenerative lesion. Treatment of underlying cause besides antiepileptic therapy.
  - If absent, it is idiopathic epilepsy and antiepileptic therapy continued.

Recurrence of a Seizure

In the patient with prior seizures or a known history of epilepsy, the evaluation is directed toward:

- **Identification of the underlying cause and precipitating factors.** Common precipitating factors are—sleep deprivation, fever, hypoglycemia, and alcohol.
- **Determination of the adequacy of** the patient's **current therapy.**
  - If no precipitating factors found, measure the plasma concentration of AED.
  - If subtherapeutic concentration: Appropriate increase in drug dosage is done.
  - If therapeutic concentration is normal: Either drug increased to maximum tolerated dose or alternate therapy is started with gradually tapering the first drug.

Laboratory Studies

- **Routine investigations:** These include serum glucose, calcium, electrolytes, renal and hepatic functions.
- **Lumbar puncture:** If indicated.
- **EEG:** May help establish the diagnosis of epilepsy, classify the seizure type, and provide evidence for the existence of a particular epilepsy syndrome.
  - The presence of electrographic seizure activity, i.e., of abnormal, repetitive, rhythmic activity having an abrupt onset and termination, clearly establishes the diagnosis.
  - The EEG findings may also be helpful in the interictal period by showing certain abnormalities that are strongly supportive of an epilepsy. Such epileptiform activity consists of bursts of abnormal discharges containing spikes or sharp waves.
  - EEG is normal in 40% of epileptic patients.
- Neuroimaging studies (MRI preferred over CT).

The differences between seizures and syncope are listed in **Table 15.30**.

TABLE 15.30: Differences between seizures and syncope.

Features	*Seizures*	*Syncope*
Immediate precipitating factor	Usually none	Emotional stress, Valsalva, orthostatic hypotension, cardiac etiologies
Premonitory symptoms	None or aura (e.g., odd odor)	Tiredness, nausea, diaphoresis, tunneling of vision
Posture at onset	Variable	Usually erect
Transition to unconsciousness	Often immediate	Gradual over seconds
Duration of unconsciousness	Minutes	Seconds
Duration of tonic or clonic movements	30–60 seconds	Never > 15 seconds
Facial appearance during event	Cyanosis, frothing at mouth	Pallor
Disorientation and sleepiness after event	Many minutes to hours	<5 minutes
Headache, muscle pain, tongue bite incontinence	Often, tongue bite—lateral	Rarely, tongue bite—tip

Treatment

Indications to Initiate Antiepileptic Drug Therapy

Antiepileptic drug therapy should be **started in any patient with recurrent seizures of unknown etiology** or a **known cause that cannot be reversed with in short time.** Risk factors associated with recurrent seizures are listed in **Box 15.21**.

Selection of AEDs **(Table 15.31)**. Certain AEDs like phenytoin and carbamazepine can worsen myoclonic seizure. Hence proper AED for proper seizure must be given.

Box 15.21: Risk factors associated with recurrent seizures.

- An abnormal neurologic examination
- Seizures presenting as status epilepticus
- Postictal Todd's paralysis
- Strong family history of seizures
- An abnormal EEG
- Abnormal CT or MRI

TABLE 15.31: Selection of antiepileptic drugs in seizures.

Seizure types	*First choice*	*Second choice*
Monotherapy for generalized-onset tonic-clonic seizures	Valproate, topiramate	Zonisamide, levetiracetam, lamotrigine phenytoin, carbamazepine
Absence seizure	Ethosuximide, valproate	Zonisamide, levetiracetam, topiramate, felbamate, clonazepam
Monotherapy for partial seizures	Carbamazepine, oxcarbazepine, phenytoin, topiramate	Lamotrigine, gabapentin, levetiracetam
Myoclonic	Valproate, levetiracetam, clonazepam	Zonisamide, topiramate
Status epilepticus	Diazepam,lorazepam	Phenytoin IV, fosphenytoin IV
Febrile convulsions	Diazepam rectal 0.5 mg/kg	
Infantile spasms	Corticotropin, corticosteroids, zonisamide	Clonazepam, nitrazepam, vigabatrin, phenobarbital

Treatment Modification

- If a treatment is modified recently, one should wait for at least four half-lives of the drug before further modifying dosage.
- If one drug is unable to control seizures then another drug should be considered when either maximum dose of the first drug is reached or the patient starts showing intolerable side effects.
- Whenever a new drug is added, the first drug is continued till the second drug controls seizures. Only after achieving adequate seizure control the first drug should be gradually withdrawn.

Indications for Discontinue Therapy

- Complete medical control of seizures for 1–5 years.
- Single seizure type, either focal or generalized.
- Normal neurologic examination (including intelligence)
- Normal EEG

  In most cases, it is preferable to reduce the dose of the drug gradually over 2–3 months.

Most recurrences occur in the first 3 months after discontinuing therapy, and patients should be advised to avoid potentially dangerous situations such as driving or swimming during this period.

Treatment of Refractory Epilepsy

- Therapy combines first-line drugs, i.e., carbamazepine, phenytoin, valproic acid and lamotrigine.
- If these drugs are unsuccessful, then the addition of a newer drug such as levetiracetam and topiramate is indicated.
- Patients with myoclonic seizures resistant to valproic acid may respond to a combination of valproic acid and ethosuximide.

Surgical Treatment of Refractory Epilepsy

- About 20–30% of patients with epilepsy are resistant to medical therapy. **Ketogenic diet**—has been advised to decrease seizure recurrence. Low carbohydrate, adequate protein, high fat has been advised.
- **Anteromedial temporal lobe** (temporal lobectomy) or a **more limited removal of the underlying hippocampus** and **amygdala** (amygdalohippocampectomy).
- Focal seizures arising from extratemporal regions may be abolished by a focal neocortical resection with precise removal of an identified lesion (lesionectomy).
- **Others:** Hemispherectomy, corpus callosotomy, etc.
- **Vagus nerve stimulation** (VNS) may be used—some of these cases, although the benefit for most patients seem to very limited.

Antiepileptic drugs for chronic use have been shown in Tables 15.32 and 15.33.

TABLE 15.32: Antiepileptic drugs for chronic use.

Type of drug		*Examples*
Na^+ channel blockers		Phenytoin, carbamazepine, oxcarbazepine, primidone, valproic acid, lamotrigine, topiramate, zonisamide, phenobarbital, gabapentin, felbamate
Ca^{2+} channel blockers		Ethosuximide, phenobarbital, zonisamide
Drugs that potentiate GABA	Increase opening time of channel	Phenobarbital
	Increase frequency of openings of channel	Diazepam, lorazepam, clonazepam
	Increase GABA in synapse	Valproic acid
	Increase GABA metabolism	Gabapentin
	Increase GABA release	Gabapentin
	Block GABA transaminase	Vigabatrin
	Block GABA transporter (GAT-1)	Valproic acid, tiagabine
	Facilitate GAD (glutamic acid decarboxylase) Increase GABA synthesis	Valproic acid
	Synaptic vesicle protein 2A binding	Levetiracetam (inhibits presynaptic calcium channels)
	AMPA agonist	Perampanel

TABLE 15.33: Antiepileptic drugs and their mechanism of action, adverse reactions, and uses.

Drug and mechanism of action	*Adverse reactions*	*Uses*
Phenytoin: Oldest nonsedative antiepileptic drug. It alters Na^+, Ca^{2+}, and K^+ conductances	Ataxia and nystagmus, cognitive impairment, hirsutism, gingival hyperplasia, coarsening of facial features, dose-dependent zero order kinetics, exacerbates absence seizures, "Fetal hydantoin syndrome"	Partial seizure, generalized (including tonic-clonic) seizures. Contraindicated in absence seizures. **Nonseizure indications** include trigeminal neuralgia, manic-depressive disorders
Carbamazepine: Tricyclic, antidepressant (bipolar) Mechanism of action, similar to phenytoin. Inhibits high-frequency repetitive firing (Na^{++})	Autoinduction of metabolism, nausea and visual disturbances, granulocyte suppression, aplastic anemia, exacerbates absence seizures	Partial seizure (including tonic-clonic) seizures. **Contraindicated in absence seizures. Nonseizure indications** include trigeminal neuralgia, manic-depressive disorders
Oxcarbazepine: Related to carbamazepine. With improved toxicity profile. Less potent than carbamazepine. Active metabolite	Hyponatremia, less hypersensitivity and induction of hepatic enzymes than with carbamazepine	
Phenobarbital: It is the oldest antiepileptic drug. Although considered one of the safest drugs, it has sedative effects Prolongs opening of Cl^- channels. Blocks excitatory GLU (AMPA) responses. Blocks Ca^{2+} currents (L, N)	Sedation, cognitive impairment, behavioral changes, induction of liver enzymes, may worsen absence and atonic seizures	Useful for partial, generalized tonic-clonic seizures, and febrile seizures
Primidone: Metabolized to phenobarbital and phenylethylmalonamide (PEMA), both active metabolites	Same as phenobarbital. Sedation occurs early. Gastrointestinal disturbances	Effective against partial and generalized tonic-clonic seizures
Valproate: Mechanism of action, similar to phenytoin. Increases levels of GABA in brain. May facilitate glutamic acid decarboxylase (GAD). Inhibits GAT-1	Elevated liver enzymes, nausea and vomiting, abdominal pain, heartburn, tremor, hair loss, syncratic, hepatotoxicity, teratogen (spina bifida)	A broad-spectrum antiseizure drug effective for partial and generalized seizures, including myoclonic and absence seizures. Nonseizure indications include migraine (prophylaxis), bipolar disorder
Ethosuximide: Reducing low-threshold Ca^{2+} channel current (T-type channel) in thalamus	Gastric distress, including pain, nausea and vomiting, lethargy and fatigue, headache, hiccups, euphoria, skin rashes	Drug of choice for absence seizures
Clonazepam: One of the most potent antiepileptic agents known	Sedation is prominent. Ataxia, behavior disorders	Long-acting drug with efficacy for absence seizures. Also effective in some cases of myoclonic seizures. Has been tried in infantile spasms
Lamotrigine: Suppresses sustained rapid firing of neurons and produces a voltage and use-dependent inactivation of sodium channels, thus its efficacy in partial seizures	Dizziness, headache, diplopia, nausea, somnolence, rash	Presently use as add-on therapy with valproic acid. Also effective in generalized and myoclonic seizures in childhood and absence seizures preferred in elderly
Topiramate: Potentiates inhibitory effects of GABA (acting at a site different from BDZs and BARBs)	Somnolence, fatigue, dizziness, cognitive slowing, paresthesia, nervousness, confusion, urolithiasis	Myoclonic seizures, migraine
Zonisamide: Sulfonamide derivative	Drowsiness, cognitive impairment, high incidence of renal stones	Effective against partial and generalized tonic-clonic seizures
Felbamate	Aplastic anemia, severe hepatitis	Third-line drug used only for refractory partial seizure cases
Vigabatrin (gamma-vinyl GABA): Irreversible inhibitor of GABA-aminotransferase	Drowsiness, dizziness, weight gain, agitation, confusion, psychosis	Use for infantile spasms, partial seizures, and contraindicated if preexisting mental illness is present
Tiagabine: GABA uptake inhibitor GAT-1	Dizziness, nervousness, tremor, difficulty concentrating, depression, asthenia, emotional liability, psychosis, skin rash	Effective against partial and generalized tonic-clonic seizures
Gabapentin: Analog of GABA that does not act on GABA receptors. Low potency	Somnolence, dizziness, ataxia, headache, tremor	Used as an adjunct in partial and generalized tonic-clonic seizures, neuropathy
Levetiracetam	Somnolence, incoordination, irritability, mood swings, psychosis	Effective for GTCS, JME. Preferred in elderly

Newer AEDs (third-generation AEDs): Carisbamate, esclicarbazepine, brivaracetam, carabersat, ganaxalone, huperzine, lacosamide, losigamone, remacemide, retigabine, rufinamide, safinamide, perampanel.

Drug-resistant epilepsy/Intractable epilepsy may be defined as failure of adequate trials of two tolerated and appropriately chosen and used antiseizure drug schedules to achieve sustained seizure freedom. Nonmedical management can be tried.

- Surgical treatments—lobar and multilobar resections, hemispherectomy, corpus callosotomy, multiple subpial transections
- Vagus nerve stimulation
- Responsive cortical stimulation
- Subcortical deep brain stimulation
- Transcranial magnetic stimulation
- Trigeminal nerve stimulation
- Ketogenic diet (high-fat, low protein) diet has demonstrated efficacy in children

Status Epilepticus

Q. Write a short essay/note on definition, complications of SE, and its emergency management.

Status epilepticus refers to **continuous seizures or repetitive, discrete seizures with impaired consciousness** in the interictal period.

Status epilepticus is an epileptic seizure of >5 minutes or more than one seizure within a 5-minute period without the patient returning to normal between them. Previous definitions used a 30-minute time limit.

Subtypes

- **Generalized convulsive status epilepticus** (GCSE), e.g., persistent, generalized electrographic seizures, coma and tonic-clonic movements.
- **Nonconvulsive status epilepticus,** e.g., persistent absence seizures or focal seizures, confusion or partially impaired consciousness, and minimal motor abnormalities.

Etiology of Status Epilepticus

See **Box 15.22**.

Box 15.22: Etiology of status epilepticus.

- Stroke, including hemorrhagic
- Low AED levels
- Alcohol withdrawal
- Anoxic brain injury
- Metabolic disturbances
- Remote brain injury/congenital malformations
- Infections
- Brain neoplasms
- Idiopathic

Clinical Features

- Self-perpetuating, GTCS or
- Series of GTCSs
- Without return to consciousness in between seizures.

Phases

- **Initial compensatory phase:** Sympathetic overdrive, increased CO, increased BP.
- **Decompensation** → homeostatic failure
  - Reduced → CO/sugar/lactate/O_2 levels leading to:
    - Cardiorespiratory collapse
    - Electrolyte imbalance
    - Rhabdomyolysis and delayed tubular necrosis
    - Hyperthermia
    - Multiorgan failure (MOF)
    - Raised ICP and cerebral edema.

Complications

These include aspiration, hypotension, cardiac arrhythmias and renal or hepatic failure.

Diagnosis

- **Diagnosis of nonconvulsive SE in critically ill patients.**
- Correlate with poorer outcome.
- EEG patterns are difficult to interpret (equivocal patterns)—criteria are **not** validated.
- A trial of rapidly acting IV AED is used to observe improvement in both clinical → EEG by several hours.

Management of Status Epilepticus (Box 15.23)

- Convulsive/nonconvulsive.
- Other available modalities:
  - Brain imaging (perfusion/metabolic imaging)
  - Intracranial monitoring with intracortical EEG
  - Brain tissue O_2 monitoring
  - Cerebral microdialysis.

Pregnancy and Epilepsy

- In approximately 50% epileptic women, the frequency of epilepsy remains the same. In about 30% it increases and in about 20% it decreases in frequency.
- Uncontrolled seizure in mother causes harm to both mother and fetus greater than the teratogenic effects of AEDs. Hence, pregnant women should be maintained on effective drug therapy.
- Due to the numerous side effects phenytoin is not used in pregnancy. Neural tube defects are associated with valproic acid and carbamazepine.

Box 15.23: Management of status epilepticus (SE).

First 5 minutes
- Check emergency ABCs
- Give O_2
- Obtain IV access
- Begin ECG monitoring
- Check finger stick glucose
- Draw blood for serum electrolytes. RFT, magnesium, calcium, phosphate, CBC, LFTs, AED levels, ABG, troponin
- Toxicology screen (urine and blood)

6–10 minutes
- Thiamine 100 mg IV; 50 mL of D50 IV unless adequate glucose known
- Lorazepam 4 mg IV over 2 minutes; if still seizing, repeat × 1 in 5 minutes
- If no rapid IV access give diazepam 20 mg PR or midazolam 10 mg intranasally, buccally or IM

10–20 minutes
- If seizures persist, begin fosphenytoin 20 mg/kg IV at 150 mg/min, with blood pressure and ECG monitoring
  Or
- Phenytoin 15–20 mg/kg at 30–50 mg/min
  Reasonable to bypass this step, or perform subsequent step simultaneous with fosphenytoin loading

10–60 minutes: One (or more) of the following four options (intubation usually necessary except for valproate):
1. Continuous IV midazolam. Load: 0.2 mg/kg; repeat 0.2–0.4 mg/kg boluses every 5 minutes until seizures stop, up to a maximum total loading dose of 2 mg/kg. Initial rate: 0.1 mg/kg/h. Continuous IV dose range: 0.05–2.9 mg/kg/h
   Or
2. Continuous IV propofol. Load: 1 mg/kg; repeat 1–2 mg/kg boluses every 3–5 minutes until seizures stop, up to maximum total loading dose of 10 mg/kg. Initial continuous IV rate: 2 mg/kg/h. Continuous IV dose range: 1–15 mg/kg/h. Avoid > 48 hours of >5 mg/kg/h (increased risk of propofol infusion syndrome)
   Or
3. IV valproate: 40 mg/kg over ~10 minutes. If still seizing, additional 20 mg/kg over ~5 minutes
   Or
4. IV phenobarbital: 20 mg/kg IV at 50–100 mg/min

60 minutes
- Continuous IV pentobarbital. Load: 5 mg/kg at up to 50 mg/min; repeat 5 mg/kg boluses until seizures stop. Initial continuous IV rate: 1 mg/kg/h. Continuous IV-dose range: 0.5–10 mg/kg/h; traditionally titrated to suppression-burst on EEG

Perform neuroimaging when convulsive activity is controlled
- Begin continuous EEG, if patient does not awaken rapidly or if continuous IV Rx is used
- Treat metabolic abnormalities and hypothermia
- Lumbar puncture and antibiotics can be considered if infection is suspected

SE not controlled even with anesthetic agents is called **super refractory SE**, for which IVIg/pulse steroid can be tried as last resort

- Carbamazepine is considered relatively safe in pregnancy, because of its low teratogenic potential. **Levetiracetam is safest drug.**
- If mother is on phenobarbital, she should be given oral vitamin K (20 mg daily) in the last 2 weeks of pregnancy, and the infant should be given an intramuscular injection of vitamin K (1 mg) at birth. This is because phenobarbital may cause a transient and reversible deficiency of vitamin K-dependent clotting factors in up to 50% of newborn infants.

NEUROINFECTIONS

Q. Classify meningitis. List the causes of meningitis.

Classifications of Meningitis

See **Box 15.24**.

Neurosyphilis

Q. Write a short essay on the clinical features and management of neurosyphilis.

- *Treponema pallidum* invades nervous system within 3-18 months (may take years to develop) after primary infection.
- **Neurosyphilis** may be asymptomatic or symptomatic. Initial event is usually in the form of asymptomatic meningitis. Later it may produce more damage. All forms of neurosyphilis have meningitis of variable severity. Secondary to meningitis, the blood vessels show endarteritis obliterans.

Asymptomatic Neurosyphilis

- Asymptomatic invasion of CNS by treponema is common and occur within few months of primary infection by *Treponema pallidum.*

Box 15.24: Classifications of meningitis.

Infective	*Noninfective (sterile)*
1. **Bacterial meningitis** – Common organisms: *Streptococcus pneumoniae, Neisseria meningitidis, Haemophilus influenzae* – Uncommon organisms: *Staphylococcus aureus, Staphylococcus epidermidis,* Group B streptococci, *Escherichia coli, Klebsiella, Proteus spp., Listeria monocytogenes.* – Rare organisms: Salmonella, Shigella, Clostridium perfringens, Neisseria gonorrhoeae 2. **Tuberculous meningitis (TBM):** *Mycobacterium tuberculosis* 3. **Viral meningitis (aseptic meningitis)** – Enteroviruses (coxsackie virus, poliovirus) – Mumps virus – Arboviruses – Human immunodeficiency virus (HIV) – Herpes simplex-2 4. **Spirochetal:** Leptospirosis, Lyme disease, syphilis 5. **Rickettsial:** Typhus fever 6. **Protozoal:** Cysticerci, amoeba, Naegleria 7. **Fungal:** *Cryptococcus neoformans, Candida, Histoplasma, Blastomyces, Coccidioides, Sporothrix*	1. **Malignant disease** – Breast cancer – Bronchial cancer – Leukemia (leukemic meningitis) – Lymphoma 2. **Subarachnoid** hemorrhage (SAH) (causes meningismus) 3. **Inflammatory disease (may be recurrent)** – Sarcoidosis – Systemic lupus erythematosus, rheumatoid arthritis – Behçet's disease – Vasculitis

- Neurosyphilis may develop in 25% cases of latent syphilis. Many of them may develop symptomatic neurosyphilis.
- Cerebrospinal fluid shows lymphocytosis with increased protein and low glucose. Antibodies in the CSF, is the most specific test for neurosyphilis. Venereal disease research laboratory test is positive.
- Treatment: Penicillin.

Symptomatic Neurosyphilis

It takes one of several forms, although mixed features are common **(Box 15.25)**.

Meningeal syphilis

- Symptoms of meningitis may develop at any time after infection, but usually occur within 2 years after primary infection.
- Symptoms:
  - These include headache, neck stiffness, seizures, altered sensorium and cranial nerve palsies. It may show skin rash on palms and soles.
  - Papilledema with symptoms of increased ICP may develop.
  - Patient is afebrile and CSF is abnormal.

Box 15.25: Major categories of symptomatic neurosyphilis.

- Meningeal syphilis
- Chronic meningovascular disease
- Parenchymatous syphilis
  - General paresis of insane
  - Tabes dorsalis

Meningovascular syphilis

- Chronic meningitis involves base of the brain, cerebral convexities and spinal leptomeninges.
- Usually presents 6–7 years after primary infection. However, it can develop as early as 6 months and as late as 10–12 years.
- It should be suspected when a young patient develops stroke (generally subacute) which results in hemiparesis, aphasia, visual loss, etc. Other features include headache, vertigo, insomnia, and psychological abnormalities.

Cerebrospinal fluid findings in neurosyphilis have been shown in **Table 15.34.**

TABLE 15.34: CSF findings in neurosyphilis.

Parameter	*Findings*
Pressure	Normal or raised
CSF fluid	Clear
Protein	Raised (100–200 mg%)
Glucose	Normal
Cell count	Mildly elevated and cells are lymphocytes
Gamma-globulin levels	Raised
Venereal disease research laboratory (VDRL)	Positive
Fluorescent treponemal antibody absorption (FTA-ABS)	Positive

Note: Gold standard test for diagnosis is VDRL from CSF. This is highly specific but only 30–70% sensitive for neurosyphilis. CSF FTA-ABS is more sensitive but not specific because false positives are common.

General paralysis of insane

- It develops about 20 years after primary infection.
- Shows generalized/diffuse brain parenchymal disease with **dementia;** hence called as general paresis of insane.
- Clinical manifestation includes personality changes, illusions, delusions, hallucinations, dementia (reduced memory), hyperactive reflexes and Argyll Robertson pupils.

Tabes dorsalis

- Tabes dorsalis is the parenchymal form of neurosyphilis characterized by **demyelination of posterior column, dorsal root and dorsal root ganglia** in the spinal cord.
- Usually develops 20–25 years after primary infection.
- **Symptoms:** Severe lightening pains in trunk and extremities, ataxia and urinary incontinence.
- **Signs:** Patchy tactile sensory loss and severe impairment of proprioception with sensory ataxia. Muscular strength is normal and tendon jerks are absent. Complications include trophic lesions such as perforating ulcers of feet and Charcot's joints. Argyll Robertson pupils may also be observed in tabes dorsalis.
- **Visceral crisis:** It consists of sudden epigastric pain with vomiting that Abadie's sign (Pinching of, or the application of firm pressure to, the Achilles tendon does not result in pain) lasts for hours. Barium studies show pylorospasm (gastric crisis). Other crisis includes intestinal crisis with diarrhea, rectal crisis with tenesmus, genitourinary crisis with strangury and pharyngeal-laryngeal crisis with gulping movements and dyspnea.
- CSF findings: (*refer* **Table 15.34**).

Treatment
- Penicillin: Drug of choice and given in the dose of 18–24 million units/day for 15–20 days.
- If patient is sensitive to penicillin: Erythromycin and tetracycline 0.5 g 6 hourly for 20–30 days.

Follow-up
- Re-examine the patient every 3 months and CSF examination at 6 months interval.
- If CSF is normal and VDRL titers are reduced, no further treatment is necessary. However, if CSF remains abnormal, patient should be treated by another full course of penicillin.

CEREBROSPINAL FLUID

- Cerebrospinal fluid is formed within the ventricles and circulates in the subarachnoid space (between arachnoid and pia matter) and in the ventricles. The total volume of CSF in adults ranges from 90 to 150 mL. It is a medium for transfer of substances from brain and spinal cord into the blood.
- **Importance of CSF examination:** Analysis of the CSF is of diagnostic importance in conditions like meningitis or primary/metastatic tumor of CNS with CSF involvement.
- **Collection of CSF:** CSF is usually obtained by lumbar puncture using a lumbar puncture needle under strict aseptic conditions.

Lumbar Puncture

Q. Write a short essay on the procedure indications, contraindications, and complications of lumbar puncture.

- Lumbar puncture is the technique **(Fig. 15.18)** done to obtain CSF sample and also provides an indirect measure of ICP.
- After local anesthetic injection, a lumbar puncture needle is inserted in the midline between lumbar spinous processes usually between L3 and L4 (3rd **lumbar space)** through the dura and into the spinal canal. In children, it is collected from the 4th lumbar space.
- Intracranial pressure can be assessed (if patients are lying on their side) and CSF obtained for analysis.
- CSF pressure is important in the diagnosis and monitoring of idiopathic intracranial hypertension.

Indications and contraindication for lumbar puncture (Box 15.26).

Complications of Lumbar Puncture

- Most common complication is **post spinal headache.** Herniation of cerebellum through the foramen magnum due to raised ICP.

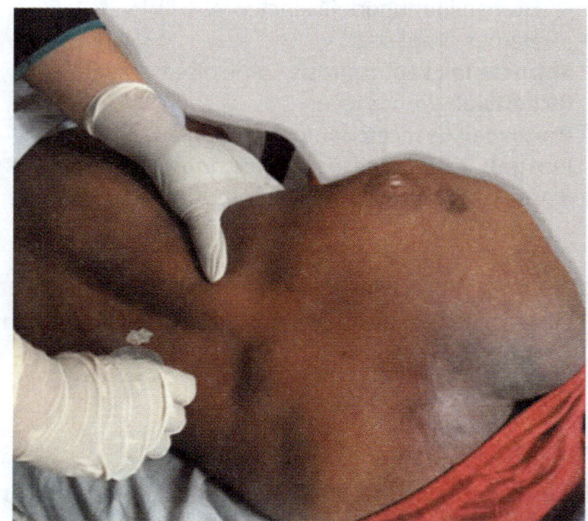

FIG. 15.18: Procedure of lumbar puncture (LP).

Box 15.26: Indications and contraindications for lumbar puncture.

Indications for lumbar puncture
- **Diagnostic indications**
  - **Infection:**
    - **Meningeal infection:** Bacterial (pyogenic, tuberculosis, syphilitic (to differentiate general paresis of insane, tabes dorsalis, and meningeal syphilis), viral, fungal
    - **Encephalitis**
  - **Subarachnoid hemorrhage**
  - **Primary or metastatic malignancy** (e.g., acute leukemia, lymphoma)
  - **Demyelinating diseases:** Multiple sclerosis and subacute sclerosing panencephalitis (SSPE)
  - **Guillain–Barré syndrome**
  - **Spinal canal blockage** leading to elevated intracranial tension (spinal cord tumors)
  - **Injecting the radiopaque dye for myelography**
- **Therapeutic indications**
  - Spinal anesthesia, epidural analgesia
  - **Intrathecal injection of chemotherapeutic drugs** for CNS prophylaxis/relapse of ALL, lymphomas
  - Therapeutic CSF drainage in cases of normal pressure hydrocephalus

Contraindications for lumbar puncture
- Raised intracranial pressure, coagulopathy
- Local infective lesion
- Bony deformities at site of puncture

- Hematoma, either extradural or subdural.
- Introduction of infection by the lumbar puncture needle through the infected skin or subcutaneous tissue.

Normal CSF findings are presented in **Table 15.35**.

- CSF osmolality and sodium level are same as that of serum
- Constituents that are in higher concentration in CSF than in blood include magnesium, chloride, H+ concentration and lactate.

TABLE 15.35: Normal CSF findings.

Constituent	*Normal value*
CSF volume	150 mL
CSF pressure	90–180 mm of water
Cell count	<5 cells, all lymphocytes, no neutrophils
CSF proteins	15–45
CSF sugar	60–80% of blood glucose

Q. Write a short note on causes of elevated CSF proteins.

Causes of low sugar in CSF: Pyogenic, tuberculous, fungal and carcinomatous meningitis.

Causes of elevated protein in CSF are presented in **Box 15.27**.

Box 15.27: Causes of elevated CSF proteins.

- Meningitis
- Brain abscess
- Brain or spinal cord tumors
- Multiple sclerosis
- Guillain–Barré syndrome
- Syphilis
- Hemorrhage
- Froin's syndrome

Q. Write a short note on xanthochromia in CSF analysis.

Xanthochromia is the yellowish appearance of CSF.

Causes: Xanthochromia is always pathological and conditions associated with it are:

- **Old SAH:** The yellow appearance is due to RBCs which may leak into the CSF during the hemorrhage. RBCs are breakdown and liberate hemoglobin which is converted into yellow bilirubin.
- Other causes are high protein in the CSF, jaundice, and Froin's syndrome.

Meningitis and Encephalitis

Q. What are the causes of meningitis? Discuss the clinical features, investigations, diagnosis, complications, and management of acute pyogenic (bacterial/meningococcal) meningitis.

Acute Bacterial (Pyogenic/Purulent) Meningitis

Q. Write a short essay/note on the common organisms causing pyogenic meningitis.

Relative frequency of various bacterial species causing meningitis varies with age.

- **Neonatal period:** Major causative agents include gram-negative bacilli (principally *Escherichia coli), Listeria monocytogenes,* and group B streptococci.
- **Infants and children:** Major causes in children beyond 1 month of age are *Haemophilus influenzae* and *Neisseria meningitidis.*
- **Adolescents and in young adults:** Meningococcus *(N. meningitidis)* is the most common pathogen.
- **Extremes of life:** *Streptococcus pneumoniae* and *L. monocytogenes.*

Causes of community acquired bacterial meningitis: Important causes are:

- *S. pneumoniae (50%):* Most common.
- *N. meningitidis* (25%): It is the only major cause of epidemics of bacterial meningitis.
- Group B *streptococci* (15%)
- *L. monocytogenes* (10%)
- *H. influenzae* (10%)

Predisposing conditions

- ***For Pneumococci:*** Other Pneumococcal infections (pneumonia, sinusitis, otitis media), splenectomy, hypogammaglobulinemia, complement deficiency.
- ***For Neisseria meningitidis:*** Complement deficiency (including properdin), B-serotype (not protected by vaccine is responsible for one-third of cases). Usually associated with petechial or purpuric skin lesions.
- ***Listeria monocytogenes:*** Important cause in neonates (<1 month), pregnant women, >60 years and immunocompromised persons.

Clinical manifestations

Q. Write a short essay/note on physical signs of meningitis.

- **Classic triad:** (1) Fever, (2) headache, and (3) nuchal rigidity.
- **Consciousness:** Vary from lethargy to coma (>75%).
- Nausea, vomiting and photophobia are common
- **Seizure/convulsions** (especially in children) may be initial presentation or present during course (20–40%).
  - **Focal:** Due to arterial ischemia, infarction, cortical venous thrombosis or focal edema.
  - **Generalized or status:** Due to hyponatremia, cerebral anoxia or toxic effects of antimicrobial drugs.

- **Classic signs of meningitis (Box 15.28).**
- **Occasionally cranial nerve palsies,** with focal neurologic deficits such as visual field defects, dysphasia, and hemiparesis may occur.
- **In meningococcus: Rash** begin as diffuse erythematous maculopapular that become petechial, found on trunk, lower limbs, mucous membrane, conjunctiva and rarely on palm and sole.
- **Raised ICP:** One of the complications of bacterial meningitis and CSF pressure may be raised to 180–400 mm H_2O. Disastrous complication of ICP is cerebral herniation.
  - Other signs: Reduced level of consciousness, papilledema, dilated poorly reactive pupil, VIth cranial palsy, decerebrate posture, Cushing reflex (bradycardia, hypertension, and irregular respiration).

Box 15.28: Classical signs of meningitis.

- Cervical rigidity/neck stiffness
- Kernig's sign: Knee pain with hip flexion
- Brudzinski's sign: Knee/hip flexion when the neck is flexed

Box 15.29: Complications of bacterial meningitis.

- Obstructive hydrocephalus
- Thrombophlebitis of leptomeningeal veins may lead to venous thrombosis, cerebral infarction, focal infection of the underlying brain parenchyma
- Chronic adhesive arachnoiditis
- Cerebral abscess
- Subdural empyema
- Focal neurologic deficits (e.g., cranial nerve palsy, hemiparesis)
- Sensorineural hearing loss
- Vasculitis of cranial vessel
- Epilepsy
- Waterhouse–Friderichsen syndrome: It results from meningitis-associated septicemia with hemorrhagic infarction of the adrenal glands and cutaneous petechiae. It occurs most often with meningococcal and pneumococcal meningitis

Complications of bacterial meningitis

See **Box 15.29**.

Diagnosis

- **By examination of the CSF:** It is usually obtained by lumbar puncture. Lumbar puncture should be postponed if there is papilledema and or focal neurologic findings suggestive of an intracranial mass lesion. It can be done only after ruling out the same by CT or MRI.
- **Blood culture:** If meningitis seems likely, blood should be sent for culture and sensitivity and empirical antimicrobial therapy should be started while the neuroimaging study is being carried out.

CSF findings in bacterial meningitis (refer ***Table 15.38****)*

Q. Write a short essay/note on CSF findings pyogenic/bacterial meningitis.

Q. Write a short essay/note on treatment of pyogenic meningitis.

Treatment

Antibiotics used in empirical therapy of bacterial meningitis and focal CNS infections.

A. *Empirical therapy (Table 15.36)*

Streptococcus pneumoniae and *Neisseria meningitidis* are common organisms. Due to emergence of penicillin and cephalosporin resistant of *S. pneumoniae* a combination therapy of 3rd or 4th generation cephalosporin (ceftriaxone, cefotaxime, cefepime) and vancomycin, plus acyclovir (HSV is a differential diagnosis) and doxycycline (tick infection) is given as empirical therapy.

TABLE 15.36: Empirical therapy for bacterial meningitis depending on the age group/predisposing factors.

Age group/predisposing factors	*Drug used*
Infants < 1 month	Ampicillin + cefotaxime
Infants 1–3 months	Ampicillin + cefotaxime/ceftriaxone
Infants >3 months and adults <55 years	Cefotaxime/ceftriaxone/cefepime + vancomycin
Adults >55 years or adult with alcohol or debilitating conditions	Ampicillin + cefotaxime/ceftriaxone/ cefepime + vancomycin
Hospital acquired, post-traumatic, post-neurosurgery, neutropenic patients or impaired cell-mediated immunity	Ampicillin + ceftazidime/meropenem + vancomycin

B. *Specific antimicrobial therapy*

- ***Neisseria meningitidis***
  - **Penicillin sensitive:** Penicillin G—250,000–300,000 U/kg/day in divided doses, Ampicillin (3 g IV TID/QID).
  - **Penicillin resistant:** Ceftriaxone 2 g IV BID/Cefotaxime 2 g IV BID.
  - 7 days IV dose are adequate.
  - All close contacts should be given chemoprophylaxis with rifampicin for 2 days or azithromycin (500 mg once) or one IM ceftriaxone (250 mg).
- *Streptococcus pneumoniae*
  - Should be tested for penicillin and cephalosporin sensitivity
  - **Penicillin sensitive:** Penicillin G
  - **Penicillin-intermediate:** Ceftriaxone/cefotaxime/cefepime
  - **Penicillin-resistant:** Ceftriaxone/cefotaxime/cefepime + vancomycin
  - 2 weeks IV is adequate.
  - Lumbar puncture is to be repeated 24–36 hours after initiation to see the response
  - Intraventricular vancomycin may be more effective than IV or intrathecal.
- **Gram-negative bacilli (except *Pseudomonas*):** Ceftriaxone/cefotaxime for 3 weeks

- ***Pseudomonas aeruginosa:*** Ceftazidime/cefepime/meropenem
- **Staphylococci spp.:**
  - **Methicillin sensitive:** Nafcillin
  - **Methicillin resistant:** Vancomycin (1 g IV TID) (IV or intraventricular)
- ***Listeria monocytogenes:*** Ampicillin for 3 weeks. Gentamicin may be added in critical ill cases. Trimethoprim and sulfamethoxazole are alternative
- ***H. influenzae***-intermediate: Ceftriaxone/cefotaxime/cefepime
- ***Streptococcus agalactiae:*** Penicillin G/ampicillin
- ***Bacteroides fragilis:*** Metronidazole
- *Fusobacterium spp.:* Metronidazole

C. *Adjunctive therapy*

- **Dexamethasone** inhibits synthesis of IL-1β and TNF-α, decrease CSF out flow resistance and stabilize blood brain barrier (BBB).
- It is to be given 20 minutes before antimicrobial therapy. It is less effective if given 6 hours after antibiotic therapy.

D. *Treatment of raised ICP*

- Elevation of head end of the bed to 30–45°, hyperventilation, and administration of mannitol.
- Duration of therapy: 7 days for *N. meningitides,* 7–10 days for *H. influenzae,* 10–14 days for *S. pneumoniae* and 3 weeks for gram-negative bacilli.

Tubercular Meningitis

Q. Describe the pathology, clinical features, investigation, complications, and treatment/management of tuberculous meningitis.

In India, tubercular meningitis (TBM) remains the most common form of meningitis.

Risk factors

- Previous history of exposure to tuberculosis or illness.
- Immunocompromised state of acquired immunodeficiency syndrome (AIDS)
- Young children.

Pathology

- Main neuropathologic finding is **basal meningeal exudates** containing mainly mononuclear cells.
- **Tubercles may** be seen on the meninges and on the surfaces of the brain.
- The **ventricles may be dilated** as a result of hydrocephalus, and the ependymal surface may be covered by **exudates.**
- **Hydrocephalus** is common in children and most develop symptoms in 2–3 weeks.
  - **Communicating type:** Common, due to blockage of basal cistern by exudates in acute phase or adhesive leptomeningitis in chronic phase.
  - **Obstructive type:** Less common, due to narrowing or occlusion of aqueduct by ependymal inflammation, tuberculomas, or obstruction of outlet of IVth ventricle.
- Arteritis can cause cerebral infarction, and basal inflammation; and fibrosis can compress cranial nerves.

Clinical features

- **Onset:** Usually subacute/chronic. Acute: children—50%, adult—14%.
- **Past history of TB:** Children—50%, adult—10%.
- **Prodromal symptoms:** Two to three weeks, vague ill health, apathy, irritability, anorexia, changes in behavior.
- **Features of meningitis:** Headache, vomiting, fever and focal neurological deficit.
- Features of raised ICP:
  - **Convulsions** (focal/generalized—20–30%).
  - **Cranial nerve palsy:** 20–30% (VIth cranial nerve).
  - **Loss of vision:** Partial/complete. Due to opticochiasmatic exudate, and arteritis.
- **Other presentation:** Hemiplegia, facial nerve palsy, optic atrophy, abnormal movement, occulomotor palsy, choroid tubercle, etc.
- **In untreated cases:** Consciousness deteriorates, pupillary abnormality, pyramidal signs due to hydrocephalus and tentorial herniation.

Complications of tubercular meningitis

See **Box 15.30.**

Box 15.30: Complications of tubercular meningitis.

- Raised intracranial pressure (ICP), cerebral edema
- Basal meningitis with cranial nerve palsy—II, III, IV, VI, and VII
- Focal neurologic deficit and seizure
- Hydrocephalus
- Tuberculoma
- Opticochiasmatic pachymeningitis: Visual loss
- Endocrine abnormality: Growth hormone and gonadotropin
- Hypothalamic disorder: Loss of control of blood pressure (BP) and temperature, delayed or precocious sexual development
- Diabetes insipidus, syndrome of inappropriate ADH secretion (SIADH)

Investigations

Q. Write a short essay/note on laboratory diagnosis and CSF findings in tuberculous meningitis.

1. **CSF study**
   - *Cytological study*
     - **Leukocyte count:** 100–500 cells/μL, rarely >1,000/cells/μL.
     - **Cell type: Lymphocytes** predominant, polymorphonuclear cells in acute stage. Hemorrhagic due to fibrinoid necrosis of vessels. No malignant cells seen.
   - *Biochemical study*
     - **Protein:** Usually 100–200 mg/100 mL. In spinal block >1 g/100 mL and xanthochromic.
     - **On standing a pellicle/cobweb formed** indicating fibrinogen—high suggestion of TBM.
     - **Glucose:** Reduced to 20–50 mg/100 mL. In most cases <40% of corresponding blood sugar, but unlike pyogenic never undetectable.
     - **Chloride:** Low value 450–600 mg/100 mL and is nonspecific indicating hypochloremia. It may be seen in bacterial, viral meningitis also.
     - **Adenosine deaminase** (ADA) produced by T lymphocytes elevated in CSF (60–100%).
   - *Microbiological study*
     - Negative with Gram stain, Indian ink stain and culture is sterile.
     - Acid-fast bacilli (AFB): AFB in smear and culture-confirmatory but number of bacteria should be >104/ml. Stained by Ziehl–Neelsen and auramine (4–40% positive).
   - **Centrifuged CSF:** The thick smear from pellicle and repeated culture enhance detection.
   - **CSF culture:** In Lowenstein–Jensen media in 4–8 weeks. It may be enhanced by liquid media like Septi-Chek AFB system or Middlebrook 7H9. Isolation is better from cisternal/ventricular CSF.
2. **Radiological investigations**
   - Chest X-ray: It may reveal miliary mottling in the lung.
   - CT scan:
     - Thickening of meninges in basal cistern (60%)
     - Hydrocephalus in 50–80% depending on duration
     - Cerebral infarct (28%) in MCA, edema (periventricular), tuberculoma (10%).
3. **Immunological methods**
   - **Antibody detection:** CSF shows antibodies against various antigens that are sensitive and are detected by ELISA and RIA.
   - Antigen detection: More specific. Antigen is detected by Latex agglutination, ELISA, etc.
   - **Molecular methods:** Amplification of specific DNA sequence by PCR used for rapid diagnosis. PCR is confirmatory and not affected by other organisms.

Management
- Antituberculous treatment (ATT) for one and a half year in uncomplicated cases is usually sufficient.
- Steroids: It is recommended to give steroids during initial 6 weeks to decrease the possibility of adhesion formation. Steroids prevent complications. There is no definite duration for which treatment might be continued, but should be judged on the basis of neuroimaging findings.
- Surgical intervention: If hydrocephalus, tuberculoma, or abscess develops. Tubercular abscess needs drainage.

Viral Meningitis/Aseptic Meningitis

- Viral infections of the meninges (meningitis) or brain parenchyma (encephalitis) often present as acute confusional states.
- Children and young adults are frequently affected.

Etiology

Common viruses include:

- **Enteroviruses** (most common, i.e., coxsackie viruses, echoviruses, and human enteroviruses): At least **two-thirds** of the cases of CSF culture-negative aseptic meningitis are due to enteroviruses.
- **Herpes simplex virus-2 (HSV-2) meningitis:** It may occur during the initial episode of genital herpes. Most cases of benign recurrent lymphocytic meningitis (previously called as Mollaret's meningitis) appear to be due to HSV
- **Arthropod-borne viruses:** These are transmitted through infected insect vectors.
- **Human immunodeficiency virus (HIV): Aseptic meningitis** is a common manifestation of primary exposure to **HIV. Cranial nerve palsies,** most commonly involving cranial nerves V, VII, and VIII are more common in HIV meningitis than in other viral infections.
- **Mumps** can also cause meningitis.

Clinical Manifestations

Fever, headache, and meningeal irritation. Other features include malaise, myalgia, anorexia, nausea and vomiting, abdominal pain, and/or diarrhea.

Laboratory Diagnosis

Q. Write short answer on CSF changes in viral meningitis.

- CSF examination:
  - Reveals lymphocytosis, mildly elevated protein and normal glucose.
  - As a rule, a **lymphocytic pleocytosis with a low glucose level** (<25 mg/dL) should **suggest** the presence of **fungal, listerial or tuberculous meningitis** or of **noninfectious disorders** (e.g., neoplastic meningitis)
- **Polymerase chain reaction (PCR):** Amplification of viral-specific DNA or RNA from CSF by PCR important method for the diagnosis of CNS viral infection.

Treatment
- **Symptomatic** and hospitalization is not required.
- **Oral or IV acyclovir** may be of benefit in patients with meningitis caused by **HSV-1 or HSV-2** and in cases of severe **EBV or VZV infection.**
- Patients with **HIV** should receive highly **active antiretroviral therapy.**

Mollaret's Meningitis

Q. Write a short note on Mollaret's meningitis.

Definition: It is a syndrome characterized by recurrent aseptic, self-limiting meningitis and presence of large typical monocytes (Mollaret cells) in the CSF.
- **Cause:** Not known, but may be due to some virus infections. Herpes simplex-2 infection must be excluded in these patients.
- **Clinical features:** Repeated self-limiting episodes of fever, meningismus and severe headache (of 2–5 days duration) separated by symptom-free intervals.

Noninfective causes of meningitis are listed in **Table 15.37**.

TABLE 15.37: Noninfective ("sterile") causes of meningitis.

Type of noninfectious meningitis	*Causes*
Carcinomatous	Leukemia, lymphoma, myeloma, melanoma, breast and lung cancer
Connective tissue disorders	Behçet's, SLE, sarcoid, rheumatoid, Sjogren's
Drugs	Azathioprine, cyclosporine, sulfasalazine
Substances injected into the subarachnoid space	Anesthetics, antibiotics, chemotherapy drugs, radiopaque contrast agents

CSF Findings in Meningitis (Table 15.38)

Q. Write a short note on compare the CSF findings of pyogenic, aseptic, and tuberculous meningitis.

TABLE 15.38: CSF findings in meningitis.

	Normal	*Acute pyogenic*	*Acute viral (aseptic)*	*Tuberculous*
Physical examination	Clear and colorless	Turbid and forms coagulum	Clear	Clear and colorless, forms cobweb on standing due to coagulation of fibrinogen
CSF pressure	60–150 mm of H_2O	Raised > 180 mm of H_2O	Raised > 250 mm of H_2O	Raised > 300 mm of H_2O
Total protein	20–40 mg/100 mL (<0.45 g/L)	>50–200 mg/100 mL	>40 mg/100 mL	50–150 mg/100 mL
Glucose	45–80 mg/100 mL (>50–60% of blood level)	0–20 mg/l00 mL (usually < 40 mg/dL)	Normal	Decreased: May be <45 mg/100 mL
Chlorides	720–750 mg/100 mL	600–700 mg/100 mL	Normal	450–600 mg/100 mL
Cells				
Polymorphs	Usually absent	1,000–5,000/mL	Absent	0–5 cells/μL
Lymphocytes	0–5 cells/μL	5–50 cells/μL	10–2,000 cells/μL	50–5,000 cells/μL
Gram stain/Ziehl–Neelsen (ZN) stain	–	Bacteria +	–	AFB + (ZN stain/auramine stain) or tuberculosis culture positive

Causes of Neck Stiffness (Box 15.31)

Q. List the causes of neck stiffness.

Encephalitis

Viral Encephalitis

- In meningitis, the infectious process and associated inflammatory response is limited largely to the meninges, whereas in encephalitis, the brain parenchyma is also involved.
- Encephalitis is characterized by nonsuppurative inflammation of brain by an inflammatory process.

Etiology (Box 15.32)

Clinical manifestations

- Acute febrile illness with evidence of meningitis and encephalitis.
- Altered level of consciousness (ranging from mild lethargy to coma), an abnormal mental state, and evidence of either focal or diffuse neurologic signs or symptoms.
- It may have hallucinations, agitation, personality change, behavioral disorders and at times a frankly psychotic state.
- Focal or generalized seizures occur in many patients with encephalitis.
- Most common focal neurological findings: Aphasia, ataxia, upper or lower motor neuron patterns of weakness, involuntary movements (e.g., myoclonic jerks, tremor), and cranial nerve deficits (e.g., ocular palsies, facial weakness).
- Involvement of the hypothalamic pituitary axis may result in temperature dysregulation, diabetes insipidus, or the development of the syndrome of inappropriate secretion of antidiuretic hormone (SIADH).

Laboratory diagnosis

1. **Cerebrospinal fluid**
   - **CSF examination:** Indistinguishable from that of viral meningitis and typically consists of lymphocytic pleocytosis, a mildly elevated protein concentration, and a normal glucose concentration.
   - **CSF PCR:** Primary diagnostic test for CNS infections caused by CMV, EBV, HHV-6 and enteroviruses.
   - **CSF culture:** Limited utility.
2. **Serologic studies and antigen defection:** Demonstration of antibodies or antigens.
3. **Brain biopsy:** Reserved for patients in whom CSF PCR studies fail to lead to a specific diagnosis, who have focal abnormalities on MRI, and who continue to show progressive clinical deterioration despite treatment with acyclovir and supportive therapy.
4. **MRI, CT and EEG.**

Box 15.31: Causes of neck stiffness.

Meningism:
- Meningitis
- Subarachnoid hemorrhage

Other conditions that mimic meningism (also resist cervical rotation):
- Cervical spondylosis
- After cervical fusion
- Parkinson's disease
- Raised intracranial pressure especially if there is impending tonsillar herniation
- Acute dystonic reaction
- Tetanus
- Strychnine poisoning

Intermittent neck stiffness is characteristic of Arnold–Chiari malformation

Box 15.32: Viruses causing encephalitis.

- Epidemics of encephalitis are caused by arboviruses
- Acute encephalitis
- Herpesvirus
  - Herpes simplex virus I (MC)
  - Varicella zoster virus
  - Epstein–Barr virus
- Arthropod-borne viruses
- West Nile virus
- Japanese encephalitis Colorado tick fever
- Others: Rabies, enteroviruses, mumps, cytomegalovirus

Management
- **General measures:** Care of the unconscious patient. Anticonvulsants may be needed. Brain edema is managed with dexamethasone 4 mg 6 hourly.
- **Herpes simplex encephalitis:** Acyclovir (10 mg/kg IV 8 hourly for 14–21 days), if instituted early.

Froin's Syndrome

Q. Write a short note on Froin's syndrome.

- Froin's syndrome describes the CSF findings in cases of complete spinal (subarachnoid) block (below the block).
- **CSF below the block** shows following features:
  - **CSF pressure:** Reduced
  - **Queckenstedt's test:** It is an outdated clinical test, formerly used for diagnosing spinal block.
  - **Physical examination:** Yellowish discoloration (xanthochromia) coagulum may form due to high protein content.
  - **Chemical examination:** Very much elevation of protein levels, sugar levels are normal or occasionally reduced if the obstruction is due to tuberculous meningitis.
  - Cytology: Normal cell count. Increased cells if the obstruction is due to tuberculous meningitis.
- **Causes of total block:**
  - Intraspinal tumors
  - Vertebral disease with compression.
  - Chronic spinal arachnoiditis.

DISEASES OF THE SPINAL CORD

Features Suggestive of Spinal Cord Involvement

See **(Box 15.33).**

Box 15.33: Features suggestive of spinal cord involvement.

- Presence of sensory deficit and/or motor weakness in both lower limbs and/or upper limbs
- Bladder and bowel involvement
- Brown–Sequard type of clinical picture
- Presence of definite sensory level

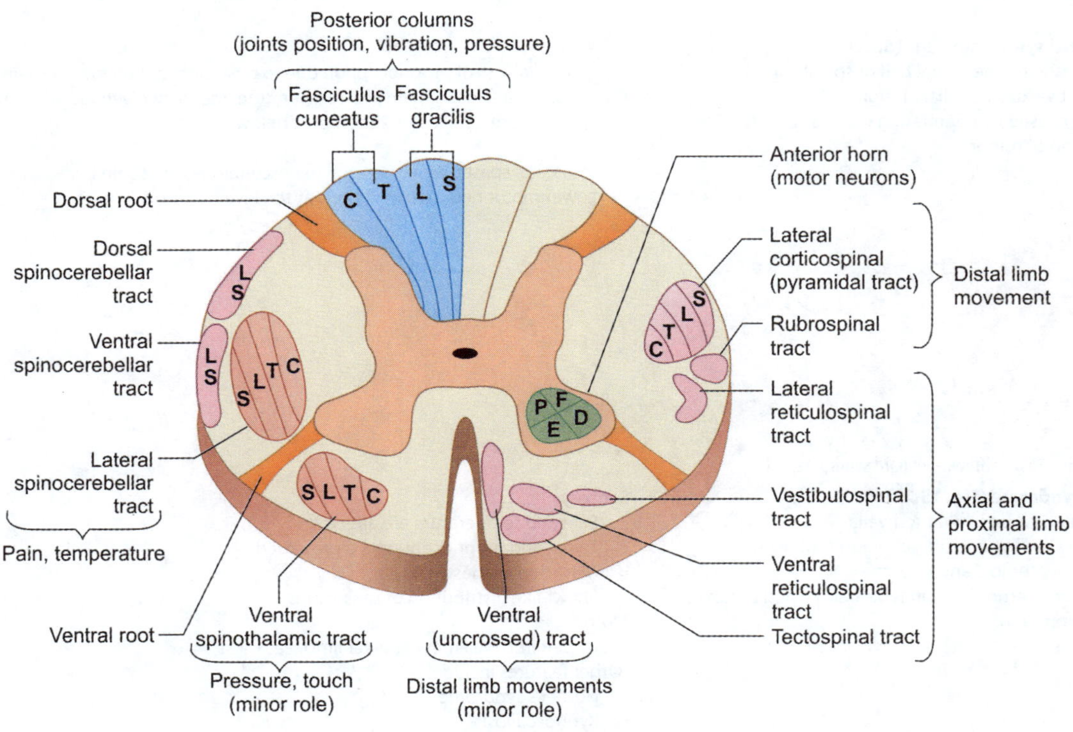

FIG. 15.19: Spinal cord anatomy.

Q. List the spinal cord syndrome with examples.

Patterns of Spinal Cord Disease (Box 15.34)

Box 15.34: Patterns of spinal cord disease.

- Complete cord transection syndrome (trauma)
- Brown–Sequard syndrome (bullet injury, multiple sclerosis)
- Central cord syndrome (syringomyelia)
- Posterior column syndrome (tabes dorsalis, Friedreich's ataxia, HIV myelopathy)
- Posterolateral cord syndrome—subacute combined degeneration of the cord (SACDC)
- Combined anterior horn cell (AHC) and pyramidal tract syndrome [amyotrophic lateral sclerosis (ALS)]
- Anterior horn cell syndrome (polio)
- Anterior cord syndrome (anterior spinal artery occlusion)
- Conus medullaris and cauda equina syndrome

Causes and Clinical Features of Spinal Cord Syndromes (Table 15.39)

TABLE 15.39: Causes and clinical features of spinal cord syndromes.

Complete cord transection (Fig. 15.20) *Causes* ➢ Trauma ➢ Metastatic carcinoma ➢ Multiple sclerosis ➢ Spinal epidural hematoma ➢ Autoimmune disorders ➢ Post-vaccinial syndromes **FIG. 15.20:** Complete cord transection.	➢ Sensory – All sensations are affected – Sensory level is usually 2 segments below the level of lesion – Segmental paresthesia occurs at the level of lesion ➢ Motor – Paraplegia due to corticospinal tract involvement – First spinal shock followed by hypertonic hyperreflexia paraplegia – Loss of abdominal and cremasteric reflexes – At the level of lesion, lower motor neuron (LMN) signs occur ➢ Autonomic – Urinary retention and constipation – Anhidrosis, trophic skin changes, vasomotor instability below the level of lesion – Sexual dysfunction can occur

Contd...

Contd...

Brown–Sequard syndrome (Fig. 15.21) ➢ Due to damage to one lateral half of spinal cord – Caused by extramedullary lesions – Usually caused by penetrating injuries (Gunshot) or tumor 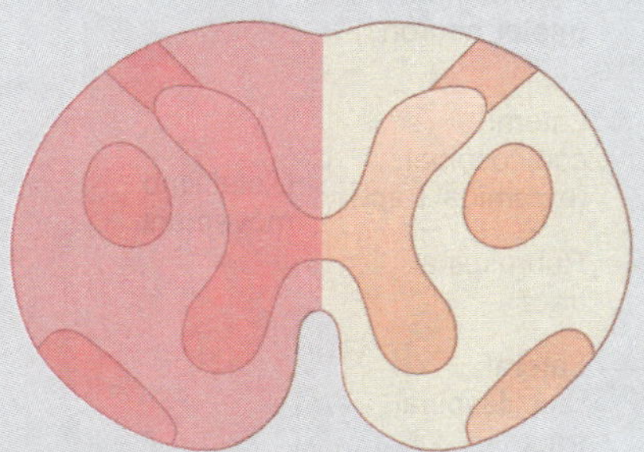 **FIG. 15.21:** Brown-Sequard syndrome.	➢ Sensory – Ipsilateral loss of proprioception due to posterior column involvement – Contralateral loss of pain and temperature due to involvement of lateral spinothalamic tract 1 or 2 segments below ➢ Motor – Ipsilateral spastic weakness due to descending corticospinal tract involvement – Lower motor neuron (LMN) signs at the level of lesion
Central cord syndrome (Fig. 15.22) ➢ Most common cause is syringomyelia ➢ Other causes are hyperextension injuries of neck, intramedullary tumors and trauma ➢ Associated with Arnold–Chiari type 1 and 2 and Dandy–Walker malformation 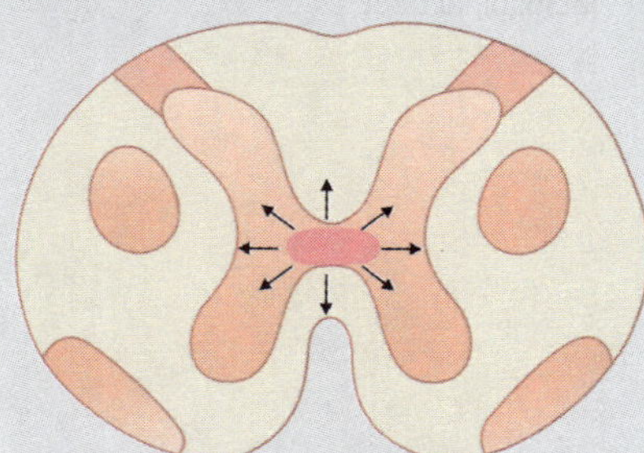 **FIG. 15.22:** Central lesions (syringomyelia).	➢ Sensory – Pain and temperature are affected – Touch and proprioception are preserved – Dissociative anesthesia – Shawl-like distribution of sensory loss ➢ Motor – Upper limb weakness > lower limb weakness ➢ Other features include – Horner's syndrome – Kyphoscoliosis – Sacral sparing – Neuropathic arthropathy of shoulder and elbow joint – Early bladder involvement (exception—syringomyelia)
Posterior column syndrome (Fig. 15.23) ➢ Occurs due to neurosyphilis, diabetes mellitus 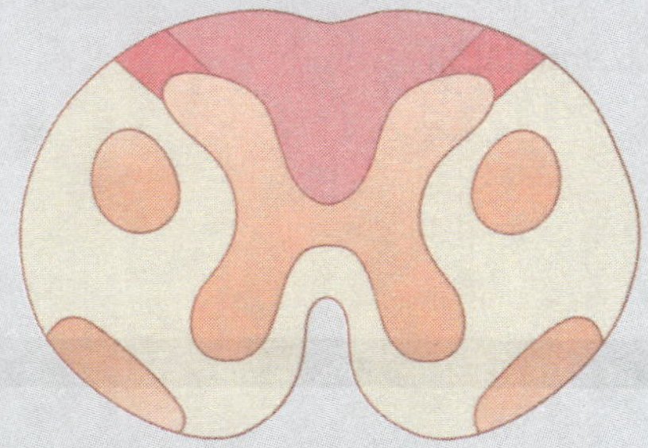 **FIG. 15.23:** Posterior column syndrome.	➢ Sensory – Impaired position and vibration sense in lower limbs – Sensory ataxia – Positive Romberg's sign, sink sign, and Lhermitte's sign ➢ Abadie's sign positive ➢ Urinary incontinence ➢ Absent knee and ankle jerk (areflexia, hypotonia) ➢ Charcot's joint ➢ Miotic and irregular pupil not reacting to light—Argyll Robertson pupil
Posterolateral column disease (Fig. 15.24) ➢ Vitamin B_{12} deficiency ➢ AIDS ➢ HTLV-associated myelopathy ➢ Cervical spondylosis 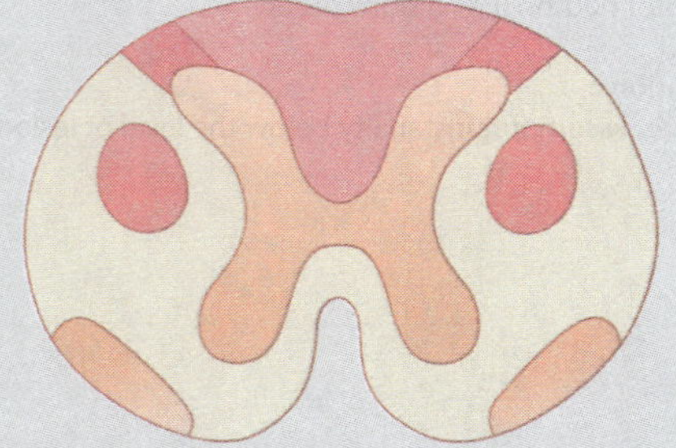 **FIG. 15.24:** Posterolateral column syndrome tabes dorsalis.	➢ Sensory – Paresthesia in feet – Loss of proprioception and vibration in legs – Sensory ataxia – Positive Romberg's sign ➢ Bladder atonia ➢ Motor – Corticospinal tract involvement—spasticity, hyperreflexia, bilateral Babinski's sign ➢ AIDS-associated dementia and spastic bladder is present ➢ HTLV-associated myelopathy—slowly progressive paraparesis and an increase in CSF IgG antibodies to HTLV1

Contd...

Contd...

Anterior horn cell syndrome (Fig. 15.25) ➢ Spinal muscular atrophy (SMA) 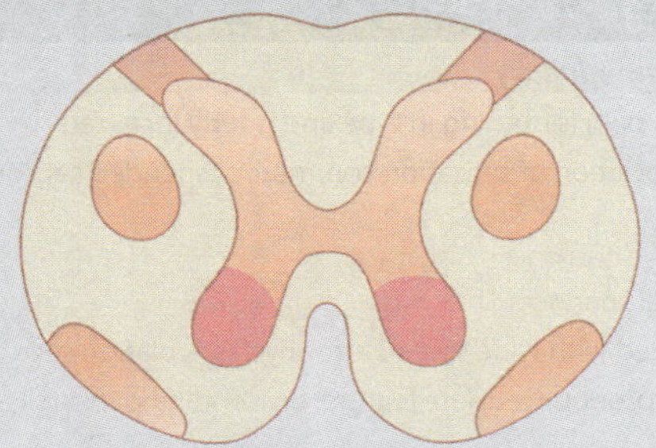 **FIG. 15.25:** Anterior horn cell syndrome.	➢ Motor – Weakness, atrophy, and fasciculations – Hypotonia with depressed reflexes – Muscles of trunk and extremities are affected ➢ Sensory system is not affected
Anterior spinal artery syndrome (Fig. 15.26) ➢ Occurs due to syphilitic arteritis, aortic dissection, atherosclerosis of aorta, systemic lupus erythematosus (SLE), AIDS, arteriovenous malformation (AVM) 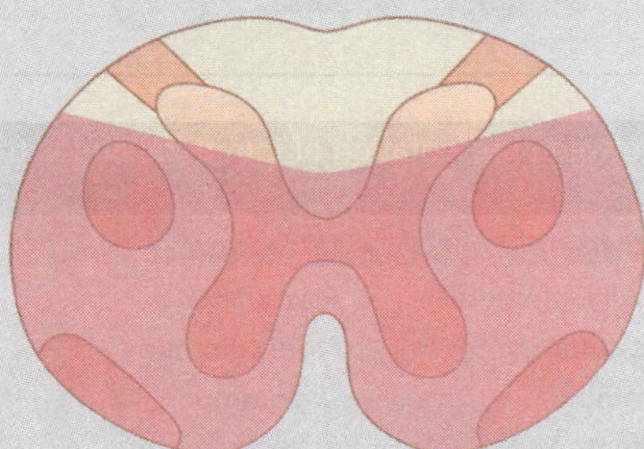 **FIG. 15.26:** Anterior spinal artery occlusion.	➢ Motor – Flaccid and areflexic paraplegia ➢ Sensory – Loss of pain and temperature – Preservation of position and vibration ➢ Autonomic – Urinary incontinence – Spinal cord infarction usually occurs in T1–T4 and L1 segment – Abrupt onset, radicular or girdle pain
Posterior spinal artery syndrome ➢ Rare	➢ Loss of proprioception and vibratory sense ➢ Pain and temperature are preserved ➢ Absence of motor deficit
Anterior horn cell and pyramidal tract (Fig. 15.27) ➢ Amyotrophic lateral sclerosis (ALS) 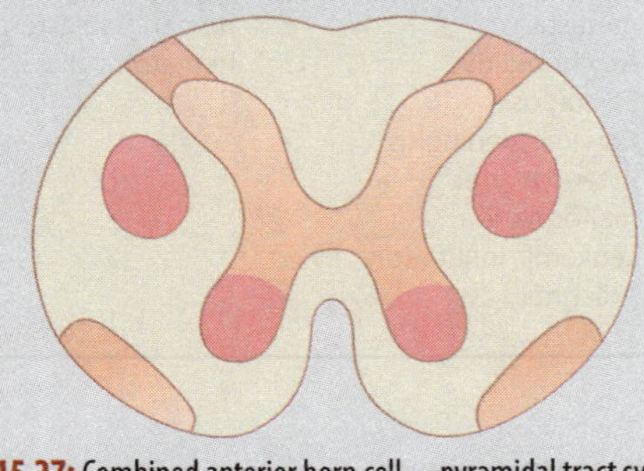 **FIG. 15.27:** Combined anterior horn cell—pyramidal tract syndrome (amyotrophic lateral sclerosis).	➢ Lower motor neuron (LMN) signs ➢ Upper motor neuron (UMN) signs ➢ Sensations preserved ➢ Onuf's nucleus spared: hence no bladder and bowel involvement

Q. List the differences between compressive and noncompressive myelopathy.

The differences between compressive and noncompressive myelopathy are presented in **Table 15.40**.

TABLE 15.40: Differences between compressive and noncompressive myelopathy.

Features	*Compressive*	*Noncompressive*
Bony deformity	+	–
Bony tenderness	+	–
Girdle-like sensation	+	–
Upper level of sensory loss	+	–
Zone of hyperesthesia	+	–
Root pain	+	–
Onset and progress	Gradual	May be acute
Symmetry	Symmetrical	Majority are asymmetrical
Flexor spasm	Common	Usually absent
Pattern of neurodeficit	U-shaped (Elsberg phenomenon)	Bilaterally symmetrical
Bladder and bowel movement	Late	Early (acute transverse myelitis)
Classical example	Tuberculosis of spine	Acute transverse myelitis, motor neuron disease (chronic)

Q. Write a short essay on differences between extramedullary and intramedullary lesions of the spinal cord.

The differences between extramedullary and intramedullary lesions of the spinal cord are listed in **Table 15.41**.

TABLE 15.41: Differences between extramedullary and intramedullary lesions of the spinal cord.

Features	*Extramedullary*	*Intramedullary*
Root pain	Early and common	Rare, pain is burning in type and poorly localized
Secondary deficit	No dissociation of sensation, contralateral loss of pain and temperature, with ipsilateral loss or proprioception	Dissociation of sensation common, suspended sensory loss
Sacral sensation	Lost (early)	Sacral sparing
Lower motor neuron (LMN) involvement	Segmental	Marked with wide spread atrophy, fasciculation seen
Upper motor neuron (UMN) involvement	Early and prominent. Ascending pattern of weakness (sacral → lumbar → thoracic → cervical)	Less pronounced, late feature, descending pattern
Reflexes	Brisk early feature	Less brisk, later feature
Autonomic involvement (bladder and bowel)	Late	Early
Trophic changes	Usually not marked	Common
Vertebral tenderness	May be sensitive to local pressure	No bony tenderness in vertebrae
Changes in CSF	Frequent	Rare

The differences between presentation of intradural and extradural lesion are presented in **Table 15.42**.

TABLE 15.42: Differences between presentation of intradural and extradural lesion.

Features	*Extradural*	*Intradural*
Mode of onset	Usually symmetrical	Asymmetrical
Root pain	Less common	More common
Spinal tenderness	Common	Uncommon
Spinal deformity	Present	Absent

Causes of Compressive Myelopathies (Table 15.43)

Q. Write a short note on common causes of compressive myelopathies.

TABLE 15.43: Causes of compressive myelopathies.

Extradural	*Intradural*	*Intramedullary*
➢ Spondylosis ➢ Disk prolapse ➢ Trauma ➢ Tumor: Metastasis, multiple myeloma ➢ Craniovertebral junction (CVJ) anomalies ➢ Fluorosis ➢ TB spine ➢ Epidural abscess ➢ Epidural hematoma	➢ Tumor: Neurofibroma, meningioma, lipoma, sarcoma ➢ metastasis ➢ Arachnoiditis ➢ Sarcoidosis ➢ Cervical meningitis ➢ Arteriovenous malformation ➢ Leukemic infiltration ➢ Arachnoid cyst	➢ Syrinx ➢ Tumor: Ependymoma, astrocytoma, hemangioblastoma, hematomyelia

Localization of the level of lesion in a compressive myelopathy

- **Distribution root pain:** Ask for specific dermatomes involved.
- **Upper border of sensory loss:** Examine the patient from below upward for demonstration of upper border of sensory loss (spinothalamic tract).
- **Girdle like sensation or sense or constriction** at the level of lesion (involvement of posterior column).
- **Zone of hyperesthesia or hyperalgesia** (zone of hyperesthesia is present just above the level of girdle like sensation, and is due to compression of posterior nerve roots.
- **Analysis of abdominal reflex:** If upper abdominal reflex is intact with loss of middle and lower one, the site of lesion is probably at T10 spinal segment.
- **Atrophy of the muscles in a segmental distribution** (due to anterior horn cells).
- **Loss of deep reflexes:** If the particular segment is involved. The reflexes will be brisk below the involved segment.
- Deformity or any swelling in the vertebra
- Tenderness in the vertebra
- The area of sweating may help (lack of sweating below the level) in localizing the level of lesion.
- The level can also be localized by X-ray of the spine, myelography, CT scan or MRI.

Beevor's Sign

- **Analysis of Beevor's sign:** It is medical sign seen in the selective weakness of the lower abdominal muscles. Rectus abdominis is innervated by the terminal branches lower six or seven thoracic spinal nerves via the lower intercostal and subcostal nerves. If a lesion lies above T6, entire rectus abdominis is weak so there is no contraction of muscle. If it is at or below T10, the upper abdominal muscular function is preserved, whereas the lower abdominal muscles are weak. Therefore, when the head is flexed against resistance (patient supine), the intact upper abdominal muscles pull the umbilicus upward and shift of umbilicus 3 cm when head flexed is considered significant.

- **Causes of Beevor's sign:**
  - Amyotrophic lateral sclerosis
  - Facioscapulohumeral muscular dystrophy (FSHD)
  - Adult form of acid maltase deficiency disease
  - Spinal cord injury
  - Myopathy

Q. List the differences between paraplegia in flexion, paraplegia in extension.

The differences between paraplegia in flexion and paraplegia in extension are listed in **Table 15.44**.

TABLE 15.44: Differences between paraplegia in flexion and paraplegia in extension.

Feature	*Paraplegia in extension*	*Paraplegia in flexion*
Definition	Lower limb muscles take an extension attitude and extensor muscles are spastic	Lower limb muscles take an attitude of flexion
Pathology	Only pyramidal tract involved	Both pyramidal and extrapyramidal tract involved. Occurs in late stage of paraplegia or progressive lesion and spinal arc is dominant
Evolution	Early	Late
Position of lower limbs	Extended	Flexed
Deep tendon reflexes	Exaggerated	Less exaggerated
Clonus	Present	Absent
Mass reflex	Absent	Present
Bladder	Precipitancy	Automatic bladder

Note: Pierre Marie–Foix test is done by firm passive plantar flexing of the toes and foot. This will result in spontaneous "withdrawal reflex", i.e., spontaneous flexion of the hip, knee and dorsiflexion of the ankle if the paraplegia is passing from extension to flexion.

Flexor Spasms

- After recovery from spinal shock, many types of innocuous or noxious cutaneous or muscle stimuli to the lower limb can elicit a prolonged, coordinated pattern of hip flexion and ankle dorsiflexion, similar to flexion withdrawal. It is attributed to increased hyperexcitability of spinal cord circuitry and lead to flexor spasms.
- Spinal cord lesions are associated with flexor spasms except for incomplete and high spinal cord lesion that usually have dominant extensor tone.

Acute and Subacute Spinal Cord Diseases

Spinal Cord Compression

Q. Write a short note on causes of extramedullary spinal cord compression.

- Spinal cord compression is one of the common neurological emergencies in clinical practice.
- **Mechanism of damage:** A space-occupying lesion within the spinal cord may damage nerve tissue either by **direct pressure** or indirectly by **interfering with blood supply.** Edema due to venous obstruction impairs neuronal function, and ischemia due to arterial obstruction may causes necrosis of the spinal cord.
- **Consequences:** During early stages, the damage is reversible but severely damaged neurons cannot recover. Hence, it is important to diagnose and treat early.
- Various causes of spinal cord compression are listed in **Box 15.35**.

Box 15.35: Causes of spinal cord compression.

Vertebral (80%)
- Vertebral body destruction by bone metastases, e.g., breast, prostate, bronchus, myeloma
- Disk and vertebral lesions: Trauma (extradural), chronic degenerative, and acute central (intervertebral) disk prolapse
- Inflammatory: Tuberculosis, Staphylococcus aureus, melioidosis

Meninges (intradural, extramedullary) (15%)
- Tumors (e.g., meningioma, neurofibroma, ependymoma, metastasis, lymphoma, leukemia)
- Inflammatory: Epidural abscess, epidural hemorrhage/hematoma

Spinal cord (intradural, intramedullary) tumors (5%)
- Extramedullary, e.g., meningioma or neurofibroma, metastasis
- Intramedullary, e.g., glioma or ependymoma

Investigations

Patients with acute or subacute spinal cord syndrome should be investigated urgently.

- MRI of spine: MRI is the investigation of choice. MRI can define the extent of compression and associated abnormality in the soft tissue.
- Plain X-rays of spine: It may show destruction of bone and soft tissue abnormalities.
- Chest X-ray: It may show evidence of systemic disease
- Myelography
- CSF: If there is complete spinal block, CSF shows a normal cell count with a raised protein causing yellow discoloration of the fluid (Froin's syndrome).
- Serum vitamin B12
- Biopsy: If a secondary tumor is causing the cord compression, needle biopsy may be established diagnosis.

Symptoms and signs of spinal cord compression

See **Box 15.36.**

Box 15.36: Symptoms and signs of spinal cord compression.

Symptoms of spinal cord compression

- **Pain:** Occurs early. Localized over the spine or in a root distribution. May be aggravated by coughing, sneezing or straining
- **Sensory:** Occurs early. Paresthesia, numbness or cold sensations (especially in the lower limbs), spread proximally to a level on the trunk
- **Motor:** Occurs late. Weakness, heaviness or stiffness of the limbs (commonly legs)
- **Sphincters:** Occurs late. Urgency or hesitancy of micturition, and retention of urine

Signs of spinal cord compression: Vary according to the level of the cord compression and the structures involved

Cervical, above C5: Frequently life threatening
- Upper motor neuron signs and sensory loss in all four limbs (quadriplegia)
- Weakness of diaphragm (phrenic nerve)

Cervical, C4–C5: Quadriplegia with preserved respiratory function

Cervical, C5–T1
- Lower motor neuron (LMN) signs and segmental sensory loss in the arms; upper motor neuron (UMN) signs in the legs
- Weakness of respiratory (intercostal) muscle

Thoracic cord
- Spastic paraplegia with a sensory level on the trunk
- Weakness of legs, sacral loss of sensation and extensor plantar responses
- Midline back pain is a useful localizing sign

Lumbar cord and Cauda equina
- Spinal cord ends at the T12/L1 spinal level. Spinal lesions below this level can cause only LMN signs by affecting the cauda equina
- L1–L2—cremasteric reflex is a cutaneous reflex useful in localization of lumbar cord disease
- L2–L4 paralyzes flexion and abduction of the thigh, weakens leg extension at the knee, and abolishes the patellar reflex
- L5–S1 paralyzes movements of the foot and ankle, flexion at the knee, and extension of the thigh, and abolishes the ankle jerk (S1)

Brown–Séquard Syndrome

Q. Write a short note on the causes and clinical manifestations of Brown–Séquard syndrome.

It refers to findings seen when the damage is confined to one side (lateral half) of the spinal cord. With compressive lesions, there is a band of pain at the level of the lesion in the distribution of the nerve roots involved by compression.

Causes: Due to extramedullary lesions, usually caused by penetrating injuries (gunshot) or tumor.

Management
- Treatment depends on the underlying lesion.
- Benign tumors should be surgically excised.
- Extradural compression due to malignancy has a poor prognosis. Useful function can be regained if treatment (e.g., radiotherapy), is started within 24 hours of the onset of severe weakness or sphincter dysfunction.
- Spinal cord compression due to tuberculosis may require surgical treatment and antituberculous chemotherapy.
- Traumatic lesions of the vertebral column needed treatment by neurosurgeon.

Clinical Features

- Sensory
  - Ipsilateral loss of proprioception due to posterior column involvement
  - Contralateral loss of pain and temperature due to involvement of lateral spinothalamic tract.
- Motor
  - Ipsilateral spastic weakness due to descending corticospinal tract involvement
  - Lower motor neuron signs at the level of lesion.

Chronic Myelopathies

Syringomyelia

Q. Write a short essay on the pathogenesis of syringomyelia.

- A syrinx is a fluid-filled cavity within the spinal cord. Syringomyelia is a **cavitary expansion of the spinal cord.** Syrinxes commonly develop in the lower cervical and high thoracic regions or in the high cervical region. They may extend proximally to the medulla or pons (syringobulbia).
- Pathogenesis: More than 50% are associated with Arnold–Chiari type I malformation characterized by herniation of cerebellar tonsils through the foramen magnum. This abnormality at the foramen magnum probably allows normal pulsatile CSF pressure waves to be transmitted to fragile tissues of the cervical cord and brainstem. This results in secondary cavity formation. There is gradually destruction of spinothalamic neurons, anterior horn cells and lateral corticospinal tracts. It leads to progressive myelopathy.
- **Classic presentation** is a central cord syndrome with dissociated sensory loss and areflexic weakness in the upper limbs.
- **Sensory loss:** Most cases begin asymmetrically with unilateral sensory loss. The sensory loss has a distribution that is "suspended" over the nape of the neck, shoulders, and upper arms (cape distribution) or in the hands.
- Neurogenic arthropathies **(Charcot's joint):** Most common in shoulder. Thoracic kyphoscoliosis is common.

- **La main succulente of syringomyelia** (subcutaneous thickening and swollen fingers)
- **Morvan's syndrome:** Progressive loss of pain sensation, ulceration, loss of soft tissues and resorption of phalanges.
- **MRI scans (Fig. 15.28):** Accurately identify syrinx cavities and associated spinal cord enlargement.
- **Treatment is surgery:** Posterior decompression of Arnold–Chiari malformation and the coperitoneal shunt to drain syrinx cavity.

Syringobulbia

It is characterized by dysphagia, nystagmus, pharyngeal and palatal weakness, asymmetric weakness and atrophy of the tongue, and loss of pain, temperature in the distribution of the trigeminal nerve (facial sensory loss resembling in distribution a **balaclava helmet),** involving the outer parts of the face but sparing the nose and mouth. This pattern of facial sensory impairment may also be known as onion-peel or onion-skin pattern.

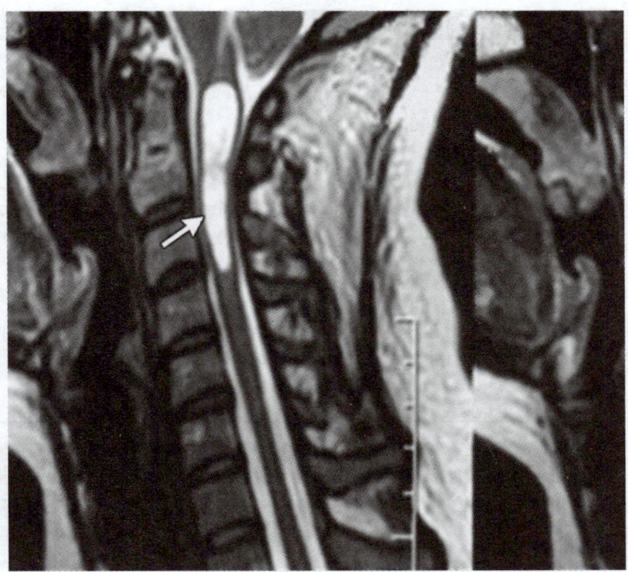

FIG. 15.28: MRI showing cervical syringomyelia.

Subacute Combined Degeneration of Cord

Q. Write a short essay on etiology, clinical features/neurological signs and management of subacute combined degeneration (SACD).

It is myelopathy that develops due to nutritional deficiency of vitamin B_{12} deficiency, including pernicious anemia.

- This treatable myelopathy presents with paresthesia in the hand and feet, early loss of vibration and position sensation, and a progressive spastic and ataxic weakness.
- Loss of reflexes due to a superimposed peripheral neuropathy in a patient who also has Babinski's sign is an important diagnostic clue.
- The myelopathy of SACD tends to be diffuse rather than focal; signs are generally symmetric and reflect predominant involvement of the posterior and lateral tracts.
- Optic atrophy and irritability prominent in advanced cases.
- **Low vitamin B_{12}** levels confirm the **diagnosis.**
- **MRI spinal cord:** Inverted V sign or rabbit ear sign due to T2 hyper intensity along posterolateral column of spinal cord.

Treatment is by replacement therapy, beginning with 100 mg of intramuscular vitamin B_{12} repeated at regular intervals or by subsequent oral treatment.

Causes of posterior column disease ***(Box 15.37)***

Q. Write a short essay on diseases affecting posterior column. Explain clinical features of any one of them.

Refer respective diseases.

Box 15.37: Causes of posterolateral column disease.

- Vitamin B_{12} deficiency
- AIDS
- HTLV-associated myelopathy
- Cervical spondylosis, hypocupremia, vitamin E deficiency

Paraplegia

Q. Write a short note on causes and differential diagnosis of spastic paraplegia.

Paraplegia is weakness or paralysis of both lower limbs, sparing the upper limbs.

Causes: It can occur in disorders of cerebrum, spinal cord, spinal roots, peripheral nerves or muscles. It is usually due to disorders of spinal cord.

Spastic Paraplegia

Spasticity is due to an upper motor neuron lesion. It is usually produced to subacute or chronic lesion. Acute lesions usually cause flaccid paralysis.

Causes of spastic paraplegia ***(Table 15.45)***

Cauda Equina Syndrome

The **epiconus** comprises the cord segment between L4 and S1, corresponding to the T12 and L1 vertebrae. The most distal bulbous part of the spinal cord (L1–L2) is called the conus medullaris. The **conus medullaris** consists of the cord segment between S2 and S5 as well as coccygeal segments. Distal to this end of the spinal cord is a collection of nerve roots (L2–L3 onward to coccygeal), which are horsetail-like in appearance called the **cauda equina (Table 15.46 and Fig. 15.29).**

TABLE 15.45: Causes of spastic paraplegia [upper motor neuron (UMN) type lesion].

A. Gradual onset	*B. Sudden onset*
Cerebral causes	
➢ Parasagittal meningioma ➢ Hydrocephalus	Thrombosis of unpaired anterior cerebral artery or superior sagittal sinus
Spinal causes	
Compressive or transverse lesion in the spinal cord: Cord compression **Noncompressive or longitudinal lesion** or systemic disease of the spinal cord ➢ Motor neuron disease (MND), e.g., amyotrophic lateral sclerosis ➢ Multiple sclerosis, Friedreich's ataxia ➢ Subacute combined degeneration (i.e., from vitamin B12 deficiency) ➢ Lathyrism, syringomyelia, Erb's spastic paraplegia, tropical spastic paraplegia ➢ Radiation myelopathy	**Compressive causes** ➢ Injury to the spinal cord (fracture-dislocation or collapse of the vertebra) ➢ Intervertebral disk prolapse ➢ Spinal epidural abscess or hematoma **Noncompressive causes** ➢ Acute transverse myelitis ➢ Thrombosis of anterior spinal artery ➢ Hematomyelia (from arteriovenous malformation, angiomas, or endarteritis)

TABLE 15.46: Differences between conus medullaris and cauda equina syndromes.

Features	*Conus medullaris syndrome*	*Cauda equina syndrome*
Presentation	Sudden and bilateral	Gradual and unilateral
Reflexes	Knee jerks preserved but ankle jerks affected	Both knee and ankle jerks affected
Radicular pain	Less severe	More severe
Low back pain	More	Less
Sensory symptoms and signs	Numbness in symmetrical and bilateral, sensory dissociation occurs. Saddle anesthesia present	Numbness is asymmetrical, may be unilateral, no necessary dissociation
Motor strength	Typically symmetric, hyperreflexic distal paresis of lower limbs	Asymmetric areflexic paraplegia
Impotence	Frequent	Less frequent
Sphincter dysfunction	Overflow urinary incontinence and fecal incontinence, tends to present early in course of disease	Urinary retention, tends to present late in course of disease

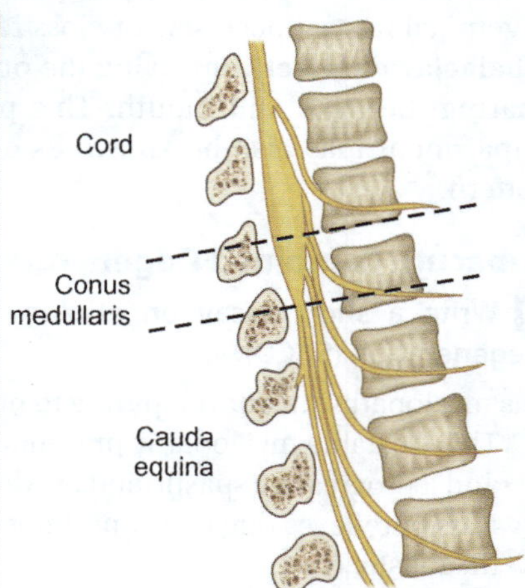

FIG. 15. 29: Cord segment—conus medullaris and cauda equina.

Q. Write a short note on differences between conus medullaris lesions and cauda equina lesions.

The differences between conus medullaris and cauda equina syndromes are listed in **Table 15.46**.

Complications of Paraplegia (Box 15.38)

Box 15.38: Complications of paraplegia.

- Pressure/bed sore
- Urinary infection and renal stones
- Fecal impaction with intestinal obstruction
- Contracture of limbs
- It may lead to death

Management of Paraplegia

- **Skin care:** Prevention of pressure sores. They develop due to loss of sensation and reduced blood supply. Following measures will be helpful.
  - Turn the patient every 2–4 hours to avoid pressure over bony prominences.
  - Keep the skin dry and clean.
  - Specially designed mattress like water or air-cushioned bed will be useful.
  - The patient should be prevented from lying on the side of the pressure sores. Needs aseptic care and may require skin grafting.
- **Bladder**
  - Aseptic intermittent catheterization. Indwelling catheter is not advisable as it predisposes to infection, reduces bladder capacity and promotes calculus formation.
  - Prompt treatment of urinary infections and maintenance of adequate fluid intake.
- **Bowel:** Laxative to prevent constipation. If fecal matter becomes hard, manual evacuation is done.
- **Paralysis**
  - Spasticity can lead to contractures and flexor spasms. Hence, regular passive movements of the limbs should be encouraged.
  - Posture should be such that flexion is prevented at joints.
  - Drug treatment of spasticity: Baclofen, diazepam and tizanidine. In severe spasticity, intrathecal baclofen via a pump or sectioning of the anterior roots (rhizotomy).
- **Rehabilitation:** Use a caliper or wheel chair and physiotherapy.

Spinal Pain

Q. Discuss the different types of spinal pain.

- **Radicular pain:**
  - It is **unilateral, lancinating, dermatomal** pain often exacerbated by cough, sneeze, or Valsalva maneuver.
  - Common with **extradural growths** (e.g., neurilemmoma which is intradural extramedullary) and rare with intramedullary lesions.
- **Vertebral pain:**
  - It is an **aching pain localized to the point of the spine involved** in the compressive process and often accompanied by point tenderness.
  - Common with **neoplastic or inflammatory extradural lesions** and infrequent with intramedullary or intradural extramedullary lesions.
- **Funicular (central) pain:**
  - It is **deep, ill-defined painful dysesthesia,** usually distant from the affected spinal cord level (and therefore of poor localizing value), probably related to dysfunction of the spinothalamic tract or posterior columns.
  - It is common with **intramedullary lesions** and very unusual with extradural lesions.
- With dysfunction of the posterior columns in the cervical region, neck flexion may elicit a sudden "electric-like" sensation down the back or into the arms **(Lhermitte's sign or Barber's chair syndrome).**
- More reliable band-like radicular pain or segmental paresthesia may occur at the level of the lesion and may be of localizing value for the appropriate spinal level.

Causes of Flaccid Paraplegia (LMN type)

- **Upper motor neuron lesion in shock stage**, i.e. sudden onset or history of long duration as in extradural transverse myelitis and spinal injury
- **Lesion involving anterior horn cells**
  - Acute anterior poliomyelitis
  - Progressive muscular atrophy (a variety of motor neuron disease)
- **Diseases affecting nerve root:** tabes dorsalis, radiculitis, GBS
- **Diseases affecting peripheral nerves**
  - Acute infective polyneuropathy (GBS)
  - High cauda equina syndrome
  - Disease of peripheral nerves involving both the lower limbs
  - Lumbar plexus injury (psoas abscess or hematoma)
- **Diseases affecting myoneural junction**
  - Myasthenia gravis (MG), Lambert–Eaton syndrome
  - Periodic paralysis due to hypo- or hyperkalemia
- **Diseases affecting muscles:** Myopathy.

Causes of Pure Motor Paraplegia

See **Box 15.39.**

Box 15.39: Causes of pure motor paraplegia.

- Hereditary spastic paraplegia
- Lathyrism
- Guillain–Barré syndrome
- Amyotrophic lateral sclerosis [motor neurone disease (MND)]
- Fluorosis
- Erb's spastic paraplegia (syphilitic)

Causes of Quadriplegia (Table 15.47)

Weakness of all the 4 limbs can occur in the lesions from cortex to C5 level of spinal cord and various lower motor neuron lesion affecting anterior horn cells, roots, peripheral nerve, neuromuscular junction and muscles.

TABLE 15.47: Causes of quadriplegia.

Upper motor neuron causes	*Lower motor neuron causes*
➢ Cerebral palsy	➢ Acute anterior poliomyelitis
➢ Bilateral brainstem lesion (glioma)	➢ Guillain–Barré syndrome
➢ Craniovertebral anomaly	➢ Peripheral neuropathy
➢ High cervical cord compression	➢ Myopathy or polymyositis
➢ Multiple sclerosis	➢ Myasthenia gravis and crisis
➢ Motor neuron disease	➢ Periodic paralysis
	➢ Snake bite, organophosphorus poisoning, etc.

Craniovertebral Junction Anomalies

Q. Discuss craniovertebral junction (CVJ) anomalies.

- **Abnormal general physical appearance:** Head may be cocked to one side, short neck and scoliosis.
- **Neurological:** Most common posterior occipital headache that worsens with neck flexion or extension. Others include myelopathy and brainstem and lower cranial nerve deficits.
- **Vascular symptoms:** Intermittent attacks of altered consciousness, confusion, transient loss of visual fields and vertigo.

Classification of CVJ anomalies is presented in Table 15.48.

Hemiplegia

Q. Discuss hemiplegia in an elderly male. Give the differential diagnosis, investigations, and its treatment.

Hemiplegia is paralysis of one side of the body. Hemiparesis is the weakness of one side of body. For differential diagnosis, investigations and its treatment, refer individual diseases.

Causes of Hemiplegia

See **Table 15.49.**

Small Muscle Wasting of the Hand (Fig. 15.30)

Q. Write a short note on wasting of small muscles of hand.

Causes of Small Muscle Wasting of the Hand

See **Box 15.40.**

MOTOR NEURON DISEASES

Q. Write a short essay/note on motor neuron disease.

Motor neuron disease (MND) is a devastating, progressive, **heterogeneous group** of **neurodegenerative** condition caused by loss of upper and lower motor neurons in the spinal cord, cranial nerve nuclei and motor cortex. There is no involvement of sensory or other nonmotor tracts. It causes progressive weakness and eventually death (usually as a result of respiratory failure or aspiration). Various types of MND are listed in **Table 15.50.**

Clinical Features

Q. Write a short answer on three neurological signs of upper and lower motor neuron disease.

There are four main clinical patterns. There is no involvement of sensory system. Hence, sensory symptoms (e.g., numbness, tingling and pain) are not present.

Amyotrophic Lateral Sclerosis

Q. Write a short essay/note on amyotrophic lateral sclerosis.

- Named by Jean Martin Charcot in 19th century. Also known as **Lou Gehrig's disease** after the famous baseball player diagnosed of ALS in 1930.
- Degeneration of the motor neuron (UMN and LMN) in motor cortex, brainstem and spinal cord.
  - **Amyotrophy:** Atrophy of muscle fibers consequent to denervation due to anterior horn cell degeneration
  - **Lateral sclerosis:** Sclerosis of the anterior and lateral corticospinal tracts which are replaced by progressive gliosis. **Epidemiology:** Incidence is 1 to 2.7/lakh, prevalence is 2.7 to 7.4/lakh
- Sex predisposition: M > F (2:1 to 7:1), (F > M in bulbar onset ALS).
- Age: Risk increases with age up to 74 years. Peak onset—6th to 7th decade (one to two decades earlier in India).
- Prognosis: 20% of patients survive for 5 years and 10% survive for 10 years.

TABLE 15.48: Craniovertebral junction anomalies.

Skeletal anomalies	*Neuraxial anomalies*
➢ Platybasia ➢ Basilar invagination (10/20) ➢ Klippel–Feil anomaly ➢ Occipitalization of atlas ➢ Atlantoaxial dislocation	➢ Arnold–Chiari malformation ➢ Dandy–Walker syndrome ➢ Occipitocervical myelomeningocele ➢ Posterior fossa cysts

TABLE 15.49: Causes of hemiplegia.

Onset	*Cause*
Acute	
➢ Stroke	Cerebral infarct (thrombotic/embolic—most common cause in elderly), intracerebral hemorrhage (hypertensive), subarachnoid hemorrhage (SAH) with intracerebral hemorrhage
➢ Trauma	Hematoma (epidural or subdural), cerebral contusion
Subacute	Meningitis, encephalitis, postseizure (Todd's paralysis)
Chronic	Cerebral metastasis, subdural hematoma, granulomas (tuberculosis—younger age, fungal), pyogenic abscesses (metastatic infection, post-traumatic), rapidly growing malignant neoplasms (e.g., glioblastoma), hypoglycemia, multiple sclerosis, slow growing neoplasms

Box 15.40: Causes of small muscle wasting of the hand.

Lesions of vertebra: Craniovertebral anomalies, vertebral metastasis
Lesions of spinal cord: Syringomyelia, cord compression by tumor
Lesion of anterior horn cell: Motor neuron disease (MND), poliomyelitis
Lesions of spinal root: Cervical cord tumor, pancoast tumor, cervical disk prolapse
Lesion of brachial plexus: Cervical rib
Lesions of peripheral nerve: Hansen's disease, carpal tunnel syndrome, lead poisoning
Diseases of muscle: Distal muscular dystrophy, polymyositis
Disuse atrophy: Therapeutic immobilization (e.g., fracture), rheumatoid arthritis, postparalytic (hemiplegia)

TABLE 15.50: Various types of motor neuron disease.

Subset of motor neurons involved	*Clinical syndromes*
Upper motor neuron + lower motor neuron	Amyotrophic lateral sclerosis
Upper motor neuron	➢ Pseudobulbar palsy ➢ Primary lateral sclerosis ➢ Familial spastic paraplegia
Lower motor neuron	➢ Bulbar palsy ➢ Spinomuscular atrophy

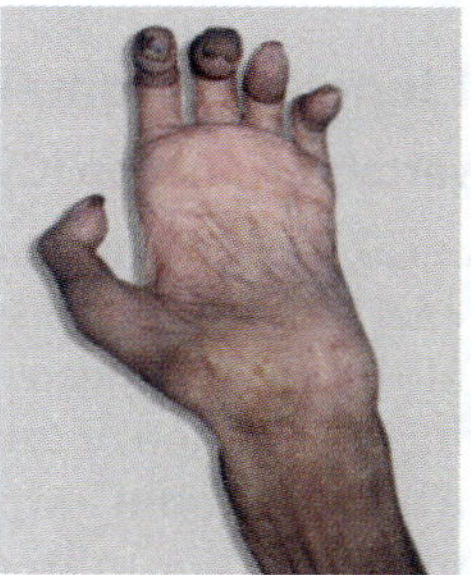

FIG. 15.30: Wasting of small muscles of hand.

Etiopathogenesis

- Undetermined etiology. Complex genetic and environmental interaction for neuronal degeneration.
- MND is usually (90–95%) sporadic.
- **Molecular pathway:** Pathological hallmarks observed in axons of MND is the ubiquitinated cytoplasmic inclusions containing the RNA processing proteins TDP43 and FUS. This indicates that protein aggregation may be involved in its pathogenesis similar to other neurodegenerative disorders. Other mechanism involved in pathogenesis may be oxidative neuronal damage, glutamate mediated excitotoxicity, mitochondrial dysfunction and impaired axonal transport.

Clinical presentation

- **Typical/spinal form** of ALS constitutes 2/3rd of cases. They present with simultaneous involvement of upper and lower motor neurons. Usually in one limb, spreading gradually. Often present with focal motor weakness of distal or proximal upper or lower limbs. The focal motor weakness spreads to contiguous muscles in the same region before involvement of another region. Then involves other limbs and trunk muscles.
- **Pseudoneurotic pattern:** Resembles neuropathy, i.e., involvement of muscles in the apparent distribution of a peripheral nerve. Fasciculations are present on wasted muscles.
- Monomelic: Involvement of one limb (as wasted leg syndrome, monomelic amyotrophy, Chopra's MND)
- Pseudopolyneuritic: Weakness in the both distal lower limbs.
- Mills hemiplegic variant: Weakness restricted to one half of the body.
- **Madras MND:** Associated sensorineural deafness, bifacial and bulbar weakness, bilateral optic atrophy in age <15 years.

Bulbar/Pseudobulbar Palsy (20%)

- Initially involves the lower cranial nerve nuclei and their supranuclear connections.
- Presents with weakness of respiratory group of muscles (e.g., dysarthria, dysphagia, nasal regurgitation of fluids and choking).
- About 10% present with bilateral upper limb weakness and wasting, flail arm of flail person in barrel syndrome.
- Head drop.
- Wasting and fasciculations of tongue seen almost in all patients **(Fig. 15.31)**.
- Cramps in the thighs, abdomen, back or even tongue.
- Nonmotor symptoms: Sleep disturbance, subtle cognitive dysfunction and mood changes.
- Rarely involved: Bladder, bowels, autonomic, extraocular movements and sensory.

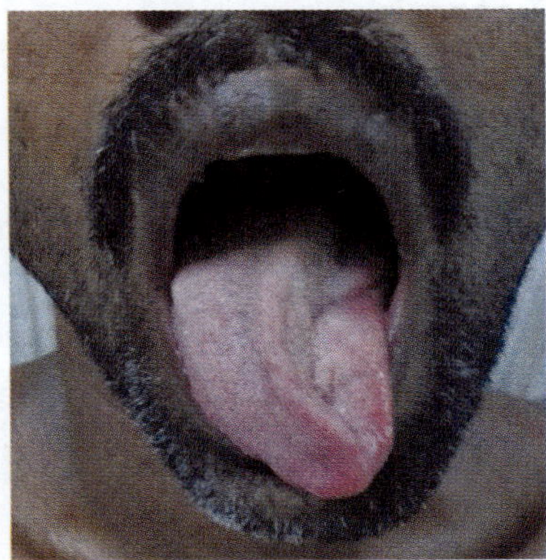

FIG. 15.31: Tongue wasting with atrophy.

Progressive Muscular Atrophy

- It presents as a pure lower motor neuron disease with symptoms of weakness, muscle wasting and fasciculation.
- Usually starts in one limb and gradually spreading to involve other adjacent spinal segments.

Primary Lateral Sclerosis (Rare 1–2%)

The least common form of MND. It involves upper motor neurons and presents with a slowly progressive tetraparesis and pseudobulbar palsy.

Diagnosis of Amyotrophic Lateral Sclerosis

- No biological marker identified so far.
- Diagnosis is largely by series of clinical and neurological examinations.
- MRI: Coronal T2WI shows bilateral symmetrical hyperintensity along corticospinal tract (thin white arrows) forming a **"wine glass appearance"** or **"garland sign"**.
- Myelogram of cervical spine (an X-ray analysis): Detects lesions in selected area of the spinal cord.
- Muscle and/or nerve biopsy.
- Electromyography and nerve conduction velocity (NCV) to measure muscle response to nervous stimulation.
    - **Split hand phenomenon:** In cases of severe changes in the thenar eminence and the relative sparing of hypothenar eminence, observed on the EMG study.

Box 15.41: Differential diagnosis of amyotrophic lateral sclerosis.

Other motor neuron diseases: Primary lateral sclerosis (UMN only), progressive muscular atrophy (LMN only), progressive bulbar palsy

Structural lesions: Cervical spondylosis, parasagittal/foramen magnum tumor, spinal cord AV malformation

Neuropathies: Chronic inflammatory demyelinating polyneuropathy (CIDP)

Myopathies: Polymyositis, inclusion body myositis

Neuromuscular junction disorder: Myasthenia gravis

Neurodegenerative diseases: Parkinson's, progressive supranuclear palsy, multiple sclerosis

Malignancy: Primary/metastasis to CNS, motor neuron syndromes with multiple myeloma, lymphoma, lung, breast

Toxic exposure: Alcohol, heavy metals

Endocrine: Hyperthyroidism, hyperparathyroidism

Infectious: HIV, CMV

Differential Diagnosis of Amyotrophic Lateral Sclerosis

As amyotrophic lateral sclerosis in untreatable, all secondary causes should be excluded **(Box 15.41)**.

Treatment

No treatment to arrest degeneration.

Drug therapy

- **Riluzole:** Dose 100 mg/day. It is a sodium channel blocker that reduces glutamate-induced excitotoxicity. Adverse drug reactions include asthenia, nausea, alterations in liver function tests, headache, abdominal pain, and tachycardia.
- **Trial drugs:** IGF-1, ceftriaxone, edaravone, tamoxifen.
- **Spasticity**
  - Baclofen 5–10 mg twice daily to three times daily.
  - Tizanidine in the dose of 2–4 mg by mouth twice daily up to a total dose of 24 mg daily.
  - Memantine starting at 5 mg daily, increasing by 5 mg a week to a maximum of 20 mg twice a day.
  - Tetrazepam 50 mg at bedtime, increasing by 25 mg a day to a maximum dose of 150 mg taken two to three times a day.

Rehabilitation

- Foot drop splint
- Finger extension splint
- Respiratory support: Tracheostomy, positive pressure ventilation, cough assisted device.
- Bulbar involvement: Gastrostomy (for feeding), speech therapy.
- Physiotherapy, speech and occupational therapy.

Prognosis

Patient usually does not survive for >3 years, though rarely patients may survive for a decade or longer.

Neurogenic Bladder

Nerve Supply of Urinary Bladder

See **Figure 15.32.**

Q. Discuss the types of neurogenic bladder.

Dysfunction of urinary bladder due to neurological disorders is known as neurogenic bladder. Various causes of neurogenic bladder are listed in **Table 15.51**.

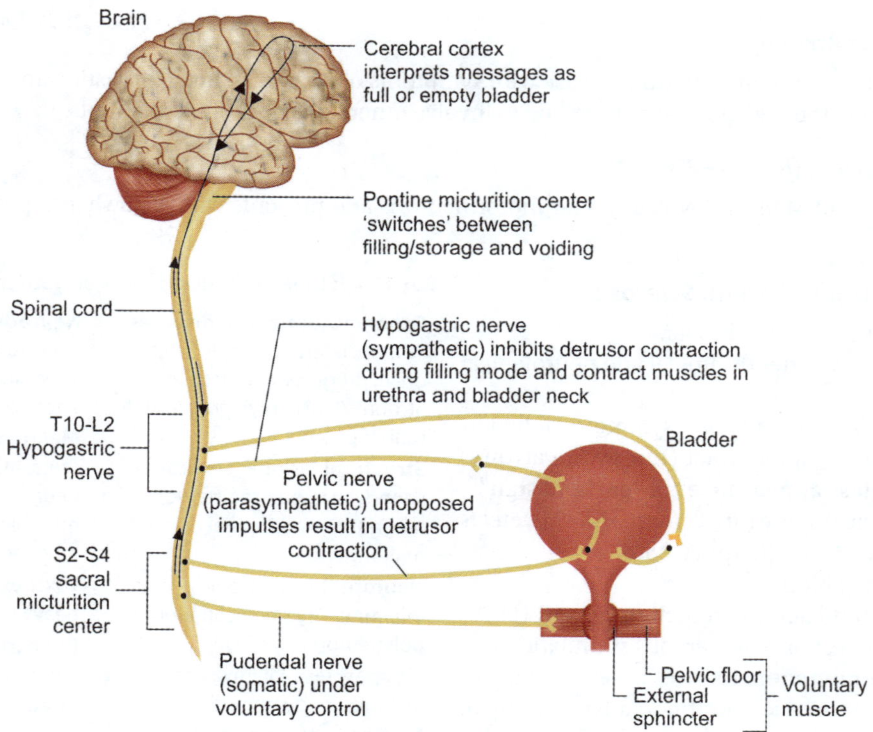

FIG. 15.32: Nerve supply of urinary bladder.

TABLE 15.51: Various causes of neurogenic bladder.

Type	Uninhibited bladder/ detrusor hyperreflexia	Automatic bladder/ Detrusor sphincter dyssynergia	Autonomous bladder/Detrusor areflexia	Sensory atonic bladder	Motor atonic bladder
Site of lesion	Suprapontine neurologic disorder, mostly frontal lobe	Upper motor neuron (UMN) disorder of the suprasacral spinal cord	Lower motor neuron (LMN) lesion at the sacral cord	LMN lesion—peripheral nerve	
Causes	Frontal tumors, parasagittal meningioma, ACA aneurysm, NPH	Spine cord trauma, compressive myelopathy, myelitis	Cauda equina syndrome, conus medullaris lesion, spinal shock	Diabetes mellitus, amyloidosis, tabes dorsalis	Lumbosacral meningomyelocele, tethered cord syndrome, lumbar canal stenosis
Bladder sensation	Preserved	Interrupted	Absent	Absent	Intact
Size of bladder	Normal	Small	Large	Large	Large
Ability to initiate voiding	Present	Absent	Absent	Present	Lost
Type of incontinence	Urge social disinhibition	Urge	Overflow	Overflow	Overflow
Residual urine	Nil	Small	Large amount	Large	Large
Anal sphincter tone	Normal	Normal	Lost	Normal	Lost
Perianal sensation	Normal	Normal	Absent	Absent	Preserved
Bulbocavernous/anal reflex	Normal	Normal	Absent	Absent	Preserved
Treatment	Anticholinergic medication	Self-intermittent catheterization	Continuous catheterization		

Transverse Myelitis

Q. Write a short note on transverse myelitis.

Transverse myelitis (TM) is an acute, usually monophasic, demyelinating inflammatory disorder affecting the spinal cord. It is characterized by acute or subacute motor, sensory and autonomic (bladder, bowel and sexual) spinal cord dysfunction.

- Myelitis refers to inflammation of the spinal cord and transverse signifies the involvement across one spinal cord level.
- Usually 1 or 2 spinal segments are affected with part or all of the cord area at that level involved.
- Varying degree of motor, sensory and autonomic disturbances are produced.

Causes of Transverse Myelitis (Table 15.52)

TABLE 15.52: Causes of transverse myelitis.

Disease	Examples
Bacterial infections	Mycoplasma pneumoniae, Lyme borreliosis, syphilis (tabes dorsalis), tuberculosis
Viral infections	Herpes simplex, herpes zoster, cytomegalovirus, Epstein–Barr virus, enteroviruses (poliomyelitis, coxsackie virus, echovirus), human T-cell, leukemia virus, human immunodeficiency virus, influenza, rabies
Postvaccination	Rabies, cowpox
Autoimmune diseases	SLE, Sjögren's syndrome, sarcoidosis, multiple sclerosis, neuromyelitis optica
Paraneoplastic syndromes	
Vascular	Thrombosis of spinal arteries, vasculitis secondary to heroin abuse, spinal arteriovenous malformation (AVM)

Q. Write a short note on clinical features of transverse myelitis.

It is usually thought to be postinfectious in origin and up to half of idiopathic cases will have a preceding respiratory or gastrointestinal illness. It is one of cause of a noncompressive spinal cord syndrome in which immune-mediated process may be responsible for neural injury of the spinal cord.

Clinical Features

- Age: It can occur at any age.
- **Symptoms develop rapidly** over several hours to several weeks which may worsen maximally within 24 hours.

Symptoms

- Lower limb weakness.
- Sensory: Sensation is diminished or absent below the level of involved spinal cord. Few patients experience tingling or numbness in the legs (subacute paraparesis). **Pain and temperature sensation are diminished.**
- **Bladder and bowel** dysfunction: It results in disturbed **sphincter control.**
- Lhermitte's sign: It is the radiation of paresthesias down the spine or limbs with neck flexion. It may be positive. It suggests intrinsic cervical spinal cord lesion.

Diagnosis

- First **exclude any mass-occupying lesion** compressing the spinal cord. Early surgical decompression results in complete recovery. MRI and CSF analysis may be useful in the diagnosis.

- **MRI:** MRI is sensitive and shows spinal cord swelling and edema with gadolinium enhancing lesions (single or multiple) at the affected level(s). MRI is also useful for excluding other treatable causes of spinal cord dysfunction (e.g., spinal cord compression).
- **CSF examination:** Shows cellular pleocytosis (usually monocytes/lymphocytes) often with polymorphs at the onset. Protein is slightly increased and IgG index is elevated. IgG index is a measure of intrathecal synthesis of immunoglobulin (Ig) and is calculated using the following formula: (CSF IgG/serum IgG)/(CSF albumin/serum albumin). Normal value is = 0.85 oligoclonal bands are usually absent.
- **Tests for exclusion of other treatable causes:** These include chest X-ray, tuberculin test, ESR, serologic tests (e.g., for mycoplasma, Lyme disease and HIV), vitamin B12 and folate levels, antinuclear antibodies (ANAs) and CSF and blood for VDRL (Venereal Diseases Research Laboratory) tests.

Treatment
- Treat the underlying cause or associated disorder. Otherwise it is mainly supportive.
- **High dose corticosteroids, intravenous immunoglobulin (IVIg) and plasmapheresis** are used in the treatment of **idiopathic cases.**
- **For severe, refractory cases:** Course of **azathioprine, methotrexate, mycophenolate, or oral cyclophosphamide.**

Outcome is variable and evolves over days. There may be no recovery. If present it may be **partial or complete** (often partial) and follows over weeks or months (1–3 months).

DISEASES OF THE PERIPHERAL NERVOUS SYSTEM

Introduction

Diseases of the PNS are common. They may affect the motor, sensory or autonomic components, either in isolation or combination. Cranial nerves III to XII share the same tissue characteristics as peripheral nerves and are prone to the same range of diseases.

Site of lesion: It may be (1) dorsal or ventral nerve root (radiculopathy), (2) brachial/lumbosacral nerve plexus (plexopathy) or (3) cranial nerves (except I and II), and other sensory, motor, autonomic or mixed nerves (neuropathy). Neuropathy is a pathological process affecting a peripheral nerve or nerves. It may be axonal, demyelinating or neoronopathy.

Classification

Peripheral nerve disorders can be broadly classified into three categories.

1. **Mononeuropathy simplex:** Signifies involvement of a single peripheral nerve [e.g., median nerve in carpal tunnel syndrome (CTS)].
2. **Mononeuropathy multiplex (now called multiple mononeuropathies):** Simultaneous or sequential several individual nerves involvement usually at random and noncontiguous (e.g., vasculitis, HIV leprosy).
3. **Polyneuropathy:** Function of numerous peripheral nerves is affected at the same time. This leads to a predominantly diffuse, distal and symmetric deficit usually commencing peripherally. It may be acute, chronic, static, progressive, relapsing or toward recovery. They are motor, sensory, sensorimotor and autonomic. They are classified into demyelinating and axonal types, depending on principal predominant pathological process. Typically, there is widespread loss of tendon reflexes with distal weakness and distal sensory loss.

Damage to peripheral nerve may affect the nerve cell body (axon) or the myelin sheath (Schwann cell), leading to axonal or demyelinating neuropathies.

Clinical Features

- **Motor nerve involvement:** It produces features of a lower motor neuron lesion.
- **Sensory nerve involvement:** It features depend on the type of sensory nerve involved; small fiber neuropathies are usually painful, present with paresthesias. Large fiber neuropathies cause sensory ataxia.
- **Autonomic involvement:** It may cause postural hypotension, disturbance of sweating, cardiac rhythm, and gastrointestinal, bladder and sexual functions. Commonly autonomic involvement complicates other neuropathies.

Diagnosis: By clinical pattern, nerve conduction/EMG, nerve biopsy, usually sural or radial, and detection of systemic or genetic disease.

Mononeuropathies

Focal involvement of a single nerve and implies a local process and may be due to direct trauma, compression or entrapment, leprosy, vascular lesions, neoplastic compression or infiltration, etc.

Peripheral Nerve Compression and Entrapment

- Nerves are susceptible to mechanical compression at a certain location (e.g., ulnar nerve at the elbow, common peroneal nerve at the head of the fibula, radial nerve at spiral groove of humerus, lateral cutaneous nerve of thigh at inguinal ligament, posterior tibial at tarsal tunnel). Focal compression or entrapment is the common cause of a mononeuropathy.
- Entrapment occurs in relatively tight anatomical passages (e.g., the carpal tunnel). At the site of compression, focal demyelination and mild degeneration of distal axonal develops.
- Predisposing causes for entrapment neuropathies include diabetes, excess alcohol or toxins, or genetic syndromes. These are recognized mainly by clinical features and diagnosis is confirmed by nerve conduction studies.
- Usually recover once the primary cause is removed, either by avoiding the precipitation of activity or by surgical decompression.

Carpal Tunnel Syndrome

Q. Write a short essay/note on carpal tunnel syndrome and its causes.

- **Common mononeuropathy** due to **entrapment of median nerve** at the wrist.
- Carpal tunnel syndrome is usually not associated with any underlying disease. However, it may be seen in: hypothyroidism, 3rd trimester of pregnancy, rheumatoid disease, amyloidosis in dialysis patients, and acromegaly.
- **Clinical features: Nocturnal pain, paresthesia/tingling on palmar aspect of hand and/or forearm and fingers.** It is usually poorly localized and not confined to the anatomical sensory territory of the nerve. At later stages, weakness and wasting of thenar muscles develop.
- **Tinel's sign** (elicited by tapping the flexor aspect of the wrist: this causes tingling and pain) and **Phalen's test** positive. (In Phalen's, the symptoms are reproduced on passive maximal flexion of wrist).
- **Treatment: Wrist splint at night** or a **local steroid injection** in mild cases. In pregnancy, CTS is self-limiting and subsides during postpartum. Definitive treatment is **surgical decompression** of the carpal tunnel.

Mononeuropathy Multiplex

- Simultaneous/sequential damage to multiple noncontiguous nerves (peripheral or cranial nerves).
- **Causes:** Ischemia caused by vasculitis (e.g., Churg-Strauss), microangiopathy in diabetes mellitus. Less common causes include HIV and hepatitis C infection, granulomatous, amyloidosis, leukemic, or neoplastic infiltration, neurofibromatosis, Hansen's disease (leprosy), toxins, paraneoplastic, and sarcoidosis.
- **Clinical features:** Symptoms will depend on the specific nerves involved. Several nerves may be affected sequentially or simultaneously, e.g., ulnar, median, radial and lateral popliteal nerves. When multifocal neuropathy is symmetrical, it is difficulty distinguishing it from polyneuropathy.
- **Treatment:** Glucocorticoids, cytotoxic agents.

The causes of peripheral nerve disorders have been shown in **Table 15.53**.

TABLE 15.53: Causes of peripheral nerve disorders.

Causes of polyneuropathy	*Causes of mononeuropathy*	*Causes of mononeuritis multiplex*
Vitamin deficiencies: Thiamine, pyridoxine, vitamin B_{12}, vitamin E **Therapeutic drugs:** Amiodarone, antibiotics (dapsone, isoniazid, metronidazole, ethambutol), antiretroviral, chemotherapy (cisplatin, vincristine, thalidomide), phenytoin **Toxins:** Alcohol, nitrous oxide (recreational use) **Infections:** HIV, leprosy **Inflammatory:** Guillain-Barré syndrome, vasculitis (e.g., polyarteritis nodosa, granulomatosis with polyangiitis, SLE), paraneoplastic (antibody-mediated) **Systemic diseases:** Diabetes, renal failure **Malignancy:** Infiltration **Genetic conditions:** Charcot-Marie-Tooth disease (CMT), familial amyloid polyneuropathy, hereditary neuralgic amyotrophy **Others:** Paraproteinemias, amyloidosis	1. **Acute:** Sustained pressure, e.g., tourniquet 2. **Chronic:** Entrapment **Causes** (according to site of compression): 1. Carpal tunnel—median nerve 2. Cubital tunnel—ulnar nerve 3. Spiral groove of humerus—radial nerve 4. Inguinal ligament—lateral cutaneous of thigh (meralgia paresthetica) 5. Neck of fibula—common peroneal nerve 6. Flexor retinaculum (tarsal tunnel)—posterior tibial nerve **Entrapment neuropathies are commonly seen in:** ➢ Endocrinal (diabetes mellitus, myxedema, acromegaly) ➢ Amyloidosis ➢ Hereditary neuropathy susceptible to pressure palsy ➢ Pregnancy ➢ Arthritis (rheumatoid)	1. Leprosy (most common) 2. Diabetes mellitus 3. Vasculitis 4. Sarcoidosis 5. Amyloidosis 6. Malignancy 7. Neurofibromatosis 8. HIV infection 9. Idiopathic multifocal motor neuropathy

Polyneuropathies (Peripheral Neuropathy)

Q. Write a short essay/note on peripheral neuropathy and its causes/etiology.

Polyneuropathy is characterized by a "length dependent" pattern, occurring first in the longest peripheral nerves and affecting the distal lower limbs before the upper limbs. Sensory symptoms and signs occur in an ascending "glove and stocking" pattern. Types of peripheral neuropathy are presented in **Figure 15.33**.

Causes: Many diseases can produce polyneuropathy **(Table 15.53)**. However, the etiology is unknown in about 50% of cases.

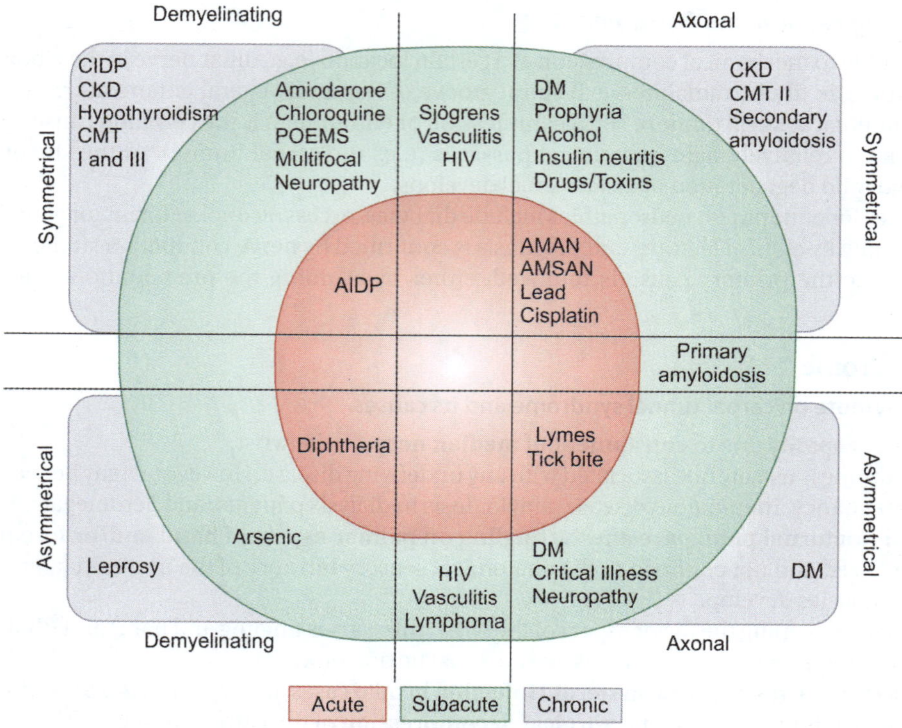

FIG. 15.33: Types of polyneuropathy.

Common causes of axonal and demyelinating chronic polyneuropathies are mentioned in **Table 15.54**.

TABLE 15.54: Common causes of axonal and demyelinating chronic polyneuropathies.

Axonal		*Demyelinating*
➢ Diabetes mellitus ➢ Alcohol ➢ Uremia ➢ Cirrhosis ➢ Amyloid ➢ Myxedema, acromegaly ➢ Paraneoplastic ➢ Deficiency states: Thiamine, pyridoxine, vitamin B_{12}, vitamin E	➢ Hereditary ➢ Infection ➢ Idiopathic ➢ Drugs and toxins: Amiodarone, antibiotics (dapsone, isoniazid, metronidazole, ethambutol), antiretrovirals, chemotherapy (cisplatin, vincristine, thalidomide), phenytoin	➢ Chronic inflammatory demyelinating polyradiculoneuropathy ➢ Multifocal motor neuropathy ➢ Paraprotein-associated demyelinating neuropathy ➢ Charcot–Marie–Tooth disease type I and type X

Q. What are causes of peripheral nerve thickening?

Causes of peripheral nerve thickening **(Box 15.42)**.

Box 15.42: Causes of peripheral nerve thickening.

- Leprosy
- Chronic inflammatory demyelinating polyneuropathy (CIDP)
- Amyloidosis
- Charcot–Marie–Tooth disease
- Neurofibromatosis
- Diabetes
- Acromegaly
- Refsum disease
- Idiopathic
- Dejerine–Sottas disease
- Relapsing Guillain–Barré syndrome

Approach to Neuropathy (Table 15.55)

TABLE 15.55: Types and causes of neuropathy.

What is the onset and temporal evolution? ➢ Acute (days to 4 weeks) ➢ Subacute (4–8 weeks) ➢ Chronic (>8 weeks)	
Acute onset	➢ Guillain–Barré syndrome ➢ Acute intermittent porphyria ➢ Critical illness polyneuropathy ➢ Thallium toxicity

Contd...

Contd...

Subacute onset	➢ Toxins or medications ➢ Nutritional deficiency ➢ Metabolic abnormality ➢ Paraneoplastic syndrome
Chronic	➢ Hereditary motor and sensory neuropathy (HMSN) ➢ Chronic inflammatory demyelinating polyneuropathy (CIDP) ➢ Chronic kidney disease (CKD)
Relapsing/remitting course	➢ Guillain–Barré syndrome ➢ CIDP ➢ HIV/AIDS ➢ Porphyria
What systems are involved? Motor (or) sensory (or) autonomic (or) mixed	
Motor symptoms	
Negative symptoms	***Positive symptoms***
➢ Weakness ➢ Wasting ➢ Loss of dexterity In the early stage, weakness in peripheral neuropathy is distal; however, early proximal weakness is a feature of demyelinating neuropathy and porphyric neuropathy.	➢ Cramps ➢ Tremors ➢ Fasciculations ➢ Spasms
Neuropathic disorders that may have only motors symptoms at presentation ➢ Motor neuron disease ➢ Lead intoxication ➢ Acute porphyria ➢ Guillain–Barré syndrome ➢ Hereditary motor neuropathy ➢ CIDP ➢ Diphtheria ➢ Brachial neuritis ➢ Diabetic lumbosacral plexus neuropathy	
Sensory symptoms	
Negative symptoms	***Positive symptoms***
Numbness, loss of sensation in hands and feet	Burning, pain, walking on cotton wool, band-like sensation on feet or trunk, stumbling, tingling, pins and needles
Large fiber neuropathy: Neuropathy of signs/ataxic neuropathy There are few symptoms (numbness, ataxia) but lots of signs (loss of vibration, joint position sense, diminished reflexes, Romberg's sign positive) Examples: ➢ Sjogren's syndrome ➢ Vitamin B_{12} neuropathy ➢ Cisplatin ➢ Pyridoxine neurotoxicity ➢ Friedreich's ataxia	**Small fiber neuropathy:** Neuropathy of symptoms Lots of symptoms (pain—burning, shock-like, stabbing, prickling, shooting, lancinating, allodynia, tight band-like pressure insensitive to heat and cold) but very few signs (loss of pain, temperature) Examples: ➢ Diabetes ➢ Amyloidosis ➢ Fabry's disease ➢ HIV ➢ Tangier's disease ➢ Hereditary sensory and autonomic neuropathy ➢ Sjogren's syndrome ➢ Chronic idiopathic small fiber sensory neuropathy
Small and large fiber neuropathy—pansensory—Global sensory loss Examples: ➢ Carcinomatous sensory neuropathy ➢ Hereditary sensory neuropathy ➢ Diabetic sensory neuropathy ➢ Vacor intoxication ➢ Xanthomatous neuropathy of primary biliary cirrhosis	
Peripheral neuropathies that are often associated with pain ➢ Cryptogenic sensory or sensorimotor neuropathy ➢ Diabetes mellitus ➢ Vasculitis ➢ Guillain–Barré syndrome ➢ Amyloidosis ➢ Toxic (arsenic, thallium) ➢ HIV related distal symmetrical polyneuropathy ➢ Fabry's disease	

Contd...

Contd...

Autonomic symptoms
Inquire if the patient has fainting spells or orthostatic light headedness, sweating abnormalities or any bowel, bladder, or sexual dysfunction Examples: **Acute** ➢ Pandysautonomia ➢ Botulism ➢ Porphyria ➢ Guillain–Barré syndrome ➢ Amiodarone ➢ Vincristine **Chronic** ➢ Amyloid ➢ Diabetes ➢ Sjogren's ➢ HSN-1 and HSN-3 ➢ Chagas ➢ Paraneoplastic

PATTENS OF NEUROPATHY

- **Pattern 1: Symmetric proximal and distal weakness with sensory loss**
  - Inflammatory demyelinating polyneuropathy (GBS and CIDP)
- **Pattern 2: Symmetric distal weakness with sensory loss**
  - Metabolic disorders, hereditary toxins, drugs
- **Pattern 3: Asymmetric distal weakness with sensory loss**
  - Multiple nerves—vasculitis
  - Single nerves/regions—compressive mononeuropathy and radiculopathy
- **Pattern 4: Asymmetric distal weakness without sensory loss**
  - Motor neuron disease—with upper motor neuron findings
  - Multifocal motor neuropathy—without upper motor neuron findings
- **Pattern 5: Asymmetric proximal and distal weakness with sensory loss**
  - Polyradiculopathy or plexopathy due to diabetes mellitus
  - Meningeal carcinomatosis
- **Pattern 6: Symmetric sensory loss without weakness**
  - Cryptogenic sensory polyneuropathy (CSPN), metabolic (diabetes and others) drugs, toxins
- **Pattern 7: Symmetric sensory loss and distal areflexia with upper motor neuron findings**
  - Vitamin B_{12} deficiency, HIV, hepatic disease
- **Pattern 8: A symmetric proprioceptive sensory loss without weakness**
  - Sensory neuronopathy (ganglionopathy)
- **Pattern 9: Autonomic symptoms and signs**
  - Neuropathies associated with autonomic dysfunction
- **Pattern 10: Syndrome of A/C ascending motor paralysis**
  - Guillain–Barré syndrome/acute idiopathic polyneuritis
  - Diphtheria
  - Porphyria
  - Triorthocresyl phosphate (TOCP) poisoning
  - Paraneoplastic
  - Post-vaccinial
- **Pattern 11: Syndrome of subacute sensory motor neuropathy**
  - Deficiency—alcoholic beriberi, pellagra, vitamin B_{12}
  - Toxins—arsenic, lead (Pb), mercury (Hg)
  - Drugs—nitrofurantoin, isoniazid (INH), dapsone, disulfiram, clioquinol
  - Uremic
  - Diabetes mellitus
  - Polyarteritis nodosa (PAN), sarcoidosis

Approach to a Patient with Neuropathy (Box 15.43)

Investigation of Peripheral Neuropathy

See **Table 15.56.**

Box 15.43: Approach to a patient with neuropathy.

Look for 6Ds

1. Distribution of the deficits
2. Duration
3. Deficits (which fibers are involved?)
4. Disease pathology (axonal or demyelinating or mixed)
5. Developmental or inherited neuropathy
6. Drug/toxin exposure

Treatment

- Depends on the underlying cause.
- Symptomatic treatment (more details refer diabetic neuropathy in Chapter 3).
- **Paresthesia:** Carbamazepine (300–1200 mg/day), amitriptyline (25–50 mg/day) or aspirin (350–1200 mg/day) pregabalin, gabapentin, duloxetine.
- **Weakness:** Physiotherapy.

TABLE 15.56: Investigation of peripheral neuropathy.

Routine tests	*Special tests*
Blood ➢ Complete blood count and peripheral smear ➢ Erythrocyte sedimentation rate ➢ C-reactive protein **Biochemical tests** ➢ Fasting blood glucose, LDH ➢ Serum protein electrophoresis ➢ Vitamin B_{12}, folate ➢ Renal function tests, liver function tests **Serology** ➢ ANA, ANCA, HIV testing **Others** ➢ Chest X-ray, USG abdomen	➢ Nerve conduction studies ➢ Vitamins E and A ➢ Nerve biopsy ➢ CSF examination ➢ Serum ACE (angiotensin-converting enzyme) ➢ Serum amyloid ➢ Genetic testing

Guillain–Barré Syndrome and other Immune-mediated Neuropathies

Q. Write a short essay/note on Guillain–Barré syndrome and diagnostic criteria for Guillain–Barré syndrome.

Guillain–Barré syndrome is a **heterogeneous group of immune-mediated conditions.**

Guillain–Barré syndrome is the most common acute, severe fulminant polyradiculopathy/polyneuropathy.

- Usually demyelinating or rarely axonal.
- Often postinfectious, postvaccinal basis
- Monophasic does not recur.

Subtypes of Guillain–Barré Syndrome (Table 15.57)

Q. What are the variants of Guillain–Barré syndrome?

TABLE 15.57: Variants of Guillain–Barré syndrome.

Common variants	*Less common variants*
➢ Acute motor and sensory axonal neuropathy (AMSAN) ➢ Acute motor axonal neuropathy (AMAN) ➢ Miller Fisher syndrome (MFS) ➢ Pure motor variants ➢ Pure sensory variants ➢ Pure dysautonomia variant ➢ Pharyngeal-cervical-brachial variant ➢ Paraparetic variant (Ropper variant)	➢ Acral paresthesias with diminished reflexes in either arms or legs ➢ Facial diplegia or abducens palsies with distal paresthesias ➢ Isolated postinfectious ophthalmoplegia ➢ Bilateral foot drop with upper limb paresthesias ➢ Acute ataxia without ophthalmoplegia ➢ Bickerstaff's brainstem encephalitis (BBE)

Etiology

Antecedent causes

- Majority of patients (70%) have preceding acute, influenza-like illness or GI infection. Infections preceding GBS may be due to ***Campylobacter jejuni,*** cytomegalovirus, EBV, herpes virus, CMV and ***Mycoplasma pneumoniae,*** or prior recent vaccination (e.g., for swine flu, influenza, rabies (old types).
- Frequently develop in patients with lymphoma, HIV seropositive, and SLE.

Immunopathogenesis

- Guillain–Barré syndrome is **an acute-onset immune-mediated demyelinating neuropathy.** Autoimmune basis for AIDP (GBS) and other subtypes. Both cellular and humoral immune mechanism causes damage. Immune response to self-antigen, infection (mentioned above under "Antecedent causes"), or vaccine induce antibody responses. Molecular mimicry, i.e., sharing of homologous epitopes between microorganism liposaccharides and nerve gangliosides (e.g., GM1), misdirect the antibodies against host peripheral nerves.
- Antiganglioside antibodies mostly to GM1 common in GBS (20–50%) and anti-GQ1b IgG antibodies seen in Miller Fisher syndrome (MFS) (>90%).

Clinical Features

- Hallmark is an **acute/rapid onset of paralysis** (predominantly motor paralysis with/without sensory) **evolving over days or weeks** with **loss of deep tendon reflexes/jerk (areflexia).**
- **Motor paralysis** predominant. Weakness beginning in the distal limbs (from lower to upper limbs) that rapidly ascends to affect proximal muscle function **("ascending paralysis").** It is more marked in legs than arms and proximally than distally. Pain in the low back, neck, and shoulder, in 50% and is often occur early. The weakness progresses proximally over few days to a maximum of 4 weeks.
- **Sensory involvement is minimal** and may precede muscle weakness. It presents as distal paresthesia or loss of pain sensation.
- Facial and respiratory muscle develops in **20–30% of cases requiring ventilatory support.**
- **No fever or constitutional symptoms** at the onset of weakness.
- Bladder dysfunction in late and severe cases.
- Clinical worsening in 4 weeks reaching a plateau and no further progression.
- Autonomic disturbances common like fluctuation of BP, postural hypotension, cardiac dysrhythmias.
- Pain—common symptom—acute/deep aching pain in weak muscles. It is self-limited.
- Physical examination shows diffuse weakness with loss of reflexes.
- Miller Fisher syndrome: It presents with ophthalmoplegia, ataxia and areflexia. Often preceded by diarrhea due to *Campylobacter jejuni* infection. Bickerstaff's brainstem encephalitis (BBE) is characterized by alteration in consciousness, paradoxical hyperreflexia, ataxia, and ophthalmoparesis.

Asbury and Cornblath criteria for GBS are presented in **Box 15.44.**

Investigations/Diagnosis

- **CSF findings:** Develop after 1 week of illness:
  - Raised protein (100–1,000 mg/dL), normal sugar, little or no pleocytosis. Cell count generally <10 cells/mm^3; rarely may be up to 50 cells/mm^3, but never above that. This is called as **albumin-cytological dissociation.**
  - CSF pleocytosis (up to 50 cells) is common in patients who have GBS and concurrent HIV infection.
- **Electrodiagnostic study:** Nerve conduction studies:
  - In mild/early stage: Normal
  - In demyelination: Prolonged distal latencies, slow conduction, velocity, conduction block, prolonged F wave latencies. Absent H-reflex.
  - In primary axonal: Reduced amplitude of compound action potential without slow conduction.
- **Antibodies:**
  - Antibodies against GQ1b, a ganglioside component of nerve are found in about 25%, usually the motor axonal form.
  - Miller Fisher syndrome: Antibodies against GQ1b (ganglioside) have 90% sensitivity.

Differential Diagnosis

Exclusion of other causes of an acute neuromuscular paralysis: For example, poliomyelitis, botulism, diphtheria, localized spinal cord syndromes or myasthenia gravis, vasculitis, toxins (organophosphates, lead), diphtheria, porphyria, spinal cord or cauda equina syndrome.

Box 15.44: Asbury and Cornblath criteria for Guillain–Barré syndrome (GBS).

Required features
- Progressive weakness in both arms and legs
- Areflexia (or hyporeflexia)

Features supportive of diagnosis
- Progression of symptoms over days to 4 weeks
- Relative symmetry
- Mild sensory signs or symptoms
- Cranial nerve involvement, especially bilateral facial weakness
- Recovery beginning 2–4 weeks after progression ceases
- Autonomic dysfunction
- Absence of fever at onset
- Typical CSF (albuminocytologic dissociation)
- EMG/nerve conduction studies (characteristic signs of a demyelinating process in the peripheral nerves)

Features casting doubt on the diagnosis
- Asymmetrical weakness
- Persistent bladder and bowel dysfunction
- Bladder or bowel dysfunction at onset
- >50 mononuclear leukocytes/mm^3 or presence of polymorphonuclear leukocytes in CSF
- Distinct sensory level

Features that rule out the diagnosis
- Hexacarbon abuse
- Abnormal porphyrin metabolism
- Recent diphtheria infection
- Lead intoxication
- Other similar conditions: poliomyelitis, botulism, hysterical paralysis, toxic neuropathy

Q. Write a short essay/note on principles of management of Guillain–Barré syndrome.

Treatment
- Early treatment, each day counts, >2 weeks of 1st motor symptoms immunotherapy not effective.
- Initiative with high dose IVIg/plasmapheresis/combination.
- **Intravenous immunoglobulin** administration has fewer side effects (0.4 g/kg daily infusion) for 5 days. GBS autoantibodies are neutralized by antibodies in IVIg. Patients should be screened for IgA deficiency because severe allergic reactions due to IgG antibodies may develop in patient with congenital IgA deficiency.
- **Plasma exchange:** 50 mL/kg, on 5 separate occasions over 1–2 weeks.
- Glucocorticoid no role.
- Full recovery in 55–69% by 1 year.
- **Worsening case:** Monitoring in intensive care unit (ICU)—blood pressure, cardiac, and nutrition. Maintenance of airway and breathing. Ventilatory support may be needed. **20-30-40 rule:** vital capacity <20 mL/kg, negative inspiratory pressure < –30 cm H_2O, maximum expiratory pressure <40 cm H_2O is an indication for intubation.
- **Supportive measures:** Deep vein thrombosis prophylaxis, tracheostomy, chest physiotherapy, skin care, bed sore, joint physiotherapy daily reassurance.

Box 15.45: Indications for plasma exchange therapy.

- Glomerulonephritis—anti-GBM disease
- Guillain–Barré syndrome
- Myasthenia gravis
- Autoimmune encephalitis
- Prerenal transplant
- Systemic vasculitis not responding adequately to immunosuppressive therapy
- Thrombotic thrombocytopenic purpura

Plasma Exchange (Plasmapheresis)

Q. Write a short note on plasma exchange (PE) therapy.

Plasma exchange (also called plasmapheresis): Plasmapheresis involves the removal of small amounts of plasma (<15% of the patient's total blood volume). It can reduce the amount of abnormal protein in the blood. Indications for PE therapy are listed in **Box 15.45**.

NEUROMUSCULAR JUNCTION DISORDERS

Myasthenia Gravis

Q. Discuss the etiology, clinical features, investigations, diagnosis, and management/treatment of myasthenia gravis (MG).

- Myasthenia gravis is an autoimmune neuromuscular junction disorder.
- Weakness and fatigue of skeletal (preferentially ocular, facial and bulbar) muscles.

Pathophysiology (Fig. 15.34)

Pathogenesis of Myasthenia Gravis

Myasthenia gravis is an autoimmune disease.

- **Antibodies:**
  - **Anti-AChR antibodies:** It is detected in about 80 to 85% of patients.
  - **Anti-MuSK antibodies:** A second group of autoantibodies against muscle-specific receptor tyrosine kinase (anti-MuSK) antibodies have been found in anti-AChR antibody negative (about 15–20%) patients.
- **Changes in thymus:** Thymus is abnormal in ~75% of patients with MG. In ~65% the thymus is "hyperplastic", with active germinal centers. In 10% of patients have thymic tumors (neoplastic). Muscle like cells (myoid cell) within thymus, bearing AChRs on their surface may serve as autoantigen and trigger immune response.

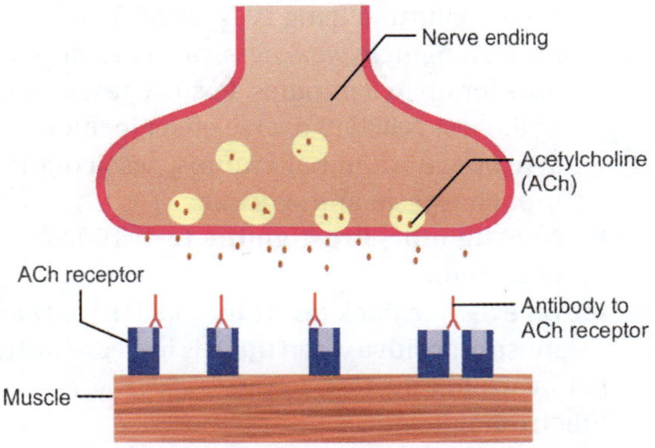

FIG. 15.34: Pathogenesis of myasthenia gravis. Antireceptor antibodies may inhibit/disturb the normal function of receptors. Autoantibodies to the acetylcholine receptor on skeletal muscle cells produce disease by blocking neuromuscular transmission and causing progressive muscle weakness.

Coexisting Autoimmune Diseases

See **Box 15.46.**

Box 15.46: Coexisting autoimmune diseases in myasthenia gravis.

- Hashimoto's thyroiditis/thyrotoxicosis (in 5–10%)
- Rheumatoid arthritis
- Pernicious anemia
- Scleroderma
- Lupus erythematosus

Clinical Features

- **Age and gender:** MG is common in women than in men (2:1). The disease presents with two peaks of incidence, below or above the age of 50, termed early-onset MG (EOMG) and late-onset MG (LOMG), respectively.
- **Cardinal feature: Fluctuating weakness (that worsens with exertion** and decrease with rest/sleep) **and fatigability of muscles**. Increase with exercise.
- **Muscle affected: Diplopia and ptosis** due to involvement of extraocular muscles. Show more focal muscle involvement (neck, shoulder, facial, jaw, respiratory, and bulbar muscles).
- **Respiratory weakness:** Respiratory muscles involvement may become so severe as to require respiratory assistance. Patient is said to be in due to diaphragmatic and intercostal muscle weakness. Aspiration may occur if the cough is ineffectual.
- **Ocular MG** when weakness is exclusive to the eyelids and extraocular muscles, and **generalized MG** when weakness extends beyond these ocular muscles.
- No sensory signs or signs of involvement of the CNS.
- **Aggravating factors:** Exertion, hot climate, infection, emotion, pregnancy, menstruation, drugs (amino glycoside phenytoin). A temporary increase in weakness may follow **vaccination, menstruation and exposure to extremes of temperature.**

Course: Variable, exacerbation and remission in early years. Remission is incomplete and temporary. Most cases have a protracted, lifelong course. Exacerbations are usually unpredictable and unprovoked.

Myasthenic Crisis

- A **rapid and severe deterioration of myasthenia** is called **"myasthenic crisis"** can bring patient to the brink of respiratory failure and **quadriparesis** in hours.
- A respiratory infection or a sedative medication with NM (neuromuscular) block may be the reason.
- It can develop at any time after the diagnosis of myasthenia.
- Anticipate if patient is restless, anxious with diaphoresis and develops tremor.
- **Require respiratory support.**

Diagnosis

- Diagnosis is based on the basis of **clinical history, physical findings** and **two-positive tests** (demonstration of autoantibodies and electrophysiological studies).
- **Serological tests:** Antibodies against AChR or MuSK.
- **Pharmacological tests:**
  - **Anticholinesterase test:** Drugs inhibiting AChE allow ACh to interact repeatedly with limited number of AChRs producing strength improvement in myasthenic muscles.
  - **Edrophonium test (Tensilon test):** Edrophonium is a rapidly acting acetylcholinesterase inhibitor. Onset of action is rapid (30 seconds) and lasts for short duration (5 minutes). It reverses of muscular weakness dramatically in myasthenia. Test dose (2 mg IV) is given to check for reactions. If there is definite improvement drop further test. If

negative further 8 mg IV is given. When the test is positive, it produces substantial improvement in weakness, ptosis, diplopia, nasal voice, etc., within 30 seconds and lasts for up to 5 minutes. Positive test is highly suggestive of MG and the sensitivity of the test is 80%. Adverse effect include nausea, diarrhea, salivation, bradycardia, syncope, abdominal cramps, fasciculation (treated with atropine—0.6 mg IV) bronchospasm and syncope.
    - **Neostigmine/Prostigmine test:** 15 mg oral neostigmine, long acting and better evaluation.
- **Ice on eyes/ice pack test (Fig. 15.35):** Apply an ice pack on eye for 3 to 5 minutes. The response is positive when there is increase in at least 2 mm of the palpebral fissure from before to after the test.
- **Electrodiagnostic:**
    - **Repeated nerve stimulation (RNS) test:** Electric shock at 2–3 second given to appropriate nerve and corresponding muscle action potential measured. In normal individuals the amplitude of the evoked muscle action potentials does not change at these rates of stimulation. However, in myasthenic patients there is a rapid reduction of >10–15% in the amplitude of the evoked responses during repetitive stimulation.
    - **Single fiber electromyogram:** Most (95%) sensitive.
- **Other tests:**
    - CT, MRI, and X-ray: to exclude thymoma.
    - CBC, ESR, RA factor, thyroid function test.
    - Pulmonary function test, fasting blood sugar, Mantoux test, ANA, etc., to exclude other diseases.
    - Screening for associated autoimmune disorders.

FIG. 15.35: Ice pack test.

Lambert–Eaton myasthenic syndrome (LEMS) differs from MG in that in LEMS antibodies are against presynaptic calcium channels, deep tendon reflexes are absent and autonomic dysfunction in present and the weakness improves with activity in LEMS. It is most commonly associated with small cell carcinoma of lung and the treatment is with aminopyridines.

Q. Write a short note on drugs used in myasthenia gravis.

Treatment

Goals: To increase the activity of acetylcholine on the remaining receptors at the NMJ. Stop the antibody mediated damage at the NMJ.

1. **Oral anticholinesterases:** Help weakness but do not change the natural history of myasthenia.
    - **Pyridostigmine:** Prolongs acetylcholine action by inhibiting cholinesterase. Onset of action is within 15–30 minutes and lasts for 3–4 hours. Dose 30–60 mg/3–4 times daily. Cholinergic crisis characterized by pallor, perspiration, pupillary constriction, paralysis, fasciculation and excessive salivation can be seen with drug over dosage. Muscarinic effects (e.g., colic and diarrhea) are treated with oral atropine/propantheline (antimuscarinic).
2. **Thymectomy**
    - **Indications:** It is an expert surgical procedure that should be carried out in (1) all patients with generalized MG between the ages of puberty and at least 55 years. (2) It may be required for thymoma to prevent spread and treat MG.
    - **Advantages:** Long-term benefit, improves prognosis, negligible medication.
3. **Immunosuppression**
    - Effective in all. Choice is guided by benefit, risk and urgency. These are used in patients who do not respond to pyridostigmine or who develop relapse on treatment.
    - For immediate: IVIg or plasmapheresis.
    - For intermediate: Glucocorticoids, cyclosporine, tacrolimus for 1–3 months.
    - For long-term: Azathioprine, mycophenolate mofetil (less commonly used) for months/years.
    - For refractory: High dose of cyclophosphamide.

The differences between myasthenic crisis and cholinergic crisis are presented in **Table 15.58**.

Treatment of myasthenic crisis

- Exacerbation of weakness due to diaphragm and intercostal involvement.
- Treat in ICU setup.
- Cause: Infection (most common), cholinergic crisis due to excess anticholinesterase dose.
- Respiratory assistance (preferably noninvasive, using BIPAP).
- Pulmonary physiotherapy.
- Plasmapheresis or IVIg.
- Stop anticholinesterase if using.

TABLE 15.58: Differences between myasthenic crisis and cholinergic crisis.

Myasthenic crisis	*Cholinergic crisis*
➤ Due to disease worsening	➤ Due to drug overdose
➤ Respiratory distress	➤ Abdominal cramps
➤ Increased pulse and blood pressure	➤ Diarrhea
➤ Poor cough	➤ Nausea and vomiting
➤ Mydriasis	➤ Excessive secretions
➤ Dysphagia	➤ Miosis
➤ Weakness	➤ Fasciculations
➤ Improve with edrophonium	➤ Weakness
➤ Treatment: Ventilatory support plus neostigmine	➤ Worsens with edrophonium
	➤ Treatment: Ventilatory support plus atropine

DISEASES OF MUSCLE

- Muscle disease is rare and may be hereditary or acquired.
- Hereditary muscle diseases include the muscular dystrophies, muscle channelopathies, metabolic myopathies (including mitochondrial diseases) and congenital myopathies.
- Skeletal muscle disease or myopathies are disorders with structural changes or functional impairment of muscle.

Muscular Dystrophies

Muscular dystrophies (hereditary myopathies) refer to a group of inherited myopathies/disorders characterized by progressive muscle weakness and wasting (due to destruction of muscle) and may be associated with cardiac and/or respiratory involvement.

Q. Write a short note on muscular dystrophies or hereditary myopathies.

Muscular dystrophy is subdivided by their mode of inheritance, age at onset, distribution of involved muscles, rate of progression, and prognosis **(Table 15.59)**.

Duchenne Muscular Dystrophy

Q. Write a short essay on Duchenne muscular dystrophy.

- Most common form of muscular dystrophy.
- Caused by a mutation of the gene responsible for producing dystrophin.
- Shows X-linked recessive inheritance and affects predominantly males.
- Duchenne dystrophy is present at birth, but the disorder usually becomes apparent between ages 3 and 5, by age 12, most patients are wheelchair dependent.
- Muscle selectively involved in order of appearance of weakness is iliopsoas, quadriceps, Gluteus-Pretibial muscles, muscles of pectoral girdle, muscles of leg and forearm (at the end).
- **Clinical features:** Use of **Gower's maneuver** while getting up for the floor, toe walking due to foot drop with associated lordotic posture and pseudo hypertrophy of the calves. Cardiomyopathy [dialated cardiomyopathy (DCM)] and mental impairment are associated features. But CHF is uncommon. Mental retardation is seen.
- **Investigations**
  - Creatine phosphokinase (CPK) levels are invariably elevated to between 20 and 100 times normal.
  - Electromyography: Features typical of myopathy.
  - Muscle biopsy: Definitive diagnosis can be established on the basis of dystrophin deficiency I in biopsied muscle tissue.
  - Gold standard: It is genetic testing.

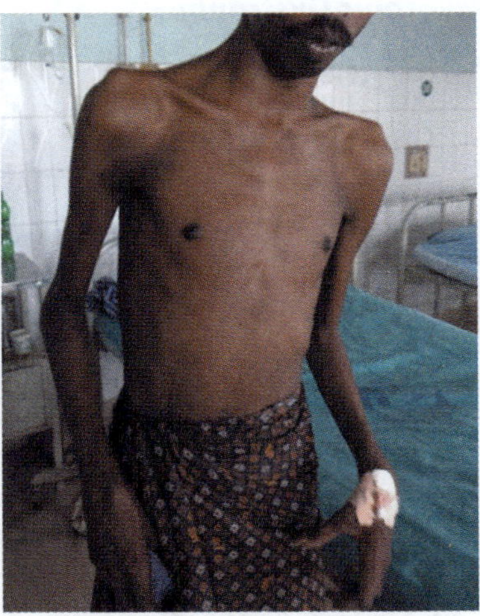

FIG. 15.36: Facioscapulohumeral dystrophy.

TABLE 15.59: Various subtypes and its features of muscular dystrophies.

Type and mode of inheritance	*Defective gene/protein*	*Onset age*	*Clinical features*
Duchenne's-XR	Dystrophin	Before 5 years	Progressive weakness of girdle muscles unable to walk after age 12, progressive kyphoscoliosis, respiratory failure in the 2nd and 3rd decades
Becker's-XR	Dystrophin	Early childhood to adult	Progressive weakness of girdle muscles, able to walk after age 15, respiratory failure may develop by 4th decade
Limb-girdle-AD/AR	Several	Early childhood to early adult	Slow progressive weakness of shoulder and hip girdle muscles
Emery–Dreifuss-XR/AD	Emerin/Lamins	Childhood to adult	Elbow contractures, humeral and peroneal weakness
Dystrophia myotonica (DM1-DM2)-AD DM1- Steinert disease DM2- Ricker syndrome	DMI: Expansion CTG repeat DM2: Expansion CCTG repeat	Childhood to adult, may be infancy if mother is affected (DM1 only)	Slowly progressive weakness of face, shoulder girdle, and foot dorsiflexion preferential proximal weakness in
Facioscapulohumeral-AD **(Fig. 15.36)**		Childhood to adult	Slowly progressive weakness of face, shoulder girdle, and foot dorsiflexion
Oculopharyngeal-AD	Expansion poly-A RNA-binding protein	5th to 6th decade	Slowly progressive weakness of extraocular, pharyngeal, and limb muscles

Becker Muscular Dystrophy

- X-linked disorder, results from defects of the same gene responsible for Duchenne dystrophy.
- Pattern of muscle wasting closely resembles that seen in Duchenne.
- It is a less severe form of disease and much less frequent than Duchenne.
- **Clinical features:** Becker patients ambulate beyond age 15, while patients with Duchenne dystrophy are typically in a wheelchair by the age of 12; allowing for a clinical distinction between Becker and Duchenne dystrophy. Cardiac involvement occurs in Becker dystrophy and may result in heart failure. Mental impairment is uncommon.
- **Investigations:** Serum CK measurement, EMG and muscle biopsy closely resemble those in Duchenne dystrophy.

Limb-Girdle Muscular Dystrophy

- Most are progressive and affect primarily the pelvic and shoulder girdle muscles. Inheritances can AR or AD and it is due to defect of sarcoglycan.
- **Clinical features:** Respiratory insufficiency from diaphragm weakness may occur. In some patients, cardiac involvement results in CHF or arrhythmias, occasional patients present with a cardiomyopathy. Intellectual function remains normal.
- **Investigations:** An elevated serum CK level, myopathic EMG findings, and muscle biopsy features indicative of myopathy.

Myotonic Dystrophy

- It is an autosomal dominant disorder and is the most common adult muscular dystrophy.
- **Clinical features:** Frontal baldness, cataracts (Christmas tree cataract), mental impairment, insulin resistance and gonadal atrophy. Hatchet like face, swan neck deformity is seen. Involvement of distal more than proximal, facial muscles and handgrip myotonia are pathognomonic features. Cardiac disturbances occur in most patients with myotonic dystrophy. Disturbances in conduction system are common. Complete heart block and sudden death may occur. Mitral valve prolapse also occurs commonly in myotonic dystrophy patients. Myotonia may improve with phenytoin, mexiletine, and quinidine.

Endocrine Myopathies

Causes of endocrine myopathies are listed in **Box 15.47**.

Box 15.47: Causes of endocrine myopathies.

- **Thyroid disorders:** Hypothyroidism, hyperthyroidism
- **Parathyroid disorders:** Hyperparathyroidism, hypoparathyroid—overt myopathy
- **Adrenal disorders:** Glucocorticoid myopathy (endogenous/exogenous) most common, Cushingoid, adrenal insufficiency, primary hyperaldosteronism (Conn's disease)
- **Vitamin deficiency:** Vitamin E, vitamin D

Q. Write a short note on causes of endocrine myopathies.

Causes of high creatinine phosphokinase **(Box 15.48)**.

Box 15.48: Causes of high creatinine phosphokinase.

- Brain injury or stroke
- Convulsions
- Delirium tremens
- Dermatomyositis or polymyositis
- Myocarditis
- Muscular dystrophies
- Myopathy
- Rhabdomyolysis
- Pulmonary and myocardial infarction
- Electric shock

Q. List the causes of high creatinine phosphokinase.

DISORDERS OF CEREBELLAR FUNCTION

- Cerebellum is an infratentorial structure in the posterior cranial fossa, attached to the brainstem by the superior, middle and inferior peduncles. The cerebellum is made up of two hemispheres separated by a midline vermis. There are three lobes anterior, posterior, and flocculonodular lobe.
- Midline lesions can produce severe gait and truncal ataxia.
- Cerebellar hemisphere lesions can produce classic ipsilateral limb ataxia (intention tremor, past pointing, and mild hypotonia).

Ataxia

Ataxia may be the result of cerebellar lesion or due to a combination of cerebellar and extracerebellar lesions.

Classification of Ataxia

See **Box 15.49.**

Box 15.49: Classification of ataxia.

Acquired or sporadic ataxias

- **Vascular:** Stroke (infarction, hemorrhage), AV malformations
- **Infectious/postinfectious diseases:** Acute cerebellitis, cerebellar abscess, postinfectious encephalomyelitis, HIV, chickenpox
- **Toxin-induced ataxias:** Alcohol, drugs (antiepileptic agents, lithium, antineoplastics, cyclosporine, metronidazole), heavy metals (mercury), 5-fluorouracil, cytosine arabinoside
- **Structural and neoplastic causes:** Gliomas, ependymoma, cerebellar tumor, meningioma, metastatic disease
- **Immune-mediated:** Multiple sclerosis, cerebellar ataxia with anti-glutamic acid decarboxylase (GAD) antibodies, paraneoplastic syndrome (small cell lung cancer, breast or ovarian cancer, and lymphoma), gluten ataxia
- **Deficiency:** Hypothyroidism, vitamin B1, vitamin B12, and vitamin E

Genetic causes

- Autosomal recessive: Friedreich's ataxia
- Autosomal dominant: Spinocerebellar ataxia

Symmetrical Cerebellar Ataxias

See **Table 15.60.**

Asymmetrical Cerebellar Ataxias

See **Table 15.61.**

Treatable Causes of Ataxia

See Box 15.50.

Clinical Features of Cerebellar Lesions

Q. Write a short note on cerebellar signs.

Cerebellar Ataxia

Q. Write a short note on cerebellar ataxia.

Lesions of the midline vermis of the cerebellum cause truncal ataxia, while lesions of the cerebellar hemispheres cause limb ataxia of the ipsilateral side.

1. **Gait ataxia**
   - Patients will tend to stand with feet well apart and are often frightened to stand.
   - Patients tend to reel to the side unilateral lesion or from side to side if central or bilateral (drunken gait) (even if supported).
   - Walking along a line of the floor (tandem gait) demonstrates minor degrees of gait ataxia.
   - Instability may increase if eyes are closed but patients do not fall. This is not a true positive Romberg's test (true positive Romberg's test is present when there is impaired joint proprioception/posterior column involvement is known as sensory ataxia).

TABLE 15.60: Types of symmetrical cerebellar ataxias.

Acute	Subacute	Chronic
➢ Drugs: Phenytoin, phenobarbitone, lithium, chemotherapeutic agents ➢ Alcohol ➢ Infectious: Acute viral cerebellitis, postinfectious ➢ Toxins: Toluene, glue, gasoline, methyl mercury	➢ Alcohol, or Nutritional (B_1, B_{12}) ➢ Paraneoplastic ➢ Antigliadin or anti-GAD antibody ➢ Prion diseases	➢ Multiple system atrophy-cerebellar type C (MSA-C) ➢ Hypothyroidism ➢ Phenytoin toxicity

TABLE 15.61: Types of asymmetrical cerebellar ataxias.

Acute	Subacute	Chronic
➢ Vascular: Cerebellar infarction or hemorrhage, subdural hematoma ➢ Infectious: Abscess	➢ Neoplastic: Glioma, metastases, lymphoma ➢ Demyelination: MS ➢ HIV related: Progressive multifocal leukoencephalopathy	➢ Congenital lesions: Arnold–Chiari malformation, Dandy–Walker syndrome

Box 15.50: Treatable causes of ataxia.

- Hypothyroidism
- Ataxia with vitamin E deficiency (AVED)
- Vitamin B_{12} deficiency
- Wilson's disease
- Ataxia with anti-gliadin antibodies and gluten senstive enteropathy
- Ataxia due to malabsorption syndromes
- Lyme disease
- Mitochondrial encephalomyopathies, aminoacidopathies, leukodystrophies, and urea cycle abnormalities

Q. Write a short note on Romberg's sign/test

- **Romberg's test is a test for sensory ataxia.**
- **Romberg's test/sign:** Patient stands upright with the feet together (touching each other) and eyes closed. When there is proprioceptive or vestibular deficit, balance is impaired only when eyes are closed, and the patient may fall if not caught. Minimal lesions can be demonstrated by asking the patient to stand on his toes with eyes closed.
- **Principle of Romberg's test:** It is based on the principle that an individual requires at least two of the three following senses to maintain balance while standing:
  - Proprioception (the ability to know one's body in space)
  - Vestibular function (the ability to know one's head position in space); and
  - Vision [which can be used to monitor (and adjust for) changes in body position].

2. **Truncal ataxia**
   - Patients cannot sit or stand unsupported and tend to fall backward.
   - It is caused by a midline cerebellar lesion, or may be a feature of post-chickenpox cerebellar syndrome.
   - Truncal tremor may be evident—constant jerking of trunk and head (titubation).
   - Lesions of the cerebellar hemisphere cause ipsilateral limb signs.
   - The outstretched arm tends to be held hyper pronated at rest and at a slightly higher level than unaffected side **(Riddoch's sign)** and rebounds upward if gently pressed downward and then suddenly released by the examiner.
   - Finger-nose and heel-knee-shin tests will demonstrate even mild limb ataxia, with terminal intention tremor and dysmetria (past pointing).
   - Limb rebound can be demonstrated by gently pushing down on outstretched arms and then suddenly releasing, causing the arm on the affected side suddenly to fly upward.
   - Pendular knee jerks and hypotonia present.
3. **Other signs** produced by cerebellar lesions/diseases
   - **Cerebellar dysarthria:** Spluttering staccato speech. Scanning dysarthria is a jerky and explosive speech with separated syllables may be demonstrated by asking the patient to repeat baby hippopotamus!
   - **Dyssynergia:** It is difficulty in carrying out complex movements. This results in breaking of an act into its components.
   - **Macrographia:** Writing may be larger than normal (contrast with micrographia of Parkinson's disease).

- **Rapid alternating movements:** Inaccuracies in rapidly repeated movements (dysdiadochokinesia). This is demonstrated by getting the patient to tap back of their own hand repeatedly with the other hand, or to tap their foot on the floor.
- **Tremor:** Unilateral or bilateral intention tremor, or a truncal tremor.
- **Nystagmus:** Coarse nystagmus, worse, on looking to the side of lesion with fast component toward the affected side.
- **Pendular knee jerk:** The reflexes are less brisk and slower in rise and fall. This produces pendular jerk at the knee. It produces three on more swings at the knee when the knee reflex is elicited with patient in sitting posture and the legs hanging from bedside.
- **Nausea and vomiting:** Sudden vomiting (without warning) after a positional change, without preceding nausea, is suggestive of a posterior fossa lesion.

Mnemonic for cerebellar signs **(Box 15.51)**.

Box 15.51: Mnemonic for cerebellar signs—DANISH.

- **D**ysdiadochokinesia and **D**ysmetria
- **A**taxia
- **N**ystagmus
- **I**ntention tremor
- **S**lurred speech
- **H**ypotonia

Hereditary Cerebellar Ataxia—Friedreich's Ataxia

- Most common form of inherited ataxia. Most common form degenerative ataxia caused by unstable trinucleotide GAA expansion in chromosome located on 9q. The protein involved is frataxin.
- It affects spinal cord—dorsal column, spinocerebellar tract, and pyramidal tract. There is also loss of dorsal root ganglion cells with depletion of large myelinated fibers in peripheral nerves.
- Age of onset usually between 8 and 16 years.

Clinical Features

- Progressive ataxia of gait (due to spinocerebellar tract involvement).
- Lower limb areflexia and later generalized areflexia.
- Leg weakness and extensor plantar responses (due to pyramidal tract involvement).
- Reduced vibration and joint position sense in lower limbs. It is due to involvement of dorsal column.
- Sensory axonal neuropathy detected on nerve conduction test.
- Other features: Dysarthria, scoliosis **(Fig. 15.37)**, nystagmus, optic atrophy, deafness, diabetes, pes cavus and cardiomyopathy.

Causes of extensor plantar response with absent ankle jerk are listed in **Box 15.52**.

Investigations

- **Nerve conduction study (NCS):** Normal conduction velocity but small or absent sensory nerve action potential (SNAP)
- CT and MRI normal cerebellar anatomy, cervical atrophy.
- DNA polymerase reaction to detect GAA expansion.

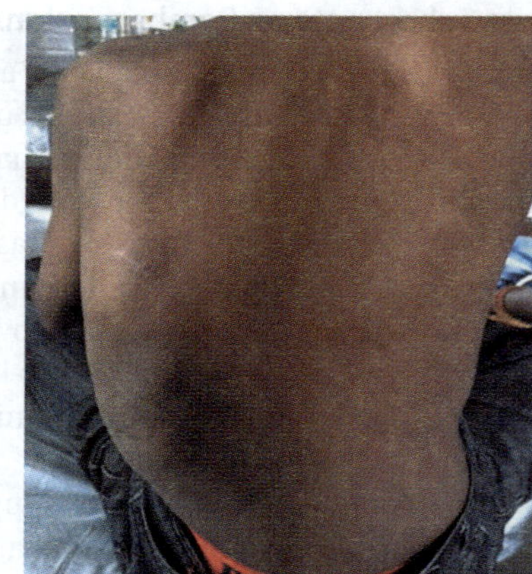

FIG. 15.37: Patient with scoliosis due to Friedreich's ataxia.

Treatment

No definite treatment, physiotherapy and occupational therapy, spasticity is treated with baclofen, orthopedic advice and surgery.

Spinocerebellar Ataxia (Late-Onset Hereditary Ataxia)

Q. Write a short note on the clinical features of spinocerebellar ataxias.

- Spinocerebellar ataxia (autosomal dominant cerebellar ataxia/ADCA) is an autosomal dominant disease that presents with slowly progressive cerebellar symptoms. Sometimes with associated optic atrophy, ophthalmoplegia, pyramidal and extrapyramidal structure.
- MRI mostly shows olivopontocerebellar atrophy.

Box 15.52: Causes of extensor plantar response with absent ankle jerk.

- Friedreich's ataxia
- Motor neuron disease (ALS)
- Taboparesis in neurosyphilis
- HIV myeloneuropathy
- Subacute combined degeneration of cord (vitamin B_{12} deficiency)
- Hypocupremic myelopathy
- Conus-cauda lesion

Sensory ataxia

It is due to severe sensory neuropathy, ganglionopathy or lesions of the posterior column of the spinal cord, e.g., Sjogren's syndrome, cisplatin, CIDP, paraneoplastic disorders, SACD, tabes dorsalis, Miller Fischer syndrome, celiac disease

- Ataxia more at night or while walking through narrow passages (coffee plantations)
- A history of falling into the sink or imbalance when splashing water on the face (wash-basin sign), passing a towel over the face or pulling a shirt over the head should also be sought

- Pseudoathetosis—"piano-playing" movements—when the patient has his arms outstretched and eyes closed, the affected arm will wander from its original position.
- Vibration and position sense are usually lost together.
- Positive Romberg's test is a hallmark of sensory ataxia.

Vestibular ataxia is due to lesion of vestibular pathways resulting in impairment and imbalance of vestibular inputs, e.g., vestibular, neuronitis, streptomycin toxicity.
- Vertigo and associated tinnitus and hearing loss
- Direction of the nystagmus in away from the lesion.

Optic ataxia was first described in a man with lesions of the posterior parietal lobe on both sides of the brain, later became known as **Balint's syndrome**.
- Among the symptoms that characterize the syndrome are a restriction of visual attention to single objects and a paucity of spontaneous eye movements.
- Patients have difficulty completing visually guided reaching tasks in the absence of other sensory cues.

Frontal lobe ataxia (Bruns ataxia) is due to involvement of subcortical small vessels, Binswanger's disease, multi-infarct state or NPH.
- The gait may appear to be a combination of awkward, magnetic (stuck to the floor), cautious, slow, and shuffling. This is also known as a frontal gait disorder, referring to the frontal lobe conditions which often cause **gait apraxia.**

The characteristic features of different types of ataxia have been shown in **Table 15.62**.

TABLE 15.62: Characteristic features of different types of ataxia.

Type of ataxia	*Cerebellar*	*Sensory*	*Frontal*
Stance and support	Wide based	Narrow based; looking down	Wide based
Velocity	Variable	Slow	Very slow
Stride	Irregular, lurching	Regular with path deviation	Short, shuffling
Romberg's	±	Unsteady; patient falls	±
Heel-Shin test	Abnormal	±	Normal
Initiation	Normal	Normal	Hesitant
Postural instability	+	+++	+++++
Falls	Late event	Frequent	Frequent
Turns	Unsteady	±	Multistepped; hesitant

MOVEMENT DISORDERS

Types of Movements

Q. Write a short note on CNS disorders characterized by involuntary movements.

- **Akathisia:** A subjective feeling of inner restlessness that is relieved by movements (e.g., crossing and uncrossing legs, rocking back and forth and pacing).
- **Asterixis:** Sudden periods of cessation of muscle contraction best seen when the patient's arms are extended in front. It is a negative myoclonus.
- **Athetosis:** Slow, sinuous, writhing movements, usually of the distal parts of the limbs.
- **Ballismus:** Wild flinging, movements that represent large amplitude proximal choreiform movements. Ballismus is often unilateral (hemiballismus).
- **Chorea:** Semipurposeful flowing movements that flit from one part of the body to another in a continuous and random pattern. Chorea can be defined as involuntary movements that are abrupt, unpredictable and nonrhythmic, resulting from a continuous random flow of muscle contractions.
- **Dyskinesia:** A general term for any excessive movement. The term dyskinesia is often used as an abbreviation for "tardive dyskinesia" (repetitive oral movements often seen in patients taking certain psychiatric medications).
- **Dystonia:** Twisting movements that are often sustained for variable periods of time with a directional preponderance resulting in posturing.

Algorithmic approach to movement disorders is given in **Flowchart 15.8**.

Q. Write a short note on myoclonus and its causes.

- **Myoclonus:** Myoclonic movements are sudden, brief, shock-like involuntary movements, which are usually positive (caused by muscle contraction), but can sometimes be negative [due to brief loss or inhibition of muscular tonus, as in asterixis—for example, when caused by hepatic encephalopathy (liver flap) or in uremic encephalopathy] **(Table 15.63)**.
- **Tics:** Tics are sudden and jerky movements, but in this case the keyword for recognition is the "stereotyped" character of the recurrent movements. Repetitive, stereotypic movements or sounds that are suppressible and that relieve a feeling of inner tension.

Tremor: Regular, oscillatory movements that may be present at rest or with action. Tremor is characterized by involuntary, rhythmic and sinusoidal alternating movements of one or more body parts.

Q. Write a short note on hemiballismus.

- **Hemiballismus:** Violent flinging movements of the limbs. It is usually unilateral, and hence called hemiballismus. Causes of some important movement disorders are listed in **Table 15.63**.

FLOWCHART 15.8: Algorithmic approach to movement disorders.

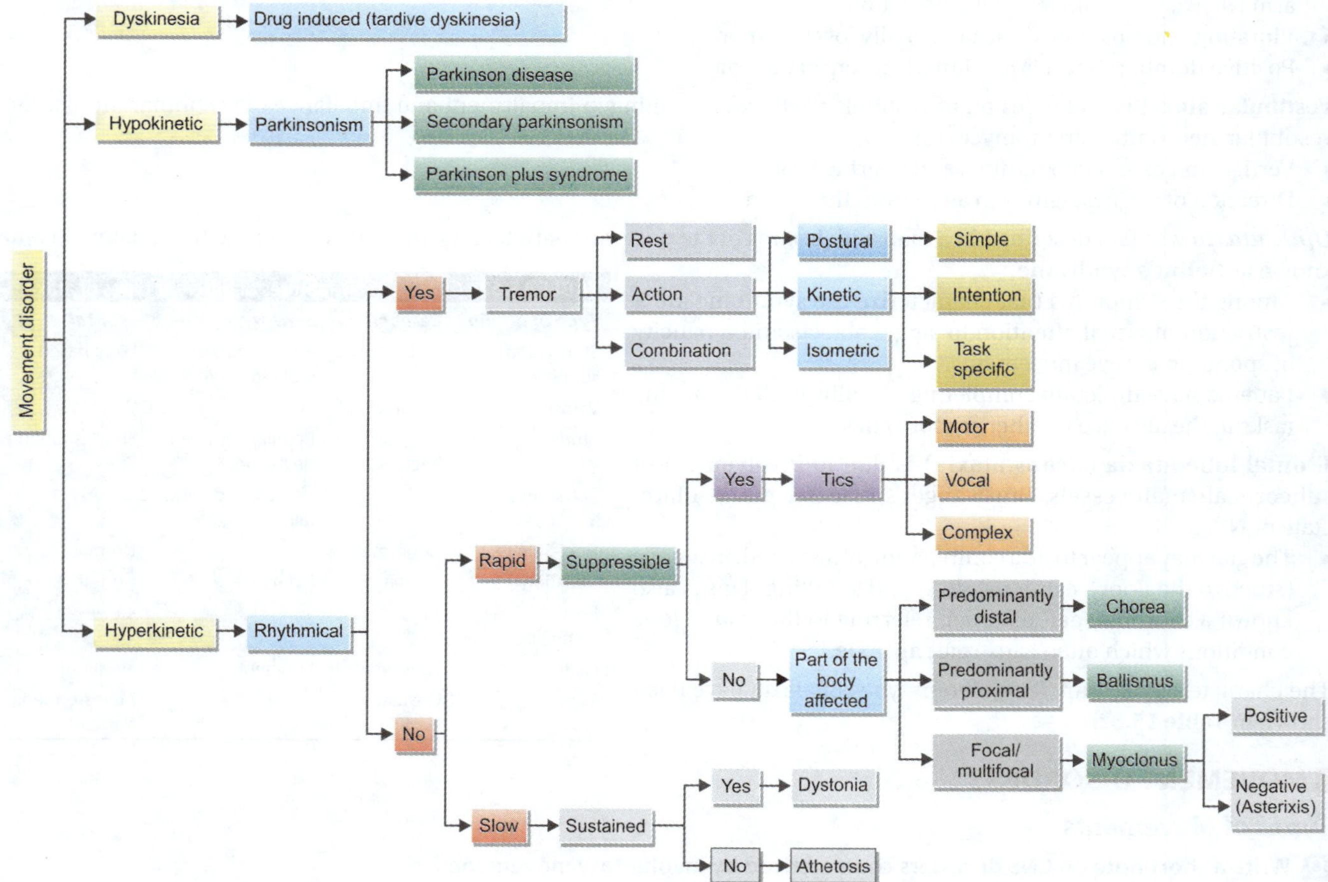

Parkinson's Disease

Q. Describe the etiology, clinical features/ manifestations, diagnosis, and management of Parkinson's disease.

Q. What is parkinsonism? How would you classify parkinsonism?

Q. Discuss the management of idiopathic parkinsonism.

Parkinsonism is a syndrome consisting of a variable combination of **tremor, rigidity, bradykinesia,** and a characteristic **disturbance of gait and posture.**

Classification of parkinsonian disorders (Flowchart 15.9): There are many causes for Parkinsonism but the most common cause is Parkinson's disease (PD).

Idiopathic Parkinson's Disease (Paralysis Agitans)

- It is a chronic, **progressive disorder** in which **idiopathic parkinsonism** occurs without evidence of more widespread neurologic involvement.
- Parkinson's disease (PD) is distinct from other parkinsonian syndromes both clinically and pathologically.
- **Age and gender:** Its incidence increases sharply with age. PD generally commences in middle or late life and average age of onset is about 60 years. Prevalence is higher in men than women (M:F = 1.5:1). It leads to progressive disability with time.

TABLE 15.63: Causes of some important movement disorders.

Name of disorder	*Causes*	*Treatment*
Asterixis	➤ Hepatic encephalopathy ➤ Uremic encephalopathy ➤ Carbon dioxide narcosis	Haloperidol, tetrabenazine
Chorea Mnemonic—CHOREA	➤ **C**horea gravidarum ➤ **H**untington's chorea ➤ **O**ral contraceptive pill and DOPA ➤ **R**heumatic chorea ➤ **E**ndocrine disorders (thyrotoxicosis) ➤ **A**rteriosclerotic or senile chorea	*Refer* later
Myoclonus	➤ Encephalitis ➤ Myoclonic epilepsy ➤ Drug overdose, hiccup ➤ Creutzfeldt–Jakob disease ➤ SSPE (subacute sclerosing panencephalitis) ➤ Anoxic encephalopathy (Lance–Adams syndrome)	Correction of underlying disease, sodium valproate (300–12,900 mg/day), clonazepam (0.5–10 mg/day)
Tremors	➤ Described later	
Hemiballismus	➤ Stroke affecting subthalamic nucleus (on contralateral side)	Haloperidol 0.5–2.5 mg TID, tetrabenazine 25–50 mg TID
Dystonia	➤ Kernicterus ➤ Previous brain injury ➤ Familial ➤ Degenerative disorders	Tetrabenazine (dopamine-depleting drug), high-dose anticholinergics, sodium valproate

FLOWCHART 15.9: Classification of parkinsonian disorders.

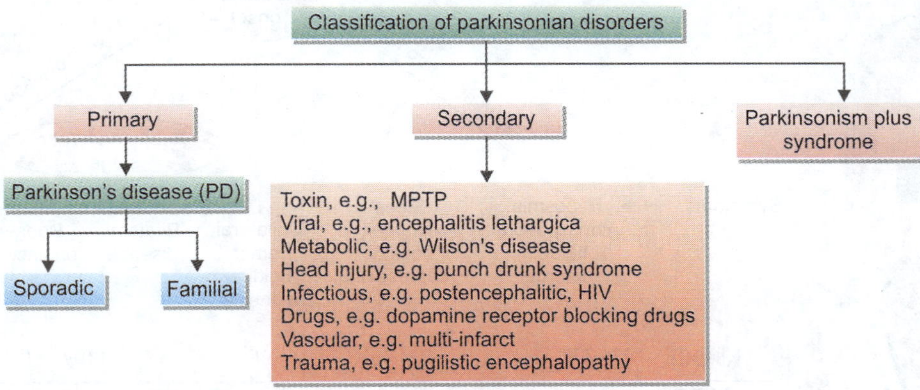

(MPTP: 1-methyl-4-phenyl-1,2,3,6-tetrahydropyridine)

Etiology

Cause of idiopathic Parkinson's disease is not known. Probably multiple interacting environmental risk factors and genetic susceptibility plays a role.

- **Environmental factors:**
  - Small increased risk with rural living and drinking well water.
  - Pesticide exposure.
  - Oxidative stress: Chemical compound 1-methyl-4-phenyl-1,2,3,6-tetrahydropyridine (MPTP) is a potent mitochondrial toxin. It causes severe Parkinsonism in young drug users of MPTP by producing oxidative stress leading to death of neuronal cell.
  - Nonsmokers have a higher risk of PD than smokers.
- **Genetic factors:** Genetic factors may play a role and several single genes causing parkinsonism have been identified.
  - **Sporadic:** Idiopathic PD is not usually familial, but there is a significant genetic component in early onset PD (onset before 40).
  - Mutations in many genes has been found in familial cases. Several genetic loci for Mendelian inherited monogenic forms of PD have been identified, designated as PARK 1–11. They are rare but cause early onset and familial PD.

Pathological features

- **Hallmark of PD: Degeneration and depletion of the pigmented dopaminergic neurons** in the substantia nigra pars compacta (SNc), reduced striatal dopamine, and the presence of α-synuclein and intracytoplasmic proteinaceous eosinophilic inclusions in nigral cells known as Lewy bodies.
- Probably environmental or genetic factors alter the α-synuclein protein, rendering it toxic. This leads to formation of Lewy body within the nigral cells. Lewy bodies are also seen in the basal ganglia, brainstem and cortex. Lewy bodies contain tangles of α-synuclein and ubiquitin. They become gradually more widespread and increase as the disease progresses.
- The loss of dopaminergic neurotransmission in the nerve cells (>80%) in the substantia nigra and other nuclei in the midbrain responsible for the symptoms of Parkinson's disease.

Clinical manifestations

A. Motor symptoms: Always asymmetrical in onset and become bilateral within a year.

- **Tremor** is an early and presenting symptom in 70% of patients.
  - Frequency is 4–6 Hz tremor and is typically **most prominent at rest** and **worsens with emotional stress.**
  - Typically tremor starts with the fingers and hands at rest.
  - Often described as pill rolling of finger and wrist, because the patient appears to be rolling something between thumb and forefinger. It often begins with rhythmic flexion-extension of the fingers, hand, or foot, or with rhythmic pronation-supination of the forearm. Initially, it may be confined to one limb or to the two limbs on one side before becoming more generalized. It also affects jaw and chin, but not the head.
  - Disappear on voluntary movement and sleep.
- **Rigidity**
  - It is a sign rather than a symptom. Increased **resistance to passive movement** is characteristic clinical feature that accounts for the flexed posture of many patients. Rigidity causes stiffness and a flexed posture.
  - Stiffness on passive limb movement is described as **"lead pipe"** rigidity because the increase in muscle tone is present throughout the range of movement. Unlike spasticity, it is not dependent on speed of movement.
  - When tremor is superimposed on the rigidity, a ratchet like jerkiness is felt, described as **"cogwheel" rigidity.**

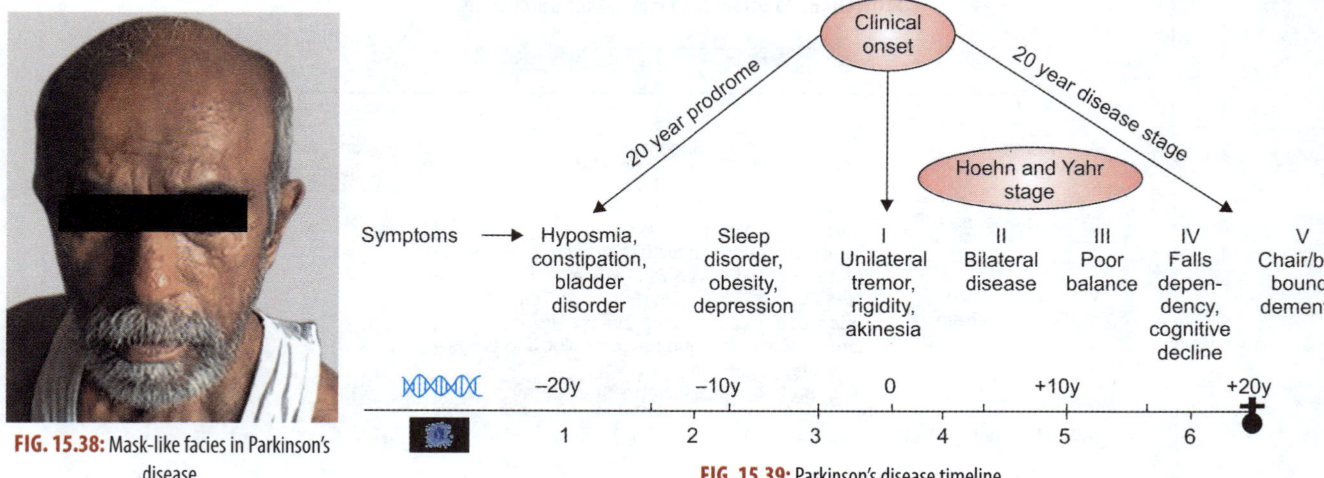

FIG. 15.38: Mask-like facies in Parkinson's disease.

FIG. 15.39: Parkinson's disease timeline.

- **Akinesia or bradykinesia**
  - Poverty/slowing of movement are the hallmark **of PD. Slowness**/difficulty of initiating **voluntary movement** and an associated **reduction in automatic movements,** such as swinging of the arms when walking.
  - There is **fixity of facial expression** (facial immobility—**mask-like face) (Fig. 15.38)**, with widened palpebral fissures and infrequent blinking.
  - Repetitive tapping (at about 2 Hz) over the glabella (Glabellar tap) produces a sustained blink response **(Myerson's sign),** in contrast to the response of normal subject. Frequency of spontaneous blinking decreases producing a serpentine stare.
  - The **combination of tremor, rigidity, and bradykinesia** results in small, tremulous, and often **illegible/difficult handwriting (micrographia).** It results in difficulty in activities such as tying shoelaces or buttoning, and difficulty rolling over in bed.
- **Postural changes:** A stooped posture is characteristic feature.
- **Gait changes:** Slow shuffling, freezing and reduced arm swing, small stride length, slow turns, festinating gait (tendency to advance rapid short steps) and catching center of gravity. Feet may be glued to floor. Postural instability and freezing may result in fall forward. Reduced eye blink.
- **Speech and swallowing:** Speech becomes softer (soft voice—hypophonia), quiet, indistinct, flat/monotonous and stuttering. Increased salivation/drooling, and dysphagia (swallowing difficulty is a late feature) which may lead to aspiration pneumonia as a terminal event.
- **Cognitive and psychiatric changes:** Cognitive impairment/dementia, depression, sleep disturbances may be present.

Parkinson's disease timeline has been shown in **Figure 15.39**.

B. Nonmotor features (Box 15.53)

Some nonmotor symptoms (NMSs) may precede the onset of more typical motor symptoms.

Box 15.53: Nonmotor symptoms of Parkinsons's disease.

Autonomic dysfunction	Neuropsychiatric	Sensory problems
• Orthostatic hypotension • Urinary incontinence • Constipation • Sexual problems	• Anxiety • Depression • Apathy • Psychosis • Dementia	• Reduces sense of smell (hyposmia) • Pain
Sleep disorders	**Rheumatological**	**Other**
• Restless legs • Insomnia • Daytime somnolence	• Frozen shoulder • Periarthritis • Swan neck deformity	• Seborrhea

Investigation/Diagnosis

- Diagnosis is made on **clinical grounds.**
- **Structural imaging** (CT or MRI) is **usually normal.**
- **Functional dopaminergic imaging:** By single-photon emission computed tomography (SPECT) or positron emission tomography (PET) is **abnormal** and shows reduced uptake of striatal dopaminergic markers, particularly in the posterior putamen. However, it is not specific for PD.
- **Dopamine transporter (DaT) imaging:** It is performed by the use of a radiolabeled ligand binding to dopaminergic terminals to know the extent of nigrostriatal cell loss. It may be rarely required to distinguish PD from other causes of tremor, or drug-induced parkinsonism **(Fig. 15.40).**

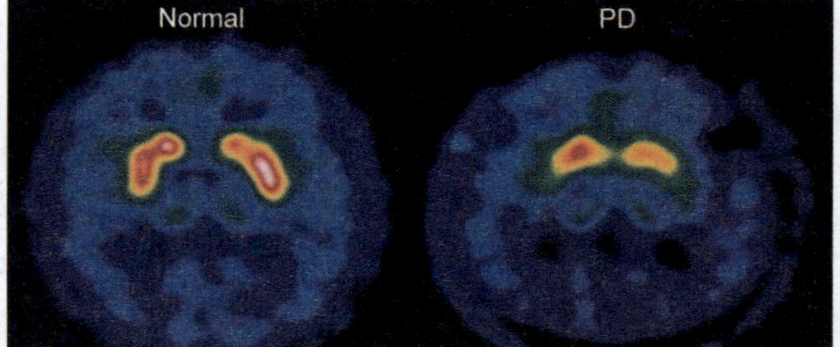

FIG. 15.40: Dopamine transporter (DaT) imaging.

Stages of Parkinson's disease **(Table 15.64).**

Q. Discuss the staging of Parkinson's disease.

Differential diagnosis

1. **Secondary parkinsonism (Box 15.54).**

Box 15.54: Causes of secondary parkinsonism.

Toxin: Manganese, 1-methyl-4-phenyl-1,2,3,6-tetrahydropyridine (MPTP), carbon monoxide, mercury, carbon disulfide, cyanide, methanol
Viral: Encephalitis lethargica, Creutzfeldt–Jakob disease
Metabolic: Wilson's disease
Head injury: Punch drunk syndrome
Infectious: Postencephalitic, HIV, SSPE, Prion diseases
Drugs: Dopamine receptor blocking drugs, reserpine, tetrabenazine, alpha-methyldopa, lithium, flunarizine, cinnarizine
Vascular: Multi-infarct, Binswanger's disease
Trauma: Pugilistic encephalopathy
Others: Parathyroid abnormalities, hypothyroidism, brain tumors, paraneoplastic, normal pressure hydrocephalus (NPH), psychogenic

TABLE 15.64: Hoehn and Yahr stage of Parkinson's disease.

Stage	Disease state
I	Unilateral involvement only, minimal or no functional impairment
II	Bilateral or midline involvement, without impairment of balance
III	First sign of impaired righting reflex, mild to moderate disability
IV	Fully developed, severely disabling disease; patient still able to walk and stand unassisted
V	Confinement to bed or wheelchair unless aided

TABLE 15.65: Parkinson plus syndromes and its features.

Syndrome	Features
Progressive supranuclear palsy (PSP, Steele–Richardson–Olszewski syndrome)	Slow ocular saccades, eyelid apraxia, and restricted eye movements with particular impairment of downward gaze and reptilian stare **(Fig. 15.41)**. Frequently experience hyperextension of the neck with early gait disturbance and falls. MRI may reveal a characteristic atrophy of the midbrain with relative preservation of the pons (the "hummingbird sign" on midsagittal images)
Multiple system atrophy (MSA) Parkinsonian (MSA-P) or striatonigral degeneration Cerebellar (MSA-C) or olivopontocerebellar atrophy Autonomic (MSA-A) form or Shy–Drager syndrome	Parkinsonism in conjunction with cerebellar signs and/or early and prominent autonomic dysfunction, usually orthostatic hypotension. Cerebellar and brainstem atrophy (the pontine "hot cross buns" sign in MSA-C)
Corticobasal ganglionic degeneration (Rebeiz–Kolodny–Richardson syndrome)	Asymmetric dystonic contractions and clumsiness of one hand coupled with cortical sensory disturbances manifest as apraxia, agnosia, focal myoclonus, or alien limb phenomenon
Dementia with Lewy bodies	Early onset dementia, visual hallucinations
Parkinsonism-dementia complex of Guam	Motor neuron disease plus Parkinson's
Guadeloupean parkinsonism	Levodopa-unresponsive parkinsonism, postural instability with early falls, and pseudobulbar palsy

Q. What are the "Parkinson plus" syndromes?

See **Table 15.65.**

Q. Write a short essay/note on drugs used in Parkinson's disease.

Treatment

A. Symptomatic pharmacologic treatment: Drug treatment in PD is symptomatic rather than curative. None of the currently available drugs are neuroprotective.

- **Anticholinergic drugs**
  - Nonselective muscarinic antagonists are helpful, especially in **relieving tremor.** For example, **trihexyphenidyl, benztropine, and orphenadrine.**
  - Treatment is started with small dose (2 mg), which is gradually built up until benefit occurs or side effects limit further increments.
  - **Adverse effects:** Urinary retention, dry mouth, blurred vision, worsening of glaucoma, constipation, confusion and hallucinosis in elderly. Hence, rarely used as first-line drugs unless patient has severe tremors. They should be avoided in patient above 65 years of age.
- **Levodopa**
  - Levodopa, the metabolic precursor of dopamine. It is the single **most effective drug** available for the treatment. It **provides symptomatic benefit** in most patients with parkinsonism and is often particularly helpful in **relieving bradykinesia.** Resolve hypokinesia and rigidity first and tremor later. Levodopa is metabolized by MAO (monoamine oxidase) and COMT (catechol-O-methyl-transferase). Its plasma half-life is around 2 hours. Early use lowers mortality rate. Combined with a dopa decarboxylase inhibitor—benserazide (co-beneldopa) or carbidopa (co-careldopa) to reduce the adverse effects (e.g., nausea and hypotension).
  - **Adverse drug reactions:**
    - Postural hypotension, fluctuations in response.
    - Mydriasis, brownish discoloration of the urine, abnormal smell, transient elevations of transaminases and BUN.
    - GIT effects: Nausea and vomiting.
    - Cardiovascular: Tachycardia, ventricular extrasystoles, atrial fibrillation.
    - Dyskinesias, behavioral disturbances.

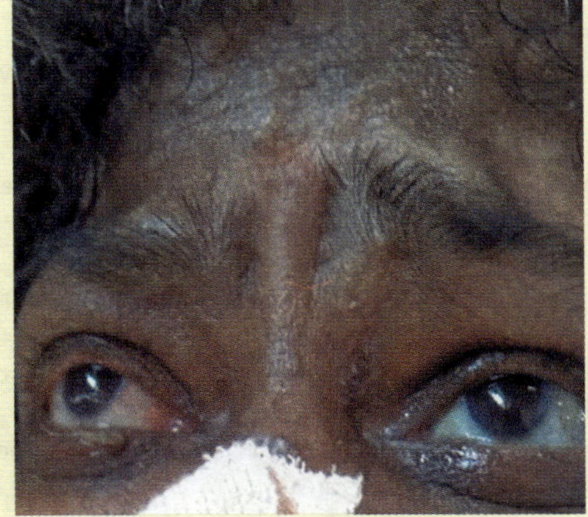

FIG. 15.41: Reptilian stare in progressive supranuclear palsy (PSP).

- **"On-off" effect:** Important late complications of levodopa therapy. It is like a light switch; without warning, all of a sudden, person goes from full control to complete reversion back to bradykinesia, tremor, etc. It lasts from 30 minutes to several hours and then get control again. The on-off phenomenon can be controlled in part by reducing dosing, intervals, administering levodopa 1 hour before meals and restricting dietary protein intake or treatment with dopamine agonists.

- **MAO-B Inhibitors**
  - Monoamine oxidase type B **facilitates breakdown of excess dopamine** in the synapse. They produce **asymptomatic motor benefit** when used as a monotherapy and **enhance the efficacy of carbidopa levodopa formulations** when used as adjuncts voided, e.g., selegiline, rasagiline.
  - The addition of selegiline, a monoamine oxidase B inhibitor, reduces the metabolic breakdown of dopamine and may slow down the degeneration in the substantia nigra.
- **Dopamine receptor agonists**
  - Dopamine receptor agonists are classified as ergot derived **(bromocriptine, pergolide and cabergoline)** or nonergot-derived **(pramipexole, ropinirole, rotigotine and apomorphine).**
  - **Side effects:** Produce impulse control disorders (e.g., pathological gambling, binge eating and hypersexuality) and daytime somnolence. Dopamine agonists are contraindicated in patients with psychotic disorders and are best avoided in those with recent myocardial infarction, severe peripheral vascular disease, or active peptic ulceration.
  - Ergot-derived agonists are no longer recommended because of rare but serious fibrotic side effects including cardiac valvular fibrosis.
  - Nonergot dopamine agonists are preferable to ergot-derived dopamine agonists. They are used as an alternative or an addition to levodopa therapy.

Q. Write a short note on COMT (Catechol-O-methyltransferase) inhibitors.

- **COMT inhibitors**
  - Catechol-O-methyl-transferase produces peripheral breakdown of levodopa (e.g., **entacapone and tolcapone).** Entacapone prolongs the duration of levodopa by decreasing its peripheral metabolism. The more potent tolcapone is less preferred because of rare but serious hepatotoxicity.
- **Dopamine facilitator**
  - **Amantadine:** It is an antiviral agent that potentiates dopaminergic function by influencing the synthesis, release, reuptake of dopamine. It has a mild antiparkinsonian effect and short-lived effect on bradykinesia. Hence, it is rarely used and are reserved for patients who are unable to tolerate other drugs. Amantadine-either alone or combined with an anticholinergic agent, helpful for mild parkinsonism. It acts by potentiating the release of endogenous dopamine.
  - **Adverse effects:** Livedo reticularis, peripheral edema, confusion and other anticholinergic effects.
- **Peripheral dopamine decarboxylase inhibitors (PDI)**
  - It does not penetrate the BBB; reduce the peripheral metabolism of levodopa. Increase plasma levels of levodopa, prolongs the plasma half-life of levodopa, increase available amounts of dopa for entry into the brain and reduce the daily requirement of levodopa by 75%. For example, **carbidopa, benserazide.**
- **Newer modalities**
  - **Transdermal delivery of Rotigotine** improves motor functions.
  - **Subcutaneous apomorphine infusion**
  - **L-dopa infusion into the duodenum**
- **Neuroprotective agents that alter pathogenesis**
  - MAO inhibitors: Selegiline and rasagiline
  - Antiexcitotoxicity drugs: Riluzole
  - Bioenergetic antioxidant agent, coenzyme Q10
  - Antiapoptotic kinase inhibitors (e.g., CEP-1347)
  - Adenosine A2A receptor antagonists (e.g., **istradefylline**).

B. Surgical Treatment

- **Indications:** Most common indications for surgery in PD are intractable tremor and drug-induced motor fluctuations or dyskinesias.
- Different surgeries are:
  - **Stereotactic surgery** (ventrolateral thalamotomy) tried in unilateral cases.
  - **Pallidotomy** improves tremor and dyskinesia
  - **Deep brain stimulation (DBS):** Stereotactic insertion of electrodes into the brain is most often performed bilaterally and simultaneously. **Best site is subthalamic nucleus.** DBS in these areas alleviates Parkinsonian motor signs particularly during the off periods and reduces troublesome dyskinesias, dystonia and motor fluctuations that result from drug administration. DBS is usually reserved for patients with medically refractory tremor or motor fluctuations.

Newer Therapies for PD

Focused ultrasound

Unilateral focused ultrasound lesioning of the STN or thalamus (in tremor-dominant forms of PD) has been found to be beneficial in some patients, particularly if the symptoms are markedly asymmetric.

Cell replacement therapies

Fetal tissue-derived cell transplants—generation dopaminergic neurons from somatic human cells and improvement in the efficacy of differentiation protocols have led to a resurgence of cell transplantation

Surgical delivery of gene therapy

MRI-guided delivery of adeno-associated viral vector serotype-2 encoding the complementary DNA for the enzyme, aromatic L-amino acid decarboxylase (VY-AADC01) into the putamen

Characteristic Features of Extrapyramidal Lesion

See **Table 15.66.**

TABLE 15.66: Characteristic features of extrapyramidal lesion.

Sign	*Site of lesion*
Resting tremor	Substantia nigra, red nucleus
Muscular rigidity	Substantia nigra, putamen
Hypokinesia	Substantia nigra, globus pallidum
Chorea	Caudate nucleus
Hemiballismus	Subthalamic nucleus
Dystonia, athetosis	Putamen

Chorea

Q. Write a short note on chorea and mention the disease which causes chorea.

General Features

- Irregular, semipurposeful, abrupt, rapid, brief, jerky, unsustained movements that flow randomly from one part of the body to another. These movements disappear during sleep.
- When choreic movements are more severe, assuming a flinging, sometimes violent, character, they are called ballism.

Causes of Chorea

See **(Box 15.55)**.

Box 15.55: Causes of chorea.

Rheumatic (Sydenham's chorea)
Huntington's chorea
Encephalitis, e.g., Japanese encephalitis, measles, mumps
Vascular, e.g., HIV-related (toxoplasmosis, progressive multifocal leukoencephalopathy, HIV encephalitis)
Immunologic, e.g., systemic lupus erythematosus, antiphospholipid antibody syndrome, paraneoplastic syndromes, acute disseminated encephalomyelopathy, celiac disease
Drugs, e.g., L-dopa, oral contraceptive, phenytoin
Degenerative disorders of the brain
Benign hereditary
Pregnancy (Chorea gravidarum)
Endocrine-metabolic dysfunction, e.g., adrenal insufficiency, hyper/hypocalcemia, hyper/hypoglycemia, hypernatremia, liver failure
Miscellaneous, e.g., anoxic encephalopathy, cerebral palsy, kernicterus, multiple sclerosis, post-traumatic

Signs in Chorea

- Involuntary protrusion and retraction of the tongue **(jack in the box)**.
- Inability to hold the hands above head with palms facing each other as it results in pronation of arms so that palms face outward **(pronator sign)**.
- Milking action of patient's fingers if asked to grasp the physician's fingers **(milk-maid sign)**.

Sydenham's Chorea (Saint Vitus Dance)

- **Most common cause of chorea in children.**
- It is self-limiting condition, nonsuppurative **complication of group A β-hemolytic streptococcal pharyngitis. It follows acute rheumatic fever** by 4–6 months. Severity varies and disorder may continue for a few months.
- It is due to molecular mimicry between streptococcal and CNS antigens. Infection by group A **β-hemolytic streptococci** in genetically predisposed individual leads to formation of cross-reactive antibodies. These antibodies disrupt the basal ganglia function. Inflammation is seen in caudate nucleus.
- **Clinical features:** It is a **neuropsychiatric disorder.** Clinical features include both **neurological abnormalities** (chorea, weakness and hypotonia) and **psychiatric disorders** (such as emotional liability, hyperactivity, distractibility, obsessions and compulsions). These abnormalities lead to inability to perform normal activities of daily living (ADL) including eating, talking, dressing, writing, walking, learning and socializing, and thus impact negatively on the child's quality of life.
- **Common sign is motor impersistence.** It can be demonstrated by an inability to sustain eye closure or tongue protrusion.
- Evaluation for valvular heart disease is a must. Antistreptolysin-O (ASLO) titers and ESR are often normal.

Treatment

Symptomatic

- **Sodium valproate** 200–600 mg TID is the first-line drug.
- If valproate is not effective, risperidone, a potent dopamine D2 receptor blocker, may be given to control chorea. The dose is 1–2 mg BID.
- Haloperidol 0.5–1.5 mg BD or TID is used occasionally.
- Other drugs include pimozide, carbamazepine, clonidine, and phenobarbital.
- Penicillin prophylaxis is necessary to reduce risk of cardiac involvement due to future streptococcal infections.

Huntington's Disease/Chorea

Q. Write a short essay on the transmission and clinical features of Huntington's disease (HD).

Huntington's disease is a progressive, fatal, highly penetrant autosomal dominant disorder characterized by motor, behavioral, and cognitive dysfunction. Onset is typically between the ages of 25 and 45 years.

Etiology

- Huntington's disease is caused by an **increase in the number of polyglutamine (CAG) repeats** (>40) in the coding sequence of the huntingtin gene located on the short arm of chromosome 4.
- The disease manifests earlier if the number of repeats is larger.
- The gene encodes the highly conserved cytoplasmic protein huntingtin, which is widely distributed in neurons throughout the CNS, but its function is not known.

Manifestations

- **Early stages:** Chorea tends to be focal or segmental, but progresses over time to involve multiple body regions. Dysarthria, gait disturbance, and oculomotor abnormalities are common features.
- **Advancing disease:** There may be a reduction in chorea and emergence of dystonia, rigidity, bradykinesia, myoclonus, and spasticity.
- HD patients eventually develop behavioral and cognitive disturbances, and the majority progress to dementia. Depression with suicidal tendencies, aggressive behavior, and psychosis can be prominent features.

Treatment

Multidisciplinary approach, with medical, neuropsychiatric, social, and genetic counseling for patients and their families.

- Medical:
  - HD chorea is self-limited and is usually not disabling.
  - Psychosis can be treated with atypical neuroleptics. Depression and anxiety are treated with appropriate antidepressant and antianxiety drugs.
  - No adequate treatment for the cognitive or motor decline.
  - Promitochondrial agents such as ubiquinone and creatine are being tested as possible disease-modifying therapies.

Tremor

Q. Write a short note on definition of tremor and mention its types with examples.

Tremor is an unintentional, **rhythmic** muscle movement involving **to-and-fro** movements (oscillations) of one or more parts of the body produced by alternating or synchronous contractions of antagonist muscles. It is the most common of all involuntary movements and can affect the hands, arms, head, face, voice, trunk, and legs.

Causes of Tremor (Box 15.56)

Box 15.56: Causes of tremor.

Physiological: Anxiety	**Drug induced:** Amphetamine, steroids
Drugs: Beta-agonists, alcohol	**Alcohol withdrawal**, liver failure
Intention tremor: Cerebellar lesion	**Mercury poisoning**
Thyrotoxicosis	Wilson's disease (wing-beating tremor)

- **Types/Nature of Tremor**
- **Resting tremor** occurs when the muscle is relaxed. For example, tremor occurring when the hands are lying on the lap or hanging next to the trunk while standing or walking. It may be shaking of the limb, even when the individual is at rest. It is usually observed only in the hand or fingers and is seen in Parkinson's disease.
- **Action tremor** is detected during any type of movement of an affected body part. There are several subtypes of action tremor.
- **Postural tremor** occurs when an individual maintains a position against gravity. For example, holding the arms outstretched.
- **Kinetic tremor** occurs during movement of a part of the body. For example, moving the wrists up and down.
- **Intention tremor** is present during a purposeful movement toward a target. For example, touching a finger to one's nose during a medical examination.
- **Task-specific tremor** occurs when performing highly skilled, goal-oriented tasks. For example, as handwriting or speaking.
- **Isometric tremor** occurs during a voluntary muscle contraction that is not accompanied by any movement.

Classification

Tremor is most commonly classified by its appearance and cause or origin.

- **Essential tremor (benign essential tremor):** It is the most common of the forms of abnormal tremor.
  - It may be mild and nonprogressive or slowly progressive. **Most commonly observed in the hands** but may involve the head, voice, tongue, legs, and trunk. Tremor of the hands is typically present as an action tremor.
  - **Triggers:** Heightened emotion, stress, fever, physical exhaustion, or low blood sugar may trigger tremors and/or increase their severity. It decreases on alcohol consumption.

- **Parkinsonian tremor** is characteristically as a resting tremor.
- **Dystonic tremor** occurs in individuals affected by dystonia. It may affect any muscle. Dystonic tremors occur irregularly and often relieved by complete rest.
- **Cerebellar tremor** is a slow tremor of the extremities that occurs at the end of a purposeful movement (intention tremor). For example, trying to press a button or touching a finger to the tip of one's nose.
  - Caused by lesions in or damage to the cerebellum, e.g., stroke, tumor, or MS. Cerebellar damage can also result in a "wing-beating" type of tremor which is a combination of rest, action, and postural tremors. Cerebellar tremor may be associated with dysarthria (speech problems), nystagmus (rapid involuntary movements of the eyes), gait problems, and postural tremor of the trunk and neck.
- **Psychogenic tremor** (functional tremor) can appear as any form of tremor movement. The characteristics may vary but generally include sudden onset and remission, increased incidence with stress. Many individuals have a conversion disorder or psychiatric disease.
- **Orthostatic tremor** detected as rhythmic muscle contractions in the legs and trunk immediately after standing.
- **Physiologic tremor** occurs in every normal individual. It may be exaggerated by strong emotion (such as anxiety or fear), physical exhaustion, etc. It is generally not caused by a neurological disease.
- Rubral tremor/Holme's tremor—seen in midbrain lesions.

ORGANIC BRAIN SYNDROME

Q. Write a short note on organic brain syndrome (OBS).

It is an abnormal mental state characterized by changes in orientation, memory, judgment and affect. It is due to diffuse impairment of brain tissue.

The two most important types of OBS are delirium (*refer* Chapter 18) and dementia is discussed in Chapter 21.

COMA

Q. How would you investigate and manage a 50-year-old patient presenting with coma?

Definitions

Consciousness

- It means the state of patient's awareness of self and environment and his responsiveness to external stimulation and inner need.
- Consciousness is maintained by two separate anatomical and physiological systems:
  - Ascending reticular activating system (ARAS) projecting from brainstem to thalamus determines arousal (the level of consciousness).
  - Cerebral cortex determines the content of consciousness.

Confusion

- Traditionally referred as **"clouding of sensorium"**.
- It denotes inability to think with customary speed, clarity and coherence, accompanied by some degree of inattentiveness and disorientation.
- Confusion results most often from process that influences the brain globally, such as toxic or metabolic disturbance or a dementia.

Drowsiness

- The inability to sustain a wakeful state without application of stimuli externally is called drowsiness.
- Slow arousal is elicited by speaking to the patient or applying a tactile stimulus.

Stupor

- A state in which the person can be aroused only by repeated vigorous stimuli is called as stupor.
- There is either absence or slow and inadequate response to spoken commands.
- It is common to find restless or stereotyped motor activity. In these patients there is a reduction in the natural shifting of positions.
- When left unstimulated, these patients quickly return to a sleep-like state.

Lethargic/Drowsiness

Patient can usually be aroused or awakened and may then appear to be in complete possession of her senses, but promptly falls asleep when left alone. It resembles normal sleepiness.
Example: High brainstem disturbances.

Obtundation

It refers to moderate reduction in the patient's level of awareness such that stimuli of mild to moderate intensity fail to arouse; when arousal does occur, the patient is slow to respond.

Coma

Coma is a condition characterized by a deep sleep like stage from which the patient cannot be aroused even with vigorous, continuous stimulation. The patient does not make any localized responses. However, the patient may grimace or show withdrawal responses to painful stimuli.

Classification of Coma

See **Box 15.57.**

Q. Write a short essay/note on causes of coma.

Box 15.57: Classification of coma.

Coma without focal signs or meningism
- **Exogenous intoxicants:** Alcohol, barbiturate, opiates
- **Endogenous metabolic disturbances:** Anoxia, hypoglycemia, diabetic ketoacidosis (DKA), hyperosmolar nonketotic state (HONK), uremia, hepatic failure, hyponatremia or hypernatremia, Addisonian crisis, carbon monoxide poisoning, myxedema
- **Severe systemic infections:** Septicemia, typhoid fever, cerebral malaria, pneumonia, peritonitis, Waterhouse–Friderichsen syndrome
- **Circulatory collapse** (shock) from any cause
- **Postseizure states**
  - Hypertensive encephalopathy
  - Hyperthermia and hypothermia
  - Concussion
  - Acute hydrocephalus

Coma with meningism
- Subarachnoid hemorrhage
- Acute bacterial meningitis
- Viral meningoencephalitis
- Neoplastic meningitis
- Parasitic meningitis
- Pituitary apoplexy

Coma with focal signs
- Hemispheral hemorrhage or massive cerebral infarction
- Brainstem infarction
- Brain abscess, subdural empyema, herpes encephalitis
- Epidural and subdural hemorrhage, brain contusion
- Brain tumor
- Miscellaneous: Thrombotic thrombocytopenic purpura (TTP), fat embolism, ADEM, cortical vein thrombosis, focal infarction caused by bacterial endocarditis

Approach to a Patient with Coma

Q. How do you proceed to investigate and manage a case of coma?

History

Inquire about history of diabetes, hypertension, head injury, convulsions, alcohol or drug use, circumstances in which patient was found, medications in hospitalized patient like anesthetics, sedatives, antiepileptic, opiates, antidepressants, and antipsychotics.

Onset of Coma

- Sudden onset of coma would suggest a vascular cause possibly SAH or brainstem involvement.
- Rapid progression from hemispheric signs to coma: Intracerebral hemorrhage.
- Protracted course: Tumor, abscess, chronic SDH.
- Altered sensorium (delirium) preceding coma, with no focal neurological deficits indicates metabolic encephalopathy.

General Examination

- **Signs of trauma:** (a) Raccoon eyes, (b) Battle's sign, and (c) CSF rhinorrhea or logorrhea
- **Blood pressure:**
  - Hypertension suggests—(a) hypertensive encephalopathy or (b) intracerebral hemorrhage
  - Hypotension suggests—(a) myocardial infarction, (b) septicemia, (c) Addison's disease, and (d) alcohol or barbiturate intoxication, (e) internal hemorrhage.
- **Pulse:** Bradycardia with periodic breathing and hypertension (Cushing reflex) suggests raised ICP.
- **Temperature:**
  - **Hypothermia** suggests—(a) alcohol or barbiturate intoxication, (b) myxedema, (c) advanced tubercular meningitis, and (d) peripheral circulatory failure
  - **Hyperthermia** suggests—(a) systemic infection, (b) meningoencephalitis, (c) heatstroke, and (d) anticholinergic drugs abuse
- **Signs of meningeal irritation:** (a) Meningitis and (b) SAH
- **Fundus:** Raised ICP (papilledema), subhyaloid hemorrhages (SAH), and hypertensive encephalopathy.
- **Smell of breath:** For ketones, alcohol, and hepatic fetor.
- **Skin inspection:**
  - Rash suggests meningococcemia, staphylococcal endocarditis, typhus, Rocky Mountain spotted fever (RMSF)
  - Excessive sweating suggests hypoglycemia or shock
  - Diffuse petechiae suggest thrombotic thrombocytopenic purpura (TTP), disseminated intravascular coagulopathy (DIC), and fat embolism.

Neurological Assessment

- Neurological assessment is done to determine the depth of coma [Glasgow coma scale (GCS)], brainstem function, and lateralization of pathology.
- Observation first without examiner intervention.
- Observe the posture of the limb, position of the eyes and head, spontaneous movement, pattern of respiration.
- Yawning and spontaneous shifting of body position indicates minimal degree of unresponsiveness.
- Multifocal myoclonus almost always indicates metabolic disorder.
- Assess responsiveness by noting patient's reaction to calling his name, or to noxious stimuli such as supraorbital or sternal pressure.

Evaluation of Severity of Coma

See **Box 15.58** and **Table 15.67.**

Q. Write a short essay/note on Edinburgh classification of coma.

Q. Write a short essay/note on Glasgow Coma Scale.

Box 15.58: Edinburgh classification of coma.

Grade 0: Fully conscious
Grade 1: Drowsy, but responds to verbal command
Grade 2: Unconscious, but responds to minimal pain stimulus
Grade 3: Unconscious, but responsive to strong pain stimulus
Grade 4: Unconscious, with no response to pain

TABLE 15.67: Glasgow Coma Scale (GCS).

Eye opening		*Best verbal response*		*Best motor response*	
				Obeys commands	6
		Oriented and converses	5	Localizes pain	5
Open spontaneously	4	Converses, but disoriented, confused	4	Exhibits flexion withdrawal	4
Open only to verbal stimuli	3	Uses inappropriate words	3	Decorticate rigidity	3
Open only to pain	2	Makes incomprehensible sounds	2	Decerebrate rigidity	2
Never open	1	No verbal response	1	No motor response	1

Maximum score = **15**
Minimum score = **3**
Coma is equal to GCS of <**8 or less**

Newer Scales for Prognosis of Coma

FOUR (Full Outline of UnResponsiveness) scale: New Coma Scale is devised in 2005, four components (eye, motor, brainstem, and respiration). Each component has maximum of score of four.

AVPU scale: Alertness, response to Verbal stimuli, response to Painful stimuli, or Unresponsive

ACDU scale: Alertness, Confusion, Drowsiness, and Unresponsiveness

Grady scale: Scale of I–V along a scale of confusion, stupor, deep stupor, abnormal posturing, and coma.

Stages of Coma

- Grade I: Individuals who respond with recognition when their name is called and **do not lapse into sleep** when left undisturbed.
- Grade II: The person lapses into sleep when undisturbed and is aroused only when **a pin is tapped gently over the chest wall.**
- Grade III: Patient who winces in response to deep pain stimulus. Deep pain stimulus **may result in abnormal postural reflexes either unilateral or bilateral.**
- Grade IV: Deep pain stimulus may result in **decorticate or decerebrate** posturing.
- Grade V: The patient who maintains a state of **flaccid unresponsiveness in spite of deep pain stimulation.**

Posture in Comatose Patient

- **Decerebrate rigidity:** It consists of opisthotonus, clenching of jaws, stiff extension of limbs with internal rotation of arms and plantar flexion of feet. Extensor posturing arises in variety of settings: Midbrain compression, cerebellar lesions, metabolic, drug intoxication, etc.
- **Decorticate rigidity:** Arms in flexion and adduction and legs extended signify lesion rostral to midbrain.
- Extensor posture of arms with weak flexor responses of legs is seen with lesions at level of vestibular nuclei.

Brainstem Reflexes (Brainstem Function)

See **Box 15.59.**

Q. Write a short note on brainstem reflexes.

As a rule, when these brainstem activities are preserved, particularly the pupil reactions and eye movements, coma must be ascribed to bilateral hemispheral disease. However, a mass in the hemispheres may cause coma and also produce herniation.

Box 15.59: Brainstem reflexes.

- Pupillary size and reactivity
- Ocular movements
- Corneal responses
- Oculovestibular reflexes
- Pattern of breathing (respiratory pattern)

Pupillary Reactions

See **Box 15.68** and **Figure 15.42.**

TABLE 15.68: Interpretation of pupillary reactions.	
Pupillary reactions	***Interpretation***
Symmetrically reactive round pupils	Exclude midbrain damage
Enlarged and unreactive pupil (>5 mm)	Intrinsic midbrain lesion (ipsilateral) or by ipsilateral mass
Oval and slightly eccentric pupils	Early midbrain or IIIrd nerve compression
Bilateral dilated and unreactive pupils	Severe midbrain damage by transtentorial herniation or anticholinergic drugs toxicity (atropine, TCA)
Dilatation of one pupil that then becomes fixed to light	Compression of the IIIrd cranial nerve and is a neurosurgical emergency
Reactive bilaterally small but not pinpoint (1–2.5 mm)	Metabolic encephalopathy or thalamic hemorrhages
Bilateral pinpoint (very small < 1 mm) but reactive pupil	Opioid or barbiturate overdose or bilateral pontine hemorrhage
Bilateral midpoint reactive pupils (i.e., normal pupils)	Metabolic comas, coma due to sedative drugs except opiates
Bilateral light fixed, dilated pupils	Cardinal sign of brain death in deep coma of any cause, but particularly in barbiturate intoxication and hypothermia

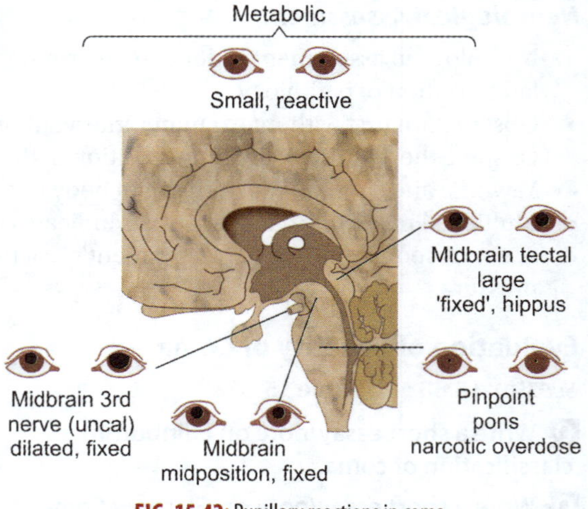

FIG. 15.42: Pupillary reactions in coma.

Eye Movements and Position (Fig. 15.43)

- In light coma of metabolic origin, eyes wander conjugately from side to side in random fashion. These movements disappear as coma deepens.
- **Adducted eye at rest:** VIth nerve palsy. If it is bilateral, it is due to raised ICT.
- **Abducted eye at rest:** IIIrd nerve palsy.
- **Conjugate deviation of eyes toward hemispheric** lesion and away from unilateral pontine lesion.
- **Downward and inward deviation of eyes:** Lesions of thalamus and upper midbrain.
- **Eyes turn toward convulsing side in focal** seizures.
- **Ocular bobbing:** It is characterized by brisk downward and slow upward movements of the eyes associated with loss of horizontal eye movements. It is diagnostic of lesions in midbrain and pons.
- **Ocular dipping:** It is characterized by slow downward followed by faster upward movement in patients with normal horizontal gaze. It indicates diffuse cortical anoxic damage and drug intoxication.
- **Disconjugate eyes (divergent ocular axes):** Brainstem lesion, e.g., skew deviation (one eye up, one eye down)
- **Oculocephalic reflex:** Also called doll's eye movement.
  - Elicited by briskly turning or tilting the head.
  - In coma of metabolic origin or due to lesions of bihemispherical structures, the response consists of conjugate movements of eyes in the opposite direction.
  - Positive response indicates: Intact oculomotor, abducent, midbrain, and pons.
  - Absent reflex indicates: Damage within brainstem. It can be also due to profound overdose of sedatives or anticonvulsants.

Oculocephalic (doll's eye)

Head to left | Central | Head to right

Head to right | Central | Eyes to left

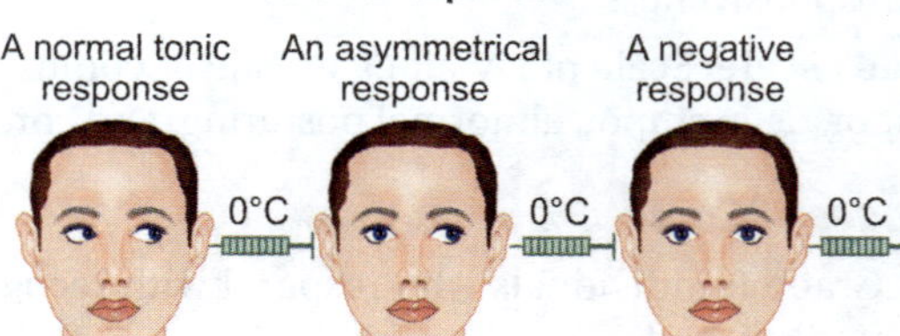

FIG. 15.43: Eye movements and position.

Oculovestibular or Caloric Test

- **Method:** Irrigate the external auditory canal with cold water.
- **Normal response:** Causes slow conjugate deviation of eyes toward irrigated ear followed in few seconds by compensatory nystagmus (i.e., fast component away from irrigated ear).
- **Interpretation:**
  - Loss of conjugate ocular movements in brainstem damage.
  - Loss of fast corrective nystagmus in metabolic or bilateral hemispheral damage. The eyes are tonically deflected to side irrigated with cold water and this position may be held for 2–3 minutes.

Respiratory Patterns (Figs. 15.44A to E)

- **Slow, shallow, regular breathing:** Metabolic or drug depression.
- **Cheyne-Stokes respiration** (alternating hyperpnea and periods of apnea): Massive supratentorial lesions, bilateral cerebral lesions and mild metabolic disturbance.

- **Central neurogenic hyperventilation:** Lesions of lower midbrain and upper pons either primary or secondary to transtentorial herniation.
- **Apneustic breathing:** Lower pontine lesions.
- **Biot's or ataxic breathing:** Lesions of dorsomedial part of medulla.
- **Agonal gasps:** Bilateral lower brainstem damage and terminal respiratory pattern.
- **Acidotic (Kussmaul) respiration** (deep, sighing hyperventilation): In diabetic ketoacidosis and uremia

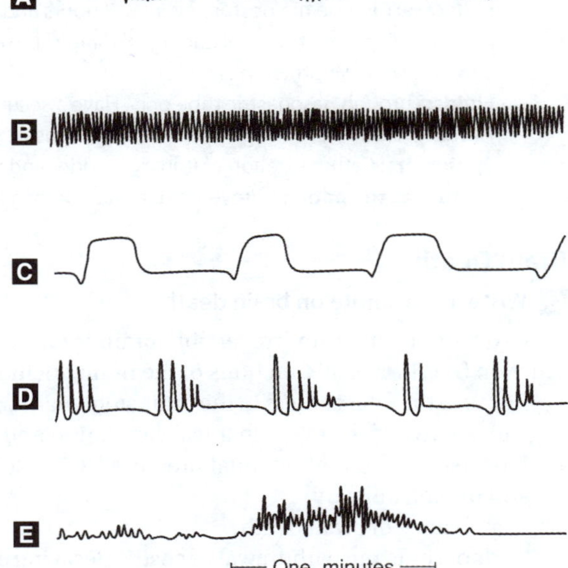

FIGS. 15.44A TO E: Respiratory patterns: (A) Cheyne-Stokes respiration; (B) Central neurogenic hyperventilation; (C) Apneustic breathing; (D) Cluster breathing; (E) Ataxic/Biot's breathing.

Laboratory Studies and Imaging

- Complete blood count
- Random blood sugar
- Renal function tests and liver function tests
- Serum electrolytes
- Urine examination for specific gravity, glucose, acetone, and protein content.
- Arterial blood gases analysis: For acidosis or high CO levels
- Chest X-ray
- ECG
- CT or MRI scan: Quick and effective in demonstrating all types of brain hemorrhage and mass lesions.
- Lumbar puncture: It should be performed in coma only after careful risk assessment. It should not be performed when there is a suspicion of an intracranial mass lesion. CSF examination may help in the diagnosis of meningoencephalitis or other infection, or in subarachnoid hemorrhage.
- EEG: It may be useful in the diagnosis of metabolic coma, encephalitis, and nonconvulsive status epilepticus.
- **Drugs screen:** Blood alcohol and salicylates, urine toxicology (e.g., screening for benzodiazepines, narcotics, amphetamines, etc.).
- Others, e.g., cerebral malaria and porphyria.

Differential Diagnosis

- **Coma vigil (vegetative state—VS):** Patient is comatose, but the eyelids are open giving the appearance of being awake. Patients can open their eyes or have random limb and head movements but there is complete absence of response to commands or to communicate. It is usually due to extensive cortical damage. Brainstem function is intact. Hence, breathing is normal without the need for mechanical ventilation. Patients may remain in this vegetative state for years. Even after 12 months if there is no recovery, it is called permanent vegetative state (PVS).
- **Minimally conscious state (MCS):** A condition in which patient have some limited/inconsistent (fluctuating) signs of awareness (unlike patients with vegetative state). These include nonreflexive response to sensory stimulation, awareness of the self or the environment, or language comprehension or expression.
- **Akinetic mutism:** It refers to a state in which the patient is partially or fully awake, but remains entirely silent and immobile. The patient does nothing voluntarily and has sleep/wake cycles and can maintain vital functions. It may be seen in bilateral frontal lobe lesions, hydrocephalus and a mass in the region of third ventricle.
- **Locked-in-state (locked-in syndrome or pseudocoma):** The patient is fully aware and alert but unable to communicate except through eye movements. There is complete paralysis except vertical eye movements and intact lid movements (blinking in ventral). This syndrome is due to extensive transverse lesions in the pontine and midbrain (infarction).
- **Conversion reaction:** Patients have normal pupils, corneal reflexes, and plantar reflexes. These patients may keep their eyes firmly closed and resist the opening of the eye by examiners. Their eyes roll up when the lids are raised. It may be due to feigned or hysterical state.
- Psychogenic coma.
- Brainstem death is discussed below.

Treatment

- **General management:** Comatose patients require careful nursing, maintenance of the airway, and breathing frequent monitoring of vital functions.
- **Specific treatment:** Diagnosis of the underlying cause/lesion should be done as early as possible and appropriate specific treatment is to be given. For example:
  - **Diabetic with hypoglycemic coma:** Administer hypertonic glucose without waiting for reports. However, bedside estimation of blood glucose and administer dextrose only if the blood glucose is below 100 mg/dL.
  - **Alcoholic with coma:** Administer glucose and vitamin B_1 100 mg intravenously, without waiting for reports.

- **Longer-term management**
  - **Skin care:** Change the posture every 2–3 hours and keep the skin clean and dry to avoid pressure/bed sores and pressure palsies.
  - **Eye care:** To prevent corneal damage (lid taping, irrigation).
  - **Oral hygiene:** Mouthwashes and suction.
  - **Fluids:** Through nasogastric tube or IV. Have a secure IV line.
  - **Feeding:** Nutrients through a fine-bore nasogastric tube.
  - **Sphincters:** Catheterization of urinary bladder and rectal evacuation.
  - **Posture of the patient:** Prevent the aspiration of gastric contents by positioning the patient in prone or lateral position.

Brain Death

Q. Write a short note on brain death.

Brain death occurs from irreversible brain injury which is sufficient to permanently eliminate all cortical and brainstem function (i.e., loss of all functions of the brain, including the brainstem).

- Because the vital centers in the brainstem maintain cardiovascular and respiratory functions, brain death is incompatible with survival despite mechanical ventilation and cardiovascular and nutritional supportive measures.
- It develops when intracranial pressure (ICP) exceeds cerebral perfusion pressure (CPP) and results in cessation of CBF and oxygen delivery.
- Significance of brain death:
  - It permits the withdrawal of costly lifesaving equipment and drugs.
  - Family can be offered the opportunity for organ donation.

Diagnosis of Brain Death

Brain death is a **clinical diagnosis.** No other tests are necessary and complete clinical examination including independent brain death determinations by two licensed physicians is conclusive.

Clinical Evaluation (Prerequisites)

- Establish known irreversible cause of coma.
- The first and foremost critical step in establishing the diagnosis of brain death is to **establish an irreversible, untreatable cause of the brain injury** (e.g., global ischemia due to cardiac arrest, intracranial bleed, and severe head injury).
- **Exclude** potentially **reversible conditions** like hypothermia, drug intoxication, poisoning, metabolic disorders (e.g., hypoglycemia, acidosis, and electrolyte imbalance). Hypothermia should also be excluded—rectal temperature must exceed 35°C.
- Achieve body temperature >36°C.
- Achieve normal systolic BP (>100 mm Hg)

Clinical Evaluation (Neuroassessment)

- **Establish coma**
- **Establish absence of brainstem reflexes**
  - Pupillary reflex (absent)
  - Eye movements
    - Oculocephalic: Absent (doll's eye movements)
    - Oculovestibular: Absent (cold caloric test)
  - Facial sensation and motor response: No corneal reflex, no jaw reflex, no grimacing to deep pressure on nail bed, supraorbital ridge or temporomandibular joint
  - Pharyngeal (gag) reflex absent
  - Tracheal (cough) reflex absent.

Establish Apnea by Apnea Test

Prerequisites for apnea test: Body temperature > 36°C, systolic blood pressure > 100 mm Hg, normal electrolytes profile, and normal $PaCO_2$ (35–45 mm Hg).

Procedure of apnea test:

- Connect a pulse oximeter and disconnect the ventilator.
- Deliver 100% O_2 by catheter through endotracheal tube at 6 L/minute.
- Observe for respiratory movement at least for 8–10 minutes.
- Discontinue testing: If BP drops to <90 mm Hg and PaO_2 decreases to 85% by pulse oximetry for 30 seconds.
- **If respiratory drive/movement** is observed after 8 minutes. Take next blood sample for blood gas studies. This indicates apnea, test result is negative.

- **Absence of respiration drive: If respiratory movements are absent** and arterial $PaCO_2$ is 60 mm Hg or 20 mm Hg increase over a baseline, normal $PaCO_2$ indicates apnea, **test** result is **positive** and **supports the clinical diagnosis of brain death.**

Ancillary Tests/Confirmatory Testing

- EEG: Electrocerebral silence absence of electrical activity during at least 30 minutes.
- Cerebral angiography: Absence of intracranial blood flow.
- PET: Glucose metabolism studies/dynamic nuclear brain scan: "Hollow skull" sign of brain death.

Documentation

Time of death is the time the arterial $PaCO_2$ reached the target value or when ancillary test officially interpreted.

DISEASES OF CRANIAL NERVES

Ist Cranial Nerve: Olfactory Nerve

Common causes of anosmia have been shown in **Box 15.60.**

Box 15.60: Common causes of anosmia.

- **Local causes**
  - Acute local inflammation
  - Heavy smoking
  - Atrophy of bulb
  - Chronic kidney diseases
- **Syndromes associated**
  - **Foster Kennedy syndrome** (anosmia, optic atrophy of one eye and contralateral eye papilledema due to tumor in brain)
  - **Pseudo-Foster Kennedy syndrome** (above features in absence of tumor)
- **Systemic causes**
  - Parkinsonism
  - Meningitis
  - Head trauma
  - Intracranial tumors
  - Endocrine diseases
    - Diabetes mellitus
    - Hypothyroidism
    - Kallmanns syndrome
    - Turners syndrome
  - Vitamin B_{12} deficiency

IInd Cranial Nerve: Optic Nerve

Clinical Examinations

Optic nerve in tested by various modalities of vision: Visual acuity, visual fields, color vision, and fundoscopy.

Visual acuity

- Snellen chart is used to measure visual acuity for distant vision.
- Visual acuity for near vision is tested by Jaeger's chart.

Pathway of optic nerve ***(Fig. 15.45)***

Q. Discuss the field defects produced and localization of lesions at various levels.

Visual fields

- Visual can be impaired by damage to the visual system anywhere from the eyes to the occipital lobes.
- One can localize the site of the lesion with considerable accuracy by mapping the visual field deficit by finger confrontation and then correlating it with the topographic anatomy of the visual pathway.
- At the optic chiasm, fibers from nasal ganglion cells decussate into the contralateral optic tract. Symmetric compression of the optic chiasm by a pituitary adenoma, meningioma, craniopharyngioma, glioma, or aneurysm results in a bitemporal hemianopia.
- A unilateral postchiasmal lesion leaves the visual acuity in each eye unaffected, although the patient may read the letters on only the left or right half of the eye chart.
- Damage to the optic radiations in the temporal lobe (Meyer's loop) produces a superior quadrantic homonymous hemianopia, whereas injury to the optic radiations in the parietal lobe results in an inferior quadrantic homonymous hemianopia.
- Lesions of the primary visual cortex give rise to dense, congruous hemianopic field defects by posterior cerebral artery infarct. They have macular sparing, because collaterals from the middle cerebral artery supply the macular representation at the tip of the occipital lobe.
- Destruction of both occipital lobes produces cortical blindness. This condition can be distinguished from bilateral prechiasmal visual loss by noting that the pupil responses and optic fundi remain normal.

Visual loss

Lesions in any areas between the retina and the visual cortex can produce visual loss. Patterns of visual field loss are shown in **Figure 15.45.**

- **Visual symptoms involving one eye:** Due to lesions anterior to the optic chiasm.
- **Transient visual loss:** It is the sudden onset of visual loss lasting < 15 minutes. It is usually due to vascular disease and may be difficult to identify whether the visual loss was monocular (carotid circulation) or binocular (vertebrobasilar circulation).

Color vision

- The retina has three classes of cones, with visual pigments of differing peak spectral sensitivity: red (560 nm), green (350 nm), and blue (430 nm).
- The red and green cone pigments are encoded on the X chromosome; the blue cone pigment on chromosome 7.

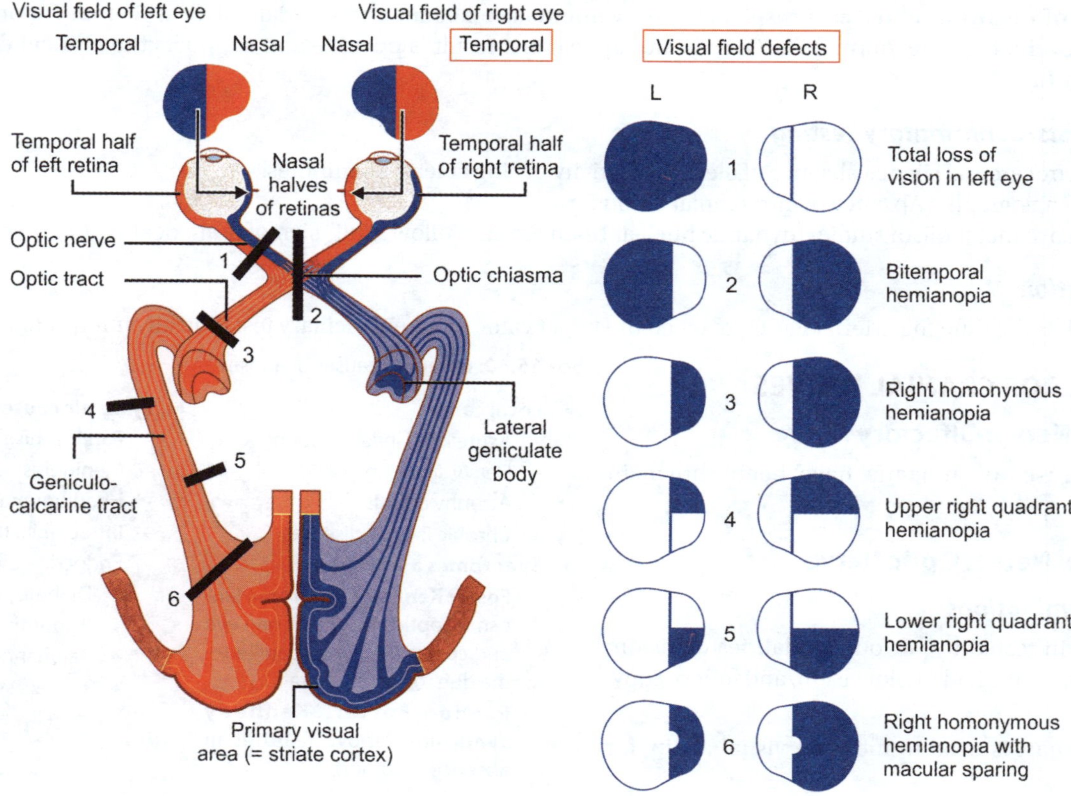

FIG. 15.45: Various visual field defects depending on the location of lesion.

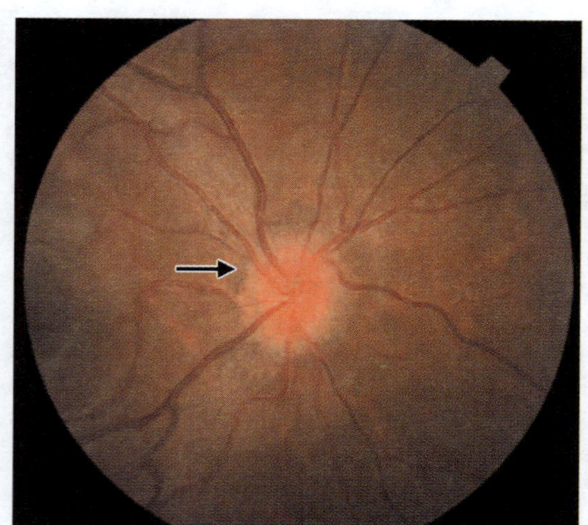

FIG. 15.46: Fundoscopy showing papilledema (arrow).

Box 15.61: Causes of papilledema.

Optic nerve damage	Raised intracranial pressure
• Demyelination (optic neuritis/papillitis) • Anterior ischemic optic neuropathy • Toxins (e.g., methanol) • Infiltration of optic disk by glioma, lymphoma, and sarcoidosis	• Cerebral mass lesion (tumor, abscess granulomas) • Obstructive hydrocephalus, diffuse brain edema • Idiopathic intracranial hypertension • Cerebral venous sinus thrombosis
Ocular blockage of venous drainage	**Systemic disorders affecting retinal vessels**
• Central retinal venous block • Cavernous sinus thrombosis	• Hypertension • Vasculitis: Giant cell arteritis and other autoimmune vasculitides • Hypercapnia, hypercalcemia • COPD (hypercapnia)

- Most common anomalies of color vision are the various types of red-green deficiency inherited as sex-linked recessive condition. Only males are affected (X-linked) and present in 8% males.
- Ishihara color plates can be used to detect red-green color blindness.
- Acquired defects of color vision occur in macular and optic nerve diseases, and due to certain drugs (e.g., ethambutol and chloroquine).

Papilledema (Fig. 15.46)

Q. List the causes of papilledema.

Papilledema is the edema (swelling) of the optic disk >3 diopters. This term has been used only for passive swelling of the optic disk secondary to raised ICP.

Causes of papilledema (Box 15.61)

It develops due to obstruction of venous outflow along with stasis of axoplasmic flow within the optic nerve. It also develops due to any cause that produces edema in the head of the optic nerve (e.g., local causes).

Argyll Robertson Pupil

Q. List the causes and eye findings in Argyll Robertson pupil.

It is the pupillary change where accommodation reflex is present but light reflex is impaired.

Findings (Box 15.62) and causes (Box 15.63)

Site of lesion: Tectum of the midbrain or peripherally in the branch of IIIrd cranial nerve.

Box 15.62: Ophthalmological findings in Argyll Robertson pupil.

- Pupils: Small, irregular, and unequal in size
- Iris: Atrophy and depigmentation
- Light reflex: Absent for direct (always) and consensual (usually stimulus)
- Accommodation reflex: Intact
- Ciliospinal reflex: Absent

Box 15.63: Causes of Argyll Robertson pupil.

- Neurosyphilis (tabes dorsalis) generally bilateral
- Diabetes
- Multiple sclerosis
- Sarcoidosis
- Tumors of pineal region

Pinpoint Pupil

Q. List the causes of pinpoint pupil.

Causes of pinpoint pupil

See **Box 15.64**.

Box 15.64: Causes of pinpoint pupil.

- Pontine hemorrhage
- Organophosphorus poisoning
- Opium poisoning
- Pilocarpine instillation
- Thalamic hemorrhage (occasionally)

Adie's Pupil

Q. Write a short note on Adie's pupil.

- Normally, pupil reaction to light is absent or markedly reduced when tested in the routine examination. However, Adie's pupil reacts slowly with prolonged maximal stimulation.
- Once the Adie's pupil reacts to accommodation, the pupil remains tonically constricted and dilates very slowly.
- **Cause:** Destruction of ciliary ganglion.

Blindness

Q. Write a short note on causes of blindness.

Causes of blindness

See **Box 15.65**.

Box 15.65: Causes of blindness.

- Cataract leading cause (47.9%)
- Glaucoma (12.3%)
- Age-related macular degeneration (AMD) (8.7%)
- Corneal opacities
- Diabetic retinopathy
- Childhood blindness
- Trachoma

Horner's Syndrome (Figs. 15.47A and B)

Q. Write a short essay/note on Horner's syndrome.

- Horner's syndrome is a syndrome complex caused by the involvement of the oculosympathetic tract.
- **Sympathetic nervous supply to the eye** consists of three-neuron pathway:
  1. Fibers through the IIIrd nerve innervate levator muscle of eyelid (Muller's muscles).
  2. Fibers through nasociliary nerve supply the blood vessels of eye.
  3. Fibers through long ciliary nerve innervate pupil.
- Damage to any part of the pathway results in Horner's syndrome.

Components of Horner's Syndrome

See **Box 15.66**.

Causes of Horner's Syndrome

- **Cerebral and brainstem lesions:** Hemispherectomy, massive cerebral infarction, brainstem demyelination
- **Cervical cord lesions:** Syringomyelia and cord tumors (e.g., ependymoma, glioma)
- **Thoracic root level:** Apical lung tumor (pancoast "tumor") or TB, cervical rib, trauma to brachial plexus
- **Sympathetic chain and carotid artery in neck:** Following thyroid/laryngeal/carotid surgery, carotid artery dissection, neoplastic infiltration, cervical sympathectomy
- **Miscellaneous:** Congenital Horner's syndrome, cluster headache (transient), idiopathic.

IIIrd, IVth, and VIth Cranial Nerves: Oculomotor, Trochlear, and Abducens Nerves

Ptosis (Fig. 15.48)

- Normal palpebral fissure 9–12 mm.
- The **narrowing of the palpebral fissures due to inability to open an upper eyelid** is called ptosis.
- Ptosis may be congenital or acquired, unilateral or bilateral, partial or complete
  - **Congenital ptosis:** It is due to bilateral congenital hypoplasia of the IIIrd nerve nuclei, and results in bilateral ptosis.
  - **Acquired ptosis:** Acquired ptosis may be unilateral or bilateral.

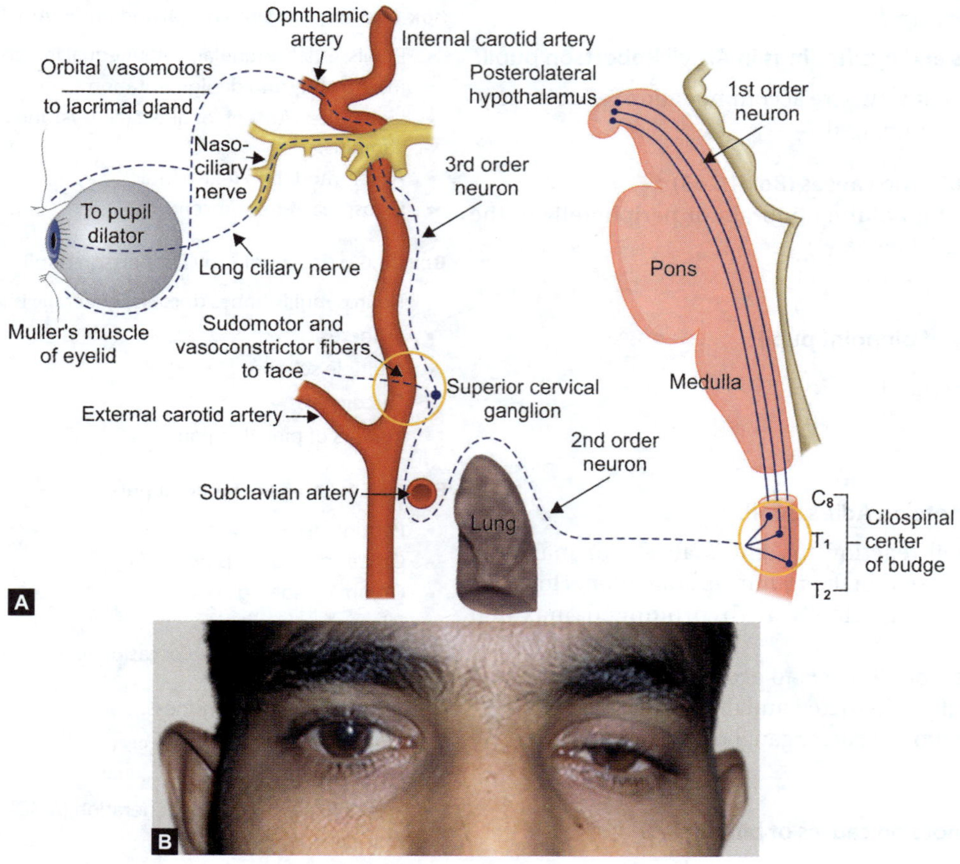

FIGS. 15.47A AND B: Left Horner's syndrome.

Causes of ptosis

Q. Write a short note on the causes of ptosis.

- **Causes for ptosis** are listed in **Tables 15.69 and 15.70**.
- **Partial ptosis:** This occurs with lesion of the cervical sympathetic pathway (Horner's syndrome) due to weakness of the tarsal muscles, innervated by cervical sympathetic nerves. The upper eyelids can however be raised voluntarily.
- **Complete ptosis:** This occurs with IIIrd nerve lesions due to paralysis of the levator palpebrae superioris, innervated by the IIIrd nerve. The patient is not able to voluntarily open the affected eye.

Ptosis and Pupillary Size

- Ptosis with a small pupil: Horner's syndrome
- Ptosis with a large pupil: IIIrd nerve palsy (compressive lesions).
- Ptosis with normal papillary size: Infarction of IIIrd nerve, myasthenia gravis, myopathies or GBS.

Ophthalmoplegia

- Ophthalmoplegia is the paralysis or weakness of the eye muscles.
- **Supranuclear ophthalmoplegia**—also called as gaze palsies. It is due to involvement of corticonuclear fibers of the IIIrd, IVth, and VIth cranial nerves.
- **Internuclear ophthalmoplegia**—due to involvement of medial longitudinal fasciculus (MLF) and paramedian pontine reticular formation (PPRF) which connect the IIIrd nerve to the contralateral VIth nerve.
- **Nuclear/Infranuclear ophthalmoplegia**—involvement of individual cranial nerves. (CN III, IV, and VI).
- **Internal ophthalmoplegia**—paralysis of constrictor pupillae and ciliary muscle.
- **External ophthalmoplegia**—paralysis of extraocular muscles.
- **Total ophthalmoplegia**—combination of external and internal ophthalmoplegia.

Box 15.66: Components of Horner's syndrome.

- Miosis due to reduced pupillodilator activity
- Partial ptosis of eyelid
- Enophthalmos
- Anhidrosis of ipsilateral half of face
- Absence of ciliospinal reflex

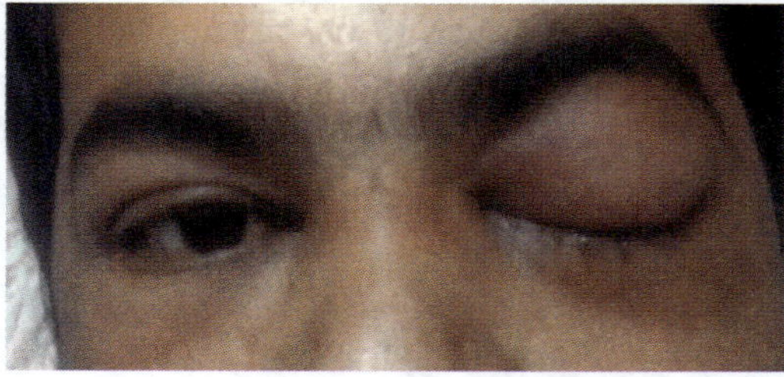

FIG. 15.48: Unilateral ptosis.

TABLE 15.69: Causes of ptosis.

1. **Congenital ptosis**	
2. **Acquired ptosis**	
Neurogenic	➤ Horner's syndrome ➤ IIIrd nerve palsy
Neuromuscular disorder	➤ Myasthenia gravis (fatigable ptosis) ➤ Poisoning (snake bite/ botulism)
Myogenic	➤ Mitochondrial myopathy ➤ Oculopharyngeal muscle dystrophy ➤ Myotonic dystrophy
Mechanical ptosis	Due to eyelid edema or tumors

TABLE 15.70: Causes of unilateral and bilateral ptosis.

Unilateral ptosis	*Bilateral ptosis*
➢ IIIrd cranial nerve lesion ➢ Lesion of cervical sympathetic pathway (Horner's syndrome) ➢ Lesions of the upper eyelid	➢ Myopathies ➢ Myasthenia gravis ➢ Bilateral Horner's syndrome ➢ Snake bite ➢ Botulism

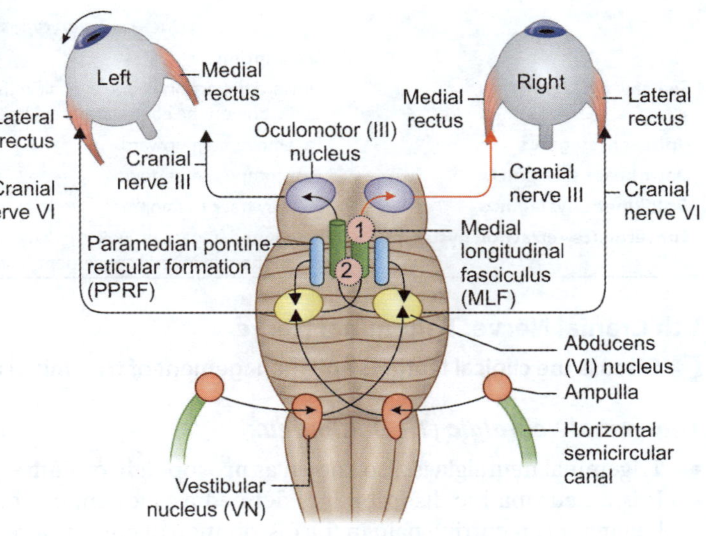

FIG. 15.49: Lesions of medial longitudinal fasciculus (MLF).

Internuclear Ophthalmoplegia (Fig. 15.49)

Q. Write a short note on internuclear ophthalmoplegia.

- It is caused by a lesion of the MLF, which carries signals from the abducens nucleus to the contralateral medial rectus oculomotor subnucleus.
- The abducens nerve and MLF coordinate conjugate horizontal eye movements with co-contraction of ipsilateral lateral rectus and contralateral medial rectus muscles.
- Classic signs of unilateral internuclear ophthalmoplegia include impaired adduction of the ipsilesional eye and abducting nystagmus of the contralateral eye.

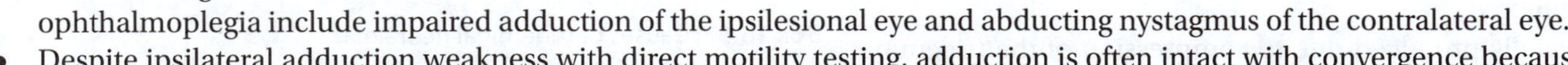

- Despite ipsilateral adduction weakness with direct motility testing, adduction is often intact with convergence because convergence signals to the medial rectus nucleus are distinct from the MLF.

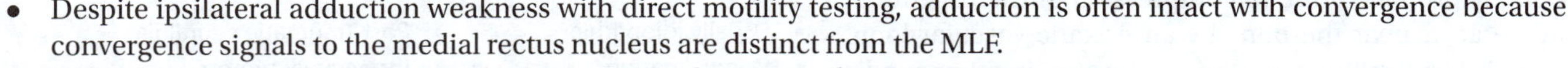

- Multiple sclerosis and microvascular brainstem ischemia are the most common causes.

Diplopia

Q. Write a short note on diplopia.

Diplopia means double vision. Most common subjective complain elicited by lesions in the oculomotor system. It occurs more frequently with lesions of the extraocular muscles or oculomotor nerves than with supranuclear lesions which result in gaze palsies.

- **Monocular diplopia**
  - The first point to clarify is whether diplopia persists in either eye after covering the fellow eye. If it does, the diagnosis is monocular diplopia.
  - The cause is usually intrinsic to the eye. For example, corneal aberrations, uncorrected refractive error, cataract, or foveal traction may give rise to monocular diplopia.
- **Binocular diplopia**
  - Diplopia alleviated by covering one eye is binocular diplopia and is caused by disruption of ocular alignment, occurs only if both eyes are open.
  - Binocular diplopia occurs from a wide range or processes. For example, infectious, neoplastic, metabolic, degenerative, inflammatory, and vascular.
  - Here two images, one real and one false are formed. The real image is closer to the eye and distinct; the false image is farther away from eye and indistinct.

Nystagmus

Q. List the causes of nystagmus.

Nystagmus is involuntary, conjugate, repetitive and rhythmic movement of eyeballs. It is a sign of disease of the retina, cerebellum and/or vestibular systems, and their connections.

Types of Nystagmus (Table 15.71)

TABLE 15.71: Types of nystagmus.

Pendular nystagmus	*Jerk nystagmus*			*Nystagmus of dissociated rhythm*
In this time of amplitude of nystagmus is equal in either directions	In this type of nystagmus, there is slow component followed by fast (jerk) component due to cortical correction.			Usually gaze-evoked nystagmus
	Horizontal	**Vertical**	**Rotatory**	
These are predominantly seen in congenital conditions especially due to visual defects from earlier years	➢ Labyrinthine disorders ➢ Cerebellar disorders ➢ Uppermost cervical lesion	➢ Never labyrinthine ➢ Cerebellar disorders ➢ Brainstem lesions ➢ Drugs like benzodiazepines, barbiturate	➢ Labyrinthine disorders ➢ Brainstem lesions	➢ MLF lesions ➢ Multiple sclerosis

Other common types of nystagmus		
	Description	**Condition seen**
See-saw nystagmus	Upward deflection of one eyeball with downward deflection on the contralateral eyeball	Suprasellar region anterior to IIIrd ventricle
Upbeat nystagmus	Fast movement upward	Lesions in the vermis of the cerebellum
Downbeat nystagmus	Fast component is down	Foramen magnum lesions
Optokinetic nystagmus	Railway track nystagmus	Deep parietal lobe lesions
Convergence-retraction nystagmus	Attempted upgaze provokes jerk nystagmus with fast component in inward convergent manner	Lesion at superior colliculus—Parinaud's syndrome

Vth Cranial Nerve: Trigeminal Nerve

Q. Discuss the clinical features and management of trigeminal neuralgia.

Trigeminal Neuralgia (Tic Douloureux)

- Trigeminal neuralgia is also known as **prosopalgia or Fothergill's disease.** Tic Douloureux means painful jerking.
- It is a neuropathic disorder. It is defined as sudden, episodes of usually unilateral, severe, brief, stabbing, intense, lancinating, recurring pain in the distribution of one or more branches of the Vth cranial nerve (trigeminal nerve).
- Middle age and later. Usually, it starts in the 6th and 7th decades and major risk factor is hypertension.

Etiology

Usually produced due to compression of the trigeminal nerve at or near the pons by an ecstatic vascular loop. Pain like trigeminal neuralgia can be seen in other conditions **(Box 15.67)**.

Box 15.67: Causes of trigeminal neuralgia.

- Usually idiopathic
- Demyelination
- Multiple sclerosis
- Petrous ridge compression
- Post-traumatic neuralgia
- Intracranial tumors
- Intracranial vascular abnormalities
- Viral etiology

Clinical features

Pain

- **Characteristics of pain:** Sudden, unilateral, intermittent (paroxysmal), sharp, shooting/knife-like/lancinating/electric shock-like. Pain rarely crosses the midline. In extreme cases, the patient will have a motionless face known as the "frozen or mask-like face". In 10–12% of cases it is bilateral and usually due to intrinsic brainstem pathology (e.g., MS) or expanding cranial tumor (acoustic schwannomas, meningiomas, epidermoids).
- **Duration of pain:** Pain is of short duration (lasting seconds), but may recur with variable frequency (may be many times a day). Attacks do not occur during sleep.
- Pain occurs along the cutaneous distribution of the Vth nerve (full or branches). Pain usually commences in the mandibular division but may spread to involve the maxillary and occasionally the ophthalmic divisions.
- Pain is precipitated by minor trauma to the trigger zones (e.g., slight touch, chewing, shaving, rinsing mouth, exposure to cold wind). Common trigger zones can be external/cutaneous (around the ala of nose, corners of lips and check) or internal/intraoral (teeth, gingivae, tongue). Trigger area on the face are so sensitive that touching or even air currents can trigger an episode.
- Neither objective signs of sensory loss nor signs of Vth nerve dysfunction can be demonstrated on examination.

Differential diagnosis

Reactivation of the varicella zoster virus is seen in older people and has predilection for ophthalmic division of the trigeminal nerve.

Treatment

- **First line of treatment: Carbamazepine** (anticonvulsant) to be started with a dose of 100–200 mg/day, increase in 2–3 weeks to 200–400 mg TID.
- **Second line of treatment:** Baclofen, lamotrigine, oxcarbazepine, phenytoin, gabapentin, pregabalin, sodium valproate.
- **Long-acting anesthetic agents:** Localized pain is managed by injecting any of the following into the particular branch of the nerve.
  - Alcohol injection
  - Peripheral glycerol injection
- **Surgery:** Indicated if drug fails or not tolerated.
  - Peripheral neurectomy (nerve avulsion)
  - Open procedures (intracranial procedures)
  - Microvascular decompression
  - Percutaneous rhizotomies
  - Gamma knife radiosurgery: Using stereotactic imaging of the trigeminal nerve root entry zone, radiation to delivered to trigeminal nerve.

VIIth Cranial Nerve: Facial Nerve

See **Figure 15.50.**

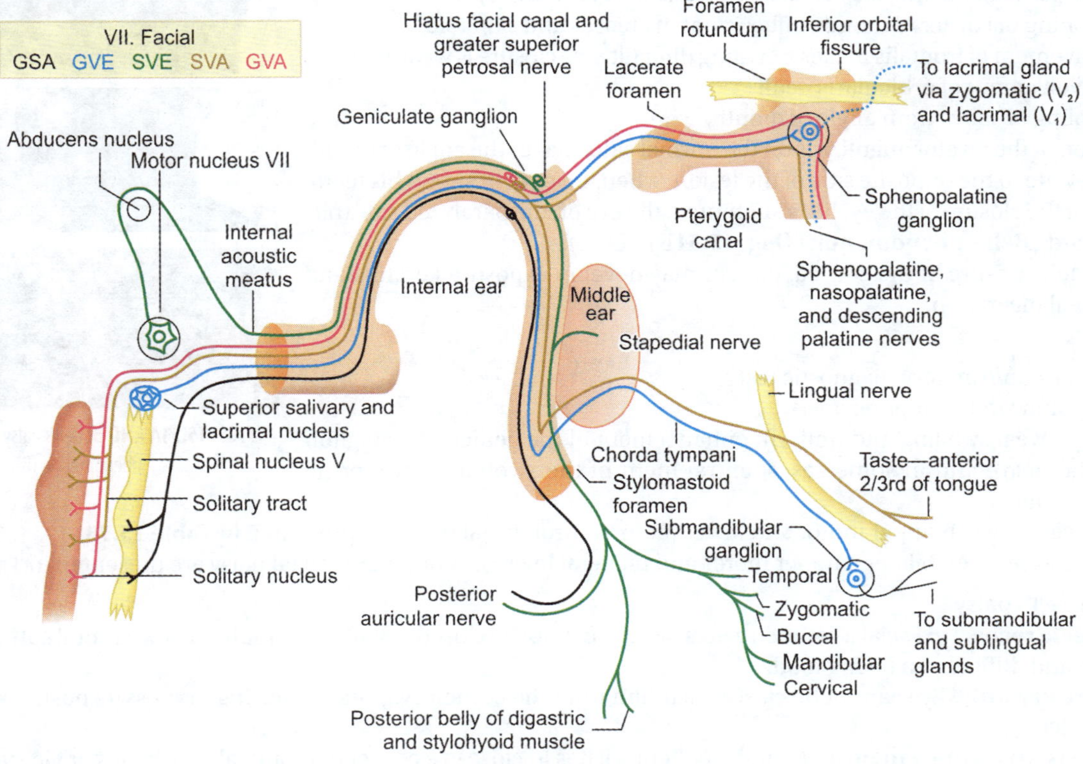

FIG. 15.50: Facial nerve anatomy.

Causes of Facial Nerve Palsy

See **Table 15.72.**

Q. List the causes of facial nerve palsy.

TABLE 15.72: Causes of facial nerve palsy.

Unilateral	*Bilateral*
Upper motor neuron ➢ Vascular (stroke) ➢ Tumor ➢ Multiple sclerosis	**Upper motor neuron** ➢ Vascular (multi-infarct dementia) ➢ Motor neuron disease
Lower motor neuron ➢ Bell's palsy ➢ Ramsay Hunt syndrome ➢ Parotid tumor ➢ Head injury ➢ Skull base tumor ➢ Basal meningitis ➢ Diabetes mellitus ➢ Hypertension ➢ Chronic suppurative otitis media	**Lower motor neuron** ➢ Guillain–Barré syndrome ➢ Sarcoidosis (uveoparotid fever) ➢ Leprosy ➢ Lyme disease ➢ Leukemia ➢ Lymphoma ➢ Moebius syndrome ➢ Melkersson–Rosenthal syndrome ➢ Toxin: Thalidomide ➢ Bilateral Bell's palsy

Bell's Palsy

Q. Discuss the etiology, clinical features, differential diagnosis, and management of Bell's palsy.

Q. Write a short essay/note on Bell's palsy.

Most common form of unilateral isolated lower motor neuron type of facial paralysis is Bell's palsy.

Pathophysiology

- Main cause of Bell's palsy is thought to be latent herpes viruses (herpes simplex virus type 1 and herpes zoster virus), which are reactivated from cranial nerve ganglia. It causes **swelling of nerve within** the tight petrous bone **facial canal.**
- Herpes zoster virus shows more aggressive biological behavior than herpes simplex virus type 1.
- Polymerase chain reaction (PCR) techniques have isolated herpes virus DNA from the facial nerve during acute palsy.
- Inflammation of the nerve initially results in a reversible neuropraxia,

Clinical manifestations

- **Race:** Slightly higher in persons of Japanese descent. Familial incidence—4.1%.
- **Age and gender:** Highest in persons aged 15–45 years. It is rare below the age of 15 and above the age of 60. No gender difference exists.
- **Onset is fairly abrupt,** with **pain around the ear** preceding the unilateral facial weakness (maximal weakness by 48 hours). Patients often describe the face as "numb" and sometimes give the history of exposure to cold.
- **Associated symptoms:** Hyperacusis, decreased production of tears and saliva, and altered taste, otalgia or aural fullness and facial or retroauricular pain.
- Less common in pregnancy but prognosis is significantly worse in pregnant women.

- **Examination:** Shows features of isolated lower motor neuron facial paralysis. On the affected side **following features are observed.** These include:
  - Paralysis of all the muscles of facial expression **(Fig. 15.51A)**.
  - Dropping of corner of mouth, effacement of creases and skin fold.
  - Involvement of frontalis makes frowning difficult. Eye closure is weak because of involvement of orbicularis oculi
  - Drooling of saliva from angle of mouth.
  - Action of the levator anguli oris on the normal side, makes the angle of mouth to deviate to the opposite side of the lesion, when the patient shows his teeth.
  - When the closure of the eyelid is attempted, the eye on the paralyzed side rolls upward **(Bell's phenomenon) (Fig. 15.51B)**.
  - Due to exposure of the cornea, patient may develop exposure keratitis and corneal ulceration.

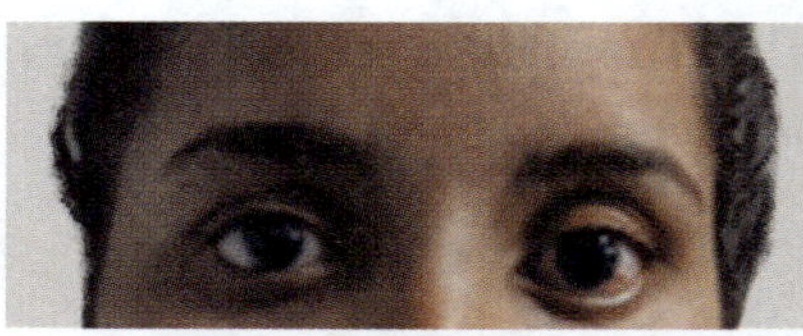

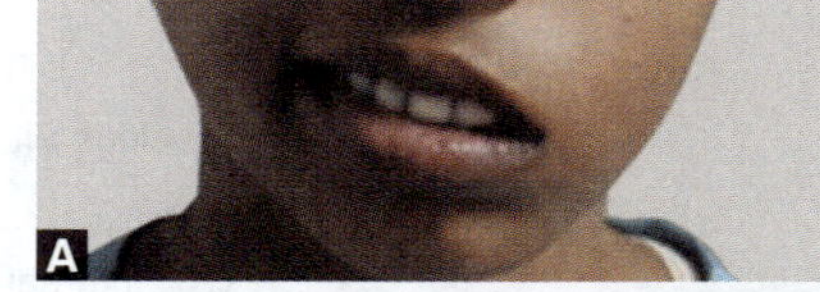

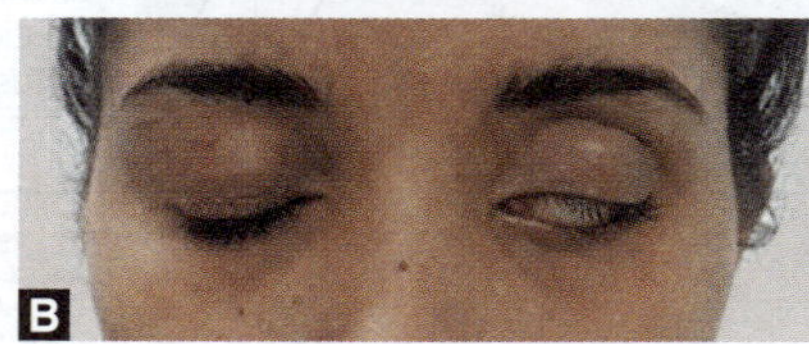

FIGS. 15.51A AND B: Bell's palsy (A) with Bell's phenomenon (B).

Investigation

- No specific confirmatory diagnostic test.
- CSF may show mild lymphocytosis.
- MRI may reveal swelling and uniform enhancement of the geniculate ganglion and facial nerve and in some cases, entrapment of the swollen nerve in the temporal bone.

The differences between upper motor and lower motor neuron facial palsy are presented in **Table 15.73**.

The differences between bilateral upper motor and bilateral lower motor neuron facial palsy are presented in **Table 15.74**.

Sequelae of Bell's palsy

- **Incomplete recovery:** Facial asymmetry persists; eye cannot be closed resulting in epiphora. A weak oral sphincter causes drooling and difficulty in taking food.
- **Exposure keratitis:** Eye cannot be closed, tear film from the cornea evaporates causing dryness, exposure keratitis and corneal ulcer.
- **Synkinesis (mass movement):** When the patient wishes to close eye corner of mouth also twitches or vice versa.
- **Tics and spasm:** Result of faulty regeneration of fibers. Involuntary movements are seen on the affected side of face.
- **Contractures:** Results from fibrosis of atrophied or fixed contraction of a group of muscles.
- **Crocodile tears (gustatory lacrimation):** Unilateral lacrimation with mastication. Due to faulty regeneration of parasympathetic fibers which now supply lacrimal gland instead of the salivary glands.
- **Frey's syndrome (gustatory sweating):** Sweating and flushing of skin over the parotid during mastication. It results from parotid surgery.
- Anomalous regeneration of the seventh nerve fibers. Originally connected with the orbicularis oculi come to innervate the orbicularis oris, closure of the lids may cause a retraction of the mouth. Jaw opening causing closure of the eyelids on the side of the facial palsy is termed **Marcus Gunn jaw-winking phenomenon.**

Treatment

- Severe facial weakness may produce inability to blink and lead to **exposure keratitis.** Use of **lubricating eye drops** may be needed, and **paper tape** to close the eye during sleep.
- Massage of weekend muscles.

Medical treatment of Bell's palsy:

- Steroids (Prednisolone) 1 mg/kg/day for 5–7 days and then tapered over the next 1 week.
- Antiviral agents: for 5–7 days.
  - Famciclovir 500 mg BD.
  - Valacyclovir 500 mg BD.
  - Acyclovir 800 mg five times a day.
- **Surgical decompression**—only if no resolution of symptoms after 2 weeks.

TABLE 15.73: Differences between upper motor neuron (UMN) and lower motor neuron (LMN) facial palsy.

UMN facial palsy	*LMN facial palsy*
Lower part of the face is involved	Both lower and upper part of the face are involved
No Bell's phenomenon	Bell's phenomenon is seen
Taste is not affected	Taste is affected
No hyperacusis	Hyperacusis may be present if nerve to stapedius is involved
Usually associated with hemiplegia	Usually not associated unless any pontine lesion is present causing crossed hemiplegia
Site of the lesion is above facial nucleus usually in the internal capsule	Usually in the nucleus or distal to the nucleus
No wasting or atrophy	Wasting or atrophy may be present

TABLE 15.74: Differences between bilateral upper motor neuron (UMN) and bilateral lower motor neuron (LMN) facial palsy.

Bilateral UMN palsy	*Bilateral LMN palsy*
➢ Emotional fibers—spared ➢ Emotional incontinence present ➢ Associated with bilateral long tract signs ➢ Jaw jerk—exaggerated ➢ Corneal reflex—present ➢ Taste sensation—spared ➢ Gag reflex—exaggerated	➢ Bell's phenomenon present ➢ Emotional fibers—affected ➢ Long tract signs—absent ➢ Jaw jerk—normal ➢ Corneal reflex—absent ➢ Taste sensation—absent

INTRACRANIAL PRESSURE

Q. Discuss the clinical manifestations and management of increased ICP.

Raised Intracranial Pressure

- Normal ICP in adults is <10–15 mm Hg. There are normal regular waves due to pulse and respiration.
- With increased pressure "pressure waves" appear. With continued rise of ICP, the perfusion pressure (PP) falls. When PP falls CBF is reduced. Electrical cortical activity fails if CBF is 20 mL/100 g/min.
- When ICP reaches MAP circulation to the brain stops.
- Raised intracranial pressure (RIP) may be caused by mass lesions, cerebral edema, obstruction to CSF circulation causing hydrocephalus, impaired CSF absorption and cerebral venous obstruction.

Common Causes of Raised Intracranial Pressure

See **Table 15.75.**

TABLE 15.75: Common causes of raised intracranial pressure.

Primary or intracranial causes	
Mass lesions ➢ **Intracranial hemorrhage** (traumatic or spontaneous): Extradural or subdural hematoma, intracerebral hemorrhage ➢ **Brain tumor:** Posterior fossa tumor or high-grade gliomas ➢ **Infective:** Cerebral abscess, tuberculomas, cysticercosis, hydatid cyst ➢ **Colloid cyst** (in ventricles)	**Disturbance of CSF circulation** ➢ **Obstructive** (noncommunicating) **hydrocephalus:** Obstruction within ventricular system ➢ **Communicating hydrocephalus:** Obstruction outside ventricular system
Diffuse brain edema or swelling ➢ Meningoencephalitis ➢ Trauma (diffuse head injury, near-drowning) ➢ Subarachnoid hemorrhage ➢ Metabolic (e.g., water intoxication) ➢ Idiopathic intracranial hypertension ➢ Postneurosurgery	**Obstruction to venous sinuses** ➢ Cerebral venous thrombosis ➢ Trauma (fractures overlying sinuses)
Secondary or extracranial causes	
➢ Hypoxia or hypercarbia (hypoventilation) ➢ Hyperpyrexia ➢ Drug and toxins (e.g., valproate sodium, lead intoxication)	➢ Hepatic failure ➢ Seizure ➢ Reye's syndrome ➢ High-attitude cerebral edema

Clinical Features

- Signs and symptoms of underlying cause.
- **Features of raised ICP (Box 15.68).**
- The speed of increase in the pressure influences presentation.
- **Acute:** If ICP has risen acutely (as in aggressive tumors), there is no time for compensatory mechanisms to develop and causes leading early symptoms, including sudden death. The pulse rate is slower, BP may be elevated (Cushing's reflex) and respiratory depression (Cushing's triad).
- **Slow:** Compensatory mechanisms develop (e.g., alteration in the volume of fluid in CSF spaces and venous sinuses) which minimize symptoms. Raised ICP of more than a few days will result in papilledema.
- VIth cranial nerve palsy: Due either to stretching of the long slender nerve or to compression against the petrous temporal bone ridge. It may be unilateral or bilateral.
- Other cranial nerve III, V, and VII may also be involved.

Box 15.68: Features of raised intracranial pressure (ICP).

- Diffuse anterior headache worse on lying/straining
- Vomiting
- Diplopia (VIth nerve involvement)
- Papilledema
- Bradycardia, raised blood pressure
- Impaired conscious level: Drowsiness and mental deterioration
- Seizures

Herniation Syndromes

Raised ICT may cause displacement and herniation of the brain. Types of herniation are presented in **Figure 15.52**.

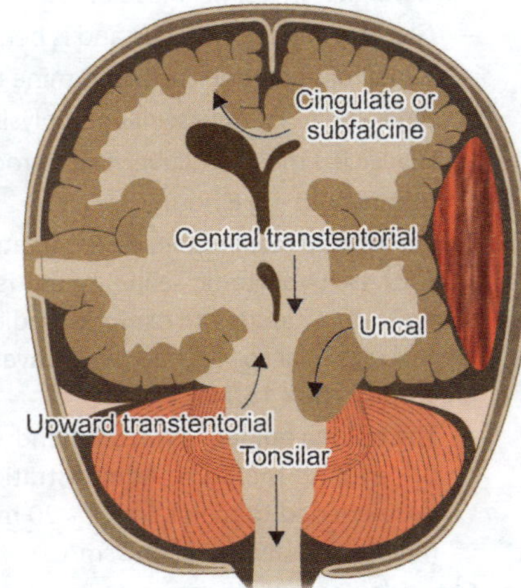

FIG. 15.52: Types of herniation.

Supratentorial Herniation

- **Uncal:** Most frequent herniation in which downward displacement of the medial temporal lobe (uncus) through the tentorium occurs.
- Results in ipsilateral pupil dilatation, decreased level of consciousness, changes in respiratory patterns, respiratory arrest, and contralateral hemiplegia.
- **Subfalcine** herniation results in opposite lower limb weakness (ACA involvement).

Central/Transtentorial Herniation

Results in loss of consciousness, small reactive pupils advancing to fixed/dilated pupils, respiratory changes leading to respiratory arrest and decorticate posturing advancing to flaccidity.

Infratentorial Herniation

Downward herniation of the cerebellar tonsils through the foramen magnum may compress the medulla oblongata (tonsillar coning) causing respiratory and cardiac arrest.

Uncal Syndrome

- Herniation of the temporal lobe (medial) transtentorially results in uncal syndrome.
- It produces drowsiness in early stages and is accompanied by unilateral pupillary dilatation.
- Sometimes due to lateral mass effect, opposite cerebral peduncle is crushed against the tentorium. This causes Babinski sign and weakness of arm and leg ipsilateral to the lesion **(Kernohan–Woltman sign).**

Investigations

- Depending on the underlying lesion/etiology.
- CT head: It may show midline shift and compression of basal cisterns.
- ICP monitoring: It is done in selected cases. For example, patients with GCS < 8 and CT scan show hematoma, contusion, edema, herniation or compressed basal cisterns.

Q. Discuss the management of increased ICP.

Treatment/Management of Increased Intracranial Pressure

Aims (Box 15.69)

- **Airway management**
- Glasgow Coma Scale < 8 requires intubation to protect airway.
- **Head positioning:** Head should be kept in midline, with around 15–30° elevation.
- **Temperature control:** Temperature can be lowered with acetaminophen and cooling blankets. Shivering prevented by neuromuscular block.
- **Hemodynamic management:** Maintain MAP > 90 mm Hg. Administer normal saline to achieve a central venous pressure of 5–10 mm Hg. Serum sodium to be maintained between 140 and 150 mmol/L.
- **Seizure management:** Prophylactic antiepileptics (phenytoin).
- **Analgesia, sedation and neuromuscular block**
  - Analgesia: Opioid like fentanyl and morphine
  - Sedation: Benzodiazepines like lorazepam and midazolam
  - Neuromuscular block: Pancuronium and vecuronium.

Box 15.69: Aims of management of increased intracranial pressure.

- Relieve the cause (e.g., surgical decompression of mass)
- Steroids to reduce vasogenic edema or shunt
- Procedure to relieve hydrocephalus
- Supportive treatment: Maintenance of fluid balance, blood pressure control, head elevation, and use of diuretics such as mannitol. Intensive care support may be required

Specific Therapy

- **Mannitol:** Osmotic diuretic
  - Mechanism: Rheologic and osmotic
  - Adverse effect: (1) intravascular volume depletion and (2) acute renal failure
- **Glycerol** acts in a similar fashion but is used less often.
  - Glycerol has caloric value and is beneficial for nutritional support.
  - Renal function does not determine the diuretic action. Hence, it can be given to patients with renal insufficiency.
  - Side effect: is intravascular hemolysis, which can be prevented by giving a low concentration (<20%) at a slow infusion rate (>1 hour).
  - Glycerol is most effective via enteroduodenal administration.
- **Frusemide:** 20 mg 8 hourly.
- **Hypertonic saline:** A more recent treatment for increased ICP is IV administration of 3–23.4% hypertonic saline. IV boluses can reduce ICP and augment CPP for several hours. Creates an osmotic gradient and draws water from the intracellular and extracellular spaces into the intravascular compartment. Potential side effects are listed in **Box 15.70**.
  - The trauma guidelines recommend: Continuous infusion of 3% saline between 0.1 and 1.0 mL/kg/h. Administration on a sliding scale, with the minimal dose needed to maintain ICP <20 mm Hg. Care to be taken while using hypertonic saline to decrease ICP, the osmolarity has to be maintained below 360 mOsm/L.

Box 15.70: Side effects of treatment by hypertonic saline in raised ICP.

- Hyperosmolar central pontine myelinolysis
- Congestive heart failure
- Subdural hematomas
- Coagulopathy (rarely)

- **Steroids: Dexamethasone** 4 mg 6 hourly. Helps only in reducing vasogenic edema around tumor, abscess or subdural hematoma. Routine administration of steroids should be avoided in patients with traumatic brain injury and raised ICP.
- **Barbiturate coma in refractory cases:** Pentobarbital 5 mg/kg lowers ICP by lowering the rate of the body's metabolic process, oxygen consumption and carbon dioxide production. Burst suppression correlates with maximal metabolic suppression.
- **Hyperventilation:** Mechanism by which hyperventilation decreases raised intracranial tension is by decreasing cerebral blood volume by vasoconstriction. **Hyperventilation** resulting in drop in $PaCO_2$ to around 25–35 decreases CBF.
- **Management of underlying cause** wherever possible or applicable.

Surgical Management

- Management of underlying cause of raised ICP.
- **Mass lesion:** Surgical decompression of mass lesion, removal of space-occupying lesion. Surgical decompression is a lifesaving procedure in which limited frontal or temporal lobectomies are done.
- **Hydrocephalus:** Ventriculoatrial or ventriculoperitoneal shunting.

TUMORS OF THE NERVOUS SYSTEM

Among CNS tumors glial tumors are the most common, accounting for 50–60% of primary brain tumors. Meningiomas account for about 25% and schwannomas for about 10%. Few primary tumors are listed in **Box 15.71**.

Box 15.71: Few common tumors of CNS.

- Astrocytoma
  - Low-grade astrocytoma
  - High-grade astrocytoma
- Oligodendrogliomas
- Ependymomas
- Medulloblastoma
- CNS lymphoma (more common in HIV patients)
- Meningiomas
- Schwannomas

Cerebellopontine Angle Tumors

Q. Write a short note on cerebellopontine angle (CP angle) tumors.

Cerebellopontine angle is an area of lateral cistern containing CSF, arachnoid tissue, cranial nerves and its associated vessels.

Box 15.72: Cerebellopontine angle tumors.

- Vestibular schwannoma/ acoustic neuroma
- Meningioma
- Cerebellar glioma

Less likely: Arachnoid cyst, nonacoustic cranial nerve schwannomas, vascular malformations, dermoids, teratomas, and lipomas.

- CP angle tumors constitute the most common posterior fossa tumors and majority of them are benign.
- Various CP angle tumors are listed in **Box 15.72**.

Clinical Features

- Most common: Progressive unilateral sensory neural hearing loss (SNHL) (retrocochlear) present in 95% of cases and often accompanied by tinnitus which is present in 65% of cases.
- Rare presentations include facial numbness or pain, earache or facial weakness, cerebellar ataxia or symptoms of hydrocephalus (headache, visual disturbance, mental status change, nausea, and vomiting).

Signs

- Ear: Normal otoscopy
- Cranial nerves:
  - 5th cranial nerve: Earliest sign is impaired corneal reflex. Motor functions are affected rarely.
  - 7th cranial nerve: Sensory first; loss of sensation in the posterior superior aspect of external auditory canal (EAC) called Hitselberger's sign. Lower motor neuron facial palsy develops later.
  - 9th and10th cranial nerve: Palsy-palatal, pharyngeal and laryngeal paralysis.
- Eyes: Nystagmus.
- Cerebellar signs present (ipsilateral).

Investigations

- **Audiological tests:** It show features of retrocochlear hearing loss (high-frequency SNHL), recruitment negative, poor speech discrimination score and presence of rollover phenomenon.
- **Acoustic reflex:** Nearly in 75% patients the stapedial reflex is lost.
- **Caloric test:** It is diminished or absent. Normal test finding does not eliminate the diagnosis.
- **Plain X-ray:** The best view is periorbital view; difference of 1 mm in the vertical height of internal acoustic meatus is significant.
- **CT scan (Fig. 15.53):** It cannot detect intermeatal tumors.
- **MRI:** With gadolinium enhancement is gold standard.

Treatment

- Surgical excision
- Radiotherapy: Stereotactic radiosurgery (gamma knife) may stop the growth of vestibular schwannoma mainly in small intracanalicular and extra canalicular lesions
- Radiosurgery is recommended in bilateral vestibular schwannomas (e.g., Morbus Recklinghausen) but only when the tumors are small.
- Annual imaging is recommended for all patients being managed conservatively for the rest of their life or until vestibular schwannoma growth is seen to a certain limit.

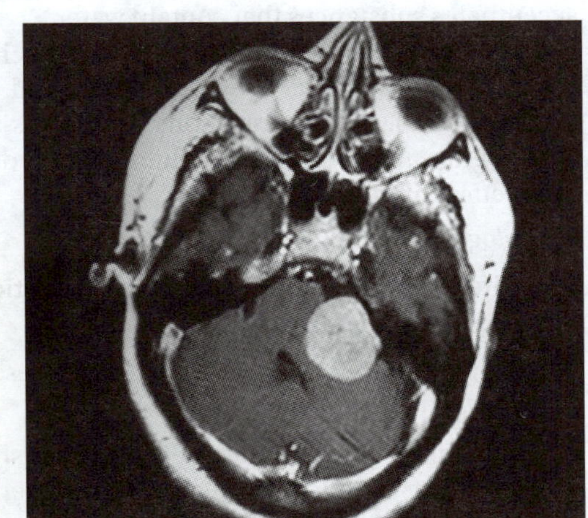

FIG. 15.53: CT showing cerebellopontine angle tumor.

Acoustic Neuroma (Schwannoma)

Q. Write a short note on acoustic neuroma.

- It is a benign tumor which arises from Schwann cells of the 8th cranial (vestibular) nerve. Majority are sporadic and unilateral.
- Common between the 4th and 6th decade of life, with a slight female preponderance.
- Site: Commonly arises near the nerve's entry point into the medulla or in the internal auditory meatus and extends into the cerebellopontine angle. Constitutes 80–90% of tumors at the cerebellopontine angle.

Clinical features: Unilateral progressive hearing impairment/loss, sometimes with tinnitus. Large tumors may manifest signs and symptoms of cerebellar and brainstem involvement.

Investigations: MRI is the investigation of choice.

Management: Total surgical excision is the treatment of choice. Stereotactic radiosurgery (radiotherapy) may be used for some tumors.

MISCELLANEOUS

Neuroimaging

Q. Write a short note on radiological investigation used in neurology.

- About 90% of neurological cases can be diagnosed by history alone, with a lesser contribution from examination and investigation.
- Investigations include assessment of structure (imaging) and function (neurophysiology).
- Neurological imaging is used for **assessment of structure.** Various techniques include X-rays (plain X-rays, CT, CT angiography, myelography, and angiography), magnetic resonance (MRI, MRA), and ultrasound (Doppler imaging of blood vessels). However, it is now possible to use imaging techniques to assess CNS function also.
- **Single-photon emission computed tomography** scanning can be used to mark CBF by using a lipid-soluble radioactive tracer. It is useful in dementia or epilepsy. Single photon emission computed tomography (SPECT) is also useful in the **diagnosis of movement disorders** (e.g., by examining dopamine activity to assess the function of the basal ganglia in patients with suspected parkinsonism).

Magnetic Resonance Imaging

Magnetic resonance imaging is an imaging technique used mainly in medical field to produce high-quality images of the inside structures of the human.

The principle of MRI is based on the presence of hydrogen atom in all human tissues. A hydrogen nucleus/atom is a proton whose electrical charge creates a local electrical field. Protons in body tissue are aligned to the magnetic axes. When protons are surrounded by a sudden strong magnetic impulses/field (as in an MRI machine), the protons are aligned along the field. Application of a radiofrequency wave at right angles to their alignment and is imaged. Then the field is suddenly reduced, and the protons resonate and spin, then revert to their normal alignment. When the magnitude and rate of energy release occurs with return to baseline alignment, images are made at different phases of relaxation. They are known as T_1, T_2, T_2 STIR, FLAIR, diffusion-weighted imaging (DWI), and other sequences. Recording is done by a coil. These intensities are used to produce images. T_1-weighted sequence accentuates substances that contain fat and T_2-weighted sequence accentuates substances that contain water.

Interpretation: In the brain, T_1-weighted images reveal the nerve connections of white matter and appear white (hyperintense), the congregations of neurons of gray matter appear gray, and cerebrospinal fluid appears dark. These are reversed in T_2-weighted imaging.

Neurological indications for MRI ***(Box 15.73)***

Box 15.73: Neurological indications for MRI.

MRI is the investigation of choice for the evaluation of all neurological disorders:
- Structural imaging: Produces high-quality soft tissue images. Useful in the investigation of disease of posterior fossa and temporal lobes, inflammatory conditions (e.g., multiple sclerosis), and in investigating epilepsy
- Magnetic resonance angiography (MRA) to study blood vessels in the neck or brain
- Functional MRI: Mainly research tools
- MR spectroscopy: Mainly research tools

Q. Write a short note on neurological indications for MRI.

Advantages and disadvantages of MRI

Advantages and disadvantages of MRI are presented in **Table 15.76.**

Contrast MRI

- Gadolinium is used as intravenous contrast to assess the vascularity in tumors and inflammatory lesions.
- Side effects: Headache, nausea, pain and sensation of cold at the injection site, dizziness, and rarely nephrogenic systemic fibrosis (fibrosis of dermis, joints and internal organs including lungs and heart). Contrast (gadolinium) imaging can worsen renal failure, so its best avoided in Acute kidney injury (AKI)/chronic kidney disease (CKD).

Special forms of MRI

- Diffusion MRI: To measure the movement or diffusion of extracellular water molecules.
- MR angiography helps us to evaluate intracranial vessels noninvasively to find for aneurysms, stenosis, or malformations.
- Magnetic resonance spectroscopy (MRS)
- Functional MRI to assess blood flow during specific tasks (e.g., speaking, remembering, and calculation).

Complications

MRI is a safe procedure. However, if a metal is present nearby serious injuries may develop when metal gets attracted to strong magnets of MRI and may act like a missile.

TABLE 15.76: Advantages and disadvantages of magnetic resonance imaging (MRI).

Advantages of MRI	*Disadvantages of MRI*
➤ High-quality soft tissue images ➤ No ionizing radiation involved ➤ Noninvasive ➤ Distinguishes between white and gray matter both in the brain and cord ➤ Spinal cord and nerve roots are directly imaged ➤ Pituitary imaging ➤ Resolution superior to CT ➤ Useful for demonstration of tumors (posterior fossa and temporal lobes), infarction, hemorrhage, MS plaques, posterior fossa, foramen magnum, and cord. Detailed and accurate evaluation of breast cancers ➤ MR angiography (MRA) images blood vessels without contrast ➤ Cardiovascular MRI: Gold standard for quantifying ventricular volumes, ejection fraction, and myocardial mass	➤ Expensive and time consuming ➤ Less widely available ➤ MRA images blood flow, not vessel anatomy ➤ Spatial resolution not as good as CT ➤ Requires experienced reader ➤ Not good for evaluation of bone cortex ➤ Claustrophobic ➤ Less effective than CT in detecting air (lungs) or gas (as in infection or bowel perforation) ➤ Contrast (gadolinium) reactions ➤ Contraindications for MRI include: Implanted cardiac pacemakers, vagus nerve stimulators, implanted cardiac defibrillator (ICD), cochlear implants, and deep brain stimulators

X-ray/CT Plain X-rays, CT, CTA

- Applications: Radiculography, myelography, intra-arterial angiography
  - X-rays: For fractures or foreign bodies
  - CT: First line for stroke
  - Intra-arterial angiography: Gold standard for vascular lesions.

Advantages: Easily available, relatively economical, and relatively quick.

Ultrasound-Doppler Studies

- Cheap, quick and noninvasive.
- B-mode and color ultrasound are useful in identifying carotid stenosis.

Radioisotope

For establishing the diagnosis, we need to do radioisotope scan, SPECT, and PET.

Q. Discuss the differential diagnosis for "ring-enhancing lesions".

It is abnormal radiological findings observed in MRI or CT scans obtained using radiocontrast. On the image, it appears as an area of decreased density surrounded by a bright rim from concentration of the enhancing contrast dye **(Fig. 15.54)**.

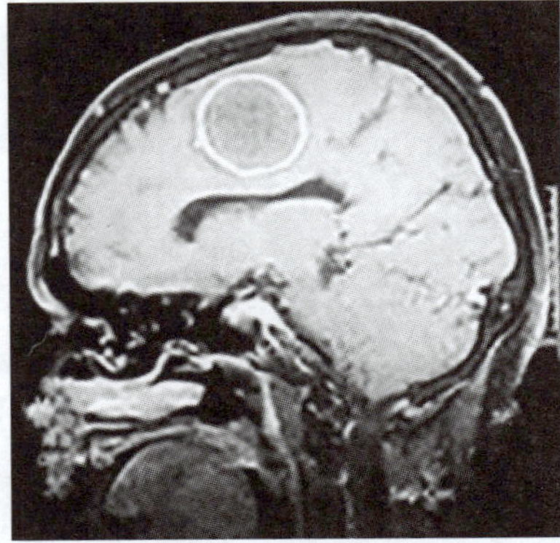

FIG. 15.54: Ring-enhancing lesion on MRI.

Causes for Ring-enhancing Lesions in the Brain

- Infections: Early brain abscess, tuberculoma, CNS toxoplasmosis, cysticercosis, fungal infections (nocardiosis, cryptococcosis), neurosyphilis.
- Inflammatory: Demyelinating disorders (MS, ADEM), sarcoidosis, Behçet's disease, Whipple's disease.
- Vascular: Cerebral venous thrombosis and several other vasculitic disorders.
- Neoplastic: Primary (e.g., glioblastoma, low-grade gliomas, CNS lymphoma) and metastasis.

Magnetic Resonance Spectroscopy

Magnetic resonance spectroscopy is a means of noninvasive physiologic imaging of the brain that measures relative levels of various tissue metabolites **(Fig. 15.55)**.

Magnetic resonance spectroscopy patterns in diseases have been shown in **Table 15.77**.

Time of Echo (TE) that conditions the number metabolites

Lactate: Resonates at 1.33 ppm
Lipids: Resonates at 1.3 ppm
Alanine: Resonates at 1.48 ppm
N-acetylaspartate (NAA): Resonates at 2.0 ppm
Glutamine/Glutamate: Resonates at 2.2–2.4 ppm
GABA: Resonates at 2.2–2.4 ppm
2-Hydroxyglutarate: Resonates at 2.25 ppm
Citrate: Resonates 2.6 ppm
Creatine: Resonates at 3.0 ppm
Choline: Resonates at 3.2 ppm
Myo-inositol: Resonates at 3.5 ppm
Glucose: Resonates at 3.43 ppm and 3.8 ppm
Mannitol: Resonates at 3.78 ppm
Water: Resonates at 4.7 ppm

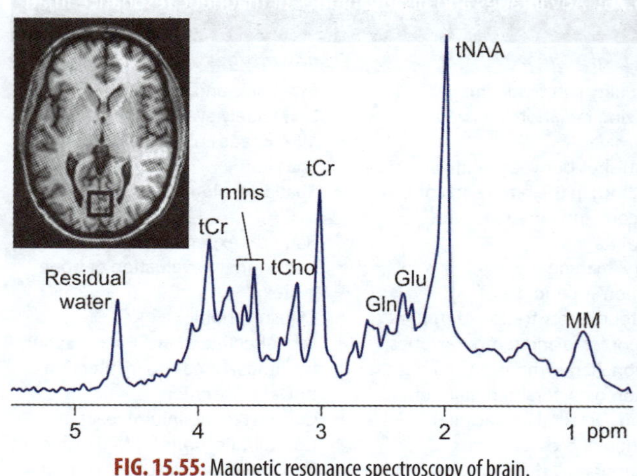

FIG. 15.55: Magnetic resonance spectroscopy of brain.

TABLE 15.77: Magnetic resonance spectroscopy (MRS) patterns of diseases.

Diseases	*MRS patterns*
Glioma	NAA and creatine decrease and choline, lipids, and lactate increase
Radiation effects	NAA, choline and creatine will all be low
Ischemia and infarction	Lactate will increase, later lipid peak appears
Infection	NAA is absent, lactate, alanine, cytosolic acid, and acetate are elevated *Note:* Choline is low or absent in toxoplasmosis, whereas it is elevated in lymphoma, helping to distinguish the two
Progressive multifocal leukoencephalopathy (PML)	Elevated myo-inositol
Canavan disease	Elevated NAA
Hepatic encephalopathy	Markedly reduced myo-inositol and choline. Glutamine is increased
Leigh's syndrome	Elevated choline, reduced NAA

Neurophysiological Testing

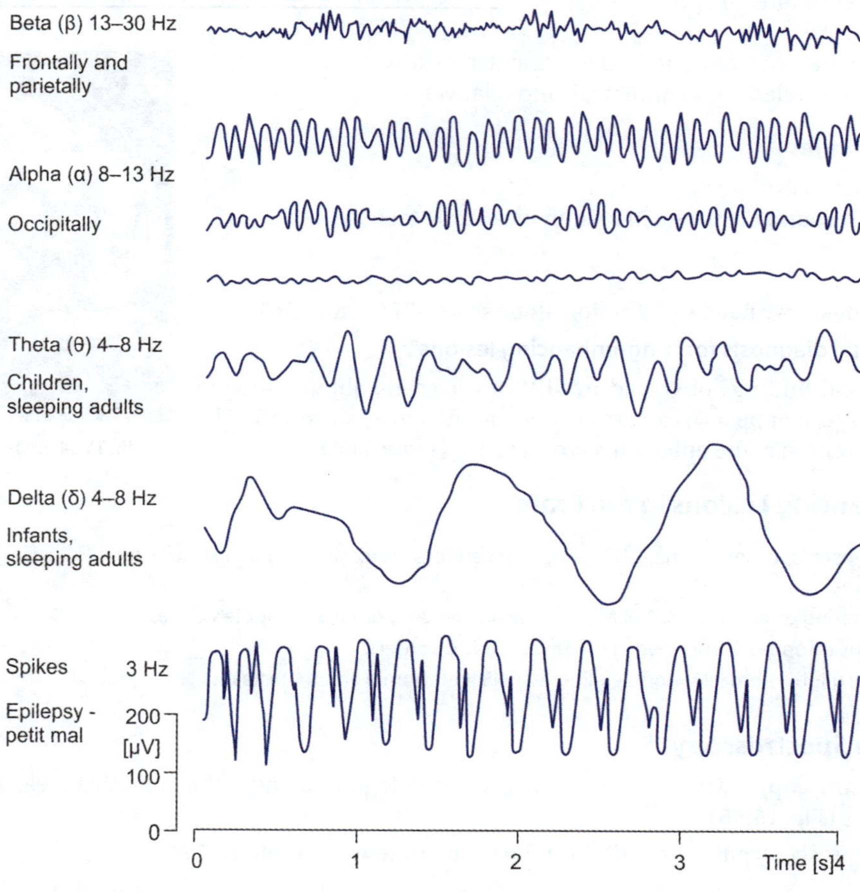

FIG. 15.56: Waves seen in electroencephalography (EEG).

Q. Write a short note on electroencephalography.

- **Electroencephalography (Fig. 15.56)**
  - The electroencephalogram recorded from scalp by placing electrodes on the scalp. It is used to detect electrical activity arising in the cerebral cortex. Rhythmic activity is recorded as waves (alpha, beta, gamma, theta, mu, and delta).
  - **Usefulness:**
    - In progressive and continuous disorders such as reduced consciousness, classification and prognosis in epilepsy and diffuse brain diseases [encephalitis, prion (Creutzfeldt-Jakob) diseases and metabolic states (e.g., hypoglycemia, hepatic coma)].

- ♦ Diagnosis of paroxysmal neurological attacks
- ♦ Differentiation between nocturnal epilepsy and parasomnias
- ♦ Diagnosis of psychogenic nonepileptic seizures
- ♦ Characterization of seizure type
- ♦ Quantification of interictal epileptiform discharge (IED) or seizure frequency
- ♦ Evaluation of candidates for epilepsy surgery.
- **Video EEG:** Useful in definitive diagnosis of epilepsy.
- **Ambulatory EEG** is analog to Holter monitor for cardiac arrhythmias.

Lathyrism

Q. Write a short note on lathyrism.

Lathyrism is a paralyzing disease caused by eating seeds of *Lathyrus sativus* (khesari dal).

Epidemiology

It is prevalent mostly people in India (e.g., Madhya Pradesh, Uttar Pradesh, Bihar and Odisha), Bangladesh, Pakistan, Nepal and Algeria.

Etiology

L. sativus (khesari dal) is a good source of protein. It is relatively cheap pulse and is consumed mostly by the poor agricultural laborer. But it contains L-ODAP (β-N-oxalyl-l-α, β-diaminopropionic acid) also called β-N-oxalylamino-L-alanine, or BOAA, which is an excitatory neurotoxin and glutamate agonist. If the diets containing > 30% of this dal is consumed over a period of 2–6 months will produce lathyrism.

Clinical Features

It affects mainly young males between 15 and 45 years of age. In humans, it mainly affects nervous system and is called neurolathyrism which produces pure motor spastic paraplegia. Sensations and sphincters are preserved.

Stages

- **Latent stage:** Patient appears healthy but when subjected to physical stress exhibits ungainly gait. If the disease is recognized at this stage, age, withdrawal of pulse from the diet will result in complete remission of disease.
- **No-stick stage:** During this stage, the patient walks with difficulty having short jerky steps but does not need the aid of a stick.
- **One-stick stage:** The patient walks with a crossed gait with a tendency to walk on toes and develops musculoskeletal stiffness. Use of a stick is necessary to maintain balance.
- **Two-stick stage:** Symptoms are more severe at this stage. Due to excessive bending of the knees and crossed legs, the patient requires support by two crutches for support. The gait is slow and clumsy and complains of easy tiredness after walking a short distance.
- **Crawler stage:** Finally spastic paralysis develops which becomes irreversible. It becomes impossible to maintain erect posture as the knee joints cannot support the weight of the body. The thigh and leg muscles become atrophied and patient crawls by throwing his weight on his hands.

Prevention

- **Vitamin C prophylaxis:** 500–1,000 mg for a week.
- **Banning the crop** if possible.
- **Removal of toxin:**
  - ▪ **Steeping method:** Soaking the pulse in hot water for 2 hours and the soaked water is drained off completely. The pulse is washed again with clean water and then drained off and dried in the sun. There will be loss of vitamins and minerals by this method.
  - ▪ **Parboiling:** Suitable for large scale operation and is similar to parboiled rice. It destroys trypsin inhibitors.

CHAPTER

16

Toxicology

CLINICAL EXAMINATION OF POISONING CASE

Q. Enumerate the clinical features in general that would help you in diagnosing the poison ingested.

Accidental or intentional poisoning produces a wide range of symptoms and signs. Therefore, meticulous history and physical examination are of paramount importance in recognizing the poisoned patient.

Initial management should be focused on acute stabilization and supportive care till the correct substance is identified. Various parameters in clinical assessment to determine the type of poisons are listed in **Table 16.1.**

TABLE 16.1: Characteristic features and the type of poisons.

Characteristics	*Type of poison*
ODOR OF POISON	
Bitter almonds	Cyanide
Acetone	Isopropyl alcohol, methanol, paraldehyde, salicylates
Alcohol	Ethanol
Wintergreen	Methyl salicylate
Garlicky/Garlic like odor	Arsenic, thallium, organophosphates
OCULAR SIGNS	
Miosis	Narcotics (except meperidine), organophosphates, muscarinic mushrooms, clonidine, phenothiazines, chloral hydrate, barbiturates (late), PCP (phencyclidine)
Mydriasis	Atropine, alcohol, cocaine, amphetamines, antihistamines, tricyclic antidepressants (TCAs), cyanide, carbon monoxide
Nystagmus	Phenytoin, barbiturates, ethanol, carbon monoxide
Lacrimation	Organophosphates, irritant gas or vapors
Retinal hyperemia	Methanol
Blurred vision	Methanol, botulism, carbon monoxide
CUTANEOUS SIGNS	
Needle tracks	Heroin, phencyclidine (PCP), amphetamines
Bullae	Carbon monoxide, barbiturates
Dry, hot skin	Anticholinergic agents, botulism
Diaphoresis	Organophosphates, nitrates, muscarinic mushrooms, aspirin, cocaine
Alopecia	Thallium, arsenic, lead, mercury
Erythema	Boric acid, mercury, cyanide, anticholinergics
Cyanosis	Central nervous system (CNS) depressant
ORAL SIGNS	
Salivation	Organophosphates, salicylates, corrosives, strychnine
Dry mouth	Amphetamines, anticholinergics, antihistamine
Burns	Corrosives, oxalate-containing plants
Gum lines	Lead, mercury, arsenic
Dysphagia	Corrosives, botulism

Contd...

Contd...

INTESTINAL SIGNS	
Cramps	Arsenic, lead, thallium, organophosphates
Epigastric tenderness	Salicylates, nonsteroidal anti-inflammatory drugs (NSAIDs)
Diarrhea	Organophosphates, antimicrobials, arsenic, iron, boric acid
Constipation	Lead, narcotics, botulism
Hematemesis	Aminophylline, corrosives, iron, salicylates
CARDIAC SIGNS	
Tachycardia	Atropine, aspirin, amphetamines, cocaine, cyclic antidepressants, theophylline
Bradycardia	Digitalis, narcotics, mushrooms, clonidine, organophosphates, β-blockers, calcium channel blockers
Hypertension	Amphetamines, LSD (lysergic acid diethylamide), cocaine, PCP
Hypotension	Phenothiazines, barbiturates, TCAs, iron, β-blockers, calcium channel blockers
RESPIRATORY SIGNS	
Bradypnea	Alcohol, narcotics, barbiturates
Tachypnea	Amphetamines, aspirin (salicylates), ethylene glycol, carbon monoxide, cyanide
CNS SIGNS	
Pulmonary edema	Hydrocarbons, heroin, organophosphates, aspirin
Ataxia	Alcohol, antidepressants, barbiturates, anticholinergics, phenytoin, narcotics
Coma	Sedatives, narcotics, barbiturates, PCP, organophosphates, salicylates, cyanide, carbon monoxide, cyclic antidepressants, lead
Hyperpyrexia	Anticholinergics, quinine, salicylates, LSD, phenothiazines, amphetamines, cocaine
Hypothermia	CNS depressant (opioids, chlorpromazine)
Muscle fasciculation	Organophosphates, theophylline
Muscle rigidity	Cyclic antidepressants, PCP, phenothiazines, haloperidol
Extrapyramidal signs	Phenothiazines, haloperidol, metoclopramide
Paresthesia	Cocaine, camphor, PCP, MSG (monosodium glutamate)
Peripheral neuropathy	Lead, arsenic, mercury, organophosphates
Altered behavior	LSD, PCP, amphetamines, cocaine, alcohol, anticholinergics, camphor
Seizures	Tricyclic antidepressants, isoniazid, selective serotonin reuptake inhibitors (SSRIs)
Metabolic acidosis	Cyanide, ethylene glycol, metformin, methanol, salicylates, iron, isoniazid
Elevated osmolal gap	Ethanol, isopropanol, methanol, ethylene glycol, isoniazid
ECG CHANGES IN COMMON POISON	
Narrow QRS tachycardia	Amphetamines Anticholinergic drugs Theophylline
Wide QRS tachycardia	Antihistamines Cocaine Propoxyphene Sodium channel blockers Tricyclic antidepressants
Bradycardia with narrow QRS	α-adrenergic blockers β-blockers Calcium channel blockers Cardiac glycosides Class Ia antiarrhythmics Sodium channel blockers
Bradycardia with wide QRS	β-blockers Calcium channel blockers
QT interval prolongation	Antihistamines Antipsychotics Class Ia antiarrhythmics Sotalol Tricyclic antidepressants Erythromycin Fluoroquinolones Halofantrine Hydroxychloroquine
RADIOPAQUE POISONS	
Radiopaque on plain X-ray (**CHIPES**—acronym)	**C**—Calcium, chlorinated compounds **H**—Heavy metals (iron, mercury, etc.) **I**—Iodinated compounds (thyroxine) **P**—Psychotropics, potassium salts, packers (cocaine/opium) **E**—Enteric-coated drugs like aspirin **S**—Salicylates

TOXIDROMES (TABLE 16.2)

Q. List the common toxidromes that are commonly encountered in clinical practice.

Based on history and clinical findings, it may be possible to define a syndrome associated with certain poisons. This is called toxidrome/toxic syndrome.

TABLE 16.2: Various toxidrome and related findings.

Toxidrome	*Vital signs*	*Mental status*	*Pupils*	*Other findings*	*Examples*
Anticholinergic (**Fig. 16.1**)	Hyperthermia, tachycardia, hypertension, tachypnea	Agitated, hallucinating	Mydriasis	Dry flushed skin, urinary retention	Antihistamines, TCAs, atropine, scopolamine, antispasmodics, trihexyphenidyl
Cholinergic (**Fig. 16.2**)	Bradycardia (muscarinic), tachycardia and hypertension (nicotinic)	Confused, coma	Miosis	**Fasciculations SLUDGE** (**S**alivation, **L**acrimation, **U**rination, **D**iarrhea, **GI** upset, **E**mesis)	Organophosphate pesticides, nerve agents—physostigmine
Hallucinogen	Hyperthermia, tachycardia, hypertension	Hallucination, synesthesia, agitation	Mydriasis	Nystagmus	PCP (phencyclidine), LSD (lysergic acid diethylamide), mescaline
Opioid	Hypothermia, bradycardia, hypotension, bradypnea	CNS depression, coma	Miosis	Hyporeflexia, pulmonary edema	Opioids (heroin, morphine, methadone, dilaudid, etc.)
Sedative-hypnotic	Hypothermia, bradycardia, hypotension, bradypnea	CNS depression, confusion, coma	Miosis	Hyporeflexia	Benzodiazepines, barbiturates, zolpidem, alcohols
Serotonin syndrome (**Fig. 16.3**)	Hyperthermia, tachycardia, hypertension, tachypnea	Confused, agitated coma	Mydriasis	Tremor, myoclonus, diaphoresis, hyperreflexia, trismus, rigidity	MAOIs, SSRIs, meperidine, dextromethorphan
Sympathomimetic (**Fig. 16.4**)	Hyperthermia, tachycardia, tachypnea	Agitated, hyperalert, paranoia	Mydriasis	Diaphoresis, tremors, hyperreflexia, seizures	Cocaine, theophylline amphetamines, pseudoephedrine

(MAOIs: monoamine oxidase inhibitors; SSRIs: selective serotonin reuptake inhibitors or serotonin specific reuptake inhibitors ; TCAs: tricyclic antidepressants)

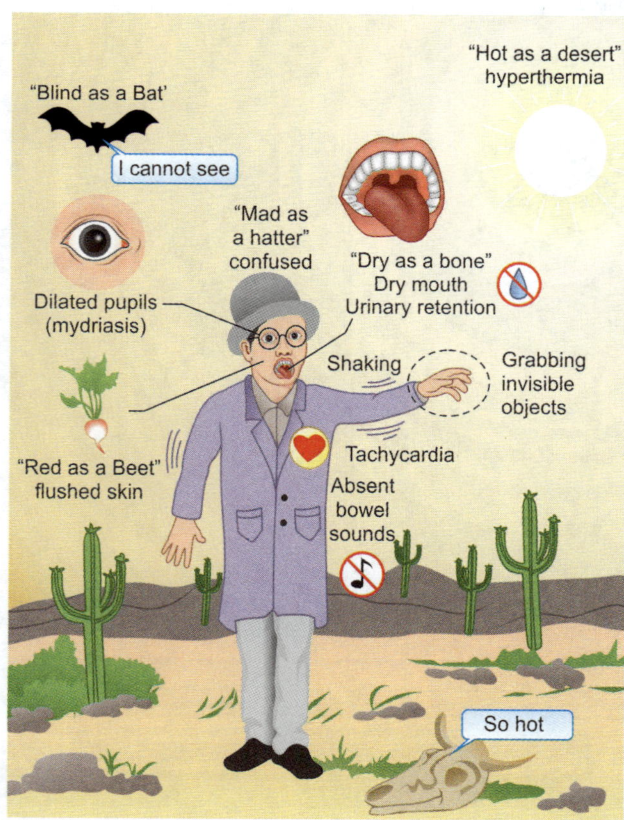

FIG. 16.1: Anticholinergic toxidrome.

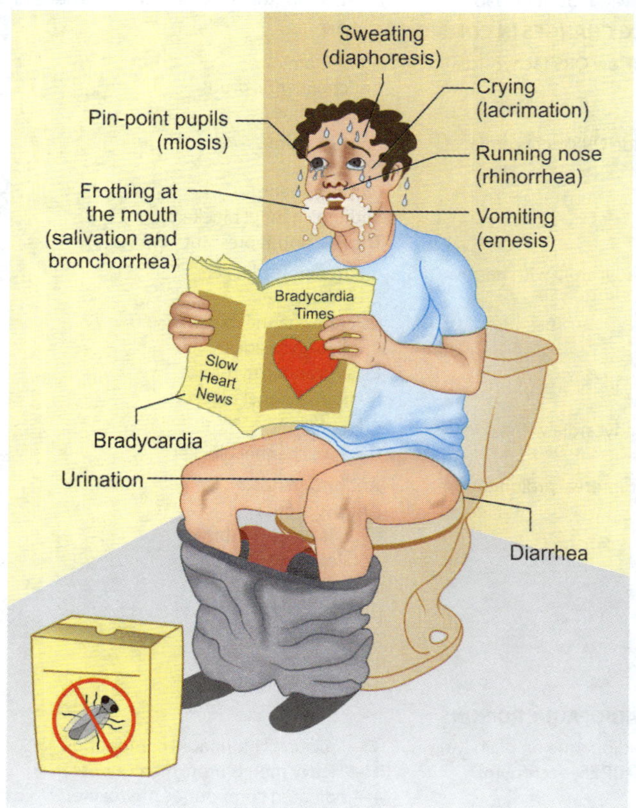

FIG. 16.2: Cholinergic toxidrome.

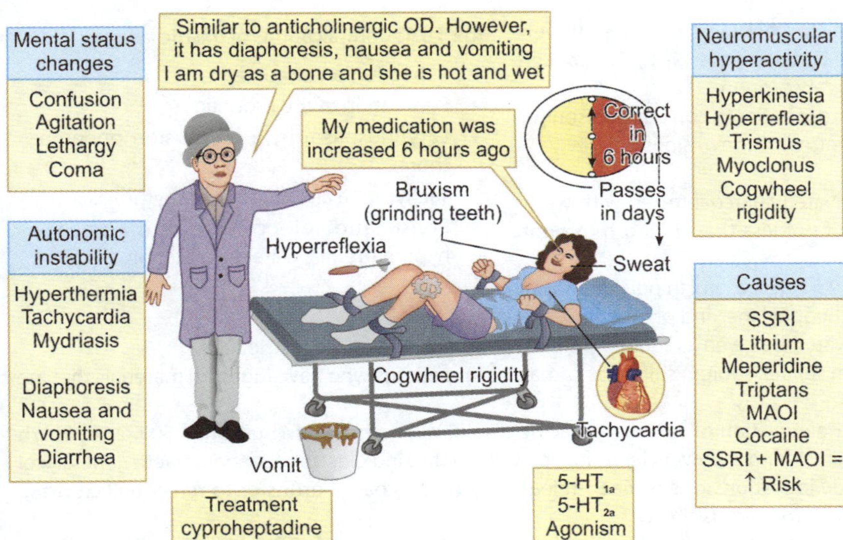

FIG. 16.3: Serotonin syndrome.
(MAOI: monoamine oxidase inhibitor; SSRI: selective serotonin reuptake inhibitor)

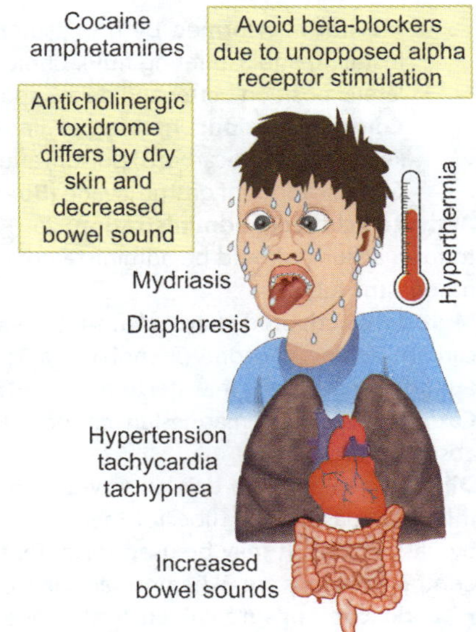

FIG. 16.4: Sympathomimetic toxidrome.

Management of Patient with Poisoning

Q. Describe the initial approach to the stabilization of the patient who presents with poisoning.

Q. Describe basic methodologies in treatment of poisoning: decontamination, supportive therapy, antidote therapy, and procedures of enhanced elimination.

Management/Treatment

Goals of Treatment

These include: (A) Support of vital signs, (B) Diagnostic testing, (C) Reduce absorption of the toxin, (D) Enhance of poison elimination, and (E) Neutralize toxin.

In the poisoned patient, diagnostic evaluation and therapeutic interventions often are initiated simultaneously.

A. Supportive Care

Patients who are seriously poisoned must receive early appropriate management. Outcome depends on appropriate nursing and supportive care, and on appropriate treatment of complications. The aims are:

- To **maintain physiologic homeostasis** till poison is eliminated from the body and the patient resumes normal physiological functions. As with any unstable or critically ill patient, the resuscitation [airway, breathing, circulation (ABC)] with basic life support takes priority.
- To **prevent and treat secondary complications:** Supportive therapy for central nervous system (e.g., cerebral edema), cardiopulmonary system (e.g., pulmonary edema, pneumonia), and renal system with proper care for coma, seizures, hypotension, bedsores, arrhythmias, sepsis, thromboembolic disease, coagulopathy, hypoxia, and acute renal failure.

B. Diagnostic testing

General tests

- Complete blood count
- Serum electrolytes, blood urea nitrogen (BUN), and creatinine
- Liver function test
- Arterial blood gas
- Electrocardiogram
- Urine pregnancy test in all women of childbearing age
- Radiographic studies—radiopaque poisons listed in **Table 16.1**

Specific tests

- Measurement of drug or toxin concentrations in body fluids (blood, urine, lavage fluid)

C. Reduce Absorption of the Toxin

Inhalational exposure: Evacuation from toxic environment and provision of supplemental oxygen.

Dermal exposure: Removal of contaminated clothing and shower or irrigation of affected site (dust before shower for dry chemical).

For eye exposure: Removal of chemicals by copious irrigation of the affected eye by up to 1 L of saline or symptomatic improvement occurs.

Oral exposure: Inducing emesis, performing gastric lavage, activated charcoal, whole bowel irrigation, cathartics.

Gastric decontamination

- **Emesis induction:** Forced emesis, if patient is awake (using saline, ipecac).
- **Gastric lavage** should be considered for life-threatening poisons that cannot be treated effectively with other therapies.
  - **Time of lavage:** Gastric lavage decreases absorption by 42% if done 20 minutes and by 16% if performed at 60 minutes.

- **Method:** Performed by first aspirating the stomach and then repetitively instilling and aspirating fluid. Choice of fluid is tap water— 5–10 mL/kg. Left lateral position better and delays spontaneous absorption.
- **Contraindication:** Unprotected airway, comatose patients, corrosive poisoning, kerosene (hydrocarbons) poison, and in patients with convulsions.
- Complications of gastric lavage **(Box 16.1)**.

Activated charcoal administration: 25–100 g activated charcoal mixed with water to form a slurry should be administered at a rate of not less than 12.5 g/h through nasogastric tube.

Multidose activated charcoal at a rate of at least 12.5 g/h is useful in poisoning with carbamazepine, dapsone, phenobarbital, quinine, theophylline, and phenytoin.

Box 16.1: Complications of gastric lavage.

- Aspiration pneumonia
- Perforation of the esophagus
- Laryngospasm/hypoxia/tension pneumothorax
- Tachycardia and cardiac dysrhythmias
- Fluid and electrolyte imbalance—hypernatremia; water intoxication

Fuller's earth (2 g/kg in water; maximum 150 g in water) be given as soon as possible per oral or via a nasogastric tube.

Cathartics: Sorbitol, magnesium citrate, magnesium sulfate, sodium sulfate as cathartics for patients who have ingested materials that are absorbed slowly.

Dilution—milk/other drinks: Advised only after the ingestion of corrosives (acids, alkali). **Whole bowel irrigation:** 1,500–2,000 mL/h through a nasogastric tube. It is performed by administering a bowel-cleansing solution containing electrolytes and polyethylene glycol by gastric tube. It may be used for potentially toxic ingestions of sustained-release or enteric-coated drugs or to remove illicit drug. Contraindications are GI hemorrhage, ileus, and hemodynamic instability.

- **Endoscopic or surgical removal** of ingested substance may be useful in rare situations (e.g., ingestion of a potentially toxic foreign body that fails to transit the gastrointestinal tract).

D. Enhance of Poison Elimination

- **Indications:** Increased elimination is possible only if
  - Drug is distributed predominantly in the ECF (extracellular fluid) and drugs that have a low protein binding.
- **Methods:** Keep a good urine output 150–200 mL/h.
  - **Alkalinization of urine using sodium bicarbonate to produce urine with a pH ≥ 7.5:** For salicylate, methotrexate, and phenobarbital poisoning.
  - **Extracorporeal removal:**
    - **Hemodialysis:** For barbiturates, salicylates, acetaminophen, valproate, alcohols, glycols.
    - **Hemoperfusion:** For theophylline, digitalis, paraquat, lipid-soluble drugs (aminoglycosides, vancomycin, and metal chelate complexes).
  - **Exchange transfusion:** Useful in cases of massive hemolysis, severe methemoglobinemia or sulfhemoglobinemia.

E. Neutralize Toxin

Antidotes may prevent absorption, bind and neutralize poisons directly, antagonize end-organ effects, or inhibit conversion to more toxic metabolites **(Table 16.3)**.

Q. Write a short note on antidote.

Neutralize toxins/poisons by toxin-specific antidotes **(Table 16.3)**.

TABLE 16.3: Toxin-specific antidotes.

Toxin/poison	*Specific antidote*	*Toxin/poison*	*Specific antidote*
Acetaminophen	N-acetylcysteine	Methanol	Ethanol, fomepizole
Anticholinergics	Physostigmine	Methemoglobinemia	Methylene blue
Benzodiazepines	Flumazenil	Glycol	Ethanol, fomepizole
Beta-blockers	Glucagon	Opioid	Naloxone
	Calcium	Oral hypoglycemics	Glucose
	Insulin + dextrose/lipid emulsion therapy	Organophosphate	Atropine/2-PAM (pralidoxime)
Calcium channel blockers	Glucagon		
	Insulin + dextrose *(hyperinsulinemia euglycemia therapy)*	Snakebites	Snake antivenom
	Calcium/lipid emulsion therapy	Sulfonylurea	Octreotide + dextrose
Carbamate	Atropine	Tricyclic antidepressants	Sodium bicarbonate
Carbone monoxide	Hyperbaric oxygen	Warfarin	Vitamin K
		Dabigatran	Idarucizumab
		Copper	Penicillamine, dimercaprol, Ca-EDTA
Cyanide	Amyl nitrite pearls Sodium nitrite (3% solution) Sodium thiosulfate (25%)	Iron	Desferrioxamine
		Lead	Ca-EDTA, dimercaprol, British anti-Lewisite (BAL)
		Mercury	DMPS (2,3-dimercapto-1-propanesulfonic acid), DMSA (meso-2, 3-dimercaptosuccinic acid), BAL
Digoxin	Digoxin antibodies	Arsenic	BAL and derivatives
Heparin	Protamine sulfate	Antimony	BAL and derivatives
Isoniazid	Pyridoxine	Botulism	Botulinum antitoxin
Datura	Physostigmine	Methemoglobinemia-causing agents (copper, nitrates, dapsone)	Methylene blue

INSECTICIDE POISONING

Q. Discuss the clinical manifestations, diagnosis, complications, and management of organophosphorus and carbamate poisoning.

Organophosphate and Carbamate Poisoning

Organophosphorus (OP) compounds are widely used as pesticides in developing countries and are a common cause of poisoning.

Classification of Organophosphate and Carbamate (Box 16.2)

Mode of intoxication: It may occur through ingestion, inhalation or dermal absorption.

Box 16.2: Classification of organophosphate and carbamate.

- **Organophosphorus**
  - **Diethyl organophosphorus:** Quinalphos, chlorpyriphos, diazinon, triazophos, phorate, dimethoate, parathion-ethyl
  - **Dimethyl organophosphorus:** Monocrotophos, dichlorvos, acephate, malathion, fenthion, methamidophos and phosphamidon
- **Carbamate:** Methomyl
- **Organochloride:** Endosulfan, endrin
- **Pyrethroids:** Cypermethrin, alpha-cypermethrin, deltamethrin, cyhalothrin
- **Neonicotinoid:** Imidacloprid, acetamiprid

Mechanism of OP Toxicity (Fig. 16.5)

- OP compounds irreversibly bind to serine-OH group at the active site of acetylcholinesterase (AChE) and phosphorylate. This inactivates the enzyme AChE.It leads to the accumulation of acetylcholine (ACh) in cholinergic synapses.
- Spontaneous hydrolysis of the OP-enzyme complex allows reactivation of the enzyme. However, loss of a chemical group from the OP-enzyme complex prevents further enzyme reactivation, a process known as **"aging"**. Aging is characterized by loss of alkyl group + strengthening of covalent bond.
- Phosphorylated AChE is very stable. Inhibition of enzyme activity → accumulation of ACh in the synapse and neuromuscular junction (NMJ). It causes overstimulation of cholinergic receptors. After aging has taken place; new enzyme needs to be synthesized before function can be restored.

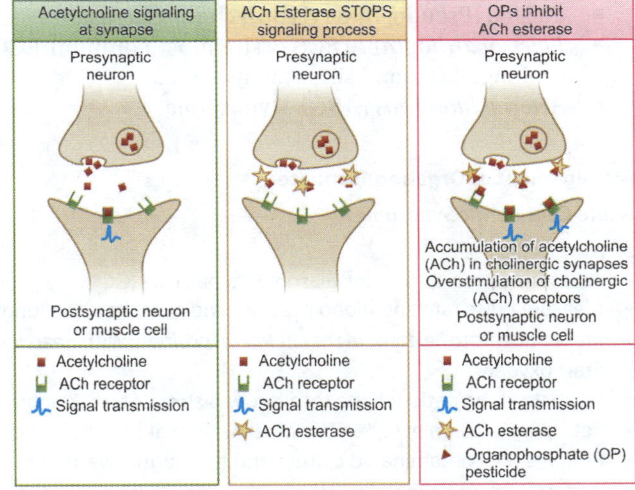

FIG. 16.5: Mechanism of organophosphorus poisoning.

Clinical Course after Acute Poisoning (Table 16.4)

Q. Write a short essay/note on clinical signs of organophosphorus poisoning.

Triphasic Illness

1. **Acute cholinergic syndrome**
   - **Onset:** Cholinergic symptoms within first 24 hours.
   - **Features (Table 16.4)**
   - SLUDGE = Salivation, Lacrimation, Urination, Defecation, Gastric Emptying
   - BBB = Bradycardia, Bronchorrhea, Bronchospasm
2. **Intermediate syndrome**
   - **Onset:** 24–96 hours after poisoning, after the cholinergic phase settles, seen in 10–40% of cases.
   - **Mechanism:** Excess Ach at NMJ causes downregulation of nicotinic receptors and muscles affected.
   - **Features:** Characterized by proximal neck muscle weakness, decreased deep tendon reflexes (DTRs), cranial nerve abnormalities (bulbar), and respiratory insufficiency
   - **Duration:** Lasts for few days to about 3 weeks.

TABLE 16.4: Clinical course after acute organophosphorus poisoning.

Time of manifestation	*Mechanism*	*Manifestation*
Acute (minutes to 24 hours): Acute cholinergic syndrome	Nicotinic receptor action	*Musculoskeletal:* Weakness, fasciculations, cramps, paralysis
		Cardiovascular: Tachycardia, hypertension
	Muscarinic receptor action	*Gastrointestinal:* Increased salivation, nausea, vomiting, abdominal pain, diarrhea, fecal incontinence *Genitourinary:* Urinary incontinence *Cardiovascular:* Bradycardia (80%), hypotension *Respiratory:* Rhinorrhea, stridor, bronchospasm, bronchorrhea, cough *Ocular:* Lacrimation, miosis

Contd...

Contd...

		Skin: Flushing, diaphoresis, cyanosis
	Central receptors	Anxiety, restless, convulsions, insomnia, tremors, respiratory depression
Delayed (24 hours to 2 weeks): Intermediate syndrome	Nicotinic receptor action	Proximal muscle weakness, hyporeflexia, bulbar weakness
	Muscarinic receptor action	Bradycardia, miosis, salivation
	Central receptors	Coma, extrapyramidal manifestation
Late (beyond 2 weeks): Delayed polyneuropathy	Peripheral neuropathy target esterase	Peripheral neuropathy

3. **OP-induced delayed polyneuropathy (OPIDN)**
   - **Onset:** 1–3 weeks after acute exposure.
   - **Mechanism:** Due to degeneration of long myelinated nerve fibers. Pure motor or sensor-motor.
   - **Features:** Characterized by cramps in the legs, numbness and paresthesia in the distal upper and lower limbs, shuffling gait, foot and wrist drop. Other features are: wasting, DTR reduced/absent, pyramidal tract signs absent.
   - **Recovery is incomplete.**

Q. Discuss the management of organophosphorus poisoning.

Diagnosis of Organophosphate Poisoning

- **Clinical diagnosis:**
  - Dreisbach's severity of OP poisoning is presented in **Table 16.5**.
- **Laboratory:**
  - Red cell cholinesterase
  - Plasma [Pseudo, Butyryl (Bu)] cholinesterase
  - *Electrocardiogram (ECG):* The most common ECG abnormality was prolonged QTc and sinus tachycardia.
  - *Arterial blood gas (ABG):* Hypoxemia.

TABLE 16.5: Dreisbach's classification showing severity of poisoning.

Grade	*Symptoms*
Mild	Nausea
Moderate	Lacrimation, salivation, miosis, fasciculation
Severe	Incontinence, apneic spells, ARDS, areflexia, seizures, coma

(ARDS: acute respiratory distress syndrome)

Management of Organophosphate

Acute Cholinergic Syndrome

Steps

- Assess and record 15-point Glasgow Coma Scale (GCS).
- Measure pulse rate and blood pressure and auscultate the lungs.
- *Make patients to lie down in the left lateral position:* With head lower than the feet.
- Start oxygen.
- Intubate, if the patient has a respiratory distress. Start atropine quickly to reduce bronchorrhea responsible for respiratory distress.
- Set-up an infusion of 0.9% normal saline. Aim at systolic blood pressure >80 mm Hg and urine output >30 mL/h.
- Remove the contaminated clothes and thoroughly wash the skin with soap and water.
- Perform gastric decontamination with gastric lavage once the patient is stabilized and within 2 hours of ingestion. Skin exposure would require irrigation of the skin with copious amounts of water and liberal use of soap. Eye exposure should be irrigated with copious amount of normal saline.
- Give activated charcoal (50 g in 200 mL) (Not much benefit due to rapid absorption of poison into blood).

Drugs Used

1. **Atropine**
   - Early use of sufficient doses of atropine is **lifesaving in patients with severe toxicity.** It reverses ACh-induced bronchospasm, bronchorrhea, bradycardia, and hypotension.
   - **When the diagnosis is uncertain:**
   - **Atropine challenge test:** To be performed, if not sure that the patient has consumed OP.
     - **Inject 0.6–1 mg IV atropine:** If pulse rate goes up by 25/minute or skin flushing develops, patient has mild or no toxicity or OP poisoning is unlikely.

Dose and mode of administration of atropine

- **Bolus**
  - Inject 1.8–3 mg (3–5 mL) of atropine bolus.
  - *Check three things after 5 minutes:* Pulse, blood pressure, and chest crepitations.
  - Aim for heart rate > 80 beats/minute, SBP > 80 mm Hg, and a clear chest.
  - If the above-mentioned objectives are not achieved, double the atropine dose every 5 minutes.
  - Review patient every 5 minutes. Once these parameters start improving, repeat last same or smaller dose of atropine. If there is persistent and satisfactory improvement in these parameters after 5 minutes, atropine infusion can be planned.

- **Atropine infusion**
  - Calculate total dose of atropine required for rapid atropinization.
  - Start hourly atropine infusion at 10–20% of total dose of atropine required for atropinization.
  - Most patients do not need > 3–5 mg/h of atropine infusion.
  - Use three-point checklist **(secretions, heart rate, pupils)** to reduce infusion rate by 20% every 4 hourly once the patient is stable. Target endpoints for atropine infusion are presented in **Box 16.3**.
  - Bronchorrhea is the most important sign for titrating dose of atropine once patient is stable.
- **Atropine toxicity = absent bowel sounds + fever + confusion/delirium**
  - Stop atropine infusion for 60 minutes, if patient has developed atropine toxicity. Restart infusion at lower rate, once the temperature comes down and the patient gets calm. If atropine is contraindicated, glycopyrrolate can be used for bronchorrhea. **Glycopyrronium bromide** can be an alternative for peripheral symptoms (0.2 mg IM stat repeated 6 hourly).

Box 16.3: Target endpoints for atropine infusion.

- Clear chest on auscultation
- Heart rate > 80 beats/minute (WHO recommends > 100 bpm)
- Systolic BP >80 mm Hg
- Pupils no longer pinpoint
- Dry axillae

Q. Write a short essay/note on pralidoxime (2-PAM).

2. **Pralidoxime (2-PAM):** Pralidoxime reactivates acetylcholinesterase enzymes by removing the phosphoryl group deposited by the organophosphate.
   - Only to treat organophosphorus poisoned patients.
   - *Bolus dose:* 30 mg/kg (i.e., 1–2 g for adults) in 100 mL normal saline over 15–30 minutes.
   - *Maintenance dose:* Continuous infusion of 8–12 mg/kg/h.
   - PAM must be given by infusion. Go slow, both for bolus and maintenance. A fast infusion can cause vomiting, hypertension, cardiac arrhythmia or a cardiac arrest.
   - Give PAM until atropine is no longer required.
3. **Benzodiazepines**
   - *Agitation and seizures:* Diazepam 10 mg slow IV push, repeated as necessary. Up to 30–40 mg diazepam per 24 hours can be given.

Supportive measures

- Mechanical ventillation, vasopressors, antibiotics, diuretics (if pulmonary edema), early enteral feeding, physiotherapy

Chronic Organophosphate Poisoning

Clinical features

- Delayed polyneuropathy (OPIDN)
- Neuropsychiatric disorder

Triorthocresyl phosphate (TOCP) poisoning associated polyneuropathy also called as **Ginger Jake Paralysis.** Owing to the consumption of ginger which was used in manufacture of bootleg alcohol and was adulterated with TOCP. It usually manifests after about 10-20 days causes distal predominant neuropathy.

Diagnosis: Clinical diagnosis, by suspicious and exclusion.

Treatment: Not established. Only supportive measures.

Carbamates

Q. Discuss management of carbamate poisoning.

- Examples: Sevin, Baygon, Lannate, carbaryl, aldicarb.
- Medicinal forms include physostigmine, pyridostigmine, and neostigmine.
- Cholinesterase inhibitors that are **structurally related to organophosphates.** Transiently and reversibly inhibit cholinesterase (<6 h). Regeneration of enzyme occurs within minutes to hours; therefore, aging does not occur.
- **Symptoms** of intoxication are similar to organophosphates, but are of shorter duration.
- Carbamates do not effectively penetrate into CNS, so **less central toxicity** and no seizures.
- Atropine therapy usually not needed for longer than 6–12 hours.
- **Avoid pralidoxime (2-PAM):** Since irreversible binding does not occur, it is not needed, and potentially can worsen some carbamate poisonings.

Organochlorine Poisoning

Q. Write a short essay on organochlorine poisoning.

Classification of Organochlorine (Box 16.4)

Acute organochlorine poisoning

- *Prodromal symptoms:* Tremor, ataxia, myoclonus, dizziness, confusion, paresthesia of mouth, nausea, vomiting.
- *Typical presentation:* **Status epilepticus** followed by respiratory failure, cardiac arrhythmias, rhabdomyolysis, and acute renal failure.

Treatment
- **Control seizure:** The same way as "status epilepticus": Benzodiazepines, phenobarbital, phenytoin.
- Prevent complications.

Subacute Organochlorine Poisoning
- **Hyperexcitability stage:** Tachycardia, tremor, hyperreflexia.
- **Treatment**
  - **Symptomatic treatment:** Anxiolytic
  - **Enhance elimination:** Cholestyramine.

Chronic Organochlorine Poisoning
- Organochlorine insecticides interfere with endocrine and reproductive systems.
- Individuals who work with the insecticides show low sperm count and motility, infertility, and abortion.
- The insecticides can be carcinogenic to animals.

Box 16.4: Classification of organochlorine.

Dichlorodiphenylmethane: DDT, methoxychlor
Hexachlorocyclohexane: Lindane
Cyclodienes
- Aldrin, chlordane, dieldrin
- Endrin, endosulfan, heptachlor
- Chlordecone (kepone): Mirex

Paraquat Poisoning

- Paraquat is a common herbicidal poison with very high case fatality (>50%).
- The toxicity is related to generation oxygen species which cause cellular damage via lipid peroxidation, activation of NF-κB, mitochondrial damage, and apoptosis.
- Ingestion of large amounts results in fulminant organ failure: pulmonary edema, cardiac, renal and hepatic failure.
- Smaller quantities mainly damage the lung and kidney. Acute kidney injury sets in rapidly. The lung involvement occurs in two phases: an acute alveolitis that occurs within 1–3 days followed by a secondary fibrosis. Severe mucosal erosions with bleeding are seen in the GIT and acute hepatitis are seen.
- There is no specific antidote available. Activated charcoal and Fuller's earth can minimize further absorption. Gastric lavage is contraindicated.
- Treatment is supportive, oxygen supplementation and nutirional support.
- Hemodialysis and hemoperfusion are imitated for renal failure.
- Immunosuppression with cyclophosphamide, MESNA, methylprednisolone and dexamethasone have been used to prevent fibrosis. Antioxidants like vitamins C and E, N-acetylcysteine, desferrioxamine, salicylic acid have also been tried.

SNAKEBITE/OPHITOXEMIA

Q. Enumerate the local poisonous snakes and describe the distinguishing marks of each. Discuss the clinical manifestations, diagnosis, and management of snakebites.

Classification of Poisonous Snakes (Box 16.5)

India recorded a staggering 1.2 million snakebite deaths in the 20-year period from 2000 to 2019 with an average of 58,000 deaths caused by snakebite annually. Around 70% of these deaths occurred in limited, low altitude, rural areas of eight states—Bihar, Jharkhand, Madhya Pradesh, Odisha, Uttar Pradesh, Andhra Pradesh (including Telangana), Rajasthan, and Gujarat. Snake may be venomous or nonvenomous. When a venomous snakebites, it may excrete venom. **Snake venom** is a **toxin (hematotoxin, neurotoxin, or cytotoxin). Composition of snake venom is mentioned in Table 16.6.**

Teeth bite marks difference between poisonous and nonpoisonous snakes (**Fig. 16.6C**).
- **Poisonous:** Two fang marks with or without marks of outer teeth.
- **Nonpoisonous:** Two fang marks with number of small teeth marks.
- Differences between poisonous and nonpoisonous snakes are described in **Figures 16.6A** and **B** and **Table 16.7**.

Box 16.5: Classification of poisonous snakes.

1. **Elapidae (neurotoxic):** Examples:
   - Common cobra/*nag* or kalsap or *Naja naja*
   - King cobra: *Raj nag* or *Naja hannah* or *Naja bungarus*
   - Krait: Subgrouped into: (a) common krait or *Bungarus caeruleus*; (b) banded krait or *Bungarus fasciatus*; (c) coral snake; (d) tiger snake; (e) mambas and (f) death adder.
2. **Viperidae (vasculotoxic):** They are grouped into:
   - **Pitiless vipers:** These include: (a) Russell's viper and (b) saw-scaled viper
   - **Pit vipers:** These include: (a) pit viper—crotalidae and (b) common green pit viper.
3. **Hydrophidae (myotoxic):** About 20 types of sea snakes are found in India. All are poisonous.

TABLE 16.6: Various components of snake venom and their actions.

Component	*Action*
Serine proteases	Hemolysis
Other proteases	Hemolysis
Phospholipase A2	Myotoxic, cardiotoxic, neurotoxic, increases vascular permeability
Hyaluronidase	Local tissue destruction
Neurotoxin	
➢ Alpha-bungarotoxin, cobrotoxin	➢ Postsynaptic inhibition
➢ Beta-bungarotoxin, crotoxin	➢ Presynaptic inhibition

Clinical Feature of Snakebite

Q. Discuss:
- **Clinical features of poisonous snakebite.**
- **Cobra bite envenomation—features and treatment.**

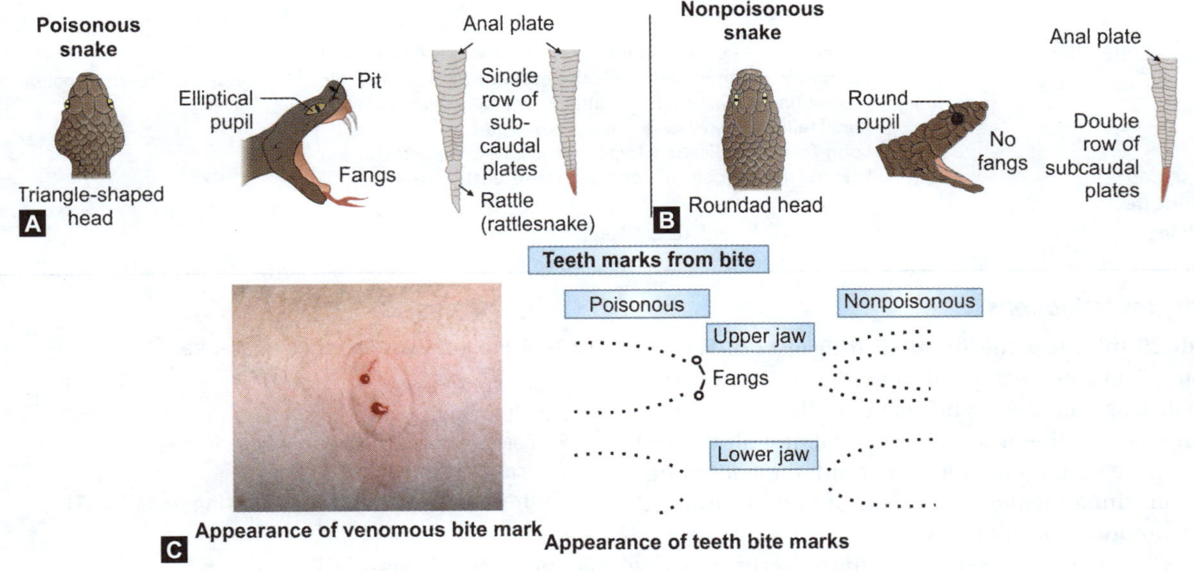

FIGS. 16.6A TO C: (A and B) Differences between poisonous and nonpoisonous snakes; (C) Teeth marks from bite.

TABLE 16.7: Differences between poisonous and nonpoisonous snakes.

Points	*Poisonous snakes*	*Nonpoisonous snakes*
1. Belly scales	*Large:* They cover the entire breadth of belly	*Small:* They never cover
2. Head scales	➢ Usually small in vipers ➢ May be large in pit vipers ➢ Cobras and Coral snakes where third labial touches the eye and nasal shields ➢ Kraits, where there is no pit and the third labial does not touch the nose and eye	Are usually large with exceptions as outlined under poisonous snakes
3. Fangs	Are hollow-like hypodermic needle	Short and solid
4. Tail	Compressed	Not markedly compressed
5. Habits	Usually nocturnal	Not so
6. Teeth bite marks	Two fang marks with or without marks of other teeth	Two fang marks with number of small teeth marks

Q. Write a short essay/note on complications of poisonous (cobra) snakebite.

Signs, symptoms and complications of snakebite are listed in **Table 16.8**.

Asymptomatic (dry bite): Significant proportion of snakebites do not result in envenomation. Patients without clinical features of local or systemic envenomation should be closely observed for 24–48 hours.

Prognosis Assessment in Snakebite

See **Box 16.6.**

TABLE 16.8: Local and systemic features/complications of snakebites.

Local features	*Systemic features*
A. Elapid bite	
Fang marks, burning pain, swelling and discoloration, serosanguineous discharge. Local symptoms are milder than in viperine bite	**Preparalytic stage:** Vomiting, headache, giddiness, weakness, and lethargy **Paralytic stage: Ptosis**, ophthalmoplegia, drowsiness, convulsion, bulbar paralysis, respiratory failure, death, paradoxical respiration: Intercostal muscle paralysis, stomach pain (Krait), submucosal hemorrhage in stomach. Neck muscle weakness **(broken neck sign)** **Krait bites:** Present in early morning with paralysis and can be **mistaken for STROKE** These symptoms can be remembered as 5 Ds and 2 Ps ➢ *5 Ds—dyspnea, dysphonia, dysarthria, diplopia, dysphagia* ➢ *2 Ps—ptosis, paralysis*
B. Viperid bite	
Rapid swelling at bite site **Discoloration** **Blister formation** **Bleeding from bite site** **Pain**	➢ **Generalized bleeding:** Epistaxis, hemoptysis, hematemesis, bleeding gums , hematuria, malena, hemorrhagic areas over skin and mucosa ➢ **Lateralizing neurological symptoms** such as asymmetrical pupils, intracranial bleed ➢ **Hypotension:** Resulting from hypovolemia/direct vasodilation ➢ **Low back pain,** indicative of early renal failure ➢ **Muscle pain:** Rhabdomyolysis

Contd...

Contd...

	➢ Parotid swelling, conjunctival edema, subconjunctival hemorrhage ➢ **Idiopathic systemic capillary leak syndrome (ISCLS)** characterized by episodes of severe hypotension, hypoalbuminemia, hemoconcentration without albuminuria ➢ **Renal failure:** Russell's viper, hump-nosed pit viper ➢ **Long-term complication:** Hypopituitarism and cardiotoxicity ➢ Saw-scaled viper generally does not cause renal failure
C. Hydrophid bite	
Local swelling **Pain**	Stiffness, myoglobinuria, renal failure

Laboratory Investigations

- **Bedside 20-minute whole blood clotting test (20-WBCT)**
  - Place 2 mL of freshly sampled venous blood in a small glass test tube and leave undisturbed for 20 minutes at ambient temperature. Gently tilt the test tube to see if the blood is still liquid; the patient has hypofibrinogenemia as a result of venom-induced consumption coagulopathy.
- *Nonspecific:* Hemogram, serum creatinine, serum amylase, creatine phosphokinase (CPK).
- Prothrombin time (PT), fibrinogen degradation product (FDP) and fibrinogen level in viper bite as it interferes with clotting mechanism.
- *LFT, ABG, and electrolyte:* For systemic manifestation.
- *Urine examination:* For proteinuria, myoglobinuria.
- *ECG:* Nonspecific changes such as bradycardia and atrioventricular (AV) block.

Box 16.6: Prognosis assessment in snakebite.

- Time of bite
- Activity at the time of bite
- First aid action taken since the bite
- Clinical examination
- **Twenty minutes whole blood clotting test (WBCT)**

Q. Describe the initial approach to the stabilization of the patient who presents with snakebite.

Management

The first aid **(Box 16.7)** being currently recommended is based around the mnemonic: **"Do it RIGHT"**.

A. Specific treatment

Antisnake venom (ASV)

Indications for ASV are presented in **Table 16.9.**

Q. Enu merate the indications and describe the pharmacology, dose, adverse reactions, hypersensitivity reactions of antisnake venom.

The classification of severity of snakebite is presented in **Table 16.10.**

- **Dosage of ASV:** Ideally administer within 4 hours but effective, if given within 24 hours:
  - In **mild cases, 5 vial (50 mL); in moderate cases, 5–10 vials; and in severe cases, 10–20 vial.**
  - Additional infusion containing 5–10 vials are infused until progression of swelling ceased and systemic symptoms are disappeared.
- **Mode of administration:** ASV is given slowly as IV injection or infusion at the rate of 2 mL/minute. ASV dilute 5–10 mL/kg body weight of normal saline or 5% dextrose and infused over 1 hour. ASV should never give locally at site of snakebite.
- No change in dose for children or pregnant women.
- *Repeat dose of ASV*
  - *in vasculotoxic or hemotoxic envenomation: Administer ASV every 6 hours until coagulation (WBCT) is restored.*
  - *in neuroparalytic or neurotoxic envenomation: Initial dose of ASV 10 vials stat as infusion to be followed by 2nd dose of 10 vials if no improvement within 1st hour (total 20 vials).*

Adverse reaction of ASV (Box 16.8): It may develop in 20% patients.

Box 16.7: First aid currently recommended for snakebite **"Do it RIGHT".**

R = Reassure the patient. Seventy percent of all snakebites are from nonvenomous species. Only 50% of bites by venomous species actually envenomate the patient

I = Immobilize in the same way as a fractured limb. Use of bandages or cloth is to hold the splints and should to block the blood supply or apply pressure. Do not compress by tight ligatures, because they can be dangerous! (Loose ligatures to block lymphatic flow can be used?)

GH = Get to Hospital immediately. Traditional remedies have NO PROVEN benefit in treating snakebite

T = Tell the physician about any systemic symptoms that develop on the way to hospital (e.g., ptosis)

TABLE 16.9: Indications for antisnake venom (ASV).

➢ **Neurotoxicity** ➢ **Bleeding/coagulopathy** – Spontaneous systemic bleeding – WBCT (20-minute whole blood clotting test) > 20 minutes – Thrombocytopenia (platelet < 100,000) ➢ **Myoglobinuria/hemoglobinuria**	➢ Cardiac toxicity ➢ Local swelling involving more than half of the bitten limb ➢ Rapid extension of swelling ➢ Development of an enlarged tender lymph node draining the bitten limb ➢ Acute renal failure

TABLE 16.10: Classification of severity of snakebite.

	Envenomation			
	Absent	***Mild***	***Moderate***	***Severe***
Fang marks	±	+	+	+
Local reaction	–	Moderate	Severe	Severe
➢ Pain	Absent	Minimum (0–15 cm)	Moderate (15–30 cm)	Severe >30 cm
➢ Local edema	Absent	+	+	+
➢ Erythema	Absent	±	+	+
➢ Ecchymosis	Absent			
Systemic features	No	No	Weakness, sweating, syncope, nausea, vomiting, thrombocytopenia	Hypotension, paresthesia, ptosis, broken neck sign, coma, pulmonary edema, respiratory failure

Box 16.8: Adverse reactions of antisnake venom (ASV).

1. *Early anaphylactic reaction* ***(Table 16.11):*** It may develop within 10 minutes to 3 hours. Patient should be monitored closely. *Treatment of anaphylactic reaction:*
   - Discontinue ASV
   - *Adrenaline:* 1:1,000 IM (0.5 mg/kg in adult and 0.01 mg/kg in children). It can be repeated every 5 minutes, if necessary.
   - *H1 antihistaminic:* IV 1 mg of chlorpheniramine maleate (CPM)
   - IV hydrocortisone
   - Once the patient has recovered, restart ASV slowly for 10–15 minutes keeping the patient under close observation. Then resume normal drip rate
2. *Late serum sickness:* Develops in 1–12 days. Characterized by fever, nausea, vomiting, diarrhea, arthritis, nephritis, myoglobinuria, etc. Treatment consists of:
   - *Oral antihistaminic:* 5-day course of oral antihistaminic. For adults—CPM 2 mg/6 hour and for children—0.25 mg/kg/day in divided dose
   - *Prednisolone:* For patient who fail to respond within 24 hours. Dose: 5 mg/6 hours in adult and 0.7 mg/kg/day in divided dose in children

TABLE 16.11: Any one of the following suggests early anaphylactic reaction.

➢ Urticaria	➢ Chills	➢ Diarrhea	➢ Hypotension
➢ Itching	➢ Nausea	➢ Abdominal cramps	➢ Bronchospasm
➢ Fever	➢ Vomiting	➢ Tachycardia	➢ Angioedema

Algorithm approach to the identification of type of snakebite is presented in **Flowchart 16.1**.

FLOWCHART 16.1: Algorithm approach for the identification of type of snake bitten by clinical syndrome in snakebite and management of the same.

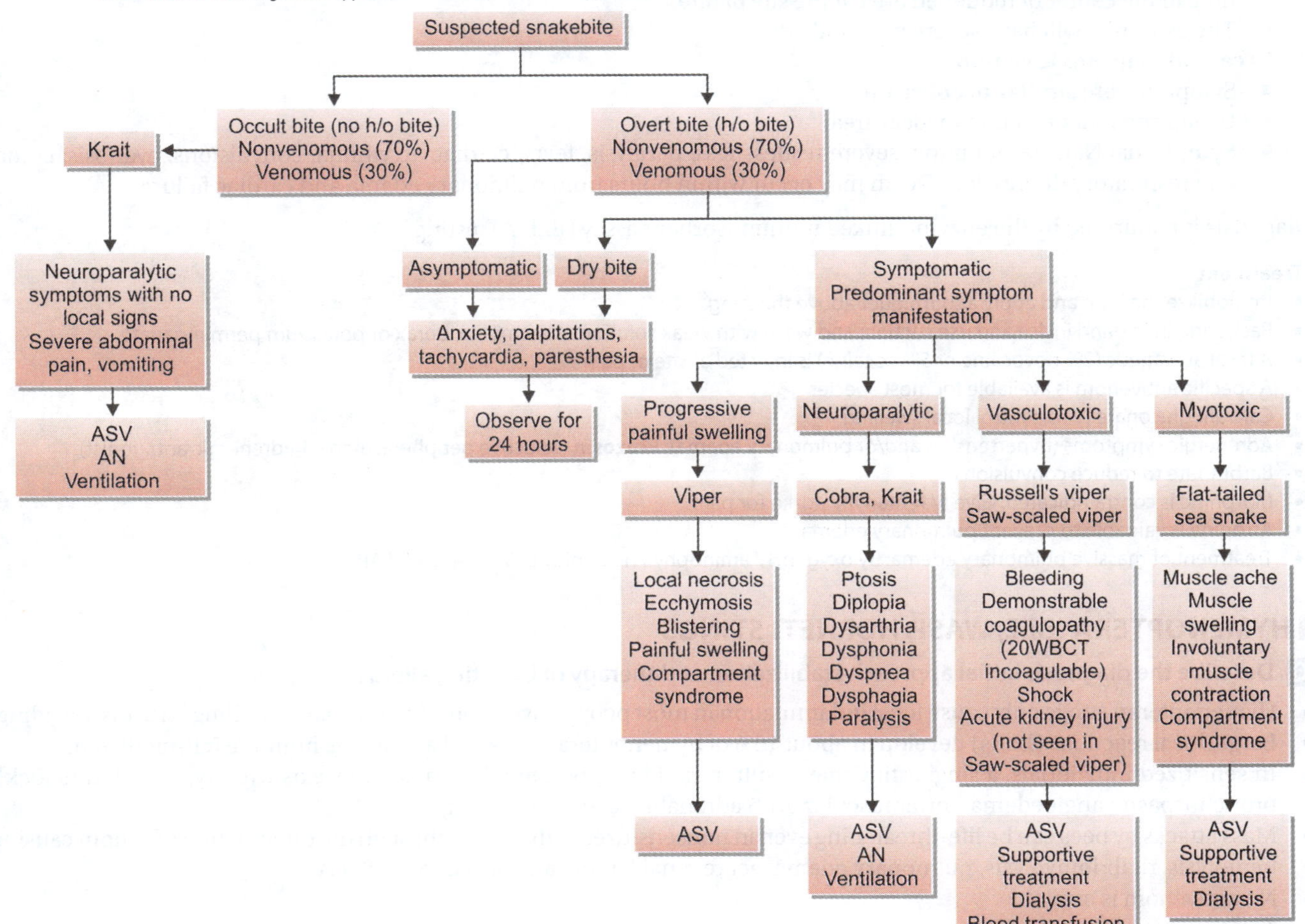

(ASV: antisnake venom; AN: atropine-neostigmine)

B. Supportive therapy
- **For coagulopathy:** If it does not reverse after ASV therapy, fresh-frozen plasma, cryoprecipitate (fibrinogen, factor VIII), fresh whole blood, platelet concentrate can be administered.
- **Management neurotoxic (neuroparalytic) envenomation**
  - ASV alone not sufficient.
  - Tracheostomy, endotracheal intubation, and mechanical ventilation.
  - ***Atropine neostigmine (AN)*** *dosage schedule: Atropine 0.6 mg followed by neostigmine (1.5 mg) to be given IV stat and repeat dose of neostigmine 0.5 mg with atropine every 30 minutes for 5 doses.* Thereafter to be given as tapering dose at 1, 2, 6 and 12 hours.
  - *Glycopyrrolate:* About 0.25 mg can be given before neostigmine in place of atropine as glycopyrrolate does not cross blood brain barrier.
- **Renal failure:** Hemodialysis/peritoneal dialysis.
- **Capillary leak syndrome:** Methylprednisolone (10 mg/kg Q8H) × 3 days.
- **Compartment syndrome:** Fasciotomy.
- **Surgical debridement of wound**
- **Care of bitten part:** Antibiotic prophylaxis and tetanus toxoid.

SCORPION BITE

Q. Describe the diagnosis, initial approach stabilization, and therapy of scorpion envenomation.

- *Scorpion venom:*
  - It is clear, colorless toxalbumin and can be classified as either neurotoxic or hemolytic.
  - Toxicity is more than snake. However, during bite only small quantity is injected.
  - Venom is strong autonomic stimulator and releases large amount of catecholamine from adrenals.
  - Mortality (except in children) is negligible, and can cause acute pancreatitis.

Signs and Symptoms

1. **In case of hemolytic venom:**
   - Reaction is predominantly local and **simulates the viper snakebite.** However, the scorpion sting bite shows only one hole in the center of reddened area at the site of bite.
   - The extremity will have severe pain and edema.
2. **In case of neurotoxic venom:**
   - Symptoms are **similar to cobra bite.**
   - Usually no mark reaction in local area.
   - **Symptoms:** Nausea, vomiting, severe restlessness, paralysis, fever, cardiac arrythmia, convulsions, cyanosis, coma, and respiratory depression. Death may occur within hours from pulmonary edema and cardiac failure.

Diagnosis is confirmed by the enzyme-linked immunosorbent assay (ELISA) testing.

Treatment
- Immobilize the limb and apply a tourniquet above the sting
- Pack sting in ice, and incise and use suction, and wash with weak solution of ammonia, borax or potassium permanganate
- A local anesthetic (2% novocaine or 5% cocaine) is injected at site of pain
- A specific antivenom is available for most species
- Calcium gluconate IV to control local swelling
- Adrenergic symptoms (hypertension and/or pulmonary edema): **Prazosin** (selective peripheral alpha-1 adrenergic antagonist)
- Barbiturate to reduce convulsions
- Morphine is contraindicated. Give IV fentanyl 1 μg/kg for pain
- Atropine is valuable to prevent pulmonary edema
- Treatment of massive pulmonary edema: By oxygen, IV aminophylline or nitroprusside, NIV/CPAP

HYMENOPTERA (BEE, WASP, HORNET) STINGS

Q. Describe the diagnosis initial approach stabilization and therapy of bee sting allergy.

- Hymenopteran stings only cause local inflammation in most people. Symptoms include pain, swelling, pruritis, bleeding.
- Large, local reactions (LLRs) develop in about 10% of hymenoptera stings and are due be immune IgE-mediated.
- In sensitized individuals, a single sting may result in rapid and potentially fatal anaphylaxis with hypotension (shock), bronchospasm, angioedema. Intramuscular 0.1% adrenaline can be lifesaving.
- Mass attacks by bees can be life-threatening even in nonsensitized individuals, through the direct action of venom causing hemolysis, rhabdomyolysis, pulmonary edema, acute renal failure, and adrenergic effects.
- No antivenom is available.
- Treatment is symptomatic.

CORROSIVE POISONING

Q. Enumerate the common corrosives used in your area and describe their toxicology, clinical features, prognosis, and approach to therapy.

- Common corrosive poisons:
  - Acids (hydrochloric, acetic, sulfuric, lactic, oxalic, carbolic)
  - Alkalis (sodium and potassium, soaps, detergents)
  - Heavy metal salts (sublimate)
  - Others: Formalin, iodine tincture

Clinical Features

- Clinical presentation of corrosive injuries in the upper gastrointestinal tract. Acids cause coagulation necrosis while alkalis cause liquefactive necrosis.
- Patient complains of oropharyngeal, epigastric, or retrosternal pain associated with dysphagia or odynophagia, and/or hypersalivation, nausea, vomiting, hematemesis. Severe forms can damage larynx, and also cause endotracheal or bronchial necrosis with mediastinitis, also perforation of stomach may occur.
- Late complications are esophageal strictures and stenosis, gastric stenosis of the antrum and pylorus, esophageal and stomach cancer.

Treatment

- Treatment mainly is to prevent the complications.
- Lavage is contraindicated.
- Upper gastrointestinal (UGI) endoscopy should be performed during the first 24 hours after ingestion in order to evaluate the extent of esophageal and gastric damage, establish prognosis, and guide therapy
- Grading of corrosive injury based on endoscopy:
  - 0: Normal mucosa
  - 1: Erythema/hyperemia
  - 2a: Superficial ulcer/erosion/friability/hemorrhage/exudates
  - 2b: Findings in 2a + deep discrete/circumferential ulcers
  - 3a: Scattered/focal necrosis (black/gray discoloration)
  - 3b: Extensive/circumferential necrosis of mucosa
- Antibiotics are recommended in grade 3 injury and suspected gastrointestinal perforation.
- Proton pump inhibitors and H2 blockers are routinely recommended.
- Nutrition is planned according to the endoscopic grade of the lesions. Patients with grade 1/2a can tolerate oral feeds and those with grade 2b/3a will require nasoenteral feeding. Patients with grade 3b lesions require gastrostomy/ jejunostomy for enteral feeding and may also require total parenteral nutrition.
- 30% of patients usually develop esophageal strictures with 2 months which will need endoscopic dilatation or surgery.

COMMON DRUG OVERDOSAGES

Q. Enumerate the commonly observed drug overdose in your area and describe their toxicology, clinical features, prognosis and approach to therapy.

Sedative Drug Poisoning

Benzodiazepines Poisoning

Q. Write a short essay/note on benzodiazepine overdose and management.

Mode of Action

- Benzodiazepines (BZDs) exert their effect via modulation of the gamma-aminobutyric acid-A (GABA-A) receptor.
- Gamma-aminobutyric acid is the main inhibitory neurotransmitter of the central nervous system.

Types (Table 16.12)

TABLE 16.12: Various categories of benzodiazepines.

Hypnotic	*Antianxiety*	*Anticonvulsant*
➤ Diazepam	➤ Diazepam	➤ Diazepam
➤ Flurazepam	➤ Chlordiazepoxide	➤ Lorazepam
➤ Nitrazepam	➤ Oxazepam	➤ Clonazepam
➤ Alprazolam	➤ Lorazepam	➤ Clobazam
➤ Temazepam	➤ Alprazolam	
➤ Triazolam		

Clinical Features of Overdosage

Oral benzodiazepines taken in overdose without a coingestant rarely cause significant toxicity. The classic presentation of a patient with an isolated BZD overdose consists of CNS depression with normal vital signs.

- **Toxic symptoms:** Sedative action on the CNS.
- **Large doses:** Neuromuscular blockade.

- **Intravenous injection:** Peripheral vasodilation, fall in BP, shock. Propylene glycol (1,2-propanediol) is the diluent used in parenteral formulations of diazepam and lorazepam which itself causes cardio- and neurotoxicity.

Of note, most intentional ingestions of BZDs involve a coingestant, the most common being *ethanol*.

Acute poisoning

- **Mild:** Drowsiness, ataxia, weakness.
- **Moderate to severe:** Vertigo, slurred speech, nystagmus, partial ptosis, lethargy, hypotension, respiratory depression, coma (stages 1 and 2).
  - **COMA (Stage 1):** Responsive to painful stimuli but not to verbal or tactile stimuli, without any disturbance in respiration or BP.
  - **COMA (Stage 2):** Unconscious, not responsive to painful stimuli, no disturbance in respiration or BP.

General Diagnostic Testing

- Check glucose, to rule out **hypoglycemia** as the cause of any alteration in mental status.
- **Acetaminophen and salicylate levels**, to rule out these common co-ingestions.
- Electrocardiogram, as it affect the QRS or QTc intervals.
- Pregnancy test in women of childbearing age.

Life Supportive Procedures and Symptomatic/Specific Treatment

- Airway, breathing and circulation
- Endotracheal intubation
- Assisted ventilation
- Supplemental oxygen intravenous fluids, inotropes, if needed.

Decontamination

Gastrointestinal decontamination with activated charcoal (AC) (usually of no benefit in cases of isolated BZD ingestion and increases the risk of aspiration).

Antidote Treatment: Flumazenil

- *Mode of action:* Competitive antagonism. Complete reversal of benzodiazepine effect with a total slow IV dose of 1 mg.
- Administered in a series of smaller doses beginning with 0.2 mg and progressively increasing by 0.1–0.2 mg every minute until a cumulative total dose of 3.5 mg is reached.
- Resedation occurs within 0.5–2 hours.
- *Side effects:* Nausea, vomiting, arrhythmias, convulsions.
- *Contraindication:* Status epilepticus.

Barbiturate Poisoning

Q. Write a short essay on clinical features and treatment of barbiturate poisoning.

- Nonselective CNS depressants.
- **Mode of action:** Direct CNS depressants bind to GABA receptors → prolongs the opening of chloride channel. Inhibits excitable cells of the CNS.

Classification

See **Table 16.13**.

TABLE 16.13: Classification of barbiturates.

Long acting (6–12 hours)	*Intermediate acting (3–6 hours)*	*Short acting (<3 hours)*	*Ultrashort acting (<15–20 minutes)*
Mephobarbital Phenobarbitone	Amobarbital Aprobarbitone Butobarbitone	Hexobarbi- tone Pentobarbitone Secobarbital	Thiopentone Methohexitone

Signs and Symptoms

See **Table 16.14**.

TABLE 16.14: Adverse and toxic effects of barbiturate poisoning.

Adverse effects	*Toxic effects*
➤ Residual depression ➤ Paradoxical excitement ➤ Hypersensitivity reactions—localized swelling of eyelid, cheek or lip, erythematous or exfoliative dermatitis ➤ Synergistic action with ethanol and antihistamines	➤ Slurred speech, ataxia, lethargy, confusion, headache, and nystagmus ➤ CNS depression, coma, shock ➤ Pupils—first constricted, later dilate becau se of hypoxia ➤ Hypothermia ➤ Cutaneous **bullae** (blisters) **(Fig. 16.7)** ➤ Death due to respiratory arrest or cardiovascular collapse

Management of Barbiturate Poisoning

- No specific antidote.
- Barbiturate poisoning is more **dangerous** than benzodiazepine poisoning.
- Management is **supportive**.
  - Cardiorespiratory support.
  - Clean the airways by thorough suctioning and insertion of oral airways.
  - If the patient is comatose, prompt intubation is strongly advocated because of worsening of respiratory failure.
  - Correction of dehydration by CVP-guided fluid therapy depending on the serum electrolytes.

- Treat hypotension by intravenous infusion of plasma expanders and vasopressors. In refractory cases, steroids are given.
- Measures to prevent absorption:
  - Gastric lavage
  - Activated charcoal is administrated orally or by nasogastric tube.
- Measures for removal of barbiturates:
  - Frequent doses of activated charcoal
  - Forced diuresis with alkalization of urine
  - Hemodialysis and hemoperfusion.

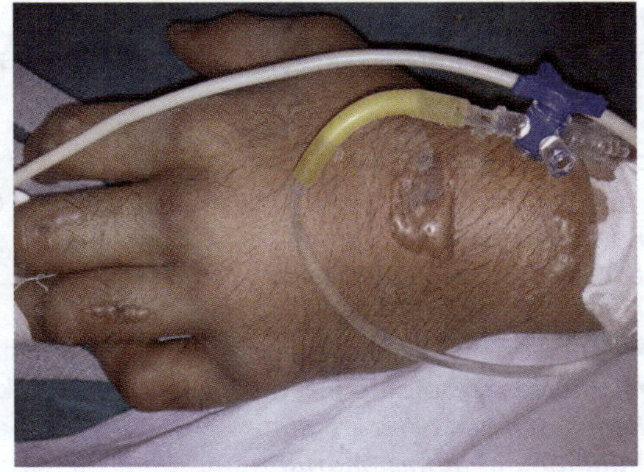

FIG. 16.7: Barbiturate blister.

Analgesic Poisoning

Paracetamol (Acetaminophen) Poisoning

Q. Write a short essay on paracetamol poisoning and its treatment.

- Toxicity unlikely to result from a single dose of <150 mg/kg in child or 7.5–10 g for adult.
- Toxicity is likely with single ingestions > 250 mg/kg or those > 12 g over a 24-hour period.
- Virtually all patients who ingest doses in excess of 350 mg/kg develop severe liver toxicity unless appropriately treated.

Mechanism of Paracetamol Toxicity (Fig. 16.8)

Toxicity is due to formation of an intermediate reactive metabolite, which binds covalently to cellular proteins, leading to cell death. This causes hepatic and occasionally renal failure. In therapeutic doses, the toxic intermediate metabolite is detoxified in reactions requiring glutathione. **With overdose, glutathione reserves become depleted**.

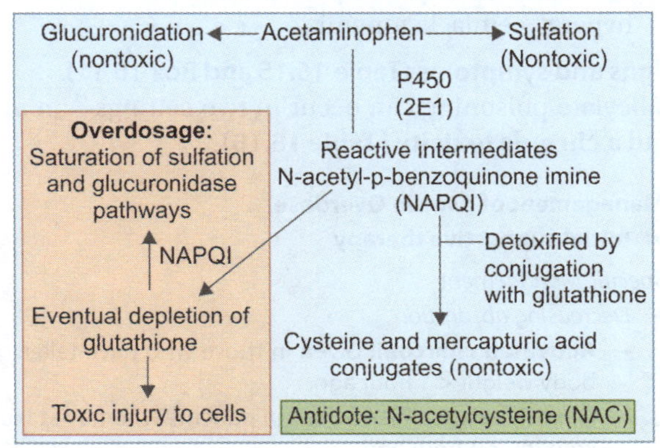

FIG. 16.8: Acetaminophen metabolism.

Clinical Manifestations of Toxicity

- **Stage I (0.5–24 hours)**
  - No symptoms; nausea, vomiting and malaise.
- **Stage II (24–72 hours)**
  - Subclinical elevations of hepatic aminotransferases (AST, ALT).
  - Right upper quadrant pain, with liver enlargement and tenderness. Elevations of prothrombin time (PT), total bilirubin, and oliguria and renal function abnormalities may become evident. Acute kidney injury is primarily **due** to acute tubular necrosis.
- **Stage III (72–96 hours)**
  - Fulminant hepatic failure; Jaundice, confusion (hepatic encephalopathy), a marked elevation in hepatic enzymes, hyperammonemia, and a bleeding diathesis, hypoglycemia, lactic acidosis, renal failure (25%), and death.
- **Stage IV (4 days to 2 weeks)**
  - Recovery phase that usually begins by day 4 and is complete by 7 days after overdose.

Treatment Options

- **Activated charcoal:** May reduce absorption by 50–90%.
- **Gastric lavage:** Only for massive ingestions (e.g., > 600 mg/kg).
- **Antidote: N-acetylcysteine (NAC) (Box 16.9)**
  - *Properties:*
    - *Mechanism of action (MOA):* A glutathione precursor.
    - Limits the formation and accumulation of NAPQI.
    - Powerful anti-inflammatory and antioxidant effects.
  - *Dosage and administration:*
    - IV infusion.
  - 150 mg/kg over 15 minutes; 50 mg/kg over next 4 hours; 100 mg/kg over next 16 hours up to 36 hours.
  - Most effective, if started within 8–10 hours after ingestion. Beyond 8 hours, NAC efficacy progressively decreases.
    - Oral N-acetylcysteine regimen consists of a 72-hour oral course given as a 140 mg/kg loading dose followed by 17 doses of 70 mg/kg every 4 hours (total dose 1,330 mg/kg).
- Alternate medication: **Oral methionine.**
- **Liver transplantation (Box 16.10)**
  It is life-saving for fulminant hepatic necrosis.

Box 16.9: Indications for N-acetylcysteine in paracetamol poisoning.

- All patients with a serum acetaminophen concentration above the possible hepatic toxicity line on the Rumack- Matthew nomogram
- Patients with an estimated ingestion of > 140 mg/kg
- Patients with an unknown time of ingestion
- Patients with a presentation > 24 hours after ingestion with elevated transaminases

Box 16.10: Indications for liver transplantation for paracetamol poisoining (King's College Criteria).

- Acidosis (pH <7.3)
- PT (prothrombin time) >100 sec
- Creatinine >3.4 mg/dL
- Grade 3 encephalopathy (or worse)

Aspirin Toxicity

Q. Write a short note on salicylates poisoning and its management.

Mechanism of toxicity

- Acetylsalicylic acid (ASA) is hydrolyzed to salicylic acid. Responsible for therapeutic and toxic effects.
- *Direct stimulation of respiratory center:* Medulla.
- *Uncouples oxidative phosphorylation:*
  - Increase in O_2 consumption and CO_2 production
  - Increase respiration leading to respiratory alkalosis.
- *Renal excretion of bicarbonate, Na and K:* Metabolic acidosis.
- *Inhibition of mitochondrial respiration:* Increase pyruvate and lactic acid → metabolic acidosis.
- Disruption of Kreb's cycle metabolism and glycolysis → hyperglycemia, ketonemia.

Signs and symptoms (Table 16.15 and Box 16.11)

Salicylate poisoning can occur in two settings—an **acute toxicity and a chronic toxicity (Table 16.16)**.

Management of Aspirin Overdose

- **Initial supportive therapy**

Specific Management

- *Decreasing absorption*
  - **Activated charcoal:** Given in those who have taken > 250 mg/kg body weight < 1 hour ago.
  - **Gastric lavage:** It is advised in patients who have taken > 500 mg/kg body < 1 hour ago.
- *Increasing drug elimination*
  - **Urinary alkalinization:**
    - Alkalinizing urine from pH 5–8 increases renal elimination of ASA from 1.3 to 100 mL/minute.
    - Serum half-life decreases from 48 to 6 hours.
    - This is done by giving an infusion of sodium bicarbonate.
  - **Hemodialysis (Box 16.12):**
    - Used in severe life-threatening overdose.
    - Aims to correct the acid-base disturbances while removing the salicylate.

TABLE 16.15: Differences between acute and chronic aspirin toxicity.

Features	*Acute*	*Chronic salicylism*
Age	Young adult	Older adults/infants
Cause	Overdose	Treatment misuse
Coingestion	Frequent	Rare
Mental status	Normal	Altered
Clinical presentation	Early	Late
Mortality	Low with treatment	High
Serum levels (mg/dL)	40 to ≥120	30 to ≥80

Box 16.11: ASPIRIN mnemonic.

- **A**ltered mental status (lethargy—coma)
- **S**weating/diaphoresis
- **P**ulmonary edema
- **I**ncreased vital signs (hypertension, increased respiratory rate, tachycardia)
- **R**inging in the ears
- **I**rritable
- **N**ausea and vomiting

TABLE 16.16: Features of salicylate poisoning.

Central nervous system	*Signs and symptoms*	*Laboratory findings*
Hyperactivity Irritability Delirium Agitation Vertigo Slurred speech Hallucination Lethargy Stupor Seizures Coma Cerebral edema	Nausea, vomiting Tinnitus, hearing loss Pulmonary edema Hyperventilation (tachypnea and/or hyperpnea) Hyperthermia Tachycardia Volume depletion Arrhythmias Diaphoresis	Respiratory alkalosis Anion gap metabolic acidosis Coagulation abnormalities Urinary ketones Hyperkalemia Hyperlactatemia (mild)

Box 16.12: Absolute indications for hemodialysis in aspirin toxicity.

- Renal failure
- Congestive heart failure
- Acute lung injury
- Persistent CNS disturbances
- Progressive deterioration in vital signs
- Severe acid-base or electrolyte imbalance, despite appropriate treatment
- Hepatic compromise with coagulopathy
- Salicylate concentration (acute) >100 mg/dL (in the absence of the above)

Cyanide Poisoning

Q. Write a short essay on management of cyanide poisoning.

Cyanide

- Present in bitter almonds (250 mg CN/100 g plant tissue), cassava (104 mg CN/100 g plant tissue), wild cherries (140-370 mg CN/100 g plant material), and other foods.
- Used extensively in industry for fumigation, electroplating, and mining activities.

Routes of exposure of cyanide is mentioned in **Box 16.13**.

Clinical Manifestations of Cyanide Poisoning

- **Onset of cyanide poisoning**
  - **Inhalation** (rapid onset, seconds to minutes), **ingestion,** and **skin contact** (delayed onset, 15-30 minutes).
- Death may occur within 6-8 minutes after inhalation of a high concentration 2-5 mg/kg of it is lethal.
- **Mechanism:** Inhibits mitochondrial cytochrome oxidase and an "asphyxiating" agent.

Box 16.13: Routes of exposure of cyanide.

- **Gas:** Inhalation (e.g., hydrogen cyanide and cyanogen chloride)
- **Liquid:** Inhalation (aerosol), ingestion, skin contact (e.g., hydrocyanic acid)
- **Solid:** Inhalation, ingestion, skin contact (e.g., cyanide salts)

- Common final pathway for cyanide intoxication is **cellular hypoxia.**
  - **Metabolic acidosis:** Nonspecific symptoms.
  - **CNS: Dizziness, nausea, vomiting, drowsiness, tetanus, trismus, hallucinations.**
  - **CVS: Dysrhythmia, hypotension.** Tachycardia and hypertension may occur transiently in early stages.
  - **Respiratory: Dyspnea, initial hyperventilation followed by hypoventilation** and **pulmonary edema.** Cyanosis not apparent, since blood is adequately oxygenated.

Laboratory Diagnosis

- **Blood cyanide levels** can be estimated, but empiric treatment is almost always required before laboratory results are available.
- **High anion gap metabolic acidosis.**
- **Arterial and venous pO_2 may be elevated.**

Treatment

- **Activated charcoal:** For alert, asymptomatic patients following ingestion.
- **Supplemental oxygen:** 100% for suspected exposure.
- Supportive care.
- **Sodium nitrite:**
  - **Mechanism: Forms methemoglobin**, competes with cytochrome oxidase for free cyanide; combines with cyanide to form cyanmethemoglobin.
  - **Dose:** (1) Adults: 300 mg IV over 5 minutes; slower if hypotension develops and (2) children: 0.12–0.33 mg/kg IV infused as above.
- **Amyl nitrite: 0.3 mL inhaled can be repeated after 3–5 minutes.** Second-line agent used when sodium nitrite is not available.
- **Sodium thiosulfate:**
  - **Mechanism:** Sulfur donor promotes rhodanese activity, detoxifies cyanide as it is released from cyanmethemoglobin. Directly detoxifies cyanide by conversion to thiocyanate; too slow to be useful as a first-line intervention.
  - **Dose:** (1) *Adults:* 12.5 g IV over 10–20 minutes following administration of sodium nitrite and (2) *Children:* 412.5 mg/kg IV over 10–20 minutes.

Hydroxocobalamin

- **Mechanism:** Direct-binding agent, **chelates cyanide.**
- **Dose:** 4–5 g IV

Dicobalt edetate is an intravenous chelator of cyanide which can be used.

Anticholinergic Toxidrome

Q. Write a short essay/note on causes of anticholinergic syndrome.

Causes of Anticholinergic Toxidrome

See **Table 16.17.**

TABLE 16.17: Various causes of anticholinergic syndrome.

Natural alkaloids	Synthetic compounds
➢ Atropine (from the plant *Atropa belladonna*/Deadly nightshade) ➢ Hyoscine (Scopolamine) (from *Hyoscyamus niger*/henbane) ➢ *Datura stramonium* (plant—Jimson weed/Angel's trumpet)	➢ *Mydriatics:* Tropicamide (eye drops) ➢ *Antisecretory antispasmodics:* Glycopyrrolate, oxybutynin ➢ *Antiparkinsonian drugs:* Benzhexol, benztropine
Semisynthetic derivatives	**Miscellaneous**
➢ Homatropine (eye drops) ➢ Tiotropium bromide	➢ Tricyclic antidepressants, e.g., amitriptyline ➢ Phenothiazines, e.g., prochlorperazine ➢ Antihistamines, e.g., cyclizine ➢ Neuroleptics, e.g., olanzapine

PLANT POISONS

Q. Enumerate the common plant poisons seen in your area and describe their toxicology, clinical features, prognosis and specific approach to detoxification.

Neurotoxic Plant Poisons

Datura Poisoning

Q. Write a short essay/note on clinical features and management of datura poisoning.

- *Datura stramonium* (jimson seed) **causes anticholinergic syndrome.** The active **toxic agents include atropine and scopolamine.** Atropine and related compounds **block acetylcholine at the receptor sites of postganglionic synapses of the cholinergic nerves.**
- **All the parts of datura plant (Figs. 16.9A and B) are poisonous,** but the seeds and fruit are the most toxic.
- **Mode of poisoning:** Most popular mode of poisoning is by mixing the seeds in sweets and given to others with the intention of thefts.

Clinical features

- Toxic symptoms often appear within 30 minutes of ingestion and last for 24–48 hours.
- Clinical features include tachycardia and the other features are described as ***"blind as a bat, mad as a hatter, red as a beet, hot as a hare, dry as a bone, the bowel and bladder lose their tone, and the heart runs alone".***
  - *Hot as a hare:* Cutaneous vasodilatation leading to anhidrotic hyperthermia.
  - *Blind as a bat:* Ciliary muscle paralysis, mydriasis, dilated pupils.

- *Dry as a bone:* Anhidrosis, dryness of mouth, urinary retention, decreased bowel motility.
- *Red as a beet:* Cutaneous vasodilatation causing flushing.
- *Mad as a hatter:* CNS arousal, agitation, delirium, hallucinations.
- In can be fatal-producing stupor, coma, and convulsions. Death is due to respiratory paralysis or cardiovascular collapse.

Management
- Gastric lavage and supportive therapy.
- Control of hyperthermia.
- Role of physostigmine, a cholinesterase inhibitor is not clear.
- Activated charcoal adsorbs the alkaloids.
- Benzodiazepines to treat agitation.

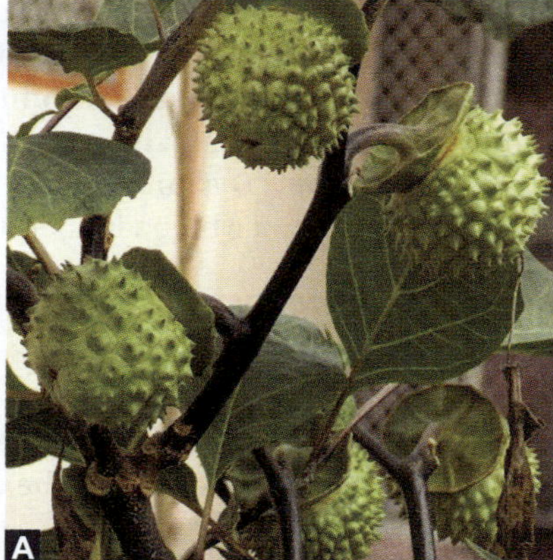

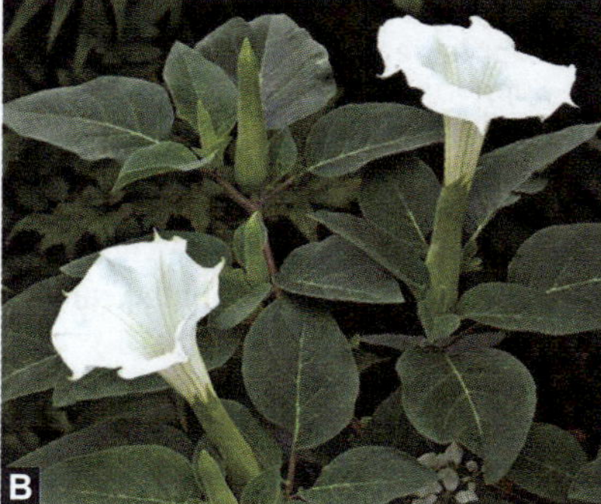

FIGS. 16.9A AND B: *Datura:* (A) Seed; (B) Flower.

Cardiotoxic Plant Poisons (Figs. 16.10A to C)

Cardiotoxic plant poisons inhibit Na^+/K^+-ATPase pump leading to overall increase in intracellular Na^+ ions and secondary increase in intracellular Ca^{2+} levels.
- *Symptoms:* On ingestion, they produce burning sensation, abdominal pain, nausea, vomiting, diarrhea, dizziness and numbness in oral and perioral region.
- Most important cardiotoxic effects are sinus bradycardia, varying degrees of heart block, ventricular ectopics, ventricular tachycardia which can be fatal.

Management of Cardiotoxicity
- Atropine 0.6 mg, orciprenaline 10 mg to maintain heart rate around 80/minute. Severe bradycardia may need pacemaker insertion.
- Sodium bicarbonate 50 mL IV 6th hourly, if ABG shows acidosis.

Gastrointestinal Toxic Plant Poisons

- *Ricinus communis* **(Fig. 16.11A)** contains ricin and *Abrus precatorius* **(Fig. 16.11B)** contains abrin.

Clinical Features

- Gastrointestinal upset, vomiting, diarrhea, abdominal pain, GI bleeding.
- Hematuria, acrocyanosis, shock, dehydration, and hemolysis.
- Abnormal liver function tests (LFTs) and renal function tests (RFTs).

Treatment: Supportive.

Opioid Poisoning

Q. Write a short essay/note on opiate overdosage, clinical features of opioid tolerance, and its management.

Opium is extracted from poppy seeds (*Papaver somniferum*) **(Fig. 16.12)**.
Opioid agonists: Morphine, heroin, hydromorphone, fentanyl, codeine.

Opioid Tolerance

- Tolerance is a **diminished responsiveness to the drug's action** that is seen with many compounds.
- Tolerance can be demonstrated by a decreased effect from a constant dose of drug or by an increase in the minimum drug dose required to produce a given level of effect.
- **Physiological tolerance** involves changes in the binding of a drug to receptors or changes in receptor transductional processes related to the drug of action. This type of tolerance **occurs** in opioids.

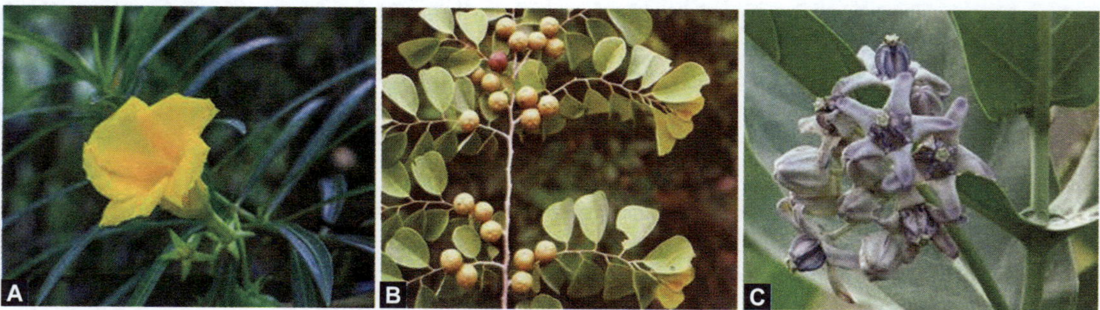

FIGS. 16.10A TO C: (A) Oleander plant; (B) *Cleistanthus collinus;* (C) *Calotropis.*

- Molecular basis of tolerance involves glutaminergic mechanisms (glutamate—excitatory amino acid neurotransmitter).
- **Physiological dependence** occurs **when the drug is necessary for normal physiological functioning**—this is demonstrated by the withdrawal reactions.
- **Withdrawal reactions** are usually the **opposite of the physiological effects** produced by the drug.

Opioid toxicity is related to opioid receptors in nonnociceptive pathways and counter-opioid responses. It is determined by genetics, organ function, and co-medications.

Acute action and withdrawal signs of opioids are listed in **Table 16.18**.

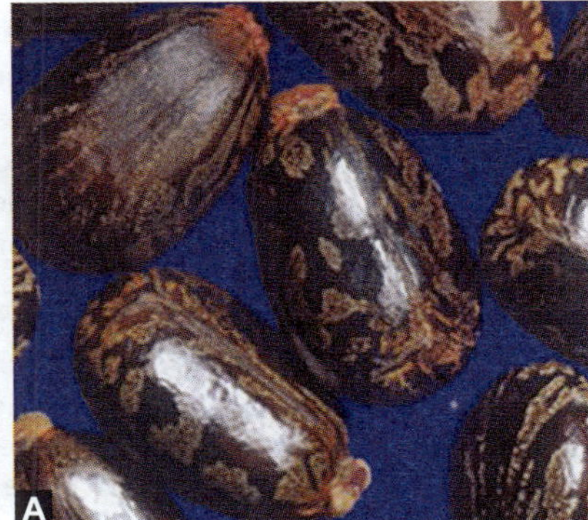
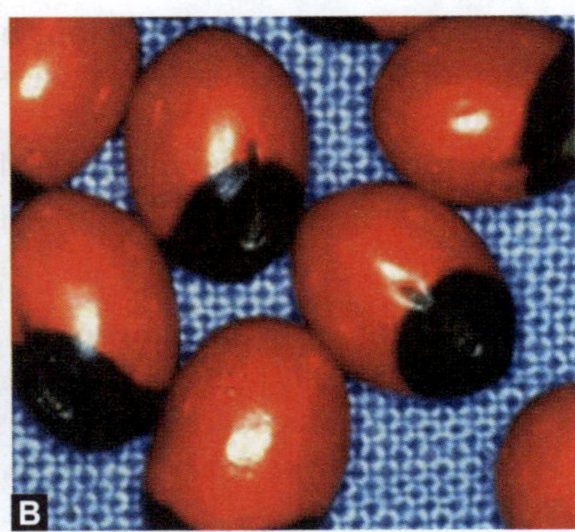

FIGS. 16.11A AND B: (A) *Ricinus communis* contains ricin; (B) *Abrus precatorius* contains abrin.

Treatment of opioid toxicity
- Ensure adequate ventilation
- Management of complications such as ARDS

Antidote—Naloxone, Naltrexone
- **MOA:** Pure opioid antagonist competes and displaces narcotics at opioid receptor sites.
- **Naloxone:** IV (preferred), IM, intratracheal, subcutaneous: 0.4–2 mg every 2–3 minutes as needed.

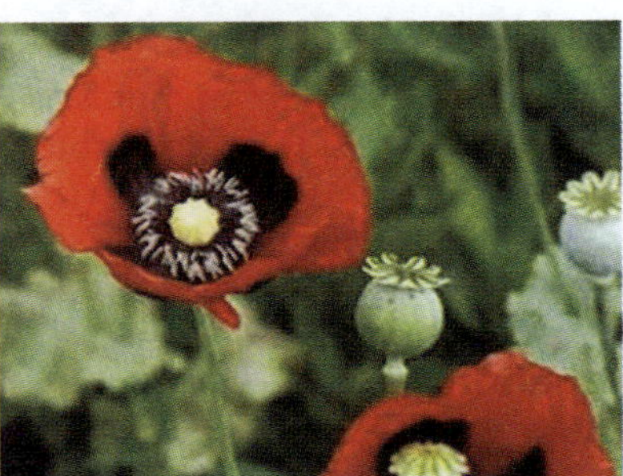

FIG. 16.12: Poppy seeds.

TABLE 16.18: Acute action and withdrawal signs of opioids.

Acute action	*Withdrawal signs*	*Acute action*	*Withdrawal signs*
➢ Analgesia ➢ Respiratory depression ➢ Euphoria ➢ Relaxation and sleep ➢ Tranquilization ➢ Decreased blood pressure	➢ Pain and irritability ➢ Hyperventilation ➢ Dysphoria and depression ➢ Restlessness and insomnia ➢ Fearfulness and hostility ➢ Increased blood pressure	➢ Constipation ➢ Pupillary constriction ➢ Hypothermia ➢ Drying of secretions ➢ Reduced sex drive ➢ Flushed and warm skin	➢ Diarrhea ➢ Pupillary dilation ➢ Hyperthermia ➢ Lacrimation, runny nose ➢ Spontaneous ejaculation ➢ Chilliness and "gooseflesh"

CARBON MONOXIDE

Q. Write a short note on carbon monoxide poisoning—signs and symptoms.

Carbon monoxide (CO) is a colorless, odorless gas generated by faulty appliances burning organic fuels. It is also present in vehicle exhaust fumes. It produces toxicity by binding with hemoglobin and cytochrome oxidase, which decreases the delivery of oxygen to tissue and inhibits cellular respiration.

Clinical Features

Acute severe CO poisoning produces nonspecific symptoms such as headache, nausea, irritability, weakness, and tachypnea. Skin changes, i.e., cherry red/pink discoloration of skin is also seen. Later, ataxia, nystagmus, drowsiness, and hyperreflexia may develop leading to coma, respiratory depression, cardiovascular collapse, and death. Myocardial ischemia/infarction, cerebral edema, and rhabdomyolysis (with myoglobinuria and renal failure) may occur. Long-term exposure can lead to Parkinsonism.

Treatment of Carbon Monoxide Poisoning

Administration of normobaric 100% oxygen is the therapy of choice for most cases, while hyperbaric oxygen therapy is reserved for severe poisonings.

ALCOHOL POISONING

Methanol Poisoning

Q Write a short note on toxicity, clinical features, and management of methanol poisoning.

- Methanol is a mild CNS depressant.
- *Metabolism:* Methanol itself is not toxic. However, its metabolites namely formaldehyde and formic acid are responsible for its toxicity.

Clinical Features

- Early clinical features are due to methanol, whereas late features are due to the methanol metabolite formic acid.
  - **Features due to methanol:** Methanol produces nausea, vomiting, abdominal pain, headache, vertigo, confusion, obtundation, convulsions, and coma.
  - **Features due to formic acid:** Metabolic acidosis and **retinal injury**. The retinal manifestations include clouding and diminished vision, dancing and flashing spots, dilated or fixed pupils, and hyperemia of the optic disc, retinal edema, and blindness.

- **Other manifestations:** Rapid breathing due to metabolic acidosis, myocardial depression, bradycardia, shock, and anuria.
- **Complication:** Putaminal necrosis producing rigidity, tremor, masked faces, and monotonous speech.

Diagnosis

- Confirmation by **measurement of serum methanol level,** which is usually > 20 mg/dL.
- Methanol-induced formic acidosis can be confirmed by a large anion gap, low serum bicarbonate, and elevated serum formate levels.
- Osmolal gap is elevated due to methanol.

Management

- **In early stages:**
  - **Gastrointestinal decontamination**
  - **Correction of systemic acidosis** with sodium bicarbonate.
- **Ethanol therapy:** Indicated in patients with visual symptoms or methanol level exceeding 20–30 mg/dL. Ethanol blocks conversion of methanol to formic acid by inhibiting alcohol dehydrogenase.
- **Hemodialysis:** Indicated (1) when methanol level exceeding 50 mg/dL, (2) those with visual signs, and (3) those with metabolic acidosis unresponsive to bicarbonate.
- **Antidote of methanol poisoning:** 4-methylpyrazole or **fomepizole (15 mg/kg IV, followed by 10 mg/kg every 12 hours)** is a direct, potent inhibitor of alcohol dehydrogenase. It may be more effective than ethanol, which is a competitive antagonist.
- **Co-factor therapy: Leucovorin 50 mg IV or folic acid 50 mg IV every 6 hours** is given in addition to ethanol or 4-methylpyrazole. It acts by enhancing the rate of degradation of formic acid to carbon dioxide.

Ethylene Glycol Poisoning

- Produces similar symptoms as methanol poisoning; however, renal failure is more common.
- Treatment is on same lines as methanol poisoning. Supplementation of thiamine and pyridoxine as cofactor therapy.

Ethanol Poisoning

- Alcohol belongs to inebriant group of neurotics class of poisons.
- Stages of alcohol intoxication:
  - Stage of excitement: Increased talkativeness, increased self-confidence, decreased sensory perception, loss of fine motor skills, slowed information processing, increased sexual desires
  - Stage of incoordination: Incordination of thought, speech, impaired judgment, confusion, slurred speech, staggering gait, dilated pupils.
  - Stage of narcosis: Deep sleep, rapid pulse, hypothermia, labored breathing, miosis → coma → death. Patients can manifest with other complications like hematemesis, pancreatitis, head injury.
- ***Management:***
  - Rule out more serious conditions such as head trauma, hypoxia, hypoglycemia, hypothermia, hepatic encephalopathy, and other metabolic derangements.
  - ABG will reveal high anion gap acidosis.
  - Gastric lavage is not helpful because of the rapid rate of absorption of ethanol from the gastrointestinal tract.
  - Dextrose saline with 100 mg thiamine has to be administered.
  - Benzodiazepines, first-generation (typical) antipsychotics and ketamine can be used to control the agitation.
  - Hemodialysis is useful for severely elevated ethanol levels and severe acidosis.
  - Post-recovery patients need psychotherapy and rehabilitation.

Aluminum Phosphide Poisoning

Q. Discuss the clinical features and management of aluminum phosphide poisoning.

Aluminum phosphide (ALP) poisoning is known worldwide, especially in developing countries such as India. Lethal dose of ALP is 1–1.5 g.

Aluminum phosphide, when ingested, liberates a lot of phosphine gas → phosphine leads to noncompetitive inhibition of the cytochrome oxidase of mitochondria, blocking the electron transfer chain and oxidative phosphorylation, producing an energy crisis in the cells.

The severe toxicity of ALP particularly affects the cardiac and vascular tissues, which manifests as profound and refractory hypotension, congestive heart failure, methemoglobinemia, myocarditis, pericarditis and subendocardial infarction, cardiac arrhythmias, lactic acidosis, and respiratory failure.

Management

It is supportive, the main objective is to provide effective oxygenation, ventilation, and circulation till phosphine is excreted. Gastric decontamination using activated charcoal, potassium permanganate, and medicated liquid paraffin have been tried. No definite antidote available.

Rodenticide Poisoning

Q. Discuss the clinical features and management of rodenticide poisoning.

Classification of Rodenticide Poisons

See **Table 16.19**.

TABLE 16.19: Classification of rodenticide poisons.

Highly toxic agents	*Moderately toxic agents*	*Less toxic agents*
LD_{50} 0–50 mg/kg body weight ➢ Strychnine ➢ Thallium ➢ Elemental phosphorus ➢ Metal phosphides ➢ Sodium monofluoroacetate ➢ Arsenic	LD_{50} 50–500 mg/kg ➢ Alpha-naphthylthiourea ➢ Cholecalciferol	LD_{50} >500 mg/kg ➢ Warfarin ➢ "Superwarfarins" or "long-acting" anticoagulant rodenticides (LAARs)—brodifacoum, bromadiolone, chlorophacinone, difenacoum, and diphacinone ➢ Bromethalin ➢ Red squill

Clinical Features

Yellow Phosphorous Poisoning

- In the first 24 hours post-ingestion, patients present with mild symptoms such as nausea and vomiting due to gastrointestinal irritation.
- In the next 24–72 hours, patients may remain asymptomatic. There may be a rise in bilirubin levels and liver enzymes at this stage.
- After 72 hours, they can manifest with acute liver failure (ALF), coagulopathy, hypotension, cardiac arrhythmias, and acute kidney injury. Central nervous system involvement occurs as confusion, psychosis, hallucinations, and coma.

Aluminium and zinc phosphide poisoning

- Early features include nausea, vomiting, and epigastric pain due to the corrosive nature of phosphides.
- There may be a garlic odor in the breath of these patients.
- Phosphine gas emitted from emesis and feces of affected.
- These features are rapidly followed by circulatory collapse, hypotension, myocarditis, pericarditis, acute pulmonary edema, and congestive heart failure.

Coumarins

- The evidence of coagulopathy occurs 24–48 hours post-consumption once all the coagulation factors are depleted below 30% of normal.
- Mild-to-severe life-threatening hemorrhage can occur, which include mucocutaneous, gastrointestinal, genitourinary, and intracranial bleeds.
- These include epistaxis, hematuria, gastrointestinal bleeding, spontaneous ecchymoses, and hematomas.
- Intracranial bleeds are associated with a high mortality.
- Paradoxical thrombosis has also been reported following LAAR toxicity. This has been attributed to depletion of protein C and S.

Management of Rodenticide Poisoning

- If there has been no bleeding, but the PT is prolonged, give vitamin K_1 10–50 mg orally two to four times a day
- For prolonged PT with less severe bleeding, give vitamin K_1 10–15 mg SC or IM
- In severe hemorrhage with prolonged prothrombin time (PT) give vitamin K_1 (phytomenadione) 20 mg by slow IV injection
- In severe bleeding, it may be necessary to give fresh frozen plasma, cryoprecipitate or fresh blood.
- N-acetylcysteine (NAC) has been used
- Extracorporeal membrane oxygenation (ECMO)
- Liver transplantation

Copper Sulfate Poisoning

Q. Discuss the clinical feature and management of copper sulfate poisoning.

- Used as insecticide (blue color copper sulfate crystals)
- The clinical features of copper sulfate poisoning include erosive gastropathy (hematemesis and melena), intravascular hemolysis, methemoglobinemia, hepatitis, acute kidney injury and rhabdomyolysis
- The management of copper sulfate:
  - Reducing absorption—dilution and neutralizing with milk
  - Chelation therapy—penicillamine/BAL.
  - Methemoglobinemia is treated with methylene blue
  - Supportive therapy—transfusion, hemodialysis, hyperbaric oxygen.

CHAPTER

17 Oncology

CELL CYCLE

Q. Describe briefly about cell cycle and its regulation?

Cell replication proceeds through a number of phases that are biochemically initiated by external stimuli and modulated by both external and internal growth controls.

Phases of Cell Cycle (Table 17.1A and Fig. 17.1)

TABLE 17.1A: Phases of cell cycle.

G0 phase		**Gap 0 or resting phase or quiescent state**	Cells are generally programmed to perform specialized functions. Cells in this state remain quiescent for variable periods, but can be recruited in cell cycle if stimulator later
Interphase	*G1 phase*	**Gap 1 or presynthetic phase**	RNA synthesis occurs, and many of the enzymes necessary for DNA synthesis are manufactured
	S phase	**DNA synthetic phase**	The cellular content of DNA doubles
	G2 phase	**Gap 2 or postsynthetic phase or premitotic phase**	Protein and RNA syntheses continue, and the microtubular precursors of the mitotic spindle are produced
M phase		**Mitosis**	Genetic material is segregated into daughter cells with the help of microtubules ➢ **Prophase:** The chromatin is condensing into chromosomes ➢ **Metaphase:** Chromosomes align at the metaphase plate ➢ **Anaphase:** Microtubules shorten resulting in chromosomal splitting ➢ **Telophase:** Decondensation of chromosomes with nuclear membrane formation

Regulators of Cell Cycle (Table 17.1B and Fig. 17.1)

TABLE 17.1B: Regulators of cell cycle.

Cyclins	➢ Synthesized during specific phases of cell cycle ➢ Appear sequentially in cell cycle in order D → E → A → B ➢ Their function is to activate CDKs
Cyclin-dependent kinases (CDK)	➢ CDKs are expressed constitutively during the cell cycle but in an inactive form ➢ They are activated by specific cyclins ➢ Their function depends on type of cyclin—CDK complex – **Cyclin D—CDK4, Cyclin D—CDK6, and Cyclin E—CDK2 complex** → phosphorylates RB, which is on-off switch of cell cycle. Phosphorylated RB activates E2F transcription factor, which is essential for transcription of genes needed for progression through S phase – **Cyclin A—CDK2 and Cyclin A—CDK1** → active in S phase – **Cyclin B—CDK1 complex** → essential for G2-M transition, it is the main mediator that propels the cell beyond prophase
CDK inhibitors	➢ They regulate the activity of Cyclin—Cdk complexes ➢ There are two classes of CDK inhibitors – **Cip/Kip family:** They inactivate complexes formed between Cyclin and CDKs (e.g., p21, p27, p57, etc.) – **INK4/ARF family:** They block the cell cycle and act as tumor suppressors (e.g., p15, p16, p18, p19). p16/INK4a binds to cyclin D—CDK4 and promotes the inhibitory effects of RB; p14/ARF increases p53 levels by inhibiting MDM2 activity

Cell Cycle Checkpoints (Table 17.1C and Fig. 17.1)

TABLE 17.1C: Cell cycle checkpoints.

G1-S checkpoint	➢ It checks for DNA damage ➢ If DNA damage is present and repairable, DNA repair mechanisms are activated ➢ If DNA damage is present but not repairable, apoptotic pathways are activated ➢ It is controlled by p53 (by inducing p21)
G2-M checkpoint	➢ It monitors the completion of DNA replication and checks whether the cell can safely initiate mitosis ➢ It is controlled by both p53 dependent (via cyclin A—CDK 2) and independent (via cdc 25) mechanisms ➢ Defect of G2-M checkpoint results in chromosomal abnormalities ➢ Cells damaged by ionizing radiation activate this checkpoint and arrest cells in G2 phase

Q. Write short essay/note on:

- **Proto-oncogene, oncogene, and tumor suppressor gene.**

Regulation of Cancer Cell Growth

Normal cell may undergo malignant transformation by corrupting any one of the normal steps involved in cell proliferation. Abnormal regulation of cell growth in cancer can occur as the result of several mechanisms. All cancers show eight fundamental changes in cell physiology. These are considered the hallmarks of cancer and include:

1. **Self-sufficiency in growth signals (activation of cell growth):**
   Cancers use multiple mechanisms to sustain their proliferation:
   - Tumors may produce growth factors for which they have receptors in an autocrine fashion.
   - Tumors may stimulate surrounding normal tissues and these normal tissues provide growth factors for the tumor.
   - Tumor may become hypersensitive to growth factors through upregulation of growth receptors or alterations of the structure of these receptors.
   - Finally, they may become independent of growth factors by the presence of somatic mutations activating downstream pathways, for example, BRAF mutations activating the mitogen-activated protein kinase (MAPK) pathway, or mutations in phosphoinositide-3-kinase (PI3K) leading to activation of the PI3K/Akt/mTOR pathway, or by altering the negative feedback loops.

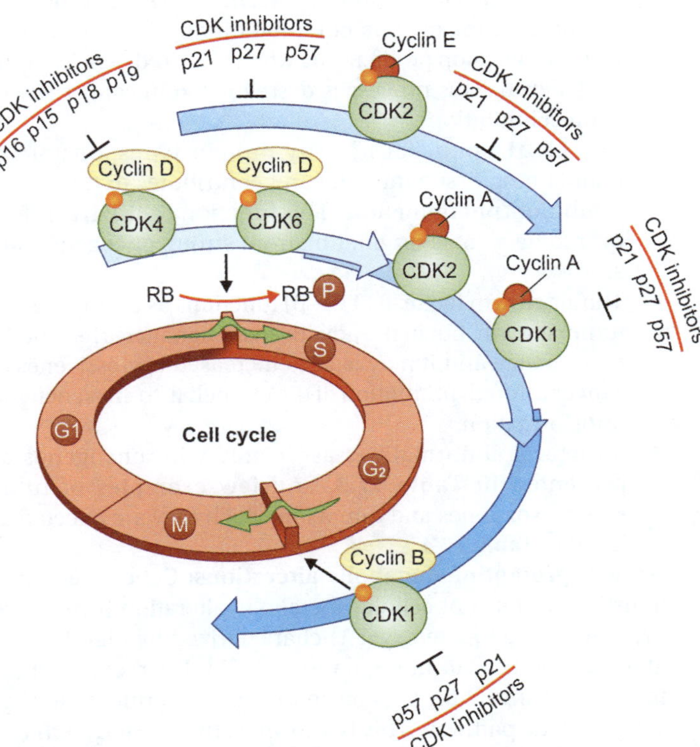

FIG. 17.1: Pictorial representation of cell cycle, cyclin-CDK complexes, CDK inhibitors, and cell cycle checkpoint.

Proto-oncogenes, Oncogenes

Proto-oncogenes are normal cellular genes, which encode a number of nuclear proteins that **regulate normal cell proliferation, differentiation, and survival**. Genes that promote **autonomous cell growth** in cancer cells are called ***oncogenes*** and are altered/mutated versions of proto-oncogenes.

Oncogenes and oncoproteins: Oncogenes can promote cell growth in the absence of normal growth-promoting/ mitogenic signals. Oncoproteins are products of oncogenes and resemble the normal products of proto-oncogenes. Oncoproteins production is not under normal regulatory control. Cells proliferate without the usual requirement for external signals and are freed from checkpoints and **growth becomes autonomous**. Oncogenes are classified depending on the function of gene product (oncoprotein) **(Table 17.2)**.

Tumor Suppressor Genes

2. **Insensitivity to growth-inhibitory signals (inhibition of tumor suppressor genes):**
   Second mechanism of carcinogenesis results from failure of growth inhibition, due to **deficiency of normal tumor suppressor genes** and **their products**. **Tumor suppressor genes (Table 17.4)** apply brakes to cell proliferation and prevent uncontrolled/abnormal cell proliferation and induce repair or self-death (apoptosis). Important tumor suppressor genes are *RB*, *p53*, *BRCA1*, and *BRCA2* genes.

- The **RB** protein is responsible for the control of the cell cycle and the switch from resting state to cell division, mainly in response to the stimuli outside of the cell. The cells that lack the RB protein do not have this control mechanism.
- The **p53** protein is also a cell cycle control protein, but it responds mainly to the intracellular stressors, and it can stop cell cycle until the abnormal processes have been corrected. the p53 protein arrests cells in the quiescent G1 and G2 phases of the cell cycle, preventing cells from entering the DNA synthetic (S) phase of the cell cycle. It can detect DNA abnormalities, such as nucleotide mismatches and DNA strand breaks, including those caused by radiation and chemotherapy. The function of p53 is thought to be critical in preserving the integrity of the cellular genome.
- The ***NF2*** gene and its product **Merlin**. Merlin is responsible for maintaining of contact inhibition through E-cadherins. Normal cells stop proliferating when a desired density of cells is achieved. This process is dysregulated in cancer (loss of contact inhibition).
- The **LKB1** epithelial polarity protein is responsible for maintaining tissue integrity and contributes to the contact inhibition phenomenon. The functional LKB1 can even overcome signals originating from strong oncogenes such as *Myc*.
- Tumor growth factor-β (**TGF-β**) functions as a suppressor of tumor growth, but in the advanced malignancies its function may change and it may lead to increased aggressiveness of cancer through promotion of the epithelial-to-mesenchymal transformation.
- Structural abnormalities associated with oncogenes are presented in **Table 17.3**. and few examples of tumor suppressor genes and tumors in which they are affected are listed in **Table 17.4**.

3. **Growth-promoting metabolic alterations:** Cancer cells show a distinctive form of cellular metabolic alteration (even in the presence of adequate oxygen) characterized by high levels of glucose uptake (via upregulation of GLUT 1 receptors) and increased conversion of glucose to lactose (fermentation) via the glycolytic pathway. This is known as the **Warburg effect** or aerobic glycolysis. Glycolytic intermediate processes are used by cancer cells for generation of nucleosides and amino acids that are essential for tumor proliferation and growth.
4. **Evasion of cell death (Apoptosis, Autophagy, and Necrosis):** ***Apoptosis*** is a programmed cell death and is one of the normal protective mechanism by which a cell with DNA damage (mutation) undergoes cell death. Mutations in the genes that regulate apoptosis may lead to neoplasm. **Examples (Table 17.5)**:

Autophagy is a natural process that allows cells to break down intracellular organelles upon exposure to stressors with help of lysosomes and recycle nutrients. It is also a protective process in case of neoplastic transformation. Cancer cells may use autophagy to recycle their nutrients and escape damaging agents. This process is regulated by PI3-kinase, AKT, and mTOR pathway and by protein Beclin-1.

Necrosis is another process of cell death in which cells increase in size and break, releasing multiple proinflammatory cytokines. Immune cells are attracted to the areas of necrosis to eliminate the remnants of cells. Cancer can use this process to induce an inflammatory proneoplastic environment, stimulate angiogenesis, and even use these cytokines to stimulate its own growth.

TABLE 17.2: Classification of oncogenes.

Classification of oncogenes	*Example/s of associated tumor/s*
Growth Factors	
PDGF **(platelet-derived growth factor)**	Nonsmall cell cancer of lung
TGF-α (tumor growth factor- alpha)	Hepatocellular cancer
Growth Factor Receptors	
EGFR **(epidermal growth factor receptor)**	Lung and gastrointestinal tumors
Her 2/neu receptor	Breast cancer
KRAS	Adenocarcinoma of colon, lung, and pancreas
NRAS	Hematopoietic tumors, melanomas
ABL	Chronic myeloid leukemia, acute lymphoblastic leukemia
Nuclear-Regulatory Proteins/Transcription Factors	
C-MYC	Burkitt's lymphoma
N-MYC	Neuroblastoma
Cell Cycle Regulators	
Cyclin D	Breast, esophageal, and liver cancers

TABLE 17.3: Structural abnormalities associated with oncogenes.

Oncogene	*Aberration*	*Neoplasm*
abl	t(9;22)	CML, AML, ALL
myc	t(8;14)	Burkitt's lymphoma, B-ALL, T-ALL
bcl-1, bcl-2	t(11;14)	B-cell lymphoma
tcl-1, tcl-2	t(11,14)	T-cell lymphoma
p53, erb-A, erb-B	t(15;17)	APML
mos, ets-2	t(8;21)	AML-M2
ets-l, sis	t(11;22)	Ewing's sarcoma
myc	t(3;8)	Renal cell carcinoma
myb	t(6;14)	Ovarian carcinoma

(CML: chronic myeloid leukemia; AML: acute myeloid leukemia; ALL: acute lymphoid leukemia; APML: acute promyelocytic leukemia)

TABLE 17.4: Few examples of tumor suppressor genes and tumors in which it is affected.

		Tumors in which gene is affected	
Gene (locus)	*Function*	*Familial*	*Sporadic*
DCC (18q)	Cell surface interaction	Not known	Colorectal cancer
Rb1 (13q)	Transcription	Retinoblastoma	Small cell carcinoma of lung
p53 (17p)	Transcription	Li-Fraumeni syndrome	Cancer of breast, colon, and lung
BRCA1(17q)	Transcription	Carcinoma breast	Carcinoma breast/ ovary
BRCA2 (13q)	Regulator/ DNA repair		
WT1 (11p)	Transcription	Wilms' tumor	Lung cancer

TABLE 17.5: Genes regulating apoptosis.

Proapoptotic genes	*Antiapoptotic genes*
Examples: Bax, bak, bok, bik, bad, bod, bid, Bcl-xS, PUMA, Noxa	***Examples:*** Bcl-2 family (Bcl-2, Bcl-xL, Bcl-w, Mcl-1, A1)
Inhibition of proapoptotic genes predisposes to cancer	Upregulation of antiapoptotic genes predisposes to cancer

5. **Limitless replicative potential:** All malignant tumors contain cells that are immortal and have limitless replicative potential.
   - **Cancer stem cells:** At least few cells in all cancers have stem cell-like properties and are called cancer stem cells.
   - **Reactivation of telomerase:** During the course of repeated cell cycles, there is progressive shortening of telomeres, making the cells vulnerable to senescence/apoptosis. The cells that are able to maintain the activity of telomerase, an enzyme that is responsible for lengthening of telomeres, can potentially proliferate uncontrollably and turn into cancer.
6. **Development of sustained angiogenesis:** Microscopic lesions rely on osmosis for delivery of nutrients, but it has been shown that early in carcinogenesis, the "angiogenic switch" occurs that promotes new blood vessel formation. Vascular endothelial growth factor A (VEGF-A) is the main protein responsible for neoangiogenesis. Its action is counterbalanced by the activity of thrombospondin-1 (TSP-1).
7. **Ability to invade and metastasize** (invasion and metastasis): Cancer cells are characterized by a unique ability of local invasion and formation of distant metastasis. E-cadherin is one of most important cell surface adhesion molecules responsible for maintaining tissue integrity. Multiple cancers express E-cadherin at a low level and express molecules implicated in cell migration such as N-cadherin at higher levels. Formation of distant metastasis is a multistep process and it consists of the following:
   - Local invasion
   - Migration into lymphatic and blood vessels
   - Spread of cancer cells through vasculature
   - Extravasation of cancer cells into tissue of remote organs
   - Growth of cancer cells in the new environment to form macroscopic tumors

   Molecular events occurring during the process of formation metastasis resemble steps of embryonic morphogenesis. The process by itself has been named **epithelial–mesenchymal transition (EMT)** and involves genes playing a physiologic role in embryogenesis such as Snail, Slug, Twist, and Zeb1/2. These genes are regulated by the intracellular oncogenic events, but they can be also influenced by microenvironmental stimuli.
8. **Ability to evade the host immune response:** The immune cells eliminate pathogens and potentially cancerous cells. Cancer cells evade this surveillance by disabling components of the immune system.

FLOWCHART 17.1: Flowchart depicting simplified scheme of molecular basis of cancer.

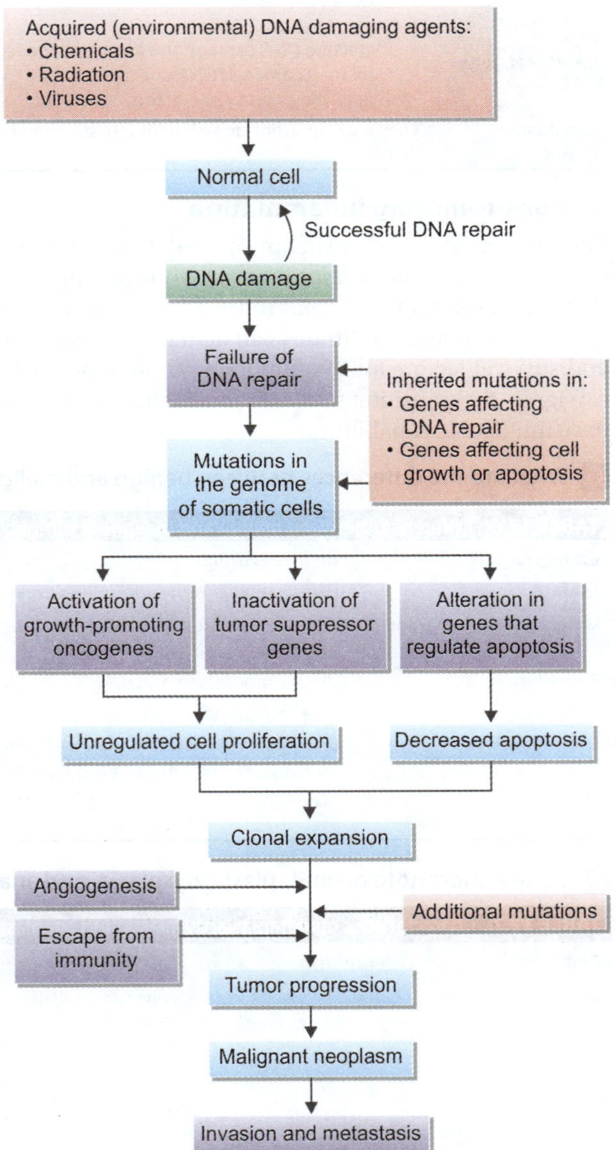

GENETIC BASIS OF TRANSFORMATION OF A NORMAL CELL INTO A MALIGNANT CELL

Q. Describe the genetic basis of selected cancers?

Molecular Basis of Cancer

1. Nonlethal genetic damage lies at the heart of carcinogenesis. Such genetic damage (or mutation) may be acquired by the action of environmental agents, such as chemicals, radiation, or viruses, or it may be inherited in the germ line **(Flowchart 17.1)**.
2. A tumor is formed by the clonal expansion of a single precursor cell that has incurred genetic damage.
3. Four classes of normal regulatory genes—the growth-promoting proto-oncogenes, the growth-inhibiting tumor suppressor genes, genes that regulate programmed cell death (apoptosis), and genes involved in DNA repair—are the principal targets of genetic damage.
4. Carcinogenesis is a multistep process at both the phenotypic and the genetic levels, resulting from the accumulation of multiple mutations.

Kinetics of tumor growth: Tumor growth depends on the size of the proliferating pool of cells and the number of cells dying spontaneously. The larger the tumor mass, the greater the percentage of nondividing and dying cells and the longer it takes for the average cell to divide.

a. The lag phase	➤ During the earliest phase of tumor development, a small mass of a tumor does not enlarge very much. ➤ During this phase, the dividing cells are accumulating various mutations. These mutations help the surviving cells improve their adaptivity to the supply of nutrients, increase the rate at which the mutated cells divide, decrease the rate of apoptosis sensitivity, provide them with invasive properties, make the mutated cells more responsiveness to host factors, and produce angiogenesis factors.
b. The log phase	➤ The tumor now shows rapid exponential growth of the tumor mass. ➤ There is a relatively high proportion of cells undergoing division, with rapidly declining rates of cell death, and the *growth fraction* (ratio of dividing to total cells) is high. ➤ This rapid growth also reflects the adaptivity of the cells and the production by the tumor cells of angiogenesis factors that induce the surrounding tissues to form new blood vessels that "feed" the tumor mass.
c. The plateau phase	➤ Tumor growth slows down as the percentage of dividing cells decreases, and a larger percentage of cells are dying. ➤ The hypotheses are that growth rates eventually plateau because of restrictions of space and nutrient availability, of limitation of blood supply, and of genetic mutations, which cause a higher death rate of cells.

Genomic Stability

The mechanisms responsible for genome stability (repair mechanisms) assure that any randomly created mutations are repaired or an abnormal cell is eliminated. In the presence of external mutagens or heritable susceptibility factors such as mutations in tumor suppressor genes, the repair mechanisms malfunction and allow abnormal cells to survive. The genes involved are caretaker genes and gatekeeper genes as described below.

Caretaker genes	They are responsible for: ➤ Detecting DNA damage and activating the repair mechanisms ➤ Repairing damaged DNA directly ➤ Inactivating mutagenic factors	Inactivation of caretaker genes leads to an increased mutation rate and increased genome instability.
Gatekeeper genes	They are responsible for inhibiting tumor growth or promoting death	A mutation in such a gene may promote the development of cancer by decreasing the DNA repair window from G1 to S phase.

Tumor-promoting Inflammation

Tumors consist not only of neoplastic cells but also of a variety of cells of the innate and adaptive immune systems. The density of immune cells and their localization within the tumor are different among different malignancies. Initially it was postulated that the presence of these cells reflected an attempt of eradication of a tumor by the immune system. Currently we know that these inflammatory infiltrates can actually promote tumorigenesis and cancer growth by providing cytokines and growth and survival factors for the tumor, by stimulating angiogenesis, and by facilitating invasion and metastasis. Inflammation can ignite the transition from a premalignant state to full malignancy, for example, by release of reactive oxygen species that have mutagenic capabilities.

Q. What are the differences between benign and malignant tumors? (Table 17.6)

TABLE 17.6: Differences between benign and malignant tumors.

Characteristic	*Benign tumors*	*Malignant tumors*
Surface	Usually regular with surrounding capsule	Usually irregular without a surrounding capsule
Differentiation/anaplasia	Well differentiated; may resemble tissue of origin	Varies from well differentiated to poorly differentiated; structure often atypical
Rate of growth	Usually progressive and slow	Erratic and may be slow to rapid
Mitotic figures	Rare and normal	Common and abnormal
Local invasion	Usually well-demarcated masses that do not invade or infiltrate surrounding normal tissues	Locally invasive, infiltrating surrounding tissue
Metastasis	Absent	Frequently present (almost all cancers metastasize except gliomas and basal cell carcinoma)

Q. Write a short note on metaplasia, dysplasia, and anaplasia? (Table 17.7)

TABLE 17.7: Characteristics of metaplasia, dysplasia, and anaplasia.

Characteristic	*Metaplasia*	*Dysplasia*	*Anaplasia*
Definition	Reversible change in which one differentiated cell type is replaced by another cell type	A loss in uniformity of the individual cells and loss of architectural orientation	An absence of differentiation
Pleomorphism	Absent	Present in low grade	Present in high grade
Reversibility	Reversible	Reversible in early stages	Irreversible
N:C ratio	Normal	Mildly increased	Grossly increased
Hyperchromatism	Absent	Present in small degree	Present in high degree
Mitotic figures	Absent	Typical mitotic figures present at abnormal places	Atypical mitotic figures at abnormal places
Examples	Barrett's esophagus	Cervical dysplasia	Carcinoma cervix

Common Cancers

Q. Describe the clinical epidemiology and inherited and modifiable risk factors for common malignancies in India. (Tables 17.8 and 17.9)

TABLE 17.8: Prevalence of cancer—World and India.

Prevalence of cancer	*World*	*India*
Most common cancer (men)	Carcinoma lung	Lip and oral cavity cancer
Most common cancer (women)	Breast cancer	Breast cancer
Most common cancer (overall—men and women)	Carcinoma lung	Breast cancer
Most common cause of cancer deaths (overall—men and women)	Carcinoma lung	Breast cancer

Source: GLOBOCAN 2020 (for updated statistics please refer GLOBOCAN fact sheet).

Risk Factors of Cancer

TABLE 17.9: Risk factors for cancer.

Intrinsic risk factors	*Nonintrinsic risk factors*	
Nonmodifiable risk factor	**Endogenous risk factors (Partially modifiable risk factors)**	**Exogenous risk factors (Modifiable risk factors)**
Refers to unavoidable spontaneous mutations that arise as a result of random errors in DNA replication	Aging Genetic susceptibility Hormones Growth factors Chronic inflammation, etc.	Exposure to radiation Exposure to carcinogens Infections Smoking Obesity Dietary imbalance Physical inactivity, etc.

Etiology of Cancer

Q. Write a note on etiological factors of cancer—genetic, chemical, infectious agents.

Genetic Predisposition (Table 17.10)

TABLE 17.10: Genetic predisposition to cancer.

Gene involved	*Syndrome associated*
Autosomal dominant cancer syndromes (mnemonic: **V**ery **R**ich, **C**ute, **N**ice **M**en **H**ereditarily **L**ike/**P**refer **F**amiliar **W**omen)*	
VHL	**V**on Hipple-Lindau syndrome (renal cell carcinomas)
RB gene	**R**etinoblastoma
PTEN	**C**owden syndrome
NF1, NF2 **PTCH**	**N**eurofibromatosis 1 and 2 Nevoid basal cell carcinoma syndrome
MEN1, RET **p16/INK4A**	**MEN** 1 and 2 Melanoma
MSH2, MLH1, MSH6	**H**ereditary nonpolyposis colon cancer
p53	**L**i-Fraumeni syndrome
LKB1	**P**eutz-Jeghers syndrome
APC	**F**amilial adenomatous polyposis
BRCA1, BRCA2	**Breast and ovarian tumors**
Autosomal recessive cancer syndromes (mnemonic: **Big FAX**)	
Bloom syndrome **F**anconi anemia **A**taxia telangiectasia **X**eroderma pigmentosum	
Familial cancers (these cancers run through the families without a clear genetic pattern of transmission)	
Breast cancer Ovarian cancer Pancreatic cancer	

*Mnemonic: adapted from Review of Pathology by Gobind Rai Garg and Sparsh Gupta (Jaypee Brothers Medical Publishers).

Chemical Carcinogenesis (Flowchart 17.2 and Table 17.11)

- It is a two-step process.
  1. **Initiation:** Initiation results from exposure of cells to a sufficient dose of a carcinogenic agent (initiator). Initiation alone, however, is not sufficient for tumor formation. Initiation causes permanent DNA damage (mutations). It is

FLOWCHART 17.2: Schematic presentation of chemical carcinogenesis.

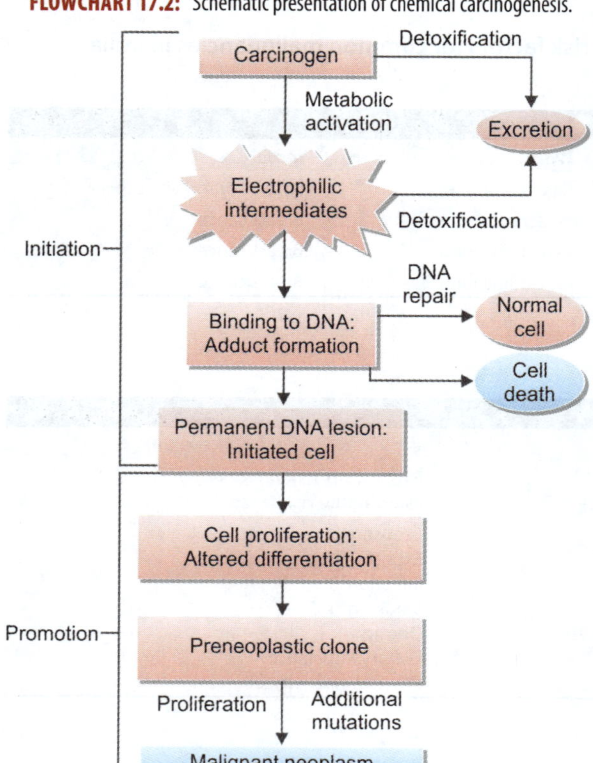

TABLE 17.11: List of carcinogenic agents and cancer associated.

Agent	*Cancer associated*
Arsenic and arsenic compounds	Lung, skin, hemangiosarcoma
Asbestos	Lung, mesothelioma; gastrointestinal tract (esophagus, stomach, large intestine)
Aromatic amines	Bladder cancer
Alkylating agents	AML, bladder cancer
Benzene	Acute myelocytic leukemia, Hodgkin's lymphoma
Beryllium compounds	Lung cancer
Chromium	Lung cancer
Cadmium	Prostate cancer
Estrogens	Breast, endometrium, liver cancers
Ethyl alcohol	Liver cancer, esophagus, and head and neck cancers
Immunosuppressive agents	Non-Hodgkin's lymphoma (NHL)
Nickel compounds	Lung cancer
Phenacetin	Renal pelvis and bladder cancer
Tobacco	Upper aerodigestive tract, bladder cancers

therefore rapid and irreversible and has "memory". It can be two types of agents (directly acting and indirectly acting agents).

Direct-acting agents	*Indirect-acting agents*
Direct-acting agents require no metabolic conversion to become carcinogenic. Most of them are weak carcinogens.	The designation *indirect-acting agent* refers to chemicals that require metabolic conversion to an *ultimate carcinogen* before they become active. *For example:* Benzopyrene and other carcinogens are formed in the high-temperature combustion of tobacco in cigarette smoking

2. **Promotion:** *Promoters can induce tumors in initiated cells, but they are nontumorigenic by themselves. The cellular changes resulting from the application of promoters do not affect DNA directly and are reversible.* Promoters enhance the proliferation of initiated cells, an effect that may contribute to the development of additional mutations in these cells.

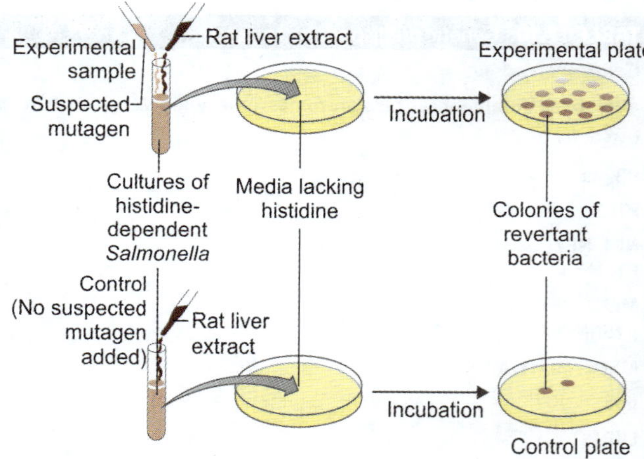

FIG. 17.2: Ames test—test for mutagenicity.

Q. Write a short note on Ames test? Test for mutagenicity (Ames test) (Fig. 17.2):

It is a biological assay to assess the mutagenic potential of chemical compounds. A positive test indicates that the chemical is mutagenic and therefore may act as a carcinogen. The Ames test uses several strains of the bacterium *Salmonella typhimurium* that carry mutations in genes involved in histidine synthesis. These strains are auxotrophic mutants, i.e., they require histidine for growth, but cannot produce it. The method tests the capability of the tested substance in creating mutations that result in a return to a "prototrophic" state, so that the cells can grow on a histidine-free medium.

Infection and Cancer (Table 17.12)

Q. Describe the relationship between infection and cancers.

Q. Describe the role of oncogenic viruses in the evolution of virus-associated malignancy.

TABLE 17.12: Infections associated with malignancy.

Organism	*Malignancy associated*	*Additional points*
Bacterial infections		
Helicobacter pylori	Gastric adenocarcinoma Gastric lymphomas [B-cell origin—MALT lymphomas t(11;18)]	
Viral infections		
ONCOGENIC RNA VIRUSES		
Human T-cell lymphotropic virus type 1	Adult T-cell leukemia/lymphoma	The product of TAX gene in HTLV-1 is responsible for transcription of host genes involved in proliferation and genomic instability by inhibiting DNA repair function
Oncogenic DNA Viruses		
1. **Human Papillomavirus**		
– HPV types 1, 2, 4, and 7	Benign squamous papilloma (wart)	Low-oncogenic risk HPV—benign lesions of squamous epithelium
– HPV-6 and HPV-11	Condylomata acuminata (genital warts) of the vulva, penis, and perianal region	
– HPV types 16 and 18	Squamous cell carcinoma of the cervix and anogenital region Oropharyngeal cancers	High-oncogenic risk HPV—malignant tumors (E6 and E7 genes are responsible for inactivation of tumor suppression genes p53 and Rb genes, respectively)
2. **Epstein-Barr Virus**	Burkitt's lymphoma Hodgkin's lymphoma Nasopharyngeal cancer	t(8;14) is responsible for Burkitt's lymphoma. Genes implicated are LMP-1 gene, EBNA-2, and vIL-10
3. **Hepatitis B and C Viruses**	Hepatocellular carcinoma	HBx gene (Hepatitis B) is responsible for the activation of growth promoting genes and inactivation of p53 gene
4. **Human Herpes Virus-8**	Kaposi's sarcoma Pleural effusion lymphoma, multicentric Castleman's disease	
5. **Merkel Cell Polyoma virus**	Merkel cell carcinoma	
Parasitic infections		
1. **Blood flukes *(Schistosoma haematobium)***	Bladder cancer	
2. **Liver flukes (*Clonorchis sinensis* and *Opisthorchis viverrini*)**	Cholangiocarcinoma	
3. ***Plasmodium falciparum***	Burkitt's lymphoma	Coexisting with EBV
Fungal infections/toxins		
1. ***Aspergillus sps.***	Esophageal cancer, hepatocellular cancer	Aflatoxins are responsible for oncogenesis

CANCER SCREENING AND PREVENTION

Q. Write a note on cancer screening (Table 17.13) and prevention (Table 17.14).

Q. Describe the need, tests involved, and their utility in the prevention of common malignancies.

Investigations

TABLE 17.13: Screening tests for cancers.

Breast cancer	Breast self-examination Clinical examination Mammography MRI (especially in young and with germline mutations in the family) Tomosynthesis
Cervical cancer	Pap smear HPV testing
Colorectal cancer	Sigmoidoscopy Fecal occult blood testing Colonoscopy Fecal DNA testing Fecal immunochemical testing CT colonography
Lung cancer	LDCT (low-dose computed tomography)
Ovarian cancer	CA-125 Transvaginal ultrasound
Prostate cancer	PSA (prostate-specific antigen) DRE (digital rectal examination)

TABLE 17.14: Cancer prevention.

Cancer vaccines (preventive)	**Hepatitis B vaccine**	Recombinant vaccine used for prevention of hepatitis B-induced HCC (total of three doses administered over 6 months—at 0, 1, and 6 months)
	HPV vaccine	Protect against acquisition of HPV infection and development of subsequent HPV-associated disease (oropharyngeal cancer, cervical cancer, vaginal cancer, vulvar cancer, and anal cancers). ***Quadrivalent HPV vaccine (Gardasil) targets*** HPV types 6, 11, 16, and 18 ***9-valent vaccine (Gardasil 9)*** targets the same HPV types as the quadrivalent vaccine (6, 11, 16, and 18) as well as types 31, 33, 45, 52, and 58 ***Bivalent vaccine (Cervarix)*** targets HPV types 16 and 18 Ideal age of immunization is before first sexual exposure **before 15 years of age:** Two doses of HPV vaccine should be given at 0 and at 6–12 months **15 years of age or older:** Three doses of HPV vaccine should be given at 0, 2, and 6 months **Immunocompromised patients:** Three doses of HPV vaccine should be given at 0, 1–2, and 6 months regardless of age Start taking early ages 9–10 2 doses / On time Ages 11–12 2 doses ✓ / Late Ages 13–14 2 doses / Late Ages 15–16 3 doses Early / On time / Late / Late
Chemo-preventive drugs	**Breast cancer**	Tamoxifen, raloxifene, and estramustine
	Colorectal cancer	Nonsteroidal anti-inflammatory drugs (NSAIDs), such as piroxicam, sulindac, and aspirin, may prevent adenoma formation or cause regression of adenomatous polyps
	Prostate cancer	Finasteride and dutasteride are 5 α-reductase inhibitors. They inhibit conversion of testosterone to dihydrotestosterone (DHT), a potent stimulator of prostate cell proliferation
Surgical prevention of cancer	**Cervical cancer**	Women with severe cervical dysplasia are treated with laser or loop electrosurgical excision or conization and occasionally even hysterectomy
	Colorectal cancer	Colectomy is used to prevent colon cancer in patients with familial polyposis or ulcerative colitis
	Breast and ovary cancer	Prophylactic bilateral mastectomy and prophylactic salpingo-oophorectomy in high-risk individuals especially BRCA1 and BRCA2 mutations

DIAGNOSIS AND STAGING OF CANCER

Q. Enumerate the list of investigations useful in diagnosis, staging, and monitoring response to treatment in a cancer patient (Table 17.15).

Q. Order and interpret diagnostic testing based on the clinical diagnosis including CBC and stool occult blood, and prostate-specific antigen.

TABLE 17.15: Investigations and evaluation in cancer patient.

Complete blood picture and peripheral smear	➢ Low hemoglobin is commonly encountered with chronic diseases like cancer ➢ High leukocyte and abnormal differential count should rise suspicion of leukemias ➢ Abnormal cells or blast in peripheral smear should be characterized and evaluated with bone marrow aspiration and biopsy ➢ Cytopenias are usually seen in patients who are on cytotoxic chemotherapies
Renal failure Hypercalcemia Anemia	➢ Usually seen in multiple myeloma
Liver function test (LFT)	➢ Conjugated bilirubin is elevated in biliary tract obstruction secondary to cancer around hepatobiliary system and periampullary carcinoma of pancreas ➢ Gamma-glutamyltransferase (GGT) elevated in hepatocellular carcinoma (HCC)
Stool occult blood	➢ Positive stool occult blood suggests GI bleeding and needs to be evaluated for source of bleeding
Urine routine	➢ Hematuria and abnormal cells in the urine may suggest pathology of genitourinary tract
Renal failure Hypocalcemia Hyperkalemia Hyperphos-phatemia	➢ Seen in tumor lysis syndrome

Contd...

Contd...

Apart from regular investigations, the following investigations are cardinal in the diagnosis and management of cancer patients	
Tumor markers (Table 17.16)	➢ Tumor markers are biochemical substance/product of malignant tumors that can be detected in the cells themselves or in serum/blood and/or body fluids ➢ Tumor markers can be a normal endogenous products produced in excess by cancer cells or products of newly switched on genes that remained quiescent in the normal cells ➢ Concentration increases with tumor progression, highest levels when tumors metastasize ➢ Include diverse molecules, such as serum proteins, oncofetal antigens, hormones, metabolites, receptors, and enzymes ➢ Tumor markers may be useful in management in certain cancers. In a particular patient, rising and falling levels of the tumor marker are usually associated with increasing or decreasing tumor burden, respectively ➢ Tumor markers help in: – Screening populations at risk – Diagnosis – Prognosis – Detection of recurrence – Monitoring response to treatment – Immunodetection of metastatic sites ***Disadvantage:*** Tumor markers are not in themselves completely specific enough for the diagnosis of malignancy. They may also be raised in few benign lesions. Few markers are specific for a single individual tumor. Most are found with different tumors of the same tissue type. They are present in higher quantities in blood from cancer patients than in blood from both healthy subjects and patients with benign diseases. However, once a malignancy has been diagnosed and shows elevated levels of a tumor marker, the marker can be used to assess response to treatment
Immunohistochemistry (IHC)	➢ IHC takes its name from the word "immuno", referring antibodies used in the procedure, and "histo", meaning tissue ➢ It involves the process of selectively identifying antigens in cells of a tissue section (specimen) with the help of specific antibodies binding against them ➢ It helps in identifying tissue of origin as well as guiding the treatment (for targeted therapy) ➢ Example: CD3 on T cells, CD117+ suggest gastrointestinal stromal tumor (GIST), Vimentin+ suggest sarcomas
Comparative genomic hybridization (CGH)	➢ It detects the amplifications and deletions of small DNA regions throughout the whole genome ➢ The tested DNA is compared to the normal one to identify the areas of DNA gains and losses. SNP (single nucleotide polymorphism) array is a form of targeted CGH that can help with detection of either absence or loss of heterozygosity ***Disadvantage:*** This method is not able to detect balanced translocations, inversions, or insertions, as these changed do not have change in copy number
Fluorescence in situ hybridization (FISH)	➢ **Fluorescence in situ hybridization** used to detect large chromosome abnormalities; however, it can detect smaller microdeletions or duplications ➢ The fluorescent labeled probes hybridize with a DNA sequence of interest and appear under the microscope as a fluorescent dot ➢ When normal chromosomes are present, two dots should be seen for each pair of chromosomes ➢ If only one is seen, it is equal to a chromosome loss; if more than two are present, it shows additional chromosomes ➢ FISH can also be used to detect translocations. Probes of two different colors are used: one for each gene of interest. Normally they should be on two different chromosomes. If translocation is present, these dots will overlap.
Next-generation sequencing (NGS)	➢ In NGS, multiple small fragments of DNA are sequenced in parallel; first the patient's purified DNA is amplified and then fragmented. The data are analyzed by computers and aligned against reference DNA; thus, the whole sequence is restored from fragments ➢ ***Third-generation sequencing*** uses the same concept, but with a single DNA molecule as a template in attempt to reduce the frequency of errors caused by amplification ➢ NGS can be applied to the whole genome (coding and noncoding DNA), exons (only coding DNA, as 85% of mutations occur in these regions), or even small regions of DNA (targeted areas genes) ➢ ***Targeted sequencing*** is faster, is less expensive, and decreases the chance for identification of VUS (variant of uncertained significance) ➢ The clinical applicability of the results of sequencing must be approached with caution: a significant number of nonpathogenic genes are identified and they must be skillfully differentiated from pathogenic genes ***Disadvantage:*** ➢ The results are compared to the results available in mutation databases, but currently available databases are not comprehensive enough ➢ Ordering of these tests is not always appropriate, especially when the results are unlikely to change the diagnosis or treatment
Gene expression profiling	**Gene expression profiling is the measurement of the activity of thousands of genes at once,** to obtain overall picture of cellular function. These profiles can, for example, distinguish between cells that are actively dividing, or show how the cells react to a particular treatment Example: **Microarrays (oligonucleotide arrays)** and **gene expressions test** (RS—Oncotype Dx) in patients with breast cancer may identify patients who are most and least likely to derive benefit from adjuvant chemotherapy
Liquid biopsy	A **liquid biopsy**, also known as **fluid biopsy** or **fluid phase biopsy**, is the sampling and analysis of nonsolid biological tissue, primarily blood. It is mainly used as a diagnostic and monitoring tool for diseases such as cancer, with the added benefit of being largely non invasive
MIBG scan	**Metaiodobenzylguanidine (MIBG)** imaging of norepinephrine transporter ➢ **Indication:** To identify metastatic and primary tumor sites for pheochromocytoma/paraganglioma, and neuroblastoma ➢ **Radiopharmaceutical:** Iobenguane sulfate, 131I-MIBG sulfate, or 123I-MIBG sulfate ➢ **Principle:** MIBG is normally concentrated by adrenergic tissues in cytoplasmic storage granules that also contain other catecholamines
Pentetreotide (octreotide) imaging	**Pentetreotide (octreotide) imaging** ➢ **Indication:** For diagnostic workup of neuroendocrine tumors that bear somatostatin receptors ➢ **Radiopharmaceutical:** Pentetreotide is a diethylenetriaminepentaacetic acid (DTPA) chelate conjugate of octreotide, which is a long-acting analog of human somatostatin. 111In is bound to the chelate. ➢ **Principle.** 111In-pentetreotide binds to somatostatin receptors (SSTRs), particularly SSTR subtype 2, throughout the body. Neuroendocrine tumors highly express these receptors and thus concentrate sufficient amounts of the radioactive agent to be seen by scintigraphy

Contd...

Contd...

PET scan (Figs. 17.3A and B)	➢ Positron emission tomography (PET) detects metabolic activity of tumor cells following injection of small amounts of radioactive tracers, such as fluorodeoxyglucose (FDG) ➢ **Uses:** – It is used for screening for (1) preliminary diagnosis, (2) accurately assess the severity and spread of cancer, (3) biopsy guidance, (4) staging, (5) prognostication, (6) therapeutic planning, and (7) judging response to therapy – PET has been found to be useful in several malignancies including melanoma, lymphoma, lung cancer, esophageal cancer, head and neck cancer, breast cancer, and thyroid cancer – Useful in diagnosing certain cardiovascular and neurolo- gical diseases because it highlights areas with increased, diminished or no metabolic activity – Also positive in patients with granulomatous diseases, like tuberculosis and sarcoidosis ➢ **Method:** – FDG is injected intravenously and is transported from the plasma to the cells by glucose transporters (GLUT 1 and GLUT 4) – It undergoes phosphorylation within the cell by the enzyme hexokinase and is converted to FDG-6-phosphate. FDG-6-phosphate is not further metabolized and gets trapped in the cell 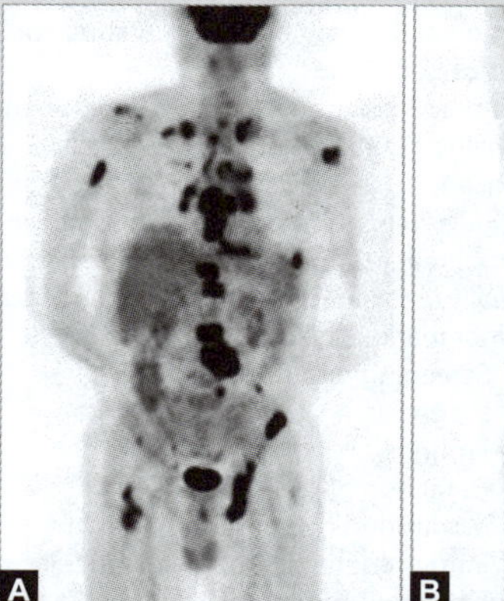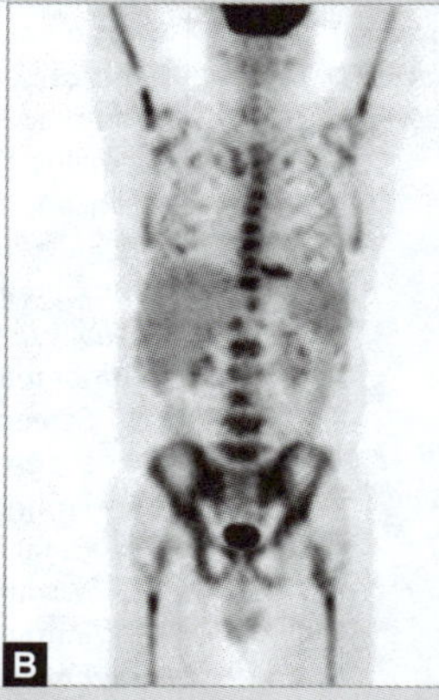 **FIGS. 17.3A AND B:** PET images of a case of non-Hodgkin's lymphoma. (A) Before chemotherapy; (B) After two cycles of doxorubicin, bleomycin, vinblastine, and dacarbazine (ABVD). ➢ Cancer cells have increased anerobic glycolysis and decreased levels of glucose-6-phosphatase. Because of this, cancer cells limit further metabolism of the tracer in cancer cells 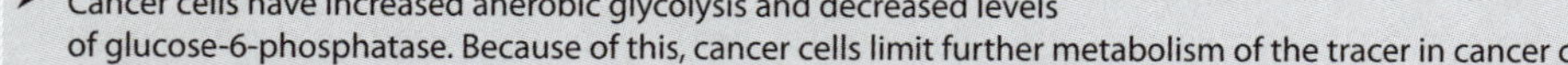 ➢ PET-CT combines the functional information from a PET scan with the anatomical information from a CT scan. It can pinpoint the exact location of abnormal activity. It is used to evaluate patients with various cancers (e.g., including lung cancer and lymphoma)
PET/CT and PET/MRI	These are the hybrid devices which combine the PET and CT/MRI in the same setting giving improved quantification and image contrast

Tumor Markers

TABLE 17.16: Common tumor markers.

Tumor marker	*Associated tumors*
	1. Enzymes
Alkaline phosphatase (ALP)	Hepatoma, secondaries in liver, ovarian, lung, gastrointestinal cancers, and Hodgkin's disease
Placental alkaline phosphatase (PLAP)	Seminoma
Prostatic acid phosphatase (PAP)	Prostate carcinoma
Neuron-specific enolase (NSE)	Small-cell carcinoma of lung, neuroblastoma
Tartrate-resistant acid phosphatase (TRAP)	Hairy cell leukemia
	2. Hormones
Human chorionic gonadotropin (hCG)	Trophoblastic tumors, nonseminomatous tumors of testis
Calcitonin	Medullary carcinoma of thyroid
Catecholamine	Pheochromocytoma
Ectopic hormones	Paraneoplastic syndromes (*see* **Table 17.33**)
	3. Oncofetal antigens
Alpha-fetoprotein	Cancer of liver, nonseminomatous germ cell tumors of testis
Carcinoembryonic antigen (CEA)	Carcinomas of the colon, pancreas, lung, and stomach. May also be elevated in cigarette smoking, peptic ulcer disease, inflammatory bowel disease, pancreatitis, hypothyroidism, cirrhosis, and biliary obstruction
	4. Carbohydrate markers/mucins and other glycoproteins
CA-125	Ovarian cancer
CA 15-3	Breast carcinoma, pancreatic, lung, ovarian, colorectal and liver cancer in some benign breast and liver diseases
CA 19-9	Pancreatic and colorectal cancer
	5. Specific proteins
Immunoglobulins	Multiple myeloma and other gammopathies
Prostate-specific antigen (PSA)	Prostate carcinoma. Other conditions include prostatitis, benign prostatic hypertrophy, prostatic trauma and after ejaculation
Ferritin	Nonspecific, Hodgkin's lymphoma, leukemia, liver, lung, and breast cancer
Thyroglobulin	Differentiated thyroid cancer
S-100	Melanoma
Inhibin A and B	Granulosa cell tumor
Catalase, profilin-1, CD59	Oral squamous cell carcinoma

Contd...

Contd...

6. Receptor markers	
Estrogen and progesterone receptors	Breast cancer as indicators for hormonal therapy
C-erbB2 (HER-2 Neu)	Coreceptor in epidermal growth factor action, overexpression associated with cancer
7. Genetic changes	
Bcr-Abl mutation	Chronic myeloid leukemia
8. New molecular markers	
p53, APC, RAS mutants in stool and serum	Carcinoma colon
p53 and RAS mutants in sputum and serum	Lung cancer
9. Mitochondrial markers	
mtDNA	Carcinoma breast, prostate, lung, thyroid, colon

Staging of Cancer

Q. Enumerate, describe, and discuss classification and staging of cancer (AJCC, FIGO, etc.).

Staging System

Cancer is often staged twice. The first rating is done before treatment and is called the clinical stage. The second rating is done after treatment, such as surgery, and is called the pathologic stage. The pathologic stage is more precise the extent of the cancer.

TNM Staging System

- The TNM staging system is most common method used for cancer staging.
- It is maintained by AJCC (American Joint Committee on Cancer) and UICC (Union for International Cancer Control).
- In this system, the letters T, N, and M describe a different area of cancer growth **(Table 17.17)**.
- Not all cancers are rated by TNM scores (exceptions include hematological cancers)

TABLE 17.17: TNM staging system.

T = Tumor	➢ The T score is a rating of the extent of the primary tumor ➢ T scores are based on the presence, size, and extension of the primary tumor – TX = primary tumor cannot be assessed – T0 = no primary tumor (It is possible to have cancer but not have a primary tumor) – Tis = there are abnormal or cancer cells without breaching the deeper layers (tumor in situ) – T1, T2, T3 there is and T4 are based on the primary tumor's size, extension, or both (varies with type of cancer)
N = Nodes	➢ The N category reflects the extent of cancer within nearby lymph nodes ➢ N scores are based on whether there is cancer in nearby lymph nodes and the number or region of nodes with cancer – NX = lymph nodes cannot be assessed – N0 = no cancer was found in the lymph nodes – N1, N2, and N3 scores are based on the number of nodes with cancer or which nodal groups have cancer (varies with type of cancer)
M = Metastasis	➢ The M category tells you if the cancer has spread to distant sites ➢ M0 means there is no cancer in distant sites ➢ M1 means there is cancer in distant sites

Stage Groups

- Each type of cancer has its own stage groups based on where the cancer has grown and spread. There are either four or five stage groups per cancer (ranked by Roman numerals starting with either stage 0 or stage I and end at stage IV).
- Stage groups for most cancers are defined by TNM scores. If TNM scores are not used, stage group are still defined by where the cancer is in the body. Some cancers that are grouped by TNM scores also use other information to define the stage groups.
- All people who meet the criteria of a stage group have a similar prognosis.
- In general, cancers that cannot spread to distant sites are rated as stage 0. Stage I includes small primary tumors that have not spread to lymph nodes. Stage II and III are larger or more extensive primary tumors with or without cancer in nearby lymph nodes. Stage IV is cancer that has spread to distant sites at diagnosis.

FIGO Staging System (Table 17.18)

It is determined by the International Federation of Gynecology and Obstetrics and used for gynecological cancers. In general, there are five stages.

TABLE 17.18: FIGO staging of gynecological cancers.

FIGO staging	
Stage 0	Carcinoma in situ
Stage I	Confined to the organ of origin
Stage II	Invasion of surrounding organs or tissue
Stage III	Spread to distant nodes or tissue within the pelvis
Stage IV	Distant metastasis(es)

Performance Status

Performance status is a measure of a patient's functional capacity. It has consistently been found to predict survival in patients with cancer, and it is used in that capacity as an entry criterion and an adjustment factor for clinical trials of anticancer therapies. A number of metrics have been developed to quantify performance status; among them, the Eastern Cooperative Oncology Group (ECOG) performance status **(Table 17.19)** and Karnofsky Performance Status (KPS) **(Table 17.20)** are the most commonly used.

TABLE 17.19: ECOG performance status.

Eastern Cooperative Oncology Group (ECOG) performance status		
Status	***Definition***	
0	Fully active Able to carry on all predisease performance without restriction	
1	Restricted in physically strenuous activity but ambulatory Able to carry out work of a light or sedentary nature, for example, office work	
2	Ambulatory and capable of all self-care; unable to carry out any work activities	Up and about more than 50% of waking hours
3	Capable of only limited self-care	Confined to bed or chair more than 50% of waking hours
4	Cannot carry on any self-care. Completely disabled	Totally confined to bed or chair
5	Dead	

TABLE 17.20: Karnofsky performance scale (KPS).

Value	***Activity and assistance***	***Signs and symptoms***	***Care required***
100	Able to perform normal activity	No signs and symptoms of disease	Care for self
90	Able to perform normal activity	Minor signs and symptoms of disease	Care for self
80	Able to perform normal activity with effort	Some signs and symptoms of disease	Care for self
70	Unable to do normal activity	–	Care for self
60	Requires occasional assistance	–	Able to care for most of personal needs
50	Requires considerable assistance	–	Requires frequent medical care
40	Disabled and requires special assistance	–	Requires special care
30	Severely disabled	–	Requires hospitalization although death not imminent
20	Very ill	–	Hospitalization and active supportive care
10	Moribund		
0	Dead		

CANCER TREATMENT

Management of Cancer Patient

Q. Describe and distinguish the difference between curative, palliative, and hospice care in patients with cancer (Table 17.21).

Q. Demonstrate an understanding and needs and preferences of patients when choosing curative and palliative therapy.

Q. Describe the therapies used in alleviating suffering in patients at the end of life (palliative therapy and hospice).

Q. Write a short note on adjuvant and neoadjuvant chemotherapy.

TABLE 17.21: Difference between curative cancer therapy, palliative cancer therapy and hospice cancer care.

Curative therapy	***Palliative therapy***	***Hospice***
Primary objective of curative treatment is to treat the disease. It may be surgery, chemotherapy, radiotherapy, targeted therapy, immunotherapy, etc. It can be defined as the proportion of patients who survive beyond the time after which the risk of treatment failure approaches zero	Palliative care is care given to improve the quality of life of patients who have a serious or life-threatening disease, such as cancer Palliative care is an approach to care that addresses the person as a whole, not just their disease Palliative care is also called comfort care, supportive care, and symptom management Palliative care can be provided either in the hospital or an outpatient clinic or a long-term care facility, or at home under the direction of a physician	Hospice is a special type of care in which medical, psychological, and spiritual support are given to patients and their loved ones when cancer therapies are no longer controlling the disease. A person's cancer treatment continues while one is receiving palliative care, but with hospice care, the focus has shifted to just relieving symptoms and providing support at the end of life The goal of hospice care is to help you live each day to the fullest by controlling pain and other symptoms, making you as comfortable as possible. It is not intended to either hasten or postpone death. The focus is on caring, not curing. If your condition improves or your cancer goes into remission, hospice care can stop and active treatment can resume

Precision medicine (also known as personalized medicine) is an emerging approach for disease treatment and prevention that takes into account individual variability in genes, environment, and lifestyle for each person.

<table>
<tr><td>Surgery</td><td>
➢ Surgical resection is often performed with curative intent, although selected patients may benefit from palliative surgery that is performed for debulking large tumor masses (e.g., ovarian cancer), increasing the efficacy of immunotherapy [e.g., renal cell carcinoma (RCC)], or relieving symptoms (e.g., mastectomy for local control in a patient with metastatic disease).
➢ Surgery can facilitate staging and guide subsequent therapeutic decisions (adjuvant treatment), including chemotherapy or radiation therapy.
➢ Surgical resection of isolated or oligometastatic sites in selected patients can improve survival. Examples include solitary brain metastases, pulmonary metastases from sarcomas, and liver metastases from colorectal cancer.
</td></tr>
<tr><td>Chemotherapy (Tables 17.22 to 17.28)</td><td>
➢ Cytotoxic chemotherapy targets all dividing cells and has broad toxicities.
➢ In patients with resectable disease, chemotherapy may be used before the surgery (neoadjuvant) or following complete resection (adjuvant).
➢ Chemotherapy is typically given in cycles of 2–4 weeks. In most regimens, IV treatment is given on the first few days of the cycle, with no further treatment until the next cycle. In other regimens, treatments are administered weekly for 2–3 weeks, with 1 week off between cycles.
➢ Curative intent chemotherapy includes neoadjuvant, adjuvant, and chemoradiation regimens in solid tumors. Chemotherapy alone is curative in many lymphomas, leukemias, and germ cell tumors.
➢ Palliative chemotherapy is used in advanced solid tumors and relapsed hematologic malignancies, with a focus on prolonging survival and improving the quality of life.
➢ Most agents have a very narrow therapeutic index, and dosing is based on body surface area (mg/m^2). Chemotherapy toxicities are variable and can be life threatening.
</td></tr>
<tr><td>Radiotherapy</td><td>
➢ Radiation is used for treatment of benign and malignant diseases. Commonly used forms of radiation include external-beam photons and electrons.
➢ Brachytherapy is an alternative method of radiation therapy, where radioactive sources are placed close to or in contact with their target tissue. Brachytherapy sources can be temporary or permanent.
➢ Radioactive substances can also be administered systemically. For instance, iodine-131 is administered orally for treating thyroid cancer, yttrium-90 microspheres are injected into the liver vasculature in hepatocellular cancer, and radium-223 is dosed intravenously in patients with prostate cancer and skeletal metastases.
➢ Radiation planning is designed to optimize precision doses of radiation to a tumor while sparing surrounding tissues.
➢ Curative intent radiotherapy is used in several settings.
➢ Neoadjuvant: Preoperative therapy intended to reduce both the extent of surgery and the risk of local relapse. Radiation in this setting is commonly administered in combination with chemotherapy.
➢ Adjuvant: Postoperative therapy intended to reduce the risk of local relapse.
➢ Definitive: High dose with curative intent.
➢ Concurrent chemoradiation: Chemotherapy with definitive radiation is associated with increased efficacy but at a cost of increased toxicity compared to either chemotherapy or radiation alone.
➢ Palliative radiotherapy is used in lower dosing to reduce symptoms, including bone pain, obstruction, bleeding, and neurologic symptoms.
➢ The total dose of radiation administered is usually divided over several days (fractionated). This allows time for normal tissue repair and increases the probability of delivering radiation to tumor cells in a radiosensitive phase of cell cycle. Radiation treatments are usually delivered either through conventional fractionation, hypofractionation, hyperfractionation, or accelerated fractionation schedules.
– Conventional fractionation consists of daily fractions typically of 1.8–2.0 Gy, usually delivered 5 days/week.
– Hypofractionation refers to the delivery of radiation divided into larger doses, with treatment once a day or less often.
– Hyperfractionation refers to the delivery of radiation divided into smaller doses per fraction, with treatments more than once per day.
– Accelerated fractionation is defined as reducing the overall duration of radiotherapy regimen without a significant change in the size of dose per fraction (by delivering more than 5 fractions/week)
</td></tr>
<tr><td>Hormonal therapy</td><td>
<table>
<tr><th>Hormonal drugs</th><th>Indication</th></tr>
<tr><td>Glucocorticoids</td><td>Combination therapy in lymphomas, brain tumors and spinal cord compression syndromes, prevention of chemotherapy-induced vomiting</td></tr>
<tr><td>Adrenal inhibitor (mitotane)</td><td>Adrenal carcinoma, Cushing's syndrome</td></tr>
<tr><td>Androgens</td><td>Breast carcinoma</td></tr>
<tr><td>Antiandrogens (bicalutamide, flutamide, nilutamide, enzalutamide, abiraterone)</td><td>Prostate cancer</td></tr>
<tr><td>Estrogens</td><td>Breast carcinoma, prostate cancer</td></tr>
<tr><td>Antiestrogens (tamoxifen, toremifene, fulvestrant)</td><td>Breast carcinoma</td></tr>
<tr><td>Aromatase inhibitors (anastrozole, letrozole, exemestane, aminoglutethimide)</td><td>Breast carcinoma (postmenopausal)</td></tr>
<tr><td>Gonadotropin-releasing hormone (GnRH) agonists (leuprolide, goserelin)</td><td>Prostate and breast cancer</td></tr>
<tr><td>Progesterone</td><td>Uterine cancer</td></tr>
</table>
</td></tr>
<tr><td>Targeted therapy (Table 17.29 and Fig. 17.4)</td><td>
➢ The advent of molecularly targeted agents has led to marked advances in the treatment of selected malignancies.
➢ The most common classes of drugs are monoclonal antibodies and receptor tyrosine kinase inhibitors (TKIs).
➢ Monoclonal antibodies (Table 17.30) are administered IV and by standard nomenclature have names that end with the stem –mab. Substems indicate the source and target of the antibody. The most common source substems in oncology include –xi—indicating a chimeric antibody (e.g., cetuximab), –zu—indicating humanized antibody (e.g., bevacizumab), and –u—indicating fully human antibodies (e.g., ipilimumab). The most common target substems include –ci—indicating circulatory system (e.g., bevacizumab), –tu—indicating tumor (e.g., cetuximab), and –li—indicating immune system (e.g., ipilimumab).
➢ TKIs are administered orally and have names that end with –ib. The most common substem is –ti—indicating tyrosine kinase inhibition (e.g., imatinib).
</td></tr>
</table>

Contd...

Contd...

Immunotherapy	Artificial stimulation of the immune system to treat cancer. Immunotherapies can be categorized as active, passive or hybrid (active and passive). ➢ Active immunotherapy directs the immune system to attack tumor cells by targeting tumor antigens. ➢ Passive immunotherapies enhance existing antitumor responses and include the use of monoclonal antibodies, lymphocytes, and cytokines. Commonly used immunotherapy targets include: ➢ **Interleukin-2 (IL-2)** was the first immunotherapy approved for treatment of human cancers. IL-2 is a T-cell growth factor that allows for expansion of T cells while maintaining their functional activity, e.g., recombinant IL-2 (**aldesleukin**). ➢ Programmed cell death–1 (PD-1) is a receptor expressed primarily on the surface of activated T cells. Binding of PD-1 to one of its ligands, PD-L1 or PD-L2, inhibits the cytotoxic T cell response. Tumor cells may co-opt this pathway to escape T cell-induced antitumor activity. The interaction between PD-1 and PD-L1 may be blocked by monoclonal antibodies against **PD-1** (nivolumab, pembrolizumab) or **PD-L1** (atezolizumab, durvalumab, avelumab). These immune checkpoint blockers have been approved for the treatment of multiple tumors including melanoma, lung cancer, bladder cancer, kidney cancer, head and neck cancer, and lymphomas. PD-L1 expression by immunohistochemistry (IHC) has been associated with response to anti-PD-1 or PD-L1 antibodies in some cancers. ➢ **Bispecific antibodies** (BITE cell—Bispecific T-cell Engagers) such as blinatumomab, which engage T cells to recognize cancer cells ➢ **Chimeric antigen receptor–T cells** (CAR-T cells) such as tisagenlecleucel and axicabtagene ciloleucel, which are specially engineered T cells capable of attacking tumor cells. They are approved for hematological malignancies derived from B cells (ALL and DLBCL) ➢ **CTLA4** is member of immunoglobulin superfamily expressed by activated T cells and results in inhibition of T reg cells. Drugs inhibiting CTLA4 include ipilimumab and tremelimumab.	
Cancer vaccines (therapeutic)	**Bacillus Calmette-Guérin (BCG) vaccine**	Live attenuated strain of *Mycobacterium bovis*, and it is given intravesically as a part to adjunctive therapy for superficial bladder cancer
	Sipuleucel-T	Dendritic cell-based cancer vaccine which enhance the T-cell response against prostatic acid phosphatase (used in castrate-resistant prostate cancer)
	GVAX	Composed of two irradiated prostate cancer cell lines that expresses granulocyte-macrophage colony-stimulating factor (GM-CSF) that promotes the activation of T cells with low affinity for self-antigens expressed by tumors
	Gp100 vaccine	Peptide vaccine with a melanocyte differentiation antigen, glycoprotein 100 (gp100). It is used in combination with high-dose IL-2 in patients with melanoma

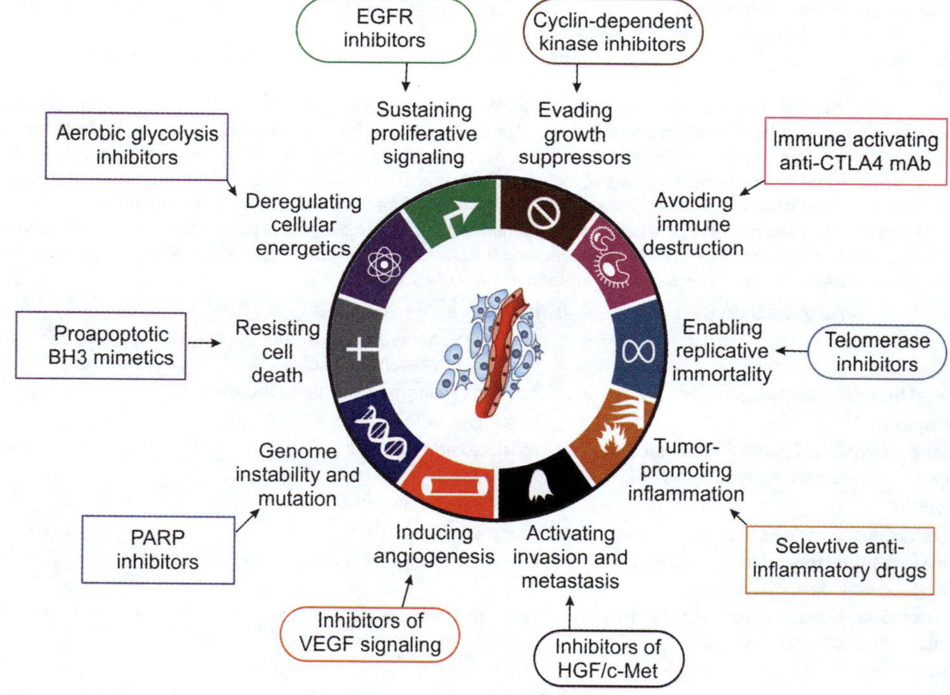

FIG. 17.4: Sites of targeted therapy.

Chemotherapeutic Agents

Q. Write a short note on classification of chemotherapeutic agents (Fig. 17.5).

Q. Write a short note on cyclophosphamide.

Q. Write a short note on cisplatin.

Q. Write a short note on methotrexate.

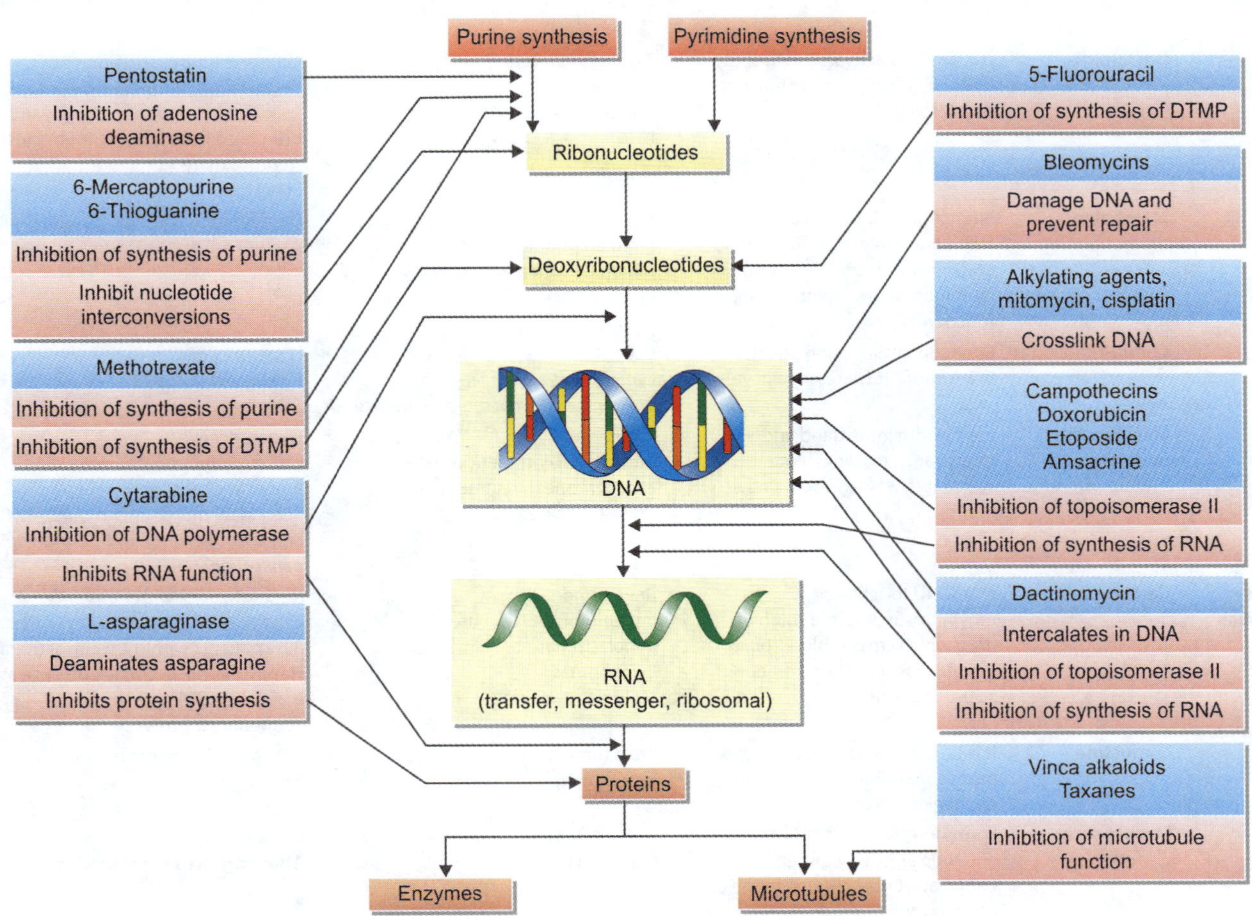

FIG. 17.5: Mechanism of action of various chemotherapeutic drugs.

TABLE 17.22: Classification of chemotherapeutic agents based on phase of cell cycle on which they act.

Cell cycle–specific drugs		***Cell cycle–nonspecific drugs***
These are effective when the cells are proliferating and act at specific phase of cell cycle		These are effective whether cells are dividing or in resting phase and can effect at any phase of cell cycle
Etoposide	G1-S phase	Alkylating agents Platinum compounds Anthracyclines Camptothecins
Antimetabolites	S phase	
Bleomycin Etoposide	G2-M phase	
Vinca alkaloids Taxanes	M phase	

TABLE 17.23: Alkylating agents.

Alkylating agents		➢ *These drugs alkylate nucleophilic groups on DNA bases (N7 of guanine is most susceptible) which lead to crosslinking of bases, abnormal base pairing, and DNA strand breakage* ➢ *These are cell cycle nonspecific drugs acting on both resting and dividing cells, can affect any stage of cell division* ***Common side effects*** *of all alkylating agents (mnemonic: BAGS):* ➢ *Bone marrow suppression* ➢ *Alopecia* ➢ *Gastrointestinal distress* ➢ *Sterility* ➢ *Secondary leukemia (leukemia and myelodysplasias)*		
Drug		***Special points***	***Common indications***	***Common adverse effects***
Nitrogen mustard	**Cyclo-phosphamide**	It is prodrug activated in liver (by Cyt P450) to 4-hydroxycyclophophamide, phosphoramide mustard and acrolein. At low doses, it is a potent immunomodulator	➢ **As anticancer agent**: Breast cancer, soft tissue sarcomas, NHL ➢ **As conditioning** regimen in HSCT ➢ **As immunosuppressant** in nephrotic syndrome, SLE, RA, Wegener's granulomatosis, PAN and other systemic vasculitis refractory ITP	➢ **Hemorrhagic cystitis** due to degradation product acrolein. It can prevented by MESNA with adequate hydration and treatment is by steroids ➢ ***Cardiotoxicity*** ➢ Syndrome of inappropriate antidiuretic hormone secretion (SIADH)

Contd...

Contd...

	Ifosfamide	It is prodrug activated in liver (by CYP450) into ifosfamide mustard and acrolein	➢ Testicular cancers ➢ Bladder cancer ➢ Soft tissue sarcomas ➢ NHL	➢ **Hemorrhagic cystitis** due to degradation product acrolein. Drug used for prevention is MESNA, and drug used for treatment is Steroids) ➢ ***Neurotoxicity*** ➢ SIADH
	Melphalan	Bifunctional alkylating agent that forms interstrand and intrastrand crosslinks with DNA, resulting in inhibition of DNA synthesis and function	➢ Multiple myeloma (as conditioning regimen prior to transplantation) ➢ Multiple myeloma (as palliative care)	➢ Dose limiting myelosuppression with nadir of 4-6 weeks
	Chlorambucil	Bifunctional alkylating agent. $T_{1/2}$ is 2-4 hours. It spares myelocytes	➢ CLL ➢ Lymphomas ➢ Waldenstrom's macroglobulinemia	➢ Hyperuricemia ➢ Pulmonary fibrosis ➢ Seizures
	Mechloretha-mine	Forms both intrastrand and interstrand crosslinks. Potent vesicant (always infuse via new IV site)	➢ Lymphomas ➢ Intrapleural, intrapericardial and intraperitoneal treatment of metastatic diseases	➢ Hyperuricemia ➢ CNS toxicity ➢ Potent vesicant ➢ Secondary malignancies (***AML****—with IV administration,* ***BCC or SCC*** *with topical application)*
Nitro-soureas	**Carmustine**	It is BCNU (bischloro-ethylnitrosurea). Lipid soluble drug which crosses blood-brain barrier, reaching concentrations >50% of plasma	➢ Brain tumors ➢ Implantable BCNU—used in glioblastomas ➢ Lymphomas ➢ Multiple myeloma	➢ Hepatotoxicity with transient elevations of transaminases in around 90% patients within 1 week of therapy ➢ **Hepatic veno-occlusive disease** in around 15–20% ➢ Pulmonary fibrosis
	Lomustine	It is CCNU (chloroethyl cyclohexyl nitrosourea). Forms intrastrand crosslinking of DNA	➢ Brain tumors ➢ Lymphomas	➢ ILD and pulmonary fibrosis ➢ **Neurotoxicity**
	Streptozocin	Forms intrastrand crosslinks of DNA. Selectively targets pancreatic beta cells due to the glucose moiety	➢ Pancreatic islet cell tumors ➢ Carcinoid tumors.	➢ Renal ➢ **Altered glucose metabolism**
Alkyl sulfonates	**Busulfan**	Bifunctional alkylating agent. Interacts with cellular thiol groups and nucleic acids to form DNA-DNA and DNA-protein crosslinks. Crosses blood-brain barrier and placental barrier	➢ CML ➢ Conditioning regimen during HSCT	➢ Interstitial pneumonitis ➢ Pulmonary fibrosis ➢ Hyperpigmentation of skin ➢ Hepatotoxic and can cause **hepatic veno-occlusive disease**
Triazines	**Procarbazine**	Hydrazine analog acting as alkylating agent. Weak MAO inhibitor. Crosses blood-brain barrier	➢ Lymphomas ➢ Brain tumor (adjuvant)	➢ To be **avoided with alcohol or tyramine**-containing foods ➢ To be **avoided in G6PD** deficiency individuals ➢ Flu-like syndrome ➢ CNS toxicity ➢ Interstitial pneumonitis
	Dacarbazine	Initially developed as a purine antimetabolite, but antitumor effect is by methylation of nucleic acids	➢ Metastatic malignant melanoma ➢ Hodgkin's lymphoma ➢ Soft tissue sarcomas ➢ Neuroblastoma	➢ Flu-like syndrome ➢ CNS toxicity ➢ **Potent vesicant**—pain and burning at the site of injection
	Temozolomide	Imidazotetrazine analog that is structurally and functionally similar to dacarbazine. Active compound is **MTIC**. Methylates guanine residues in DNA but do not crosslink DNA strands. Oral bioavailability is 100%. Crosses blood-brain barrier	➢ Brain tumors ➢ Metastatic melanoma	➢ Myelosuppression is dose limiting ➢ Photosensitivity ➢ Mild elevation of hepatic transaminases
Ethylen-imines	**Thio-TEPA**	Crosslinks DNA leading to inhibition of synthesis of DNA, RNA, and proteins	➢ HSCT for brain tumors ➢ Leptomeningeal metastasis (intrathecal)	➢ CNS—intracranial hemorrhage, seizures ➢ Hepatitis ➢ Contact dermatitis ➢ Hemorrhagic cystitis
	Hexamethyl-melamine	Highest concentrations are attained in tissues with high fat content	➢ Ovarian cancer (advanced or recurrent disease)	➢ Neurotoxicity (may be reduced with vitamin B_6 supplementation) ➢ Flu-like syndrome

TABLE 17.24: Platinum compounds.

Platinum compounds	➢ *They have similar mechanism of action of alkylating agents* ➢ *They use platinum compounds instead of alkyl group to form dimers in DNA* ➢ *Covalently binds to DNA at N-7 position of guanine and adenine. Reacts with two different sites of DNA producing crosslinks (90% intra-strand links).* ➢ *Also binds to nuclear and cytoplasmic proteins resulting in cytotoxic effects.* ➢ *All are administered only by IV route.* ***Common adverse effects:*** – *Nausea and vomiting* – *Bone marrow suppression* – *Ototoxicity, nephrotoxicity, and neurotoxicity*		
Drug	***Special points***	***Common indications***	***Common adverse effects***
Cisplatin	Highest concentrations in liver and kidneys. Hydration prior and post administration of drug	➢ Testicular cancer ➢ Ovarian cancer ➢ Bladder cancer ➢ Head and neck cancer ➢ Esophageal cancer ➢ SCLC and NSCLC ➢ NHL ➢ Trophoblastic neoplasm	➢ ***Coomb's positive hemolytic anemia*** ➢ Nephrotoxicity (dose related and reversible; hypomagnesemia, hypocalcemia and hypokalemia are common) ➢ Neurotoxicity (sensory neuropathy) ➢ Ototoxicity (high frequency hearing loss and tinnitus) ➢ Ocular toxicity (optic neuritis, papilledema, and cerebral blindness) ➢ Nausea and vomiting (acute and delayed) ➢ **Vascular events like MI, CVA,** etc. ➢ Azoospermia, impotence, and sterility ➢ *SIADH*
Oxaliplatin	Third-generation platinum compound. Prolonged terminal half life of 240 hours	➢ Colorectal cancer (in combination of 5-FU and leucovorin) ➢ Pancreatic cancer ➢ Gastric ➢ Gastroesophageal cancer	➢ Neurotoxicity: ***Acute toxicity***—sensory neuropathy occurs usually 1–3 days after therapy; ***Chronic toxicity***—dose dependent—proprioception and neurosensory function. As compared to cisplatin, oxaliplatin induced neuropathy is reversible and returns to normal within 3–4 months of discontinuation of therapy ➢ ***Autoimmune thrombocytopenia, AIHA, and TTP*** have also been reported ➢ Hepatotoxicity with sinusoidal injury seen ➢ ***RPLS—reversible posterior leukoencephalopathy*** is seen rarely
Carboplatin	Crosses blood-brain barrier and enters CSF	➢ Ovarian cancer ➢ Germ cell tumors ➢ Head and neck cancers ➢ SCLC and NSCLC ➢ Endometrial cancer	➢ Thrombocytopenia is more pronounced ➢ Nephrotoxicity (Peripheral neuropathy)

TABLE 17.25: Anti-metabolites.

Antimetabolites		➢ *These drugs act in S phase of cell cycle* ➢ *Only dividing cells are responsive to these drugs* ➢ *They have additional immunosuppressive properties* ***Common adverse effects:*** – *Myelosuppression* – *Mucositis* – *Allergy/skin rash*		
Drug		***Special points***	***Common indications***	***Common adverse effects***
Folic acid analogs (Requires intracellular polyglutamation by folyl polyglutamate synthase—FPGS for its cytotoxic activity. All of these are predominantly excreted by kidneys)	**Methotrexate**	Mechanism of action is by inhibition of DHFR (reducing folate levels), inhibition of de novo thymidylate synthesis, inhibition of de novo purine synthesis and incorporation of dUTP into DNA, resulting in inhibition of DNA synthesis and function. Drugs used to treat overdose are **leucovorin, thymidine and gucarpidase**	**As anticancer agent** ➢ Head and neck cancer ➢ Choriocarcinoma ➢ Osteogenic sarcoma ➢ ALL ➢ Primary CNS lymphoma **Noncancerous indications:** ➢ Rheumatoid arthritis ➢ Crohn's disease ➢ Abortion (MTP) ➢ Ectopic pregnancy ➢ Psoriasis	➢ Renal failure ➢ Liver toxicity ➢ Pneumonitis ➢ ***Chemical arachnoiditis*** ➢ Acute cerebral dysfunction ➢ Menstrual irregularities
	Pemetrexed	Mechanism of action is by inhibition of folate-dependent enzyme thymidylate synthase and DHFR. All the patients require **folic acid and vitamin B_{12} supplementation**	➢ NSCLC (note that pemetrexed is not to be used in SCLC) ➢ Mesothelioma	Hand foot syndrome Mucositis
	Pralatrexate	Mechanism is similar to methotrexate. Only IV route. All the patients require **folic acid and vitamin B_{12} supplementation**	➢ Peripheral T-cell lymphoma	➢ Myelosuppression ➢ Mucositis

Contd...

Contd...

Purine analogs	**6-MP**	Requires intracellular phosphorylation by enzyme HGPRT to the cytotoxic monophosphate form. MOA is mainly by inhibition of purine synthesis by inhibiting enzymes PRPP (phophoribosyl pyrophosphate amidotransferase) and inhibition of DNA/RNA synthesis by incorporation of thiopurine triphosphate nucleotides. **Metabolized by xanthine oxidase in liver**	➢ ALL **Noncancerous indications:** ➢ Crohn's disease ➢ Ulcerative colitis	➢ Allopurinol inhibits xanthine oxidase and hence enhances toxicity of 6-MP ➢ Hepatotoxicity ➢ Mutagenic ➢ **Teratogenic** ➢ **Carcinogenic** ➢ Immunosuppression
	6- TG	Similar to 6-MP. But**, no need of dose adjustment with renal or hepatic failure. Not metabolized by xanthine oxidase** and hence no drug interaction with allopurinol	➢ ALL ➢ AML ➢ CML **Noncancerous indications:** ➢ Crohn's disease ➢ Ulcerative colitis ➢ Psoriasis	➢ Same as side effects of 6-MP
	Cladribine	Purine deoxyadenosine analog with **high specificity for lymphoid cells**. Antitumor activity on both dividing and resting cells. MOA **include DNA synthesis inhibition, depletion of NAD and induction of apoptosis**. Crosses blood-brain barrier. Usually given **as 7 day continuous IV infusion**	➢ Hairy cell leukemia ➢ Chronic lymphocytic leukemia (CLL) ➢ NHL (low grade)	➢ Immunosuppression ➢ **Fever (due to cytokine release)** ➢ Tumor lysis syndrome (**All patients should receive prophylactic allopurinol**)
	Fludarabine	Analog of arabinofuranosyl adenosine with **high specificity to lymphoid cells. Inhibits DNA chain extension, DNA polymerases alpha and beta, and promotes apoptosis**	➢ CLL ➢ NHL ➢ Cutaneous T-cell lymphoma	➢ **Autoimmune hemolytic anemia** ➢ **Drug-induced aplastic anemia** ➢ Immunosuppression with decrease in CD4 and CD8 cells ➢ **Fever (due to cytokine release)** ➢ **Tumor lysis syndrome**
	Clofarabine	MOA is similar to cladribine. Also, it inhibits **DNA polymerases alpha, beta, and gamma**	➢ Pediatric relapsed/ refractory ALL	➢ Immunosuppression ➢ **Capillary leak syndrome** ➢ Renal toxicity ➢ Liver toxicity ➢ Cardiac toxicity
Pyrimidine	**Fluorouracil (5-FU)**	Cell cycle-specific drug acting in S phase of cell cycle. Inhibits thymidylate synthase, DNA synthesis, and RNA translation. Active metabolites FdUMP, FdUTP, and FUTP highest concentration in GI mucosa, bone marrow, and liver. Penetrates third space fluid collections and crosses blood-brain barrier. 90% of drug cleared in urine and lungs. Leucovorin enhances the antitumor activity and toxicity	➢ GI malignancies ➢ Head and neck cancer ➢ Breast cancer ➢ Ovarian tumors ➢ Topical use for skin cancers	➢ Hand-foot syndrome (palmar-plantar erythrodysesthesia)—incidence can be reduced by prophylactic usage of vitamin B_6, Celecoxib and Nicotine patch ➢ Ocular problems (blepharitis, tear duct stenosis, conjunctivitis) ➢ Neurological symptoms ➢ Cardiac symptoms (chest pain with ECG changes)
	Capecetabine	Prodrug of 5 FU. It is activated into active form in liver and tumor tissue. **Contraindicated in DPD deficiency** (dihydropyrimidine dehydrogenase deficiency)	➢ Breast (metastatic) ➢ Colorectal cancers ➢ GI cancers	➢ Diltiazem can prevent capecitabine-induced **coronary vasospasm** and chest pain ➢ Hepatotoxicity
	Cytarabine	It is activated into active metabolite ara-CTP. Incorporation of ara-CTP results in chain termination and inhibition of DNA synthesis. Also it inhibits DNA polymerases alpha, beta, and gamma. Good CSF penetration	➢ AML ➢ ALL ➢ CML ➢ NHL ➢ Leptomeningeal carcinomatosis	➢ Hepatic dysfunction ➢ Acute pancreatitis ➢ **Ara-C syndrome** (allergic reaction in pediatric population—it is characterized by fever, myalgia, malaise, bone pain, skin rash, conjunctivitis, and occasional chest pain) ➢ Pulmonary complications ➢ Skin changes ➢ Eye toxicity (conjunctivitis and keratitis)
	Gemcitabine	It requires intracellular activation by deoxycytidine kinase to form active metabolite gemcitabine triphosphate. MOA is by inhibition of DNA polymerases alpha, beta, and gamma; alterations in RNA processing and mRNA translation	➢ Pancreatic cancer ➢ NSCLC ➢ Breast cancer ➢ Ovarian cancer ➢ Bladder cancer ➢ Lymphomas	➢ Flu-like syndrome ➢ Renal microangiopathy (HUS, TTP) ➢ Radiation recall dermatitis

Contd...

Contd...

	5-azacytidine	Converted into active metabolite azacitidine triphosphate, which is incorporated into RNA and DNA. Incorporation into DNA results inhibition of methyltransferases, which in turn leads to loss of DNA methylation and gene reactivation. Aberrantly silenced genes like tumor suppressor genes are reactivated	➢ MDS ➢ CMML	➢ Myelosuppression ➢ Peripheral edema ➢ GI toxicity ➢ Renal toxicity
	Decitabine	Converted into active metabolite decitabine triphosphate. MOA—similar to 5-azacytidine	➢ MDS	➢ Similar to 5- azacytidine

TABLE 17.26: Mitotic spindle inhibitors.

Mitotic spindle inhibitors		➢ They act at M phase of cell cycle ➢ Plant-derived alkaloids **Adverse effects:** - Myelosuppression - SIADH (vinca alkaloids) - Vesicants (vinca alkaloids) - Hypersensitivity, alopecia, and nail changes (especially Taxanes) - Neuropathy (predominantly sensory neuropathy)		
Drug		***Special points***	***Common indications***	***Common adverse effects***
Vinca alkaloids Plant alkaloid derivatives (from *Catharanthus roseus)*	**Vincristine**	Inhibits tubulin polymerization, disrupting formation of microtubules during mitosis	➢ ALL ➢ Lymphomas ➢ Soft tissue sarcomas ➢ Wilms' tumor ➢ Neuroblastoma	➢ Constipation and paralytic ileus ➢ SIADH ➢ Azoospermia and amenorrhea
	Vinblastine	Same as vincristine	➢ Testicular tumors ➢ Hodgkin's lymphoma (ABVD regimen) ➢ Breast cancer ➢ Kaposi's sarcoma ➢ Renal cell carcinoma	➢ Raynaud's syndrome in combination with bleomycin ➢ Hypertension ➢ Vascular events—MI, stroke, and Raynaud's syndrome
	Vinorelbine	Semisynthetic alkaloid of Vinblastine	➢ NSCLC ➢ Breast cancer ➢ Ovarian cancer	➢ Similar to vinblastine ➢ Lesser incidence of vascular events
Taxanes	**Paclitaxel**	Enhances tubulin polymerization leading to inhibition of mitosis. It is radiosensitizing agent	➢ Ovarian cancer ➢ Breast cancer ➢ Lung cancer ➢ Esophageal cancer ➢ Head and neck cancer	➢ Cardiotoxicity (arrhythmias) ➢ Onycholysis
	Docetaxel	MOA is similar to paclitaxel	➢ Breast cancer ➢ NSCLC ➢ Prostate cancer ➢ Gastric cancer ➢ Head and neck cancers	➢ Fluid retention syndrome ➢ Brown discoloration of finger nails ➢ Vesicant
	Cabazitaxel	Binds to tubulin and promotes its assembly into microtubule while simultaneously inhibiting disassembly, thus inhibiting mitotic and interphase cellular functions	➢ Hormone-refractory metastatic prostate cancer	➢ Cardiac arrhythmias
Others	**Ixabepilone**	Binds directly to beta tubulin subunits on microtubule leading to inhibition of normal microtubule dynamics. Exhibits activity against drug-resistant tumors	➢ Metastatic taxane resistant breast cancer	➢ Hypersensitivity reactions ➢ Neurotoxicity ➢ Myalgias ➢ Fatigue
	Eribulin	Inhibits microtubule growth by sequestering tubulin in non-productive aggregates with no effect on microtubule shortening. Active against taxane-resistant tumor lines	➢ Metastatic refractory breast cancer ➢ Metastatic liposarcoma	➢ QT prolongation ➢ Myelosuppression ➢ Peripheral neuropathy
	Estramustine	Nor-nitrogen mustard conjugate of estradiol without alkylating agent properties. Mainly works by inhibiting microtubule structure and function	➢ Hormone-refractory metastatic prostate cancer	➢ Gynecomastia ➢ Diarrhea ➢ Cardiovascular complications ➢ Skin rash

TABLE 17.27: Topoisomerase inhibitors.

Topoisomerase inhibitors		***Common adverse effects:*** ➢ ***Myelosuppression*** ➢ ***Alopecia***		
Drug		***Special points***	***Common indications***	***Common adverse effects***
Camptothecins	**Irinotecan**	Active form is SN-38 metabolite. Binds and stabilizes topoisomerase I and results in double-strand DNA breaks. Colorectal tumors have higher levels of topoisomerase I	➢ Colorectal cancer ➢ NSCLC ➢ SCLC	➢ Diarrhea* ➢ Asthenia ➢ Elevation of liver enzymes
	Topotecan	MOA—similar to irinotecan	➢ Ovarian cancer ➢ SCLC ➢ Cervical cancer	Microscopic hematuria Headache and myalgias
Epipodophyllotoxins	**Etoposide**	Cell cycle-specific agent with activity in late S and G2 phases. Inhibits topoisomerase II. Associated with early secondary malignancies (especially AML associated with t(11; 23) which develops within 2–3 years of treatment)	➢ Germ cell tumors ➢ SCLC ➢ NSCLC ➢ NHL and HL ➢ Gastric cancer	➢ Metallic taste ➢ Radiation recall skin changes
	Teniposide	MOA—similar to etoposide	➢ ALL (refractory state)	➢ GI side effects ➢ Hypotension ➢ Hypersensitivity

*Early-onset diarrhea which occurs withing 24 hours of therapy is due to cholinergic excess and managed by atropine, whereas late-onset diarrhea is managed with antimotility agents.

TABLE 17.28: Antitumor antibiotics.

Antitumor antibiotics		***Common adverse effects:*** ➢ ***Myelosuppression*** ➢ ***Cardiotoxicity (especially anthracyclines)**** ➢ ***Mucositis, nail changes, and alopecia*** ➢ ***Potent vesicants***		
Drug		***Special points***	***Common indications***	***Additional adverse effects***
Anthracyclines	**Doxorubicin**	Intercalates into DNA resulting in inhibition of DNA synthesis and function. Inhibits opoisomerase II and also results in formation of cytotoxic oxygen-free radicals. Also inhibits DNA-dependent RNA polymerases	➢ Breast cancer ➢ HL and NHL ➢ Soft tissue sarcomas ➢ Ovarian cancer ➢ SCLC and NSCLC ➢ Wilms' tumor ➢ Neuroblastoma ➢ ALL	➢ Hyperpigmentation ➢ Radiation recall phenomenon ➢ Red-orange discoloration of urine
	Daunorubicin	Similar to doxorubicin	➢ AML ➢ ALL	➢ Similar to doxorubicin
	Mitoxantrone	Similar to doxorubicin	➢ Hormone-refractory prostate cancer ➢ AML ➢ Breast cancer ➢ NHL	➢ Blue discoloration of fingernails and sclera ➢ Secondary AML
Others	**Dactinomycin**	Preferentially binds to guanine-cytosine base pairs. Formation of oxygen-free radicals results in single- and double-stranded DNA breaks and subsequent inhibition of DNA synthesis and function	➢ Rhabdomyosarcoma ➢ Germ cell tumors ➢ Wilms' tumor ➢ Ewing's sarcoma ➢ Gestational trophoblastic diseases	➢ Hyperpigmentation ➢ Radiation recall syndrome
	Bleomycin	Contains DNA-binding region and iron-binding region. Iron is absolutely necessary as cofactor for free radical generation and bleomycin cytotoxic activity. It causes single- and double-stranded DNA breaks	➢ HL and NHL ➢ Germ cell tumors ➢ Head and neck tumors ➢ SCC of skin, cervix, and vulva	➢ Maintain a low FiO_2 in order to avoid pulmonary toxicity ➢ Skin reactions ➢ Pulmonary toxicity ➢ Hypersensitivity inform of fever and chills ➢ Vascular events (MI, stroke, Raynaud's phenomenon, etc.)
	Mitomycin	Acts as alkylating agent crosslinking DNA and also inhibits DNA-dependent RNA polymerase	➢ Gastric cancer ➢ Breast cancer ➢ Superficial bladder cancer ➢ Anal cancer ➢ Head and neck cancer	➢ Hemolytic uremic syndrome/MAHA ➢ Interstitial pneumonia ➢ Hepatic veno-occlusive disease ➢ Chemical cystitis and bladder contraction

***Cardiotoxicity:** Acute cardiotoxicity—myocarditis, pericarditis, arrhythmias; chronic cardiotoxicity—dilated cardiomyopathy; risk of cardiotoxicity increases with cumulative dose of >450 mg/m^2.

Targeted Therapy

Q. Write short essay/note on various types of targeted therapy in cancer patients.

TABLE 17.29: Targeted therapy agents.

Group	*Drug*	*Common indications*
ALK (Anaplastic lymphoma kinase) inhibitors	**Alectinib**	NSCLC
	Ceritinib	NSCLC
	Crizotinib	NSCLC
BCL2 inhibitors	**Venetoclax**	CLL with 17p deletion
BCR-ABL inhibitors	**Bosutinib**	CML
	Dasatinib	CML, Ph+ ALL
	Imatinib	CML, GIST, Dermatofibrosarcoma protuberans, MDS, ALL Ph+
	Nilotinib	CML
	Ponatinib	CML (T315I mutant)
BRAF, MEK inhibitors	**Cobimetinib**	Melanoma
	Dabrafenib	Melanoma
	Trametinib	Melanoma
	Vemurafenib	Melanoma
BTK inhibitors	**Ibrutinib**	Mantle cell lymphoma, CLL, Waldenström's macroglobulinemia
CDK (Cyclin-dependent kinase) 4/6 inhibitors	**Palbociclib**	ER-positive, HER2-negative advanced breast cancer
EGFR (Epidermal growth factor receptor) inhibitors	**Afatinib**	Metastatic NSCLC
	Erlotinib	Locally advanced or metastatic NSCLC pancreatic cancer
	Gefitinib	Metastatic NSCLC
	Osimertinib	Epidermal growth factor receptor (EGFR) T790M mutation-positive NSCLC
HDAC (Histone deacetylase) inhibitors:	**Belinostat**	Relapsed or refractory peripheral T-cell lymphoma
	Panobinostat	Multiple myeloma
	Romidepsin	Cutaneous T-cell lymphoma (CTCL), peripheral T-cell lymphoma (PTCL)
	Vorinostat	Cutaneous T-cell lymphoma
HER2 (Human epidermal growth factor receptor 2) inhibitors	**Lapatinib**	Breast cancer
	Neratinib	Breast cancer
JAK (Janus-associated kinase) inhibitors	**Ruxolitinib**	Myelofibrosis, polycythemia vera
mTOR (Mammalian target of rapamycin) inhibitors	**Everolimus**	HER2-negative breast cancer, PNET, NET, RCC, renal angiomyolipoma
	Temsirolimus	Advanced renal cell carcinoma
PARP [Poly (ADP-ribose) polymerase] inhibitors	**Olaparib**	BRCA-mutated advanced ovarian cancer and breast cancer
	Rucaparib	BRCA-mutated advanced ovarian cancer and breast cancer
PI3Kδ (Phosphatidylinositol 3-kinase delta) inhibitors	**Idelalisib**	Relapsed CLL, in combination with rituximab, relapsed follicular B-cell NHL (FL), relapsed small lymphocytic lymphoma (SLL)
Proteasome inhibitors	**Bortezomib**	Multiple myeloma, mantle cell lymphoma
	Carfilzomib	Multiple myeloma
	Ixazomib	Multiple myeloma
SMO (Smoothened)/Hedgehog pathway inhibitors	**Sonidegib**	Locally advanced basal cell carcinoma (BCC)
	Vismodegib	Metastatic or locally advanced BCC
VEGFR (Vascular endothelial growth factor receptor) inhibitors	**Axitinib**	Advanced renal cell carcinoma
	Cabozantinib	Advanced renal cell carcinoma, medullary thyroid cancer
	Lenvatinib	Radioactive iodine refractory differentiated thyroid cancer; renal cell carcinoma
	Pazopanib	Advanced renal cell carcinoma, advanced soft tissue sarcoma
	Regorafenib	Metastatic colorectal cancer, metastatic GIST
	Sorafenib	Metastatic renal cell carcinoma; unresectable hepatocellular carcinoma
	Sunitinib	Metastatic renal cell carcinoma; GIST after progression on imatinib; progressive pancreatic neuroendocrine tumors

TABLE 17.30: Monoclonal antibodies.

Drug	*Target*	*Common indications*	*Adverse effects*
Ado-trastuzumab emtansine	HER2-targeted antibody-drug conjugate	Metastatic breast cancer	Hepatotoxicity, pneumonitis
Alemtuzumab	CD52	T-cell prolymphocytic leukemia; relapsed or refractory B-cell CLL	Significant immunosuppression

Contd...

Contd...

Atezolizumab	PD-L1	Urothelial carcinoma and nonsmall cell lung cancer	Immune-mediated adverse events such as pneumonitis, colitis, endocrinopathies, encephalitis, etc.
Bevacizumab	VEGF	Advanced colorectal cancer, nonsquamous NSCLC, glioblastoma, cervical cancer, ovarian cancer, fallopian tube cancer, primary peritoneal carcinoma	Thromboembolism Hypertension (severe in 15%), proteinuria, bleeding (especially epistaxis or GI)
Blinatumomab	Bispecific CD19-directed CD3 T-cell engager	Philadelphia chromosome-negative relapsed or refractory B-cell precursor ALL	Cytokine release syndrome
Brentuximab vedotin (Antibody-drug conjugate)	CD30-specific chimeric IgG1 antibody	Refractory Hodgkin's lymphoma and refractory systemic anaplastic large cell lymphoma	Myelosuppression Neuropathy
Cetuximab	EGFR (HER1, ErbB-1)	Metastatic colon cancer	Severe infusion reactions characterized by rapid onset of airway obstruction, hypotension, and/or cardiac arrest
Daratumumab	CD38	Multiple myeloma	Severe infusion reactions
Dinutuximab	Qlycolipid GD2	Neuroblastoma	Severe infusion reactions, pain (severe neuropathic pain in the majority of patients; administer intravenous opioid prior to, during, and for 2 hours following completion of the infusion)
Elotuzumab	SLAMF7	Multiple myeloma	Severe infusion reactions
Ipilimumab	CTLA-4	Unresectable or metastatic melanoma	Immune-mediated adverse effects
Necitumumab	EGFR	NSCLC	Severe infusion reactions, hypomagnesemia
Nivolumab	PD-1	Unresectable or metastatic melanoma as a single agent or in combination with ipilimumab, metastatic NSCLC, advanced renal cell carcinoma, classical Hodgkin's lymphoma	Immune-mediated adverse events such as pneumonitis, colitis, endocrinopathies, encephalitis, hepatitis, nephritis
Obinutuzumab	CD20	CLL	Tumor lysis syndrome
Ofatumumab	CD20	CLL	Prolonged severe neutropenia
Panitumumab	EGFR	Metastatic colorectal cancer	Severe dermatologic toxicity
Pembrolizumab	PD-1	Metastatic melanoma, metastatic NSCLC	Immune-mediated adverse events such as pneumonitis, colitis, endocrinopathies, hepatitis, nephritis
Pertuzumab	HER2	HER2-positive metastatic breast cancer	Left ventricular dysfunction
Ramucirumab	VEGFR2	Advanced gastric or gastroesophageal junction adenocarcinoma, metastatic NSCLC, metastatic colorectal cancer	Hemorrhage and GI perforation
Rituximab	CD20	CD20-positive, B-cell NHL, CLL, rheumatoid arthritis, microscopic polyangiitis, Wegener's granulomatosis	Severe mucocutaneous reactions, serious cardiac arrhythmias
Siltuximab	IL-6	Multicentric Castleman's disease (MCD)	Infections, pruritus, weight gain
Trastuzumab	HER2	Breast cancer, stomach cancer	Cardiomyopathy

The currently approved conjugated antibodies have been shown in **Box 17.1**.

Q. Write a short note on immunosuppressive drugs.

- **These drugs inhibit cellular and/or humoral immunity response and have major role in organ transplantation and autoimmune diseases. List of immunosuppressive drugs useful in cancer management are enumerated in Box 17.2.**

Box 17.1: Conjugated antibodies.

Conjugated antibodies currently approved
- Radio-conjugated antibodies
  - Tositumomab
  - Ibritumomab
  - Both used against refractory lymphomas
- Toxin-conjugated antibody
  - Gemtuzumab ozogamicin
  - Used against AML

Box 17.2: Immunosuppressive drugs.

Immunosuppressive drugs
- Calcineurin inhibitors (specific R cell inhibitors): For example, cyclosporine, tacrolimus
- Antiproliferative drugs (cytotoxic drugs): Azathioprine, cyclophosphamide, methotrexate, chlorambucil, mycophenolate mofetil (MMF)
- Glucocorticoids: Prednisolone and others
- Antibodies: Muromonab CD3, antithymocyte globulin (ATG), Rho (D) immunoglobulin

PAIN ASSESSMENT AND MANAGEMENT

Q. Describe and assess pain and suffering objectively in a patient with cancer.

Q. Describe and enumerate the indications, use, side effects of narcotics in pain alleviation in patients with cancer.

Assessment of Pain

1. Careful pain history (site of pain, onset, acute or chronic, constant or intermittent, provoking and alleviating factors, and associated symptoms)
2. Quality of the pain (nociceptive somatic, nociceptive visceral, and neuropathic pain)
3. Impact on daily activities
4. The pain interventions already tried and their level of effectiveness
5. Screen for history of alcohol or drug dependence
6. Evaluation for depression
7. Physical examination.

Scaling of pain (Wong-Baker FACES pain rating scale) (Fig. 17.6):

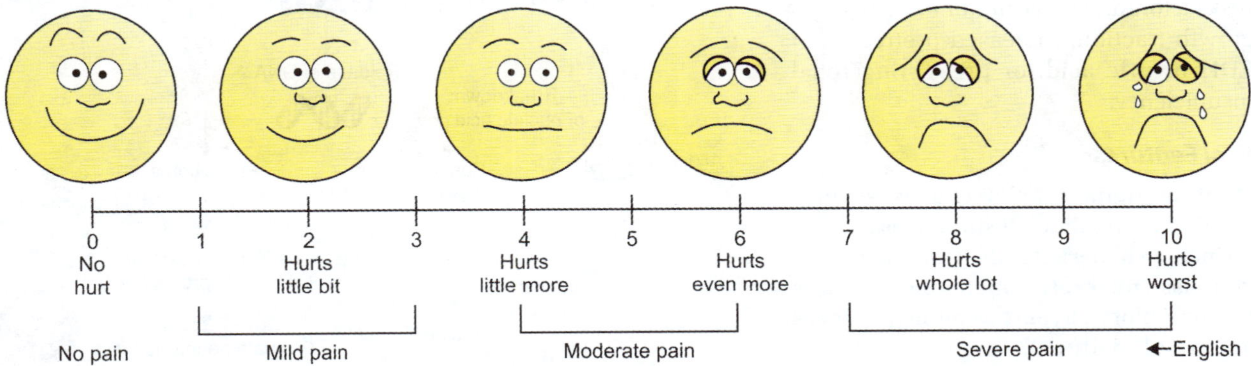

FIG. 17.6: Wong-Baker FACES pain rating scale.

Cancer Pain Management (Fig. 17.7 and Table 17.31)

Pain is a highly prevalent symptom in patients with cancer. Adequate pain relief can be achieved in 90% of patients when treatment guidelines for cancer pain are followed.

Common Side Effects of Narcotics (Opioids)

1. Gastrointestinal: Constipation, nausea, and vomiting
2. CNS: Sedation, confusion, and myoclonus
3. Urinary retention
4. Tolerance
5. Drug addiction and abuse

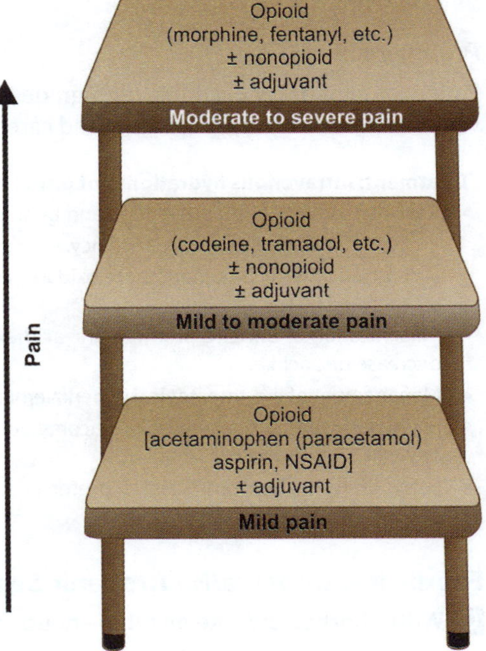

FIG.17.7: WHO pain ladder.

ONCOLOGIC EMERGENCIES

Q. Write short note on:

- **Emergency conditions related to tumors. (Table 17.32)**
- **Clinical features and treatment of tumor lysis syndrome.**

Tumor Lysis Syndrome (TLS) (Fig. 17.8)

Tumor lysis syndrome (TLS) is treatment related complication.
It can develop 1–5 days postchemotherapy treatment of leukemias and lymphomas.

- Metabolic triad of **hyperuricemia, hyperkalemia, hyperphosphatemia**.
- It can also lead to **renal failure and hypocalcemia** as secondary complications.
- It is due to release of the breakdown products of dying tumor cells. Chemotherapeutic agents cause cell lysis and cell death with release of intracellular components into the bloodstream.
- Breakdown of nucleic acid, catabolism of hypoxanthine and xanthine lead to elevated uric acid.

TABLE 17.31: Levels of pain and management.

Level of pain	Treatment recommended	Commonly used drugs
Level 1 (mild pain)	Nonopioid ± adjuvant	Acetaminophen Aspirin NSAIDs
Level 2 (mild to moderate pain)	Opioid ± nonopioid ± adjuvant	Opioids used are codeine, tramadol, etc.
Level 3 (moderate to severe pain)	Opioid ± nonopioid ± adjuvant	Opioid used are morphine, fentanyl, etc.

TABLE 17.32: Oncologic emergencies.

Metabolic or hormonal problems	Treatment related	Pressure or obstruction
➢ Hypercalcemia ➢ Syndrome of inappropriate antidiuretic hormone secretion (SIADH) ➢ Lactic acidosis ➢ Hypoglycemia ➢ Adrenal insufficiency	➢ Tumor lysis syndrome ➢ Human antibody infusion reactions ➢ Febrile neutropenia ➢ Thrombocytopenia ➢ Pulmonary infiltrates ➢ Hemorrhagic cystitis ➢ Hyperviscosity syndrome ➢ Disseminated intravascular coagulation ➢ Hypersensitivity reactions to antineoplastic drugs	➢ Superior vena cava syndrome ➢ Epidural spinal cord compression ➢ Pericardial effusion/cardiac tamponade ➢ Intestinal obstruction ➢ Urinary obstruction

- Potassium and phosphate are present at high levels in cytoplasm.
- Risk factors are: Large tumor burden, high-growth fraction, increased pretreatment LDH or uric acid, or preexisting renal insufficiency.

Clinical Features

Lysis of malignant cells causes several metabolic abnormalities/disturbances.

These include **hyperkalemia** (leads to cardiac arrhythmias), **hyperphosphatemia** (produces acute renal failure), **hyperuricemia** (produces acute renal failure), hyperuricosuria, **hypocalcemia** (results in seizures, muscle cramps, tetany, and arrhythmia), and consequent acute uric acid nephropathy and renal failure.

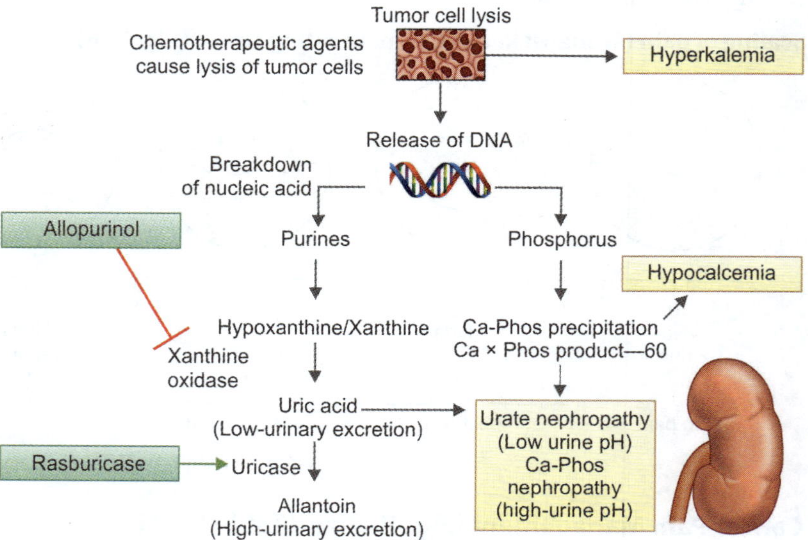

FIG. 17.8: Mechanism of tumor lysis.

Prophylaxis

Patient at high risk: Leukemia, high-grade lymphoma, rapidly proliferating bulky solid tumor (e.g., small cell) must receive vigorous prehydration, allopurinol and careful metabolic monitoring.

Treatment: Intravenous hydration is of prime importance.

- **Rasburicase** (works for prevention and treatment)
  - Contraindicated in G6PD deficiency.
  - Rasburicase (recombinant urate oxidase) converts uric acid into allantoin, which is an inactive and soluble metabolite and is easily excreted by the kidneys.
- Alkalinization of urine to promote uric acid excretion is controversial (it may worsen hypocalemic tetany). Allopurinol can be used to decrease uric acid.
- Management of life-threatening hyperkalemia with antihyperkalemic measures.
- For hypocalcemia, infuse calcium gluconate under ECG monitoring. Hyperphosphatemia can be treated by giving aluminum hydroxide orally or hemodialysis.
- Early dialysis (hemodialysis is preferred) is required when uric acid >10 mg/dL, phosphorus >10 mg/dL or creatinine >10 mg/dL.

Febrile Neutropenia/Neutropenic Sepsis/Neutropenic Fever

Q. Write short essay/note on febrile neutropenia.

- Neutropenia (decrease of neutrophils below normal range) is a common complication of malignancy. It can occur secondary to chemotherapy, radiotherapy (if large amounts of bone marrow are irradiated) or as a component of pancytopenia due to infiltration of the bone marrow by malignancy.
- Neutropenic fever is defined as a fever/pyrexia of 38.3°C for >1 hour in a patient with a neutrophil count <500/mm^3. The risk of sepsis is dependent on the severity and duration of neutropenia and the presence of other risk factors (e.g., intravenous or bladder catheters).

Clinical Features

- The typical presentation is with high fever. Neutropenic patients are prone to bacterial and fungal infection, most often from endogenous source (e.g., enteric bowel flora). Carefully examine for potential foci of infection. However, examination usually does not define the primary source of the infection. Signs and symptoms of infection may be minimal, particularly in patients receiving corticosteroids.
- Apart from fever, patients may also have nonspecific symptoms (e.g., nausea, diarrhea, drowsiness, breathlessness).
- Hypotension is a bad prognostic feature and may lead to systemic circulatory shutdown and organ failure.

Investigations

Full blood count, cultures (urine, sputum, stool depending on the case), chest X-ray, and swabs for culture (throat, central line, wound). Before antibiotic therapy, two sets of blood cultures from a peripheral vein and any indwelling venous catheters should be sent.

Treatment

Upon initial evaluation, each patient should be assessed for risk of complications from severe infection. Appropriate risk assessment may determine the type of empiric therapy (oral vs IV), duration of antibiotic therapy, and determination of inpatient versus outpatient management. Patients are classified into high-risk and low-risk groups.

Low-risk group	*High-risk group*
➢ Anticipated brief (<7-day duration) period of neutropenia ➢ ANC > 100/µL and absolute monocyte count > 100/µL ➢ Normal findings on chest radiograph ➢ Outpatient status at the time of fever onset ➢ No associated acute comorbid illness ➢ No hepatic or renal insufficiency ➢ Early evidence of bone marrow recovery	➢ Anticipated, prolonged (>7-day duration), and profound neutropenia (ANC < 100/µL) following cytotoxic chemotherapy ➢ Significant medical comorbidities, including hypotension, pneumonia, new-onset abdominal pain, or neurologic changes

- Antibiotics **(Flowchart 17.3)**.
- Antifungal: If there is no response for antibiotics after 72–96 hours, treatment with amphotericin B or voriconazole should be given to cover fungal infection.
- Growth factors: G-CSF, GM-CSF are given to improve the blood counts.
- Other supportive therapy: Patients with signs of systemic illness, such as tachycardia, hypotension, oliguria require urgent admission and resuscitation with intravenous fluids to restore circulatory function. Other supportive therapy includes inotrope therapy, ventilation or hemofiltration.

FLOWCHART 17.3: Algorithm for the antibiotic.

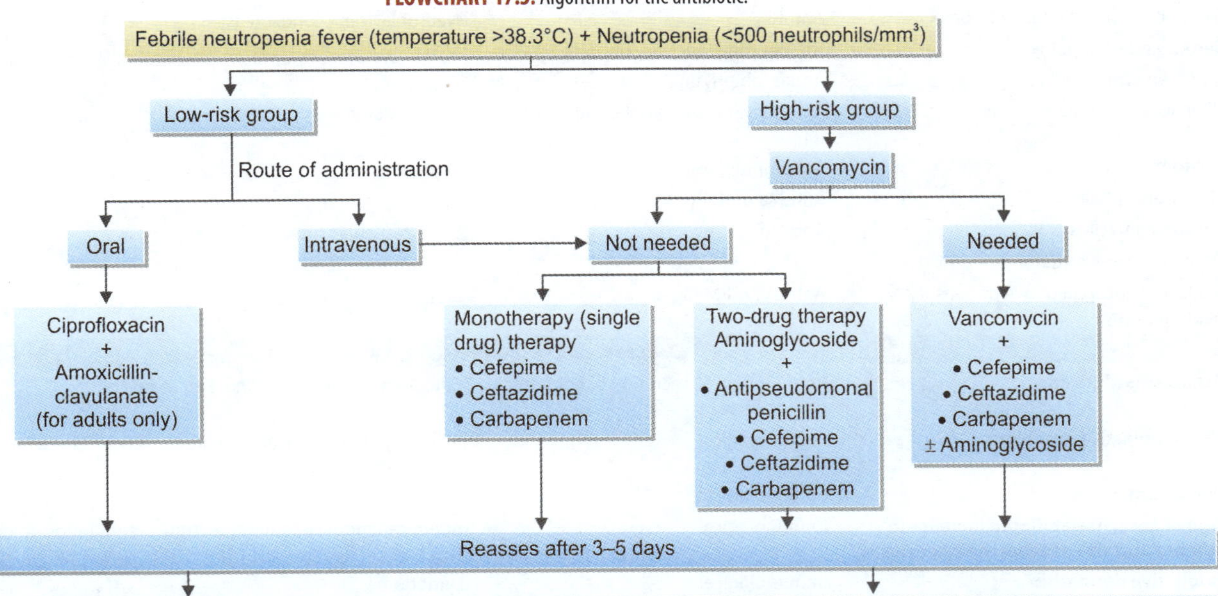

Prophylactic fluoroquinolones

- It is given to high-risk and intermediate-risk groups (consists of patients receiving high-dose chemotherapy and those with hematological malignancy) in which the anticipated duration of neutropenia is >7 days.
- Prophylactic fluoroquinolones are not indicated in patients with solid tumors undergoing standard outpatient cyclical chemotherapy in which the anticipated duration of neutropenia is <7 days, because it may lead to microbial resistance.

PARANEOPLASTIC SYNDROMES

Q. Write a short essay/note on paraneoplastic syndromes.

Definition: Paraneoplastic syndromes are **symptom complexes in cancer patients** which are **not directly related to mass effects or invasion or metastasis or by the secretion of hormones indigenous to the tissue of origin**.

Frequency: Though they occur in 10–15% of patients, it is important because:

- **May be the first manifestation** of an occult neoplasm.
- **May be mistaken for metastatic disease** leading to inappropriate treatment.
- May present clinical problems which **may be fatal**.
- Certain tumor products causing paraneoplastic syndromes may be **useful in monitoring recurrence** in patients who had surgical resections or are undergoing chemotherapy or radiation therapy.

Some paraneoplastic syndromes, their mechanism, and common cancer causing them are listed in **Table 17.33**.

TABLE 17.33: Paraneoplastic syndromes.

Clinical syndromes	*Cause/mechanism*	*Associated cancer (example)*
	1. Endocrinopathies	
Cushing's syndrome	ACTH or ACTH-like substance	Small-cell carcinoma of lung (SCLC)
Syndrome due to inappropriate antidiuretic hormone secretion	Antidiuretic hormone or atrial natriuretic hormones	Small-cell carcinoma of lung
Hypercalcemia	Parathyroid hormone-related protein (PTHRP), TGF-α, TNF, IL-1	Squamous cell carcinoma of lung
		Renal carcinoma
Carcinoid syndrome	Serotonin, bradykinin	Bronchial carcinoid
Hypoglycemia	Insulin or insulin-like substance	Fibrosarcoma
Polycythemia	Erythropoietin	Renal carcinoma, hepatocellular carcinoma
	2. Neurologic (neuromyopathic) syndromes	
Cerebellar degeneration	Anti-Yo, Anti-Tr, Anti-Ri	Ovary, breast, uterus, Hodgkin's disease, SCLC
LEMS	Antivoltage-gated calcium channel	SCLC
Opsoclonus-myoclonus syndrome	Anti-Ri	Neuroblastoma, lung, breast
Sensory neuronopathy	Antineuronal nuclear antibody-3	SCLC
Stiff-man syndrome	Antiamphiphysin	Breast, SCLC
Retinal degeneration	Antirecoverin, antibipolar cells of the retina	SCLC, melanoma
Neuromyotonia	Antiamphiphysin	Thymoma
Limbic encephalitis	Anti-Ma proteins	SCLC
Encephalomyelitis	Anti-Hu	SCLC, testicular, breast
Dermatopolymyositis	-	SCLC, others
Multifocal encephalomyelitis/sensory neuronopathy	Anti-CV2/CRMP5	Lung, uterus, ovary
	3. Cutaneous syndromes	
Acanthosis nigricans	Immunological; secretion of epidermal growth factor	Carcinoma of stomach, lung, and uterus
Paraneoplastic pemphigus	Immunological	B-cell lymphoproliferative disorders (80%), CLL, Castleman, disease, thymoma
Dermatomyositis	Immunological	Bronchogenic, breast carcinoma
Sign of Leser-Trelat (Rapid increase in number and size of seborrheic keratosis)	Immunological	Adenocarcinoma (stomach, rectum, breast, lungs, colon)
Exfoliative dermatitis	Immunological	Lymphoma
Acquired diffuse palmoplantar keratoderma (Fig. 17.9)	Immunological	Cancers of breast, lung, stomach, and leukemia
Bazex syndrome (Acrokeratosis paraneoplastica)(Fig. 17.10)	Immunological	Squamous cell carcinoma of the upper aerodigestive tract
Pityriasis rotunda	Immunological	Hepatocellular, gastric and prostate cancer, leukemia, lymphoma

Contd...

Contd...

Paget's disease		Invasive breast carcinoma
Erythema gyratum repens	Immunological	Transitional carcinoma of the kidney and adenocarcinoma of lung, breast, and esophagus
Sweet's syndrome		Leukemia
Pyoderma gangrenosum		AML, CML, myeloma
Necrolytic migratory erythema		Glucagonoma
4. Changes in osseous, articular, and soft tissue		
Hypertrophic osteoarthropathy and clubbing of the fingers	Not known	Bronchogenic carcinoma
5. Vascular and hematologic syndromes		
Venous thrombosis (Trousseau's syndrome)	Tumor products like mucins which activate clotting	Pancreatic carcinoma
		Bronchogenic carcinoma
Disseminated intravascular coagulation	Procoagulant substance: Cytoplasmic granules (e.g., acute promyelocytic leukemia cells), or mucus (adenocarcinomas)	Acute promyelocytic leukemia, prostatic adenocarcinomas
Nonbacterial thrombotic endocarditis	Hypercoagulability	Advanced mucus-secreting adenocarcinomas
6. Renal syndromes		
Nephrotic syndrome	Tumor antigens, immune complexes	Various cancers
7. Amyloidosis		
Primary amyloidosis	Immunological (AL-amyloid light chain protein)	Multiple myeloma
Secondary amyloidosis	AA (amyloid associated) protein	Renal cell carcinoma

(ACTH: adrenocorticotropic hormone; IL: interleukin; TGF: transforming growth factor; TNF: tumor necrosis factor)

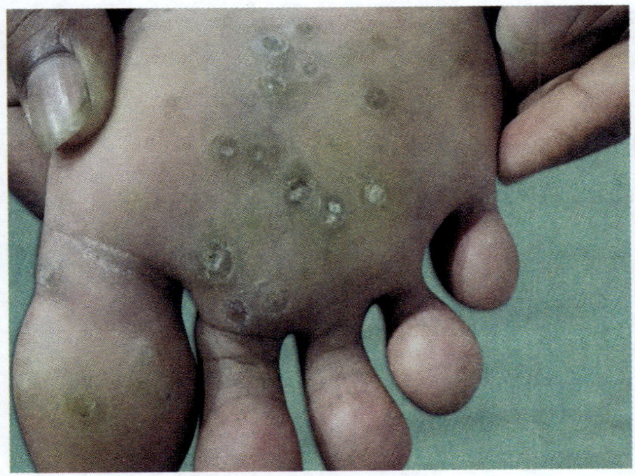

FIG. 17.9: Palmoplantar keratoderma.

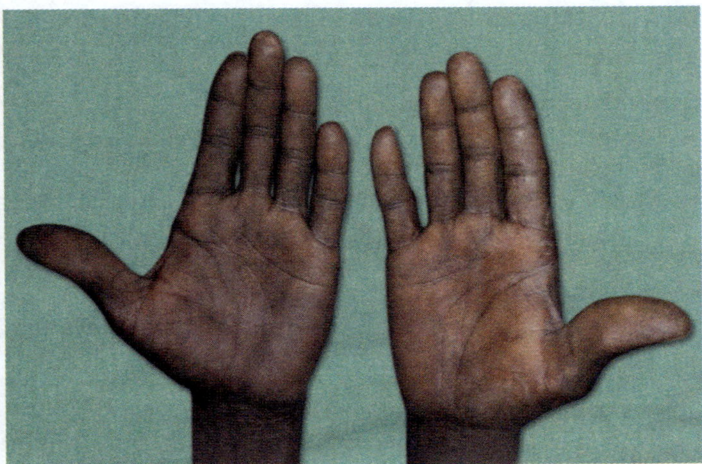

FIG. 17.10: Bazex syndrome.

CHAPTER

18

Psychiatry

Classificatory Systems in Psychiatry

	ICD-11: International Classification of Diseases	DSM-5: Diagnostic and Statistical Manual
Published by	WHO in 2018	American Psychiatric Association in 2013
Disorders included	All medical disorders in 26 chapters Psychiatric disorders classified in Chapter 6	Psychiatric disorders only

Q. Describe and discuss important signs and symptoms of common mental disorders.

Mental Status Examination (Systemic Examination in Psychiatry)

It involves the following areas:

General Appearance and Behavior

- Grooming: Note whether the patient is well-groomed or has poor hygiene, e.g., overdressed for the occasion/unkempt
- Posture (e.g., drooping of shoulders)
- Facial expressions, e.g., happy, sad, *Otto Veraguth sign* (increased forehead marking seen in depression), worried, excess perspiration, and tensed voice (signs of anxiety)
- Eye to eye contact made or not
- Attitude towards examiner (e.g., co-operative/hostile/agitated)
- Psychomotor activity: Motor execution of psychic events (e.g., restlessness/retardation)

Speech

Assess fluency, speed, volume, and tone

Example: Slow and low tone speech in depression, excessive and high tone speech in mania

Thought Abnormalities

- **Thought formation**—Is the speech coherent? Or is there loosening of association? (Suggests schizophrenia)
- **Thought possession**—Ask the patient if the thoughts are his own or if it is controlled by an external source. It can be:
  - *Thought insertion*—Someone else's thoughts are being put in one's mind.
  - *Thought withdrawal*—One's thoughts are being removed from one's mind.
  - *Thought broadcast*—Many people are getting to know one's thoughts.
- **Thought stream**—Speed: increased (flight of ideas), decreased (inhibition, slowing of thinking).
- **Thought continuity**—Perseveration (repetition beyond the point of relevance), thought block.
- **Thought content**—Determined by asking "What are your main concerns?" Look for presence of ***delusions, obsessions.***

Q. Define delusion. Give examples.

Delusion

It is a false belief held with strong conviction despite superior evidence to the contrary (strongly held false beliefs). It is a disorder of thought content.

Types of delusion:

- **Persecutory**, e.g., belief that others are out to harm me
- **Grandiose**, e.g., belief that one has special powers or status (suggests mania)

- **Nihilistic**, e.g., conviction that "My head is missing", "I have no body", "I am dead".
- **Erotomanic** delusion (e.g., believing a movie star secretly loves them)
- **Somatic** delusion (e.g., believing head is filled with air/worms—parasitosis)
- Delusion of **reference** (e.g., belief that the story in a book is referring to them)
- Delusion of **control/passivity** (e.g., believing one's thoughts and movements are controlled by aliens).
- Other delusions are delusion of jealousy/infidelity/guilt/misinterpretation/parasitosis, hypochondriacal delusion, fantastic/bizarre delusion

In contrast, ***overvalued ideas*** are strongly held but not fixed.

Q. Define obsession.

Obsessions

These are persistent, recurrent, unwanted thoughts/ideas/impulses/images that seem to invade a person's consciousness and hence cause marked anxiety/distress. Theme of obsessions can be of following types:

- *Cleanliness*: Fears of contamination
- *Symmetry and numbers*: Reading the same line for a particular number of times
- *Forbidden or taboo thoughts*: Aggressive, sexual, and religious obsessions
- *Harm* (e.g., thoughts about harm on oneself or others)

Mood and Affect

- **Mood** *(subjective long-term emotional state):* Ask the patient how he feels, e.g., sad/happy/anxious/tensed/worried
- **Affect** *(objective short-lived emotional state)* is assessed by observing facial expression, posture, movements, e.g., depressed/elated/anhedonic (inability to experience pressure from previously pleasurable activities)
- Elevated mood with excess energy and reduced need for sleep (suggests mania)
  Feeling guilty or hopeless (suggests depression). Note whether patient has thoughts of self-harm? If so, enquire about plans.
  Feeling excessively worried about many things (suggests anxiety).

Perceptual Abnormalities

Assess for presence of hallucination or illusion.

Q. Define hallucination. Give examples.

Hallucination

- It is perception in the absence of corresponding external stimuli, i.e., sensory experiences of stimuli that is not actually present. It is a disorder of thought perception.
- It can occur in any sensory modality; most common in psychiatric disorders being *auditory* (thought echo, command hallucination, running commentary) and most common in organic psychiatric disorders being *visual* (e.g., seeing "visions", Lilliputian hallucination).
- Other types include *tactile* (cocaine bug); superficial/kinesthetic/visceral, olfactory, gustatory, and complex hallucinations.
- In narcolepsy two specific hallucinations are seen. *Hypnagogic*: They occur when falling asleep. *Hypnopompic*: They occur on waking.
  Table 18.1 shows the differences between true perception, hallucination, and mental imagery.

TABLE 18.1: Differences between true perception, hallucination, and mental imagery.

	Source of stimuli	*Individual's awareness of source of stimuli*
True perception	Comes from external world	Realizes as coming from outside
True hallucination	Comes from within (one's own mind)	Considers it real and as coming from external world
Mental imagery	Comes from within	Realizes as coming from within

Pseudohallucination: Phenomenon lying in between true hallucination and mental imagery

- Hare described it as hallucination with insight
- Jasper described it as hallucination occurring in inner subjective space
- Kandensky described it as mental imagery that is clear

In contrast, **illusions** are misperceptions of real external stimuli (e.g., mistaking a shrub for a person in poor light)

Cognitive Functions

- ***Level of consciousness and alertness:*** Important in case of delirium (**Table 18.2**)
  Normal consciousness: Alert, vigilant, and lucid
- ***Orientation to time, place, and person*** (e.g., ask what time is it? Where are you now? Ability to recognize family members)

TABLE 18.2: Abnormalities of consciousness.

Quantitative	*Qualitative*
➢ Clouding ➢ Drowsy: Drifts to sleep if not actively stimulated ➢ Sopor/obtundation: Constant stimulation even for minimal response ➢ Coma: Complete unawareness, cannot be aroused	➢ Twilight: Disruption of continuity ➢ Oneiroid: Dream-like state ➢ Stupor: Akinesia + mutism in awake, alert patient ➢ Delirium: Altered sensorium

- ***Attention and concentration:*** It is assessed by serial subtraction test (100 - 7) in which the patient is asked to subtract 7 from 100 and then 7 from the answer and so on.
- ***Memory***

Q. Discuss how is memory tested clinically?

Based on length of storage of memory

- ***Registration/Immediate***: It is judged by asking the patient to repeat simple new information (e.g., name and address) **immediately** after hearing it. It is dependent on attention and concentration.
- ***Recent***: It is judged by asking the patient to repeat simple new information (as mentioned above) **after an interval of 1-2 minutes** during which time the patient's attention should be diverted elsewhere **or 24 hours recall.**
- ***Remote***: It is judged by asking the patient to recall past events (>24 hours).

Based on type of information

- ***Implicit/Procedural memory:*** It does not require conscious attention to recall (e.g., memory for procedures, skills, and habits).
- ***Explicit/Declarative memory:*** It requires conscious attention to recall. It can be further classified into **episodic memory** (for specific events and contexts) and **semantic memory** (for vocabulary and concepts).

Structure involved in memory	*Function*
Cortical:	
• Frontal lobe	Immediate and working memory
• Temporal and parietal lobe	Auditory-visual memory
• Cerebellum	Procedural memory
Subcortical:	
• Medial temporal lobe	
– Hippocampus	Consolidation: Convert short-term memories to long-term memories
– Amygdala	Emotional memories
• Diencephalic structures: Thalamus, mamillary body	Registration of memory

Intellectual Ability

It can be assessed by asking about general knowledge, calculation, and vocabulary.

Abstract Ability

It can be assessed using similarity test (e.g., What is the similarity between chair and table) and proverb test (ability to understand inner meaning of a proverb).

Judgment

It can be assessed by giving a certain test situation and asking how would the patient respond, e.g., What would you do if you found an addressed letter on road.

Insight

It refers to patients understanding of one's illness, its cause, and the need for treatment. Lack of insight, i.e., failure to accept that one is ill and/or in need of treatment and is a feature of psychotic disorders. Grading of insight described in color box.

Table 18.3 shows the mini-mental state examination.

Grading of Insight

- Grade a: Complete denial of illness
- Grade b: Slight awareness of being ill and needing help, but denying it at the same time
- Grade c: Aware of being ill, but blaming it on others, external factors or on organic factors
- Grade d: Aware of being ill, but attributing it to internal unknown factors
- Grade e: Intellectual insight—aware of being ill and that the symptoms are due to disturbance in thoughts/feelings/behavior but unable to apply this knowledge to current/future experiences
- Grade f: True emotional insight—aware of being ill and that the symptoms are due to disturbance in thoughts/feelings/behavior and also is able to apply this knowledge to bring about changes in behavior.

TABLE 18.3: Mini-mental state examination.

Component assessed	*Test score/total score*
1. Orientation: **Time**, day, date, month, year **Place**: Room/floor/building, city, district, state, country	 -/5 -/5
2. Registration: Examiner presents three names of unrelated objects that the patient is asked to repeat immediately, e.g., apple, Sunday, blue	-/3
3. Attention and calculation *Serial subtraction* of 7 from the answer starting from 100, to continue up to five steps, e.g., 93, 84, 77, 70, 63 OR Spell *WORLD backwards*, e.g., DLROW	-/5
4. Recall: Patient is asked to recall the three words given during registration assessment	-/3
5. Language: a. *Naming* any two objects (e.g., book and table) b. *Repeat the sentence* "No, ifs, ands or buts" c. *Follow a three stage command*, e.g., "Pick the paper from table, crumble it and throw in the dustbin" d. *Read and obey the command*, e.g., "Close your eyes" e. *Writing a sentence*	 -/2 -/1 -/3 -/1 -/1
6. Copy an *intersecting pentagon*	-/1
Final Score	-/30
MMSE Scoring ➢ ≥24: No cognitive impairment ➢ 18–23: Mild cognitive impairment ➢ ≤17: Severe cognitive impairment	

PSYCHOPHARMACOLOGY

Drugs used in psychiatry:

- Antipsychotics: For psychosis
- Antidepressants: For depression
- Mood stabilizers: For bipolar affective disorders
- Antianxiety drugs: For anxiety disorders

Q. Write short note on antipsychotic drugs.

Classification of Antipsychotics Drugs (Table 18.4)

Typical antipsychotics/first generation:
- Phenothiazines (chlorpromazine, perphenazine, fluphenazine, and thioridazine)
- Thioxanthenes (flupentixol and zuclopenthixol)
- Butyrophenones (haloperidol and droperidol)

Atypical antipsychotics/second generation:
- Aripiprazole, asenapine, brexpiprazole, cariprazine, clozapine, iloperidone, lurasidone, olanzapine, paliperidone, pimavanserin, quetiapine, risperidone, and ziprasidone

Mechanism of action of most first and second-generation antipsychotics: It appears to be postsynaptic blockade of brain dopamine D2 receptors. ***Exceptions:***
- Aripiprazole and brexpiprazole are D2 receptor partial agonists
  - Cariprazine is a D3-preferring D3/D2 receptor partial agonist
  - Pimavanserin is a serotonin 5HT2A inverse agonist and antagonist with no dopamine D2 affinity

Antipsychotic Drugs and their Action (Fig. 18.1)

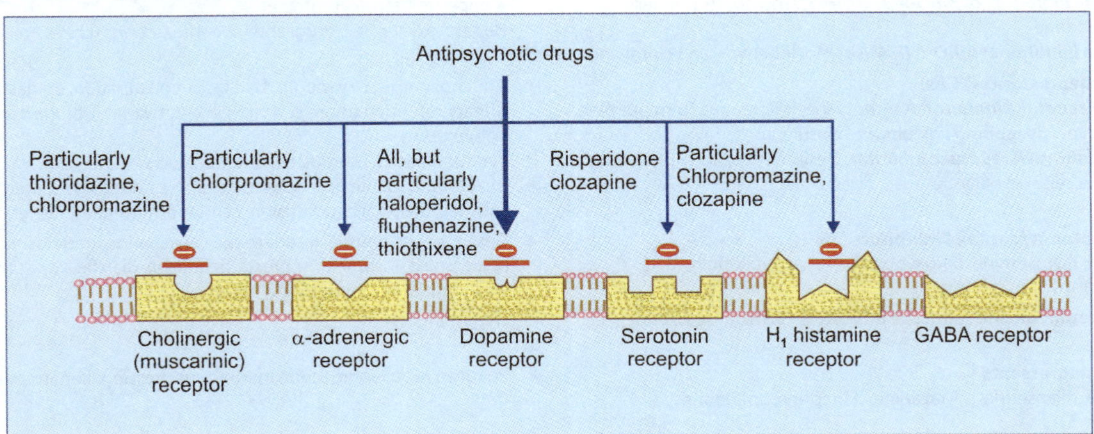

FIG. 18.1: Antipsychotic drugs and their action.

Indications

- **Psychomotor agitation:** High-potency APMs (haloperidol) parenteral.
- **Schizophrenia:** Treatment of choice for acute psychotic episodes and for prophylaxis
- **Other psychotic disorders:** Treatment of psychotic disorders due to general medical conditions and substances, delusional disorder, brief psychotic disorder, schizophreniform disorder, and other rarer psychotic disorders.
- **Mood disorders:** Treatment of agitation and psychosis during mood episodes.
- **Sedation:** Useful when benzodiazepines are contraindicated (especially in older patients) or as an adjunct during anesthesia.
- **Movement disorders:** Treatment of choice for Huntington disease and Tourette disorder.

TABLE 18.4: Differences between typical and atypical neuroleptic drugs.

	Typical neuroleptic	*Atypical neuroleptic*
Mode of action	D2 antagonist	5-HT2A antagonist D2 antagonist + Rapid D2 dissociation
Other effect	Antagonism of H1, M1, alpha-1 receptor, among other	Antagonism of H1, M1, 5-HT2c, alpha 1 receptor, among other
Effect on schizophrenia symptoms	Improvement in positive symptoms	Improvement in both positive and negative symptoms
EPS, TD, hyperprolactinemia	Pronounced	Less
Metabolic side effects	Few	Marked
Mood stabilizing property	Less	More

(EPS: extrapyramidal symptoms; TD: tardive dyskinesia)

General Adverse Effects

- **Sedation:** Due to the antihistaminic activity.
- **Hypotension:** Effect is due to alpha-adrenergic blockade and is most common with low potency antipsychotic medications.
- **Anticholinergic symptoms:** Dry mouth, blurred vision, urinary hesitancy, constipation, bradycardia, confusion, and delirium.
- **Endocrine effects:** Gynecomastia, galactorrhea, and amenorrhea (secondary to hyperprolactinemia).
- **Dermal and ocular syndromes:** Photosensitivity, abnormal pigmentation, and cataracts. Thioridazine can cause retinitis pigmentosa.

- **Cardiac conduction abnormalities:** Ziprasidone prolongs QT interval.
- **Agranulocytosis:** Clozapine
- **Movement syndromes:** Tardive dyskinesia (TD)
- **Extrapyramidal syndromes (EPS):** Newer APMs cause minimal or no EPS. Low-potency APMs (e.g., chlorpromazine, thioridazine) cause less EPS than higher-potency APMs, but has more sedative effects.
- **Metabolic syndrome:** Weight gain, diabetes, and dyslipidemia
- **Cholestatic jaundice**
- **Neuroleptic malignant syndrome**

Q. Write short note on:
- Antidepressants/newer antidepressants
- Tricyclic antidepressants
- Selective serotonin reuptake inhibitors (SSRIs)

Table 18.5 shows the various types of antidepressants and their side effects.

TABLE 18.5: Various types of antidepressants and their side effects.

Group and drug	*Side effects*
Monoamine oxidase (MAO) inhibitors ➢ ***Irreversible inhibitors of MAO-A and B:*** Isocarboxazide, phenelzine, tranylcypromine ➢ ***Reversible inhibitor of MAO-A (RIMA)s:*** Moclobemide and clorgyline	➢ ↑ appetite (phenelzine) ➢ ↓ appetite (tranylcypromine) ➢ Hepatotoxicity, SLE, drug, and food interactions (cheese reaction)
Tricyclic antidepressants (TCAs) ➢ ***NA + 5 HT reuptake inhibitor***: Amitriptyline, imipramine, trimipramine, clomipramine, doxepin, dothiepin, and dosulepin ➢ ***Predominantly NA reuptake inhibitor***: Desipramine, nortriptyline, amoxapine, reboxetine	➢ Anticholinergic: Dry mouth, bad taste, constipation, epigastric fullness, urinary retention (more common in elderly male), blurred vision, and palpitation ➢ Sedation, mental confusion, and weakness ➢ Increased appetite and weight, sweating, fine tremors, precipitation of seizures, postural hypotension, cardiac arrhythmias, rashes, and jaundice
Selective serotonin reuptake inhibitors (SSRIs) ➢ Fluoxetine, fluvoxamine, paroxetine, sertraline, citalopram, and escitalopram	➢ Gastric upset, nausea, interfere with ejaculation, nervousness, restlessness, insomnia, anorexia, headache, diarrhea, epistaxis, ecchymosis, and serotonin syndrome
Selective norepinephrine reuptake inhibitors (SNRIs): Duloxetine, venlafaxine	➢ Hypertension
Atypical antidepressants ➢ Trazodone, mianserine, mirtazapine, tianeptine, amineptine, and bupropion	➢ Priapism (trazodone), bone marrow suppression, hepatotoxicity
NMDA (glutamate) antagonists: Ketamine	➢ Psychosis

Serotonin Syndrome

- Life-threatening condition associated with increased serotonergic activity in the central nervous system most often due to SSRI overdose.
- Symptoms are diaphoresis, tachycardia, hyperthermia, hypertension, vomiting, diarrhea, tremor, muscle rigidity, myoclonus, hyperreflexia, and bilateral Babinski sign.
- Treatment involves stopping of all serotonergic agents, supportive care to normalize vital signs, hyperthermia and autonomic instability, sedation with benzodiazepines, and administration of serotonin antagonists (Cyproheptadine).

Cheese Reaction

- Cheese, beer, wine, meat, fish, yeast (contain large amount of tyramine and other indirectly acting amines) → these escape degradation in intestinal wall and liver due to irreversible block of MAO → reach to circulation and displace large amount of noradrenaline from loaded nerves → hypertensive crises (CVA, encephalopathy)
- Treatment: IV phentolamine, prazosin

If antidepressants are given for bipolar depression, they should be combined with a mood-stabilizing drug (mentioned below) to avoid "switching" the patients into (hypo) mania.

Mood-stabilizing Agents

They help in bringing the mood back to normal.

The main drugs consist of lithium, sodium valproate, divalproex, and carbamazepine. Others include lamotrigine, gabapentin, topiramate, olanzapine, quetiapine, and risperidone.

Q. Write short note on lithium and its side effects.

Lithium (Lithium Carbonate)

Indications

- It is the first-line medication for the treatment of mania.
- It is used for both treatment and prophylaxis of mood episodes in bipolar affective disorder.

- Adjunctive treatment of resistant depression in combination with tricyclic antidepressants.
- Treatment of schizoaffective disorders.
- It has antisuicidal properties.
- Other uses: Cluster headache, gout, ulcerative colitis, and neutropenia.

Mechanism of action

- Lithium partly replaces sodium and is nearly equally distributed in and outside the cell: This affects ionic fluxes across the brain cells.
- It decreases the release of NA and DA without affecting 5 HT release.
- It inhibits hydrolysis of inositol monophosphate.

It has a narrow therapeutic range. Hence, a regular blood monitoring is needed to maintain a plasma level of **0.6–1.2 mmol/L.**

Side effects

- **Dose-related: Tremor, convulsions,** gastrointestinal distress (nausea, vomiting), and headache.
- **Acne and weight gain:** Long-term use may result in weight gain, interfere with patient compliance and exacerbate psoriasis.
- **Cardiac conduction:** Prolonged **QRS, heart blocks, T wave inversions,** and ECG changes usually benign.
- **Hypothyroidism, nephrogenic diabetes insipidus,** increased calcium and parathormone, and renal failure.
- Teratogenicity: Associated with **Ebstein's anomaly**, and should not be given during the first trimester of pregnancy.
- Leukocytosis: Usually occurs and seems to be benign.

Divalproex

- Treatment of choice for rapid-cycling bipolar disorder, or when lithium cannot be used.
- Time course of treatment response is similar to lithium.
- **Side effects:** Sedation, cognitive impairment, tremor, GI distress, and hepatotoxicity.
- **Teratogenicity:** Associated with **spina bifida**.

Carbamazepine

- Second-line choice for treatment of bipolar disorder when **Lithium** and **Divalproex** are ineffective or contraindicated.
- **Side effects: Agranulocytosis** hematologic toxicity, hyponatremia, and hepatotoxicity.

Gabapentin

Q. Write short note on gabapentin.

This lipophilic GABA derivative crosses to the blood brain-barrier and enhances GABA release but does not act as agonist at GABA receptor. It is used primarily to treat focal seizures and neuropathic pain, and can also be used for bipolar disorders.

Sodium Valproate and Olanzapine

- They can be used both as prophylaxis in bipolar disorder, and as second-line alternative to lithium.
- **Side effects:** Valproate can cause birth defects and, hence, should not be given to women of child-bearing age. Olanzapine can produce weight gain.

Anxiolytic (Antianxiety) Medications (Table 18.6)

Q. Write short notes on anxiolytic (antianxiety) medications.

TABLE 18.6: Antianxiety drugs.

Benzodiazepine	*Azapirones*	*Others*
• Clonazepam • Alprazolam • Lorazepam • Nitrazepam • Diazepam • Oxazepam • Chlordiazepoxide	• Buspirone • Gepirone • Ipsapirone	• Beta blocker: Propranolol • Antihistaminics: Hydroxyzine • SSRIs and other antidepressant drugs

Indications for anxiolytic (antianxiety) medications:

- Panic disorder: Alprazolam, SSRIs, imipramine, and clonazepam decrease frequency and intensity
- Generalized anxiety disorder: Venlafaxine, other SSRIs, and buspirone decrease overall anxiety
- Social phobia: SSRIs and buspirone decrease fear associated with social situations
- Adjustment disorder with anxious mood: Benzodiazepines with supportive psychotherapy
- Obsessive compulsive disorder: SSRIs and clomipramine decrease obsession thinking

Features of Benzodiazepines:

- Mechanism: Bind to specific CNS receptors that modulate **GABA** transmission
- Commonly used for the treatment of anxiety, insomnia, and for alcohol withdrawal symptoms
- First choice for **emergency treatment of acute anxiety and severe mania**
- **Alprazolam** is the first choice for **panic attack**
- **Chlordiazepoxide** is used for prevention of **alcohol withdrawal**
- Benzodiazepines that do not interact with **P450: lorazepam, oxazepam,** and **temazepam**
- **Zolpidem:** Used in initial insomnia-t ½ 2–3 hours. Side effects include headache, nausea, dry mouth, etc.
- **Zopiclone:** Also acts on GABA receptors, and has short duration of action
- **Suredone, bretazenil, imidazenil, alpidem, and abecarnil:** Anxiolytic as well as anticonvulsant

Adverse effects:

- Sedation, disinhibition, tolerance, withdrawal, abuse potential, and possible teratogenicity
- Impairment of cognitive and motor performance

Features of Buspirone:

- It is used for the treatment of generalized anxiety disorder and social phobia
- Lag time of about **1 week** before clinical response
- **No additive effect** with **alcohol** or **sedative-hypnotics**
- No withdrawal syndrome
- No sedation or cognitive impairment
- Headache may occur

ELECTROCONVULSIVE THERAPY

Q. Write short note on electroconvulsive therapy.

Electroconvulsive therapy (ECT) is a procedure in which electrical stimuli is used to induce seizures.

Procedure for Modern ECT

- Obtain written informed consent
- Preanesthetic work-up
- Withholding drugs that can raise seizure threshold, NPO for 12 hours prior to procedure
- Premedication with anticholinergics to decrease secretions
- Administration of muscle relaxant (to prevent trauma to muscles and bones) and short-acting anesthetic agent
- **Electrode placement:** Electrodes are placed at the temporal fossa, 2.5–4 cm (1–1.5 inches) above the line joining the tragus of the ear and the lateral canthus of the eye.
- A brief electrical stimulus is delivered and seizure activity is noted mechanically via isolated limb and electrically via EEG.

Types of electroconvulsive therapy (ECT):

- **Direct:** ECT without general anesthesia which has been prohibited and hence not practised
- **Modified:** Use general anesthesia and muscle relaxants
- **Unilateral ECT:** Right unilateral (RUL) has less cognitive effect, may be less clinically effective
- **Bilateral ECT:** Most common, most effective, most cognitive dysfunction

Mechanism of Action

Alteration in levels of neurotransmitters, neuromodulators, e.g., increase in brain-derived natriuretic factor (BDNF).

Indications

Q. Write short note on indications for ECT.

- **Severe depression:** When a rapid antidepressant response is needed (e.g., due to failure to eat or drink in depressive stupor; high suicide risk), previous history of good response to ECT, patient preference, and suicidal ideas.
- **Failure to respond to drug treatments** or patient is not able to tolerate side effects of drugs (e.g., puerperal depressive disorder or postpartum psychosis.
- **Catatonic schizophrenia**
- **Resistant OCD**
- **Neuroleptic malignant syndrome**
- **Intractable seizure**
- **Parkinson's disease (rigidity, bradykinesia)**

Contraindications

- **Absolute:** None
- **Relative:**
  - Increased intracranial pressure (ICP)
  - Cardiovascular diseases: Recent MI, coronary artery disease, hypertension, aneurysms, and arrhythmias
  - Cerebrovascular disease: Recent strokes, space-occupying lesions, and aneurysms
  - Severe pulmonary diseases: Tuberculosis, pneumonia, and asthma
  - Deep vein thrombosis (DVT)
  - High risk pregnancy

- **Risks and side effects:** ECT is safe with few side effects.
  - Impairment of cognition: Period of confusion immediately after ECT and generally lasts for few minutes to several hours.
  - Memory loss: May forget weeks/months before treatment, during treatment, or after treatment has stopped. Usually improves within a couple of months. Permanent loss of memory is rare.
  - Myalgia, dislocation, and fractures
  - Medical complications: Nausea, vomiting, headache, aspiration, and jaw pain.

Q. Write short note on types of psychotherapy.

PSYCHOTHERAPY

It mainly can be classified into three types:

Supportive

- It focusses on enhancing stress coping mechanisms and strengthening defenses to bring about emotional equilibrium.
- There is no cause finding or an intent to change the personality.
- It is used in the management of adjustment disorder.

Reconstructive

- It focuses on finding out the root cause of a problem in personality and attempts at personality reconstruction.
- Based on Sigmund Freud's principles of psychoanalysis: Making the patient aware of repressed unconscious conflicts, teaching them skills for better personality development
- Classical psychoanalysis and brief psychodynamic therapy are the two types
- It is less commonly used in the current days.

Re-educative

- It focusses on modifying patients' thinking (cognitive), behavior or both (combined)
- It aims at restructuring cognitive distortions with no much emphasis on cause finding and has been given specific names based on methods used, such as:
  - ***Systematic desensitization*** in phobia and OCD where in systematic exposure to phobic stimuli is done followed by use of relaxation techniques to desensitize the patient. It is based on the principle of exposure decreases fear and avoidance increases fear.
  - ***Graded exposure and response prevention*** in phobia and OCD: It is similar to systematic desensitization; however, no relaxation techniques are used.
  - ***Cognitive behavior therapy*** for depression wherein negative schemas, cognitive distortions 7 automatic thoughts are addressed.
  - ***Eye-movement desensitization reprocessing*** is used for PTSD.
  - ***Aversive therapy*** used in paraphilias, wherein aversive stimuli is applied to decrease the undesired behavior.

TABLE 18.7: Differentiating between psychosis and neurosis.

	Psychosis	*Neurosis*
Insight/Reality contact/ Illness awareness	Absent	Present
Delusions/hallucinations	Present	Absent
Neurotransmitter involved	Dopamine	Serotonin
Pharmacotherapy of choice	Antipsychotics	Selective serotonin reuptake inhibitor
Interpersonal behavior	Marked disturbance	Preserved
Empathy	Absent	Present
Examples	Schizophrenia	Anxiety, phobia, depression

CLINICAL PSYCHIATRY: APPROACH TO DIAGNOSIS IN PSYCHIATRY

Q. Write short essay on differences between psychosis and neurosis.

See **Table 18.7.**

PSYCHOSIS (FIG. 18.2)

- Psychosis is a symptom or feature of mental illness characterized by radical changes in personality, impaired functioning, and thoughts that are distorted or nonexistent.
- It is an abnormal condition of the mind described as involving a **'loss of contact with reality'**.
- Psychosis is not pathognomonic of psychiatric disorder. It is a nonspecific cluster of signs and symptoms that may occur in medical, neurologic, and surgical disorders or as a

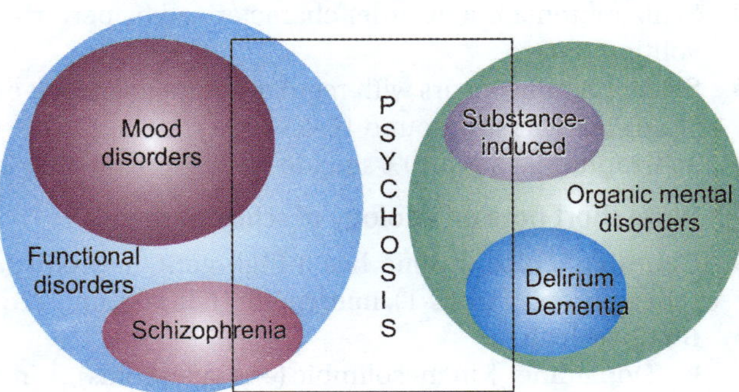

FIG. 18.2: Relationship of various psychological disorders.

consequence of pharmacologic treatment, substance abuse, or the withdrawal of drugs and alcohol.
- **Classification of psychoses:** Organic or functional:
  - **Organic psychotic disorders** are caused by structural defects or physiologic dysfunction of the brain, e.g., brain tumor.
  - **Functional disorders** have no identifiable cause, e.g., schizophrenia or bipolar disorder.
- **Lack of insight** refers to failure to accept that one is ill and/or in need of treatment and is characteristic of acute psychosis.
- Specific psychotic symptoms include delusions, hallucinations, ideas of reference, and disorders of thought.

TABLE 18.8: Differentiating between functional and organic psychosis.

	Functional psychosis	*Organic psychosis*
Demonstrable underlying **cause**	Absent	Present
Predominant type of **hallucination**	Auditory	Visual
Sensorium	Intact	Altered
Onset	Gradual	Acute
Focal neurological deficit	Usually absent	Usually present
Example	Schizophrenia	Delirium

Q. Write short essay on distinction between an organic and functional psychosis.

Table 18.8 shows the differentiation between functional and organic psychosis.

Functional psychosis can be affective or nonaffective **(Table 18.9)**. **Table 18.10** shows the differences between schizophrenia and delusional disorders.

TABLE 18.9: Differences between nonaffective and affective psychosis.

	Nonaffective psychosis	*Affective psychosis*
Mood symptoms	Not predominant	Predominant
Includes	➢ Schizophrenia ➢ Delusional disorder	➢ Bipolar disorder ➢ Schizoaffective disorder

TABLE 18.10: Differentiating between schizophrenia and delusional disorder.

	Schizophrenia	*Delusional disorder*
Delusions	Present	Present
Hallucinations	Present	Absent
Behavior	Abnormal	Normal
Socio-occupational functioning	Impaired	Intact

Based on **duration of symptoms schizophrenia-like disorders** can be further differentiated as:
- <1 month: Acute and transient psychotic disorder/brief psychotic disorder
- 1–6 months: Schizophreniform disorder
- >6 months: Schizophrenia

Affective psychosis can be further differentiated as **(Table 18.11)**:

TABLE 18.11: Differences between bipolar and schizophreniform disorders.

	Bipolar disorder	*Schizophreniform disorder*
Episodes	Mania/depression ± Psychosis (Psychotic symptoms; delusions are usually mood congruent)	Mania/depression + Psychosis
Intervening period	Normal	Psychotic symptoms always present

PSYCHOTIC DISORDERS

Psychotic disorders were also called as:
- Demence Precoce: Benedict Morel
- Dementia Praecox, Manic depressive illness: Emil Kraeplin
- Eugene Bleuler coined the term schizophrenia

SCHIZOPHRENIA

Q. Write short essay/note on schizophrenia.

- Schizophrenia is a disorder characterized by perturbations of language, perception, thinking, social activity, affect, and volition.
- Schizophrenia occurs with regular frequency nearly everywhere in the world in **1% of population** and begins mainly in young age (mostly around 16–25 years).
- Schizophrenia has a 10% suicide rate (approximately one-third attempt suicide).

Q. Write short note on etiology of schizophrenia.

- **Genetic:** Schizophrenia has a high genetic predisposition, involving many susceptibility genes, e.g., disrupted in schizophrenia (DISC-1), neuregulin (NRG-1), and 22q deletion.
- **Biochemical:**
  - Dopamine: ↑ in mesolimbic (+ve symptoms), ↓ in mesocortical (–ve symptoms)
  - Serotonin increase: Responsible for +ve and –ve symptoms
  - Norepinephrine decrease: Responsible for –ve symptoms

- **Neuropathological:** ↑ size of ventricles, ↓ size of limbic system, basal ganglia
- **Environmental:** Maternal exposure to infection (influenza, rubella), advanced paternal age, winter birth, urban birth and upbringing, stressful life events, cannabis use, obstetric complications, and developmental abnormalities.
- **Abnormal family dynamics:** Negative expressed emotions in family lead to early relapse.
- **Psychological stresses:** Episodes of acute schizophrenia may be precipitated by social stress, adverse life events, and cannabis (which increase dopamine turnover and sensitivity).
- ***Schizophrenia syndrome***: It is characterized by temporal lobe epilepsy, Huntington's chorea, cerebral tumors, and demyelinating diseases. This is known as **symptomatic schizophrenia**.

Q. Write short essay/note on clinical features of schizophrenia.

DSM-5 diagnostic criteria for schizophrenia: Patient must have at least two of five symptoms for 6 months, with at least 1-month of active symptoms.

Table 18.12 shows the positive and negative symptoms of schizophrenia.

TABLE 18.12: Positive and negative symptoms of schizophrenia.

Positive symptoms	*Negative symptoms*
➢ **Delusions** ➢ **Hallucinations** ➢ **Disorganized/bizarre behavior:** Aggressive/agitated, odd clothing or appearance, odd social behavior, and repetitive stereotyped behavior ➢ **Disorganized thought/speech:** Loosening of association, formal thought disorders, neologisms, and conceptual disorganization	➢ **Alogia:** "Lack of words," including poverty of speech and of speech content in response to a question ➢ **Affective flattening/blunting:** Lack of expressive gestures ➢ **Alexithymia**: Inability to describe and express emotions ➢ **Avolition:** Loss of drive ➢ **Apathy:** Lack of concern ➢ **Anhedonia:** Loss of interest in previously pleasurable activities ➢ **Asociality**: Diminished social engagement, few friends, activities, interests; impaired intimacy ➢ **Attention impairment**

Q. Write short note on Eugen Bleuler's criteria for the diagnosis of schizophrenia.

***Eugene Bleuler's 4A's/primary symptoms of schizophrenia*:**

1. **Autism**: Self-absorbed, totally engrossed in own thoughts, not concerned of external stimuli
2. **Association loosening**: Loss of logical sequence of thought, disconnected thoughts
3. **Ambivalence**: Inability to choose between 2 opposite *thoughts* (Ambitendency: Inability to choose between 2 opposite *action*, do/do not)
4. **Affective blunting**/(Snap prop): Decreased expression of feelings

TABLE 18.13: Kurt Schneider's 11 first rank symptoms of schizophrenia.

3 Thought phenomenon 1. Thought insertion 2. Thought withdrawal 3. Thought broadcasting **3 Made phenomenon** 1. Made impulse 2. Made volition 3. Made affect	**3 Disorders of perception;** auditory hallucinations 1. 1st person (Thought Echo) 2. 2nd person (Command Hallucination) 3. 3rd person (Running commentary) **2 Special phenomenon** 1. Somatic passivity 2. Delusional perception

Q. Write short note on Schneider's first rank symptoms of schizophrenia.

See **Table 18.13.**

Q. Write short note on subtypes of schizophrenia.

Major Subtypes of Schizophrenia

1. **Paranoid schizophrenia:**
   - Most common type of schizophrenia, has good prognosis
   - Predominant features include: Delusions and hallucinations that are persecutory/grandiose or of reference/control
2. **Disorganized (Hebephrenic) schizophrenia:**
   - Predominant features of disorganization of behavior, speech, affect, volition
   - Marked thought disorder, incoherence, loosening of associations
   - Emotional disturbances—blunted effect, and **senseless giggling**
3. **Catatonic schizophrenia** has marked disturbance of motor behaviors:

   Clinical forms:
   - Excited catatonia: Increase in psychomotor activity (restlessness, agitation, excitement aggressiveness) and increase in speech production
   - Stuporous (retarded) catatonia: Extreme retardation of psychomotor function
   - Catatonia alternating between excitement and stupor: Features of both the above forms
4. **Simple schizophrenia:** Has predominant negative symptoms
5. **Schizophrenia undifferentiated type:** Meets criteria for schizophrenia. Do not meet criteria for other schizophrenia types.

Note: *Subtyping of schizophrenia has been removed in DSM-5/ICD-11 versions*

ICD-11 Course Specifiers for Schizophrenia

- 1st episode: No past episodes
- Multiple episodes: At least 1 past episode with significant remission of symptoms between current and last episode
- Continuous: No remission of symptoms, illness present for >1 year

Typical **stages** of schizophrenia: Prodromal phase, active phase, and residual phase **(Table 18.14)**.

TABLE 18.14: Types of schizophrenia.

Characteristic	*Type I*	*Type II*
Predominant symptoms	Positive	Negative
Onset	Acute	Insidious
Premorbid functioning	Good	Poor
Cognition	Intact	Impaired
Changes in brain	Increased dopamine in mesolimbic pathway	Ventriculomegaly on CT
Reversibility	Reversible	Irreversible
Response to treatment with antipsychotics	Good	Poor
Prognosis	Good	Poor

Investigation of schizophrenia

- Full neurological examination: Gait and motor
- Cognitive examination: MMSE
- Blood: Complete blood count, liver function tests, renal function tests, thyroid functions tests, and glucose
- Urine drug screen
- EEG if suspicion of temporal lobe epilepsy
- Brain imaging findings:
  - CT: Lateral and third ventricular enlargement, reduction in cortical volume
  - MRI: Increased cerebral ventricles
  - PET: Hypoactivity of the frontal lobes

Q. Write short essay on management/treatment of schizophrenia/psychosis.

Management of schizophrenia

Hospital admission is necessary for a first episode to permit a full physical and psychiatric assessment.

Indications for hospital admission

Indications include suicidal tendencies, violent behavior, severe psychosis, severe depression, catatonic schizophrenia, noncompliance and failure of outpatient treatment.

Drug treatment

Antipsychotics (atypicals preferred) + Benzodiazepines is the mainstay in acute phase of treatment.

Psychological treatment

It is an essential component of management in maintenance phase of treatment.

- Psychoeducation can prevent relapse by enhancing insight.
- Cognitive remediation to challenge delusions.
- Social skill training: Improve relationship.
- Behavioral: Positive reinforcement of desirable behavior.
- Family therapy: To reduce expressed emotion (EE). (High EE include hostility, over involvement, critical comments from family; hence reduce relapse rate).

Social treatment

- After the control of an acute episode of schizophrenia, social rehabilitation may be needed.
- Patients with chronic schizophrenia may need long-term, supervised accommodation.

Other treatments

- Rehabilitation to enhance self-care, compliance and insight.
- ECT (electroconvulsive therapy) is for catatonic schizophrenia.

Prognosis

- **Rules of quarters:** Complete remission (25%), good recovery (25%), partial recovery (25%), and downhill course (25%).
- **Good prognostic factors:** Late onset, female gender, married, and presence of precipitating event

OTHER PSYCHOTIC DISORDERS

Schizophreniform Disorder (>1 Month but <6 Months)

- **Presenting symptoms:** Same as in schizophrenia (hallucinations, delusions, disorganized speech, grossly disorganized or catatonic behavior, negative symptoms, social and/or occupational dysfunction).
- **Difference from schizophrenia:** Symptoms are present > 1 month but < 6 months and most of the patients return to their baseline level of functioning.

Treatment

- Must assess whether the patient needs hospitalization, to assure safety of patient and/or others.
- Antipsychotic medication is indicated for a 3–6-month course.
- Individual psychotherapy

Schizoaffective Disorder

- **Presenting symptoms:** Mood disorders (major depressive episode, manic episode, or mixed episode) + psychosis (schizophrenia).
- Delusions or hallucinations for at least 2 weeks in the absence of mood symptoms.
- **Prognosis:** Better prognosis than patients with schizophrenia. Worse prognosis than patients with affective (mood) disorders.

Treatment

Antidepressant medications and/or anticonvulsants to control the mood/symptoms. If these are not effective, consider the use of antipsychotic medications to help control the ongoing symptoms.

MOOD DISORDERS

Q. Write short essay on:
- **Mood/affective disorders and its classification.**
- **Bipolar affective disorders.**

- Mood or affective disorders are among the most common diagnoses in psychiatry.
- Mood refers to a pervasive and sustained emotional state (as differentiated from affect, which is immediately expressed and observed emotion).
- Mood disorders are characterized by a disturbance of mood and behavior.
- It can either be unipolar (depression/mania) or bipolar.

Categories/Classification of Mood Disorder (Table 18.15 and Fig. 18.3)

- **Unipolar depression:** Only one end of the emotion spectrum and characterized by one or more episodes of low mood and associated symptoms (depression form).
- **Dysthymic disorder:** Characterized by chronic low-grade depressed mood without sufficient other symptoms to count as "clinically significant" or "major" depression.
- **Bipolar disorder:** Cycling between both ends of the emotion spectrum and characterized by episodes of elevated mood interspersed with episodes of depression (both manic and depression).

Mood (affective) disorders can be classified into **primary and secondary**.
- In **primary** affective disorder, the affective episodes (mania or depression) are **not secondary to any other psychiatric** or physical illness.
- In **secondary** affective disorder, the affective episodes **are secondary to another psychiatric or physical illness.**

TABLE 18.15: Classification of mood disorder.

Unipolar	*Bipolar*	*Mood disorders with known etiology*
Major depressive disorder	Bipolar I disorder	Substance-induced mood disorder
Dysthymic disorder	Bipolar II disorder	Mood disorder due to general medical condition
	Cyclothymic disorder	Depression, mania, bipolar disorders, depression—affect, mood, and syndrome

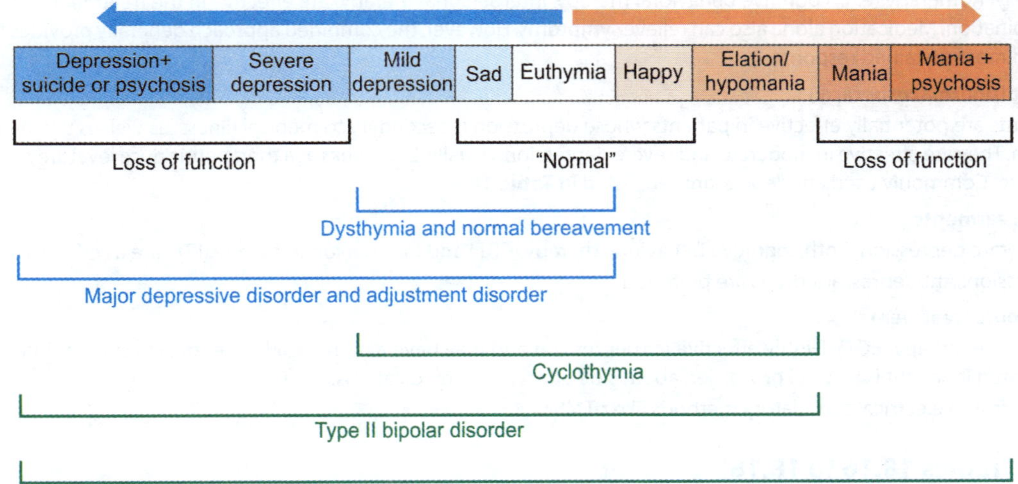

FIG. 18.3: Spectrum of mood disorder.

Unipolar Depression/Major Depressive Disorder

Q. Write short essay/note on depression, its clinical features and management.

- Depressive disorders are characterized by persistent low mood, loss of interest, and reduced energy that usually impairs day-to-day functioning.
- It is more common in middle-aged females.
- **Number of episodes:**
    - ***Single episode*** of major depression.
    - ***Recurrent:*** Two or more episodes of major depression.
    - ***Persistent depressive disorder*** (dysthymia): Low mood persisting for more than 2 years
- Risk of suicide in an individual with a depressive disorder is 10 times more than that in the general population.

Etiology

- ***Trimonoaminergic depletion***: Reduced levels of serotonin, epinephrine, and dopamine are seen in depression
- ***HPA axis dysfunction:*** Evident through blunted response to dexamethasone suppression test
- ***Hypothyroidism***
- ***Pathology of left side of the brain:*** Predominantly involving prefrontal cortex, amygdala, hippocampus, and anterior cingulate cortex
- ***Aaron T Beck's cognitive triad of depression:*** Negative thoughts about self (worthlessness), environment (helplessness), and future (hopelessness)

Major depressive disorder is characterized by one or more major episodes of depression **(Box 18.1)**.

Q. Write short note on reactive depression.

Reactive depression is a type of clinical depression that is precipitated by events in the individuals life (to be differentiated from normal grief) arising as a consequence of severe traumatic events in life (e.g., the loss of home in a fire). Reactive depression becomes a clinical concern if the depression lasts too long without signs of recovery or if the depression becomes too deep (e.g., leading to suicidal feelings). Most of the time, reactive depression resolves itself.

Melancholic/endogenous depression:

- Depression that occurs in the absence of external life stressors
- Mostly seen in elderly
- Characterized by severe anhedonia, severe vegetative symptoms (early morning awakening, decreased appetite), profound guilt, and suicidal thoughts

Box 18.1: Diagnostic criteria for major depressive episode.

General criteria for a major depressive episode require five or more of the below symptoms to be present for at least 2 weeks; one symptom must be ***depressed mood or loss of interest or pleasure.*** *The symptoms must also cause* ***distress or impairment.***

- **Mood:** Depressed mood most of the day, nearly every day (dysphoria)
- **Interest:** Marked decrease in interest and pleasure in most activities (anhedonia)
- **Energy:** Fatigue or low energy nearly everyday
- **Concentration:** Decreased concentration or increased indecisiveness
- **Sleep:** Insomnia or hypersomnia
- **Appetite:** Increased or decreased appetite or weight gain or loss
- **Psychomotor:** Psychomotor agitation or retardation
- **Guilt:** Feelings of worthlessness or inappropriate guilt
- **Suicidality:** Recurrent thoughts of death, suicidal ideation, suicidal plan, and suicide attempt

Treatment of depression

Both drug and psychotherapy (e.g., cognitive behavioral therapy, interpersonal therapy) are effective in the treatment of depression either alone or in combination. Medication alone also can relieve symptoms. However, the combined approach generally provides the patient with the quickest and most sustained response.

Drug treatment (pharmacotherapy)

All antidepressants are potentially effective in patients whose depression is secondary to medical illness, as well as those in whom it is the primary problem. They are effective in moderate and severe depression. Usually, 2–6 weeks at a therapeutic dose level are needed to observe a clinical response. Commonly used antidepressants are listed in **Table 18.5**.

Psychological treatments

- Mild-to-moderate depression: Both cognitive behavioral therapy (CBT) and interpersonal therapy (IPT) are as effective.
- Severe depression: Antidepressant drugs are preferred.

Nonpharmacologic treatments

- Electroconvulsive therapy (ECT): Highly effective for depression and may have a more rapid onset of action than drug treatments. ECT may be indicated if patient is suicidal or worried about side effects from medications.
- Other magnetic and electrical stimulatory methods like r-TMS

Acute Mania (Tables 18.16 to 18.18)

Q. Write short essay/note on clinical features of mania.

Mania is an abnormally elevated mood state.

TABLE 18.16: Clinical features of acute mania.

Changes in mood	Changes in speech	Changes in thinking	Changes in perceptions
Cheerfulness, irritability, excitability, exhilaration, hostility, anxious	Rapid, pressured speech, talkativeness, clang associations	Distractibility, flight of ideas, creative/disjointed/racing/expansive thoughts	Inflated self-esteem, feeling superior, hallucinations, paranoia
Increased energy and activity Little fatigue despite decreased need for sleep, increased productivity, doing several things at once, making lots of plans, taking on too many responsibilities, restlessness, difficulty staying still		**Impaired judgment** Lack of insight, inappropriate humor and behaviors, impulsive or thrill-seeking behaviors: increased alcohol consumption; financial extravagance; dangerous driving; sexual promiscuity	**Increased social behavior** Unnecessary phone calls, increased sexual activity, talkative and sociable, indiscretions in eating habits

TABLE 18.17: Diagnostic criteria for manic episode.

Three to four of the following criteria are required during the elevated mood period.

1. Self-esteem: Highly inflated, grandiosity
2. Sleep: Decreased need for sleep, rested after only a few hours
3. Speech: Pressured
4. Thoughts: Racing thoughts and flight of ideas
5. Attention: Easy distractibility
6. Activity: Increased goal-directed activity
7. Hedonism: High excess involvement in pleasurable activities (sex, spending, travel)

TABLE 18.18: Elevated mood: It has four stages depending on severity of manic episodes.

Stage	*Features*
1. Euphoria (Stage I) Hypomania	Increased sense of psychological well-being and happiness not in keeping with ongoing events
2. Elation (Stage II)	Moderate elevation of mood with increased psychomotor activity
3. Exaltation (Stage III)	Intense elation of mood with delusions of Grandeur
4. Ecstasy (Stage IV)	Severe elevation of mood, intense sense of rapture, or blissfulness seen in delirious or stuporous mania

Treatment of Mania

- Hospitalization: To avoid injury to self/others, to control agitation and to ensure medication compliance
- Mood stabilizing agents (discussed earlier)
- Antipsychotics
- Electroconvulsive therapy (ECT) (discussed earlier)

Bipolar Disorder

Q. Write short essay on bipolar affective disorders.

Bipolar disorder is characterized by episodes of elevated mood interspersed with episodes of depression (both manic and depressive).

- Elevated mood when mild or short-lived (4 days) is known as hypomania, or when severe or chronic (at least 1 week), is called mania.
- The lifetime risk of developing bipolar disorder is about 1–2%. The lifetime risk of suicide is about 5–10%.
- **Types:** As per DSM-5, bipolar disorders are divided into: bipolar I disorder, bipolar II disorder, cyclothymic disorder, substance/medication-induced bipolar disorder, and bipolar disorder due to another medical condition.
  - **Bipolar I disorder:** It is characterized by the occurrence of one or more manic or mixed episodes (usually), and usually one or more major *depressive* episodes.
  - **Bipolar II disorder:** It is characterized by the occurrence of one or more major depressive episodes, at least one *hypomanic* episode and without any manic or mixed episode.

Management and Prognosis of Bipolar Disorders

- Mood stabilizing agents (discussed earlier) + Antipsychotics/Antidepressants
- Electroconvulsive therapy (ECT) (discussed earlier)

Cyclothymic Disorder

Q. Write short note on features of cyclothymia.

It is characterized by:

- Chronically fluctuating mood states; periods of hypomania and depression
- Duration of at least 2 years in adults and 1 year in adolescents and children
- Individual is not without symptoms for more than 2 months at a time.
- There are no major depressive, manic, or mixed episodes during the initial 2 years. After the initial 2 years, there may be superimposed manic, mixed, or depressive episodes.

NEUROTIC DISORDERS

Neurotic disorders can be:

- Anxiety symptom predominant
- Somatic symptom predominant
- After stress/trauma
- Dissociative disorders

Anxiety Predominant Disorders

	Generalized anxiety disorder	*Panic disorder*	*Phobia*
Anxiety symptoms	Continuous	Episodic	Episodic; on exposure to phobic stimulus

Types of Phobia

- **Specific phobia**: Fear of specific situation/object
- **Social phobia**: Fear of socially demanding situations
- **Agoraphobia**: Fear of places from where escape is difficult

Disorders Occurring After Trauma/Stress

Following sudden, life-threatening trauma/stress		After gradual routine life stress
Symptom duration <1 month	Symptom duration >1 month	
Acute stress reaction	**Post-traumatic stress disorder**	**Adjustment disorder**

Dissociative Disorders

- Dissociative **amnesia:** Patchy loss of autobiographical memory
- Dissociative **fugue:** Amnesia + travel, attains new identity
- Dissociative **identity disorder:** ≥2 identities in a person at a time
- **De-personalization** and **derealization** disorder: "As if" change in person/environment respectively.

Somatic Symptom Predominant Disorders

- Preoccupation with symptoms: **Somatization**/somatic symptom disorder
- Preoccupation with pain: **Somatoform pain** disorder
- Preoccupation with diagnosis: **Hypochondriasis**/illness anxiety disorder
- Preoccupation with imagined defect: **Body dysmorphic disorder**

Based on Symptom Production

		Conscious	
Symptom production	***Unconscious***	***With motive***	***Without motive***
Example	**Somatoform disorder** **Dissociative disorder**	**Malingering**	**Factitious disorder**

ANXIETY DISORDERS

- Anxiety disorders are characterized by unrealistic, irrational fear or anxiety of disabling intensity, worrisome thoughts, avoidance behavior, and the somatic symptoms of autonomic arousal.
- Anxiety is a syndrome with psychological (insecurity, worry, apprehension) and physiologic (sympathetic activation) components. Patients with anxiety may also have depression.

Q. Write short notes on types of anxiety disorder.

See **Table 18.19.**

Generalized Anxiety Disorder (GAD)

- It is a chronic state associated with uncontrollable excessive and free floating anxiety and worry persisting for minimum 6 months.
- **Symptoms:** It is associated with somatic symptoms of muscle tension and bowel disturbance, sleep disturbance, and difficulty concentrating or mind going blank.

TABLE 18.19: Differences between anxiety disorders.

Characteristics	*Generalized anxiety disorder*	*Panic disorder*	*Phobic anxiety disorder*
Occurrence	Persistent	Paroxysmal	Situational
Symptoms	Persistent	Episodic	On exposure
Cognitions	Worry	Fear of symptoms	Fear of situation
Behavior	Agitation	Escape	Avoidance

Panic (Paroxysmal) Disorder

- Panic disorder is defined as the occurrence of recurrent unexpected attacks of intense anxiety that include marked physical symptoms, such as tachycardia, chest pain, hyperventilation, dizziness, trembling, numbness, and sweating.
- Panic disorder may occur with or without agoraphobia (avoidance of situations where a person may feel trapped and unable to escape). A discrete period of intense fear or discomfort which develops abruptly and reaches a peak within 10 minutes. In between the attacks, patient is free from anxiety.

- Age of onset for panic disorder varies but lies between late adolescence and mid-30s.
- Patients have persistent concern of having attack and they worry about the implications of attack.

Phobic Anxiety Disorder

- A phobia is an *abnormal or excessive, persistent and disproportionate fear of an object or situation* that presents little or no actual danger to the person. It causes avoidance of it (e.g., excessive fear of dying in an air crash leading to avoidance of flying). Phobic responses can develop to general medical procedures, such as venipuncture.
- **Specific phobias:** It is characterized by clinically significant anxiety provoked by exposure of specific feared object or situation, often leading to avoidance.
- **Social phobia:** It is characterized by clinically significant anxiety provoked by exposure to certain types of social or performance situation, which people are exposed to unfamiliar people or to scrutiny by others.
- **Agoraphobia:** It is generalized phobia (marked fear) of going out alone or being in crowded places. Thus, avoid being alone or being in a public place (e.g., bridges, tunnels, crowds, etc.).

List of phobias:
- Claustrophobia: Fear of being in constricted, confined spaces
- Aerophobia: Fear of flying
- Arachnophobia: Fear of spiders
- Zoophobia: Fear of animals
- Aquaphobia: Fear of water
- Acrophobia: Fear of heights

Q. Mention the differential diagnosis of anxiety disorders.

Physical illness which mimic anxiety disorder: Hyperthyroidism, pheochromocytoma, hypoglycemia, paroxysmal atrial arrhythmias, alcohol withdrawal, and temporal lobe epilepsy.

Q. Write short notes on management of anxiety disorders.

***Psychological treatment*:**
- Explanation and reassurance
- Specific treatment may be necessary. Treatments include relaxation training, graded exposure (desensitization) to feared situations for phobic disorders, flooding and implosive therapy and CBT (cognitive behavioral therapy).

***Drug treatment*:**

Drugs of choice are antidepressants (SSRI). Benzodiazepines are useful in the short-term but long-term use can result in dependence. When somatic symptoms are prominent, β-blocker (e.g., propranolol) may be used.

Post-traumatic Stress Disorder

Q. Write short notes on post-traumatic stress disorder (PTSD).

- It is characterized by the re-experiencing (recurrent bouts) of an extremely traumatic event accompanied by the symptoms of increased arousal and by avoidance of stimuli associated with trauma.
- The traumatic event (e.g., a military experience, a physical or sexual assault, a motor vehicle accident, a natural disaster) involved may have caused death or near death experience or serious injury to self or others.
- Typically, patients re-experience the traumatic event (e.g., nightmares, flashbacks intrusive recollections), engage in avoidance of trauma or talk of trauma, or recollections of stimuli associated with the sentinel trauma. Patients experience increased autonomic reactivity, such as hypervigilance, irritability, insomnia startle responses, etc.

Classification of PTSD

- ***Acute PTSD***: Symptoms begin within 3 months of trauma or the duration of symptoms is less than 3 months.
- ***Chronic (or delayed) PTSD***: Symptoms start more than 3 months after trauma (delayed) or persist for 3 months or longer.
- ***With delayed onset***: 6 months have passed between the traumatic event and the onset of symptoms.

DISSOCIATIVE DISORDER

Q. Write short notes on dissociative disorder.

- It was formerly called **hysteria** (dissociative disorder) and this old term was replaced in DSM-IV and ICD-10 by new term dissociative disorder. More common in women and children.
- Definition: Dissociative disorder is a syndrome characterized by a loss or distortion of neurological function which cannot be fully explained by organic disease.
- Psychological functions commonly affected include conscious awareness and memory. Physical functions affected (conversion) include changes in sensory or motor function. These changes may resemble lesions in the motor or sensory nervous system.

Etiology

- Unconscious psychological process: Patient lacks insight into nature of symptoms. It is maladaptive way of coping with an unresolved psychological conflict by becoming ill.
- An association of this disorder with adverse childhood experiences, including physical and sexual abuse, is being observed.

Clinical Features

- Primary gain: Keeps internal conflicts outside patient's awareness.
- Secondary gain: Benefits received from being "sick".
- *La belle indifference:* Patient seems unconcerned about impairment.
- Gait disturbance
- Loss of function in limbs
- Aphonia
- Pseudoseizures (nonepileptic seizures)
- Sensory loss
- Blindness

Management/Treatment of Dissociative Disorder

- Physical and psychiatric examination to exclude organic disease.
- Explanation and reassurance.
- Resistant cases: Abreaction under hypnosis or small IV dose of penthanol.

CONVERSION DISORDER

It is called functional neurological symptom disorder in DSM-5.

Etiology: Unresolved psychological conflict is **converted** acutely and unconsciously into sensorimotor neurological symptoms → maladaptive coping mechanism.

Treatment: Psychodynamic therapy—resolution of psychological conflict.

SOMATOFORM DISORDERS

These disorders have somatic symptoms which are not explained by a medical condition (medically unexplained symptoms), nor better diagnosed as part of a depressive or anxiety disorder.

Symptom Production

- If **unconscious**—comes under **somatoform disorders**
- If **conscious with motive** to obtain benefit is called as **malingering.**
- If conscious but **done without motive—factitious disorder/Munchausen syndrome**.

FACTITIOUS DISORDER

It is an uncommon disorder characterized by the repeated and deliberate production of the signs or symptoms of disease to gain medical care, e.g., dipping of thermometers into hot drinks to fake a fever.

Munchausen's Syndrome

Q. Write short notes on Munchausen's syndrome.

- It is a rare, severe, chronic form of factitious disorder named after the *German Baron von Munchausen*, who was legendary for his inventive lying.
- He traveled widely, sometimes visiting several hospitals in one day. Patient frequently changes his name, with history of doctor shopping.
- These patients are memorable because they present so dramatically. They usually seek medical attention at night when junior doctors or residents are on duty. They fabricate a convincing history and present to the doctor with dramatic symptoms of a medical emergency. They persuade an inexperienced doctor to undertake investigations or initiate treatment including exploratory surgery.
- Abdomen may show several scar marks ("surgical battlefield") due to previous operations.

Management

- Gentle and firm confrontation with clear evidence of the fabrication of illness.
- Psychological support.
- Recognition of the condition to avoid further iatrogenic harm.

OBSESSIVE-COMPULSIVE DISORDER

Q. Write short notes on obsessive-compulsive disorder.

Obsessive-compulsive disorder (OCD) is characterized by obsessive, recurrent, unwanted thoughts (which cause marked anxiety) and by compulsions (which serve to neutralize or relieve anxiety).

- **Obsessions:** These are persistent *thoughts, ideas, impulses, or images* that seem to invade a person's consciousness.
- **Compulsions:** Repetitive behaviors (e.g., handwashing, ordering, checking) or mental acts (e.g., praying, counting, repeating words silently) that the individual feels driven to perform in response to an obsession.

Etiology

Cortico-striatal-thalamo-cortical circuit dysfunction.

Types

People have symptoms like:

- Cleaning: Fears of contamination
- Symmetry: Arranging items symmetrically and repeating, ordering, and counting compulsions
- Forbidden or taboo thoughts: Aggressive, sexual, and religious obsessions.
- Harm (e.g., thoughts about harm on oneself or others).

Management

It usually responds to some degree to antidepressant drugs (SSRIs—paroxetine, citalopram, or escitalopram and SNRI—clomipramine) and to psychotherapy (behavioral, supportive). However, relapses are common and it often becomes chronic.

Cingulotomy/capsulotomy can be used in refractory cases.

Other OCD-related Disorders

- Trichotillomania
- Skin picking/excoriation disorder
- Hoarding disorder: Difficulty in disposing items regardless of its value
- Body dysmorphic disorder

IMPULSE CONTROL DISORDERS

Q. Write short essay/note on impulse disorders.

- Impulsive disorder is defined as a sudden and irresistible force which compels a person to do some action without motive or forethought. A normal person always tries to analyze his actions whether they are consistent with law or not. Once he realizes that his action may be contrary to law he stops it.
- But in impulsive disorder, a person is not able to control himself. Examples:
  - Kleptomania: An irresistible desire to steal things usually of low value.
  - Pyromania: An irresistible desire to set things on fire.
  - Mutilomania: An irresistible impulse to maim animals.
  - Dipsomania: An irresistible impulse to drink at periodic intervals.
  - Sexual impulses: All sexual perversions.
  - Homicidal impulses: To kill some persons.
  - Suicidal impulses: To commit suicide. Impulses are quite commonly seen in various mental disorders like depression, schizophrenia, mania, etc.
  - Trichotillomania: It is an irresistible desire to pull out one's own hair.
  - Oniomania: Compulsive desire to shop (shopping addiction).

ORGANIC MENTAL DISORDERS (TABLE 18.20)

TABLE 18.20: Organic mental disorders.

Characteristic	*Delirium*	*Dementia*	*Amnestic disorder*
Onset	Acute	Chronic	Chronic
Course	Fluctuating	Progressive	Progressive
Sensorium	Altered	Clear	Clear
Cognitive functions affected	Multiple: ➤ Poor attention and concentration: Recent memory affected ➤ Remote memory normal	Multiple: ➤ Amnesia (Remote + recent) ➤ Apraxia ➤ Agnosia ➤ Aphasia ➤ Loss of executive functions	Only memory affected Recent > remote

Contd...

Contd...

Confabulations (filling up gaps in memory)	Absent	Absent	Present
Psychotic symptoms	➢ Present ➢ Fleeting paranoid delusions ➢ Transient visual hallucinations	➢ Present ➢ Fixed paranoid delusions ➢ Auditory, visual hallucinations	Absent
Cause	Metabolic, infective, endocrine, drug intoxication/withdrawal	➢ Reversible: Depression, NPH, B_{12} deficiency, hypothyroidism ➢ Irreversible: Alzheimer's, vascular, Lewy body, frontotemporal	B_{12} deficiency: Korsakoff's amnestic syndrome
Management	Treat the underlying cause	Antidementia drugs	B_{12} supplementations

DELIRIUM

Q. Write short essay/notes on definition, causes, clinical features (clinical recognition), and initial management of delirium.

Definition

It is an acute organic mental disorder characterized by confusion, restlessness, incoherence, inattention, anxiety, or hallucinations which may be reversible with treatment.

Clinical Features

- **Acute course:** Sudden onset, short episode.
- Global impairment of cognitive functions (memory, attention, orientation, thinking, etc.).
- Fluctuating course.
- **Cardinal features:**
  - Clouding of consciousness, impaired alertness, awareness, and attention.
  - Variability in state of arousal.
  - Reduced responsiveness is interspersed with periods of excited outbursts.
  - Sleep/wake cycle disrupted.
- Impaired perception: Misperceives surrounding and attendants, hallucinations.
- Disturbance of emotion: Agitation, fear, depression, and anxiety.
- Psychomotor changes: Hyperactivity, restlessness, and repetitive (plucking, tossing).

Predisposing and precipitating factors of delirium are shown in **Table 18.21** and causes of delirium are shown in **Table 18.22.**

TABLE 18.21: Predisposing and precipitating factors of delirium.

Predisposing	*Precipitating*
➢ Diseases of brain: Dementia, stroke, and past severe head injury ➢ Drugs: Sedatives and anticholinergics ➢ Impairments of special senses: Sight and hearing ➢ Multiple severe illnesses ➢ Malnutrition	➢ **Iatrogenic**: Unpleasant environmental change, invasive procedures, new medications, trauma, dehydration, ongoing malnutrition, and elimination malfunction ➢ **Illnesses:** Infections, intracranial pathologies, impaired organ function, abnormal metabolite function, pain, and drug withdrawal

TABLE 18.22: Causes of delirium.

➢ Metabolic causes: - Hypoxia, CO_2 narcosis - Hypoglycemia - Hepatic encephalopathy - H_2O and electrolyte imbalance	➢ Endocrine causes: - Hypo- and hyperpituitarism - Hypo- and hyperthyroidism - Hypo- and hyperparathyroidism - Hypo- and hyperadrenalism
➢ Drugs and poisons: - Digitalis - Alcohol - Tricycle antidepressants - Salicylates, penicillin, etc.	➢ Intracranial causes: - Epilepsy - Head injury - Meningitis - Migraine
➢ Nutritional deficiencies: - Thiamin, niacin - Proteins	➢ Miscellaneous: - Postoperative states - Sleep deprivation - Acute and chronic systemic infections - Febrile delirium in children

Investigations

If cause is not obvious: Complete blood count, urine analysis, blood glucose, blood urea, serum electrolytes, liver and renal function tests, arterial blood gases, thyroid function test, X-ray chest, ECG, CSF, VDRL, HIV-testing, EEG, and cranial CT scan or MRI scan.

Management: Identify the cause and treat it accordingly
- Chlorpromazine (50–100 mg 8th hourly) or haloperidol (5–10 mg 8th hourly) are the drugs of choices except in delirium tremens, where benzodiazepines (BZDs) or diazepam 10–20 mg 6th hourly is preferred.
- Also give supportive medical and nursing care.

Q. Write short notes on differences between delirium, dementia, and psychosis.

Differences between delirium, dementia, and psychosis are shown in **Table 18.23**.

TABLE 18.23: Differences between delirium, dementia and psychosis.

Condition	*Onset*	*Pattern*	*Orientation*	*Attention*	*Memory*	*Duration*
Delirium	Acute	Fluctuating	Usually impaired	Impaired/fluctuating	Impaired	Hours or days
Dementia	Insidious	Progressive	Normal or impaired	~Normal	Impaired	Months or years
Psychosis	Variable	Variable	~Normal	Normal or impaired	Normal or impaired	Variable

SUBSTANCE USE DISORDERS

Q. Write short notes on substance use, its effects, and treatment.

- **Substance use includes harmful use, dependence, effects of intoxication and withdrawal**
- ***Harmful use*:** Substance use pattern that causes harm to individual's physical/mental health or has caused harm to others through the behavioral changes.
- ***Dependence*:** Due to continuous use of substance, individual has become dependent on the substance and unable to regulate the pattern of his use. Manifestation can either psychological or physiological.
- Psychological manifestations can be seen as craving (strong desire to use the substance), loss of control in using substance, continuing use despite harmful consequences, and prioritizing substance use while neglecting alternate activities for pleasure.
- Physiological manifestations can be seen by symptoms of tolerance and withdrawal.
- ***Tolerance*:** It is defined by either of the following:
  - A need for markedly increased amounts of the substance to achieve intoxication or desired effect.
  - A markedly diminished effect with continued use of the same amount of the substance.
- ***Substance intoxication*:** Reversible, substance-specific syndrome caused by the recent ingestion of or exposure to a substance.
- ***Substance withdrawal*:** Characteristic substance-specific, maladaptive behavioral change, with physiologic and cognitive concomitants, caused by the cessation of or reduction in heavy and prolonged substance use.

Risk Factors/Etiology (Table 18.24)

- **Family history:** Parental drug use, marital conflict, and disturbed family environment.
- **Physiology:** Individuals who are innately more tolerant to substance.
- **Developmental history:** Poor parenting, childhood physical and sexual abuse.
- **Environmental:** Peer pressure, economic disadvantage, and social isolation. Availability and access to drugs.
- **Psychiatric illness:** Conduct disorder, depression, and bipolar disorder.
- **Age group:** Highest prevalence of substance abuse is between 18 and 22 years of age. Experimentation with gateway drugs may start as early as preadolescence.

TABLE 18.24: Common symptoms and signs of substance abuse.

Symptoms	*Signs*
➤ Frequent absences from school or workplace ➤ Depression/anxiety ➤ Epigastric distress, diarrhea ➤ Sleep disorders ➤ Sexual dysfunction ➤ Frequent trauma/injury	➤ Tremors ➤ Tachycardia ➤ Labile hypertension ➤ Conjunctival injection ➤ Odor of alcohol on breath in alcohol use ➤ Tender hepatomegaly

Investigations and Diagnosis

Diagnosis may be apparent from the history or may be made when the patient presents with a complication.

Laboratory Toxicology

- **Breath, blood, and urine examination:** Screen for types of substances of abuse and its concentrations.
- **Intravenous drug abuse workup:**
  - HIV, hepatitis B, hepatitis C, and tuberculosis.
  - Drug screening of samples of urine or blood will help in confirming the diagnosis.
- Other laboratory studies for evidence of systemic damage from substance use.

Treatment of Substance-related Disorders

Biological treatment: Pharmacologic intervention to ameliorate psychological or physical symptoms.

- **Agonist substitution:** Safe drug with a similar chemical composition as the abused drug, e.g., methadone for heroin addiction.
- **Antagonistic treatment:** Drugs that blo Treatment of Substance-related Disorders ck or counteract the positive effects of substances, e.g., naltrexone for opiate and alcohol problems.
- **Aversive treatment:** Drugs that make the injection of abused substances extremely unpleasant, e.g., disulfiram for alcoholism and silver nitrate for nicotine addiction.

Psychosocial treatment

- Community support programs: These are strongly encouraged.
- Emotional reassurance and providing a structured and secure environment.
- Components of comprehensive treatment and prevention programs: Individual and group therapy, aversion therapy and convert sensitization, contingency management, community reinforcement, relapse prevention, and preventative efforts via education.

Main Categories of Substances

- **Depressants:** Result in behavioral sedation (e.g., alcohol, sedatives, anxiolytic, and hypnotic drugs).
- **Stimulants:** Increase alertness and elevate mood (e.g., cocaine, nicotine, caffeine, and amphetamines).
- **Opiates:** Primarily produce analgesia and euphoria (e.g., heroin, morphine, codeine, and brown sugar).
- **Hallucinogens:** Alter sensory perception [e.g., marijuana (cannabis), lysergic acid diethylamide, phencyclidine]
- **Club/rave party drugs**: Cause anterograde amnesia (e.g., gamma hexane butyrate, flunitrazepam, and ketamine)
- **Other drugs of abuse:** Includes volatile solvents, anabolic steroids, and medications.

NICOTINE

Nicotine withdrawal: Symptoms in chronic users appear about 30 minutes after every dose. These include confusion, anxiety, restlessness, insomnia, depression, frustration and anger, nightmares, and headache.

Treatment of Tobacco Use Disorder

- **Smoking cessation**
- Cognitive behavioral therapy (CBT)
- Nicotine gum or lozenge, transdermal patch, and nasal spray inhalers
- Medication:
  - **Bupropion:** It is an antidepressant which is chemically unrelated to tricyclic antidepressants or SSRIs. Dose 150 mg po twice a day.
  - **Varenicline and cytisine:** It is an alpha-4 beta-2 nicotinic receptor partial agonist more effective than nicotine and bupropion. Dose 1 mg po bid.

ALCOHOL

Consumption of alcohol when associated with social, psychological, and physical problems constitutes alcohol use disorder.

Etiology

Alcohol is a central nervous system depressant. It influences several neurotransmitter systems, mainly GABA (inhibition of behavior) but also glutamate system and serotonin system.

Alcohol Dependence

It is characterized by a problematic pattern of alcohol use leading to clinically significant impairment or distress, as manifested by multiple psychosocial, behavioral, or physiologic features.

Features of alcohol dependence

- Loss of control: Engaging in risky behaviors while under the influence.
- Compulsive preoccupation: Worrying compulsively about getting a "fix" and spending a lot of their time thinking about the drug.
- Continued use of alcohol despite negative consequences: Losing control of the ability to monitor how much and how often the user takes their drug.
- Loss of motivation: Losing interest in activities that the user enjoyed prior to addiction.
- Desire to stop drinking, but inability to do so.
- Excessive time spent getting or using alcohol, or recovering from its effects.
- Craving, or preoccupation with drinking.
- Problems stemming from alcohol use; ignoring those problems; drinking despite obvious hazards, including physical danger.
- Retreating from important work, family, or social activities and roles.
- Tolerance: The need to drink more and more alcohol to feel the same effects, or the ability to drink more than other people without getting drunk.
- Withdrawal symptoms: After stopping or cutting back on drinking, symptoms are anxiety, sweating, trembling, trouble sleeping, nausea or vomiting, and, in severe cases, physical seizures and hallucinations. The person may drink to relieve or avoid such symptoms.

Q. Write short notes on consequences/complications of alcohol harmful use/dependence.

Consequences of alcohol harmful use/dependence

Neuropsychiatric

- Depression, suicide
- Alcohol relieves anxiety in the short term, dependence can develop in long-term use
- Alcoholic hallucinosis: auditory hallucinations
- Alcoholic "blackouts": Amnesia for events that occurred during bouts of intoxication in very heavy alcoholic drinkers.
- **Alcohol withdrawal** (discussed below): Maximum symptoms usually develop 2–3 days after the last drink and can produce seizures ("rum fits").
- **Delirium tremens:** It is a form of delirium found with severe alcohol withdrawal.
- Neurological: Peripheral neuropathy, dementia, cerebral hemorrhage, cerebellar degeneration, Marchiafava-Bignami syndrome, subacute combined degeneration of the cord myopathy, ventricular enlargement, and cognitive impairment.
- Wernicke's encephalopathy: Global confusion, nystagmus, ophthalmoplegia, and ataxia
- Korsakoff's syndrome: Short-term memory deficits, confabulation
- **Alcoholic dementia:** It is a global cognitive impairment which may resemble Alzheimer's disease. It does not progress and may improve if the patient abstains from alcohol.
- **Indirect effects on brain:** It may be due to head injury subdural hematoma, hypoglycemia, and encephalopathy.

Medical

- Hepatic: Fatty change and cirrhosis, hepatocellular carcinoma
- Gastrointestinal: Esophagitis, esophageal varices, Mallory-Weiss syndrome, esophageal carcinoma, gastritis, malabsorption, pancreatitis, and parotid enlargement
- Skin: Palmar erythema, spider naevi, Dupuytren's contractures, and telangiectasias
- Cardiac: Cardiomyopathy and hypertension
- Respiratory: Pneumonia and tuberculosis
- Musculoskeletal: Myopathy and fractures
- Endocrine and metabolic: Pseudo-Cushing's syndrome, hypoglycemia, and gout
- Reproductive: Hypogonadism, infertility, and fetal alcohol syndrome

Social: Absenteeism from work, unemployment, marital discord, child abuse, financial difficulties, violence, and traffic offences.

Investigations and Diagnosis

Laboratory detection of alcohol abuse:

- **Breath, blood, and urine examination:** Screen for alcohol.
- **Gamma-glutamyl transpeptidase (GGT):** It is most sensitive for alcohol abuse and is raised in patients with alcohol abuse.
- **MCV (mean corpuscular volume):** Raised, but is less sensitive than GGT.
- **Carbohydrate-deficient transferrin level:** Elevated and is highly specific in the absence of liver disease.
- **Phosphatidylethanol (PEth)**—concentration greater than 20 ng/dL is evidence of intoxication; it can detect excessive alcohol intake within a 2-week period.
- **Others:** Alanine aminotransferase (ALT), aspartate aminotransferase (AST), and lactate dehydrogenase (LDH).

CAGE questionnaire: Affirmative answers to any two of the following questions (or to the last question alone) are suggestive of alcohol abuse.

- Have you ever felt that you should **Cut** down your drinking?
- Have you ever felt **Annoyed** by others criticizing your drinking?
- Have you ever felt **Guilty** about your drinking?
- Have you ever had a morning drink (**Eye**-opener) after hangover?

Treatment

It involves management of intoxication phase, withdrawal phase, and rehabilitation.

Alcohol Intoxication

Features of Acute Alcoholic Intoxication

- Ataxia, slurred speech, emotional incontinence, and aggression
- Hypotension, gastritis, hypoglycemia, collapse, respiratory depression, coma, and death
- Disturbances in emotional and behavioral state
- Medical symptoms: Due to hypoglycemia, aspiration of vomit, respiratory depression
- Complication of other medical problems
- Accidents, injuries developed in fights

Q. Write short note on treatment of acute alcoholic intoxication.

Treatment of acute alcoholic intoxication

- Maintain patent airway and prevent aspiration of vomitus. Tracheal intubation and positive pressure respiration may be needed. Do not use analeptics because they may precipitate convulsions.
- Maintain fluid and electrolyte balance.
- Hypoglycemia is corrected by glucose infusion.
- Thiamine 100 mg in 500 mL glucose solution infused intravenously.

Note: Gastric lavage is helpful only when the patient is brought immediately after alcohol ingestion.

Alcohol Withdrawal

Q. Write short note on clinical features of alcohol withdrawal syndrome.

Alcohol withdrawal is characterized by sudden exhibition of central nervous system excitation.

Clinical Features

They occur 6–8 hours after the reduction of ethanol intake and may last for 2–7 days.

- **Minor withdrawal symptoms:**
  - Psychological: Restlessness, anxiety, panic attacks, insomnia, and tremors (the shakes)
  - Autonomic: Tachycardia, palpitations, sweating/diaphoresis, hypertension, pupil dilatation, nausea, vomiting, and hyper-reflexia
  - Others: Gastrointestinal upset, anorexia, and headache
  - They resolve within 24–28 hours.
- **Alcoholic hallucinosis:**
  - These are hallucinations appear within 8–12 hours of abstinence and disappear within 48–72 hours.
  - Usually these hallucinations are visual. In contrast to delirium tremens, it is not associated with clouding of the sensorium.
- **Withdrawal seizures**

Q. Write short note on causes and management of convulsions in alcoholics.

  - These seizures (**"rum fits"**) are generalized tonic-clonic convulsions. These develop usually 12–24 hours after the last drink, but may develop after only 2 hours of abstinence.
  - About 3% of chronic alcoholics develop withdrawal-associated seizures and, about 3% of them may develop status epilepticus.
  - About 30% of patients, who develop delirium tremors, give a history of preceding alcohol withdrawal seizures.
- **Delirium tremens**

Q. Write short note on delirium tremens.

  - It usually develops between 24 and 72 hours after the last drink and last for about 1–5 days. If early alcohol withdrawal is not treated, about 5% will progress to delirium tremens.
  - **Clinical features:**
    - These include agitation, visual hallucinations (Lilliputian/macroscopic), illusions, delusions, tachycardia, hypertension, diaphoresis, and dilated pupils.
    - Dehydration may occur as a result of diaphoresis, hyperthermia, vomiting, and tachypnea.
    - **Other features:** Hypokalemia, hypomagnesemia, and hypophosphatemia.
  - Death occurs in about 5% of patients, usually due to arrhythmias, pneumonia, or electrolyte imbalance.

Management of alcohol withdrawal syndrome

- Maintain patent airway and breathing.
- Thiamine 100 mg in 500 mL glucose solution infused intravenously after withdrawing appropriate blood samples since in alcoholics, the thiamine will be depleted and the TPP would not be present as a result, in patients with altered sensorium for prevention of progress to Wernicke Korsakoff psychosis.
- Maintain fluid and electrolyte balance.
- **Mild cases of withdrawal:** Provide supportive care, such as reassurance and nursing care (monitoring of vital sings).
- **Benzodiazepines (nitrazepam, diazepam, and lorazepam):** For patients with moderate to severe withdrawal. They also control seizures.
- **β-blockers:** It may reduce anxiety and tremors.
- **Anticonvulsants:** Such as phenytoin, valproic acid, carbamazepine, and levetiracetam are of little value in treating or preventing alcohol withdrawal seizures.
- **Management of associated conditions:** Such as pneumonia, electrolyte imbalances, GI bleed, liver failure, pancreatitis, neurological injury, and trauma.

Rehabilitation

Aims at relapse prevention by using the pharmacotherapy and psychotherapy.

Drugs used for relapse prevention in alcohol dependence:
- **First-line medications:** Naltrexone and acamprosate
- **Second-line medications:** Disulfiram, topiramate, gabapentin, baclofen, and nalmefene

- **Disulfiram**
  - Disulfiram is **inhibitor of enzyme aldehyde dehydrogenase (ALDH)** and blocks the conversion of acetaldehyde (derived from alcohol) to acetic acid, thus increasing the levels of toxic substance, acetaldehyde in the body.
  - When alcohol is consumed while on disulfiram, acetaldehyde accumulates in tissues and blood and produces distressing symptoms (aldehyde syndrome). These unpleasant symptoms include flushing, burning sensation, throbbing headache, perspiration, uneasiness, palpitations, nausea, postural faintness, and, in some cases, circulatory collapse. Duration of symptoms (1–4 hours) depends on the amount of alcohol consumed.
  - **Side effects:** Infrequent and include rashes, metallic taste, nervousness, and malaise. Very rarely myocardial infarction, congestive heart failure, respiratory depression, convulsions, and death may develop.
  - **Dosage:** Oral 250–500 mg/daily.
- **Naltrexone:**
  - It is an opioid-receptor antagonist. It reduces alcohol craving, number of drinking days, and chances of resumed heavy drinking.
  - **Dose:** Oral 50 mg/day in a single dose.
  - **Side effects:** Nausea decreased appetite, fatigue, and headache.
- **Acamprosate:**
  - It is a weak N-methyl-D-aspartate (NMDA) receptor antagonist with modest GABA A receptor antagonist. It normalizes the dysregulated NMDA-mediated glutamatergic excitation that occurs in alcohol withdrawal and early abstinence. It reduces relapse of the drinking behavior.
  - **Dose:** Oral 666 mg given thrice a day. It is available in 333 mg enteric-coated tablet.
  - **Side effects:** Diarrhea, dizziness, and headache.

EATING DISORDERS

Type	*Anorexia nervosa*	*Bulimia nervosa*	*Binge eating disorder*
Symptoms	• Avoidance • Binge • Compensation	• Binge • Compensation	Binge only
Weight	Underweight	Normal weight	Overweight

Anorexia Nervosa

Q. Write short note on anorexia nervosa (AN) and its management.

Etiology: Unknown but probably includes genetic, environmental, psychologic, and cultural factors.

Onset: Average age is 17 years, often associated with emotional stressors, particularly conflicts with parents about independence and sexual conflicts. Very late-onset anorexia nervosa has a poorer prognosis.

Clinical Features

- **Avoidance of high calorie food** and restricted food intake because of intense fear of gaining weight or becoming fat
- **Compensatory behaviors:** Excessive exercise routine, self-induced vomiting or use of laxatives/diuretics/enemas
- **Marked weight loss:** Refusal to maintain body weight at or above a minimally normal weight for age and height.
- **Distortion of body image** so that patients regard themselves as fat even when they appear grossly underweight, significant amount of time spent examining and denigrating self for perceived signs of excess weight, great concern with appearance, and denial of emaciated condition.
- In postmenarcheal females, **amenorrhea**, i.e., the absence of at least three consecutive menstrual cycles.
- Excessive interest in food-related activities (other than eating).
- Obsessive-compulsive symptoms and depressive symptoms.

Major Subtypes

- **Restricting type:** Fasting, introverted, decreased risk of substance abuse, family conflict is covert.
- **Bulimic type:** Binge eating or purging, more volatile, family frequently disengaged, prone to substance abuse.

Physical Examination

- **Signs of malnutrition:** Emaciation, hypotension, bradycardia, lanugo (i.e., fine hair on the trunk), and peripheral edema.
- **Signs of purging:** Eroded dental enamel caused by emesis and scarred or scratched hands from self-gagging to induce emesis. Parotid abscess and dental caries—because of keeping food in mouth for long time.
- Evidence of medical conditions due to abnormal diets, starvation, and purging.

Diagnostic Tests

- **Signs of malnutrition:** Normochromic normocytic anemia, abnormal electrolytes, and elevated liver enzymes
- **Signs of purging:** Metabolic alkalosis, hypochloremia, and hypokalemia due to emesis. Metabolic acidosis caused by laxative abuse.
- **Hormonal abnormalities:**
  - Elevated growth hormone and plasma cortisol levels and reduced gonadotropin levels (along with low FSH, LH, estrogen, and testosterone).
  - T3 may be reduced, but T4 and TSH are often normal.
  - Increased corticotrophin CSF levels.

Course and Outcome

- About 20–30% of restricting anorexics eventually develop binge eating within the first 5 years of onset.
- These illnesses have a chronicity of 5–10%.
- Generally favorable outcome is achieved in 60–70% of patients at 5–7-year outcome.
- Long-term mortality rate of individuals hospitalized for anorexia nervosa is 10%, due to the effects of starvation and purging or suicide.

Treatment
- Initial treatment should be correction of significant physiologic consequences of starvation with hospitalization if necessary.
- Behavioral therapy should be initiated, with rewards or punishments based on absolute weight, not on eating behaviors.
- Family therapy designed to reduce conflicts about control by parents.
- Antidepressants when comorbid depression is present.

Bulimia Nervosa

Q. Write short note on bulimia nervosa.

Occurs at 1:9 male-to-female ratio.

Etiology: Psychologic conflict regarding guilt, helplessness, self-control, and body image may be predisposing factor.

Onset: During late adolescence or early adulthood and often follows a period of dieting.

Clinical Features

- Recurrent episodes of **binge eating**
- Obsession with dieting but followed by binge eating of high-calorie foods.
- Absence of self-control over eating during binges.
- Binges are associated with emotional stress and followed by feelings of guilt, self-recrimination and compensatory behaviors.
- Recurrent, inappropriate compensatory behavior: **Self-induced vomiting, purgation** or dieting after binges.
- Self-castigation for mild weight gain or binges. Attempts to conceal binge-eating or purging, or lies about behaviors.
- **Weight maintained** within normal range.

Major Subtypes

- **Purging type:** Self-induced vomiting or use of laxatives, diuretics, or enemas.
- **Nonpurging type:** Use of other compensatory mechanisms, such as fasting or excessive exercise.

Physical Examination

- Calluses on the dorsal surface of their hands (self-induced vomiting), dental erosion and caries, esophageal erosion, lanugo hair, enlarged parotid glands (chipmunk face secondary to increased amylase), bradycardia, hypotension, and arrhythmias (secondary to hypokalemia).
- **Associated problems:** Depression, substance abuse, and impulsivity (kleptomania).
- **Comorbid disorders:** Borderline personality disorder is present in 50% of patients.

Diagnostic Tests: Evidence of Laxative or Diuretic Abuse

- ***Course:*** It may be chronic or intermittent.
- ***Outcome:*** Prognosis of bulimia is better than anorexia.
  - Favorable prognostic indicators: Younger age at onset, higher social class, and family history of alcohol abuse.

Differences between anorexia and bulimia are shown in **Table 18.25**.

Treatment
- Antidepressants (SSRI).
- Cognitive and behavioral therapy.
- Psychodynamic psychotherapies are useful for borderline personality traits.

TABLE 18.25: Differences between anorexia and bulimia.	
Anorexia nervosa	***Bulimia nervosa***
➢ Denies abnormal eating behavior ➢ Introverted ➢ Turns away food in order to cope ➢ Preoccupation with losing more and more weight	➢ Recognizes abnormal eating behavior ➢ Extroverted ➢ Turns to food in order to cope ➢ Preoccupation with attaining an "ideal" but often unrealistic weight

SLEEP DISORDERS

Disturbed sleep is one of the most frequent health complaints.

Sleep disorders can be of various types:

- Dyssomnias: Insomnia and hypersomnia
- Parasomnias:
  - NREM parasomnias: Somnambulism, somniloquy, sleep terrors, and bruxism (teeth grinding)
  - REM parasomnias: Night mares, REM behavioral disorder
- Narcolepsy, Kleine Levin syndrome
- Circadian rhythm disorders
- Sleep-related movement disorders: RLS and PLMD
- Obstructive sleep apnea, upper airway resistance syndrome

Major categories of sleep disorders as per DSM IV:

- **Dyssomnias:** Sleeping disorder that makes it difficult to get to sleep, or to stay sleeping.
- **Parasomnias**
- **Neurological/ psychiatric disorders**

Q. Write short notes on insomnia.

Insomnia is the complaint of ***inability to sleep*** long enough or maintain sleep despite the patient having adequate amount of time to devote to sleep. It is associated with impairment of daytime functioning or mood symptoms.

Insomnia can be classified according to the nature of sleep disruption and the duration of the complaint. Most insomnia patients present with two or more of these symptoms.

- **Sleep onset insomnia:** Difficulty falling asleep.
- **Sleep maintenance insomnia:** Frequent or sustained awakenings.
- **Sleep offset insomnia:** Early morning awakenings or frequent nocturnal awakenings.

Common causes of insomnia

Primary sleep disorders:

- Idiopathic insomnia
- Periodic leg movements
- Restless legs syndrome

Secondary sleep disorders:

- **Psychiatric or psychological problems:** Mood disorders (e.g., mania, depressive, and anxiety disorders); delirium and dementia
- **Use or misuse of drug/substance abuse:** Consumption or discontinuation of drugs/substances. Withdrawal of addictive drug (e.g., alcohol and benzodiazepines); stimulant drugs (e.g., caffeine, nicotine, and amphetamines); prescribed drugs (corticosteroids and dopamine agonists)
- **Physical/medical disorders:** Chronic pain (e.g., carpal tunnel syndrome); nocturia (e.g., prostatism); malnutrition, chronic obstructive pulmonary disease, asthma, menopause, and neurologic disorders.

Consequences

- Depression may cause insomnia, and insomnia may cause depression.
- Can heighten the perception of pain.
- May be associated with:
  - Development of endocrine disturbances.
  - Increased risk for hypertension or cardiovascular disease.
  - Increased risk for motor vehicle accidents and occupational errors.

Treatment

- **Behavioral therapy** is effective but may be time-consuming. These include: Relaxation techniques and cognitive behavior therapy.
- Other measures include: Decreasing alcohol intake, to have early supper, daily exercise, and hot bath prior to going to bed and routine going to bed at the same time.
- **Pharmacologic treatment:**
  - Benzodiazepines (e.g., temazepam, triazolam, estazolam, and eszopiclone) for sleep-maintenance insomnia.
  - Nonbenzodiazepines (e.g., zolpidem, zolpidem-controlled release zaleplon, zopiclone or eszopiclone) for both sleep-onset and sleep-maintenance insomnia.
  - Melatonin agonist (e.g., ramelteon) for sleep onset insomnia.
  - Antihistamines (e.g., diphenhydramine and promethazine) and antidepressants (e.g., amitriptyline, trimipramine, trazodone, and mirtazapine).

Q. Write short notes on parasomnias.

It consists of various uncommon disruptive sleep-related disorders with abnormal unpleasant or undesirable behaviors or experiences that occur during sleep, entry to sleep, or arousal from sleep **(Table 18.26)**.

Treatment

- **Avoid:** Caffeine or alcohol and drugs, such as serotonin reuptake inhibitors and MAO inhibitors.
- **Remove dangerous objects** from the environment of sleep.
- **Pharmacologic therapy:** These include clonazepam, tricyclic antidepressants, dopamine agonists or levodopa, melatonin, and carbamazepine.

TABLE 18.26: Types and features of parasomnias.

NREM sleep-associated parasomnias	
Confusional arousals	Sudden arousals, associated with confusion and disorientation
Sleep terrors	Sudden arousal with fearful agitated behavior, often with screaming or crying; patient may be disoriented, unresponsive to the environment and typically do not remember the event afterward
Sleepwalking	Arousal with complex motor behavior, walking, running, talking, and eating
Others	Somniloquy (sleep talking), bruxism (teeth grinding)
REM sleep-associated parasomnias	
Nightmare disorder	Recurrent, disturbing dreams not associated with autonomic activity or amnesia
REM sleep behavior disorder (RBD)	Abnormal persistence of muscle tone during REM sleep, permitting vigorous movements while dreaming. Also includes screaming, punching, and kicking for up to several minutes, sometimes resulting in injury to the patient or bed partner

NARCOLEPSY

Q. Write short notes on narcolepsy.

Etiology

- Loss of orexin (hypocretin) signaling
- Strong genetic/HLA association: HLADQB1*0602 haplotype is present in 95% of patients with cataplexy and in 96% of those with orexin deficiency.

Clinical Features

The classic "narcolepsy tetrad" consists of four main clinical features.

1. **Excessive daytime sleepiness (EDS)** occurring almost daily for at least 3 months that interferes with functioning **plus three specific symptoms** related to an intrusion of REM sleep characteristics. Sleep attack is the most common symptom.
2. **Cataplexy** (*pathognomonic sign*): Sudden weakness or loss of muscle tone without loss of consciousness, usually precipitated by loud noise, laughter, or other intense emotions.
3. **Hypnagogic/hypnopompic hallucinations: Hypnagogic hallucinations** (hallucinations occur as the patient is going to sleep) or **hypnopompic hallucinations** (hallucinations upon awakening).
4. **Sleep paralysis:** Muscle paralysis upon awakening. It consists of episodes up to several minutes in duration of inability to move and occasionally feeling unable to breathe despite being awake. Fragmented sleep is classically seen in patients.

Diagnosis

- **Electrographic evidence/multiple sleep latency test:** Demonstration of rapid transition from wakefulness to sleep and shortened REM sleep onset is confirmatory for the diagnosis. A mean sleep latency of ≤8 minutes and two or more sleep onset REM periods (SOREMPs) on a multiple sleep latency test (MSLT) is performed using standard techniques.
- HLA testing may also be useful.
- Cerebrospinal fluid (CSF) hypocretin-1 concentration is low.

Treatment

Mainly symptomatic: Forced naps at a regular time of day is usually the treatment of choice.

Psychostimulants:

- **Wake-promoting therapeutics: Modafinil** is the drug of choice, principally because it has few side effects and has low addiction potential. Older drugs such as methylphenidate or methamphetamine or dextroamphetamine are used as alternatives, particularly in refractory patients.
- **Tricyclic antidepressants** (TCAs) help to suppress the REM sleep (e.g., protriptyline, imipramine, and clomipramine) or the selective serotonin reuptake inhibitors (SSRIs) [e.g., fluoxetine (10–20 mg/d)] or selective norepinephrine reuptake inhibitors (e.g., venlafaxine) can improve cataplexy.
- **Gamma hydroxybutyrate** (GHB) is effective in reducing daytime cataplectic episodes.
- **Sodium oxybate,** a sodium salt of GHB alone or combined with modafinil, can reduce sleep disruption significantly. It is administered at night to help consolidate REM sleep and increase slow-wave sleep. It significantly reduces daytime sleepiness and also improves cataplexy.
- **Pitolisant**, a histamine H3 receptor inverse agonist, is effective treatment for cataplexy and daytime sleepiness.
- Others: Selegiline, clomipramine, fluoxetine, and venlafaxine.

Q. Write short notes on circadian rhythm sleep disorders.

- Circadian rhythm sleep disorders (CRSDs) are mainly due to alterations of the circadian time-keeping system or asynchrony between the endogenous circadian rhythm and external factors that affect the timing or duration of sleep.
- Wake-sleep schedule disorders fall into two categories:
  1. Primary malfunction of the biologic clock per se
  2. Secondary malfunction due to environmental effects on the underlying clock.

Example: Shift work type: Night shift or shift changes

Jet Lag Disorder is associated with excessive daytime sleepiness, sleep onset insomnia, and frequent arousals from sleep, especially in the latter half of the night. Transient symptoms of difficulty falling asleep at the appropriate time and daytime sleepiness following rapid change in time zones altering the timing of exogenous light stimuli.

Diagnosis

- Made by **history** and a **sleep diaries**.
- **Actigraphy:** Based on a wrist-mounted motion detector worn as an outpatient for at least 7 days. It can help in quantify time spent asleep.

Treatment of the Primary Circadian Rhythm Disorders

- **Chronotherapy:**
  - Useful in delayed sleep phase type of circadian rhythm disorders.
  - Patient delays the onset of sleep by a few hours every day and sleeps only the predetermined number of hours until the onset of sleep occurs at the desired time.
- **Phototherapy:** Bright light therapy:
  - Patient sits at a prescribed distance from a bright light with an illuminance of greater than 2,500 lux at that distance for 2–3 hours in the morning.
- **Pharmacologic therapy:**
  - **Melatonin** 3 mg given 4–5 hours before the desired time of sleep onset. Useful in patients with delayed sleep phase.
- **For jet lag:**
  - Behavioral strategies (good sleep hygiene), shifting sleep, and wake times gradually before travel to conform to the destination's time zone and avoiding bright light exposure before bedtime.
  - Melatonin administered before bedtime in the new time zone.

Q. Write short notes on sleep-related movement disorders.

These include restless leg syndrome and periodic limb movement disorder.

Restless Leg Syndrome (Willis-Ekbom Disease)

It is characterized by urge to move legs and patient usually complains of a variety of uncomfortable sensations in the legs (e.g., pins and needles, creeping or crawling sensations, aching, itching, stabbing, heaviness, tension, burning, or coldness).

- Symptoms are usually experienced during periods of prolonged rest or inactivity.
- Symptoms are typically relieved only by movement or stimulation of the legs.
- The discomfort appears more prominent during evening and between midnight and 4 AM.
- May disrupt sleep initiation.

Types

- **Primary or idiopathic:** Inherited as an autosomal dominant disorder.
- **Secondary:** To other causes, including **iron deficiency**, pregnancy, varicose vein or venous reflux, uremia, or folate deficiency, peripheral neuropathy, radiculopathy rheumatoid arthritis, etc. It often develops suddenly and may be daily from the very beginning.

Treatment

- Treatment of the underlying condition.
- **First-line drugs:** Dopamine agonists (e.g., pramipexole, carbidopa/levodopa or pergolide, and ropinirole) are the treatments of choice.
- **Other drugs** include quinine levodopa preparations, gabapentin, opiate agonists (e.g., oxycodone, codeine, propoxyphene oxycodone, or methadone), benzodiazepines (e.g., clonazepam which often assists in staying asleep and reducing awakenings from the movements) may also be effective. Anticonvulsants, such as gabapentin, often helpful in patients with painful sensations.

Periodic Limb Movement Disorder

- It is a repetitive, stereotyped limb movement and consists of 0.5- to 5.0-s extensions of the great toe and dorsiflexion of the foot.

- It occurs/recurs every 20–40 seconds during NREM sleep and each episode lasts from minutes to hours.
- Movements often disrupt sleep and lead to daytime sleepiness.

Treatment
Dopaminergic medications or benzodiazepines.

SEXUAL DISORDERS

It includes sexual dysfunction, paraphilia, and gender identity disorder.

Q. Write short notes on sexual dysfunctions: based on phases of sexual cycle.

- ***Desire disorders***:
  - Decreased—frigidity/hypoactive sexual desire disorder
  - Increased—satyriasis (male), nymphomaniac (female)
- ***Arousal disorders***: Erectile dysfunction (organic/psychological), female sexual arousal disorder
- ***Orgasm disorders***: Premature ejaculation, female orgasm disorder
- ***Resolution disorders***: Post-coital dysphoria

Q. Write short notes on paraphilias.

See **Table 18.27.**

TABLE 18.27: Paraphilia—abnormality in sexual preference.

	Deviation in sexual object	
Deviation in sexual act: Sexual pleasure attained by	***Animate***	***Inanimate***
➢ ***Sadism***—inflicting pain on others ➢ ***Masochism***—feeling pain inflicted by partner ➢ ***Voyeurism***—watching others grooming/getting intimate ➢ ***Exhibitionism***—showing private parts to unexpecting individual ➢ ***Frotteurism***—rubbing genitals against clothed individual	➢ ***Pedophilia***—child ➢ ***Bestiality/zoophilia***—animal ➢ ***Necrophilia***—cadavers	➢ ***Fetishism***—shoes, stockings, etc. ➢ ***Transvestite fetishism***—cross dress *for sexual pleasure*

Q. Write short notes on gender identity disorders (DSM-IV).

- It has been renamed as gender dysphoria in DSM-5 and as gender incongruence in ICD-11.
- ICD-11 considers gender identity disorder as a sexual health disorder and not a psychiatric disorder.
- It refers to presence of incongruence/dissatisfaction with allotted/biological sex + persistent desire to be identified as member of opposite sex.
- It can be further classified as:
- Transexualism is the severe form and they can be offered sex reassignment surgery along with hormonal therapy.
- Removal of male external genitalia and reconstruction of female external genitalia and vice-versa is the procedure followed in sex reassignment surgery.

Feature	*Dual role transvestism*	*Transexualism*
Cross dressing *to be identified as member of opposite sex*	Present	Present
Desire for sex change therapy	Absent	Present

PERSONALITY DISORDERS

Personality: Enduring pattern of behavior, cognition, and emotions that makes every individual unique.
Personality disorder: Problems with understanding self and others, thus causing interpersonal dysfunction.

Q. Write short notes on clinical features of personality disorders.

See **Table 18.28.**

TABLE 18.28: Classification of personality disorders (DSM-5) and their characteristic features.

Cluster A *Odd, eccentric*	*Cluster B* *Dramatic, emotional*	*Cluster C* *Anxious, fearful*
➢ ***Schizoid*** (emotionally detached) ➢ ***Schizotypal*** (magical thinking, speech oddities) ➢ ***Paranoid*** (extreme suspiciousness)	➢ ***Borderline*** (unstable relationships, mood swings) ➢ ***Histrionic*** (need to center of attraction) ➢ ***Narcissistic*** (self-centered) ➢ ***Antisocial*** (break rules and laws)	➢ ***Anxious-avoidant*** (sensitive to rejection) ➢ ***Dependent*** (need reassurance) ➢ ***Anankastic*** (perfectionist)

Management of personality disorders includes both pharmacological methods (like antidepressants, antipsychotics and mood stabilizers) as well as psychotherapy. Dialectic behavior therapy is used for borderline personality disorder.

CHILD PSYCHIATRY

It includes the following disorders:

- Neurodevelopmental disorders: Intellectual disability, specific learning disability
- Disruptive behavioral disorders of childhood: Oppositional defiant disorder, conduct disorder
- ADHD, Tourette's syndrome
- Autism spectrum disorders
- Disruptive mood dysregulation disorder

INTELLECTUAL DISABILITY

Q. Write short notes on intellectual disability (ID).

- It was called mental retardation in ICD-10. It has been renamed as intellectual disability in DSM-5 and ICD-11 calls it disorders of intellectual development.
- Normal intelligence is defined as: IQ 90–110
- Dull normal intelligence: IQ 80–89
- Borderline intelligence: IQ 70–79

Table 18.29 shows the classification based on severity of intellectual disability.

TABLE 18.29: Classification based on severity of intellectual disability.

Feature	*ICD10*	*ICD11/DSM-5*
Severity assessed by	Intelligence quotient	Adaptive functioning
Mild	50–69	2–3 SD below mean
Moderate	35–49	3–4 SD below mean
Severe	20–34	> 4 SD below mean
Profound	<20	

Etiology

Genetic disorders like Down syndrome and Fragile X syndrome are the most common causes of intellectual disability. Other causes include metabolic and chromosomal disorders, obstetric complications, and nutritional and infective causes.

Clinical Features

These include physical stigmata of respective chromosomal anomaly like wide spaced eyes, microcephaly, short stature, etc., slow to learn, below average intelligence.

Investigations

- Blood and urine work up to look for inborn errors of metabolism
- Neuroimaging and karyotyping to establish the cause of ID
- Intelligence assessment

Management

It includes behavior therapies like contingency management, life skills training, use of antipsychotics to control aggression, etc.

Specific learning disability includes:

- **Dyslexia:** Difficulty in reading
- **Dysgraphia:** Difficulty in writing
- **Dyscalculia:** Difficulty in arithmetics

Management: Training with the help of special educator

Q. Write short notes on disruptive behavioral disorders of childhood.

See **Table 18.30**.

TABLE 18.30: Disruptive behavioral disorders of childhood.

Features	*Oppositional defiant disorder*	*Conduct disorder*
Angry, irritable, and revengeful	Present	Present
Disobedient behavior, out of keeping with child's developmental age	Persistent ≥6 months	Persistent ≥12 months
Abusive behavior	Verbal	Verbal and physical
Violation of others rights (theft, destruction of property, fire setting, and torturing animals)	Usually not seen	Present

ATTENTION DEFICIT HYPERACTIVITY DISORDER

Q. Write short notes on attention deficit hyperactivity disorder.

- It is a disorder characterized by triad of hyperactivity, impulsivity, attention deficit manifesting at ≥2 contexts and having its onset before 12 years of age. It is more common in boys.
- Etiology: Abnormality in information processing due to involvement of cortico-striato-thalamo-cortical loop
- Clinical features include—inability to wait for their turn or to sit at one place, poor concentration, losing things easily, poor scholastic performance despite normal IQ, etc.
- Management includes pharmacotherapy stimulants like methylphenidate and dextroamphetamine and nonstimulants like atomoxetine, clonidine, and behavioral techniques like attention enhancing tasks, social skills training, and behavior therapy.

Tic/Tourette Disorder

- Tourette syndrome (TS) is a neurological disorder characterized by repetitive, stereotyped, involuntary movements and vocalizations called tics.
- It can be of four types:
  1. Vocal tics: Throat clearing, grunting
  2. Motor tics: Eye blinking, head nodding
  3. Coprolalia: Blurting obscene words
  4. Palilalia: Repeating words
- It can be managed by using antipsychotics like risperidone and haloperidol. Clonidine can also be used.
- Behavioral techniques include habit reversal and others.

AUTISTIC SPECTRUM DISORDER

Q. Write short notes on autism spectrum disorders.

- It was previously called pervasive developmental disorders to describe a group of disorders that shared similar clinical features, i.e., abnormalities in reciprocal communication and repetitive stereotyped behaviors as core features.
- Clinical features include self-absorbed child with poor eye to eye contact, lack of social smile, delayed milestones, problems in attachment with parents and others, repetitive hand wringing, banging, etc.
- Management is mainly with psychotherapy (social skills training, speech and communication, behavioral) and antipsychotics like risperidone and aripiprazole.

Q. Write short notes on mood disorders seen in children.

Childhood Depression

- It can also be called as anaclitic depression.
- Clinical features differ from that in adults that it can present with school refusal, frequent anger outburst, and recurrent somatic complaints.
- Fluoxetine is the antidepressant approved for use.

Disruptive Mood Dysregulation Syndrome

- Characterized by presence of temper outbursts which can be expressed verbally/physically, are out of keeping with the situation and in excess than that expected for child's developmental age.
- Seen in children of age 6–18 years
- Temper outbursts occur ≥3 times/week for at least 12 months, in at least two different settings (school, home, etc.)
- Management is with pharmacotherapy (SSRI, stimulants, etc.) and psychotherapy (CBT).

GERIATRIC PSYCHIATRY

- All the psychiatric disorders can occur in the elderly too.
- They might vary in their presentation due to significant overlap of symptoms of dementia and other medical comorbidities.
- Due to altered bodily response of the drug, management of the illness varies from adult psychiatry.
- Common psychiatric disorders in elderly are:
  - Geriatric depression/melancholic depression (described under depression): Sertraline may be beneficial especially in those with cardiac comorbidities.
  - Old age psychosis: Features of late-onset schizophrenia may be seen including paranoid ideations.
- Management depends on management of comorbidities, avoid polypharmacy, adequate palliative care, slower titration of drug dosage, active watch for side-effects, and supportive psychotherapy.

PUERPERAL DISORDERS

Three common psychiatric disorders occur after childbirth.

1. **Postpartum blues:** These are characterized by irritability, labile mood, and tearfulness. Symptoms start soon after childbirth, and peak by about the fourth day and then resolve.
2. **Postpartum depression:** It develops in 10–15% of women within a month of delivery and is characterized by guilt, anhedonia, and suicidal thoughts. It is managed with antidepressants, ECT.
3. **Puerperal psychosis**

Q. Write short note on puerperal psychosis.

- It is a rare disorder occurring in perhaps less than 1 or 2 per 1,000 deliveries. It is more common in primiparous than multiparous women.
- Symptoms generally appear abruptly within about 3 days to several weeks after delivery.
- Rarely serious complication, such as a manic or depressive psychosis may develop. It may be associated with a personal or familial history of bipolar disorder.
- Management is with antidepressants, antipsychotics, and ECT.
- Hospitalization is generally indicated.
- Most women recover but have an increased (25%) risk of developing puerperal psychosis in the next pregnancy, and a 50% lifetime risk.

EMERGENCIES IN PSYCHIATRY

Q. Enumerate and describe the recognition and clinical presentation of psychiatric emergencies. Describe the initial stabilization and management of psychiatric emergencies.

It can be broadly classified as behaviors manifesting with harm to self/others, acute effects of substance use, and acute psychosis/mania.

Suicide, Deliberate Self Harm

- It is an act leading to intentional death.
- September 10 is observed as World Suicide Prevention Day by WHO and International Association for suicide prevention as an awareness creating tool regarding the preventability of suicide.
- Suicide has become one of the leading causes of preventable deaths.
- Mental Health Care Act, 2017 has decriminalized suicide by stating that any individual committing suicide shall be presumed to be under severe stress, unless proven otherwise.

Emil Durkheim described three ***types of suicide***:

1. Egoistic: Due to lack of integration into society, e.g., person with poor support committing suicide
2. Altruistic: Due to excessive integration into society, e.g., committing suicide for the sake of a celebrity
3. Anomic: Due to rejection of integration into society, e.g., committing suicide due to debts

Risk Factors

- Middle-aged men
- Poor family and social support
- Single/unmarried/divorced
- Recent loss in relationship, occupation, and finance
- Medical comorbidities: Long-standing illness, end-stage diseases
- Psychiatric comorbidities: Depression, substance use, and schizophrenia
- Previous suicide attempt
- Family history of suicide
- Postmortem studies have found low-levels of 5-hydroxyindoleacetic acid in those who completed suicide

Early warning signs of suicidal intent:

- Writing a suicide note
- Making a will
- Transferring money to the account of family member
- Transferring one's responsibility
- Indicating that this is my last visit and after this all the problems will be solved
- Procuring/collecting harmful substances (gun, knife, and insecticides)
- Visiting the site to inspect and find out the timings when human traffic will be lower
- Expressing feelings of hopelessness, worthlessness
- Indulging in harmful behavior: Driving with high speeds, excessive substance intake

Management

- Suicidal risk assessment: Assess for risk factors and early warning signs. Hopelessness carries a high risk
- IP care is advisable for an individual with high suicidal risk.
- 24-hour supervision while ensuring a safe environment (keep away any objects that can be used to harm oneself).
- Complete diagnostic evaluation for medical and psychiatric comorbidities and their management.
- Clozapine and lithium are the two drugs with antisuicidal properties.
- Antidepressants and mood stabilizers can be used in comorbid depressive disorder.
- Intranasal/IV Esketamine/ECT also has been used for rapid control of symptoms
- Provision of psychological and emotional support through supportive, cognitive behavioral psychotherapy, and family therapy

Acute Agitation

Agitation refers to a state of sudden behavioral activation. It can occur as a symptom of psychiatric disorders (mania, substance intoxication/withdrawal), depression, schizophrenia, dissociative disorders or due to organic causes (delirium, catastrophic reaction in dementia, and head injury).

Management includes:

- Evaluation for organic causes
- Ensure safety of patient and the examiner: Examination in open room which is free of objects that can be used to harm.
- Oral/IV drugs: Benzodiazepines (lorazepam and diazepam) and antipsychotics (haloperidol)
- Use of physical restraints if required
- Monitoring vitals and detailed evaluation once the patient is calm.

PSYCHOSOMATIC DISORDER

Q. Write short note on psychosomatic disorder.

Psychosomatic disorder is characterized by presence of organic pathology, but is altered by psychological influence. It includes those disorders which are either initiated or exacerbated by the presence of meaningful psychosocial environmental stressors.

Classical psychosomatic illnesses:
- Bronchial asthma
- Ulcerative colitis
- Peptic ulcer
- Neurodermatitis
- Thyrotoxicosis
- Rheumatic arthritis
- Essential hypertension

COMMUNITY PSYCHIATRY

Q. Write short note on National Mental Health Programme (NMHP), 1982.

Objectives

- To ensure availability and accessibility of minimum mental health care for all in foreseeable future, particularly to most vulnerable and underprivileged section of population.
- Encourage application of mental health knowledge in general health care and social development.
- Promote community participation in mental health service development and stimulate efforts toward self-help in community.

Strategies

- Integration of mental health care with primary health care (training PHC doctors in diagnosis and treatment of common psychiatric disorders like depression and insomnia).
- Strengthening tertiary care institutions for treatment of mental health disorders.
- Eradicating stigmatization of mentally ill patients (through awareness campaigns) and protecting their rights through regulatory institutions like central and state mental health authorities.
  NMHP is implemented through District Mental Health Program (DMHP) and School Mental Health Program (SMHP).

Activities in ***District Mental Health Program***:
- Training of medical, paramedical personnel, and community leaders
- Community mental health care through existing infrastructure of health services
- Information, education, and communication activities

Activities in ***School Mental Health Program***: Training school teachers by providing:
- Knowledge and skills to identify emotional, conduct in students
- System to refer students with psychological problems to DMHP team for evaluation and treatment
- Skills to promote life skills among students

FORENSIC PSYCHIATRY

Confidentiality in Psychiatry

- Mental healthcare professional has the duty to maintain confidentiality with respect to information providing during diagnosis and treatment of mental illness.
- However, maintaining confidentiality is exempted when the information is required for treatment, in legal issues, to prevent harm to others or for public safety.

Q. Write short note on criminal responsibility of mentally ill.

- If the act occurred as a product of mental illness, individual with mental illness in not criminally responsible, if at the time of committing the act he was unable to understand the nature and consequences of the act or that the act is wrong or contrary to law. This is also called the insanity defense.
- McNaghten's rule states that unless proven otherwise, every person shall be considered to be of sane mind which shall be decided by the jury.
- Insanity is punishable if he was of sound mind at the time of committing the act (i.e., during lucid interval, remission phase of episodic illness)
- Acts committed under intoxication of substance/hypnotization cannot stand for legal defense as the person was aware of the consequences while initiating the act.

Q. Write short note on civil responsibility of mentally ill.

- During lucid intervals of psychiatric disorder when he is able to understand the consequences of the act, one can exercise his civil rights of making a will to dispose one's assets, to give witness, and also can make a contract. However, these are subject to courts discretion.

- Individual with profound intellectual disability/dementia cannot hold a driving license.
- A marriage shall be void and eligible for divorce if at the time of marriage, either of the party was incapable of giving valid consent or has been suffering from such severity of illness that interferes with usual course of marriage and procreation.

Q. Write short note on Mental Health Care Act, 2017.

It has replaced the Mental Health Care (MHC) bill of 2013, wherein previous assurance-based approach has been changed to right-based approach. Its main features include:
- It recognizes the rights of mentally ill by recognizing capacity of individual to make mental healthcare decisions, making regulations for hospitalization (independent and supported), and use of restraints.
- Advanced directive: An individual has the right to choose how he wants to be treated for mental illness.
- Nominated representative: Every individual can appoint his representative who would take decisions on his behalf in case he loses his capacity to make mental health decisions.
- Central and state mental health authorities to protect the rights of mentally ill.
- Decriminalizing suicide: Any person attempting suicide shall be presumed to be under severe stress and hence should not be punished.
- Prohibition of ECT in minors and prohibition of direct ECT
- Rules for establishing Mental Health Establishments

Child Abuse

- Abuse is defined by tissue damage, neglect, sexual exploitation, and mental cruelty.
- It is mandatorily reportable offense.
- Treating physician will be charged for criminal offense if not reported.
- Duties of treating physician include: To report the offense and to protect the child
- Clinical features that should raise the index of suspicion: Broken bones in 1st year of life, STD in young children, soft tissue injuries, and nonaccidental burns.

POCSO: Prevention of Children from Sexual Offences Act, 2012 has been framed to protect the child from such offenses.

Penetrative and aggravated penetrative sexual assault have a punishment of minimum 10 and 20 years life imprisonment + fine, respectively, whereas sexual assault and aggravated sexual assault have a punishment of fine + imprisonment for 3–5 years and 5–7 years, respectively.

MISCELLANEOUS TOPICS

Important Names in Psychiatry
- Johann Christian Reil: Coined the term "Psychiatry", Father of Psychiatry
- Philippe Pinel: Unchaining and humane treatment of mentally ill
- Sigmund Freud: Father of Psychoanalysis, interpretation of dreams, structure of mind
- Ugo Cerlitti and Bini: ECT
- John Cade: Lithium

Terminologies
- **Rapport:** Meaningful and therapeutic relation between patient and healthcare provider
- **Empathy:** Ability to understand what and how others feel
- **Stigma:** Sign of disgrace that sets a person apart from others
- **Stereotype:** Generalized belief about a particular group/class of people
- **Prejudice:** Affective feeling toward an individual solely based on his group membership

BREAKING BAD NEWS

Q. Discuss SPIKES protocol for breaking bad news.

SPIKES protocol is followed for breaking bad news.
- **S**: Setting up and starting the conversation
- **P**: Elicit patient/family members perception
- **I**: Invite them to ask what they would want to know
- **K**: Provide knowledge in small pieces
- **E**: Recognize and empathize with their emotions
- **S**: Set out strategy of plan of action and summarize the gist of the conversation

DOCTOR–PATIENT RELATIONSHIP

Q. Write short note on four models of doctor–patient relationship.

	Decision-making responsibility	*Level of disclosure of medical information*
Paternalistic/autocratic	Doctor	Minimal
Deliberative	Doctor > patient	Selective
Interpretative	Patient > doctor	Major
Informative	Patient	Complete

Learning

Q. Explain the theories and process of learning.

Learning: Process by which behavioral changes occur.

- ***Ivan Pavlov's*** classical conditioning using dog experiment:
  - Neutral stimulus (bell) + Unconditioned stimulus (food) = Unconditioned response (drool)
  - After conditioning, neutral stimulus becomes conditioned stimulus to produce conditioned response (drool).
- ***Skinner's***: Operant conditioning using rats and pigeons:
  - Operant chamber in which food was delivered when animal pressed the lever. This was used to describe the effect of reinforcement and punishment on behavioral change.

CHAPTER

19

Genetics

COMMON GENETIC AND CHROMOSOMAL DISORDERS

Q. Write short essay/note on various types (classification) of chromosomal disorders/aberrations.

Classification of Chromosomal Disorders (Box 19.1)

Box 19.1: Types of chromosomal abnormality.

Numerical abnormalities

Aneuploidy
- Monosomy
- Trisomy
- Tetrasomy

Polyploidy
- Triploidy
- Tetraploidy

Structural abnormalities
- Translocations (exchange)
- Deletions (loss)
- Duplications
- Insertions
- Inversions
- Nondisjunction
- Ring chromosome

Isochromosomes

Mixoploidy
- Mosaicism
- Chimerism

Numerical Chromosomal Aberrations

Normal cells are **diploid** containing 46 chromosomes, 22 pairs of autosomes and 1 pair of sex chromosomes. The 23 chromosomes (22 autosomes and one sex chromosome) constitute a **haploid**. Any exact multiple of the haploid number is called **euploid**.

Types of numerical aberrations

Aneuploidy: It is defined as a **chromosome number that is not a multiple of 23** (the normal haploid number). It is caused by either loss or gain of one or more chromosomes. Aneuploidy may result from **nondisjunction or anaphase lag**.

- **Trisomy:** Numerical abnormalities with the presence of **one extra chromosome** are referred to as trisomy (2n + 1). It may involve either **sex chromosomes or autosomes**. *Examples:* Down syndrome (patients have three copies of chromosome 21, i.e., 47 XX, +21, hence Down syndrome is often known as trisomy 21), Patau syndrome (trisomy 13; 47 XY, +13), and Edwards syndrome (trisomy 18; 47 XY, +18).
- **Monosomy:** Numerical abnormalities with the **absence or loss of one chromosome** (2n – 1) are referred to as monosomy. It may involve autosomes or sex chromosomes. Monosomy of autosomes is almost incompatible with survival. Example for monosomy of sex chromosomes is Turner syndrome **(45 XO)** instead of normal XX (46 XX).

Polyploidy: It is chromosome number that is a multiple greater than two of the haploid number (multiples of haploid number 23). Triploidy is three times the haploid number (69), tetraploidy is four times the haploid number (92). Polyploidy is incompatible with life and usually results in spontaneous abortion.

Causes of numerical aberrations

- Numerical aberrations can occur during meiosis and/or mitosis. These errors are due to nondisjunction and anaphase lag.
- **Nondisjunction:** It is failure of paired chromosomes to separate during meiosis or mitosis. Meiotic nondisjunction is the most common cause.
- **Anaphase lag:** Anaphase lag results in the loss of a chromosome during meiosis or mitosis.

Structural Chromosomal Aberrations (Box 19.1)

Q. Discuss chromosomal translocations with examples.

- **What is reciprocal translocation?**
- **Write a note on Robertsonian translocation.**

Structural chromosomal aberrations may occur either during **mitosis** or **meiosis**.

Causes of structural alterations: It may occur spontaneously at a low rate and is increased by exposure to environmental mutagens, such as chemicals and ionizing radiation.

Types of Structural/Chromosomal Aberrations (Figs. 19.1A to H)

Translocations: It is a structural alteration between two chromosomes in which a **segment of one chromosome gets detached and is transferred to another chromosome**. There are two types of translocations.

1. **Balanced reciprocal translocations:** It is characterized by single break in each of the two chromosomes with exchange of genetic material distal to the break. There is no loss of genetic material. A balanced reciprocal translocation between the long arm of chromosome 5 and the short arm of chromosome 10 would be written *46, XX, t (5; 10) (q31; p14)*.
   - **Simple translocation:** In this case, terminal segment of a chromosome is integrated at one end of a nonhomologous region. Simple translocations are rather rare.
   - **Shift:** In shift, an intercalary segment of a chromosome is integrated within a nonhomologous chromosome.
2. **Robertsonian translocation/centric fusion:**
   - This results from the breakage of two acrocentric chromosomes (i.e., chromosome **13, 14, 15, 21, 22)** at or close to their centromeres and subsequent fusion of their long arms.
   - The short arms of each chromosome are lost, this being of no clinical importance as they contain genes only for ribosomal RNA, for which there are multiple copies on various other chromosomes.
   - The total chromosome number is reduced to **45**.
   - The overall incidence of this translocation is 1 in 1,000, the most common being 13q14q.
   - The major practical importance is that this can predispose to the birth of babies with Down syndrome.

Inversion: When a segment of chromosome is oriented in the reverse direction, such segment said to be inverted and the phenomenon is termed as inversion.

Isochromosomes: They are formed **due to faulty centromere division**. Normally, centromeres divide in a plane parallel to long axis of the chromosome. If a centromere divides in a plane transverse to the long axis, it results in pair of isochromosomes. One pair consists of two short arms and the other of two long arms.

Deletion: It is **the loss of a part of a chromosome**. It is of two types namely: (1) interstitial (middle) and (2) terminal (rare).

- **Interstitial deletion:** It occurs when there are two breaks within a chromosome arm. This is followed by loss of the chromosomal material between the breaks and fusion of the broken ends of the remaining portion of the chromosome. It has to be specified in which region(s) and at what bands the breaks have occurred. For example, *46, XY, del (16) (p11.2p13.1)* describes breakpoints in the short arm of chromosome 16 at 16p11.2 and 16p13.1 with loss of material between breaks.
- **Terminal deletion:** It results from a single break at the terminal part in a chromosome arm, producing a shortened chromosome bearing a deletion and a fragment with no centromere. The fragment is then lost at the next cell division.

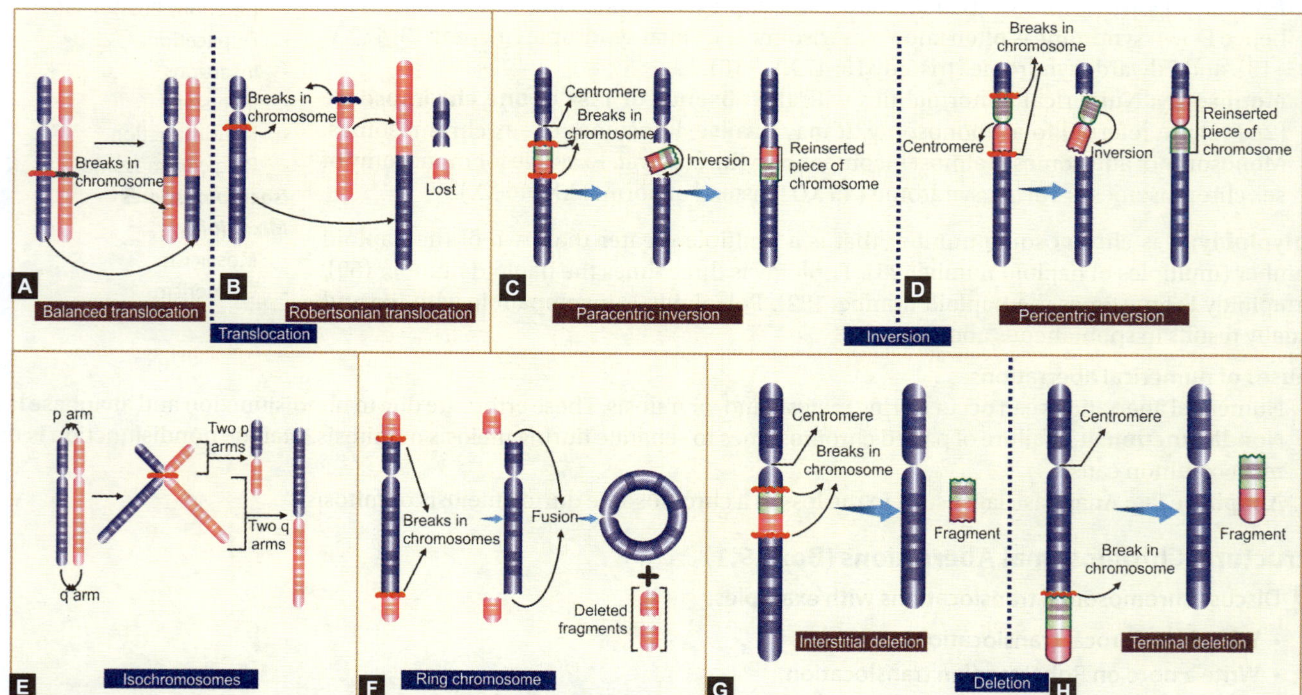

FIGS. 19.1A TO H: Types of structural abnormalities of chromosome.

Ring chromosome: It is a **special form of deletion**. Ring chromosomes are formed by a break at both the ends of a chromosome with fusion of the damaged ends.

Insertion: It is a form of **nonreciprocal translocation** in which a fragment of chromosome is transferred and inserted into a nonhomologous chromosome.

Mixoploidy

Mosaicism: Defined as the presence in an individual, or in a tissue, of two or more cell lines that differ in their genetic constitution but are derived from a single zygote, i.e., they have the same genetic origin. Seen in Down syndrome (1–2%) and Duchenne muscular dystrophy.

Chimerism: Defined as the presence in an individual, or in a tissue, of two or more cell lines that are derived from more than one zygote, i.e., they have different genetic origin.

DOWN SYNDROME (TRISOMY 21)

Q. Write short essay/note on Down syndrome and its clinical features.

The best known and most common chromosome related syndrome. Formerly known as "Mongolism".
It is the most common chromosomal disorder and is a leading cause *of mental retardation.* The incidence of Down syndrome in newborns is about 1 in 700 live births.

Etiology and Pathogenesis

- **Maternal age:** It has a **strong influence** on the incidence of trisomy 21. Children of older mothers have much greater risk of having Down syndrome. The risk for mothers < 25 years of age to have the trisomy is about 1 in 1,500 births. At 40 years of age, 1 in 100 births. At 45 years, 1 in 40 births.
- **Other factors:** Increased incidence may be associated with exposure of mother to pesticides, electromagnetic fields, anesthetic drugs, alcohol, and caffeine.

Mechanism of trisomy 21: The three copies of chromosome 21 in somatic cells cause Down syndrome. It may be due to:
1. About 95% of these individuals have *nondisjunction* during the first meiotic division of gametogenesis.
2. *Robertsonian translocation* of an extra long arm of chromosome 21 to another acrocentric chromosome causes about 5% of cases.
3. About 1% *mosaicism* having two different cell lines, one with normal chromosomal constitution and the other with an extra chromosome 21.

Clinical Features (Fig. 19.2)

Craniofacial and Skeletal Features

- Flat face and occiput, with a low-bridged nose, reduced interpupillary distance and oblique palpebral fissures.
- Epicanthal folds of the eyes impart an almond shape to the eyes and an oriental appearance (obsolete term mongolism).
- A speckled appearance of the iris (Brushfield spots), enlarged and malformed ears.
- A protruding furrowed tongue (macroglossia), which typically lacks a central fissure and protrudes through an open mouth (scrotal tongue).
- Broad, short neck, brachycephaly, Simian crease-single palmar flexion crease (50% cases), clinodactyly-incurved fifth finger with hypoplastic mid phalanx (60%), short stature, hypotonia and space between the first and second toes (sandal gap).

Brain: Mild to moderate intellectual **disability**, attention-deficit hyperactivity disorder, autism, dementia, atlantoaxial dislocation.

Heart: Congenital **cardiac anomalies** are responsible for the majority of the deaths in infancy and early childhood. The genetic band in 21q22 critical region is considered responsible for the cardiac anomalies. Complete atrioventricular septal defect (CAVSD)—37%, ventricular septal defect (VSD)—31%, atrial septal defect (ASD)—15%, partial atrioventricular septal defect (PAVSD)—6%, and patent ductus arteriosus (PDA)—4%.

Gastrointestinal tract: It may show esophageal/duodenal stenosis or atresia, imperforate anus and Hirschsprung disease (megacolon).

Genitourinary: Hypospadias, cryptorchidism. Males are infertile due to impaired spermatogenesis.

Immune system: Affected children are susceptible to infections due to defective immunity.

Endocrine system: Antithyroid antibodies may cause hypothyroidism and type 1 diabetes.

Hematologic disorders: They have increased risk of acute myeloid or lymphoblastic leukemia. Polycythemia, macrocytosis, leukopenia, and leukemia (acute megakaryoblastic, and acute lymphoblastic).

Other features: Refractive errors, strabismus, sensory neural hearing loss, obesity, obstructive sleep apnea, palmoplantar hyperkeratosis, juvenile idiopathic arthritis.

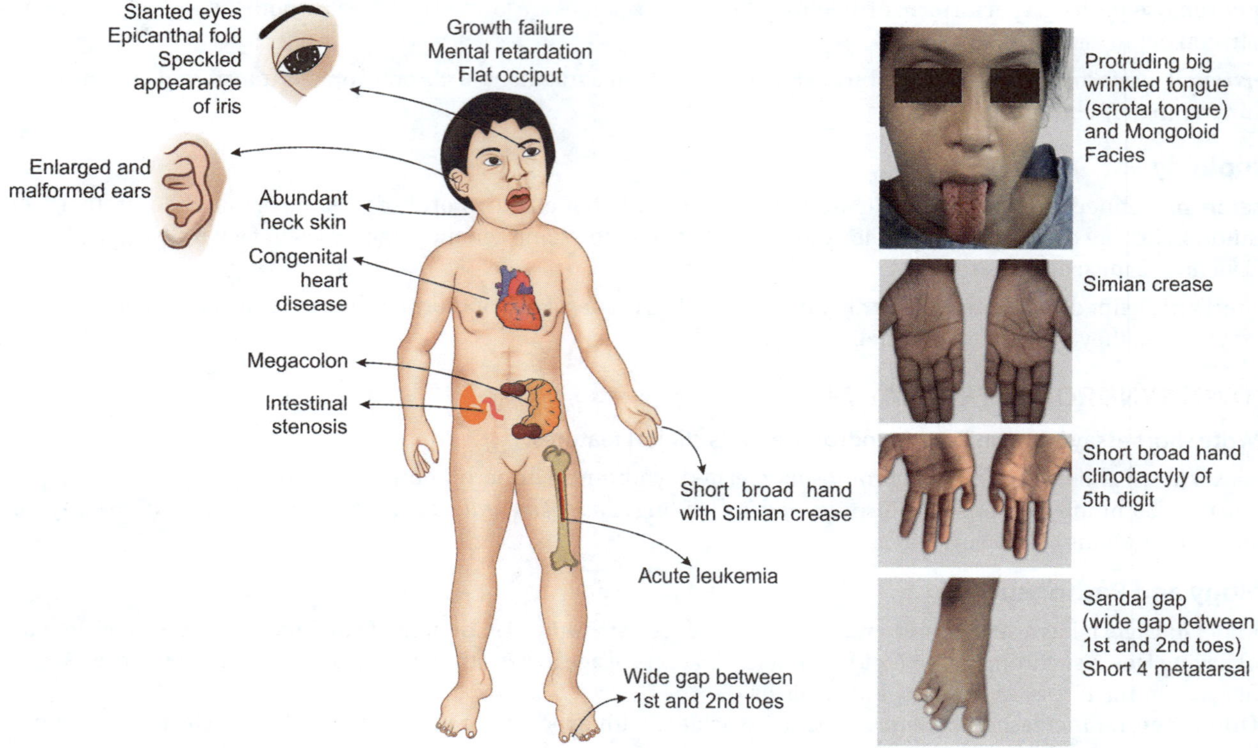

FIG. 19.2: Major clinical features of Down syndrome.

Down syndrome screens are mentioned in **Box 19.2**.

Box 19.2: Down syndrome screens.

- **Triple screen (75% sensitive):** Maternal serum alpha- fetoprotein, estriol, and human chorionic gonadotropin.
- **Quad screen (79% sensitive):** Maternal serum alpha-feto-protein, estriol, human chorionic gonadotropin, and high inhibin-alpha (INHA).
- **Nuchal translucency/free beta-hCG>/PAPPA screen (91% sensitive):** Ultrasound to measure nuchal translucency in addition to the free Beta-hCG and PAPPA (pregnancy-associated plasma protein A).
- **The full integrated test** (first-trimester nuchal translucency and PAPPA plus second-trimester quadruple markers) detects 85% of Down syndrome fetuses.

KLINEFELTER SYNDROME

Q. Write short essay/note on Klinefelter syndrome.

It is an important genetic cause of male hypogonadism and is associated with reduced spermatogenesis and male infertility.

Pathogenesis

- Most patients with Klinefelter syndrome have one extra X chromosome (47, XXY karyotype). It is due to *nondisjunction* of X chromosome during meiosis.
- A minority is mosaic (e.g., 46, XY/47, XXY) or has more than two X chromosomes (e.g., 48, XXXY) and one or more Y chromosomes.

Clinical Features (Fig. 19.3)

- Klinefelter syndrome is usually diagnosed after puberty.
- Most patients are **tall and thin** with relatively long legs (eunuchoid body habitus). Mental retardation is uncommon, although average intelligence quotient (IQ) is reduced.
- At puberty, **testes and penis remain small with lack of secondary male characteristics**.
  - Female characteristics develop which include a **high-pitched/deep voice, gynecomastia,** and a **female pattern of pubic hair**. Sparse facial, body and sexual hair.
  - **Azoospermia** results in infertility.

All of these changes are due to hypogonadism and reduced levels of testosterone.

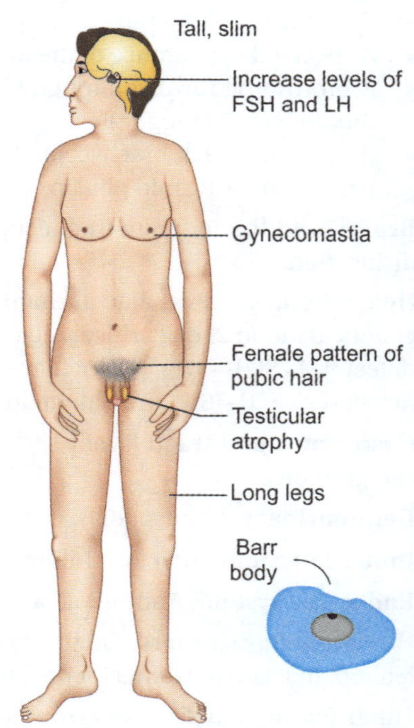

FIG. 19.3: Clinical features of Klinefelter syndrome.

Diagnosis

- **Buccal smear for Barr body:** Extra X chromosome may be seen as a Barr body on buccal smears.
- **Nuclear sexing of leukocytes: Neutrophils** in the peripheral smear may also be examined for nuclear sexing. In a normal female (XX), the neutrophils in a peripheral smear show a drumstick which is counterpart of Barr body in buccal smear. One extra drumstick is found in males with *Klinefelter syndrome* (XXY).
- Chromosomal analysis
- *Hormonal status:*
  - Follicle-stimulating hormone (FSH) and luteinizing hormone (LH) are remarkably high.
  - *Testosterone:* Low to low-normal level.
  - The ratio of estrogens and testosterone determines the degree of feminization.

Complications of Klinefelter syndrome are listed in **Box 19.3**.

Box 19.3: Complications of Klinefelter syndrome.

- Increased **risk of breast carcinoma** in 47, XXY (relative risk exceeding 200 times).
- **Endocrine complications:** Diabetes mellitus, hypothyroidism and hypoparathyroidism.
- **Autoimmune diseases:** Systemic lupus erythematosus, Sjögren's syndrome and rheumatoid arthritis.
- Decreased bone density:
  - Increased risk of ischemic heart disease, mitral valve prolapse, lower extremity varicose veins, venous stasis ulcers, and deep venous thrombosis and pulmonary embolism
  - Extragonadal germ cell cancer and non-Hodgkin lymphoma occur in more frequency

Management

- *Testosterone:* It should be started at puberty (around 12 years age) and increasing its dosage sufficient to maintain serum concentrations of testosterone, estradiol, FSH, and LH appropriate to the age. It promotes normal body proportions and development of normal secondary sex characteristics. However, it does not affect infertility, gynecomastia, and atrophy of testis. It decreases the long-term complications such as breast cancer, autoimmune disease, and osteoporosis.
- Speech therapy.
- Physiotherapy for hypotonia or delayed motor skills.

TURNER SYNDROME

Q. Write short essay/note on Turner syndrome.

- Turner syndrome is a sex chromosomal abnormality. Turner syndrome is characterized by a spectrum of abnormalities due to **complete or partial monosomy of the X chromosome** in a phenotypic female.
- It is characterized by hypogonadism and is the **most common sex chromosome abnormality in females.**

Karyotypic Abnormalities

- *Missing of an entire X chromosome:* This resulting in a 45, X karyotype due to *nondisjunction* of X chromosomes during meiosis. Genetic constitution hence becomes 45 XO.
- *Structural abnormalities of the X chromosomes:* These includes isochromosome of the long arm, translocations, ring chromosome, and deletions (Xp/Xq).
- *Mosaics:* The mosaic patients have combination of a 45, X cell population along with one or more karyotypically normal or abnormal cell types. *Examples:* (1) 45, X/46, XX; (2) 45, X/46, XY. It is known as mosaic Turner syndrome.

Clinical Features (Fig. 19.4)

Turner syndrome is usually not discovered before puberty. It presents with **failure to develop normal secondary sex characteristics.** Important diagnostic features are:

- **Adult women** with **short stature** (<5 feet tall) **primary amenorrhea and sterility**. Raised FSH levels are noted.
- *Other features are:*
  - **Webbed neck,** and **low posterior hairline,** wide/increased carrying angle at the elbows (**cubitus valgus**), **Madelung deformity** of the forearm and wrist, broad chest (**shield chest**) with widely spaced nipples and hyperconvex fingernails.
  - The **genitalia remains infantile, breast development is inadequate,** and there is little pubic hair. The ovaries are converted to fibrous streaks. Lack of secondary sexual characteristics.

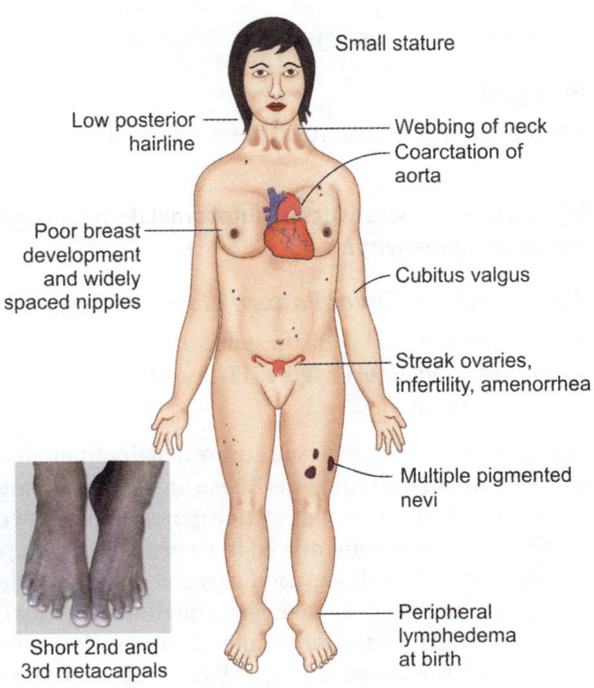

FIG. 19.4: Clinical features of Turner syndrome.

- Pigmented nevi and pilomatricoma as the age advances.
- Congenital lymphedema, short fourth metacarpals and/or metatarsals, horsehoe kidney, osteoporosis.
- **Cardiovascular anomalies** such as congenital heart disease particularly **coarctation of the aorta** or **bicuspid aortic valve** may be present. Aortic dissection or rupture is a common cause of death. Systemic hypertension is seen in 30% of cases. No mental retardation.

INTELLECTUAL DISABILITY

Q. Write short note on mental retardation and its causes.

Definition: It is a neurodevelopmental disorder that begins in childhood and is characterized by limitations in both intelligence and adaptive skills, affecting at least one of three adaptive domains (conceptual, social, and practical), with varying severity. Earlier was termed as mental retardation.

Causes of Intellectual Disability

See **Box 19.4.**

Box 19.4: Causes of intellectual disability.

- Genetic and chromosomal disorders, e.g., Down syndrome and fragile X syndrome
- *CNS lesions:*
  - Hydrocephalus
  - Microcephaly
  - Cerebral palsy
  - Post-traumatic, postmeningitic and postencephalitic states
  - Birth trauma, kernicterus
- *Environmental causes:*
  - *Associated intrauterine infections:* Congenital infections, congenital rubella syndrome, cytomegalovirus, and other viruses
  - *Intrauterine exposure to toxins and other insults:* Alcohol, hypoxia or malnutrition
  - *Postnatal causes:* Exposure to toxins, infection, and heavy metals
- Metabolic disease, e.g., cretinism, phenylketonuria, mucopolysaccharides, inborn errors of metabolism (e.g., glycogen storage diseases)

Assessment of Degree of Intellectual disability

Adaptive function: Impaired functioning in at least **one** of the following three domains, affecting participation in multiple everyday settings: conceptual domain, social domain, and practical domain. The American Psychiatric Association's DSM-5 categorizes adaptive impairment from mild to profound.

Intellectual function: It is assessed by IQ testing **(Table 19.1).**

$$IQ = \frac{\text{Mental age}}{\text{Chronological age}}$$

TABLE 19.1: Intellectual disability by IQ range.

Severity of mental retardation	*IQ range*
Mild	50–55 to 70
Moderate	35–40 to 50–55
Severe	20–25 to 35–40
Profound	Below 20–25

INHERITANCE

Inheritance patterns are classified as either monogenic (Mendelian and non-Mendelian) or polygenic.

Single-Gene or Monogenic Disorders/Mendelian Disorders

Genetic disorders that result from mutations in single gene are called as single-gene or monogenic (Mendelian) disorders. This type of inheritance is called *Mendelian inheritance.*

Polygenic

Examples: Hypertension, diabetes—caused by the cumulative and interactive effects of genetic variation in more than one gene.

Q. List the characteristics of autosomal dominant inheritance with examples. What do you mean by penetrance and variable expressivity?

Autosomal Dominant Pattern of Inheritance

- It is determined by the presence of one abnormal gene on one of the autosomes (chromosomes 1-22)
- Disease is in **heterozygotes** (These disorders generally manifest when one of the two homologous (paired) chromosomes carries a mutant gene).

The general characteristics of autosomal dominant inheritance:

- **Location of mutant gene:** These are found on **autosomes.**
- **Required number of defective genes:** Only **one copy of the mutant** (abnormal) **gene** is required for effects.
- The disorder is **transmitted in a vertical (parent to child) pattern, appearing in multiple generations.**
- **Sex affected:** Males and females are equally affected.
- **Pattern of inheritance: Every affected individual has one affected parent.**
- Unaffected individuals (family members who do not manifest the trait) do not pass the disorder to their children.
- **Risks of transmission (Figs. 19.5A to C) to children (offspring):** Affected males and females have an equal risk of passing on the disorder to children.

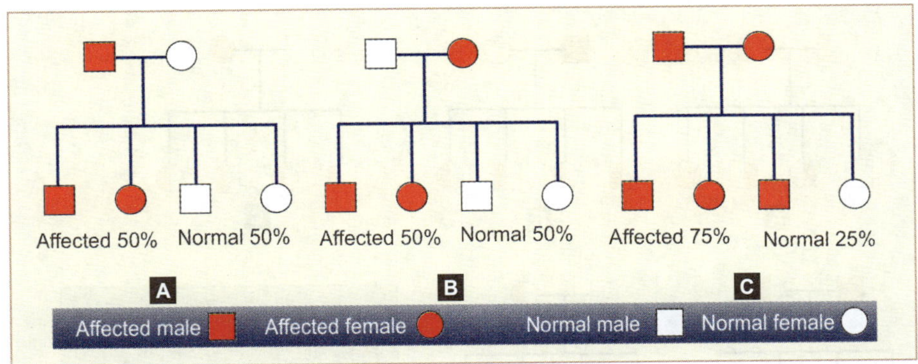

FIGS. 19.5A TO C: Pedigree illustrating autosomal dominant transmission. (A and B) One parent is affected; (C) Both parents are affected. Note that both males and females are affected equally.

- ***When only one parent is affected and other is normal:*** An affected individual has a 50% (1 in 2) chance of passing on the deleterious genes for *each* pregnancy, and therefore of having a child affected by the disorder. This is called as the **recurrence risk** for the disorder.
- ***When both parents are affected:*** It has 75% chance of children being affected and a 25% chance to be normal.

- Finding of **male-to-male transmission** essentially confirms autosomal dominant inheritance.
- Examples of autosomal dominant and autosomal recessive disorders are listed in **Table 19.2**.

TABLE 19.2: Examples of autosomal dominant and autosomal recessive disorders.

System	*Autosomal dominant disorder*	*Autosomal recessive disorder*
Nervous	Huntington disease Neurofibromatosis Tuberous sclerosis Myotonic dystrophy	Friedreich's ataxia Spinal muscular atrophy Ataxia telangiectasia
Skeletal/ Dermatological	Marfan syndrome Achondroplasia Osteogenesis imperfecta Noonan syndrome	Alkaptonuria Ehlers-Danlos syndrome Albinism
Metabolic	Familial hypercholesterolemia Intermittent porphyria	Cystic fibrosis, phenylketonuria, lysosomal storage diseases, galactosemia, hemochromatosis, glycogen storage diseases, alkaptonuria
Hematopoietic	Hereditary spherocytosis von Willebrand disease	Sickle cell anemia, thalassemia Homocystinuria
Renal	Polycystic kidney disease	Congenital adrenal hyperplasia
Gastrointestinal	Familial polyposis coli	Wilson's disease Dubin-Johnson syndrome
Pulmonary		Alpha-1 antitrypsin deficiency Cystic fibrosis

- **Additional properties:**
  - **Penetrance:** Penetrance is the percentage of individuals with the mutation who present with clinical symptoms.
    - **With complete penetrance,** all individuals show clinical symptoms.
    - **With incomplete penetrance** or **reduced penetrance,** only some individuals show disease and in **nonpenetrance** (gene is not expressed at all) individuals may not show any symptoms.
    - For example, *retinoblastoma:* AD malignant eye tumor is a good example of reduced penetrance. About 10% of the obligate carriers of the RB susceptibility gene (affected parent and affected child or children) do not have the disease.
  - **Variable expressivity:** It refers to variations in expression (qualitatively or quantitatively) of severity of the same disorder among individuals (even within the same family), who have the abnormal gene. In some, the disorder may be mild and in others it may show significant symptoms. Penetrance may be complete, but severity of disease can vary greatly. Well-studied example is **neurofibromatosis type 1, or von Recklinghausen disease**.

Q. Discuss autosomal recessive inheritance with examples.

Autosomal Recessive Pattern of Inheritance

- Autosomal recessive inheritance involves mutations in both copies of a gene.
- These disorders generally manifest when both the homologous chromosomes carry mutant genes (**homozygous** state).

The general features of these disorders are:

- **Location of mutant gene:** These genes are located on **autosomes**.
- **Required number of defective gene:** Symptoms of the disease appear only when an individual has **two copies** of the mutant gene. The heterozygote state is called as a carrier. In the carrier state, the product of the normal gene is able to compensate for the mutant allele and is hence the patients are asymptomatic.
- **Horizontal transmission:** The observation of multiple affected members of kindred in the same generation, but no affected family members in other generations.
- **Pattern of inheritance:** For a child to be at risk, both parents must be having at least one copy of the mutant gene. *Almost all inborn errors of metabolism are autosomal recessive disorders.*

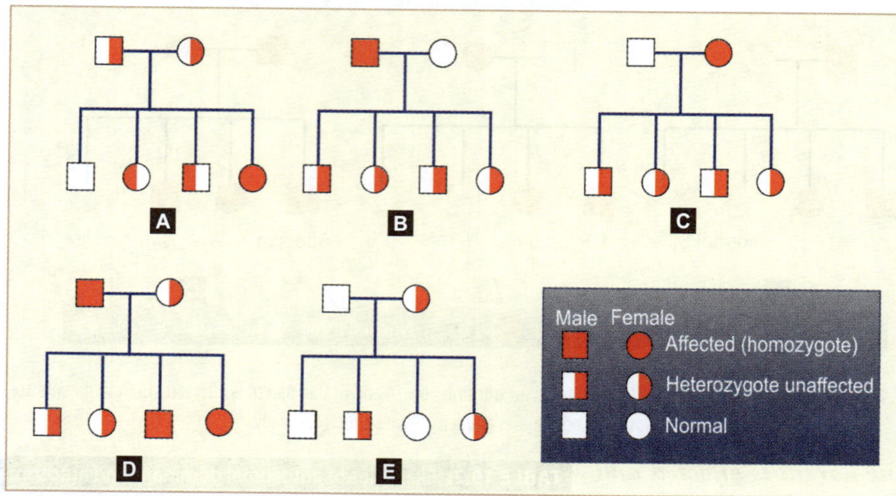

FIGS. 19.6A TO E: Pedigree illustrating mechanism of autosomal recessive transmission. (A) Both parents are unaffected heterozygotes; (B and C) One parent is sufferer (homozygous) and other is normal; (D) One parent is sufferer and other is unaffected heterozygote; (E) One parent is normal and other is an unaffected heterozygote.

- **Sex affected:** Males and females being equally affected, though some traits exhibit different expression in males and females (ovarian cancer, hypospadias).
- **Consanguineous marriage:** It is common predisposing factor.
- Recurrence risk of 25% for parents with a previous affected child.
- **Risks of transmission (Figs. 19.6A to E) to children (offspring):**
  - ***When both parents are heterozygous for the condition:*** Heterozygous parents carry one mutated gene and normal gene. When two ***heterozygotes*** mate, 25% of the children will be affected, 50% will be unaffected heterozygotes and 25% will be normal.
  - ***When one parent is affected and the other is normal:*** All the children will be unaffected heterozygote.
  - ***When one parent is affected and the other is heterozygote:*** The chances are that 50% of children will be unaffected heterozygote and 50% homozygous affected.
  - ***When one parent is normal and the other is heterozygote:*** This may result in 50% unaffected heterozygote carriers and 50% normal children.
- If the frequency of an autosomal recessive disease is known, then frequency of the heterozygote or carrier state can be calculated from the *Hardy-Weinberg formula:* $p^2 + 2pq + q^2 = 1$, where p is the frequency of one of a pair of alleles and q is the frequency of the other.

Examples of autosomal dominant and autosomal recessive disorders are listed in **Table 19.2**.

X-Linked Pattern of Inheritance

Q. Discuss X-linked inheritance with examples.

Almost all sex-linked Mendelian disorders are X-linked. Males with mutations affecting the Y-linked genes are usually infertile.

Expression of an X-linked disorder is different in males and females. Though X-linked disorders may be inherited either as dominant or recessive, almost all X-linked disorders have recessive pattern of inheritance.

Characteristics of X-linked inheritance:

- Males are more commonly and more severely affected than females.
- **Female carriers** are generally unaffected, or if affected, they are affected more mildly than males.
- Affected males will have only carrier daughters.
- Carrier women have a 25% risk for having an affected son, a 25% risk for a carrier daughter, and a 50% chance for a child that does not inherit the mutated X-linked gene.

X-linked Recessive Traits

- **Location of mutant gene:** Mutant gene is on the X chromosome and there is no male-to-male transmission.
- **Required number of defective gene:** One copy of mutant gene is required for the manifestation of disease in males, but two copies of the mutant gene are needed in females.
- **Sex affected:** Males are more frequently affected and manifest disease than females; daughters of affected male are all asymptomatic carriers. In many diseases, males do not survive.
- **Pattern of inheritance (Figs. 19.7A to D):** Transmission is through female carrier (heterozygous). Mothers are always carriers and all their sons are affected. The disease is never passed from father to son.

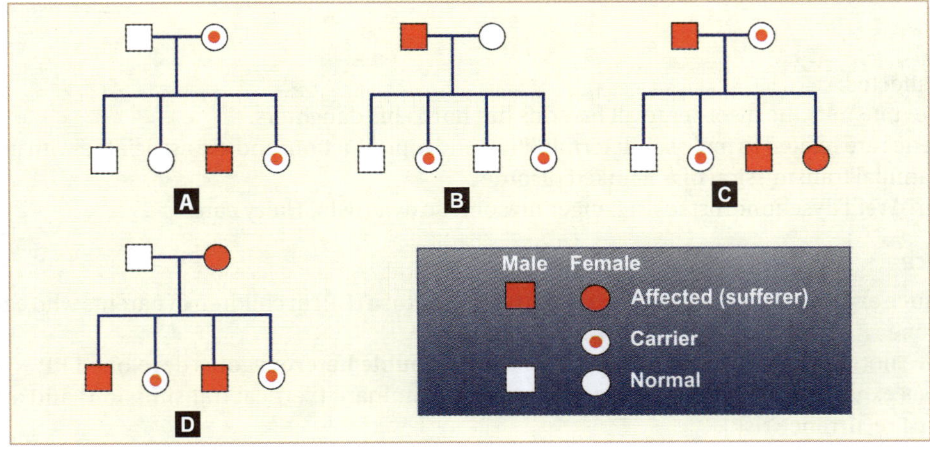

FIGS. 19.7A TO D: Mode of X-linked recessive transmission. Note the absence of male-to-male transmission. (A) Male is normal and female is a carrier; (B) Male is sufferer and female is normal; (C) Male is a sufferer and female is a carrier; (D) Male is normal and female is a sufferer.

- Very rarely, a female can develop the disease due to:
  - Female having Turner syndrome (XO) with only one X chromosome.
  - Presence of testicular feminization syndrome.
  - Father with mutation in X chromosome and a carrier female.
  - Affected father and carrier mother.
  - Inactivation of normal X chromosome in most cells (Lyon hypothesis).

Examples of X-linked recessive disorders are shown in **Table 19.3**.

TABLE 19.3: Examples of X-linked recessive disorders.

System	*Related X-linked recessive disease*
Musculoskeletal	Duchenne and Beckers muscular dystrophy
Blood	Hemophilia A and B
	Glucose-6-phosphate dehydrogenase deficiency Wiskott-Aldrich syndrome
Immune	Agammaglobulinemia
Metabolic	Diabetes insipidus, Hunter disease, Lesch-Nyhan
Nervous	Fragile-X syndrome, retinitis pigmentosa, color blindness

X-linked Dominant Conditions

- Disorders are relatively uncommon (very rare). For example, vitamin D resistance rickets, Alport's syndrome, Rett syndrome
- **Location of mutant gene:** It is located on the X chromosome and there is no transmission from affected male to son. This is because the son's "normal" X chromosome is from mother.
- **Required number of defective gene:** One copy of mutant gene is required for its effect.
  - Often lethal in males and so may be transmitted only in the female line.
  - Often lethal in affected males and they have affected mothers.
  - There is no carrier state as the disease will manifest, even if single chromosome has abnormal gene.
  - These are more frequent in females than in males.
- **Risks of transmission to children (offspring) (Figs. 19.8A to C):**
  - ***When female is affected and the male is normal:*** They transmit the disorder to 50% of their sons and 50% of their daughters.
  - ***When male is affected and the female is normal:*** They transmit to all their daughters but none to their sons. All daughters of an affected father develop disease because the daughter gets abnormal X from the father.
  - ***When both male and female are affected:*** All the females will be affected and half of males will be affected.

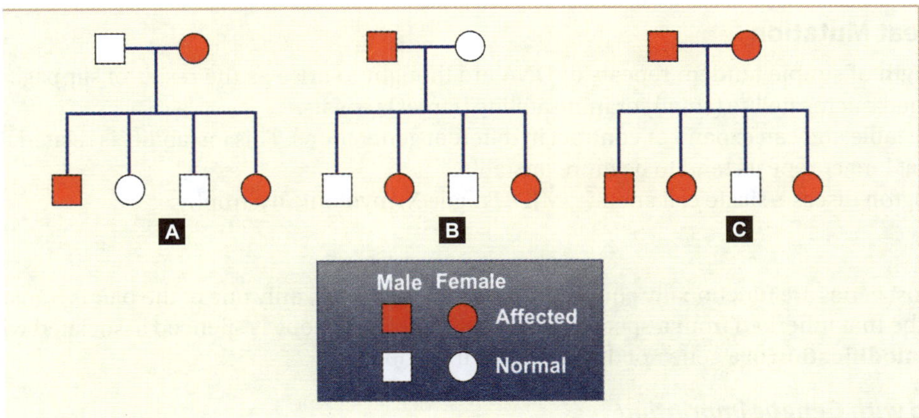

FIGS. 19.8A TO C: X-linked dominant transmission. Only females are affected. Usually males who inherit the mutant allele die in utero. (A) Normal male and female affected (sufferer); (B) Affected male and normal female; (C) Both male and female are affected.

Y-linked Diseases

Characterized by:

- Only males are affected.
- An affected male transmits the disorder to all his sons but not to his daughters.
- Most Y-linked genes are related to male sex determination and reproduction, and are associated with infertility. Therefore, it is rare to see familial transmission of a Y-linked disorder.
- For example, Leri-Weill dyschondrosteosis, Langer mesomelic dwarfism, Hairy ears.

Digenic Inheritance

- Digenic inheritance explains the occurrence of **retinitis pigmentosa** (RP) in children of parents who each carry a different RP-associated gene.
- Both parents have normal vision, but the offspring who were **double heterozygotes** developed RP.
- Digenic pedigrees exhibit characteristics of both autosomal dominant (vertical transmission) and autosomal recessive inheritance (1 in 4 recurrence risk).
- Other disorders with digenic inheritance—Bardet-Biedl syndrome, Hirschsprung disease, Long QT syndrome.

Mitochondrial Inheritance

- An individual's mitochondrial genome is entirely derived from the mother.
- Examples include Leber optic atrophy, **MELAS** (myopathy, encephalopathy, lactic acidosis, and stroke-like episodes), **MERRF** (myoclonic epilepsy associated with ragged red fibers), and **Kearns-Sayre syndrome** (ophthalmoplegia, pigmentary retinopathy, and cardiomyopathy).

Pseudodominant Inheritance

Pseudodominant inheritance of a recessive trait in two generations of a family without consanguinity mimics a dominant pattern. Pseudodominant inheritance of hereditary hemochromatosis (HH), an autosomal recessive disorder, can be attributed to the high carrier frequency of HFE alleles in individuals of European descent. In this case, the father is homozygous for the mutated alleles and the mother is the carrier of the genetic mutation; therefore, there are 50% chances that the offspring will inherit mutated genes from both the parents and will have hemochromatosis.

Triplet Repeat Expansion Disorders

- Caused by expansion in the number of three-base-pair repeats.
- An error in replication can result in expansion of that number, referred to as **premutation**.
- There is a clinical correlation to the size of the expansion, with a greater expansion causing more severe and/or earlier age of onset for the disease. The observation of increasing severity of disease and early age of onset in subsequent generations is termed **genetic anticipation** and is a defining characteristic of triplet repeat expansion disorders.
- Examples of triplet repeat expansion disorders are listed in **Table 19.4**.

TABLE 19.4: Examples of triplet repeat expansion disorders.

Disease	*Triplet repeated*	*Disease*	*Triplet repeated*
Huntington	CAG	Fragile X syndrome (FRAXA)	CGG
Myotonic dystrophy	CTG	FXTAS (Fragile X-associated tremor/ataxia syndrome)	CGG
X-linked spinal and bulbar muscular atrophy	CAG	Machado-Joseph disease (MJD)	CAG
Spinocerebellar ataxia type I	CAG	Friedreich's ataxia	GAA

Simple Tandem Repeat Mutation

- Variations in the length of simple tandem repeats of DNA are thought to arise as the result of slippage of DNA during meiosis and are termed microsatellite (small) or minisatellite (larger) repeats.
- These repeats are unstable and can expand or contract in different generations. This instability is related to the size of the original repeat, in that longer repeats tend to be more unstable.
- For example, Huntington disease, sickle cell anemia, MJD, Fragile X, myotonic dystrophy.

Genetic Imprinting

- The two copies of most genes are functionally equivalent. In a small number, only one of the pair is transcribed.
- The active gene will be that inherited from a specific parent, and the other copy is silenced associated with methylation of DNA **(epigenetic modification** of a gene not due to a DNA mutation).

Conditions Associated with Genetic Imprinting

- **Prader-Willi syndrome** with paternal chromosome deletion.
- **Angelman syndrome** with maternal chromosome deletion.

- Uniparental disomy (UPD): Rare occurrence of a child inheriting both copies of a chromosome from the same parent is another genetic mechanism that can cause Prader-Willi and Angelman syndromes.
- Other conditions associated with imprinting are Beckwith-Wiedemann syndrome and Russell-Silver syndrome, Duchenne muscular dystrophy (DMD) in females and epigenetic silencing in oncogenesis, e.g., colon cancer 3p21 MLH1.

Pleiotropy

- Genes that exert effects on multiple aspects of physiology or anatomy are pleiotropic.
- *For example:* Marfan syndrome (affects eye, the skeleton, and the cardiovascular system), cystic fibrosis (affects sweat glands, lungs, pancreas, and genitourinary system), osteogenesis imperfecta (affects bones, teeth, and sclera), sickle cell anemia (affects RBCs, bone, and spleen).

Locus Heterogeneity

- Disease that can be caused by mutations at different loci in different families is said to exhibit locus heterogeneity.
- *Osteogenesis imperfecta (OI):* Subunits of procollagen triple helix are encoded by two genes, one on chromosome 17 and the other on chromosome 7. Mutation in either of these genes can alter the structure of the collagen molecules and lead to OI, disease states are often indistinguishable.

Polymorphisms

- A polymorphism is defined as one that exists with a population frequency of >1%.
- Most common polymorphisms are neutral but some cause subtle changes in gene expression or in protein structure and function. For example, cystic fibrosis, hemochromatosis, alpha-1 antitrypsin deficiency, spinomuscular dystrophy.

GENE THERAPY

Q. Write short note on gene therapy.

Definition: Gene therapy is the insertion of genes into an individual's cells and tissues to treat a disease, such as a hereditary disease in which a deleterious mutant allele is replaced with a functional one.

To be effective, the gene therapy requires methods that ensure the safe, efficient and stable introduction of genes into human cells. Gene therapy uses genes to treat or prevent disease. First done on September 14, 1990 for Ashanthi DeSilva suffering from SCID where the missing gene introduced through processed WBC.

Approaches for Correcting Faulty Genes

- A normal gene may be inserted into a nonspecific location to replace a nonfunctional gene.
- An abnormal gene could be swapped through homologous recombination.
- Repair through selective reverse mutation.
- The regulation of a particular gene could be altered.

Types of Gene Therapy

The cells in the body can be divided into two main categories: (1) somatic cells and (2) germ cells.

- **Somatic cell therapy:** It involves delivering a correcting gene to somatic cells in the affected tissues. Somatic cells are the nonreproductive cells and its therapeutic effect ends with the individual receiving it and is not passed on to the future generations. Hence, somatic cell therapy is considered as a safer approach. This type of gene therapy is used for disorders such as cystic fibrosis, muscular dystrophy, cancers, and certain infectious diseases.
- **Germ cell therapy:** In germ cell therapy, germ cells (egg or sperms) are used and it results in permanent changes that are passed on to the future generations. Thus, it offers the possibility of permanently eliminating some diseases from a particular family and ultimately from the population. It is not accepted at present due to ethical reasons.

Arguments for Germline Gene Therapy

- *Medical utility:* The potential of a true "cure".
- *Medical necessity:* May be only way to cure some diseases.
- *Prophylactic efficacy:* Better to prevent a disease rather than to treat pathology.
- *Parental autonomy:* Parents can make choices about what is best for their children.
- Easier, more effective than somatic gene therapy.
- Eradication of disease in future generations.
- *Part of being human:* Supporting human improvement.

Forms of Gene Therapy

There are two basic forms of somatic gene therapy: (1) *ex vivo* and (2) *in vivo.*

1. ***Ex vivo:*** Transfer of gene in cultured cells and finally these cultured cells are reintroduced into patients.
2. ***In vivo:*** Delivery of genes into cells of particular tissues. The gene may be transferred by a viral vector or by a nonviral method. This is most often used technique.

Vectors in Gene Therapy

The most common form of gene therapy involves insertion of normal gene into the genome with the help of certain carriers called **vectors**. These vectors can be divided into two main types: (1) viral and (2) nonviral vectors.

Viral vectors: The various viruses include retroviruses, adenoviruses, adeno-associated viruses, and herpes simplex viruses.

Nonviral methods: Gene delivery can also be carried by nonviral methods. These have some advantages. They do not elicit an immune response, safer and simpler to use and allow large-scale production. The nonviral methods include: direct inoculation/naked DNA, liposomal-mediated DNA transfer, gene gun method, and dendrimers. Pure DNA constructs and lipoplexes are used for in vivo transfer while bone marrow cells are used for ex vivo transfer.

Problems/Limitations of Gene Therapy

- **Short-lived nature of gene therapy**. Hence, patients will have to undergo multiple rounds of gene therapy.
- **Immunotoxicity:** Gene therapy may stimulate the immune response against introduced gene and reduce the effectiveness of gene therapy.
- **Problems with viral vectors:** Viral vectors may sometimes cause potential problems to the patient like: toxicity and inflammatory responses. In addition, the viral vector, once inside the patient, may recover its ability to cause disease.
- **Gene silencing**—repression of promoter
- **Multifactorial disorders:** Genetic disorders due to single gene mutations usually show best response to gene therapy. Unfortunately, some the most commonly occurring disorders (e.g., atherosclerosis, hypertension, diabetes, Alzheimer's disease, and rheumatoid arthritis) are multifactorial and are difficult to treat effectively using gene therapy.
- **Phenotoxicity**—complications arising from overexpression or ectopic expression of the transgene
- **Risk of inducing a tumor (insertional mutagenesis):** If the gene is integrated in the wrong place in the genome (e.g., in a tumor suppressor gene), it could induce a tumor.
- **Risk of death:** Deaths have occurred due to gene therapy.

TABLE 19.5: Therapeutic application of gene therapy.

Disease	*Gene therapy trials*
Inherited single gene disorders—to provide a normally functioning gene	
Severe combined immunodeficiency	Adenosine deaminase (ADA)
Cystic fibrosis	CFTR—Cystic fibrosis transmembrane regulator
Familial hypercholesterolemia	LDL receptor
Emphysema	Alpha-1 antitrypsin
Hemophilia B	Factor IX
Thalassemia	Alpha- or beta-globin
Sickle cell anemia	Beta-globin
Duchenne muscular dystrophy	Dystrophin
Cancer therapy—to augment the immune response/to direct tumor lysis	
Nasopharyngeal cancer	P53
Melanoma	Tumor necrosis factor
Retinoblastoma and mesothelioma	Thymidine kinase (Suicide gene therapy)
Antibody delivery—not been used clinically	

Therapeutic Applications (Table 19.5)

- Not been approved for clinical use.
- Trials are being conducted on using gene therapy in the treatment of various genetic disorders, cancers, infectious diseases, and other diseases such as Alzheimer's disease and atherosclerosis.

HUMAN GENOME PROJECT

Q. Write short note on human genome and human genome project.

Introduction

Genome: A **genome** is the entire DNA in an organism, including its genes. The human genome is estimated to contain 30,000–40,000 genes that are divided among the 23 chromosomes. The 23 different chromosomes, 22 are autosomes (numbered 1–22) and 1 pair of sex chromosomes (X and Y). The functions of over 50% of discovered genes are not known.

Gene mapping: It is the process of identifying and sequencing each and every human gene of the human genome. The map of the human genome provides a picture of locations, and structures of genes.

- **Genetic mapping** (linkage analysis): A genetic map describes the order of genes and defines the position of a gene relative to other loci on the same chromosome.
- **Physical mapping:** Physical mapping indicates the position of genes in a chromosome, which is determined by physical distances (measured in base pairs) between genes.

  Organisms and their genomic size are presented in **Table 19.6**.

TABLE 19.6: Organisms and their genomic size.

Organism	*Genomic size in base pairs*
Epstein-Barr virus	0.172×10^6
Bacteria *(E. coli)*	4.6×10^6
Yeast	12.1×10^6
Nematode worm *(C. elegans)*	95.5×10^6
Fruit fly	180×10^6
Human	3200×10^6

(E. coli: Escherichia coli; C. elegans: Caenorhabditis elegans)

The **human genome project (HGP)** is an international scientific research project to understand the genomes of humans and other organisms. It was started in 1990 under **Dr James D Watson** at the United States National Institute of Health. In addition to the United States, the international consortium comprised geneticists in the United Kingdom, France, Germany, Japan, China, and India.

Goals of Human Genome Project

- Understand and **identify all genes** of the human genome.
- Determine the **human DNA sequence:** The primary focus of the HGP was to obtain DNA sequence for the entire human genome. The goal was to map all genes of the human genome and also to map human inherited diseases. Thus included creation of genetic maps, development of physical maps, and determination of the complete human DNA sequence.
- **Develop software for large-scale DNA analysis,** store all found information in databases and improve tools for data analysis.
- Transfer-related technologies to the private sector
- **Collect and distribute data**
- **Study the ethical, legal, and social issues** (ELSI) of **genetic research** that may arise from the project.

Components involved in human genome are diagrammatically shown in **Figure 19.9**.

All humans have unique gene sequences. Therefore, the data published by the HGP does not represent the exact sequence of each and every individual's genome. It is the combined genome of a small number of anonymous donors. The HGP genome is a scaffold for future work in identifying differences among individuals.

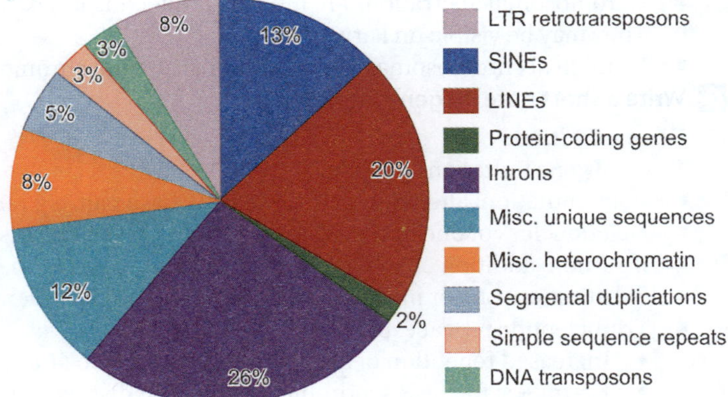

FIG. 19.9: Components of human genome.

Uses of Human Genome Project

Human genome project will shed light on a wide range of basic questions, to identify the number of genes in humans, how cells work, how living things evolved, how single cells develop into complex creatures, and what exactly happens when we become ill. The understanding of the genome provides clues for:

1. **Etiology** of cancers, Alzheimer's disease, etc.
2. Defining the **pathogenesis** of a disease and to study the disease processes at molecular level.
3. **Susceptibility** of an individual to a variety of illnesses, e.g., carcinoma breast, disorders of hemostasis, liver diseases, cystic fibrosis, etc.
4. Predict new ways **to prevent** a number of diseases that affect the human beings.
5. To **diagnose and treat** disease. Target genes for treatment and management of diseases.
6. *Human development and anthropology:* Analysis of similarities between DNA sequences from different organisms helps to **study evolution**.
7. **Researcher:** By visiting the human genome database on the Worldwide Web, researcher can examine what other scientists have written about the gene.

Ethical Issues (Box 19.5)

Human genome project helps to identify disease-causing genes, thereby can lead to improvements in diagnosis, treatment, and prevention. It is estimated that most individuals harbor several serious recessive genes. However, completion of the human genome sequence and determination of the association of genetic defects with disease has raised many new issues with implications for the individual and mankind.

Box 19.5: Ethical issues in human genome project (HGP).

- Fairness in the use of genetic information
- Privacy and confidentiality
- Psychological impact and stigmatization
- Genetic testing
- Reproductive issues
- Education, standards, and quality control
- Commercialization
- Conceptual and philosophical implications.

GENETIC MUTATIONS

Mutations are alterations in the genome of a cell.

Mechanism:

- As a result of errors during DNA replication or cell division
- Ineffective DNA repair mechanisms
- Damage to DNA caused by endogenous and exogenous toxins

Types of mutations:

- Mutations according to affected cell population

- Chromosomal aberrations
- Gene mutations

A. **Based on the affected cells**
  - Germline mutation (gametic mutation):
    - Mutations in the cells from which egg or sperm cells develop
    - These mutations can, therefore, be passed on to offspring.
  - Somatic mutation:
    - Acquired mutations that are present only in certain somatic cells
    - Primarily affect only one allele of a gene
    - Do not occur in the germline and therefore cannot be passed on to offspring via the ovum or sperm
    - Almost all malignancies are preceded by a somatic mutation.

B. **Chromosomal aberrations**
  - Chromosomal aberrations are mutations affecting large segments of DNA
  - They may be visible on karyogram
  - Numerical chromosomal aberrations or structural chromosomal aberrations (discussed earlier)

Q. Write a short note on gene mutations.

C. **Gene mutations**

  Types of gene mutations include:
  - Point mutation: alteration of a single DNA base pair, e.g., sickle-cell disease
  - Deletion: loss of one or more base pairs, e.g., cystic fibrosis
  - Insertion: addition of one or more base pairs, e.g., beta-thalassemia
  - Substitution: one or more base pairs are replaced by different base pairs
  - Trinucleotide repeat expansion:
    - Increased repetition of base triplets that leads to faulty protein synthesis or folding
    - Examples: fragile X syndrome, Huntington disease, myotonic dystrophy.

Gene mutations can be classified based on the outcome:

- *Frameshift mutation:*
  - Shift in the reading frame caused by insertion or deletion of a number of nucleotides not divisible by 3, which leads to modified amino acid coding in the gene segments downstream.
  - It results in the synthesis of shorter or longer proteins that have a modified function or are dysfunctional.
  - Examples: Tay-Sachs disease, Duchenne muscular dystrophy
- *In-frame deletion or insertion:*
  - Deletion or insertion of three, six, nine, or more base pairs (always in triplets!), without a shift in the reading frame, but with deletion or insertion of one, two, three, or more amino acids in the protein during translation
- *Silent mutation:*
  - Altered codon, which codes for the identical amino acid
- *Nonsense mutation:*
  - Formation of a stop codon, which leads to alterations in the splicing process and early termination of translation
- *Missense mutation:*
  - Altered codon, which codes for a different amino acid
  - Example: sickle cell disease (glutamic acid → valine)
  - Considered as "conservative" missense mutation when the new amino acid is similar in chemical structure to the original amino acid
- *Splice mutation:*
  - Alterations (especially point mutations) in the nucleotide sequences required for splicing (e.g., on the exon-intron border or at the junction) that lead to defective mRNA and shortened proteins
  - Examples: some types of β-thalassemia, dementia, cancers, and epilepsy
- Dominant negative mutation:
  - A gene mutation that results in nonfunctional protein that impairs the function of protein produced by the wild-type allele in heterozygotes

MISCELLANEOUS

Q. Write short note on proteomics/proteome.

Proteome

- The term proteome is derived from proteins expressed by a genome. It refers to all the proteins produced by an organism and proteins are the functional units. Thus, the proteome represents full sets of proteins produced by the body and is similar to the term genome for the entire set of genes. Human body contains more than 2 million different proteins, each having different functions.

- Proteomics is the study of the proteome (full set/entire library of proteins in a cell type or tissue) and its variation/relationship to disease.
- Amino acids are the basic units of proteins and are very small. Each amino acid consists of atoms ranging from 7 to 24 and cannot be identified under even the powerful microscopes.
- *Uses:* Proteomic technologies play an important role in drug discovery, diagnostics, and molecular medicine. When a defective protein-causing particular diseases are found, new drugs can be developed to either alter the shape of a defective protein or mimic a missing one.

Epigenetics

Q. Write a short note on epigenetics.

Definition: Epigenetics is a **reversible, heritable change/alteration** in gene expression which occurs without mutation and is unrelated to gene nucleotide sequence. Epigenomics is the study of epigenetics. Epigenetic alterations are associated with cancers and other diseases. Unlike genetic changes in cancer, epigenetic changes are reversible.

- In normal cells, the majority of the genome is not expressed. Some portions of the genome are silenced by DNA methylation and histone modifications.
- In some tumors, epigenetic changes may directly contribute to tumor development. Epigenetic changes involve post-translational modifications of histones and DNA methylation, both of which affect gene expression.
- In cancer cells, there is global DNA hypomethylation and selective promoter-localized hypermethylation.

Examples

1. **Silencing genes by hypermethylation** (epigenetic mechanism)
   a. *Tumor suppressor genes:* Examples: p53 can be indirectly inactivated through silencing ARF by hypermethylation. This hypermethylated ARF prevents inhibition of the MDM2 oncogenic protein and the enhancement of p53 degradation; *BRCA1* in breast cancer and VHL in renal cell carcinomas.
   b. *DNA repair genes:* Mismatch-repair gene *MLH1* in colorectal cancer.
2. **Hypomethylation:** The genome of cancer cells may also undergo global DNA hypomethylation. Gene hypomethylation can cause chromosomal instability, derepression of growth regulatory genes, and overexpression of antiapoptotic genes, which may induce tumors.

Clinical Applications

- Use of epigenetic tumor markers.
- Use of epigenetic therapeutic agents (e.g., azacitidine, decitabine, vorinostat) in the treatment of myelodysplastic syndromes (MDS) and lymphoma.

Pharmacogenomics

Q. Write short note on pharmacogenomics and pharmacogenetics.

- Pharmacogenetics or pharmacogenomics is the study of interaction between genetics and therapeutic drugs.
- Pharmacogenetics is the study of unexpected drug response result and to look for a genetic cause.
- Pharmacogenomics is the study of identifying genetic differences within a population that explain certain observed responses to a drug or susceptibility to a health problem.

Applications

- To develop a drug that has maximum therapeutic effect and produces least damage to adjacent healthy cells.
- To prescribe drugs depending on the patient's genetic profile so as to reduce the adverse reactions.
- To determine the accurate dosage.
- To determine drug responses in the treatment of cardiac, respiratory, and psychiatric conditions.
- To develop targeted therapy (e.g., psychiatry, dementia, cardiac conditions) and in the treatment of breast cancer (testing for HER2 receptor for response to trastuzumab) and other cancers (e.g., testing for BCR-ABL for response to imatinib in CML; testing for epidermal growth factor receptor response to gefitinib and erlotinib in lung cancer).

List of chromosomal disorders are presented in Table 19.7.

TABLE 19.7: List of chromosomal disorders.

Chromosome	*Abnormality*	*Disease association*
X	XO	Turner syndrome
Y	XXY	Klinefelter syndrome
Y	XYY	Double Y syndrome

Contd...

Contd...

Y	XXX	Trisomy X syndrome
Y	Xp21 deletion	Duchenne/Becker syndrome congenital adrenal hypoplasia, chronic granulomatus disease
1	1p (somatic) monosomy trisomy	Neuroblastoma
2	Monosomy trisomy 2q	Growth rerdation, developmental and mental delay, and minor physical abnormalities
3	Monosomy trisomy (somatic)	Non-Hodgkin lymphoma
4	Monosomy trisomy (somatic)	Acute nonlymphocytic leukemia (ANLL)
5	5p deletion	Cri du chat; Lejeune syndrome
5	5q (somatic) monosomy trisomy	Myelodysplastic syndrome
6	Monosomy trisomy (somatic)	Clear-cell sarcoma
7	7q 11.23 deletion	William's syndrome
8	Monosomy trisomy	Myelodysplastic syndrome; Warkany syndrome; chronic myelogenous leukemia
9	Trisomy	Complete trisomy 9 syndrome: mosaic trisomy 9 syndrome
10	Monosomy trisomy (somatic)	ALL or ANLL
11	11p-	Aniridia: Wilms tumor
11	Monosomy (somatic) trisomy	Myeloid lineages affected (ANLL, MDS)
12	Monosomy trisomy (somatic)	CLL, Juvenile granulosa cell tumor (JGCT)
13	13q14 deletion	Retinoblastoma
13	Monosomy trisomy	Patau syndrome
14	Monosomy trisomy (somatic)	Myeloid disorders (MDS, ANLL, atypical CML)
15	15q11-q13 deletion monosomy	Prader-Willi, Angelman syndrome
15	Trisomy (somatic)	Myeloid and lymphoid lineages affected, e.g., MDS, ANLL, ALL, CLL
16	16q13.3 deletion monosomy trisomy (somatic)	Rubinstein-Taybi, papillary renal cell carcinomas (malignant)
17	17p-(somatic)	17p syndrome in myeloid malignancies
17	Monosomy trisomy (somatic)	Renal cortical adenomas
18	Monosomy trisomy	Edwards syndrome
19	Trisomy, deletion	
20	20p-	Trisomy 20p syndrome
20	20q-	MDS, ANLL, polycythemia vera, chronic neutrophilic leukemia
20	Monosomy trisomy (somatic)	Papillary renal cell carcinomas (malignant)
21	Monosomy trisomy	Down syndrome
22	22q11.2 deletion	DiGeorge syndrome, velocardiofacial syndrome, conotruncal anomaly face syndrome, CML-reciprocal translocation 9:22 Opitz G/BBB syndrome, Cayler cardiofacial syndrome
22	Monosomy trisomy	Complete trisomy 22 syndrome

GENETIC TESTING

Indications of genetic testing are listed in Table 19.8.

TABLE 19.8: Indications of genetic testing.

Indications for germ line mutation testing	Indications for analysis of genetic alteration
➢ *Perinatal analysis* – >35-year old mother – Previous child with genetic abnormalities – Family history – Mother having a known recessive gene or balanced translocation or X-linked genetic disorders – Triple test abnormal – Fetal abnormalities in USG ➢ *Postnatal analysis* – Multiple congenital anomalies – Unexplained mental retardation – Suspected aneuploidy/unbalanced autosome/sex chromosomal abnormality – Multiple spontaneous abortions	➢ *Diagnosis and management of cancer* – Identifying tumor suppressor gene or identifying cytogenetic alteration – Identifying clonal proliferation confirming neoplasm – Identification of mutations that can alter direct therapeutic choices – Determination of therapeutic efficacy ➢ *Diagnosis and management of infectious disease* – Microorganism-specific genetic material to identify and diagnose genetic material – Identification of genetic changes associated with drug resistance – Determination of treatment efficacy

Genome-wide Association Study

- Genome-wide association studies (GWASs) test hundreds of thousands of genes simultaneously and are used in genetics research to associate specific genetic variations with particular diseases.
- It involves scanning the genomes from many different people and looking for genetic markers that can be used to predict the presence of a disease.

POLYMERASE CHAIN REACTION AND ITS APPLICATIONS

Q. Write short essay/note on polymerase chain reaction (PCR).

Kary Mullis discovered polymerase chain reaction in 1983. PCR is a method employed to amplify minute amount of DNA within a few hours. This technique consists of selective amplification of specific target nucleic acid sequences from total DNA by using primers specific for the target region to be amplified.

Basic Steps

- **Denaturation:** In this step, the double-stranded template DNA is denatured by heat (temperature of around 92–96°C) into single-stranded DNA.
- **Annealing:** DNA primers of interest are added along with the four basic deoxynucleotides and the solution is cooled. It causes binding of DNA probes to their specific target regions of the single-stranded DNA at a temperature of around 50–65°C.
- **Extension:** The primers are extended at a temperature of around 68–78°C in the presence of DNA polymerase, dNTPs and Mg^{2+} ions. The newly synthesized DNA strand acts as a template for the next cycle. This cycle is repeated several times (around 25–30 times) and produces millions of copies of the original specific target DNA. To retain the activity of DNA polymerase enzyme at such high denaturation temperature, *Taq* DNA polymerase, extracted from a microorganism *(Thermus aquaticus)* is used in the PCR reaction.

Applications of Polymerase Chain Reaction

Polymerase chain reaction is the starting test used in most of the molecular genetic tests.

- *Diagnosis of hereditary/genetic diseases:* In genetic disorders, genetic mutations can be detected by PCR alone (e.g., Huntington disease), PCR followed by digestion with restriction endonucleases (e.g., diagnosis of spinal muscular atrophy), PCR followed by dot-blot hybridization (e.g., thalassemia mutation detection), PCR followed by capillary electrophoresis for genotyping (e.g., detection of triplet repeat disorders).
- *Sequencing:* It is used as first step for DNA amplification for all methods of DNA sequencing.
- *Detection of pathogens:* To detect small quantities of pathogen DNA (e.g., PCR for *Mycobacterium tuberculosis),* to detect viruses, (including use of reverse transcriptase enzyme for RNA viruses), and real-time PCR (RT-PCR) for quantification of viral load, e.g., hepatitis B and C, human immunodeficiency virus (HIV).
- *Forensic genetics:* To identify DNA sequences that are unique to each individual.

Reverse transcriptase PCR (RT-PCR): Initial step is to convert RNA to complementary DNA and rest of the process is same as PCR. It is used to quantify the amount/number of copies of input DNA/RNA.

Real-time PCR: This technique, quantifies the PCR product in "real-time". It is used to quantify the amount/number of copies of input DNA/RNA.

Immunoblot (Western Blot)

It is a test to detect antibodies. According to molecular weight, the microbial proteins are separated by polyacrylamide gel electrophoresis (PAGE). They are transferred (blotted) on to a nitrocellulose membrane, which is incubated with serum of patient. Binding of specific antibody is detected with an enzyme—anti-immunoglobulin conjugate (similar to in ELISA), and specificity is confirmed by its location on the membrane. The test is a highly specific and can be used to confirm the results of less specific tests such as ELISA.

Lysosomal Storage Disorders

Classification of Lysosomal Storage Disorders

The classification of lysosomal storage disorders has been shown in **Table 19.9**.

TABLE 19.9: Classification of lysosomal storage disorders.

Disorder	*Underlying defect*
Mucopolysaccharidoses	Defective metabolism of glycosaminoglycans
Sphingolipidoses and sulfatidoses	Defective degradation of sphingolipids and their components
Glycogen storage diseases	Defective degradation of glycogen
Oligosaccharidoses	Defective degradation of the glycan portion of glycoproteins
Mucolipidoses	Defective degradation of acid mucopolysaccharides, sphingolipids and/or glycolipids

Mucopolysaccharidoses

The various types of mucopolysaccharidoses have been shown in **Table 19.10**.

MPS I (Hurler Syndrome)

- **Head/face:** Prominence of the forehead, broad nose with a flattened nasal bridge, enlargement and protrusion of the tongue, chronic hearing loss, corneal clouding, retinal degeneration or glaucoma; tonsillar/adenoidal hypertrophy (predispose the child to URI), sleep apnea.
- **Heart:** Cardiomyopathy with asymmetric hypertrophy of the ventricular septum, thickening of the aortic and mitral valves, which progress to valvular insufficiency.
- **Abdomen:** Hepatosplenomegaly results in a protuberant abdomen.
- **Neurological:** Mental retardation.

TABLE 19.10: Various types of mucopolysaccharidoses (MPSs).

Type of disorder	*Enzyme deficiency*
MPS I (Hurler syndrome, Hurler-Scheie syndrome, Scheie syndrome)	α-L-iduronidase
MPS II (Hunter syndrome)	Iduronate-2-sulfatase
MPS III (Sanfilippo disease)	
➢ Type A	Heparan *N*-sulfatase
➢ Type B	α-*N*-acetylglucosaminidase
➢ Type C	α-glucosaminide N-acetyltransferase
MPS IV (Morquio disease)	
➢ Type A	Acetylgalactosamine-6-sulfatase
➢ Type B	β-galactosidase
MPS VI (Maroteaux-Lamy disease)	Arylsulfatase B
MPS VII (Sly disease)	β-glucuronidase

MPS II (Hunter Syndrome)

- Initial symptoms starts at 2–4 years of age with progressive growth delays, resulting in short stature.
- **Head/face:** Macrocephaly, delayed tooth eruption, progressive hearing loss, thickening of the lips, tongue, and nostrils.
- **Heart:** Thickening of the heart valves leading to a decline in cardiac function.
- **Lungs:** Obstructive airway disease.
- **Abdomen:** Hepatosplenomegaly.
- **Skeletal:** Short neck and broad chest, joint stiffness, with restriction of movements.
- **Neurological:** Hydrocephalus, mental retardation, and seizures.

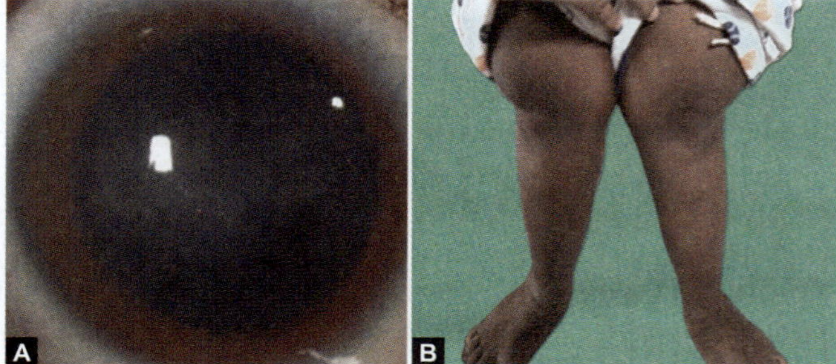

FIGS. 19.10A AND B: (A) Corneal clouding seen in Hurler and Morquio syndrome; (B) Knock knees in Morquio syndrome.

MPS IV (Morquio Syndrome)

- Widely spaced teeth, corneal clouding **(Fig. 19.10A)**, hearing loss, enlarged heart.
- **Abnormal skeletal development:** Scoliosis, hypermobile joints, large fingers, knock-knees **(Fig. 19.10B)**, short trunk with pectus carinatum, bell-shaped chest (ribs flared), severe growth retardation (82–115 cm), odontoid hypoplasia, compression of spinal cord (cervical myelopathy), and dwarfism.

Phenylketonuria (PKU)

- Autosomal recessive disease, due to deficiency of enzyme *phenylalanine hydroxylase* causing failure to convert phenylalanine to tyrosine.
- Developmental delay, mental retardation, seizures, eczema, blue eyes, hyperactivity, aggressive behavior, blond hair and musty/mousy odor.

Galactosemia

Autosomal recessive disease due to deficiency of the enzyme *galactose-1-phosphate uridyltransferase.* It is due to ingestion of galactose (lactose).

- Liver failure (hypoglycemia, bilirubinemia), hepatosplenomegaly
- Renal tubular disorder (acidosis, glycosuria, albuminuria)
- Lethargy, feeding intolerance, failure to thrive, cataracts
- Learning disorders in older children—mental retardation
- About 25% will develop sepsis (*E. coli*) in first 1–2 weeks, if untreated → death.

DIGEORGE SYNDROME

Q. Write a short note on DiGeorge syndrome.

DiGeorge syndrome (DGS) is a constellation of signs and symptoms associated with defective development of the pharyngeal pouch system. Most cases are caused by a **heterozygous chromosomal deletion at 22q11.2**. Chromosome 22q11.2 deletion syndrome (22qDS) includes DGS and other similar syndromes, such as velocardiofacial syndrome.

The classic triad of features of DGS on presentation is **conotruncal cardiac anomalies, hypoplastic thymus, and hypocalcemia (resulting from parathyroid hypoplasia)**.

Cardiac anomalies
- Interrupted aortic arch
- Truncus arteriosus
- Tetralogy of Fallot
- Atrial or ventricular septal defects

Hypocalcemia: Hypocalcemia, resulting from underdevelopment of the parathyroid glands and may present with jitteriness, tetany, or seizures, with low serum calcium, elevated serum phosphorus, and very low parathyroid hormone levels.

Hypoplastic/aplastic thymus: The thymus is absent in patients with complete DGS. In patients with partial DGS, the thymus is present, although it is often reported as hypoplastic.

Immunodeficiency: Immunodeficiency is common in patients with DGS and can range from recurrent sinopulmonary infections (termed partial DGS) to severe combined immunodeficiency (SCID)

GENETIC COUNSELING

Q. Write a short note on genetic counseling.

Genetic counseling is the process of helping people understand and adapt to the medical, psychological, and familial implications of genetic contributions to disease. This process integrates:
- Collection of a detailed family history, interpretation of the family history with the medical history to assess the chance of disease occurrence or recurrence
- Education of the patient and family regarding the inheritance, testing, management, risk reduction, available resources and research regarding the condition
- Counseling to promote informed choices and appropriate interventions

Genetic counseling can be conducted from preconception to old age. This includes preconception and prenatal counseling about the potential health of a baby, genetic evaluation of a neonate with birth defects or a toddler with developmental delay.

Family history: The initial step in assessing inherited risk for many chronic conditions is collecting data related to the family history.
Key factors that suggest the presence of a genetic disorder include the following:
- Multiple affected individuals in multiple generations from either side of the individual's family.
- Occurrence of the disease at an earlier age than usual.
- Close degree of relatedness (i.e., first- or second-degree relative) between affected relatives and the individual.

Once the family history is collected, it is used with the medical history to assess the possibility of an inherited etiology and to identify the chance of disease occurrence or recurrence.

Once an objective risk figure has been determined, the genetic counselor can provide explanations of penetrance and expressivity and apply these to the patient's family history and **assess personal risk**.

Risk modification: The genetic counseling session also provides information about risk modification strategies (if available) that may be appropriate for the patient and/or family. This may involve more aggressive screening (earlier, more frequent), lifestyle or dietary modifications, and medical or surgical interventions.
Examples include:
- **Familial cancer syndromes**: A patient with hereditary breast and ovarian cancer syndrome is at risk for both types of cancers and may have earlier mammography and clinical breast examinations and prophylactic surgeries.
- **Prenatal counseling**: Testing for the partner may be indicated for autosomal recessive conditions when a couple is referred for prenatal counseling.

Q. Write a short note on enzyme replacement therapy.

- **Enzyme replacement therapy** (**ERT**) is a type of treament which replaces an enzyme that is deficient or absent in the body. Enzymes can be made by recombinant DNA technology and can be given by intravenous injection.
- ERT has also been successful in treating SCID caused by an adenosine deaminase (ADA) deficiency.

Enzyme replacement therapy for diseases has been shown in **Table 19.11**.

TABLE 19.11: Enzyme replacement therapy for diseases.

Disease	*Enzyme therapy*
Fabry disease	Agalsidase beta
Gaucher disease	Imiglucerase
MPS I	Laronidase
MPS II	Idursulfase
MPS IVA	Elosulfase alfa
MPS VI	Galsulfase
Pompe disease	Alglucosidase alfa (160-L bioreactor)

CHAPTER

20

Immunology

INTRODUCTION

Immune system is defined as the body's defense system that protects against pathogenic microorganisms and noninfectious foreign substances.

Immune system is the third line of defense against infection **(Fig. 20.1).** Innate and adaptive are the two types of immune response.

DUALITY OF IMMUNE SYSTEM

Humoral (Antibody-mediated) Immunity

- It involves production of antibodies against foreign antigens, by a subset of lymphocytes called B-cells. These B cells are stimulated to form plasma cells and they secrete antibodies.
- Humoral immunity is involved in defense against bacteria, bacterial toxins, and viruses that circulate freely in body fluids, before they enter cells. They are also responsible for certain reactions against transplanted tissue.

Cell-mediated Immunity

Q. Write short note on cell-mediated immunity.

- It involves specialized set of lymphocytes called T-cells that recognize foreign antigens on the surface of cells, organisms, or tissues: Helper T-cells and cytotoxic T-cells.
- Defense against:
  - Bacteria and viruses which lie inside the host cells and are not accessible to antibodies.
  - Fungi, protozoa, and helminths, cancer cells, transplanted tissue.

Antigens

Most of the antigens are proteins or large polysaccharides from a foreign microbes or nonmicrobes.

- **Microbes:** The antigens may be capsules, cell walls, toxins, viral capsids, flagella, etc.
- **Nonmicrobes:** These antigens include pollen, egg white, serum proteins, and surface molecules of red blood cell and transplanted tissue.

  Lipids and nucleic acids become antigen only when combined with proteins or polysaccharides.

Nonspecific defense mechanisms		Specific defense mechanisms (immune system)
First line of defense	Second line of defense	Third line of defense
• Skin • Mucous membranes • Secretions of skin and mucous membranes	• Phagocytic white blood cells • Antimicrobial proteins • The inflammatory response	• Lymphocytes • Antibodies

FIG. 20.1: Nonspecific and specific defense mechanisms.

Haptens

These are small foreign molecules which are not antigenic by themselves. They become antigenic when coupled to a carrier molecule. Once antibodies are formed they will recognize haptens.

Epitope

Epitope represents a small part of an antigen that interacts with an antibody. Each antigen may have one to several epitopes. Each epitope is recognized by a different antibody.

Antibodies

Q. Briefly discuss immunoglobulins and its functions.

- Antibodies (immunoglobulins) are proteins which recognize and bind to a particular antigen with very high specificity.
- These are produced in response to exposure to the antigen.
- One virus or microbe may have several antigenic determinant sites. Each site may bind to different antibodies.
- Each antibody possess at least two identical sites which bind to an antigen. These sites are called as antigen-binding sites.
- Valence of an antibody: It is the number of antigen-binding sites in antibody and most antibodies are bivalent.

Antibody structure

- Monomer: It is an antibody molecule having a flexible Y-shape with four protein chains, i.e., two identical light chains and two identical heavy chains.
- Variable regions: These are two sections at the end of the Y's arms. They contain the antigen-binding sites (F_{ab}). They are identical on the same antibody, but vary from one antibody to another.
- Constant regions: They represent the stem of monomer and lower parts of Y arms.
  - F_c regions: They are regions on the stem of monomer and are important because they can bind to complement or cells.
  - F_{ab} region: For antigen binding.

Immunoglobulin classes *(Table 20.1)*

Functions of immunoglobulins/antibodies

- **Act as opsonins:** Immunoglobulins coat bacterial surface and act as opsonins. This facilitates phagocytosis by cells possessing F_c receptors (e.g., neutrophils).
- **Antibody-dependent cell-mediated cytotoxicity (ADCC):** In this, antibodies bind to microbes via their F_{ab} region. Cytotoxic NK cells attach via F_c receptors and kill these organisms by release of toxic substances called perforins.
- **Activation of complement system:** Binding of antibodies to antigen can trigger activation of the classical complement pathway. Complement components can function as opsonins (C3b component), aid in phagocytosis, chemotaxis (recruitment of leukocytes by C3a and C5a), and cause death of microbes (by MAC-membrane attack complex C5–9).
- **Neutralization:** Some antibodies may directly neutralize the biological activity of their antigen target or toxins released by bacteria. This is an important feature of IgA antibodies at mucosal surfaces.
- **Processing of antigen:** Antibodies present on B lymphocytes help in internalization of antigen and further processing it for presentation to other cells.
- **Agglutination:** IgM antibodies help in agglutination of particulate matter including bacteria and viruses.
- **Immobilization of microbes:** Antibodies against bacterial cilia or flagella may immobilize their movement and ability to escape the phagocytosis.
- **Protection of mucosal surface:** This is observed with IgA type of antibodies.

TABLE 20.1: Features of immunoglobulin classes.

Features	*IgG*	*IgM*	*IgA*	*IgD*	*IgE*
Structure	Monomer	Pentamer, hexamer	Dimer	Monomer	Monomer
Subtypes	G1, G2, G3, G4	Other chains: J chain	Al, A2		
Percentage serum antibodies	75–85% (IgG1 = 45–53%, IgG2 = 11–15%)	5–10%	7–15%, (IgA1 = 11–14% IgA2 = 1– 4%)	0.04%	0.003%
Location	Blood, lymph, intestine	Blood, lymph, B cell surface (monomer)	Secretions (tears, saliva, intestine, milk), blood, and lymph	B-cell surface, blood, and lymph	Bound to mast cells and basophils throughout body
Half-life in serum	23 days	5 days	6 days	3 days	2.5 days
Complement fixation	Yes (classical, alternate)	Yes (classical)	No	Alternate pathway	No
Placental transfer	Yes	No	No	No	No
Known functions	Enhances phagocytosis, neutralizes toxins and viruses, protects fetus and newborn	First antibodies produced during an infection. Effective against microbes and agglutinating antigens	Localized protection of mucosal surfaces. Provides immunity to infant digestive tract	In serum function is unknown. On B-cell surface, initiate immune response. Marker of mature B-cell	Allergic reactions and antiparasitic action

- **Immune-complex formation:** Antibodies combine with antigen to form immune complexes. The size of these immune complexes varies depending upon the ratio between antigens and antibodies. Larger immune complexes can be removed by the phagocytic cells in the reticuloendothelial (RE) system.
- **Transplacental passage:** Maternal antibodies can pass through placenta from mother to fetus conferring immunity to the fetus.

CYTOKINES

Q. Write short note on cytokines.

The immune response involves multiple interactions between many cells. These cells are lymphocytes, dendritic cells, macrophages, other inflammatory cells (e.g., neutrophils), and endothelial cells. Few of these interactions are due to cell-to-cell contact. However, many interactions and effector functions of leukocytes are mediated by short-acting soluble proteins: multipurpose chemical messengers called **cytokines.** Cytokines which mediate communications between leukocytes are called **interleukins.**

Mode of action: Cytokines exert their effect by binding to specific receptors on target cells. They may act by three ways.

1. Autocrine when the cytokines act on the same cells which secrete them.
2. Paracrine when cytokines are produced by one cell type which act on adjacent/nearby target cells.
3. Endocrine when the cytokines secreted into the circulation act on target cells at a site distant from their site of synthesis.

Interleukins

- They are produced by and signal between white cells which mediate endocrine communication at a site distant from their site of synthesis.
- **Source:** Activated macrophages.
- **Effects:** Fever, bone marrow release of neutrophils into circulation (leukocytosis), B-cell proliferation, antibody production, and production of IL-2 by T-cells. Interleukin-2 (IL-2) stimulates the proliferation of activated B-cells, T-cells, and NK cells.

Tumor necrosis factor-α

- **Source:** TNF-α is produced by activated macrophages in response to infection by bacteria and other microbes.
- **Effects:** Fever, cachexia (pathologic state characterized by weight loss and anorexia seen in neoplastic diseases and some chronic infections), anorexia, shock, enhanced leukocyte cytotoxicity, enhanced NK-cell function, acute phase protein synthesis, proinflammatory cytokine induction, increases apoptosis, and expression of cytokines and adhesion molecules.
- Important cytokines and their functions are given below:

Cytokines	*Family*	*Main source*	*Function*
IL-1β	IL-1	Macrophages, monocytes	Pro-inflammation, proliferation, apoptosis, differentiation
IL-4	IL-4	T_H-cells	Anti-inflammation, T-cell and B-cell proliferation, B-cell differentiation
IL-6	IL-6	Macrophages, T-cells, adipocytes	Pro-inflammation, differentiation, cytokine production
IL-8	CXC	Macrophages, epithelial cells, endothelial cells	Pro-inflammation, chemotaxis, angiogenesis
IL-10	IL-10	Macrophages, T-cells, B-cells	Anti-inflammation, inhibition of the pro-inflammatory cytokines
IL-12	IL-12	Dendritic cells, macrophages, neutrophils	Pro-inflammation, cells differentiation, induces acute phase proteins
IL-11	IL-6	Fibroblasts, neurons, epithelial cells	Anti-inflammation, differentiation, induces acute phase proteins
TNF-α	TNF	Macrophages, NK cells, CD4+ lymphocytes, adipocyte	Pro-inflammation, cytokines production, cell proliferation apoptosis, anti-infection
IFN-γ	INF	T-cells, NK cells	Pro-inflammation, innate, adaptive immunity, antiviral activity
GM-CSF	IL-4	T-cells, macrophages, fibroblasts	Pro-inflammation, macrophage activation, increases neutrophil and monocyte function
TGF-b	TGF	Macrophages, T-cells	Anti-inflammation, inhibition of pro-inflammatory cytokine production

Interferons

Q. Write short note on interferons.

- They are critical cytokines that play a key role in defense against viral infections and other intracellular microbes (e.g., *Toxoplasma gondii).* This group includes interferon-α (IFN-α), interferon-β (IFN-β), and interferon-γ (IFN-γ).
- **Source:**
  - These are produced by a wide range of cells, when attacked by viruses and other non-self-pathogenic antigens.
  - IFN-γ is released by T cells and NK cells.

Erythrocyte Sedimentation Rate

Q. Write short note on erythrocyte sedimentation rate (ESR).

- It is the rate at which red blood cells (RBCs) settle down when anticoagulated whole blood is allowed to stand.
- RBCs have net negative charge on their surface and do not aggregate but tend to repel each other. Plasma proteins have positive charge and neutralize the surface negative charge called Zeta potential of red cells.

Factors Affecting ESR

Plasma factors: Increase in certain plasma proteins (especially fibrinogen), reduces the repulsive forces between the red blood cells and cause them to stack together like tyres, or rouleaux. Rouleaux have more mass/surface area ratio than single red cells, and therefore sediment faster and increase the ESR.

- An accelerated ESR is favored by elevated levels of fibrinogen, globulins, and cholesterol (which increase the positive charge of plasma) whereas albumin and lecithin retard ESR.
- Elevated fibrinogen and raised ESR are also observed in pregnancy, old age, and end-stage renal disease.
- In acute inflammation ESR and acute phase reactants are raised.
- ESR is increased in conditions associated with monoclonal (multiple myeloma) or polyclonal (chronic infections like tuberculosis) increase in immunoglobulins. In systemic lupus erythematosus (SLE), ESR is raised but CRP may be normal.

Red cell factors: The sedimentation rate is directly proportional to the weight of the cell aggregates and inversely proportional to the surface area. ESR may be low if plasma proteins are low or red cell morphology is abnormal making rouleaux formation impossible.

- Anemia increases the ESR and polycythemia decreases it.
- Microcytes sedimentation is slower than macrocytes.
- Red cells with an abnormal or irregular shape, such as sickle cells or spherocytes, do not exhibit rouleaux formation and have low ESR.

Normal range: For men 1–10 mm 1st hour and for women 5–20 mm 1st hour.

Acute Phase Reactants/Proteins (Fig. 20.2)

Q. Write short note on acute phase reactants.

Acute phase proteins are produced by liver in response to inflammatory stimuli.

- **ESR** (discussed above)
- **C-reactive protein:** C-reactive protein (CRP) plays an important role in host defense and stimulates repair and regeneration. CRP is an acute phase reactant produced in the liver.
  - It opsonizes invading pathogens.
  - CRP increases (may be up to 1,000-fold) within 6 hours of acute inflammation. Levels fall within a few days after the inflammation subsides. Sequential measurement of CRP is useful in monitoring disease activity.
  - In some inflammatory diseases there may be normal or slight elevations of CRP concentration despite unequivocal evidence of active inflammation. These include SLE, systemic sclerosis, ulcerative colitis, and leukemia. However, existing infection in these conditions is associated with significantly raised levels of CRP.
  - It is to be noted that intercurrent infection does not cause a significant CRP response in these conditions.
- **Procalcitonin** is a 14.5 kDa peptide, a sensitive marker of bacterial infections. It can guide regarding the progression of infections, especially for pneumonia and sepsis. Levels of procalcitonin can be used to guide antibiotic therapy.
- **Ferritin:** During malignancy and infection, ferritin concentrations are elevated. Organisms like pseudomonas cause ferritin levels to drop because they have virulence factor siderophores (pyoverdine and pyocyanin) that chelate and import iron.
- **Haptoglobin:** It is a scavenger protein that has antioxidant, antimicrobial, and anti-inflammatory properties. The levels of haptoglobin decrease during intravascular hemolysis and its levels increase during inflammation.
- **Serum amyloid A** plays a role in host defense and stimulates repair and regeneration. In chronic inflammation, it may contribute to the development of amyloidosis.

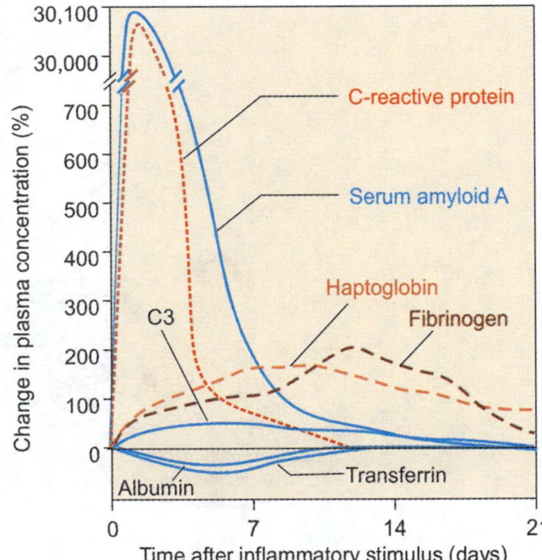

FIG. 20.2: Various acute phase reactants and their levels in inflammation.

- **Fibrinogen** plays an essential role in wound healing.
- **α_1-antitrypsin and α_1-antichymotrypsin:** They control inflammation by neutralizing the enzymes produced by activated neutrophils and prevent tissue destruction.
- **Hepcidin** increases during inflammation causing anemia of chronic disease.
- **Albumin:** Albumin is a negative APP, and its production is decreased to conserve amino acids for positive APPs.
- **Transferrin**: Transferrin is a negative APP. Macrophages internalize transferrin to sequester iron and inhibit microbial iron scavenging.
- Others: Ceruloplasmin, Alpha2-macroglobulin, Alpha1-antichymotrypsins, and manganese superoxide dismutase.

COMPLEMENT SYSTEM

Q. Write short note on the complement system.

- The complement system is a group of plasma proteins (β globulins), major source being the liver. C1q produced mainly by bone marrow derived cells like macrophages and dendritic cells.
- They are proteases and are important in both inflammation and immunity.

Pathways of Complement System Activation (Fig. 20.3)

The decisive step in complement activation is the proteolysis of the third component, C3. Cleavage of C3 can occur by any one of three pathways:

1. **Classical pathway:** It is activated by **antigen-antibody** (Ag-Ab) complexes in which C1 binds to antibody (IgM or IgG), acute phase proteins, charged molecules, and apoptotic or necrotic cell debris.
2. **Alternative pathway:** This pathway is antibody-independent.
   - It is activated by binding of C3 directly to microbial surface molecules [e.g., endotoxin, or lipopolysaccharides (LPS)], complex polysaccharides, cobra venom, and "altered self" such as tumor cells, **in the absence of antibody.** They **cleave C3 to C3b.**
   - **C3b** in the presence of **factors B and D generates C3bBb** (alternative pathway C3 convertase).
   - **C3bBb is labile** and **degraded by factors I** and H, but **stabilized by properdin** and can subsequently activate C3.
   - This results in persistent and prolonged C3 activation and hypocomplementemia. In addition, decreased synthesis of C3 by the liver is also responsible for hypocomplementemia.
3. **Lectin pathway:** It directly activates C1 when plasma mannose-binding lectin (MBL) binds to mannose on microbes.

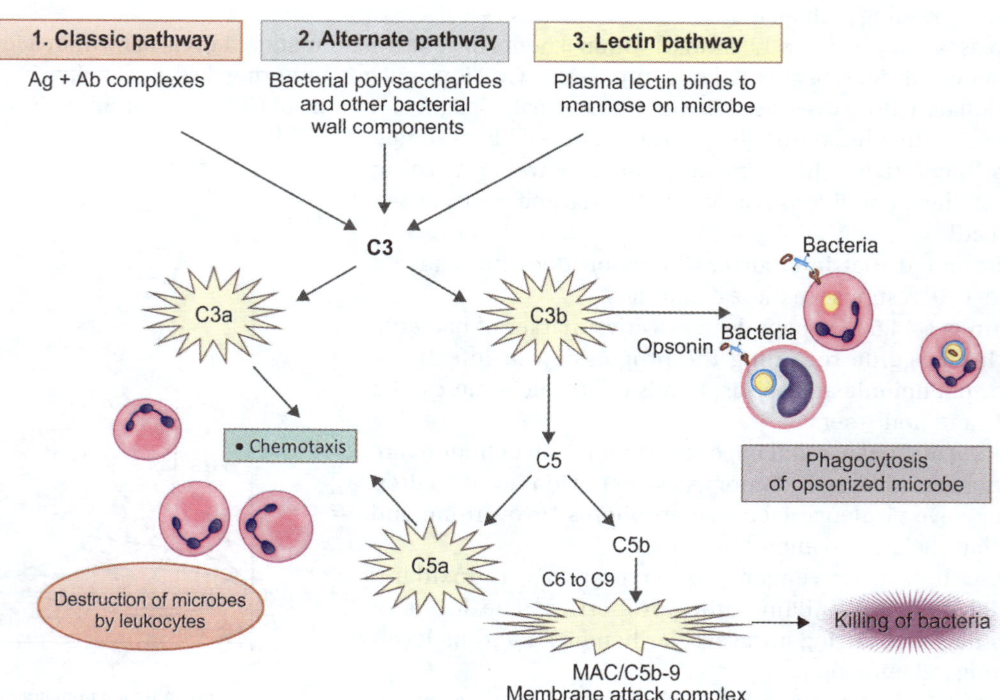

FIG. 20.3: Different pathways of activation and functions of the complement system. All pathways of activation lead to cleavage of C3.

Complement System and Disease (Table 20.2)

TABLE 20.2: Genetic deficiencies of plasma complement components and associated clinical findings.

Deficiency	*Infection*	*Autoimmune disease*
Classical pathway		
C1q	Pneumococcal B/M, other pyogenic	SLE, GN, DV/DLE
Clrs	Other pyogenic pneumococcal B/M, DGI	SLE GN
C4	Other pyogenic	SLE, GN, other AD
C2	Other pyogenic, pneumococcal B/M, meningococcal M	SLE, GN, DV/DLE, other AD
C3	Other pyogenic Pneumococcal B/M, meningococcal M	GN, DV/DLE, SLE, other AD
C5, C6, C7, C8, C9	Meningococcal M, DGI, other pyogenic	SLE, GN, other AD
Lectin pathway		
MBL	Other pyogenic, fungal, HIV	SLE
MASP-2	Pneumococcal pneumonia	SLE
Alternative pathway		
Factor D	DGI, meningococcal M, other pyogenic	
Control proteins		
C1 INH	Hereditary angioedema	SLE
Factor I	Other pyogenic, meningococcal M, pneumococcal B/M	
Factor H	Meningococcal B/M, other pyogenic	GN, HUS, SLE
Properdin	Meningococcal M, pneumococcal B/M, other pyogenic	DV/DLE
C4-binding protein		Other AD

(B/M: bacteremia or meningitis; DGI: disseminated gonococcal infection; DV/DLE: dermal vasculitis or typical discoid lupus erythematosus; GN: glomerulonephritis in various forms, often membranoproliferative; HIV: human immunodeficiency virus; HUS: hemolytic-uremic syndrome; M: meningitis; MASP: MBL-associated serine protease; MBL: mannose-binding lectin; other AD: autoimmune disease (almost all possible diagnoses have been reported); other pyogenic: serious deep or systemic infection due to, or typically caused by, a pyogenic bacterium (abscess, osteomyelitis, pneumonia, bacteremia other than pneumococcal, meningitis other than meningococcal or pneumococcal, cellulitis, myopericarditis, and peritonitis); SLE: typical systemic lupus erythematosus or an SLE-like syndrome without characteristic serologic findings)

Major Histocompatibility Complex

Q. Write short note on HLA system/major histocompatibility complex (MHC).

All human cells express a series of molecules on their surfaces that are recognized by other individuals as foreign antigens. It was found that major histocompatibility antigens are the important antigens involved in the rejection of transplanted organs. These antigens are encoded by a segment of **chromosome 6 (6p21.3)** known as the major histocompatibility complex.

Significance of MHC/HLA System

Q. List diseases associated with HLA-B27.

- **In transplantation:** HLA typing is prerequisite in selecting appropriate donor and recipient combinations for transplantation.
- **Regulations of cell-to-cell interaction:** During immune response (immune response genes).
- Defense against viral infections.
- **HLA and disease association (Table 20.3):** HLA alleles confer a state of susceptibility, or risk, for disease. Many diseases are known to be associated with certain HLA alleles. The diseases associated with the HLA locus can be broadly categorized as mentioned in **Table 20.3.**

TABLE 20.3: Diseases showing positive HLA antigen association.

System	*Disease*	*HLA antigen*	*Relative risk*
Rheumatologic	➢ Ankylosing spondylitis	B27	90.0
	➢ Reiter syndrome	B27	37.0
	➢ Acute anterior uveitis	B27	8.2
	➢ Reactive arthritis	B27	18.0
	➢ Psoriatic arthritis	B27 B38	10.7 9.1
	➢ Juvenile rheumatoid arthritis	B27	3.9
	➢ Juvenile rheumatoid arthritis (pauciarticular)	DR5	3.3
	➢ Rheumatoid arthritis	DR4/Dw4	6.0
	➢ Sjögren syndrome	Dw3	10.0
	➢ Systemic lupus erythematosus	DR3	2.6
Gastrointestinal	➢ Gluten-sensitive enteropathy	DR3	12.0

Contd...

Contd...

	➢ Chronic active hepatitis	DR3	6.8
	➢ Ulcerative colitis	B5	3.8
	➢ IgA deficiency	DR3	13.0
Hematologic	➢ Idiopathic hemochromatosis	A3 B14	6.7 2.7
	➢ Pernicious anemia	A3, B14	90.0
	➢ Hodgkin disease	DR5 DP3	5.0 2.0
Dermatologic	➢ Dermatitis herpetiformis	DR3	17.3
	➢ Psoriasis vulgaris	Cw3	7.5
	➢ Psoriasis vulgaris (Japanese)	Cw6	8.5
	➢ Pemphigus vulgaris (Jewish)	DR4	24.0
	➢ Behçet disease (White)	A26	4.8
	➢ Behçet disease (Japanese)	B5 B51	3.8 12.4
Endocrine	➢ Diabetes mellitus, type 1	DR4 DR3	6/7 5.0
	➢ Graves' disease	DR2 BfF1 + B8 DR3	0.25 15.0 2.5 3.7
	➢ Graves' disease (Japanese)	B35 DR3	4.4 3.7
	➢ Addison disease	Dw3	10.5
	➢ Subacute thyroiditis	B35	13.7
	➢ Hashimoto thyroiditis	DR5	3.0
	➢ Congenital adrenal hyperplasia	B47	15.4
Neurologic	➢ Myasthenia gravis	B8	3.0
	➢ Multiple sclerosis	DR2/Dw2	6.0
	➢ Narcolepsy	DR2, DQ6	130.0
Psychiatric	➢ Bipolar disorder	B16	2.3
	➢ Schizophrenia	A28	2.3
Renal	➢ Idiopathic membranous nephropathy	DR3	5.7
	➢ Goodpasture syndrome	DR2	16.0
	➢ Minimal change disease	DR7	4.2
	➢ IgA nephropathy (French, Japanese)	DR4	3.1
	➢ Gold/penicillamine nephropathy	DR3	14.0
	➢ Polycystic kidney disease	B5	2.6
Infectious	➢ Tuberculoid leprosy (Asians)	B8	6.8
	➢ Paralytic polio	B16	4.3
	➢ Low versus high response vaccinia	Cw3	12.7
	➢ Falciparum malaria, severe	B53	0.4/0.5
	➢ Progression to AIDS	B35	2–3
Others	➢ Birdshot retinochoriodopathy (BSRC)	HLA-A29	80–98
	➢ Cervical cancer	DR11-DQ3	2–3

IMMUNODEFICIENCY

Immunodeficiency may be primary or secondary.

Primary Immunodeficiency Diseases (Box 20.1)

Classification of Primary Immunodeficiency Diseases

Q. Classify primary immunodeficiency disorders.

Primary immunodeficiency diseases (PIDs) are classified into eight major categories according to the component of the immune system primarily involved **(Box 20.1)**. Common components, their frequency, and their susceptibility in primary immunodeficiency are presented in **Table 20.4.**

Box 20.1: Classification of primary immunodeficiency diseases.

- Combined T-cell and B-cell immunodeficiencies
- Predominantly antibody deficiencies
- Other well-defined immunodeficiency syndromes
- Diseases of immune dysregulation
- Congenital defects of phagocyte number and function
- Defects in innate immunity
- Autoinflammatory disorders
- Complement deficiencies

TABLE 20.4: Common components, their frequency, and their susceptibility in primary immunodeficiency.

Class (Deficiency)	*Relative frequency*	*Susceptibility*	*Treatment*
B lymphocytes	50%	Bacterial infections	Immunoglobulin injection
Combined B and T lymphocytes	10-20%	Viral, bacterial, fungal, and protozoal	Bone marrow transplant
Phagocytes	18%	Bacterial infections	Antibiotics and cytokines
Complement	2%	Bacterial infections and autoimmunity	Infusion of complement components

Warning Signs for Suspicion of Primary Immunodeficiency Disorders (Table 20.5)

TABLE 20.5: Warning signs for suspicion of primary immunodeficiency disorders (PID).

➢ Four or more new ear infections within 1 year	➢ Recurrent, deep skin or organ abscesses
➢ Two or more serious sinus infections within 1 year	➢ Persistent thrush in mouth or fungal infection on skin
➢ Two or more months on antibiotics with little effect	➢ Need for intravenous antibiotics to clear infections
➢ Two or more pneumonias within 1 year	➢ Two or more deep-seated infections including septicemia
➢ Failure of an infant to gain weight or grow normally	➢ A family history of PID

Antibody Deficiencies

Q. Write short note on B-cell (antibody) immunodeficiency disorders.

- Constitute 70% of PIDs.
- Recurrent pyogenic infections starting after 6–12 months. Main types of antibody deficiencies are listed in **Box 20.2.**

Box 20.2: Main types of antibody deficiencies.

- X-linked and autosomal recessive agammaglobulinemia
- Common variable immunodeficiency
- IgA deficiency
- IgG subclass deficiency
- Transient hypogammaglobulinemia of infancy
- Selective antibody deficiency
- Associated to other immunodeficiencies (Job syndrome, hyper-IgM)

X-linked agammaglobulinemia (XLA) (Bruton agammaglobulinemia)

Q. Write short note on XLA.

- Described as the "prototypical antibody deficiency" and is the first immunodeficiency described.
- **Bruton tyrosine kinase** *(Btk)* is necessary for the growth and the maturation of B-cell precursors. It is deficient in this disease.
- **Xq21.3–22** (>300 mutations).
- **B-lymphocytes are decreased,** <1% CD19 or CD20-positive lymphocytes.
- Tonsils are small, no palpable lymph node.
- **Autosomal recessive transmission** due to mutation in the genes of the surface bound μ heavy chain, λ5, and Igα.

Clinical features: Little Boys With Big Infections!

- Symptoms appear at 6–9 months of age (after loss of maternal Ig).
- **Sites of infection:** Mucous membranes, ear (otitis media), lungs (bronchitis/pneumonia), blood (sepsis), gut (giardia, or enterovirus), skin, eyes, and meningitis.
- Typical bacterial infections include *Haemophilus influenzae* and *Streptococcus pneumoniae.*
- Also seen: Neutropenia, malignancy in older patients, and renal and joint involvements.

Prevention of infections in patients with PID involves avoidance measures, vaccination, prophylactic antibiotics, immune globulin therapy.

Common Variable Immunodeficiency (CVID)

Q. Write short note on common variable immunodeficiency.

- Diagnosis depends on the exclusion of other causes of antibody deficiencies.
- Incidence: 1/10,000–1/50,000 (second or third decade)
- Decrease in IgG, A +/–M. B-Cells are normal or decreased.

Clinical features

- CVID has a tendency to autoantibody formation.
- Chronic pulmonary infections, chronic giardiasis, intestinal malabsorption, atrophic gastritis, and pernicious anemia.
- T-cell immunity may be deficient.
- Increased risk of lymphoreticular and gastrointestinal malignancies.

IgA deficiency

- Incidence: 1/700 Caucasians but symptoms in <33%.
- Presents with recurrent respiratory infections and chronic diarrhea. Associated conditions with IgA deficiency are listed in **Box 20.3.**

Box 20.3: Associated conditions with IgA deficiency.

- Common variable immunodeficiency (CVID)
- Deficiency of IgG2 (IgG4, E) and poor response to polysaccharide antigens
- Ataxia-telangiectasia
- Risk of asthma and autoimmune diseases (RA, vitiligo, thyroiditis)
- Auto and allo anti-IgA antibodies (MG!).

IgG subclass deficiencies

- Normal total serum IgG levels with subnormal levels of one or more IgG subclasses.
- Mutations in heavy chain genes on 14q32.3 (γ1, 2, 3, 4).
- IgG1: Lead to a decrease in total serum IgG.
- IgG2: Most common IgG subclass deficient in children. Frequently associated with poor response to polysaccharide antigens and IgA deficiency.
- IgG3: Most common IgG subclass deficient in adults.
- IgG4: Levels vary widely in normal people.

Transient hypogammaglobulinemia of infancy

- Decrease of the maternal IgG transferred to the fetus during pregnancy but delayed Ig production (IgM, IgG, and IgA).
- Normal range after 36 months.
- Normal response to vaccination.

Selective antibody deficiencies

- Normal total serum levels of IgG and IgM but failure to respond to certain antigens (polysaccharide antigens).
- Asymptomatic or recurrent sinopulmonary infections.
- Found in sickle cell anemia, asplenia, Wiskott-Aldrich syndrome, and DiGeorge syndrome.

Hyper-IgM syndrome

- Deficit in IgM: IgG switch. Elevated IgM levels and a deficiency in IgG, IgA and IgE.
- The most frequent deficit concerns CD154 on CD4+ T-cell (Xq26.3–27.1).

The hyper-IgE syndrome (Job syndrome)

- Recurrent abscesses, eczema, dysmorphy, eosinophilia, and high serum levels of IgE.
- Autosomal dominant and sporadic cases.

Cell-mediated (T-cell) Immunodeficiency (Box 20.4)

Q. Write short note on T-cell (cell-mediated) immunodeficiency disorders.

Box 20.4: T-cell (cell-mediated) immunodeficiency disorders.

- DiGeorge syndrome
- Defect in CD3/TCR
- Defect in signaling
- Defect in cytokine production as IL-2 and IFN gamma
- Defect in cytokine response

Combined Immunodeficiencies (Box 20.5)

Severe combined immunodeficiency (SCID)

Q. Write short note on severe combined immunodeficiency.

- Failure to thrive.
- Onset of infections in the neonatal period.
- Opportunistic infections, chronic or recurrent thrush, chronic rashes, and chronic or recurrent diarrhea.
- Lack of lymphoid tissue including thymus, tonsils, and lymph nodes.
- Characteristic abnormality in adenosine deaminase deficient SCID includes cupping at the end of the ribs demonstrated on a chest radiograph and an absent thymic shadow.
- Common: *Pneumocystis jirovecii* infection, or persistent oral or diaper candidiasis.

Box 20.5: Combined immunodeficiency disorders.

- Severe combined immunodeficiency (SCID)
- Omenn syndrome
- Adenosine deaminase deficiency (ADA)
- Ataxia-telangiectasia (AT) syndrome
- Wiskott-Aldrich syndrome (WAS)
- EBV-associated immunodeficiency (Duncan's syndrome)

ADA (adenosine deaminase deficiency) SCID: Profound lymphopenia (<500/mm^3); skeletal abnormalities, including chondro-osseous dysplasia (flared costochondral junctions and bone-in-bone anomalies in vertebrae); and deficiency of all types of lymphocytes.

Omenn syndrome

It is a rare autosomal recessive disease usually presenting in neonatal period, characterized by symptoms of SCID associated with other findings like erythroderma, lymphadenopathy, hepatosplenomegaly, and eosinophilia.

Treatment

- Pneumocystis prophylaxis with trimethoprim-sulfamethoxazole.
- Replacement IgG therapy. Enzyme replacement therapy [e.g., polyethylene glycol-adenosine deaminase (PEG-ADA)].
- Patients should only be transfused with irradiated blood products and should not receive any live vaccines.

Q. List the clinical features of DiGeorge syndrome.

Features of DiGeorge syndrome (congenital thymic aplasia) are mentioned in **Box 20.6.**

Wiskott-Aldrich syndrome (WAS)

Q. Write short note on Wiskott-Aldrich syndrome.

- X-linked recessive disease.
- Immunodeficiency, microplatelet thrombocytopenia, and eczema.
- Mutations of the gene encoding WASP at X11p.
- **Low IgM, normal IgA and IgG, and high IgE.**

Ataxia-Telangiectasia

Q. Write short note on ataxia-telangiectasia.

- Autosomal recessive.
- Progressive cerebellar ataxia, abnormal eye movements, oculocutaneous telangiectasias, and immune deficiency. Also characterized by recurrent sinopulmonary infections, bronchiectasis, and interstitial lung disease.
- Vascular malformations (telangiectasia).
- IgA and IgG2 deficiency. T-cell function is variably depressed.
- Gene responsible on **chromosome 11q22.3.**
- Increased serum alfa fetoprotein is diagnostic.
- Prone for various malignancies (lymphomas, breast cancer, and acute leukemias).

Box 20.6: DiGeorge syndrome (congenital thymic aplasia).

- Defective development in thymus and parathyroid that develop from third and fourth pharyngeal pouch.
- Thymic hypoplasia leading to variable immunodeficiency.
- Characteristic facies. Deletion in 22q11 in >80%.
- **Acronym—CATCH 22**
  - **C**ardiac abnormality (commonly interrupted aortic arch, truncus arteriosus and tetralogy of Fallot)
  - **A**bnormal facies
  - **T**hymic aplasia
  - **C**left palate
  - **H**ypocalcemia/hypoparathyroidism

Phagocyte Deficiencies

- Chronic granulomatous disease (CGD)
- Leukocyte adhesion deficiency (LAD I)
- **Chediak-Higashi syndrome,** autosomal recessive condition, is characterized by oculocutaneous albinism, easy bruising, abnormal functions of the natural killer cells, and recurrent pyogenic infections and is a result of a mutation in the lysosomal trafficking regulator (*LYST*) gene.
- IL-12/IFNg pathway deficiencies.
- Chronic or cyclic neutropenia.

Diseases of Immune Dysregulation

Four groups of diseases are included in this category.

1. Familial hemophagocytic lymphohistiocytosis (FHL) that includes perforin deficiency. HLH secondary to autoimmune diseases is called macrophage activation syndrome.
2. UNC13D (Munc13-4) deficiency
3. Syntaxin 11 deficiency and STXBP2 (Munc18-2) deficiency
4. Autoimmune lymphoproliferative syndrome (ALPS).

Q. List the clinical features of IgG4-related diseases.

Immunoglobulin G4-related Disease (IgG4-RD)

IgG4-RD is an immune-mediated fibroinflammatory condition affecting multiple organs.

The hallmarks of IgG4-RD are dense lymphoplasmacytic infiltrations with predominance of IgG4-positive plasma cells in the affected tissue, as accompanied by some degree of fibrosis and obliterative phlebitis and increased number of eosinophils.

Clinical Manifestations

Four main clinical phenotypes have been identified.

1. Group 1: Pancreato-hepato-biliary disease
2. Group 2: Retroperitoneal fibrosis/aortitis
3. Group 3: Head and neck limited disease
4. Group 4: Classic Mikulicz syndrome with systemic involvement.

Common manifestations of IgG4-RD include the following, type 1 autoimmune pancreatitis and IgG4-related sclerosing cholangitis, Mikulicz disease, Riedel's thyroiditis, interstitial pneumonitis, and tubulointerstitial nephritis.

Tissue biopsy is the gold standard for the diagnosis which reveals tumor-like swelling of involved organs, a lymphoplasmacytic infiltrate enriched in IgG4-positive plasma cells, variable degree of fibrosis that has a characteristic **"storiform"** pattern. In addition elevated serum concentrations of IgG4 are found in 60–70% of patients.

Treatment

- Glucocorticoids-prednisone
- Rituximab, azathioprine, and methotrexate.

Q. Discuss the clinical presentation and management of cytokine release syndrome.

Cytokine Release Syndrome

Cytokine release syndrome (CRS) is an acute systemic inflammatory syndrome characterized by fever and multiple organ dysfunction that can be triggered by a variety of factors such as infections and certain drugs. It is associated with chimeric antigen receptor (CAR)-T cell therapy, therapeutic antibodies, and haploidentical allogenic transplantation.

CRS was reported in the setting of haploidentical donor stem cell transplantation, graft-versus-host disease. Cytokine storm due to massive T cell stimulation is also a proposed pathomechanism of severe viral infections such as influenza, SARS 2-COVID-19.

Clinical Manifestations

- Include fever, which may be accompanied by fatigue, headache, diarrhea, and arthralgia.
- Mild CRS can progress to a more severe syndrome which may include hypotension, hypoxia, and uncontrolled systemic inflammatory response with circulatory collapse, vascular leakage, cardiac dysfunction, and multiorgan system failure.

Treatment

- Mild CRS of any cause, symptomatic treatment with antihistamines, antipyretics, and fluids
- For severe CRS caused by CART-T cell therapy, initial treatment with tocilizumab plus a corticosteroid rather than single agent alone appears beneficial. Tocilizumab should be given intravenously over 1 hour as follows, patients <30 kg 12 mg/kg, patients >30 kg 8 mg/kg; total tocilizumab dose should not exceed 800 mg. Steroid therapy includes hydrocortisone 100 mg every 8 hours, dexamethasone 10 mg four times daily or methylprednisolone 1 mg/kg/day until there is improvement in CRS.

Q. List the diagnostic criteria of hemophagocytic lymphohistiocytosis.

Hemophagocytic Lymphohistiocytosis

Hemophagocytic lymphohistiocytosis (HLH) is an aggressive and life-threatening syndrome of excessive immune activation. It is most common in infants and young children but can affect patients of any age, with or without a predisposing familial condition. The term **macrophage activation syndrome (MAS)** refers to a form of HLH that occurs primarily in patients with juvenile idiopathic arthritis or other rheumatologic diseases.

Genetic defect: Mutations at familial hemophagocytic lymphohistiocytosis (FHL) loci include PRF1/Perforin, UNC13D/Munc13-4, STX11/Syntaxin11.

Clinical Features

Diagnostic Criteria of HLH-2004

The diagnosis of HLH can be established if one of either 1 or 2 below is fulfilled:

1. A molecular diagnosis consistent with HLH is made.
2. Diagnostic criteria for HLH are fulfilled (5 of the 8 criteria below):
   - Fever
   - Splenomegaly
   - Cytopenias (affecting >2–3 lineages in the peripheral blood):
     - Hemoglobin <9 g/dL(in infants <4 weeks of age, hemoglobin <10 g/dL)
     - Platelets <100 × 109/L
     - Neutrophils <1.0 × 109/L
   - Hypertriglyceridemia (fasting triglycerides >265 mg/dL) and /or hypofibrinogenemia (fibrinogen <150 mg/ dL)
   - Hemophagocytosis in bone marrow, spleen, or lymph nodes
   - Low or absent NK-cell activity
   - Ferritin >500 ng/mL
   - Elevated soluble CD25 (i.e., sIL2R) two standard deviations above age-adjusted laboratory specific norms.

Treatment

- Among patients who are acutely ill or deteriorating, HLH-94-based therapy includes etoposide and dexamethasone given as tapering doses over 8 weeks, with intrathecal methotrexate and hydrocortisone for those with central nervous system involvement.
- Patients should receive supportive care like transfusions of red blood cells, platelets, and fresh frozen plasma.
- Hematopoietic cell transplantation (HCT) following induction therapy is recommended.
- Refractory or recurrent HLH—emapalumab (interferon gamma blocking antibody) and alemtuzumab (anti-CD52 antibody) can be tried.

HYPERSENSITIVITY REACTIONS

Q. List the types of hypersensitivity reactions.

Immunologically mediated reactions (hypersensitivity reactions) that may produce in tissue damage are summarized in **Figure 20.4 and Table 20.6.**

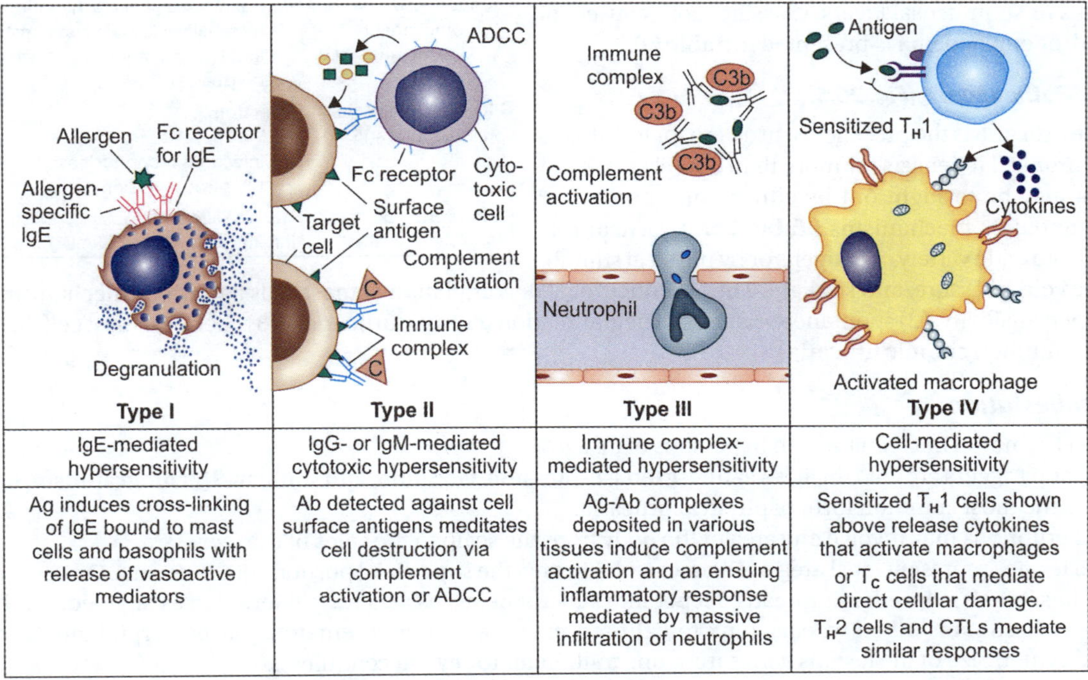

FIG. 20.4: Features of hypersensitivity reactions (Gell and Coombs classification).

TABLE 20.6: Characteristic features of hypersensitivity reactions.

Type	*I (immediate)*	*II (cytotoxic)*	*III (immune complex)*	*IV (delayed)*
Antigens	Pollens, molds, mites, food drugs and parasites	Cell surface or tissue bound	Exogenous (viruses, bacteria, fungi, parasites) autoantigens	Cell/tissue bound
Mediators	IgE and mast cells	IgG, IgM, and complement	IgG, IgM, IgA, and complement	Cytotoxic T-cells, activated macrophage
Time taken for reaction to develop	5–10 minutes	6–36 hours	4–12 hours	48–72 hours
Pathological feature	Edema, vasodilatation, mast cell degranulation, eosinophils	Antibody-mediated damage to target cells	Acute inflammatory reaction (neutrophils), vasculitis	➢ Perivascular inflammation, mononuclear cells, fibrin ➢ Granulomas: Caseation and necrosis in TB
Prototype disorder/diseases produced	➢ Asthma (extrinsic) ➢ Anaphylaxis (systemic and localized) ➢ Urticaria, eczema ➢ Angioedema ➢ Allergic rhinitis ➢ Food allergies	➢ Autoimmune hemolytic anemia, transfusion reactions, hemolytic disease of newborn ➢ Goodpasture's syndrome ➢ Pernicious anemia ➢ Myasthenia gravis	Autoimmune diseases (e.g., SLE, glomerulonephritis, rheumatoid arthritis), serum sickness, Arthus reaction	➢ Tuberculosis ➢ Contact dermatitis ➢ Leprosy ➢ Transplant rejection
Diagnostic tests	➢ Skin-prick tests ➢ Specific IgE in serum	➢ Coombs test ➢ Indirect immunofluorescence	Immune complexes, complement levels	➢ Skin test—erythema induration (e.g., tuberculin test)
Treatment	➢ Antigen avoidance ➢ Antihistamines, corticoste-roids (usually topical) ➢ Leukotriene receptor antago-nists ➢ Sodium cromoglicate ➢ Epinephrine (adrenaline) for life-threatening anaphylaxis	➢ Exchange transfusion ➢ Plasmapheresis ➢ Immunosuppressives/ cytotoxic drugs	➢ Corticosteroids ➢ Immunosuppressives/ cytotoxic drugs ➢ Plasmapheresis ➢ Anti-TNF antibody, anti-B-cell antibody, anti-CTLA-4 antibody	➢ Immunosuppressives ➢ Corticosteroids, removal of antigen

Urticaria ("Hives")

Q. Write short essay/note on urticaria or hives or nettle rash.

Urticaria (also known as hives) is produced due to localized edema of dermis secondary to a temporary increase in capillary permeability. The term angioedema is used if edema involves subcutaneous or submucosal layers. Classification (causes) of urticaria and/or angioedema is presented in **Table 20.7**.

TABLE 20.7: Classification of urticaria and/or angioedema.

Immunologic:	**Nonimmunologic reactions:**
➤ Autoimmune ➤ Immunoglobulin E (IgE)-dependent ➤ Immune complex-mediated ➤ Complement-kinin dependent	➤ Direct mast cell-releasing agents (opiates, antibiotics, curare, D-tubocurarine, radiocontrast media) ➤ Vasoactive stimuli ➤ Agents that alter arachidonic acid metabolism (aspirin and nonsteroidal anti-inflammatory agents, azo dyes, and benzoates)
Physical: Heat, cold, pressure, sun, and water	**Infection:** ➤ Viral hepatitis ➤ Infectious mononucleosis ➤ HIV seroconversion
Idiopathic	**Drugs:** Salicylates, opiates, nonsteroidal anti-inflammatory drugs (NSAIDs), antibiotics

Etiology and Pathogenesis (Fig. 20.5)

Types: Acute urticaria is the presence of urticaria for less than 6 weeks and chronic if it persists for more than 6 weeks.

- Urticaria may be brought out by either immunologic or nonimmunologic mechanisms **(Table 20.7)**. Urticaria is triggered by a wide variety of antigens or by physical stimuli, including cold, pressure, and sunlight. They produce local degranulation of mast cells by various mechanism such as (1) type I hypersensitivity, (2) spontaneous mast cell degranulation (chronic urticarial), (3) chemical mast cell degranulation, (4) autoimmunity (chronic urticaria).

Clinical Manifestation

- Urticaria is common and can be seen in persons of all ages.
- The common triggers are cold, heat, sweating, exercise, pressure, vibration, and sunlight. **Dermographism**, literally "skin writing," is the most common form of physical urticaria.
- Urticarial eruptions may involve any area of the body from the scalp to the soles of the feet.
- Urticarial lesions represent local area of edema involving only the superficial portions of the dermis. On certain body sites (e.g., the lips, hands), the edema spreads deeper into subcutaneous tissue and is referred to as angioedema.
- They are well-circumscribed wheals, pink to light red in color, with erythematous raised serpiginous borders and a blanched center. Size of the lesions varies from one millimeter to several centimeters.
- Almost always pruritic and individual wheals come and go within 24 hours and those lesions lasting up to 6 weeks are called as acute urticaria. If the urticaria recurs over a period of 6 weeks or more it is known as chronic urticaria.
- When individual lesions last more than 36–48 hours and leave postinflammatory hyperpigmentation or palpable purpura, it is called as urticarial vasculitis.
- Urticaria may be associated with headache, dizziness, nausea, vomiting, abdominal pain, diarrhea, and arthralgias.

Management

- Management of urticaria depends on its severity and the duration.
- Mild urticaria limited to the skin: Antihistamines (diphenhydramine) or the newer nonsedating agents (terfenadine, cetirizine, and loratadine).
- Severe urticaria: Short-term corticosteroids (up to 1 mg/kg).
- Chronic urticaria: Finding the cause and remove the causative antigen. Antihistamines, omalizumab and cyclosporine for 8–16 weeks, may be beneficial.

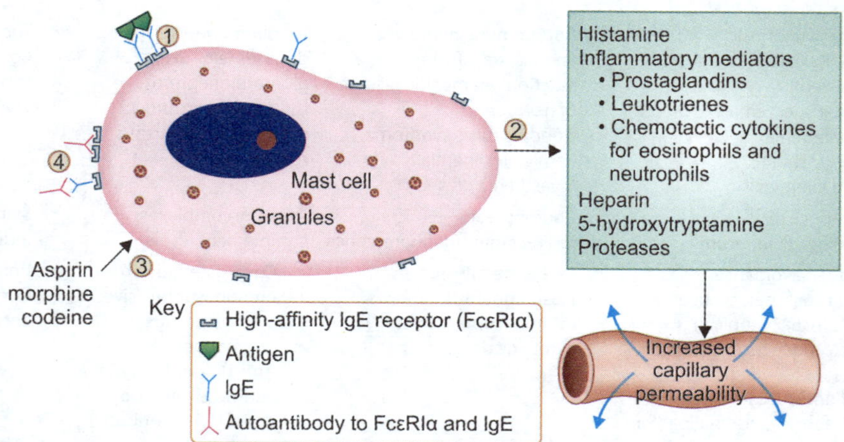

FIG. 20.5: Pathogenesis of urticaria. Mast cell degranulation can occur by different mechanism. (1) Type I hypersensitivity. (2) Spontaneous mast cell degranulation (chronic urticarial). (3) Chemical mast cell degranulation. (4) Autoimmunity (chronic urticaria).

Allergy

Q. Define allergy. List atopic disorders.

- Allergy is defined as a hypersensitivity reaction induced by exposure to an otherwise harmless exogenous substance (known as an allergen), generally environmental.
- In an allergic reaction, initial exposure to allergen triggers the production of specific IgE antibodies by activated B-cells. These IgE antibodies bind to the surface of mast cells via high-affinity IgE receptors.
- The first dose of allergen (priming dose) sensitizes the immunologic system (B lymphocyte). On re-exposure, the allergen (shocking dose) binds to membrane-bound IgE which activates the mast cells, releasing vasoactive mediators (the early phase response), and causing a type I hypersensitivity reaction and the symptoms of allergy. This may be followed by late phase reaction and is mediated by basophils, eosinophils, and macrophages.
- Examples: Asthma, anaphylaxis, rhinitis, urticaria, angioedema, eczema, and food hypersensitivity.

Angioedema

Q. Write short essay/note on the clinical features and treatment of angioedema.

Angioedema is defined as a well-demarcated localized edema involving the deeper layers of the skin, including the subcutaneous tissue and submucosal tissues.

Etiology

It is an IgE-mediated reaction that causes direct release of histamine from the mast cells. It follows a variety of allergens. It may develop due to insect sting, drug reaction, food allergy, and exposure to other biological products. Rarely, angiotensin-converting enzyme (ACE) inhibitors may produce angioedema due to increased levels of bradykinin. Most of the cases are idiopathic.

C1-esterase Inhibitor Deficiency

C1 esterase (C1INH) inhibitor is a complement protein that inhibits spontaneous activation of classical complement pathway. C1 esterase inhibitor also regulates kinin cascade, activation of which increases local bradykinin levels and produces local pain and swelling. Both C1-esterase inhibitor and C1 levels are low. C1INH deficiency produces bradykinin. Deficiency of C1INH may be hereditary or acquired disorder.

- **Hereditary angioedema:** It is an autosomal dominant disorder, is due to C1 esterase inhibitor (C1INH) deficiency. Angioedema develops either spontaneously or following infection or injury (e.g., dental injury). Onset is usually in early childhood. The attacks become worse at puberty and usually its frequency and severity decreases after the age of 50 years and may even disappear totally. Diagnosis is confirmed by low levels of C1-esterase inhibitor (in 85% cases) or dysfunctional C1-esterase inhibitor (in 15% cases).
- Mutations in chromosome 11; Autosomal dominant inheritance.
  - Type I C1ID: 85% patients have no detectable protein.
  - Type II C1ID: 15% patients have dysfunctional protein
- **Acquired C1INH deficiency:** It presents in a manner similar to the hereditary angioedema but the onset occurs in the fifth and sixth decades of life. It is due to appearance of an autoantibody. It may occur with B-cell lymphoma, multiple myeloma, Waldenstrom's macroglobulinemia, and chronic lymphocytic leukemia.

Clinical Features

- It may occur at any age but most common in young adults.
- It presents with well-defined, nonpitting swelling, usually nonpruritic. It may be associated with urticaria lesions.
- Angioedema up to 6 weeks is called acute and if it lasts beyond 6 weeks is called chronic.
- It may involve any area of the body but often affects periorbital area, lips **(Fig. 20.6)**, and genital areas.
- Angioedema of the upper respiratory tract may cause laryngeal obstruction which may be life-threatening.
- Involvement of gastrointestinal system may produce abdominal colic, with or without nausea and vomiting.
- Angioedema does not produce residual discoloration unless there is extravasation of RBCs.

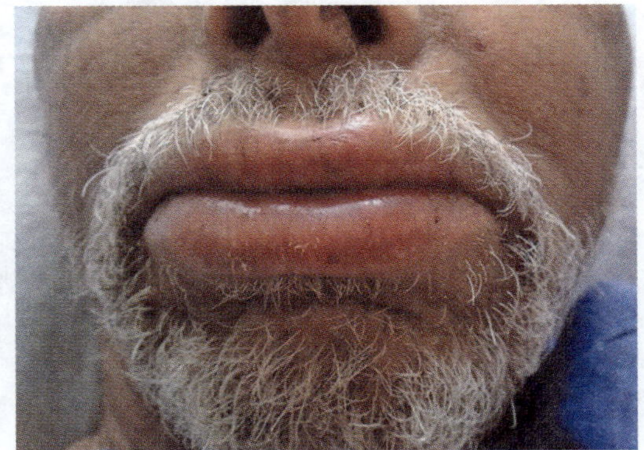

FIG. 20.6: Angioedema.

Treatment

- Identification of the etiologic factor(s) and remove the offending agent if possible.
- Antihistamines to control the lesions, e.g., diphenhydramine cetirizine, desloratadine.

- Observe for any evidence of airway obstruction and if present manage in a fashion similar to those with anaphylaxis.
- Acute attack should be controlled with epinephrine.
- Chronic angioedema not responding to maximal dosages of antihistamines, glucocorticosteroids and other immunomodulating agents (e.g., methotrexate, cyclosporine) may be considered.
- During severe attacks of hereditary angioedema due to C1INH deficiency, fresh frozen plasma is lifesaving as it provides C1-esterase inhibitor. Danazol is useful to prevent episodes of hereditary angioedema.
- Newer therapy for hereditary angioedema: Purified C1 inhibitor concentrate, recombinant C1INH—**Conestat alfa,** bradykinin receptor antagonist—**Icatibant** and kallikrein inhibitor—**Ecallantide.**

Systemic Anaphylaxis

Q. Write short note on anaphylactic reactions (anaphylaxis).

Q. Discuss the causes and treatment/management of anaphylactic shock.

Definition: Systemic anaphylaxis is a life-threatening form of immediate (appears within minutes after systemic exposure to specific antigen) type I hypersensitivity reaction mediated by IgE. It is a systemic response that develops when mast cells (possibly basophils) are provoked to secrete mediators with potent vasoactive and smooth muscle contractile activities.

Causes

It occurs in sensitized individuals and requires prior sensitization to inciting antigen, either alone or in combination with a hapten. It usually occurs when allergen is administered parenterally and it is less likely after oral ingestion, inhalation, or cutaneous or ocular topical contact. The causes of systemic anaphylactic reactions are listed in **Box 20.7**.

Anaphylaxis may be triggered by extremely small doses of antigen, e.g., the minute dose used in skin testing for various forms of allergies.

Box 20.7: Causes of systemic anaphylactic reactions.

Anaphylaxis: IgE-mediated mast cell degranulation

1. **Proteins:**
   - Foreign proteins (e.g., antisera)
   - Foods (peanuts, fish and shellfish, egg, milk, and soya products)
   - Food additives (aspartame, monosodium glutamate)
2. **Drugs:**
   - Antibiotics (penicillins, cephalosporins tetracyclines, trimethoprim-sulfamethoxazole, vancomycin, and nitrofurantoin)
   - Chemotherapeutic agents
   - Hormones (e.g., insulin, vasopressin, and parathormone)
   - Enzymes (chymotrypsin, penicillinase, and streptokinase)
   - Intravenous anesthetic agents (suxamethonium and propofol)
   - Latex
3. **Biological agents:**
   - Blood
   - Tetanus, rabies, and diphtheria antitoxins
   - Antithymocyte globulin
   - Vaccines
4. **Insect bites and stings:**
   - Honey bee (bee venom)
   - Wasps (wasp venom)

Mechanism (Fig. 20.7)

- **Initial exposure to antigen:** The sensitizing antigen (allergen) from its site of entry is presented to T-cells which

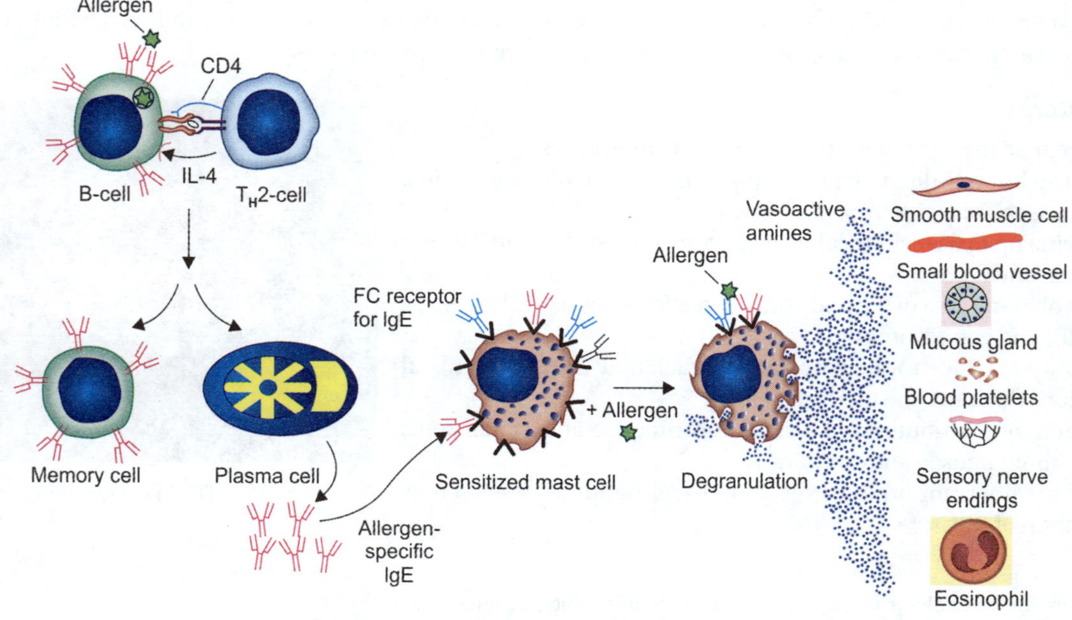

FIG. 20.7: Mechanism of systemic anaphylaxis.

differentiate into T_H2 cells. IL-13 secreted by T_H2 cells **enhances IgE production by B-cells. IgE gets attached to mast cells and basophils.**

- **During subsequent exposure to antigen,** the antigen (allergen) binds to the IgE antibodies previously bound to the mast cells and produces IgE-induced degranulation of mast cells and basophils. It results in the liberation of a number of mediators **(Table 20.8)**. Mediators released by mast cells include preformed mediators (stored in secretory granules) and secondary mediators (newly synthesized products). They are responsible for the pathogenesis of an anaphylactic reaction **(Table 20.8)**.

TABLE 20.8: Mast cell mediators in anaphylactic reactions.

Preformed mediators (primary mediators)	*Secondary (newly synthesized) mediators*
1. Vasoactive amines: Histamine 2. Enzymes: Neutral proteases (chymase, tryptase) and several acid hydrolases 3. Proteoglycans: These include heparin (anticoagulant), and chondroitin sulfate 4. Eosinophil chemotactic factor 5. Neutrophil chemotactic factor	1. Lipid mediators: • Leukotrienes B_4, C_4, and D_4. • Prostaglandin D_2 • Platelet-activating factor (PAF) 2. Cytokines: TNF, IL-1, IL-4 and chemokines

Anaphylactoid Reactions (Pseudo-allergic Reactions/Non-IgE-mediated)

Q. Write short note on anaphylactoid reactions.

- They are indistinguishable from anaphylactic reactions.
- Most non-IgE-dependent foreign agents do not require antigen processing (sensitization) and can elicit a mast cell activation response on first antigenic exposure itself. However, they may be associated with IgG and IgM antibodies and not IgE. These antibodies activate the complement system through classical pathway and produce activated complement components and may cause direct release of preformed mediators from mast cells and basophils.
- Short lived because involves only degranulation of mast cells and not cytokine synthesis.
- Causes: *Refer* **Box 20.8.**

Box 20.8: Anaphylactoid reactions (Pseudo-allergic reactions/non-IgE-mediated).

Anaphylactoid: Non-IgE-mediated mast cell degranulation

1. **Drugs:**
    - Aspirin and nonsteroidal anti-inflammatory drugs (NSAIDs)
    - Vancomycin
    - Narcotics (e.g., codeine, morphine, opiates)
    - Radiocontrast media/dye
2. **Physical:**
    - Exercise
    - Exposure to cold
3. **Autoimmune**
4. **Narcotics/vancomycin**
5. **Idiopathic**

Clinical Features (Tables 20.9 and 20.10)

The anaphylactic response appears within minutes after systemic exposure to specific antigen.

TABLE 20.9: Clinical features of systemic anaphylaxis.

Cutaneous	*Respiratory*
➢ Itching (pruritus) ➢ Hives (urticaria) ➢ Skin erythema with or without angioedema ➢ Flushing ➢ Insect stings	➢ Intense bronchospasm resulting in respiratory distress ➢ Dyspnea and wheeze ➢ Laryngeal edema resulting in hoarseness and laryngeal obstruction ➢ Pulmonary edema
Gastrointestinal	***Cardiovascular***
➢ Nausea ➢ Vomiting ➢ Abdominal cramps ➢ Diarrhea	➢ Tachycardia ➢ Hypotension ➢ Arrhythmias ➢ Shock and collapse
Central nervous system	
➢ Confusion ➢ Feeling of impending doom ➢ Apprehension ➢ Metallic taste ➢ Altered levels of consciousness	**Biphasic anaphylaxis** is recurrence of symptoms that develops following the apparent resolution of the initial anaphylactic episode with no additional exposure to the causative agent.

TABLE 20.10: Clinical features of systemic anaphylaxis depending on severity.

Severity	*Features*
Mild	Cutaneous features only: Pruritus, erythema, urticaria or mild angioedema
Moderate	The above plus more severe angioedema and/or vomiting, abdominal pain and/or mild dyspnea or tightening of throat
Severe	The above plus respiratory difficulty (laryngeal edema or asthma) and/or hypotension

Diagnostic Criteria for Anaphylaxis

Anaphylaxis is likely when one of the following three criteria occurs:

1. Acute skin and/or mucosal symptoms (e.g., hives, pruritus, flushing, lip/tongue/uvula swelling) and one of the following:
    a. Respiratory symptoms (e.g., wheezing, stridor, shortness of breath, and hypoxia)
    b. Hypotension or associated end-organ dysfunction (e.g., hypotonia, syncope, and incontinence)
2. Exposure to probable allergen and two or more of the following:
    a. Skin/mucosal tissue involvement
    b. Respiratory symptoms
    c. Hypotension or end-organ dysfunction
    d. Persistent gastrointestinal symptoms (e.g., emesis and abdominal pain)
3. Decreased blood pressure after exposure to known allergen for the patient:
    a. Adults: Systolic blood pressure <90 mm Hg or $>30\%$ decrease in systolic blood pressure
    b. Infants and children: Hypotension for age or $>30\%$ decrease in systolic blood pressure

Q. Write short note on treatment of anaphylaxis. List lifesaving drugs used in anaphylactic shock.

Treatment

Anaphylaxis is an acute medical emergency and its early recognition is imperative, since death occurs within minutes to hours after the first symptoms.

- **Prevent further contact with allergen,** e.g., removal of bee sting.
- **Ensure airway patency:** Fatal outcomes in anaphylaxis are mainly due to either airway constriction or hypotension.
- **Oxygen alone via a nasal catheter or with nebulized salbutamol/albuterol,** oxygen 4–6 L/min.
  - If progressive hypoxia develops, either endotracheal intubation or tracheostomy with intermittent positive ventilation is required for oxygen delivery.
- **Administer adrenaline (epinephrine) intramuscularly** into the thigh and is the most critical drug to administer. Earlier administration during the course of an anaphylactic event is better.
  - Adult: 0.3–0.5 mg (0.3–0.5 mL of a 1:1,000 solution) IM in the lateral thigh, repeated at 10- to 15-minute intervals if necessary.
  - Child: 1:1,000 dilution at 0.01 mg/kg or 0.1–0.3 mL administered IM in the lateral thigh, repeated at 10- to 15-minute intervals if necessary.
  - 0.5 mL of 1:1,000 solution sublingually in cases of major airway compromise or hypotension.
  - 3–5 mL of 1:10,000 solution via central line.
  - 3–5 mL of 1:10,000 solution diluted with 10 mL of normal saline via endotracheal tube.
  - For protracted symptoms that require multiple doses of epinephrine, an IV epinephrine drip may be useful; the infusion is titrated to maintain adequate BP.
- **Administer antihistamines:** They may prevent the progression of urticaria and pruritus, but does not reverse hypotension or tissue edema by directly opposing effects of mast cell activation, e.g., chlorphenamine 10 mg IM or slow IV injection, diphenhydramine, 50–100 mg IM or IV.
- **Administer corticosteroids:** Hydrocortisone 200 mg IV stat (not effective for the acute event as it takes 4 hours to act; but alleviate recurrence of bronchospasm, urticaria, and hypotension).
- **Glucagon** could reverse refractory bronchospasm and hypotension in patients who are taking β-adrenergic antagonists. Recommended dosage is 1–5 mg intravenously bolus slowly over 5 minutes followed by an infusion at 5–15 µg/min titrated to clinical response.
- **Provide supportive treatments:**
  - Bronchodilators: They relieve bronchospasm, e.g., nebulized β_2-agonists/salbutamol and aminophylline, 0.25–0.5 g IV.
  - Hypotension: Immediately put patient in the Trendelenburg position (prevent progression to anaphylactic shock). Shock is treated with intravenous fluids (if needed with dopamine) to restore or maintain blood pressure. **ECMO** has been tried.

Non-IgE-mediated (idiopathic) anaphylaxis: Usually presents slowly over a few hours. Begins with pruritus of the palms and soles, then progresses to general pruritus, erythema, and urticaria, with diarrhea, abdominal pain, and hypotension. Respiratory symptoms are rare.

Allergen Immunotherapy or Desensitization

- Subcutaneously incremental doses of allergen are given at 1–2 weekly intervals until the top dose is reached. Sublingual immunotherapy has been practiced too.
- Useful for prevention of atopy/anaphylaxis.

Acute Serum Sickness

Q. Write short note on serum sickness.

- It is a systemic immune complex-mediated disease (type III hypersensitivity reaction).
- It was a frequent sequelae to the administration of large amounts of foreign serum (e.g., serum from immunized horses used for protection against diphtheria). But nowadays it is infrequent.
- IgG is produced when a foreign antigen is injected in large quantities. They form soluble immune (antigen-antibody) complexes.

Mechanism: Introduction of antigen → body's immune system responds by synthesizing antibodies after 4–10 days → antibody reacts with antigen, forming soluble complexes that may diffuse into vascular walls and may initiate activation of complement → complement-containing immune complexes generate influx of leukocytes into vessel walls—proteolytic enzymes that can mediate tissue damage are released → immune complex deposition + inflammatory responses are responsible for vasculitic lesions seen.

Clinical Features

Fever, urticaria (at the site of injection), joint pains (arthralgias), lymph node enlargement, and proteinuria appear during this phase. Wherever immune complexes deposit the tissue damage is similar **(Box 20.9)**.

Treatment

Treatment of acute serum sickness is shown in **Box 20.10.**

AUTOIMMUNITY

Q. Write short essay/note on autoimmunity.

Definition: Autoimmunity is defined as an immune reaction in which body produces autoantibodies and immunologically competent T-lymphocytes against self-antigens.

Mechanisms of Autoimmunity (Fig. 20.8)

Genetic Factors

Role of susceptibility genes: Most autoimmune diseases are complex multigenic disorders and genetic factors have an important role.

- **Runs in families:** The incidence is greater in monozygotic than in dizygotic twins.
- **Association with HLA genes:** Most significant.

Environmental Factors

Role of infections

A variety of microbes may trigger autoimmunity by several mechanisms.

- **Molecular mimicry:** Few viruses and microbes may express antigens that have the antigenic structure similar to self-antigens. Immune responses against them may cross-react with self-tissue and this phenomenon is known as molecular mimicry. Example: **Rheumatic heart disease,** in which antibodies formed against streptococcal bacterial proteins, cross-react with myocardial proteins and cause myocarditis. Molecular mimicry between microbial proteins and host tissues is also found in *Klebsiella* and HLA-B27 in ankylosing spondylitis, Coxsackievirus and glutamic acid decarboxylase in insulin-dependent (type l) diabetes mellitus, rheumatoid arthritis, and multiple sclerosis.
- **Breakdown of anergy:** Tissue necrosis and inflammation produced by microbial infections can cause **up-regulation of co-stimulatory molecules** on APCs. This may favor breakdown of anergy and activation of T-cells.
- **Immune dysregulation:** Normally, T-cells regulate any autoreactive T- and B-cells that have survived clonal deletion. Dysregulation of T-cell function can lead to loss of control and the development of autoimmune disease, e.g., immunodeficiency diseases such as hypogammaglobulinemia and HIV infection are commonly associated with autoimmune phenomena.

Other environmental factors

- **Ultraviolet radiation**
- **Cigarette smoking**
- **Local tissue injury/damage:** Some autoantigens are hidden within the cells or tissues in immunologically privileged sites (e.g., brain or the anterior chamber of the eye). Therefore, the lymphoid cells remain in a state of immunologic ignorance. In this state, lymphoid cells are neither activated nor anergized to proteins expressed by these immunologically privileged sites. If the tissue in the privileged site is damaged by trauma or inflammation or tumor, the antigens may be released. These antigens can evoke an autoimmune response, e.g., Dressler's syndrome is an acute pericarditis developing in a patient with myocardial infarction secondary to the production of antimyocardial antibodies, development of insulin-dependent diabetes in association of Coxsackie virus infection, multiple sclerosis, and sympathetic ophthalmia.
- **Drugs:** T-cell bypass is a mechanism by which T-cells help autoreactivation of B-cells instead of suppressing them, e.g., include drug-induced autoimmune responses such as quinine-induced thrombocytopenia.
- **Hormones.**

Box 20.9: Lesion produced in acute serum sickness.

- Vasculitis—inflammatory lesion in blood vessels.
- Glomerulonephritis—inflammatory lesion in renal glomeruli.
- Arthritis—inflammatory lesion in the joints.

Box 20.10: Treatment of acute serum sickness.

- Corticosteroid creams or ointments: Relieve discomfort from itching and rash.
- Antihistamines: May reduce the length of illness and itching.
- NSAIDs: May relieve joint pain.
- Paracetamol: Helpful in relieving fever and muscle pain.
- Medications causing problem should be stopped and future use should be avoided.

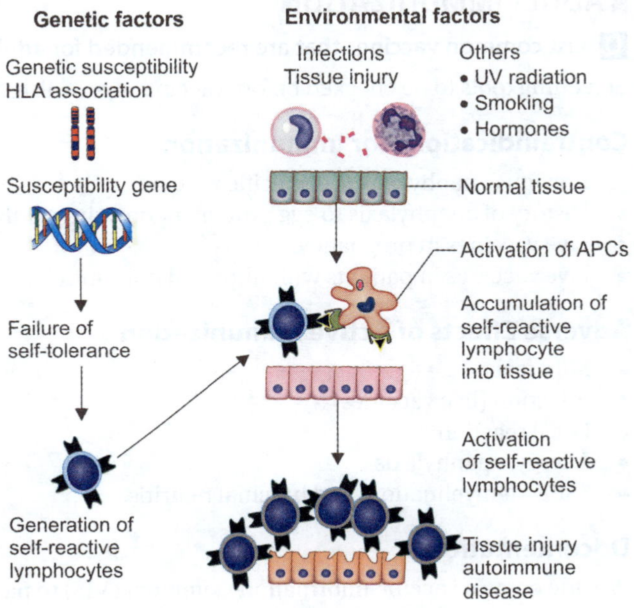

FIG. 20.8: Pathogenesis of autoimmunity.

Classification of autoimmune disorders is presented in **Table 20.11.**

TABLE 20.11: Classification of autoimmune disorders.	
Organ specific autoimmune diseases	***Systemic autoimmune diseases***
➢ Type I diabetes mellitus ➢ Goodpasture syndrome ➢ Multiple sclerosis ➢ Grave's disease ➢ Hashimoto's thyroiditis ➢ Autoimmune pernicious anemia ➢ Autoimmune Addison's disease ➢ Vitiligo ➢ Myasthenia gravis	➢ Rheumatoid arthritis ➢ Scleroderma ➢ Systemic lupus erythematosus ➢ Primary Sjögren syndrome ➢ Polymyositis

Therapy of Autoimmune Disease

- Control of symptoms (e.g., nonsteroidal anti-inflammatory drugs for joint pains, fever, etc., in SLE; β-blockers in patients with thyrotoxic features).
- Specific replacement therapy where the organ has been completely destroyed (e.g., thyroid hormone replacement in hypothyroidism).
- Immunosuppressive therapy including corticosteroids, cytotoxic drugs in different forms, different regimens, and different routes.
- Newer and experimental forms of therapy including immunomodulation, e.g., plasmapheresis, intravenous immunoglobulin therapy, and cyclosporin.

ADULT IMMUNIZATION

Q. List common vaccines that are recommended for adults.

Screening tools to be checked before vaccination are listed in **Box 20.11.**

Box 20.11: Utilize screening tools; H-A-L-O.

- **H**ealth condition
- **A**ge
- **L**ifestyle
- **O**ccupation

Contraindications for Immunization

- Previous anaphylaxis to a specific vaccine
- History of anaphylaxis to egg protein, neomycin (MMR)
- Live vaccines in pregnancy
- Live vaccines in patients with impaired immunity.

Adverse Effects of Active Immunization

- Mild fever
- Infection (live vaccines)
- Local reaction
- Allergy/anaphylaxis
- SSPE, demyelination, and brachial neuritis.

Documentation

Provide copy of vaccine information statement (VIS) to patient/documents to be maintained.

- Date of vaccination and next dose
- Vaccine manufacturer
- Lot number
- Dose and site of vaccine
- Vaccinator's initials

The Advisory Committee on Immunization Practices (ACIP) adult immunization, age-based recommendations in India, is presented in **Table 20.12.**

TABLE 20.12: Adult immunization, age-based recommendations in India, 2020.

Vaccine/Age group	*19–26 years*	*27–49 years*	*50–59 years*	*60–64 years*	*>65 years*
Tetanus, diphtheria, pertussis (Tdap)	Substitute one time dose of Tdap with Td, then booster with Td every 10 years				Td booster every 10 years
Human papilloma vaccine	3 doses				
Varicella	2 doses				
Zoster				1 dose	
Measles, mumps, and rubella	1 or 2 doses		1 dose		
Influenza			1 dose annually		
Pneumococcal (polysaccharide)	1 or 2 doses				1 dose
Hepatitis A	2 doses				
Hepatitis B	3 doses				
Meningococcal	1 or more doses				

Recommended if some risk factor is present; All persons who meet the age criteria; No recommendation

Adult immunization based on medical and other indications in India is presented in **Table 20.13.**

TABLE 20. 13: Adult immunization based on medical and other indications in India, 2020.

Indication		*Immunocompromised conditions (Excluding HIV)*	*HIV infection with CD4 count*		*Diabetes, heart disease, chronic lung disease*	*Asplenia (excluding elective splenectomy disease)*		*Kidney failure, end-stage renal disease, on hemodialysis*	
Vaccine	*Pregnancy*		*<200 cells/uL*	*≥200 cells/uL*			*Chronic liver disease*		*Health-care professionals*
Tetanus, diphtheria, pertussis (Tdap)	Td	Substitute one time dose of Tdap with Td, then booster with Td every 10 years							
Human papilloma vaccine		3 doses for females through age 26 years							
Varicella	Contraindication	2 doses							
Zoster	Contraindication	1 dose							
Measles, mumps, and rubella	Contraindication	1 or 2 doses							
Influenza		1 dose annually							1 dose
Pneumococcal (polysaccharide)		1 or 2 doses							
Hepatitis A	2 doses								
Hepatitis B									
Meningococcal	1 or more doses								

Recommended if some risk factor is present; All persons who meet the age criteria; Contraindication

Vaccination details are presented in **Table 20.14.**

TABLE 20.14: Vaccination details.

Vaccine	*Recommendation*	*Booster*	*Route*	*Dose*	*Special population/efficacy*
Diphtheria, tetanus, pertussis	18–64 years Three dose series at 0 and 4 weeks, the third 6–12 months after second	Tdap every 10 years	Intramuscular	0.5 mL	92% efficacy. Pregnant women—1 dose in second or third trimester
Measles, mumps, and rubella	>18 years of age should receive at least one dose of MMR if there is no serologic proof of immunity	No	Subcutaneous		Pregnancy to be avoided for at least 4 weeks after vaccination
Influenza	Annual, single dose	Annual	Intramuscular Nasal spray	0.5 mL, 0.25 mL into each nostril	➢ People aged >50 years ➢ Chronic obstructive pulmonary disease (COPD) ➢ Cardiac diseases ➢ Diabetes mellitus, cancer ➢ Immunodeficiency, renal disease ➢ Hemoglobinopathies ➢ Pregnant women ➢ Healthcare providers ➢ Adult household contacts ➢ Travelers to endemic area
Pneumococcal polysaccharide vaccine (PPSV23) and conjugate vaccine (PCV13)	Single dose Aged above 65 years	Can be repeated after 5 years	Intramuscular	0.5 mL	➢ Anatomic asplenia ➢ Sickle cell disease ➢ Immunocompromised persons ➢ Pregnant women with high-risk conditions
Hepatitis B	For immunocompetent adults, administered at 0, 1, and 6 months	A booster if anti-HBs levels decline to <10 mIU/mL and <100 mIU/mL in patients on dialysis	Intramuscular	1 mL (20 µg)	Protection (anti-HBs antibody titer of 10 mIU/mL or higher) after recombinant vaccine After first dose—20–30%. After second dose—75–80%. After third doses—90–95%
Hepatitis A	Two doses of 1 mL at 6 month interval		Intramuscular	1 mL	Only recommended in: ➢ People who travel to endemic area of hepatitis A ➢ Persons who work with HAV-infected primates or with HAV in a laboratory ➢ Who receive clotting factor concentrates ➢ Food handlers ➢ Chronic liver disease/CKD awaiting transplant ➢ Men who have sex with men

Contd...

Contd...

Varicella	<13 years—1 dose; ->13 years—2 doses. Interval between 2 doses should be 4–8 weeks		Subcutaneous	0.5 mL	Healthcare workers; family contacts of immunocompromised persons; high risk of exposure (e.g., teachers, day care employees, military personnel, and international travelers)
Human papilloma virus	Gardasil vaccine, 3 doses—at 0, 2, and 6 months Cervarix vaccine, 3 doses IM—at 0, 1, and 6 months		Intramuscular	0.5 mL	Woman age 26 years or younger or a man age 21 years or younger. The immunization must precede the sexual debut Age for initiation for vaccination to be 10–12 years (females) and 9–12 years (males)
Meningococcal meningitis	Single dose	Nil	Intramuscular	0.5 mL	During an outbreak (HCW, laboratory worker, close contacts). During interepidemic period. To travelers, pilgrims (quadrivalent), people attending fairs and festivals (bivalent 10–14 days prior)
Herpes zoster	Single dose	Nil	Subcutaneous	0.65 mL	➢ Recommended for persons >60 years ➢ High risk for developing recurrent herpes zoster, such as: - Patients with chronic medical conditions (CKD, diabetes mellitus, rheumatoid arthritis, and chronic pulmonary disease) - Persons who are likely to have severe immunosuppression in near future
Haemophilus influenzae type b (Hib)			Intramuscular	0.5 mL	Not recommended for routine practice
Typhoid: ➢ Live oral Ty21a vaccine ➢ Injectable Vi polysaccharide vaccine, and ➢ Vi-rEPA vaccine		Every 5 years			Not recommended for routine practice
Cholera	Two separate doses, 1–6 weeks apart for those aged over 6 years	No	Oral		85–90% protection

AMYLOIDOSIS

Q. Discuss the classification, clinical features and management of amyloidosis.

Definition: Amyloidosis is a group of acquired and hereditary disorders characterized by extracellular deposition of insoluble polymeric **proteins** fibrils in tissues and organs.

Classification of Amyloidosis (Table 20.15)

TABLE 20.15: Classification of amyloidosis.

Category	*Precursor protein*	*Fibril protein*	*Associated disease/(s)*
A. Systemic (generalized) amyloidosis			
1. Immunocyte dyscrasias with amyloidosis (primary amyloidosis)	Immunoglobulin light chains (mainly λ)	AL	Multiple myeloma, other plasma cell dyscrasias
2. Reactive systemic amyloidosis (secondary amyloidosis)	Serum amyloid associated (SAA)	AA	Chronic inflammatory process
3. Hemodialysis-associated amyloidosis	β_2-microglobulin	$A\beta_2m$	Chronic renal failure
B. Hereditary or familial amyloidosis			
1. Familial Mediterranean fever	SAA	AA	
2. Familial amyloidotic neuropathies 3. Systemic senile amyloidosis	Transthyretin	ATTR	
C. Localized amyloidosis			
1. Senile cerebral	Amyloid precursor protein (APP)	Aβ	Alzheimer disease
2. Endocrine			
• Thyroid	Calcitonin	A Cal	Medullary carcinoma
• Islets of Langerhans	Islet amyloid peptide	AIAPP	Type 2 diabetes

Clinical Features

- It is usually a rapidly progressive disease. The clinical features depend on the organs involved.
- **Nonspecific symptoms:** These include fatigue and weight loss.

- **Renal amyloidosis:** Kidneys are affected in about 70% of patients. It usually presents with proteinuria (often in the nephrotic range), hypoalbuminemia, secondary hypercholesterolemia, and edema or anasarca.
- **Cardiac amyloidosis:** The heart is the second most commonly (50%) affected organ and may show concentric thickening of ventricles and diastolic dysfunction, leading to a restrictive cardiomyopathy. It may present with heart failure.
- **Neuropathies:** Autonomic dysfunction with gastrointestinal motility disturbances (diarrhea, constipation) and peripheral sensory neuropathies are relatively common. Carpal tunnel syndrome with weakness and paresthesia of the hands may be an early presenting feature.
- **Macroglossia (Fig. 20.9A):** Enlarged tongue is pathognomonic of AL amyloidosis that may be found in ~10% of patients.
- **Amyloidosis of liver:** It causes cholestasis and hepatomegaly.
- **Amyloidosis of spleen:** It may produce functional hyposplenism in the absence of significant splenomegaly.
- **Cutaneous amyloidosis:** It can produce:
  - Easy bruising due to amyloid deposits in capillaries or due to deficiency of clotting factor X, which can bind to amyloid fibrils.
  - Cutaneous ecchymosis especially around the eyes and can produce "raccoon-eye" sign **(Fig. 20.9B)**.
- **Other findings:** These include nail dystrophy, alopecia, and amyloid arthropathy with thickening of synovial membranes in wrists and shoulders.

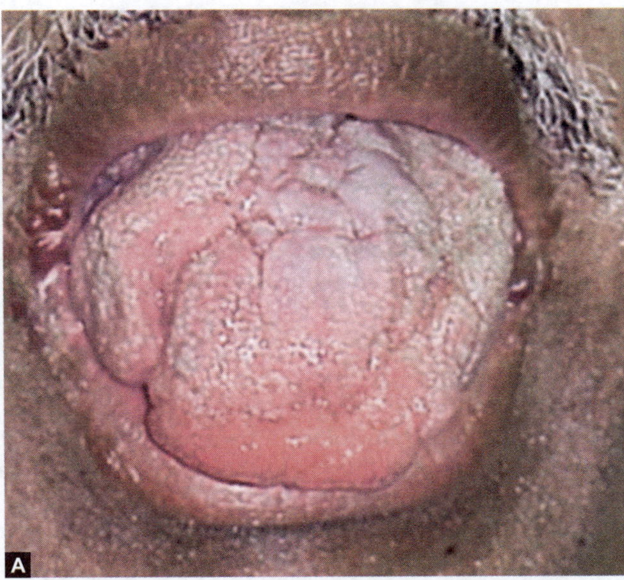

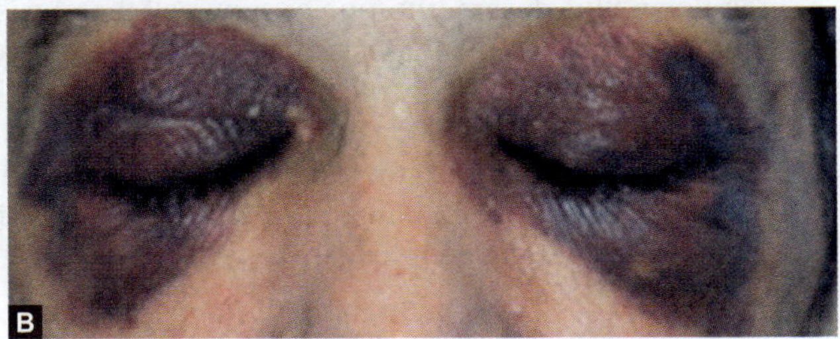

FIGS. 20.9A AND B: (A) Macroglossia; (B) Racoon eyes in amyloidosis.

Diagnosis

- Key feature for diagnosis of AL amyloidosis is the identification of the underlying B-lymphoproliferative process and clonal light chain.
- Serum protein electrophoresis (SPEP) and urine protein electrophoresis (UPEP) are NOT useful screening tests. However, more than 90% of cases show serum or urine monoclonal LC or whole immunoglobulin by immunofixation electrophoresis of serum (SIFE) or urine (UIFE).

Heredofamilial Amyloidosis

1. Familial Mediterranean Fever

- **Autosomal recessive** disorder.
- Characterized by recurrent attacks of fever accompanied with inflammation of serosal surfaces (peritoneum, pleura, and synovial membrane).

2. Familial Amyloidotic Neuropathies

- Familial amyloidotic neuropathies are characterized by **deposition of amyloid in peripheral and autonomic nerves** and the **fibrils are made up of mutant TTRs.**
- **ATTR (transthyretin associated)** amyloidosis is transmitted as autosomal dominant disease.
- Clinically, they present with peripheral sensorimotor and autonomic neuropathy and symptoms of autonomic dysfunction, diarrhea, and weight loss. Renal involvement is less common than with AL amyloidosis. Macroglossia does not develop.

Hemodialysis-associated (Dialysis Related) Amyloidosis

- Patients with **chronic renal failure** (ESRD) **on long-term hemodialysis** have high **levels of β_2-microglobulin** in the serum because it cannot be filtered through dialysis membrane and gets deposited as amyloid. Its incidence appears to be decreasing with newer high-flow dialysis techniques.
- It produces rheumatologic manifestations and usually presents with carpal tunnel syndrome, persistent joint effusions, spondyloarthropathy, or cystic bone lesions.

Other Amyloids

- **Cerebral amyloidosis:** Brain is a common site of amyloid deposition, though it is not directly affected in any form of acquired systemic amyloidosis.
- **Alzheimer's disease:** Intracerebral and cerebrovascular amyloid deposits are found in Alzheimer's disease. Most cases are sporadic.
- **Transmissible spongiform encephalopathy:** In hereditary spongiform encephalopathies, several amyloid plaques are observed.

FLOWCHART. 20.1: Guidelines for the treatment of newly diagnosed primary amyloidosis.

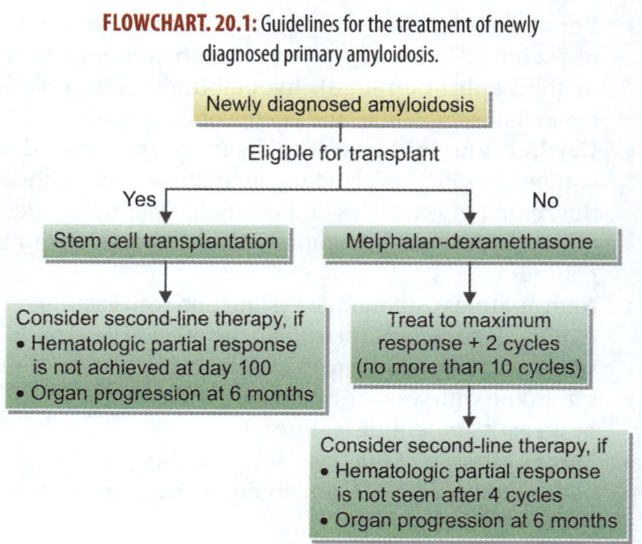

Treatment

- **Aim of treatment:** To support the function of affected organs and, in acquired amyloidosis, treatment of the associated primary disorder to prevent further amyloid deposition.
- **Treatment of underlying disorder:** Treatment of any underlying inflammatory source or infection may produce regression of existing amyloid deposits. Chemotherapy with melphalan plus dexamethasone or stem cell therapy is useful in AL amyloidosis. Guidelines for the treatment of newly diagnosed primary amyloidosis are presented in **Flowchart 20.1.**
- Second-line chemotherapy includes thalidomide/lenalidomide, bortezomib, carfilzomib plus dexamethasone.
- Colchicine may be useful in familial Mediterranean fever.
- Nephrotic syndrome and congestive cardiac failure are treated with the relevant therapies.
- Hereditary transthyretin amyloidosis: In ATTR amyloidosis, where transthyretin is mainly produced in the liver, liver transplantation is the definitive therapy.

CHAPTER

21

Geriatrics

GERIATRICS

- It is essentially the field of medicine dedicated to providing care for the elderly.
- Geriatricians are physicians who have special training to better understand the unique needs of older adults, which is why they typically prescribe care for adults 65 and older.
- The United Nations (UN) has agreed for a cutoff of 60+ years to refer to the older population.

GERONTOLOGY

- A gerontologist studies the problems of aging from a broader perspective. Not only our medical issues, but all the various problems faced by seniors and the elderly.
- Both are involved with addressing issues related to the aging process, but while geriatric professionals provide immediate care for older adults, gerontologists are focused on studying the aging process in general.

The difference between gerontology and geriatrics has been shown in **Figure 21.1**.

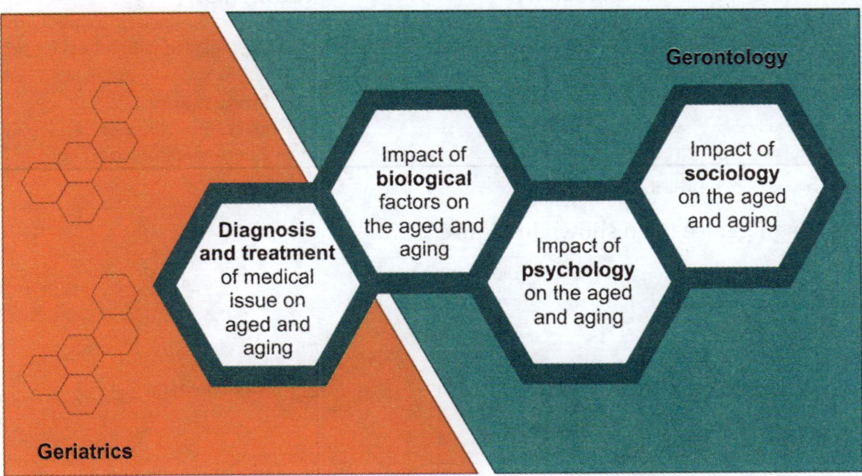

FIG. 21.1: Difference between gerontology and geriatrics.

BIOLOGY OF AGING

Aging

Q. What is aging?

Definition: Aging can be defined as a gradual, insidious, and progressive decline in structure and function which begins to unfold after the achievement of sexual maturity. Various mechanisms that cause and counteract cellular aging are shown in **Figure 21.2**.

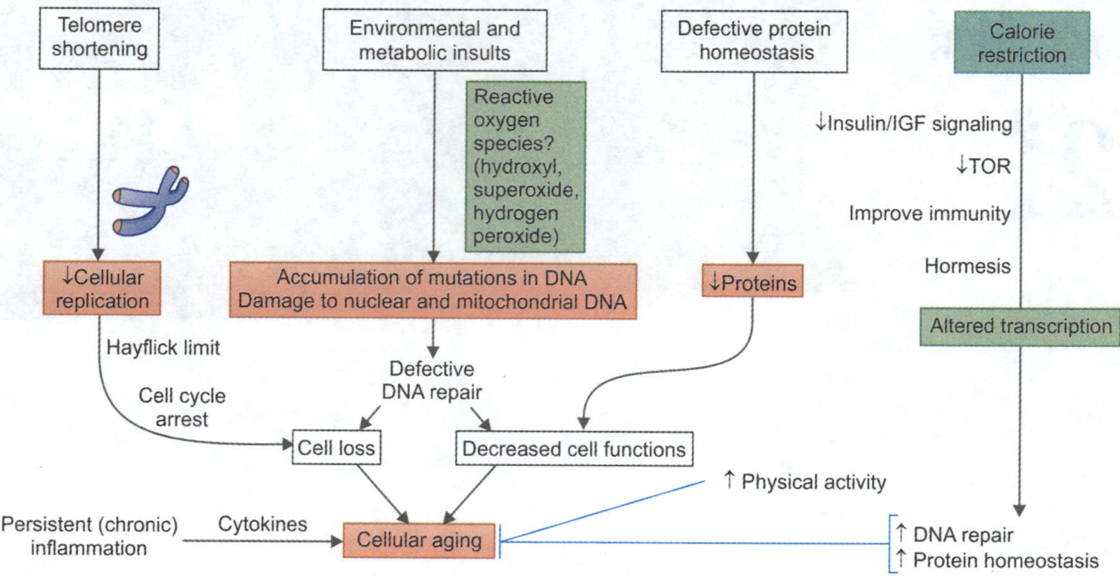

FIG. 21.2: Mechanisms of cellular aging and that counteract cellular aging.
(IGF: insulin-like growth factor; TOR: target of rapamycin)

Theories of Aging

Q. List the common theories of aging.

The common theories of aging have been shown in **Table 21.1**.

TABLE 21.1: Common theories of aging.

Stochastic Aging is caused by external forces acting on the body cells and there are ways to slow down the process	**Nonstochastic** Aging is internally regulated by a biological time clock and nothing can change it	**Psychological** Attempt to explain behavior, roles and relationships in the aging process
Free radical theory Cells and damaged by free radicals which lead to aging	**Programmed aging theory** A biological clock controls cell behavior and life span	**Disengagement theory** Older adults and society mutually withdraw from each other. The aging person becomes more introspective and self-focused
Somatic mutation theory Chromosomes are damaged by exposure to toxins or radiation	**Pacemaker theory** Neurochromosomes (brain) regulated development and aging throughout the life span	**Activity theory** Continuing the social activities of middle age or those activities must be replaced with others for successful aging
Wear and tear theory Damage from everyday wear eventually exceeds the body's ability to repair itself	**Immunological theory** Changes in the immune system are responsible for the effects of aging	**Continuity theory** Personality and behavior develop over a lifetime and are key to how a person adjusts to aging

Remember, no single theory is universally accepted as THE theory of aging

The biological hallmarks of aging have been shown in **Figure 21.3.**

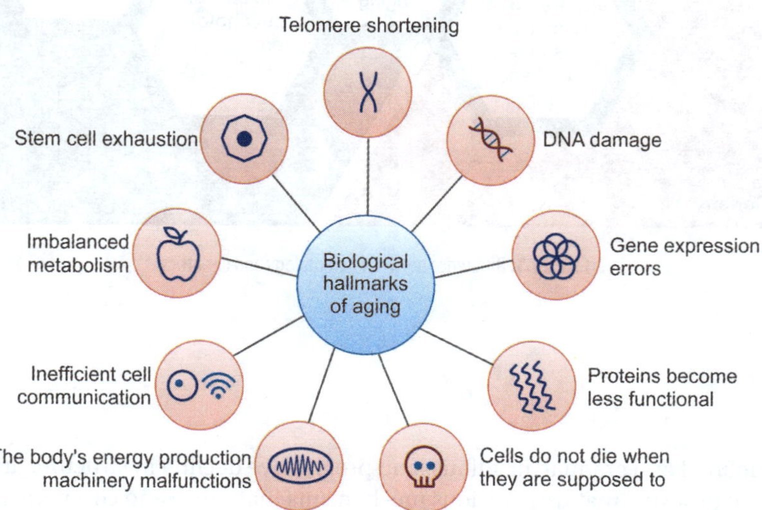

FIG. 21.3: Biological hallmarks of aging.

Q. Describe and discuss the epidemiology, pathogenesis, clinical evolution, presentation, and course of common diseases in the elderly.

Q. Describe health problems of aged population.

Changes in Physiologic Function with Age

The changes in physiologic function with age have been shown in **Table 21.2**.

TABLE 21.2: Changes in physiologic function with age.

Organ system	*Age-related change*
Cardiovascular	➢ Impaired contractile function and baroreceptor function ➢ Decreased conductivity and ventricular filling ➢ Increased systolic blood pressure
Respiratory	➢ Decreased lung elasticity, decreased maximal breathing capacity, decreased number of cilia and diminished mucus clearance, decreased arterial PO_2 ➢ Diminished cough reflex and diminished number of functional alveoli
Gastrointestinal	Decreased esophageal and colonic motility
Renal	➢ Decreased renal blood flow and glomerular filtration rate ➢ Kidney size decreases by 20–30% by age 90
Bladder	Decline in bladder capacity from about 500–600 to about 250 mL
Immune	➢ Decreased cell-mediated immunity, decreased T-cell number, decreased T-helper cells ➢ Increased T-suppressor cells, increased autoimmunity ➢ Loss of memory cells ➢ Decline in antibody titers to known antigens
Endocrine	➢ Decreased hormonal responses to stimulation and decreased androgens and estrogens ➢ Impaired glucose tolerance and impaired norepinephrine responses
Autonomic nervous	➢ Impaired response to fluid deprivation ➢ Decline in baroreceptor reflex ➢ Increased susceptibility to hypothermia
Neurologic	➢ Decreased vibratory sense and decreased proprioception ➢ Slowed neuronal transmission
Special senses	➢ Presbyopia ➢ Lens opacification ➢ Decreased hearing, taste, and smell
Musculoskeletal	Sarcopenia (reduced muscle mass and contractile force)
Integumentary changes	➢ Decreased skin elasticity-wrinkling, senile purpura ➢ Increased dryness ➢ Thickened nails ➢ Thinning of hair (baldness) ➢ Decreased subcutaneous fat

Factors which make assessment/treatment of elderly different are presented in **Box 21.1**.

Box 21.1: What makes the assessment/treatment of elderly different?

- Individuals become more dissimilar as they grow.
- Abrupt decline in any system is always due to disease and not due to normal aging.
- Multiple pathology
- Missing symptoms (e.g., angina in an elderly patient with osteoarthritis—may not manifest)
- Masking symptoms (e.g., history of fall and fracture neck of femur in an elderly female-masked a coexistent hemiparesis due to an internal capsule infarct.)

Atypical Disease Presentations in Older Adults

Atypical disease presentations in older adults have been shown in **Table 21.3**.

TABLE 21.3: Atypical disease presentations in older adults.

Diagnosis	*Potential presenting symptoms and signs*	*Diagnosis*	*Potential presenting symptoms and signs*
Myocardial infarction	➢ Altered mental status ➢ Fatigue ➢ Fever ➢ Functional decline	Malignancy	➢ Altered mental status ➢ Fever ➢ Pathologic fracture
Infection	➢ Altered mental status ➢ Functional decline ➢ Hypothermia	Pulmonary embolus	➢ Altered mental status ➢ Fatigue ➢ Fever ➢ Syncope

Contd...

Contd...

Hyperthyroidism	➤ Altered mental status ➤ Anorexia ➤ Atrial fibrillation ➤ Chest pain ➤ Constipation ➤ Fatigue ➤ Weight gain	Vitamin deficiency	➤ Altered mental status ➤ Ataxia ➤ Dementia ➤ Fatigue
Depression	➤ Cognitive impairment ➤ Failure to thrive ➤ Functional decline	Fecal impaction	➤ Altered mental status ➤ Chest pain ➤ Diarrhea ➤ Urinary incontinence
Electrolyte disturbance	➤ Altered mental status ➤ Falls ➤ Fatigue ➤ Personality changes	Aortic stenosis	➤ Altered mental status ➤ Fatigue

COMPREHENSIVE GERIATRIC ASSESSMENT

Q. What is comprehensive geriatric assessment (CGA)? Perform multidimensional geriatric assessment that includes medical, psychosocial and functional components.

- Comprehensive geriatric assessment is a multidimensional, multidisciplinary, diagnostic and therapeutic process conducted to determine the medical, mental, and functional problems of older people with frailty so that a coordinated and integrated plan for treatment and follow-up can be developed (**Table 21.4**).
  Domains assessed and considered in the multidimensional approach of CGA are shown in **Figure 21.4**.
  Basic activities of daily living (BADLs) and instrumental activities of daily living (IADLs) are presented in **Table 21.5**. The Barthel Index of Activities of Daily Living (Barthel Index) and Lawton's Instrumental Activities of Daily Living (IADL) can be used to determine the **functional status**.
- Such assessments may be done by a geriatrician working independently, or as part of an interdisciplinary team that often include specially trained nurses (RNs), occupational therapists (OTs), physical therapists (PTs), social workers (SWs), dietitians, speech language pathologists (SLPs), and specialty pharmacists.
  How to identify elderly patients who would benefit from such an assessment (i.e., the frail elderly)?
  Strongly consider if they have three or more of the "Red flags" listed in **Box 21.2**. These red flags are indications to do CGA.

TABLE 21.4: Systematic comprehensive geriatric evaluation of an older person.

Medical evaluation PLUS	*Additional assessment*
Standard medical history PLUS	➤ Slow the pace of history taking ➤ Ensure the patient can hear ➤ Obtain collateral history ➤ Ask about functional independence ➤ Ask a full drug history

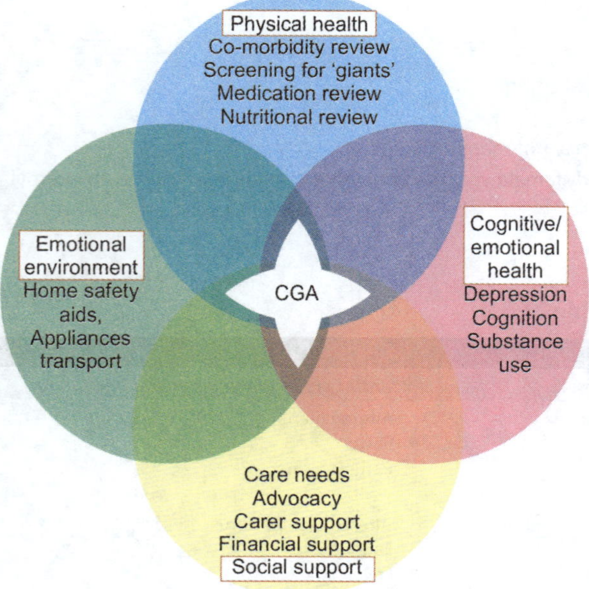

FIG. 21.4: Components of comprehensive geriatric assessment (CGA).

TABLE 21.5: Basic activities of daily living (BADLs) and instrumental activities of daily living (IADLs).

Basic activities of daily living	*Instrumental activities of daily living*
BADLS are fundamental activities such as personal cares which are basic to independent living. Loss of BADLs places a heavy burden on the caregivers and is a marker of complete dependence. ➤ Toileting, self-hygiene, bathing, grooming, dressing, feeding, and ambulation (stairs too). ➤ For each of the questions, inquire whether the person can perform it independently, whether he/she needs assistance or he/she is completely caregiver dependent	IADLs are complex tasks which enable an older adult to live independently and safely. They are not necessary for fundamental existence in the way that BADLs are necessary, but are an indicator of functional independence. Assessment of IADLs is useful during baseline and follow-up assessments among older adults. Loss of IADLs may be the first indication of deterioration in an older adult. ➤ Complex tasks and roles they do at home ➤ Shopping, meal planning and preparation, housekeeping, laundry, transit, financial management, using a telephone, medication management and driving

Box 21.2: Indications for doing comprehensive geriatric assessments (Red Flags).

- >75 years
- Needs help with BADLs/IADLs by caregiver
- Lives alone
- Falls
- Delirium/confusion
- Incontinence
- >2 admissions to acute care hospital/year
- "Failure to thrive"

TABLE 21.6: Objective measures of physical function.

➢ Timed up-and-go test **(Fig. 21.5)**	>30 s: fall risk
➢ 6-meter walk	<5.8 s
➢ Gait speed	>6.0 s
➢ 6-minute walk	<300 m: mortality
	<400 m: functional impairment

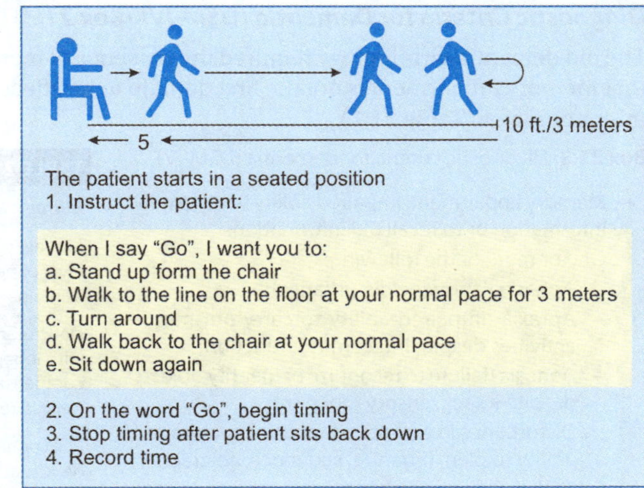

FIG. 21.5: Timed up-and-go test.

Objective Measures of Physical Function

The objective measures of physical function have been shown in **Table 21.6**.

COMMON CLINICAL PROBLEMS OF AGING

Geriatric Giants (Fig. 21.6)

- It is a term coined by Sir Bernard Isaacs. He recognized that multiple illness of the senior years needed a broader perspective in socioeconomic and medical terms.
- "Geriatric giants" or the four I's:
  - Immobility
  - Instability
  - Incontinence
  - Impairment of intellect
    - Cognitive impairment
    - Delirium
    - Depression
- Newer geriatric giants
  - Frailty
  - Sarcopenia
  - The "anorexia of aging"
  - Mild cognitive impairment (MCI)
- Giants refer to the principal chronic disabilities of old age that have an impact on physical, mental, and social domains of older adults. Many of these conditions are often wrongly perceived to be an unavoidable part of old age. However, they can be improved.

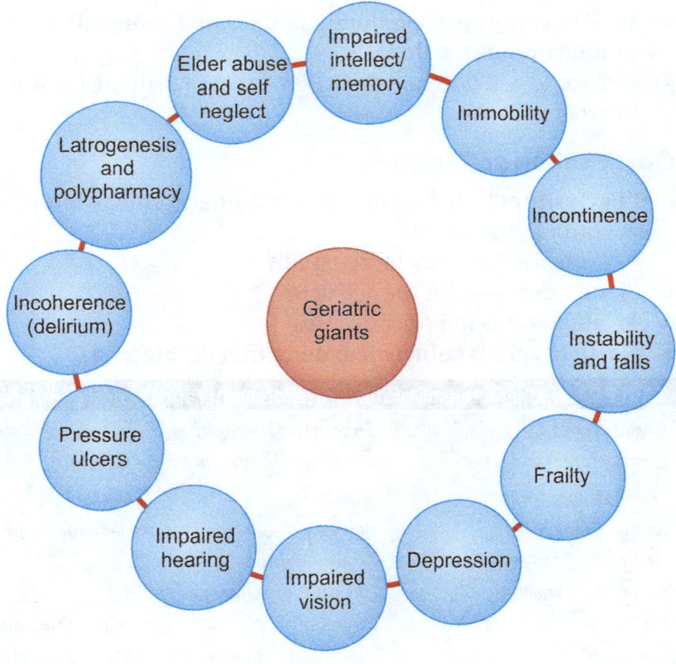

FIG. 21.6: Modern geriatric giants.

Dementia

Q. List the common causes of dementia.

Dementia is typically progressive and nonreversible. It affects 5–10% of those >65 years and 20–25% >85 years.

- Alzheimer's disease (AD) was the most common type of dementia in India constituting about 45–50%, the prevalence of vascular dementia was found to be 25% in India as against 5% in the West.
- While mean age of dementia patients was around 65 years in India, it was 75 years in the West.
- Hypertension, diabetes, cardiovascular diseases, and stroke are among the chief causes for a higher rate of vascular dementia in India.

Diagnostic Criteria for Dementia (DSM-IV) (Box 21.3)

The old dementia terminology required the presence of memory impairment for all of the dementias. It has been recognized that memory impairment is not the first domain to be affected. Hence, DSM-5 has subgrouped neurocognitive disorder into minor or major **(Table 21.7)**.

Box 21.3: Diagnostic criteria for dementia (DSM-IV).

- Memory impairment: Impaired ability to learn new information or to recall old information.
- One or more of the following:
  - Aphasia (language disturbance)
  - Apraxia (impaired ability to carry out motor activities despite intact motor function)
  - Agnosia (failure to recognize or identify objects despite intact sensory function)
  - Disturbance in executive functioning-impaired ability to plan, organize, sequence, abstract.
- Cognitive deficits result in functional impairment (social/occupational).
- Cognitive deficits do not occur exclusively during a delirium.
- NOT due to other medical or psychiatric conditions.

TABLE 21.7: DSM-5 subgroups of neurocognitive disorder.

Minor neurocognitive disorder (DSM-5)	*Major neurocognitive disorder (DSM-5)*
Modest cognitive decline from a previous level of performance in one or more of the domains	Substantial cognitive decline from a previous level of performance in one or more of the domains
Deficits are insufficient to interfere with independence, but greater effort, compensatory strategies, or accommodation may be required to maintain independence	Deficits are sufficient to interfere with independence
The cognitive deficits do not occur exclusively in the context of a delirium. The cognitive deficits are not primarily attributable to another mental disorder	
Cognitive domains: ➢ **Learning and memory** ➢ **Complex attention** ➢ **Language**	➢ **Perceptual motor** ➢ **Executive function** ➢ **Social cognition**

Mild Cognitive Impairment/Prodromal Dementia

- It is a condition in which there is mild memory impairment alone (1.5 standard deviations below that of age matched controls) in the absence of global cognitive decline or functional disabilities; it can only be diagnosed by sophisticated neuropsychiatric testing. **It does not meet criteria for dementia.**
- When memory loss predominates, termed **Amnestic MCI,** while if other domains affected with memory being intact its termed **nonamnestic MCI**
- Dementia will develop about 30% of those with MCI within 3 years. The remainders have stable, MCIs that do not appear to progress.

Classification of Dementia

- **"Early onset"**—before the age of 60, often familial, more common for frontotemporal dementia (FTD)
  - Strong genetic link
  - Tends to progress more rapidly
- **"Late onset"**—after the age of 60
  - Represents majority of cases
- **Cortical versus subcortical dementia (Table 21.8)**

TABLE 21.8: Characteristic of subcortical dementia and cortical dementia.

Characteristic	*Subcortical dementia*	*Cortical dementia*
Primary functional lesion	Impaired information processing	Domain-specific deficits (aphasia, apraxia, agnosia)
Speed of cognition	Slow	Normal
Memory deficit	Retrieval (recall aided by cues and recognition)	Encoding/storage (poor recognition memory)
Neuropsychiatric symptoms	Apathy, depression	Depression less common
Motor abnormalities	Dysarthria, extrapyramidal	Uncommon, gegenhalten
Pathology	Prominent changes in striatum and thalamus	Prominent changes in cortical association areas
Examples	Huntington's disease, acquired immunodeficiency syndrome (AIDS) dementia complex, progressive supranuclear palsy	Alzheimer's and Creutzfeldt–Jakob disease

Causes of Dementia (Box 21.4)

Box 21.4: Causes of dementia.

Degenerative/inherited
- Alzheimer's disease (60–70%)
- Neurodegenerative disorders: Frontotemporal dementia (including Pick's disease), Lewy body disease, Parkinson's disease, Huntington's disease

Vascular dementia (10–20%): Diffuse small vessel disease
Neoplastic: Primary/secondary deposits
Traumatic: Chronic subdural hematoma, posthead injury
Infections: Creutzfeldt–Jakob disease, human immunodeficiency virus (HIV), syphilis
Toxic/nutritional: Alcohol, thiamine deficiency, vitamin B_{12} deficiency
Prion diseases
Reversible dementia

Modifiable/Reversible Causes of Dementia

The modifiable/reversible causes of dementia have been shown in **Table 21.9**.

Q. List the reversible causes of dementia.

TABLE 21.9: Modifiable causes of dementia.

		Mnemonic—DEMENTIA
➤ Depression so-called "Pseudodementia" ➤ Electrolyte disorders (hyponatremia, hypercalcemia, etc.) ➤ Hypothyroidism ➤ Late-onset psychosis ➤ Medication side effects (e.g., sedatives, anticonvulsants, antihypertensives, anticholinergics, first-generation neuroleptics) ➤ Ethanol overuse/misuse	➤ Vitamin deficiencies (B_{12}, folate) ➤ Obstructive sleep apnea ➤ Normal pressure hydrocephalus (reverse with shunting) ➤ Brain tumor (postresection) ➤ Subdural hematoma (SDH) ➤ Subacute CNS infections (i.e., meningitis, encephalitis, syphilis)	D = Drugs, Delirium E = Emotions (such as depression) and Endocrine disorders M = Metabolic disturbances E = Eye and Ear impairments N = Nutritional disorders T = Tumors, Toxicity, Trauma to head I = Infectious diseases A = Alcohol, Arteriosclerosis

Alzheimer's Disease

Q. Write a short essay/note on Alzheimer's disease.

Introduction and Definition

- Alzheimer's disease is the most common cause of dementia in the world. It is the most common cause of dementia above the age of 40.
- In India: Most common cause of dementia is AD (60–80%) followed by vascular and dementia with Lewy bodies (DLBs).

Etiology

- **Genetic factors**
  - Genetic factors play an important role and about 15% of AD is familial. Familial cases may be of two main groups: (1) early-onset disease with autosomal dominant mode of inheritance and (2) a later-onset group with polygenic inheritance.
  - **Mutations:** It can occur in several genes.
    - Point mutation in **amyloid precursor protein (APP)** can cause AD.
    - Mutations in the gene **presenilin 1 (PS1) and presenilin 2 (PS2)**. PS1 mutations are implicated in over 50% of families with familial AD.
    - The inheritance of one of the alleles of apolipoprotein-ε4 (apo-ε4) is associated with an increased risk of AD.
- **Environmental risk factors**
  - **Age:** If is the main risk factor and incidence of AD increases exponentially with age.
  - **Female gender** may also be a risk factor independent of the greater longevity of women.
  - **Head trauma and vascular risk factors.**
  - According to some studies, long-term consumption of **NSAIDs** and acetaminophen has shown protection.

Pathology

- Biochemically characterized by a deficiency of acetylcholine, with cortex, amygdala, hippocampus all affected
- Basal nucleus of Meynert depleted of acetylcholine-containing neurons
- In minority of cases, there is an autosomal dominant inheritance linked to chromosomes 1, 14, or 21 (early onset)
- Apolipoprotein E gene, coded on chromosome 19, when homozygous for allele E4, increases the risk for late-onset AD.

Clinical Features

Q. Write a short essay/note on clinical features of Alzheimer's disease.

The main clinical features are:

- **Memory impairment/loss:** Early recent (short-term) memory loss is key feature of AD.
- **Language problem:** It is the next common symptom, common being anomia and difficulty with word finding is characteristic.
- **Apraxia:** It is impaired ability to carry out skilled, complex, organized motor activities.
- **Agnosia:** It is failure to recognize familiar objects (e.g., clothing, places or people).
- **Frontal executive function:** It is impairment of organizing, planning, and sequencing.
- **Parietal presentation:** Visuospatial difficulties and difficulty with orientation in space.
- **Myoclonic jerks** (sudden brief contractions of various muscles or the whole body) may occur spontaneously or in response to physical or auditory stimulation. This phenomenon raises the possibility of Creutzfeldt–Jakob disease (CJD), but the course of AD is much more prolonged.

- **Generalized seizures** may also occur.
- Death usually results from malnutrition, secondary infections, or heart disease.
- The typical duration of AD is 8–10 years, but the course can range from 1 to 25 years.
- Course of the disease
  - **Mild** [Mini-Mental State Examination (MMSE) 20–24]—primarily memory and visuospatial deficits, mild executive functioning impairment
  - **Moderate** (MMSE 11–20)—more pronounced aphasia, apraxia, loss of IADLs, may need increased assistance with BADLs, often exhibiting neuropsychiatric symptoms
  - **Severe** (MMSE 0–10)—severe language disturbances, pronounced neuropsychiatric manifestations, neurological symptoms (rigidity, incontinence, dysphagia, gait disturbance)
  - **Death** 8-12 years after the diagnosis
  - **Institutionalization** common with increasing neuropsychiatric symptoms, loss of BADLs, caregiver stress

Diagnostic Criteria for Alzheimer's Disease

The diagnostic criteria for AD have been shown in **Box 21.5**.

Investigations

Investigation is aimed at excluding other treatable causes of dementia.

- Neuroimaging studies [computed tomography (CT) and magnetic resonance imaging (MRI)] are not specific for AD and may be normal early in the course of the disease. As AD progresses, diffuse cortical atrophy becomes apparent, and detailed MRI scans show atrophy of the hippocampus.
- Positron emission tomography (PET) scan: It is the test of choice. It shows hypoperfusion in bilateral perietotemporal cortex.
- Cerebrospinal fluid (CSF) markers: (1) raised tau proteins, (2) low beta-42 amyloid, and (3) elevated ceramide level.
- Routine investigations: Blood chemistry, a complete blood count, tests for syphilis, serum levels of vitamin B_{12}, and thyroid functions.

Box 21.5: Diagnostic criteria for Alzheimer's disease.

- Memory impairment
- One or more of the following:
  - Aphasia
  - Apraxia
  - Agnosia
  - Disturbance in executive functioning.

Treatment for Alzheimer's Disease

There is no specific treatment and the primary focus is on long-term amelioration of associated behavioral and neurologic problems

Drugs used (Table 21.10): Donepezil, rivastigmine, galantamine, and tacrine are cholinesterase inhibitors. Patients with AD have reduced cerebral content of choline acetyltransferase, which leads to a decrease in acetylcholine synthesis and impaired cortical cholinergic function

- Memantine appears to act by blocking overexcited N-methyl-D-aspartate (NMDA) channels
- Statins may have protective effect on dementia especially vascular. Antioxidants (vitamin E, selegiline), estrogen replacement, *Ginkgo biloba* have been tried
- Mild-to-moderate depression is common in the early stages of AD and responds to antidepressants. Selective serotonin reuptake inhibitors (SSRIs) are commonly used due to their low anticholinergic side effects
- Recommend psychotherapy, exercise, pleasurable activities, support groups, memory aids
- Minimize changes in caregivers/environment
- Music therapy is gaining strength as evidence-based intervention for treatment of anxiety

TABLE 21.10: Drugs used for Alzheimer's disease and their adverse reactions.

Donepezil	Initial dose 5 mg at bedtime Titrate to 10 mg once daily at 4–6 weeks For moderate to severe dementia, may titrate to 23 mg at 3 months	Nausea, vomiting, diarrhea, muscle cramps
Galantamine	Initial dose 4 mg twice a day Titrate to 8 mg twice a day at 4 weeks Titrate to 12 mg twice a day at 4 weeks	Nausea, vomiting, agitation, sleep disturbances
Rivastigmine	Initial dose 1.5 mg twice daily for 2 weeks Increase in increments of 1.5 mg twice daily every 2 weeks if well tolerated Maximum dose 12 mg a day	Nausea, vomiting, diarrhea, headache, dizziness
Memantine N-methyl-D-aspartate (NMDA) receptor antagonist—glutamate receptor antagonist)	Initial dose 5 mg daily, at 1-week increase to 5 mg twice a day, in another week increase to 5 mg in the morning and 10 mg in the evening, and in another week increase to target dose of 10 mg twice a day	Dizziness, confusion, hallucination, agitation

Contd...

Contd...

Other drugs available	Newer developmental agents:
➢ **Selegiline**—selective monoamine oxidase B (MAO-B) inhibitor (10 mg/day) ➢ **Vitamin E (alpha-tocopherol)**—2,000 international units/day ➢ Citicoline ➢ Cerebrolysin ➢ Estrogen replacement ➢ *Ginkgo biloba* ➢ Statins	➢ Immunization against β-amyloid ➢ Huprine X—acetylcholinesterase inhibitor ➢ Xanomeline patch—M1/M4 muscarinic receptor agonist ➢ AIT-082 (purine hypoxanthine derivative)—increases neurotransmission ➢ Cyclooxygenase-2 (COX-2) inhibitors—neuroinflammation therapy ➢ Protease inhibitors—target gamma-secretases to prevent amyloid formation

Note: Do not routinely prescribe or continue acetylcholineterase inhihitors or NMDA antagonists in patients with advanced dementia

Vascular Dementia (Multi-infarct Dementia)

Q. Discuss the clinical features of vascular dementia.

- Second most common cause of dementia. Found in 15–30% of patients with dementia.
- **Risk factors:** Male sex, advanced age, diabetes, hypertension and/or other cardiovascular disorders.
- **Abrupt onset** of symptoms followed by **stepwise deterioration.**
- Findings on neurologic examination consistent with prior stroke(s), infarcts on cerebral imaging.
- **Focal neurologic symptoms:** Pseudobulbar palsy, dysarthria, and dysphagia are most common.

NINDS-AIREN Criteria for Vascular Dementia

All the following criteria should be present:

- Dementia
- Focal signs on examination + evidence of cerebrovascular disease by CT or MRI.

A relationship of the two above, with dementia within 3 months of a recognized stroke and/or abrupt deterioration in fluctuation, or fluctuating stepwise progression of cognitive deficits.

Physical examination

- May show increased tone (especially in the legs), exaggerated deep tendon reflexes, and Babinski responses.
- Examination may reveal carotid bruits, fundoscopic abnormalities, and enlarged heart.
- Gait apraxia ("magnetic" gait) may be seen.
- MRI may reveal hyperintensities and focal atrophy suggestive of old infarctions.

Types of Vascular Cognitive Impairment

The types of vascular cognitive impairment have been shown in **Box 21.6**.

Box 21.6: Types of vascular cognitive impairment.

1. Vascular cognitive impairment, no dementia (VCIND)
2. Vascular dementia (VaD)
   - Poststroke dementia (PSD), defined as dementia manifesting within 6 months after a stroke
   - Subcortical ischemic vascular dementia (SIVaD)
   - Multi-infarct (cortical) dementia
3. Mixed vascular cognitive impairment (VCI) plus Alzheimer's disease (AD)

Treatment

- Control of risk factors such as hypertension, smoking, diabetes, hyperlipidemia
- Antiplatelets/statins
- Correction of sources of emboli, endarterectomy, and anticoagulant therapy

Frontotemporal Dementia

Q. Write short essay on the clinical features of frontotemporal dementia.

- Characterized by focal atrophy of the frontal and temporal lobes in the absence of Alzheimer's pathology.
- **Pick's disease** was the first recognized subtype of FTD, one that is characterized pathologically by the presence of Pick's bodies (silver staining intracytoplasmic inclusions) in the neocortex and hippocampus.
- Clinically, presents initially with **language abnormalities** and **behavioral disturbances**.
- Occurs between the ages of 35 and 75 years, and only rarely after age 75; the mean age of onset is the 6th decade.
- Both sexes are equally affected.
- "Walnut brain"—as there is profound loss of matter in the frontal lobes, to a slightly lesser degree in the temporal lobes, in comparison with relatively preserved parietal and occipital lobes.

Genetics of Frontotemporal Dementia

- 45% of patients have a family member affected.
- Up to 18% of these have an abnormality on the short arm of chromosome 17 localized near gene for the microtubule-associated protein, *tau*.

Box 21.7 lists the core diagnostic features and **Table 21.11** lists the supportive diagnostic features of FTD.

Box 21.7: Core diagnostic features of frontotemporal dementia (FTD).

- Insidious onset and gradual progression
- Early decline in social interpersonal conduct
- Early impairment in regulation of personal conduct
- Early emotional blunting
- Early loss of insight

TABLE 21.11: Supportive diagnostic features of frontotemporal dementia.

Behavioral disorder	***Speech and language deficits***
➢ Decline in personal hygiene and grooming ➢ Mental rigidity and inflexibility ➢ Distractibility and impersistence ➢ Utilization behavior hyperorality and dietary changes ➢ Perseverations and stereotyped behavior	➢ Altered speech output (aspontaneity and economy of speech) ➢ Stereotype speech ➢ Echolalia ➢ Perseverations ➢ Mutism
Physical signs	***Investigations***
➢ Primitive reflexes; at least one of grasp, snout and sucking ➢ Incontinence ➢ Akinesia, rigidity and tremor (rarely) ➢ Low and labile blood pressure	➢ **Neuropsychology:** Significant impairment on frontal lobe tests in the absence of severe amnesia, aphasia or perceptuospatial disorder ➢ Electroencephalography (**EEG**)**:** Normal despite clinically evident dementia ➢ **Brain imaging** (structural or functional) predominant frontal and/or temporal abnormality

Dementia with Lewy Bodies

- Most common dementia syndrome associated with parkinsonism.
- Second most common form of neurodegenerative dementia after AD.
- For a probable diagnosis **(Box 21.8)** of Lewy body disease, need at least two of the following:
  - Fluctuating cognition with pronounced variations in attention and alertness
  - Recurrent **visual hallucinations** which are typically well-formed and detailed
  - Spontaneous motor features of parkinsonism

Box 21.8: Features supporting the diagnosis of dementia with Lewy bodies.

- Syncope or transient loss of consciousness (LOC)
- Neuroleptic sensitivity (i.e., new shuffling gait, tardive dyskinesia)
- Systematized delusions
- Hallucinations in other modalities (i.e., smell, hearing, taste)
- Falls

Parkinson's Disease

- **Cardinal motor features**
  - Bradykinesia and akinesia
  - Rigidity
  - Resting tremor
  - Postural instability
- Dementia typically occurs in the last half of the clinical course of Parkinson's disease, whereas it is often one of the presenting features of DLB.

Pick's Disease and Creutzfeldt–Jakob Disease

Salient features of Pick's disease and CJD are presented in **Table 21.12**.

TABLE 21.12: Salient features of Pick's disease and Creutzfeldt–Jakob disease.

Pick's disease	***Creutzfeldt–Jakob disease***
➢ Subtype of frontal lobe dementia ➢ Pick bodies (silver staining intracytoplasmic inclusions in neocortex and hippocampus) ➢ Language abnormalities ➢ Logorrhea (abundant unfocused speech) ➢ Echolalia (spontaneous repetition of words/phrases) ➢ Palilalia (compulsive repetition of phrases)	➢ Rapid onset and deterioration ➢ Motor deficits ➢ Seizures ➢ Slowing and periodic complexes on EEG ➢ Myoclonic activity

Normal Pressure Hydrocephalus

It is a condition of pathologically enlarged ventricular size with normal opening pressures on lumbar puncture, clinically presents with a triad of dementia, gait disturbance, and urinary incontinence **(Adams triad**—"wet, wobbly, and wacky" triad) reversible by the placement of a ventriculoperitoneal shunt.

Cognitive Testing

- **Mini-mental state examination** tests a broad range of cognitive functions including orientation, recall, attention, calculation, language manipulation, and constructional praxis. Scores can be classified as: no cognitive impairment = 24–30; MCI = 18–23; severe cognitive impairment = 0–17.
- **Montreal cognitive assessment** (MoCA) is a 30-point test that is more sensitive for the detection of MCI, and it includes items that sample a wider range of cognitive domains, including memory, language, attention, visuospatial, and executive functions.
- **Mini-Cog** combines clock drawing and three item memory test.
- **Saint Louis University Mental Status** (SLUMS).

Delirium in the Elderly

Definition: It is an acute syndrome of transient, reversible cognitive dysfunction *(details discussed in Chapter 18)*.

Management

Prevention is the best medicine

- Eliminate extra medications, reverse metabolic abnormalities, hydration, and nutrition
- Education of patients and family
- Reorientation by staff, family, sitters, clocks, calendars
- Remove nonessential lines and tubes
- Drug therapy:
  - Delirium that causes injury to the patient or others should be treated with medications
  - The most common medications used are neuroleptics (haloperidol, risperidone, olanzapine)
  - Benzodiazepines (lorazepam) often are used for withdrawal states
  - Thiamine, cyanocobalamin supplementation

Depression

- Depression is the most common psychiatric illness in the elderly. Although common, it is not a natural part of aging.
- The prevalence in community dwelling elders ranges from 8 to 15%; it raises to as much as 30% of those in long-term care facilities. Depression and suicide are common in the elderly (especially older males; those over 75, have the same risk of suicide as 20–24 years old depressed males).
- Depression is NOT present in ALL older adults, but is under recognized and under treated.

Bereavement or grief reaction is commonly misdiagnosed as depression. A normal grief reaction after the death of a spouse or a loved one lasts about 2 months in time, with the mourning process being complete in <2 years. Feelings of sadness and preoccupation with the deceased are not helped by antidepressant medications during this time of mourning.

Treatment of depression in the elderly is discussed in Chapter 18.

The characteristics of depression, delirium, and dementia have been shown in **Table 21.13**.

TABLE 21.13: Characteristics of depression, delirium, and dementia.

	Depression	*Delirium*	*Dementia*
Onset	Weeks to months	Hours to days	Months to years
Mood	Low/apathetic	Fluctuates	Fluctuates
Course	Chronic; responds to treatment	Acute; responds to treatment	Chronic, with deterioration over time
Self-awareness	Likely to be concerned about memory impairment	May be aware of changes in cognition; fluctuates	Likely to hide or be unaware of cognitive deficits
Activities of daily living (ADLs)	May neglect basic self-care	May be intact or impaired	May be intact early, impaired as disease progresses
Instrumental activities of daily living (IADLs)	May be intact or impaired	May be intact or impaired	May be intact early, impaired before ADLs as disease progresses

Incontinence

Involuntary loss of urine or stool in sufficient amount or frequency to constitute a social and/or health problem.

Urinary Incontinence

- Urinary incontinence is defined as the involuntary loss of urine. It is a heterogeneous condition that ranges in severity from dribbling small amounts of urine to continuous urinary incontinence.
- The prevalence increases with age, but it is not a part of normal aging. It affects about 25–30% of community dwelling older women and 10–15% of community dwelling older men, 50% of nursing home residents; often associated with dementia, fecal incontinence, inability to walk, and transfer independently.

- Consequences:
  - Social stigmata—leads to restricted activities and depression
  - Medical complications—skin breakdown, increased urinary tract infections
  - Institutionalization—urinary incontinence is the second leading cause of nursing home placement.

Reversible Conditions Associated with Urinary Incontinence

Potentially reversible causes of urinary incontinence are listed in **Box 21.9**. Medications causing incontinence are listed in **Box 21.10**.

Box 21.9: Potentially reversible causes.

"DIAPPERS"	DRIP
D—**D**elirium	D—**D**elirium
I—**I**nfection	R—**R**estricted mobility, **R**estraint
A—**A**trophic vaginitis or urethritis	I—**I**nfection, **I**nflammation, **I**mpaction
P—**P**harmaceuticals	P—**P**olyuria, **P**haramaceuticals
P—**P**sychological disorders	
E—**E**ndocrine disorders	
R—**R**estricted mobility	
S—**S**tool impaction	

Box 21.10: Medications causing incontinence.

- Diuretics
- Anticholinergics: Antihistamines, antipsychotics, antidepressants
- Sedatives/hypnotics
- Alcohol
- Narcotics
- α-adrenergic agonists/antagonists
- Calcium channel blockers

Categories of Incontinence

- **Urge incontinence:** Other names: Detrusor hyperactivity, detrusor instability, irritable bladder, spastic bladder.
  - Most common cause of urinary incontinence >75 years of age.
  - Abrupt desire to void cannot be suppressed.
  - Usually idiopathic.
  - **Causes:** Infection, tumor, stones, atrophic vaginitis or urethritis, stroke, Parkinson's disease, dementia.
- **Stress incontinence:**
  - Most common type in women <75 years old.
  - Occurs with increase in abdominal pressure; cough, sneeze, etc.
  - Hypermotility of bladder neck and urethra; associated with aging, hormonal changes, trauma of childbirth or pelvic surgery (85% of cases).
  - Intrinsic sphincter problems: Due to pelvic/incontinence surgery, pelvic radiation, trauma, neurogenic causes (15% of cases).
- **Overflow incontinence:**
  - Overdistention of bladder.
  - Bladder outlet obstruction; stricture, benign prostatic enlargement (BPH), cystocele, fecal impaction.
  - Noncontractile bladder (hypoactive detrusor or atonic bladder), diabetes, multiple sclerosis, spinal injury, medications.
- **Functional incontinence:**
  - Does not involve lower urinary tract.
  - Result of psychological, cognitive or physical impairment.

A recently defined syndrome, **overactive bladder,** includes urinary frequency (more than eight voids per 24 hours), nocturia (awakening at night from sleep to void), and urgency (the acute need to void), with or without incontinence is prevalent in around 31% women 75 years and older and 42% men 75 years and older.

Treatment Options in Urinary Incontinence (Flowchart 21.1)

General treatment options in urinary incontinence are mentioned in **Box 21.11**.

Pharmacological interventions:

- **Urge incontinence:** Oxybutynin, propantheline, imipramine.
- **Stress incontinence:** Phenylpropanolamine, pseudoephedrine, estrogen (orally, transdermally or transvaginally).

FLOWCHART 21.1: Approach to urinary incontinence.

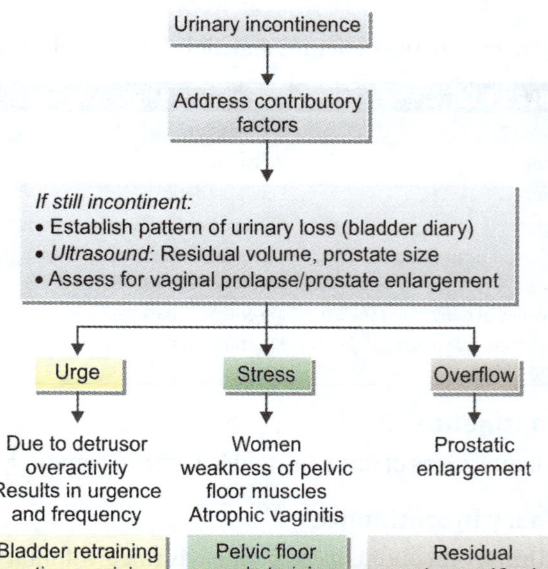

Box 21.11: General treatment options in urinary incontinence.

- Reduce amount and timing of fluid intake
- Avoid bladder stimulants (caffeine)
- Use diuretics judiciously (not before bed)
- Reduce physical barriers to toilet (use bedside commode)
- Bladder training
- Patient education
- Scheduled voiding
- Positive reinforcement
- Pelvic floor exercises (Kegel exercises)
- Biofeedback
- Caregiver interventions: Scheduled toileting, habit training, prompted voiding

Surgical interventions:
- **Urethral hypermotility:** Marshall–Marchetti–Krantz procedure, needle neck suspension.
- **Intrinsic sphincter deficiency:** Sling procedure.

Other interventions:
- Other interventions have been shown in **Box 21.12**.

Box 21.12: Other interventions in urinary incontinence.

- Pessaries
- Periurethral bulking agents (periurethral injection of collagen, fat or silicone)
- Diapers or pads
- Chronic catheterization
  - Perurethral or suprapubic
  - Indwelling or intermittent

Falls in the Elderly

Q. Describe and discuss the etiopathogenesis, clinical presentation, identification, functional changes, acute care, stabilization, management, and rehabilitation of falls in the elderly.

About 30% of individuals over 65 years of age fall each year. About 10–15% of falls result in serious injury and they are the cause of >90% of hip fractures in this age group. Factors causing falls in elderly are listed in **Flowchart 21.2**.

FLOWCHART 21.2: Factors causing falls and their effects in elderly.

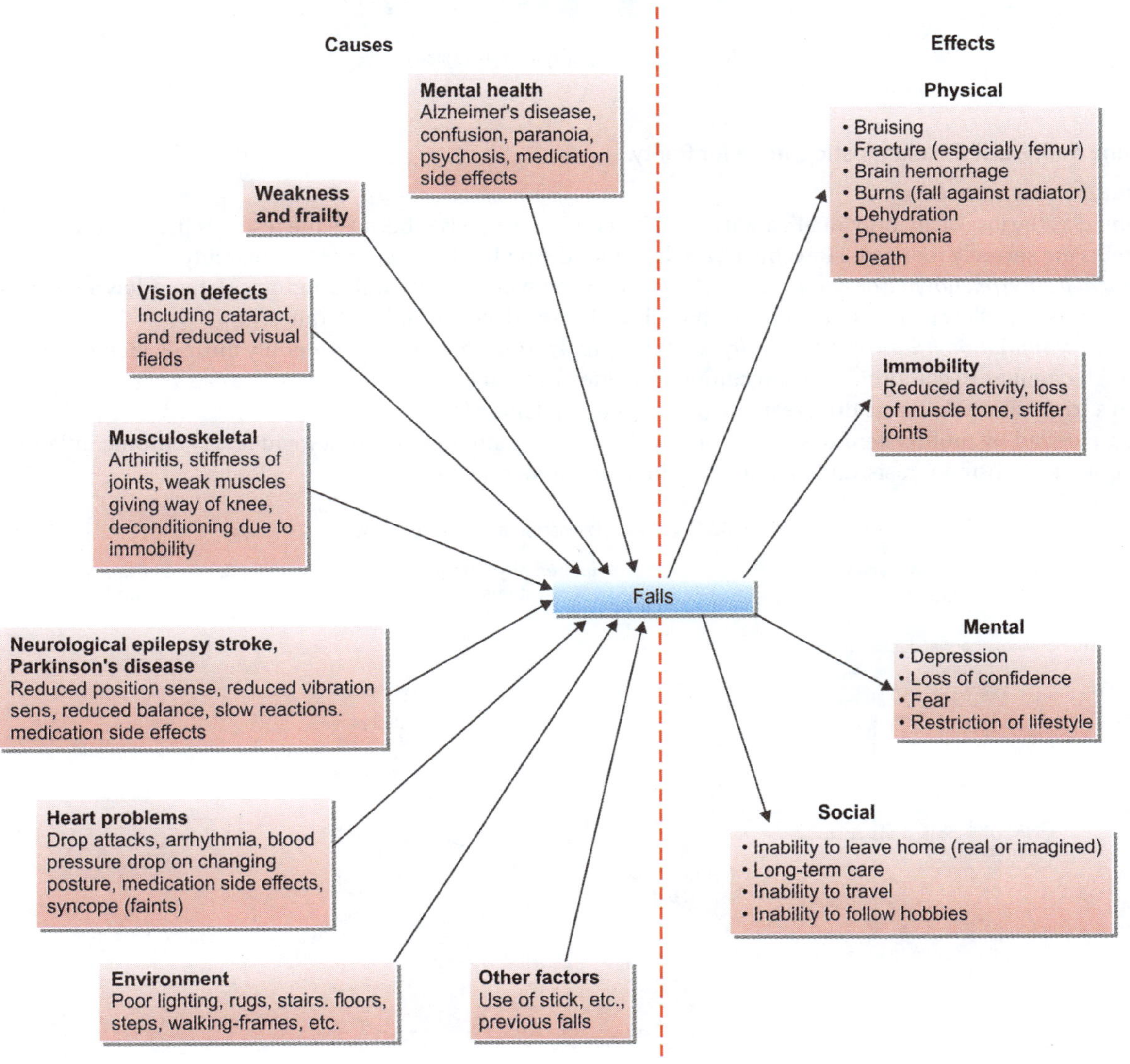

Fall risk factors and targeted interventions have been shown in **Table 21.14**.

TABLE 21.14: Fall risk factors and targeted interventions.

Risk factor	*Targeted intervention*
Postural hypotension	Behavioral recommendations, such as hand clenching, elevation of head of bed; discontinuation or substitution of high-risk medications
Use of benzodiazepine or sedative-hypnotic agent	Education about sleep hygiene; discontinuation or substitution of medications
Use of multiple prescription medications	Review of medications
Environmental hazards	Appropriate changes; installation of safety equipment (e.g., grab bars)
Gait impairment	Gait training, assistive devices, balance or strengthening exercises
Impairment in transfer or balance	Balance exercises, training in transfers, environmental alterations (e.g., grab bars)
Impairment in leg or arm muscle strength or limb range of motion	Exercise with resistance bands or putty, with graduated increases in resistance

The multidisciplinary approach to prevent falls has been shown in **Figure 21.7**.

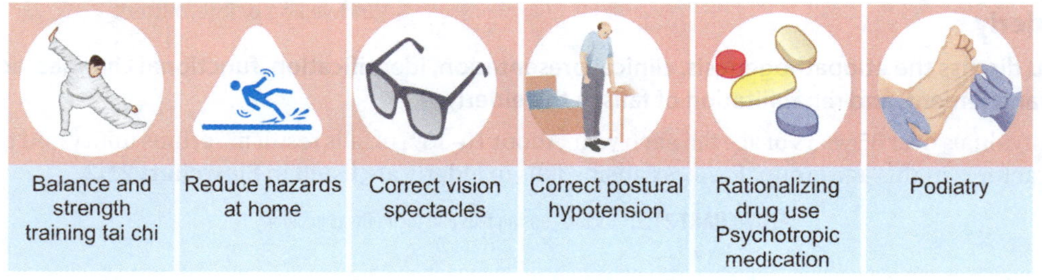

FIG. 21.7: Multidisciplinary approach to prevent falls.

Frailty

Q. Define frailty. List the diagnostic criteria for frailty.

- **Frailty = Loss of reserve**
- Defined as the loss of an individual's ability to withstand minor stresses because the reserves in function of several organ systems are severely reduced. **Flowchart 21.3** describes the pathophysiological basis of frailty.
- *Physical frailty/phenotypic or syndromic frailty* captures the specific signs and symptoms (fatigue, low activity, weakness, weight loss, and slow gait) of older adults who vulnerable to adverse health outcomes.
- *Deficit accumulation frailty or index frailty* is a conceptual framework that helps identify the frail, vulnerable older adults through cumulative comorbidities and cumulative illnesses as frail.
- Even a trivial illness/adverse drug reaction (ADR) → organ failure/death.
- Characterized by multisystem dysregulation involving four main domains that include: (1) chronic inflammation, (2) sarcopenia, (3) osteoporosis, and (4) alteration in neuroendocrine function.

FLOWCHART 21.3: Pathophysiological basis of frailty.

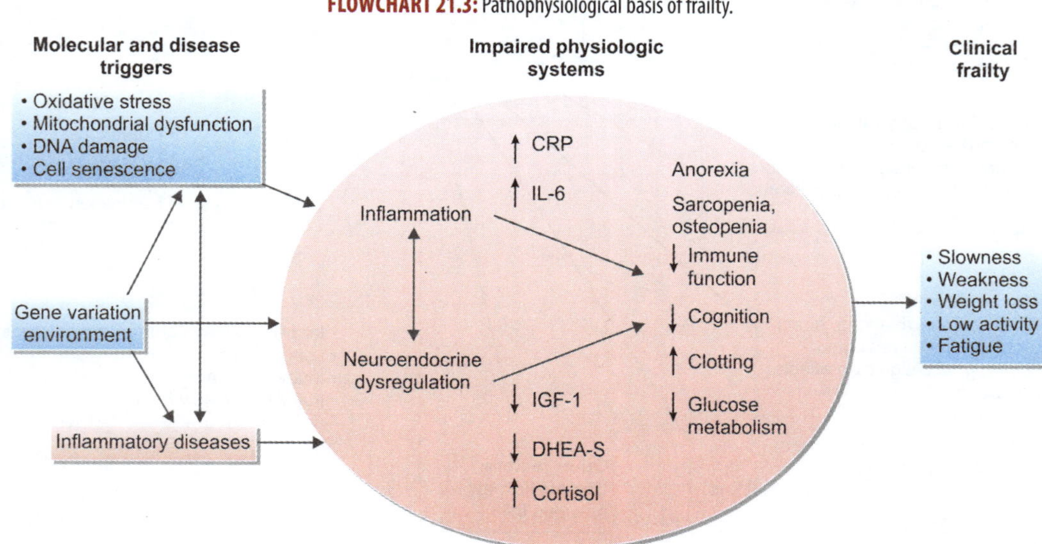

- **Fried frailty score** non-frail (score 0), pre-frail (score 1–2) and frail (score 3–5).
  - Weight loss (≥5% of body weight in last year)
  - Exhaustion (positive response to questions regarding effort required for activity)
  - Weakness (decreased grip strength)
  - Slow walking speed (gait speed) (>6–7 seconds to walk 15 feet)
  - Decreased physical activity (kcals spent per week: males expending <383 kcals and females <270 kcals)

Treatment
- Address the precipitating acute illness
- Address the underlying loss of reserve
- Exercise—improve musculoskeletal function, balance and aerobic capacity
- Medication review and deprescribing
- Nutritional support to improve lost weight

Q. Discuss failure to thrive, sarcopenia, and anorexia of aging.

Failure to Thrive

- It is a syndrome of weight loss, decreased appetite, poor nutrition, and inactivity, often accompanied by dehydration, depressive symptoms, impaired immune function, and low cholesterol.
- Affects following four main domains:
  - Functional: BADL/IADL
  - Malnutrition: Weight trend, body mass index (BMI), lymphocytes, and albumin
  - Depression: ± Geriatric Depression Scale (GDS)
  - Cognition: Confusion Assessment Method (CAM), standardized MMSE

Management
- Interdisciplinary assessment and care planning
- Treat the cause

Sarcopenia

- Age-related loss of muscle mass
- Increases the risk for falls, fractures, dependency, use of hospital services, institutionalization, poor quality of life, and mortality
- Assessment
  - 5-item SARC-F (**s**trength, **a**ssistance in walking, **r**ise from a chair, **c**limb stairs, and **f**alls) score

Management
- Protein supplementation
- Resistance exercises

Anorexia of Aging

- The multifactorial decrease in appetite and/or food intake that occurs in late life
- Specific geriatric syndrome that can lead to malnutrition if not appropriately diagnosed and treated
- **Features:**
  - Body wasting (cachexia and sarcopenia)
  - Poor endurance
  - Reduced physical performance
  - Slow gait speed
  - Impaired mobility
- Impacts survival independent of age, gender, and multimorbidity
- Age-related reduction in smell and taste perception → alters food palatability and diet variety
- Decreased gastrointestinal muscle tone and motility
- Causes constipation and flatulence
- **Risk factors:**
  - Functional impairment
  - Chronic medical conditions
  - Polypharmacy
  - Environmental factors—physical limitations causing mobility problems
  - Poor dentition/dentures
  - Depression—refusal to eat
  - Economic inequality
  - Social Isolation—living alone/living in old age home
- **Assessment**—the Simplified Nutritional Assessment Questionnaire (SNAQ) and Functional Assessment of Anorexia and Cachexia Therapy (FAACT) shortened 12-question version questionnaire

Management
- Address reversible contributing factors/comorbidities
- Prescription review
- Improve food texture and palatability
- Protein supplementation—1–1.2 g/kg body weight

Multimorbidity and Polypharmacy

- **Multimorbidity:** The coexistence of ≥2 chronic conditions, where one is not necessarily more central than the others.
- **Polypharmacy:** Administration of more medications than clinically indicated, representing unnecessary drug use, i.e., ≥5 drugs during a 3-month period.

- *Appropriate polypharmacy:* Prescribing for an individual for complex conditions or for multiple conditions in circumstances where medicines use has been optimized and where the medicines are prescribed according to best evidence.
- *Problematic polypharmacy:* The prescribing of multiple (medicines) inappropriately, or where the intended benefit of the [medicines are] not realized.

GUIDELINES FOR DRUG THERAPY IN THE ELDERLY (BOX 21.13)

There are several reasons for the greater incidence of iatrogenic drug reactions in the elderly, the most important of which is the high number of medications that are taken by elders, especially those with multiple comorbidities.

Box 21.13: Guidelines for drug therapy in the elderly.

Recommended approach

- Use nonpharmacologic approaches whenever possible. Avoid *routine* use of "as needed" drugs for sleep, anxiety, pain.
- Choose the drug with the least toxic potential. Substitute less toxic alternatives whenever possible (antacid or sucralfate for an H_2-blocker or proton pump inhibitors, metamucil or kaopectate for imodium, scheduled acetaminophen regimen for pain management).
- Reduce the dosage. "Start low and go slow". Start with 25–50% of the standard dose of psychoactive drugs in the elderly. Titrate the drug slowly.
- Set realistic endpoints: Titrate to improvement, not elimination of symptoms. Keep the regimen simple. Regularly reassess the medication list. Re-evaluate long-time drug use because the patient is changing.
- Review over-the-counter medication use.
- **Deprescribing**—discontinuing a therapy prescribed for an indication that no longer exists, discontinuing therapy with side effects that may be contributing to frailty symptoms, substituting a therapy with a potentially safer agent.

Medication optimization is defined as 'a person-centered approach to safe and effective medicines use, to ensure people obtain the best possible outcomes from their medicines. Medicine optimization applies to people who may or may not take their medicines effectively. Shared decision-making is an essential part of evidence-based medicine, seeking to use the best available evidence to guide decisions about the care of the individual patient, taking into account of their needs, preferences and values'.

Q. Enumerate and describe the social problems in the elderly including isolation, abuse, change in family structure and their impact on health.

Elder Abuse

- More than a million people world over aged 65 or older have been injured, exploited, or otherwise mistreated by someone on whom they depended for care or protection. Neglect is the most common form of abuse followed by financial and emotional abuse.
- Elder abuse can be suspected when the patient exhibits behavioral changes in the presence of the caregiver, delays between occurrence of injuries and sought treatment, inconsistencies between an observed injury and associated explanation, lack of appropriate clothing or hygiene, and not filling prescriptions.
- Many elders with cognitive impairment become targets of financial abuse.
- Abuse and self-neglect has increased risk of mortality.
- **Who are the abusers?**
  - Domestic elder abuse (caregivers/distant relatives)
  - Institutional elder abuse
  - Self-abuse/neglect
- **Reasons for abuse**
  - Caregiver stress/burnout
  - Impairment of dependent elder (i.e., dementia)
  - Transgenerational "cycle of violence"
  - Material or other gain
- About half of the elderly population in the country face some form of abuse, more in case of women than men

Major Forms of Abuse

1. **Physical and sexual abuse:** Any act of violence or rough treatment, whether or not actual physical injury results, e.g., slapping, punching, kicking, pinching, burning, restraints.
2. **Emotional and psychological abuse:** Any act that diminishes dignity and self-worth, e.g., confinement, isolation, verbal assault, humiliation, and infantilization.
3. **Financial abuse and material exploitation:** Any improper conduct that results in monetary or personal loss for the older adult.

4. **Abandonment and neglect**
   - Active neglect: Intentional (deliberate) withholding of basic necessities and/or care for physical or mental health.
   - Passive neglect: Not providing basic necessities and care. There is no conscious attempt to inflict distress.
5. **Medical abuse:** Any medical procedure or treatment done without the permission of the older person or their Power of Attorney or substitute decision maker.

Indicators of abuse are listed in **Box 21.14**.

Box 21.14: Indicators of abuse.

- Unexplained physical injury
- Unexplained malnutrition/decubitus ulcers
- Unkempt appearance
- Failure of a medical condition to improve or the continued presence of pain
- Fear of certain family members, friends, or caregivers
- The older person is largely ignored or treated passively by caregivers or others
- Caregivers who are entirely ignorant of the medical problems or treatments for the older person they are directly caring for.

CHAPTER

22

Dermatology, Venereology and Leprosy

INTRODUCTION

Description of Primary Skin Lesions (Fig. 22.1)

Q. Define primary/secondary skin lesions and give examples.

Lesion	Description	Lesion	Description
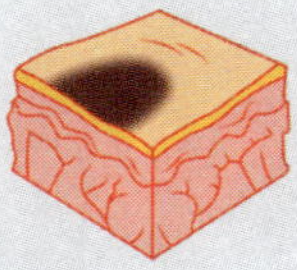 Macule	*Description:* A circumscribed flat, colored lesion, <2 cm in diameter, with sharp borders, not raised above the surface of the surrounding skin. *Examples:* Freckle, rashes of rickettsial infections, rubella	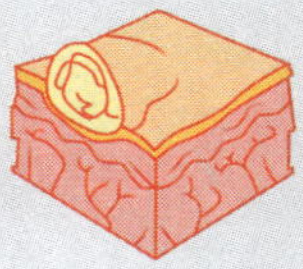 Vesicle	*Description:* A small, fluid-filled lesion, <0.5 cm in diameter, raised above the plane of surrounding skin. *Examples:* Herpes infections, acute allergic contact dermatitis, dermatitis herpetiformis
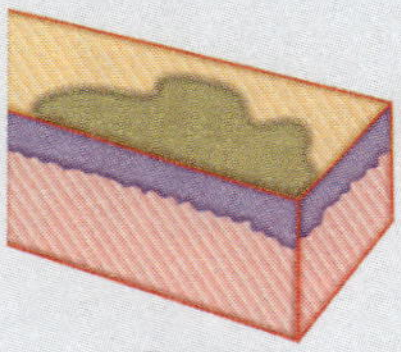 Patch	*Description:* A large (>2 cm) flat lesion with a color different from that of surrounding skin. *Example:* Vitiligo	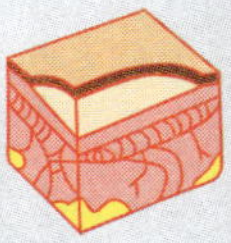 Bulla	*Description:* A fluid-filled, raised, often translucent lesion >0.5 cm in diameter. *Examples:* Burns, pemphigus vulgaris, bullous pemphigoid
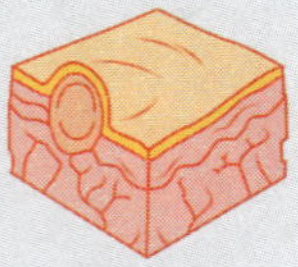 Papule	*Description:* A small, solid, <0.5 cm in diameter, without fluid, lesion raised above the surface of the surrounding skin with sharp borders. *Examples:* Nevi, warts, lichen planus, seborrheic and actinic keratosis	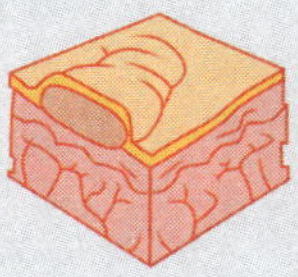 Wheal	*Description:* An evanescent elevated lesion with erythema and edema frequently with central pallor. *Example:* Urticaria
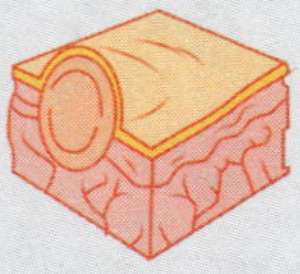 Nodule, tumor	*Description* *Nodule:* A palpable, large (0.5–5.0 cm), firm/solid lesion with distinct border raised above the surface of the surrounding skin. *Tumor:* A solid, raised growth >5 cm in diameter. *Examples:* Cysts, lipomas, fibromas	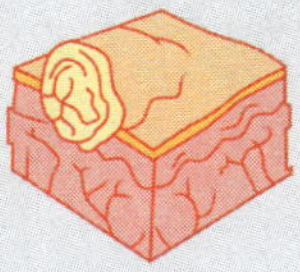 Pustule	*Description:* A vesicle filled with pus (leukocytes). *Example:* Folliculitis
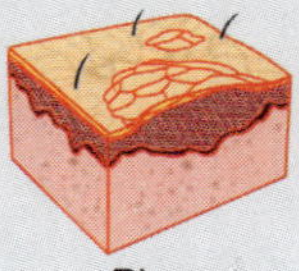 Plaque	*Description:* A large (>1 cm), flat-topped, raised area of skin *Examples:* Psoriasis, granuloma annulare	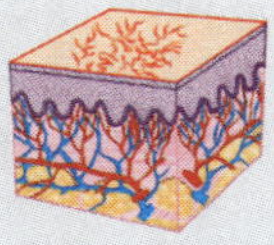 Telangiectasia	*Description:* A visible dilatation of small cutaneous blood vessels *Example:* Hereditary hemorrhagic telangiectasia

FIG. 22.1: Schematic representation of common primary skin lesions.

Description of Secondary Skin Lesions (Fig. 22.2)

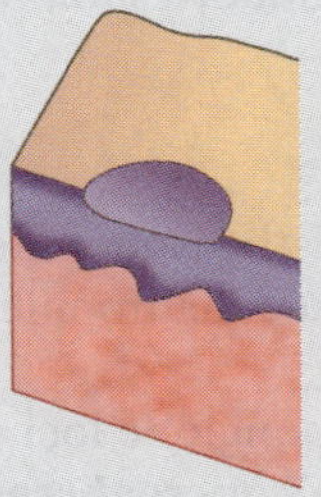 Erosion	*Description:* Partial loss of epidermis, which will heal without scaring	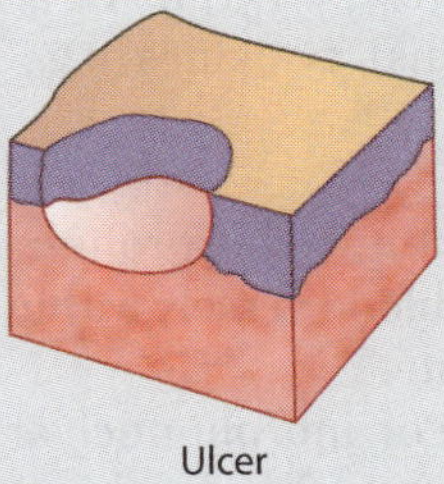 Ulcer	*Description:* Full thickness loss of epidermis and some dermis, which will heal with scaring
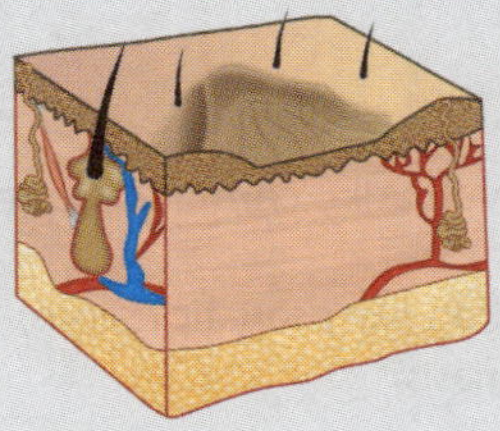 Atrophy	*Description:* Depression of the surface due to thinning of the epidermis or dermis	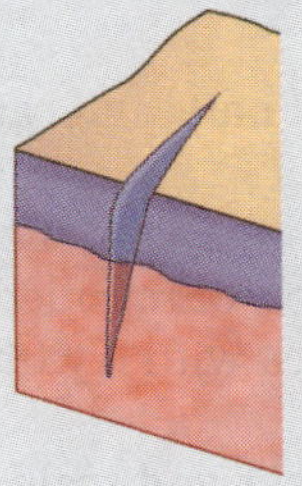 Fissure	*Description:* Linear split in the epidermis or dermis at an orifice (angle of the mouth or anus)
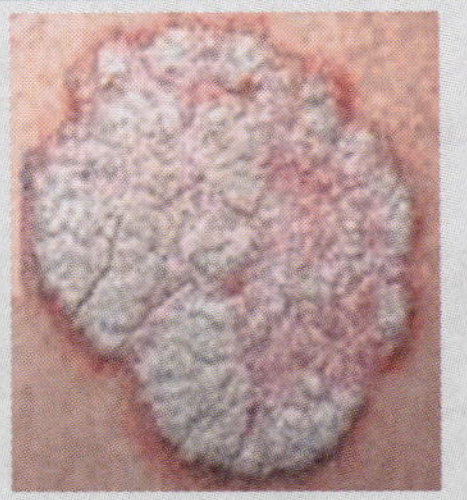 Scale	*Description:* Dry/flaky surface due to abnormal stratum corneum with accumulation of or increased shedding of keratinocytes *Example:* Psoriasis	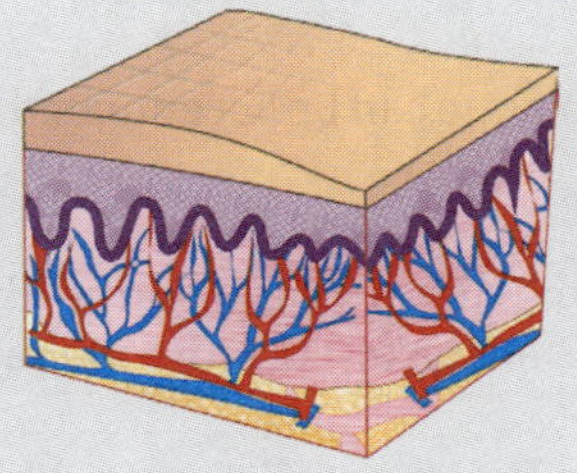 Lichenification	*Description:* Thickening of the epidermis with exaggerated skin markings. *Example:* Lichen planus

FIG. 22.2: Schematic representation of common secondary skin lesions.

PAPULOSQUAMOUS DISORDERS

Psoriasis

Q. Discuss the types and describe the various modalities of treatment of psoriasis including topical, systemic, drugs, and phototherapy.

It is a noninfectious, chronic papulosquamous, T-cell-mediated inflammatory skin disorder and is one of the most common skin diseases. It usually follows a relapsing and remitting course.

- **Gender:** It equally affects males and females.
- **Age:** It occurs in two peaks of age.
  i. Early onset (age 16–22) is more common and often has a positive family history. It has an increased prevalence of the **human leukocyte antigen (HLA) group Cw6.**
  ii. Late onset (peaks at age 55–60 years) has no HLA association.

Etiology

The exact etiology of psoriasis is not known.

- **Genetic factors:** The genetic component is complex and polygenic. There is a clear genetic predisposition (with a positive family history in >50% of patients) in association with certain environmental triggers. Nine susceptibility genes have been identified *(PSORS1* to *PSORS9),* most important being *PSORS1 (on* chromosome 6p21.3).
- **Environmental factors:** Several environmental triggers produce psoriasis in a genetically predisposed individual. These include infections, stress, physical injury, trauma, smoking, alcohol, and drugs.

Pathogenesis

- Psoriasis results from **interactions of genetic and environmental factors**. There is a shortened cell cycle time for keratinocytes (36 hours compared with 311 hours in normal skin) and a decreased turnover time of the epidermis (4 days from basal cell layer to stratum corneum, compared with 27 days in normal skin).
- Available evidence suggests that cells in genetically susceptible individuals, triggering factors activate the antigen-presenting cells (dendritic/Langerhans), which in turn activate CD4+ T_H1 and T_H17 cells via interleukin (IL)-12 and

IL-23, respectively and these T cells enter the skin and accumulate in the epidermis. These T cells secrete mediators [tumor necrosis factor (TNF)-α and interferon-γ by T_H1; IL-17A, 17F and 22 by T_H17], which activate keratinocytes to produce antimicrobial peptides (e.g., β-defensins), cytokines (e.g., TNF-α, IL-1β, and IL-6) and chemokines.

Pathology

- Increased epidermal cell proliferation (hyperproliferation of keratinocytes): Proliferation of the subepidermal vasculature leads to dilated, tortuous blood vessels within the dermal papillae surrounded by a mixed neutrophilic and lymphohistiocytic perivascular infiltrate.
- Dense inflammatory cell infiltrates. Polymorphonuclear abscesses may be seen within mildly spongiotic foci of the superficial epidermis **(spongiform pustules)** and within the parakeratotic stratum corneum **(Munro's microabscesses).**

Clinical Features

- Psoriasis can involve the **skin, scalp, and nails** and can present with different clinical patterns.
- Clinically, skin lesions are characterized by well-defined pink-red, sharply demarcated macules, papules, or rounded plaques that are usually covered by silvery scales with a whitish halo around lesions **(Woronoff's sign).**
- It predominantly affects **extensor surfaces** and scalp, and has a chronic fluctuating course. *There is increased association of psoriasis with HIV infection.*
- **Grattage test:** Scales in a psoriatic plaque can be accentuated by grating with a glass slide.
- **Auspitz sign:** Three steps—
  - *Step 1*: Gently scrape lesion with a glass slide—this accentuates the silvery scales (Grattage test positive). Scrape off all the scales
  - *Step 2*: Continue to scrape the lesion—a glistening white adherent membrane (**Burkley's membrane**) appears
  - *Step 3*: On removing the membrane, punctate bleeding points become visible—positive Auspitz sign.

Box 22.1: Types of psoriasis.

- Plaque psoriasis (psoriasis vulgaris), chronic plaque psoriasis
- Guttate psoriasis (small rain drop-like psoriatic lesions)
- Inverse psoriasis (flexural psoriasis)
- Localized pustular psoriasis
- Generalized pustular psoriasis
- Palmoplantar psoriasis
- Erythrodermic psoriasis
- Von Zumbusch psoriasis (pustular + erythroderma)

Types of Psoriasis

See **Box 22.1**.

Plaque Psoriasis (Psoriasis Vulgaris), Chronic Plaque Psoriasis

- It is most common form and accounts for 90% of cases.
- Lesions (**Figs. 22.3A and B**):
  - Symmetrically distributed plaques involving the scalp, extensor surfaces of the elbows, knees, gluteal cleft, lower back, ears and back. Plaques 1–10 cm in diameter with raised, well-defined margins
  - Thick silvery scales frequently present (although bathing may remove scale)
  - Classically asymptomatic, although some patients report pruritus, irritation, or pain
  - Pitting of nail plates and involvement of intertriginous areas (umbilicus and intergluteal cleft) may occur.
  - Psoriatic lesions can be induced in susceptible individuals by minor local injury/trauma, a process known as the **Koebner phenomenon** (**Fig. 22.4**).
- **Exacerbating factors**: Drugs (lithium, β-blockers, chloroquine, NSAIDs, ACE inhibitors, and terbinafine), infections (bacterial and viral), and ethanol abuse.

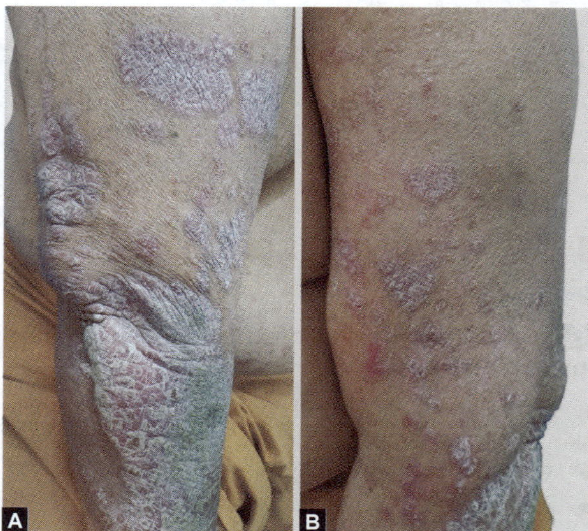

FIGS. 22.3A AND B: Skin lesion of psoriasis.

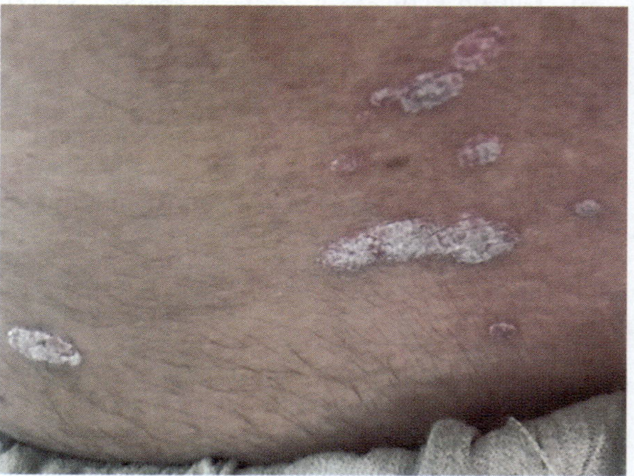

FIG. 22.4: Koebner phenomenon in psoriasis.

Associated Features of Psoriasis

- **Nails (Fig. 22.5):** Involvement is common and may be observed up to 50% of patients with psoriasis. These include—(a) "thimble pitting" of the nail plate, (b) distal separation of the nail plate from the nail bed (onycholysis), (c) yellow-brown discoloration underneath the nail plate ("oil drop" sign), (d) subungual hyperkeratosis, and (e) thickening of the nail (onychodystrophy).

- **For diagnosis of nail involvement:** More than six nails should be involved with each nail having >20 pits.
- **Psoriatic arthropathy:** It may be seen in 5–10% of psoriatic patients. It usually develops several years after appearance of skin lesions and most of these will have nail changes. It is a form of chronic seronegative spondyloarthropathy (discussed in Chapter 9).
- **Others:** It may be associated with comorbidities such as ulcerative colitis, Crohn's disease, coronary artery disease, metabolic syndrome, and lymphoma.

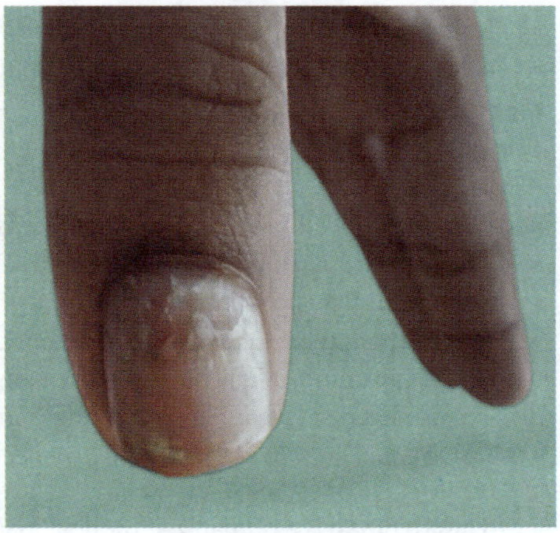

FIG. 22.5: Nail changes in psoriasis.

Investigations and Diagnosis

In most cases, the diagnosis can be made based on the history and physical examination alone. Biopsy is seldom necessary.

Management of psoriasis

Treatment depends on the type, location, and extent of disease.

General management

- Education, explanation, reassurance, and instructions are important.
- Instructed to avoid excess drying or irritation of skin and to maintain adequate hydration of skin

Treatment can be divided into four broad categories namely—(1) topical agents, (2) ultraviolet (UV) therapies, (3) systemic agents, and (4) biological therapies.

Treatment of psoriasis vulgaris: A three step approach.

Step 1: Topical treatments

- **Emollients/moisturizers:** Petroleum jelly and thick creams, especially effective when applied after hydrating bath or shower
- **Topical corticosteroids:** These are mainstay for treatment. Moderate to high potency ointments (e.g., betamethasone 0.5%) ± occlusion by tape or plastic wrap are recommended for thick plaques on extensor surfaces, whereas low-potency ointments (e.g., 0.05% fluocinonide) are usually sufficient for face and intertriginous areas.
- **Coal tar:** Usually used in conjunction with steroids, although can be used alone
- **Calcipotriene and Calcitriol:** Vitamin D_3 analog that affects growth and differentiation of keratinocytes
- **Tazarotene:** Topical retinoid (vitamin A derivative)
- **Topical calcineurin inhibitors**: Topical **tacrolimus and pimecrolimus**
- **Salicylic acid**: Keratolytic that softens and removes scale from plaques, allowing topical meds to penetrate
- Topical anthralin

Q. Discuss PUVA (psoralen and ultraviolet A) therapy in psoriasis.

Step 2: Phototherapy: *Effect likely through immunomodulatory properties*

- **Sunlight**: Careful sun exposure may improve psoriasis, but sunburn may exacerbate it.
- **UVB (295–320 nm) radiation:** Erythema inducing doses (3–5×/week until remission) are used for moderate to extensive disease, alone or in combination with topical tar.
- **UVB narrow band (311 nm)**: It has been shown to be more effective than the broader band in some studies, inducing more apoptosis of T-cells.
- **Psoralen and ultraviolet A:** Photochemotherapy with oral psoralen (8-methoxypsoralen) followed by exposure to UVA (320–400 nm) radiation is used for moderate-to-severe disease when UVB fails. It is effective (75% of patients note marked improvement), but increases risk for cataract, pigmentation, premature skin aging, and skin cancer. Psoralens are natural photosensitizers found in many plants. Psoralen molecules intercalate between the two strands of DNA and on excitation with ultraviolet A (UVA), photons cross-link the DNA strands. It is thus a pro-drug, which after oral administration is distributed throughout the body, but only activated in skin that is exposed to UVA. Other uses of PUVA include vitiligo, mycosis fungoides, atopic dermatitis, and senile pruritus. Risk of skin cancer and folate deficiency is associated with PUVA therapy.
- **High-energy 308-nm excimer laser:** It treats only involved skin and allows higher doses to be delivered to the plaques, compared with traditional phototherapy.
- Two regimens used commonly are:
  1. *Goeckerman regimen:* UVB + coal tar
  2. *Ingram regimen:* Coal tar + UVB + dithranol

Step 3: Systemic therapy

- **Methotrexate:** It is effective in severe psoriasis, psoriatic arthritis, and psoriatic nail disease.
- **Acitretin:** Vitamin A analog used for treatment of severe psoriasis, especially pustular and erythrodermic variants. It is a teratogen and pregnancy is contraindicated for 3 years after discontinuing the drug. It may be used in combination with UVB or PUVA.

- **Cyclosporine:** T-cell suppressor indicated for severe psoriasis not responsive to other agents
- **Apremilast**, a phosphodiesterase 4 inhibitor, is indicated for the treatment of moderate-to-severe plaque psoriasis.

Biologics, immunomodulatory drugs

- **Etanercept**: Recombinant TNF-alpha inhibitor, approved for treatment of psoriatic arthritis and for adults with moderate-to-severe plaque psoriasis
- **Alefacept:** Recombinant protein that binds to CD2 receptor on T-lymphocytes
- **Efalizumab**: It is monoclonal antibody to CD11a. It is approved for moderate-to-severe plaque psoriasis
- **Infliximab:** TNF-alpha inhibitor
- Human interleukin-12/23 monoclonal antibody:
  - **Ustekinumab,** a fully human monoclonal antibody against the p40 subunit of IL-12 and IL-23, is effective.
  - **Guselkumab** is a human immunoglobulin G1 (IgG1) lambda monoclonal antibody that binds to the p19 subunit of IL-23.
- *Monoclonal antibody against the p40 molecule shared by IL-12 and IL-23*: For example, **briakinumab** is effective in moderate and severe psoriasis.
- **Risankizumab** is a humanized monoclonal antibody directed against the p19 subunit of IL-23 and IL-39.
- **Brodalumab** (an anti-IL-17 receptor antibody) and ixekizumab (an anti-IL-17 monoclonal antibody) can also be effective in psoriasis.

Newer treatment options:

- **Climatotherapy** (bathing in sea water in combination with sun exposure)
- **Balneophototherapy** (salt water baths with artificial UV exposure)

Lichen Planus

Q. Describe the clinical features and treatment modalities for lichen planus.

Lichen planus is a pruritic inflammatory dermatosis that is commonly associated with mucosal involvement. It may affect the skin (cutaneous lichen planus), oral cavity (oral lichen planus), genitalia (penile or vulvar lichen planus), scalp (lichen planopilaris), nails, or esophagus.

Etiology

Autoimmune: An autoimmune mechanism is suspected because of its association with hepatitis C, inflammatory bowel disease, primary biliary cirrhosis, autoimmune hepatitis, hepatitis B, alopecia areata, myasthenia gravis, and thymoma. There are similarities with graft-versus-host disease (GVHD). Drugs, such as thiazides, INH, allopurinol, angiotensin-converting enzyme (ACE) inhibitors, and antimalarials, can produce lichenoid eruptions.

Clinical Features

Age and gender: Lichen planus affects women more than men (at a ratio of 3:2) and occurs most often in middle-aged adults.

Characteristics of lesion

- **Skin lesions (Figs. 22.6A and B):**
  - The typical rash of lichen planus is well described by the "5 P's": Well-defined **pruritic, planar, purple, polygonal papules, or plaques.**
  - **Sites involved:** Flexor surfaces especially wrists, flanks, medial thighs, shins of tibia, glans penis, nails, scalp, and oral mucosa.
  - There may be a characteristic fine lacy white pattern (network) on the surface of lesions **(Wickham's striae).**
  - **Koebner's phenomenon** is observed.
  - After lesions subside, post-lichen hyperpigmentation occurs.
- **Mucous membrane:** Involvement is common (30–70%) and prominent symptom is of severe pain rather than itch. The mouth is the most commonly affected. It can also affect genital and other mucosal surfaces.
- **Nail involvement:** Occurs in about 10% and causes a thinning of the nail with longitudinal ridges and may progress to complete loss of the nail plate **(pterygium formation) (Fig. 22.7)**.
- **Scalp involvement:** Lichen planopilaris is the specific name given to lichen planus on the scalp that may cause permanent, scarring alopecia.

Diagnosis

Histological changes: Characteristic histological changes include—(1) hyperkeratosis with thickening of the granular cell layer, (2) basal cell degeneration, and (3) dense, band-like T-lymphocyte infiltrate at the dermal-epidermal junction, with affinity for the epidermis (epidermotropism). The dermoepidermal junction becomes ragged and appears "saw-toothed". The basal layer shows liquefactive degeneration with colloid (apoptotic) bodies, **Colloid or Civatte bodies** in the upper dermis.

Prognosis

It is usually self-limiting and often clears by 18 months but can recur at intervals.

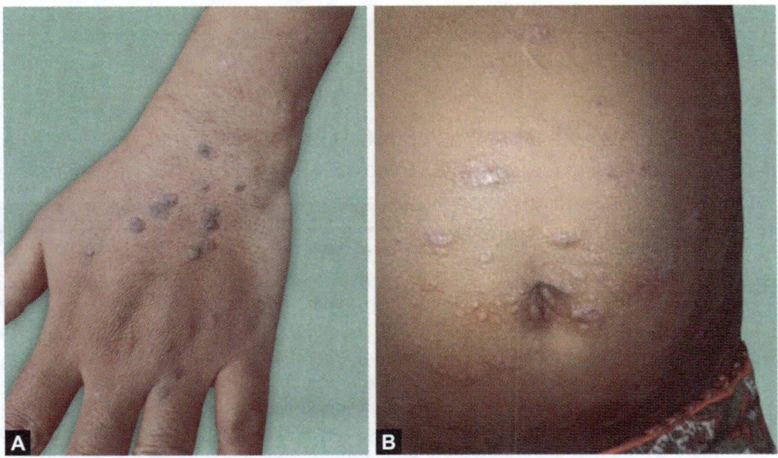

FIGS. 22.6A AND B: Skin lesions in lichen planus.

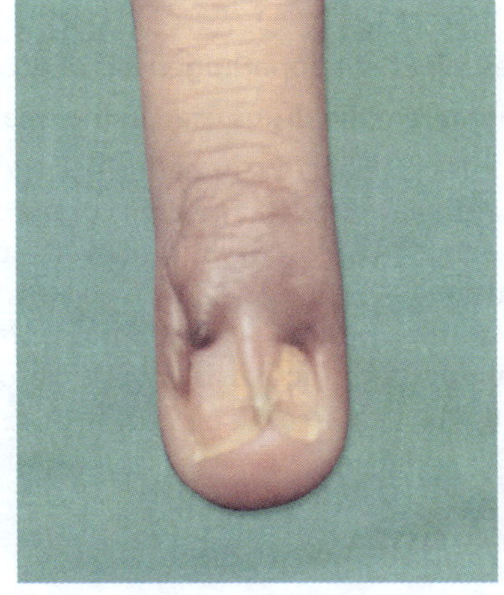
FIG. 22.7: Nail changes (pterygium formation) in lichen planus.

Complications of Lichen Planus (Box 22.2)

Management

- Treatment is symptomatic.
- *Topical corticosteroids*: Potent local corticosteroids (e.g., 0.05% clobetasol propionate, 0.1% triamcinolone ointment, twice daily for 2–4 weeks) are helpful in patients with limited disease. Oral lesions may require high-potency steroids given as an ointment, gel, or mouthwash. Topical 0.1% tacrolimus ointment or pimecrolimus may be very useful for painful oral disease unresponsive to steroids.
- *Oral therapy*: Short courses of systemic corticosteroids (oral prednisolone 30 mg daily for 2–4 weeks) are sometimes required for extensive disease.
- Widespread lichen planus may require UVB, PUVA, or UVA1 and in resistant cases, retinoids or immunosuppressants such as azathioprine and ciclosporin may be helpful.
- Hydroxychloroquine and dapsone have also been tried.

Acanthosis Nigricans

Q. Write short note on acanthosis nigricans (AN).

It is a skin lesion marked by thickened, verrucous (warty) hyperpigmentation of the skin with a velvety texture (**Fig. 22.8**) predominantly of the flexural areas (axillae, skin folds of the neck, groin, and anogenital regions) including the lips.

- In 80% of cases, it is associated with benign conditions [most commonly with obesity, **insulin resistance**, and diabetes, and drugs such as nicotinic acid, fusidic acid, stilbestrol, oral contraceptive pills (OCPs)] and develops gradually, usually during childhood or puberty. They are associated with very high levels of insulin owing to insulin resistance. Obesity-associated AN is sometimes termed "pseudoacanthosis nigricans".
- In the remaining cases, it arises in association with underlying cancers (most commonly *gastrointestinal adenocarcinomas)*, usually in middle-aged and older individuals. In this setting, it occurs as a paraneoplastic phenomenon caused by growth factors released from tumors. Other tumors producing this are Wilm's tumor and malignant tumors of bronchus, pancreas, ovary, bile duct, gallbladder, breast, and thyroid.

Associated thickening of palms with accentuated dermatoglyphics is called **Tripe palms. Acrochordons (skin tags) may be present.**

Treatment

- Treat any underlying disease/malignancy.
- Weight loss is advised in the obese.
- Topical or oral retinoids (0.5 mg/kg per day) may be helpful.

Few may benefit from metformin, oral isotretinoin, topical retinoic acid, topical salicylic acid, and oral fish oil.

Box 22.2: Complications of lichen planus (LP).

- Squamous cell carcinoma in oral ulcerative lesions
- Cicatricial alopecia in scalp LP
- Postinflammatory hyperpigmentation

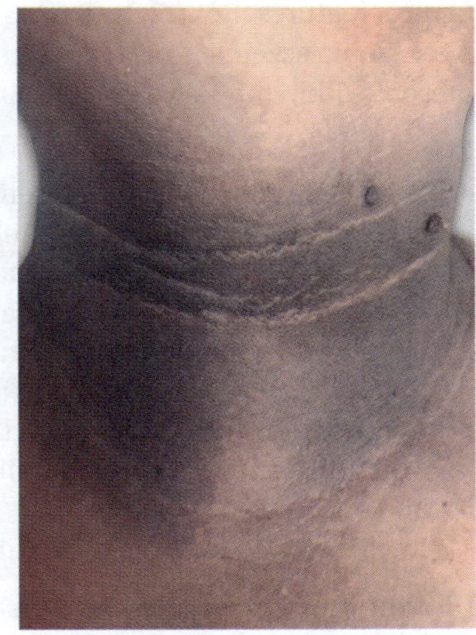
FIG. 22.8: Skin lesions of acanthosis nigricans.

Eczema

Q. Describe the etiopathogenesis of eczema. Classify and grade eczema.

Q. Enumerate the drugs used in the treatment of eczema.

Eczema is catarrhal inflammation of a sensitive skin, synonymous with the term dermatitis. Eczema is not a specific disease entity and may develop as a final common response of the skin to several causes. These causes may be either exogenous or endogenous in origin. It presents with spectrum of clinical presentation from acute through to chronic. Acute type is histologically characterized by spongiosis (intercellular edema of the epidermis) and intraepidermal vesiculation (producing multilocular blisters). Chronic eczema shows more epidermal thickening (acanthosis).

TABLE 22.1: Classification of eczema.

Endogenous	*Exogenous*
➢ Atopic eczema ➢ Discoid eczema (nummular eczema) ➢ Seborrheic eczema ➢ Hand eczema ➢ Venous ("gravitational")/ Asteatotic eczema ➢ Pityriasis alba, pompholyx	➢ Contact eczema: – Irritant – Allergic ➢ Photosensitive eczema ➢ Lichen simplex/ nodular prurigo ➢ Infective dermatitis

Classification of Eczema

See **Table 22.1**.

Atopic Dermatitis

Q. Write short essay/answer on atopic dermatitis.

Atopic dermatitis (AD) is an endogenous type of eczema that develops in individuals who are "atopic" and is the cutaneous expression of the atopic state. Atopic state is characterized by a family history of asthma, allergic rhinitis, or eczema.

Etiology

The exact pathophysiology is partially defined in atopic dermatitis.

- **Genetic factors:** Atopic eczema is a genetically complex familial disease and often associated with positive family history of atopic disease (90% concordance in monozygotic twins but only 20% in dizygotic twins).
- **Environmental allergens:** Atopy is characterized by generalized and prolonged hypersensitivity to common environmental antigens (e.g., pollen, food, animal hair, and house dust mite). Atopic individuals develop one or more of a group of diseases such as asthma, hay fever, food and other allergies, and atopic eczema.
- **Epidermal barrier impairment:** It is a major and perhaps primary factor in atopic eczema. It was observed in Caucasian individuals that loss of function mutations in the epidermal barrier protein filaggrin can predispose to atopic eczema. *Filaggrin* is coded by *FLG* gene on chromosome 1q21.

Exacerbating factors: Factors that can exacerbate eczema include—

- **Infection:** Infection in the skin or systemic infection can exacerbate atopic eczema. Paradoxically, lack of infection (in infancy) may allow eczema to develop **("hygiene hypothesis").**
- **Irritants:** Such as strong detergents, chemicals, and woolen clothes
- **Severe anxiety or stress** in some individuals
- **Others:** Cat and dog fur, food allergens, dairy products, or eggs

Box 22.3: Clinical features of atopic dermatitis.

- Family history of atopy (asthma, allergic rhinitis, food allergies, or eczema)
- Itching and scratching
- Lichenification of skin (in adults)
- Dry skin (xeroderma)
- Course:
  - Characterized by exacerbations and remissions
  - Lasts for >6 weeks

Clinical features (Box 22.3)

Age: Atopic eczema is most commonly seen among young children. About 50% present within the 1st year of life, and 80% present by 5 years of age.

Character of lesion (Fig. 22.9)

- Primary lesions include erythematous macules, papules, and vesicles, which can coalesce to form patches and plaques. **The most common presentation** is extremely **itchy erythematous scaly patches** accompanied by scratching.
- The symptom of itch is so central in the pathogenesis that atopic dermatitis is described as **"the itch that rashes and not the rash that itches".**
- It may also present as widespread cutaneous dryness (roughness).
- **Acute lesions** can produce small vesicles. In severe cases, secondary lesions from infection or excoriation (due to scratching) may be marked by weeping and crusting.
- **In chronic lesions,** repeated rubbing produces lichenification.

Distribution of lesion: Varies with age—

- Lesions are usually found in the periorbital area and the **flexor areas such as in front of the elbows and ankles,** behind the knees (popliteal fossae) and around the neck.
- In **infants, eczema** usually starts on the **face** before spreading to the body.

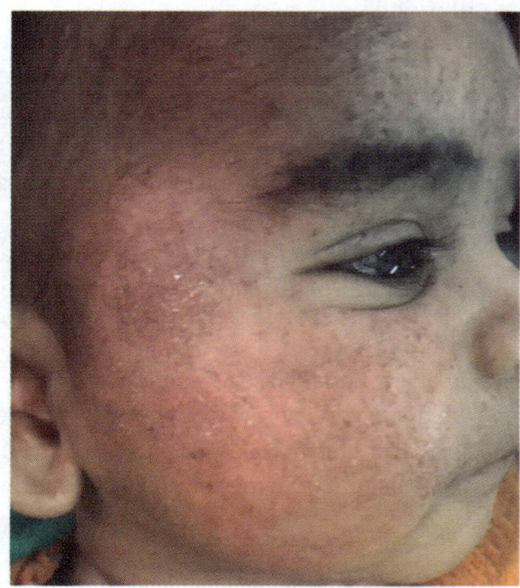

FIG. 22.9: Skin lesions of atopic dermatitis.

Cutaneous and vascular stigmata of atopic dermatitis (Table 22.2)

Diagnosis: It is made based on—(1) morphologic features, (2) the distribution of the lesions, and (3) a family and personal history of atopy. About 80% of patients may have high serum IgE levels or high specific IgE levels to certain ingested or inhaled antigens and a blood eosinophilia. Hanifin and Rajka criteria are used for diagnosis.

TABLE 22.2: Cutaneous and vascular stigmata of atopic dermatitis.

Cutaneous stigmata	*Vascular stigmata*
➢ **Dennie–Morgan** infraorbital fold ➢ Pityriasis alba ➢ Keratosis pilaris ➢ **Hertoghe's sign**—thinning of the lateral eyebrows	➢ **Headlight sign**—perinasal and periorbital pallor ➢ **White dermographism (Fig. 22.10)**—blanching of the skin at the site of stroking with a blunt instrument—causes edema and obscures color of underlying vessels

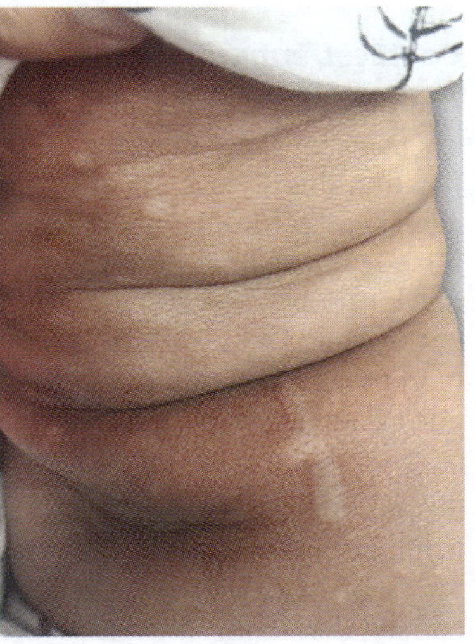

FIG. 22.10: Dermographism seen in urticaria and atopic dermatitis.

Complications of Atopic Eczema (Box 22.4)

Box 22.4: Complications of atopic eczema.

Secondary infection
- *Bacterial*: *Staphylococcus aureus* is most common
- *Viral*: For example, viral warts and *Molluscum contagiosum*, especially if treated with topical corticosteroids. Herpes simplex virus (HSV) can cause severe widespread eruption (eczema herpeticum).

Increased susceptibility to irritants due to defective barrier function

Increased susceptibility to allergy:
- Food allergy mainly in infants, e.g., egg, cow's milk, protein, fish, and wheat may cause an urticarial eruption.

Management

General measures:

Atopic eczema—
- Education, explanation, and reassurance
- Avoidance of contact with skin irritants (especially soaps or furry animals), heat, and dryness. Advised to wear cotton clothes
- **Emollients for moisturizing:** Emollients are used to moisturize, lubricate, protect, and soften skin
- **Topical anti-inflammatory agents:**
  - **Topical corticosteroid ointments:** They should be used judiciously. Depending on the potency, topical corticosteroids can be divided into five groups (**Box 22.5**). Mid-potency topical glucocorticosteroids are used in most treatment regimens.
  - **Topical immunomodulators:** These include two macrolide immunosuppressant namely tacrolimus ointment (0.1% for 3–4 weeks), and pimecrolimus cream (1% for 3–4 weeks).

The "triple" combination of topical steroid, emollients, and bath oil and soap substitute (e.g., aqueous cream) is usually helpful.

- **Adjunct therapies:**
  - **Oral antihistamines:** Control of pruritus is most often achieved by use of antihistamines. These include fexofenadine, 180 mg every morning, and hydroxyzine hydrochloride 10–25 mg at nighttime.
  - **Bandaging:** Paste bandaging may be used for lichenified eczema of the limbs. It helps absorption of topical treatment and also acts as a barrier to prevent scratching.
  - **Prompt treatment of secondary infection by antibiotics:** Secondary infection of eczema may lead to exacerbation of atopic dermatitis. The causative agent for secondary infection should be identified by culture and treated with appropriate systemic antibiotics.
- **Phototherapy:**
  - **Narrow-band-UVB phototherapy:** Ultraviolet radiation (UVR) treatment—most commonly narrow-band ultraviolet B is used.
  - **Psoralen and ultraviolet A (PUVA)**

Box 22.5: Classification of topical corticosteroids by potency.

Potency	*Class*	*Topical corticosteroid*	*Formulation*
Ultrahigh	I	Clobetasol propionate	Cream, 0.05%
		Diflorasone diacetate	Ointment, 0.05%
High	II	Amcinonide	Ointment, 0.1%
		Betamethasone dipropionate	Ointment, 0.05%
		Desoximetasone	Cream or ointment, 0.025%
		Fluocinonide	Cream, ointment or gel, 0.05%
		Halcinonide	Cream, 0.1%
	III	Betamethasone dipropionate	Cream, 0.05%
		Betamethasone valerate	Ointment, 0.1%
		Diflorasone diacetate	Cream, 0.05%
		Triamcinolone acetonide	Ointment, 0.1%
Moderate	IV	Desoximetasone	Cream, 0.05%
		Fluocinolone acetonide	Ointment, 0.025%
		Fludroxycortide	Ointment, 0.05%
		Hydrocortisone valerate	Ointment, 0.2%
		Triamcinolone acetonide	Cream, 0.1%
	V	Betamethasone dipropionate	Lotion, 0.02%
		Betamethasone valerate	Cream, 0.1%
		Fluocinolone acetonide	Cream, 0.25%
		Fludroxycortide	Cream, 0.05%
		Hydrocortisone butyrate	Cream, 0.1%
		Hydrocortisone valerate	Cream, 0.2%
		Triamcinolone acetonide	Lotion, 0.1%
Low	VI	Betamethasone valerate	Lotion, 0.05%
		Desonide	Cream, 0.05%
		Fluocinolone acetonide	Solution, 0.01%
	VII	Dexamethasone sodium phosphate	Cream, 0.1%
		Hydrocortisone acetate	Cream, 1%
		Methylprednisolone acetate	Cream, 0.25%

- **Systemic therapy:**
  - Systemic glucocorticosteroids should be given for severe exacerbations that do not respond to topical therapy. Generally, oral prednisolone is given in the dose of 0.5–1 mg/kg/day.
  - *Use of cyclosporin*: Cyclosporin is an immunosuppressant that inhibits production of interleukin-2 by T lymphocytes.

Contact Dermatitis

Allergic Contact Eczema (Figs. 22.11A and B)

This develops as a manifestation of delayed hypersensitivity reaction following contact with antigens or haptens. Many agents can cause allergic contact eczema and common agents include nickel in costume jewelry and buckles (e.g., eczema of the earlobes and umbilicus), chromate in cement (eczema of the hands and foot), and latex in surgical rubber gloves (eczema of the hands and wrist). Allergy persists indefinitely and eczema develops at sites of contact of allergen.

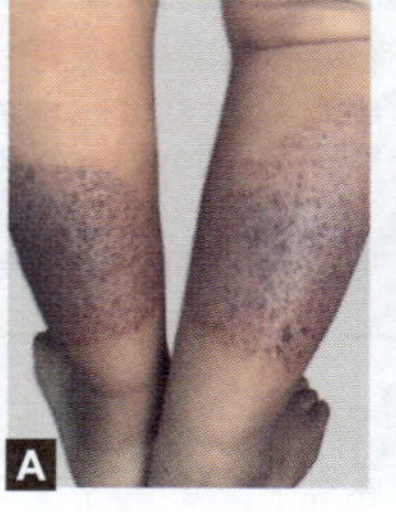

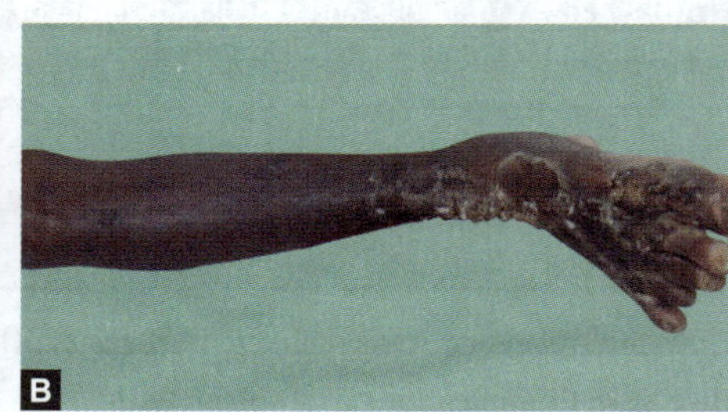

FIGS. 22.11A AND B: (A) Skin lesions of symmetrical atopic dermatitis; (B) Chronic contact dermatitis.

During the acute phase, lesions show edema, erythema, and vesicle formation. Later, vesicles rupture producing oozing and papules and plaques appear. In the chronic phase, scaling, lichenification, and excoriations predominate.

Irritant Contact Eczema

This type of eczema can occur in any individual and the injury is due to an inherent characteristic of compound-irritant contact dermatitis. It usually develops on the hands after repeated exposures to irritants (e.g., detergents, soaps or bleach, alkalis, and acids) and is common in housewives, cleaners, hairdressers, mechanics, and nurses. The lesions may be acute (wet and edematous) with strong irritants or chronic (dry, thickened, and scaly) with weak irritants.

Treatment of contact dermatitis

- Identify and avoid the contact with causative agent/irritants and use of protective gloves or clothing. In extreme cases, even changing of occupation or hobbies may be needed.
- Treatment with high-potency topical glucocorticoids
- In cases where systemic therapy is indicated, daily oral prednisone beginning at 1 mg/kg, but usually 60 mg/day is given. It should be tapered over 2–3 weeks.

Seborrheic Dermatitis

Seborrheic dermatitis is a common, chronic disorder, characterized by red scaly patches or plaques.

Etiology: It is due to *Pityrosporum ovale* (also called *Malassezia furfur* in its hyphal form).

Sites of involvement: Seborrheic dermatitis affects body sites rich in sebaceous glands.

- **Scalp:** It most commonly affects the scalp (recognized as severe dandruff).
- **Facial region:** On the face, it affects the nasolabial folds, eyebrows, eyelids, and glabella. Scaling of the external auditory canal and the postauricular areas often show maceration and tenderness.
- Other sites include central chest, axilla, groin, submammary folds, and gluteal cleft.

Clinical features: Three age groups are affected by seborrheic dermatitis.

i. **In neonates**: It presents as yellowish thick crusts on the scalp **(cradle cap),** face, or groin. Normally, it improves spontaneously after a few weeks.
2. **In young adults (especially males)**: The rash is more persistent and presents as an erythematous scaling along the sides of the nose, in the eyebrows, around the eyes, and in the scalp (dandruff). It is more common in patients with **Parkinson's disease,** in those who have had cerebrovascular accidents, and in those with **HIV infection** (especially with CD4 cell count $<400/mm^3$).
3. **In elderly people**: It can be more severe and progress to involve large areas of the body.

Treatment of seborrheic dermatitis:

Treatment is suppressive rather than curative.

- A **combination of low-potency topical glucocorticoids** (e.g. 1% hydrocortisone applied twice daily) with a **topical antifungal cream** (e.g., miconazole or ketoconazole or Ciclopirox olamine cream applied twice daily) is often effective. Topical 0.1% tacrolimus ointment or pimecrolimus cream can also be effective.
- **Antipityrosporal agents,** such as ketoconazole shampoo and arachis oil, are useful for the scalp and beard areas. Emollients and a soap substitute may be used as adjuncts. High-potency topical glucocorticoids (betamethasone or clobetasol) are effective in cases with severe scalp involvement. However, they should not be used on the face because they may be associated with steroid-induced rosacea or atrophy.

Pityriasis Versicolor (Tinea Versicolor)

Q. Write short essay/note on pityriasis versicolor (tinea versicolor).

- Pityriasis versicolor is a relatively common persistent, superficial skin condition caused by a common commensal lipophilic yeast—**Malassezia furfur** (also known as pityrosporum ovale). The yeast is a normal inhabitant of the skin.
- **Predisposing factor:** Infection is more frequent in warmer, humid climates, and is usually more severe and persistent in the immunocompromised individuals.
- **Appearance of skin lesion (Fig. 22.12):** Typical lesion is round, scaly, oval macules on the upper trunk. It is usually hypopigmented (on dark skin) but occasionally hyperpigmented (on light skin). Hypopigmentation is more obvious after sun exposure and tanning. Sometimes, it may have raised erythematous margins. Inappropriate use of topical steroids causes spread of the lesion.
- **Sites affected** are upper back, shoulders, and chest but it also affects upper arms, neck, and rarely on the face. The lesions are more extensive in patients in tropics.
- **Other diseases associated with tinea versicolor:** Cushing's syndrome, hyperhidrosis, and altered immune status (e.g., HIV).

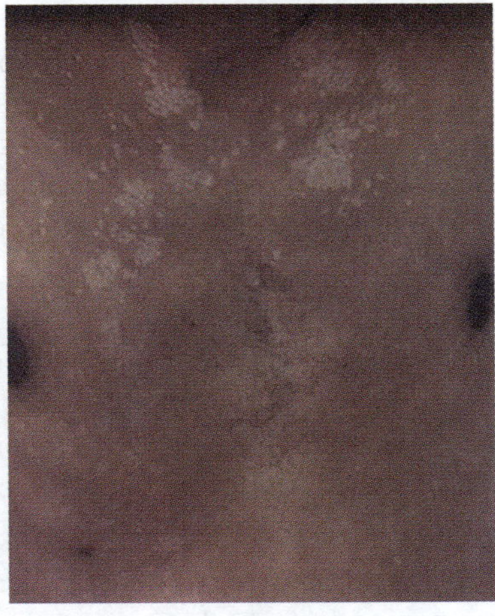

FIG. 22.12: Skin lesions of pityriasis versicolor (tinea versicolor).

Diagnosis

The diagnosis can be confirmed by:
- **Skin scraping:** It shows characteristic ***"spaghetti and meatballs"*** appearance.
- **Wood's light examination:** It shows some pigment (yellow fluorescence) in skin regions involved by tinea versicolor whereas in vitiligo, there is total loss of pigment in the affected areas.

Treatment

Topical antifungals
- Selenium sulfide or 2% ketoconazole shampoo to be applied to the affected areas of the body and removed after 30–60 minutes and repeated daily for 1 week. In resistant cases, overnight application may be useful.
- Topical imidazole (miconazole, clotrimazole, and ketoconazole) cream twice daily for 10 days

Oral antifungals

Oral itraconazole (100 mg twice daily for 1 week) is given in resistant cases. The pigmentation takes months to recover even after successful treatment. Others include ketoconazole (200 mg daily for 10 days or 400 mg/day for 2 days, though less effective), and fluconazole (150–300 mg weekly for 2–4 weeks). The condition may recur but can be retreated.

BLISTERING (BULLOUS) DISORDERS OF SKIN

Blistering skin diseases (BSDs) are skin conditions characterized by blister formation. A blister is an accumulation of fluid between cells of the epidermis or upper dermis (**Fig. 22.13**). Causes of blister formation may be genetic, physical, inflammatory, immunologic, and as a reaction to drugs. Blistering disorders are mostly due to autoimmune mechanism.

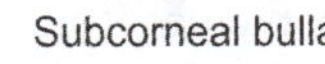

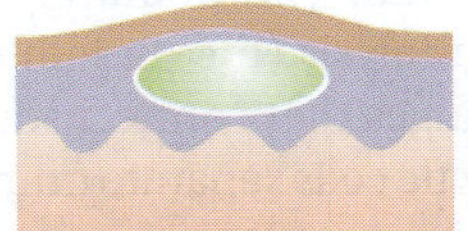

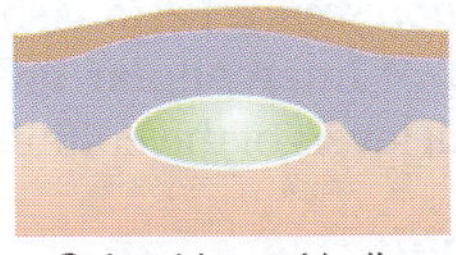

FIG. 22.13: Location of bullae and few associated diseases.

Types of Blistering Diseases (Box 22.6)

Box 22.6: Types of blistering diseases.

Genetic blistering diseases: (1) Epidermolysis bullosa and (2) Hailey–Hailey disease (benign familial pemphigus)

Immunobullous diseases:
- **Intraepidermal immunobullous diseases:** (1) Pemphigus vulgaris (PV), (2) pemphigus vegetans, (3) pemphigus foliaceus, (4) pemphigus erythematosus, and (5) paraneoplastic PV
- **Subepidermal immunobullous diseases:** (1) Bullous pemphigoid, (2) pemphigoid gestationis, (3) linear IgA disease, (4) epidermolysis bullosa acquisita, and (5) dermatitis herpetiformis

Pemphigus Vulgaris

Q. Write short essay/note on etiology, clinical features, diagnosis, and treatment of pemphigus vulgaris.

Pemphigus vulgaris (PV) is a potentially fatal mucocutaneous blistering disease.

Etiology

- **Autoimmunity:** It is thought to be an autoimmune disorder. Patients with PV have IgG4 autoantibodies directed against desmosomal protein desmoglein-1 and -3 (belong to the cadherin family of calcium-dependent adhesion molecules). Desmoglein-1 and -3 are expressed in skin and mucosal surfaces. IgG4 autoantibodies are responsible for blister formation and their titer correlates with disease activity.
- **Drug-induced pemphigus:** Pemphigus may also be drug induced (e.g., sulfonamides, penicillins, and antiepileptic drugs).

Clinical features

- **Age and gender:** It predominates in patients between the fourth and sixth decades of life and both sexes are affected equally.
- **Lesions:** They typically begin on mucosal surfaces and often progress to involve the skin. Lesions consist of fragile, flaccid blisters that rupture to produce erosions in mucous membranes and skin.

Oral cavity

- **Characteristic of lesion:** Mucosal involvement (especially oral ulceration) is the most common (up to 75% of cases) presenting sign. Lesions consist of fragile, flaccid blisters that rupture to produce erosions in mucous membranes.
- **Sites:** Lesions within the oral cavity can be seen anywhere and are most often found in areas subjected to friction trauma (e.g., cheek mucosa, tongue, palate, and lower lip).

Skin lesions

- **Sites:** Typically involves scalp, face, neck, trunk, and intertriginous areas (axilla and groin).
- Skin lesions follow oral lesion and appear as **nonitchy flaccid blisters filled with clear fluid** that arises on normal skin. Blistering usually becomes widespread and is fragile. They **rapidly denude/rupture** giving rise to painful **erythematous and weeping erosions.** Erosions are often large. Intact blisters may be sparse.

Q. Write short essay/note on Nikolsky's sign.

Nikolsky's sign: It is positive. It is elicited by applying gentle manual sliding pressure to the affected skin (e.g., where a blister is located, or rub sideways over the perilesional skin or normal skin with a cotton swab or finger). A positive response is indicated by extension of the blister and/or separation of the epidermis in the area immediately and is known as Nikolsky's sign. This sign is not specific to pemphigus but is also seen in toxic epidermal necrolysis (TEN), Stevens-Johnson syndrome, staphylococcal-scalded skin syndrome, bullous impetigo, and epidermolysis bullosa. This sign is usually negative in bullous pemphigoid.

Bulla-spread phenomenon: Gentle pressure on an intact bulla forces the fluid to spread under the skin away from the site of pressure (also called ***Asboe–Hansen sign, or the "indirect Nikolsky" or "Nikolsky II" sign***).

Diagnosis

- *Skin biopsy*: Microscopically, it shows suprabasal blister due to suprabasilar (immediately above the basal cell layer) acantholysis (the dissolution or lysis of the intercellular bridges that connect squamous epithelial cells). Acantholytic cells separate from one another, lose their polyhedral shape, and appear round (tombstone appearance).
- *Direct immunofluorescence*: Lesions show a characteristic net-like pattern of intercellular IgG deposits. IgG is usually seen at all levels of the epithelium.

Treatment

- Anesthetic mouth lozenges to reduce the pain of mouth ulcers
- Fluids and electrolytes balance and nutritional support, if required
- Antibiotics to control secondary infections

Patients with moderate-to-severe PV:

- **Systemic glucocorticoids:** These are mainstay of treatment to inhibit production of the autoantibodies. These usually started on oral prednisone, 1 mg/kg/day as an early morning dose.
- **Immunosuppressive agents:** If new lesions continue to appear after 1–2 weeks of treatment with prednisone, the dose is to be increased and/or combined with other immunosuppressive agents such as azathioprine, mycophenolate mofetil, or cyclosporin, or cyclophosphamide.
- **Immunoglobulins:** One course of intravenous immunoglobulin (400 mg/kg/day for 5 days) may be a safe and effective treatment for cases resistant to steroids.

Severe/treatment-resistant disease:

Plasmapheresis [six high-volume exchanges (i.e., 2–3 L per exchange) over ~2 weeks], **IV immunoglobulin** (IVIg) (2 g/kg over 3–5 days every 6–8 weeks), or **rituximab** (375 mg/m^2 per week × 4, or 1,000 mg on days 1 and 15). The duration of therapy varies according to the level of disease activity.

Bullous Pemphigoid

Q. Write short essay/note on:

- **Bullous pemphigoid or pemphigoid**
- **Etiology, clinical features, diagnosis, and treatment of bullous pemphigoid.**

Bullous pemphigoid (BP) is the most common autoimmune subepidermal blistering disease. Mucosal involvement is rare.

Age and gender: It occurs in elderly in the fifth to seventh decades, with an average age of onset of 65 years. Males and females are equally affected.

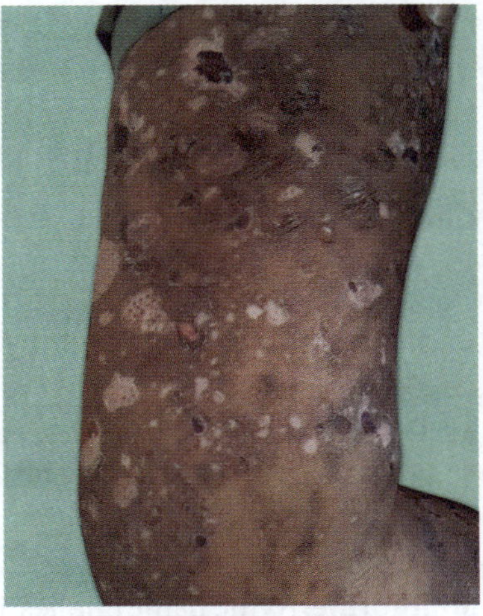

FIG. 22.14: Bullous pemphigoid.

Etiopathogenesis

Bullous pemphigoid is caused by autoantibodies against specialized proteins that are involved in adherence of basal keratinocytes to the basement membrane. These linking proteins are called **hemidesmosomes** and the so-called bullous pemphigoid antigens (BPAGs) are components of these hemidesmosomes.

Clinical features

Bullae (Fig. 22.14): Patient usually presents with large tense bullae anywhere on the skin but often involve flexor surfaces of the arms and legs, axilla, groin, and abdomen. The bullae may be centered on an erythematous or urticated skin. The bullae may contain hemorrhagic fluid. Pemphigoid can be very itchy. Mucosal ulceration is uncommon and when seen, it is of minor clinical significance. Nontraumatized bullae usually heal without scarring.

Diagnosis

Skin biopsy: Biopsies of skin lesion show subepidermal blisters with an eosinophil-rich inflammatory infiltrate at sites of vesicle formation and in perivascular areas.

Direct immunofluorescence: It shows linear deposits of **IgG and C3 at the dermoepidermal junction.**

Treatment

- Patients with local or mild disease can sometimes be controlled with the application of very potent topical steroids to all sites in frail elderly patients. Occasionally, it can be controlled by oral dapsone or high-dose oral minocycline or tetracyclines.
- The mainstay of treatment is systemic **glucocorticoid** (oral prednisolone 30–60 mg daily). Patients with more extensive lesions respond to systemic glucocorticoids either alone or in combination with immunosuppressive agents. Immunosuppressive agents include azathioprine, mycophenolate mofetil, or cyclophosphamide.

Intravenous immunoglobulin as a steroid-sparing therapy in BP may also be useful.

Dermatitis Herpetiformis

Q. Write short note on dermatitis herpetiformis.

- It is characterized by intensely itchy, chronic papulovesicular eruption distributed symmetrically on extensor surfaces.
- **Age:** It may start at any age. Most commonly, it occurs in 2nd, 3rd, and 4th decades of life.
- **Skin biopsy:** If a vesicle can be biopsied before it is scratched away, the microscopic examination shows a subepidermal blister, with dermal papillary collections of neutrophils (microabscesses).
- **DIF (direct immunofluorescence):** Granular **IgA** deposits in normal-appearing skin are diagnostic for DH.
- Most DH patients (not all) have an associated **gluten-sensitive enteropathy.** So, associated antiendomyseal antibodies are positive.

Treatment

- The rash responds rapidly to **dapsone** therapy.
- Gluten-free diet works very slowly.

REACTIVE DISORDERS OF SKIN

Erythema Multiforme

Q. Write short essay/note on precipitating causes, clinical manifestations, and management of erythema multiforme.

- Erythema multiforme (EM) is an uncommon acute, self-limiting, recurrent cutaneous and/or mucocutaneous blistering eruption that occurs in individuals of any age.
- Eruptions are characterized by target-shaped plaques commonly over extremities and face.

Causes

Erythema multiforme can be triggered by variety of factors (**Box 22.7**).

Box 22.7: Precipitating factors in erythema multiforme.

1. **Infections:**
   - Viral, e.g., herpes simplex, Orf, infectious mononucleosis, hepatitis B, and HIV
   - *Mycoplasma* and other bacterial infections (e.g., typhoid)
   - Fungal, e.g., histoplasmosis and coccidioidomycosis
   - Rickettsia
2. **Exposure to drugs:**
   For example, sulfonamides, penicillins, barbiturates salicylates, hydantoins, antimalarials, and carbamazepine
3. **Systemic disease:**
   - Sarcoidosis
   - Malignancy (carcinomas and lymphomas)
   - Collagen vascular diseases [Systemic lupus erythematosus (Rowell's syndrome), Wegener's granulomatosis, dermatomyositis, and polyarteritis nodosa]
4. **Other:** Radiotherapy, pregnancy

Pathogenesis

Immune-mediated disease: It is characterized by keratinocyte injury caused by CD8+ cytotoxic T lymphocytes in the skin. The CD8+ cytotoxic T cells are found in the central portion of the lesions, and CD4+ helper T cell and Langerhans cells are found in the peripheral portions. The epidermal antigens causing the disease are not known.

Classification

See **Box 22.8**.

Box 22.8: Classification of erythema multiforme (EM).

- **EM Minor**: Cutaneous without mucous involvement
- **EM Major (EMM)**: Cutaneous + mucous involvement
- **Mucosal EM**: Fuch's ectodermosis pluriorificialis
- **HAEM**: Herpes-associated EM
- **MPAEM**: Mycoplasma-associated EM

Clinical Features of Erythema Multiforme

- Male:Female = 3:2
- Occurs in the young/adolescents
- About 50% of patients give history of preceding herpetic infection.
- Associated with HLA - DQB1 * 0301 Allele

Elementary skin lesions

Multiforme: As the name implies, it presents with a diverse array of lesions (multiforme), including macules, papules, vesicles, and bullae.

Distribution of skin lesions (topography)

- Lesions are symmetrical, acral, and centripetal in distribution
- *Extensor aspect*: Extremities > face > neck > trunk
- Predilection to sun-exposed areas/Koebnerization present.

Characteristic lesion

Q. Write short essay/note on target lesions, iris lesions, and bull's eye lesions of erythema multiforme.

- **Classic target lesion (Fig. 22.15):** It consists of **three concentric distinct zones/rings** of different colors—a **dark central circular dusky red** (darker red) zone is surrounded by an **intermediate light rim** (white), which in turn is encircled by a **outermost red zone** (iris lesions). Central circular zone may show bulla formation or crust. The lesion may resemble a **"bull's eye"**.
- Larger lesions show central bulla and marginal ring of vesicles: **Herpes iris of Bateman.**

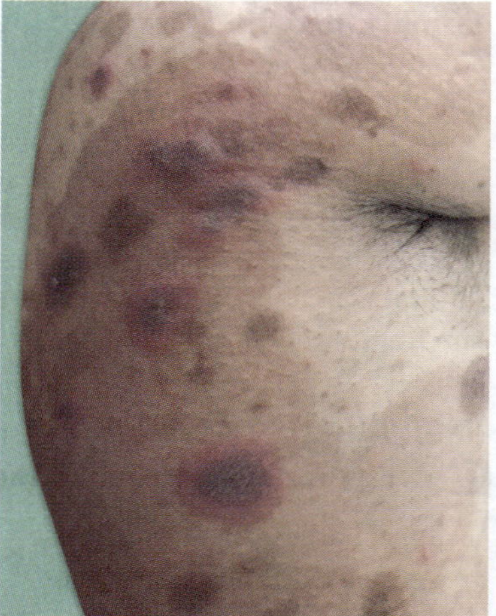

FIG. 22.15: Erythema multiforme with target lesion.

Mucosal lesions

Mucosal (oral mucosa) involvement is usually absent and, when present, lesions are few in number and mildly symptomatic.

Stevens–Johnson Syndrome (Figs. 22.16A to C)

Q. Write short essay/note on Stevens–Johnson syndrome.

- Stevens–Johnson syndrome (SJS) is a rare, acute, and life-threatening mucocutaneous disease with systemic involvement and is nearly always drug-related.
- SJS is a "minor form of TEN" with <10% body surface area (BSA) detachment
- *Overlapping Stevens–Johnson syndrome/toxic epidermal necrolysis (SJS/TEN)*: Detachment of 10–30% BSA
- *Toxic epidermal necrolysis (TEN)*: **Detachment of >30% BSA**

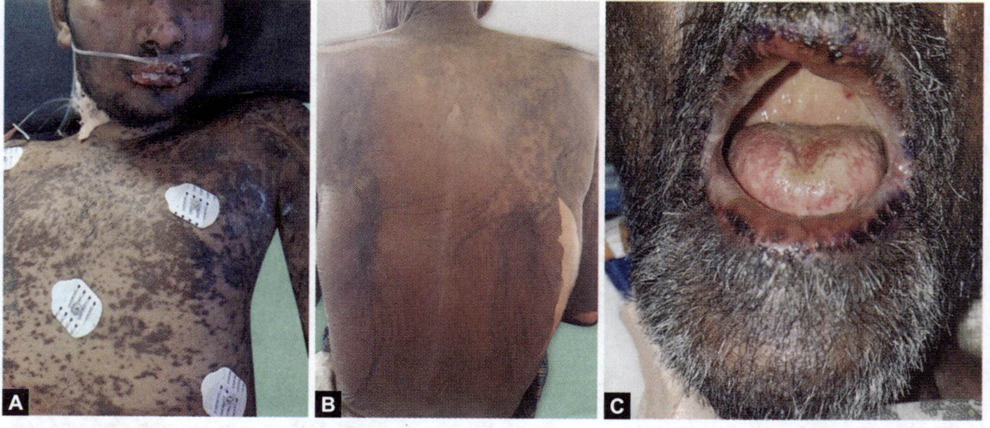

FIGS. 22.16A TO C: (A) Stevens–Johnson syndrome (SJS)/toxic epidermal necrolysis (TEN); (B) Toxic epidermal necrolysis; (C) Oral lesions in SJS/TEN.

Clinical features of Stevens-Johnson syndrome are listed in **Table 22.3**.

Mortality rate in SJS: 1–5%

TABLE 22.3: Clinical signs and symptoms of Stevens–Johnson syndrome/toxic epidermal necrolysis.

Cutaneous	*Mucous membrane*[a]	*Extracutaneous*
Initial phase: ➢ Erythematous, dusky red, flat, and atypical targetoid macules ➢ Symmetrical lesions distributed on the face/trunk/proximal part of limbs. It can spread to entire body *Later phase*: ➢ Lesions progressively coalesce and evolve into flaccid blisters ➢ Detachment of epidermis	➢ *Ocular:* Edema of eyelid, redness, photophobia, discharge, lacrimation, and corneal scarring ➢ *Buccal:* Erosive hemorrhagic lesions, grayish–white pseudomembranes, and crust on lips ➢ *Genital:* Erosive hemorrhagic lesions and painful urination	➢ *Nonspecific*: Fever, pain, and weakness ➢ *Respiratory*[b]: Respiratory distress ➢ *Gastrointestinal*: Diarrhea, nausea, malabsorption, and perforation of colon, melena ➢ *Renal*[b]: Proteinuria, hematuria, and microalbuminuria

a—normally involves at least two sites; *b*—lower occurrence in SJS compared to TEN

Toxic Epidermal Necrolysis (Lyell's Syndrome)

Q. Write short essay/note on toxic epidermal necrolysis.

- Toxic epidermal necrolysis is characterized by diffuse necrosis and sloughing of skin and mucosal epithelial surfaces. It begins with severe mucosal erosions and progresses to diffuse, generalized detachment of the skin epidermis.
- Nikolsky sign often positive, i.e., sliding pressure from a finger on normal-looking epidermis dislodges the epidermis.
- No target lesions seen
- *Mortality rate in TEN*: High (30%)

Management

Treatment of Erythema Multiforme

- Management of the precipitating factors/causes. If a drug is suspected, it must be discontinued and precipitating infection should be treated.
- Treatment of EM otherwise is nonspecific.
- Severe cases may require systemic corticosteroids.
- Oral acyclovir early reduces the number and duration of lesions.
- Chronic antiviral treatment with acyclovir (400 mg twice daily for 6 months) in herpes-associated outbreaks in patients with recurrent erythema multiforme

Treatment of SJS (Stevens–Johnson syndrome) and TEN (toxic epidermal necrolysis)

- Maintain the fluid and electrolyte balance
- Manage oral mucosal lesions with mouthwashes. Topical anesthetics may reduce pain and allow the patient to take in fluids
- Area of denuded skin should be covered with compresses of saline
- ***Systemic corticosteroid** is **contraindicated** in Stevens–Johnson syndrome*
- Treatment of toxic epidermal necrolysis is very difficult, but intravenous immune globulin (2–3 g/kg over a period of 2–5 days) may improve the prognosis.

DRESS Syndrome

Q. Write a short note on DRESS syndrome.

"Drug reaction with eosinophilia and systemic symptoms"

It is potentially life-threatening drug-induced, hypersensitivity reaction that includes skin eruption, hematologic abnormalities, lymphadenopathy, and internal organ damage.

Etiology and Risk Factors

Frequently reported		*Also reported*	
➢ **Antiepileptics (carbamazepine, lamotrigine, phenytoin, phenobarbital)** ➢ **Allopurinol**	➢ **Sulfonamides** ➢ Dapsone ➢ Minocycline ➢ Vancomycin	➢ Phenindione ➢ Beta lactams ➢ Olanzapine ➢ Febuxostat (DRESS with renal involvement)	➢ Nevirapine ➢ Oxcarbazepine ➢ Strontium ranelate ➢ Lenalidomide

Clinical Features

Systemic symptoms:

- 2–6 weeks after the initiation of the offending drug
- Fever (38–40°)
- Malaise
- *Lymphadenopathy*: Tender and slightly enlarged. Biopsy shows features of viral lymphadenopathy or benign lymphoid hyperplasia.

Visceral involvement: At least one organ involved in 90% patients—

- *Liver*: Hepatomegaly, jaundice, and asymptomatic hepatitis
- *Kidney*: Acute interstitial nephritis
- *Lung*: Nonspecific symptoms (cough, fever, and tachypnea/dyspnea). CXR/CT—evidence of interstitial pneumonitis and/or pleural effusion
- *Cardiac*: Eosinophilic myocarditis and pericarditis
- *Gastrointestinal tract (GIT)*: Diarrhea, mucosal erosions, bleeding, and pancreatitis
- *Thyroid*: Autoimmune thyroiditis
- *Nervous system*: Encephalitis, meningitis, and polyneuritis
- Myositis and increase in CPK
- *Eye*: Uveitis
- It rarely has been associated with shock/multiorgan failure and DIC.

Skin:

- Starts as a morbilliform eruption and progresses rapidly to a diffuse/confluent erythema with follicular accentuation
- DRESS is likely when the eruption involves >50% of BSA and/or includes two or more of facial edema/infiltrated lesions/scaling and purpura. Percentage of BSA involved is a marker of disease severity.
- In 20–30%, erythema can progress to exfoliative dermatitis.
- Face, upper part of trunk and extremities involved initially.
- Facial edema in 50% cases. It is symmetric, persistent, and associated with erythema.
- *Mucosa*: Inflamed, usually at one site only, does not progress to erosions.

Laboratory Features

Complete blood count (CBC)	Leukocytosis Peripheral eosinophilia Atypical lymphocytosis
Liver function test (LFT)	Alanine aminotransferase > 2 times the upper limit Alkaline phosphatase >1.5 times the upper limit
Renal function test (RFT)	Moderate increase in serum creatinine Low-grade proteinuria Abnormal urinary sediment with eosinophils
Serology	To exclude viral hepatitis in cases with deranged LFTs
Skin biopsy	Mild spongiosis, lymphocytic infiltrate in the superficial dermis with eosinophils and dermal edema

Management

- **Drug withdrawal and avoidance of introducing new medications during the course**
- Fluid, electrolyte, and nutritional support
- Warm, humid environment, and skincare with warm baths/wet dressings and emollients
- Patients without evidence of renal/pulmonary involvement and only modest elevation of liver transaminases (<3 times) can be treated symptomatically.
  - **For pruritus and skin inflammation, high-potency topical steroids (betamethasone, clobetasol, fluocinonide, halobetasol) are applied 2 times/day for 1 week.**
- Patients with severe organ involvement:
  - *Acute hepatitis*: Withdrawal of offending drug and follow-up by serial LFT. Liver transplant in cases of acute liver failure.
  - **Moderate-to-high dose of systemic corticosteroids in severe lung involvement** (dyspnea, abnormal CXR, and hypoxemia) and severe renal involvement (creatinine >150% basal level, proteinuria, or hematuria).
    Given till clinical improvement or normalization of laboratories and then tapered over 8–12 weeks.
- **Cyclosporine: Second-line therapy for those who do not respond to steroids or if steroids are contraindicated.**

PIGMENTARY DISORDERS OF SKIN

Hypopigmentation

Q. List the differential diagnosis of hypopigmented cutaneous lesions/hypopigmentation.

Causes of Hypopigmentation

See **Box 22.9**.

Box 22.9: Causes of hypopigmentation and/or depigmentation.

Genetic
- Albinism
- Piebaldism
- Phenylketonuria
- Waardenburg's syndrome
- Chediak-Higashi syndrome
- Tuberous sclerosis

Endocrine
- Hypopituitarism

Chemical
- Contact with substituted phenols (in rubber industry) Chloroquine and hydroxychloroquine

Postinflammatory
- Eczema
- Pityriasis alba
- Psoriasis
- Sarcoidosis
- Lupus erythematosus
- Lichen sclerosus et atrophicus
- Cryotherapy

Infections
- Leprosy
- Pityriasis versicolor
- Syphilis, yaws and pinta

Tumors
- Halo nevus
- Malignant melanoma

Miscellaneous
- Vitiligo
- Idiopathic guttate hypomelanosis

Vitiligo

Q. Write short note on etiology, clinical features, and treatment of vitiligo.

Vitiligo is a common, slowly progressive acquired condition caused by focal loss of melanocytes within the skin resulting in the development of well-circumscribed patches of hypopigmentation (**Figs. 22.17A to C**).

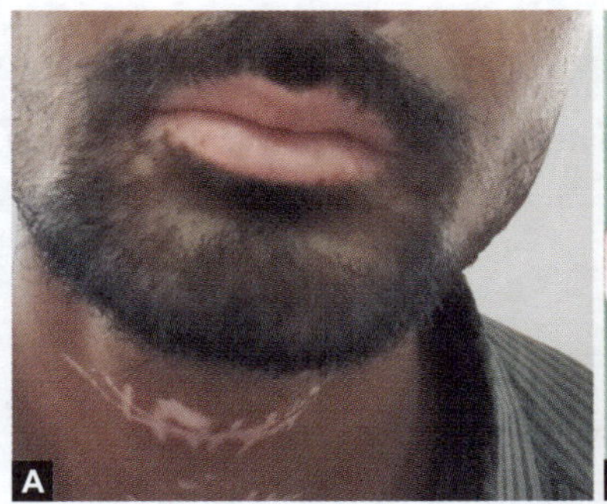
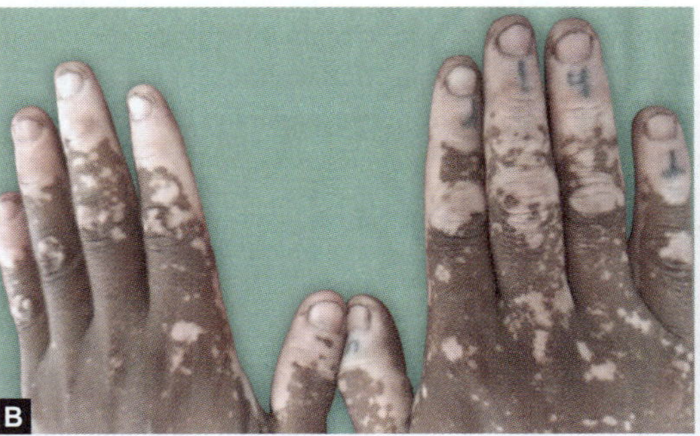
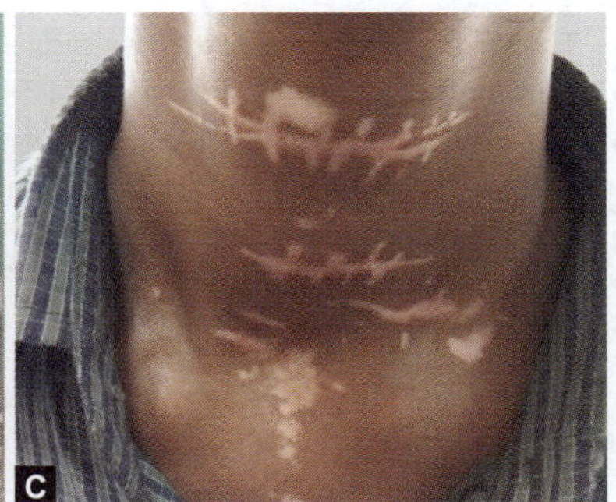

FIGS. 22.17A TO C: (A) Vitiligo; (B) Acral vitiligo; (C) Koebner phenomenon in vitiligo.

Classification

See **Box 22.10**

Box 22.10: Classification of vitiligo.

Localized
- **Focal vitiligo:** One or more macules in one area not clearly in a segment
- **Segmental vitiligo:** Number of macules in unilateral segment of the body (stops abruptly at midline)
- **Mucosal vitiligo:** Affects lips, oral cavity, and genitalia

Generalized
- **Acrofacial vitiligo:** Lesions on the acral (hand and feet) and face (perioral)
- **Vitiligo vulgaris:** Multiple macules bilaterally symmetrically scattered
- **Lip–tip vitiligo:** Tips of digits and lips only
- **Mixed:** Any combination of the above
- **Universal vitiligo:** Complete or near complete depigmentation of the body

Clinical Features

Nonsegmental vitiligo (NSV)

- It presents as small, depigmented macule that may enlarge and coalesce into larger patches.
- NSV is further divided into subtypes based upon the distribution of skin lesions (i.e., generalized, acral or acrofacial, mucosal, localized, universal, and mixed pattern).
- It is often symmetrical and occurs mainly around body orifices (around the eyes, nose, lips, and genitalia), hands, feet, flexor surface of the wrists, ankles, elbows, knees, and major body folds.
- The hair of the scalp, beard, eyebrows, and lashes (leukotrichia) may also show depigmentation.
- **Vitiligo fulminans/galloping vitiligo:** Rapid downhill course with rapid progression of skin lesions
- Patients are very susceptible to sunburn.
- Nonsegmental vitiligo can spread by **Koebner phenomenon (Fig. 22.17C).** *Other skin conditions that spread by Koebner phenomenon include psoriasis, molluscum contagiosum, warts, EM, and lichen planus.*

Segmental vitiligo

It is **restricted to one part** of the body. The patches of depigmentation are sharply defined. Spotty perifollicular pigment may be seen within the depigmentation. **Sensation in the depigmented patches is normal** (unlike in tuberculoid leprosy). Wood's light examination shows the contrast between pigmented and nonpigmented skin.

Trichrome vitiligo (vitiligo gradate): Presence of tan-colored zone in-between normal skin and the depigmented macule. Sometimes, a fourth color dark brown is present at sites of perifollicular repigmentation–**quadrichrome vitiligo.**

Association of vitiligo with other diseases

See **Box 22.11**.

Box 22.11: Vitiligo association with other diseases.

- Autoimmune thyroiditis
- Addison's disease
- Pernicious anemia
- Diabetes mellitus
- **Vogt–Koyanagi–Harada syndrome**: Vitiligo, poliosis, uveitis, alopecia, meningismus, and hearing difficulties
- **Alezzandrini syndrome:** Unilateral facial vitiligo, unilateral retinal degeneration, poliosis, and hearing loss
- **Kabuki syndrome:** Developmental delay, facial dysmorphism, skeletal and visceral anomalies

Management
- Protect the patches from excessive sun exposure with clothing or sunscreen to avoid sunburn.
- **Treatment:** Often unsatisfactory

Topical treatment

It includes the use of potent topical corticosteroids and topical immunomodulators (e.g., calcineurin-inhibitors tacrolimus 0.1% ointment especially on the face).

Phototherapy
- Topical psoralen plus ultraviolet-A (UV-A) phototherapy (PUVA therapy) is a most effective repigmentary treatment available for nonsegmental generalized vitiligo.
- *Narrow-band UVB (NB-UVB) phototherapy*: It is the treatment of choice for active, generalized vitiligo. Cosmetic results are better and side effects are less than PUVA.

- Topical application of corticosteroids along with UVA exposure is often effective.
- Autologous melanocyte transfer is effective for treating stable, focal vitiligo.
- Extensive vitiligo may be treated with removal of pigment from the remaining normally pigmented skin by using bleaching creams (e.g., monobenzylether of hydroquinone and 4-methoxy-phenol).
- Human placental extract and calcipotriol have been tried.
- **Systemic treatment (Box 22.12)**
- **Surgical treatment (Box 22.13)**

Pityriasis Alba

- Common skin disorder in children that is usually evident before puberty.
- **Cause:** Not known, however, there is often a history of atopy.

Clinical Features

Hypopigmented patches or macules with slight scale, mainly on the face and less frequently on the neck, trunk, and extremities. No permanent damage to the skin. Often improves after puberty.

Treatment: Use of lubricants and mild topical steroids

Box 22.12: Systemic treatment for vitiligo.

- Psoralen and UV-A
- Corticosteroids
- Immunomodulators (cyclosporine, levamisole, and azathioprine)
- Phenylalanine plus UV-A
- Khellin
- Antioxidants
- Monobenzyl ether of hydroquinone (monobenzone)

Box 22.13: Surgical treatment for vitiligo.

- Punch grafting
- Split skin thickness grafting
- Blister grafting
- Melanocyte culture and transplantation
- Tattooing

Inherited Hypopigmentation Disorders

Q. Write short note on inherited hypopigmentation disorders.

Albinism

- Autosomal recessive inherited disorder
- Genetic defect in melanin synthesis and normal melanocyte number and structure
- Mutation in tyrosinase gene
- Affected individual will be born with white hair and skin and blue eyes (retinal pigment epithelium involved).
- Selenium deficiency in the setting of total parental nutrition can lead to **pseudoalbinism.**

Piebaldism

- Rare autosomal dominant disease
- Congenital **white forelock**
- Hyperpigmented macules within the amelanotic macules and normally pigmented skin are characteristic.

Waardenburg syndrome

Autosomal dominant disorder characterized by white forelock, heterochromia iridis, and hypomelanotic macules.

Conditions Associated with Increased Pigmentation (Box 22.14)

Q. List the differential diagnosis for hyperpigmentation.

Box 22.14: Conditions associated with increased pigmentation.

- Melasma
- Freckles (ephelides)
- Lentigines (NAME syndrome and Leopard syndrome)
- Peutz–Jeghers syndrome

Systemic Diseases Causing Hyperpigmentation (Table 22.4)

TABLE 22.4: Systemic diseases causing hyperpigmentation.

Causes of increased melanin production		
Acquired	***Congenital/Inherited***	***Non-melanin causes***
➢ Melasma ➢ Post-inflammatory pigmentation ➢ Solar lentigines ➢ Ephelides ➢ Lichen planus ➢ Fixed drug eruption ➢ Erythromelanosis follicularis faciei et colli ➢ Pellagra ➢ Poikiloderma of Civatte ➢ Riehl's melanosis	➢ Mongolian spots ➢ Nevus of Ota ➢ Nevus of Ito ➢ Spindle cell naevus ➢ Blue nevus ➢ Halo nevus ➢ Café au lait ➢ Peutz-Jeghers syndrome ➢ Albright syndrome	➢ Primary hemochromatosis ➢ Hepatic cirrhosis ➢ Chronic renal failure ➢ Alkaptonuria ➢ Lamellar ichthyosis ➢ Epidermolytic hyperkeratosis ➢ Drug and heavy metal toxicity ➢ Canthaxanthin ➢ Pituitary tumors

SKIN TUMORS

Q. Write short essay/answer on benign, premalignant conditions of the skin.

Benign and Premalignant Lesions of Skin (Table 22.5)

TABLE 22.5: Benign and premalignant lesions of skin.

Benign conditions		*Premalignant conditions*
➢ Ephelide	➢ Seborrheic keratosis	➢ Bowen's disease
➢ Melanocytic nevi	➢ Squamous cell papilloma	➢ Keratoacanthoma
➢ Granuloma telangiectaticum	➢ Warts	➢ Marjolin's ulcer
➢ Hemangioma of skin	➢ Skin tags (acrochordons)	➢ Paget's disease of the nipple
➢ Dermatofibroma	➢ Pyogenic granuloma	➢ Senile keratosis/actinic keratosis
➢ Papilloma	➢ Keloids	➢ Erythroplasia of Queyrat

Malignant Skin Tumors

Q. Write short essay/answer on common malignant skin tumors.

Malignant tumor of skin is the most common malignancy in fair-skinned populations.

Categories

See **Table 22.6**.

TABLE 22.6: List of malignant skin tumors.

Common malignant tumors	*Uncommon malignant tumors*
➢ Basal cell carcinoma ➢ Squamous cell carcinoma and its precursor Bowen's diseases	➢ Primary: - Malignant melanoma - Cutaneous T-cell lymphomas (e.g., mycosis fungoides) - Kaposi sarcoma - Apocrine carcinoma of the skin ➢ Metastasis

Etiology and Pathogenesis of Skin Malignancy

- **Sun exposure**: UVR (ultraviolet radiation) is the main environmental risk factor for skin cancer.
- **Genetic predispositions:**
  - Xeroderma pigmentosum
  - Basal cell nevus (Gorlin's) syndrome
- **Cutaneous immune surveillance:** Immunosuppressed organ transplant recipients have an increased risk of skin cancer, particularly SCC (squamous cell carcinoma). Patients who have received high numbers of PUVA treatments (>150), which are immunosuppressive, are also at increased risk of skin cancer, particularly SCC.
- **Chronic inflammation:** It is also a risk factor for SCC, which may arise in chronic skin ulcers/scars.

Basal Cell Carcinoma (Rodent Ulcer)

Basal cell carcinomas (BCC) are the most common slow-growing **invasive** malignant skin tumor that rarely metastasizes.

Types of Basal Cell Carcinoma

See **Box 22.15**.

Box 22.15: Types of basal cell carcinoma (BCC).

- Superficial BCC
- Nodular BCC, rodent type (most common type—75%)
- Pigmented BCC
- Sclerosing or morphea form BCC
- Metaphysical
- Recurrent BCC
- Cystic BCC

Clinical Presentation

- Incidence of BCCs increases with age on exposed sites and males are more commonly affected.
- **Sites:** Occur at **sun-exposed sites** and in fair-skinned people. Usual site is **above a line drawn from angle of mouth to the pinna of the ear.**
- Appear as a slow-growing **pearly papules** or nodule (or rarely be cystic), often containing prominent, dilated subepidermal blood vessels (telangiectasia).
- Advanced tumors **may ulcerate** to form a crater with a rolled, pearly edge. They **locally invade and erode the underlying bone or facial sinuses like a rodent** and are known as **rodent ulcers.** Crusting and bleeding in the center of the tumor is frequently seen.
- They are 10–20 times more common in the chronically immunosuppressed solid organ transplant recipients.

Management/Treatment

Basal cell carcinoma rarely metastasizes. Hence, a metastatic work-up is usually not required.

- **Surgical therapy:**
  - **Surgical excision** with controlled borders is often the treatment of choice and recurrence rates are lowest.
  - **Mohs' micrographic surgery**
- **Nonsurgical therapies:**
  - Topical photodynamic therapy and topical 5% imiquimod cream and 5-fluorouracil
  - *Cryotherapy*: It is a destructive treatment that uses liquid nitrogen
  - Radiotherapy
  - Hedgehog pathway inhibitors (vismodegib) for advanced inoperable BCC
  - *Curettage and cautery*: Occasionally can be used in older patients

Squamous Cell Carcinoma

- **Second most common skin cancer** arising **on sun-exposed sites**
- More aggressive than basal cell carcinoma, as it can metastasize if left untreated.
- **Sex:** More **common in** elderly **men** than in women
- **Clinical presentation:** Appear as sharply defined, red, scaling plaques

Risk Factors

See **Box 22.16.**

Box 22.16: Risk factors for squamous cell carcinoma of skin.

- *Precursors of SCC*: Solar/actinic keratoses or Bowen's disease
- *Industrial carcinogens*: Tars and oils
- Chronic nonhealing skin ulcers, e.g., chronic osteomyelitis
- Old burn scars (e.g., Marjolin's ulcers)
- Ingestion of arsenicals
- Ionizing radiation or previous X-ray therapy
- Tobacco and betel nut chewing in the oral cavity
- Chronic venous ulcers and discoid lupus erythematosus

Clinical Features

- **Sites:** Usually occurs on chronically sun-exposed portions of the skin, such as bald scalp, tops of ears, face, lower lip, and back of hands.
- **Appearance:** Depends on histological grading. Well-differentiated tumors present as keratotic nodules, whereas poorly differentiated tumors tend to be ill defined and infiltrative, often-warty nodule or plaque that may ulcerate.
- **Behavior:** They can grow very rapidly. SCC has metastatic potential.

Management

- **Early diagnosis** is important. **Regional lymph nodes** should be routinely examined particularly for high-risk tumors arising on lips, ears, perigenital regions, or tumor developing at sites of chronic ulceration, burn scars, or sites of previous radiotherapy.
- **Complete surgical excision** is the usual treatment of choice. Excision with a 3–4-mm margin has a cure rate of about 90–95% for most SCC.
- **Other options:**
  - *Curettage and cautery*: Curettage should be avoided and is reserved for small, low-risk lesions
  - *Radiotherapy*: If surgery is not feasible
  - **Medical management** is not usually considered for invasive SCC. These include photodynamic therapy, systemic retinoids, imiquimod and other immunomodulators, new formulations of 5-fluorouracil, diclofenac in hyaluronic acid gel, and ingenol mebutate.

Malignant Melanoma

Malignant melanoma is a **relatively common** and most serious malignant tumor of epidermal melanocytes. Melanoma has metastatic potential, which can occur early and it causes deaths even in young individual.

Etiology and Pathogenesis

Predisposing factors

A. **Sun exposure:**
   - **Melanomas most commonly develop on sun-exposed surfaces,** particularly the upper back in men and the back and legs in women.
   - **Lightly pigmented** (pale/fair skinned) **individuals** are at **greater risk** than darkly pigmented individuals. Other environmental factors may also contribute to risk.

B. **Inherited genes:**
   About 10–15% of melanomas are familial and the genetic abnormalities are:
   Mutations in tumor suppressor gene: *CDKN2A* gene, RB gene, PTEN gene, mutations of NRAS and BRAF

C. **Other risk factors:** These include multiple melanocytic nevi (>50), sun sensitivity, immunosuppression, giant congenital melanocytic nevi, lentigo maligna, and a family history of malignant melanoma.

Box 22.17: Classification of malignant melanoma of skin.

- **Melanoma without metastatic potential (noninvasive):**
  - Melanoma in situ
  - Lentigo maligna
- **Melanoma with invasive potential:**
  - Superficial spreading melanoma
  - Nodular melanoma
  - Acral lentiginous melanoma
  - Lentigo maligna melanoma
  - Subungual melanoma

Clinical Features

Age and gender: It can occur at any age and either sex, but typically affects the leg in females and back in males. It is rare before puberty.

Sites

- **Skin:** It is the most common site and may develop in the trunk, leg, face, sole, palm, and nail beds.
- **Other sites:** Oral and anogenital mucosal surfaces, esophagus, leptomeninges, eye, and the substantia nigra

Classification of Malignant Melanoma of Skin (Box 22.17)

Clinical signs that help to distinguish malignant from benign moles are presented in **Table 22.7**.

TABLE 22.7: Clinical criteria for the diagnosis of malignant melanoma.

ABCDE features of malignant melanoma:	
Asymmetry of mole	**D**iameter >6 mm
Border irregularity	**E**levation irregular
Color variegation	(+ Loss of skin markings)
The Glasgow 7-point checklist	
Major criteria	***Minor criteria***
➢ Change in size	➢ Diameter >6 mm
➢ Change in shape	➢ Inflammation
➢ Change in color	➢ Mild itch or altered sensation
	➢ Oozing or bleeding

Management/Treatment
- **Surgical excision:** For local disease, surgical excision is the only curative treatment.
  - **Metastatic disease:** If there is sentinel node metastasis, surgical resection of lymph nodes, isolated limb perfusion, radiotherapy, immunotherapy (peginterferon α-2b, ipilimumab (anti-CTLA-4), vemurafenib, dabrafenib (BRAF inhibitor), trametinib (MEK inhibitor), pembrolizumab (PD-1 blocker), and chemotherapy may be required.

Mycosis Fungoides

Mycosis fungoides (MF) is a cutaneous lymphoma of mature CD4+ T-cells. This is the most common cutaneous T-cell lymphoma. Not all cutaneous T-cell lymphomas are MF.
- Incidence—3 per million (0.29 per 100,000 population in USA) and 2% of all new cases of NHL
- Age—Older adults (55–60 years)
- Male:Female—2:1

Clinical Features

Mycosis fungoides patches are usually distributed in sun-shielded areas such as those covered by a bathing suit or intertriginous regions. The cardinal features of MF are infiltration of epidermis and then dermis by atypical cerebriform lymphoid cells—**Pautrier's microabscess.** It is a chronic, slowly progressive disease that evolves from patch stage to plaque stage and subsequently to nodule/tumor stage. A diagnosis of **Sézary syndrome** is made when there is high number of these cells circulating in the peripheral blood in the presence of a lymphadenopathy and cutaneous erythroderma occupying >80% of the body surface area.

Chemotherapy, retinoids, electron beam therapy, and photochemotherapy are used in the treatment.

PHAKOMATOSES

Neurocutaneous Syndromes

Q. Write short note on neurocutaneous syndromes.

- They are group of inherited syndromes characterized by involvement of the brain and skin (sometimes retina).
- Phakomatoses (or neuro-oculocutaneous syndromes) are multisystem disorders that have characteristic central nervous system, ocular and cutaneous lesions (embryologically all originate from ectoderm) of variable severity.

Common Neurocutaneous Syndromes (Box 22.18)

Box 22.18: Common neurocutaneous syndromes.

- Neurofibromatosis I and II
- Tuberous sclerosis
- Von Hippel–Lindau disease
- Sturge–Weber syndrome
- Klippel–Trenaunay–Weber syndrome
- Osler–Weber–Rendu syndrome
- Wyburn–Mason syndrome
- Linear sebaceous nevus syndrome
- Neurocutaneous melanosis
- Waardenburg syndrome type 1 and 2
- Fabry's disease
- Lentiginosis, deafness, and cardiopathy syndrome
- Hypomelanosis of Ito
- Ataxia–telangiectasia (Louis–Bar syndrome)
- Xeroderma pigmentosum (**Fig. 22.18**)
- Cockayne's syndrome
- Rothmund–Thomson syndrome
- Sjögren–Larsson syndrome
- Neuroichthyosis
- Werner syndrome and Progeria
- Incontinentia pigmenti
- Neurocutaneous melanosis
- Retinal-neurocutaneous cavernous hemangioma syndrome (Weskamp–Cotlier syndrome)

Neurofibromatosis Type 1

Q. Write short note on neurofibromatosis.

- *Synonyms*: von Recklinghausen disease and Watson disease
- An autosomal-dominant neurogenetic disorder
- NF1 affects about 1 in 3000 people. Neurofibromatosis type I (NF1) is caused by mutation in the neurofibromin gene located on chromosome 17, at the band q11.2.

Diagnostic Criteria for Neurofibromatosis Type 1 (Box 22.19)

Box 22.19: Diagnostic criteria for neurofibromatosis type 1.

Two or more of the following clinical features must be present:
- Six or more café-au-lait macules of >5 mm in greatest diameter in prepubertal individuals, and >15 mm in greatest diameter in postpubertal individuals
- Two or more neurofibromas of any type (**Fig. 22.19**) or one plexiform neurofibroma
- Freckling in the axillary or inguinal regions
- Optic glioma
- Two or more iris hamartomas (Lisch nodules) (**Fig. 22.20**)
- Distinctive bony lesion, such as sphenoid dysplasia, or thinning of the long bone cortex with or without pseudoarthrosis
- A first-degree relative (parent, sibling, or offspring) with NF1 based on the above criteria

Three subtypes of neurofibromas exist: Cutaneous, subcutaneous, and plexiform. Freckles can be present since birth or sometimes appear later in life especially in the intertriginous region **(Crowe's sign).**

Button hole sign: Molluscum fibrosum—small, superficial, soft, skin-colored to darker, dome-shaped nodules, which can be pushed through a defect in the skin.

Neurofibromatosis Type 2

- Neurofibromatosis type 2 (NF2) is associated with abnormalities of the *NF2* gene, which is located on chromosome 22.
- The *NF2* gene produces merlin, also known as schwannomin, a cell membrane-related protein that acts as a tumor suppressor. NF2 has an estimated birth frequency of 1 in 33,000 to 40,000.

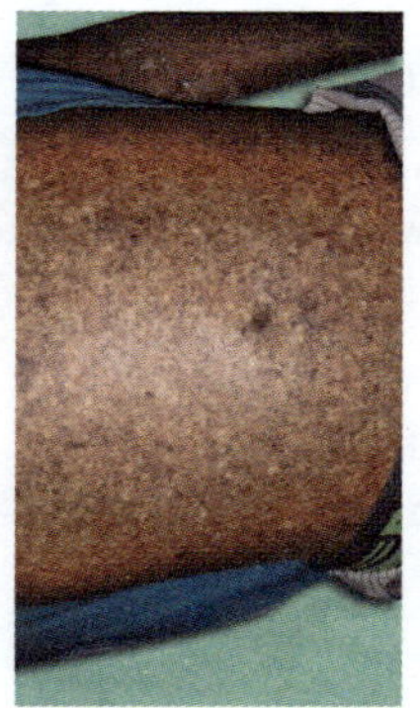

FIG. 22.18: Xeroderma pigmentosum.

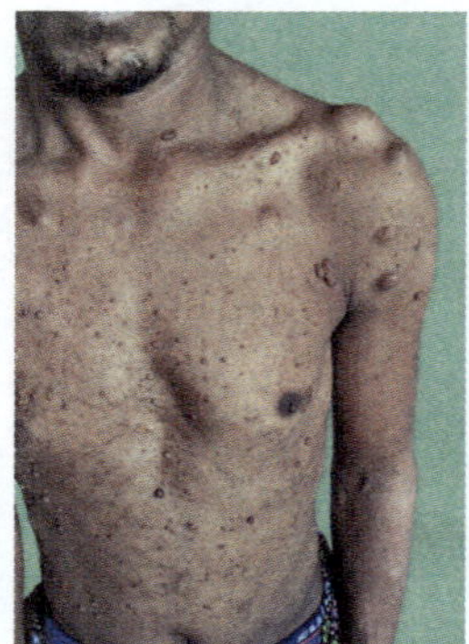

FIG. 22.19: Neurofibromatosis.

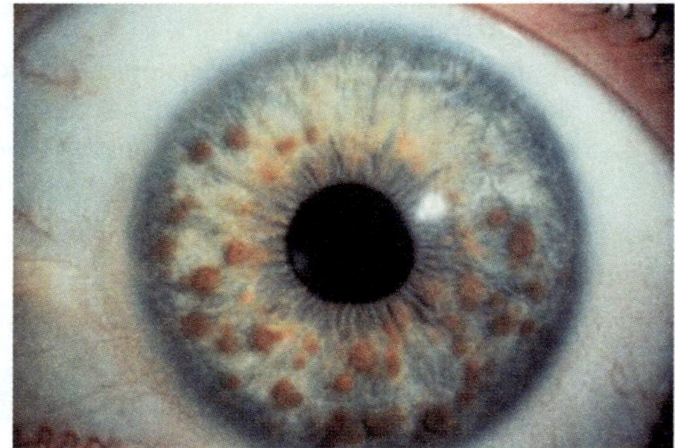

FIG. 22.20: Iris nodules (Lisch nodules) in neurofibromatosis.

Diagnostic criteria for NF2 are listed in Box 22.20.

Box 22.20: Diagnostic criteria for neurofibromatosis type 2.

- Bilateral vestibular schwannomas
- A first-degree relative with NF2 and:
  - Unilateral vestibular schwannoma or
  - Any two of—meningioma, schwannoma, glioma, neurofibroma, and posterior subcapsular lenticular opacities*
- Unilateral vestibular schwannoma and
  - Any two of—meningioma, schwannoma, glioma, neurofibroma, and posterior subcapsular lenticular opacities*
- Multiple meningiomas and
  - Unilateral vestibular schwannoma or
  - Any two of—schwannoma, glioma, neurofibroma, and cataract

*Any two of = Two individual tumors or cataract.

Tuberous Sclerosis

Q. Write short note on tuberous sclerosis.

- Tuberous sclerosis complex is an inherited neurocutaneous disorder characterized by pleomorphic features involving many organ systems, including multiple benign hamartomas of the brain, eyes, heart, lung, liver, kidney, and skin.
- It is called as **Bourneville disease**, as it was first described by him in 1880.
- Clinical triad of Vogt—**EPI-LOI-A:** Epilepsy, low intelligence, and adenoma sebaceum (**Fig. 22.21A**).
- Incidence—1 in 6,000–9,000
- Dominant inheritance but a high frequency of spontaneous mutation

Diagnostic criteria for tuberous sclerosis complex are given in **Table 22.8**.

TABLE 22.8: Diagnostic criteria for tuberous sclerosis complex (TSC).

Major features	***Minor features***
➢ Facial angiofibromas or forehead plaque	➢ Multiple randomly distributed pits in dental enamel
➢ Nontraumatic ungual or periungual fibroma	➢ Hamartomatous rectal polyps
➢ Hypomelanotic macules (more than three) (**Fig. 22.21B**)	➢ Bone cysts
➢ Shagreen patch (connective tissue nevus) (**Fig. 22.21C**)	➢ Cerebral white matter migration lines
➢ Multiple retinal nodular hamartomas	➢ Gingival fibromas
➢ Cortical tuber	➢ Non-renal hamartoma
➢ Subependymal nodule	➢ Retinal achromic patch
➢ Subependymal giant cell astrocytoma	➢ "Confetti" skin lesions
➢ Cardiac rhabdomyoma—single or multiple	➢ Multiple renal cysts
➢ Lymphangiomyomatosis	
➢ Renal angiomyolipoma	
Definite TSC: Either two major features or one major feature with two minor features Probable TSC: One major feature and one minor feature Possible TSC: Either one major feature or two or more minor features	

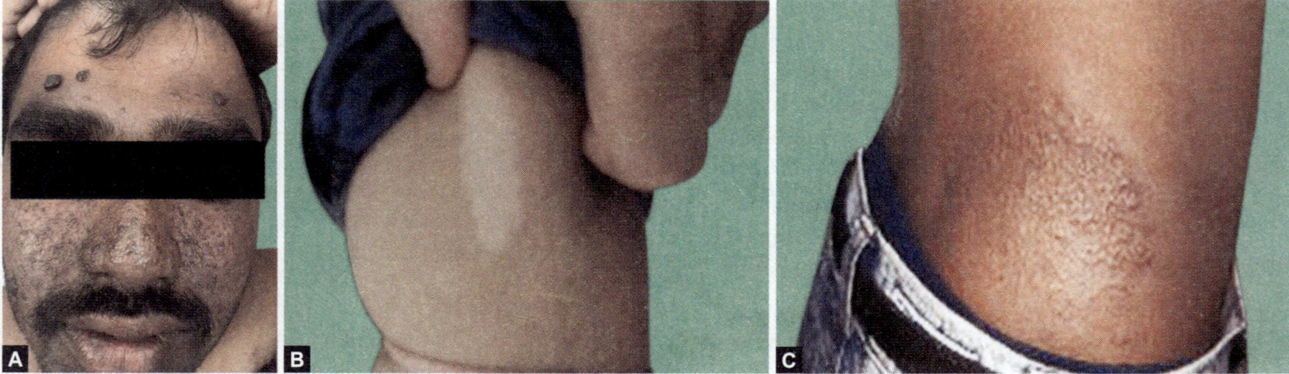

FIGS. 22.21A TO C: (A) Adenoma sebaceum; (B) Ash leaf-shaped macule is a hypopigmented macule oval at one end and pointed at the opposite end; (C) Shagreen patches.

Café-au-lait Macules

Q. Write short note on café-au-lait macules (CALMs).

- These are well-circumscribed, evenly pigmented macules (**Fig. 22.22**); size ranges from 1 to 2 mm to >20 cm.
- Microscopically shows increased melanin in both melanocytes and basal keratinocytes.
- In McCune-Albright syndrome, CALM may have a block-like distribution with midline demarcation and an irregular, jagged outline ("coast of Maine").
- In NF1, there is more numbers of CALM and has more widespread distribution (with the exception of segmental NF1), which is "typical" based on their regular borders, smooth ("coast of California") and uniform pigmentation. In adults, the presence of six or more café-au-lait macules is highly suggestive of NF1.
- In fair-skinned infants, they may be difficult to detect on routine physical examination, but are accentuated with examination under a Wood's lamp.
- CALMs may be observed in tuberous sclerosis, ataxia telangiectasia, Bloom's syndrome, and Watson's syndrome.

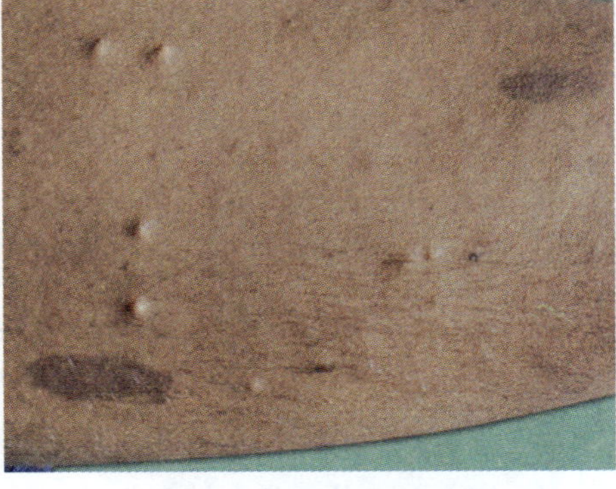

FIG. 22.22: Café-au-lait macules (CALMs).

TABLE 22.9: Factors that induce or exacerbate acne vulgaris (secondary acne).

- **Endocrine causes:** Polycystic ovary syndrome, Cushing's syndrome, congenital adrenal hyperplasia, androgen-secreting tumors of adrenals, ovary and testis, and acromegaly
- **Drugs:**
  - **Glucocorticoids:** Systemic and local agents
  - **Hormones:** Adrenocorticotropic hormone, testosterone, gonadotropins, and oral contraceptives
  - **Halides:** Iodides and bromides
  - **Anabolic:** Danazol and stanozolol
  - **Anticonvulsants/antiepileptics:** Phenytoin, carbamazepine, topiramate, gabapentin, and lithium
  - **Antidepressants:** Amitriptyline, lithium, and sertraline
  - **Antituberculous:** Isoniazid and rifampicin
  - **Chemotherapeutic agents:** Dactinomycin, pentostatin, and gefitinib
  - **Antineoplastic drugs:** Epidermal growth factor receptor (EGFR) inhibitor, and cetuximab
  - **Antiviral:** Ritonavir and ganciclovir
  - **Vitamins:** B_6 and B_{12}
- **Occupational exposures:** To cutting oils, chlorinated aromatic hydrocarbons, and coal tars
- **Conditions favoring occlusion of sebaceous glands**, e.g., heavy clothing, greasy cosmetics, and tropical climates
- **Genetic factors**

DISORDERS OF SKIN APPENDAGES

Acne Vulgaris

Q. Write short note on etiology, clinical features, and management of acne vulgaris.

- Acne is a multifactorial disease characterized by abnormalities in sebum production, follicular desquamation, bacterial proliferation, and inflammation.
- **Age and gender:** It starts after puberty and is seen primarily in teenagers (12–20 years of age) and young adults. 85% adolescents experience it. Prevalence of comedones in adolescents approaches 100%. But, it can persist into the thirties and forties, particularly in females. It affects both males and females, although males tend to have more severe disease.

Cutibacterium acnes, Staphylococcus epidermis, and *Malassezia furfur* induce inflammation and induce follicular epidermal proliferation.

Clinical Features (Table 22.9)

- **Sites:** Most common location for acne is the face (**Fig. 22.23**), but it may involve the chest and back (trunk).
- Greasiness of the skin (seborrhea) is often observed.
- **Type of lesions:** The hallmark is the **comedone.**

Microcomedone

- *Hyperkeratotic plug made of sebum and keratin in follicular canal*
- These comedones may be noninflammatory or inflammatory type (open or closed comedones)
- Open comedones (blackheads) appear as black papules due to the keratin debris and closed comedones (white heads) usually have no visible follicular opening. Inflammatory papules, nodules, and cysts may arise from comedones.

Sequelae: Most cases remain mild and do not lead to scarring. Few may develop large inflammatory cysts and nodules and may heal by significant scarring. Solid facial edema (Morbihan's disease) is a rare complication of acne that presents as facial soft-tissue edema and erythema. Postinflammatory hyperpigmentation and bacterial folliculitis can be seen.

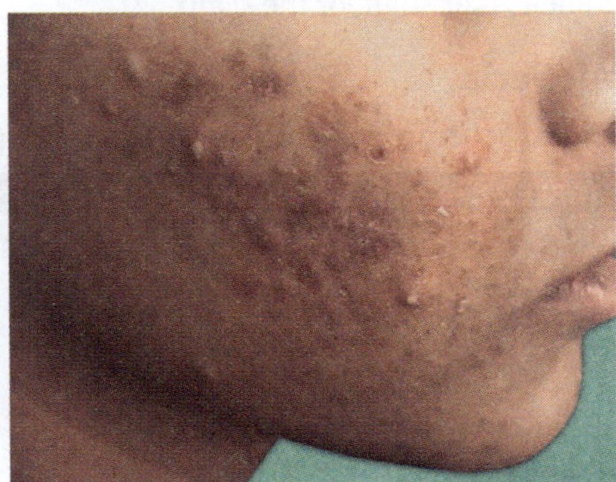

FIG. 22.23: Acne vulgaris.

Grading of acne

- *Grade 1*: Comedones. They are of two types—open and closed. Open comedones are due to plugging of the pilosebaceous orifice by sebum on the skin surface. Closed comedones are due to keratin and sebum plugging the pilosebaceous orifice below the skin surface.
- *Grade 2*: Inflammatory lesions present as a small papule with erythema.
- *Grade 3*: Pustules
- *Grade 4*: Many pustules coalesce to form nodules and cysts

Clinical variants

- **Acne conglobata** is rare and commonly affects adult males. It is a severe form of acne characterized by numerous comedones, large abscesses with sinuses, grouped inflammatory nodules associated with suppuration. It may be associated with **hidradenitis suppurativa** (a chronic, inflammatory disorder of apocrine glands, mainly affecting axillae and groins), folliculitis, and pilonidal sinus.
- **Acne fulminans** is a rare, severe variant of acne, usually affecting the trunk in adolescent males. It presents with fever, arthralgias, and systemic inflammation, with leukocytosis and raised plasma viscosity.
- **Acne excoriée** (also known as "picker's acne") is self-inflicted excoriations produced by compulsive picking of pre-existing or imagined acne lesions. It is usually observed in teenage girls with psychological problems.
- **SAPHO syndrome:** Synovitis, Acne, Pustulosis, Hyperostosis, and Osteitis syndrome
- **Acne venenata:** Contact with acnegenic chemicals can produce comedones. For example, chlorinated hydrocarbons, cutting oils, petroleum oil, and coal tar
- **Acne aestivalis** (Mallorca acne): It is rare and seen in females 25–40 years. It starts in spring and resolves by fall characterized by small papules on cheeks, neck, and upper body. Comedones and pustules are sparse or absent.

Management

Mild-to-moderate disease

Local therapy:

- Areas affected with acne should be kept clean by regular washing with soap and water. However, vigorous scrubbing may cause mechanical rupture of comedones.
- Topical agents such as benzoyl peroxide (most cost-effective therapy), retinoids [tretinoin (most potent keratolytic agent), adapalene (less irritating), or tazarotene], or salicylic acid should be used.
- *Topical antibacterial agents*: Inflammatory acne responds to topical antibacterial agents such as azelaic acid, topical erythromycin, or clindamycin.
- Topical Dapsone

Systemic therapy:

- *Antibiotics*: Moderate inflammatory acne will benefit from the addition of systemic therapy such as oral tetracycline (oxytetracycline or lymecycline), doxycycline (200 mg/day), or minocycline (200 mg/day) for 3–6 months.
- *Hormonal therapy*: These include estrogen-containing oral contraceptives or a combined estrogen/anti-androgen (such as cyproterone acetate) contraceptive.

Moderate-to-severe disease

- **Isotretinoin:** Moderate-to-severe acne or if there is no adequate response to 6 months of therapy with the other therapies (combined systemic and topical approaches), patients should be considered for isotretinoin (13-*cis*-retinoic acid).
  - **Mechanism of action:** It decreases sebaceous gland size and sebum excretion, decreases follicular hypercornification and reduces *P. acnes* colonization.
  - **Side effects:** Oral isotretinoin is teratogenic (prevent pregnancy while taking isotretinoin), and possibly associated risk for severe depression, pseudotumor cerebri and other significant side effects.

Other treatments and physical measures:

- **For inflamed acne nodules or cysts:** They may require intralesional injections of **triamcinolone acetonide or** incision and drainage, **or** excision under local anesthesia.
- **Scarring:** Prevention of scarring by adequate treatment of active acne. Keloid scars respond to intralesional steroid injection and/or silicone dressings. Other measures for scarring include carbon dioxide laser, microdermabrasion, chemical peeling, or localized excision.
- **UVB phototherapy:** They are rarely used in patients with inflammatory acne who are unable to use conventional therapy, such as isotretinoin.

HAIR DISORDERS

Q. List the causes of alopecia.

Alopecia: Alopecia is defined as "absence or loss of hair". It is a chronic disorder secondary to the disease of either the hair follicle, hair shaft, or the scalp.

Alopecia

Classification and Causes of Alopecia (Table 22.10)

TABLE 22.10: Classification and causes of alopecia.

Localized	*Diffuse*
Nonscarring	
A. **Abnormality of cycling:** - Alopecia areata - Syphilitic alopecia B. **Production decline:** - Androgenetic alopecia - Triangular alopecia C. **Hair breakage:** - Trichotillomania - Tinea capitis - Traction alopecia - Primary or acquired hair shaft abnormality	A. **Abnormality of cycling:** - Alopecia areata - Telogen effluvium - Anagen effluvium - Loose anagen syndrome B. **Hair shaft abnormality:** - Hair breakage - Unruly hair C. **Failure of follicle production:** - Congenital universal atrichia - Atrichia with papular lesions - Hereditary vitamin-D-resistant rickets

Contd...

Contd...

	Androgenetic, hypothyroidism, hyperthyroidism, hypopituitarism, diabetes mellitus, HIV, nutritional (especially iron) deficiency, liver disease, postpartum, alopecia areata, syphilis, drug-induced (e.g., chemotherapy and retinoids)
Scarring	
A. **Lymphocytic:** - Chronic cutaneous lupus erythematosus, discoid lupus erythematosus (DLE) - Lichen planopilaris - Classic pseudopelade of Brocq - Alopecia mucinosa B. **Neutrophilic:** - Folliculitis decalvans - Dissecting folliculitis/cellulitis C. **Mixed:** - Folliculitis (acne) keloidalis - Folliculitis (acne) necrotica - Erosive pustular dermatitis	➢ Discoid lupus erythematosus ➢ Radiotherapy ➢ Folliculitis decalvans ➢ Lichen planus

Alopecia Areata

Definition: Rapid and complete loss of hair in one or most often several round or oval patches, usually on the scalp (**Fig. 22.24**), bearded area, eyebrows, eye lashes, and less commonly on other hairy areas of the body.

Approximately 1.7% of the population will experience an episode of alopecia areata during their lifetime.

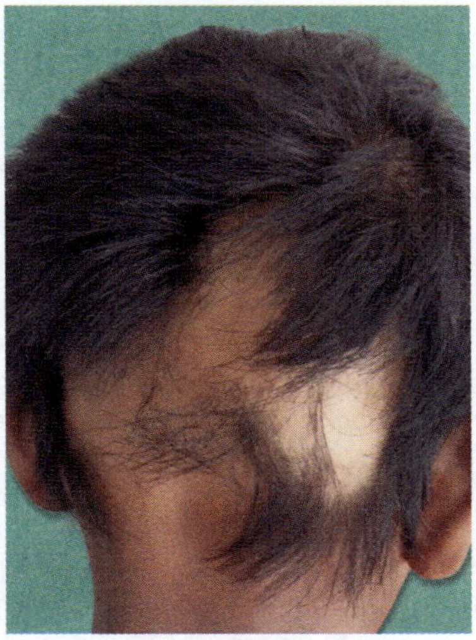

FIG. 22.24: Alopecia areata.

Etiology

It is an autoimmune disease:

- Mediated by the cellular arm (T-cell and macrophages)
- Modified by genetic factors (HLA-R4, DR11, and DQ7)

Stages of Alopecia Areata (Box 22.21)

Box 22.21: Stages of alopecia areata.

- Acute hair loss
- Persistent (chronic) baldness
- Partial telogen to anagen conversion (incomplete recovery)
- Normal recovery

Clinical features

- Rapid and complete loss of hair in one or several patches (**Fig. 22.24**)
- *Site*: Scalp, bearded area, eyebrows, eyelashes, and less commonly other areas of body
- *Size*: Patches of 1–5 cm in diameter
- **Exclamation point hairs,** short broken hairs for which the proximal end of the hair is narrower than the distal end, are pathognomonic finding in alopecia areata.

Alopecia totalis is a more advanced form of alopecia areata, which results in total loss of all hair on the scalp.

Alopecia universalis is the most advanced form of alopecia areata, which results in total loss of all hair on the body, including eyelashes and eyebrows.

Alopecia barbae is alopecia areata that is localized to the beard area. It can be a single bald patch or more extensive hair loss across the whole of the beard area.

Androgenetic Alopecia (Fig. 22.25)

- It is a thinning of the hair to an almost transparent state in both men and women.
- It is hereditary.
- In both men and women, it is linked to having an excess of male hormones (androgens) around the hair follicles, which can block hair growth.
- Women are more likely to develop androgenic alopecia after menopause, when they have fewer female hormones.

Investigations

- *Blood investigations*: Complete blood count, serum ferritin, blood sugar, renal and liver function, hormones (thyroid, FSH, LH, and testosterone), vitamin B_{12}, and vitamin D
- *Trichometric analysis*: The folliscope can magnify these images by up to 100 times, giving doctors a detailed look at hair, hair follicles, and the scalp

- Fungal culture
- Punch biopsy—used to distinguish between the types of cicatricial, or scarring, alopecia.
- *Daily hair counts*:
  - Useful for quantitative assessment of the actual number of hairs shed daily in patients with complaints of excessive shedding. Collect for 14 consecutive days
  - Average daily loss—30–70 hairs/day
  - If >70 hairs—microscopic examination is done to detect pathology

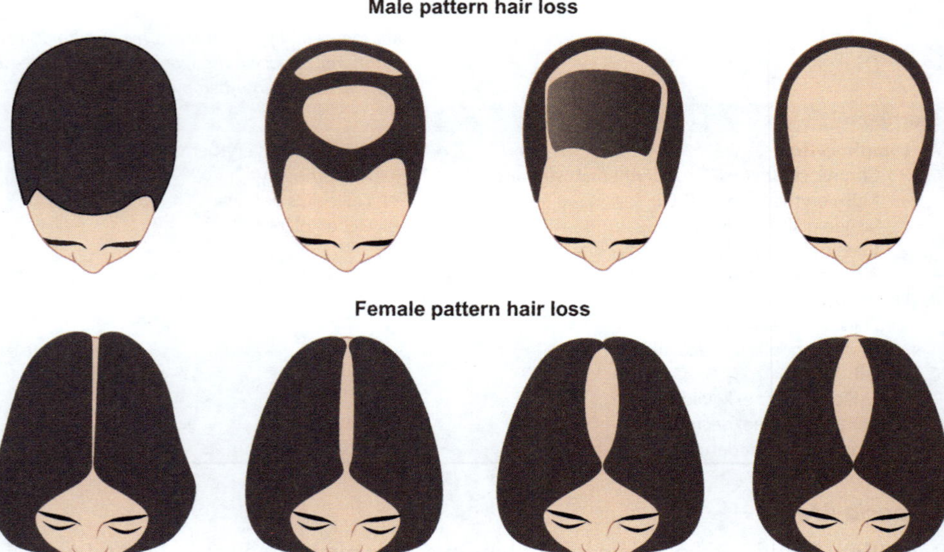

FIG. 22.25: Male and female pattern of hair loss.

Treatment
- Many cases of hair loss are temporary, for example, due to chemotherapy, or they are a natural part of aging and do not need treatment.
- If hair loss is caused by an infection or another condition, treating the underlying problem may help to prevent further hair loss
- Spontaneous recovery is extremely common for patchy alopecia areata.
- *Steroid*: Both local (intralesional and topical) and systemic (in short course)
- *Topical 1% anthralin cream*: Applied for 15–20 minutes and then shampooed off the treated side
- *5% topical minoxidil*: As a single agent or as an adjuvant with topical anthralin
- PUVA
- *Contact sensitizer*: Squaric acid dibutylester, diphencyprone, and dinitrochlorobenzene
- *Finasteride*: It acts by preventing the hormone testosterone being converted to the hormone dihydrotestosterone (DHT). DHT causes the hair follicles to shrink, so blocking its production allows the hair follicles to regain their normal size.
- Psychological support
- Hair transplantation is a surgical technique that removes hair follicles from one part of the body, called the "donor site", to a bald or balding part of the body known as the "recipient site". The technique is primarily used to treat male pattern baldness.
- Follicular unit transplantation (FUT) is a hair restoration technique, also known as the strip procedure, where a patient's hair is transplanted in naturally occurring groups of 1–4 hairs, called follicular units.

LEG ULCERS

Q. Write short note on causes of nonhealing leg ulcer.

Ulceration of the skin is defined as complete epidermal loss. It results in exposure of dermal (or deeper) layers.

Causes of Leg Ulcers (Table 22.11 and Fig. 22.26)

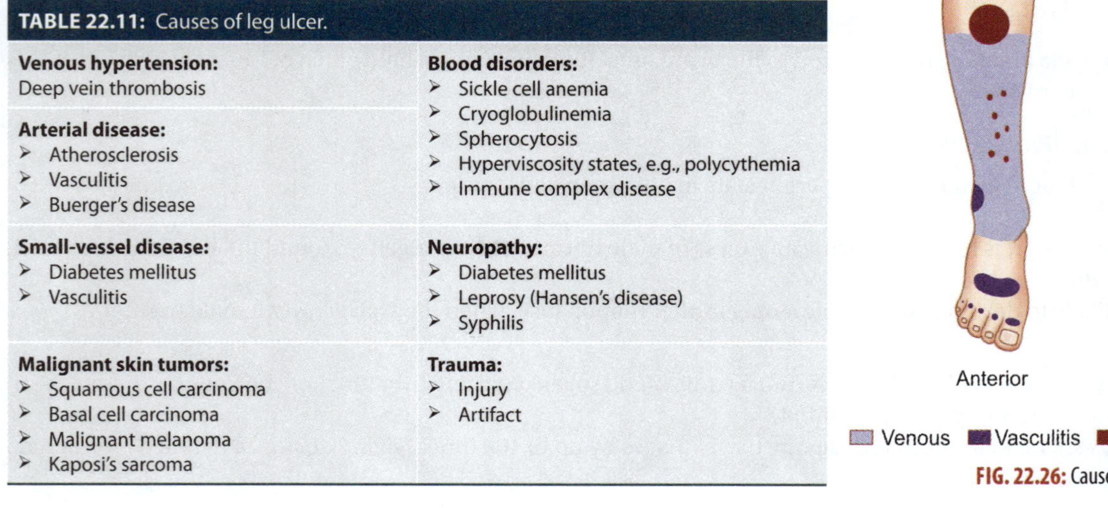

TABLE 22.11: Causes of leg ulcer.

Venous hypertension: Deep vein thrombosis	**Blood disorders:** ➢ Sickle cell anemia ➢ Cryoglobulinemia ➢ Spherocytosis ➢ Hyperviscosity states, e.g., polycythemia ➢ Immune complex disease
Arterial disease: ➢ Atherosclerosis ➢ Vasculitis ➢ Buerger's disease	
Small-vessel disease: ➢ Diabetes mellitus ➢ Vasculitis	**Neuropathy:** ➢ Diabetes mellitus ➢ Leprosy (Hansen's disease) ➢ Syphilis
Malignant skin tumors: ➢ Squamous cell carcinoma ➢ Basal cell carcinoma ➢ Malignant melanoma ➢ Kaposi's sarcoma	**Trauma:** ➢ Injury ➢ Artifact

FIG. 22.26: Causes of leg ulcers.

XEROSTOMIA

Q. Write short note on xerostomia.

- Normal healthy adults daily produce about 1,500 mL of saliva.
- Xerostomia is characterized by dry mouth and may be due to decrease in the production of saliva.

Effects of Xerostomia

- Symptoms may be minor or may hamper activities of daily living.
- May produce burning sensation in mouth, difficulty in eating, chewing, and swallowing
- May produce tooth decay, bad breath, candida infection, and viral infections (e.g., herpes simplex)

Etiology

- **Anticholinergic drugs** (reduce volume of saliva): For example, anticholinergics, antidepressants, antipsychotics, antiemetics, antihistamines, antihypertensives, antiparkinsonian drugs, antispasmodics, and diuretics.
- **Sympathomimetic drugs** (produce viscous saliva): For example, amphetamines, appetite suppressants, decongestants, and bronchodilators
- **Systemic diseases:** Addison's disease, Alzheimer's diseases, salivary gland infection, Sjögren's syndrome, alcoholic cirrhosis, diabetes mellitus, HIV/AIDS, radiation to head and neck region (e.g., for cancer therapy), and severe dehydration.
- **Other causes:** Elderly individuals, sleep-related xerostomia (due to mouth breathing during sleep).

Management

- Stop the offending drug
- Frequent sips of water and teeth brushing
- **Oral hygiene:** Chlorhexidine rinses
- **Artificial salivary substitutes:** They act as lubricant and protective and not as substitutes for digestive and enzymatic actions (e.g., sodium carboxymethyl cellulose, potassium dihydrogen orthophosphate, and sorbitol).
- **Cholinergic agonists:**
  - *Pilocarpine and cevimeline*: It should be cautiously used in patients with cardiovascular disease and chronic respiratory conditions. They are contraindicated in patients with uncontrolled asthma, angle-closure (narrow angle) glaucoma, and liver disease.

PRURITUS

Q. Write short essay/note on pruritus/generalized pruritus and its causes.

The terms "itch" and "pruritus" are used synonymously; however, "pruritus" is often used for generalized itch.

Definition: Itch is an unpleasant cutaneous sensation that leads to scratching or rubbing.

Causes (Box 22.22 and Table 22.12)

Box 22.22: Dermatological causes of pruritus.

- Atopic dermatitis
- Scabies
- Xerosis
- Lichen simplex chronicus
- Contact dermatitis
- Insect bites
- Sunburn
- Ichthyoses
- Dermatitis herpetiformis
- Psoriasis
- Lichen planus
- Fungal infections
- Pediculosis
- Plaster of Paris casts

TABLE 22.12: Systemic causes of pruritus.

Autoimmune: ➢ Dermatitis herpetiformis ➢ Dermatomyositis	**Hepatobiliary:** ➢ Biliary cirrhosis ➢ Drug-induced cholestasis
Hematological: ➢ Hemochromatosis ➢ Mastocytosis ➢ Polycythemia vera	**Metabolic and endocrine:** ➢ Carcinoid syndrome ➢ Chronic renal disease ➢ Diabetes mellitus
Infectious diseases: ➢ AIDS ➢ Infectious hepatitis ➢ Parasitic diseases (e.g., giardiasis and ascariasis)	**Malignancy:** ➢ Leukemia and lymphoma ➢ Multiple myeloma ➢ Solid tumors with paraneoplastic syndrome
Neurologic: ➢ Cerebral abscess ➢ Cerebral tumor	**Others:** ➢ Drug ➢ Pregnancy

Management/Treatment

General measures:

- Avoid soap
- Control of xerosis with moisturizers and humidification of indoor environment

Specific measures:

- Establish the diagnosis and treat the underlying skin or systemic disease
- If a clear-cut diagnosis is not possible, various nonspecific measures can be used for symptom control. It is necessary to reassess intermittently in order to avoid missing the diagnosis.
- UVB (ultraviolet B) phototherapy in chronic kidney disease
- Ursodeoxycholic acid (UDCA) in cholestasis
- Cholestyramine, rifampicin, and opioid antagonists (e.g., naltrexone) in primary biliary cirrhosis
- Corticosteroids in Hodgkin's disease
- Paroxetine (selective serotonin reuptake inhibitor) in itching as paraneoplastic manifestation of malignancies

Symptomatic measures:

- These include sedation, often with H1 antagonist antihistamines, emollients, and counter-irritants (such as topical menthol-containing preparations).
- *Intractable cases*: Phototherapy, low-dose tricyclic antidepressants (e.g., amitriptyline), or gabapentin may help.

Complications of pruritus:

- Prurigo nodularis is a variant of lichen simplex chronicus in which nodules develop at the site of scratching.
- Local infection due to scratching
- Lichen simplex chronicus is localized skin thickening produced due to intense scratching.

PANNICULITIS

- Panniculitis is an inflammatory reaction in the subcutaneous fat tissue.
- Panniculitis may preferentially affect—(1) the lobules of fat (lobular panniculitis with necrosis and purpura) or (2) the connective tissue that separates fat into lobules (septal panniculitis).

Erythema Nodosum

Q. Write short essay/note on the etiology, clinical features, diagnosis, and treatment of erythema nodosum.

- Erythema nodosum (septal panniculitis) is the most common form of panniculitis.
- It is also called subacute migratory panniculitis of Vilanova and Piñol.

Etiology

Factors provoking erythema nodosum: Occurrence of erythema nodosum is often associated with provoking factors (**Box 22.23**). Most often, it is idiopathic without any identifiable underlying cause.

Box 22.23: Triggering factors associated with erythema nodosum.

Infections:
- Bacteria, e.g., **β-hemolytic streptococci,** mycobacteria (usually primary **tuberculosis,** leprosy), *Brucella, Mycoplasma, Rickettsia, Chlamydia, Salmonella, and Yersinia*
- Viruses, e.g., hepatitis B and infectious mononucleosis
- Fungi, e.g., coccidioidomycosis, histoplasmosis, and blastomycosis
- Parasitic, e.g., amebiasis and giardiasis

Drug administration, e.g., **sulfonamides,** sulfonylureas, and oral contraceptives

Systemic disease, e.g., **sarcoidosis,** inflammatory bowel disease, and Behcet's disease

Malignancies: Lymphoma, leukemia, and renal cell carcinoma.

Idiopathic: >50% cases

Clinical Features

Age and gender: Age 20–30 years but any age group may be affected. Female-to-male ratio is 3–6:1.

*Lesions (**Table 22.13 and Fig. 22.27**)*

TABLE 22.13: Features of lesions erythema nodosum.

➤ Sudden onset	➤ Undergo color changes as advance in the duration
➤ Symmetrical	➤ Resolve without scarring or atrophy
➤ Painful	➤ Associated with pyrexia, malaise, headache, and arthralgias
➤ Erythematous	➤ Recurrent episodes are known
➤ Warm	
➤ Nonulcerated nodules/plaques	
➤ Knees, shins, and feet may be at thighs, arms, and face	

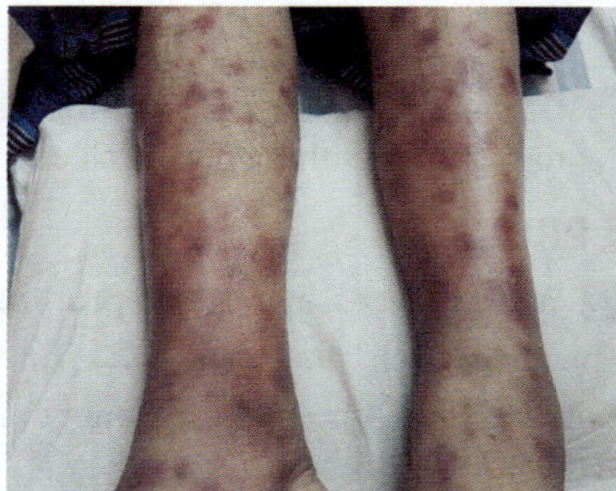

FIG. 22.27: Erythema nodosum on both legs.

Diagnosis

- Most often based on clinical presentation
- **Deep wedge biopsy** including the subcutis is usually required for histologic diagnosis. Histologically shows inflammation of the connective tissue septa in the subcutaneous fat tissue (septal panniculitis). Vasculitis is not observed.
- **Identification of triggering factors causing erythema nodosum:**
  - Complete blood count (CBC) with differential ESR (erythrocyte sedimentation rate) and C-reactive protein level
  - *Evaluation for β-hemolytic streptococcal infection*: Throat culture for group A streptococci, rapid antigen test, anti-streptolysin-O titer, and polymerase chain reaction assay
  - Chest radiograph, e.g., to detect tuberculosis and sarcoidosis—Mantoux test
  - Stool examination for ova and parasite, e.g., in patients with GIT symptoms
  - Evaluation for inflammatory bowel disease in patient with symptoms of IBD

Treatment
- Identify and remove/treat any underlying cause (treatment of tuberculosis/IBD/sarcoid).
- Bed rest, leg elevation, and analgesics with NSAIDs may produce symptomatic relief. However, avoid NSAIDs, if secondary to Crohn disease because they may trigger a flare-up the underlying Crohn disease.
- Systemic corticosteroids must be avoided in cases with infection and malignancy.
- Dapsone and potassium iodide orally (400–900 mg/day) have been effective for stubborn disease (if NSAIDs do not relieve pain or the lesions persist) for symptomatic relief. Recalcitrant, chronic, or recurring EN is treated with thalidomide, colchicine, and hydroxychloroquine.

LEPROSY

Q. Classify and describe the epidemiology, etiology, microbiology pathogenesis and clinical presentations and diagnostic features of leprosy.

Definition: Leprosy (Hansen's disease) is a **chronic, granulomatous,** slowly progressive, destructive infection affecting skin and nerves, caused by *Mycobacterium leprae*.

Epidemiology

- The WHO launched a 5-year "Global Leprosy Strategy 2016–2020" in April, 2016 titled "accelerating towards a leprosy-free world".
- In India, the National Leprosy Eradication Programme (NLEP) is the centrally sponsored health scheme of the Ministry of Health and Family Welfare, Government of India.
- India continues to account for 60% of new cases reported globally each year and is among the 22 "global priority countries" that contribute 95% of world numbers of leprosy warranting a sustained effort to bring the numbers down.
    - **Mode of transmission:** (1) Inoculation/inhalation and (2) Intimate contact
    - **Incubation period:** Generally 2–7 years

Bacteriological Considerations

- *Mycobacterium leprae* is an acid and alcohol fast, intracellular bacillus.
- Lepra bacilli survive and grow better at a temperature below that of the internal organs (close to 30°C rather than 37°C). Hence, it affects sites such as skin, peripheral nerves, the mucosa of the upper airways, and other tissues (bone, eyes, testis, and some viscera).
- *Mycobacterium leprae* can be grown in the footpads of mice and **nine-banded armadillos. Cannot be cultured** on artificial media or in cell culture.

Classification (Fig. 22.28)

In the early stage, disease may be indeterminate and may either spontaneously undergo remission or develop into overt leprosy.

A. **Ridley and Jopling (1966) classification:** It depends on the clinicopathological spectrum of the disease, which is **determined by the immune resistance of the host.**
    - **Tuberculoid leprosy (TT):** It is the polar form that has maximal immune response. It is characterized by single or few sharply demarcated skin lesions with predominant peripheral nerve involvement. The bacilli are usually absent or difficult to demonstrate.
    - **Borderline tuberculoid (BT):** In this type, the immune response falls between BB and TT.
    - **Borderline leprosy (BB):** It exactly falls between two polar forms of leprosy.
    - **Borderline lepromatous (BL)** has the immune response that falls between BB and LL.
    - **Lepromatous leprosy (LL):** It is the other polar form with least immune response. This is characterized by extensive, diffuse, and bilaterally symmetrical skin lesions that contain numerous bacilli. The peripheral nerves are better preserved than in the tuberculoid form.
    - **Indeterminate type:** When the biopsy sample shows definite diagnostic evidence of leprosy (both nerve involvement and acid-fast bacilli) but clinically not fitting to the leprosy spectrum.

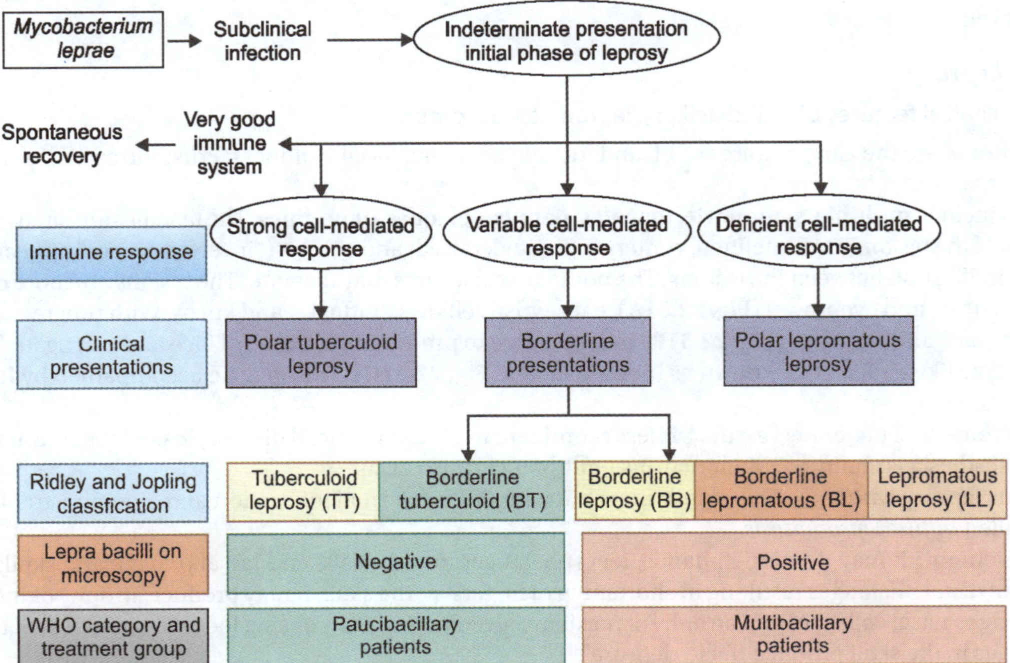

FIG. 22.28: Classification of leprosy.

B. **WHO classification:**
- *Paucibacillary*: All cases of tuberculoid leprosy and some cases of borderline type
- *Multibacillary*: All cases of lepromatous leprosy and some cases of borderline type bacilli are present in large numbers, and hence the term multibacillary (MB).

Clinical Features

Tuberculoid Leprosy

Q. Discuss the clinical features of tuberculoid leprosy.

- **Skin lesions:** The early features consist of one or few, localized, well-demarcated, dry, elevated, **hypoesthetic, red or hypopigmented** macules (**Fig. 22.29A**). Later, the lesions become larger, margins elevated and circinate or gyrate. Fully developed lesions are anesthetic and show loss of sweat glands and hair follicles.
- **Nerve involvement** occurs early and is **the dominating feature** in tuberculoid leprosy. It is usually asymmetric and the involved nerves (**Fig. 22.29B**) are thickened and palpable. Routinely, the nerves such as ulnar, peroneal (lateral popliteal), and greater auricular nerves should be palpated. Sometimes, TT may present with only nerve involvement without any skin lesions **(neural leprosy or pure neuritic leprosy).** Consequences (complications) of nerve involvement are:
  - **Sensory nerve involvement** produces sensory dysfunctions such as glove and stocking anesthesia (more common in LL), chronic nonhealing, plantar ulcers, and repeated injuries to hands and feet (leading to **autoamputation** of fingers or toes).
  - **Motor nerve involvement** produces muscle weakness, wasting, and later paralysis followed by contractures. Nerves involved and their consequences are as follows:
    - **Ulnar nerve:** Claw hand (main en griffe) (**Fig. 22.30**)
    - **Median nerve:** Ape hand (main de singe)
    - **Lateral popliteal nerve:** Foot drop
    - **Posterior tibial nerve:** Claw toes or hammer toes
  - **Autonomic involvement** produces anhidrosis or hyperhidrosis
  - **Cranial nerve involvement:** Facial nerve is commonly affected and results in facial paralysis, lagophthalmos, exposure keratitis, and corneal ulcerations (may lead to blindness). Trigeminal nerve involvement may develop early causing loss of corneal reflex. Greater auricular nerve (**Fig. 22.29B**), supraorbital, supratrochlear, and infraorbital nerves are also thickened.

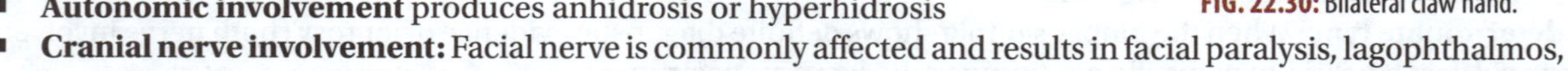

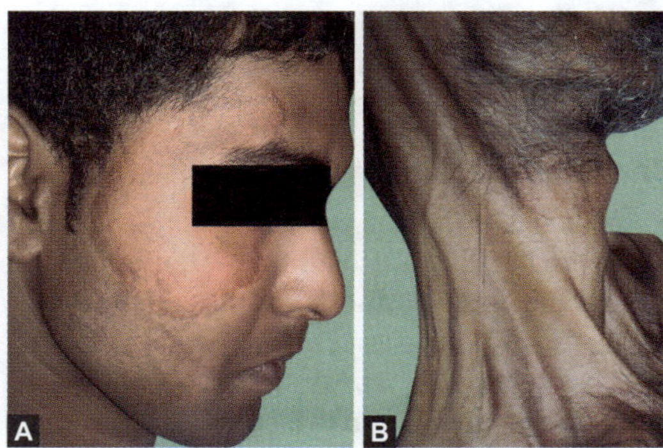

FIGS. 22.29A AND B: Lesions of tuberculoid leprosy: (A) Hypopigmented macules on face; (B) Visible greater auricular nerve thickening.

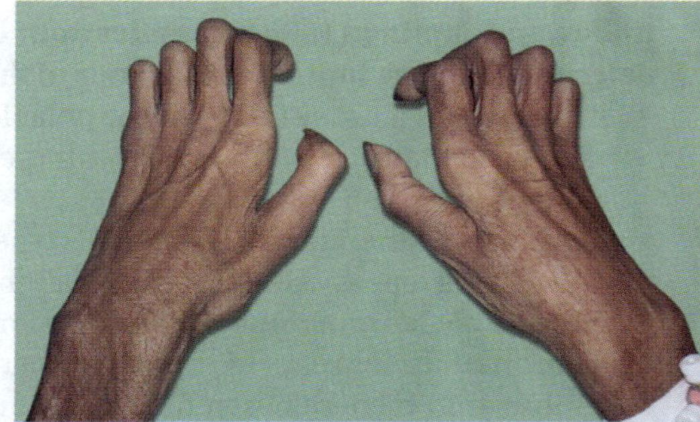

FIG. 22.30: Bilateral claw hand.

Lepromatous Leprosy

Q. Discuss the clinical features of multibacillary/lepromatous leprosy.

- **Nasal symptoms** are the early features of LL and include anosmia, nasal stuffiness, crust formation, and blood-stained nasal discharge.
- **Skin lesions** include **multiple, symmetric, macules, papules,** plaques, **or nodules**. The macules are often hypopigmented. The borders of the lesions are ill-defined, centers indurated, raised, and convex ("inverted saucer" appearance). There is also diffuse infiltration between the lesions. The nodular skin lesions may ulcerate. The lesions are more common on the face (cheeks, nose, and eyebrows) (**Fig. 22.31A**), ears, wrists, elbows, buttocks, and knees. With progression, the nodular lesions in the face and ear lobes (**Fig. 22.31B**) may coalesce to produce thickening of face and corrugated forehead. This produces a lion-like appearance known as **leonine facies** (**Fig. 22.31C**). This may be accompanied by loss of eyebrows and eyelashes.
- **Nerve involvement** of major nerve trunks is less prominent in LL. In advanced disease, **loss of sensation with** "glove and stocking" anesthesia is common. Mononeuritis multiplex can also occur.
- Lepromatous leprosy without visible skin lesions but with diffuse dermal infiltration and a demonstrable thickening of dermis is called *diffuse lepromatosis*.
- **Bone involvement:** It may develop in hands, feet (phalanges, metatarsals, and tarsal bones), and skull. It causes slow absorption of distal phalanges resulting in shortening of fingers. In the skull, it may produce atrophy of the anterior nasal spine (leading to nasal collapse) and atrophy of maxillary alveolar process (causing loosening and loss of upper incisors). These changes in the skull produce "facies leprosa".

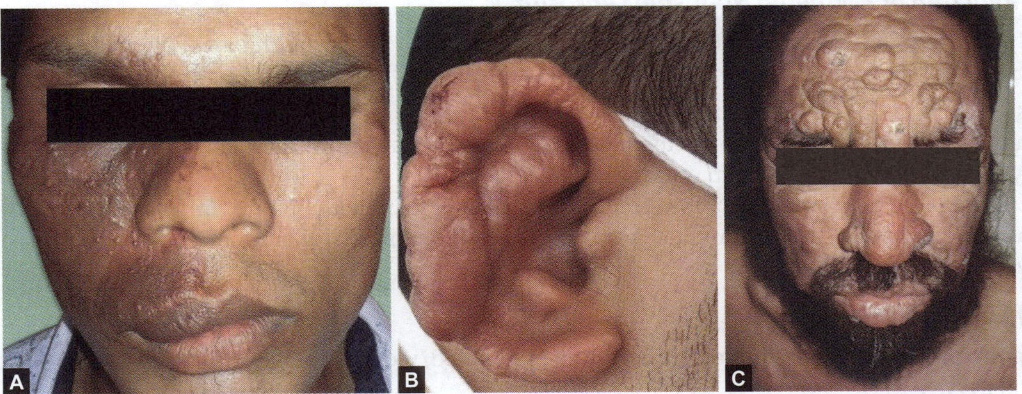

FIGS. 22.31A TO C: Lesions of lepromatous leprosy: (A) Facial involvement; (B) Nodular lesions on ear; (C) Leonine facies.

- **Other features:**
  - **Bilateral edema** of legs and ankles
  - **Saddle nose:** Swollen and broad nose, septal perforation, and nasal collapses produce saddle nose deformity.
  - **Teeth:** Loosening of upper incisor teeth, which may later fall off
  - **Anterior chamber of the eye** involvement results in keratitis, iridocyclitis, and **blindness.**
  - **Upper airways:** Chronic nasal discharge, laryngitis, palatal perforation, and hoarseness (voice change).
  - **Testes:** Usually severely involved, leading to destruction of the seminiferous tubules, testicular atrophy, impotence, infertility, and gynecomastia.
  - **Painless lymphadenopathy** involving inguinal and axillary lymph nodes
  - **Renal lesions:** Secondary glomerulonephritis, interstitial nephritis, pyelonephritis, and renal amyloidosis

Q. **Enumerate and describe the complications of leprosy and its management.**

Complications of lepromatous leprosy are summarized in **Table 22.14**.

TABLE 22.14: Complications of lepromatous leprosy.

- **Permanent nerve damage with sensory loss** (usually begins in extremities):
  - Leading to skin ulcers
  - "Glove and stocking" anesthesia
  - Mononeuritis multiplex
- **Infection of skin ulcers**
- **Disfiguration of the face** (leonine facies)
- **Eye damage:** Keratitis, iridocyclitis, and blindness
- **Upper airways:**
  - *Nasal damage*: Anosmia, nasal stuffiness, crust formation, and blood-stained nasal discharge
  - Laryngitis, palatal perforation, and hoarseness (voice change)
- **Muscle weakness:** Claw-like hands or an inability to flex the feet
- **Bone involvement:**
  - *Hands and feet*: Slow absorption of distal phalanges (shortening of fingers)
  - *Skull*: Nasal collapse and atrophy of maxillary alveolar process, saddle nose
- **Testes:** Testicular atrophy, impotence, infertility, and gynecomastia
- **Renal lesions:** Secondary glomerulonephritis, interstitial nephritis, pyelonephritis, and renal amyloidosis

Borderline Leprosy

Clinical features are poorly defined and these overlap with features of other subtypes.

Reactions in Leprosy or Lepra Reactions

Immunity in leprosy may change spontaneously or following treatment. The course of leprosy may be interrupted by lepra reactions, which comprise several common immunologically mediated inflammatory states. There are two types of lepra reactions. Both types of reactions can occur in untreated patients, but more often develop as complications of chemotherapy.

Type I Lepra Reaction

Q. **Enumerate, describe, and identify lepra reactions and supportive measures and therapy of lepra reactions.**

Borderline leprosy (BT, BB, or BL) is the **most unstable form of leprosy** where **immune status may shift up or down and** type I reaction occurs in 50% of these patients. These are delayed hypersensitivity reactions and may be of two types: **Downgrading reaction and reversal reaction.**

1. **Downgrading reaction:** If type I lepra reactions precede the initiation of appropriate antimicrobial therapy, they are termed as downgrading reactions. It is associated with decrease of immunity and histologically the disease moves (usually from borderline) toward lepromatous leprosy.
2. **Upgrading/reversal reaction:** If type I lepra reactions occur after the initiation of antimicrobial therapy, they are termed as reversal reactions. It is associated with improved immunity and histologically the disease moves (usually from borderline) toward tuberculoid leprosy. It develops usually in the 1st month or year after the initiation of therapy but may also occur after several years.

Manifestations: Existing skin lesions (i.e., macules, papules, and plaques) develop classic signs of inflammation in the form of erythema and swelling and new skin lesions may appear. Peripheral nerves inflammation (i.e., neuritis) causes pain and exquisitely tenderness of nerves. Irreversible nerve damage may occur suddenly (24 hours) unless the reaction is treated promptly.

Type 2 Lepra Reaction or Erythema Nodosum Leprosum

It occurs mostly in lepromatous leprosy (BL/LL) particularly within 2 years of institution of chemotherapy. It develops due to widespread immune-complex deposition (type III hypersensitivity reactions) and overproduction of tumor necrosis factor (TNF-α).

Manifestations

- **Crops** of painful, tender inflamed, red, subcutaneous papules or plaque (on the face and limbs) that resolve spontaneously in a few days to a week but new crops may appear.
- Severe reactions may be accompanied by low-grade fever, malaise, lymphadenopathy symptoms of neuritis, and arthralgia.
- **Other features** include uveitis, iritis, orchitis, myositis, glomerulonephritis, edema, anemia, leukocytosis, and abnormal liver function tests.

Diagnosis of Leprosy

- **Clinical diagnosis** is by cardinal signs of leprosy: Hypopigmented/reddish patches with loss of sensation and thickening of peripheral nerves
- **Slit-skin smears:** The smears are made from skin lesions (earlobes and dorsum of the ring or middle finger) by scraped-incision method and the dermal material (fluid obtained) on to a glass slide and stained for acid-fast bacilli (AFB). It is useful in borderline lepromatous (BL) and LL.
- **Nasal secretions** for AFB from LL show numerous bacilli.
- **Lepromin test:** Lepromin is an antigen extract of dead *M. leprae*. The test is performed like the tuberculin test by intradermal injection of lepromin but is read after 4 weeks. It is **not a diagnostic test** for leprosy. It is **used for classifying** the leprosy based on the immune response. It is **interpreted** as follows:
  - **Lepromatous leprosy** shows **negative lepromin test** due to suppression of cell-mediated immunity.
  - **Tuberculoid leprosy** shows **positive lepromin test** because of delayed hypersensitivity reaction.
  - **Borderline leprosy:** Negative or weakly positive responses
- **Skin biopsy:** Involvement of peripheral nerves in a skin biopsy taken from the affected area is pathognomonic, even in the absence of bacilli. Lepra bacilli can be demonstrated in LL and BL types by Fite–Ferraco stain.
- **Serological test** is not sensitive or specific enough for diagnosis.
  - Hypergammaglobulinemia is common in LL and can give false-positive serological tests (VDRL, rheumatoid factor, and antinuclear antibodies).
  - IgM antibodies to PGL-1 (phenolic glycolipid-1) may be found in 95% of LL and in 60% of TT. However, these antibodies may also be present in normal individuals.
- **PCR testing** for *M. leprae* DNA: Detection of *M. leprae* DNA is possible in all types of leprosy using the polymerase chain reaction, but not sensitive or specific enough for diagnosis. It can be used to assess the efficacy of treatment.

Q. Enumerate the indications and describe the pharmacology, administration, and adverse reaction of pharmacotherapies for various classes of leprosy based on national guidelines.

Q. Describe the treatment of leprosy based on the World Health Organization (WHO) guidelines.

Multibacillary leprosy (MB): Duration of treatment is 1 year/12 months

- **Regimen 1:**
  - Dapsone 2 mg/kg daily (maximum 100 mg)
  - Clofazimine 50 mg daily or 100 mg three times a week
  - Rifampicin, 450 mg (for patients <35 kg) or 600 mg (for patients <35 kg), on 2 consecutive days in a month
- **Regimen 2:**
  - Dapsone 100 mg daily (self-administered)
  - Clofazimine 50 mg daily (self-administered) + 300 mg once a month (supervised)
  - Rifampicin 600 mg once a month (supervised)

Paucibacillary leprosy (PB): Duration of treatment is 6 months

- Dapsone 100 mg given daily
- Rifampicin 600 mg is given once a month under supervision.
- Clofazimine 50 mg daily (self-administered) + 300 mg once a month (supervised) -- New addition in 2020

Treatment

Drugs

- Main drugs available include dapsone (100 mg), rifampicin (600 mg), clofazimine (100 mg), ethionamide (500 mg), and thiacetazone (150 mg). Other drugs effective against leprosy are ofloxacin, minocycline, and clarithromycin.
- **Side effects** of various drugs are as follows:
  - **Dapsone:** Hemolysis, agranulocytosis, hepatitis, and exfoliative dermatitis (**Box 22.24**)
  - **Clofazimine:** They are mainly found in the skin (e.g., reddish pigmentation of skin and ichthyosis) and intestinal tract (e.g., diarrhea and cramping abdominal pain).

Box 22.24: Dapsone resistance cases.

- Clofazimine alone, or
- Clofazimine + ethionamide 500 mg daily and rifampicin given on the first 2 days of each month

Treatment regimens for leprosy

There are two recommended regimens for multibacillary and one for paucibacillary leprosy (**Table 22.15**).

TABLE 22.15: Treatment (WHO) regimens for leprosy.

Drug	*Indication*	*Mechanism*	*Side effects*
Rifampin	Paucibacillary, multibacillary	Bactericidal, RNA-Pol inhibitor	GI: abdominal pain, nausea, vomiting, diarrhea Dermatologic: pruritus, rash Renal: acute renal failure pseudohematuria Hepatic: transient liver dysfunction, jaundice, induction of P450 enzymes
Dapsone	Paucibacillary, multibacillary	Bacteriostatic, antifolate	Dermatologic: rash Hematologic: agranulocytosis, hemolysis (severe if G6PD deficient), methemoglobinemia Other: drug fever
Clofazimine	Paucibacillary, multibacillary	Bacteriostatic, binds *M. leprae* DNA	Dermatologic: skin pigmentation that often resolves with drug cessation GI: nausea, vomiting, diarrhea
Ofloxacin	Single-lesion paucibacillary	Bactericidal, DNA gyrase inhibitor	GI: nausea Dermatologic: rash, pruritus, photosensitivity CNS: seizures, headache, dizziness
Minocycline	Single-lesion paucibacillary	Bacteriostatic, inhibits protein synthesis via 30S	GI: nausea, vomiting, diarrhea, hepatotoxicity Dermatologic: photosensitivity Other: dental staining; therefore contraindicated in pregnant women, neonates, children <8 years old

(CNS: central nervous system; GI: gastrointestinal)

Box 22.25: Treatment of lepra reactions.

During lepra reactions, the chemotherapy for leprosy is maintained.

1. *Type 1 lepra reaction (reversal reaction)*:
   - **Mild cases:** Aspirin 600 mg 6 hourly
   - **Severe cases:** Start with prednisone 40–80 mg daily and reduce gradually over 3–9 months
2. *Type 2 lepra reaction (erythema nodosum leprosum)*:
   - **Mild cases:** Aspirin 600 mg 6 hourly
   - **Severe cases:** Prednisone 1 mg/kg/day. If there is no response to steroids, add clofazimine (300 mg/ day) or thalidomide (100 mg 4 times daily). The doses are slowly reduced over 1–3 months. If there is involvement of eyes, 1% hydrocortisone drops or ointment and 1% atropine drops is given.

ECTOPARASITES

Ectoparasites are parasites that live on the surface of its host.

SCABIES

Q. Discuss the clinical features and management of scabies.

Scabies is an intensely itchy rash caused by the ectoparasitic mite, *Sarcoptes scabiei* var. *hominis*.

Age: It is most common in **children and young adults** but can occur at any age group.

Mode of Transmission

- **Person-to-person contact:** Scabies is a highly contagious. Newly fertilized female mites are transmitted from person to person by prolonged close/intimate personal contact (e.g., within households or institutions) with the skin and by sexual contact. This transmission is facilitated by social crowding, poor hygiene, and multiple sexual partners. In the absence of host contact, the mites usually die within a day or so. About 15–20 minutes of close contact with an infected individual is necessary for transfer of the mites from one individual to another.
- **Through contaminated clothes:** Transfer through clothes and bedding contaminated by infested patient immediately beforehand.

Clinical Features

- Scabies clinically present with itchy red papules (or occasionally vesicles and pustules). Itching/pruritus are worse at night.
- **Distribution of lesions:** It often suggests the diagnosis. Skin lesions can occur anywhere but rare on the face and scalp, except in infants. Sites of predilection are—(1) between the web spaces of the fingers (**Fig. 22.32A**) and toes, (2) on the palms and soles (more commonly in small children), (3) around the wrists and axillae, on the male genitalia (**Fig. 22.32B**), and around the nipples and umbilicus. **Circle of Hebra** is an imaginary circle intersecting sites of predilection and includes areolae, axillae, elbow flexures, wrists, finger webs, umbilicus, lower abdomen, and genitalia.

- **Pruritus/itching** is a prominent feature and usually intense and worse (most severe) at night and after a hot shower. The itching develops a few days after infestation. It may develop within a few hours, if the mite is infested for second time. It develops in the trunk and limbs, and usually not affects the scalp.
- **Generalized rash** of scabies appears as tiny red intensely itchy bumps on the limbs and trunk. It is due to an allergic reaction to the mites and their products. It may develop several weeks to develop after initial infestation.
- **Nodules:** Presence of itchy lumps or nodules in the armpits and groins or along the shaft of the penis is highly suggestive of scabies. Nodules may persist for several weeks or longer even after the successful eradication of living mite.
- **Acropustulosis:** Blisters and pustules on the palms and soles of infants with scabies.

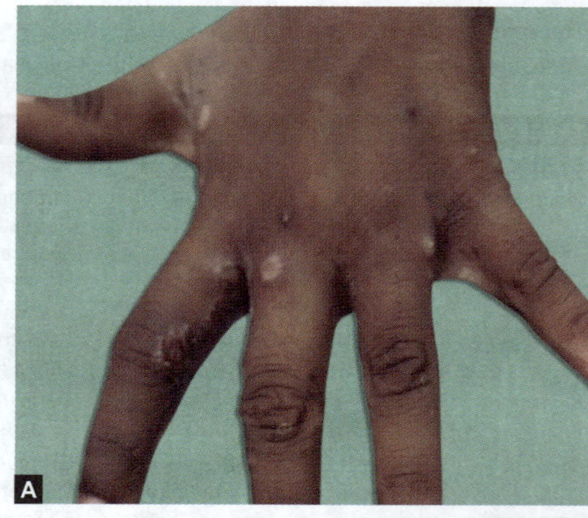

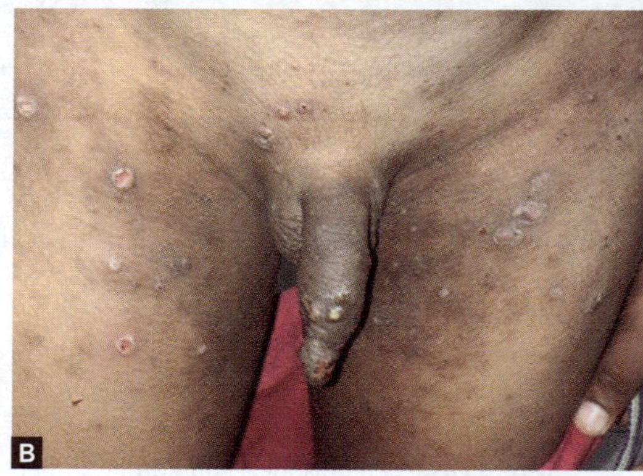

FIGS. 22.32A AND B: (A) Scabies involving the web spaces of the fingers; (B) Genital region of male.

Pathognomonic sign: It is the presence of **linear or curved skin burrows** in which the mites live. However, these are not always seen. Burrows are seen as dark wavy lines in the epidermis and measure up to 15 mm. Typical burrows may be only a few in number. Hence, they are often missed, if the skin has been scratched or become secondarily infected or if there is eczema. Microscopic examination of the contents of a burrow may show many mites, eggs, or mite feces (scybala).

Complication: Excoriations and secondary bacterial infection may develop in the skin rash. Secondary infection of lesions of scabies due to nephritogenic streptococci may complicate the rash leading to poststreptococcal glomerulonephritis.

Diagnosis

- **Clinical grounds:** Scabies should be considered on the basis of clinical presentation and history. Diagnosis can be made in patients with itching and symmetrical skin lesions in characteristic distribution/locations. It may be obvious if there is a history of household/close contact with an affected patient.
- **Confirmation of scabies:** It is by **identifying the scabietic burrow** and **visualizing the mite**. Burrows should be unroofed with a sterile needle or scalpel blade. The skin scrapings of a lesion should be examined microscopically (by a potassium hydroxide preparation) for the mite and/or its eggs and its fecal pellets. Microscopic examination of clear adhesive tape lifted from lesions and skin biopsy also may be useful for diagnosis.
- **Dermoscopy**: The characteristic finding is a dark and triangular shape that represents the head of the mite within a burrow ("delta wing" sign).

Q. Write short note on crusted scabies/Norwegian scabies.

Crusted or Norwegian Scabies

- Crusted scabies, Boeck scabies, keratotic scabies, or Norwegian scabies is clinical variant of scabies characterized by hyperinfestation (huge numbers) of *Sarcoptes scabiei* mites in the skin.
- It is named Norwegian scabies because of its initial description in Norwegian patients with leprosy.
- **Predisposing conditions:** Patients are highly infectious. The number of mites rapidly increases (hyperinfestation) due to impaired immune response, lack of pruritus or patient's with neurological disorders with physical inability to scratch. Disorders predisposing to crusted scabies are listed in **Table 22.16**. It may be associated with HLA-A11. Transmission through fomites can occur because mites survive on the sloughed skin in environment.
- **Clinical features:** Patient presents with marked thickening and crusting of the skin (hyperkeratotic crusted lesions) particulars on the hands. However, entire body including the face and scalp is often involved. Nails often show hyperkeratosis. Pruritus is minimal or absent.

Disorders predisposing to crusted scabies are shown in **Table 22.16**.

TABLE 22.16: Disorders predisposing to crusted scabies.

Disorders with defective T-cell response: AIDS, lymphoma, organ transplantation, and T-cell leukemia	**Neurological disorders:** Parkinson's disease, tabes dorsalis, and syringomyelia
Physical debilities: Critical illness and kwashiorkor	**Mental debilitation:** Down's syndrome and mental retardation
Reduced sensation: Leprosy	**Metabolic disorder:** Diabetes mellitus

Q. Discuss management of scabies/drugs used to treat scabies.

Treatment

Principles of Scabies Treatment

- Topical treatment of the patient and all asymptomatic close contacts (family members/physical contacts) should be done simultaneously to ensure eradication.
- Include a scabicidal and a keratolytic in the treatment.
- To avoid reinfection, washing, or cleaning of recently worn clothes (including underclothing) and bed linen (preferably at 60°C) is recommended.

Topical Treatment

- **Areas of application:** Scabicides are applied thinly and thoroughly to all over the skin below the neck (including the genitalia, palms and soles, and under the nails). Reapply topical scabicide to the hands, if patient washed it during the treatment period.
- **Duration of treatment:** Usually, effectively treated scabies infestations become noninfectious within a day. However, even after successful treatment, pruritus/itching and rash may remain even up to 4 weeks. Unnecessary retreatment may cause contact dermatitis.
- **Repetition of application:** Topical application should be repeated after 1 week.

Topical Scabicide

These include—(i) precipitated sulfur 2–10% in petrolatum, (ii) benzyl benzoate 10–25%, (iii) crotamiton 10%, (iv) Lindane (gamma benzene hexachloride) 1%, (v) permethrin 5%, and (vi) malathion 0.5%.

Oral Therapy

Ivermectin

- **Dose:**
  - Single oral dose 200 µg/kg in otherwise healthy individuals and side effects are rare.
  - Two doses of oral ivermectin (200 µg/kg, as 2 doses 2 weeks apart) are easy to use and as effective as topical therapy. Two doses are indicated in crusted scabies or Norwegian scabies. The toxic effects with two doses are insignificant.

Oral antihistamines can alleviate the hypersensitivity response.

LICE INFECTION

Q. Write a short essay/note on pediculosis.

Lice are blood-sucking ectoparasites and can infest human in three ways:

1. **Head lice (pediculosis capitis):**
   - Infestation with the head louse, *Pediculus humanus capitis,* is common worldwide.
   - **Age and gender:** Predominantly affects children and more common in females.
   - **Spread:**
     - It is highly contagious and spread by direct head-to-head contact and is associated with overcrowding.
     - It may be indirectly spread through hats, clothes, or pillow covers.
   - **Clinical presentation:** Head lice usually presents with scalp itch that leads to scratching, scalp excoriations, secondary infection (important cause of impetigo) and cervical lymphadenopathy. Itching may produce sleep disturbances and difficulties in concentration and the affected children may perform poorly in school.
   - **Diagnosis:**
     - Confirmed by identifying the living louse or nymph or empty egg cases ("nits" look like whitish shells stuck to the hair shaft on the scalp and are difficult to dislodge)

Treatment

- Apply **malathion or permethrin or carbaryl or phenothrin in lotion or aqueous formulations**, twice at an interval of 7–10 days (with a contact time of 12 hours). If treatment with one fails, a different insecticide is used for the next course. Rotational treatments within a community can avoid resistance. Treatment is usually repeated after 7 days.
- Regular "wet-combing" (physical removal of live lice by regular combing of conditioned wet hair, metal nit combs may help remove the eggs) is less effective than pharmacological applications.
- Apply Vaseline to eyelashes/brows twice daily for at least a fortnight.
- **Resistant cases:** Use oral ivermectin (400 µg/kg as two doses 1 week apart)
- Treatment of secondary bacterial infection if present

2. **Body lice (Pediculosis corporis)**
   - Body lice are ectoparasites similar to head lice but they live on clothing (e.g., seams), and feed on the skin.
   - **Predisposing factors** include poor hygiene, poverty, neglect, and overcrowded conditions. It is rare in developed countries (except in homeless and vagrants).
   - **Spread:** By direct contact or sharing infested clothing. The lice and eggs are commonly found on the clothing but are rarely observed on the skin of the patient.

- **Clinical presentation:** It presents with itch, excoriations, and secondary infection. Sometimes, there may be postinflammatory hyperpigmentation of the skin.

Treatment: By malathion or permethrin. Dry cleaning and high temperature washing or insecticide treatment for the clothes is helpful.

3. **Pubic lice (Crab lice or Phthiriasis pubis):**
   - Pubic louse *(Phthirus pubis)* is a bloodsucking insect that attaches tightly to the pubic hair.
   - **Mode of transmission:** Usually, it is sexually acquired (direct contact) and transferred only by close bodily contact. The lice lay its eggs (nits) at hair bases and usually hatch within a week.
   - **Clinical presentation:** It may be asymptomatic or presents with severe itching, especially at night. It usually infests public hair and occasionally other hairy areas (eyebrows, eyelashes, and the beard). Lice can be seen near the base of the hair with eggs.

Treatment: Similar to head lice and the treatment of choice is malathion or carbaryl in an aqueous base. They are applied on two occasions to the whole body, because it can also infest body hair. All sexual contacts (patient's partner) should also be treated. Patient should be screened for other sexually transmitted diseases. Infestation of the eyelashes and eyebrows is treated with application of white soft paraffin three times daily for 1–2 weeks.

SEXUALLY TRANSMITTED INFECTIONS

Sexually transmitted diseases (STDs) are a group of communicable diseases that are transmitted predominantly by sexual contact and caused by a wide range of bacterial, viral, protozoal, and fungal agents and ectoparasites (**Table 22.17**).

TABLE 22.17: Sexually transmitted infections.

Bacterial agents:	Viral agents:
➤ *Neisseria gonorrhoeae* ➤ *Chlamydia trachomatis* ➤ *Haemophilus ducreyi* ➤ *Mycoplasma hominis* ➤ *Ureaplasma urealyticum* ➤ *Calymmatobacterium granulomatis* ➤ *Shigella* species ➤ Group B *Streptococcus* ➤ Bacterial vaginitis associated organisms	➤ Human (alpha) herpesvirus ➤ Human (beta) herpesvirus ➤ Hepatitis B virus ➤ Human papillomavirus ➤ Molluscum contagiosum virus ➤ Human immunodeficiency virus
Protozoal agents: ➤ *Entamoeba histolytica* ➤ *Giardia lamblia* ➤ *Trichomonas vaginalis*	**Fungal agents:** *Candida albicans* **Ectoparasites:** ➤ *Phthirus pubis* ➤ *Sarcoptes scabiei*

Gonorrhea

Q. Write short note on gonorrhea/acute gonococcal urethritis.

Definition: Gonorrhea is a sexually transmitted infection (STI) due to the gram-negative diplococcus, *Neisseria gonorrhoeae*. It commonly infects columnar epithelium in the lower genital tract (cervicitis and urethritis), rectum (proctitis), and eye (conjunctivitis).

Mode of transmission: Genital–genital, genital–anorectal, or orogenital or oroanal contact or from mother to child transmission during delivery

Incubation period: Usually 2–10 days following exposure

Clinical Features

- **Gonococcal infections in men: Acute urethritis** is the most common clinical manifestation and presents with urethral discharge and dysuria usually without urinary frequency or urgency. On examination, urethra shows mucopurulent discharge that may be accompanied by erythema of the urethral meatus.
- **Gonococcal infections in women:** Gonococcal cervicitis and vaginitis present with symptoms related to endocervical and urethral infection and include scant vaginal discharge and dysuria. Gonococci may infect the urethra, paraurethral glands/ducts, and Bartholin's glands/ducts. It may be asymptomatic in up to 80% of women.
- **Anorectal and pharyngeal gonorrhea** are usually asymptomatic.
- **Ocular gonorrhea:** Gonococcal conjunctivitis is an uncommon. It may present with purulent discharge from the eye(s), inflammation of the conjunctivae and edema of the eyelids, pain, and photophobia. Gonococcal ophthalmia neonatorum also presents with purulent conjunctivitis and edema of the eyelids. Conjunctivitis must be treated early to prevent corneal damage.
- **Disseminated gonococcal infection (DGI):** Dissemination can result in gonococcal bacteremia and is rare and develops in women with asymptomatic genital infection. Symptoms include arthritis of one or more joints (asymmetric and migratory), pustular skin lesions, fever, and tenosynovitis. Gonococcal endocarditis or meningitis may rarely occur.
- **Acute perihepatitis (Fitz–Hugh–Curtis syndrome)** is a rare complication of PID, and is thought to occur through direct extension of *N. gonorrhoeae* from fallopian tube to liver capsule and peritoneum along the paracolic gutters. Patients present with sharp, pleuritic right upper quadrant pain.

Diagnosis

- **Gram staining and culture** of urethral exudates, genital, rectal, pharyngeal, or ocular secretions show gram-negative intracellular monococci and diplococci.
- **Sterile pyuria:** Urine may show polymorphonuclear leukocytes with a negative urine culture report.
- **Nucleic acid probe tests:** Nucleic acid amplification tests (NAATs) are more sensitive than culture. They can be performed on urine samples, swabs from endocervix, urethra, rectum, and pharynx.

- Direct antigen detection by fluorescein-conjugated monoclonal antibodies and direct fluorescence microscopy
- Enzyme-linked immunoassays for the detection of gonococcal antigen
- Blood cultures in disseminated disease.

Complications

If untreated infection can develop following complications:

- **In females:** It causes pelvic inflammatory disease PID (pelvic inflammatory disease). Local complications such as endometritis, salpingitis, tubo-ovarian abscess, bartholinitis, peritonitis, and perihepatitis
- **In male patients:** Periurethritis, epididymitis epididymo-orchitis, and prostatitis
- **Newborns:** Ophthalmia neonatorum in newborns

Treatment of Gonorrhea

See **Box 22.26.**

Box 22.26: Treatment of gonorrhea.

- One of the following regimens is recommended at present:
  - Cefixime 400 mg orally (single dose)
  - Ceftriaxone 250 mg intramuscularly (single dose)
  - Spectinomycin 2 g intramuscularly (single dose)
- If quinolone and azithromycin resistance is not a problem:
  - Ciprofloxacin 500 mg orally (single dose)
  - Ofloxacin 400 mg orally (single dose)
  - Levofloxacin 250 mg orally (single dose)
  - Azithromycin 2 g orally (single dose)
- For epididymo-orchitis, doxycycline 100 mg twice daily for 14 days along with one dose of ceftriaxone or ciprofloxacin

Nongonococcal Urethritis

Q. List the etiology and drugs used in nongonococcal urethritis.

Etiology

See **Table 22.18.**

TABLE 22.18: Causes of nongonococcal urethritis.

Chlamydia trachomatis (15–40%)	*Mycoplasma genitalium (15–25%)*
Others (20–50%): ➤ *Trichomonas vaginalis* ➤ *Ureaplasma urealiticum* ➤ Herpes simplex virus (in absence of skin lesions) ➤ Adenovirus ➤ Haemophilus	*Miscellaneous*: In association with urinary tract infection, bacterial prostatitis, urethral stricture, phimosis, secondary to instrumentation of the urethra, congenital abnormalities, chemical irritation, and tumors

Signs and Symptoms

Symptoms and signs of gonococcal urethritis and nongonococcal urethritis are similar but differ significantly in severity.

Diagnosis

- **Gram staining** of **discharge or sediment** of first voided urine (symptomatic/asymptomatic)
- Direct fluorescence assay
- Enzyme immunoassay
- Hybridization assay
- Nucleic acid amplification tests

Treatment

STD treatment guidelines from the CDC, 2010 and the WHO recommends:

- **Doxycycline 100 mg twice daily** for 7 days, **or**
- **Azithromycin 1 g orally**

Alternatives

- Erythromycin base 500 mg four times for 7 days, or
- Ofloxacin 300 mg twice daily for 7 days, or
- Levofloxacin 500 mg once daily for 7 days

General features

- All sex partners in last 60 days should be evaluated and treated
- Sexual abstinence till completion of treatment
- Patients should be reviewed 2–3 weeks after treatment to confirm resolution of symptoms and treatment of sexual contacts
- Patients should be checked for other STIs including syphilis and HIV. Results of tests should be checked during review.

Chancroid

Q. Write short essay/note on clinical features and treatment of chancroid.

- Chancroid or soft chancre is an acute sexually transmitted infection caused by *Haemophilus ducreyi*. It is characterized by painful genital ulcerations and inguinal adenitis.
- The genital ulceration in chancroid increases the efficiency of transmission and the degree of susceptibility to HIV in infection.
- Coinfection with *Treponema pallidum* and herpes simplex is observed in 10% of cases.

Clinical Features

- *Incubation period*: Usually 3–10 days
- Infection is acquired due to a break in the epithelium during sexual contact with an infected individual
- **Lesions in the external genitalia:**
  - **Sites of lesions:** Prepuce and frenulum in men and vaginal entrance and the perineum in women. At the site of inoculation (the external genitalia), an initial erythematous papule appears, which then breaks down within 2–3 days into a classic chancroidal ulcer.

- **Characteristics of ulcer:** The chancroid ulcer is superficial, circumscribed, and painful. Ulcers have ragged and undermined edges, and necrotic base bleeds easily and generally not indurated. Ulcer may be single. If multiple, they may merge to form giant serpiginous ulcer.
- **Lymphadenopathy:** About 50% of patients develop enlarged, painful, and tender inguinal lymph nodes (usually unilateral). The involved nodes become matted and progress to form large unilocular buboes, which suppurate.

Diagnosis

- It is based on the microscopic identification and culture isolation of *Haemophilus ducreyi* in scrapings from ulcer or pus from bubo.
- Polymerase chain reaction (PCR) technique not commercially available
- Detection of antibody to *H. ducreyi* using EIA may be useful.

Treatment of chancroid (Box 22.27)

Sex partners of chancroid patients should be examined and treated, if they had sexual contact with the patient during the 10 days preceding the patient's onset of symptoms. This is regardless of whether they have symptoms of the disease or not.

Box 22.27: Treatment options for chancroid.

- Azithromycin, 1 g orally, as a single dose, or
- Ceftriaxone, 250 mg by intramuscular injection as a single dose, or
- Ciprofloxacin, 500 mg orally, twice daily for 3 days, or
- Erythromycin base, 500 mg orally 4 times daily for 7 days

CHLAMYDIAL INFECTIONS

Chlamydial infections may be asymptomatic or cause:

- **In male:** Urethritis, epididymitis, and prostatitis. Untreated infection can cause infertility and reactive arthritis.
- **In female:** Cervicitis and salpingitis. Most of the infected females are asymptomatic and are likely to develop complications such as PID, infertility, or ectopic pregnancy.

Lymphogranuloma Venereum

Q. Write a short note on lymphogranuloma venereum (LGV).

It is a sexually transmitted disease caused by *Chlamydia trachomatis* (types LGV 1, 2, and 3).

Clinical Features

- **Incubation period:** 3–30 days.
- **Stages:** Three characteristic stages—
  1. **Primary genital lesion:** LGV starts as an asymptomatic small painless papule at the site of inoculation (external genitalia) and tends to ulcerate.
  2. **Regional lymphadenopathy:** Within a few days to weeks, the ulcers heal and regional lymphadenopathy (usually unilateral) develops. The lymph nodes are initially discrete painful and fixed and the overlying skin appears dusky and erythematous.
  3. **Buboes:** Later in the course, the lymph nodes may become matted, fluctuant (buboes), and rupture. The overlying skin becomes thinned, inflamed, and fixed. Finally, multiple draining fistulae may occur. Extensive enlargement of inguinal lymph nodes above and below the inguinal ligament **("groove sign")** can develop.
- **Other features:**
  - Acute LGV can also cause proctitis with perirectal abscesses, which may resemble anorectal Crohn's disease.
  - **Chronic phase:** Chronic infection may produce extensive scarring, abscess and sinus formation. The destruction of local lymph nodes can produce lymphedema of the genitalia.
  - **Constitutional symptoms:** These include fever, chills, headache, anorexia, meningismus, myalgia, and arthralgia.

Diagnosis

- **Detection of nucleic acid (DNA):** Direct immunofluorescent antibody and nucleic acid amplification tests are positive, which should be confirmed by real-time PCR for LGV-specific DNA.
- **Isolation of the LGV (L1–3 serotypes) strain of Chlamydia:** Tissue culture from swab obtained from ulcer-aspirated bubo pus, rectum, urethra, endocervix, or from other infected tissue is the most specific test; however, sensitivity is only 75–85%.
- **Serological tests:** Microimmunofluorescence (micro-IF) test and complement fixation test (CF) to detect antibodies
- Frei skin test is not useful.

Treatment (Box 22.28)

- Early treatment is necessary to prevent the chronic phase.
- Fluctuant buboes should be aspirated with a syringe and needle.
- Surgical drainage or reconstructive surgery may be sometimes needed.

Box 22.28: Treatment options for lymphogranuloma venereum.

- Doxycycline, 100 mg orally, twice daily for 14 days, or
- Erythromycin, 500 mg orally, 4 times daily for 14 days, or
- Tetracycline, 500 mg orally, 4 times daily for 14 days

GRANULOMA INGUINALE (DONOVANOSIS)

Q. Write short note on granuloma inguinale (donovanosis).

Granuloma inguinale is a genital ulcerative disease caused due to intracellular gram-negative bacterium *Klebsiella granulomatis* formerly known as *Calymmatobacterium granulomatis* (Donovan bodies).

Incubation period: 3–40 days

Clinical Features (Genital Lesions)

- Painless and progressive ulcerative lesions without regional lymphadenopathy
- Genital lesions are highly vascular, produce "beefy red appearance", and bleed easily on touch. However, it can also produce hypertrophic granulomatous, necrotic, or sclerotic lesions.

Diagnosis

Microscopy examination of material from the lesion (tissue crush preparation or biopsy) shows dark staining intracellular bipolar-staining Donovan bodies. The causative organism is difficult to culture.

Treatment

- Treatment will prevent the progression of lesions. Treatment should be continued until all lesions have completely epithelialized.
- Treatment with antibiotics is needed for at least 3 weeks. Effective regimens are presented in **Box 22.29**.

Box 22.29: Treatment options for granuloma inguinale.

- Azithromycin, 1 g orally on the 1st day, then 500 mg orally, once a day, or
- Doxycycline, 100 mg orally, twice daily, or
- Erythromycin, 500 mg orally, 4 times daily, or
- Tetracycline, 500 mg orally, 4 times daily, or
- Trimethoprim 80 mg/sulfamethoxazole 400 mg, 2 tablets orally, twice daily

SYPHILIS

Q. Classify syphilis based on the presentation and clinical manifestations.

Syphilis (lues) is a **chronic,** systemic infection **caused by spirochete *Treponema pallidum*,** which is usually **sexually transmitted.**

Spirochetes are gram-negative and slender corkscrew shaped.

Source of Infection

Contact with an open infectious lesion of **primary or secondary syphilis**. Lesions in the mucous membranes or skin of the genital organs, rectum, mouth, fingers, or nipples. These lesions include chancre, mucous patch, skin rash, or condylomata lata.

Mode of Transmission

- **Sexual contact:** It is the usual mode of spread.
- **Transplacental transmission:** From mother with active disease to the fetus (during pregnancy) → congenital syphilis
- **Blood transfusion**
- **Direct contact** with the open lesion is rare mode of transmission.
  Transmission from a mother to her fetus and rarely by blood transfusion is possible for several years following infection.
- *Treponema pallidum* can penetrate intact mucous membranes or abraded skin rapidly and gain entry into the lymphatics and bloodstream and produce systemic infection.

Classification (Table 22.19 and Fig. 22.33)

TABLE 22.19: Classification of syphilis.

Acquired syphilis	*Congenital syphilis*
➤ Primary syphilis ➤ Secondary syphilis ➤ Latent syphilis ➤ Late syphilis (tertiary): – Late latent – Benign tertiary – Quaternary syphilis (cardiovascular and neurosyphilis)	➤ Intrauterine death and perinatal death ➤ Early (infantile) ➤ Late (tardive)

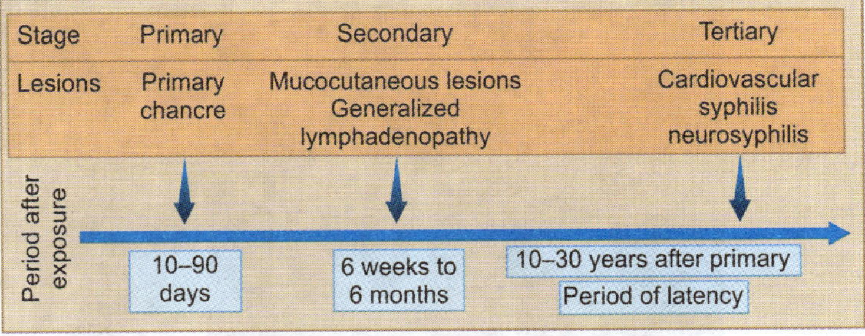

FIG. 22.33: Course of syphilis (if untreated).

Acquired Syphilis

Primary syphilis

Primary chancre: It is the classical lesion of primary syphilis.

- **Location:** The primary chancre develops at the site of inoculation.
  - **In males: Penis or scrotum** in males (in heterosexual) and in homosexual males, it may occur in the anal canal, rectum, fingers, or within the mouth.
  - **In females: Cervix, vulva,** and **vaginal** wall
- Primary chancre (**Fig. 22.34**) is single, firm, **non-tender (painless)**, slightly raised, **red papule** (chancre) up to several centimeters in diameter. It rapidly becomes eroded to create a clean-based shallow ulcer. Because of the induration surrounding the ulcer, it is designated as **hard chancre.**

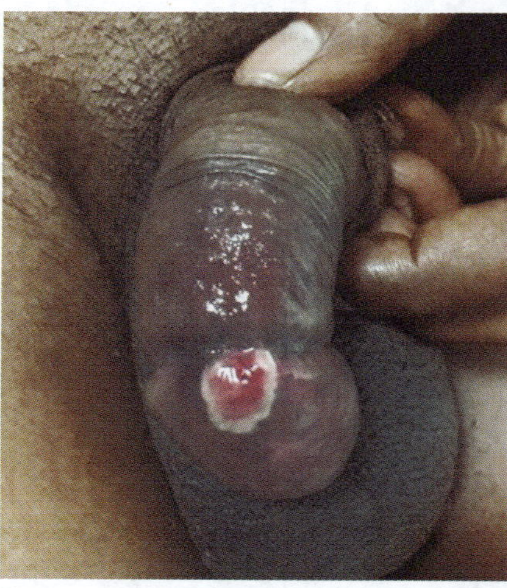

FIG. 22.34: Primary chancre in primary acquired syphilis.

Regional lymphadenitis: Usually accompanies the primary chancre within 1 week of the onset of the lesion.

- The lymph nodes are firm, rubbery, mobile, nonsuppurative, painless, and nontender.
- Chancres on external genitalia and anus produce bilateral inguinal lymphadenopathy, whereas those on cervix and vagina cause iliac or perirectal lymphadenopathy.

Fate: Even without therapy, the primary chancre heals within 4–6 weeks, but the lymphadenopathy may persist for months.

- Primary syphilis in HIV-positive patients is often asymptomatic and they frequently present with secondary or latent syphilis.

Secondary syphilis

Secondary syphilis develops 4–10 weeks after the primary chancre in approximately 75% of untreated patients. Its manifestations are due to systemic spread and proliferation of the spirochetes within the skin and mucocutaneous tissues. It starts with symptoms of generalized infection such as malaise, sore throat, headache, low-grade fever, and arthralgia.

Lesions

Mucocutaneous lesions: These are painless and superficial lesions and contain spirochetes and are infectious.

- **Skin rashes (75%):** They begin as **discrete red-brown macules** <5 mm in diameter. They are generalized symmetrical and nonirritable but more frequent on the trunk and proximal limbs. These macular lesions may progress to a scaly/pustular/annular or necrotic ulcers, which frequently involve the palms (**Fig. 22.35A and B**) and soles. The lesions are initially red, changing to a "gun-metal" gray as they resolve.
- **Condylomata lata (10%)** (**Fig. 23.35B**): These are **broad-based,** moist, pink, or gray-white, **elevated plaques** (papules coalescing to plaques), **highly** infectious containing numerous spirochetes. They are seen in moist, warm, intertriginous areas of the skin, such as the **anogenital region (perineum, vulva, and scrotum)**, inner thighs, and axillae.
- **Mucosal lesions (30%):** These usually occur in the mucous membranes of **oral cavity (lip, oral** mucosa, tongue, palate, and pharynx) **or** vulva, vagina, or glans penis **as silvery-gray superficial** mucosal **erosions**. They are surrounded by a red serpiginous periphery and are usually painless. Rarely, they may coalesce to produce characteristic "snail track" ulcers in the mouth.
- These lesions contain numerous *T. pallidum* and are the **highly infectious. Microscopy:** Similar to primary chancre, i.e., infiltration by plasma cells and endarteritis obliterans.

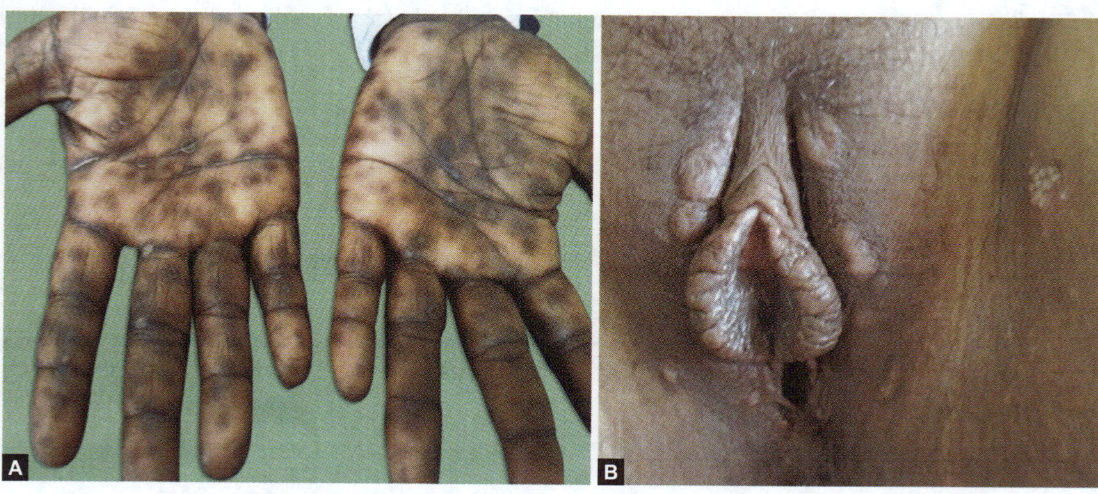

FIGS. 22.35A AND B: (A) Symmetrical skin rashes of secondary syphilis on palm; (B) Condyloma lata.

Generalized painless lymphadenopathy: Generalized, firm nontender lymphadenopathy (shotty) occurs in about 50% of patients. They involve especially **epitrochlear nodes** and show plenty of spirochetes. Mild fever, malaise, and weight loss are common in secondary syphilis, which may last for several weeks. The lesions subside even without treatment.

Less common manifestations include meningitis, cranial nerve palsies, anterior or posterior uveitis, hepatitis, gastritis, glomerulonephritis (proteinuria, nephrotic syndrome, or hemorrhagic glomerulonephritis), or arthritis and periostitis.

Latent syphilis

Without treatment, the clinical manifestations of secondary syphilis will resolve over 3–12 weeks. In an untreated (about 30%) patient during this phase, there is no evidence of clinical disease but it shows the presence of positive syphilis serology or the diagnostic cerebrospinal fluid (CSF) abnormalities of neurosyphilis. This is known as latent syphilis and is divided into:

- *Early latency (within 1 year of infection):* During this period, syphilis may be transmitted sexually.
- *Late latency (begins at 1 year of infection)*: During this period, the patient is no longer sexually infectious. Pregnant women with latent syphilis may infect the fetus in utero.

Late (tertiary) syphilis

- **Late latent syphilis:**
  - This phase may persist for many years or for life.
  - No symptoms or signs of syphilis
  - More than 60% of patients suffer little or no ill health even without treatment.
- **Benign tertiary (gummatous) syphilis:**
  - It is called benign because of its response to therapy rather than its clinical manifestations.
  - It may develop after 3–10 years after initial infection.
  - *Structures involved*: Skin (frequently at sites of trauma as nodules or ulcers), mucous membranes (mouth, pharynx, larynx, or nasal septum appears as punched-out ulcers), bone (e.g., skull, tibia, fibula, and clavicle) muscle, or viscera (e.g., liver hepar lobatum and spleen).
  - *Characteristic feature*: It is a chronic granulomatous (sometimes ulcerating) lesion called a gumma, which may be single or multiple.
  - *Consequences*: Healing with scar formation may damage the function of the structure involved.
- **Quaternary syphilis**: **Neurosyphilis and cardiovascular syphilis may coexist and sometimes called as quaternary syphilis.**
  - *Cardiovascular syphilis*:
    - It may present many years after initial infection.
    - Most **frequently involves the aorta** (the ascending aorta aortic valve and/or the coronary ostia, the aortic arch) and known as syphilitic aortitis
    - Clinical features include angina, features of aortic incompetence, and aortic aneurysm.
  - **Neurosyphilis** (discussed in Chapter 15).

Congenital Syphilis (Box 22.30)

Q. Write short note on congenial syphilis.

- ***Transplacental transmission*:** *T. pallidum* can cross placenta and spread from infected **mother to the fetus** (during pregnancy).
- Transmission occurs, when **mother is suffering from primary or secondary syphilis** (when the spirochetes are abundant). Because routine serologic testing for syphilis is done in all pregnancies, congenital syphilis is rare.

Box 22.30: Stigmata of congenital syphilis.

- Hutchinson's incisors (anterior–posterior thickening with notch on narrowed cutting edge)
- Mulberry molars (imperfectly formed cusps/deficient dental enamel)
- High-arched palate
- Maxillary hypoplasia
- Saddle nose
- Rhagades (radiating scars around mouth, nose, and anus following rash)
- Salt and pepper scars on retina (from choroiditis)
- Corneal scars (from interstitial keratitis)
- Sabre tibia (from periostitis)
- Bossing of frontal and parietal bones (healed periosteal nodes)

Manifestations

It can be divided into:

- **Intrauterine death and perinatal death**
- **Early (infantile) congenital syphilis:** It manifests within the **first 2 years of life** and often manifested by **nasal discharge** (rhinitis) and congestion (**snuffles**). They resemble features of secondary syphilis.
  - A desquamating or bullous eruption/rash can lead to epidermal sloughing of the skin, mainly in the hands, feet, around the mouth, and anus. It also may show condyloma lata.
  - *Skeletal abnormalities*: Syphilitic osteochondritis (inflammation of bone and cartilage is more distinctive in the nose → produces characteristic saddle nose deformity); syphilitic periostitis (involves the tibia and leads to anterior bowing or saber shin)
  - Others organs involved are **liver** (diffuse fibrosis) and **lung** (airless-**pneumonia alba**).

- **Late (tardive) congenital syphilis:**
  - Manifests 2 years after birth, and about 50% of untreated children with neonatal syphilis will develop late manifestations and take the form of "stigmata" relating to early damage to developing structures, particularly teeth and long bones.
  - Distinctive manifestation in Hutchinson's triad are—(1) interstitial keratitis, (2) Hutchinson's teeth, and (3) eighth-nerve deafness. Other features include Clutton's joints, neurosyphilis, gummatous periostitis, destruction of palate, and nasal septum. Cardiovascular involvement is rare. Stigmata of congenital syphilis are listed in **Box 22.30**.

Laboratory Diagnosis

Q. Write short note/essay on:

- Tests for diagnosis of syphilis
- Serological tests for syphilis
- Venereal Diseases Research Laboratory (VDRL) test

Demonstration of Treponema Pallidum

- **Dark-field microcopy:** Most sensitive and specific method is identification in serum collected from primary chancres, or from moist or eroded mucous lesions in secondary syphilis by dark-field microscopy. It shows drifting rotary motion (corkscrew) of *Treponema pallidum*. Patients with either primary or secondary disease are highly infectious.
- **Direct fluorescent antibody *T. pallidum* (DFA-TP) test**: In fixed smears from the chancre, it is important for diagnosis in primary syphilis.
- Microscopic demonstration of *Treponema pallidum* in tissues stained by appropriate stains and PCR are also useful.

Serological Tests

- **Nontreponemal antibody (nonspecific) tests:** These tests measure antibody to cardiolipin, a phospholipid presents in both host tissues and *T. pallidum*.
  These tests include:
  - **Venereal Diseases Research Laboratory (VDRL) test**
  - Rapid plasma reagin (RPR) test
- **Treponemal (specific) antibody tests:** They measure antibodies, which react with *T. pallidum*.
- Significance—
  - Used for confirmation. They are highly specific for treponemal disease. However, they do not differentiate between syphilis and other treponemal infection (e.g., as yaws).
  - In most of the patients, these tests usually remain positive for life, regardless of treatment or disease activity. However, 15–25% of patients treated in primary stage become nonreactive after 2–3 years.
  - Various tests include:
    - Treponemal antigen-based enzyme immunoassay (EIA) for IgG and IgM
    - *T. pallidum* hemagglutination assay (TPHA)
    - *T. pallidum* particle agglutination assay (TPPA)
    - Fluorescent treponemal antibody absorption (FTA-ABS) test

Examination of CSF: In benign tertiary and cardiovascular syphilis, CSF should be examined because of coexistence of asymptomatic neurological disease. CSF should be examined in neurosyphilis and in both early and late congenital syphilis.

Other tests: Chest X-ray, electrocardiogram (ECG), and echocardiogram are necessary in cardiovascular syphilis. Biopsy may be necessary to diagnose gumma.

Q. Enumerate the indications and describe the pharmacology, administration, and adverse reaction of pharmacotherapies for syphilis.

Management (Table 22.20)

- **Patients allergic to penicillin:** In primary, secondary, and early latent syphilis, these patients should be given tetracycline or doxycycline for 2 weeks and in late latent syphilis, it should be given for 4 weeks.
- **Ceftriaxone:** It may be given in the dose of 1 g once a day for 10–14 days.
- **Azithromycin:** Single dose of 2 g is also effective except in homosexual men and during pregnancy.
- **Response to treatment** is considered as satisfactory, if there is a four-fold decrease in nontreponemal titers at 3–6 months in all stages of syphilis.
- **Neurosyphilis:** It should be followed up with lumbar puncture and evaluation of CSF every 6 months until the cell count is normal. If after 6 months the cell count is not decreased, retreatment should be given.

TABLE 22.20: Management of syphilis.

Stage of syphilis	Drug	Regimen
Primary	Procaine penicillin	600,000 units IM/day for 12 days
	Oxytetracycline	500 mg orally four times/day for 15 days
	Doxycycline	100 mg orally two times/day for 15 days
	Benzathine penicillin	2.4 mega (million) units IM single dose (1.2 million units in each buttock)
Secondary	Procaine penicillin	600,000 units IM once daily for 15 days
	Benzathine penicillin	2.4 million units IM single dose
Early latent	Benzathine penicillin	2.4 million units IM single dose
Late latent/tertiary and cardiovascular syphilis	Benzathine penicillin	2.4 million units IM weekly for 3 weeks
Neurosyphilis	Crystalline penicillin	18–24 million units/day for 10–14 days
	Procaine penicillin PLUS probenecid	2.4 million units/day IM for 10–14 days + 500 mg QID for 10–14 days

(IM: intramuscular)

Treatment reactions

- **Anaphylaxis:** Penicillin is a common cause.
- **Jarisch–Herxheimer reaction:**
  - Treatment of syphilitic patients having a high bacterial load by antibiotics can cause a massive release of endotoxins, and cytokine causing Jarisch–Herxheimer reaction.
  - Jarisch–Herxheimer reaction is an acute febrile reaction that follows after (about 8 hours after the first injection) any therapy for syphilis. It is characterized by headache, myalgia, malaise, mild fever, rigors, and other symptoms that usually resolve within the first 24 hours.
  - It is common in early syphilis and rare in late syphilis.
  - It may induce fetal distress or premature labor in pregnancy. This concern should not prevent or delay therapy. It may be severe and worsen the clinical manifestations in cardiovascular or neurosyphilis.
  - Penicillin should not be withheld because of the Jarisch–Herxheimer reaction. Because, it is not dose dependent and there is no point in giving a smaller dose.
  - Prednisolone 10–20 mg orally three times daily for 3 days given for 24 hours prior to therapy may prevent the reaction.

APPROACH TO A CASE OF GENITAL ULCER [GENITAL ULCER DISEASE (GUD)]

Definition: Genital ulcer is defined as ulcerative, erosive, pustular, or vesicular lesions on the genitalia with or without lymphadenopathy.

Etiology (Table 22.21)

TABLE 22.21: Causes of genital ulcer disease.

STD-related etiologies and organisms	
Genital herpes	*Herpes simplex virus type 1 and type 2*
Primary syphilis	*Treponema pallidum var. pallidum*
Chancroid	*Haemophilus ducreyi*
Lymphogranuloma venereum (LGV)	*Chlamydia trachomatis serovars L1-L3*
Granuloma inguinale (Donovanosis)	*Calymmatobacterium granulomatis* now called *Klebsiella granulomatis*
Non-STD-related etiologies	
Non-STD infectious	Candida, CMV, EBV, Mycobacteria, *Staphylococcus*
Noninfectious	Bechet's, Reiter's, cancer, trauma, aphthous, and fixed drug eruptions
No etiological agent is found in 20–50% of genital ulcer disease (GUD)	

(CMV: cytomegalovirus; EBV: Epstein–Barr virus; STD: sexually transmitted disease)

Features and differential diagnosis of genital ulcer disease are presented in **Table 22.22**.

TABLE 22.22: Differential diagnosis of a few genital ulcer diseases.

Characteristic	Syphilis	Herpes (Fig. 22.36)	Chancroid	LGV	Donovanosis
Primary lesion	Papule	Vesicle	Pustule	Papule, vesicle, and pustule	Papule
Number of lesions	Usually 1	Multiple	Multiple	Single	Variable
Diameter	5–15 mm	1–2 mm	Variable	2–10 mm	Variable
Edges	Sharply demarcated elevated	Erythematous and polycyclic	Undermined and ragged	Elevated, round, or oval	Elevated, irregular
Depth	Superficial or deep	Superficial	Excavated	Superficial or deep	Elevated
Base	Smooth and nonpurulent covered with serous exudate	Erythematous	Purulent and dirty gray base	Variable	Red velvety, bleeds easily
Induration	Button hole	None	Not indurated	Not indurated	Not indurated
Pain	Absent	Present	Present	Absent	Absent
Lymph nodes	Bilateral nontender, firm, lead shot, and nonsuppurative	Bilateral tender, firm, nonsuppurative	Unilateral, tender, suppurative, and unilocular	Unilateral, tender, suppurative, and multilocular	None pseudobubo seen

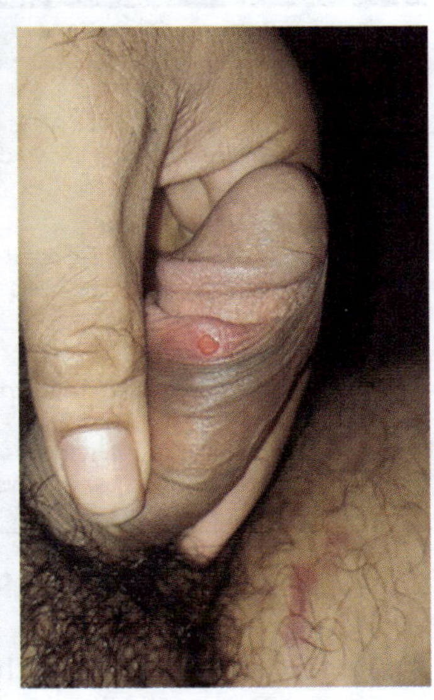

FIG. 22.36: Herpetic penile ulcer.

CHAPTER

23 Clinical Pharmacology

INTRODUCTION

- Drug metabolism that varies on genetic basis is often called polymorphic drug metabolism **(Table 23.1)**.
- **Pharmacogenetics:** It is the study of individual gene-drug interactions, usually one or two genes that have a dominant effect on a drug response.
- **Pharmacogenomics** is the study of genomic influence on drug response.

TABLE 23.1: Genetic polymorphisms in drug metabolism.

Defect	*Enzyme involved*	*Drug*	*Consequences*
Oxidation	CYP2D6	Codeine	Reduced analgesia
Oxidation	Aldehyde dehydrogenase	Ethanol	Facial flushing, hypotension, tachycardia, nausea, vomiting
N-Acetylation	*N*-acetyltransferase	Isoniazid	Peripheral neuropathy
Ester hydrolysis	Plasma cholinesterase	Succinylcholine	Prolonged apnea
Oxidation	CYP2C9	Warfarin	Bleeding

ADVERSE DRUG REACTION

Definition: An unwanted or harmful reaction experienced following the administration of a drug or a combination of drugs under normal conditions of use and suspected to be related to the drug.

Adverse drug reaction (ADR) could be trivial or serious or fatal.

Classification of Adverse Drug Reaction (Table 23.2)

TABLE 23.2: Classification of adverse drug reactions (ADRs).

➢ ***Type A*** **(Augmented) reactions** – are predictable, often dose-dependent, and related to the pharmacokinetics (PK) of the drug – comprise up to 80% of all ADRs – e.g., hepatic failure due to overdose of acetaminophen, sedative side effects of antihistamines	➢ ***Type D*** **(Delayed) reactions** – are time related, uncommon, become apparent sometime after use of the drug – e.g., carcinogenesis, tardive dyskinesia, teratogenesis
➢ ***Type B*** **(Bizarre) reactions** – are unpredictable and are not related to the dose or the drug's PK – account for 10–15% of all ADRs	➢ ***Type E*** **(End of use) reactions** – are withdrawal, uncommon and occur soon after withdrawal of the drug – e.g., withdrawal syndrome with opiates/benzodiazepines
➢ ***Type C*** **(Chronic) reactions** – are chronic, dose related and time related, uncommon and related to cumulative dose – e.g., hypothalamic-pituitary-adrenal axis suppression by corticosteroids, osteonecrosis of the jaw with bisphosphonates	➢ ***Type F*** **(Failure) reactions** – are common, dose-dependant and caused by drug interactions – Cause an unexpected failure of therapy – e.g., inadequate dosage of an oral contraceptive when used with an enzyme inducer, resistance to antimicrobial agents

Severity of Adverse Drug Reaction

- **Minor:** No need of therapy, antidote or hospitalization.
- **Moderate:** Requires drug change, specific treatment, hospitalization.
- **Severe:** Potentially life-threatening, permanent damage and prolonged hospitalization.
- **Lethal:** Directly or indirectly leads to death.

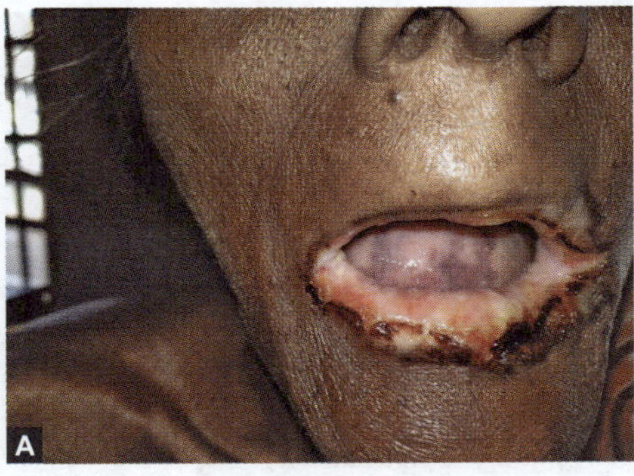
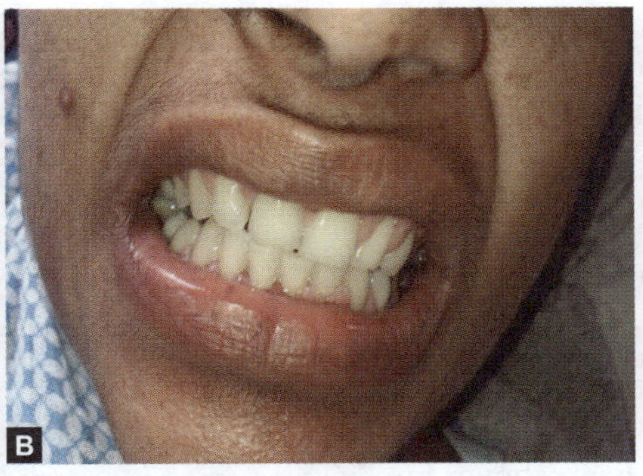
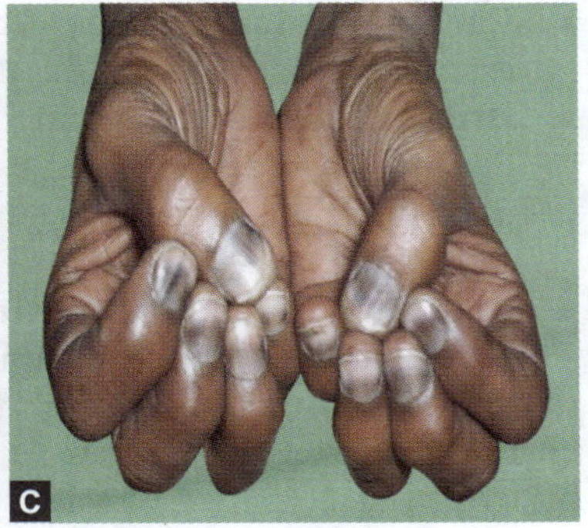

FIGS. 23.1A TO C: (A) Mucositis induced by anticancer drug; (B) Phenytoin-induced gum hyperplasia; (C) Zidovudine-induced nail pigmentation.

Types of Adverse Drug Reaction

- **Side effects:**
  - Unavoidable, predictable, decreased dose results in amelioration.
  - ***Occurs as extension of the same therapeutic effect***, e.g., atropine as antisecretory in preanesthetic medication → dry mouth, mucositis induced by anticancer drug **(Fig. 23.1A)**.
  - ***Occurs as a distinctly different effect***, e.g., promethazine as antiallergic—sedation, phenytoin-induced gum hyperplasia **(Fig. 23.1B)**, zidovudine-induced nail pigmentation **(Fig. 23.1C)**.
  - Estrogen as antiovulatory → nausea.
  - ***Side effect exploited for a therapeutic use***, e.g., codeine (antitussive) constipating action used in diarrhea.
    - Sulfonylureas (tested as antibacterial) were found to decrease blood glucose.

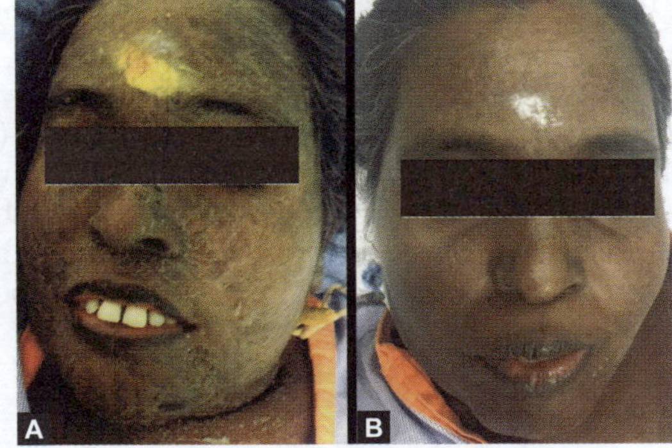

FIGS. 23.2A AND B: Drug rash with eosinophilia and systemic symptoms (DRESS) syndrome: (A) Presteroid therapy; (B) Poststeroid therapy.

- **Secondary effects:** Indirect effect of therapy. For example, intestinal microflora killed by tetracycline causing superinfection, corticosteroids decrease immunity causing oral candidiasis.
- **Toxic effects:** Overdose or prolonged use. Examples of toxic effects, overdosage or prolonged use includes atropine delirium, paracetamol → hepatic necrosis, barbiturates → coma, and morphine → respiratory failure.
- **Intolerance:** It is opposite of tolerance and characterized by increased sensitivity to low doses. Examples, few doses of carbamazepine → ataxia, single dose of triflupromazine → muscular dystonia.
- **Idiosyncrasy:** Genetically determined atypical or bizarre effect. Examples, barbiturate → excitement and mental confusion, streptomycin → deafness with single dose.
- **Drug reaction with eosinophilia and systemic symptoms (DRESS)** is a rare, potentially life-threatening, drug-induced hypersensitivity reaction that includes skin eruption, hematologic abnormalities (eosinophilia, atypical lymphocytosis), lymphadenopathy, and internal organ involvement (liver, kidney, lung). Common drugs associated are phenytoin, olanzapine, sulfonamides, febuxostat, dapsone, and vancomycin **(Figs. 23.2A and B)**.
- **Drug allergy or hypersensitivity:** Immunologically mediated, independent of dose and occurs in a small proportion of patients. Prior sensitization is required and occurs after 1–2 weeks after first dose. Drug acts as an antigen or hapten. Chemically-related drugs may show cross-sensitivity. Same drug can cause different allergic reactions in different individuals. Types of allergy include:
  - ***Type I***: Urticaria **(Fig. 23.3)**, angioedema, asthma, anaphylactic shock.
  - ***Type II***: Thrombocytopenia, agranulocytosis, aplastic anemia, systemic lupus erythematosus (SLE).
  - ***Type III***: Arthralgia, lymphadenopathy, Stevens-Johnson syndrome.
  - ***Type IV***: Contact dermatitis, fever, photosensitization, e.g., penicillin, sulfonamides, carbamazepine, and methyldopa.
- **Photosensitivity:**
  - ***Phototoxic***: Drug accumulates in skin → absorbs light → photochemical reaction → photobiological reaction → tissue damage. Example, erythema, edema, blistering with *tetracyclines.*
  - ***Photoallergic***: Drug → cell-mediated immune response → contact dermatitis on exposure to light, e.g., sulfonamides, griseofulvin.
- **Drug dependence:** Can be psychological and physical dependence.
- **Teratogenicity:** Drug use in pregnancy affects fetus. Examples, thalidomide → phocomelia, phenytoin → cleft palate.

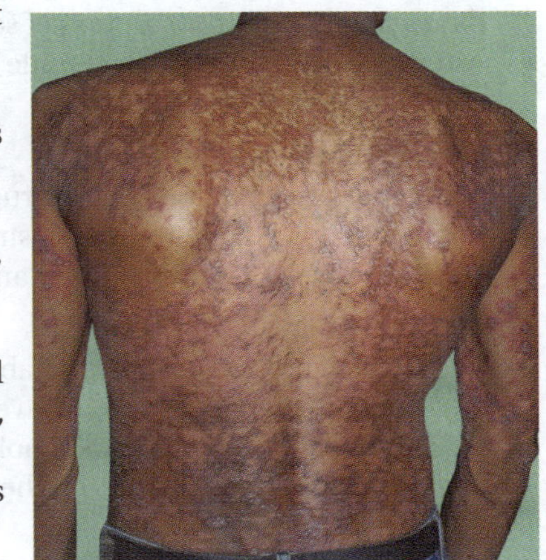

FIG. 23.3: Nevirapine-induced rash.

- **Carcinogenicity and mutagenicity:** For example, anticancer drugs, estrogens.
- **Drug-induced diseases/iatrogenic diseases:** Examples, salicylates → peptic ulcer, phenothiazine → Parkinsonism, isoniazid (INH) → hepatitis.
- **Drug withdrawal reaction:** Examples, propranolol → hypertension, acute adrenal insufficiency following withdrawal of corticosteroids.

The management of ADR has been shown in **Table 23.3**.

The ways of preventing ADR are listed in **Box 23.1**.

TABLE 23.3: Management of adverse drug reaction.

Evaluation	*Supportive care*	*Enhancing elimination*
➢ Airway	➢ Respiratory	➢ Activated charcoal
➢ Breathing	➢ Cardiovascular	➢ Forced alkaline diuresis
➢ Circulation	➢ Central nervous system (CNS)	➢ Hemodialysis/perfusion
➢ Degree of consciousness		
➢ History of exposure/ ingestion		
➢ Physical examination		
Decontamination	***Diagnostic studies***	***Antidotes***
➢ Gastric lavage	➢ Blood tests	➢ Organophosphates—atropine, oximes
➢ Induction of emesis	➢ Electrocardiogram (ECG)	➢ Morphine—naloxone
➢ Activated charcoal	➢ X-rays	➢ Benzodiazepines—flumazenil
➢ Other decontamination	➢ Specific drug levels	➢ Paracetamol—*N*-acetylcysteine

Box 23.1: Prevention of adverse drug reaction.

- Avoid inappropriate drugs in the context of clinical condition
- Use right dose, route, frequency-based on patient variables
- Elicit medication history; consider untoward incidents
- Elicit history of allergies (higher chances in patients with allergic diseases)
- Rule out drug interactions
- Adopt right technique, e.g., slow IV injection of aminophylline
- Carry out appropriate monitoring, e.g., prothrombin time (PT) with warfarin; drug levels

DRUG INTERACTION

Definition: A measurable modification (in magnitude and/or duration) of the action of one drug by prior or concomitant administration of another substance, including prescription, nonprescription (including complementary medicines) drugs, food, alcohol, cigarette smoking or diagnostic tests.

Outcomes of drug interaction are listed in **Box 23.2**.

Box 23.2: Outcomes of drug interaction.

- Loss of therapeutic effect
- Toxicity
- Unexpected increase in pharmacological activity
- Beneficial effects, e.g., additive and potentiation (intended) or antagonism (unintended)
- Chemical or physical interaction, e.g., intravenous incompatibility in fluid or syringes mixture

Mechanism of Drug Interaction

Pharmacokinetic Interaction

Altered gastrointestinal tract (GIT) absorption:

- **Altered pH:** The nonionized form of a drug is more lipid soluble and more readily absorbed from GIT than the ionized form does. For example, antacids and H_2 blockers change gastric pH—decrease the dissolution of ketoconazole which requires acidic pH. Therefore, these drugs must be separated by at least 2 hours in the time of administration of both.
- **Altered intestinal bacterial flora:** In patients receiving digoxin, 40% or more of the administered dose is metabolized by the intestinal flora. If patients simultaneous take antibiotics which destroy the intestinal flora, digoxin toxicity can occur.
- **Complexation or chelation:** Tetracycline interacts with iron preparations → unabsorbable complexes. Decrease absorption of ciprofloxacin by 85% due to chelation, if given along with antacids.
- **Drug-induced mucosal damage:** Antineoplastic agents, e.g., cyclophosphamide, vincristine, procarbazine → mucosal damage and inhibit absorption of several drugs, e.g., digoxin.
- **Altered motility:** Metoclopramide (antiemetic) → increase absorption of cyclosporine due to the increase of stomach emptying time.

Displaced protein binding:

- It depends on the affinity of the drug to bind to plasma protein.
- Phenytoin is highly bound to plasma protein (90%), tolbutamide (96%), and warfarin (99%). Drugs that displace these agents are aspirin, sulfonamides, and phenylbutazone.

Altered metabolism:

- The effect of one drug on the metabolism of the other is well documented. The liver is the major site of drug metabolism but other organs can also be involved, e.g., white blood cell (WBC), skin, lung, and GIT.
- CYP450 family is the major metabolizing enzyme in phase I (oxidation process).
- Therefore, the effect of drugs on the rate of metabolism of others can involve the following examples:
  - ***Enzyme induction:***
    - A drug may induce the enzyme that is responsible for the metabolism of another drug or even itself, e.g., carbamazepine (antiepileptic drug) increases its own metabolism.

- ♦ Phenytoin increases hepatic metabolism of theophylline → leading to decrease its level, reduces its action and vice versa.
- ■ ***Enzyme inhibition:***
  - ♦ It is characterized by reduction of the rate of metabolism of a drug by another drug. This leads to increased concentration of the target drug and thereby increases its toxicity.
  - ♦ Inhibition of the enzyme may be caused by the competition on its binding sites. This shortens the onset of action (may be within 24 hours).
  - ♦ Example, erythromycin inhibit metabolism of astemizole and terfenadine → raises the serum concentration of the antihistaminic and thereby increasing the cardiotoxicity which may be life-threatening.

First-Pass Metabolism

- Administration of drug by oral route increases its metabolism in the liver and GIT. This causes loss of a part of the drug dose and decreases its action.
- This is more evident when such drug is an enzyme inducer or inhibitor.
- By increasing its first pass metabolism, rifampin reduces serum concentration of verapamil level. Also, rifampin induces the hepatic metabolism of verapamil.

Renal Excretion

Active tubular secretion:
- It occurs in the proximal tubules (a portion of renal tubules).
- The drug combines with a specific protein and reaches the proximal tubules.
- When drug X has a competitive reactivity to the protein responsible for the active transport of drug Y, drug X will cause toxicity of Y due to a decrease in drug excretion of Y (increased concentration of Y).
- For example, probenecid → decreases tubular secretion of methotrexate.

Passive tubular reabsorption:
- In the tubules, excretion and reabsorption of drugs is by passive diffusion and is regulated by concentration and lipid solubility.
- For example, sodium bicarbonate—increases lithium clearance and decreases its action.

Pharmacodynamic Interaction

- It indicates that there is alteration of the drug action without change in its serum concentration by pharmacokinetic factors.
- For example, **synergism** means = 1 + 1 = 3, **additive** means = 1 + 1 = 2, **potentiation** means = 1 + 0 = 2, and **antagonism** means = 1 + 1 = 0 or 0.5.

Prevention of Drug Interaction

- Monitoring therapy and making adjustments.
- Monitoring blood level of some drugs with narrow therapeutic index, e.g., digoxin, anticancer agents, etc.
- Monitoring of some parameters may help to detect the early events of interaction or toxicity. For example, with warfarin treatment, it is necessary to monitor the prothrombin time to adjust drug dosages.
- Increase the interest in case report studies to report different possibilities of drug interaction.

DRUGS AND LIVER

Common drugs metabolized in liver are mentioned in **Table 23.4**.

TABLE 23.4: Common drugs metabolized in the liver.

Type of conjugation	*Endogenous reactant*	*Examples*
Glucuronidation	Uridine diphosphate (UDP)-glucuronic acid	Nitrophenol, morphine, acetaminophen, diazepam, N-hydroxydapsone, sulfathiazole, digitoxin, digoxin
Acetylation	Acetyl-CoA	Sulfonamides, isoniazid, clonazepam, dapsone, mescaline
Glutathione conjugation	Glutathione (GSH)	Acetaminophen, ethacrynic acid, bromobenzene
Glycine conjugation	Glycine	Salicylic acid, benzoic acid, cholic acid, deoxycholic acid
Sulfation	Phosphoadenosyl phosphosulfate	Estrone, aniline, phenol, 3-hydroxycoumarin, acetaminophen, methyldopa
Methylation	S-adenosylmethionine	Dopamine, epinephrine, pyridine, histamine, thiouracil
Water conjugation	Water	Carbamazepine

Cirrhotic Patients with Portosystemic Shunts

- Blood from intestines bypasses the liver, delivering much more of orally administered drugs to the systemic circulation. Thus, systemic bioavailability of orally administered high clearance drugs is much greater.
- *Hepatic impairment*:
  - ■ Research has shown reduced drug-metabolizing enzyme (CYP and conjugation reactions) in cirrhotics which worsen disease severity (Child-Pugh score), but with large variability!

- Preferentially recommend conjugatively metabolized agents in cirrhotics
- In the absence of recommended doses:
  - *Child-Pugh A*: Reduce maintenance to 50%
  - *Child-Pugh B*: Reduce maintenance to 25%
  - *Child-Pugh C*: Use drugs proven safe, or drugs with level monitoring available.

DRUGS AND KIDNEY

Dosing of Drugs in Renal Failure

- Without careful dosing and therapeutic drug monitoring in patients with renal dysfunction, accumulation of drugs/toxic metabolites can occur. Drug dosing has to be adjusted to the calculated glomerular filtration rate (GFR).
- Renal disease affects the pharmacokinetic as well as pharmacodynamic (PD) effect of drugs.
- Uremia can alter drug disposition, protein binding, pharmacokinetics (PK), PD and can also increase sensitivity to drugs.

Effect of Renal Failure on Bioavailability

- Absorption of drugs in patients with renal disorders could be inhibited by gastrointestinal disturbances seen in uremia (nausea, vomiting, and diarrhea), uremic gastritis, and pancreatitis.
- Edema of GIT can occur with nephrotic syndrome and impair absorption.
- Gastric motility can be impaired by uremia.
- Uremia can also increase gastric ammonia and lead to increased gastric pH thus affecting drugs that require acidic pH for absorption (e.g., ferrous sulfate).
- First-pass effect is reduced in patients with renal disease (therefore, absorption of drugs with high first-pass effect is increased, e.g., propranolol).

Effect of Renal Failure on Protein Binding and Volume of Distribution

- The effect of a drug is related to the amount of free or unbound drug available to target tissues.
- Also, hypoalbuminemia is common to patients with renal failure. Therefore, highly protein binding drug has fewer albumins to cling to. This is especially important with phenytoin.

Elimination

- As kidney disease progresses, the kidney's ability to excrete uremic toxins decreases as does its ability to eliminate certain drugs.
- Kidney eliminates primarily through filtration or active secretion.
- Drugs with low protein binding are filtered more readily.
- Large molecules (molecular weight > 20,000 daltons) are not readily filtered due to its size.

Drug Removed by Dialysis

- Removal by dialysis is specific to each drug.
- *Factors affecting removal*: Type of machine, membrane surface area, pore size, flow rates.
- Dialysis is sometimes used to remove excess drug in an overdose situation.

DRUG USAGE IN PREGNANCY

- The safety of approximately 50% of medications for the mother and fetus remains unknown.
- Pharmacokinetics are profoundly affected by pregnancy-associated physiological changes and dose adjustments are sometimes necessary for optimal clinical outcome.

Current Categories for Drug Use in Pregnancy (FDA) (Table 23.5)

Few drugs contraindicated during pregnancy and those which have teratogenic effects are listed in **Table 23.6**. Common problems in pregnancy and drugs that can be safely used in these cases are mentioned in **Table 23.7**.

CLINICAL TRIALS BASIC CONCEPTS

Clinical trial is an experimental epidemiological method. It is an interventional study on individuals, usually on patients.

Objectives of Clinical Trials

- Intervention trials determine whether experimental treatments are safe and effective under controlled environments.
- Observation trials address health issues in large groups of people in natural settings.

TABLE 23.5: Current categories for drug use in pregnancy.

Category	*Description*
A	Adequate, well-controlled studies in humans show no risk to the fetus (e.g., magnesium sulfate)
B	No well-controlled studies have been conducted in humans. Animal studies show no risk to the fetus (e.g., amoxicillin, amoxicillin + clavulanic acid, cefotaxime, methyldopa, metronidazole, erythromycin)
C	No well-controlled studies have been conducted in humans. Animal studies have shown an adverse effect on the fetus (e.g., diclofenac, rifampicin, fluoroquinolones, aminoglycosides, glyburide)
D	Human studies have demonstrated a risk to the fetus. However, the benefits of therapy may outweigh the potential harm [e.g., tetracyclines, phenytoin, valproic acid, carbamazepine, angiotensin-converting enzyme (ACE) inhibitors]
X	Controlled studies in animals or humans have demonstrated fetal abnormalities. The use of the product is contraindicated in women who are or may become pregnant (e.g., thalidomide, oral contraceptive pills, misoprostol)

TABLE 23.6: List of few drugs contraindicated during pregnancy and those which have teratogenic effects.

Drug	*Side effects*
Tetracycline	Yellow staining of the primary or deciduous teeth and diminished growth of the long bones
Phenytoin	Fetal hydantoin syndrome consisting of intrauterine growth retardation (IUGR), microcephaly, mental retardation, distal phalangeal hypoplasia
Retinoic acid	Craniofacial dysmorphisms, cleft palate, thymic aplasia, and neural tube defects
Thalidomide	Meromelia, absence of the limbs to rudimentary limbs to abnormally shortened limbs
Alcohol	IUGR, small head, small eyes or short eye openings, or a poorly developed philtrum and congenital heart disease
Nicotine	Intrauterine growth retardation
Warfarin	Nasal hypoplasia and a depressed nasal bridge, stippled epiphysis; termed fetal warfarin syndrome
Estrogen and androgens	Genital tract malformations
Chloramphenicol	Gray baby syndrome

TABLE 23.7: Common problems in pregnancy and drugs that can be safely used.

Common problems in pregnancy	*Drugs that can be safely used*
Nausea and vomiting	Pyridoxine, meclizine diphenhydramine
Constipation	Mild purgative-like senna
Peptic ulcer	Sucralfate, H_2 blockers
Hematopoietic (iron and folic acid deficiency)	Iron and folic acid
Urinary tract infections	Ampicillin, amoxicillin, cefuroxime axetil
Other infections	β-lactam antibiotics, cephalosporins
Malaria	Chloroquine, quinine, proguanil
Amoebiasis	Metronidazole and diloxanide furoate
Worm infestation	Piperazine citrate, pyrantel pamoate
Fungal infection	Miconazole, clotrimazole, nystatin
Human immunodeficiency virus (HIV) infection	None of the anti-HIV drugs are safe, except zidovudine and nevirapine
Tuberculosis	INH and ethambutol are safe. If third drug is needed, then rifampicin
Diabetes mellitus	Insulin
Hypothyroidism	Thyroxine
Thyrotoxicosis	Propylthiouracil
Hypertension	α-methyldopa, in emergency—hydralazine, β-blockers—labetalol, atenolol
Thromboembolic disease	Heparin
Headache and inflammatory condition	Paracetamol, avoid other nonsteroidal anti-inflammatory drugs (NSAIDs)
Epilepsy	Sodium valproate and phenytoin to be avoided, carbamazepine in lower dose can be used
Migraine	Paracetamol, propranolol, amitriptyline
Antidepressants	Amitriptyline and imipramine

TABLE 23.8: Levels of evidence.

Level of evidence (LOE)	*Description*
Level I	Evidence from a **systematic review or meta-analysis** of all relevant RCTs (randomized controlled trials) or evidence-based clinical practice guidelines based on systematic reviews of RCTs or three or more RCTs of good quality that have similar results
Level II	Evidence obtained from at least one well-designed **RCT** (e.g., large multisite RCT)
Level III	Evidence obtained from well-designed **controlled trials without randomization** (i.e., quasi-experimental)
Level IV	Evidence from well-designed **case-control or cohort studies**
Level V	Evidence from systematic reviews of descriptive and qualitative studies (metasynthesis)
Level VI	Evidence from a single descriptive or qualitative study
Level VII	Evidence from the opinion of authorities and/or reports of expert committees

TABLE 23.9: Features of observational and experimental studies.

Observational studies	*Experimental studies*
Cross-sectional, case series, case-control studies, cohort studies ➢ Identify participants ➢ Observe and record characteristics ➢ Look for associations	Before and after studies, comparative trials (controlled or head to head), randomized trials ➢ Identify participants ➢ Place in common context ➢ Intervene ➢ Observe/evaluate effects of intervention

Levels of Evidence (Table 23.8)

Levels of evidence (sometimes called hierarchy of evidence) are assigned to studies based on the methodological quality of their design, validity, and applicability to patient care. These decisions give the "grade (or strength) of recommendation".

Features of observational and experimental studies are mentioned in **Table 23.9**.

Types of Study

The types of study have been shown in **Table 23.10**.

TABLE 23.10: Types of study with its pros and cons.

Types of study	*Description*	*Pros*	*Cons*
RCT (randomized controlled trial)	An experimental comparison study where participants are allocated to treatment/intervention or control/placebo groups using a random mechanism. Best for studying the effect of an intervention	Unbiased distribution of confounders. Blinding more likely. Randomization facilitates statistical analysis	*Expensive*: Time and money. Volunteer bias Ethically problematic at times
Crossover trial	A controlled trial where each participant has both therapies, i.e., randomized to treatment A first then starts treatment B	All participants serve as own controls and error variance is reduced, thus reducing sample size needed. All participants receive treatment (at least some of the time). Statistical tests assuming randomization can be used. Blinding can be maintained	All participants receive placebo or alternative treatment at some point. Washout period lengthy or unknown. Cannot be used for treatments with permanent effects
Cohort study	Data obtained from groups who have already been exposed, or not exposed, to the factor of interest. No allocation of exposure is made by the researcher. Best for studying effects of *risk factors on an outcome*	Ethically safe Participants can be matched Can establish timing and directionality of events Eligibility criteria and outcome assessments can be standardized	Controls may be difficult to identify. Exposure may be linked to a hidden confounder. Blinding is difficult For rare disease, large sample sizes or long follow-up necessary
Case-control study	Patients with a certain outcome or disease and an appropriate group of controls, without the outcome or disease, are selected (usually with somematching); then information is obtained on whether the subjects have been exposed to the factor under investigation	Quick and cheap as fewer people needed than cross-sectional studies. Only feasible method for very rare disorders or those with long lag between exposure and outcome	Reliance on recall or records to determine exposure status confounders Selection of control groups is difficult. *Potential bias*: Recall, selection
Cross-sectional study	Examines the relationship between (1) diseases/other health-related characteristics and (2) other variables of interest as they exist in defined population at one time. Exposure and outcomes both measured at the same time. Quantifies prevalence, risk, or diagnostic test accuracy	Cheap and simple. Ethically safe	Establishes association at most, not causality Recall bias, social desirability bias, Researcher's (Neyman) bias. Group sizes may be unequal. Confounders may be unequally distributed

Phases of Clinical Trials

Most trials that involve new drugs go through a series of steps:
- Experiments in the laboratory.
- Once deemed safe, go through 1–4 phases.
  - **Phase I:** Small group (20–80) for 1st time to evaluate safety, determine safe dosage range and identify side effects.
  - **Phase II:** Treatment given to larger group (100–300) to confirm effectiveness, monitor side effects, and further evaluate safety.
  - **Phase III:** Treatment given to even larger group (1,000–3,000) to fulfill all of phase II objectives and compare it to other commonly used treatments and collect data that will allow it to be used safely.
  - **Phase IV (postmarketing surveillance):** Done after treatment has been marketed—studies continue to test treatment to collect data about effects in various populations and side effects from long-term use.

Informed Consent

Informed consent document will be obtained from the participants in the study population after explaining them fully about: (1) the purpose; (2) duration; (3) required procedures; (4) expectations; (5) risks and benefits; (6) adverse effects of the trial if any, and (7) participants rights.

It is a continuous process throughout the study of learning of key facts by participants about a clinical trial. It also explains the rights of the participant. It is not a contract and the participant can withdraw from the trial at any time.

Ethical Aspects

- Participants are human beings with a motive to help the researcher and society.
- Researcher should never be overenthusiastic in his intervention to get his results while dealing with participants.
- Informed consent is not having a legal binding on the patients. It is a communication document.

Random Allocation

The participants in the study population are randomly allocated into two groups (arms) using random number tables to avoid selection and confounding biases.

Purpose of randomization: This elimination of allocation bias will greatly enhance the validity of the trial.

Blinding

The investigator, the participant and sometimes even the evaluator are all kept unaware (blinded) of the outcomes of the trial and secrecy is maintained to improve the validity.

Purpose of blinding: Blinding or masking is done to eliminate: (1) investigator bias; (2) evaluation bias and (3) Hawthorne effect.

Types of Blinding

The types of blinding have shown in **Table 23.11**.

TABLE 23.11: Types of blinding and their descriptions.

Types	*Description*
Unblinded or open label	All parties are aware of the treatment the participant receives
Single blind or single-masked	Only the participant is unaware of the treatment they receive
Double blind or double-masked	The participant and the clinicians/data collectors are unaware of the treatment the participant receives
Triple blind	Participant, clinicians/data collectors and outcome adjudicators/data analysts are all unaware of the treatment the participant receives

Unblinding

In emergencies and life-threatening situations for participants, unblinding can be done.

Assessment Criteria

- Whether the outcomes or endpoints are single or multiple, subjective or objective, uniform and similar type of evaluation of endpoints for both the groups is to be carried out.
- Subjectivity of the outcome, e.g., reduction of pain, may lead to observer error and poor assessment.
- Double blinding eliminates observer bias to a large extent.

Intention-to-Treat Principle

Whole of the experimental population including nonparticipants, once randomized, whether they are participating or not in the trial, have to be considered for evaluation as our intention is to treat all the people randomized.

Placebo Effect or Attention Bias

Psychological relief of symptoms, not true biological relief, is often reported. Neurophysiologically there is a increase of dopamine and opiods in people experiencing placebo effects.

Nocebo Effect

- These are adverse events produced by negative expectations. These are observed not only in everyday clinical practice, but also in clinical trials.
- Neurophysiologically there in decrease in dopamine, but increase in cortisol and CCK in people experiencing nocebo effect.
- These nonspecific side-effects distress patients, add to the burden of their illness, and increase the costs of their care.
- They may lead to nonadherence, cause physicians to discontinue what is otherwise an appropriate therapy or prompt attempts to treat these side-effects with additional drug.

Hawthorne Effect

- Sometimes the participants in comparison group may exaggerate the effects/outcomes to please the investigator or when they like the study or for some other reasons. Investigator does more frequent follow-up of exposed group in order to establish the cause.
- This will affect the assessment unless controlled.

CHAPTER

24

Emergencies in Medical Practice

CASE 1: MANAGEMENT OF SEVERE HYPERKALEMIA

History

An 80-year-old male found collapsed at home, incontinent of urine and feces. He is a known case of HTN and CCF; he is on enalapril for HTN, spironolactone and metoprolol for CCF.

Examination

Patient is confused and combative.

Vitals:

BP: 78/60 mm Hg PR: 75 bpm RR: 32/min SpO_2: 91%

GCS: 13

Investigations

pH: 7.23 K^+: 7.0 Blood glucose: 189 mg/dL

ECG:

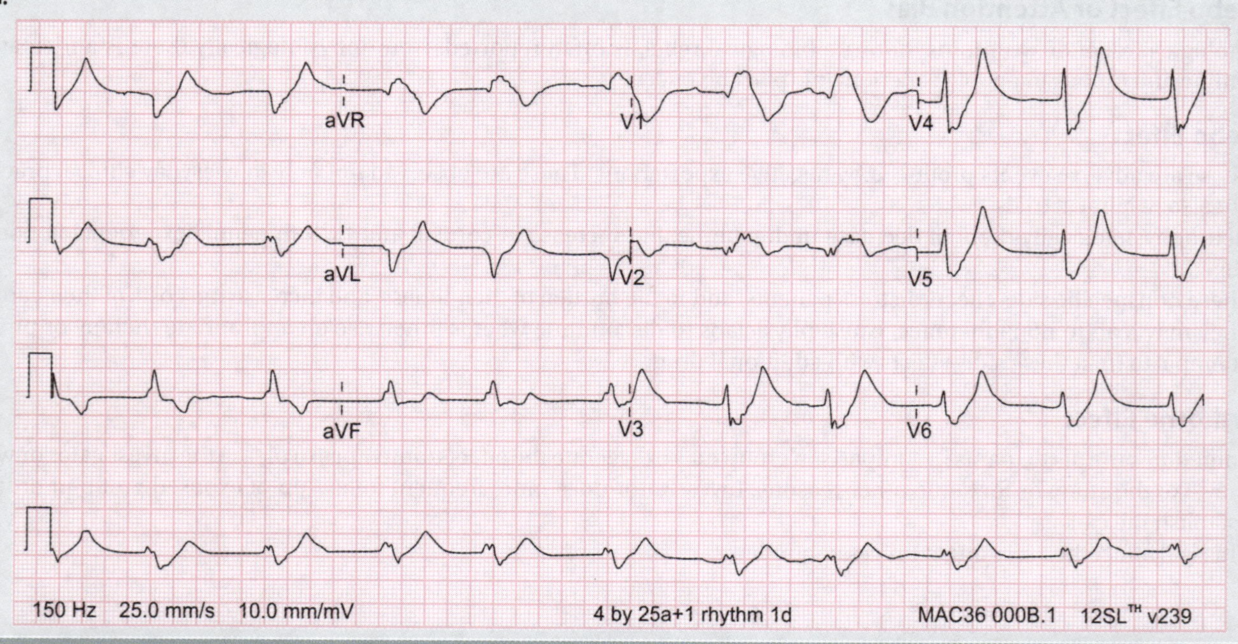

Management

Immediate antagonism of cardiac effects of hyperkalemia: **Membrane stabilization**	Calcium gluconate 10%, 10 mL slow IV over 10 minutes Calcium chloride 3–4 mL
Rapid reduction in plasma K^+ by redistribution into the cells	IV 50 mL of 50% dextrose + 10 units of regular insulin 10–20 mg of nebulized albuterol in 4 mL NS inhaled over 10 minutes
Removal of K^+ from the body	Ion exchange resin: Sodium polystyrene sulfonate 15–30 g powder—given in a premade suspension with 33% sorbitol, IV furosemide and NS, hemodialysis

CASE 2: METABOLIC ACIDOSIS

History

A 56-year-old man with a history of alcohol use presents with a 4-day history of severe abdominal pain, nausea, and vomiting.

Examination

Vitals:
BP: 80/50 mm Hg   Epigastric tenderness +

Investigations

Electrolytes:	**Serum biochemistry:**	**Arterial blood gas:**
Na: 132 Cl: 92 HCO_3: 16	Creatinine: 1.5 Amylase: 400 Lipase: 250	pH: 7.28 PCO_2: 34 mm Hg PO_2: 88 mm Hg HCO_3: 16.3 mEq/dL

Identify and treat the underlying cause
Determine ΔAG

Management

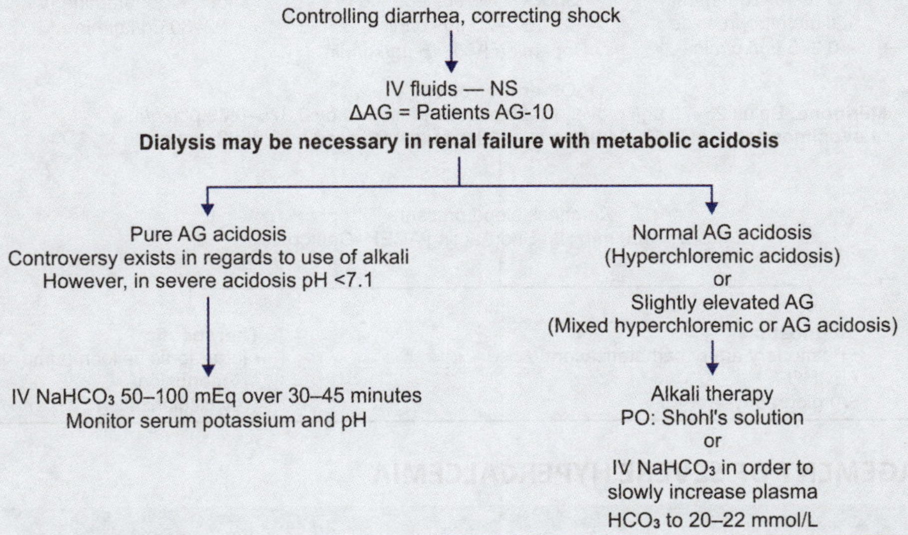

Controlling diarrhea, correcting shock
↓
IV fluids — NS
ΔAG = Patients AG-10
Dialysis may be necessary in renal failure with metabolic acidosis

- Pure AG acidosis
  Controversy exists in regards to use of alkali
  However, in severe acidosis pH <7.1
  ↓
  IV $NaHCO_3$ 50–100 mEq over 30–45 minutes
  Monitor serum potassium and pH

- Normal AG acidosis
  (Hyperchloremic acidosis)
  or
  Slightly elevated AG
  (Mixed hyperchloremic or AG acidosis)
  ↓
  Alkali therapy
  PO: Shohl's solution
  or
  IV $NaHCO_3$ in order to slowly increase plasma HCO_3 to 20–22 mmol/L

CASE 3: HYPOGLYCEMIA

History

A 32-year-old patient with altered level of consciousness. History of mellitus, on insulin.

Examination

GCS: 10 (E 3, V3, M4)
Vitals:
Pulse: 72 bpm   BP: 100/56 mm Hg SpO_2: 98%

Investigations

Blood sugar: 32 mg/dL

Management

Mild	***Severe***
If detected early, and patient is able to take and tolerate orally, carbohydrates orally in an easily absorbable form should be given.	Dextrose 75 mL of 20% dextrose IV Oral carbohydrate to be given as soon as the patient is able to eat Glucagon 0.5–1 mg SC/IM Octreotide Identify and treat the cause: ➢ Adjusting the dose of OHA, insulin ➢ Changing the timing of insulin injection

CASE 4: MANAGEMENT OF ACUTE PULMONARY EDEMA

History

A 62-year-old elderly male patient came with complaints of sudden severe shortness of breath.
Past history: MI—6 months back

Examination	
Patient is sitting leaning forward. He is pale, distressed, and sweaty. Productive pink tinged frothy sputum. **Vitals:** Pulse: 140 bpm BP: 200/110 mm Hg RR: 38/min SpO_2: 78%	Bilateral pedal edema present upto ankle level **Cardiovascular system:** Gallop rhythm **Respiratory System:** Basal crepitations present bilaterally

Management

Monitor vitals
Oxygen: Noninvasive positive pressure ventilation or intubation and mechanical ventilation
Furosemide 0.5–1 mg/kg IV bolus
Morphine 2–4 mg IV

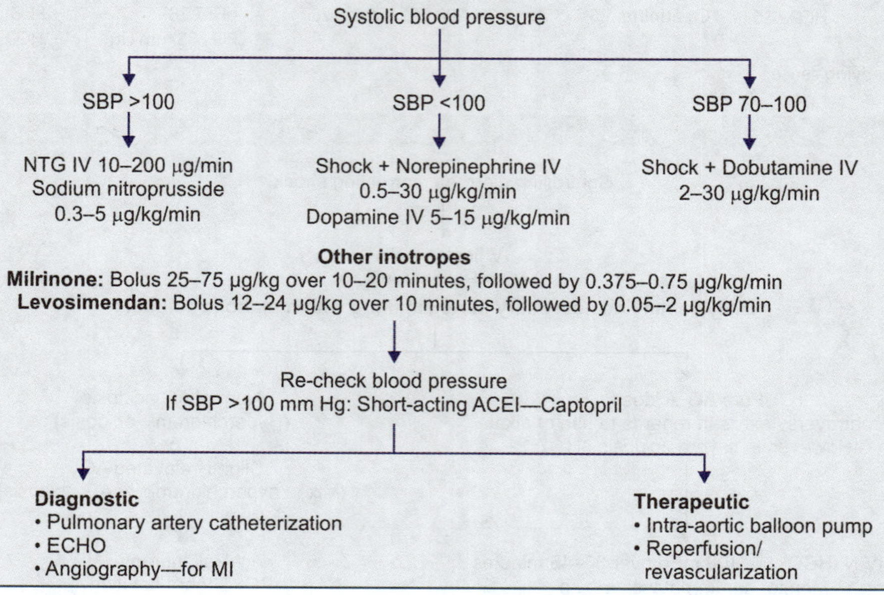

Systolic blood pressure

- SBP >100 → NTG IV 10–200 µg/min; Sodium nitroprusside 0.3–5 µg/kg/min
- SBP <100 → Shock + Norepinephrine IV 0.5–30 µg/kg/min; Dopamine IV 5–15 µg/kg/min
- SBP 70–100 → Shock + Dobutamine IV 2–30 µg/kg/min

Other inotropes
Milrinone: Bolus 25–75 µg/kg over 10–20 minutes, followed by 0.375–0.75 µg/kg/min
Levosimendan: Bolus 12–24 µg/kg over 10 minutes, followed by 0.05–2 µg/kg/min

↓

Re-check blood pressure
If SBP >100 mm Hg: Short-acting ACEI—Captopril

Diagnostic
- Pulmonary artery catheterization
- ECHO
- Angiography—for MI

Therapeutic
- Intra-aortic balloon pump
- Reperfusion/revascularization

CASE 5: MANAGEMENT OF SEVERE HYPERCALCEMIA

History

An 80-year-old woman presented with vomiting, diarrhea, fatigue, malaise, generalized abdominal pain, and weight loss. K/c/o metastatic breast cancer.

Examination

Vitals:
Pulse: 98 bpm BP: 90/70 mm Hg RR: 14/min
Per abdomen: Generalized abdominal tenderness present

Investigations

Serum calcium > 11 mg/dL

Management	
Intravenous normal saline	4–6 L may be required over first 24 hours
Bisphosphonates	Inhibit bone resorption: ➢ Zoledronic acid 4 mg IV over 30 minute ➢ Pamidronate 60–90 mg IV over 2–4 hours ➢ Ibandronate 2 mg IV over 2 hours
Calcitonin	Increases calcium excretion; 100 U; 3 times/day; IM/SC for first 24–48 hours
Gallium nitrate	➢ 200 mg/m² IV daily for 5 days ➢ Alternative to bisphosphonates ➢ Nephrotoxic
Dialysis	

CASE 6: TENSION PNEUMOTHORAX

History

A 23-year-old man presents with a single gunshot wound to the right side of his chest.

Examination	
Patient is conscious. Central cyanosis **Vitals:** Pulse: Palpable, rapid, thready BP: 90/60 mm Hg RR: 30/min, rapidly progressing dyspnea	**Respiratory system:** Trachea deviated to the left Jugular veins are distended Palpable crepitus Decreased chest movements on right side Percussion—hyper-resonance on right side Decreased/Absent breath sounds and vocal resonance on right side

Investigations

Chest X-ray

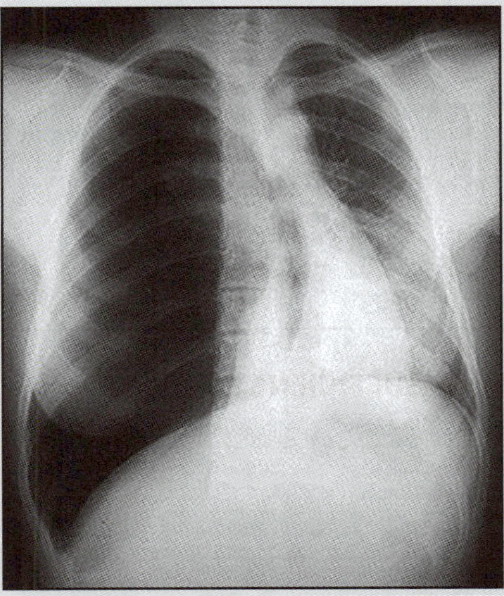

Management

Insertion of wide bore needle into pleural space through the anterior 2nd ICS. Needle is left in place till a thoracostomy tube is inserted
OR
Insertion of a wide bore plastic cannula, attached to a long rubber tubing, end of which is placed underwater

↓

Insertion of intercostal drainage tube in 4th/5th/6th ICS in mid-axillary line connected to an underwater seal or one way Heimlich valve

CASE 7: MYXEDEMA COMA

History

A 47-year-old female patient known case of hypothyroidism presented with complaints of falls, leg edema and pain, drowsiness, headaches, and shortness of breath.

Examination

Vitals:
Pulse: 50 bpm BP: 90/70 mm Hg
RR: 20/min

Periorbital edema is present.
Nonpitting edema is present.
Central nervous system: Delayed tendon reflexes

Investigations

Thyroid function:	Na^+: 121 mEq/L	**Other investigations required:**
Free T3: 0.05 ng/dL (0.93–1.7)	K^+: 4.2 mEq/L	T4, CPK, ABG, RBS, sepsis screening
TSH: 30.12 µIU/mL (0.27–5.0)	Cl^-: 87 mEq/L	

Management

Treatment must be initiated even before biochemical confirmation of diagnosis
Monitor vitals—temperature
Levothyroxine 500 µg IV bolus or **Tri-iodothyronine** 10–25 µg every 8–12 hourly IV; followed by oral levothyroxine 50–100 µg daily
Hydrocortisone 100 mg IV TID
Slow rewarming
Cautious use of **IV fluids**: Hypotonic fluids to be avoided because they can increase water retention.
Broad spectrum antibiotics
High flow oxygen
Identify and treat the cause

CASE 8: THYROTOXIC CRISIS/THYROID STORM

History

A 39-year-old woman presented with a 3-month history of increased sweating and palpitations with weight loss of 7 kg. She had family history of thyroid disease.

Examination

Vitals:
Pulse: 122 bpm BP: 130/80 mm Hg RR: 20/min
Warm and moist skin. Her thyroid gland is enlarged bilaterally. Bilateral exophthalmos present.
S/E: CVS: Tachycardia present PA: Generalized abdominal tenderness

Investigations			
T4—12.00 ng/dL (0.73–1.84)	T3—1173.00 ng/dL (123–211 ng/dL)	TSH < 0.018 ulU/mL	T3, T4, TSH, sepsis screen, LFT, ECG

Management

Rehydrate
Propranolol: Given orally: 60–80 mg 4 times a day. IV: 1–5 mg 4 times a day
Propylthiouracil: Loading dose: 500–1000 mg followed by maintainance dose of 250 mg 4th hourly oral or via NG tube
Carbimazole: 15–30 mg stat followed by 15 mg TID
Lugol's iodine: 10 drops TID—1 hour after PTU/carbimazole
Sodium ipodate: 500 mg/day orally
Hydrocortisone: 200 mg IV bolus followed by 100 mg every 8th hourly
Oxygen, IV fluids, external cooling
Identify and treat the cause
Antibiotics if infection is present.

CASE 9: ACUTE ADRENAL INSUFFICIENCY

History

A 38-year-old female is admitted for complaints of progressive fatigue for 2 weeks. She also complains of nausea and vomiting. History of loss of 8 kg in the past 2 weeks. History of recent onset of breathlessness.

Examination

Vitals: Pulse: 134 bpm BP: 80/40 mm Hg RR: 18/min Temperature: 99°F	Appears pale, dehydrated, and malnourished **Systemic examination:** Unremarkable

Investigations

Na: 120 mmol/L K: 5.9 mmol/L	Hb: 12.4 g/dL WBC: 11,600 and mild eosinophilia

Management

Monitor vitals
Rehydration
Normal saline IV infusion: 1 L/hr with continuous cardiac monitoring
Draw blood for plasma cortisol and blood sugars
Hydrocortisone: 100 mg IV bolus, followed by 100 mg 6th hourly for the first 24 hours and continue parenterally till patient can take orally.
Treat hypoglycemia and hyperkalemia
Treat the precipitating cause

CASE 10: COMA

Investigations

CBC, RBS, electrolytes LFT, RFT, ABG, blood culture, CXR, ECG, CT scan, drug screen if indicated

Management

General measures	***Specific treatment***	***Long-term management***
➢ Monitor vitals ➢ Protect the airway: Oropharyngeal airway/intubation if needed ➢ Avoid secondary insults to the brain like hypoxia, hypoglycemia, and hypotension ➢ Secure IV access: Hypotonic IV fluids with close monitoring	➢ Hypoglycemic coma: Thiamine followed by dextrose ➢ Fever and meningismus indicate urgent need for CSF analysis followed by IV antibiotics	➢ Frequent change of position every 2–3 hourly to avoid bedsores ➢ Lid taping ➢ Catheterization ➢ Prevent aspiration by positioning the patient left lateral

CASE 11: SNAKE BITE

A 24-year-old farmer brought to the casualty with history of snakebite 3 hours back.

Management

- Reassure the patient
- Immobilize the bitten limb
- **Investigations:** Whole blood clotting time (**WBCT),** CBC, coagulation screen, RFT, electrolytes, CPK, ECG, URE, FDP, fibrinogen level
- Monitor vitals
- Input/output (I/O) charting
- Secure IV access
- ASV if indicated:
  - Mild cases: 5 vials
  - Moderate cases: 5–10 vials
  - Severe cases: 10–20 vials
- Given as IV infusion in 5–10 mL/kg of NS and given over 1 hour
- **Never give locally at the site of snakebite**
- Keep adrenaline ready in case of anaphylaxis
- For coagulopathy: FFP/cryoprecipitate/platelet concentrate

- In case of neurotoxic snake bite: If there is respiratory failure or bulbar paralysis:
  - Intubation and mechanical ventilation
  - Give injection glycopyrrolate 0.25 mg
  - Followed injection neostigmine IV infusion 50–100 mg/kg/4 hours
- Antibiotic prophylaxis
- Antitetanus prophylaxis
- Renal failure managed with hemodialysis

CASE 12: HYPOVOLEMIA

History

A 50-year-old male is brought in an ambulance, following road traffic accident 45 minutes prior, with a penetrating injury to the thigh.

Investigations

Hemoglobin, hematocrit, BUN, creatinine, electrolytes, ABG, urinary sodium

Management

Monitor vitals
Secure IV line
Strict I/O charting
Mild hypovolemia can be treated with oral hydration.
Severe hypovolemia requires intravenous hydration, give isotonic normal saline – 0.9 % NaCl (154 mM Na^+).
Calculation of free water deficit:

$$\text{Free water deficit} = \text{Total body water} \times \frac{[\text{plasma sodium}-1]}{140}$$

50% of this calculated deficit is given over the first 24 hours and the remaining over the next 24 hours.
Patients with bicarbonate loss and metabolic acidosis may need IV bicarbonate.
Patients with severe hemorrhage should receive red cell transfusion without increasing hematocrit >35%.
Identify and treat the cause of hypovolemia.

CASE 13: MANAGEMENT OF SHOCK

History

A 25-year-old male patient is admitted to ICU with 3 days old perforation. History of chills and fever is present.

Examination

Mental status is altered, restless
Vitals:
Pulse: 130 bpm BP: 80/60 mm Hg RR: 40/min
Skin—warmed and flushed

Investigations

Hemoglobin, hematocrit, sepsis screen, LFT, RFT, electrolytes, ABG

Management

Secure IV access
Assess GCS, qSOFA score
Oxygen/intubation and mechanical ventilation if needed, e.g., GCS <8

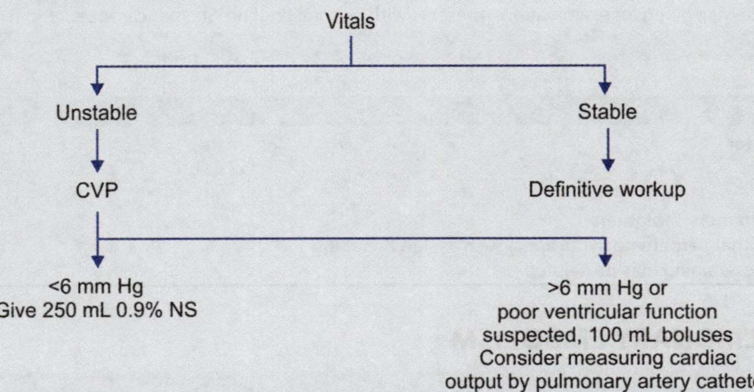

Monitor vitals, I/O charting, peripheral perfusion
Optimize Hb: Transfuse red cells
Achieve target BP: Inotropes once the hypovolemia is corrected
- Dobutamine: 2–8 µg/kg/min
- Adrenaline: 1–8 µg/kg/min

➢ Refractory hypotension: Add Inj. Hydrocortisone 50 mg IV Q6H

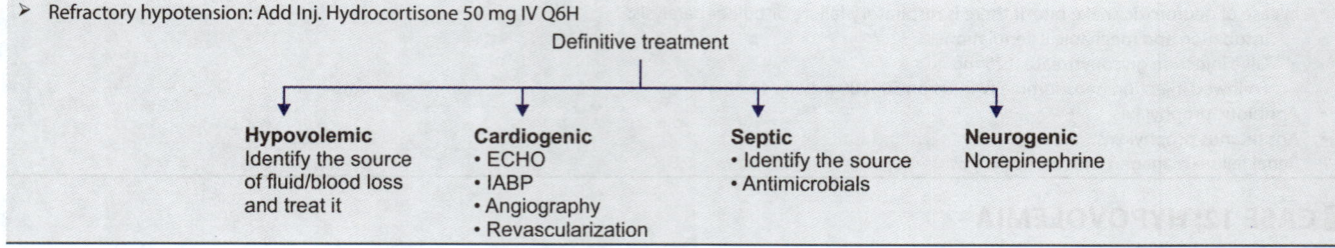

CASE 14: ISCHEMIC STROKE

History

A 41-year-old male patient, alcoholic, k/c/o hypertension presents to casualty with chief complaint of right sided weakness, slurred speech, and loss of balance. Symptoms began 90 minutes prior to arrival.

Examination

Vitals:		**CNS:**	
Pulse: 88 bpm, irregular	BP: 178/90 mm Hg	Right side facial weakness	Power is reduced on right side
RR: 18/min	GCS—11/15	No sensory deficit on right side	Plantar extensor on right side

Investigations

Plain CT brain, RBS, electrolytes, ECG, suspected AF → thyroid function tests, ECHO

Management

General measures	Airway—ensure airway patency Breathing—O_2 if SpO_2 is < 95% Circulation—check PR, BP. Secure IV access. Treat abnormalities with IV fluids/antiarrhythmias/inotropes Look for hypoglycemia and treat accordingly
IV thrombolytics	Intravenous rtPA within 3 hours of onset of ischemic stroke Dose: 0.9 mg/kg → 10% of total dose as IV bolus, remaining as IV infusion over 60 minutes
Endovascular mechanical thrombectomy	If IV thrombolysis is contraindicated or has failed
Antiplatelets	Aspirin 75–150 mg OD
Statins	Atorvastatin, rosuvastatin 10–20 mg OD
Medical support	Catheterization RT feeding Treat fever with antipyretics, surface cooling Pneumatic compression stockings Prevent bedsores and contractures Initiate secondary preventive measures
Rehabilitation	Early physiotherapy, occupational/speech therapy

CASE 15: HYPERVENTILATION

History

A 21-year-old girl, k/c/o anxiety disorder, going for examinations, presents with perioral tingling. She has carpopedal spasms.

Investigation

ABG

Management

Identify and treat the initiating factor
Reassurance
Rebreathing into a closed bag
If there is associated palpitations/tremors: β-blockers
Identifying and eliminating habits that perpetuate hypocapnia such as sigh breathing
Breathing exercises, diaphragmatic retaining may be helpful.

CASE 16: ACUTE PULMONARY EMBOLISM

History

A 71-year-old woman bedridden for last 4 days following fall and trauma to right hip is brought to emergency with complaints of sudden onset of dyspnea and dizziness.

Examination

Vitals:		Diaphoresis present
Pulse: 124 bpm	BP: 118/90 mm Hg	Right lower limb edema present extending from mid-thigh to foot
RR: 28/min	SpO_2: 84%	Calf muscle tenderness present

Investigations

ECG, CXR, 2D ECHO, D-dimer, pulmonary angiography

Management

Supportive measures	Oxygen and IV fluids
Anticoagulation	**Unfractionated heparin:** 80 U/kg bolus → 18 U/kg/hr with aPTT monitoring. (Platelet count to be monitored at least every 3rd day) **LMWH:** Subcutaneously (should not be discontinued until INR is >2 for at least 24 hours) **Warfarin:** 5 mg/day—started on day 1 with INR monitoring Fondaparinux **Others:** Rivaroxaban, Apixaban, Argatroban, Ximelagatran *Note:* Anticoagulation to be continued for at least 6 months
Thrombolysis	Indication: Acute massive pulmonary embolism with cardiogenic shock. 100 mg rtPA IV infusion over 2 hours
Surgical therapy	Surgical embolectomy Caval filter

CASE 17: HEMOPTYSIS

History

A 40-year-old male chronic smoker, with past history of tuberculosis, presents with history of hemoptysis, 3 episodes in the last 1 day.

Examination

Vitals:
Pulse: 100 bpm BP: 100/60 mm Hg Clubbing +
Respiratory system: Coarse crepitations in right infraclavicular area

Investigations

Blood grouping, cross matching, CBC, PT/INR, CXR

Management

Measure vitals
Patient should be positioned upright or bleeding side down.
Secure airway—intubation with double lumen ET tube is preferable.
Secure IV access: Large bore IV cannula
Administer IV fluids or blood transfusion, if needed
Vasopressin 0.2 to 0.4 U/min IV

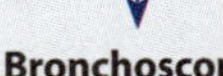

Bronchoscopy
- Rigid bronchoscopy is preferable.
- Fiberoptic bronchoscopy may be used for cold saline lavage.
- Topical thrombin
- Laser photocoagulation
- Balloon catheter can be inflated proximally in the bleeding bronchus.

↓

Endovascular embolization
OR
Emergency surgery

CASE 18: HYPERTENSIVE EMERGENCY/CRISIS

History

A 69-year-old male patient presented with complaints of chest tightness and shortness of breath, k/c/o DM for the last 10 years and is a chronic smoker. History of hypertension, not on treatment.

Examination

Vitals: Pulse: 110 bpm BP: 230/120 mm Hg	**S/E:** CVS: S3 gallop, No murmur RS: Bi-basal fine inspiratory crackles

Management

Reduce the MAP by no more than 25% within minutes—2 hours
Continuous monitoring of BP

Labetalol	2 mg/min IV; maximum of 300 mg In acute renal failure, subarachnoid hemorrhage, intracranial bleed, and acute aortic dissection
Nitroglycerine	0.6–1.2 mg/hr IV In acute pulmonary edema, acute coronary syndrome, IC bleed

Sodium nitroprusside	0.3–1 μg/kg/min IV Drug of choice for hypertensive encephalopathy
Nicardipine	5 mg/hr IV titrate by 2.5 mg/hr at 5–15-minute intervals → Maximum 15 mg/hr
Esmolol	80–500 μg/kg over 1 minute → 50–300 μg/kg/min IV
Hydralazine	10–50 mg at 30 minute intervals

CASE 19: SEVERE DEHYDRATION

History

A 23-year-old male, presented with history of vomiting 5–6 episodes/day and diarrhea 6–7 episodes/day for the last 2 days.

Clinical features

Sunken eyes, dry tongue, skin pinch going back slowly. BP is 80 mm Hg systolic.

Investigations

Electrolytes, urea, creatinine, RBS

Management

Secure IV access
Monitor vitals
I/O chartings
IV fluids started immediately—RL + 5% dextrose or normal saline
ORS can be given as soon as the patient is able to take orally (5 mL/kg/hr).
Reclassify dehydration and treat accordingly
Daily fluid requirement:
- Up to 10 kg: 100 mL/kg
- 10–20 kg: 50 mL/kg
- >20 kg: 20 mL/kg

	30 mL/kg	***70 mL/kg***
<12 months	1 hour	5 hours
>12 months	30 minutes	2.5 hours

CASE 20: CARDIAC ARREST

Immediate identification of cardiac arrest and activation of emergency response system

↓

Early CPR (30:2)

↓

Basic life support:
Circulation: Chest compression → push hard – push fast
Airway: Clear the airway—head tilt, chin lift; jaw thrust; sweep finger inside oral cavity; Heimlich maneuver
Breathing: Mouth to mouth

↓

Advanced cardiac life support:
Circulation: IV access, attach cardiac monitors, assess the rhythm and defibrillate
Airway: Face mask, Ambu bag, oropharyngeal airway, laryngeal mask airway, endotracheal tube
Breathing: Supplement oxygen

Drugs:
Adrenaline, vasopressin, amiodarone, magnesium sulfate, atropine

↓

Defibrillation:
Shockable rhythms are ventricular fibrillation and pulseless ventricular tachycardia

↓

Postresuscitation care:
Mild therapeutic hypothermia for resuscitated cardiac arrest victims who are hemodynamically stable but remain comatose

↓

Long-term management:
Identify and treat the cause
Example: Implantable cardioverter defibrillator in Brugada syndrome
Initiating antiarrythmics

CASE 21: VENTRICULAR FIBRILLATION

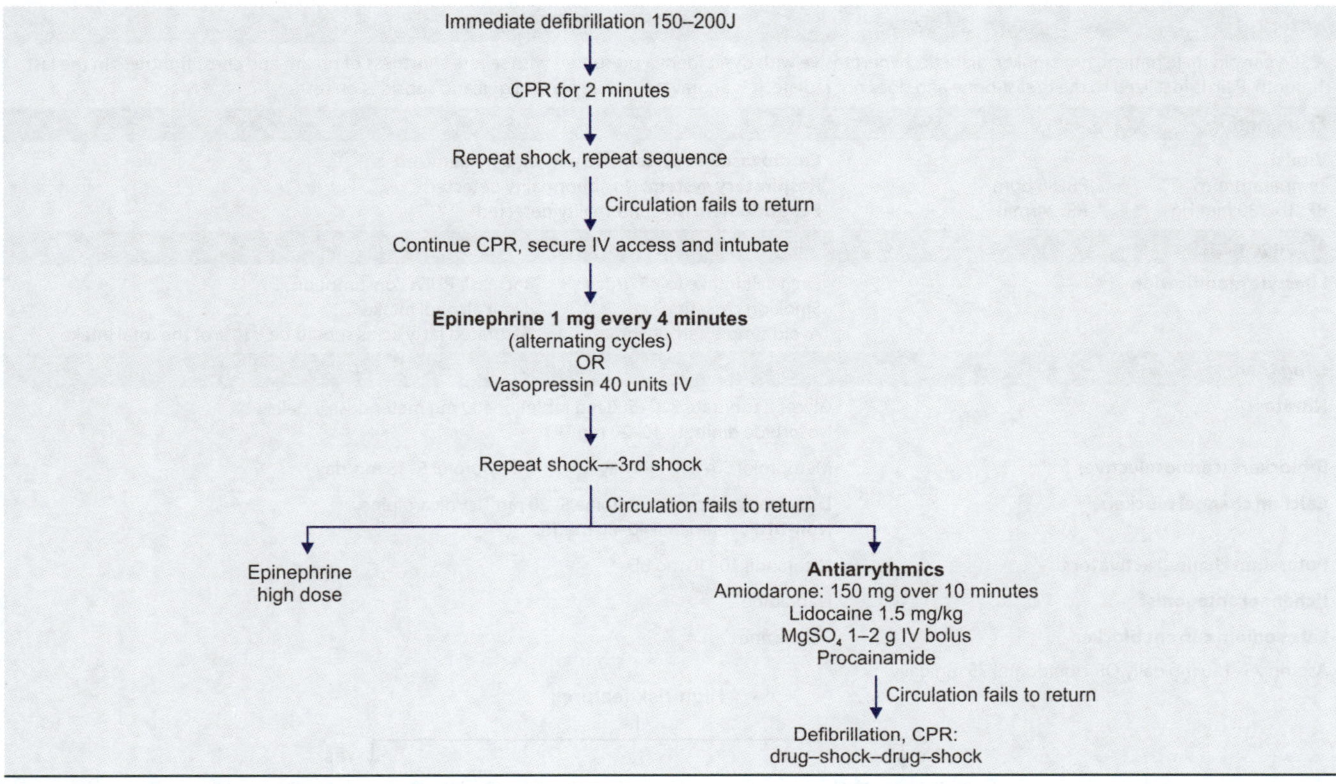

CASE 22: UPPER GASTROINTESTINAL BLEED

History

A 45-year-old male, k/c/o alcoholic liver disease, presents with 4 episodes of vomiting, fresh blood present.

Investigations

CBC, electrolytes, LFT, urea, PT/INR, blood grouping and cross-matching

Management

NPO
Secure IV access
Monitor vitals, I/O charting
Restore blood volume: IV fluids/blood transfusion if needed
IV PPI 80 mg bolus → 8 mg/hr infusion
Suspected variceal bleed

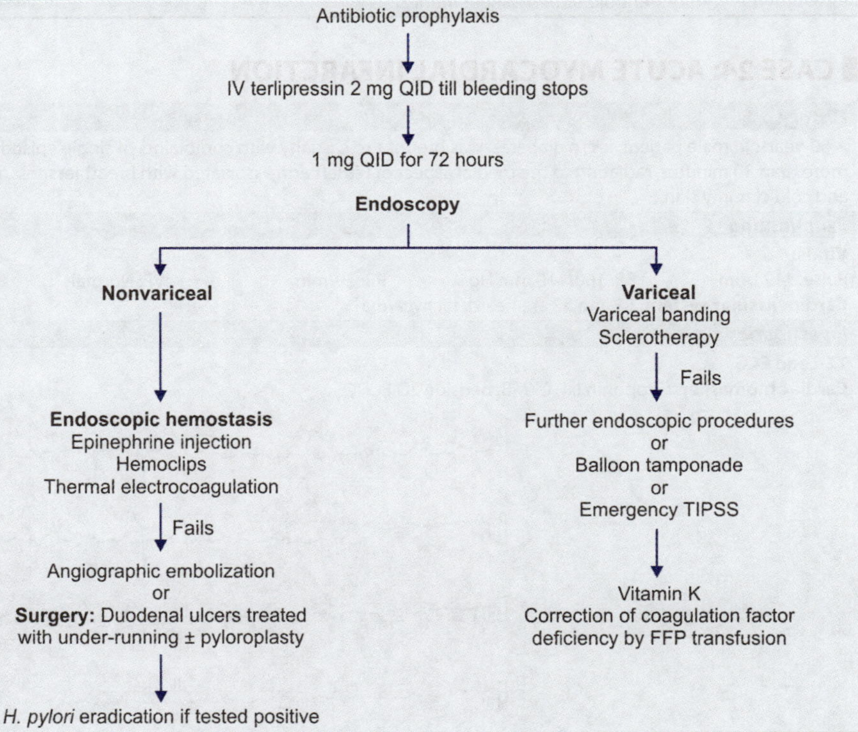

Antibiotic prophylaxis
↓
IV terlipressin 2 mg QID till bleeding stops
↓
1 mg QID for 72 hours

Endoscopy

Nonvariceal
↓
Endoscopic hemostasis
Epinephrine injection
Hemoclips
Thermal electrocoagulation
↓ Fails
Angiographic embolization
or
Surgery: Duodenal ulcers treated with under-running ± pyloroplasty
↓
H. pylori eradication if tested positive

Variceal
Variceal banding
Sclerotherapy
↓ Fails
Further endoscopic procedures
or
Balloon tamponade
or
Emergency TIPSS
↓
Vitamin K
Correction of coagulation factor deficiency by FFP transfusion

CASE 23: MANAGEMENT OF ANGINA

History

A 58-year-old male patient, nonsmoker, diabetic, hypertensive with dyslipidemia presented with severe shortness of breath and chest tightness in the last 1 month. Pain is localized to the breast bone and does not radiate. It is aggravated while playing golf and subsides on rest.

Examination

Vitals:		**Cardiovascular system:** No abnormality detected
Temperature: 37°C	PR: 88 bpm	**Respiratory system:** No abnormality detected
BP: 162/80 mm Hg	RR: 24/min	**Per abdomen:** No abnormality detected

Management

Lifestyle modification	Limit salt intake to <5 g/day	Increase PUFA consumption
	Smoking cessation	Limit alcohol intake
	Avoid simple carbohydrate	Saturated fatty acids should be <10% of the total intake

Drug therapy

Nitrates	Glyceryl trinitrate 300–500 mg tablet or 400 mg meter dose inhaler Isosorbide dinitrate 10–20 mg TID
β-blockers (cardioselective)	Metoprolol 50–200 mg/day Bisoprolol 5–15 mg/day
Calcium channel blockers	**Dihydropyridines:** Nifedipine 5–20 mg TID, nicardipine **Non-DHP:** Verapamil 40–80 mg TID
Potassium channel activators	Nicorandil 10–30 mg BD
I_f channel antagonist	Ivabradine
Late sodium current blocker	Ranolazine

Aspirin 75–150 mg daily OR clopidogrel 75 mg daily.

High-risk features

- No → Symptoms controlled
  - Yes → Continue medical therapy, Periodic stress assessment
  - No → Coronary angiography
- Yes → Coronary angiography → Anatomy suitable for revascularization → PCI / CABG

CASE 24: ACUTE MYOCARDIAL INFARCTION

History

A 60-year-old male patient, k/c/o diabetes, was brought to casualty with complaints of single episode of sudden, rapid onset, severe chest pain, lasting more than 30 minutes, radiating to the medial aspect of his left arm associated with breathlessness, nausea, heavy perspiration, lightheadedness, fever, and cold clammy skin.

Examination

Vitals:

Pulse: 112 bpm BP: 160/110 mm Hg RR: 20/min JVP: Normal

Cardiovascular system: S1 and S2 are heard, tachycardia

Investigations

12-Lead ECG

Cardiac biomarkers: Troponin I, T, CKMB, bedside 2D ECHO

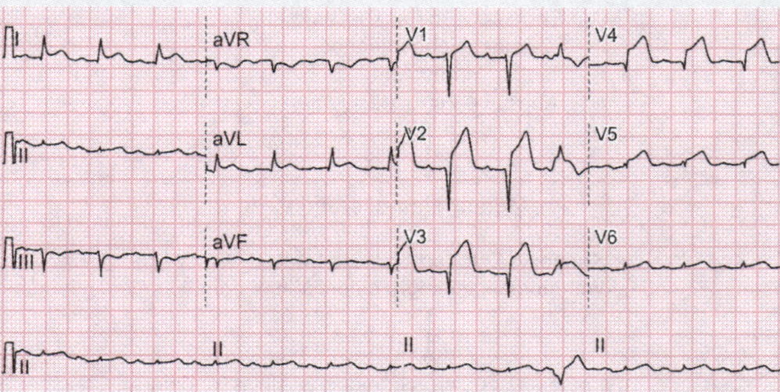

Management
Monitor vitals and oxygen saturation Administer oxygen via mask or nasal cannula **Nitrates:** Glyceryl trinitrate 300–500 µg sublingually ↓ If pain persists after 3 doses given 5 minutes apart IV NTG 5–10 µg/min (maintain SBP >40 mm Hg) **Morphine:** 2–5 mg IV—analgesia **Antiplatelets:** ➢ Aspirin: 325 mg nonenteric formulations → 75–100 mg/day ➢ Clopidogrel: 300 mg orally → 75 mg/day ➢ Others: Oral—prasugrel, ticagrelor ➢ IV—abciximab, eptifibatide, tirofiban **Anticoagulants:** ➢ Unfractionated heparin ➢ Low-molecular-weight heparin ➢ Direct thrombin inhibitor—bivalirudin ➢ Factor Xa inhibitor—fondaparinux β-blockers unless contraindicated; ACEI; high dose statins **Specific treatment:** ➢ **Thrombolytic therapy**—for ST elevation MI. Not recommended in unstable angina and NSTEMI ➢ **Coronary interventions**—percutaneous coronary interventions, coronary artery bypass graft

CASE 25: ORGANOPHOSPHATE POISONING

History			
A 27-year-old male brought to casualty at 1:00 am with history of sudden loss of consciousness in his room after having a family quarrel. History of 4 episodes of vomiting and incontinence of urine and feces.			
Examination			
Vitals: Temperature: 102°F BP: 90/70 mm Hg **GCS:** 7 (1, 2, 4)	 Pulse: 100 bpm RR: 28/min, shallow	**Central nervous system:** Pupils: Bilateral pinpoint, nonreacting Power: Grade I **Per abdomen:** Bowel sounds are exaggerated	 Tone: Increased Plantar: Nonelicitable
Investigations			
LFT, ABG, ECG, electrolytes, glucose, amylase			
Management			
Prevent further exposure—remove contaminate clothing, wash the skin thoroughly with soap and water, irrigate eyes Airway cleared of excessive secretions → high flow oxygen IV access → 0.9% NS infusion Monitor vitals, SpO_2, auscultate the lungs. Ventilatory support, if needed Gastric lavage with activated charcoal if the patient presents within 1 hour of ingestion, Foley catheterization			

Atropine bolus	***Atropine infusion***
Start at 1.8–3 mg IV bolus; aim for HR > 80 bpm, SBP > 80 mm Hg and a clear chest If not achieved—double the dose every 5 minutes till there is satisfactory improvement	Start infusion at 20% of total dose of atropine required for atropinization Bronchorrhea is the most import sign for titrating the dose
Pralidoxime	Bolus: 30–45 mg/kg over 30 minutes followed by infusion: 8–12 mg/kg/hr Give PAM until atropine is no longer required
Benzodiazepines	Reduces agitation, seizures, fasciculations Sedation during ventilation
Intensive cardiorespiratory monitoring and support **Others:** $MgSO_4$, $NaHCO_3$, clonidine, hemodialysis	

CASE 26: MANAGEMENT OF ANAPHYLAXIS

History	
A 12-year-old boy is brought to the emergency department after being stung by a bee. Initially complained of localized pain and swelling, but 15 minutes later he began to complain of shortness of breath, weakness, and dizziness.	
Examination	
Vitals: Pulse: 120 bpm BP: 68/46 mm Hg RR: 39/min	He has generalized urticaria **Respiratory system:** Mild wheeze bilaterally **Cardiovascular system:** Tachycardia present **Per abdomen:** No abnormality detected

Management
Prevent further contact with the antigen Ensure airway patency **Supportive measures:** ➤ **Oxygen** ➤ IV fluids ➤ B_2 agonist **Drug therapy:** ➤ **Adrenaline:** 0.01 mg/kg (maximum dose of 0.5 mg) per single dose. Injected intramuscularly into the mid-outer thigh (vastus lateralis muscle) ➤ **Antihistamines:** – Chlorphenamine—10 mg IM/slow IV – Diphenhydramine IM/IV ➤ **Corticosteroids:** Hydrocortisone 200 mg IV stat

CASE 27: MANAGEMENT OF ACUTE SEVERE ASTHMA

History			
A 16-year-old female patient complains of acute onset of difficulty in breathing. Symptoms increase on exposure to cold. Positive family history.			
Examination			
Vitals:			
Pulse: 126 bpm	BP: 148/86 mm Hg	RR: 54/min	SpO_2: 88 at room air
Respiratory system: Expiratory wheeze noted			
Investigations			
ABG **PaO_2:** Low due to hypoxia **$PaCO_2$:** Low due to hyperventilation Normal or rising $PaCO_2$ is a sign of impending respiratory failure			
Management			
Oxygen	*Bronchodilators*	*Systemic corticosteroids*	*Other*
High concentration (60%) **oxygen** via mask ventilation Maintain saturation >92%	**Nebulized salbutamol** 5 mg OR **Terbutaline** 2.5 mg to be administered immediately and repeated if required Can be followed up with **nebulized ipratropium bromide** 0.5 mg if required	**Hydrocortisone sodium succinate** 200 mg IV at presentation and repeated 4–6th hourly for 24 hours	**Aminophylline** IV infusion may be beneficial, but requires cardiac monitoring **$MgSO_4$**—IV bronchodilator **Antibiotics** are given only if there are signs of respiratory infection
Indications for assisted ventilation	Coma Respiratory arrest Deterioration in ABG—PaO_2 <60 mm Hg and falling, $PaCO_2$ >45 mm Hg and rising, pH <7.3 and falling Exhaustion, confusion, drowsiness		

CASE 28: DIABETIC KETOACIDOSIS

History			
A 32-year-old male patient, k/c/o type 1 diabetes mellitus, was taken to casualty with complaints of drowsiness, fever, diffuse abdominal pain and vomiting.			
Examination			
Patient appears confused. **Vitals:** Temperature: 39°C PR: 104 bpm BP: 100/70 mm Hg RR: 24/min	Dry mucous membranes	Poor skin turgor	Rales in right lower chest
Investigations			
Arterial blood gas: pCO_2: 17 mm Hg pH: 7.12 HCO_3: 5.6 mEq/L **Urinalysis:** Glucose: 4+ Ketone: 3+	**Biochemistry:** Blood glucose: 420 mg/dL Blood urea nitrogen: 16 mg/dL Creatinine: 1.1 mg/dL **Electrolytes** Na: 139 mEq/dL Cl: 112 mEq/dL HCO2: 11.2 mEq/L K: 5.0 mEq/dL		
Management			
Confirm the diagnosis Monitor vitals and maintain hourly input/output monitoring Send investigations—Na, K, HCO_3, phosphate, Mg, ABG, RFT Monitor capillary glucose 1–2 hourly, electrolytes 4th hourly for the first 24 hours			

Fluids	Insulin	Potassium
0.9% NS 10–20 mL/kg/hr 0.45% NS at 250–500 mL/hr **Replacement:** 1 L over 60 minutes followed by 1 L over 2 hours 1 L over 4 hours 1 L over next 4 hours 1 L over 6 hours Change over to 0.45% NS + 5% glucose when plasma glucose reaches 250 mg/dL	Short-acting insulin IV bolus 0.1 U/kg ↓ IV infusion at 0.1 U/kg/hr Increase 2–3-fold if no response by 2–4 hours Initiate subcutaneous insulin at least 2 hours prior to interruption of insulin infusion	**Serum potassium 3.5–5.2 mEq/L:** Replace with 10 mEq/hr or 20–30 mEq/L of infusion fluid **Serum potassium <3.5 mEq/L:** Replace with 40–80 mEq/hr. Do not administer insulin until potassium is corrected.

CASE 29: STATUS EPILEPTICUS

History

A 65-year-old male, k/c/o epilepsy, presents with a generalized tonic-clonic seizure for the last 30 minutes and loss of bladder control and difficulty in speech.

Management

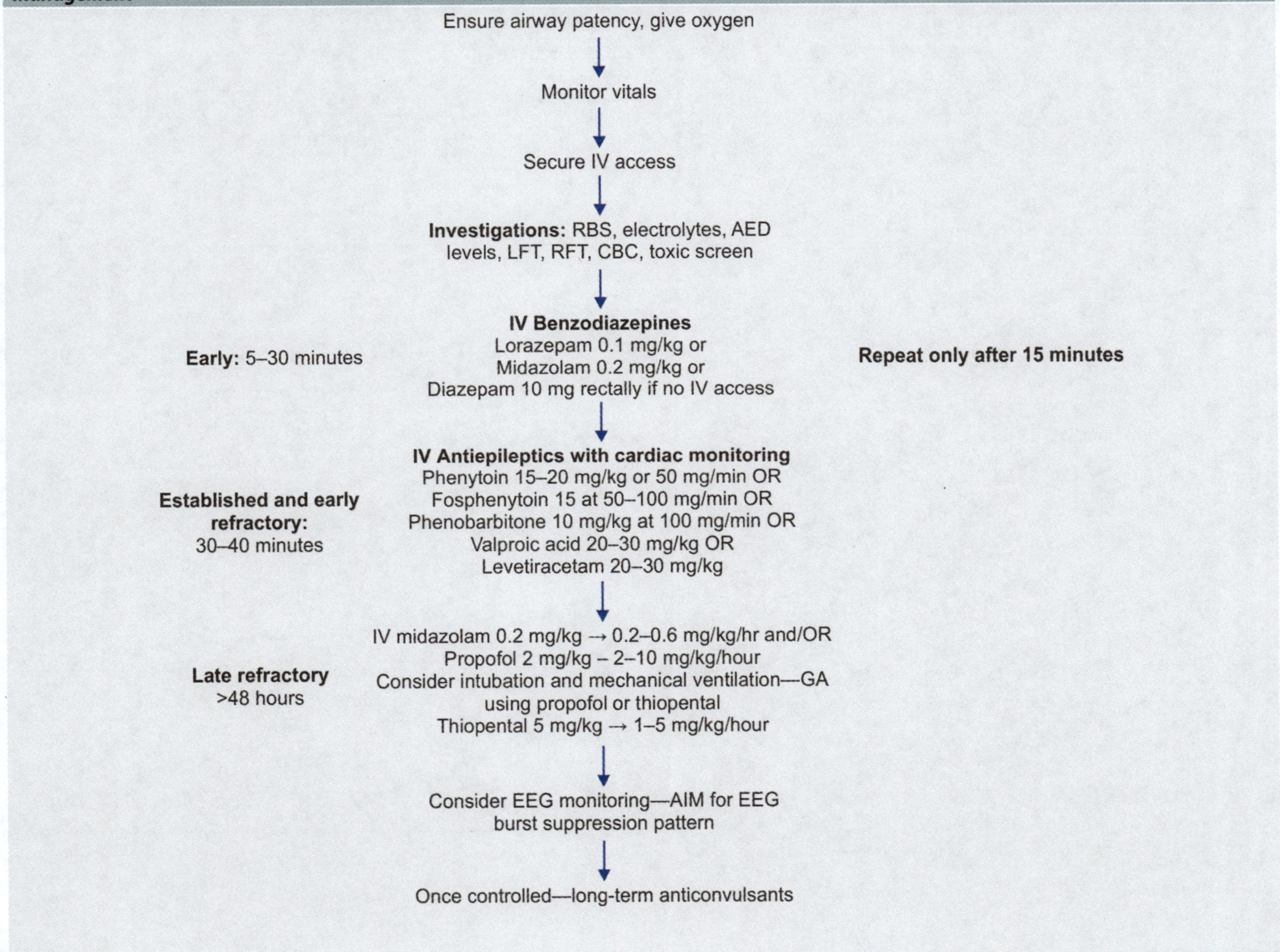

Ensure airway patency, give oxygen

↓

Monitor vitals

↓

Secure IV access

↓

Investigations: RBS, electrolytes, AED levels, LFT, RFT, CBC, toxic screen

↓

Early: 5–30 minutes

IV Benzodiazepines
Lorazepam 0.1 mg/kg or
Midazolam 0.2 mg/kg or
Diazepam 10 mg rectally if no IV access

Repeat only after 15 minutes

↓

Established and early refractory: 30–40 minutes

IV Antiepileptics with cardiac monitoring
Phenytoin 15–20 mg/kg or 50 mg/min OR
Fosphenytoin 15 at 50–100 mg/min OR
Phenobarbitone 10 mg/kg at 100 mg/min OR
Valproic acid 20–30 mg/kg OR
Levetiracetam 20–30 mg/kg

↓

Late refractory >48 hours

IV midazolam 0.2 mg/kg → 0.2–0.6 mg/kg/hr and/OR
Propofol 2 mg/kg – 2–10 mg/kg/hour
Consider intubation and mechanical ventilation—GA using propofol or thiopental
Thiopental 5 mg/kg → 1–5 mg/kg/hour

↓

Consider EEG monitoring—AIM for EEG burst suppression pattern

↓

Once controlled—long-term anticonvulsants

Appendix

LABORATORY VALUES OF CLINICAL IMPORTANCE

In this appendix, tables of reference values of some important common laboratory investigations are provided which will help in interpreting the results during examinations as well as during clinician's practice. The term "reference values" has replaced older terminology "normal values/ranges". A variety of factors can influence reference values and it varies between laboratories depending on the laboratory methods, mode of standardization, and other factors. This is especially the case with enzyme assays. The reference or "normal" ranges given in this appendix may, therefore, not be appropriate for all laboratories and they should only be used as general guidelines. Hence, reference values provided by the laboratory performing the test should be used in the interpretation of laboratory results. Most clinical laboratories and all medical and scientific journals use SI system. Since, conventional units are still used in many laboratories of developing countries, in this section, laboratory values are given in both conventional and international units. Many analytes are measured in either serum (the supernatant of clotted blood) or plasma (the supernatant of anticoagulated blood).

The laboratory reference values in this appendix is divided into different section namely: (1) hematology and coagulation (**Table A1.1**), (2) clinical chemistry of blood (**Table A1.2**), (3) lipid profile (**Table A1.3**), (4) urea and electrolytes (**Table A1.4**), (5) thyroid function tests (**Table A1.5**), (6) urine (**Table A1.6**), (7) cerebrospinal fluid (**Table A1.7**), and short list of routinely used formulas in medicine (**Table A1.8**).

Hematology and Coagulation (Table A1.1)

TABLE A1.1: Hematology and coagulation.

Component (specimen)	*Reference value*	
	Conventional	*SI units*
RBCs and hemoglobin		
RBC count ➢ Males ➢ Females	 4.5–5.5 × 10^{12}/L (mean 5.0 × 10^{12}/L) 3.8–4.8 × 10^{12}/L (mean 4.3 × 10^{12}/L)	
RBC diameter	6.7–7.7 µm (mean 7.2 µm)	
RBC indices (absolute values) ➢ Mean corpuscular volume (MCV) ➢ Mean corpuscular hemoglobin (MCH) ➢ Mean corpuscular hemoglobin concentration (MCHC) ➢ Red cell distribution width (RDW)	 82–100 fL 27–32 pg 31–35 g/dL 11.5–14.0%	
RBC lifespan	120 days	
Erythrocyte sedimentation rate (ESR) (Whole blood) ➢ Westergren, 1st hour - Males - Females - Children	 0–15 mm 1st hour 0–20 mm 1st hour 0–10 mm 1st hour	
➢ Wintrobe, 1st hour - Males - Females	 0–9 mm 1st hour 0–20 mm 1st hour	
Ferritin (serum) ➢ Males ➢ Females	 20–300 ng/mL 15–200 ng/mL	 20–300 µg/L 15–200 µg/L
Folate (serum)	3–20 µg/L	3–20 ng/mL
Hematocrit (PCV) ➢ Males ➢ Females ➢ Neonate (cord blood)	 38–47% 36–46% 45–70%	

Contd...

Contd...

Component (specimen)	Reference value	
	Conventional	SI units
Hemoglobin (Hb) ➤ Adult hemoglobin (HbA) ➤ Males ➤ Females ➤ Hemoglobin A_2 (HbA_2) ➤ Hemoglobin, fetal (HbF) in adults ➤ HbF, children under 6 months	 95–98% 13.0–17.0 g/dL 12.0–15.0 g/dL 1.5–3.5% <0–2% <5%	
➤ Iron, total (serum) ➤ Total iron binding capacity (TIBC) ➤ Transferrin saturation	80–180 µg/dL 250–425 µg/dL 20–45%	7–25 µmol/L 45–73 µmol/L 0.20–0.45
Osmotic fragility ➤ Slight hemolysis ➤ Complete hemolysis ➤ Mean corpuscular fragility	 at 0.45–0.39 g/dL NaCl at 0.33–0.36 g/dL NaCl 0.4–0.45 g/dL NaCl	
Reticulocytes ➤ Adults ➤ Infants ➤ Newborn (cord blood)	 0.5–2.5% 2–6% 1–7%	
Transferrin saturation ➤ Male ➤ Female	 25–56% 14–51%	
Vitamin B_{12} (serum) ➤ Body stores ➤ Daily requirement ➤ Serum level	 10–12 mg 2–3 µg 280–1,000 pg/mL	
Autohemolysis test (whole blood)	0.4–4.50%	0.004–0.045
Autohemolysis test with glucose (whole blood)	0.3–0.7%	0.003–0.007
Leukocytes		
Differential leukocyte count (DLC) ➤ P (polymorphs or neutrophils) ➤ L (lymphocytes) ➤ M (monocytes) ➤ E (eosinophils) ➤ B (basophils)	 40–70% (2,000–7,500/µL) 20–40% (1,500–4,000/µL) 2–10% (200–800/µL) 1–6% (40–450/µL) <1% (10–100/µL)	
Total leukocyte count (TLC) ➤ Adults ➤ Infants (full term, at birth) ➤ Infants (1 year)	 4,000–11,000/µL 10,000–25,000/µL 6,000–16,000/µL	
Platelets and coagulation		
Bleeding time (BT) ➤ Ivy's method ➤ Template method	2–7 minutes 2–9 minutes	
Clot retraction time (clotted blood) ➤ Qualitative ➤ Quantitative	Visible in 60 minutes (complete in <24 hours) 48–64% (55%)	
Clotting time (CT) ➤ Lee and White method	4–11 minutes	
D-dimer (plasma)	220–740 ng/mL	
Fibrinogen (plasma)	200–400 mg/dL	
Fibrin split (or degradation) products (FSP or FDP)	<10 µg/mL	
Partial thromboplastin time with kaolin (PTTK) or activated partial thromboplastin time (APTT/aAPTT)	30–40 seconds	
Platelet count	150,000–450,000/µL	
Prothrombin time (PT) (Quick's one stage method)	11–16 seconds	
Thrombin time (TT)	15–19 seconds (control ± 2 seconds)	

(PCV: packed cell volume; RBC: red blood cells)

Clinical Chemistry of Blood (Table A1.2)

TABLE A1.2: Clinical chemistry of blood.

Component	Specimen	Reference value	
		Conventional	***SI units***
Alpha fetoprotein (AFP), adults	Serum	0–8.5 ng/mL	0–8.5 μg/L
Aminotransferases (transaminases) ➢ Aspartate (AST, SGOT) ➢ Alanine (ALT, SGPT)	 Serum Serum	 12–38 U/L 7–41 U/L	 0.20–0.65 μkat/L 0.12–0.70 μkat/L
Amylase	Serum	20–96 U/L	0.34–1.6 μkat/L
Bilirubin ➢ Total ➢ Direct (conjugated) ➢ Indirect (unconjugated)	Serum	 0.3–1.3 mg/dL 0.1–0.4 mg/dL 0.2–0.9 mg/dL	 5.1–22 μmol/L 1.7–6.8 μmol/L 3.4–15.2 μmol/L
CA-125	Serum	0–35 U/mL	0–35 Ku/L
Calcium—ionized	Whole blood	4.5–5.3 mg/dL	1.12–1.32 mmol/L
Calcium—total	Serum	8.7–10.2 mg/dL	2.2–2.6 mmol/L
Chloride	Serum	102–109 mEq/L	102–109 mmol/L
C-reactive proteins	Serum	0.2–3.0 mg/L	0.2–3.0 mg/L
Creatine kinase (CK), total ➢ Males ➢ Females	Serum	51–294 U/L 39–238 IU/L	0.87–5.0 μkat/L 0.66–4.0 μkat/L
Creatine kinase MB (CKMB)	Serum	0–5.5 ng/mL	0–5.5 μg/L
Gamma glutamyl transpeptidase (transferase) (γ-GT)	Serum	9–58 IU/L	0.15–1.00 μmol/L
Glucose (fasting) ➢ Normal ➢ Impaired fasting glucose (IFG) ➢ Diabetes mellitus	Plasma	 70–100 mg/dL 101–125 mg/dL >126 mg/dL	 <5.6 mmol/L 5.6–6.9 mmol/L >7.0 mmol/L
Glucose (2-hour postprandial) ➢ Normal ➢ Impaired glucose tolerance (IGT) ➢ Diabetes mellitus	Plasma	 <140 mg/dL 140–200 mg/dL >200 mg/dL	 <7.8 mmol/L 7.8–11.1 mmol/L >11.1 mmol/L
Glycated hemoglobin (HbA_{1c})	Whole blood	4.0–6.0%	20–42 mmol/mol Hb
Lactate dehydrogenase (LDH)	Serum	115–221 U/L	2.0–3.8 μkat/L
Muramidase	Serum	5–20 μg/mL	
5-nucleotidase	Serum	0–11 U/L	0.02–0.19 μkat/L
Phosphatases ➢ Acid phosphatase ➢ Alkaline phosphatase	Serum	 0–5.5 U/L 33–96 U/L	 0.90 μkat/L 0.56–1.63 μkat/L
Prostate-specific antigen (PSA)	Serum	0–4.0 ng/mL	0–4.0 μg/L
Proteins—total ➢ Albumin ➢ Globulins ➢ Albumin/globulin ratio	Serum	6.7–8.6 g/dL 3.5–5.5 g/dL 2.0–3.5 g/dL 1.5–3 : 1	67–86 g/L 35–55 g/L 20–35 g/L
Rheumatoid factor	Serum	<15 IU/mL	< 15 kIU/L
Troponins, cardiac (cTn) ➢ Troponin I (cTnI) ➢ Troponin T (cTnT)	 Serum Serum	 0–0.08 ng/mL 0–0.01 ng/mL	 0–0.8 μg/L 0–0.1 μg/L
Blood urea nitrogen (BUN)	Blood	7–20 mg/dL	2.5–7.1 mmol/L
Uric acid ➢ Males ➢ Females	Serum	 3.1–7.0 mg/dL 2.5–5.6 mg/dL	 0.18–0.41 μmol/L 0.15–0.33 μmol/L

(SGOT: serum glutamic oxaloacetic transaminase; SGPT: serum glutamic pyruvic transaminase)

Lipid Profile (Table A1.3)

TABLE A1.3: Lipid profile.

Component	*Reference value*	
	Conventional	*SI units*
Total serum cholesterol		
➢ Desirable for adults	<200 mg/dL	<5.17 mmol/L
➢ Borderline high	200–239 mg/dL	5.17–6.18 mmol/L
➢ High undesirable	>240 mg/dL	>6.21 mmol/L
LDL cholesterol		
➢ Desirable range	100–130 mg/dL	<3.34 mmol/L
➢ Borderline high	130–159 mg/dL	3.36–4.11 mmol/L
➢ High	160–189 mg/dL	4.11–4.20 mmol/L
➢ Very high	>190 mg/dL	>4.21 mmol/L
HDL cholesterol		
➢ Low	<40 mg/dL	<1.03 mmol/L
➢ High, protective range	>60 mg/dL	>1.55 mmol/L
Triglycerides	<160 mg/dL	<2.26 mmol/L

(HDL: high-density lipoprotein; LDL: low-density lipoprotein)

Renal Function Tests (Table A1.4)

TABLE A1.4: Urea and electrolytes.

Analyte	*Reference value*	
	Conventional	*SI units*
Sodium	136–146 mEq/L	136–146 mmol/L
Potassium	3.5–5.0 mEq/L	3.5–5.0 mmol/L
Chloride	95–107 mEq/L	95–107 mmol/L
Urea	20–40 mg/dL	3.3–6.6 mmol/L
Creatinine	0.6–1.2 mg/dL	53–106 μmol/L

Thyroid Function Tests (Table A1.5)

TABLE A1.5: Thyroid function tests.

Thyroid function tests	*Specimen*	*Reference value*	
		Conventional	*SI units*
Radioactive iodine uptake (RAIU) 24 hours		5–30%	
Thyroxine (T4) total	Serum	5.4–11.7 μg/dL	70–151 nmol/L
Tri-iodothyronine (T3) total	Serum	77–135 ng/dL	1.2–2.1 nmol/L
Thyroid stimulating hormone (TSH)	Serum	0.4–4.25 μg/mL	0.4–4.25 mU/L

Urine (Table A1.6)

TABLE A1.6: Normal urine values.

Component	*Reference value*
Volume—24 hours	600–1,800 mL (variable)
pH	5.0–9.0
Specific gravity, quantitative (random)	1.002–1.028 (average 1.018)
Protein—24 hours urine	<150 mg/day
Protein, qualitative (random)	Negative
Glucose, quantitative—24 hours urine	50–300 mg/day
Glucose, qualitative (random)	Negative
Urobilinogen—24 hours urine	1.0–3.5 mg/day
Microalbuminuria (24 hours)	0–30 mg/24 hours (0–0.03 g/day) (0–30 μg/mg creatinine) (0–0.03 g/g creatinine)

Cerebrospinal Fluid (Table A1.7)

TABLE A1.7: Normal values of cerebrospinal fluid.

Component	Reference value	
	Conventional	*SI units*
CSF volume	120–150 mL	
Appearance	Clear and colorless	
CSF pressure	60–150 mm water	
pH	7.31–7.34	
Total proteins	20–40 mg/dL	0.14–0.45 g/L
Glucose	40–80 mg/dL	2.3–4.5 mmol/L
Chlorides	720–750 mg/dL	
Cells ➢ Polymorphs ➢ Lymphocytes	 Usually absent 0–5/μL	

(CSF: cerebrospinal fluid)

Short List of Routinely Used Formulae in Medicine (Table A1.8)

TABLE A1.8: Short list of routinely used formulae in medicine.

Electrolyte disorders	
Plasma osmolality	2 Na^+ (mEq/L) + serum glucose (mg/dL)/18 + BUN (mg/dL)/2.8
Corrected sodium	Increase Na^+ by 1.6 mEq/L for each 100 mg% of serum glucose (when serum glucose >100 mg%)
Total body sodium deficit	(Desired sodium – measured sodium) x Body weight x [0.6 (men) or 0.5 (women)]
Potassium deficit	1 mmol/L decrease → approximately 200–400 mmol loss of total body K^+
Urine-plasma electrolyte ratio (in chronic hyponatremia)	Urinary (sodium + potassium)/plasma sodium ➢ >1 (fluid restriction up to <500 mL/day) ➢ =1 (500–700 mL/day) ➢ <1 (fluid restriction up to 1 L)
Water deficit (in hypernatremia)	Water deficit = (plasma sodium – 140) x TBW/140
TTKG (trans-tubular potassium gradient) in hypokalemia	Urinary potassium x plasma osmolality/serum potassium x urinary osmolality ➢ >4 indicates renal loss of potassium
Corrected calcium	0.8 x (4 – serum albumin) + serum calcium
Acid base disorders	
Anion gap (serum)	(Sodium + potassium) – (bicarbonate + chloride) ➢ 8–16 mEq/L (old methods) ➢ 5–11 mEq/L (new techniques)
Urine anion gap	Urine sodium + potassium – chloride ➢ –25 to –50 (normal range)
Delta ratio	(Serum anion gap – 12)/(24 – serum bicarbonate) ➢ <0.4 hyperchloremic normal anion gap acidosis ➢ <1 high AG and normal AG acidosis ➢ >2 high AG acidosis and a concurrent metabolic alkalosis
Respiratory acidosis	Acute: 10 increase in pCO_2 → 1 increase in bicarbonate Chronic: 10 increase in pCO_2 → 4 increase in bicarbonate
Respiratory alkalosis	Acute: 10 decrease in pCO_2 → 2 decrease in bicarbonate Chronic: 10 decrease in pCO_2 → 5 decrease in bicarbonate
Metabolic acidosis	pCO_2 = 1.5 (bicarbonate) + 8 ± 2
Metabolic alkalosis	10 increase in bicarbonate → pCO_2 increases by 6
Nephrology	
Renal failure index	Urine Na/(Urine Cr/PCr)
Cockcroft-Gault GFR	(140 – Age) × (Body weight in kg) × (0.85 if female)/(72 × Cr)
Fractional excretion of sodium (FENa)	(Serum Cr × Urine Na)/(Serum Na × Urine Cr)%

Contd...

Contd...

Hematology	
Corrected reticulocyte count	Reticulocyte % × (Hb/15)
Reticulocyte production index	= Corrected reticulocyte count/maturation time ➢ At a hemoglobin of 15, the maturation time = 1 day ➢ At a hemoglobin of 12, the maturation time = 1.5 days ➢ At a hemoglobin of 8, the maturation time = 2 days ➢ At a hemoglobin of 5, the maturation time = 2.5 days
Mentzer index	(MCV, in fL) divided by (RBC, in millions per µL) ➢ <13, thalassemia is said to be more likely
Parenteral iron in iron deficiency anemia	[2.3 x body weight (kg) x Hb deficit (gm/dL)] + 1,000 mg (to replenish stores)
Respiratory system	
A-a gradient	$PAO_2 - PaO_2$ ($PAO_2 = (FiO_2 \times 713) - PaCO_2/0.8$; PaO_2 is obtained from the ABG)
Cardiology	
Corrected QT	QT interval / √(RR interval) (Bazzett's formula)
MAP	Systolic BP + (2 × diastolic BP)/3
Miscellaneous	
BMI	W/H^2 (W = weight in kg and H = Height in meters)

(BMI: body mass index; BUN: blood urea nitrogen; GFR: glomerular filtration rate; MAP: mean arterial pressures; MCV: mean corpuscular volume; RBC: red blood cells)

Index

Page numbers followed by *b* refer to box, *f* refer to figure, *fc* refer to flowchart, and *t* refer to table, respectively.

A

B

C

D

E

G

H

I

N

O

P

Q

R

S

T

U

V

W

X

Y

Z